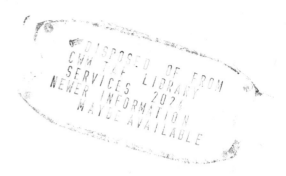

TEXTBOOK OF PEDIATRIC CRITICAL CARE

TEXTBOOK OF PEDIATRIC CRITICAL CARE

Peter R. Holbrook, M.D.

Professor, Anesthesiology and Pediatrics
George Washington University School of Medicine;
Director, Intensive Care Unit and
Chairman, Department of Critical Care Medicine
Children's National Medical Center
Washington, D.C.

W. B. SAUNDERS COMPANY
Harcourt Brace Jovanovich, Inc.

Philadelphia London Toronto Montreal Sydney Tokyo

W. B. SAUNDERS COMPANY
Harcourt Brace Jovanovich, Inc.

The Curtis Center
Independence Square West
Philadelphia, Pennsylvania 19106

Library of Congress Cataloging-in-Publication Data
Textbook of pediatric critical care / [edited by] Peter R. Holbrook.
p.   cm.
ISBN   0–7216–2352–2
1. Pediatric intensive care.   I. Holbrook, Peter R. [DNLM: 1. Critical Care—in infancy & childhood. WS 366 T3553]
RJ370.T46 1993
618.92′0025—dc20
DNLM/DLC   92-45006

Textbook of Pediatric Critical Care   ISBN   0–7216–2352–2

Printed in Mexico.

Last digit is the print number: 9   8   7   6   5   4   3   2   1

To medical professionals throughout the world who devote their lives to the care of critically ill children

To the beneficiaries of critical care, some of whom are Robin, Shannon, Channing, Megan, Bobby, Miko, Jennifer, Kelly, and Benjamin

To the memories and the families of those for whom our efforts were not enough, some of whom are Carl, Adrian, Suzie, Timothy, Joshua, Gregory, Darlyssa, Michael, Jose, Tershea, and Hunt

To Henry, Behle, Ashley, Lara, and Matt

To Lucy

Contributors

Richard J. Andrassy, M.D.

A. G. McNeese Professor of Surgery and Pediatrics, University of Texas Medical School; Hermann Children's Hospital; M. D. Anderson Cancer Center; Lyndon B. Johnson Hospital; Texas Children's Hospital; St. Luke's Episcopal Hospital, Houston, Texas.

Chapter 14: Nutritional Failure and Therapy

Raymond R. Arons, Dr. P.H.

Adjunct Assistant Professor, School of Public Health, Columbia University; Director, Office of Case Mix Studies, The Presbyterian Hospital in the City of New York at the Columbia Presbyterian Medical Center, New York, New York.

Chapter 95: Clinical, Economic, and Political
    Implications of Critical Care

Robert J. Attorri, M.D.

Assistant Professor of Surgery, University of Medicine and Dentistry of New Jersey; Cooper Hospital/University Medical Center, Camden, New Jersey.

Chapter 87: Burns in Children

Gerard T. Berry, M.D.

Associate Professor of Pediatrics, University of Pennsylvania School of Medicine; Senior Physician, Division of Metabolism, Children's Hospital of Philadelphia, Philadelphia, Pennsylvania.

Chapter 60: Disorders of Intermediary Metabolism

Glenn H. Bock, M.D.

Associate Professor of Pediatrics, George Washington University School of Medicine; Vice Chairman, Department of Nephrology, Children's National Medical Center, Washington, District of Columbia.

Chapter 53: Diagnosis and Management of Acute Renal
    Failure in the Critical Care Unit

Desmond Bohn, M.B., B.Ch., F.R.C.P.(C).

Associate Professor of Anesthesia and Pediatrics, University of Toronto; Assistant Director, Pediatric Intensive Care Unit, The Hospital for Sick Children, Toronto, Ontario, Canada.

Chapter 41: Cardiopulmonary Interactions

Linda M. Bradley, M.D.

Assistant Professor of Pediatrics, George Washington University School of Medicine and Health Sciences; Department of Cardiology, Children's National Medical Center, Washington, District of Columbia.

Chapter 34: Chest Vasculature

Gordon L. Bray, M.D.

Associate Professor, Department of Pediatrics, George Washington University School of Medicine and Health Sciences; Director, Coagulation Disorders Program, Department of Hematology, Oncology, Children's National Medical Center, Washington, District of Columbia.

Chapter 64: Inherited and Acquired Disorders of
    Hemostasis

Joseph A. Carcillo, M.D.

Assistant Professor, Anesthesia and Critical Care, Children's Hospital of Pittsburgh, Pittsburgh, Pennsylvania.

Chapter 3: Mechanisms of Cellular Communication and
    Signal Transduction
Chapter 12: Management of Pediatric Septic Shock

Leticia Castillo, M.D.

Instructor in Pediatrics, Harvard Medical School; Assistant in Pediatrics, Massachusetts General Hospital, Boston, Massachusetts.

Chapter 59: Endocrine Disorders

Bart Chernow, M.D.

Physician-in-Chief, Department of Medicine, Sinai Hospital of Baltimore; Professor of Medicine, Anesthesia, and Critical Care, Johns Hopkins University School of Medicine, Baltimore, Maryland.

Chapter 59: Endocrine Disorders

Koteswara Rao Chundu, M.D.

Assistant Professor of Anesthesiology and Pediatric Medicine, George Washington University; Member of Attending Staff, Department of Critical Care Medicine, Children's National Medical Center, Washington, District of Columbia.

Chapter 97: Research in Critical Care

J. Perren Cobb, M.D.

Clinical Associate, Critical Care Medicine Department, National Institutes of Health, Bethesda, Maryland.

Chapter 70: Nosocomial Infections in the Practice of Pediatric Critical Care

Arthur Cooper, M.D.

Associate Professor of Clinical Surgery, College of Physicians and Surgeons, Columbia University; Chief, Pediatric Surgical Critical Care, Harlem Hospital Center, New York, New York.

Chapter 85: Critical Management of Chest, Abdomen, and Extremity Trauma

Thomas O. Crawford, M.D.

Attending Physician, Assistant Professor of Neurology, Johns Hopkins University; Johns Hopkins Hospital, Baltimore, Maryland.

Chapter 24: Respiratory Failure and Other Complications of Neuromuscular Disease

Robert E. Cunnion, M.D.

Senior Investigator, Critical Care Medicine Department, National Institutes of Health, Bethesda, Maryland.

Chapter 2: Mechanisms of Inflammation

Robert L. Danner, M.D.

Senior Investigator, Critical Care Medicine Department, National Institutes of Health, Bethesda, Maryland; Assistant Clinical Professor of Medicine, Georgetown University, Washington, District of Columbia; Attending Physician, Critical Care Medicine Department, Warren G. Magnusen Clinical Center, National Institute of Health, Bethesda, Maryland.

Chapter 70: Nosocomial Infections in the Practice of Pediatric Critical Care

Ronald Day, M.D.

Assistant Professor of Pediatric Cardiology, University of Utah, Primary Children's Medical Center, Salt Lake City, Utah.

Chapter 33: Congenital Heart Disease

J. Michael Dean, M.D.

Associate Professor of Pediatrics and Chief, Division of Critical Care, Department of Pediatrics, University of Utah School of Medicine; Director, Pediatric Intensive Care Unit, Primary Children's Medical Center, Salt Lake City, Utah.

Chapter 5: Basic Mechanisms of Resuscitation

Louis DePalma, M.D.

Associate Professor of Pathology and Assistant Professor of Pediatrics, George Washington University School of Medicine; Assistant Director, Hematology/Blood Bank, Children's National Medical Center, Washington, District of Columbia.

Chapter 63: Transfusion Therapy in the Pediatric Intensive Care Unit

Roger E. Dionne, Pharm.D.

Clinical Instructor, Tufts University School of Medicine, Department of Pediatrics; Pediatric Clinical Pharmacy Specialist, New England Medical Center, Department of Pharmacy, Boston, Massachusetts.

Chapter 74: Pharmacokinetics-Pharmacodynamics: Drug Delivery and Therapeutic Drug Monitoring

E. Dobyns, M.D.

Fellow in Critical Care, The Children's Hospital; Assistant Professor of Pediatrics, University of Colorado Health Sciences Center, Department of Pediatrics, The Children's Hospital, Denver, Colorado.

Chapter 11: Neonatal Sepsis

Lee W. Doty, J.D.

Vice President and General Counsel, Children's National Medical Center, Washington, District of Columbia.

Chapter 91: Legal Considerations

Craig E. Downs, D.O.

Director, Pediatric Critical Care Center, St. John's Regional Health Center, Springfield, Missouri.

Chapter 7: Resuscitation of the Child

Lynn F. Duffy, M.D.

Assistant Professor of Pediatrics, George Washington University School of Medicine; Attending Physician, Department of Gastroenterology and Nutrition, Children's National Medical Center, Washington, District of Columbia.

Chapter 57: Gastrointestinal Dysfunction and Failure

Howard Eigen, M.D.

Professor of Pediatrics, Indiana University School of Medicine; Director, Section of Pediatric Pulmonology and Critical Care, James Whitcomb Riley Hospital for Children, Indianapolis, Indiana.

Chapter 38: Respiratory Monitoring
Chapter 46: Lower Airway Disease

Mary Beth Fasano, M.D.

Fellow, Division of Immunology, Department of Pediatrics, Johns Hopkins Hospital, Baltimore, Maryland.

Chapter 4: Pathophysiology of the Immune System

Alan I. Fields, M.D.

Professor of Anesthesiology and Associate Professor of Pediatrics, George Washington University School of Medicine; Associate Director, Pediatric Intensive Care Unit, Children's National Medical Center, Washington, District of Columbia.

Chapter 9: Drowning and Near-Drowning

Karla M. Gerberding, M.D.

Clinical Assistant Professor of Pediatrics, Indiana University School of Medicine; James Whitcomb Riley Hospital for Children, Indianapolis, Indiana.

Chapter 46: Lower Airway Disease

Jacqueline J. Glover, Ph.D.

Director, Program in Bioethics, Department of Health Care Sciences, George Washington University; Philosopher-in-Residence, Children's National Medical Center, Washington, District of Columbia.

Chapter 92: Ethical Considerations

Philip C. Guzzetta, M.D.

Professor of Surgery and Pediatrics, George Washington University; Attending Surgeon, Children's National Medical Center, Washington, District of Columbia.

Chapter 55: Renal Transplantation

Theresa A. Hantsch, M.D.

Fellow in Pediatric Critical Care Medicine, University of California, San Francisco, California.

Chapter 30: Congestive Heart Failure

Burton H. Harris, M.D.

The Orvar Swenson Professor of Pediatric Surgery, Tufts University School of Medicine; Chief, Division of Pediatric Surgery, New England Medical Center; Director, Kiwanis Pediatric Trauma Institute, New England Medical Center, Boston, Massachusetts.

Chapter 8: Resuscitation of the Critically Injured Child

Carol Gannon Hartman, M.S.N., R.N.

Clinical Nurse III, Children's National Medical Center, Washington, District of Columbia.

Chapter 94: Organ Donation

Mary Fran Hazinski, M.S.N., R.N., F.A.A.N.

Clinical Assistant, Vanderbilt University School of Medicine; Clinical Specialist, Division of Trauma, Departments of Surgery and Pediatrics, Vanderbilt University Medical Center, Nashville, Tennessee.

Chapter 98: Physician-Nurse Interaction in the Intensive Care Unit

Marc B. Hershenson, M.D.

Assistant Professor of Pediatrics, University of Chicago; Attending Physician, Wyler Children's Hospital, Chicago, Illinois.

Chapter 48: Diseases of the Chest Wall

Keith D. Herzog, M.D.

Attending Physician, Holy Redeemer Hospital and Medical Center, Meadowbrook, Pennsylvania.

Chapter 73: Immunodeficient States in Children

Alan Hill, M.D., Ph.D.

Professor, Department of Pediatrics, University of British Columbia; Head, Division of Neurology, British Columbia's Children's Hospital, Vancouver, British Columbia, Canada.

Chapter 18: Hypoxic-Ischemic Cerebral Injury in the Newborn

Peter R. Holbrook, M.D.

Professor, Anesthesiology and Pediatrics, George Washington University School of Medicine; Director, Intensive Care Unit and Chairman, Department of Critical Care Medicine, Children's National Medical Center, Washington, District of Columbia.

Chapter 9: Drowning and Near-Drowning
Chapter 10: Sudden Unexpected Death
Chapter 61: Acid-Base Disorders
Chapter 82: Heat Syndromes
Chapter 83: Cold Syndromes
Chapter 89: Disaster Management for Children
Chapter 90: Pediatric Critical Care Transport
Chapter 92: Ethical Considerations
Chapter 93: Death

Deidre G. Holley, M.B., B.S.

Cardiology Fellow, Children's National Medical Center, Washington, District of Columbia.

Chapter 27: Cardiovascular Monitoring and Evaluation

Constance S. Houck, M.D.

Instructor in Anesthesia (Pediatrics), Harvard Medical School; Assistant in Anesthesia, The Children's Hospital, Boston, Massachusetts.

Chapter 39: Access to the Airway
Chapter 76: Anesthetic Agents—Actions and Toxicity

Allen I. Hyman, M.D.

Professor of Anesthesiology and Director of Education, Department of Anesthesiology, College of Physicians and Surgeons, Columbia University; Attending Anesthesiologist, Columbia University, New York, New York.

Chapter 95: Clinical, Economic, and Political Implications of Critical Care

Marshall L. Jacobs, M.D.

Associate Professor of Surgery, University of Pennsylvania; Associate Surgeon, Division of Cardiothoracic Surgery; Director, Cardiac Transplantation Program, Children's Hospital of Philadelphia, Philadelphia, Pennsylvania.

   Chapter 32: Cardiac Transplantation

Hector E. James, M.D.

Clinical Professor of Neurosurgery and Pediatrics, School of Medicine, University of California; Vice-Chairman, Department of Neurosciences, Children's Hospital of San Diego; Senior Staff, Children's Hospital; Consulting Staff, UCSD Medical Center, San Diego, California.

   Chapter 21: Head Trauma

Barbara A. Jantausch, M.D.

Assistant Professor of Pediatrics, The George Washington University Medical Center; Attending Physician, Infectious Diseases, Children's National Medical Center, Washington, District of Columbia.

   Chapter 20: Intracranial Infections

Dennis L. Johnson, M.D.

Associate Professor, George Washington University; Children's National Medical Center, Rockville, Maryland.

   Chapter 22: Spinal Cord Injury in Children

Michael V. Johnston, M.D.

Professor and Haller Scholar of Neurology and Pediatrics, Johns Hopkins University School of Medicine; Kennedy Krieger Institute and Johns Hopkins Hospital, Baltimore, Maryland.

   Chapter 23: Neuroexcitatory Syndromes

Mireille B. Karda, M.D.

Assistant Professor of Pediatrics, George Washington University School of Medicine and Health Sciences; Attending Physician, Department of Pediatric Medicine, Washington, District of Columbia.

   Chapter 86: Child Abuse and Neglect: A Critical Care
   Challenge

Robert K. Kanter, M.D.

Associate Professor of Pediatrics, University of North Carolina at Chapel Hill; University of North Carolina Hospital, Chapel Hill, North Carolina.

   Chapter 51: Neuromuscular Disorders

Robert Katz, M.D.

Associate Professor of Pediatrics and Director, Pediatric Intensive Care Unit, Division of Pediatric Pulmonary/Critical Care, University of New Mexico School of Medicine; Associate Professor of Pediatrics, University of New Mexico School of Medicine; Director, Pediatric Intensive Care Unit, University Hospital, Albuquerque, New Mexico.

   Chapter 50: Bronchopulmonary Dysplasia in the
   Pediatric Intensive Care Unit

Karen L. Kaucic, M.D.

Fellow, Department of Hematology/Oncology, Children's National Medical Center, Washington, District of Columbia.

   Chapter 66: Bone Marrow Transplantation

Benny Kerzner, M.D.

Professor of Pediatrics, George Washington University School of Medicine; Chairman, Department of Pediatrics and Nutrition, Children's National Medical Center, Washington, District of Columbia.

   Chapter 56: Hepatic Failure
   Chapter 57: Gastrointestinal Dysfunction and Failure

William Keyes, M.D., Ph.D.

Active Staff, Pediatric Intensive Care Unit, Scottish Rite Children's Medical Center, Atlanta, Georgia.

   Chapter 77: Sedatives and Analgesics
   Chapter 78: Neuromuscular Blockers

Stephen A. Klem, M.D.

Assistant Professor, Departments of Anesthesiology and Pediatrics, University of Missouri–Kansas City School of Medicine; Associate Director, Pediatric Intensive Care Unit, Children's Mercy Hospital, Kansas City, Missouri.

   Chapter 28: Cardiovascular Support—Mechanical

Bernice R. Krafchik, M.B., Ch.B., F.R.C.P.(C)

Associate Professor of Pediatrics, University of Toronto Faculty of Medicine; Sick Children's Hospital, Toronto, Ontario, Canada.

   Chapter 67: Dermatologic Diseases

Laurie A. Latchaw, M.D.

Assistant Professor of Surgery, Tufts University School of Medicine; Assistant Surgeon, New England Medical Center— The Floating Hospital for Infants and Children, Boston, Massachusetts.

   Chapter 8: Resuscitation of the Critically Injured Child

James J. Logan, M.D.

Instructor of Pediatrics, Division of Pediatric Pulmonology, Department of Pediatrics, University of Alabama at Birmingham; Attending Physician, The Children's Hospital of Alabama, Birmingham, Alabama.

   Chapter 47: Lung Parenchyma

Naomi L. C. Luban, M.D.

Professor of Pediatrics and Pathology, George Washington University School of Medicine; Director, Hematology/Blood Bank; Attending Hematologist, Children's National Medical Center, Washington, District of Columbia.

   Chapter 63: Transfusion Therapy in the Pediatric
   Intensive Care Unit

Johan Lundgren, M.D.
Attending Physician, Department of Paediatrics, University Hospital, Lund, Sweden.
Chapter 1: Mechanisms of Hypoxia-Ischemia

Gerard R. Martin, M.D.
Associate Professor of Pediatrics, George Washington University School of Medicine and Health Sciences; Director of Echocardiography, Children's National Medical Center, Washington, District of Columbia.
Chapter 27: Cardiovascular Monitoring and Evaluation

Lynn D. Martin, M.D.
Assistant Professor, Departments of Anesthesiology/Critical Care, Medicine, and Pediatrics, Johns Hopkins University School of Medicine; Attending Physician, Pediatric Anesthesia, ECMO, Pediatric Intensive Care Unit, Johns Hopkins Hospital, Baltimore, Maryland.
Chapter 37: Maturation of the Respiratory System

Henry Masur, M.D.
Professor of Clinical Medicine, George Washington University Medical Center; Chief, Critical Care Medicine Department, Clinical Center, National Institutes of Health, Bethesda, Maryland.
Chapter 71: Principles of Antimicrobial Therapy

John McCloskey, M.D.
Professor, Department of Anesthesiology and Critical Care Medicine, Johns Hopkins Hospital, Baltimore, Maryland.
Chapter 4: Pathophysiology of the Immune System

James H. McCrory, M.D.
Pediatric Critical Care Medicine, St. John's Regional Health Center, Springfield, Missouri.
Chapter 7: Resuscitation of the Child

Bennie McWilliams, M.D.
Associate Professor of Pediatrics, Division of Pediatric Pulmonary/Critical Care; Director, Pulmonary Diagnostic Laboratory, University of New Mexico School of Medicine, Albuquerque, New Mexico.
Chapter 50: Bronchopulmonary Dysplasia in the Pediatric Intensive Care Unit

Tyrone Melvin, M.D.
Assistant Professor of Pediatrics, Oregon Health Sciences University; Clinical Assistant, Professor of Pediatrics, University of Illinois College of Medicine, Urbana, Illinois.
Chapter 58: Fluid and Electrolyte Therapy

Brenda J. Milo, R.N.
Clinical Nurse Investigator, Office of Case Mix Studies, The Presbyterian Hospital in the City of New York, New York.
Chapter 95: Clinical, Economic, and Political Implications of Critical Care

Richard B. Mink, M.D.
Assistant Professor of Pediatrics, St. Louis University School of Medicine; Attending Physician, Department of Pediatrics, Cardinal Glennon Children's Hospital, St. Louis, Missouri.
Chapter 13: Hypoxic-Ischemic Injuries
Chapter 19: Hypoxic-Ischemic Encephalopathy in the Child

Katsuyuki Miyasaka, M.D.
Director of Pathophysiology Research Laboratory, National Children's Medical Research Center; Anesthetist-in-Chief, Department of Anesthesia and Intensive Care Unit, National Children's Hospital, Tokyo, Japan.
Chapter 40: Mechanical Ventilation

Parvathi Mohan, M.B.B.S., M.D.
Assistant Professor of Pediatrics, George Washington University; Attending Physician, Department of Gastroenterology and Nutrition, Children's National Medical Center, Washington, District of Columbia.
Chapter 56: Hepatic Failure

Phillip Moore, M.D.
Fellow in Pediatric Cardiology, University of California, San Francisco; Attending Physician, University of California, San Francisco Affiliated Hospitals, San Francisco, California.
Chapter 35: Acquired Heart Disease

Catherine A. Musemeche, M.D.
Assistant Professor of Surgery, The University of Texas Medical School; Attending Physician, University Children's Hospital at Hermann M.D. Anderson Hospital and Lyndon B. Johnson General Hospital, Houston, Texas.
Chapter 14: Nutritional Failure and Therapy

Vinay M. Nadkarni, M.D.
Director, Pediatric Critical Care, Medical Center of Delaware; Assistant Professor of Pediatrics, Jefferson Medical College; Director, Pediatric Critical Care, Christiana Hospital, Newark, Delaware; Pediatric Staff, Division of Pediatric Critical Care, A. I. duPont Institute, Wilmington, Delaware.
Chapter 15: Multiple Organ System Failure

Kurt Newman, M.D.
Associate Professor of Surgery and Pediatrics, George Washington University School of Medicine; Attending Surgeon, Children's National Medical Center, Washington, District of Columbia.
Chapter 88: Electrical Injuries in Children

David G. Nichols, M.D.

Asssociate Professor, Departments of Anesthesiology/Critical Care Medicine and Pediatrics, Johns Hopkins University School of Medicine; Director, Pediatric Intensive Care Unit, Johns Hopkins Hospital, Baltimore, Maryland.

  Chapter 37: Maturation of the Respiratory System

William I. Norwood, M.D., Ph.D.

Professor of Surgery, University of Pennsylvania; Chief, Division of Cardiothoracic Surgery, Children's Hospital of Philadelphia, Philadelphia, Pennsylvania.

  Chapter 32: Cardiac Transplantation

Daniel A. Notterman, M.D.

Associate Professor of Pediatrics, Clinical Pharmacology and Surgery (Pediatrics) and Director, Division of Pediatric Critical Care Medicine, New York Hospital—Cornell Medical Center, New York, New York.

  Chapter 29: Cardiovascular Support—Pharmacologic

Frederick P. Ognibene, M.D.

Assistant Clinical Professor of Medicine, George Washington University School of Medicine and Health Sciences, Washington, District of Columbia; Senior Investigator, Head, Pediatric Section, Critical Care Medicine Department, National Institutes of Health; Senior Investigator and Head, Pediatric Section, Critical Care Medicine Department, National Institutes of Health, Bethesda, Maryland.

  Chapter 65: Oncologic Issues

Jose Ramon C. Ongkingco, M.D.

Senior Fellow, Department of Nephrology, Children's National Medical Center, George Washington University School of Medicine, Washington, District of Columbia.

  Chapter 53: Diagnosis and Management of Acute Renal Failure in the Critical Care Unit

P. Pearl O'Rourke, M.D.

Associate Professor, Anesthesia (Pediatrics), University of Washington; Director, Pediatric Intensive Care Unit, Children's Hospital; Codirector, ECMO Program, Children's Hospital, Seattle, Washington.

  Chapter 42: Extracorporeal Techniques

Lavdena A. Orr, M.D.

Assistant Professor, Department of Pediatrics, George Washington University Schools of Medicine and Health Sciences; Associate, Pediatric Medicine, Children's National Medical Center, Washington, District of Columbia.

  Chapter 86: Child Abuse and Neglect: A Critical Care Challenge

Kristan M. Outwater, M.D.

Assistant Professor of Pediatrics, Tufts University School of Medicine; Associate Director, Pediatric Critical Care Services, New England Medical Center, Boston, Massachusetts.

  Chapter 84: Intensive Care Management of the Traumatized Child

Margaret M. Parker, M.D.

Associate Professor of Pediatrics, Pediatric Critical Care, SUNY at Stony Brook, Stony Brook, New York.

  Chapter 31: Cardiogenic Shock

J. Alan Paschall, M.D.

Assistant Professor of Pediatrics, Oregon Health Sciences University; Director, Pediatric Critical Care, Doernbecher Children's Hospital, Oregon Health Sciences University, Portland, Oregon.

  Chapter 58: Fluid and Electrolyte Therapy

Anthony L. Pearson-Shaver, M.D.

Assistant Professor of Pediatrics, Medical College of Georgia, University Hospital of Augusta, and Walton Rehabilitation Hospital, Augusta, Georgia.

  Chapter 79: Evaluation of the Poisoned Child
  Chapter 80: Specific Poisoning Agents

George J. Peckham, M.D.

Professor of Pediatrics, Department of Pediatrics, University of Pennsylvania School of Medicine; Attending Physician, Children's Hospital of Philadelphia, Philadelphia, Pennsylvania.

  Chapter 6: Resuscitation of the Newborn

Philip A. Pizzo, M.D.

Professor of Pediatrics, Uniformed Services University of the Health Sciences; Chief, Department of Pediatrics, and Head, Infectious Disease Section, National Cancer Institute, National Institutes of Health, Bethesda, Maryland.

  Chapter 65: Oncologic Issues

Murray M. Pollack, M.D.

Professor, Departments of Anesthesiology and Pediatrics, George Washington University School of Medicine and Health Sciences; Director, Health Services and Clinical Research, Children's Research Institute; Associate Director, Pediatric Intensive Care Unit, Children's National Medical Center, Washington, District of Columbia.

  Chapter 96: Outcome Analysis

Neil S. Prose, M.D.

Assistant Professor of Medicine (Dermatology) and Pediatrics, Duke University Medical Center; Attending Physician, Duke University Medical Center, Durham, North Carolina.

  Chapter 67: Dermatologic Diseases

Ralph R. Quinones, M.D.
Assistant Professor of Pediatrics, The George Washington University School of Medicine; Director, Bone Marrow Transplantation, Department of Hematology/Oncology, Children's National Medical Center, Washington, District of Columbia.
Chapter 66: Bone Marrow Transplantation

Tamara A. Rakusan, M.D., Ph.D.
Assistant Professor of Pediatrics, The George Washington University School of Medicine; Director, Special Immunology Service, Children's National Medical Center, Washington, District of Columbia.
Chapter 73: Immunodeficient States in Children

Carl B. Ramsey, M.D.
Fellow, Pediatric Critical Care Medicine, Children's National Medical Center; Affiliated with George Washington Medical University, Washington, District of Columbia.
Chapter 82: Heat Syndromes
Chapter 90: Pediatric Critical Care Transport

Judson G. Randolph, M.D.
Professor Emeritus, George Washington University; Former Surgeon-in-Chief, Children's National Medical Center, Washington, District of Columbia.
Chapter 87: Burns in Children

Gregory H. Reaman, M.D.
Professor of Pediatrics, The George Washington University School of Medicine and Health Sciences; Chairman, Department of Hematology—Oncology, Children's National Medical Center, Washington, District of Columbia.
Chapter 62: Hematologic Disorders

James L. Robotham, M.D.
Professor, Anesthesiology and Critical Care Medicine, Johns Hopkins University School of Medicine; Director, Pulmonary Anesthesiology Research Laboratory, Francis Scott Key Hospital, Baltimore, Maryland.
Chapter 37: Maturation of the Respiratory System

William J. Rodriguez, M.D., Ph.D.
Professor, Department of Pediatrics, George Washington University School of Medicine; Chairman, Department of Infectious Disease, Children's National Medical Center, Washington, District of Columbia.
Chapter 69: Prevention of Nosocomial Infection

Roger N. Ruckman, M.D.
Professor of Pediatrics, George Washington University School of Medicine and Health Care Sciences; Senior Attending Cardiologist, Children's National Medical Center; Director, Pediatric Cardiology Fellowship Training Program, George

Washington University Medical Center, Washington, District of Columbia.
Chapter 26: Development and Maturation of the Cardiovascular System

Edward J. Ruley, M.D.
Professor of Pediatrics, George Washington University School of Medicine; Chairman, Department of Nephrology, Children's National Medical Center, Washington, District of Columbia.
Chapter 54: Hypertension

Barbara B. Sands, R.N.
Clinical Nurse Specialist and Heart Transplant Coordinator, Division of Cardiothoracic Surgery, Children's Hospital of Philadelphia, Philadelphia, Pennsylvania.
Chapter 32: Cardiac Transplantation

Rosemarie Scully, M.S.N.
Psychiatric Liaison Nurse Specialist, Children's National Medical Center, Washington, District of Columbia.
Chapter 68: Psychiatric Aspects of Critical Care

Nita L. Seibel, M.D.
Assistant Professor, George Washington University School of Medicine; Attending Physician, Department of Hematology/Oncology, Children's National Medical Center, Washington, District of Columbia.
Chapter 62: Hematologic Disorders

Frank E. Shafer, M.D.
Associate Hematologist, Children's Hospital Oakland, Oakland, California.
Chapter 62: Hematologic Disorders

Bo K. Siesjö, M.D., Ph.D.
Professor, Laboratory for Experimental Brain Research, Experimental Research Center, University Hospital, Lund, Sweden.
Chapter 1: Mechanisms of Hypoxia-Ischemia

Nalini Singh-Naz, M.D.
Associate Professor of Pediatrics, George Washington University School of Medicine and Health Sciences; Medical Director of Epidemiology and Senior Attending Physician, Department of Infectious Diseases, Children's National Medical Center, Washington, District of Columbia.
Chapter 69: Prevention of Nosocomial Infection

Scott J. Soifer, M.D.
Associate Professor of Pediatrics, Critical Care Medicine and Cardiology, University of California; Director, Division of

Pediatric Critical Care Medicine, University of California, San Francisco, California.
> Chapter 30: Congestive Heart Failure
> Chapter 35: Acquired Heart Disease

Charles A. Stanley, M.D.

Professor of Pediatrics, University of Pennsylvania School of Medicine; Senior Endocrinologist, Endocrine/Diabetes Division, Children's Hospital of Philadelphia, Philadelphia, Pennsylvania.
> Chapter 60: Disorders of Intermediary Metabolism

Curt M. Steinhart, M.D.

Associate Professor of Pediatrics, Surgery, and Anesthesiology, Medical College of Georgia; Director, Pediatric Intensive Care Unit, MCG Hospital and Clinics; Director, Pediatric Intensive Care Unit, University Hospital, Augusta, Georgia.
> Chapter 79: Evaluation of the Poisoned Child
> Chapter 80: Specific Poisoning Agents

Elizabeth C. Suddaby, M.S.N., R.N., C.C.T.C.

Heart Transplant Coordinator, Children's National Medical Center, Washington, District of Columbia.
> Chapter 94: Organ Donation

Anthony F. Suffredini, M.D.

Senior Investigator, Critical Care Medicine Department, National Institutes of Health, Bethesda, Maryland.
> Chapter 2: Mechanisms of Inflammation

Gregory M. Susla, Pharm.D.

Critical Care Pharmacist, Pharmacy Department, Warren G. Magnuson Clinical Center, National Institutes of Health, Bethesda, Maryland.
> Chapter 74: Pharmacokinetics-Pharmacodynamics: Drug Delivery and Therapeutic Drug Monitoring

Paul S. Thornton, M.B., B.Ch., M.R.C.P.I.

Instructor in Pediatrics, University of Pennsylvania School of Medicine; Exchange Fellow, The Hospital for Sick Children, London, England, and Endocrine/Diabetes Division, Children's Hospital of Philadelphia, Philadelphia, Pennsylvania.
> Chapter 60: Disorders of Intermediary Metabolism

James W. Thorp, Capt., M.C., U.S.N.

Head, Health Monitoring Division, Diving Medicine Naval Medical Research Institute; Neonatologist, National Naval Medical Center, Bethesda, Maryland.
> Chapter 43: Hyperbaric Oxygen Therapy

Samuel J. Tilden, M.S., M.D.

Associate Professor of Pediatrics and Anesthesiology and Director, Division of Pediatric Critical Care Medicine, University of Alabama at Birmingham; Director, Pediatric Intensive Care Unit, The Children's Hospital of Alabama, Birmingham, Alabama.
> Chapter 47: Lung Parenchyma

Orrawin Trocki, M.S., R.D.

Clinical Dietician, Children's National Medical Center, Washington, District of Columbia.
> Chapter 87: Burns in Children

Michael R. Uhing, M.D.

Research Fellow, Division of Neonatology, University of Illinois at Chicago, Chicago, Illinois.
> Chapter 49: Respiratory Disease in the Newborn

Victoria L. Vetter, M.D.

Associate Professor of Pediatrics, University of Pennsylvania School of Medicine; Senior Cardiologist and Director, Electrocardiography and Electrophysiology Laboratories, Children's Hospital of Philadelphia, Philadelphia, Pennsylvania.
> Chapter 36: Arrhythmias

Dharmapuri Vidyasagar, M.D.

Professor of Pediatrics, Department of Pediatrics, and Director of Neonatology, University of Illinois at Chicago, Chicago, Illinois.
> Chapter 49: Respiratory Disease in the Newborn

Joseph J. Volpe, M.D.

Bronson Crothers Professor of Neurology, Harvard Medical School; Neurologist-in-Chief, Children's Hospital, Boston, Massachusetts.
> Chapter 18: Hypoxic-Ischemic Cerebral Injury in the Newborn

Thomas L. Walsh, M.D.

Associate Professor, Psychiatry and Behavioral Sciences and Pediatrics, George Washington University School of Medicine; Senior Attending Physician, Children's National Medical Center, Washington, District of Columbia.
> Chapter 68: Psychiatric Aspects of Critical Care

S. Webb, M.D.

Fellow, Department of Critical Care, The Children's Hospital, Denver, Colorado; Assistant Professor of Pediatrics, Division of Pediatric Critical Care, Medical University of South Carolina, Charleston, South Carolina.
> Chapter 11: Neonatal Sepsis

Richard E. Weibley, M.D., M.P.M.

Associate Professor of Pediatrics, University of South Florida; Medical Director, Pediatric Intensive Care Unit; Vice-Chief,

Department of Pediatrics, Children's Medical Center, Tampa General Hospital, Tampa, Florida.
Chapter 45: Disorders of the Proximal Airway

Kathryn Weise, M.D.
Assistant Professor, Department of Pediatrics, University of Virginia School of Medicine; Attending Physician, Pediatric Intensive Care Unit, University of Virginia Children's Medical Center, Charlottesville, Virginia.
Chapter 75: Receptor Physiology

David F. Westenkirchner, M.D.
Clinical Assistant Professor of Pediatrics, Section of Pediatric Pulmonology and Intensive Care, Department of Pediatrics, College of Medicine, Indiana University Medical Center; Associate Medical Director, Intensive Care Unit, Medical Director, Emergency Room, Riley Hospital for Children, Indianapolis, Indiana.
Chapter 38: Respiratory Monitoring

Randall C. Wetzel, M.B., B.S.
Associate Professor, Departments of Anesthesiology/Critical Care Medicine, and Pediatrics, Johns Hopkins University School of Medicine; Chief, Division of Pediatric Anesthesia, The Johns Hopkins Hospital, Baltimore, Maryland.
Chapter 37: Maturation of the Respiratory System

Jonathan M. Whitfield, M.B., Ch.B., F.R.C.P.(C), F.C.C.P.
Associate Professor of Pediatrics, University of Colorado Health Sciences Center; Director, Children's Hospital Emergency Transport Service, Denver, Colorado; Director of Neonatal and Pediatric Critical Care, Baylor University Medical Center, Dallas, Texas.
Chapter 11: Neonatal Sepsis

Bernhard L. Wiedermann, M.D.
Associate Professor of Pediatrics, The George Washington University School of Medicine and Health Sciences; Attending Physician in Infectious Diseases and Director, Pediatric Residency Training Program, Children's National Medical Center, Washington, District of Columbia.
Chapter 72: Characteristics of Pathogenic Microbes and Infectious Syndromes

James D. Wilkinson, M.D.
Assistant Professor of Anesthesiology and Pediatrics, The George Washington University School of Medicine; Attending Physician, Department of Critical Care Medicine, and Medical Director, Intermediate Intensive Care Unit, Children's National Medical Center, Washington, District of Columbia.
Chapter 52: Oxygen Transport

Roberta G. Williams, M.D.
Professor, Department of Pediatrics; Chief, Division of Cardiology, UCLA Medical Center, Los Angeles, California.
Chapter 33: Congenital Heart Disease

Jerry A. Winkelstein, M.D.
Professor of Pediatrics, The Johns Hopkins University School of Medicine; Director, Division of Allergy and Immunology, Department of Pediatrics, Johns Hopkins Hospital, Baltimore, Maryland.
Chapter 4: Pathophysiology of the Immune System

Muriel D. Wolf, M.D.
Associate Professor of Pediatrics, George Washington University School of Medicine; Associate Medical Director, General Pediatric Ambulatory Center and Senior Attending in Pediatrics and Cardiology, Children's National Medical Center, Washington, District of Columbia.
Chapter 81: Envenomation

Ido Yatsiv, M.D.
Director, Pediatric Intensive Care Unit, Department of Pediatrics, Hadassah Medical Center, Jerusalem, Israel.
Chapter 16: Central Nervous System Evaluation and Monitoring
Chapter 17: Central Nervous System Support Techniques
Chapter 25: Postoperative Neurosurgical Management

Aaron R. Zucker, M.D.
Associate Professor of Pediatrics and Director, Section of Pediatric Critical Care, Wyler Children's Hospital, University of Chicago, Chicago, Illinois.
Chapter 44: Pharmacologic Adjuncts to Mechanical Ventilation in the Adult Respiratory Distress Syndrome in Children

Preface

Now comes pediatric critical care bringing a new way of looking at the critically ill child: comprehensive, integrated, and outcome-focused. The breadth of critical care is the breadth of critical illness and is limited only by death or wellness. The depth of critical care ranges from intranuclear to societal levels. It encompasses physiology, pharmacology, cardiology, and pulmonary medicine. Critical care is not anesthesiology, neonatology, traumatology, nor cardiac surgery—but, it involves all of these specialties.

The field emerged from practical management issues of resuscitation, monitoring, concentration of resources, and bedside titration of therapy. These remain cornerstones but are supplemented by considerations of pansystemic conditions like sepsis, nutritional and multiple organ system failure, and even death itself. Outcome prediction, intercellular communication, economics, and interaction of the health care givers at the bedside are new considerations.

The target organ remains the brain, while cardiovascular and pulmonary support are mainstays. The recognition that the return to homeostasis of all the organ systems is essential to achieve a satisfactory outcome of the patient characterizes modern critical care thought. That all body systems are interactive is axiomatic.

The *Textbook of Pediatric Critical Care* is a humble effort to assist the care giver in his or her pursuits. It is comprehensive and integrative and has the luxury of drawing on the expertise of superb authors from around the world. No chapter is less important than another. They should all be read. I am indebted to the authors for their efforts.

PETER R. HOLBROOK, M.D.

Acknowledgments

No book is possible without the efforts of many people other than the editor. I specifically thank the staff of W.B. Saunders—Richard Zorab, Hazel N. Hacker, Marjory I. Fraser, Bill Preston, and Sandra Valkhoff; my office manager Sallie Brodus and her assistant Marcia Howard; my fellows and colleagues who assisted in many ways; and my family who bear the brunt of all the things I do.

PETER R. HOLBROOK, M.D.

Contents

III Pansystemic Illness

IV Organ System Failure

Central Nervous System

Cardiovascular System

Respiratory System

Renal System

Digestive System

Mechanisms of Hypoxia-Ischemia*

Johan Lundgren, M.D., and Bo K. Siesjö, M.D., Ph.D.

Hypoxic-ischemic injury is commonplace in the intensive care unit. Although the effects of this injury are pansystemic, the clinical outcome is determined by the impact of the insult on the brain. This chapter discusses mechanisms for brain cell damage following hypoxia-ischemia.

PATHOPHYSIOLOGY

Coupling Among Adenosine Triphosphate Production, Ion Transport, and Biosynthetic Work

The normal function of brain cells depends, to a relatively unique extent, on an abundant supply of oxygen and glucose. This is because neurons, and probably also glia cells, have an unusually high energy dependence, which is related, at least in part, to constant leakage and repumping of ions across their membranes.[1-6] Directly or indirectly, all cellular work is done at the expense of adenosine triphosphate (ATP) formed during glycolysis in the cytoplasm (a minor part) or during oxidative phosphorylation in the mitochondria (the major fraction). The participation of ATP in ion transport is illustrated in Figure 1–1. The ATP fuels the Na^+/K^+ and the Ca^{2+}/H^+ transporters, which achieve the coupled efflux of $3Na^+$ and uptake of $2K^+$ and the efflux of Ca^{2+} in exchange for $2H^+$, respectively. The ATP-driven Na^+/K^+ transport is electrogenic, exporting a positive charge. The balance of charge requires that a negative ion, probably Cl^-, is also extruded. Extrusion of (extra) Na^+ and of Cl^- also leads to export of water. In this sense, the Na^+,K^+-ATPase (adenosine triphosphatase) helps regulate cell volume.

An indirect ATP dependence is shown by ion translo-

cators that export ions, notably Ca^{2+} and H^+, at the expense of the Na^+ gradient created by the Na^+,K^+-ATPase. The Na^+/Ca^{2+} exchanger is electrogenic, exporting $1Ca^{2+}$ in exchange for $3Na^+$. This means that the rate (and direction) of Na^+/Ca^{2+} exchange depends on both the Na^+ gradient and the membrane potential. Under certain circumstances, the exchanger can be reversed and become responsible for loading cells with calcium. Export of H^+ also occurs by ionic exchange in which the Na^+ gradient is used to expel H^+ by an electroneutral exchanger, which operates to maintain intracellular pH (pH_i) at around 7.0.

Normally, ATP-driven transport matches spontaneous leakage of Na^+ and Ca^{2+} into the cell and of K^+ out of the cell. Leakage occurs via conductance channels, which may be selective or unselective (see further on), or via ion translocators (antiporters or symporters). These translocators are proteins that can shuttle ions or molecules between extra- and intracellular fluids. They may be electrogenic (e.g., catalyzing $3Na^+/Ca^{2+}$ exchange; see earlier) or electroneutral. The latter encompass symport mechanisms, translocating $1Na^+$ and $1Cl^-$ or $1Na^+$, $1K^+$, and $2Cl^-$. In principle, loss of ion homeostasis can occur either because there is a shortage of ATP or because leakage is enhanced. Activation of conductance pathways occurs during enhanced functional activity and during seizures. Less is known about increased flux catalyzed by membrane-bound ion translocators, but conceivably such translocators are activated in disease.

Although ion transport may consume about 50% of the energy produced within the tissue, the remainder must be used to support biosynthetic tasks, which encompass reactions that achieve synthesis of lipids, proteins, and ribonucleic acid (RNA) following their degradation or loss from the cell. This principle can be exemplified by turnover in the two major phospholipid cycles in the cell (Fig. 1–2). Thus, though the breakdown of both phosphatidylinositol bisphosphate (PIP_2) and other phospholipids is thermodynamically spontaneous, resynthesis of the original phospholipid molecules re-

*This work was supported by the Swedish Medical Research Council (Grants No. 14X-263 and No. 12X-7123), the National Institute of Health of the United States Public Health Service (Grant No. 5. ROI NS-07838), and the Margarethahemmet Society.

quires ATP or the equivalent amount of another nucleoside triphosphate.

Although phospholipids probably have an unusually rapid turnover, the principles are the same for all macromolecules and macromolecular assemblies: The molecules are degraded in thermodynamically spontaneous reactions; hence, ATP is required to maintain cellular structure (and function). However, degradation of structure is not due to loss of energy for resynthesis alone, since conditions prevailing in energy-deprived tissues may enhance the rate of degradation. For example, although agonists acting on receptors coupled to phospholipase C accelerate breakdown of PIP_2 (and PIP), calcium can accelerate deacylation of other phospholipids. Calcium has a similar effect on protein breakdown (see further on).

Types of Tissue Hypoxia

Since the major part of ATP production occurs via oxidative phosphorylation, tissue hypoxia causes damage to cells by hindering ATP production. As shown in Figure 1–3, a reduction of oxygen availability at tissue level (hypoxia) can have several causes. We can distinguish between arterial hypoxia and ischemia. The former results from reduction of either arterial Po_2 (hypoxic hypoxia) or hemoglobin concentration (anemic hypoxia). Unless complicated by cardiac failure or hypotension, hypoxia usually leads to a rise in cerebral blood flow (CBF). If such complications are present, CBF will fall from its increased hyperemic value. This situation— that is, hypoxia with restricted hyperemia—may be detrimental even if CBF has not decreased to less than normal. This is because O_2 availability is determined by the product of CBF and O_2 content. For example, if CBF falls from a hyperemic value of 200% of control to normal values, O_2 availability will decrease to 50% of its hyperemic value.

A reduction of blood flow to values that produce symptoms of oxygen deficiency is conveniently called ischemia. Complete ischemia is encountered in cardiac arrest. This is the only situation that leads to anoxia— that is, to complete lack of oxygen at the cellular level. Incomplete ischemia is more common, particularly since it characterizes focal ischemia of the stroke type. In complete and near-complete ischemia, there is reduced (or no) delivery, not only of oxygen but also of substrate. As will be discussed further on, continued supply of the major substrate (i.e., glucose) may improve survival or "wreck the machinery," depending on the degree of energy failure. The beneficial effect can be explained in terms of the survival value of the ATP produced when the extra glucose is metabolized glycolytically. However, since anaerobic glycolysis produces lactate⁻ plus H⁺, it may lead to excessive acidosis. This is probably why hyperglycemia, which triggers additional production of lactic acid, may be harmful. As will also be discussed further on, a persisting blood flow with continued oxygen delivery may theoretically trigger the production of reactive oxygen species.

The term asphyxia is used to denote a situation in

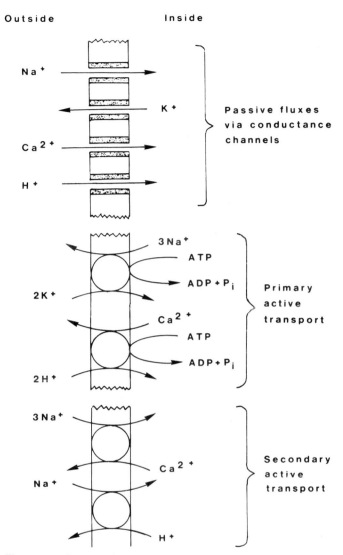

Figure 1–1. Diagram illustrating passive fluxes of Na⁺, K⁺, Ca²⁺, and H⁺ ions; primary ATP-driven active transport; and secondary ATP-dependent active transport with extrusion of Ca²⁺ and H⁺ ions occurring at the expense of the Na⁺ gradient.

which reduction of tissue oxygen tension is combined with a rise in carbon dioxide tension. In adults, the primary cause is usually respiratory insufficiency. It should be emphasized, however, that hypoxia-hypercapnia is often associated with hypotension. Thus there is often a component of relative or absolute ischemia in the syndrome denoted by the term asphyxia.

Metabolic Events in Hypoxia-Ischemia

The primary and most damaging event in hypoxia-ischemia is ATP depletion. However, though cell death is the end result of ATP depletion, this depletion may not be the direct cause of the damage incurred. This is because energy failure triggers a series of events that hasten the breakdown of cell structure and elicit unfavorable reactions. The type and degree of perturbation

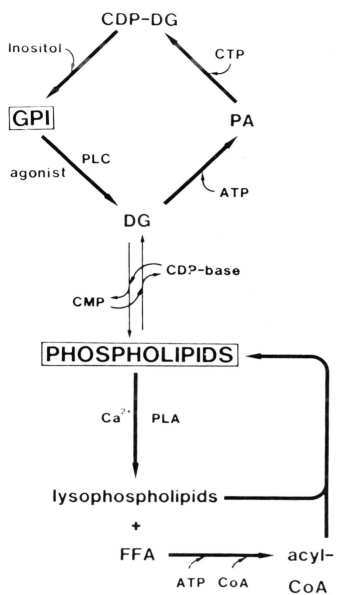

Figure 1–2. Diagram illustrating degradation-resynthesis of phospholipids under normal conditions. Inosine phosphoglyceride (*GPI*) is broken down by an agonist-activated phospholipase C (PLC); other phospholipids are broken down by a calcium-activated phospholipase A (PLA); and energy (*ATP* and *CTP*) is needed to resynthesize the original phospholipids. DG = diacylglyceride; PA = phosphatidic acid; FFA = free fatty acid; ATP = adenosine triphosphate; CTP = cytidine triphosphate. (Modified from Wieloch T and Siesjö BK: Ischemic brain injury: the importance of calcium, lipolytic activities, and free fatty acids. Pathol Biol 30:269, 1982.)

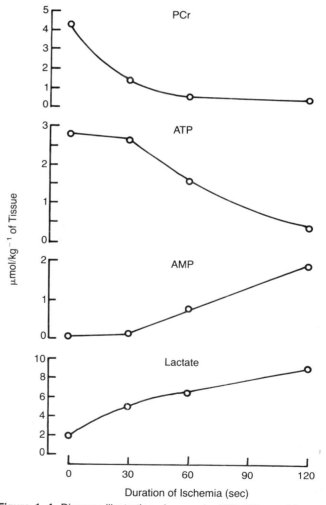

Figure 1–3. Schematic illustration showing the factors determining oxygen availability. CBF = cerebral blood flow. (From Siesjö BK: Brain Energy Metabolism. Copyright 1978. Reprinted by permission of John Wiley & Sons, Ltd., Bath.)

transport or biosynthetic work can be performed only at the expense of available stores of phosphocreatine (PCr) and ATP or the glycolytically formed ATP. As shown in Figure 1–4, the decrease in PCr and ATP is

of cell metabolism depend to a large extent on the severity of the hypoxia and its characteristics. The following section will describe events in complete or near-complete ischemia, concentrating on energy metabolism, loss of ion homeostasis, and changes in lipid constituents.

Energy Metabolism

Following cessation of CBF, oxygen tension decreases toward zero within a few seconds. Thereafter, active

Figure 1–4. Diagram illustrating changes in ATP, PCr, and lactate content of rat cerebral cortex during the initial phase of complete ischemia. PCr = phosphocreatine; ATP = adenosine triphosphate; AMP = adenosine monophosphate. (Data from Nordström CH and Siesjö BK: Influence of phenobarbital on changes in the metabolites of the energy reserve of the cerebral cortex following complete ischemia. Acta Physiol Scand 104:271, 1978.)

rapid. After a sudden interruption of circulation, PCr concentration approaches zero within the first minute, and ATP falls close to its minimal value after 2 minutes.[7-9] During that period, ATP is formed from PCr via the creatine kinase equilibrium and during anaerobic glycolysis. During ischemia, when ATP is hydrolyzed to yield adenosine diphosphate (ADP) and adenosine monophosphate (AMP), the latter is degraded to purine nucleosides and bases, including hypoxanthine. This has two effects. First, the size of the adenine nucleotide pool (ATP + ADP + AMP) decreases. Since resynthesis of nucleotides is slow, the pool size and the ATP concentration may remain reduced for many hours, even if recirculation is achieved. Second, once oxygen supply is restored, hypoxanthine may be metabolized to superoxide anion ($\cdot O_2^-$), a free radical.[10]

During complete ischemia, the amount of lactate formed is proportional to the preischemic stores of glycogen and glucose.[11] Since the glucose store varies with the preischemic plasma glucose concentration, hypoglycemia is associated with a reduced lactate content in tissue, and hyperglycemia is associated with an increased tissue lactate content. If some flow remains, additional lactate may be formed from the glucose delivered. Since glucose supply is limited by the reduction in flow, however, acceleration of glycolysis requires a raised plasma glucose concentration. This is why hyperglycemia may lead to grossly exaggerated lactic acidosis. Two factors are thus required to yield excessive degrees of acidosis: (1) sufficient energy deprivation to cause massive stimulation of glycolysis and (2) a plasma glucose concentration that is sufficiently raised to overcome the flow limitation of glucose supply.

A somewhat different situation is encountered in arterial hypoxia (or asphyxia)—that is, in situations of tissue hypoxia in which CBF is not reduced. In this case, the severity of the lactic acidosis depends on the reduction in phosphorylation potential rather than on plasma glucose concentration.[12] Plasma glucose concentration seems to modulate the lactic acidosis only if it is reduced to low levels, since hypoglycemia can prevent excessive acidosis from occurring at low phosphorylation potentials.[13]

Ion Homeostasis

Complete ischemia leads to rapid and extensive loss of ion homeostasis.[14, 15] In the rat, changes in extracellular ion concentrations show two phases. During the first 1 to 2 minutes, extracellular K^+ (K^+_e) increases slowly to 10 to 15 mM, whereas Ca^{2+}_e, Na^+_e, and Cl^-_e remain essentially unaltered. The second phase is characterized by rapid efflux of K^+ from cells and uptake of Ca^{2+}, Na^+, and Cl^-. At the same time, extracellular fluid volume decreases to about 50% of control, reflecting cell swelling. The latter is probably due to uptake of Na^+ and Cl^-, with osmotically obligated water.

The phase 2 ionic shifts suggest that a major, unspecific ion conductance is activated. The mechanisms may be as follows:[16, 17] At the onset of ischemia, a K^+ conductance is activated, causing loss of potassium from cells and a slow rise in K^+_e. When K^+_e reaches a certain value, presynaptic endings depolarize and release excitatory transmitters, notably glutamate. These transmitters activate two major receptor types, each gating unspecific cation channels.[18-20] The first, specifically activated by amino-3-hydroxy-5-methyl-isoxazole-4-propionate (AMPA), gates a channel permeable to both Na^+ and K^+, whereas the second, selectively activated by N-methyl-D-aspartate (NMDA), gates a channel permeable to calcium as well (Fig. 1–5). These two channels may be at least partly responsible for the "shock" opening of ion conductances observed during ischemia. The NMDA-gated channel is normally blocked by Mg^{2+} in a voltage-dependent manner, meaning that the block is relieved when the membrane depolarizes. Since activation of AMPA receptors gives rise to Na^+ influx and depolarization, it obviously also sets the stage for Ca^{2+} influx (see also Chapter 26).

Evidence exists that rapid ion fluxes during ischemia reflect a marked increase in ion permeability.[5] Such an increase could be caused by release of excitatory amino acids (EAAs). However, it is also possible that a certain degree of depolarization, or a rise in Ca^{2+}_i, causes unspecific channels to open. Whatever the explanation, it is likely that energy-deprived cells maintain "leaky" membranes. Re-establishment of ionic gradients is possible only if ATP is resupplied to achieve ion pumping and reuptake of transmitters. ATP failure and loss of ion homeostasis are probably mutually reinforcing occurrences, explaining the "avalanche" character of events once energy production is critically reduced.

If CBF is reduced gradually, electrical failure with cessation of electroencephalographic activity occurs at a higher threshold (CBF 15 to 20 ml/100 g^{-1}/min^{-1}) than that associated with loss of ion homeostasis (CBF 10 to 15 ml/100 g^{-1}/min^{-1}).[21-23] The first threshold probably reflects the activation of a K^+ conductance, causing postsynaptic hyperpolarization, whereas the second threshold represents rapid loss of ionic homeostasis. Interestingly, if a spreading depression (SD) is elicited in the brain of a normal animal, one observes ionic shifts resembling those occurring in ischemia.[5, 14] In SD, however, these shifts are spontaneously reversible. It is tempting to assume that the SD is elicited by release of glutamate or a related EAA, which triggers activation of unspecific cation channels, and that the termination of the event is related to ATP-fueled ion transport and glutamate reuptake.

Clearly, since loss of ion homeostasis is detrimental, it would be advantageous to therapeutically prolong phase 1. At present, this is difficult to do pharmacologically. The delay to depolarization during ischemia depends on the preischemic metabolic rate and the nutritional state. For example, preischemic hyperglycemia prolongs the duration of phase 1.[5] However, maintained glucose delivery carries a serious disadvantage because it produces additional lactate⁻ and H^+, further reducing pH_e and pH_i.

Acid-Base Changes

Many cellular reactions lead to production of H^+. For example, H^+ is produced when ATP is broken down to

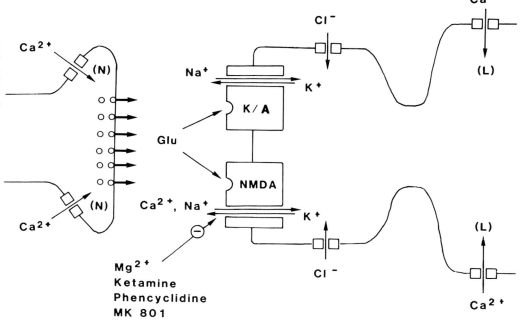

Figure 1–5. Diagram illustrating voltage-sensitive calcium channels (presynaptic N type, and dendrite or cell-soma localized L and T types) and postsynaptic agonist-operated ones. The postsynaptic AMPA ($\approx$K/A)–operated channel is assumed to gate a channel permeable to Na^+ and K^+, whereas the NMDA-operated channel is permeable to Ca^{2+} as well. K/A = kainic acid; NMDA = N-methyl-D-aspartate. (Data from Siesjö BK: The role of calcium in cell death. *In*: Price DL, Aguayo AJ, and Thoenen H [eds]: Neurodegenerative Disorders: Mechanisms and Prospects for Therapy. New York, John Wiley & Sons, in press, 1992.)

ADP and P_i, and when free fatty acids (FFAs) accumulate.[24] Most of the H^+ produced during ischemia-hypoxia is associated with lactate$^-$.[17] If the level of ATP falls, some extra H^+ is generated, but this is usually much less than that associated with lactate. It should also be recalled that the hydrolysis of PCr *consumes* H^+.

Changes in pH_i during ischemia have been derived by calculation from CO_2 data,[25, 26] by umbelliferone histochemistry,[27, 28] and by ^{31}P-NMR (nuclear magnetic resonance) imaging.[29, 30] Figure 1–6 shows that in normoglycemic rats, pH_i falls to about 6.1 during ischemia and recovers during the first 30 to 60 minutes of recirculation. As predicted by Ljunggren and associates,[11] pre-ischemic hypoglycemia reduces and hyperglycemia exaggerates the reduction in pH_i and pH_e.[17, 26]

It has been proposed that H^+ becomes compartmentalized during complete ischemia and that intraglial pH becomes extremely acid (pH 5.2) in hyperglycemic animals, whereas neurons and extracellular fluid have a pH that is about 1 unit higher.[31] Direct microelectrode measurement confirms the presence of a very acid compartment in the ischemic brain, at least in excessively hyperglycemic animals.[32] This is a controversial issue, though, and additional data are required to reveal whether major compartmentalization occurs during ischemia.[17]

Changes in Lipid Constituents

Inspection of Figure 1–2 makes it clear that ischemia must lead to breakdown of phospholipids, with accumulation of FFAs. It has also been repeatedly documented that ischemia is associated with increased tissue concentration of FFAs and diacylglycerides,[33–36] as well

as with reduced concentrations of PIP_2 and PIP.[37] The changes observed are probably secondary to activation of both phospholipase A_2 and phospholipase C, as well as plasmalogenases.

Clearly, extensive degradation of membranes of phospholipase activity could be harmful. However, there are also secondary effects from the phospholipase activity. The increased levels of FFAs persist for some time during recirculation when oxygen supply is resumed.[35, 36] This predictably sets the stage for oxidative metabolism of arachidonic acid by cyclooxygenase and lipoxygenase.[1] Such an arachidonic acid cascade has been shown to occur.[38, 39] The potential consequences of the accumulation of arachidonic acid metabolites are discussed further on.

TYPES OF ISCHEMIC/HYPOXIC BRAIN DAMAGE

A useful subdivision of ischemic brain damage is into global and focal types. Global damage results from cardiac arrest or systemic disorders such as arterial hypotension or hypoxia. Focal damage results from either obstruction of arteries, such as the middle cerebral artery, or from trauma. Global ischemia jeopardizes the survival of the organism. In survivors, ischemia is therefore usually of brief duration. In contrast, focal ischemia is often permanent. However, recanalization of occluded arteries may make stroke a transient insult. This sets the stage for so-called reperfusion damage—that is, damage exacerbated by the (sudden) return of oxygen to a previously energy-compromised tissue.

Brief ischemia-hypoxia often gives rise to neuronal damage, which typically is localized to selectively vul-

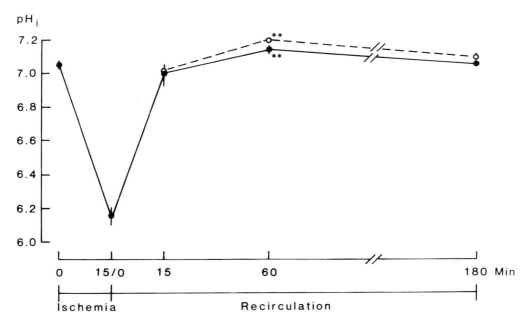

Figure 1–6. Diagram illustrating calculated pH; during and after normoglycemic ischemia. (Data from von Hahnwehr R, et al: extra- and intracellular pH during near-complete forebrain ischemia in the rat. J Neurochem 46:331, 1986 and Smith ML, et al: Changes in extra- and intracellular pH in the brain during and following ischemia in hyperglycemic and in moderately hypoglycemic rats. J Cereb Blood Flow Metab 6:574, 1986.)

nerable neurons, encompassing cells in the middle cortical layers, the CA1 sector of the hippocampus, the dentate hilar region, the dorsolateral crescent of the caudoputamen, and some thalamic nuclei.[40–42] Selective neuronal vulnerability is also the hallmark of hypoglycemic and epileptic brain damage.[43]

The typical lesion in stroke is infarction—that is, pan-necrotic destruction of nerve and glia cells, as well as vascular tissue.[41] The transition between selective neuronal vulnerability and infarction is a gradual one. Usually, ischemia of increased duration favors infarctions, as do preischemic hyperglycemia and hyperthermia.[16] In other cases, typically those leading to reduction of blood flow due to arterial hypotension, the damage is of the boundary zone type—that is, it affects neurons in the areas situated between the distribution territories of the major cerebral arteries.[41]

MECHANISMS OF ISCHEMIC BRAIN DAMAGE

Current hypotheses are centered around (1) the potentially harmful effects of the loss of ion homeostasis, particularly of calcium homeostasis and (2) the acidosis and the presumed generation of free radicals.

Calcium-related Damage

As discussed elsewhere,[44, 45] it has been assumed for close to 20 years that calcium mediates anoxic-ischemic cell death. The original hypothesis was proposed to explain damage to ischemic hearts[46] and dystrophic muscle,[47] but the hypothesis has subsequently become more general, encompassing cell death in a variety of conditions that lead to an enhanced plasma membrane permeability.[48] When calcium "overload" was assumed

to explain ischemic, hypoglycemic, and epileptic brain damage, it was proposed that cells that are preferentially affected are those having high membrane conductances to calcium.[1]

Calcium was originally assumed to cause cell damage by mitochondrial overload. Typically, when ischemic tissue underwent recirculation after long periods of ischemia, calcium would enter the tissue from the blood and be sequestered in the re-energized mitochondria. This would then cause mitochondrial failure and secondary tissue damage. At present, more emphasis is put on other calcium-triggered events.[20, 44] This is partly because calcium-mediated cell damage may occur even though the ischemia is too brief to give rise to mitochondrial damage during the immediate period following ischemia.

Evidence that calcium mediates cell damage from excessive glutamate exposure and anoxia has been obtained in in vitro exposure, and anoxia has been obtained in in vitro experiments on primary neuronal cultures.[20, 49, 50] Thus cells are much less sensitive to these insults if studied in calcium-free media, and damage is enhanced if the calcium concentration is increased. Such experiments also suggest that a major entry pathway for calcium is provided by NMDA-gated channels. Thus, NMDA antagonists ameliorate or prevent damage due to EAA exposure or anoxia. Blockers of voltage sensitive calcium channels (VSCCs) have a much less pronounced effect.[51] Interestingly, under certain conditions, NMDA antagonists could ameliorate damage even when given *after* the exposure to EAAs, suggesting a hysteresis with enhanced calcium influx following the insult. This was also evident in experiments on cultured granular cells from the cerebellum, since removal of calcium from the medium *after* the insult ameliorated cell damage.[52] In this case, however, neither glutamate nor calcium antagonists had a similar effect.

Figure 1–7 illustrates the cascade of calcium-related events that are elicited by energy failure and the potentially adverse reactions that result from this cascade.[16]

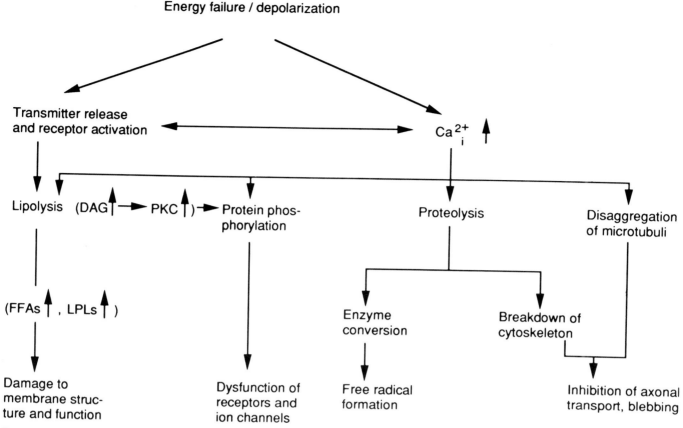

Figure 1–7. Schematic diagram illustrating the cascade of presumed calcium-related pathologic events. Since lipolysis occurs also by phospholipase C activity, a rise in Ca^{2+}_i may not be the dominant cause of the accumulation of FFAs. DAG = diacylglyceride; PKC = protein kinase C; FFAs = free fatty acids; LPLs = lysophospholipids. (From Siesjö BK: The role of calcium in cell death. *In*: Price DL, Aguayo AJ, and Thoenen H [eds]: Neurodegenerative Disorders: Mechanisms and Prospects for Therapy. New York, John Wiley & Sons, in press, 1992. Reprinted by permission of John Wiley & Sons, Ltd.)

As observed, these events encompass enhanced lipolysis, proteolysis, and protein phosphorylation, as well as disaggregation of microtubuli. Not only do lipolytic events lead to accumulation of FFAs and, potentially, to production of harmful levels of cyclooxygenase and lipoxygenase products but they also lead to formation of diacylglycerides, which trigger activation and translocation of protein kinase C.[53, 54] As discussed further on, such activation-translocation may, if sustained, contribute to slowly maturing damage. Proteolysis and disaggregation of microtubuli may interact to yield extensive dissolution of the cytoskeleton, which can cause "blebbing" of the plasma membrane and thereby pathologic enhancement of the plasma membrane permeability.[55, 56] The importance of proteolytic events is underscored by the amelioration of ischemic brain damage by leupeptine, a protease inhibitor.[57]

Some confusion has arisen from the fact that NMDA antagonists have little or no effect on brain damage caused by global or forebrain ischemia, whereas they have a very significant effect in ameliorating damage due to experimental stroke. The following hypothesis has been proposed to explain these seemingly discrepant results.[45] NMDA antagonists cannot prevent calcium influx in a situation (complete or near-complete ischemia) in which multiple calcium conductances are activated and no energy is available to extrude calcium. However, when energy metabolism is compromised rather than deranged (as in the penumbra zone of a stroke lesion), such antagonists are efficacious because they prevent calcium influx through a major entry route, allowing the ATP produced to balance fluxes via other routes. Probably this is also the situation prevailing during hypoxia-ischemia, and one can anticipate that NMDA antagonists could be useful tools to protect the brain during asphyxia. This hypothesis is supported by results suggesting that the ischemic penumbra shows irregularly occurring calcium transients that, when summed up, could be what cause an extension of the focus into the penumbra zone.[58]

Previous data showed that flunarizine, an unspecific calcium blocker, could ameliorate damage caused by complete or near-complete ischemia, even when given after the ischemic transient event.[59] An even more pronounced effect has recently been reported for an AMPA receptor blocker.[60] These results can be explained if one assumes that transient ischemia causes membrane damage and an increased calcium cycling, which is secondary to "fast" excitation due to enhanced Na^+ influx via channels that, at least in part, are gated by AMPA receptors. Thus, though NMDA-gated calcium channels play a role in focal ischemia, AMPA receptor–coupled Na^+ influx could be instrumental in giving delayed neuronal damage after transient ischemia.

Acidosis and Free Radical Production

Preischemic hyperglycemia is known to exaggerate damage caused by dense, transient ischemia.[1, 3, 61, 62] Its adverse effects, which are probably related to enhanced intra- and extracellular acidosis, encompass an increased tendency toward seizures following the ischemic event, accentuated edema, and damage to additional brain areas, such as substantia nigra pars reticulata (SNPR). It is less clear if hyperglycemia exerts such effects in permanent focal ischemia.[58] If acidosis persists in hypoxic-ischemic tissue, several adverse mechanisms can be envisaged.[3] First, since a lowering of pH toward 6.0 markedly reduces oxidative phosphorylation of mitochondria, ATP production will be essentially blocked. Thus acidosis will enhance damage that is secondary to ATP depletion. Second, since acidosis stimulates regulation of pH_i by Na^+/H^+ exchange, it can enhance Na^+ influx. This can lead to one of two adverse effects: (1) it may predispose to cell edema or (2) it may cause additional Ca^{2+} influx. The first effect would result if Na^+/H^+ exchange is coupled to Cl^-/HCO_3^- exchange or if Cl^- influx occurs by other routes. The second effect could be the result if conditions favor calcium influx by $3Na^+/Ca^{2+}$ exchange—that is, if a reversal of the exchanger causes calcium to accumulate in the cell.

If acidosis does not persist—that is, if recirculation occurs but damage nevertheless is observed, other mechanisms must be invoked. Obviously, the mechanisms sought are those that are triggered by the accentuated acidosis and that cause cell damage at a time when the acidosis is no longer present. One such mechanism is loss of inhibitory control with induction of seizures in the recovery period following transient ischemia. It has been proposed (and indeed established) that hypoxia-ischemia preferentially destroys GABAergic cells.[63, 64] A more direct link to seizure induction was demonstrated when hyperglycemic rats, which almost invariably show postischemic seizures, were found to experience damage to GABAergic systems, including that encompassing the SNPR.[65, 66] This structure (SNPR) gates an important inhibitory system, exerting control of excitatory influences.[67] One may envisage, therefore, that cell necrosis in SNPR reflects loss of GABAergic tonus from the striatum and that more widespread loss of GABAergic inhibition leads to seizures, which then become the direct cause of secondary brain damage.[68] However, one must then assume that such a loss does not necessarily lead to an increase in metabolic rate.[69]

Although the role of ATP failure in hypoxic-ischemic damage is unequivocal, and the mediation of loss of calcium homeostasis and acidosis is highly likely, the participation of free radicals is more speculative. Theoretically, hypoxia-ischemia should, particularly if followed by reperfusion, lead to enhanced production of free radicals.[1, 70–73] This is because (1) reduction of oxygen at the cytochrome a_1a_3 step would favor univalent reduction of oxygen, (2) auto-oxidation of catecholamines and other compounds is likely to occur during recirculation, (3) the metabolism of arachidonic acid by cyclooxygenase and lipoxygenase is accompanied by production of free radicals, and (4) calcium loading of cells can cause the proteolytic conversion of xanthine dehydrogenase to xanthine oxidase, the latter oxidizing hypoxanthine to O_2^-. Although it has been assumed for many years that free radical production contributes to ischemic brain damage, it has turned out to be difficult to unequivocally demonstrate that such a link exists.[16] With the advent of new technologies, it has been shown that ischemia with reperfusion is followed by production of reactive oxygen species and also that the damage incurred is ameliorated by established free radical scavengers.[74, 75] It has been difficult to explain, though, that other results are negative. The discrepancies can be explained by a hypothesis that predicts that ischemia of brief duration primarily causes neuronal damage, secondary to a loss of calcium homeostasis, whereas free radicals enter as important mediators of ischemic damage following long periods of ischemia, whether followed by reperfusion or not.[45]

It is in this context that marked acidosis may play a role. Thus acidosis is known to enhance free radical production, at least in part by releasing pro-oxidant iron from protein bindings.[76–78] Iron binding to transferrin occurs according to the reaction:[79]

$$Fe^{3+} + HCO_3^- + H_3TFn \leftrightarrow FE\text{-}TFn\text{-}HCO_3^- + 3H^+$$

Thus release of iron at low pH is secondary to protonic attack on the HCO_3^- (or CO_3^{2-}) bridge through which iron is bound to the protein. This is not an exclusive mechanism for iron release, however, since acidosis is also known to release iron from ferritin.[80] Furthermore, release of iron may not be the only mechanism whereby acidosis accelerates free radical reactions, since acidosis shifts the reaction

$$\bullet O_2H \leftrightarrow H^+ + \bullet O_2^- \quad (pK' = 4.8)$$

to the left. Since the hydrated form of superoxide anions ($\bullet O_2H$) is more lipid-soluble and a stronger pro-oxidant than $\bullet O_2^-$, acidosis may act by increasing the toxicity of produced $\bullet O_2^-$.[81]

At present, the hypothesis of acidosis-related damage secondary to enhanced production of free radicals is speculative, and additional data are required to either validate the hypothesis or refute it.

It is now clear that acidosis may not be responsible for damage caused by less severe but more protracted hypoxia-ischemia, but such damage may nonetheless involve free radicals. For example, free radical scavengers have been reported to ameliorate damage caused by permanent occlusion of one middle cerebral artery in rats.[53] It seems likely, therefore, that formation of free radicals can occur even if excessive acidosis is not present (see Chapters 21 and 22).

References

1. Siesjö BK: Cell damage in the brain: A speculative synthesis. J Cereb Blood Flow Metab 1:155, 1981.

2. Siesjö BK: Cerebral circulation and metabolism. J Neurosurg 60(5):883, 1984.

3. Siesjö BK: Acidosis and ischemic brain damage. Neurochem Pathol 9:31, 1988.

4. Astrup J: Energy-requiring cell functions in the ischemic brain. J Neurosurg 56:482, 1982.

5. Hansen AJ: Effects of anoxia on ion distribution in the brain. Physiol Rev 65(1):101, 1985.

6. Erecińska M and Silver IA: ATP and brain function. J Cereb Blood Flow Metab 9:2, 1989.

7. Lowry OH, Passoneau JV, Hasselberger FX, et al: Effect of ischemia on known substrates and cofactors of the glycolytic pathway. J Biol Chem 239:18, 1964.

8. Nilsson B, Norberg K, Nordström CH, et al: Rate of energy utilization in the cerebral cortex of rats. Acta Physiol Scand 93:569, 1975.

9. Nordström CH and Siesjö BK: Influence of phenobarbital on changes in the metabolites of the energy reserve of the cerebral cortex following complete ischemia. Acta Physiol Scand 104:271, 1978.

10. McCord JM: Oxygen-derived free radicals in postischemic tissue injury. N Engl J Med 312:159, 1985.

11. Ljunggren B, Norberg K, and Siesjö BK: Influence of tissue acidosis upon restitution of brain energy metabolism following total ischemia. Brain Res 77:173, 1974.

12. Salford LG, Plum F, and Siesjö BK: Graded hypoxia-oligemia in rat brain. Arch Neurol 29:227, 1973.

13. Gardiner M, Smith ML, Kögström E, et al: Influence of blood glucose concentration on brain lactate accumulation during severe hypoxia and subsequent recovery of brain energy metabolism. J Cereb Blood Flow Metab 2:429, 1982.

14. Nicholson C: Dynamics of the brain cell microenvironment. Neurosci Res Program Bull 18:177, 1980.

15. Hansen AJ Effects of anoxia on ion distribution in the brain. Physiol Rev 65(1):101, 1985.

16. Siesjö BK, Agardh CD, and Bengtsson F: Free radicals and brain damage. Cerebrovasc Brain Metab Rev 1:165, 1989.

17. Siesjö BK, Ekholm A, Katsura K, et al: Acid-base changes during complete brain ischemia. Stroke 21 (Suppl III):194, 1990.

18. Fagg GE: L-Glutamate, excitatory amino acid receptors and brain functions. Trends Neurosci 8:207, 1985.

19. Cotman CW, Iversen LL: Excitatory amino acids in the brain—focus on NMDA receptors. Trends Neurosci 10:236, 1987.

20. Choi DW: Calcium-mediated neurotoxicity: Relationship to specific channel types and role in ischemic damage. Trends Neurosci 11:465, 1988.

21. Branston NM, Symon L, Crockard HA, et al: Relationship between the cortical evoked potential and local cortical blood flow following acute middle cerebral artery occlusion in the baboon. Exp Neurol 45:195, 1974.

22. Astrup J, Symon L, Braton NM, et al: Cortical evoked potential and extracellular K^+ and H^+ at critical levels of brain ischemia. Stroke 8:51, 1977.

23. Astrup J, Siesjö BK, and Symon L: Thresholds in cerebral ischemia—the ischemic penumbra. Stroke 12:723, 1981.

24. Hochachka PW and Mommsen TP: Protons and anaerobiosis. Science 219:1391, 1983.

25. von Hahnwehr R, Smith ML, and Siesjö BK: Extra- and intracellular pH during near-complete forebrain ischemia in the rat. J Neurochem 46:331, 1986.

26. Smith ML, von Hanwehr R, and Siesjö BK: Changes in extra- and intracellular pH in the brain during and following ischemia in hyperglycemic and in moderately hypoglycemic rats. J Cereb Blood Flow Metab 6:574, 1986.

27. Sundt TMJ and Anderson RE: Umbelliferone as an intracellular pH-sensitive fluorescent indicator and blood-brain barrier probe: Instrumentation, calibration, and analysis. J Neurophysiol 44:60, 1980.

28. Paschen W, Djriicic B, Mies G, et al: Lactate and pH in the brain: Association and dissociation in different pathophysiological states. J Neurochem 48:154, 1987.

29. Chopp M, Welch KMA, Tidwell CD, et al: Global cerebral ischemia and intracellular pH during hyperglycemia and hypoglycemia in cats. Stroke 19:1383, 1988.

30. Behar KL, Rothman DL, and Hossmann KA: NMR spectroscopic investigation of the recovery of energy and acid-base homeostasis in the cat brain after prolonged ischemia. J Cereb Blood Flow Metab 9:655, 1989.

31. Kraig RP, Pulsinelli WA, and Plum F: Carbonic acid buffer changes during complete brain ischemia. Am J Physiol 250:R348, 1986.

32. Kraig RP and Chesler M: Astrocytic acidosis in hyperglycemic and complete ischemia. J Cereb Blood Flow Metab 10:104, 1990.

33. Bazan NG: Free arachidonic acid and other lipids in the nervous system during early ischemia and after electroshock. Adv Exp Med Biol 72:317, 1976.

34. DeMedio G, Garacci G, Horrocks L, et al: The effect of transient ischemia on fatty acid and lipid metabolism in the gerbil brain. Ital J Biochem 29:412, 1980.

35. Yoshida S, Inoh S, Asano T, et al: Effect of transient ischemia on free fatty acids and phospholipids in the gerbil. J Neurosurg 53:323, 1980.

36. Rehncrona S, Westerberg E, Åkesson B, et al: Brain cortical fatty acids and phospholipids during and following complete and severe incomplete ischemia. J Neurochem 38:84, 1982.

37. Abe K, Yuki S, and Kogure K: Strong attenuation of ischemic and postischemic brain edema in rats by a novel free radical scavenger. Stroke 19:480, 1988.

38. Gaudet RJ, Alam I, and Levine L: Accumulation of cyclooxygenase products of arachidonic acid metabolism in gerbil brain during reperfusion after bilateral common carotid artery occlusion. J Neurochem 35(3):653, 1981.

39. Moskowitz MA, Kiwak KH, Heikimian K, et al: Synthesis of compounds with properties of leukotrienes C_4 and D_4 in gerbil brains after ischemia and reperfusion. Science 224:886, 1984.

40. Pulsinelli WA, Brierley JB, and Plum F: Temporal profile of neuronal damage in a model of transient forebrain ischemia. Ann Neurol 11:491, 1982.

41. Brierly JB and Graham DI: Hypoxia and vascular disorders of the central nervous system. In Adams JH, Corsellis JAN, and Duncan LW (eds): Greenfield's Neuropathology. London, Edward Arnold, 1984, pp 125–207.

42. Wieloch T: Neurochemical correlates to selective neuronal vulnerability. Prog Brain Res 63:69, 1985.

43. Auer RN and Siesjö BK: Biological differences between ischemia, hypoglycemia and epilepsy. Ann Neurol 24:699, 1988.

44. Siesjö BK: Historical overview. Calcium, ischemia, and death of brain cells. Ann NY Acad Sci 522:638, 1988.

45. Siesjö BK, Bengtsson F, Grampp W, et al: Calcium, excitotoxins, and neuronal death in the brain. Ann NY Acad Sci 568:234, 1989.

46. Fleckenstein A, Janke J, Doring HJ, et al: Myocardial fiber necrosis due to intracellular CA overload—a new principle in cardiac hypertrophy. Rec Stud Cardiac Struct Metab 4:563–568, 1974.

47. Wrogemann K and Pena SDJ: Mitochondrial calcium overload: A general mechanism for cell necrosis in muscle diseases. Lancet 1:672, 1976.

48. Schanne FAX, Kane AB, Young EE, et al: Calcium dependence of toxic cell death: A final common pathway. Science 206:700, 1979.

49. Choi DW: Glutamate neurotoxicity in cortical cell culture is calcium dependent. Neurosci Lett 58:293, 1985.

50. Rothman SM and Olney JW: Glutamate and the pathophyiology of hypoxic-ischemic brain damage. Ann Neurol 19:105, 1986.

51. Choi DW: Methods for antagonizing glutamate neurotoxicity. Cerebrovasc Brain Metab Rev 2:105, 1990.

52. Manev H, Favaron M, Guidotti A, et al: Delayed increase of Ca^{2+} influx elicited by glutamate: Role in neuronal death. Mol Pharmacol 36(1):106, 1989.

53. Martz D, Rayos G, Schielke GP, et al: Allopurinol and dimethylthiourea reduce brain infarction following middle cerebral artery occlusion in the rat. Stroke 20:488, 1989.

54. Nishizuka Y: Studies and perspectives of protein kinase C. Science 233:305, 1986.

55. Langer GA, Frank JS, and Philipson KD: Ultrastructure and calcium exchange of the sarcolemma, sarcoplasmatic reticulum and mitochondria of the myocardium. Pharmacol Ther 16:331, 1982.

56. Nicotera P, Hartzell P, Davis G, et al: The formation of plasma membrane blebs in hepatocytes exposed to agents that increase cytosolic Ca^{2+} is mediated by the activation of a non-lysosomal proteolytic system. FEBS 209:139, 1986.

57. Lee KS, Frank S, Vanderklish P, et al: Inhibition of proteolysis protects hippocampal neurons from ischemia. Proc Natl Acad Sci USA 88:7233, 1991.
58. Nedergaard M: Mechanisms of brain damage in focal cerebral ischemia. Acta Neurol Scand 77:1, 1988.
59. Deshpande JK and Wieloch T: Flunarizine, a calcium entry blocker, ameliorates ischemic brain damage in the rat. Anesthesiology 64:215, 1986.
60. Sheardown MJ, Nielsen EO, Hansen AJ, et al: 2,3-Dihydroxy-6-nitro-7-sulfamoyl-benzo (F) quinoxaline: A neuroprotectant for cerebral ischemia. Science 2:247:571, 1990.
61. Meyers RE: Lactic acid accumulation as a cause of brain edema and cerebral necrosis resulting from oxygen deprivation. In Korobkin R and Guilleminault G (eds): Advances in Perinatal Neurology. New York, Spectrum, 1979, pp. 85–114.
62. Plum F: What causes infarction in ischemic brain? The Robert Wartenburg lecture. Neurology 33:222, 1983.
63. Sloper JJ, Johnson P, and Powell TPS: Selective degeneration of interneurons in the motor cortex of infant monkeys following controlled hypoxia: a possible cause of epilepsy. Brain Res 198:204, 1980.
64. Francis A and Pulsinelli W: The response of GABAergic and cholinergic neurons to transient cerebral ischemia. Brain Res 243:271, 1982.
65. Smith ML, Kalimo H, Warner DS, et al: Morphological lesions in the brain preceding the development of postischemic seizures. Acta Neuropathol (Berlin) 76:253, 1988.
66. Folbergrovö J, Smith ML, Inamura K, et al: Decrease of glutamate decarboxylase activity in substantia nigra and caudoputamen following transient hyperglycemic ischemia in the rat. J Cereb Blood Flow Metab 9:897, 1989.
67. Gale K: GABA in epilepsy: The pharmacologic basis. Epilepsia 30 (Suppl 3):S1, 1989.
68. Lundgren J, Smith M, and Siesjö BK: Influence of moderate hypothermia on ischemic brain damage incurred under hyperglycemic conditions. Exp Brain Res 84:91–101, 1991.
69. Kozuka M, Smith ML, and Siesjö BK: Preischemic hyperglycemia enhances postischemic depression of cerebral metabolic rate. J Cereb Blood Flow Metab 9:478, 1989.
70. Demopoulos HB, Flamm ES, Seligman ML, et al: Molecular pathology of lipids in CNS membranes. In Jöbsis F (ed): Oxygen and Physiological Function. Dallas, Professional Informational Library, 1977, pp 491–508.
71. Flamm ES, Demoupolos HB, Seligman ML, et al: Free radicals in cerebral ischemia. Stroke 9:445, 1978.
72. Kogure K, Arai H, Abe K, et al: Free radical damage of the brain following ischemia. Prog Brain Res 63:237, 1985.
73. Watson BD and Ginsburg MD: Mechanisms of lipid peroxidation potentiated by ischemia in brain. In Halliwell B (ed): Oxygen radicals and tissue injury. Proceedings of an Upjohn symposium. Bethesda, MD, FASEB, 1988, pp 81–91.
74. Patt A, Harken AH, Burton LK, et al: Xanthine oxidase-derived hydrogen peroxide contributes to ischemia reperfusion-induced edema in gerbil brains. J Clin Invest 81:1556, 1988.
75. Hall ED: Lazaroids: Efficacy and anti-oxidant mechanism in experimental cerebral ischemia. In Kriegelstein J and Oberpichler H (eds): Pharmacology of Cerebral Ischemia. Stuttgart, F.R.G., Wissenschaftliche Verlagsgesellschaft, 1990, pp. 343–350.
76. Barber AA and Bernheim F: Lipid peroxidation: Its measurement, occurrence and significance in animal tissues. Adv Gerontol Res 2:355, 1967.
77. Siesjö BK, Bendek G, Koide T, et al: Influence of acidosis on lipid peroxidation in brain tissues in vitro. J Cereb Blood Flow Metab 5:253, 1985.
78. Rehcrona S, Nielsen Haugh H, and Siesjö BK: Enhancement of iron-catalyzed free radical formation by acidosis in brain homogenates: Difference in effect by lactic acid and CO_2. J Cereb Blood Flow Metab 9:65, 1989.
79. Aisen P: Some physico-chemical aspects of iron metabolism. Ciba Found Symp 51:1, 1979
80. Halliwell B: Oxidants and human disease: Some new concepts. FASEB J 1:358, 1985.
81. Gebicki JM and Bielski BHJ: Comparison of the capacities of the perhydroxyl and superoxide radicals to initiate chain oxidation of linoleic acid. J Am Chem Soc 103:7020, 1981.

Mechanisms of Inflammation*

Anthony F. Suffredini, M.D., and
Robert E. Cunnion, M.D.

Inflammation is the dynamic complex of reactions occurring in blood vessels and adjacent tissues in response to physical, chemical, or biologic agents. As described in classical times by Celsus, the four cardinal clinical signs are rubor, calor, tumor, and dolor—redness, warmth, swelling, and pain. Sometimes a fifth cardinal sign, functio laesa—loss of function—is added.[1] Redness and warmth result from the increased amount of blood in the affected tissue; swelling results from vascular congestion and extravascular exudation of fluids; and pain results from changes in osmotic pressure, alterations in pH, and mechanical stimulation of nerve endings. Inflammation may be acute, lasting only a few days to a few weeks and having a clear termination, or it may be chronic, lasting months or years, with the host's tissues responding in a manner insufficient to overcome completely the persisting effects of the inciting agent.

The cornerstone of the inflammatory response is recruitment of phagocytic leukocytes from bone marrow and other sites and their migration to local tissues. This complicated process entails aggregation and adherence of phagocytic cells to vascular endothelium, their passage through the endothelial layer, and their infiltration into perivascular tissues. An effective inflammatory response depends on the ability of phagocytes to adhere, deform, and respond to chemical signals with directed locomotion. Normal and pathologic functioning of the immune system (phagocytes, T lymphocytes, B lymphocytes, and their humoral products) are discussed in Chapter 4. The subject of this chapter, by contrast, is inflammation per se, the mechanisms through which injurious agents engender vascular and cellular responses by activating plasma protease systems, and cell-generated inflammatory mediators (Table 2–1). This general overview will emphasize acute inflammation as it pertains to common pediatric critical care problems, such as serious infection, shock, and ischemia.

The clinical manifestations of many inflammatory responses are organ-specific (e.g., diffuse alveolar damage in acute lung disease). Nonetheless, tissues have in common certain basic mechanisms of cellular injury and in-

flammation, which together constitute a complex network of interrelated processes. In vitro studies permit elucidation of the effects of particular molecules on particular target cells. In vivo, however, it is rarely possible to be confident of a complete understanding of all the biologic effects of a particular molecule. Cells receive multiple influences, and the net effect on cell function depends on the cell type, the concentrations of various mediators, and a variety of other factors.[2, 3] Interactions among inflammatory mediators may be complementary or antagonistic and are further influenced by counterregulatory mechanisms. Inflammation is a rapidly evolving investigative field, and advances in understanding inflammatory cascades, mediators, and mechanisms may serve to identify targets for therapeutic manipulations.

Those caring for sick children should be familiar with mechanisms of inflammation because they are fundamental to the pathogenesis of shock syndromes, multiple organ system failure, and critical illness in general. In critically ill children, normal inflammatory responses may be altered by infection, immunocompromised states, and anti-inflammatory or immunosuppressive therapies.[4]

VASCULAR AND CELLULAR RESPONSES TO INJURY

Overview

Septic shock exemplifies a severe systemic response to infection in which multiple inflammatory processes lead to cell injury and cell death in multiple organs. Histologically, it is manifested by cell swelling and necrosis, intracellular and interstitial edema, deposition of thrombi and fibrin aggregates, hemorrhage, disruption of connective tissue matrices, fibrosis, and infiltration of organ parenchyma by inflammatory cells.[5, 6] The degree of histologic abnormality depends in part on the type, duration, and severity of the injurious process, as well as on the susceptibility of tissues and cells to noxious influences. Cell homeostasis and viability are threatened by a number of factors: alterations in cell membrane integrity, abnormalities of aerobic respiration that limit adenosine triphosphate production and impair ionic and osmotic pumps and other membrane functions, inhibi-

*All material in this chapter is in the public domain, with the exception of any borrowed figures or tables.

Table 2–1. MAJOR COMPONENTS OF THE ACUTE
INFLAMMATORY RESPONSE

Responses to Injury
Vascular
Cellular

Inflammatory Mediators
Plasma protease systems
Contact activation
Hemostatic and fibrinolytic
Complement
Cell-generated
Reactive oxygen species
Eicosanoids
Platelet-activating factors
Vasoactive amines
Neurogenic inflammation
Peptide regulatory molecules
Cytokines
Growth factors

tion of synthesis of enzymes and structural proteins, and alterations in the genetic integrity of the cell.[7, 8] All of these processes occur to varying degrees after an inflammatory insult.

The response of vascularized tissue to injury is nonspecific and includes vascular dilatation, increased vessel wall permeability, exudation of plasma proteins, and infiltration of leukocytes.[9] Clinically, there are wide variations in the relative prominence of each of these responses (e.g., lack of significant neutrophil infiltration in patients with neutropenia). Molecules that enhance blood flow, alter the permeability of the vascular endothelium, or induce the migration of inflammatory cells from blood into tissues are considered acute inflammatory mediators.[10, 11] Some of these mediators are released from plasma or cells in direct response to inflammatory stimuli. Others are released secondarily, after toxins, bacteria, or ischemia have directly killed cells.[12] Biologic effects of the major mediators of inflammation are summarized in Table 2–2.

Inflammation and repair are inextricably associated. Damaged cells are regenerated or replaced by connective tissue.[14] Cells and tissues have, in addition, a complex system of endogenous anti-inflammatory responses that limit the acute inflammatory events. After a particular noxious stimulus (e.g., acute bacterial pneumonia), the consequences of inflammation and repair usually are adaptive; the offending agent is destroyed and tissues are repaired with minimal fibrosis. Unfortunately, the consequences of inflammation sometimes are maladaptive, with progressive cell damage, cell death, and compromise of organ function (e.g., adult respiratory distress syndrome).

Vascular Responses

The anatomic changes associated with inflammatory alterations in vascular size and flow have been well characterized.[9, 12] Following an inflammatory stimulus, arterioles transiently constrict and then dilate, resulting in augmented flow and recruitment of additional microvascular beds in the involved area. These changes in

vascular smooth muscle tone are mediated in part by the opposing actions of endothelin, a potent vasoconstrictor, and endothelium-derived relaxing factor, an endogenous nitrate and potent vasodilator.[15] Changes occur in the integrity of the vascular endothelium, leading to exudation of fluid and plasma proteins into the interstitium. These fluid and protein shifts increase interstitial osmotic pressure. Blood viscosity increases, sludging of intravascular cellular components follows, and ultimately local blood flow decreases.[9, 12, 16]

Three types of changes that increase vascular permeability in animal models have been described.[9, 17] The first type, *immediate-transient* permeability change, is maximal within 5 to 10 minutes of the stimulus and wanes over 15 to 30 minutes. The change is elicited by certain mediators (e.g., histamine) that act on small and medium-sized venules and is characterized histologically

Table 2–2. BIOLOGIC EFFECTS OF THE MAJOR
MEDIATORS OF INFLAMMATION*

Vasodilatation
Vasoactive amines (histamine, serotonin)
Kinins
Eicosanoids (PGD_2, PGE_2, and PGI_2, LTC_4, LTD_4, and LTE_4)
Endothelium-derived relaxing factor

Altered Vascular Permeability
Vasoactive amines (histamine, serotonin)
Anaphylatoxins (C3a, C5a)
Bradykinin
Platelet-activating factors
LTC_4, LTD_4, and LTE_4
Lysosomal constituents (cationic proteins and neutral proteases)
Fibrinopeptides
Oxygen radicals
IL-1
TNF

Augmented Leukocyte-Endothelial Cell Interaction
C5a
LTB_4
IL-1
TNF
Chemotactic peptides
Platelet-activating factors
Endotoxin

Neutrophil and Monocyte-Macrophage Chemotaxis
C5a
Leukotrienes (LTB_4, LTD_4, and LTE_4)
Hydroxyeicosatetranoic acid (HETE)
Hydroperoxyeicosatetranoic acid (HPETE)
Platelet-activating factors
Lysosomal constituents (cationic proteins)
Bacterial products
IL-1
TNF
IL-8

Tissue Damage
Contents of granules and lysosomes from infiltrating cells
Reactive oxygen species
Phospholipase products

Healing and Control of the Inflammatory Reaction
Inactivators of chemotactic factors
Antiproteinases
Anticytokines
Oxygen radical scavengers and antioxidants
Growth factors

*Adapted from references 10, 12, and 13.

by contraction of the endothelial cells and an increase in the gap between endothelial cells.[16, 18] The second type, *immediate-sustained* permeability change, occurs in arterioles, capillaries, and venules of animals with severe injuries (e.g., burns) that cause endothelial cell necrosis. The significantly increased permeability persists for hours to days, continuing until the original injury is repaired. The third type, *delayed-prolonged* leakage, is characterized by delayed-onset permeability changes in venules and capillaries that last for hours or days following thermal injury, bacterial toxemia, or type IV (delayed) hypersensitivity reactions.[12] Vessels in different tissues and organs, though morphologically similar, may vary in their sensitivity to factors causing increased permeability.[16] Thus varying degrees of altered permeability may be present even within a single organ after an injury.

Cellular Responses

Cellular events in inflammation include activation and interaction of endothelial cells and phagocytic leukocytes, primarily neutrophils and monocytes-macrophages. The process of leukocyte accumulation at a site of injury is initiated by leukocyte margination. As stasis of flow develops, leukocytes preferentially orient themselves along the vascular endothelium and become adherent. The process of adhesion depends on the appearance of specific receptors on activated leukocytes and endothelial cells.[19, 20] Endothelial cells activated by endotoxin or cytokines (e.g., interleukin-1 [IL-1], tumor necrosis factor [TNF]) express specialized cell surface molecules, including endothelial leukocyte adhesion molecule and intracellular adhesion molecule. They appear to be important in the early stages of neutrophil adherence.[13] The leukocytes subsequently migrate through the vascular wall to the interstitium and perivascular tissue.[21] Leukocytes accumulate at sites of injury to phagocytose bacteria and necrotic debris. The degree of their response may serve to limit or prolong inflammation.

Activated leukocytes, like activated endothelial cells, express several specific cell adhesion molecules, including those of the CD11/CD18 complex. CD11a/CD18 is a lymphocyte-associated antigen, whereas CD11b/CD18 and CD11c/CD18 are complement receptors. CD11b/CD18 also serves as a receptor for factor X, fibrinogen, and microorganism recognition.[20, 22] Antibodies to these cell adhesion molecules ameliorate injury in experimental models of myocardial ischemia and hemorrhagic shock.[22]

Migration of neutrophils through the vascular wall occurs within the first 24 hours after an insult, followed by monocyte migration at 24 to 48 hours. Occasionally, lymphocytes or eosinophils may be the predominant infiltrating cells.[12] Migration depends on the presence of specific leukocyte receptors for chemotactic agents. These agents activate the leukocytes and result in unidirectional migration toward the attractants.[23] For neutrophils these chemical attractants include both endogenous and exogenous molecules, including soluble bacterial products, complement components (e.g., C5a), arachidonate metabolites (e.g., leukotriene B$_4$), and certain cytokines (e.g., interleukin-8).[21, 24, 25] Monocyte chemotactic factors include C5a, fibrinopeptide, cytokines, platelet-derived growth factor (PDGF), transforming growth factor β (TGFβ), and breakdown products of collagen.[12, 25] Leukocyte activation occurs in a series of steps. Receptor-ligand binding activates protein G (see Chapter 4), which activates phospholipase C, which hydrolyzes membrane phospholipids. This generates inositol trisphosphate, which releases intracellular calcium stores, affecting actin regulatory proteins and diacylglycerol. Diacylglycerol activates protein kinase C, a key component in leukocyte secretion and degranulation.[21, 23]

Phagocytosis and intracellular degradation of noxious or infectious agents require recognition (through IgG opsonins and the complement component C3b) and attachment of the leukocyte to the offending agent.[21] Following this attachment, engulfment occurs by fusion with lysosomal granules and formation of the phagolysosome. Extracellular release of phagocytic cell products may occur by leakage, by reverse endocytosis, or following cell death. Proinflammatory mediators released in this process include lysosomal enzymes, O$_2$-derived active metabolites, and arachidonate metabolites.[26] Phagocytosis and degranulation are accompanied by biochemical events similar to those already noted for the process of chemotaxis. Release of intracellular calcium stores also activates phospholipase A$_2$, which generates arachidonic acid metabolites from membrane phospholipids.

The degradation of ingested material or killing of bacteria by the phagocyte occurs by oxygen-dependent mechanisms (an H$_2$O$_2$-myeloperoxidase-halide system in neutrophils and an H$_2$O$_2$-myeloperoxidase-independent system in macrophages).[27] This degradation is associated with a burst of oxygen consumption, an increase in glucose oxidation, and production of reactive oxygen metabolites. When no oxidative burst is present, bacteria can be killed by oxygen-independent mechanisms, involving several constituents of the leukocyte granules, especially bacterial permeability increasing protein, lysozymal enzymes, and lactoferrin.[21, 26] Table 2-3 summarizes the major neutrophil granule constituents and neutrophil-derived inflammatory mediators, and Table 2-4 summarizes the major inflammatory mediators secreted from monocytes-macrophages.

Inflammatory Mediators

Molecules that mediate the response of vascularized tissue to injury and lead to increased blood flow, altered permeability, plasma exudation, and leukocyte infiltration of the interstitium and perivascular area are inflammatory mediators. These chemical substances originate from plasma, activated cells, or damaged tissues and act upon inflammatory cells in a variety of ways. *Autocrine* effects occur when a cell's secretory product interacts with a receptor on the same cell. *Paracrine* effects occur when a cell's product affects another cell in close proximity. *Endocrine* pathways are active when the secretory

Table 2–3. NEUTROPHIL GRANULE CONSTITUENTS AND INFLAMMATORY MEDIATORS*

Primary (Azurophilic) Granules
Neutral serine proteases (degrade collagen, connective tissue, and circulating proteins)
Acid hydrolases (degrade enzymes, break sulfhydryl bonds of proteins increasing susceptibility to oxidation)
Myeloperoxidase (catalyzes peroxidase reaction)
Antimicrobial proteins

Secondary (Specific) Granules
Lactoferrin (promotes neutrophil adhesiveness, facilitates hydroxyl radical formation)
Cytochrome b (superoxide production)
f-Met-Leu-Phe receptor (chemotaxis)
CR3 receptor (adhesiveness and margination)
Laminin receptor (extracellular matrix interaction)
Plasminogen activator
Complement activator (generates opsonins and chemoattractants)
Monocyte chemoattractant
Degradative enzymes

Membrane-associated Enzymes
Phospholipase (arachidonic acid metabolites)
Platelet-activating factor synthetic enzymes
NADPH-oxidase system (reactive oxygen intermediates)

Cytokines
IL-1, IL-6, IL-8
TNF

*Adapted from references 21, 24, and 26 in part.

product circulates in the blood and acts as a hormone affecting another cell distant from its site of production. Two major groups of inflammatory mediators are the products of circulating plasma protease systems and the mediators generated by endothelial and phagocytic cells.

Plasma Protease Systems

The three major plasma protease systems are the contact activation system (kinin-generating or surface-mediated defense reaction), the coagulation-fibrinolysis system, and the complement system. These plasma systems generate molecules that cause vasodilatation, increased vascular permeability, and leukocyte migration. The inflammatory cascades involved in kinin generation, coagulation, fibrinolysis, and complement activation are interconnected by common initiating molecules. Hageman factor (factor XII), either directly or through secondary processes, can activate all three protease systems, as well as neutrophils.[29] Plasmin, generated by contact activation or by tissue plasminogen, can activate the third component of complement and can initiate the generation of bradykinin.[29] Intricate feedback phenomena within these inflammatory cascades control and limit their degree of activation.

Contact Activation System. This surface-mediated defense reaction results from the transformation of three zymogens (factor XI, factor XII, and prekallikrein) into active serine proteases (factor XIa, factor XIIa, and kallikrein). The process is initiated when factor XII binds to a negatively charged surface such as collagen, basement membrane, or endotoxin. This binding, in turn, activates factor XI and prekallikrein.[29] These activations require the presence of a nonenzymatic cofac-

tor, high molecular weight kininogen. Enzymes capable of activating the system are contained in endothelial cells and mast cells.[30]

These active serine proteases initiate and amplify several important host defense mechanisms, including (1) activation by factor XIIa of the classical complement pathway via the first component of complement C1; (2) initiation by factor XIa of the intrinsic coagulation pathway and by factor Va of the extrinsic coagulation pathway; (3) activation of plasminogen by kallikrein, initiating fibrinolysis; (4) activation by kallikrein of

Table 2–4. SECRETORY PRODUCTS OF MONONUCLEAR PHAGOCYTES IMPORTANT IN INFLAMMATORY RESPONSES*

Polypeptide Hormones
Cytokines (IL-1, IL-6, IL-8, TNF)
α- and (?) γ-Interferons
Platelet-derived growth factors
Fibroblast growth factors
Fibroblast-activating factors
TGF β
Insulin-like growth factors (somatomedins)
Colony stimulating factors for granulocytes and monocytes
Complement Components
Classical pathway (C1–C5)
Alternate pathway (properdin and factors B and D)
Complement inhibitors (C3b inactivator)
Active fragments generated by monocyte proteases (C3a, C3b, C5a)
Coagulation Factors
Intrinsic pathway (factors V, IX, and X, prothrombin)
Extrinsic pathway (factor VII)
Surface activities (tissue factor, prothrombinase)
Fibrinolytic activities (plasminogen activator)
Antithrombolytic activities (plasminogen activator inhibitor, plasmin inhibitor)
Other Enzymes
Neutral proteases (plasminogen activator, elastase, collagenase, angiotensin convertase)
Lipases (lipoprotein lipase, phospholipase A_2)
Glucosaminidase (lysozyme)
Lysosomal acid hydrolases (proteases, lipases, deoxyribonucleases and ribonucleases, phosphatases, glycosidases, sulfatases)
Deaminase (arginase)
Enzyme and Cytokine Inhibitors
Protease inhibitors (α_2-macroglobulin, α_1-antiproteinase, plasminogen activator inhibitor, plasmin inhibitors, collagenase inhibitors)
Phospholipase inhibitors (lipomodulin)
Inhibitors of IL-1 and TNF
Cell Adhesion Proteins and Extracellular Matrix Proteins
Fibronectin
Thrombospondin
Chondroitin sulfate
Gelatin-binding protein
Bioactive Lipids
Cyclooxygenase products (PGE_2 and $PGF_{2\alpha}$, prostacyclin, thromboxane)
Lipoxygenase products (LTB_4, LTC, LTD, and LTE)
Platelet-activating factors
Reactive Oxygen and Nitrogen Intermediates
Superoxide anion
Hydroxyl radical
Hydrogen peroxide
Hypohalous acids
Nitrites and nitrates

*Modified from Nathan CF: Secretory products of macrophages. J Clin Invest 79:319, 1987. Copyright permission of the American Society of Clinical Investigation.

neutrophil chemotaxis, superoxide production, and release of elastase; and (5) generation by kallikrein of bradykinin from high molecular weight kininogen.[29] Bradykinin is a remarkably potent peptide that produces vasodilatation, increased vascular permeability, contraction of smooth muscle, margination and infiltration of leukocytes, and stimulation of the production of arachidonic acid metabolites.[31] Tissue kallikreins are potent kinin-generating enzymes that may have a role in organ-specific inflammatory reactions.[31]

Control mechanisms that serve to limit the activity of these activated proteases include several plasma protease inhibitors: C1-inhibitor (C1-inh), α_2-macroglobulin, and α_1-proteinase inhibitor (α_1-antitrypsin).[29] Activation of the contact system can be assayed in sepsis and shock by measuring activated proteins in plasma or by measuring changes in inhibitors or in inhibitor-activated component complexes (C1-inh, factor XII–C1-inh, kallikrein–α_2-macroglobulin, and kallikrein–C1-inh).[29-31] However, it should be kept in mind that activation of the contact system may be confined to local microvascular beds and may not be reflected by changes in activity of peripheral contact system components.

Hemostatic and Fibrinolytic Systems. One consequence of injury to vascular endothelium is activation of platelets and plasma serine proteases. The initiating step in this process is factor XII activation, which ultimately results in conversion of fibrinogen to fibrin via thrombin (factor II). Control of fibrin generation during inflammation or tissue repair depends on intricate balances among thrombogenic factors and protective mechanisms that regulate thrombus formation and fibrinolysis. Thrombi consist of fibrin, erythrocytes, platelets, and leukocytes attracted by chemotactic factors from platelets. Thrombogenic factors include endothelial damage, platelet aggregation, protease activation, and stasis of flow. Antithrombotic protective factors include maintenance or restoration of the integrity of the endothelial cell surface, neutralization of activated coagulation factors by protease inhibitors, dilution of coagulation factors and platelet aggregates by blood flow, and the fibrinolytic system.[32]

When endothelial cells are damaged, their basement membranes and associated collagen are exposed to circulating platelets and proteases, which are activated through a complex series of reactions to form fibrin aggregates and thrombi. Platelet adhesion to the subendothelial structures depends on the presence of von Willebrand factor. After exposure to collagen, adenosine diphosphate (ADP), epinephrine, or thromboxane A_2, platelets release their granule contents, which include serotonin, ADP, fibronectin, thrombospondin, platelet factor 4, β-thromboglobulin, PDGF, fibrinogen, acid hydrolases, high molecular weight kininogen, α_1-antitrypsin, and α_2-macroglobulin.[33] Collagen, thromboxane A_2, thrombin, platelet-activating factors, and ADP induce platelet aggregation through a mechanism entailing calcium mobilization in the platelet cytoplasm. Activated platelets change in shape and facilitate clot formation through the interaction of platelet lipoproteins and coagulation factors II, V, VIII, IX, and X.[32, 33]

Two pathways result in activation of thrombin to convert fibrinogen (factor I) to fibrin.[34] The intrinsic pathway is initiated by contact of factor XII with vascular surfaces following endothelial damage. Activated factor XII (factor XIIa) converts factor XI from its inactive zymogen precursor to factor XIa, which converts factor IX to its active form, factor IXa. In conjunction with factor VIII, factor IXa activates factor X. This last factor can also be activated by the extrinsic pathway, which is initiated by the release of tissue thromboplastin from damaged endothelium or from other damaged tissues. In the presence of calcium, factor V, and platelet phospholipid, tissue thromboplastin activates factor II (prothrombin) to form thrombin, which then converts fibrinogen to fibrin. Several feedback loops serve to enhance or inhibit these cascades. Circulating plasma inhibitors, which serve to limit the effects of the activated proteases, include C1-inh (for factor VIIIa, factor XIIa, and kallikrein), α_1-antitrypsin (for factor XIa), antithrombin III (for factors IIa, IIc, IXa, and Xa), and α_2-macroglobulin (as a general backup inhibitor).[35]

The lack of thrombogenicity of intact endothelium depends on the presence of factors that bind or modify the activity of thrombin, inhibit platelet aggregation, or induce fibrinolysis.[34, 36] Endothelial cell–derived prostacyclin and lipoxygenase products inhibit platelet aggregation. Two glycosaminoglycans inhibit blood coagulation. The first, thrombomodulin, inhibits thrombin and facilitates activation of protein C, which inactivates factors Va and VIIIa and stimulates release of tissue plasminogen activator from endothelial cells.[37] The second, heparan sulfate, facilitates inhibition of thrombin, factor IXa, and factor Xa by circulating antithrombin III.[32] Table 2–5 provides a summary of endothelial cell products that are important in inflammatory responses.

Fibrinolysis occurs on the surface of the fibrin clot through the action of plasminogen activators derived from endothelial cells (tissue plasminogen activator) or other tissues (urokinase or urinary plasminogen activator) or through the action of factor XIIa (activated through the contact activation system).[41] Plasminogen activators convert plasminogen to plasmin, an activated enzyme that lyses fibrin clots. An alternative pathway of fibrinolysis is via proteolytic enzymes, released from leukocytes attracted by chemotactic products of platelets.[32] Inhibitors of fibrinolysis, derived from endothelial cells (plasminogen activator inhibitor) or from the liver, circulate in the blood[35] (see also Chapter 62).

The Complement System. The complement cascade consists of 20 circulating serine proteases that are activated by cells, immunoglobulins, or microorganisms. The proteolytic cleavage products of complement interact to produce important proinflammatory fragments (including the anaphylatoxins C3a and C5a) that bind to specific high-affinity receptors on neutrophils, monocytes-macrophages, mast cells, platelets, and smooth muscle cells. These interactions promote the release of other inflammatory mediators (histamine, serotonin, hydrolytic enzymes, platelet activating factors, IL-1, TNF, arachidonic acid metabolites, activated oxygen products, and chemotactic factors), enhance neutrophil adhesion to endothelial cells, and cause smooth muscle contrac-

Table 2–5. ENDOTHELIAL PRODUCTS IMPORTANT IN THE INFLAMMATORY RESPONSE*

Antithrombotic Molecules
  Prostacyclin
  Tissue plasminogen activator
  Heparan sulfate
  Proteins C and S
  Thrombomodulin
Procoagulant Molecules
  von Willebrand factor
  Tissue factor
  Plasminogen activator inhibitor
  Factor V
Modulation of Blood Flow and Vascular Reactivity
  Endothelium-derived relaxing factor
  Endothelin
  Prostacyclin
  Platelet-derived growth factors
Regulation of Inflammation and Immunity
  IL-1, IL-6, IL-8
  Adhesion molecules
  Colony stimulating factors
  Platelet-derived growth factors
  Antioxidants
Extracellular Matrix–Connective Tissue Components
  Collagen
  Thrombospondin
  Fibronectin
  Elastin
  Glycosaminoglycans
  Laminin
  Collagenases
Regulation of Cell Growth
  Stimulators (Platelet-derived growth factors, colony stimulating
    factors, fibroblast growth factor)
  Inhibitors (heparin-like inhibitor of smooth muscle cells, TGFβ)
Inactivators of Vasoactive Substances
  Angiotensin converting enzyme
  Angiotensinases A and C

*Adapted from references 13, 38, 39, and 40.

tion.[42, 43] In plasma, C5a is converted by peptidases to C5a des Arg, which in the presence of the serum factor cochemotaxin is a potent chemotactic molecule.[43] The anaphylatoxins are thus important mediators, directly and through other molecules, in altering vascular permeability and inducing leukocyte chemotaxis. Complement products are also important opsonins, mediating the lysis and death of target cells.

The complement cascade is activated by either the classical or the alternate pathway.[42] The classical pathway is activated by interaction of the first component of complement (C1) with antigen-antibody complexes. This is initiated by the binding of the C1q subunit of C1 to the Fc receptors of immunoglobulin (primarily IgG 1, IgG 2, IgG 3, or IgM). The activated product, C1 esterase, in turn, activates C4 and C2 to form a complex C4bC2a (also called *C3 convertase*). This complex cleaves and activates C3 to C3a and C3b fragments. C3b binds to C3 convertase to form C5 convertase, which then cleaves and activates C5 to C5a and C5b fragments. Thus the early portion of the complement cascade generates potent proinflammatory C3a and C5a fragments. The C5b fragment activates the later portion of the cascade by interacting with C6, C7, C8, and C9 to form the membrane attack complex. This activated complement sequence can insert itself into lipid bilayers,

forming transmembrane channels. These functional holes alter the permeability of cells or microorganisms, resulting in their death.[44]

The alternate pathway of complement activation occurs via the binding of C3 or C3b to substances such as endotoxin, fungi, bacteria, aggregated immunoglobulins, or complex polysaccharides. The activated C3 forms a complex with two proteins, factors B and D, which serves as the C3 convertase. When stabilized by a third protein, properdin, this complex acts as a C5a convertase.[42]

In addition to the the classical and alternate pathways, C3a and C5a can be activated by plasmin, bacterial proteases, or tissue proteases.[43] Thus in some inflammatory states, complement products can play a central role in initiating inflammation. Several circulating and membrane-associated proteins, such as C1-inh, serve as counterregulatory mechanisms to control the generation of activated fragments and to protect host cells from the injurious effects of activated complement fragments. The importance of these counterregulatory mechanisms is illustrated by hereditary angioedema, in which congenital or acquired reduction in functional C1-inh leads to recurrent episodes of complement-mediated angioedema.[45]

Deficiencies of early complement components (C1 to C5) are associated with autoimmune phenomena such as glomerulonephritis and systemic lupus erythematosus. Deficiencies of late components (C5 to C8) are associated with recurrent *Neisseria* infections.[45]

Cell-Generated Mediators of Inflammation

Injury Resulting from Reactive Oxygen Species. A free radical is a molecule that contains one or more unpaired electrons in its outer orbit because of the gain or loss of an electron.[46] This results in a highly unstable molecule that can react with a variety of substrates. Biologically important free radicals include those centered around hydrogen, carbon, sulfur, nitrogen, and oxygen.[47] Oxygen-derived free radical molecules are of particular importance in acute inflammatory responses and tissue injury. These reactive oxygen species are generated by neutrophils, monocyte-macrophages, and eosinophils during normal cell metabolism and especially during inflammatory responses.[46] Oxygen radicals are involved in a number of pathogenetic processes, including ischemia-reflow states (reperfusion injury), certain drug- and toxin-induced injuries, radiation injury, bronchopulmonary dysplasia, and adult respiratory distress syndrome.[47]

During normal aerobic metabolism, oxygen is reduced to water in the cell by the acceptance of four electrons in a reaction catalyzed by mitochondrial and mixed-function oxidases.[46] Copper and iron ions are important catalysts in free radical reactions because of their ability to accept or donate single electrons.[47] Partial reduction of oxygen results in the formation of highly reactive intermediates: superoxide, hydrogen peroxide, and hydroxyl radical. During normal cell metabolism, these potentially toxic oxidants are confined to active oxidase sites in the mitochondria, endoplasmic reticulum, peroxisomes, and cytoplasm.[27] Protective mechanisms to limit the toxic effects of these molecules on the cell include specific neutralizing enzymes and antioxidants. Superoxide dismutase converts superoxide to hydrogen peroxide; both catalase and glutathione peroxidase convert hydrogen peroxide to water. Antioxidants include vitamin E, cysteine, transferrin, and ceruloplasmin.[27, 48]

Formation of reactive oxygen species is accelerated by a variety of agents, including certain chemicals, radiation, hyperoxia, tumor destruction, killing of microbes by phagocytosis, and reperfusion after tissue ischemia.[46] Reactive oxygen species can alter the structure and function of proteins, lipids, and carbohydrates. Additionally, reactive oxygen species can generate additional oxygen radicals and amplify their destructive potential through autocatalysis.[48]

Oxidant injury can result when the rate of formation of reactive oxygen intermediates increases or the function of antioxidant cell defenses decreases.[49] The toxicities of some agents, like paraquat or bleomycin, are directly related to the generation of oxygen radicals.[49] A more common cause of increased oxygen radical formation is the respiratory burst that occurs in phagocytic cells following exposure to inflammatory stimuli.[50] During the respiratory burst, the univalent reduction of oxygen generates superoxide and hydrogen peroxide. In addition, the reduction of superoxide and hydrogen peroxide generates hydroxyl radicals.[51] In the presence of myeloperoxidase, hydrogen peroxide oxidizes halides to hypohalous acids, which are oxidants that react vigorously with a variety of biologic substrates (e.g., amino acids, thiols, nucleotides, and polyenoic acids).[51] Hypohalous acids do not accumulate in the cell but react with ammonia or amines to generate another group of oxidants termed *chloramines*. Hypohalous acids and chloramines are both potentially cytotoxic.[51]

In addition to release of oxygen radicals into phagocytic vacuoles, which facilitates the killing of microorganisms, oxygen radicals are released outside the cell even without cell lysis.[26] Tissue injury may ensue from their oxidant effects on phospholipids and proteins of cell membranes. Oxidation of methionyl residues may result in inactivation of proteinases. This may potentiate injury—for example, by altering α_1-antiproteinase, which allows unopposed effects of neutrophil elastase, a proteolytic enzyme important in the development of tissue injury.[52]

The mechanism of cell injury caused by reactive oxygen species results from complicated interactions among short-lived reactive oxygen moieties (primarily hypohalous acids and chloramines), proteolytic enzymes, and antioxidant and antiproteinase systems in the cell.[27, 49, 51] The mechanisms of cell injury appear to depend in part on the generation of hydroxyl radicals and other oxidizing species more potent than superoxide or hydrogen peroxide.[49, 51] Hydroxyl radicals can initiate the peroxidative decomposition of inner mitochondrial membranes, as well as cause breakage of deoxyribonucleic acid (DNA) strands.[49] Carbohydrates may be depolymerized and nucleotides damaged. The resultant chromosomal damage may inhibit cellular protein synthesis.[48] Membrane fatty acids may be oxidized to generate lipid peroxyl radicals, initiating an autocatalytic process (lipid peroxidation) that can destroy unsaturated fatty acids of cellular membranes.[48, 49]

Injury from neutrophil-derived oxidants can be potentiated by inactivation by oxidants of antiproteinases (e.g., α_1-antiproteinases, α_2-macroglobulin, and secretory leukoproteinase inhibitor), which allows the activity of proteolytic enzymes (e.g., elastase, collagenase, and gelatinase) to proceed unopposed.[51] Further, inactive proteolytic enzymes can be activated by oxidants and can then attack other antiproteinases (e.g., plasminogen-activator inhibitor), further amplifying the inflammatory response.[51] Normally, regulation of neutrophil influx and replacement of dysfunctional antiproteinases by local synthesis permit containment of the inflammatory response and of cell damage within a local area.[51]

A number of antioxidants with potential therapeutic applications have been evaluated experimentally. They include dimethyl sulfoxide, acetylcysteine, and liposomally encased formulations of catalase and superoxide dismutase.[27]

Prostaglandins, Leukotrienes, and Other Eicosanoids. Arachidonic acid, an essential fatty acid, is a component of all cellular membranes. Following cell stimulation, phospholipases A_2, C, and D release arachidonic acid from membrane phospholipids. There are three major enzymatic pathways, distributed throughout various cells and tissues, for arachidonic acid oxygenation: lipoxygenase, monooxygenase (P_{450}), and cyclooxygenase.[53] They insert oxygen into various positions in the arachidonate molecule, rapidly producing a large number of prostaglandins, leukotrienes, and other eicosanoids with a broad spectrum of biologic activity (Fig. 2–1). Leukocytes, mast cells, platelets, endothelial cells, and epithelial cells of different organs all generate eicosanoids in sufficient quantity to influence other inflammatory cells.[54] Eicosanoids serve an essential role in inflammation by mediating alterations in vascular tone, permeability, leukocyte infiltration, and other cell-generated inflammatory responses. Additionally, many eicosanoids have effects on nonvascular smooth muscle, causing alterations in airway caliber and platelet function.[54] The biologic effects of the eicosanoids are controlled at several levels, including transcriptional and translational control of the enzymes required for their synthesis and of their cell receptors.[53] Prostaglandins regulate the synthesis of cyclic adenosine monophosphate by activating or inhibiting adenylate cyclase, resulting in alterations in intracellular calcium. Most tissues have enzymes that degrade the eicosanoids to inactive products.[53]

Cyclooxygenase is a membrane-bound enzyme that catalyzes the formation of prostaglandin endoperoxides (PGG_2 and PGH_2), the precursors of thromboxane (TxA_2), prostacyclin (PGI_2), and prostaglandins D_2, E_2, and $F_{2\alpha}$ (PGD_2, PGE_2, and $PGF_{2\alpha}$).[55, 56] TxA_2 is a potent, short-lived vasoconstrictor synthesized in platelets by thromboxane synthetase. Additionally, it is a powerful inducer of platelet aggregation and platelet granule release.[55] PGI_2 is a potent vasodilator generated by vascular endothelium and vascular smooth muscle and requires the activation of protein kinase C.[56] PGI_2, PGD_2, and PGE_2 antagonize the platelet-aggregating

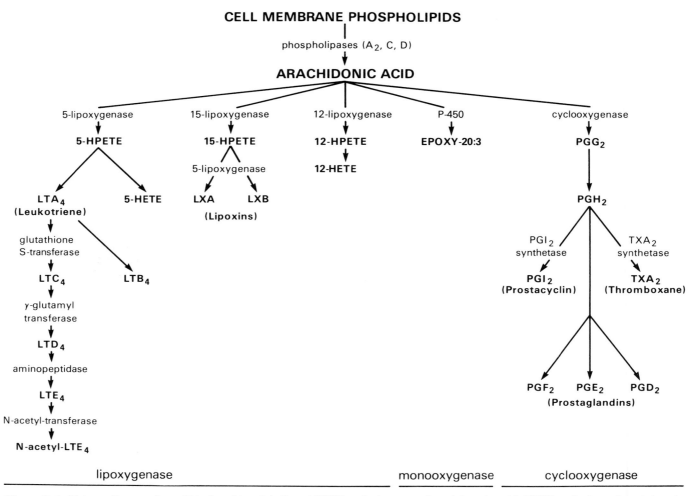

CELL MEMBRANE PHOSPHOLIPIDS

phospholipases (A_2, C, D)

ARACHIDONIC ACID

5-lipoxygenase	15-lipoxygenase	12-lipoxygenase	P-450	cyclooxygenase
5-HPETE	**15-HPETE**	**12-HPETE**	**EPOXY-20:3**	**PGG₂**

5-lipoxygenase

12-HETE

LTA₄ (Leukotriene)   5-HETE   LXA   LXB (Lipoxins)

PGH₂

glutathione S-transferase

PGI₂ synthetase   TXA₂ synthetase

LTC₄   LTB₄

PGI₂ (Prostacyclin)   TXA₂ (Thromboxane)

γ-glutamyl transferase

LTD₄

aminopeptidase

LTE₄

PGF₂   PGE₂   PGD₂ (Prostaglandins)

N-acetyl-transferase

N-acetyl-LTE₄

lipoxygenase   monooxygenase   cyclooxygenase

Figure 2–1. Major pathways of arachidonic acid metabolism. HPETE = hydroperoxyeicosatetranoic acid; HETE = hydroxyeicosatetranoic acid.

effects of TxA₂.[40] PGD₂ is found in mast cells and has a wide spectrum of activities, including (in addition to inhibition of platelet aggregation) vasodilatation, pulmonary vasoconstriction, and increased airway reactivity.[53, 54] PGD₂, in conjunction with PGE₂, potentiates the activities of histamine and bradykinin on vascular permeability.[53] Macrophages are the major source of PGE₂; it functions as a regulator of cell growth and inflammatory responses.[57] PGF₂α is a pulmonary vasoconstrictor and a potent bronchoconstrictor.[54, 55]

The lipoxygenases are a family of three different cytosolic enzymes that insert oxygen into arachidonic acid at the 5, 12, or 15 positions. Lipoxygenase products cause alterations in vascular permeability, chemotaxis of leukocytes, and constriction of vascular and bronchial smooth muscle.[58]

Neutrophils, monocytes-macrophages, and mast cells use the 5-lipoxygenase pathway to generate leukotrienes, a family of molecules that serves an important role in systemic and local immunologic reactions, inflammation, shock, and trauma.[59, 60] The first 5-lipoxygenase product, leukotriene A₄ (LTA₄), is an unstable metabolite. LTA₄ is converted to leukotriene B₄ (LTB₄) or

conjugated with glutathione to leukotriene C₄ (LTC₄), the precursor of leukotriene D₄ (LTD₄) and leukotriene E₄ (LTE₄). The cysteinyl-containing leukotrienes (LTC₄, LTD₄, and LTE₄), formerly termed the *slow reacting substance of anaphylaxis,* constrict smooth muscle of the vasculature, lung, and gut and are capable of increasing venule permeability.[58] LTB₄ is a neutrophil chemotactic factor and causes neutrophil aggregation, enzyme release, superoxide generation, and cell adhesion.[60] Additionally, LTB₄ has a role in the activation of lymphocytes and eosinophils.[60] LTC₄ and LTD₄ are myotropic, causing bronchoconstriction, coronary and cerebral arteriolar constriction, and in some animal species myocardial depression.[54, 59, 60]

Another family of molecules, lipoxins, are derived from the action of either 5- or 15-lipoxygenases on arachidonate. Their potential roles in human inflammation include regulation of cell activation, chemotaxis, smooth muscle contraction, and vasodilatation.[58] The 15-lipoxygenase pathway is found primarily in eosinophils, endothelial cells, and epithelial cells and is a major pathway of arachidonate metabolism in the lung. In addition to generating lipoxins, it also converts arachidonate to 15-hydroperoxyeicosatetranoic acid (15-HPETE). 15-HPETE alters host immune responses and modulates other oxygenation enzymes.[40, 53]

12-Lipoxygenase, found predominantly in platelets and leukocytes, forms 12-hydroxyeicosatetranoic acid (12-HETE) and 12-HPETE.[53] These products induce secretion of neutrophil-specific granules, cause chemotaxis, and increase IgE release by mast cells.

The monooxygenase (cytochrome P_{450}) system, located primarily in lung and liver, is active in oxygenating a variety of lipophilic compounds, such as arachidonate and its metabolites.[53] The products of this pathway are called ω and $\omega 1$ oxygenated products. Monooxygenase products, through their capacity to regulate Na,K-ATPase, act to modulate vascular smooth muscle reactivity and local blood flow.[53]

Inflammatory cells vary in the predominant eicosanoid species produced.[54, 56] Neutrophils primarily produce PGE_2, LTB_4, and 5-HETE, whereas monocytes produce PGE_2, LTB_4, LTC_4, and TxA_2.[56] Alveolar macrophages appear to produce greater amounts of LTB_4 and 5-HETE than do peripheral blood monocytes.[56] Platelets produce TxA_2 and 12-HETE, whereas vascular endothelial cells produce PGD_2, PGE_2, $PGF_{2\alpha}$, PGI_2, and 15-HETE.[54, 56] Cells may require interactions with other cell types to synthesize eicosanoids because of the selective distribution of key enzymes such as 5-lipoxygenase.[60] Endothelial cells employ prostaglandin endoperoxides produced by platelets to synthesize PGI_2 and LTA_4 produced by neutrophils to synthesize leukotrienes.[56, 60]

Eicosanoids have been implicated in the pathogenesis of a number of human diseases. Lipoxygenase products can be detected in the pulmonary secretions of patients with asthma (LTB_4, LTC_4, LTD_4, and LTE_4), adult respiratory distress syndrome (LTB_4, LTD_4, and LTE_4), and neonatal hypoxemia and pulmonary hypertension (LTC_4 and LTD_4).[54]

Platelet-Activating Factors. PAFs, like the eicosanoids, are metabolites of cell membrane phospholipids that have important biologic activities. PAFs and eicosanoids are not preformed and stored but are rapidly generated after cell stimulation. PAF is the historic and functional name given to a family of acetylated phosphoglycerides released from IgE-stimulated basophils that result in platelet aggregation. However, the biologic functions of this family of molecules are considerably more diverse than platelet aggregation alone. A variety of cells—including phagocytic leukocytes, platelets, and endothelial cells—produce PAF, and it serves as an important mediator of normal physiology and pathophysiologic states.[61, 62]

PAF is synthesized by two different pathways.[61, 63] The first involves structural modification of membrane lipids. This endogenous pathway is probably the route for synthesis of PAF during hypersensitivity reactions and inflammatory responses. The second is de novo synthesis, which appears to be the route of PAF synthesis during normal physiologic processes. PAF responses are controlled in part by specific receptors that act through G proteins and activation of adenyl cyclase. Inactivation occurs by removal of acetyl groups from the parent molecule.[61]

The known cellular effects of PAF include aggregation and degranulation of platelets and neutrophils, stimulation of chemotaxis, increased superoxide formation, adherence of neutrophils to endothelial cells, increased protein phosphorylation, activation of protein kinase C, increased arachidonate metabolism with generation of TxA_2 and LTB_4, and increased production of TNF.[61, 63] PAF and arachidonate are released from a common precursor, and some PAF responses may be mediated by lipoxygenase or cyclooxygenase products.

Experimental administration of PAF to animals by intravenous injection induces a number of inflammatory events, including neutropenia and platelet aggregation and sequestration.[62, 63] Following intradermal injection of PAF, vasoconstriction at the site is followed by erythema and pruritus. PAF induces contraction of endothelial cells in postcapillary venules, resulting in increased vascular permeability. This latter effect is independent of other mediators known to cause changes in vascular permeability and is synergistic with the effects of other mediators such as histamine or neutrophil products. PAF is a potent inducer of airway microvascular leakage and bronchoconstriction and has been detected in plasma and bronchoalveolar lavage fluid from patients with asthma.[63] Intradermal or subcutaneous injections of PAF result in leukocyte infiltration of the perivascular area, and large doses result in a severe vasculitis with tissue destruction. In vivo, PAF has a role in normal and abnormal physiologic responses through its capacities to contract smooth muscle and endothelial cells and to stimulate the release of eicosanoids and other potent inflammatory mediators.[62]

Some PAF antagonists have been developed by structural modification of the PAF molecule, whereas others are natural compounds. These substances inhibit binding of PAF to platelets or to lung receptors and may have potential therapeutic uses.[63]

Vasoactive Amines. Histamine and serotonin are vasoactive amines with important roles in early inflammatory responses. Histamine, formed by the decarboxylation of the amino acid histidine, is stored in the granules of mast cells, basophils, and platelets. Its release is induced by physical agents, IgE, the anaphylatoxins C3a and C5a, substance P, or histamine-releasing activities from lymphocytes, phagocytes, or endothelial cells.[64] Serotonin, synthesized from tryptophan, is found in the dense granules of platelets, as well as in neurons of the central nervous system.[33] When stimulated by epinephrine, ADP, collagen, or thrombin, platelets undergo conformational changes and degranulation, releasing a wide variety of inflammatory mediators, including histamine and serotonin. Serotonin has both stimulant and inhibitory influences on smooth muscle; its effects vary significantly among species.

Both of these vasoactive amines are stored and are immediately available upon stimulation. Histamine and serotonin are potent vasodilators and increase the permeability of postcapillary venules.[64] Histamine mediates early inflammatory responses and immediate IgE-mediated hypersensitivity reactions.[64] Serotonin potentiates platelet aggregation, alters vascular tone, and enhances the adherence of neutrophils to endothelial cells.[33]

Neurogenic Inflammation. The neuropeptides are a novel class of inflammatory mediators with important regulatory effects on pulmonary, gastrointestinal, cardiovascular, neural, and endocrine function. Three neural systems affect smooth muscle tone in the lung and gastrointestinal tract: the cholinergic, the adrenergic, and the nonadrenergic-noncholinergic (formerly termed *peptidergic*) pathways.[65] Neuropeptides may act as neurotransmitters, alone or in conjunction with classic cholinergic or adrenergic mediators. As such, neuropeptides have major effects on smooth muscle tone, blood flow, vascular permeability, and mucous secretion.[65]

Receptors for neuropeptides such as vasoactive intestinal peptide (VIP) are found on neutrophils, eosinophils, and mononuclear cells.[66] In addition to having proinflammatory effects, VIP can inhibit inflammatory cell function and antagonize inflammatory mediators such as histamine, $PGF_{2\alpha}$, and leukotrienes C_4 and D_4.[66] VIP is found in high concentrations in lung, in which it is localized in efferent nerves. Its capacities to produce bronchodilatation, vasodilatation, and increased airway mucous secretion are consistent with a major role for VIP in the pathogenesis of asthma.[65]

Peptide histidine methionine (PHM) is present in the same nerves as VIP and has similar effects.[65] VIP and PHM normally counteract the bronchoconstrictive effect of acetylcholine. During asthma, peptidases from inflammatory cells may increase the degradation of VIP and PHM, resulting in unopposed bronchoconstriction.[65]

Substance P is localized to unmyelinated sensory fibers (C fibers) in the airways.[65] Its effects include bronchoconstriction, increased production of airway secretions, increased microvascular permeability, and chemotactic effects on inflammatory cells.[65] Calcitonin gene-related peptide, which may be stored along with with substance P, is a potent vasodilator and bronchoconstrictor.[65] Other neuropeptides that may have significant roles in airway and other inflammatory responses include neurokinin A, neuropeptides K and Y, cholecystokinin octapeptide, somatostatin, and enkephalins.[65]

Peptide Regulatory Molecules. Peptide regulatory factors are molecules weighing less than 80 kDa with short or intermediate durations of action and specific high-affinity cell surface receptors.[66a] These molecules, which affect cell differentiation and proliferation, include cytokines (which have immunomodulatory effects) and growth factors (which modulate proliferation of nonimmunologic cells). The functional distinction between the two groups of peptides often is blurred by similarities; cytokines often act on nonimmunologic cells.[66a]

Cytokines. Cytokines are soluble proteins with a broad range of activities in normal and pathophysiologic states.[67] This class of mediators includes molecules that were originally defined by their cell of origin (i.e., monokines from monocytes or lymphokines from lymphocytes) or by their target cells (i.e., interleukins for leukocytes). These molecules mediate many aspects of inflammation through their effects on leukocyte and endothelial activation. In addition they have major roles in the regulation of growth and differentiation of lymphoid and hematopoietic cells. Because of their potent effects on the immune system, control of cytokine production and activities has important therapeutic potential. Cytokine actions are characterized by pleiotropy (diversity of function) and redundancy (functions of one cytokine often overlap with those of other cytokines).[2]

Cytokines are synthesized not only by immunologic effector cells but also by nonimmunologic tissues.[68] Some cytokines serve primarily as growth factors (e.g., TGF β), whereas others have primarily proinflammatory activity (e.g., IL-1 or TNF). In general, those cytokines with proinflammatory activity are induced by a stimulus (e.g., endotoxin or complement) rather than constantly expressed and stored intracellularly. These agents are low molecular weight molecules (less than 80 kDa), often glycosylated, and are potent even in picomolar concentrations.[66a] Cytokines may be secreted or may remain cell-associated and expressed on the cell surface. They bind to specific high-affinity receptors on target cells in an autocrine, paracrine, or endocrine fashion. Despite differing structures and cell receptors, individual cytokines frequently have overlapping activities, presumably based on induction of DNA expression for production of common cell proteins.[2] The effects of cytokines on target cells can be amplified through induction of further cytokine release by the target cells (i.e., a cytokine network or cascade).[68, 69] The interactions of these molecules on target cells may be additive, synergistic, or antagonistic. A summary of major cytokines and their roles in inflammation is provided in Table 2–6.

Many features of acute inflammation are mediated by the effects of cytokines on endothelial cells and phagocytic leukocytes. Cytokines that have a major role in acute inflammatory responses include IL-1, γ-interferon, TNF, IL-6, and IL-8. These molecules have properties that directly or indirectly result in altered endothelial permeability and vasoreactivity and in leukocyte activation and accumulation.

IL-1 is synthesized by multiple cell types, including monocytes, lymphocytes, and endothelial cells.[70] Two distinct genes produce IL-1α or IL-1β, which have similar biologic activities despite limited homology between amino acid sequences. The former is largely membrane-bound, whereas the latter can be detected in circulating blood after an appropriate stimulus.[70] Both molecular species of IL-1 serve as primary mediators of the acute phase response, a constellation of systemic responses that develop after infection or injury.[71] These responses include fever, hepatic synthesis of acute phase proteins, release of stress hormones, release of amino acids from skeletal muscle, and activation of neutrophils, lymphocytes, and endothelial and phagocytic cells.[72]

γ-Interferon is a major immunomodulatory cytokine produced by activated T lymphocytes. It interacts with a variety of cells, including monocytes-macrophages and lymphocytes.[73] Its actions include activation of macrophages for enhanced phagocytosis, activation and growth enhancement of T and B cells, induction of class I and class II major histocompatibility complex antigen expression, and expression of adhesion molecules by endothelial cells.[13, 39]

TNFα is synthesized primarily by monocytes and

Table 2–6. KNOWN BIOLOGIC EFFECTS OF THE MAJOR CYTOKINES

	IFN α	IFN β	IFN γ	TNF α	LT	IL-1	IL-2	IL-3	IL-4	IL-5	IL-6	IL-7	IL-8	G CSF	M CSF	GM CSF	TGF β
Induces cellular antiviral state	+	+	+	+	+	+											+
Mitogenic for various cells			+	+	+	+	+	+	+	+	−	+			+	+	+/−
Cytostatic for various cells	+	+	+	+	+	+					+						+/−
Cytostatic for tumor cells	+	+	+	+	+	+											
Activates macrophages			+	+	+		+		+						+	+	
Stimulates granulocyte activity				+	+	+		+							+	+	
Stimulates eosinophil activity				+		−									−	+	
Stimulates NK activity	−			−		−	+	+									
Stimulates LAK activity	+		+/−	−			+										
Enhances MHC class I	Inhib	Inhib	+	+	+		+	+						−			Inhib
Enhances MHC class II	+/−	+/−	+	−	−	−		Inhib	+/−								−
Activates B cells									B cell + +	Mice + +							
Stimulates B cell proliferation	+	+	+	+/−	+	+	+		+	Mice +/−	+	+					Inhib
Stimulates B cell differentiation	+		+	+/−	+	+	+	+		Mice +/−	+						Inhib
Stimulates isotype selection			IgG₂ₐ +						IgG₁,IgE +	IgA +							IgA +
Induces IgE receptors on B cells									+								
Activates T cells	Inhib	? +				+	+		+		+						
Stimulates T cell proliferation		−		+		+	+		+		+	+				+	Inhib
Stimulates T cell differentiation							+				+						Inhib
Induces ICAM-1			+	+		+	+										
Induces chemotactic migration of cell				+									+			+/−	+/−
Activates endothelial cells			+	+	+	+											
Stimulates production of ECM proteins				+		+											+
Stimulates osteoclastic bone resorption				+	+	+											+/−
Induces membrane formation						+/−											
Induces fever	+	+	+	+	+	+					+						
Induces acute phase proteins			+	+		+					+						
Adjuvanticity			+	+	+	+	+	+									
Stimulates angiogenesis in vivo			+	Inhib									+				+
Antitumor activity	+	+	+	+	+	+	+	+									
Stimulates in vivo hematopoiesis							+							+		+	

*Adapted with permission from Balkwill FR and Burke F: The cytokine network. Immunol Today 10:299, 1989.

†= biologic effect present; − = biologic effect lacking; inhib = inhibitory effect; IFN = interferon; TNF = tumor necrosis factor; LT = lymphotoxin (TNFβ); IL = interleukin; GCSF = granulocyte colony stimulating factor; MCSF = monocyte colony stimulating factor; GMCSF = granulocyte-monocyte colony stimulating factor; TGF = transforming growth factor; NK = natural killer cell; LAK = lymphokine-activated cell; MHC = major histocompatibility complex; Ig = immunoglobulin; ICAM = intracellular adhesion molecule; ECM = extracellular matrix.

macrophages. Like IL-1, TNF is a major mediator of acute inflammatory responses to infection and tissue injury;[74] it can be measured in the circulation after acute infection or injury.[71] An endogenous pyrogen, it has potent effects on metabolism and is a major mediator of cachexia.[74] Its pleiotropic effects include enhancement of macrophage and neutrophil chemotaxis, increased neutrophil adhesion, degranulation and release of lysozyme, increased phagocytic and cytotoxic activity, and free radical production by leukocytes.[74] TNF-mediated cytotoxicity depends on G protein activation of phospholipases, free radical generation, and damage to DNA by endonucleases.[75] Like IL-1, TNF amplifies the inflammatory response by inducing release of other cytokines such as IL-6.[74]

IL-1 and TNF act on endothelial cells in six identifiable ways.[13, 39] First, they induce release of procoagulant molecules (plasminogen activator inhibitor, tissue factor, and von Willebrand factor) while inhibiting the protein C anticoagulation system through decreased thrombomodulin expression. The net result is the development of a more thrombogenic endothelial surface. Second, they cause release of PGI_2, a powerful vasodilator and platelet inhibitor. Third, they cause increased expression of leukocyte adhesion molecules on the endothelium of postcapillary venules. Fourth, IL-1 and TNF induce PAF release. Fifth, they increase endothelial synthesis of other cytokines (IL-1, IL-6, IL-8, and granulocyte and granulocyte-monocyte colony stimulating factors), which recruit and activate leukocytes at the site of endothelial cell damage. Sixth, they activate phospholipase A_2, resulting in synthesis of prostaglandins and leukotrienes.[13, 39, 74] Thus the net effect of IL-1 and TNF release on endothelial cell function is to produce conditions favoring altered vasoreactivity, thrombosis, and leukocyte adhesion, which are critical elements in the acute inflammatory response. TNF effects are additive to those of IL-1.[13] During recovery from acute inflammation, both IL-1 and TNF stimulate fibroblast proliferation and collagen and protein synthesis.[12, 68, 69]

IL-6, synthesized by several different cell types, including monocytes-macrophages, fibroblasts, and endothelial cells, is a major regulator of acute phase protein release by the liver,[71, 76] a property also shared by IL-1 and TNF. Acute phase proteins that increase include C-reactive protein, serum amyloid A, fibrinogen, haptoglobin, α_1-antiproteinase, α_1-antichymotrypsin, ceruloplasmin C3, α_2-antiplasmin, C1-inh, and α_1-acid glycoprotein. During the acute phase response, synthesis of transferrin and albumin decreases.[76] In addition to these effects, IL-6 enhances the proliferation of hematopoietic progenitors and, like IL-1 and TNF, mediates the production of fever.[76]

IL-8 is expressed by several cell types, including monocytes-macrophages and endothelial cells, following stimulation by endotoxin, TNFα, or IL-1β.[24, 77] Neutrophil exposure to IL-8 in vitro results in several proinflammatory effects, including neutrophil chemotaxis, degranulation, and expression of cell surface markers.[24] IL-8 is part of a novel superfamily of cytokines identified in activated T cells, macrophages, and fibroblasts.[78] IL-8 has sequence homology with peptides from platelet α-granules such as platelet basic protein, connective tissue–activating peptide III, platelet factor 4, and macrophage inflammatory protein 2.[24] These inflammatory proteins function in the regulation of inflammation and cell growth.[78]

Because of their pivotal role in inflammation, cytokines are a promising focus of research into new therapeutic interventions.[79] The synthesis and release of proinflammatory cytokines such as IL-1 or TNF can be altered by pretreatment with corticosteroids, pentoxifylline, or cyclooxygenase inhibitors.[57, 70] Soluble receptors and inhibitors appear in urine and serum after the release of IL-1 and TNF, and these molecules may serve a role in limiting the physiologic responses to these cytokines.[80–82] Although acute cytokine levels have been shown to correlate with organ damage in sepsis and burns, it is important to remember that these mediators are part of the normal response to stress, infection, and tissue injury.[71] Under some circumstances, their effects are beneficial and necessary for the host's antimicrobial defenses,[83] and they may be used therapeutically as adjuvants to enhance host immune responses against malignancies.[71, 84] In other circumstances (e.g., septic shock), acute cytokine release may be associated with organ damage. Development of therapies that limit cytokine effects (e.g., monoclonal anticytokine antibodies) could be of potential benefit in such conditions.[71, 82, 84]

Growth Factors. The repair of damaged tissue is a complex phenomenon that involves controlled growth of parenchymal and connective tissue and synthesis of extracellular matrix proteins.[12] Growth factors stimulate cell migration, differentiation, and tissue remodeling and affect the ability of fibroblasts, blood vessels, and epithelial cells to undergo DNA synthesis.[3, 14]

Epidermal growth factor is a mitogen for epithelial cells and fibroblasts.[85] PDGF is stored in platelet α-granules or secreted by monocyte-macrophages, endothelium, and smooth muscle cells. It causes migration and proliferation of fibroblasts and smooth muscle cells. PDGF is chemotactic for monocytes and neutrophils and is a potent vasoconstrictor.[86] Fibroblast growth factor (also called *heparin binding protein I or II*) is elaborated by activated macrophages (acidic fibroblast growth factor) or neural tissue (basic fibroblast growth factor) and is necessary for angiogenesis.[3, 87] TGF α is homologous with epidermal growth factor and produces many of the same biologic activities, including in vivo angiogenesis and mitogenesis of fibroblasts and endothelium.[85] TGF β is produced by platelets, endothelium, macrophages, and T cells. It is a growth inhibitor that stimulates fibroblast chemotaxis and the production of collagen and fibronectin.[88] On cells of mesenchymal origin, its effects on proliferation or activation of the cell may be stimulatory or inhibitory, depending on the concomitant effects of other growth factors on that cell.[88]

Hematopoietic growth factors stimulate bone marrow precursors, potentiate neutrophil responses, and influence the migration and proliferation of endothelial cells and fibroblast precursors.[89, 90] These factors include multicolony stimulating factor (also known as IL-3), which is pluripotent for stem cells and granulocyte, monocyte, or granulocyte-monocyte colony stimulating factors. In addition to effects on marrow progenitor cells, granulocyte-monocyte colony stimulating factor is a potent activator of neutrophils, eosinophils, and macrophages. It induces neutrophil phagocytic activity, at least in part through an increase in cell surface adhesion molecules. Granulocyte colony stimulating factor is a potent stimulator of superoxide production and phagocytosis, and monocyte colony stimulating factor activates mature macrophages and enhances cell cytotoxicity.[90] Clinical applications of hematopoietic growth factors include shortening the duration of myelosuppression after chemotherapy, treating cytopenias, and improving bone marrow transplant engraftment.[91]

ANTI-INFLAMMATORY DRUGS

Glucocorticoids

Adrenal glucocorticoids represent the single most effective class of drugs for the therapy of diseases of inflammation.[92] Oral or intravenous administration of glucocorticoids causes marked decreases within 4 to 6 hours in the numbers of circulating basophils and eosinophils. The numbers of circulating lymphocytes are reduced to a lesser extent, but there are profound alterations in lymphocyte function, including inhibition of the production of IL-1, IL-2, and γ-interferon. Macrophages and monocytes are exquisitely sensitive to glucocorticoids, which interfere with cell activation and hence inhibit production of cytokines. Glucocorticoid administration increases the number of circulating neutrophils, reflecting decreased egress from the blood, decreased vascular margination, and increased production by the bone marrow.[93] Notwithstanding the increased number of circulating neutrophils, there is inhibition of the accumulation of neutrophils at sites of inflammation, probably because of alterations in neutrophil adhesion and migration factors.

Through undefined mechanisms, glucocorticoids also decrease vascular permeability in response to inflammatory stimuli such as vasoactive amines and eicosanoids.[92, 93] Glucocorticoid administration also inhibits phospholipase A_2 activity, limiting arachidonic acid availability for eicosanoid synthesis. Hence, formation of prostaglandins and leukotrienes is inhibited. Complement production appears to be resistant to glucocorticoids.[93] With prolonged administration of glucocorticoids, there is delay in wound healing resulting from its effects on angiogenesis, fibroplasia, and other elements of tissue repair.

Glucocorticoids have unequivocal benefit in a wide variety of allergic and autoimmune diseases. Unfortunately, despite their usefulness in specific inflammatory diseases, glucocorticoids do not appear to reduce mortality in the most common life-threatening illnesses—for example, septic shock and adult respiratory distress syndrome.[94, 95]

Aspirin and Other Nonsteroidal Anti-Inflammatory Agents

As a general rule, the clinically useful nonsteroidal anti-inflammatory agents (i.e., aspirin, indomethacin, and ibuprofen) all inhibit cyclooxygenase activity and decrease the synthesis of TxA_2, PGI_2, PGD_2, PGE_2, and $PGF_{2\alpha}$.[40, 96] These cyclooxygenase products cause erythema and fever but generally do not by themselves cause edema or tissue injury. Consequently, their value in acute inflammation lies principally in relieving symptoms. These agents also acetylate the cyclooxygenase in platelets—irreversibly with aspirin and reversibly with indomethacin or ibuprofen. This serves to inhibit platelet TxA_2 production; hence, aspirin is therapeutically effective in adult diseases such as myocardial infarction, pregnancy-induced hypertension, and transient ischemic attacks.[40] Inhibition of cyclooxygenase products can lead to increased formation of leukotrienes, perhaps because of the increased availability of arachidonate. Nonsteroidal agents have a variety of in vitro effects on neutrophil function, but it is not clear whether they are clinically relevant.[96] Selective 5-lipoxygenase inhibitors and leukotriene-receptor antagonists are becoming available investigatively as anti-inflammatory agents.[53, 97]

EFFECTS OF AGE ON INFLAMMATION

The immune system in the newborn is not fully mature, and certain aspects of the inflammatory response may be limited. These immature host responses may serve to increase the neonate's risk of infection (see also Chapter 11).

Alterations in phagocytic cell function in the newborn have been reviewed recently.[98–100] Compared with older children and adults, granulocytes from neonates have (1) less serum chemotactic activity; (2) decreased responsiveness to chemotactic factors, resulting in impaired adherence, impaired chemotaxis, and increased intracellular calcium; (3) abnormalities of deformation and aggregation, which are important for chemotaxis; (4) abnormal distribution of ligand binding sites and lower expression of adhesion molecules; and (5) less myeloperoxidase. Conflicting data exist regarding the occurrence in neonates of (1) impaired phagocytosis of gram-negative organisms by stimulated neutrophils, possibly related to immature forms or maturational defects; (2) decreased lactoferrin levels; (3) altered actin cytoskeletal polymerization; (4) increased respiratory burst activity, which may predispose the host to auto-oxidative cell damage; and (5) decreased production of superoxide and hydroxyl radicals.[98, 99]

The monocytes-macrophages of newborns also exhibit functional defects, which include (1) impaired antibody responses due to impaired antigen presentation by macrophages, (2) poor resistance to facultative intracellular organisms due to maturational delay in macrophage activation, and (3) weak oxidative burst upon stimulation due to limited availability of fibronectin for opsonization. The capacity of neonates to secrete cytokines (IL-1, γ-interferon, and TNF) in general appears to be comparable to adults.[99] Conflicting data exist regarding the impairment of neonatal monocyte-macrophage phagocytosis, oxygen radical generation, antimicrobial activity, response to chemotactins, and migratory activity.[99-101]

Maternal complement components do not cross the placenta.[102] In term neonates, C3 and C4 are 50 to 75% of maternal levels, whereas C8 and C9 are only 10% of maternal levels.[102] Preterm and low birth weight infants have lower levels of complement than do term infants; by 3 months of age most infants have complement levels within the normal adult range.[99, 102] The decreased opsonic activity of neonatal serum may result in part from relatively low C3, factor B, and other complement component levels and may contribute to an increased risk of infection.[102]

CONCLUSION

Despite rapid developments in the scientific understanding of inflammation at the molecular level, the capacity of physicians to manipulate inflammation therapeutically remains sorely limited. Inflammatory processes are so intricately interregulated that perturbation of one component invariably induces counterregulatory changes in several other components. Agents such as corticosteroids, though extremely useful in a variety of specific inflammatory diseases, do not appear to reduce mortality in the most common life-threatening illnesses—for example, septic shock and adult respiratory distress syndrome.[94, 95] Nonetheless there are solid grounds for optimism. In much the same way that monoclonal antiendotoxin antibodies have been shown to reduce mortality in adult septic shock,[103] there is abundant therapeutic potential in monoclonal antibodies directed against other exogenous mediators and against endogenous inflammatory mediators—for example, monoclonal anti-TNF antibodies.[104] Investigators are actively seeking inflammatory receptor antagonists, analogues, membrane-stabilizing agents, selective enzyme inhibitors, immunologic adjuvants, and other biologic response modifiers to augment or inhibit specific steps in inflammatory pathways. With time, it should become possible to stimulate specifically the adaptive inflammatory responses that enhance control of infection, while diminishing the generalized and maladaptive inflammatory responses that lead to organ system failure and death.

References

1. Weissman G: Inflammation: Historical perspective. In: Gallin JI, Goldstein IM, and Snyderman R (eds): Inflammation: Basic Principles and Clinical Correlates. New York, Raven Press, 1988, pp 5–8.
2. Balkwill FR and Burke F: The cytokine network. Immunol Today 10:299, 1989.
3. Sporn MB and Roberts AB: Peptide growth factors are multifunctional. Nature 332:217, 1988.
4. Parrillo JE and Masur H (eds): The Critically Ill Immunosuppressed Patient: Diagnosis and Management. Rockville, Aspen Publishers, 1987, pp i–600.
5. Coalson JJ: Pathology of sepsis, septic shock, and multiple organ failure. In: Sibbald WJ and Sprung CL (eds): Perspectives on Sepsis and Septic Shock. Fullerton, Society of Critical Care Medicine, 1986, pp 27–59.
6. McGovern VJ: Shock revisited. Pathol Annu 19:15, 1984.
7. Cotran RS, Kumar V, and Robbins SL: Cellular injury and adaptation. In: Robbins' Pathologic Basis of Disease, 4th ed. Philadelphia, WB Saunders, 1989, pp 1–38.
8. Macknight ADC: Cellular response to injury. In: Staub NC and Taylor AE (eds): Edema. New York, Raven Press, 1984, pp 489–520.
9. Ryan GB and Majno G: Acute inflammation: A review. Am J Pathol 86:185, 1977.
10. Larsen GL and Henson PM: Mediators of inflammation. Annu Rev Immunol 1:335, 1983.
11. Wilhelm DL: Mechanisms responsible for increased vascular permeability in acute inflammation. Agents Actions 3:297, 1973.
12. Cotran RS, Kumar V, and Robbins SL: Inflammation and repair. In: Robbins' Pathologic Basis of Disease, 4th ed. Philadelphia, WB Saunders, 1989, pp 39–86.
13. Pober JS and Cotran RS: Cytokines and endothelial cell biology. Physiol Rev 70:427, 1990.
14. King RJ, Jones MB, and Minoo P: Regulation of lung cell proliferation by polypeptide growth factors. Am J Physiol (Lung Cell Mol Physiol 1) 257:L23, 1989.
15. Brenner BM, Troy JL, and Ballermann BJ: Endothelium-dependent vascular responses: Mediators and mechanisms. J Clin Invest 84:1373, 1989.
16. Hurley JV: Inflammation. In: Staub NC and Taylor AE (eds): Edema. New York, Raven Press, 1984, pp 463–488.
17. Cotran RS and Majno G: A light and electron microscope analysis of vascular injury. Ann NY Acad Sci 116:750, 1964.
18. Joris I, Majno G, Corey EJ, et al: The mechanism of vascular leakage induced by leukotriene E₄: Endothelial contraction. Am J Pathol 126:19, 1987.
19. Harlan JM: Consequences of leukocyte-vessel wall interactions in inflammatory and immune reactions. Semin Thromb Hemost 13:434, 1987.
20. Ward PA and Marks RM: The acute inflammatory reaction. Curr Opin Immunol 2:5, 1989.
21. Gallin JI: The neutrophil. In: Samter M, Talmage DW, Frank MM et al (eds): Immunological Diseases, 4th ed. Boston, Little, Brown, 1988, pp 737–788.
22. Patarroyo M and Makgoba MW: Leucocyte adhesion to cells in immune and inflammatory responses. Lancet 2:1139, 1989.
23. Sandbourg RR and Smolen JE: Early biochemical events in leucocyte activation. Lab Invest 59:300, 1988.
24. Baggiolini M, Walz A, and Kunkel SL: Neutrophil-activating peptide-1/interleukin 8, a novel cytokine that activates neutrophils. J Clin Invest 84:1045, 1989.
25. Hugli TE: Chemotaxis. Curr Opin Immunol 2:19, 1989.
26. Henson PM, Henson JE, Fittschen C, et al: Phagocytic cells: Degranulation and secretion. In: Galiin JI, Goldstein IM, and Snyderman R (eds): Inflammation: Basic Principles and Clinical Correlates. New York, Raven Press, 1988, pp 363–390.
27. Henson PM and Johnston RB: Tissue injury in inflammation: Oxidants, proteinases, and cationic proteins. J Clin Invest 79:669, 1987.
28. Nathan CF: Secretory products of macrophages. J Clin Invest 79:319, 1987.
29. Colman RW: Surface-mediated defense reactions: The plasma contact activation system. J Clin Invest 73:1249, 1984.
30. Kozin F and Cochrane CG: The contact activation system of plasma: Biochemistry and pathophysiology. In: Gallin JI, Goldstein IM, and Snyderman R (eds): Inflammation: Basic Principles and Clinical Correlates. New York, Raven Press, 1988, pp 101–120.
31. Proud D and Kaplan AP: Kinin formation: Mechanisms and role in inflammatory disorders. Annu Rev Immunol 6:49, 1988.
32. Hirsh J, Salzman EW, Marder VJ, et al: Overview of the thrombolytic process and therapy. In: Colman RW, Marder VJ, Salzman EW, et al (eds): Hemostasis and Thrombosis: Basic Principles and Clinical Practice, 2nd ed. Philadelphia, JB Lippincott, 1987, pp 1063–1072.
33. Weksler B: Platelets. In: Gallin JI, Goldstein IM, and Snyderman R (eds): Inflammation: Basic Principles and Clinical Correlates. New York, Raven Press, 1988, pp 543–557.

34. Colman RW, Marder VJ, Salzman EW, et al: Overview of hemostasis. *In:* Colman RW, Marder VJ, Salzman EW, et al (eds): Hemostasis and Thrombosis: Basic Principles and Clinical Practice, 2nd ed. Philadelphia, JB Lippincott, 1987, pp 3–18.

35. Harpel PC: Blood proteolytic enzyme inhibitors: Their role in modulating blood coagulation and fibrinolytic enzyme pathways. *In:* Colman RW, Marder VJ, Salzman EW, et al (eds): Hemostasis and Thrombosis: Basic Principles and Clinical Practice, 2nd ed. Philadelphia, JB Lippincott, 1987, pp 219–234.

36. Gerlach A, Esposito C, and Stern DM: Modulation of the endothelial hemostatic properties: An active role in the host response. Annu Rev Med 41:15, 1990.

37. Schafer AI: Focusing of the clot: Normal and pathologic mechanisms. Annu Rev Med 38:211, 1987.

38. Jaffe E: Endothelial cells. *In:* Gallin JI, Goldstein IM, and Snyderman R (eds): Inflammation: Basic Principles and Clinical Correlates. New York, Raven Press, 1988, pp 559–576.

39. Mantovani A and Dejana E: Cytokines as communication signals between leukocytes and endothelial cells. Immunol Today 10:370, 1989.

40. Vane JR, Änggard EE, and Botting RM: Regulatory functions of the vascular endothelium. N Engl J Med 323:27, 1990.

41. Francis CW and Marder VJ: Concepts of clot lysis. Annu Rev Med 37:187, 1986.

42. Müller-Eberhard HJ: Complement: Chemistry and pathways. *In:* Gallin JI, Goldstein IM, and Snyderman R (eds): Inflammation: Basic Principles and Clinical Correlates. New York, Raven Press, 1988, pp 21–53.

43. Goldstein IM: Complement: Biologically active products. *In:* Gallin JI, Goldstein IM, and Snyderman R (eds): Inflammation: Basic Principles and Clinical Correlates. New York, Raven Press, 1988, pp 55–74.

44. Müller-Eberhard HJ: The membrane attack complex. Annu Rev Immunol 4:503, 1986.

45. Fries LF and Frank MM: Complement and related proteins: Inherited deficiencies. *In:* Gallin JI, Goldstein IM, and Snyderman R (eds): Inflammation: Basic Principles and Clinical Correlates. New York, Raven Press, 1988, pp 89–100.

46. Klebanoff SJ: Phagocytic cells: Products of oxygen metabolism. *In:* Gallin JI, Goldstein IM, and Snyderman R (eds): Inflammation: Basic Principles and Clinical Correlates. New York, Raven Press, 1988, pp 391–444.

47. Halliwell B: Oxidants and human disease: Some new concepts. FASEB J 1:358, 1987.

48. Southorn PA and Powis G: Free radicals in medicine. I: Chemical nature and biologic reactions. II: Involvement in human disease. Mayo Clin Proc 63:381, 1988.

49. Farber JL, Kyle ME, and Coleman JB: Mechanisms of cell injury by activated oxygen species. Lab Invest 62:670, 1990.

50. Clark RA: The human neutrophil respiratory burst oxidase. J Infect Dis 161:1140, 1990.

51. Weiss SJ: Tissue destruction by neutrophils. N Engl J Med 320:365, 1989.

52. Janoff A: Elastase in tissue injury. Annu Rev Med 36:207, 1985.

53. Holtzman MJ: Arachidonic acid metabolism: Implications of biological chemistry for lung function and disease. Am Rev Respir Dis 143:188, 1991.

54. Burrall BA, Payan DG, and Goetzl EJ: Arachidonic acid-derived mediators of hypersensitivity and inflammation. *In:* Middleton E, Reed CE, Ellis EF, et al (eds): Allergy: Principles and Practice. St. Louis, CV Mosby, 1988, pp 164–178.

55. Vane JR and Botting RM: Prostaglandins, prostacyclin, thromboxane, and leukotrienes. The arachidonic acid cascade. *In:* Fuhrman BP and Shoemaker WC (eds): Critical Care Medicine: State of the Art, Vol 10. Fullerton, Society of Critical Care Medicine, 1989, pp 1–24.

56. Parker CW and Stenson WF: Prostaglandins and leukotrienes. Curr Opin Immunol 2:28, 1989.

57. Kunkel SL, Remick DG, Streiter RMN, et al: Mechanisms that regulate the production and effects of tumor necrosis factor α. Crit Rev Immunol 9:93, 1989.

58. Samuelsson B, Dahlen SE, Lindgren JA, et al: Leukotrienes and lipoxins: Structures, biosynthesis, and biological effects. Science 237:1171, 1987.

59. Feuerstein G and Hallenbeck JM: Leukotrienes in health and disease. FASEB J 1:186, 1987.

60. Lewis RA, Austen KF, and Soberman RJ: Leukotrienes and other products of the 5-lipoxygenase pathway: Biochemistry and relation to pathobiology in human disease. N Engl J Med 323:645, 1990.

61. Snyder F: Platelet-activating factor and related acetylated lipids as potent biologically active cellular mediators. Am J Physiol (Cell Physiol 28) 259:C697, 1990.

62. Pinckard RN, Ludwig JC, and McManus LM: Platelet activating factors. *In:* Gallin JI, Goldstein IM, and Snyderman R (eds): Inflammation: Basic Principles and Clinical Correlates. New York, Raven Press, 1988, pp 139–167.

63. Chung KF and Barnes PJ: Platelet-activating factor and asthma. *In:* Kaliner MA, Barnes PJ, and Persson CGA (eds): Asthma: Its Pathology and Treatment. New York, Marcel Dekker, 1990, pp 267–300.

64. White MV and Kaliner MA: Histamine. *In:* Gallin JI, Goldstein IM, and Snyderman R (eds): Inflammation: Basic Principles and Clinical Correlates. New York, Raven Press, 1988, pp 169–193.

65. Barnes PJ: Neuropeptides and asthma. Am Rev Respir Dis 143:S28, 1991.

66. Said SI: Neuropeptides (VIP and tachykinins): VIP as a modulator of lung inflammation and airway constriction. Am Rev Respir Dis 143:S22, 1991.

66a. Green AR: Peptide regulatory factors: Multifunctional mediators of cellular growth and differentiation. Lancet 2:705, 1989.

67. Kelso A: Cytokines: Structure, function, and synthesis. Curr Opin Immunol 2:215, 1989.

68. Kelly J: Cytokines of the lung. Am Rev Respir Dis 141:765, 1990.

69. Elias JA, Freundlich B, Kern JA, et al: Cytokine networks in the regulation of inflammation and fibrosis in the lung. Chest 97:1439, 1990.

70. Dinarello CA: Interleukin-1 and the effects of cyclooxygenase inhibitors on biological activities. Bull NY Acad Med 65:80, 1989.

71. Fong Y, Moldawer LL, Shires GT, et al: The biologic characteristics of cytokines and their implication in surgical injury. Surg Gynecol Obstet 170:363, 1990.

72. Dinarello CA: Interleukin-1 and the pathogenesis of the acute-phase response. N Engl J Med 311:1413, 1984.

73. Dinarello CA and Mier JW: Lymphokines. N Engl J Med 317:940, 1987.

74. Beutler B and Cerami A: The biology of cachectin/TNF—a primary mediator of the host response. Annu Rev Immunol 7:625, 1989.

75. Larrick JW and Wright SC: Cytotoxic mechanism of tumor necrosis factor α. FASEB J 4:3215, 1990.

76. Heinrich PC, Castell JV, and Andus T: Interleukin-6 and the acute phase response. Biochem J 265:621, 1990.

77. Bazzoni F, Cassatella MA, Rossi F, et al: Phagocytosing neutrophils produce and release high amounts of the neutrophil-activating peptide 1 / interleukin 8. J Exp Med 173:771, 1991.

78. Wolpe SD and Cerami A: Macrophage inflammatory proteins q1 and 2: members of a superfamily of cytokines. FASEB J 3:2565, 1989.

79. Larrick JW: Native interleukin 1 inhibitors. Immunol Today 10:61, 1989.

80. Arend WP and Dayer JM: Cytokines and cytokine inhibitors or antagonists in rheumatoid arthritis. Arthritis Rheum 33:305, 1990.

81. Spinas GA, Bloesch D, Kaufmann MT, et al: Induction of plasma inhibitors of interleukin-1 and TNFα activity by endotoxin administration to normal humans. Am J Physiol (Regul Integrative Comp Physiol 28) 259:R993, 1990.

82. Ohlsson K, Bjork P, Bergenfeldt M, et al: Interleukin-1 receptor antagonist reduces mortality from endotoxin shock. Nature 348:550, 1990.

83. Cross AS, Sadoff JC, Kelly N, et al: Pretreatment with recombinant murine tumor necrosis factor α/cachectin and murine interleukin 1α protects mice from lethal bacterial infection. J Exp Med 169:2021, 1989.

84. Heath AW: Cytokines and infection. Curr Opin Immunol 2:380, 1990.

85. Waterfield MD: Epidermal growth factor and related molecules. Lancet 1:1243, 1989.

86. Ross R: Platelet-derived growth factor. Annu Rev Med 38:71, 1987.

87. Folkman J and Klagsbrun M: Angiogenic factors. Science 235:442, 1987.
88. Wahl SM, McCartney-Francis N, and Mergenhagen SE: Inflammatory and immunomodulatory role of TGFβ. Immunol Today 10:258, 1989.
89. Metcalf D: Haemopoietic growth factors. Lancet 1:825, 1989.
90. Sieff CA: Biology and clinical aspects of the hematopoietic growth factors. Annu Rev Med 41:483, 1990.
91. Robinson BE and Quesenberry PJ: Hematopoietic growth factors: Overview and clinical applications, Part III. Am J Med Sci 300:311, 1990.
92. Schleimer RP: Glucocorticosteroids: Their mechanisms of action and use in allergic diseases. *In:* Middleton E, Reed CE, Ellis EF, et al (eds): Allergy: Principles and Practice. St. Louis, CV Mosby, 1988, pp 739–765.
93. Bowen DL and Fauci AS: Adrenal corticosteroids. *In:* Gallin JI, Goldstein IM, and Snyderman R (eds): Inflammation: Basic Principles and Clinical Correlates. New York, Raven Press, 1988, pp 877–910.
94. Bernard GR, Luce JM, Sprung CL, et al: High-dose corticosteroids in patients with the adult respiratory distress syndrome. N Engl J Med 317:1565, 1987.
95. Bone RC, Fisher CJ, Clemmer TP, et al: A controlled clinical trial of high-dose methylprednisolone in the treatment of severe sepsis and septic shock. N Engl J Med 317:653, 1987.
96. Goldstein IM: Agents that interfere with arachidonic acid metabolism. *In:* Gallin JI, Goldstein IM, and Snyderman R (eds): Inflammation: Basic Principles and Clinical Correlates. New York, Raven Press, 1988, pp 935–946.
97. Snyder DW and Fleisch JH: Leukotriene receptor antagonists as potential therapeutic agents. Annu Rev Pharmacol Toxicol 29:123, 1989.
98. Abramson JS, Wheeler JG, and Quie PG: The polymorphonuclear phagocyte system. *In:* Steihm ER (ed): Immunologic Disorders in Infants and Children, 3rd ed. Philadelphia, WB Saunders, 1989, pp 68–80.
99. Burgio GR, Ugazio AG, and Notarangelo LD: Immunology of the neonate. Curr Opin Immunol 2:770, 1990.
100. Douglas SD, Hassan NF, and Blaese RM: The mononuclear phagocyte system. *In:* Steihm ER (ed): Immunologic Disorders in Infants and Children, 3rd ed. Philadelphia, WB Saunders, 1989, pp 81–96.
101. Johnston RB: Monocytes and macrophages. N Engl J Med 318:747, 1988.
102. Berger M and Frank MM: The serum complement system. *In:* Steihm ER (ed): Immunologic Disorders in Infants and Children, 3rd ed. Philadelphia, WB Saunders, 1989, pp 97–115.
103. Ziegler EJ, Fisher CJ, Sprung CL, et al: Treatment of gram-negative bacteremia and septic shock with HA-1A human monoclonal antibody against endotoxin. N Engl J Med 324:429, 1991.
104. Larrick JW: Antibody inhibition of the immunoinflammatory cascade. J Crit Care 4:211, 1989.

Mechanisms of Cellular Communication and Signal Transduction

Joseph A. Carcillo, M.D.

The principles of practice in critical care medicine are based on an understanding of physiology and pharmacology. Initially, both fields were conceptualized in "macro" terms. For example, the heart was visualized as a pump that pulsed blood through a series of distensible tubes known as the systemic vasculature. Congestive heart disease was described in terms of "pump failure" and increased "afterload." Researchers in pharmacology responded to this definition of pathophysiology with the development of pharmacotherapeutic agents that increased cardiac muscle fiber shortening velocity or relaxed vascular smooth muscle. In the 1960s, investigators in the field of pharmacology discovered the existence of receptors, and the search for a "micro" understanding of physiology and therapeutics began.

Research on the molecular and cellular basis of disease and therapeutics has dominated medical literature in recent years. The study of signal transduction in biologic systems has particular significance to critical care medicine. This field concentrates on the mechanisms by which hormones, drugs, macromolecules, and mediators elicit cellular responses under physiologic and pathophysiologic conditions. This chapter discusses the role of signal transduction in the cell and the significance of molecular physiology and pharmacology to bedside practice in the pediatric intensive care unit.

COMMUNICATION ACROSS THE CELL MEMBRANE

The cell membrane is a semifluid structure composed of a phospholipid bilayer with a hydrophobic core and hydrophilic surfaces. This selectively permeable structure is occupied by protein molecules that span the membrane in the form of ion channels, ion pumps, receptors, transport systems, and enzymes. The remarkable fluidity of this system allows these proteins to exist in a dynamic state, migrating to locations within and on the surface of the membrane, providing the first line of

cellular communication and signal transduction with myriad mechanistic possibilities. One mechanism by which macromolecules, including glucose and amino acids, can be transported across this membrane is through active transport or carrier-mediated systems. The most studied of these systems are the glucose transporters, which demonstrate three mechanisms: (1) facilitated (nonactive) sugar transport; (2) the hormone-sensitive, insulin-dependent D-glucose carrier found in muscle and adipocytes; and (3) the sodium-dependent cotransporter found at the mucosal surface of the small intestine and renal proximal tubule (Fig. 3–1).[1] The insulin-mediated transporter system allows for hormonal control of glucose metabolism through receptor-mediated mechanisms. In this system, insulin binds to its receptor, thereby activating tyrosine kinase and a system of second messengers, which leads to translocation of the carrier protein from an intracellular pool to the

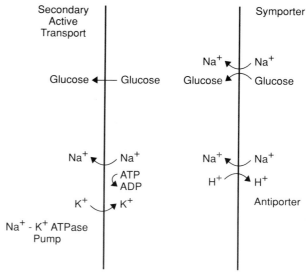

Figure 3–1. Carrier-mediated mechanisms. Secondary active transport, symporter, and antiporter.

membrane. The sodium-dependent cotransporter is an example of secondary active transport. The serosal Na, K⁺-ATPase pump is located at the blood or peritubular side of the cell. As it uses adenosine triphosphate (ATP) to bring in two K^+ ions for every three Na^+ ions released, an electrochemical gradient is created in which Na^+ ions from the mucosal side are brought into the cell. Glucose follows this chemical gradient, giving the name *sodium-dependent cotransporter*. This is known as a *symporter* system because the solute moves in the same direction as the Na^+ molecules. When the solute moves in the opposite direction of Na^+, such as occurs with the H^+ ion, the system is known as an *antiporter* or *countertransporter*.

Macromolecules may also move across the cell membrane via the mechanism of receptor endocytosis (Fig. 3–2).[2] One notable example is low-density lipoprotein. In this mechanism, the receptor, a glycoprotein, attaches with specific affinity to its ligand. The receptor-ligand complex then migrates along the membrane to a localized region known as a *fuzzy pit* (named for its appearance on electron microscopy). The pit invaginates into a coated vesicle that can then migrate inside the cell through the endoplasmic reticulum and the trans-Golgi network. The protein clathrin appears to be responsible for the "coated" appearance of the pit and its vesicles. This protein facilitates the process by concentrating receptors and increasing the efficiency of their delivery into the cell. Once inside the endosomal apparatus, the ligand can be processed. Low-density lipoprotein and its internalized receptor, for example, may give signals that control hydroxymethylglutaryl-coreductase activity and cholesterol biosynthesis. Elucidation of defects in this process and its relationship to familial hypercholesterolemia was the basis for the work done by Goldstein and Brown and their colleagues, for which they received a Nobel Prize.[3] Endocytosis by noncoated vesicles (lack of clathrin) is the pathway of nonfacilitated internalization of toxins and virus and a few notable receptor exceptions.[4]

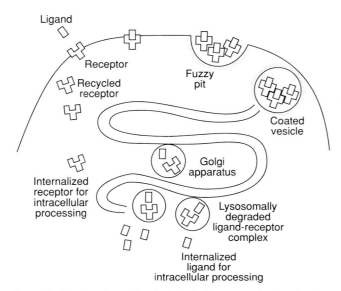

Figure 3–2. Receptor endocytosis. Significant mechanism for internalization of ligands and control of cell surface receptor numbers.

Receptor endocytosis is the most significant mechanism for control of receptor numbers in the cell membrane. This process is under control of the signal transduction system of the cell itself. For example, in the case of agonist stimulation, endocytosis increases and transcytosis decreases, with a resultant decrease in receptor number on the membrane surface that is known as *down-regulation*. Antagonist or decreased agonist stimulation results in increased transcytosis and decreased endocytosis, leading to increased receptor numbers or *up-regulation*. This process can be under the control of the hormone system. For example, thyroid and cortisol hormones both increase β-adrenergic receptor up-regulation. This observation has been offered as support for the use of steroids during β-agonist stimulation in children with asthma.

Receptor endocytosis is also the mechanism by which the "receptor" itself can become a signal in the signal transduction process. Notably, the thyroid receptor and the steroid receptor have been shown to undergo conformational changes upon binding to their respective hormones, which allows them to bind to deoxyribonucleic acid (DNA). Receptor internalization is necessary for this process to be effected. The newly identified adhesion proteins, which have significance in intercellular communication in morphogenesis and inflammation, are hypothesized to occur through such endocytotic mechanisms as well.

Endocytosis is a physiologically "slow" process occurring over minutes to hours. When cellular responses occur in fractions of seconds, the receptor-mediated second-messenger systems or ion channels, or both, are the means of signal transduction across the cell membrane. The receptor is a glycoprotein that spans the cell membrane with extracellular, intramembrane, and cytosolic domains. For any given type of receptor, subtypes may be defined. For example, the adrenergic receptors, which bind catecholamines, are defined according to their effect on catalytic subunits. There are three groups: the β₁- and β₂-adrenergic receptors, which activate adenylate cyclase; the α₂-adrenergic receptor, which inhibits adenylate cyclase; and the α₁-adrenergic receptor, which activates phospholipase C. The muscarinic receptors, which bind acetylcholine, have been differentiated into five types on the basis of pharmacologic features. Most recently, subtypes are being defined on the basis of gene sequences. The site of binding to the receptor can affect affinity. For example, the adrenergic antagonists bind more substantially to the hydrophobic domain, whereas the agonists bind to the hydrophilic domain. This results in a receptor ligand dissociation constant for epinephrine or isoproterenol of 2 to 3μM, whereas the dissociation constant for propranolol is 0.0012 μM. Application of this knowledge has been lifesaving in children in whom bradycardia or asystole develops after treatment with intravenous propranolol for supraventricular tachycardia. As much as an ampule of isoproterenol may be required to displace the competitive antagonist.

Each receptor is coupled to its catalytic unit or enzyme, (which provides the second messenger) by a G protein.[5, 6] These proteins, previously referred to as N for nucleotide proteins, have had their name changed because they bind guanosine triphosphate (GTP). At present, there have been five G proteins described. G_s (stimulatory) stimulates adenylate cyclase (β_1-receptor), G_i (inhibitory) inhibits adenylate cyclase (α_2-, M receptors), G_t (transducin) regulates rhodopsin-mediated cyclic guanosine monophosphate phophodiesterase activity, G_o may effect calcium channels, G_k effects potassium channels, and G_p (phospholipase C) has been purported to stimulate phospholipase C activity, but this has not been proved (α_1-, M receptors). The ternary complex model of receptor binding is based on the "collision coupling theory" (Fig. 3–3). According to this explanation, the agonist-bound receptor interacts with the guanosine diphosphate (GDP)-bound G_s protein, "opening" a GTP binding site. GTP is exchanged for GDP on the α-subunit of the G protein and this, in turn, activates the catalytic unit C, which in this case is an adenyl cyclase, to produce cyclic adenosine monophosphate (cAMP) as a second messenger. The activation of the G protein–catalytic subunit is a catalytic event, as the agonist-bound receptor dissociates from the complex. Although the "collision" is transient, activation of adenylate cyclase continues until the intrinsic guanosine triphosphatase (GTPase) activity on the α-subunit of the G_s protein metabolizes all GTP to GDP. This allows significant amplification of the system. Each released agonist-receptor complex can go on to interact with 10 G_s–adenylate cyclase molecules, and each activated G protein–catalytic unit complex produces 100 cAMP molecules before the intrinsic GTPase activity stops the process. Thus each agonist molecule produces 10^3 second-messenger molecules. Agonists that attain this full degree of amplification are "full agonists" and include drugs such as epinephrine, norepinephrine, and isoproterenol. The partial agonists phenylephrine and dopamine elicit a less than maximal response, because fewer receptors are activated. The better the agonist, the greater the coupling of receptors to G_s.[7]

Two toxins have specific effects on the G_s and G_i proteins. Cholera toxin covalently modifies the G_s protein, transferring the adenosine diphosphate (ADP)–ribose moiety of nicotinamide adenine dinucleotide to α_s, causing persistent stimulation of adenyl cyclase. Similarly, pertussis toxin modifies the G_i protein through ADP ribosylation of α_i. Both toxins have been purported to mediate their pathologic effects on physiologic secretion processes through these mechanisms.

G-proteins couple ion channels as well. Ion channels are protein structures that are divided into two classifications: voltage-sensitive channels, which are opened in response to an appropriate change in membrane action potential, and receptor-operated channels, which are opened in response to agonist receptor stimulation (Fig. 3–4).[8, 9] In addition, some channels are both voltage- and receptor-regulated. · In most excitable cells with voltage-sensitive ion channels, the action potential is composed of three ion fluxes. The first is the rapid influx of Na^+ through the sodium channel.[10] This depolarization, in turn, opens the voltage-sensitive slow inward Ca^{2+} channel, allowing for a plateau phase in repolarization. The slow influx of Ca^{2+} ion into the cytosol is the so-called electromechanical coupling step in signal transduction. The Ca^{2+} ion is the signal transduced into the cell on a millisecond time scale. The action potential is terminated when the voltage-sensitive K^+ channel is activated. This channel, which purportedly is coupled to G_k, mediates an outward current of K^+ ions, which repolarizes the cell. This K^+ channel participates in setting the resting membrane potential of the cell. The ATP-dependent Na^+, K^+-ATPase pump is responsible for maintaining the resting potential.

Receptor-operated channels depend on the interaction between cell surface receptors and specific neurotransmitters, including norepinephrine and acetylcholine. Activation of these receptors can also modulate ion conductance in the voltage-sensitive channels. At present, three Ca^{2+} channels have been characterized: the L or slow channel, the T or fast channel, and the N or neuronal channel. The L channel, which is the channel responsible for calcium influx during voltage-sensitive depolarization of cardiac muscle, is also receptor-mediated and sensitive to the G_s-coupled β_1-agonist. Calcium channel blockers can also bind to the L channel and modulate the voltage-sensitive process.[11] Thus, the distinction of voltage- versus receptor-operated ion channels may have considerable overlap.

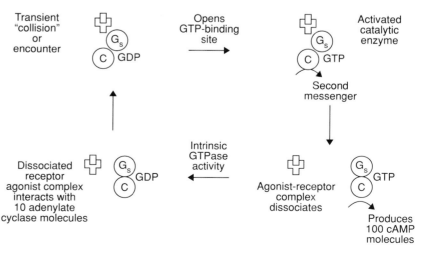

Figure 3–3. The ternary complex model of receptor binding. The interactions of receptor, agonist, G-protein, GDP, GTP, and the catalytic enzyme allow for amplification of second messenger production.

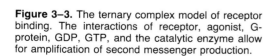

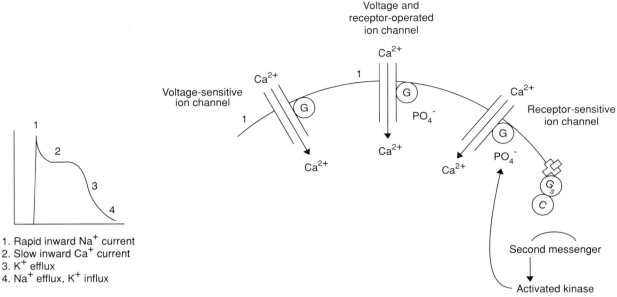

1. Rapid inward Na^+ current
2. Slow inward Ca^+ current
3. K^+ efflux
4. Na^+ efflux, K^+ influx

Figure 3–4. Voltage and receptor-operated ion channels.

RECEPTORS, ION CHANNELS, SECOND MESSENGERS, AND THE CALCIUM MESSENGER SYSTEM

Calcium is the messenger of cell function (Fig. 3–5).[12] Receptor-mediated second-messenger systems and ion channels all lead to rapidly increased intracellular (Ca^{2+}) concentrations. This ion activates enzymes to respond in milliseconds. This occurs through two groups of enzymes—the calcium-dependent and the calmodulin-dependent enzymes. Calmodulin is a protein that undergoes a conformational change when binding to Ca^{2+} ions. This, in turn, activates the associated enzyme. Unfortunately, increased Ca^{2+} has limitations as an ideal messenger. First and foremost, it is a toxic ion at concentrations similar to those required to activate these dependent enzyme systems.[13] The extracellular calcium ion concentration is 10^{-3} M, whereas normal intracellular calcium concentration is maintained at 10^{-7} M or submicromolar levels. The low physiologic level of cytosolic calcium is accomplished through a network of intracellular calcium-binding proteins, buffering by the endoplasmic or sarcoplasmic reticulum and mitochondria, and a group of calcium-extruding pumps including the Ca^{2+}-ATPase and the Na^+-Ca^{2+} exchange pumps. These mechanisms of calcium extrusion are more ATP-dependent/mole than are the calcium influx mechanisms. When these processes are overwhelmed, increased calcium concentrations become toxic to the cell. Mitochondrial function is most sensitive to this process. For this reason, the cell developed a system in which the increase in intracellular calcium ions was at most transient.

Nature's answer to continued cellular response to a transient calcium message has been found in the remarkable phosphate ion. The addition of this ion to multiple substrates, including enzymes, receptors, ion channels, and nucleic acids, is known as phosphorylation. This is a process of covalent modification. In formation of this chemical bond, the modified substrate enjoys a change in structure, with a new, lower energy state. This change in structure, in turn, leads to a change in function. The enzymes that carry out phosphorylation are known as kinases. The key to function in signal transduction lies in the effects of this kinase system. Kinases are generally named according to their catalysts. For example, there are Ca^{2+}-dependent kinases, Ca^{2+}-calmodulin–dependent kinases, cAMP-dependent ki-

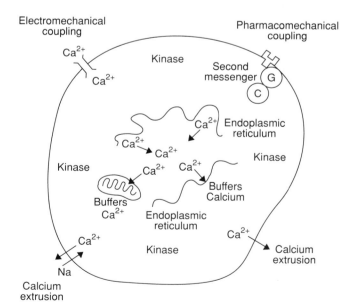

Figure 3–5. The calcium messenger system—voltage or receptor mediated mechanisms increase intracellular Ca^{2+} through ion channel opening or through release from the endoplasmic reticulum. This increase in calcium activates kinase and other enzyme systems leading to altered cellular function. Calcium ion is then buffered by mitochondria and endoplasmic reticulum and extruded by Ca^{2+} pumps and exchangers. Further function may occur at near-normal calcium concentration as a result of kinase functions.

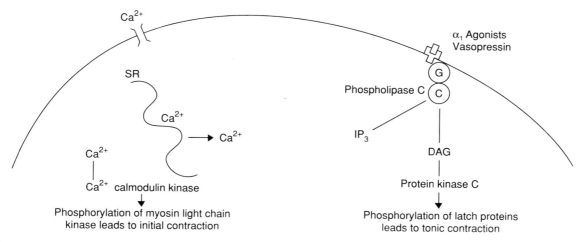

Figure 3–6. Proposed mechanism for phasic and tonic contraction in vascular tissue through α-adrenergic and vasopressin receptors. (SR = sarcoplasmic reticulum.)

nases (protein kinase A), cGMP-dependent kinases (protein kinase G), and the phospholipase C–derived diacylglycerol (DAG)-dependent kinase (protein kinase C).

Receptor-agonist interactions or depolarization-induced calcium channel opening or both lead immediately to increased intracellular Ca^{2+} ion concentrations and the production of second messengers. These, in turn, activate the kinase system. Through phosphorylation, the kinases modify the Ca^{2+}-dependent enzymes so that they can be activated at intracellular calcium concentrations of 10^{-6} to 10^{-7} M, the normal physiologic level of the resting cytosol. This allows continued stimulation of these enzymes without generation of toxic Ca^{2+} concentrations. Other kinases may phosphorylate channels in an open position, G proteins to effect coupling changes or receptors to effect further responses. This can allow a continued response beyond the initial stimulus. Phosphatases (enzymes responsible for dephosphorylation) in turn allow control of the kinase system by dephosphorylating the substrates effected by the kinase system.

Cardiac and vascular tissue are two good models to illustrate the specific details of signal transduction and the calcium messenger system. According to currently accepted modeling, during vasoconstriction the adrenergic agonist norepinephrine binds to the α_1-adrenoceptor. This, through a proposed but unproven G_p-coupled mechanism, activates membrane-bound phospholipase C activity. Phospholipase C hydrolyzes the cell membrane lipid phosphotidyl inositol, yielding a series of metabolites, including the second messengers inosine phosphorylase 3 (IP3), inositol-3,4,5-triphosphate and DAG.[14, 15] IP3 causes an immediate release of calcium ions from the sarcoplasmic reticulum. This increased intracellular calcium ion concentration is proposed to activate Ca^{2+}- and calmodulin-dependent kinases, including myosin light chain kinase, which may participate in phosphorylation of filament proteins and initial contraction. If long-term continued response or tonic contraction is to be achieved without increasing toxic Ca^{2+} ion release from the sarcoplasmic reticulum, phosphorylation must allow for contraction to continue at physi-

ologic cytosolic calcium levels. DAG has the remarkable ability to activate the enzyme protein kinase C precisely by lowering the threshold of calcium ion–induced activation to resting physiologic levels. It is proposed that protein kinase C and other activated hormones may, in turn, phosphorylate the latch proteins and lead to tonic contraction (Fig. 3–6). Phosphorylation of the receptor-regulated calcium channel may also occur, further allowing regulation of calcium influx. Feedback inhibition of contraction may also be mediated by protein kinase C. For example, this kinase phosphorylates and activates IP3 phosphomonoesterase, which hydrolyzes the IP3 second messenger. Once tonic contraction has occurred at physiologic calcium levels, there may be little need for further release of calcium from the sarcoplasmic reticulum. The phosphoinositide pathway provides myriad inositol phosphates with significant biologic functions in signal transduction. However, for the sake of simplicity in this chapter, we have concentrated on IP3 and DAG.[16]

Relaxation in vascular tissue or vasodilatation is mediated by decreasing intracellular calcium, dephosphorylating contractile elements, and phosphorylating Ca^{2+} uptake mechanisms in vascular tissue. This is proposed to be mediated through cGMP- and cAMP-dependent kinases. Nitrate vasodilators, atrial natriuretic factor (ANF), and acetylcholine activate guanylate cyclase to release cGMP. Nitrates activate particulate guanylate cyclase, ANF activates soluble guanylate cyclase, and acetylcholine causes release of an "endothelial-derived relaxant factor," which activates guanylate cyclase.[17] The β_2-agonists, including isoproterenol, activate adenylate cyclase, with presumed coupling with G_s protein, to produce the second-messenger cAMP. Activation of the cGMP- and cAMP-dependent kinases increases calcium extrusion from the cell through activation of ion pumps, as well as increased uptake into the sarcoplasmic reticulum. In addition, these kinases may inhibit phospholipase C–mediated production of IP3 and DAG. Vasodilatation may also be induced by agents, including minoxidil, which facilitate outward K^+ ion current, causing membrane hyperpolarization or repolarization.[18]

This, in turn, closes the calcium ion channel to calcium influx and decreases intracellular calcium concentrations.

Cardiac tissue is functionally distinct from vascular tissue. Cardiac muscle must contract in a controlled, rapid-phase pattern (0.6 seconds or less), rather than the tonic pattern of vascular smooth muscle. Evolution has achieved this function with receptor-mediated voltage-sensitive ion channels and a specialized calcium messenger system (Fig. 3–7).[19] Calcium-dependent automatic cells in the sinoatrial node produce an action potential that is propagated by the previously described ion channels. In the contractile heart cell, the activated sodium channel results in a rapid influx of sodium ions with a change in resting membrane potential from -90 Mv to $+20$ Mv. This activates the slow calcium or L-type channel.[20] The influx of calcium ions activates the sarcoplasmic reticulum to release a large pool of calcium ions, increasing intracellular calcium concentration to 1 μM. This changes the conformation of calcium–troponin C, resulting in a shift of troponin I, troponin T, and tropomyosin to a location that allows cross-bridges to attach to specific sites on actin. The activated sarcoplasmic reticulum calcium–ATPase pump then pumps calcium from troponin C back into the sarcoplasmic reticulum, causing relaxation and diastole when intracellular calcium levels drop to 100 nM. The calcium ions are stored in the sarcoplasmic reticulum until the next event. The "trigger" calcium ions that had entered through the calcium channel are extruded by a calcium-calmodulin–sensitive sarcolemmal ATPase pump and the sodium-calcium exchange system. The prevention of further influx of calcium ion is attained by potassium channel–induced closing of the calcium channel during repolarization and diastole.

The voltage-sensitive ion channel calcium messenger system is under control of receptor and G protein mechanisms.[21] The β_1-adrenergic agonists and sympathetic adrenergic neurotransmitters activate adenylate cyclase to produce cAMP. CAMP-dependent kinase (protein kinase A) has two prominent functions. Protein kinase A phosphorylates the calcium channel in a more open position, increasing levels of triggering calcium ions during depolarization-induced calcium channel opening. This, in turn, increases velocity of contraction. CAMP also improves diastole and relaxation. Protein kinase A phosphorylates an 11-kDa protein called phospholamban, which, in turn, releases its inhibitory effects on the calcium ATPase pump. This results in more rapid uptake of cytosolic calcium into the sarcoplasmic reticulum. This salutary effect on relaxation is further orchestrated by protein kinase A–mediated phosphorylation of troponin I, which lowers the affinity of troponin C for calcium. Calcium calmodulin kinase and protein kinase C also phosphorylate phospholamban, emphasizing the importance of the kinase systems in controlling the calcium messenger system in cardiac tissue.

The acetylcholine-mediated parasympathetic system has negative modulatory effects on the calcium messenger system in the heart.[22-24] The potassium channel is coupled to the G_k protein.[25] Acetylcholine stimulates the G_k protein and opens the potassium channel. In the

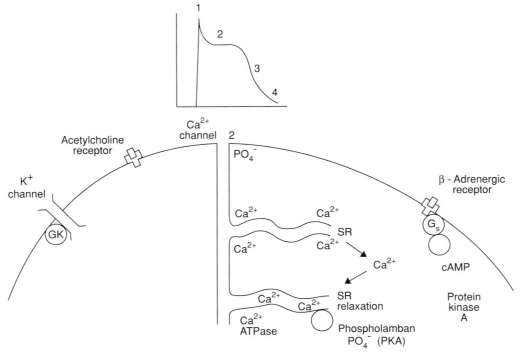

Figure 3–7. Proposed model for voltage and β_1-adrenegic receptor-mediated cardiac phasic contraction. Depolarization opens the voltage sensitive calcium channel and triggers release of calcium ions from sarcoplasmic reticulum, leading to contraction. Calcium ions are immediately extruded by the sarcolemmal ATPase pump, leading to diastole. The β-adrenergic receptor-mediated production of cAMP leads to phosphorylation of the calcium channel and the phospholamban protein. This leads to improved contraction and relaxation. The acetylcholine-mediated potassium channel negatively modulates this system.

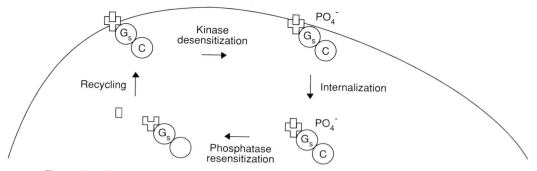

Figure 3–8. Proposed model for kinase-mediated desensitization of the β-adrenergic receptor.

presence of acetylcholine, repolarization may occur to a more hyperpolarized membrane potential. Opening of the calcium channel is dependent on the resting membrane potential. Under conditions in which the membrane is hyperpolarized by acetylcholine-mediated potassium channel activity, the calcium channel does not open to its usual degree during depolarization, nor is it as effectively maintained in an open position by β_1-agonist–induced phosphorylation. The result is decreased intracellular calcium during depolarization with decreased contractility. The parasympathetic–mediated potassium channels can also decrease heart rate through hyperpolarization of pacemaker cells.

The role of the phospholipase C second-messenger system in cardiac tissue is unknown at present, but it does not contribute as significantly to contraction in cardiac muscle as it does in vascular muscle. This observation underlines the evolutionary prowess of signal transduction in the cardiovascular system. Cardiac and vascular tissue develop from a common origin to a physiologically perfect balance. The adenylate cyclase–mediated system increases cardiac contractility and vasodilatation—the perfect combination for increased cardiac output. Similarly, the sympathetic and parasympathetic systems are well complemented. Vagal stimulation results in diminished heart rate, contractility, and vascular tone through potassium-mediated mechanisms. Sympathetic stimulation results in increased heart rate, contractility, and vascular tone, accomplished by using two different second-messenger systems to increase cytosolic calcium, adenylate cyclase in cardiac muscle, and phospholipase C in vascular muscle.

The role of the calcium messenger and kinase systems goes beyond mediation of short-term functional responses to long-term adaptation and alteration of the signal transduction mechanism itself. This is illustrated by examination of the response of the cell to long-term receptor stimulation. Cells that are exposed to continued agonists undergo receptor down-regulation. This may occur as "homologous" or "heterologous" desensitization. Homologous desensitization occurs, for example, when a cell loses responsiveness to a β_2-adrenergic agonist but can still respond to other agents that stimulate adenylate cyclase. In cell-free homogenates, this occurs within 1 to 3 minutes of exposure to catecholamines. Heterologous desensitization occurs when the cell shows declining responsiveness to all agents that

mediate their effect through adenylate cyclase. This occurs after the more rapid homologous desensitization step. Experiments show that desensitization occurs as a result of receptor internalization through endocytosis. Removal of the β_2-agonist results in the rapid appearance of receptors with adenylate cyclase–coupled activity. However, very prolonged exposure of cells to agonist may result in loss of receptors, requiring new protein synthesis for resensitization. Recent evidence suggests that this desensitization process may be mediated by a β-adrenergic receptor kinase that phosphorylates the adenylate cyclase–coupled receptor, priming it for internalization (Fig. 3–8). This has led to a model of desensitization that holds that the kinase system modulates long-term response to agonists. This suggestion has been further supported by the finding of glucocorticoid-responsive elements in the β_2-adrenergic receptor gene. This would provide a mechanism by which glucocorticoid-induced signal transduction could moderate synthesis of new β_2-receptors after prolonged desensitization.

SIGNAL TRANSDUCTION INTO THE NUCLEUS: THE THIRD MESSENGER

Receptor-mediated ion channels and second-messenger systems can transduce signals, and the calcium messenger and kinase systems can elicit cellular responses within seconds to minutes. However, experience suggests that signals also may affect long-term function and perhaps alter the phenotype of the cell and its signal transduction apparatus. Testing of this hypothesis requires the development of techniques in molecular biology to examine the role of the nucleus and the gene in signal transduction.

The nucleus is surrounded by a membrane and so, again, would require specialized mechanisms to transduce cytosolic signals into the nuclear "cytosol" or nuclear plasma. Once inside the nucleus, signals would ultimately interact directly or indirectly with nucleic acids. DNA is the genetic structure and code of the cell. The double helix structure of DNA has the ability to uncoil into two single-stranded substrates. Depending on the presence of enzymes (DNA polymerase or ribonucleic acid [RNA] polymerase), the single strand may be transcribed to synthesize a mirror image DNA or RNA single strand. RNA is the genetic message from the DNA genetic code. This strand of total RNA is arranged in sets of three bases, which are known as codons. This RNA molecule is spliced to yield messenger RNA (mRNA). The mRNA is transported by transfer RNA to ribosomal RNA in the cytoplasm in which each codon is translated into an amino acid, which is, in turn, assembled into new proteins. Since receptors, ion channels, kinases, and clathrin are proteins, it is logical that signal-induced alterations in DNA transcription, RNA translation, or protein synthesis might alter long-term cellular response. In addition, it is possible that synthesis of other proteins could allow signals to induce the cell to new functions.

The segment of DNA that is transcribed to synthesize RNA for the production of a specific protein is called the gene. Its expression is controlled by other segments of the DNA sequence, which may be in close *(cis)* or remote *(trans)* vicinity (Fig. 3–9). The promoter is the region of DNA in close proximity to the gene that can bind polymerase and begin transcription. These sequences can be activated by nucleoprotein binding and are also known as responsive elements. Gene expression can be described as inducible when outside signals activate these regulatory elements, or they can be tissue-specific when changes in cell cycle control transcription.[26] In either case, nucleoprotein interactions are theorized to be essential.

The discovery of the retrovirus and oncogenes allowed insight into the role of the nucleus in signal transduction.[27] *Oncogene* was the name given to the genes that were inserted into transformed cells after infection with various retroviruses. It was hypothesized that if the transfer of genes into cells could cause the cells to lose control of their growth, the protein products of these genes might be responsible for tumorigenesis. Interestingly, it was observed that oncogenes were also expressed in normal, uninfected, nontransformed cells as part of the normal growth process. In this case, these genes were called *proto-oncogenes*. It was then theorized that the oncogene protein products, or oncoproteins, were proteins with normal physiologic functions, which if overproduced could lead to overproliferation. Identification of the oncoproteins was consistent with this hypothesis. The *sis-PDGF* (platelet derived growth factor) and *int-1* oncoprotein products were found in secretory vesicles and were proposed to be a growth factor and ligand for the membrane receptor; *erb B-EGF* receptor and *Fms–CSF-1* receptor proteins were found in the plasma membrane and were proposed to be the

growth factor receptors with protein-tyrosine kinase activity; the *src* and *abl* proteins were found in the inner face of the cell membrane with protein-tyrosine kinase activity; and the *ras* protein was found to have intrinsic binding activity to the α-subunit of the G protein and hence was proposed to function in signal transduction, GTP binding, and hydrolysis. This was a dramatic demonstration that components of the signal transduction apparatus could affect cell function, at least in the arena of growth.

The identification of the oncoproteins *jun, fos,* and *myc* revealed (1) a nuclear location, (2) DNA binding, and (3) transcriptional regulation. These oncoproteins were the best candidates for examination of the role of the nucleus in signal transduction. It was soon discovered that a number of agonists that were not classically considered to mediate cell growth could activate expression of these oncogenes. This inducible gene expression was associated with agents, including catecholamines, that increased intracellular calcium and activated protein kinase C. It was further found that during oncogene induction, PDGF activated protein kinase C. Using phorbol ester, it was shown that activation of protein kinase C led to phosphorylation of the AP-1 binding site nucleoprotein complex. These observations suggested two important premises: first, that nuclear expression might be affected during signal transduction and second that this might occur as a result of the kinase system. This postulate was a remarkable parallel to known cytosolic events.

Investigation of the *fos* protein has now further established this concept. Activation of the *fos* gene in rat brain by an epileptogenic agonist causes expression of *fos* mRNA and synthesis of the *fos* protein.[29] Within 1 hour, this protein is transported back into the nucleus, where it binds to DNA.[30] In other experiments, the *fos* protein and the *jun* protein have both been shown to bind at the regulatory element AP-1 binding site. Although either protein alone may bind to this site, the formation of a heterodimeric complex of these proteins results in a 30-fold increase in the binding affinity of this nucleoprotein complex. This is accomplished through binding of leucine repeats in each protein in what has been recently referred to as the *leucine zipper* (Fig. 3–10).[23, 31, 32, 33, 53] Both proteins are expressed in response to a number of agonists, and the nucleoprotein complex may occur up to 8 hours after stimulation. It has been suggested that a cascade of such complexes could regulate overlapping patterns of gene expression of pheno-

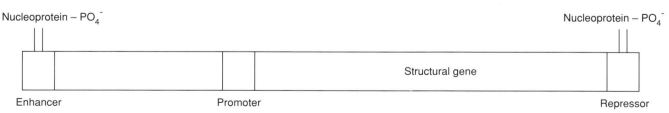

Figure 3–9. Induction of gene expression is thought to occur when nucleoproteins bind to specific DNA elements known as enhancers or repressors. This binding process directly affects promotor-mediated gene expression. Phosphorylation is proposed to activate nucleoprotein-DNA interactions during signal transduction–induced gene expression. The thyroid and steroid hormone receptors have been shown to bind to hormone-responsive elements (HRE) that induce gene expression.

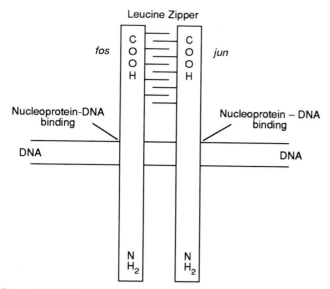

Figure 3–10. The leucine zipper hypothesis: The observation that the *fos* and *jun* proteins form a heterodimeric complex with DNA has led to this new model for nucleoprotein binding and transcriptional activation, which allows for a myriad of interactions and may be the basis for a "third messenger" in signal transduction.

type. These protein complexes may provide a "third messenger" in signal transduction.

Gene expression can also be induced directly by the signal transduction process without the "third messenger." This is the case with the steroid and thyroid receptors and their hormone ligands.[34] Each receptor undergoes a conformational change upon binding the hormone that enables DNA binding. These receptors attach to regulatory elements in the DNA sequence and transform normally hormone-unresponsive genes into hormone-responsive genes. These "hormone regulatory elements" are enhancers. Interestingly, it appears that this process of gene activation is normally repressed at the receptor level. Neither the steroid binding domain nor the DNA binding domain of the receptor is required for enhancement. Rather it seems that the hormone-binding region of the receptor prevents DNA binding and that the hormone or ligand association stops this inhibition. This mechanism of receptor-mediated gene expression remains to be identified in other systems.

SIGNAL TRANSDUCTION AND RIBONUCLEIC ACID

The role of signal transduction at the post-transcriptional level is less well studied. This would include the post-transcriptional production of cytoplasmic mRNA as well as the fate of this mRNA. This depends on its relative stability as well as on its translation. This has been elucidated in the life cycle of mRNA, which codes for ferritin and the transferrin receptor. The cell required evolution of a mechanism to control levels of iron because this element has a tendency to catalyze reactions that produce cytotoxic hydroxyl radicals. Iron is internalized by endocytosis of the bound transferrin

receptor. In the endosome, it is released from the receptor into the cytosol in which it may be used or sequestered into ferritin. The expression of the receptor and ferritin is regulated by the amount of available iron. When extracellular iron is high, the receptor numbers decrease and the amount of ferritin increases, whereas when iron levels are low, the receptor numbers increase and the ferritin level decreases. This appears to be regulated by a protein known as the iron-responsive element-binding protein. This protein binds to the *cis*-acting element in ferritin and transferrin receptor mRNA. When iron levels are low, the protein develops a high-affinity state, and when levels are high, it develops a low-affinity state. This is theorized to be controlled by reversible iron-mediated oxidation-reduction of one or more disulfides in the binding protein. In the iron-limited high-affinity state, the protein binds the iron-responsive element, causing no mRNA translation of ferritin mRNA and no mRNA degradation of transferrin receptor mRNA. In the iron-rich low-affinity state, the protein does not bind, allowing mRNA translation of ferritin mRNA and degradation of transferrin receptor mRNA.[35]

ACUTE AND CHRONIC EFFECTS OF SIGNAL TRANSDUCTION: THE LONG-TERM PHENOTYPIC RESPONSE OF THE CELL TO ITS ENVIRONMENT

The establishment of gene expression as an integral part of signal transduction suggests that agonists may alter cellular phenotype as well. Returning again to cardiovascular tissue as a model to illustrate this concept, the role of various agonists can be explained. Catecholamines and angiotensin II have been examined in their role in gene expression. Norepinephrine and angiotension both induce the phospholipase C–mediated second-messenger system and protein kinase C activity. Both agonists have been shown to activate *fos* mRNA expression in cardiovascular tissue. In addition, myosin gene expression has been similarly induced by α_1-agonist stimulation in cardiac cells. This suggests that the third-messenger hypothesis may apply to the cardiovascular system. In particular, it is well known that cardiac tissue responds with hypertrophy to the prolonged high renin and catecholamine state of pressure overload. This process would hold that the third-messenger *fos* protein complex might alter future gene expression. The increased production of myosin might be one such example.

Returning to the initial illustration of signal transduction in cardiac and vascular tissue, it would be proposed that long-term agonist stimulation results in chronic responses that include not only receptor down-regulation and alteration of the signal transduction system but also fundamental alterations in gene expression, which can affect basic cell function. Figure 3–11 illustrates this model of acute and long-term cellular response to signals from the external environment.

Stimulation of the G protein–coupled second-messenger systems and calcium ion channels leads to increased

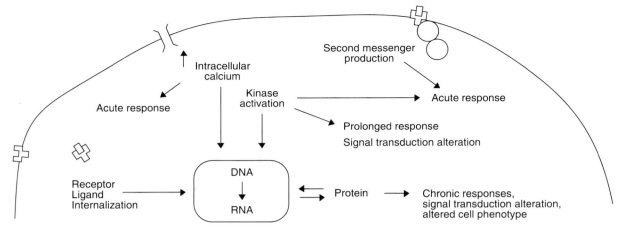

Figure 3–11. A proposed model of signal transduction in the cell by which acute, long-term, and chronic responses to stimuli may occur. Alterations in various steps in this scheme can be the basis of abnormal responses to therapy as well as disease itself.

intracellular calcium and kinase activation. This increase in intracellular calcium mediates an immediate acute cellular response in the cytosol and perhaps in the nucleus as well. The activation of kinases allows the acute response to continue at normal cytosolic levels of calcium and in addition shifts the cell into an altered signal transduction process with phosphorylation of receptors, ion channels, and enzyme systems. The kinases may also phosphorylate nucleoproteins that have been in association with DNA regulatory elements or newly associated nucleoprotein complexes to induce gene expression. In the case of the *fos* and *jun* genes, the newly synthesized proteins may migrate back into the nucleus to bind to other regulatory elements. This binding process might serve many hypothetical functions. For example, it may serve as a master "switch," transforming the cell to function with a chronic response, such as prolonged tonic contraction in vascular tissue, or it may effect other regulatory elements to new functions, such as myosin production and hypertrophy in cardiac tissue. Alternatively, it could perhaps induce gene expression of proteins that further alter the signal transduction process and start the process again, such as seen with induction of receptor genes to produce more receptors after prolonged agonist stimulation and receptor degradation.

PHYSIOLOGIC AND PHARMACOLOGIC PRINCIPLES OF CELLULAR COMMUNICATION AND SIGNAL TRANSDUCTION AT THE BEDSIDE

Five principles should be integrated when applying basic understanding of cellular communication and signal transduction to clinical care of the critically ill child: (1) Therapeutic agonists can mediate beneficial effects by acting on specific organs; however, each agent influences multiple tissues and organ systems; (2) pharmacotherapeutic agents may produce distinct responses when employed as acute or chronic therapies; (3) long-term drug therapy may alter cellular response in a manner that causes a fundamental change in organ function; (4) alterations in signal transduction may be the basis of cellular dysfunction and drug insensitivity in disease states; and (5) varied responses to drug therapy may be observed as components of signal transduction evolve during development.

Therapeutic agents are discussed, for the most part, in terms of their beneficial effects on specific organ function. However, it is clear that most agents affect many organs and tissues. As discussed, single receptors may have multiple ligands. For example, multiple agonists may stimulate a β_1-, β_2-, or α_1-adrenergic receptor. In addition, single ligands may have multiple receptors.[36] For example, two thyroid receptors have been isolated. This has been hypothesized to confer several potential advantages. These receptors could be expressed in a tissue-specific fashion, responding differently to thyroid metabolites, or perhaps even providing different enhancers that interact with distinct regulatory elements. The degree to which any one drug might affect various tissue types and organs could then be dependent on tissue distribution of receptor numbers or possibly even relative binding affinities. The significance of this principle to disease states is illustrated by the newly recognized "spill-over" receptor state. In this scenario, increased levels of an agonist may "spill over" and stimulate receptors that are not generally considered ligands at usual agonist concentrations. For example, patients with acromegaly and growth hormone excess have been noted to have galactorrhea despite normal prolactin levels. This occurs because the excess growth hormone interacts with the lactogenic receptor, a process that does not occur under physiologic conditions. In critical care medicine, the use of agonists to excessive quantities could have similar outcomes, recruiting receptors or tissue that is usually unaffected by the given agonist at lower doses.

These principles have been used in approaching several clinical problems. Digoxin binds with the α-subunit of the Na, K-ATPase pump and inhibits sodium efflux. This, in turn, activates the sodium-calcium exchange system to pump out three sodium ions for each incoming calcium ion. This increases intracellular calcium concentration and results in increased tension and a positive inotropic effect. Extrapolating that diaphragmatic muscle could also benefit from this process, investigators have shown that digoxin similarly improves contractility, suggesting that patients with diaphragmatic fatigue may benefit from this therapy.[37] The use of nitroglycerin as a potentially selective coronary, pulmonary, or systemic arterial vasodilator has recently been tried. At low doses, the continuous infusion of nitroglycerin has been used in adults to improve myocardial perfusion during angina. It has now been shown in children that intermediate doses can decrease pulmonary artery hypertension postoperatively in patients with congenital heart disease.[38] Further increase in infusion rate mediates systemic vasodilatation. This presumably occurs on the basis of relative differences in receptor numbers, affinities, or coupling in these tissues.

In addition to affecting multiple tissues, pharmacotherapeutic agents may also elicit different responses with short- or long-term use. Desensitization occurs within minutes of exposure of cells to agonists; however, clinically significant insensitivity rarely occurs in children before hours or days have elapsed. Investigators have recently examined this phenomenon in patients receiving nitroglycerin infusions. Since this particular agonist relies on the generation of nitrosothiol to activate guanylate cyclase, they reasoned that increased availability of sulfhydryl groups for this reaction might inhibit the desensitization process. Using N-acetylcysteine, investigators have now shown that sensitivity to nitrates can be restored after chronic nitroglycerin infusion.[39, 40] Other approaches to desensitization include the use of combinations of lower infusion concentrations or intermittent use of higher concentration infusions of a single inotrope or vasodilator (such as dobutamine or nitroprusside), or both. In patients in whom insensitivity is refractory, the thyroid and steroid hormone status should be ascertained, as both hormones may coordinate up-regulation of receptors and improve cellular responsiveness.

The phenomenon of down-regulation provides an explanation for the observation that there are no set agonist levels that can be expected to elicit a given effect as time goes on in the intensive care unit. For example, the mixed β- and α-adrenergic agonist dopamine is classically represented as a β-agonist in the range of 5 to 10 μ/kg/min and as an α-agonist at greater than 10 μg/kg/min. However, with receptor down-regulation, the concentration levels required to attain a given outcome variable could change. In addition, with significant desensitization, the use of full agonists, rather than partial agonists, may be required—for example, norepinephrine or epinephrine, rather than dopamine.

The role of the calcium messenger system in acute and long-term response also requires consideration. The use of calcium as an inotropic or vasoactive drug has recently been limited to the scenario in which hypocalcemia or hyperkalemia exists. This is because overwhelming of the cell's calcium extrusion and buffering mechanisms leads to cytotoxicity. Inotropes and vasopressors may be used, as they allow the cell's protective mechanisms to function. However, excessive, prolonged concentrations of these agents have been hypothesized

to have a deleterious effect on the calcium status of the cell. Indirect evidence for this school of thought is based on the remarkable failure of inotropes and the success of β-blockers and calcium channel blockers in improving outcome in patients with the cardiomyopathies of congestive heart disease. This has led to the conventional wisdom that adequate but minimal levels of agents that increase intracellular calcium, including inotropic and vasoactive infusions, should be used to attain an effective outcome.

Long-term treatment with pharmacotherapeutic agents can change cell function and alter the patient's responses. Psychotherapeutic agents have demonstrated this in the clinical setting, frequently requiring several weeks to mediate beneficial outcome. Patients may arrive in the intensive care unit receiving chronic drug therapy, or, as chronic critical care residents, they may require long-term infusion and drug therapy. It is hypothesized that such alterations involve induction of gene expression. At present, the only indirect evidence for this process occurring as a result of critical care medicine is in a case report of ventricular hypertrophy with prolonged vasoactive infusion. This could be potentially induced by activation of *jun, fos,* and myosin genes.

More commonly, alterations in signal transduction and patient responsiveness in the intensive care unit occur as the result of disease.

It is becoming increasingly apparent that the pathophysiologic consequences of disease processes are frequently the result of alterations in signal transduction; cystic fibrosis is now being examined as a possible defect in chlorine channel phosphorylation,[41, 42] and pseudohypoparathyroidism is being investigated as a genetically determined deficiency in the α-subunit of protein G_s. Genetically determined types of diabetes mellitus have been characterized as having changes in G proteins, as well as specific receptors (one that affects mRNA expression and another that affects binding by interfering with receptor insertion into the plasma membrane)[7, 55]; and the genetically determined hypertrophic cardiomyopathies that include idiopathic hypertrophic subaortic stenosis have been shown to have an increased density of voltage-sensitive ion channels in the heart.[43] Alterations in receptors and G proteins have similarly been documented in a host of acquired disease states, including sepsis, congestive heart failure, hypo- and hyperthyroidism, and in steroid treatment.[40, 44, 45, 54] Returning to cardiovascular tissue as our model to illustrate the effect of disease on signal transduction and the influence of this understanding on therapy, we examine three disease states: ischemic heart disease, vascular failure in sepsis, and cardiac dysfunction in congestive heart failure.

Focal ischemic heart disease is quite rare, but global ischemia secondary to cardiopulmonary bypass is a daily phenomenon in pediatric intensive care. Global ischemia results in decreased ATP stores in cardiac tissue. As previously mentioned, the calcium extrusion mechanisms are more ATP-dependent than is the calcium influx mechanism in cardiac cells. This results in altered signal transduction as intracellular calcium stores increase. Physiologically, this is recognized as an altered relaxation state during diastole. Left atrial pressure readings reveal high filling pressure for a given left ventricular end-diastolic volume, and cardiac output commonly requires support to maintain perfusion and optimal outcome. Given the choice between inotropy or vasodilators, the use of guanylate cyclase agonists, such as nitroglycerin and nitroprusside, has several theoretic advantages. Since cGMP enhances calcium extrusion from cardiac cells, these agents might decrease intracellular calcium concentration, improve diastolic function and cardiac performance, and reverse the cycle of calcium toxicity. In addition, as vasodilators, these agents may mediate coronary artery relaxation, improving coronary artery perfusion, and decrease aortic impedance, reducing afterload and myocardial oxygen requirements. It would appear that cGMP-mediated agonists could be beneficial in the presence or absence of inotropic support when coming off the cardiopulmonary bypass pump.

The use of calcium infusion had once been a popular therapy for these children. Its beneficial effect was seen in terms of inotropy, blood pressure, and restoration of rhythm. However, its physiology may have been based on the use of cardioplegic solution, which left the heart in a potassium-toxic state. According to the American Heart Association Advanced Pediatric Life Support (APLS) guidelines, the only remaining indications for calcium infusion are in hyperkalemia and hypocalcemia. Ischemic cardiac tissue is actually rendered more arrhythmogenic by calcium when hyperkalemia is not present. Again in the ischemic state, because of increased intracellular calcium and diminished sodium potassium ATPase function, resting membrane potential is less negative. Atrial or ventricular cells that show no physiologic spontaneous automaticity can, when partially depolarized, develop automaticity and become ectopic foci. Since intracellular calcium concentration increases the amplitude and upstroke velocity of automatic cells, the use of calcium infusion may exacerbate the automaticity of these ischemic cells, leading to increased arrhythmogenicity.

Vascular failure remains a leading cause of death in children with sepsis and septic shock. This is associated with a profound insensitivity of the systemic vasculature to α-adrenergic agonists. This phenomenon has been studied in an animal model of insensitivity to α_1-adrenergic agonists in which the aorta is similarly insensitive in vitro. This vessel showed a significant reduction in α_1-adrenergic receptor numbers, norepinephrine-induced phosphoinositide hydrolysis, calcium flux, and protein phosphorylation.[46] Since no vasoactive agents were infused in this animal model, it appears that this generalized down-regulation of signal transduction could occur as a result of a high endogenous catecholamine state or because of an unidentified pathologic mediator or mediators of sepsis. At present, conventional thought prefers the latter mechanism because in the high-catecholamine state of acute congestive heart failure without sepsis there is no vascular unresponsiveness to adrenergic stimulation. This vascular unresponsiveness has been shown in vitro in the isolated organ bath, suggesting that the alterations in the signal transduction system are intrinsic and not reversible simply by removing the

mediator. Recognizing that a significant decrease in the signal transduction apparatus of α_1-agonist–mediated vasoconstriction exists, the clinician may form a clinical approach. The use of volume may be more beneficial in maintaining perfusion pressure than the use of adrenergic agents. However, vasopressors are still required if systemic vascular resistance becomes too low. It is not known whether or not the use of the α-adrenergic agonists contribute to further down-regulation. At present no clinical studies have attempted to up-regulate this second-messenger system.

Congestive heart failure can present in its acute or chronic stage in children in the pediatric intensive care unit. This disease nicely illustrates the numerous concepts discussed in this chapter.[47, 56] Acute heart failure results in baroreflex-mediated activation of the sympathetic nervous and renin-angiotensin systems.[48] Interactions of catecholamine and angiotensin with their receptor-mediated signal transduction systems result in salt and water retention, vasoconstriction, and increased heart rate and contractility. These mechanisms maintain cardiac output and blood pressure. Any excessive increase in arterial or atrial pressure leads to baroreflex-mediated inhibition of the sympathetic nervous system and release of the ANF. This guanylate cyclase–activating hormone opposes the vasoactive effect of circulating norepinephrine and opposes further adrenergic-mediated activation of the renin-angiotensin system.

In some children, such as those with uncorrected complex congenital heart disease or severe bronchopulmonary dysplasia, heart failure persists into a chronic stage. Continued overactivation of the sympathetic and renin-angiotensin second-messenger systems may result in modification of the signal transduction mechanisms and the cardiomyopathy of overload. The first stage is marked by loss of sensitivity of the atrial and arterial baroceptors, with resultant overactivation of β_1-adrenergic receptors and vasoconstrictor activity and progressive loss of vasodilator response. This is accompanied by a progressive down-regulation of β_1-receptors, as well as a reduction in the G_s:G_i ratio. Despite these alterations, abnormalities in intracellular calcium are also purported to exist because of excessive adrenergic stimulation. In addition, within an hour of acute pressure overload, c-fos and c-myc are transiently induced, with ensuing expression of fetal isoforms of several contractile proteins, including actin and tropomyosin. Induction of gene expression is associated with further alterations in the phenotype of the cardiac cell.

With continued overload, the ventricle becomes dilated and then begins to hypertrophy. This may unload the cells by adding new sarcomeres, decreasing the rate of mechanical energy expenditure/cell. However, this compensatory mechanism becomes deleterious over time, as it is not accompanied by an increase in mitochondrion or capillary numbers. This increase in the ratio of myofibrils:ATP eventually leads to greater imbalance between energy demand and supply. This may further exacerbate abnormal calcium metabolism.

Changes in the molecular structure of the proteins synthesized during the hypertrophic response may further affect cardiac function. Increased expression of V3 myosin heavy chains (low myosin ATPase activity) leads to reduced shortening velocity and a negative inotropic effect but improved mechanical efficiency in rat ventricles. Humans synthesize only the slow myosin isoforms in ventricular tissues, but a similar change in left atrial tissue has been shown. In addition, new myosin and actin isoforms are synthesized as overload continues. Abnormalities in proteins involved in calcium metabolism have also been reported. Relaxation is diminished in vitro in papillary muscle from cardiac transplant recipients with dilated and hypertrophic cardiomyopathy. Although this could be secondary to chronic ATP imbalance, animal models suggest a reduced concentration of calcium ATPase molecules in the sarcoplasmic reticulum and reduced calcium sensitivity of the sodium-calcium exchanger. In addition, altered isoforms of ion channels may result in delayed inactivation of L-type calcium channels as well as attenuation of the potassium channels, resulting in prolongation of the action potential. This could further contribute to abnormal diastolic function, as well as potential arrhythmogenicity. The end stage of cardiomyopathy of overload is dominated by fibrosis of the heart. Initial synthesis of collagen, perhaps to minimize dilatation and relieve wall stress, eventually leads to replacement of cardiac cells with fibrosis, which is once again an acute response with long-term deleterious effects.

In formulating a therapeutic approach to congestive heart failure without knowledge of alterations in signal transduction, investigators first used β_1-agonists, as well as phosphodiesterase inhibitors, to attempt to increase cAMP levels. This therapeutic approach was based on the concept that cardiomyopathy, as a disease of cardiac output, should improve if this parameter were increased. Surprisingly, this strategy did not decrease mortality and may have had arrhythmogenic consequences.[46] With more detailed understanding of signal transduction, investigators hypothesized that down-regulation of β-adrenergic receptors and cAMP levels was in some way protective of the myocardium. This produced a novel approach to cardiomyopathy. Targeting baroreceptor insensitivity as the major pathologic consequence of the disease process, the hallmarks of therapy became digoxin and the angiotensin-converting enzyme inhibitors. Digitalis may improve function by activating the atrial and arterial baroreceptors, whereas the converting enzyme inhibitors decrease the inhibiting effects of angiotensin II on sensitivity. In addition, adult patients with chronic heart failure have been further treated with β-blockers to diminish long-term effects of sympathetic stimulation.[49, 57] These strategies have resulted in increased numbers of adrenergic receptors and G_s protein in tissues from patients with congestive heart failure. More importantly, outcome has improved in this disease.

Developmental influences of signal transduction must always be considered when using pharmacotherapeutic agents in treating disease in infants and children. Developmental effects have been illustrated in fetal rats in which angiotensin II receptors appear in novel tissues (including skeletal muscle and connective tissues), then decrease by 80% 1 day after birth, and disappear during adulthood.[49, 50] Studies have also shown that G protein levels and function may be regulated during development.[51, 52] The clinical consequence of the influence of development on the response of cells to signals is no more dramatically illustrated than in the dire consequence discovered when using calcium channel blockers in children less than 1 year of age. The initial use of verapamil as a treatment of supraventricular tachycardia in infants resulted in reports of asystole, thereby proving a contraindication for the drug in children less than 1 year of age. A similar increased sensitivity of children to intravenous β-blockers has led to the recommendation that digoxin be used as the initial drug of choice for supraventricular tachycardia without congestive heart failure. Propranolol can be used, if necessary, with judicious clinical acumen and isoproterenol at the bedside. These findings emphasize the necessity for careful examination of adult therapies when contemplating their use in the pediatric intensive care setting.

One explanation for these observations is the known lack of complete sympathetic innervation in ventricular tissue during the first 6 months of life in canine and feline tissue. With a relative predominance of parasympathetic and potassium channel activity, the blocking of calcium channels could have significant consequences. This knowledge has importance in the use of inotropic agents as well. For example, the use of dopamine before the age of 6 months may not be as effective in increasing cardiac output as the use of the direct-acting catecholamine epinephrine. This can be explained on the basis of dopamine's mechanism of action. Dopamine causes the release of norepinephrine from secretory vesicles. If sympathetic innervation is not developed, this effect would be lacking. This has led to the recommendation that direct-acting agents be used in children younger than 6 months of age who are not responding to dopamine. In this case, understanding of signal transduction and its developmental influences allows improved therapy.

CONCLUSION

Understanding the cellular and molecular basis of physiology and pharmacology and the application of the principles of intracellular communication and signal transduction allow a sophisticated therapeutic approach to the critically ill child. No child responds to therapeutic agents in the same manner over time, and each patient may differ in the response to therapeutic agents according to age and disease state. The benefits of therapeutic strategies depend on the contribution of these factors in the critically ill child.

References

1. Silverman M: Molecular biology of the Na + -D glucose transporter. Hosp Pract 2:188, 1986.
2. Stahl P and Schwartz AL: Receptor mediated endocytosis. J Clin Invest 77:657, 1986.
3. Goldstein JL, Brown MS, Anderson RGW, et al: Receptor endocytosis. Ann Rev Cell Biol 1:1, 1985.

4. Brodsky FM: Living with clathrin: Its role in intracellular membrane traffic. Science 246:1390, 1988.
5. Dophin AC: Nucleotide binding proteins in signal transduction and disease. Trends in Neurosciences 10:53, 1987.
6. Mayorga LJ, Diaz R, and Stahl PD: Regulatory role of GTP binding protein in endocytosis. 244:1475, 1989.
7. Levitski A: From epinephrine to cyclic AMP. Science 241:800, 1989.
8. Catteral WA: Structure and function of voltage sensitive ion channels. Science 242:50, 1988.
9. Miller RJ: Calcium channels and neuronal function. Science 230:186, 1987.
10. Benos DJ: The biology of amiloride sensitive sodium channels. Hosp Pract April 15, 1989, pp. 149–164.
11. Schwartz A: Calcium antagonists: Review and perspective on mechanism of action. Am J Cardiol 64:31, 1989.
12. Rasmussen H and Parrott PR: Calcium messenger system: An integrated view. Physiol Rev 65:938, 1984.
13. Scharfman HE and Schwartzkoin PA: Protection of dentate hilar cells from prolonged stimulation by intracellular calcium chelation. Science 245:217, 1989.
14. Berridge MJ: Inositol trisphosphate and diacylglycerol as second messengers. Biochem J 220:345, 1985.
15. Michell RH: Inositol phopholipid break down as a step in adrenergic stimulus response coupling. Clin Sci 68(10):435, 1985.
16. Majerus PW, Connolly TM, Dechmyn H, et al: Metabolism of phosphoinositide derived second messenger molecules. Science 274:1519, 1986.
17. Vanhoutte PM: Modulation of vascular smooth muscle contraction by the endothelium. Ann Rev Physiol 48:307, 1980.
18. Stander NB, Quagh JM, and Davis NM: Hyperpolarizing vasodilators activate ATP-sensitive K+ channels in arterial smooth muscle. Science 245:177, 1989.
19. Bridge JHB, Spitzer KW, and Ershler PR: Relaxation of isolated ventricular cardiomyocytes by a voltage dependent process. Science 240:823, 1988.
20. Nabauer M, Callevaert G, Cleeman L, et al: Regulation of calcium release is gated by calcium current. Science 244:808, 1989.
21. Yatani A and Brown AM: Rapid B-adrenergic modulation of cardiac calcium channel current by a fast G-protein pathway. Science 245:71, 1989.
22. Cerbai E, Klockner U, and Isutey G: The α subunit of the GTP binding protein activates muscarinic potassium channel of the atrium. Science 240:1787, 1988.
23. Difranceso D, Ducouset R, and Robinson R: Muscarinic modulation of cardiac rate at low acetylcholine concentration. Science 244:763, 1989.
24. Otera AS, Britweisser GE, and Stabo G: Activation of muscarinic potassium current by ATP in atrial cells. Science 242:443, 1989.
25. Yatani A, Codina J, Brown A, et al: Direct activation of mammalian atrial muscarinic potassium channels by GTP regulatory protein GK. Science 235:207, 1987.
26. Maniatis T, Goodbourn S, and Fischer JA: Regulation of induceable and tissue specific gene expression. Science 236:1238, 1987.
27. Bishop JM: The molecular genetics of cancer. Science 235:305, 1987.
28. Nishizuka Y: The role of protein kinase C in cell surface signal transduction and tumor production. Nature 308:693, 1984.
29. Morgan JI, Cohen DR, Hempstead JC, et al: Mapping of c-fos expression in the central nervous system after seizure. Science 257:192, 1987.
30. Sagar SM, Sharp FR, and Curran T: Expression of a c-fos protein in brain: Metabolic mapping at the cellular level. Science 240:1328, 1988.
31. O'Shea EK, Rutkowski R, Stafford WF, et al: Preferential heterodimeric formation by isolated leucine zippers from fos and jun. Science 245:646, 1989.
32. Turner R and Tjian R: Leucine repeats and an adjacent DNA binding domain mediate the formation of functional c-fos c-jun heterodimers. Science 243:1689, 1989.
33. Vinson CR, Sigler P, and McKnight SL: Scissor grip model for DNA recognition by a family of leucine zipper proteins. Science 245:911, 1989.
34. Evans RM: The steroid and thyroid hormone receptor superfamily. Science 241:839, 1988.
35. Klausner RO and Harfand JB: Cis trans models for post-transcriptional gene regulation. Science 246:370, 1989.
36. Hart CE, Forstron JW, and Kelly JD: Two classes of PDGF receptor recognize different isoforms of PDGF. Science 24:1520, 1988.
37. Aubier M, Murciano D, Viires N, et al: Effects of digoxin on diaphragmatic strength. Am Rev Respir Dis 135:544, 1987.
38. Ilbawi MN, Idriss FS, and DeLeon SY: Hemodynamic effects of intravenous nitroglycerin in pediatric patients after heart surgery. Circulation 72:101, 1985.
39. May DC, Popna JJ, and Black WH: In vivo induction and reversal of nitroglycerin tolerance in coronary arteries. N Engl J Med 317(13):805, 1987.
40. Packer M, Lee WH, and Kessler PD: Prevention and reversal of nitrate tolerance in patients with congestive heart failure. N Engl J Med 317:799, 1987.
41. Dubinsky WP: The physiology of epithelial chloride channels. Hosp Pract 1:69, 1989.
42. Landschultz WH, Johnson PF, and McKnight JL: The leucine zipper: A hypothetical structure common to a new class of DNA binding proteins. Science 421:1763, 1988.
43. Braunwald E: Hypertrophic cardiomyopathy—continued progress. N Engl J Med 320:12 and 301, 1989.
44. Lefkowitz RJ and Caron MG: Adrenergic receptors: Molecular mechanisms of clinically relevant regulation. Clin Res 33(3):395, 1985.
45. Lefkowitz RJ, Caron MG, and Stiles GL: Clinical mechanisms of receptor regulation. N Engl J Med 310(24):1570, 1984.
46. Roth BL, Suba EA, Carcillo JA, et al: Alterations in hepatic and aortic phospholipase C coupled receptors and signal transduction in rat intraperitoneal sepsis. In: Roth BL, Nielson TB, and McKee AE (eds): Molecular and Cellular Mechanisms of Septic Shock. New York, Alan R Liss, 1989, p 41.
47. Cohn JN: Inotropic therapy for heart failure. Paradise postponed. N Engl J Med 320(11):729, 1989.
48. Packer M: Neurohormonal interactions and adaptation in congestive heart failure. Circulation 77(4):721, 1988.
49. Dzau VJ: Circulatory versus local renin angiotensin system in cardiovascular homeostasis. Circulation 77(Suppl I): I-9, 1988.
50. Millan MA, Carvallo P, and Izumi S: Novel sites of expression of functional angiotensin II receptors in the late gestation fetus. 242:1340, 1989.
51. Steinberg SF, Drugge E, Bilezikiar JP, et al: Developmental alterations in atrial myocyte nucleotide binding proteins. Science 230:1130, 1985.
52. Stromgen JC: Developmental biology of T cell receptors. Science 247:943, 1989.
53. Gentz R, Rausche FJ, Abate C, et al: Parallel association of fos and jun leucine zipper juxtaposes DNA binding domains. Science 243:1695, 1989.
54. Insel PA and Rausia LA: G-protein and cardiovascular disease. Circulation 78:1511, 1988.
55. Kahn CR and Goldobesh BS: Molecular defects in insulin action. Science 245:13, 1989.
56. Katz AM: Cardiomyopathy of overload. N Engl J Med 322(2):100, 1990.
57. Packer M: Combined beta-adrenergic and calcium entry blockade in angina pectoris. N Engl J Med 320(11):709, 1989.

Pathophysiology of the Immune System

Mary Beth Fasano, M.D., John McCloskey, M.D., and Jerry A. Winkelstein, M.D.

The immune system is composed of a wide variety of cells and their secretory products, which share the important functions of recognizing foreign antigens and reacting against them. When the individual components of the immune system function normally and are successfully integrated, they play a critical role in the host's defense against infection and the generation of a normal inflammatory response. In contrast, when the immune system fails to recognize foreign antigens, when it fails to discriminate between "self" and foreign antigens, or when it initiates an abnormal or uncontrolled inflammatory response, a variety of pathologic conditions can result.

This chapter will review the normal physiology of the immune system, discuss the ways in which abnormalities in immune function can contribute to the immunopathogenesis of a variety of clinically significant disorders, and give specific examples of the immunopathologic disorders that are likely to be encountered in the intensive care unit.

COMPONENTS OF THE NORMAL IMMUNE SYSTEM

B Lymphocytes

The development of B lymphocytes occurs largely in the bone marrow and is a two-stage process (Fig. 4–1). In the first stage, a wide variety of different clones are generated by a series of immunoglobulin gene rearrangements that are independent of antigenic stimulation. Once the immunoglobulin heavy chain genes have become rearranged, cytoplasmic immunoglobulin is produced, and the cells have reached the pre-B cell stage. Further differentiation involves the rearrangement of immunoglobulin light chain genes and is associated with the expression of IgM and IgD on the cell surface. Each such B cell has specificity for a single antigen. The second stage of B cell differentiation is initiated when an antigen binds to the specific antibody expressed on the surface of a B lymphocyte, and the B cell proliferates to form a clone of progeny cells, each possessing an identical antibody specificity. These cells then differentiate into plasma cells, which secrete either IgM, IgG, IgA, or IgE. Most antigens are T-dependent—that is, optimal B-cell differentiation into plasma cells requires the presence of T helper lymphocytes. However, there are a few antigens, such as bacterial capsular polysaccharides, that are T-independent—that is, they are able to trigger terminal B cell differentiation without an absolute requirement for T lymphocytes. In either case, T helper (T_H) (CD4+) and T suppressor (T_s) (CD8+) lymphocytes are important modulators of B cell function, influencing the magnitude, the duration, and the quality (affinity and class distribution) of the antibody response.

There are five classes of immunoglobulins: IgG, IgM, IgA, IgE, and IgD. Each class possesses features in common with the others; in spite of their similarities, however, each class has some unique structural and functional characteristics. There are minor differences in the amino acid sequence of the heavy chain, differences in the number and location of disulfide bonds, and differences in the amount of carbohydrate. Immunoglobulins function in host defense through a variety of mechanisms, including opsonization of foreign microorganisms, activation of serum complement, neutralization of toxins, neutralization of viruses, and inhibition of microbial attachment to mucosal surfaces. IgM is the first immunoglobulin produced in an immune response and is an efficient activator of complement. IgG is the predominant serum immunoglobulin; it is actively transported across the placenta, possesses opsonic activity, and activates complement. IgA is the major immunoglobulin secreted onto mucosal surfaces; it has as its major roles the prevention of microbial adherence to mucosal surfaces and the clearance and disposal of antigens. IgE is a mediator of allergic disease.

T Lymphocytes

T lymphocytes not only are effectors of cell-mediated immunity but also modulate the functions of B lympho-

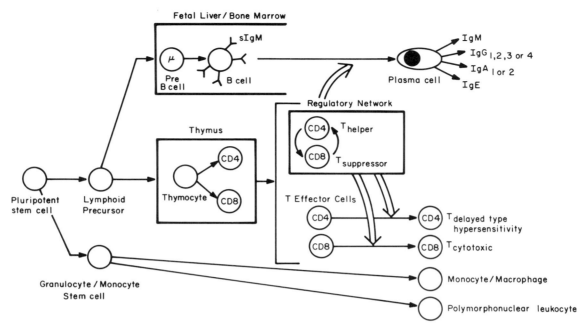

Figure 4–1. The cells of the immune system.

cytes, T lymphocytes, and nonlymphoid cells such as monocytes (see Fig. 4–1). Differentiation of T lymphocytes occurs within the thymus. In a manner analogous to that occurring in the B lymphocyte lineage, T lymphocyte clones with a wide variety of antigenic specificities are generated without the presence of antigen by rearrangements of T cell antigen receptor genes and the subsequent expression of the T cell receptor on the cell surface. The diverse effector and regulatory functions of T lymphocytes are carried out by distinct lymphocyte subpopulations. A second differentiation process, operating in addition to the process that generates antigenic specificity, causes individual T lymphocytes to mature along functionally distinct pathways. These T lymphocyte subpopulations have characteristic patterns of cell surface membrane proteins, which presumably are related to functional activities. For example, the subset of T lymphocytes that positively modulates immune responses (helper T lymphocytes, T_H) bear the cell surface protein CD4. A related but distinct T lymphocyte subpopulation, which also bears CD4, is responsible for delayed-type hypersensitivity responses (T_{DTH}). A subset of T lymphocytes bearing the cell surface protein CD8 has the ability to negatively modulate immune responses (suppressor T lymphocytes, T_S). Another subset, also bearing CD8, has the ability to function as cytotoxic effectors in cell-mediated immunity (cytotoxic T lymphocytes, T_C).

T lymphocyte regulatory functions are carried out mainly by the release of soluble protein mediators, lymphokines. A rapidly increasing number of lymphokines has been identified in recent years. Although all of their functions have not yet been fully elucidated, it is known that some lymphokines stimulate B and T lymphocyte proliferation and differentiation (e.g., interleukin [IL]-1, IL-2), some lead to the activation of monocytes (e.g., IL-1, IL-6), and still others stimulate

proliferation of precursors for a variety of hematopoietic cells (e.g., IL-1, IL-4, IL-6). Other lymphokines preferentially lead to the activation of specific classes of immunoglobulin-secreting cells (e.g., IgA or IgE producers IL-4, IL-5). The repertoire of lymphokines secreted by T_H cells differs from the repertoire secreted by T_S cells, accounting in part for their functional differences.

Cytotoxic effector T lymphocytes (T_C) can kill target cells such as virus-infected host cells, tumor cells, or the cells of a histoincompatible tissue graft. T_C cells reversibly bind to their targets by means of the T cell antigen receptor as well as several other cell surface molecules. Once a T_C-target conjugate is formed, the T_C cell reorganizes its cytoplasm to concentrate cytoplasmic granules for attack at the point of contact. Lytic molecules are released onto the surface of the target cell, leading to lysis of the target.

Phagocytic Cells

Phagocytic cells possess the ability to ingest foreign antigens such as microorganisms. Although many phagocytic cells are mobile and can move from the blood stream through tissues to a site of inflammation or microbial invasion, other phagocytic cells are fixed in the sinusoids of the blood stream and the lymphatic system in which they clear microorganisms and other particulate matter from the circulation. Neutrophils arise in the bone marrow, circulate in the blood stream, and migrate into tissues, in which they are the first line of defense against local infections. Monocytes also arise from stem cells in the bone marrow, circulate in the blood stream, and migrate to the tissues in which they undergo morphologic and functional maturation to become macrophages. Monocytes-macrophages not only participate as effector cells in host defense and inflammation but also present antigen to lymphoid cells and thus play an important role in the generation of a normal immune response.

In order to function properly, phagocytes must attach to a substrate (adherence), move through tissues toward the site of microbial invasion (chemotaxis), attach to opsonized microbes and ingest them, and finally kill the microbes (intracellular killing).

Adherence to a substrate is a necessary prerequisite for phagocytic cells to move. For example, phagocytes circulating in the blood stream must adhere to vascular endothelium before they can egress from the blood stream. Similarly, once in the tissues, phagocytic cells adhere to tissue substrates as they crawl toward the site of microbial invasion or inflammation. The adherence of phagocytic cells is mediated by a family of cell surface glycoproteins including CR3 (a receptor for the major cleavage fragment of the third component of complement, iC3b), LFA-1, and p150,95. This adherence is enhanced by a number of soluble mediators, including C5a, thromboxane A_2, and leukotrienes.

The directed movement of phagocytic cells toward a chemical stimulus is termed *chemotaxis*. A variety of substances act as chemoattractants. One of the more important stimuli is C5a. In addition, bacteria can release their own chemotactic peptides. Finally, a variety of prostaglandins, monocyte-derived factors (monokines), and lymphokines possess chemotactic activity. Together, these chemotactic stimuli cause phagocytic cells to migrate to and accumulate at sites of infection or tissue injury.

Once phagocytic cells reach the site of microbial invasion, they ingest microbes that have been opsonized with either IgG or C3b. Receptors for these opsonins exist on phagocytic cells, allowing them to serve as ligands to bind the microbe to the phagocytic cell. Ingestion occurs by a process in which the phagocytic cell membrane circumferentially surrounds the opsonized particle, leading to its internalization in a phagocytic vacuole.

The process of intracellular killing begins soon after the phagosome has been internalized. Both primary (azurophilic) and secondary (specific) granules can fuse with the phagosome. A number of antimicrobial substances are thereby introduced into the phagosome. These substances include lysozyme, lactoferrin, acid hydrolases, and cationic proteins. Perhaps the most important, however, is the myeloperoxidase-H_2O_2-halide system. Upon ingestion of microorganisms, molecular oxygen is reduced to superoxide. The superoxide, in turn, undergoes further reactions, leading to the generation of reduced oxygen derivatives such as hydrogen peroxide and hydroxyl radicals. The net effect of these toxic derivatives of reduced molecular oxygen is to kill the microorganisms within the phagocytic vacuole.

The Complement System

The majority of the biologically significant effects of the complement system are mediated by the third component (C3) and the terminal components (C5 to C9) (Fig. 4–2). However, in order to subserve their biologic functions, C3 and C5 to C9 must first be activated via either the classical or the alternative pathway.

In the classical pathway, antigen-antibody complexes composed of either IgG or IgM activate the first component of complement (C1). C1 is a trimolecular complex composed of C1q, C1r, and C1s. It is the C1q that binds to the Fc portion of the immunoglobulin molecule and as a consequence activates C1r, which, in turn, activates the C1s. Activated C1s then cleaves C4 and C2, and the larger cleavage products of each combine to form the classical pathway C3-cleaving enzyme, C4b, 2a. In contrast to the classical pathway, activation of the alternative pathway can occur without the presence of specific antibody. Apparently, fluid phase C3 binds factor B, allowing its cleavage by factor D. The larger cleavage product, Bb, can then associate with C3 to form a low-grade, C3-cleaving enzyme, C3,Bb. This enzyme is responsible for the continuous generation of small amounts of nascent C3b, which possesses a reactive thiol ester that allows it to covalently bind to molecules on the surface of suitable cells. Bound C3b then forms a complex with native factor B, which, in turn, is cleaved by factor D to create a new and highly efficient particle-bound C3-cleaving enzyme, C3b,Bb. Properdin acts to stabilize this C3b,Bb complex.

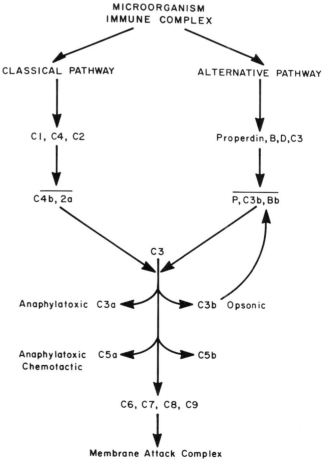

Figure 4–2. The complement system.

Whether C3 is activated via the classical or the alternative pathway, two fragments of unequal size are produced, C3a and C3b. The activation of C3 represents an amplification step, since hundreds of C3 molecules can be cleaved by a single C3-convertase. C3a is released into the fluid phase in which it can act as an anaphylatoxin. Most of the C3b is also released into the fluid phase in which it is rapidly inactivated by hydrolysis. Some C3b, however, binds covalently to the surface of the activating cells or to the immune complex, thereby acting as an opsonin or combining with either of the two C3-cleaving enzymes to create C5-cleaving enzymes.

Activation of C5 creates a small cleavage product, C5a, and a large cleavage product, C5b. C5a is released into the fluid phase in which, like C3a, it can act as an anaphylatoxin. In addition, C5a possesses potent chemotactic activity. Nascent C5b can combine with native C6 to initiate the formation of the membrane attack complex, a multimolecular assembly of C5b, C6, C7, C8, and C9. This complex inserts into cell membranes and is responsible for the cytolytic and bacteriolytic-bactericidal actions of complement.

If the activation of C3 and C5 to C9 were to proceed in an uncontrolled fashion, it could result in the generation of excessive amounts of the phlogistic fragments of complement and immunopathologic damage to the host. However, a number of mechanisms control the assembly and expression of the C3- and C5-convertases. For example, the enzymatic actions of C1r and C1s are inhibited by a control protein, C1 esterase inhibitor. Thus in the usual situation, the assembly and expression of the C3 cleaving enzymes proceed in a controlled fashion and are limited to the immediate vicinity of the initiating substance.

INTEGRATION OF THE IMMUNE RESPONSE

Dozens of cells and hundreds of molecules constitute the normal immune system. Successfully integrated and functioning together, B lymphocytes, T lymphocytes, phagocytic cells, and the complement system collectively play a critical role in the generation of a normal immune response. Although it is beyond the scope of this chapter to review all aspects of an integrated immune response, there are selected aspects that deserve emphasis. For example, individual components of one functional compartment rarely function in isolation from the others. T cells positively and negatively influence the production of antibody by B cells. The products of B cells, antibodies, are efficient activators of the complement system. The products of complement activation (specifically C3 cleavage products) can, in turn, modulate B cell function. Similarly, one of the consequences of complement activation is to deposit opsonically active C3b on bacterial surfaces, but the opsonic potential of C3b cannot be fulfilled if phagocytic cells bearing receptors for C3b on their surface are not present. Finally, the ability to generate a normal humoral immune response depends on macrophages to process and present antigen in an appropriate immunogenic form to B cells and T cells.

Thus the induction and expression of a normal immune response depend on cooperation among a variety of individual components. Conversely, abnormal function of one component may have consequences for the others.

Another important feature of the immune response that deserves emphasis is that many of its functions can be served by more than one component. For example, both IgG and C3b can act as opsonins. Similarly, though C5a is a potent chemotactic factor, a variety of other soluble mediators, such as certain lymphokines, prostaglandins, and bacterial peptides, also possess chemotactic activity. Conversely, a single component or cell of the immune system may subserve a number of related but distinct functions. For example, cells of the monocyte-macrophage series not only function in the efferent arm of the immune response by ingesting and killing microorganisms but also function in the afferent arm by ingesting and processing antigen for presentation to lymphocytes. Similarly, antibody molecules have a number of different roles to play in a normal immune response, since the same molecule not only can act directly as an opsonin but also can activate the complement system and initiate its diverse activities.

Finally, the immune system is also characterized by complex systems of regulation. Some networks, such as T helper and T suppressor cells, act to limit the duration and magnitude of the antibody response. Similarly, there are inhibitors of complement activation, such as C1 esterase inhibitor, that limit the degree to which immune complexes and C1 can activate the rest of the complement cascade. Thus the immune system is carefully modulated in order to prevent uncontrolled expression of its defensive and inflammatory functions.

PATHOPHYSIOLOGIC MECHANISMS OF IMMUNODEFICIENCY

In recent years there has been a growing appreciation that immunodeficiency plays an important role in a wide variety of clinically significant disorders. The number of primary immunodeficiency diseases has grown, and many are more common than previously thought. In addition, a secondary immunodeficiency—acquired immunodeficiency syndrome—has begun to reach epidemic proportions. Finally, it has become clear that significant immunodeficiency also accompanies a variety of other conditions, such as malignancies. Since details regarding the individual immunodeficiency diseases are covered elsewhere (see Chapter 73), this chapter will address some of the pathophysiologic mechanisms by which immunodeficiency arises.

Primary Immunodeficiency Diseases

There are more than 50 different primary immunodeficiency diseases that affect every functional compartment of the immune system. Although the majority are genetically determined and inherited as mendelian traits, some clearly are not. Although originally identified in infants and young children, it is clear that some primary immunodeficiency diseases may not become clinically apparent until adolescence or adult life. Similarly, although the first primary immunodeficiency diseases to be identified had the most severe clinical expression, many others are associated with less severe clinical signs and symptoms.

Those primary immunodeficiency diseases that are genetically determined are best viewed as inborn errors of metabolism not unlike any other. In some instances, the defect results in the accumulation of a metabolite in immunologically active cells and interferes significantly with their function. For example, one form of severe combined immunodeficiency disease is caused by an autosomal recessive deficiency of adenosine deaminase, an enzyme important in the purine salvage pathway. The enzyme defect results in the accumulation of purine metabolites, such as deoxyadenosine, which are toxic for lymphocytes. In other instances, the metabolic defect results in the failure to produce a protein necessary for normal immune function. For example, most of the complement deficiency diseases are characterized by a marked decrease in the serum levels of the individual component (<1%) secondary to a pretranslational defect in synthesis. In still other instances, the defect results in the arrested development of the immunologically active cell. For example, in X-linked agammaglobulinemia, the defect appears to interfere with the normal development of B cells. Although pre-B cells are present in the bone marrow of these patients, B cells and plasma cells are lacking in the blood and tissues.

Immunodeficiency Secondary to Viral Infections

A number of viral infections cause some degree of immunosuppression. However, the degree of immunosuppression, the type of immunosuppression, and the frequency with which immunosuppression occurs vary, depending on the type of virus and the developmental age or genetic background of the host, or both.

Most viral infections are self-limited, and if there is immunosuppression it, too, is of brief duration. For example, the clinical manifestations of measles virus infection commonly last for only a few days to 1 week, and measles virus can be cultured from peripheral blood mononuclear cells for only a short time after the onset of the rash. The immunologic changes that occur after measles virus infection are characterized by depressed delayed–type hypersensitivity skin reactions in vivo and decreased mitogen-induced proliferative responses of lymphocytes in vitro. Even though these changes in immune function can persist for several weeks after the acute infection has terminated, they too are ultimately self-limited.

In contrast to the transient nature of the immunosuppression seen in some viral infections, there are some viruses that cause a sustained and significant immunodeficiency. Perhaps the best example is seen in human immunodeficiency virus infection. This retrovirus infects CD4-positive T lymphocytes; in fact, the receptor on the T lymphocyte for the virus is the CD4 molecule. In the majority of individuals, the initial infection is either asymptomatic or self-limited and resembles a "flu-like" illness followed by a variable period of latency. Reactivation of the virus some months or years later is characterized by a variety of immunologic abnormalities, including delayed-type hypersensitivity skin test anergy, decreased in vitro proliferative responses of T cells to mitogens and antigens, and decreased numbers of CD4-positive lymphocytes. The accompanying immunodeficiency is sustained and progressive and ultimately results in a marked increased susceptibility to other bacterial, viral, and fungal infections.

In some instances, a virus causes a secondary immunodeficiency only at a critical point in development. Before an effective vaccine was developed, rubella infection in the first trimester of pregnancy often resulted in infection of the fetus and disrupted organogenesis. The so-called rubella syndrome was usually characterized by microcephaly, mental retardation, congenital cataracts, and congenital heart disease. In addition, in some children the consequences of intrauterine rubella infection included a dysgammaglobulinemia (decreased IgG and IgA increased IgM) that was sustained for the life of the child, a consequence of rubella infection that is not seen when infection occurs postnatally.

In other instances, the viral infection causes a significant and sustained immunodeficiency only in a subset of genetically susceptible hosts. For example, in most individuals, Epstein-Barr virus infection is not accompanied by a significant secondary immunodeficiency. However, in individuals who have the X-linked lymphoproliferative syndrome, Epstein-Barr viral infection may result in a variety of serious immunopathologic consequences, which include acquired agammaglobulinemia, as well as aplastic pancytopenia, neutropenia, and B cell lymphomas. The immunopathologic consequences vary from one patient to another even within the same kindred. In the case of acquired hypogammaglobulinemia, the immunodeficiency is long-lasting and is usually accompanied by an increased susceptibility to infection.

Immunodeficiency Secondary to Drugs

Patients with immunosuppression secondary to pharmacotherapy are encountered frequently in the intensive care unit. For a number of these individuals, immunosuppression is a major part of their therapy, whereas other patients experience immunosuppression as a deleterious side effect.

Cytotoxic Drugs

As the use of antineoplastic drugs evolved, it became evident that a majority of these agents caused immunosuppression. This effect upon the immune system led to the use of these drugs for conditions (e.g., transplant rejection, autoimmune disease) in which immunsuppression is an integral part of therapy. These drugs can be classified into several groups: steroids, alkylating agents, antimetabolites, and purine antagonists.

Corticosteroids affect the immune system by several mechanisms. Their primary effect involves altering the transcription of messenger ribonucleic acid (mRNA). Steroids enter cells and bind to intracytoplasmic receptors. These complexes subsequently penetrate the nuclei, bind to deoxyribonucleic acid (DNA), and modify the transcription of mRNA. In macrophages and monocytes, this leads to an inhibition of IL-1 formation and an attenuation in the immune response, since IL-1 stimulates the production of lymphokines. Steroids also produce an anti-inflammatory effect by inducing lipocortin, which is an inhibitor of phospholipase A_2, the enzyme necessary for the production of arachidonic acid. The final mechanism by which steroids inhibit the immune system is by direct lysis of a small subpopulation of activated lymphocytes.

Cyclophosphamide, an alkylating agent, transfers an alkyl group to DNA, which causes breakage and cross-linking of the DNA during cell division. This leads to an arrest in cell replication of rapidly dividing cells such as those in the immune system.

Methotrexate, an antimetabolite, is a competitive inhibitor of dihydrofolate reductase. Inhibition of this enzyme leads to impaired synthesis of tetrahydrofolate, which is necessary for the production of thymidine. The decrease in thymidine production leads to impaired DNA synthesis and eventually impaired cell replication.

Azathioprine, a purine antagonist, exerts its primary effect on the immune system by inhibiting the de novo and salvage pathways of purine synthesis. The decrease in purine production inhibits the synthesis of DNA and RNA. Azathioprine may also cause a delayed cytotoxicity by the incorporation of its metabolite, 6-thioguanine, into DNA. Like cyclophosphamide, this incorporation causes increased DNA breakage and cross-linking during cell replication. Finally, azathioprine appears to block antigen recognition by alkylating thiol groups on T cell surface membranes. Although azathioprine affects lymphocytes in general, it appears to have more of an effect on T cells than on B cells.

All of these drugs have proved to be effective immunosuppressive agents. However, their effects on the immune system are nonspecific; they not only affect T and B lymphocyte replication but also affect other leukocytes, red blood cells, platelets, and mucosal epithelium.

Cyclosporine

Since the late 1970s, cyclosporine has been an integral part of therapy for conditions requiring immunosuppression. Unlike the cytotoxic drugs, cyclosporine has specific effects on the immune system. Its primary role involves the inhibition of IL-2 synthesis by helper T cells. This inhibition in IL-2 production impairs the activation and replication of helper and cytotoxic T cells. However, it does not have an effect on suppressor T cells. Although its primary effects are on T cells, cyclosporine does affect B cells to a small degree and also inhibits the production of IL-1 by macrophages.

Antilymphocyte Globulin

Unlike the previously mentioned immunosuppressive agents, antilymphocyte globulin (ALG) is not a drug but is an antiserum directed against lymphocytes. When administered to a patient, ALG causes a rapid depletion of circulatory T lymphocytes while sparing B and natural killer cells.

Orthoclone OKT3

Like ALG, OKT3 is an antibody directed against lymphocytes. Unlike ALG, it is a monoclonal antibody directed against the T3 (CD3) complex on the surface of mature post-thymic T lymphocytes. The actions of OKT3 are mediated by its attachment to the subunits of the T3 complex, which blocks recognition of class I and class II major histocompatibility antigens. Once it is attached to the T3 complex, it has three effects: It causes rapid clearance of T cells by the reticuloendothelial system; it may cause removal of the T3 complex from the T cell membrane without causing depletion of the cell from the circulation; and it may inhibit functioning of sessile T cells located within an allograft.

Other Drugs

There are a wide variety of other drugs administered in the intensive care unit that can cause immunosuppression on the basis of bone marrow suppression. To name all of them is beyond the scope of this chapter; however, a few general classes of drugs that can cause bone marrow suppression include antibiotics (e.g., chloramphenicol and sulfa drugs) and antiseizure medications (e.g., valproic acid and carbamazepine). Fortunately, these side effects do not occur very often, and in many cases they are reversible. There are also some drugs that have somewhat more selective effects on the immune system. For example, phenytoin causes a decrease in serum IgA, and there is some evidence that diazepam inhibits phagocytosis and killing by polymorphonuclear leukocytes and monocytes.

PATHOPHYSIOLOGIC MECHANISMS OF HYPERSENSITIVITY

Normally, the immune response works to the host's advantage. In some instances, however, the host's immune response may actually result in destructive changes to tissues. The term *hypersensitivity* is often used to describe a normal immune response that occurs in an exaggerated or inappropriate form, causing tissue damage and other inflammatory reactions. Most of these hypersensitivity reactions or immunologic diseases can be classified by the type of effector mechanism primarily responsible for the destructive changes. The most widely used classification system is that described by Gell and Coombs in 1963.[1] They described four types of hypersensitivity (Fig. 4–3). Although still a useful classification, these reactions often overlap and it has become increasingly apparent that some hypersensitivity diseases often involve multiple components of the immune system whether directed against self or foreign antigens. Each of these types of hypersensitivity, individually or in concert, results in the pathogenesis of clinically im-

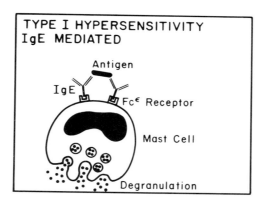

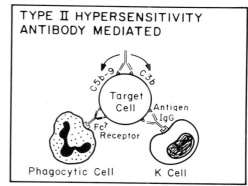

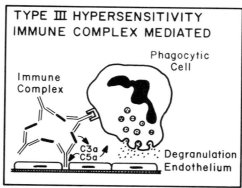

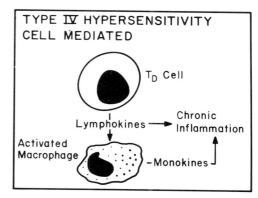

Figure 4–3. Hypersensitivity reactions.

portant immunopathologic disorders that may be encountered in the intensive care setting (Table 4–1). These disorders may range from the relatively benign picture of allergic rhinitis to serious conditions such as asthma, systemic anaphylaxis, hemolytic disease of the newborn, graft versus host disease, or systemic lupus erythematosus.

Type I Immediate Hypersensitivity

Type I hypersensitivity, or immediate hypersensitivity, occurs when specific IgE bound to mast cells becomes cross-linked via antigen, resulting in mast cell degranulation and the release of preformed and newly synthesized inflammatory mediators. Upon initial exposure to an allergen (e.g., pollen), B lymphocytes are stimulated to produce IgE. This process requires T helper cells and is regulated by T suppressor cells. Specific IgE is produced primarily at the site of allergen entry (usually mucosal surfaces) and then "sensitizes" local mast cells by binding to receptors on the cell surface specific for the Fc portion of the IgE heavy chain (Fc^E receptors) (Fig. 4–3). In addition to local sensitization, IgE also circulates and binds to Fc^E receptors on basophils and tissue-fixed mast cells throughout the body. The mast cell represents a very heterogeneous population of cells that, along with basophils, express high-affinity Fc^E receptors and are the main effectors of IgE-mediated reactions. Upon re-exposure to specific antigen, the mast cells and basophils coated with specific IgE are triggered to release the biologically active mediators that are responsible for the clinical expression of type I hypersensitivity reactions. In addition to IgE-mediated triggering, mast cell degranulation can also be brought about by a variety of other physical and chemical stimuli, such as hyperosmolarity, the anaphylatoxins C3a and C5a, and drugs such as synthetic adrenocorticotropic hormone, codeine, and morphine. Whether triggered by IgE or by other nonspecific mechanisms, mast cell degranulation is a complex energy-dependent

Table 4–1. CLINICAL EXAMPLES OF HYPERSENSITIVITY REACTIONS

Type of Hypersensitivity	Clinical Disorders Encountered in Intensive Care Unit
Type I: IgE-mediated	Asthma Drug reactions Food reactions Insect sting reactions
Type II: Antibody-mediated	Transfusion reactions Hemolytic disease of the newborn Hyperacute graft rejection Myasthenia gravis Graves' disease Autoimmune anemia and thrombocytopenia
Type III: Immune complex-mediated	Systemic lupus erythematosus Membranoproliferative glomerulonephritis Serum sickness
Type IV: Cell-mediated	Graft versus host disease Graft rejection Sarcoidosis Tuberculous granulomas

process, requiring calcium influx, increases in cyclic adenosine monophosphate, activation of methyltransferases, and hydrolysis of phosphatidylinositides.

There are three sources of mediators generated by mast cell degranulation: preformed (primary) molecules that act immediately after release, newly synthesized (secondary) mediators, and constituents of the granule matrix that act for a prolonged period after degranulation (late phase allergic reactions).

Primary mediators are contained within mast cell granules and include substances such as histamine, eosinophil chemotactic factor of anaphylaxis, and neutrophil chemotactic factors. Histamine exerts a wide range of biologic activities mediated primarily via interaction with two specific cell surface receptors termed H_1 and H_2 receptors. Histamine, acting through its H_1 receptor, leads to contraction of airway and gastrointestinal smooth muscle as well as increased vascular permeability and vasodilatation. The histamine present in human skin mast cells, acting through its H_1 receptor, is responsible for the wheal and flare reaction seen with allergy skin testing. The H_1 receptors are blocked by the classic antihistamines such as diphenhydramine. Histamine, through H_2 receptors, also has the capacity to promote gastric acid secretion from parietal cells and increase mucus production. In addition, H_2 receptors are involved with enhancing C3b (CR1) receptor expression on human eosinophils, enhancing neutrophil and eosinophil chemokinesis and augmenting T suppressor cell activity. The H_2 receptors are blocked by cimetidine. A number of chemotactic factors are also released from human mast cells (e.g., eosinophil chemotactic factor of anaphylaxis and neutrophil chemotactic factor) and result in the accumulation of a variety of cells at the site of mast cell activation. These factors are of particular interest, as they help elicit a second phase of inflammation, beginning hours after the initial antigen challenge, that is mediated by the influx of neutrophils and eosinophils. This second wave of inflammation, or late phase response, contributes to the pathogenesis of chronic allergic conditions such as asthma, eczema, and urticaria.

The secondary or newly synthesized mediators are molecules derived from arachidonic acid and formed after mast cell triggering. Arachidonic acid may be metabolized by two pathways. The cyclooxygenase pathway yields the primary prostaglandins (PGD_2, PGE_2, and $PGF_{2\alpha}$), prostacyclin (PGI_2), and thromboxane A_2. PGD_2, the most abundant of these mediators, causes increased vasodilatation and vasopermeability in addition to bronchoconstriction at a potency ten times that of histamine. The other cyclooxygenase products also exert their primary effects on the microvasculature and bronchial smooth muscle. Arachidonic acid may also be metabolized by lipoxygenase enzymes generating eicosanoids, including the leukotrienes (LTs). Leukotrienes that are generated by the 5'-lipoxygenase pathway play an especially important role in hypersensitivity reactions. Originally referred to as slow-reacting substance of anaphylaxis, the leukotrienes LTC_4, LTD_4, and LTE_4 are capable of constricting airways and altering vascular permeability. Another lipoxygenase product, LTB_4, is chemotactic and chemokinetic for neutrophils and eosinophils and enhances the expression of C3b receptors on these cells.

The third type of mediator released by mast cell degranulation is the granule-matrix–associated molecules, which include heparin, chymotrypsin, trypsin, and inflammatory factors of anaphylaxis. They are unique in that they remain in macromolecular association after release from the mast cell and exert a more delayed effect as they are slowly released from the matrix. It has been postulated that these molecules play a role in the pathogenesis of the late phase reaction. Allergic late phase reactions are IgE-dependent responses that are delayed in time. Occurring anywhere from 3 to 8 hours after allergen exposure, they are manifested histologically by an initial infiltration of eosinophils, basophils, and neutrophils, followed hours later by the influx of lymphocytes and monocytes-macrophages. Clinically this may be manifested by airway hyperreactivity and chronic inflammation in the asthmatic individual and by nasal congestion hours after allergen exposure in individuals with allergic rhinitis.

Immediate-type hypersensitivity can present clinically as a local phenomenon in diseases such as allergic rhinitis and asthma or systemically as anaphylaxis following an insect sting, drug ingestion, or food ingestion. The pathologic changes seen in these conditions can be attributed to the mediators released from mast cells and basophils. Treatment of these diseases is therefore directed at either inhibiting mast cell degranulation or blocking the effects of the various mediators once degranulation has occurred.

Type II Hypersensitivity

Type II hypersensitivity, or antibody-mediated hypersensitivity, is characterized by antibody directed against antigens present on the surface of cells or other tissue components (see Fig. 4–3). Tissue damage then results when the antibody interacts with molecules of the complement system (complement-dependent reactions) or with a variety of effector cells. Immunopathologic states can also result when antibody reacts with an antigen that performs a vital function or that serves as a surface receptor and thus blocks or neutralizes these biologically active molecules.

Antibodies responsible for type II hypersensitivity are usually of the IgG or IgM class. The antigens they recognize can include blood group antigens on the red blood cell surface (transfusion reactions, hemolytic disease of the newborn, autoimmune hemolytic anemia), drug or drug metabolites absorbed to cell membranes (drug-induced hemolytic anemia or thrombocytopenia purpura), blood group or class I major histocompatibility complex (MHC) antigens on tissue grafts (hyperacute graft rejection), glomerular basement membrane glycoprotein (Goodpasture's syndrome), or receptors on cell surfaces (myasthenia gravis, Graves' disease).

In some type II hypersensitivity reactions, antibody combined with the cell surface antigen activates the classical pathway of complement, resulting in the activation of C3 and C5 to C9 and the generation of their phlogistic activities. If C3b is deposited on the host cell's surface, the cell is opsonized, making it susceptible to phagocytosis by macrophages and neutrophils. Chemotactic stimuli provided by C5a result in the attraction of macrophages and neutrophils to the area. The tissue damage that ensues results from the inability of neutrophils to effectively ingest large targets; granular and lysosomal contents are nevertheless released, causing damage to neighboring tissue. Finally, in some instances the generation of the membrane attack complex (C5b to C9) can cause cell damage or lysis.

Another form of antibody-mediated cell injury does not specifically involve complement activation but instead is mediated by effector cells that have in common the presence of an Fc receptor for IgG. In addition to macrophages and neutrophils, a distinct population of lymphocytes called natural killer cells can mediate cell damage. These lymphocytes are morphologically defined as large granular lymphocytes. This cell can also demonstrate spontaneous cytotoxicity against certain target cells without the need for antibody. Following Fc receptor–mediated binding of effector cells to target cells, lytic attack occurs. Reactive oxygen intermediates (e.g., H_2O_2) appear to play a major role in this step. This process, often referred to as antibody-dependent cellular cytotoxicity, can be enhanced by C3 fragments (C3bi, C3d), γ-interferon, and tumor necrosis factor (TNF).

A number of clinically relevant immunopathologic reactions are mediated by type II hypersensitivity. For example, antibodies to ABO blood system antigens are usually of the IgM class and cause agglutination, complement activation, and intravascular hemolysis (i.e., transfusion reactions). In the case of hemolytic disease of the newborn resulting from rhesus (Rh) incompatibility, maternal anti-Rh IgG antibodies formed during a previous pregnancy cross the placenta and lead to red blood cell destruction in the fetus. Although cell-mediated immunity is the major effector in graft rejection, antibodies can also be involved, as is seen most frequently in grafts that are connected directly to the host's blood supply, such as kidney grafts. Hyperacute renal graft rejection can occur via type II hypersensitivity mechanisms when the transplant recipient has preformed antibodies directed against the graft, usually those to A1 or B blood group substances or to transplantation antigens.

Finally, antibody-mediated reactions against cells can cause disease even when cytotoxicity is not involved. An example of this is myasthenia gravis, a disease associated with IgG antibodies directed against acetylcholine (ACh) receptors at the neuromuscular junction. The antibodies against ACh receptors not only block available receptors but also seem to accelerate receptor degradation. The ability of ACh to depolarize muscle is therefore diminished, and patients experience extreme muscle weakness. Cell-receptor modulation by antibody can also be seen in patients with Graves' disease. An antibody, termed *long-acting thyroid stimulator,* binds to thyrotropin receptors and, rather than diminish function of the affected cell, stimulates thyroid hormone secretion.

Type III Hypersensitivity

Type III hypersensitivity, or immune complex–mediated hypersensitivity, results from the formation of immune complexes that are not cleared effectively from the circulation and become deposited in host tissues (see Fig. 4–3). This ultimately results in local tissue damage or systemic inflammatory responses, or both.

Immune complex formation is the consequence of a normal host response and occurs whenever an antibody and antigen combine. These complexes, however, are usually removed from the body by wandering or fixed phagocytic cells of the reticuloendothelial system. Under normal conditions, immune complexes can be processed or cleared by a variety of related mechanisms. First, immune complexes composed of IgG or that have C3b fixed to them can be ingested by phagocytic cells as would any other opsonized "particle." In addition, circulating immune complexes bearing C3b can fix to erythrocytes through CR1 receptors on the erythrocyte surface. The immune complexes are then carried by the erythrocyte to organs of the reticuloendothelial system (RES), such as the liver, in which the immune complexes are picked off the erythrocytes and the erythrocytes are returned to the circulation. Finally, activation of C3 and the fixation of C3b to immune complexes help prevent their precipitation and maintain them in solution.

The manner and efficiency in which immune complexes are processed depend on a number of variables. They may include the quantity of immune complexes being produced, their size, the ratio of antigen to antibody, the type of antigen, the class of antibody, and its affinity. Under normal conditions, immune complexes are efficiently cleared or processed, or both, by cells of the RES. Under a variety of circumstances, however, immune complexes may not be handled properly and may contribute to the pathogenesis of disease. In some situations, such as a chronic infectious disease (e.g., subacute bacterial endocarditis or hepatitis), the production of immune complexes may outstrip the ability of the RES to handle them. In other circumstances, such as in some autoimmune diseases (e.g., systemic lupus erythematosus [SLE]) the continued production of an autoantibody to self-antigens leads to the continued production of complexes and ultimately their deposition in tissues. Finally, in still other instances, circulating antibody combines with foreign antigens deposited in specific tissues to produce local immune complexes and organ-specific disease (e.g., farmer's lung).

The deposition or persistence, or both, of immune complexes in tissues is followed by an inflammatory reaction, which, in turn, is largely responsible for the clinical signs of immune-complex disease. Immune complexes are potent activators of the classical complement pathway, leading to the generation of anaphylatoxic, chemotactic, and opsonic activities. As a consequence of complement activation, the presence of immune complexes in tissues leads to increased vascular permeability, the accumulation of extravascular fluid, and an ingress of phagocytic cells. As a result, the accumulation of immune complexes in tissues such as the kidney, lung, or joints may result in an inflammatory reaction that is detrimental to the host.

Immune complex–mediated inflammation has been implicated in the pathogenesis of a wide variety of infectious diseases and rheumatic disorders. Some of the more common manifestations include the nephritis seen in chronic hepatitis or subacute bacterial endocarditis; the arthritis seen in SLE, rheumatoid arthritis, and cryoglobulinemia; and the vasculitis that accompanies SLE and polyarteritis.

Type IV Hypersensitivity

Type IV hypersensitivity, or delayed-type hypersensitivity, is mediated by sensitized T lymphocytes and macrophages (i.e., cell-mediated hypersensitivity) and does not specifically involve antibody (see Fig. 4–3).

Traditionally there have been four types of experimentally induced delayed hypersensitivity reactions, which were initially classified based on the type of skin reaction that occurs and the time interval involved after antigen exposure. However, it is likely that they are not completely distinct reactions and that many clinically significant type IV hypersensitivity reactions possess elements of more than one type, including the following: (1) Cutaneous basophil hypersensitivity or Jones-Mote hypersensitivity is manifested by skin edema that is maximal at 24 hours after antigen challenge. Histologically this is characterized by a basophilic infiltrate under the epidermis. (2) Contact hypersensitivity, which is a predominantly epidermal reaction occurring at a cutaneous site of contact with allergen (e.g., nickel, poison ivy, poison oak), is usually maximal at 48 hours. Histologically, there is an initial mononuclear cell infiltration of the epidermis, accompanied by edema and microvesicle formation. (3) Tuberculin reactions occur at the site of intradermal antigen injection and peak at 48 to 72 hours. This reaction is characterized by a dermal infiltration of lymphocytes and monocytes. (4) Granulomatous reactions occur as a result of the presence of persistent antigen in macrophages. Granulomatous lesions are characterized by a core of epithelioid cells and macrophages and occasionally multinucleate giant cells surrounded by a cuff of lymphocytes and fibrosis. Granulomatous delayed-type hypersensitivity is manifested in a number of chronic diseases, including tuberculosis, leprosy, leishmaniasis, and schistosomiasis. These diseases are all characterized by infectious agents that present a chronic antigenic stimulus to the host.

During initial contact with an antigen, memory T cells become sensitized and remain in the circulation for an extended period. Upon rechallenge with antigen, these T cells are stimulated to divide and produce a series of lymphokines, including IL-1, TNFα, interferon (IFN) γ, macrophage chemotactic factor, and migration inhibiting factor. These lymphokines exert a variety of inflammatory effects, including the recruitment of macrophages to a local site, their activation, and their maintenance at the site. Activated macrophages are responsible for the ongoing inflammation and tissue injury that then ensues. Although the initial stimulus for lymphokine production is immunologically specific, the ensuing inflammatory and cytoxic response is not.

Another form of cell-mediated immunity that results in tissue destruction involves cytotoxic T lymphocytes, which directly lyse antigen-bearing cells. This type of damage is entirely antigen-specific and involves direct interaction between antigen receptors on the T cell surface and membrane-associated antigens on the target cell. These may be foreign human leukocyte antigens or antigens associated with tumors or viruses. Cytotoxic T cells are able to elicit their tissue destruction without antibody and complement; however, the susceptible target cell must display both antigen and self-major histocompatibility complex products, and the cells must come into direct contact. Cytotoxic T cells are usually small lymphocytes within the CD8 + subpopulation and lack Fc receptors for IgG. Examples of this type of reaction resulting in an immunopathologic disease include graft versus host disease, allograft rejection, and the destruction seen with lymphocyte choriomeningitis virus. It is also felt that the tissue destruction associated with many autoimmune diseases, such as rheumatoid arthritis, may occur via this mechanism.

References

General References

Cooper MD: B-lymphocytes: Normal development and function. N Engl J Med 317:1452, 1987.

Frank MM: The complement system in host defense and inflammation. Rev Infect Dis 1:483, 1979.

Ghan GL, Gruber SA, Skjei KL, et al: Principles of immunosuppression. Crit Care Clin 4:841, 1990.

Gilbert-Barness EF and Barness LA: Pathology of transplant rejection and immunosuppressive therapy: Part II—pathologic effects of immunosuppressive therapy. Adv Pediatr 37:329, 1990.

Gleichmann E, Kimber I, and Purchase IFH: Immunotoxicology: Suppressive and stimulatory effects of drugs and environmental chemicals on the immune system. Arch Toxicol 63:257, 1989.

Griffin DE: Immunologic abnormalities accompanying acute and chronic virus infections. Rev Inf Dis, in press.

Kaliner M: Asthma and mast cell activation. J Allergy Clin Immunol 83:510, 1989.

Malech HL and Gallin JI: Neutrophils in human diseases. N Engl J Med 317:687, 1987.

Nossal GJV: The basic components of the immune system. N Engl J Med 316:1320, 1987.

Royer HD and Reinherz EL: T-lymphocytes: Ontogeny, function, and relevance to clinical disorders. N Engl J Med 317:1136, 1987.

Schifferli JA and Taylor RP: Physiological and pathological aspects of circulating immune complexes. Kid Internat 35:993, 1989.

Serafin WE and Austen KJ: Mediators of immediate hypersensitivity reactions. N Engl J Med 317:30, 1987.

II Resuscitation

Basic Mechanisms of Resuscitation

J. Michael Dean, M.D.

"Let one the mouth, and either nostril close,
While through the other the bellows gently blows.
Thus the pure air with steady force convey,
To put the flaccid lungs again in play.
Should bellows not be found, or found too late,
Let some kind soul with willing mouth inflate;
Then downward, though but lightly, press the chest,
And let th' inflated air be upward prest "[1]

HISTORY

Cardiopulmonary resuscitation (CPR) has been the subject of intense study for many years, with attempts at patient revival described many centuries ago. Galen attempted respiratory support with a bellows device in the 2nd century, and Vesalius pursued ventilatory support in the 16th century.[2] In the 18th century, the Society for the Recovery of Persons Apparently Drowned was formed, changing its name in 1775 to the Royal Humane Society for the Apparently Dead. This organization described various methods of resuscitation and sought to promote attempts at patient revival following sudden death. Initial attempts centered around provision of electrical shock to a dead patient. In 1797 their report concluded "The success of the Royal Humane Society has corrected popular prejudice and proved that persons, provided that no fatal laceration ensued, may be restored to life."[3] At the same time, it became a recommendation that the lungs be inflated during these electrical attempts at resuscitation. Attempts at artificial respiration included endotracheal tubes and tracheostomy devices even in the 18th century. Proceedings of the Royal Humane Society eventually included recommendations that sternal compressions be used to help deflate the lungs. Thus, we see a progression from electrical therapy to provision of ventilation, and perhaps accidentally to provision of circulatory support with sternal compressions. The fact that these efforts were often successful is suggested by numerous historical writings, including claims that nearly a thousand patients were saved in a 20-year period by the societies based in Amsterdam and London.[4]

In the 19th century, open chest cardiac massage was used for patient revival, with intermittent success. In the early 20th century, defibrillation was developed, though success in humans was not reported until 1947. Finally, closed chest cardiac massage was reintroduced into clinical practice, having been virtually lacking for more than a century. In 1960, Kouwenhoven, Jude, and colleagues published their classic papers describing the combination of closed chest cardiac massage, artificial respiration, and electrical defibrillation in adult humans.[5, 6] The history is reviewed in more detail by DeBard[7] and Kouwenhoven and Langworthy.[8]

Although efforts by scholars such as Galen and Vesalius generally failed, the modern intensive care unit uses CPR on a regular basis with a fair degree of technical success. Specific details concerning resuscitation of newborns, infants, and children will be presented in the chapters that follow. The purpose of this chapter is to provide the reader with a cohesive scientific model of the basic underlying mechanisms by which blood flow and organ perfusion are generated during CPR. Although research in this area remains unfinished, a picture has emerged that should permit the reader to understand why a specific mechanical maneuver might be beneficial or why a specific drug strategy should be used during CPR, as well as answer a host of other questions about this complex subject. Although the technical details and written guidelines will change in the future, it is hoped that this model will continue to serve the reader throughout those changes.

MECHANISM OF BLOOD FLOW DURING CARDIOPULMONARY RESUSCITATION

During CPR, the goal of therapy is to reverse the cardiac arrest and restore blood flow to the body tissues. Vital organ blood flow during cardiac massage is ob-

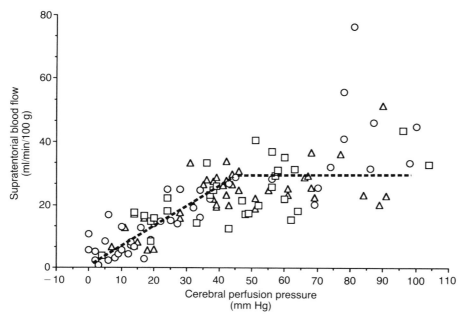

Figure 5–1. Supratentorial cerebral blood flow is plotted against mean cerebral perfusion pressure (aortic minus sagittal sinus pressure) in 2-week-old swine subjected to conventional CPR using 30% duty cycle compressions at 150 per minute (triangles) or 100 per minute (squares), or 60% duty cycle compressions at 100 per minute (circles). Cerebral autoregulation is intact, as flow is relatively constant when cerebral perfusion pressure exceeds 40 to 50 mm Hg. Below this pressure, flow becomes pressure passive and decreases linearly. During CPR, it is important to achieve cerebral perfusion pressures in excess of 40 to 50 mm Hg.

viously necessary if the patient is to survive in the long run. Simplistically, effective CPR produces an adequate cerebral and myocardial perfusion gradient to provide flow. Figures 5–1 and 5–2 demonstrate the relationship of cerebral and myocardial blood flow to their respective perfusion pressures. These data show that the major determinant of vital organ flow during prolonged CPR is the perfusion pressure calculated in the same manner as during spontaneous circulation. Cerebral autoregulation is strikingly intact during CPR if adequate perfusion pressure is generated.

When internal cardiac massage is provided, the heart is physically squeezed by the rescuer. It is likely that the mechanism of blood flow generation is similar to spontaneous contraction of the heart. When Jude and Kouwenhoven revived the concept of external cardiac massage, they understood the mechanism of blood flow

to be an extension of the events occurring during internal massage. Namely, they hypothesized that the heart was physically squeezed between the sternum and the vertebral column, thus providing blood flow in a manner identical to spontaneous circulation. This hypothesis received little early support from physiologic data in humans, which failed to demonstrate the pressure gradients that one would expect with cardiac pumping.[9–11] Laboratory studies both supported and refuted the hypothesis. However, the cardiac compression concept was not seriously challenged until the 1970s when Criley noted that in human patients vigorous coughing was capable of supporting the circulation during ventricular fibrillation.[12–14] This has been corroborated in other publications[15–18] and refined by Criley and associates.[19] This finding demonstrated beyond question that a noncardiac compression mechanism *could* generate blood

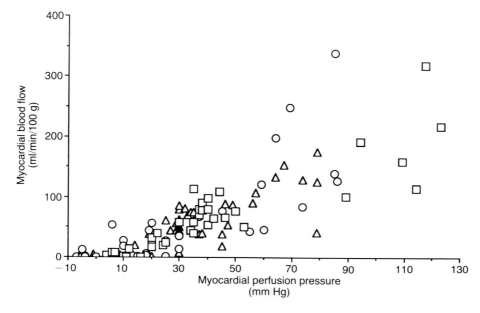

Figure 5–2. Myocardial blood flow is plotted against myocardial perfusion pressure (aortic minus right atrial) during the relaxation or diastolic phase of conventional CPR in 2-week-old swine using 30% duty cycle compressions at 150 per minute (triangles) or 100 per minute (squares), or 60% duty cycle compressions at 100 per minute (circles). When myocardial perfusion pressure exceeds 30 to 40 mm Hg, coronary blood flow exceeds 50 ml/min/100 g, and successful resuscitation is more likely.

flow during CPR. This was more a rediscovery than news, since Crile and Dolley had reached this conclusion in 1906, writing "Pressing upon the thorax itself, would effect a certain amount of circulation, if no heart existed and a system of vessels, one having valves and the other not, replaced it, and in the dead animal pressure upon the thorax alone is capable of producing an artificial circulation. This is by no means accomplished by its action upon the heart solely, but by its action upon all the large vessels—arteries, veins, and capillaries together."[20]

The cardiac compression model does not explain several clinical observations. When the chest is mechanically damaged by multiple rib fractures, producing a flail chest, chest compressions are generally ineffective during CPR. Yet this is a situation in which the heart ought to be optimally compressed, since the sternum and vertebral column are more closely approximated than normal. At the other extreme, emphysematous patients are technically able to be resuscitated with external chest compressions. The heart is unlikely to be directly compressed in this situation because of the barrel chest configuration seen in advanced emphysema. Deep inspiration enhances subsequent generated pressures, whereas it should make cardiac compression less efficient. Finally, repetitive attempts to measure pressures in the heart have failed to demonstrate the required pressure gradients during external chest compressions.

In 1980, Rudikoff and coworkers provided compelling evidence that fluctuations of intrathoracic pressure were involved in generation of blood flow during CPR.[21] The "thoracic pump" model assumes that intrathoracic pressures are increased in an essentially uniform manner during compressions, and the gradient for forward flow exists between the intrathoracic and extrathoracic arteries. Competent venous valves, at least at the jugular level,[22] prevent transmission of the intrathoracic venous pressure to extrathoracic veins, thus permitting a mechanism for net forward flow. During relaxation, intrathoracic pressure drops, and refill of the "thoracic pump" then occurs. In this model, the heart is essentially a passive conduit. Echocardiographic data have been obtained to support[23] and refute[24, 25] competence of the mitral valve during external compression, but a recent study has demonstrated that the mitral valve can open and close from intrathoracic pressure fluctuations.[26] Several investigators have shown that the mitral valve may be competent with rapid, high-velocity or high-compressive force CPR but incompetent in the same animal preparations at lower compression forces.[27, 28] It is clear that echocardiographic "proofs" of either the cardiac compression or thoracic pump model have failed to resolve the controversy.

The thoracic pump and cardiac compression models have important predicted behaviors that affect the optimum manner in which to apply cardiac massage in the clinical situation. If cardiac compression is the major mechanism responsible for forward flow during resuscitation, ejection will cease once the heart has been compressed. The duration of compression should be kept minimal beyond this compression, and increasing the compression rate should increase the total forward flow. In contrast, however, the thoracic pump mechanism is relatively unaffected by compression rate and is exquisitely sensitive to compression duration. These predictions have been studied in depth by Halperin and colleagues.[26, 29–31] Their experimental data in dogs clearly support the thoracic pump as the predominant mechanism of flow. The clinical ramifications are that the duration of compression should be a focus of attention by the clinician. Prolonged compression duration has been recommended.[32] Conversely, some investigators believe that cardiac compression is at least a contributor to forward flow and recommend increases in compression rate.[23, 33, 34] The most recent American Heart Association guidelines included an increase in compression rate, which reflected the cardiac compression "school."[35] Increased compression rates, however, also increase the duration of compression when human rescuers are involved because it is not easy to prolong compressions effectively at low compression rates. Thus, the 1986 recommendations were considered to improve blood flow regardless of predominant mechanism.[36]

The mechanism of flow has particular importance for pediatricians who deal with patients who have cardiac shunt lesions, such as an infant with pulmonary atresia who is dependent on a Blalock-Taussig shunt for pulmonary blood flow (Fig. 5–3). If the cardiac compression mechanism is predominant, as shown in the upper portion of Figure 5–3, pressure gradients will develop during compressions, which will permit pulmonary blood flow to occur. In contrast, if the thoracic pump mechanism is predominant, as shown in the lower portion of Figure 5–3, no gradient will develop for blood flow to the pulmonary vasculature. As a result, blood will not be oxygenated and CO_2 will not be excreted. If we knew unequivocally that blood flow is dependent on the thoracic pump, there would be a clear rationale for open chest cardiac massage in infants and children with such cardiac lesions.

LABORATORY INVESTIGATIONS OF CARDIOPULMONARY RESUSCITATION

Although clinicians have pursued CPR with anecdotal success, laboratory investigators encountered some difficulty demonstrating the efficacy of CPR in animal models (primarily canine). Although our understanding about the mechanism of CPR has been improved by these studies, confusion about clinical applicability remains. This discussion will concern adult and pediatric studies, both in animal models and in human patients.

Adult Studies

External cardiac massage is much less effective than a spontaneously beating heart, and vital organ perfusion is markedly decreased during CPR. Numerous studies have demonstrated very poor results with conventional external cardiac massage in dogs, with myocardial blood flow ranging between 4 and 20% of prearrest flow.[37–41]

$P_{PA} < P_{RV}$

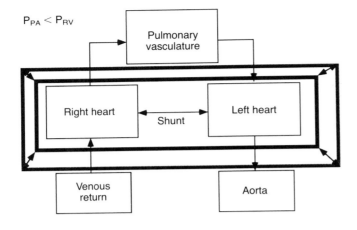

$P_{PA} = P_{RV}$

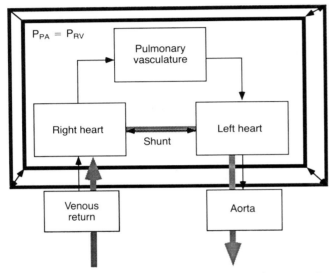

Figure 5–3. Schematic diagram showing the effect of pump mechanism on pulmonary blood flow during cardiopulmonary resuscitation in patients with shunt dependent pulmonary blood flow. The upper portion shows a cardiac compression pump mechanism in which the right and left heart are subjected to pressure changes but the pulmonary vasculature is not. The right ventricular pressure exceeds pulmonary artery pressure and thus blood flows into the pulmonary vascular bed. This is the normal situation as well as the operative mechanism during open chest cardiopulmonary resuscitation. In the lower portion, the thoracic pump mechanism is shown, which includes the pulmonary vasculature within the pump mechanism. In this situation, the pressure in the pulmonary artery is identical to the right heart, and there is no gradient for blood flow to occur to the lungs. However, the intrathoracic—extrathoracic pressure gradient does maintain forward flow from the thorax. The effect is to have effective systemic flow generation without any pulmonary blood flow.

This amount of coronary perfusion is likely to be inadequate for restoration of myocardial function.[42, 43]

One might consider several ways (Fig. 5–4) to improve these results.[44] First, assuming a predominant thoracic pump mechanism, increasing the intrathoracic pressure would increase pump output. Second, the blood volume could be increased, which would facilitate refill of the pump. Third, the vascular compliance could be reduced, which would enhance venous return. This maneuver would also divert blood flow from splanchnic beds to vital organs, and increased relaxation (diastolic) aortic pressure would improve coronary perfusion.

Several mechanical methods were developed to increase intrathoracic pressure more efficiently. Two such methods are simultaneous compression-ventilation CPR (SCV-CPR) and CPR with continuous abdominal binding. SCV-CPR improves blood flow during CPR in animal models[37, 45–47] but has not provided an obvious advantage in human resuscitation.[48] Similarly, abdominal binding has improved blood flow in some animal studies[49–53] but has failed to gain a clinical role because its efficacy is unclear in humans.[54] One might argue that dogs are simply a poor model in which to develop CPR methods for humans, but hemodynamic observations in adult humans are actually quite similar to those observed in experimental canine studies.[55]

An obvious way to improve pump function is performance of open chest massage, which assures the operator the ability to selectively pressurize the cardiac chambers. Despite the technical difficulties of thoracotomy, the technique continues to be regarded as a serious alternative to closed chest CPR[56–66] in a variety of settings. However, survival has not been improved in most instances,[67, 68] and the technique is associated with complications, both obvious and subtle.[69] In the cardiac surgical patient who is in the immediate postoperative setting, the technique is simpler and may merit serious consideration.[67, 70]

Rapid volume expansion during CPR has also been studied. Following rapid infusion of 1 l of fluid in a canine CPR model, total forward output increased dramatically. Unfortunately, coronary and cerebral flow decreased with volume infusion[39] because right atrial and intracranial pressures dramatically increased and impaired vital organ perfusion. Less dramatic fluid administration improves resuscitation rates, however.[71] Another approach to increase pump refill is *interposed* compression of the abdomen (not continuous abdominal binding), which pushes blood from abdominal venous capacitance vessels into the thorax during the relaxation phase of the thoracic pump.[72] In humans,[73] this technique appears to have promise, increasing the rate of resuscitation among adult study patients.

The administration of vasoconstrictive agents will reduce vascular compliance, raise perfusion pressures during the relaxation phase of CPR, and may further divert precious blood flow to the brain and heart at the expense of less vital organs. Epinephrine, norepinephrine, phenylephrine, and methoxamine have been extensively studied in this regard,[41, 74–92] and in general these agents improve blood flow during CPR in a variety of animal models.

A less obvious approach to improving arterial perfusion pressure of the brain and heart is the use of an intra-aortic balloon pump with constant inflation of the balloon. This has been studied in dogs and is effective,[93] but there are very large technical limitations on applicability of this technique in children. However, intra-aortic counterpulsation balloons are being used increasingly in infants and children with selected conditions, and in such children the technique may be useful.

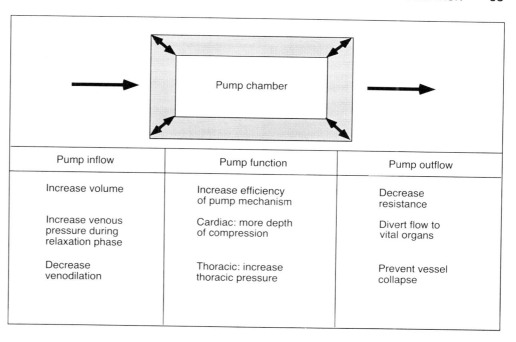

Figure 5–4. Possible ways to optimize pump function during cardiopulmonary resuscitation. Pump inflow, function, and outflow can be improved by various maneuvers that are shown in the diagram. Interventions that improve pump refill or outflow will be beneficial regardless of the operative pump mechanism.

Pump inflow	Pump function	Pump outflow
Increase volume	Increase efficiency of pump mechanism	Decrease resistance
Increase venous pressure during relaxation phase	Cardiac: more depth of compression	Divert flow to vital organs
Decrease venodilation	Thoracic: increase thoracic pressure	Prevent vessel collapse

Immature Animal Studies

The extrapolation of results from adult animal or human studies to infants and children is problematic. Fleisher and colleagues[62] devised an infant canine model and found that there was very low blood flow with conventional closed chest cardiac resuscitation in puppies. Open chest resuscitation was relatively effective.

There are difficulties interpreting these data because the chest configuration of dogs is unlike humans. The anteroposterior dimension of the canine chest is larger than the lateral dimension, which is opposite that of the human chest configuration. This results in a potentially negative thoracic ejection during early compression,[94] as shown in Figure 5–5. This would cause a threshold of chest compression beneath which no blood flow would be generated (Fig. 5–6). Indeed, such a threshold phenomenon was previously noted in adult dog studies by Babbs and colleagues.[95] In infant piglets, the chest has a nearly circular shape, eliminating such a threshold phenomenon. Indeed, Schleien and colleagues demonstrated that conventional closed chest cardiac massage yielded excellent blood flow to heart and brain during prolonged periods.[74] In the same model, using SCV-CPR failed to improve blood flow,[96] which suggests either that the predominant mechanism of blood flow is cardiac compression or alternatively that intrathoracic pressure generation is adequate in this model with conventional external chest compressions. Cerebral perfusion pressure appears to correlate with a prolonged compression duration in this model,[97] consistent with the thoracic pump model. However, measured cerebral and myocardial blood flow is improved with a shorter compression (30% versus 60% of total cycle time) when CPR is provided for a prolonged period (unpublished data). At the time of this writing, it remains unclear whether either the cardiac or thoracic pump model

predominates in this infant swine model, and it is possible that both mechanisms contribute to forward blood flow during CPR in these studies.

SYMPATHOMIMETIC DRUGS

It is worthwhile to return to the seminal writings of Crile and Dolley who wrote in 1906, "By adding to cardiac massage artificial respiration and intravenous saline infusion, resuscitations were in a slightly greater proportion successful. The same procedures, with the addition of adrenalin to the intravenous saline infusion,

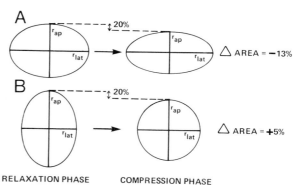

Figure 5–5. Changes in area of ellipses with constant circumference. Each ellipse is labeled with the anteroposterior (ap) and lateral (lat) radii, and a 20% anteroposterior compression is applied. Indicated change in area is equal to the relaxed area minus compressed area. *A*, Initial anteroposterior/lateral ratio = 0.7, and compression leads to positive ejection because relaxed area minus compressed area is negative. *B*, Initial anteroposterior/lateral ratio = 1.4, and compression toward a circular shape results in an increase in area. (Reproduced with permission from Dean JM, Koehler RC, Schleien CL, et al: Age-related changes in chest geometry during cardiopulmonary resuscitation. J Appl Physiol 62[6]:2212, 1987.)

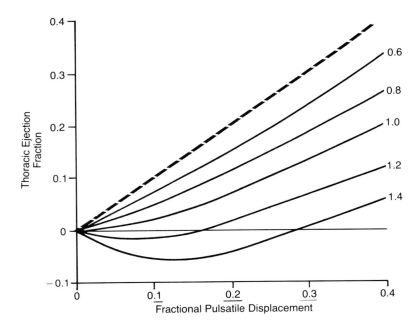

Figure 5–6. Predicted thoracic ejection fraction as a function of fractional pulsatile (piston) displacement. In these curves, total anteroposterior fractional displacement is equal to pulsatile displacement, since permanent deformity of the chest is not considered. Each line represents a different thoracic index, shown on right. *Dashed line* = limit of an infinitely wide rectangular sheet. As thoracic index increases, a threshold phenomenon becomes evident for generating positive ejection. (Reproduced with permission from Dean JM, Koehler RC, Schleien CL, et al: Age-related changes in chest geometry during cardiopulmonary resuscitation. J Appl Physiol 62[6]:2212, 1989.)

were markedly more successful in the deaths from asphyxia. . . ."[20] These prescient observations summarize the current approach to resuscitation. Epinephrine is the mainstay of drug therapy during CPR. It has not always been so, however, and we will briefly review the reasons for the importance of epinephrine (or possibly other α-adrenergic drugs).

Epinephrine was long noted to improve ventricular fibrillation by converting it to a coarser pattern, which, in turn, seemed clinically to be more susceptible to defibrillation. This was regarded as a primary effect on the electrical activity of the heart, which was attributed to β-sympathetic effects of the drug. However, it has been convincingly demonstrated that the important effect of epinephrine is related to α-adrenergic stimulation.[98] The beneficial effects of the drug relate to increased vascular tone and resultant increases in coronary and cerebral perfusion during CPR.[41] The improved coronary blood flow results in a higher likelihood of defibrillation.

Epinephrine is now the primary sympathomimetic resuscitation drug recommended for asystole, idioventricular rhythms, other bradyarrhythmias, and electromechanical dissociation. Our understanding of CPR has improved by simplification, as we now recognize that resolution of these arrhythmias during CPR depends much more on overall generation of coronary blood flow than on sophisticated pharmacologic actions on the myocardium or the conduction system. Understanding that epinephrine improves the mechanics that underlie vital organ perfusion during external cardiac massage during CPR[41] is perhaps the major breakthrough of the past decade.

Epinephrine is known to have several other effects on the myocardium that might be disadvantageous in the setting of reduced cardiac output. The major problem is that myocardial oxygen consumption may be increased by this drug at a time when blood delivery is subopti-

mal.[82] Phenylephrine has been shown to be less effective[75] or equally effective[79, 99] in animals and is equally effective in humans[91] when compared with epinephrine. Methoxamine may also be as effective as epinephrine in humans.[81] It seems clear that all these agents are effective vasoconstrictors, and the influence of stimulating myocardial oxygen consumption during CPR is relatively minor. In brain, epinephrine does not appear to exert a harmful effect when compared with phenylephrine,[99] suggesting that β-receptor–mediated increases in cerebral oxygen consumption do not occur during epinephrine administration.

The main controversy about epinephrine is no longer whether it should be used but rather how much should be used. This has been a subject of intense experimental investigation.[76, 78, 80, 89, 100–102] It is the author's opinion that the bulk of evidence supports significantly increasing the dose of epinephrine used during CPR. In addition, studies using a continuous drip instead of bolus administration have yielded better results[74, 94, 96, 97, 99] during prolonged CPR, and this mode of administration should be carefully considered.

ACIDOSIS, CARBON DIOXIDE, AND SODIUM BICARBONATE

Development of metabolic and respiratory acidosis is a prominent and well-known occurrence during cardiopulmonary resuscitation. There are at least two mechanisms by which pH is lowered (Fig. 5–7). First, decreased delivery of oxygen to the tissues leads to anaerobic metabolism, production of lactic acid, and a resultant metabolic acidosis. Second, decreased delivery of blood from the tissues to the lungs leads to increased CO_2 tension in the tissues, causing a respiratory acidosis.

Although neither of these concepts should be a revelation to the reader, recent studies have resurrected the

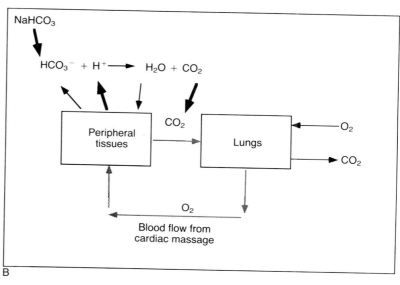

Figure 5–7. Schematic diagram illustrating the effect of sodium bicarbonate administration during cardiopulmonary resuscitation. In *A*, the normal situation is shown. In this scenario, carbon dioxide is formed by tissue buffering of hydrogen ion, which is produced in relatively small quantities under aerobic conditions. The CO_2 is easily carried to the lungs via the normal cardiac output and excreted via ventilation. In *B*, blood flow is greatly decreased as would occur during external cardiac massage. Because of decreased oxygen delivery more tissues are under anaerobic conditions, and hydrogen ion concentration rises. Tissue buffering mechanisms produce CO_2, which cannot be removed adequately from the tissues because of the low blood flow. Administration of sodium bicarbonate exacerbates this situation by increasing the CO_2-producing buffering in the tissues, and respiratory acidosis increases. Upon restoration of the circulation, this respiratory acidosis will be resolved and a metabolic alkalosis will frequently ensue if sodium bicarbonate has been administered.

important issues surrounding the importance of acidosis during CPR, the proper use of sodium bicarbonate, and whether other buffers might be superior to sodium bicarbonate during CPR. First, it has been confirmed that CO_2 build-up occurs in tissues during CPR, leading to a significant venoarterial gradient in blood CO_2 tensions.[103–106] It is likely that administration of sodium bicarbonate or other CO_2-producing buffer agents will worsen this tissue CO_2 retention, thereby worsening the tissue pH rather than ameliorating tissue acidosis. This has been demonstrated in several studies.[105, 107] The mechanism of myocardial acidosis remains unclear,[108] however, and administration of non–CO_2-producing buffers has not been demonstrated to be superior to sodium bicarbonate.[109, 110]

In the author's opinion, the prudent clinician will reserve sodium bicarbonate therapy for situations in which ventilation is assured, blood gas measurements have been obtained, and the duration of CPR has been prolonged. There is little evidence that acidosis per se prevents resuscitation, and several controlled studies have clearly demonstrated that sodium bicarbonate is either unhelpful or harmful during CPR in both animal experiments and human patients.[105, 107, 111–113] Following

restoration of the circulation, buffer therapy should be based on arterial blood gas measurements.

AMERICAN HEART ASSOCIATION GUIDELINES

The Emergency Cardiac Care (ECC) Committee of the American Heart Association meets on a regular basis to develop guidelines that provide standards for teaching lay and professional personnel about CPR. These guidelines have been published in 1974, 1980, and 1986; the next revision is anticipated by 1993. The goal of this effort is to provide guidelines, not rigid rules, that will permit all concerned individuals to have a common understanding of a starting place. In the 1986 publication, the Committee wrote "Thus, there is no intent to limit the adoption of new advances as they emerge; deviations from these standards and guidelines may occur when a trained physician proficient in CPR and ECC recognizes that such is in the best interests of the patient."[36] Readers of this textbook should heed these words, as critical care physicians are experts in this field and should deviate from the written guidelines in any instance in which it is appropriate.

The 1986 guidelines contained several significant changes related to medical professionals. First, the compression and ventilation rates were altered to reflect physiologic differences between adults and children. Ventilation is no longer interposed on a fixed basis after endotracheal intubation; instead, ventilation is delivered at an age-appropriate rate following intubation. The compression rate was increased for both adults and children. This would increase forward flow based on a cardiac compression model (recall that such a pump is rate-dependent); it would also increase flow based on a thoracic pump model because a longer duty cycle is delivered by human rescuers when the rate is increased. This is due to the difficulty of sustaining the compression duration at lower rates. Thus, despite continued controversy about the mechanism of blood flow during CPR, the compression rate increase would be expected to improve vital organ perfusion during CPR. Second, recommendations concerning the use of sodium bicarbonate, calcium salts, and atropine were drastically changed. These drugs were considered overused, and indications for their use were sharply delineated. Third, a more aggressive stance was taken on rapid intravenous access and use of the intraosseous route.[114-120] Fourth, hand placement for pediatric compressions was changed to a lower position, reflecting a persuasive argument by Orlowski.[121] Finally, issues of legal protection for rescuers were discussed at more length. Since the publication of the guidelines, the American Heart Association has published guidelines concerning protection of rescuers from infectious diseases carried by cardiac arrest victims. This reflects increased recognition of the legal and actual health risks that are taken by rescuers.

The American Heart Association also promulgates course material aimed at the public and health care professionals. The adult Advanced Cardiac Life Support (ACLS) and Pediatric Advanced Life Support (PALS) courses are aimed primarily at physicians and other health care professionals who practice in critical care settings. These courses are designed to deal with technical issues of resuscitation and are not intended to be comprehensive courses in emergency or critical care medicine or pediatrics. The PALS course is particularly valuable for nonpediatricians who must occasionally deal with cardiorespiratory emergencies in infants and children. The course has been criticized for not including numerous pediatric topics such as trauma management, but it is a particularly effective course with a very specific goal: teaching pediatric resuscitation. The American Academy of Pediatrics and American College of Emergency Physicians produce a course entitled Advanced Pediatric Life Support (APLS), which deals with numerous topics in pediatric emergency medicine. This course does not emphasize resuscitation per se, and thus a combination of PALS and APLS should be used in order to provide a complete review for physicians and nurses interested in these subjects.

References

1. Scherlis L: Poetical Version of the Rules of the Humane Society for recovering drowned persons. Crit Care Med 9:430, 1981.
2. Baker A: Artificial respiration, the history of an idea. Med Hist 15:336, 1971.
3. Julian DG: Cardiac resuscitation in the eighteenth century. Heart Lung 4:46, 1975.
4. Bartecchi CE: Cardiopulmonary resuscitation—an element of sophistication in the 18th century. Am Heart J 100(4):580, 1980.
5. Kouwenhoven WB, Jude JR, and Knickerbocker GG: Closed-chest cardiac massage. JAMA 173:1064, 1960.
6. Jude JR, Kouwenhoven WB, Ing DR, et al: Cardiac arrest: Report of application of external cardiac massage on 118 patients. JAMA 178:85, 1961.
7. DeBard ML: The history of cardiopulmonary resuscitation. Ann Emerg Med 9(5):273, 1980.
8. Kouwenhoven WB and Langworthy OR: Cardiopulmonary resuscitation: An account of forty-five years of research. Johns Hopkins Med J 132(3):186, 1973.
9. Mackenzie G, Taylor S, McDonald A, et al: Hemodynamic effects of external cardiac compression. Lancet 1:1342, 1964.
10. Weale FE and Rothwell-Jackson RL: The efficiency of cardiac massage. Lancet 1:990, 1962.
11. Thomsen JE, Stenlund RR, and Rowe GG. Intracardiac pressures during closed-chest cardiac massage. JAMA 205:116, 1968.
12. Criley JM, Blaufuss AH, and Kissel GL: Self-administered cardiopulmonary resuscitation by cough-induced cardiac compression. Trans Am Clin Climatol Assoc 87:138, 1976.
13. Criley JM, Blaufuss AH, and Kissel GL: Cough-induced cardiac compression. Self-administered form of cardiopulmonary resuscitation. JAMA 236(11):1246, 1976.
14. Niemann JT, Rosborough JP, Hausknecht M, et al: Pressure-synchronized cineangiography during experimental cardiopulmonary resuscitation. Circulation 64(5):985, 1981.
15. Bircher N, Safar P, Eshel G, et al: Cerebral and hemodynamic variables during cough-induced CPR in dogs. Crit Care Med 10(2):104, 1982.
16. Miller B, Lesnefsky E, Heyborne T, et al: Cough-cardiopulmonary resuscitation in the cardiac catheterization laboratory: Hemodynamics during an episode of prolonged hypotensive ventricular tachycardia. Cathet Cardiovasc Diagn 18(3):168, 1989.
17. Niemann JT, Rosborough JP, Niskanen RA, et al: Mechanical "cough" cardiopulmonary resuscitation during cardiac arrest in dogs. Am J Cardiol 55(1):199, 1985.
18. Schultz DD and Olivas GS. The use of cough cardiopulmonary resuscitation in clinical practice. Heart Lung 15(3):273, 1986.
19. Criley JM, Niemann JT, Rosborough JP, et al: Modifications of cardiopulmonary resuscitation based on the cough. Circulation 74(Suppl IV):42, 1986.
20. Crile G and Dolley DH: An experimental research into the resuscitation of dogs killed by anesthetics and asphyxia. J Exp Med 8:713, 1906.
21. Rudikoff MT, Maughan WL, Effron M, et al: Mechanisms of blood flow during cardiopulmonary resuscitation. Circulation 61(2):345, 1980.
22. Fisher J, Vaghaiwalla F, Tsitlik J, et al: Determinants and clinical significance of jugular venous valve competence. Circulation 65(1):188, 1982.
23. Deshmukh HG, Weil MH, Gudipati CV, et al: Mechanism of blood flow generated by precordial compression during CPR. I:Studies on closed chest precordial compression. Chest 95(5):1092, 1989.
24. Rich S, Wix HL, and Shapiro EP: Clinical assessment of heart chamber size and valve motion during cardiopulmonary resuscitation by two-dimensional echocardiography. Am Heart J 102:368, 1981.
25. Werner JA, Greene HL, Janko CL, et al: Visualization of cardiac valve motion in man during external chest compression using two-dimensional echocardiography: Implications regarding the mechanism of blood flow. Circulation 63(6):1417, 1981.
26. Halperin HR, Weiss JL, Guerci AD, et al: Cyclic elevation of intrathoracic pressure can close the mitral valve during cardiac arrest in dogs. Circulation 78:754, 1988.
27. Feneley MP, Maier GW, Gaynor JW, et al: Sequence of mitral valve motion and transmitral blood flow during manual cardiopulmonary resuscitation in dogs. Circulation 76(2):363, 1987.
28. Hackl W, Simon P, Mauritz W, et al: Echocardiographic assessment of mitral valve function during mechanical cardiopulmonary resuscitation in pigs. Anesth Analg 70(4):350, 1990.

29. Halperin HR, Tsitlik JE, Guerci AD, et al: Determinants of blood flow to vital organs during cardiopulmonary resuscitation in dogs. Circulation 73(3):539, 1986.
30. Halperin HR, Guerci AD, Chandra N, et al: Vest inflation without simultaneous ventilation during cardiac arrest in dogs: Improved survival from prolonged cardiopulmonary resuscitation. Circulation 74(6):1407, 1986.
31. Halperin HR, Tsitlik JE, Beyar R, et al: Intrathoracic pressure fluctuations move blood during CPR: Comparison of hemodynamic data with predictions from a mathematical model. Ann Biomed Eng 15(3–4):385, 1987.
32. Taylor GJ, Tucker WM, Greene HL, et al: Importance of prolonged compression during cardiopulmonary resuscitation in man. N Engl J Med 296(26):1515, 1977.
33. Babbs CF, Bircher N, Burkett DE, et al: Effect of thoracic venting on arterial pressure, and flow during external cardiopulmonary resuscitation in animals. Crit Care Med 9(11):785, 1981.
34. Maier GW, Tyson GSJ, Olsen CO, et al: The physiology of external cardiac massage: High-impulse cardiopulmonary resuscitation. Circulation 70(1):86, 1984.
35. Maier GW, Newton JJ, Wolfe JA, et al: The influence of manual chest compression rate on hemodynamic support during cardiac arrest: High-impulse cardiopulmonary resuscitation. Circulation 74(Suppl IV):51, 1986.
36. Anonymous: Standards and Guidelines for Cardiopulmonary Resuscitation (CPR) and Emergency Cardiac Care (ECC). JAMA 255(21):2905, 1986.
37. Luce JM, Ross BK, O'Quin RJ, et al: Regional blood flow during cardiopulmonary resuscitation in dogs using simultaneous and nonsimultaneous compression and ventilation. Circulation 67(2):258, 1983.
38. Voorhees WD III, Ralston SH, and Babbs CF: Regional blood flow during cardiopulmonary resuscitation with abdominal counterpulsation in dogs. Am J Emerg Med 2(2):123, 1984.
39. Ditchey RV and Lindenfeld J: Potential adverse effects of volume loading on perfusion of vital organs during closed-chest resuscitation. Circulation 69(1):181, 1984.
40. Ralston SH, Voorhees WD, and Babbs CF: Intrapulmonary epinephrine during prolonged cardiopulmonary resuscitation: improved regional blood flow and resuscitation in dogs. Ann Emerg Med 13(2):79, 1984.
41. Michael JR, Guerci AD, Koehler RC, et al: Mechanisms by which epinephrine augments cerebral and myocardial perfusion during cardiopulmonary resuscitation in dogs. Circulation 69(4):822, 1984.
42. Sanders AB, Kern KB, Atlas M, et al: Importance of the duration of inadequate coronary perfusion pressure on resuscitation from cardiac arrest. J Am Coll Cardiol 6(1):113, 1985.
43. Paradis NA, Martin GB, Rivers EP, et al: Coronary perfusion pressure and the return of spontaneous circulation in human cardiopulmonary resuscitation. JAMA 263(8):1106, 1990.
44. Wise RA and Summers WR: Cardiopulmonary resuscitation. In: Dantzker D (ed): Cardiopulmonary Critical Care. Orlando, Grune & Stratton, 1986, p 335.
45. Chandra N, Rudikoff M, and Weisfeldt ML: Simultaneous chest compression and ventilation at high airway pressure during cardiopulmonary resuscitation. Lancet 1(8161):175, 1980.
46. Chandra N, Weisfeldt ML, Tsitlik J, et al: Augmentation of carotid flow during cardiopulmonary resuscitation by ventilation at high airway pressure simultaneous with chest compression. Am J Cardiol 48(6):1053, 1981.
47. Koehler RC, Chandra N, Guerci AD, et al: Augmentation of cerebral perfusion by simultaneous chest compression and lung inflation with abdominal binding after cardiac arrest in dogs. Circulation 67(2):266, 1983.
48. Krischer JP, Fine EG, Weisfeldt ML, et al: Comparison of prehospital conventional and simultaneous compression-ventilation cardiopulmonary resuscitation. Crit Care Med 17(12):1263, 1989.
49. Babbs CF and Blevins WE: Abdominal binding and counterpulsation in cardiopulmonary resuscitation. Crit Care Clin 2(2):319, 1986.
50. Bucur I: Abdominal binding during cardiopulmonary resuscitation (Letter). JAMA 248(7):827, 1982.
51. Chandra N, Snyder LD, and Weisfeldt ML: Abdominal binding during cardiopulmonary resuscitation in man. JAMA 246(4):351, 1981.
52. Niemann JT, Rosborough JP, Ung S, et al: Hemodynamic effects of continuous abdominal binding during cardiac arrest and resuscitation. Am J Cardiol 53(2):269, 1984.
53. Niemann JT, Rosborough JP, and Criley JM: Continuous external counterpressure during closed-chest resuscitation: A critical appraisal of the military antishock trouser garment and abdominal binder. Circulation 74(Suppl IV):102, 1986.
54. Swenson RD, Weaver WD, Niskanen RA, et al: Hemodynamics in humans during conventional and experimental methods of cardiopulmonary resuscitation. Circulation 78(3):630, 1988.
55. Chandra NC, Tsitlik JE, Halperin HR, et al: Observations of hemodynamics during human cardiopulmonary resuscitation. Crit Care Med 18(9):929, 1990.
56. Alifimoff JK: Open versus closed chest cardiac massage in non-traumatic cardiac arrest. Resuscitation 15(1):13, 1987.
57. Arai T, Dote K, Tsukahara I, et al: Cerebral blood flow during conventional, new and open-chest cardio-pulmonary resuscitation in dogs. Resuscitation 12(2):147, 1984.
58. Bircher N and Safar P: Manual open-chest cardiopulmonary resuscitation. Ann Emerg Med 13:770, 1984.
59. Del Guercio L: Open chest cardiac massage: An overview. Resuscitation 15(1):9, 1987.
60. Eldor J, Frankel DZ, and Davidson JT: Open chest cardiac massage: A review. Resuscitation 16(3):155, 1988.
61. Ewer MS, Ali MK, and Frazier OH: Open chest resuscitation for cardiopulmonary arrest related to mechanical impairment of circulation: A report of two cases. Crit Care Med 10(3):198, 1982.
62. Fleisher G, Sagy M, Swedlow DB, et al: Open- versus closed-chest cardiac compressions in a canine model of pediatric cardiopulmonary resuscitation. Am J Emerg Med 3(4):305, 1985.
63. Heller MB: Open-chest cardiac massage: The possible rebirth of an old procedure. Postgrad Med 87(8):189, 1990.
64. Kern KB, Sanders AB, and Ewy GA: Open-chest cardiac massage after closed-chest compression in a canine model: When to intervene. Resuscitation 15(1):51, 1987.
65. Robertson C: Open-chest cardiac massage for non-traumatic cardiac arrest. Arch Emerg Med 4(4):207, 1987.
66. Sanders AB, Kern KB, and Ewy GA: Open chest massage for resuscitation from cardiac arrest (Editorial). Resuscitation 16(3):153, 1988.
67. Blakeman B: Open cardiac resuscitation: A surgeon's viewpoint. Postgrad Med 87(1):247, 1990.
68. Geehr EC, Lewis FR, and Auerbach PS: Failure of open-heart massage to improve survival after prehospital nontraumatic cardiac arrest (Letter). N Engl J Med 314(18):1189, 1986.
69. Herz BL: Open-chest cardiac massage esophageal trauma (Letter). Am J Emerg Med 5(2):179, 1987.
70. Raman J, Saldanha RF, Branch JM, et al: Open cardiac compression in the postoperative cardiac intensive care unit. Anaesth Intensive Care 17(2):129, 1989.
71. Sanders AB, Kern KB, Fonken S, et al: The role of bicarbonate and fluid loading in improving resuscitation from prolonged cardiac arrest with rapid manual chest compression CPR. Ann Emerg Med 19(1):1, 1990.
72. Beyar R, Kishon Y, Kimmel E, et al: Intrathoracic and abdominal pressure variations as an efficient method for cardiopulmonary resuscitation: Studies in dogs compared with computer model results. Cardiovasc Res 19(6):335, 1985.
73. Ward KR, Sullivan RJ, Zelenak RR, et al: A comparison of interposed abdominal compression CPR and standard CPR by monitoring end-tidal P_{CO_2}. Ann Emerg Med 18(8):831, 1989.
74. Schleien CL, Dean JM, Koehler RC, et al: Effect of epinephrine on cerebral and myocardial perfusion in an infant animal preparation of cardiopulmonary resuscitation. Circulation 73(4):809, 1986.
75. Brown CG, Birinyi F, Werman HA, et al: The comparative effects of epinephrine versus phenylephrine on regional cerebral blood flow during cardiopulmonary resuscitation. Resuscitation 14(3):171, 1986.
76. Brown CG, Werman HA, Davis EA, et al: Comparative effect of graded doses of epinephrine on regional brain blood flow during CPR in a swine model. Ann Emerg Med 15(10):1138, 1986.
77. Brown CG, Davis EA, Werman HA, et al: Methoxamine versus epinephrine on regional cerebral blood flow during cardiopulmonary resuscitation. Crit Care Med 15(7):682, 1987.

78. Brown CG, Werman HA, Davis EA, et al: The effects of graded doses of epinephrine on regional myocardial blood flow during cardiopulmonary resuscitation in swine. Circulation 75(2):491, 1987.
79. Brillman J, Sanders A, Otto CW, et al: Comparison of epinephrine and phenylephrine for resuscitation and neurologic outcome of cardiac arrest in dogs. Ann Emerg Med 16(1):11, 1987.
80. Ditchey RV and Lindenfeld J: Failure of epinephrine to improve the balance between myocardial oxygen supply and demand during closed-chest resuscitation in dogs. Circulation 78(2):382, 1988.
81. Turner LM, Parsons M, Luetkemeyer RC, et al: A comparison of epinephrine and methoxamine for resuscitation from electro-mechanical dissociation in human beings. Ann Emerg Med 17(5):443, 1988.
82. Brown CG, Taylor RB, Werman HA, et al: Myocardial oxygen delivery/consumption during cardiopulmonary resuscitation: A comparison of epinephrine and phenylephrine. Ann Emerg Med 17(4):302, 1988.
83. Lindner KH, Ahnefeld FW, and Bowdler IM: The effect of epinephrine on hemodynamics, acid-base status and potassium during spontaneous circulation and cardiopulmonary resuscitation. Resuscitation 16(4):251, 1988.
84. Brown CG, Taylor RB, Werman HA, et al: Effect of standard doses of epinephrine on myocardial oxygen delivery and utilization during cardiopulmonary resuscitation. Crit Care Med 16(5):536, 1988.
85. Lindner KH, Ahnefeld FW, and Bowdler IM: Comparison of epinephrine and dopamine during cardiopulmonary resuscitation. Intensive Care Med 15(7):432, 1989.
86. Brown CG, Robinson LA, Jenkins J, et al: The effect of norepinephrine versus epinephrine on regional cerebral blood flow during cardiopulmonary resuscitation. Am J Emerg Med 7(3):278, 1989.
87. Lindner KH, Ahnefeld FW, Schuermann W, et al: Epinephrine and norepinephrine in cardiopulmonary resuscitation: Effects on myocardial oxygen delivery and consumption. Chest 97(6):1458, 1990.
88. Lindner KH, Ahnefeld FW, Schuermann W, et al: The effect of adrenaline and noradrenaline on the oxygen supply of the myocardium during cardiopulmonary resuscitation. Anaesthetist 38(5):245, 1989.
89. Hoekstra JW, Van LP, Neumar R, et al: Effect of high dose norepinephrine versus epinephrine on cerebral and myocardial blood flow during CPR. Resuscitation 19(3):227, 1990.
90. Martin GB, Gentile NT, Paradis NA: Effect of epinephrine on end-tidal carbon dioxide monitoring during CPR. Ann Emerg Med 19(4):396, 1990.
91. Silfvast T, Saarnivaara L, Kinnunen A, et al: Comparison of adrenaline and phenylephrine in out-of-hospital cardiopulmonary resuscitation: A double-blind study. Acta Anaesthesiol Scand 29(6):610, 1985.
92. Otto CW, Yakaitis RW, and Ewy GA: Effect of epinephrine on defibrillation in ischemic ventricular fibrillation. Am J Emerg Med 3(4):285, 1985.
93. Wesley RJ and Morgan DB: Effect of continuous intra-aortic balloon inflation in canine open chest cardiopulmonary resuscitation. Crit Care Med 18(6):630, 1990.
94. Dean JM, Koehler RC, Schleien CL, et al: Age-related changes in chest geometry during cardiopulmonary resuscitation. J Appl Physiol 62(6):2212, 1987.
95. Babbs CF, Voorhees WD, Fitzgerald KR, et al: Relationship of blood pressure and flow during CPR to chest compression amplitude: Evidence for an effective compression threshold. Ann Emerg Med 12(9):527, 1983.
96. Berkowitz ID, Chantarojanasiri T, Koehler RC, et al: Blood flow during cardiopulmonary resuscitation with simultaneous compression and ventilation in infant pigs. Pediatr Res 26(6):558, 1989.
97. Dean JM, Koehler RC, Schleien CL, et al: Age-related effects of compression rate and duration in cardiopulmonary resuscitation. J Appl Physiol 68(2):554, 1990.
98. Otto CW, Yakaitis RW, Redding JS, et al: Comparison of dopamine, dobutamine, and epinephrine in CPR. Crit Care Med 9(9):640, 1981.
99. Schleien CL, Koehler RC, Gervais H, et al: Organ blood flow and somatosensory-evoked potentials during and after cardiopulmonary resuscitation with epinephrine or phenylephrine. Circulation 79(6):1332, 1989.
100. Goetting MG and Paradis NA: High dose epinephrine in refractory pediatric cardiac arrest. Crit Care Med 17(12):1258, 1989.
101. Gonzalez ER, Ornato JP, Garnett AR, et al: Dose-dependent vasopressor response to epinephrine during CPR in human beings. Ann Emerg Med 18(9):920, 1989.
102. Koscove EM and Paradis NA: Successful resuscitation from cardiac arrest using high-dose epinephrine therapy: Report of two cases. JAMA 259(20):3031, 1988.
103. Weil MH, Rackow EC, Trevino R, et al: Difference in acid-base state between venous and arterial blood during cardiopulmonary resuscitation. N Engl J Med 315(3):153, 1986.
104. Nowak RM, Martin GB, Carden DL, et al: Selective venous hypercarbia during human CPR: Implications regarding blood flow. Ann Emerg Med 16(5):527, 1987.
105. Imai T, Kon N, Kunimoto F, et al: Exacerbation of hypercapnia and acidosis of central venous blood and tissue following administration of sodium bicarbonate during cardiopulmonary resuscitation. Jpn Circ J 53(4):298, 1989.
106. Grundler W, Weil MH, Rackow EC, et al: Selective acidosis in venous blood during human cardiopulmonary resuscitation: A preliminary report. Crit Care Med 13(11):886, 1985.
107. von Planta M, Gudipati C, Weil MH, et al: Effects of tromethamine and sodium bicarbonate buffers during cardiac resuscitation. J Clin Pharmacol 28(7):594, 1988.
108. von Planta M, Weil MH, Gazmuri RJ, et al: Myocardial acidosis associated with CO_2 production during cardiac arrest and resuscitation. Circulation 80(3):684, 1989.
109. Kette F, Weil MH, von Planta M, et al: Buffer agents do not reverse intramyocardial acidosis during cardiac resuscitation. Circulation 81(5):1660, 1990.
110. Gazmuri RJ, von Planta M, Weil MH, et al: Cardiac effects of carbon dioxide-consuming and carbon dioxide-generating buffers during cardiopulmonary resuscitation. J Am Coll Cardiol 15(2):482, 1990.
111. Lindner KH, Ahnefeld FW, Dick W, et al: Sodium bicarbonate administration in cardiopulmonary resuscitation: Results of an animal experimental study. Anaesthetist 34(1):37, 1985.
112. Guerci AD, Chandra N, Johnson E, et al: Failure of sodium bicarbonate to improve resuscitation from ventricular fibrillation in dogs. Circulation 74(Suppl IV):75, 1986.
113. Makisalo HJ, Soini HO, Nordin AJ, et al: Effects of bicarbonate therapy on tissue oxygenation during resuscitation of hemorrhagic shock. Crit Care Med 17(11):1170, 1989.
114. Zimmerman JJ, Coyne M, and Logsdon M: Implementation of intraosseous infusion technique by aeromedical transport programs. J Trauma 29(5):687, 1989.
115. Spivey WH, Lathers CM, Malone DR, et al: Comparison of intraosseous, central, and peripheral routes of sodium bicarbonate administration during CPR in pigs. Ann Emerg Med 14(12):1135, 1985.
116. McNamara RM, Spivey WH, and Sussman C: Pediatric resuscitation without an intravenous line. Am J Emerg Med 4(1):31, 1986.
117. Kramer GC, Walsh JC, Hands RD, et al: Resuscitation of hemorrhage with intraosseous infusion of hypertonic saline/dextran. Braz J Med Biol Res 22(2):283, 1989.
118. Kanter RK, Zimmerman JJ, Strauss RH, et al: Pediatric emergency intravenous access. Evaluation of a protocol. Am J Dis Child 140(2):132, 1986.
119. Glaeser PW, Losek JD, Nelson DB, et al: Pediatric intraosseous infusions: Impact on vascular access time. Am J Emerg Med 6(4):330, 1988.
120. Brunette DD and Fischer R: Intravascular access in pediatric cardiac arrest. Am J Emerg Med 6(6):577, 1988.
121. Orlowski JP: Optimum position for external cardiac compression in infants and young children. Ann Emerg Med 15(6):667, 1986.

Resuscitation of the Newborn

George J. Peckham, M.D.

During the human life cycle, there is probably no time that resuscitation is more needed, more predictable, or of greater efficacy than during the neonatal period, especially in the first few minutes after birth. The reanimation of the newly born infant can be truly viewed as a normal part of the birth process, rather than a rarely applied intensive care technique for a medical emergency. Despite these realizations, the orientation in many of the more than 5,000 hospitals that deliver babies in the United States is toward the "routine" delivery of a normal baby.

The statistics do not support a complacent approach. For example, 1% of deliveries are of babies weighing less than 1500 gm, 80% of whom require resuscitation. In addition, it is estimated that about 6% of deliveries involve problems related to fetal compromise, leading to meconium aspiration, persistent pulmonary hypertension, shock, or other sequelae of intrauterine asphyxia. That translates to about a quarter of a million newborns who require resuscitation that if not immediately and effectively provided, can result in mortality and morbidity involving lifelong medical and developmental disabilities. When viewed in this perspective, readily available and skillful resuscitation of the newborn can be seen as a major public health program aimed at reducing the incidence of neurodevelopmental problems on a large scale. This requires that *every* hospital provide well-trained personnel and appropriate equipment for *every* baby's birth at *every* hour of the day or night on *every* day of the week. This should be a personal professional, as well as institutional, commitment that is an essential element of all obstetric services.

MATERNAL-PLACENTAL PHYSIOLOGY

The fetal-placental unit is a structure created de novo within the mother at the time of conception. It is a "foreign" antigen that is tolerated by the host in most cases for 38 to 42 weeks of gestation. The functioning of this new entity is highly dependent upon the quality of the uterine attachment and blood flow and is compromised by ischemia, infarction, or infection of the placental tissue. Most of the transfer of oxygen, carbon dioxide, hydrogen ion, other metabolites, and metabolic waste products takes place in the intervillous space. It is in this important area that the maternal and fetal blood come in closest approximation and, by either pressure gradients or active and passive mechanisms, transfer substances to and from the fetus.

The efficiency of this critical interphase is dependent on several maternal factors, including (1) uterine blood flow, (2) oxygen-carrying capacity, (3) plasma level of metabolites, (4) presence of microbiologic organisms, (5) placental attachment, and (6) other less well defined aspects of maternal health status. Disruptions that occur in each of these physiologic areas lead to a compromise of placental functioning that will, in turn, threaten fetal well-being. These disruptions can be expressed in clinical terms as prenatal risk factors:

Uterine Blood Flow
- Chronic hypertension
- Pre-eclampsia
- Toxemia
- Smoking
- Drug abuse
- Acute hypotension

Oxygen-carrying Capacity
- Anemia
- Rh or ABO sensitization
- Heart disease

Plasma Level Of Metabolism
- Diabetes
- Renal disease
- Jaundice
- Drug therapy
- Electrolyte disturbances

Presence of Microbiologic Agents
- Teratogenic: rubella, cytomegalovirus, toxoplasmosis
- Fetal infection: hepatitis, human immunodeficiency virus, listeriosis
- Intrapartum: chorioamnionitis, herpes, group B streptococci

Placental Attachment and Function
- Placenta previa
- Abruptio placenta
- Preterm labor
- Postmaturity

Other Health Factors
- Age of mother
- Nutrition
- Socioeconomic factors
- Prenatal care

FETAL PHYSIOLOGY

Features of the fetal physiology that need to be focused on as a knowledge base for the resuscitation of a newborn primarily involve the unique aspects of the circulatory system and both its intrauterine and extra-uterine adaptive (or maladaptive) mechanisms.[1] The normal fetus is in a state of hypoxia and relative hyper-capnea and hypotension when compared with the extra-uterine cardiopulmonary status of the newborn. These "abnormalities" serve a positive function by stimulating constriction of the pulmonary vasculature and thereby facilitating blood flow from the right atrium to the left atrium through the foramen ovale and from the pulmonary circulation to the lower resistance systemic circulation via the patent ductus arteriosus. The efficiency of this pattern of circulation is further enhanced by the fact that the blood returning to the right atrium from the placenta, in which it is oxygenated, preferentially flows to the left atrium through the foramen ovale and then into the left ventricle, from which it is pumped into the ascending aorta. This highly oxygenated blood is then delivered first to the high-priority organs of the heart and brain. The deoxygenated fetal blood returning to the right atrium primarily flows across the tricuspid valve and then into the pulmonary circulation with much of it going into the distal aorta via the patent ductus arteriosus. This less oxygenated blood flows to "lower priority" organs such as the kidneys, gut, and musculo-skeletal system.

As gestational life progresses, this pattern of blood flow is reinforced by the maintenance of a high level of pulmonary vascular resistance through the increased muscularity of the pulmonary vessels and precapillary, arterioles. These vessels react constrictively to decreasing Po_2, increasing CO_2, and acidosis. When intrauterine asphyxia takes place, causing an alteration in one or more of these factors, pulmonary vasoconstriction is accentuated. This, in turn, elevates the right ventricular end-diastolic pressure, producing an increase in right-to-left shunting of oxygenated blood across the foramen ovale into the left side of the circulation. The net result of this important adaptive maneuver is an "autotransfusion" of oxygenated blood away from the pulmonary circuit into the systemic circulation of the fetus. When the various stimuli remain over a protracted period, the muscular layer of the pulmonary vessels hypertrophies, setting up a situation for the persistence of the fetal blood flow pattern after the infant is born.

INTRAUTERINE ASPHYXIA

Asphyxia in the fetus usually involves multiple factors that are often interactive in a vicious cycle, sometimes to the point of overcoming the adaptive mechanisms already described.[2] It is a process involving (1) hypoxia, (2) hypercarbia, (3) acidosis, and (4) hypotension. Each of these clinical conditions has to be understood and dealt with both separately and synergistically in order to have a resuscitation plan that is therapeutically rational and hopefully successful. When the exchange of oxygen and carbon dioxide across the intervillous space becomes impaired because of placental dysfunction caused by a number of maternal risk factors, a series of events takes place at the cellular level, resulting in organic acidosis from anaerobic metabolism, intracellular acidosis from the diffusion of high levels of carbon dioxide into the cell and, eventually, poor tissue perfusion because of the impaired cardiac function caused by the acidosis and depletion of myocardial catecholamines. The resultant hypotension accentuates the acidosis and the vicious cycle ensues.

The overall effect of severe asphyxia is to produce multiorgan problems. The pulmonary vasculature remains constricted, and right-to-left shunting persists at the foramen ovale and ductus arteriosus. The brain undergoes a loss of autoregulation of cerebral blood flow with resultant edema, ischemia, or hemorrhage. The severe acidosis and catecholamine depletion of the myocardium result in decreased cardiac contractility, which can be associated with subendocardial infarction and papillary muscle dysfunction, causing atrioventricular valve regurgitation. The reduced perfusion to the liver can result in hepatocellular necrosis; the kidney can sustain acute tubular necrosis; and the gut can develop atony, producing ileus or full-blown enterocolitis.

In the fetus, asphyxia can be manifested by bradycardia or the loss of beat-to-beat variability on the fetal cardiogram, or both. At the time of birth, the infant can present with meconium staining, apnea, cyanosis, bradycardia, and areflexia. Although a poorly functioning placenta may be able to partially compensate for the acid-base derangements, once the baby is delivered, immediate and effective resuscitation must be initiated within seconds. The personnel and equipment should provide life support well before the 1-minute Apgar score.

Preparation for Resuscitation in the Delivery Room

The key features of delivery room resuscitation are (1) anticipation of need, (2) special environment, (3) all necessary equipment, and (4) a team of skilled professionals. All four of these components must be fully operational in every setting in which deliveries take place no matter what the size or remoteness of the obstetric service.[3, 4]

The need for immediate life support can often be anticipated from the maternal history in which certain risk factors for prematurity or fetal asphyxia can be elicited (see earlier). This can provide the lead time in which the team can be alerted and the environment and equipment prepared and tested. A separate area either within or immediately adjacent to the delivery room should be set up exclusively and permanently for delivery room resuscitation. It should have facilities for oxygen, compressed air, and suction and should be well lighted. It should have a radiant warmer[5] and a procedure table. The equipment should include the following:

Suction Equipment
- Vacuum regulator
- Bulb syringe
- Meconium aspiration adapter

Bag and Mask Equipment
- Oxygen-air blender
- Flow meter
- Self-inflating bag with pop-off valve and oxygen reservoir
- Anesthesia bag with an adjustable valve and a pressure gauge
- Cushioned-rim face masks: term and premature sizes
- Oral airways

Intubation Equipment
- Laryngoscope with No. 0 and No. 1 blades
- Endotracheal tubes: 2.5-, 3.0-, 3.5-mm
- Stylet

Miscellaneous Equipment
- Scissors
- Stethoscope
- Heart rate monitor (preferable)

Supplies
- Suction catheters
- Feeding tube (No. 8 French)
- Adhesive tape
- Syringes
- Needles
- Umbilical artery catheterization set
- Umbilical artery catheters: Nos. 3.5 and 5 French

Skill Development of Neonatal Resuscitation Team

The fact that resuscitation is relatively frequent is a special consideration when implementing a program of resuscitation for the newborn. It needs to be provided in a skilled manner within seconds of delivery at all times. If death or lifelong damage to the infant is to be avoided, there must be at least one person present at every delivery who is skilled in the basic steps of resuscitation. In the case of an unanticipated problem, this may be a nurse who is competent in performing all the steps up to and including chest compression. The physician should be readily available in house to be notified when it is apparent that intubation and medications will be required. However, in the case of high-risk deliveries (and ideally for all deliveries) two skilled individuals, one of whom can intubate and administer

medications, should be present in the delivery room prior to the delivery. To accomplish this rather formidable yet necessary task requires an organized educational approach for the entire staff of the delivery room, the nurseries, and any other health professionals from other areas of the hospital who will be called upon to assist in the resuscitation of a newborn.

Such an educational program should emphasize skills based on knowledge in a teamwork format in which all persons will be competent to perform those techniques that are within their level of responsibility. The procedures that are taught should have an: evaluation → decision → action → evaluation → decision → action interaction for each step of the resuscitative process. The three basic areas of evaluation involve (1) respiratory effort, (2) heart rate, and (3) color. The decisions are based on a yes-no status or different levels of heart rate. The actions to be taken need to be precisely defined and taught in a hands-on skill-development format and evaluated by a performance checklist of the steps that need to be successfully accomplished by each student. Once the initial task of teaching all existing staff members has been accomplished, the educational program should become an integral part of the orientation of new personnel and should be given as a refresher course or as a "resuscitation drill" on a periodic basis in order to maintain skills. A course that achieves these objectives is sponsored by the American Heart Association and the American Academy of Pediatrics.[6]

Initial Steps

The initial steps in resuscitation are in fact actions that should be performed on all babies immediately upon delivery. They are procedures that can be performed by every health professional in the delivery room and, when done proficiently, can often prevent the need for further resuscitative intervention. The initial steps follow:

- Prevention of heat loss
- Positioning
- Suctioning
- Stimulation
- Evaluation

A newly delivered infant must make a rapid adjustment from an environment at body temperature to one that is 20 to 25° F colder in the delivery room. In addition, the infant is covered with amniotic fluid and blood, which contributes to the evaporative heat loss. Therefore the newborn should be immediately wrapped in towels, transferred to a preheated radiant warmer, and dried off, with the wet towel being discarded. The next step is to place the infant on his or her back with the neck slightly extended to open the airway. A rolled towel placed under the shoulders may facilitate achieving the correct position. At this point, the mouth should be suctioned, followed by each nare. Care should be taken not to stimulate the posterior pharynx to avoid severe bradycardia from a vagal reflex. The infant is usually stimulated to breathe with the preceding maneuvers. If further stimulation is needed, however, it should be restricted to rubbing the trunk or flicking the baby's heels. At this point about 20 seconds have elapsed, and the infant should be evaluated for:

- Respiratory effort
- Heart rate
- Color
- Presence of meconium

If after adequate stimulation the infant is apneic or gasping, positive pressure ventilation (PPV) should be given either by bag and mask or bag and endotracheal tube. Once ventilation is established, the heart rate should be auscultated and if it is less than 100 bpm, PPV should be continued. If it is greater than 100 bpm and the infant is breathing spontaneously, color should be observed for central cyanosis. If present, 100% free flowing oxygen should be supplied. When meconium-stained amniotic fluid is noted or particulate meconium is suctioned from the mouth, the baby should be immediately intubated and suction applied to the endotracheal tube as it is withdrawn. The preceding steps should then be taken. It should be noted that the passage of meconium in utero is a sign of intrauterine asphyxia, and special vigilance is necessary in the delivery room and the nursery. It is important that a plan be in effect at *all* deliveries for how to deal with the need for endotracheal intubation of an infant born at risk of meconium aspiration. To be truly effective, the procedure must be performed in the first few seconds of life in situations in which the passage of meconium is before the first breath and often not anticipated.

Bag and Mask Ventilation

Apnea, gasping, or a heart rate less than 100 bpm is an absolute indication for PPV. In most situations, this can be provided initially by bag and mask ventilation, but to be effective a knowledge of the equipment and skill in its use is required. There are two types of bags used for infant PPV. One is the so-called anesthesia bag, which is composed of a flow-inflating bag with a gas inlet and a patient outlet to which the mask or endotracheal tube is attached. In addition, there should be a flow control valve and a pressure gauge. This type of anesthesia bag requires a tight seal with the face mask and an appropriate flow rate of gas into the bag and proper control of the flow control valve in order to maintain proper inflation of the bag. The advantages of this type of bag are that it assures a tight seal of the face mask, provides for the delivery of 100% oxygen or any amount dialed in at the blender, and permits any inflation pressure that would be required with the level monitored by the attached pressure gauge.

The second type of bag is the self-inflating bag, which returns to an inflated state after each positive pressure compression. The bag has an air inlet and an oxygen inlet at the end and a patient outlet on the front to which the mask or endotracheal tube is attached. The valve assembly is attached to this end. It opens to allow the air-oxygen mixture to enter when the bag is squeezed during inhalation and closes during exhalation to prevent the patient's rebreathing air that is expired into the bag. There is usually a pop-off valve set at about 30 to 35 cm H_2O, and on some models there is an attachment for a pressure gauge. Since most infants require 100% oxygen during resuscitation, an oxygen reservoir should be attached to the air inlet part to avoid drawing in room air, keeping the mixture at 100% oxygen or any other percentage supplied by the blender.

No matter which type of bag setup is used, it is always important to check each component of the equipment prior to its use. It also should be noted that free flowing oxygen can be given with the anesthesia bag, but the O_2-air mixture flows reliably in the self-inflating bag only during the short period that the bag is compressed.

It is essential that a tight seal be created with the face mask; therefore, a cushioned design is preferred because the rim conforms to the shape of the infant's face with less pressure and less chance of damaging the infant's eyes and face. An array of mask sizes should be available at each delivery.

Once the decision to provide PPV is made, a tight seal with the face mask should be assured and several inflations should be performed while observing for chest wall movement and having an assistant auscultate for breath sounds bilaterally. If it is decided to create an airway with an endotracheal tube, the procedure must be performed quickly by a skilled person. Since properly applied bag and mask ventilation can produce effective PPV, repeated and perhaps traumatic attempts at intubation should not be undertaken. Once proper inflation of the lung is assured, a ventilatory rate of 40 to 60 breaths/minute should be established. It is felt by some clinicians that the higher rate initially will blow off carbon dioxide and correct the respiratory acidosis and perhaps enhance dilatation of the pulmonary vasculature. The initial inflations of the lung may require a positive inspiratory pressure as high as 40 cm H_2O. When there is aspiration of amniotic fluid or poor pulmonary compliance from asphyxia, a level of 30 to 40 cm H_2O might need to be maintained until there is evidence of improvement. However, for most premature infants and term newborns without lung disease, an inflating pressure of 15 to 20 cm H_2O is usually sufficient for effective PPV. An orogastric tube should be inserted as soon as possible after establishing an effective ventilatory pattern in order to reduce distention of the stomach, which frequently occurs with bag and mask ventilation.

The failure to achieve good ventilation may be due to the following:

- Poor seal of face mask
- Incorrectly placed endotracheal tube
- Obstruction of airway from improper head position
- Presence of secretions in airway
- Need for higher inflating pressure
- Excessive air in the stomach

PPV can be discontinued when the heart rate has stabilized at greater than 100 bpm and respirations are spontaneous and regular. Free flowing oxygen should be continued until there is no longer central cyanosis.

Chest Compressions

The heart rate will improve in most situations of bradycardia in the delivery room when effective PPV with 100% oxygen is provided. However, if after 15 to 30 seconds of PPV, the heart rate remains low, there is clinical evidence of severe impairment of myocardial contractility produced by the intrauterine asphyxia. When the heart rate is less than 60 bpm or remains at 60 to 80 bpm without increasing, cardiac compressions should be initiated in order to maintain an adequate circulation and thereby prevent ongoing acidosis and tissue hypoxia. The procedure involves two, and ideally three, individuals—one to continue PPV by either mask or endotracheal tube, another to perform the chest compressions, and a third person to monitor the strength and rate of the pulse, auscultate the heart rate and breath sounds, and prepare and administer medications if they are needed as the resuscitation continues.

The technique of chest compression for the newborn (and infant up to about 1 year of age) involves two approaches, depending upon the size of the infant in relation to the size of the hands of the operator. The initial step is to locate the position at the lower third of the sternum at which the pressure will be applied. This can be most practically identified by drawing an imaginary line connecting the nipples and placing the area for compression on the sternum just below that line but above the xyphoid.[7] The first technique involves encircling the hands around the thorax and placing the thumbs such that the sternum is depressed about 0.5 to 0.75 in. The pressure should be well localized to the lower third of the sternum and care should be taken to avoid squeezing the ribs, which makes the process less effective and runs the risk of fracturing ribs and perhaps producing a pneumothorax. The second technique involves applying pressure on the lower third of the sternum with the tips of the index and middle fingers. The fingers should be perpendicular to the sternum in order for the technique to be both efficacious and safe. Care should be taken to keep the fingertips on the sternum and avoid a bouncing or stabbing type of motion. The other hand should support the infant's back so that the heart is most effectively compressed between the sternum and the spine. The rate of chest compression should be about 120/minute. An assistant should palpate the right axillary artery pulse to evaluate the effectiveness and rate of cardiac "activity" produced by the chest compressions. When the spontaneous heart rate is greater than 80 bpm and the peripheral pulse is full, chest compression can be stopped, but PPV should be continued until the heart rate remains steady at greater than 100 bpm.

Endotracheal Intubation

The insertion of an endotracheal tube is a procedure that requires eye-hand coordination and cannot be taught by a textbook. However, the indications, equipment, and comments about teaching the technique can be discussed. During the initial stages of resuscitation in the delivery room, PPV can be achieved effectively for most infants using bag and mask ventilation.[8] However, endotracheal intubation is required in the following situations:

- Tracheal suctioning of meconium
- Suspected diaphragmatic hernia
- Bag and mask ventilation is ineffective
- Prolonged mechanical ventilation needed

The frequency with which these conditions occur makes it mandatory that every hospital's delivery room have all the necessary equipment for endotracheal intubation readily available, as well as the personnel skilled in performing the procedure.

The equipment and supplies needed for all endotracheal intubations include the following:

- Laryngoscopes with extra bulbs and batteries
- No. 0 (preterm) and No. 1 (term) straight blades
- Endotracheal tubes (uniform diameter): sizes 2.5-mm, 3.0-mm, 3.5-mm, and 4.0-mm internal diameter
- Stylet

The following should be immediately available:

- Suction catheter
- Bag and mask with adapter for attachment to endotracheal tube
- Scissors
- Adhesive tape

Prior to performing the intubation, a series of preparatory steps should be taken. The correct-sized endotracheal tube should be selected based on the guide provided in Table 6–1.

When the appropriate-sized tube is selected, it should be shortened to 13 cm in length, and the endotracheal tube connector should be replaced. Most of the tubes currently manufactured are of relatively firm consistency and have a natural curve. However, some operators prefer the rigidity and curvature provided by a stylet. Care must be taken to assure that the tip does not protrude beyond the end of the endotracheal tube and that the stylet is secured in place so that it does not advance during intubation. The appropriate laryngoscope blade should be attached, and the light bulb should be checked. It is also helpful to have the suction catheter attached to the vacuum regulator and strips of adhesive tape readily available to the person performing the intubation. The bag and mask apparatus should also be immediately available for connection to the endotracheal tube and for test ventilations to observe chest wall

Table 6–1. CHOOSING THE CORRECT-SIZED ENDOTRACHEAL TUBE

Tube Size (Internal Diameter [mm])	Infant's Weight	Gestational Age
2.5	<1000 g	<28 wk
3.0	1000–2000 g	28–34 wk
3.5	2000–3000 g	34–38 wk
3.5–4.0	>3000 g	>38 wk

movement and auscultate air entry. A major feature of learning and performing endotracheal intubation is the ability to recognize the key anatomic landmarks:

- Base of tongue
- Epiglottis
- Vocal cords
- Esophagus

The next step in the learning process is a knowledge of the relationship of the laryngoscope's blade tip to those anatomic structures. Finally, it is necessary to know the corrective maneuvers to take in order to visualize the glottis and place the endotracheal tube in the correct position.[6]

The performance of endotracheal intubation in the newborn is a two-person procedure. The operator checks the equipment and performs the intubation. The assistant arranges the supplies, assists in suctioning the airway, auscultates the heart rate and breath sounds, provides free flowing oxygen during intubation and bag and mask ventilation prior to and after intubation attempts, and can sometimes assist in bringing the glottis into view by putting light pressure on the neck over the larynx. If the airway is not successfully intubated within 20 seconds, or if severe bradycardia develops, the procedure should be stopped and ventilation provided by bag and mask until the infant's condition is stabilized. Correct position of the endotracheal tube should be confirmed by observation of symmetric chest wall movement and auscultation of the chest for bilateral air entry and over the stomach for lack of air flow there.

When meconium is present, the endotracheal intubation should be performed immediately after suctioning the meconium from the mouth, which should preferably be done by the obstetrician at the time the head is delivered. When the endotracheal tube is properly placed, it should be attached to a wall suction plastic adapter that connects directly to the endotracheal tube connector. Suction is applied continuously as the endotracheal tube is steadily withdrawn. This procedure can be repeated judiciously until the trachea appears to have been cleared.

Medications

Most delivery room resuscitations do not progress to the point that medications are required. When they are needed, however, it is important that each member of the resuscitation team be well versed in the protocol for the drugs to be used, the sequence in which they are to be administered, and the concentration, dosage, and preparation of each drug, as well as the route of administration. At the Emergency Cardiac Care conference of the American Heart Association in 1985, new standards for medications to be used in neonatal resuscitation were elucidated.[4] Epinephrine became the first-line drug when PPV and cardiac compression failed to produce effective myocardial function. The use of sodium bicarbonate is deferred until there is evidence of metabolic acidosis and PPV has been well established. This is because the chemical breakdown of sodium bicarbonate results in CO_2 and water. The CO_2 is readily diffusible across cell membranes and the blood-brain barrier and will cause a tissue acidosis even though the hydrogen ions in the blood are being buffered. This paradoxic action of sodium bicarbonate is particularly enhanced when it is administered in the early stages of resuscitation before adequate PPV has been established[9] (see also Chapter 5). In addition, the high osmolality of the sodium bicarbonate solution has been implicated as one cause of intracranial hemorrhage and cerebral edema in premature and asphyxiated newborns. Volume expanders are advised for use only in situations in which there is evidence of reduced circulating blood volume from hemorrhage or other causes. Many cases of hypotension in the newborn at the time of delivery are thought to be secondary to the effects of asphyxia on myocardial function. Additional volume under that condition could put a further load on an already failing heart. Dopamine has been recommended as an adrenergic agent that will improve cardiac output and renal perfusion during the transition from acute resuscitation to stabilization of the asphyxiated infant. Naloxone remains a drug of choice because of its efficacy in reversing respiratory depression secondary to the administration of a narcotic medication to the mother during labor. It has a low level of toxicity but should not be administered to infants of narcotic-addicted mothers because of the risk of inducing withdrawal seizures. The algorithm for administration of medications is shown in Figure 6–1.

Atropine is no longer recommended for use in neonatal resuscitation because it increases the heart rate by its parasympatholytic effects without producing a concomitant improvement in myocardial contractility. This results in a greater oxygen consumption by the myocardium without enhanced cardiac output and coronary blood flow. Calcium and glucose are also no longer recommended as resuscitation drugs for the newborn. They should be used only as supplements when serum calcium and glucose levels are abnormally low.

The recommended route of administration of medications in the delivery room is via an umbilical vein catheter placed a few centimeters below skin level. However, endotracheal instillation of epinephrine is recommended, rather than the highly dangerous intracardiac injections.[10] This route can also be used for naloxone. Unfortunately, there have been no large scale studies of the pharmacokinetics of this form of drug administration in different clinical conditions of the newborn.

The concentration, dosage, route of administration, and precautions for the medications for neonatal resuscitation are summarized in Figure 6–2.

Special Considerations

The most common conditions requiring resuscitation in the delivery room are prematurity, asphyxia, meconium aspiration, and respiratory depression. However, there are a few other conditions that require special diagnostic alertness and therapeutic action.

Medications
Epinephrine
Volume Expander
Sodium
  Bicarbonate

Dopamine

Naloxone
Hydrochloride

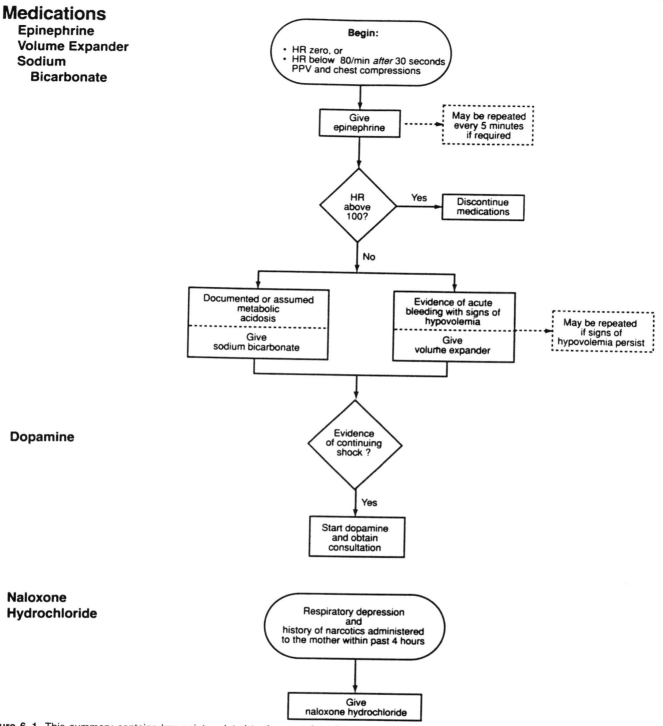

Figure 6–1. This summary contains key points related to the use of medications during neonatal resuscitation. (From Textbook of Neonatal Resuscitation, © 1987, 1990, American Heart Association. By permission of the American Heart Association, Inc.)

Diaphragmatic Hernia

The chief clinical features of diaphragmatic hernia are a depressed (scaphoid) abdomen because of the lack of a hemidiaphragm and the migration of the abdominal organs into the thorax. Upon recognizing these features, it is important to immediately insert an endotracheal tube as well as a nasogastric catheter to prevent disten-tion of the bowel located in the chest, which if air-filled could compress the normal lung as well as the mediastinal structures.

Choanal Atresia

At the time of initial suctioning in all babies it is important to be aware of the patency of both nostrils.

Medications for Neonatal Resuscitation

Medication	Concentration to Administer	Preparation	Dosage/ Route*	Total Dose/Infant			Rate/Precautions
Epinephrine	1:10,000	1 mL	0.1–0.3 mL/kg I.V. or E.T.	**weight** 1 kg 2 kg 3 kg 4 kg		**total mL's** 0.1– 0.3 mL 0.2– 0.6 mL 0.3– 0.9 mL 0.4– 1.2 mL	Give rapidly
Volume Expanders	Whole Blood 5% Albumin Normal Saline Ringer's Lactate	40 mL	10 mL/kg I.V.	**weight** 1 kg 2 kg 3 kg 4 kg		**total mL's** 10 mL 20 mL 30 mL 40 mL	Give over 5–10 min
Sodium Bicarbonate	0.5 mEq/mL (4.2% solution)	20 mL or two 10-mL prefilled syringes	2 mEq/kg I.V.	**weight** 1 kg 2 kg 3 kg 4 kg	**total dose** 2 mEq 4 mEq 6 mEq 8 mEq	**total mL's** 4 mL 8 mL 12 mL 16 mL	Give *slowly*, over at least 2 min Give only if infant being effectively ventilated
Naloxone	0.4 mg/mL	1 mL	0.1 mg/kg (0.25 mL/kg) I.V., E.T., I.M., S.Q.	**weight** 1 kg 2 kg 3 kg 4 kg	**total dose** 0.1 mg 0.2 mg 0.3 mg 0.4 mg	**total mL's** 0.25 mL 0.50 mL 0.75 mL 1.00 mL	Give rapidly I.V., E.T. preferred I.M., S.Q. acceptable
	1.0 mg/mL	1 mL	0.1 mg/kg (0.1 mL/kg) I.V., E.T., I.M., S.Q.	1 kg 2 kg 3 kg 4 kg	0.1 mg 0.2 mg 0.3 mg 0.4 mg	0.1 mL 0.2 mL 0.3 mL 0.4 mL	
Dopamine	$6 \times \dfrac{\text{weight (kg)} \times \text{desired dose (mcg/kg/min)}}{\text{desired fluid (mL/hr)}} = $ mg of dopamine per 100 mL of solution		Begin at 5 mcg/kg/min (may increase to 20 mcg/kg/min if necessary) I.V.	**weight** 1 kg 2 kg 3 kg 4 kg		**total mcg/min** 5–20 mcg/min 10–40 mcg/min 15–60 mcg/min 20–80 mcg/min	Give as a continuous infusion using an infusion pump Monitor HR and BP closely Seek consultation

From: *Textbook of Neonatal Resuscitation*
© 1987, 1990 American Heart Association   *I.M. — Intramuscular; E.T. — Endotracheal; I.V. — Intravenous; S.Q. — Subcutaneous

Figure 6–2. Medications for neonatal resuscitation. I.M. = intramuscular; E.T. = endotracheal; I.V. = intravenous; S.Q. = subcutaneous. (From Textbook of Neonatal Resuscitation, © 1987, 1990, American Heart Association. By permission of the American Heart Association, Inc.)

If the passage of the catheter is obstructed on one or both sides, the tentative diagnosis of choanal atresia should be made, and an oral airway immediately inserted. This may later be replaced by an endotracheal tube when the diagnosis is confirmed and surgery is to be performed.

Pierre-Robin Syndrome

This is a congenital anomaly in which the growth of the mandible is delayed but the tongue is of normal size. Because of the small jaw, the tongue is pushed against the posterior pharynx, causing obstruction of the

Table 6–2. STEPS IN NEONATAL RESUSCITATION

Evaluation	Decision	Action
Respiratory effort	Regular respirations	Observe
	Apnea, gasping	PPV*
Heart rate	>100 bpm	Observe
	<100 bpm	PPV
	60–100 bpm and increasing	PPV
	60–80 bpm and not increasing	PPV and chest compression
	<60 bpm	PPV and chest compression
Color	Pink or peripheral cyanosis	Observe
	Central cyanosis	Provide oxygen

*PPV = positive pressure ventilation.

airway. The tongue needs to be pushed out of the way by an oral airway. If this does not immediately relieve the respiratory difficulties, an endotracheal tube should be inserted to provide a patent airway until further definitive action can be taken.

SUMMARY

The systematic approach to neonatal resuscitation begins with the cycle (Table 6–2):

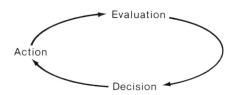

By keeping the decision-making process to a few clear-cut alternatives, all members of the team can anticipate the next step and assist each other in helping the baby through a smoothly run and effective resuscitation. This algorithm is presented in Figure 6–3.

The current approach to a rational therapeutic protocol for neonatal resuscitation has been greatly simplified into the following choices:

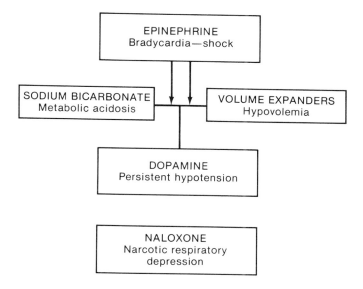

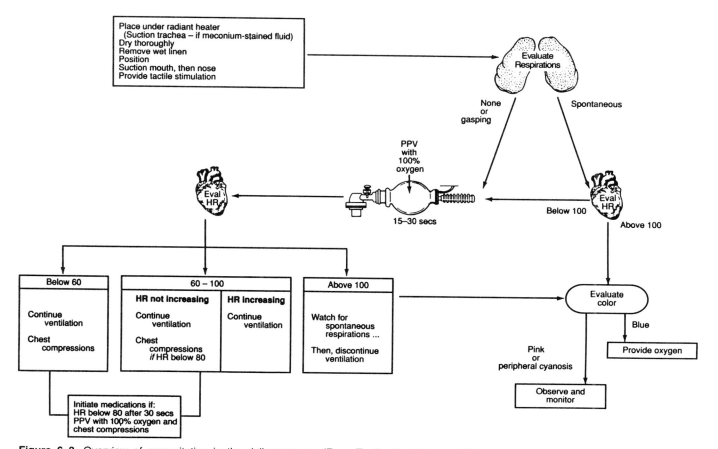

Figure 6–3. Overview of resuscitation in the delivery room. (From Textbook of Neonatal Resuscitation, © 1987, 1990, American Heart Association. By permission of the American Heart Association, Inc.)

Although the choices of resuscitation medications are now more limited, the clinical judgment as to when hypovolemia or metabolic acidosis is present, without the benefit of invasive measures, remains a difficult one. It represents the best possible decision in an environment of urgency and uncertainty and cannot be defined by textbooks or dictated by standards of care.

There remains a large void in the scientific basis upon which more clear-cut therapeutic protocols for neonatal resuscitation should be based. Well-designed, randomized, large scale clinical trials that systematically compare therapies currently in use or of potential benefit to the critically ill newborn are greatly needed.[1] Since these therapies need to be provided in an emergency setting, the incorporation of well-defined protocols into settings that have ongoing data management systems would provide a relatively low cost—high yield means for assembling this important clinical information on a large number of infants. However, a priority must be created for supporting the organization and implementation of such multicenter collaborative studies to provide the best means of giving life support for the infant at risk.

Another area of ongoing uncertainty involves both the clinical and ethical parameters that define when resuscitation should not be provided or should be discontinued.[11] Many critically ill or extremely premature infants are born with little warning and to be effective, their resuscitation must be initiated within seconds. This situation provides the setting for serious ethical problems that can have lifelong consequences. Until more precise prognostic indicators are available, the clinician is best guided by the following ethical imperatives: (1) provide care based on benefit to the patient; (2) when in doubt, support life; (3) provide full intensive care while there is life—avoid prolonging the process of dying; (4) avoid using "possibilities" of adverse long-term outcomes as a basis for making decisions about immediate life-threatening situations that are usually responsive to emergency measures (see also Chapter 92).

A large agenda of problems remain to be addressed in this critical area of medicine. Hopefully, clearer insight will emerge as we approach the next millennium.

References

1. Stevenson DK, Frankel LR, and Benitz WE: Immediate management of the asphyxiated infant: Facilitating the cardiorespiratory transition from fetus to newborn. J Perinatol 7(3):221, 1987.
2. Woods JR, Jr: Birth asphyxia: Pathophysiologic events and fetal adaptive changes. Clin Perinatol 10(2):473, 1983.
3. American Academy of Pediatrics–American College of Obstetricians and Gynecologists: Guidelines of Perinatal Care. Chicago, American Academy of Pediatrics, 1989.
4. Standards and Guidelines for Cardiopulmonary Resuscitation (CPR) and Emergency Cardiac Care (ECC). JAMA 255(21):2905, 1986.
5. Schubring C: Temperature regulation in healthy and resuscitated newborns immediately after birth. J Perinatol Med 14(1):27, 1986.
6. American Heart Association–American Academy of Pediatrics: Textbook of Neonatal Resuscitation. Dallas, 1990.
7. Phillips GW and Zideman DA: Relation of infant heart to sternum: Its significance in cardiopulmonary resuscitation. Lancet 1(8488):1024, 1986.
8. Lissauer TJ and Steer PJ: The relation between the need for intubation at birth, abnormal cardiotocograms in labor and cord artery blood gas and pH values. Br J Obstet Gynaecol 93(10):1060, 1986.
9. Zaritsky A: Drug therapy of cardiopulmonary resuscitation in children. Drugs 37(3):356, 1989.
10. Lindemann R: Resuscitation of the newborn. Endotracheal administration of epinephrine. Acta Paediatr Scand 73(2):210, 1984.
11. Lantos JD, Miles SH, Silverstein MD, et al: Survival after cardiopulmonary resuscitation in babies of very low birthweight: Is CPR futile therapy? N Engl J Med 318(2):91, 1988.

Resuscitation of the Child

James H. McCrory, M.D., and Craig E. Downs, D.O.

The death of a child is a deeply disturbing event that can be felt throughout an entire community. As clinicians, it reminds us of the fragility of childhood, of the importance of families, and of our limitations as therapists. At the same time, it challenges us to expand our capabilities in reducing childhood illnesses and injury.

Assuming responsibility for the resuscitation of a child is a complex and often frustrating task. It involves not only the selection and sequencing of medical interventions but also multiple humanistic, ethical, educational, and legal considerations. The care of the child has to be individualized and balanced with the needs and expectations of the family, as well as with the expertise of the medical staff. Advanced training of the latter is necessary for rapid deployment and collaboration during the critical period. When successful, resuscitation leads to reanimation of the whole child and to recovery of many years of meaningful life. When unsuccessful, attention must instead be focused on the needs of the family in dealing with a poor outcome, resulting in either the death of their child or survival with profound impairment.

Infant and childhood mortality data reveal the scope of the problem. In the United States in 1988, there were 3,909,510 births and 38,910 deaths in children less than 1 year of age, so that the infant mortality rate was 10 deaths/1,000 live births (995.3 deaths/100,000 live births).[1] Two thirds of these deaths occurred in the first 28 days of life. In addition, 7,429 deaths took place in children between 1 and 4 years of age, 4,357 deaths occurred in children between 5 and 9 years of age, and 4,568 deaths occurred in children between 10 and 14 years of age, so that there were 55,264 deaths before the age of 15 years.

Traditionally, death has been defined as the permanent cessation of cardiopulmonary function. After the onset of apnea and pulselessness, however, there is a brief period before hypoxia and ischemia cause permanent disruption of cellular metabolism. Once cellular injury cascades to a point of irreversibility, either an immediate or delayed death occurs. In the former, resuscitative efforts are unable to re-establish spontaneous circulation. In the latter, perfusion is temporarily restored, but critical dysfunction of one or more organ systems precludes recovery. The pattern of ensuing complications varies and reflects the pattern of hypoxic-ischemic damage sustained. In these situations, the clinical manifestations can include recurrent cardiac arrests, anoxic encephalopathy with profound cortical impairment or brain death, acute pulmonary injury, disseminated intravascular coagulation, anasarca, acute tubular necrosis, hepatic failure, intestinal necrosis, sepsis, and multiple organ failure.

The primary goal of resuscitation is to restore spontaneous circulation before this point of irreversibility is reached. Secondary attention is then shifted to diagnosing and treating the underlying cause and to predicting and enhancing the degree of neurologic recovery. Efforts at cerebral resuscitation, however, have been disappointing[2-6] and underscore the importance of anticipating and preventing the arrest when possible in order to eliminate subsequent hypoxic-ischemic damage.

Over the past 2 decades, emergency medical services in the United States have begun evolving to meet the needs of the child in arrest or impending arrest. Changes include the training of lay people in basic life support, the establishment of 911 and other systems for rapid communication, the development of prehospital care by paramedic services, the staffing of adult and pediatric emergency departments, the development of air transport and hospital-to-hospital referral networks, and the regionalization of pediatric intensive care units. Some selective results have been encouraging. Two studies on submersion injuries have shown good neurologic recovery in 72% and 67%, respectively, in the subset of children who survived after receiving life support in the field.[7, 8] The prognosis is still poor, however, for out-of-hospital arrests in children who, upon arrival to the emergency department, require cardiac massage,[9] cardiotonic medications,[7] or greater than 25 minutes of cardiopulmonary resuscitation.[8]

CARDIOPULMONARY RESUSCITATION

Changes in skin color, loss of consciousness, apnea, and pulselessness are the obvious signs of cardiopulmonary arrest. Electrocardiographic monitoring reveals a terminal rhythm: asystole, ventricular fibrillation, electrical mechanical dissociation, or wide idioventricular complexes.

Maintenance of oxygen delivery to both the myocardium and the central nervous system begins with basic life support, which can be initiated by a bystander without any equipment. After establishing unresponsiveness and calling for help, two slow breaths are given while observing for chest rise. Lack of chest rise indicates either air leakage from a poor seal or airway obstruction. The head is repositioned using a chin lift and a head tilt in order to relieve obstruction caused by prolapse of the tongue and soft tissue into the hypopharynx. Hyperextension of the head is avoided because it collapses the trachea near the cricoid ring, which is the narrowest portion of an infant's airway.

Failure to obtain chest rise after proper head repositioning and repeated ventilation with a tight seal indicates obstruction from a foreign body. If the patient is not breathing spontaneously, an artificial cough can be produced in order to expel the object. Heimlich's maneuver consists of quick upward abdominal thrusts made by a fisted hand placed just above the umbilicus and covered by the other hand. In some cases, as many as 8 to 12 thrusts have been reported before the object was expelled. When the patient is less than 1 year old, there has been concern that this procedure may produce hepatosplenic injury. In this age group, the American Heart Association recommends four back blows, followed by four chest thrusts if necessary.[10] In a medical setting, however, direct laryngoscopy with removal of the object using Magill's forceps may be the more appropriate approach.

Once chest rise is observed, carotid pulses in adults or brachial pulses in infants are checked. If they are lacking, chest compressions deep enough to generate a pulse are begun with a 5:1 ratio of compression: ventilation, at a rate of 80 to 100/min in adults and children and 100 to 120/min in newborns.

Mouth-to-mouth ventilations deliver an FiO$_2$ of 15 to 18%. Closed chest compressions can produce a cardiac output of 15 to 20% of normal. When these basic maneuvers fail to restore spontaneous circulation, advanced life support techniques are indicated. The main goal of most interventions is increased oxygen delivery to the myocardium. Coronary blood flow is determined by the coronary perfusion pressure, which is the difference between the systemic mean arterial pressure and the central venous pressure.

In an arrest state, increasing systemic vascular resistance improves coronary perfusion, albeit at the expense of oxygen delivery to peripheral tissues. α-Adrenergic agonists have been traditionally used for this purpose. Redding showed that pure α agents, such as methoxamine and phenylephrine, are as effective as epinephrine in restoring spontaneous circulation after cardiac arrest from anoxia, whereas isoproterenol is ineffective.[11] The implication is that the primary importance of epinephrine in an arrest is its α effect, not its β$_1$ effect of enhancing contractility and dromotropism.

In regard to coronary perfusion, removal of carbon dioxide is equal in importance to delivery of oxygen. Recent studies of pH and PcO$_2$ in coronary venous blood and within the myocardium during an arrest have shown the initial acidosis to be primarily respiratory.[12] Formerly, it was thought that rapidly correcting meta-

bolic acidosis would lead to an improvement in contractility. Now it is thought that administration of sodium bicarbonate to tissues in which PcO$_2$ is not adequately removed worsens intramyocardial acidosis and further depresses activity. Hence, the role of sodium bicarbonate in resuscitation has become controversial.[13]

Failure to regain spontaneous circulation after adequate ventilation and oxygenation with an FiO$_2$ of 100% through an endotracheal tube and after standard administration of epinephrine leads to a reassessment to look for both respiratory and circulatory complications. Important complications of intubation and positive-pressure ventilation include obstruction by mucous plug, tube displacement into the esophagus or right mainstem bronchus, and tension pneumothorax. Circulatory complications can include cardiac tamponade, fine ventricular fibrillation, and electrical mechanical dissociation.

The presence of chest rise and breath sounds eliminates the possibility of esophageal intubation and mucous plug causing total obstruction in most patients. In young infants, however, insufflation of the esophagus can produce both a chest rise and transmitted breath sounds so that direct laryngoscopy is often necessary to reaffirm the proper position of the endotracheal tube. If there is still no improvement, needle thoracentesis of the right and left sides of the chest rapidly rules out tension pneumothorax as the cause. If there is still no improvement, a needle pericardiocentesis can exclude cardiac tamponade as the reason for lack of spontaneous circulation.

If the problem is fine ventricular fibrillation that is resistant to defibrillation attempts, consideration is given to the use of epinephrine to convert the pattern from fine to coarse. Bretylium administration is also considered. For asystole, some consultants recommend a trial of defibrillation to rule out fine ventricular fibrillation masquerading as asystole. If electrical mechanical dissociation is present, the problem is probably end-stage myocardial anoxia, but treatable causes such as hypovolemia and cardiac tamponade also need to be considered.

Table 7–1 lists 31 standard interventions used in

Table 7–1. STANDARD INTERVENTIONS

Airway	Circulation
Head tilt	Chest compressions
Chin lift	Oxygen
Jaw thrust	Trendelenburg positioning
Abdominal compressions	Electrocardiographic monitoring
Back blows	Vascular access:
Finger sweeps	Peripheral
Pharyngeal suctioning	Central
Nasopharyngeal airway	Intraosseous
Oropharyngeal airway	Volume expansion
Endotracheal intubation	Inotropic agents
Needle cricothyrotomy	Chronotropic agents
	Dromotropic agents
Breathing	Afterload modulators
	Acid-base buffers
Mouth-to-mouth	Calcium-potassium balance
Mouth-to-face mask	Cardioversion-defibrillation
Bag-valve-mask device	Pericardiocentesis
Mechanical ventilation	
Thoracentesis	

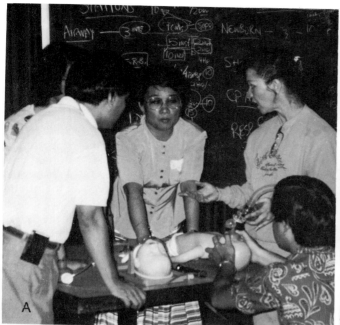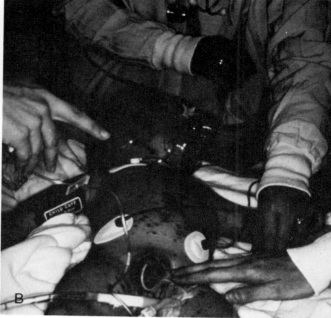

Figure 7–1. *A,* Mock arrests are useful in training personnel in cooperative decision-making and are designed to simulate critical situations. The dominant person, who assumes leadership and initiates action in each of the groups, can be recognized by authoritative hand gestures. *B,* The quiet contributions of others are also noticeable in maintaining the airway, in assessing oxygenation and ventilation continuously, in diagnosing shock by monitoring pulses, and in eliciting and redirecting the leader's thoughts. (Photographs courtesy of Doug Campbell, Jose Martinez, Children's Hospital of Manila, and Lucian DeNicola.)

cardiopulmonary resuscitation. The process of arriving at these standards was one of consensus under the auspices of various national and international organizations. In the 1960s and 1970s, the American Heart Association assumed a leadership role in this area by providing a forum to review existing research and clinical experience every 6 years. The results are published as standards and guidelines.[10]

The value of this approach is in the codification and dissemination of existing knowledge about resuscitation. Critics readily point to the flaw in this methodology: Formulation of many of the standards is often arbitrary when there is no scientific data to guide the decision. Paradoxically, however, the controversy over such standards has generated much valuable clinical and laboratory research, which continues to change and modify the approaches taken to resuscitation.

MANAGING THE ARREST

In order for collaborative efforts to flow smoothly, forethought must be given to the refinement of group performance in critical situations. Division of the group into specific roles is important for the accomplishment of multiple tasks, but it heightens the need for communication of ideas and priorities. Sequencing is as important as selection when deciding which of the 31 standard interventions are needed. Once chosen, each intervention needs to be performed in an automatic, almost reflexive fashion.

Perseveration and delay can occur from faulty assessment, conflicting choices of intervention, unclarified

priorities, unfamiliarity with age-related variations in equipment sizes and medication dosages, and psychologic barriers in confronting a critically ill child. The dominant person in the group emerges either to begin the resuscitation or to encourage others to do so. Resolution of the preceding problems depends not only on the leader's personal knowledge but also on the leader's ability to elicit the group's knowledge and the group's ability to redirect the leader when necessary.

This interaction of technical and cognitive skills performed by a group requires preparation and practice. (Fig. 7–1). In the 1980s, educational advances were made in the evolution of two national courses: the Advanced Pediatric Life Support Course (APLS) and the Pediatric Advanced Life Support Course (PALS).[14–16] Both 2-day courses teach resuscitation skills but vary in areas of emphasis: the APLS course elaborates on the first 20 minutes of stabilization involved in multiple causes that lead to arrest (e.g., trauma, seizure, coma, diabetic ketoacidosis, poisonings, meningitis, asthma), whereas the PALS course stresses variations in the management of respiratory failure and shock as the two final common pathways leading to arrest. Despite the differences in content, both courses are changing the methodology of clinicians in their approach to critically ill children, as well as the methodology of teaching resuscitation in general.

RAPID CARDIOPULMONARY ASSESSMENT

To prevent childhood morbidity and mortality from impending arrests, the early signs and symptoms of respiratory failure and shock need to be recognized and appropriate supportive care initiated. The assessment begins with the initial inspection of the patient, followed by palpation of peripheral pulses and auscultation of breath sounds. This physiologically oriented examination precedes the usual documentation of vital signs. With practice, the 30 items listed in Table 7–2 can be evaluated in a matter of seconds.

Airway

The first priority in resuscitation is the airway, which must be open and stable, regardless of the cause of the underlying illness. The patency of the airway is primarily determined by the adequacy of ventilation and is categorized into one of three functional conditions: (1) normal, (2) maintainable by simple maneuvers, or (3) unmaintainable without intubation. Simple maneuvers include head or jaw positioning, suctioning, pharyngeal airways, and positive-pressure ventilation via bag-valve-mask devices. After each maneuver, the adequacy of ventilation must be reassessed before going on to the next step. If these simple maneuvers fail to provide sufficient ventilation, a rapid oral intubation should be performed by the person at the scene most skilled in management of pediatric airways.

Breathing

Under normal circumstances, chemoreceptors in the respiratory center stimulate a respiratory drive sufficient to maintain an arterial pressure of oxygen greater than 80 mm Hg, an arterial carbon dioxide pressure close to 40 mm Hg, and a pH close to 7.4. This balance is accomplished by modulating the respiratory rate and the tidal volume.

Clinically, oxygenation is assessed by the color of skin and mucous membranes, whereas ventilation is assessed by chest rise, inspiratory breath sounds, and respiratory drive. When ventilation is being assisted, mild hyperventilation produces apnea, which signifies the moment at which the hypercapnic drive is lost. An arterial blood gas measurement performed at this time usually reveals a P_{CO_2} of 33 to 34 mm Hg, unless there is an underlying metabolic acidosis, hypoxemia, or reason for central nervous system hyperventilation.

Circulation

Clinically, perfusion is assessed by evaluating the skin, central nervous system, extremities, urinary output, and cardiovascular system. In regard to the latter, palpation of peripheral pulses rapidly gives information about heart rate, rhythm, stroke volume, blood pressure, and systemic vascular resistance. In low–cardiac output states, poor capillary refill and lack of peripheral pulses indicate diminished stroke volume. These signs precede hypotension, which occurs late in infants and children in shock.

Perfusion is directly related to cardiac output, which equals the heart rate times the stroke volume. Physiologically, the main determinants of stroke volume are preload, contractility, and afterload. Medically, improvement of the cardiac output is achieved by modulating heart rate, preload, afterload, and contractility.

Delivery of Oxygen to Tissues

Oxygen delivery from the atmosphere to the mitochondria for the production of high-energy phosphates is a complex sequence of events. It involves ventilation, diffusion, hemoglobin, cardiac output, metabolic rate, and numerous other factors. Mathematically, oxygen delivery is expressed as the product of the content of arterial oxygen and cardiac output. Respiratory failure, anemia, and problems with hemoglobin dissociation lower the content of arterial oxygen. Shock lowers cardiac output.

Clinically, problems with oxygen delivery are most prominent in signs involving the skin, central nervous system, and muscle tone. In regard to skin color, pink areas indicate good perfusion with saturated hemoglobin, pallor indicates ischemia or anemia, and cyanosis indicates the presence of desaturated hemoglobin from either hypoxemia or increased extraction in a low-flow state. Mottling represents all of these processes occurring at once and changes in pattern as the capillary beds open and close.

Analogous to the variability of mottling over time are the changes in mental status observed as cortical perfusion deteriorates: The infant's responses change from

Table 7–2. RAPID CARDIOPULMONARY ASSESSMENT

Airway	Delivery of Oxygen to Tissues
Normal	
Maintainable	Central nervous system
by simple maneuvers	Recognizes parents
Unmaintainable—	No recognition
intubation required	Combative
Breathing	Withdraws from pain
	Posturing
Work of breathing	No response to pain
Normal	Fluctuating level of
Increased	consciousness and
Decreased	responsiveness
Chest rise–inspiratory	Skin
breath sounds	Pink
Normal	Blue
Diminished	Pale
Lacking	Mottled
Circulation	Muscles
	Normal tone
Palpation of peripheral pulses	Flaccid
Bounding	
Normal	
Diminished	
Lacking	
Capillary refill	
<2 sec	
>2 sec	
Toe temperature	
Warm	
Cold	

being alert, to not recognizing parents, to being combative, to being unresponsive to pain. There is a danger of underdiagnosing early shock if the clinician becomes falsely reassured by the child's best neurologic response and ignores the significance of the fluctuating level of consciousness. Instead, intermittent intervals of failure to respond to venipuncture and other painful procedures can alert the clinician to the poor status of cerebral blood flow.

Muscle tone becomes affected both by poor oxygen delivery to the muscles and by central nervous system depression. The child's general appearance is one of prostration with minimal movement and an apathetic facies. With time, hypotonia progresses to flaccidity.

ESTABLISHMENT OF PRIORITIES

The rapid cardiopulmonary assessment leads to placement of the patient into one of the following six physiologic categories: (1) stable, (2) early respiratory failure, (3) late respiratory failure, (4) normotensive shock, (5) hypotensive shock, or (6) cardiopulmonary failure (Fig. 7–2). The diagnostic work-up of a stable patient can proceed in a leisurely fashion, but supportive care must precede definitive diagnosis and therapy in the unstable patient. Selection and timing of the initial interventions depend upon the nature and degree of the physiologic instability.

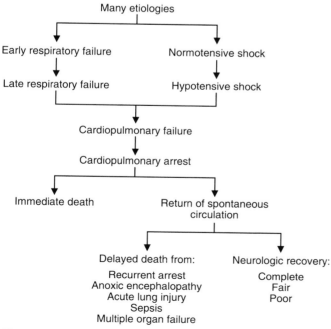

PATHOPHYSIOLOGY OF PEDIATRIC ARRESTS:
THE FINAL COMMON PATHWAYS

Figure 7–2. Recognition of the child in impending arrest depends on the rapid cardiopulmonary assessment (see Table 7–2), whereas the selection and sequencing of interventions (see Table 7–1) depends on the physiologic categories listed above.

Respiratory Failure

Alterations in airway and breathing lead to failure in oxygenation and ventilation. Clinically, respiratory failure is easy to recognize when visible changes in mental status and the effort of breathing occur. In early respiratory failure from pulmonary or neuromuscular diseases, the patient is alert and anxious. There is an increased effort of breathing, as evidenced by flaring, retractions, and use of accessory muscles. In late respiratory failure, hypoxemia and hypercapnia produce central nervous system depression, resulting in failure to recognize parents, loss of head control, poor muscle tone, and loss of consciousness.

The approach to the patient is determined by the rapid assessment. In early respiratory failure, it is important to respect the child's position of comfort and to maintain the comfort of parental contact. The approach to the patient should minimize or eliminate additional burdens of stress, including separation from parents, taking of rectal temperatures, and the performance of oral examinations, venipunctures, and radiographic procedures. Increased FiO_2 is administered in a manner acceptable to the child. Transcutaneous pulse oximetry provides a rapid, noninvasive method of quantifying oxygenation and can be used to help titrate the amount of FiO_2 necessary to correct hypoxemia. Oral intake should be restricted to minimize the risk of aspiration, particularly if the child may later need intubation. The stress of hypothermia or hyperthermia must be avoided. Finally, in late respiratory failure, the parent and child are separated when the child no longer recognizes the parent and invasive procedures are indicated to re-establish normal oxygenation and ventilation.

Once the child is stabilized, further therapy is directed by specific physiologic, etiologic, and anatomic considerations. Arterial blood gas determinations not only confirm the diagnosis of respiratory failure but also further define the primary problem in terms of oxygenation, ventilation, acid-base balance, carboxyhemoglobinemia, or methemoglobinemia, or combinations of these conditions. Infectious, congenital, congestive, allergic, traumatic, metabolic, iatrogenic, and chronic causes need to be considered. Anatomically, the primary problem may originate in the central nervous system, neuromuscular apparatus, or pulmonary tract.

Shock

Shock is the failure of the cardiovascular system to perfuse the other organ systems. Low cardiac output results in decreased delivery of oxygen and glucose to the tissues and in the accumulation of toxic waste products, particularly carbon dioxide and hydrogen ions. Despite low cardiac output, blood pressure can remain normal in the early phases of shock because of an increase in systemic vascular resistance.

Early diagnosis of normotensive shock in children depends on recognizing signs of poor perfusion of the skin, central nervous system, and muscles. Hemodynamically, tachycardia is a compensatory mechanism for diminished stroke volume from hypovolemia and loss of preload. Other signs of a decreased stroke volume include loss of peripheral pulses, prolonged time of capillary refill, and cool extremities. Weil has pointed out the correlation between cardiac output and extremity temperature, but the prognostic significance of this finding was also well known to his mentor, Hippocrates: Εν τοισιν οξεσι νουσημασι ψυξισ ακρωτηριων κακον. ("In acute diseases, coldness of the extremities is bad.").[17]

When hypotension does occur, it is a late and often premorbid sign. In one series, the mortality rate for septic shock with hypotension was 55%.[18, 19] Regardless of cause, the hemodynamics of the hypotensive phase of shock are similar.[20] The interventions chosen to restore perfusion, however, are dependent upon the causes and mechanisms responsible for producing the low cardiac output state. Volume expansion to restore preload and ventricular filling are important in circumstances involving an absolute or relative hypovolemia. Such causes point to abnormal fluid losses or distribution problems, respectively. Vasoactive infusions, in contrast, are selected in cardiogenic forms of shock in order to modulate contractility, heart rate, or afterload (see also Chapters 11 and 12).

The priorities in shock are strikingly different from those in respiratory failure. Vascular access is of primary importance, whether the initial therapy is volume expansion or vasoactive infusions. When percutaneous peripheral access is not readily attainable, the three safest alternatives are intraosseous needle, percutaneous catheterization of the femoral vein, and cutdown of the lower saphenous vein. In more experienced hands, consideration can be given to percutaneous cannulation of internal jugular or subclavian veins, with the concomitant risks of hemothorax and pneumothorax.

The timing and amount of volume expander administered are critical in order to re-establish perfusion before irreversible tissue ischemia occurs. Aliquots of 10 to 20 ml/kg can be safely given over 1 to 5 minutes in most patients, with two important exceptions: patients in cardiogenic shock and premature infants at risk for intraventricular hemorrhage.

Response to volume expansion is assessed immediately. Improvements in heart rate, blood pressure, and peripheral pulses are important initial responses, but continued volume expansion is necessary until improvement in perfusion of the central nervous system, skin, and kidneys is also observed. This may require 60 to 100 ml/kg or more over a brief period. Concern for the risk of fluid overload has to be balanced with concern for the risk of death from hypoperfusion: pulmonary edema is readily manageable, whereas multiple organ failure is often fatal.

Although less common, cardiogenic shock needs to be recognized and approached differently from absolute or relative hypovolemia. Hepatomegaly, venous engorgement, rales, and a gallop rhythm all point to the difference in volume status in these patients. The history reveals no abnormal fluid losses. Cardiomegaly on chest radiograph confirms the diagnosis and points to the importance of inotropic or chronotropic therapy instead of multiple volume expansions.

Cardiopulmonary Failure

Immediately prior to an arrest, it is impossible to distinguish respiratory failure from shock. The clinical picture is one of poor oxygen delivery to all tissues. Extreme signs are present, including loss of consciousness, profound cyanosis, no distal pulses, no capillary refill, irregular respirations, hypotension, and bradycardia.

Airway and breathing maneuvers will usually improve the heart rate and blood pressure. Once oxygenation and ventilation are re-established, perfusion is reassessed. In respiratory failure, perfusion rapidly returns toward normal, whereas in shock, perfusion only partially improves.

SPECIAL PEDIATRIC CONSIDERATIONS

From the didactic standpoint, the mnemonic "ABC" is helpful in reinforcing the basic priorities of *airway, breathing,* and *circulation* for the beginning student. Variations from these priorities are dictated according to the patient's physiologic status, the circumstances of the scene, the cause of the disease process, and other age-related problems. For instance, in an adult who has a witnessed arrest, a quick look for ventricular fibrillation and rapid defibrillation supersedes consideration of airway and breathing. In a child whose arrest is witnessed by medical personnel, a brief period of hyperventilation with 100% FiO_2 by a bag-valve-mask device and monitoring for the return of a normal heart rate is a reasonable alternative to immediate initiation of chest compression. This section will briefly mention some specific refinements in selection and timing of resuscitative interventions for various common pediatric situations.

Full Stomach Precautions

Acute lung injury from regurgitation of gastric contents ranges from mild, asymptomatic aspiration to fatal forms of adult respiratory distress syndrome. Cricoid pressure during intubation (the Sellick maneuver) minimizes the risk of aspiration from regurgitation and enhances visualization of the vocal chords. A large-bore suction device should be readily available to evacuate the oropharynx in case of regurgitation (see also Chapter 39).

Arrests in Infants with Tracheostomies

Infants with tracheostomies are at high risk for total airway obstruction from a mucous plug. Their developmental disadvantages include small tracheal diameter, ineffective cough, and inability to cry or go for help. Prevention of arrests in these infants requires continuous direct or indirect monitoring by someone trained in suctioning and changing the tracheostomy tube.

Intubating the Struggling Child

The conscious child or the unconscious child with intact reflexes will naturally resist intubation in order to protect the airway. The risks of intubation in this situation include aspiration and trauma. The use of rapid sedation and muscle relaxation is preferred if personnel trained in the administration of these medications to children are available.

Intubating the Child in Shock

Shock ultimately ends in hypoperfusion to the medulla, leading to a change in respiratory rhythm from tachypnea to irregular respirations to gasping to apnea. The resulting bradycardia and asystole is often impossible to reverse, even if apnea is witnessed. Intubation of the child in early shock, however, can diminish the cardiac output by two mechanisms: (1) positive-pressure ventilation impedes venous return and (2) presedation suppresses the sympathetic nervous system centrally. Consequently, the compensatory mechanisms of tachycardia and increased systemic vascular resistance become impaired. In the initial approach to shock, oxygenation and ventilation should be monitored continuously, with preparation undertaken to intubate when necessary (see Fig. 7–1B). If perfusion improves with initial interventions, intubation may not be necessary. If perfusion remains unchanged or deteriorates, intubation should be performed before impaired perfusion to the brain stem results in changes in the respiratory rhythm.

Arrests while Child Is Intubated

When heart rate, blood pressure, and perfusion suddenly deteriorate in a patient who is intubated and on positive-pressure ventilation, the diagnoses of tension pneumothorax and complications of the endotracheal tube must be rapidly excluded. Displacement of the tube into the esophagus causes a gurgling sound on inspiration that is audible without a stethoscope. Either direct laryngoscopy to confirm the position or replacement of the tube is indicated. Obstruction, in contrast, causes an audible rush of air to escape through the pop-off valve of a bag-valve device or causes the alarm on a ventilator's high-pressure monitor to go off. If suctioning fails to relieve the obstruction rapidly, the tube is removed and bag-valve-mask ventilation is resumed.

If these maneuvers fail to restore circulation, tension pneumothorax is likely. In newborns, tension pneumothorax causes a mediastinal shift and torsion on the great vessels, which can rapidly impede both venous return and cardiac output. Asymmetry of chest rise and tracheal deviation may be subtle. Transmitted breath sounds in small infants preclude reliance upon unilateral diminution of breath sounds. Clinical suspicion of pneumothorax is confirmed by chest radiograph, transillumination, or thoracentesis. If bradycardia is present, the latter is the procedure of choice.

Coma with Increased Intracranial Pressure

When pupillary changes and posturing point to impending cerebral herniation, the need for endotracheal intubation for hyperventilation has to be balanced against the risk of increased intracranial pressure elicited by a gag reflex during laryngoscopy. Hyperventilation can sometimes be maintained by spontaneous respirations or a bag-valve-mask device until personnel skilled in rapid-sequence induction with pentothal and a muscle relaxant can perform the procedure (see Chapter 39).

Trauma

Immobilization of the spine for suspected injury is a priority that has implications important to airway management. Head tilt is contraindicated in suspected cervical trauma; chin lift or jaw thrust should be used instead. In children, blunt trauma is more common than injury from penetrating objects, so shock from occult bleeding needs to be anticipated and diagnosed. Common sites of hemorrhage include lacerations of liver and spleen, hemothorax, and fractures of the femur and pelvis.

Burns of the Face and Neck

Indications for endotracheal intubation include protecting the airway, treating respiratory failure, and administering FiO_2 100% for carboxyhemoglobinemia. Intubation is best performed before the edematous phase of burns distorts the anatomy and threatens the airway within the first few hours.

Septic Shock

The early phase of sepsis differs significantly from other forms of shock. The low cardiac output phase is preceded by a hyperdynamic phase, which is characterized by increased cardiac output and decreased systemic vascular resistance. The pulses are bounding, the diastolic pressure is low, and the extremities are warm and well perfused, hence the term *warm shock*. Despite the perfusion, however, oxygen utilization by the tissues is decreased from a variety of mechanisms. The presence of fever usually simplifies the determination of the cause of shock in these patients. The diagnostic challenge, however, is distinguishing benign forms of fever from the early stage of fulminating septic shock, in which the child is usually still ambulatory and appears relatively well. When compensatory mechanisms become overwhelmed, signs of low cardiac output develop suddenly. Before then, a few petechiae may be the only clue to the significance of the fever and hyperdynamic state in early septic shock (see also Chapters 11 and 12).

Table 7–3. REPORTED CASES OF PROLONGED SUBMERSION WITH GOOD OUTCOME*

Reference	Age/Sex	Estimated Submersion Time	Water Temperature	Body Core Temperature	Duration of Resuscitation	Outcome
1. Haukebo 1960	38 yo† M	15 min	−4 to −5° C	?	Open-chest massage 5–10 min	Good
2. Kvittinger 1963	5 yo M	22 min	Ice	24° C @ 4½ hr	160 min	Good
3. Ohlsson 1964	3 yo M	20 min	Stream in Nov in Sweden	27° C @ 80 min	35 min (10 min ECC)‡	Good to fair
4. King 1964	21 yo M	17 min	April in Melbourne	32° C at 4 hr	No ECC	Good
5. Devillota 1973	1 yo M	20 min	Swimming pool in Feb in Madrid Air temp: 11° C high, 0.6° C low	27.8° C @ 2 hr	50 min	Good
6. Hunt 1974	5 yo M	30 min	Ice	27° C	No ECC	Good
7. Siebke 1975	5 yo M	40 min	Ice	24° C	67 min	Good
8. Imbach 1975	2 yo M	20 min	5–7° C	32.5° C @ 4 hr	1 hr	Good
9. Klarskov 1976	6 yo M	15–20 min	2–3° C	21° C	80 min (21 min ECC)	Good
10. Theilade 1977	6 yo M	25 min	4° C	31.8° C	40 min	Good
11. Scientific American	18 yo M	38 min	Ice	?	2 hr	Good
12. Jessen 1978	6 yo M	15–20 min	2–3° C	21° C	15 min	Good
13. Sekar 1980	23 yo F§	25 min	Ice	28.8° C	45 min	Good
14. Young 1980	7 yo M	15 min	Ice	27° C	2¼ hr	Good
15. Nugent 1980	3 10/12 yo M	12–15 min	Swimming pool Dec in Maryland (probably ice)	23° C	60 min	Good to fair
16. Genoni 1982	29 yo F	20 min	10° C	28° C	25 min	Good
17. Newsweek 1984	4 yo M	20 min	Ice	29° C	60 min	Good

*From Orlowski, JP: Drowning, near-drowning, and ice water submersions. Pediatr Clin North Am 34(1)75, 1987.
†YO = years old; M = male.
‡ECC = emergency cardiac care.
§F = female.
Cases of good neurologic recovery after prolonged resuscitation for out-of-hospital arrests have been individually reported. The true incidence of such cases is unknown, as is the incidence of poor recovery after ice water submersion.

OUTCOME

Two types of clinical studies have reported outcome after arrests: Individual case reports and single-institution reviews of multiple cases. Orlowski summarized 17 reports of good neurologic recovery after prolonged resuscitation for cold water submersion, 13 of which were in subjects less than 20 years of age (Table 7–3).[21] Zaritsky tabulated results from 1,026 childhood arrests in 14 series, ranging from 9 to 219 cases (Table 7–4).[22] The literature on near drowning gives additional descriptions of out-of-hospital arrests.[23–39]

Comparison and detailed analysis of these reports is limited because of a lack of standard definitions and the

Table 7–4. LITERATURE SURVEYS OF OUTCOME AFTER PEDIATRIC ARRESTS*

Study	Patient Source	Number of Patients by Type of Arrest			Survival to Discharge (%)		Survivors with Poor Neurologic Outcome (%)
		Respiratory	CRA†	NR‡	Overall	CRA	
1. Eisenberg	Out of hospital	—	119	—	—	7	NR
2. Lewis	Hospital	16	58	—	28	15.5	35
3. Wark	Hospital	—	—	41	42	NR	NR
4. Rosenberg	Emergency room	—	26	—	—	15	NR
5. Ehrlich	Hospital	—	—	219	47	NR	NR
6. DeBard	Hospital	—	—	44	55	NR	NR
7. Ludwig	Hospital	—	—	130	55	NR	NR
8. Nichols	Out of hospital	—	—	13	23	NR	0
9. Nichols	Hospital	—	—	34	44	NR	0
10. Friesen	In and out of hospital	—	66	—	—	9	30
11. Torphy	Emergency room	—	91	—	—	3.5	60
12. O'Rourke	Out of hospital	—	34	—	—	21	100
13. Gillis	Hospital	9	33	—	17	9	14
14. Zaritsky	Hospital	40	53	—	34	9.4	NR

*From Zaritsky A: Cardiopulmonary resuscitation in children. Clin Chest Med 84(4):561, 1987.
†CRA = cardiorespiratory arrest.
‡NR = not reported.
Single-institution reviews show a variety of neurologic outcomes, when reported. Differences in clinical definitions and types of arrests make comparison of data difficult. The poorest outcome is reported in out-of-hospital arrests that are apneic and pulseless on arrival to the emergency department.

Table 7–5. PROGNOSTIC FACTORS INFLUENCING OUTCOME IN PEDIATRIC ARRESTS

Favorable	Unfavorable
In hospital	Out of hospital
Respiratory	Cardiorespiratory
Bradycardia	Asystole
Witnessed	Unwitnessed
Hypothermia	Normothermia
Basic life support (BLS) only	Advanced life support (ALS) required
Pulses return in field	Pulseless in emergency room
No cardiotonic medications	More than two doses of epinephrine
No underlying disease	Chronic illness

variability in reporting basic parameters, such as the location of the arrest, the type of the arrest, and the classification of outcome. The collective importance of these studies is in the description of prognostic indicators predictive of outcome (Table 7–5). Such indicators can be helpful in dealing with the two primary ethical issues of resuscitation: (1) when to discontinue resuscitation efforts in the acute setting, and (2) when to discontinue prolonged life support efforts when survival with severe anoxic encephalopathy is the most likely outcome.

Given the gravity of these decisions, some authors have pointed to the desirability of absolute indicators that predict outcome with 100% certainty.[7] The problem with this approach is that current studies that define absolute indicators are small. The true incidence of good recovery after prolonged resuscitation is unknown. Given the occasional survivor with good recovery after prolonged resuscitation, there may indeed be no absolute indicators of either survival or good neurologic recovery.

In reality, these decisions must be made despite the restraints of limited knowledge. To guide clinical decision-making in the future, one approach could be to set arbitrary time limits based on data from known cases and consensus among experienced clinicians. Another approach could be to test the known predictive indicators prospectively in a large group of patients, then devise a formula for when to stop the life support effort. Both of these approaches have flaws: The first is arbitrary and authoritarian, and the second could be more valid scientifically but difficult to study and perhaps clinically impractical to use.

A more immediate and practical approach is to identify the decision-making process undertaken by the physician in charge so that it can be understood, examined, and challenged by those involved, including the family, the nurses, the public, and other professionals. The physician's primary responsibility is for supervising the medical care being rendered to the child. The secondary responsibility is for counseling the family and the hospital staff involved.

Initiating Resuscitation

Without specific advance directives, the assumption is made that resuscitative efforts are wanted. In most

situations, the physician does not make the decision to initiate resuscitation. Instead, resuscitation is usually begun by a bystander, a paramedic, a nurse, or other allied personnel, with a physician assuming responsibility for the situation as soon as possible. The physician's first responsibility to the child in full arrest is to assess the adequacy of standard interventions in assisting oxygenation, ventilation, and perfusion and then to recognize complications and gather data regarding the prognosis. Once the physician is assured that standard interventions are being appropriately implemented, a brief conference is held with immediately assembled family members to inform them of the child's condition, the efforts being undertaken, and the prognosis. This time is also used to take a brief history to try to further clarify the diagnosis and prognosis.

Terminating Resuscitation

If the child fails to respond to standard interventions, the physician must decide to continue these interventions for a reasonable length of time, based upon the working prognosis, or to attempt nonstandard interventions, depending upon the clinical setting and the family's wishes. Elaborate counseling to determine the family's wishes is not possible at this time, but the physician is in a position to listen to any spontaneously volunteered requests to "do everything possible" versus "stop if meaningful survival is not likely." In the emergency department, the partially assembled family is usually in a state of shock, and it may be unclear who the natural parents are, who the legal guardian is, or who has the moral authority within the family. True consensus cannot be obtained, so the weight given to family requests made in this situation has to be individualized.

Discontinuing Prolonged Life Support

For the child who responds to resuscitation, parental counseling about immediate prognosis is important: The distinction needs to be made between return of spontaneous circulation versus return of neurologic function after hypoxic-ischemic injury, and the physician's limited ability to influence the latter needs to be clarified. Depending on the situation, emphasis may need to be placed on the likelihood of recurrent cardiac arrests, brain death, or other fatal complications.

When survival appears likely, the degree of neurologic recovery becomes the key issue. Possibilities include complete recovery, minor impairment, major deficits, and survival in a persistent vegetative state. In the normothermic patient, quality of survival is related to the duration of resuscitation required to restore circulation. Once restored, sequential neurologic examinations are probably the most sensitive predictor of recovery[40] (see Chapters 18 and 19).

Deep, painful stimuli are used to elicit signs of minimal return of cortical function. These signs include purposeful withdrawal of extremities, eye opening, grimacing, and head turning. Slightly higher cortical function is necessary for localizing and combating painful stimuli, responding to voice command, recognizing parents, and following objects visually. When any of these signs are present 6 to 72 hours after restoration of circulation, chances are favorable for good neurologic recovery. During the assessment, there must be no suppressant effects from hypothermia, hypotension, sedatives, or muscle relaxants.

Survival in a persistent vegetative state or other profound impairment is the most likely prognosis when the child's best neurologic examination during this time period indicates only brain stem recovery. In such cases, a respiratory drive is present, along with some combination of pupillary, corneal, oculocephalic, and gag reflexes, but there is generalized flaccidity and lack of cortical function. Deep, painful stimuli elicit either no response or generalized spasticity.

Despite the presence of spontaneous respirations, the child may still be dependent upon mechanical ventilation and vasoactive infusions for life support. Oftentimes, cardiopulmonary functions become stable and slowly improve over days to weeks so that dependence upon life support is not permanent. The therapeutic dilemma becomes whether to withdraw life support to avoid a probable poor outcome or to prolong life support with the hope that there will be a delayed neurologic recovery. In such a situation, the prognosis of profound neurologic impairment can be made only with an element of uncertainty because of sporadic reports of good neurologic recovery after prolonged arrests and without rapid recovery of cortical function. In addition to the gaps in the data defining neurologic recovery after prolonged arrest, the dilemma is heightened by the sudden onset of a tragic illness or injury in a previously healthy child.

Despite these uncertainties, many physicians are now willing to enter into joint family-physician decisions to withdraw life support when anoxic encephalopathy is severe. The process needs to be guided by decisions that are in the child's best interest and that are obtained by a full consensus of the family and medical personnel. The latter need to recognize that the family has the right to hope for their child's improvement and has the ultimate decision in judging what constitutes good neurologic recovery. The process usually involves neurodiagnostic tests and second opinions to confirm the relative hopelessness of the situation. If there are conflicting opinions, consultation with the hospital ethics committee can be helpful. Nurses, respiratory therapists, and other involved hospital personnel also need to be included in the decision-making process, both to act as child and family advocates and to address their own feelings (see also Chapter 92).

Counseling needs to be not only open and direct but also sensitive and noncoercive in guiding the family to the final decision. The physician needs to be willing to follow either path: prolonged support for the child or care and comfort after withdrawing selected therapies. One parent's silence may mean disapproval of withdrawing support or lack of understanding of the issues involved. Conversely, the presence of both parents at the child's side when the physician withdraws support

demonstrates their involvement and consent and can obviate the need to request their signatures on written statements. Parents must also be prepared for the possibility of agonal activity, increased spasticity, and prolonged survival after withdrawal of support (see also Chapter 92).

Grieving

As the hopelessness of an individual situation becomes apparent and death draws near, the sensitivity of the physician's approach is important to the grieving family coping with difficult issues. They must deal with feelings of disbelief, anger, guilt, and depression, while simultaneously confronting decisions about withdrawal of support, organ donation, autopsy, and burial.

Access to the child should be unrestricted as much as possible and actively encouraged if there is any reluctance. Once invasive procedures have been performed, parents can be allowed to enter the room, even during a resuscitation procedure. The importance of their presence at the moment of cessation of cardiopulmonary function and the time spent holding the child immediately thereafter can be inferred from the experience of one mother who was denied such an opportunity. Months later, she confided to other parents that she could not begin grieving because of the difficulty she was having conceptualizing her child's death: When she returned home from shopping, she learned her child had died and was transferred from an emergency department to a funeral home.

Upon the death of a child, family, friends, and society have ritualized approaches to help the parents through the immediate grieving process. Two to 6 weeks later, though, it becomes uncomfortable for most people to talk about the child. The topic becomes taboo and parents often feel abandoned. A conference with the physician can be important, both to clear up any remaining questions about diagnosis or medical care and to guide them to appropriate literature, individuals, or groups comfortable with the ongoing process of grieving. Organizations such as Compassionate Friends provide safe opportunities for parents to express and explore the depths of their grief, as well as for physicians to become aware of the complexity of these issues.[41]

ETIOLOGY

This chapter has described how to differentiate respiratory failure from shock and how to establish a working diagnosis and a presumptive cause during a resuscitation procedure. Understanding etiology is also important in designing strategies and programs to prevent childhood mortality. Epidemiologic studies of childhood mortality examine the vital statistics for a community, particularly the certificates of birth and death. Analysis of deaths of infants less than 1 year of age leads to an appreciation of the most common causes in the various pediatric age groups (Table 7–6). As already stated, two thirds of the 38,910 infant deaths that

Table 7–6. SELECTED CAUSES OF INFANT MORTALITY IN THE UNITED STATES IN 1988*

All causes	38,910	(100%)
Congenital anomalies	8,141	(21%)
Perinatal conditions not separately listed	6,128	(15.7%)
Sudden infant death syndrome	5,476	(14.1%)
Other newborn respiratory conditions	3,588	(9.2%)
Short gestation and low birth weight	3,268	(8.4%)
Respiratory distress syndrome of newborn	3,181	(8.2%)
Diseases of respiratory system	1,219	(3.1%)
Accidents and adverse effects	936	(2.4%)
Infections specific to the perinatal period	878	(2.3%)
Intrauterine hypoxia–birth asphyxia	777	(1.9%)
Homicide, including child battering	315	(0.8%)
Birth trauma	216	(0.6%)
Certain gastrointestinal diseases	186	(0.5%)
Human immunovirus infection	81	(0.2%)
All other causes	4,520	(11.6%)

*Modified from Wegman ME: Annual summary of vital statistics–1989. Pediatrics 86(6):845, 1990. Reproduced by permission of Pediatrics.

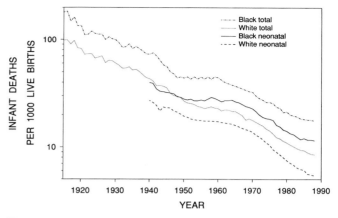

Figure 7–3. Infant and neonatal mortality rates, by race, in the United States from 1915 to 1988. (From Wegman ME: Annual summary of vital statistics—1989. Pediatrics 86[6]:844, 846, 1990. Reproduced by permission of Pediatrics.)

occurred in 1988 took place in the first 28 days of life and reflect the leading neonatal problems: prematurity and related conditions, congenital anomalies, obstetric conditions, birth asphyxia, and perinatal infections.[1] Dollfus showed the ongoing impact of low birth weight on mortality: 32.5% of 1,790 deaths between 28 and 364 days occurred in infants who weighed less than 2,500 gm at birth.[42] Beyond the first 28 days, sudden infant death syndrome was the leading cause of death. Accidents, including child abuse, accounted for 3.2% of the deaths in infants but prevail as the leading cause of mortality after the first year of life through adolescence.[1] Note also the presence of only 81 reported deaths due to acquired immunodeficiency syndrome in 1988.

CHALLENGES

The greatest gains in pediatric resuscitation in the past 10 years have occurred not in the discovery of new resuscitative techniques but in the education of large numbers of paramedics, nurses, and physicians in recognizing critically ill children and meeting their needs with a few well-timed interventions. This process needs to be refined on an ongoing basis, with research aimed at the hypotheses involved in select interventions. Laboratory research needs to be directed toward defining the optimal method for enhancing cardiac output during resuscitation and correlating the results with improvement in neurologic recovery. Clinical research needs to define the value of nonstandard forms of resuscitation, such as the use of higher dosages of epinephrine, as well as to describe in greater detail the outcome of survivors. The latter involves determining the true incidence of survival with good neurologic recovery after prolonged resuscitation and the predictive value of the known prognostic indicators.

The impact of advances in childhood resuscitation and life support on infant mortality is unknown. Figure 7–3 shows the continued improvement in infant and neonatal mortality in the United States since 1915, as well as the ongoing discrepancy in survival between black and white infants. Figure 7–4 places this progress in perspective with other developed nations. The 1988 infant mortality rates in Japan, Sweden, and France are 4.8, 5.8, and 7.7%, respectively.[1] The United States ranks 21st of the 28 countries with populations greater than 2.5 million and infant mortality rates less than 15%. These figures indicate the need for further development of programs for prevention of fatal childhood diseases, in addition to improvement in crisis management. In the United States, better prenatal care and accident prevention obviously deserve priority.

Beyond these needs, there are other unexplored challenges in terms of using current knowledge and resources to reach greater numbers of critically ill children. In 1988, the United Nations International Children's Emergency Fund (UNICEF) estimated that there were 14

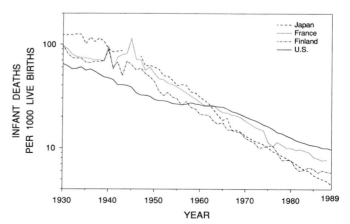

Figure 7–4. Infant mortality rates in selected countries from 1930 to 1988. (From Wegman ME: Annual summary of vital statistics—1989. Pediatrics 86[6]:844, 846, 1990. Reproduced by permission of Pediatrics.)

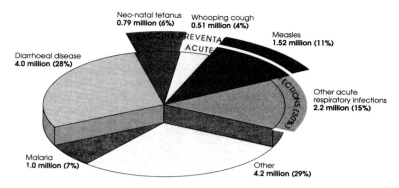

Figure 7–5. Annual deaths of children under age 5 globally by main causes. In 1988, WHO and UNICEF estimated that there were more than 14 million childhood deaths, nearly two thirds of which are accounted for by just four specific causes: diarrhea, respiratory infections, measles, and neonatal tetanus. The great majority of these deaths could now be prevented at very low cost. For the purposes of this chart, one cause has been allocated for each child death. In practice, children often die of multiple causes, and malnutrition is a contributory cause in approximately one third of all deaths in children. Notice the growing importance of respiratory failure and hypovolemic shock as the three vaccine preventable causes become better controlled. (From UNICEF: The State of the World's Children, 1990. New York, UNICEF, 1990.)

million deaths in children less than 5 years of age. In some developing areas, infant mortality rates range from 266/1,000 to 300/1,000 or 3 of every 10 children. The magnitude of these problems is overwhelming on initial review and points to the need for a perspective and understanding of international issues in childhood survival, as well as thoughtful priorities developed by leaders in public health.

Figure 7–5 illustrates the major causes of childhood mortality. For the purposes of this chart, each child was assigned only one cause of death. Malnutrition was a contributory cause in approximately one third of the 14 million childhood deaths.[43] Three vaccine-preventable diseases (neonatal tetanus, whooping cough, and measles) accounted for 2.82 million deaths in 1988. Malaria is still an important cause of death (1 million, 7%). The growing specter of acquired immunodeficiency syndrome is not yet apparent in these data. Diarrheal diseases remain the largest single problem, accounting for 4 million (28%) deaths, followed by non–vaccine preventable causes of acute respiratory infections (2.2 million, 15%). The 11,000 deaths/day from diarrheal diseases contrasts sharply with the 360 to 500 deaths/year in the United States currently reported,[44, 45] but it is similar to the experience in the United States in 1915, when the infant mortality rate was 100/1,000 live births, and diarrheal diseases accounted for one third of this mortality.[4, &6]

UNICEF, the World Health Organization (WHO), and United Nations Educational, Scientific, and Cultural Organization (UNESCO) have issued a communications challenge to distribute fundamental health facts to all families by the year 2000 in the publication *Facts for Life*.[47] Ten essential areas are outlined: birth spacing, prenatal care, breast-feeding, monitoring child growth, immunizations, diarrhea control, acute respiratory infections, sanitation, malaria, and acquired immunodeficiency syndrome (Fig. 7–6). Female literacy has been added as an 11th item that is critical in disseminating this knowledge and in empowering people to act.

Governments and voluntary organizations are forming alliances to meet these challenges. In 1988, the United States Agency for International Development spent $169,868,000 on child survival programs.[48] Although this sum ranks the United States as a major contributor to UNICEF's Expanded Programme for Immunization and WHO's Center for Diarrheal Diseases, it is only equivalent to the annual education budget for a municipality

of 300,000 individuals in the United States. In order for immunizations and oral rehydration solutions to become universally available, childhood survival programs need to become a priority politically and to receive appropriate funding. The United Nations continues its child advocacy role by articulating the rights of children, by proposing plans of action for child survival, and by providing political forums to enhance the visibility of these issues.[49, 50]

Despite the ongoing challenges, some results are encouraging, as indicated by the improving statistics that estimate the probability of dying before age 5 years (Fig. 7–7). In developed countries, the continuum of care for the critically ill child from the field to the emergency department to the intensive care unit to rehabilitation is still in an early stage and undergoing refinement. In developing countries, pediatric care and public health measures are evolving in a parallel fashion. Have medical personnel in developed countries learned anything about childhood resuscitation that is applicable to situations faced by medical and public health personnel in developing areas? Are there any low-cost, high-impact resuscitation procedures that can improve child-

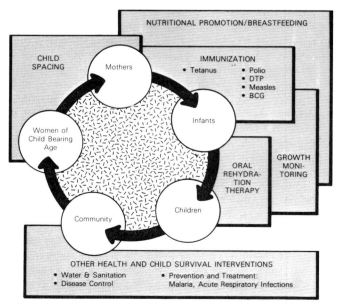

Figure 7–6. Essential areas of education, prevention, and treatment for all children. (From Child Survival: A Third Report to the Congress on the USAID Program.)

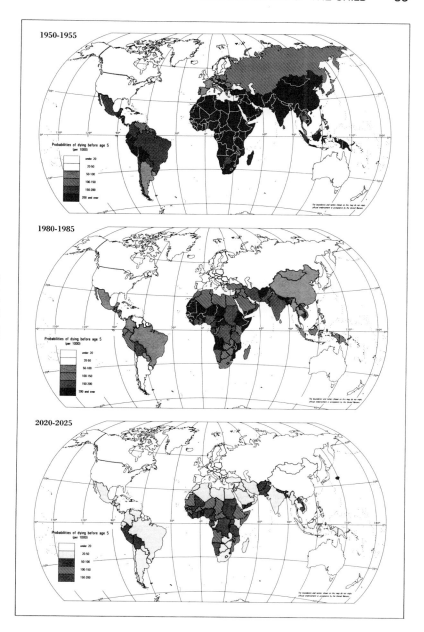

Figure 7–7. Looking ahead: Estimated probabilities of dying before age 5. (*Note:* Figures shown are the probabilities of dying before age 5 per 1,000 births. *Source:* Mortality of Children Under Age Five: Estimates and Projections, 1950–2025 [United Nations publication, Sales No. E.88.XIII.4] Maps No. 3444.1–3444.3, United Nations, July 1987.)

hood mortality and morbidity without the expensive burden of intensive care units? What are the educational and programmatic needs of pediatric departments in developing areas and how do they interrelate with maternal and child health needs addressed by public health agencies?

Answers to these questions require an understanding of the priorities of health care in developing areas and of the complementary nature between pediatric and public health agencies. Globally, control of vaccine-preventable diseases, improved nutrition, diarrheal control by better sanitation and expanded access to oral rehydration therapy, and treatment of acute respiratory infections are the main priorities. As the three vaccine-preventable diseases shown in Figure 7–5 come under better control, two problems emerge: hypovolemic shock and respiratory failure. The 245.8 million people in the United States represent only 4.8% of the earth's population of 5.1 billion. Yet, within that population, neonatology, pediatric critical care medicine, pediatric emergency medicine, and pediatric trauma services have emerged with advances in understanding the pathophysiology and the medical systems approach to critically ill children. What are the international implications of these advances?

References

1. Wegman ME: Annual Summary of Vital Statistics–1989. Pediatrics 86(6):835, 1990.
2. Abramson NS, Safar P, Deitre K, et al: Brain Resuscitation Clinical Trial (BRCT) I Study Group: Randomized clinical study of thiopental loading in comatose cardiac arrest survivors. N Engl J Med 314:397, 1986.

3. Nussbaum E and Maggi JC: Pentobarbital therapy does not improve neurologic outcome in nearly drowned, flaccid-comatose children. Pediatrics 81(5):630, 1988.

4. Abramson NS, Sutton-Tyrrell K, Safar P, et al: A randomized clinical study of a calcium-entry blocker (lidoflazine) in the treatment of comatose survivors of cardiac arrest. N Engl J Med 324(18):324, 1991.

5. Steinbereithner K, Schindler I, Budka H, et al: Nimodipine does not reduce brain damage after ventricular fibrillation in an acute pig model. Crit Care Med 16(4):386, 1988.

6. Reich H, Safar P, Angelos M, et al: Failure of a multifaceted anti-reoxygenation injury therapy to ameliorate brain damage after ventricular fibrillation (VF) cardiac arrest of minutes in dogs. Crit Care Med 16(4):387, 1988.

7. Nichter MA and Everett PB: Childhood near-drowning: Is cardiopulmonary resuscitation always indicated? Crit Care Med 17(10):993, 1989.

8. Quan L, Wentz KR, Gore EJ, et al: Outcome and predictors of outcome in pediatric submersion victims receiving prehospital care in King County, Wash Pediatr 86(4):586, 1990.

9. O'Rourke PP: Outcome of children who are apneic and pulseless in the emergency room. Crit Care Med 14(5):466, 1986.

10. Standards and Guidelines for Cardiopulmonary Resuscitation (CPR) and Emergency Cardiac Care (ECC): JAMA 255:2954, 1986.

11. Redding JS and Pearson BM: Evaluation of drugs for cardiac resuscitation. Anesthesiology 24(2):203, 1963.

12. Gazmuri RJ, Planta MV, Weil MH, et al: Absence of acidemia in arterial blood after 12 minutes of cardiac arrest (abstract). Crit Care Med 16(4):385, 1988.

13. Dantzker DR: Cardiopulmonary Critical Care. Philadelphia, WB Saunders, 1991, p 410.

14. Bushore M: Advanced Pediatric Life Support. Elk Grove, IL, American Academy of Pediatrics and American College of Emergency Physicians, 1989.

15. Chameides L: Textbook of Pediatric Advanced Life Support. Dallas, American Heart Association and American Academy of Pediatrics, 1988.

16. Seidel JS and Burkett DL: Instructor's Manual for Pediatric Advanced Life Support. Dallas, American Heart Association and American Academy of Pediatrics, 1988.

17. Coar: The Aphorisms of Hippocrates. 1822: Aphorism 1, Section 7, page 189. London: AJ Valpy: Red Lion Court, Fleet Street.16 Reprinted 1982: The Classics of Medicine Library, Division of Gryphon Editions, Birmingham AL, PO Box 76108, private printing.

18. Pollack MM, Fields AI, and Ruttimann UE: Sequential cardiopulmonary variables of infants and children in septic shock. Crit Care Med 12(7):554, 1984.

19. Pollack MM, Fields AI, and Ruttimann UE: Sequential cardiopulmonary variables of infants and children in septic shock. Crit Care Med 12(7):554, 1984.

20. Carcillo JA, Pollack MM, Ruttimann UE, et al: Sequential physiologic interactions in pediatric cardiogenic and septic shock. Crit Care Med 17(1):12, 1989.

21. Orlowski JP: Drowning, near-drowning, and ice-water submersions. Pediatr Clin North Am 34(1):75, 1987.

22. Zaritsky A: Cardiopulmonary resuscitation in children. Clin Chest Med 8(4):561, 1987.

23. Allman FD, Nelson WD, Pacentine GA, et al: Outcome following cardiopulmonary resuscitation in severe pediatric near-drowning. Am J Dis Child 140:571, 1986.

24. Bohn DJ, Biggar WD, Smith CR, et al: Influence of hypothermia, barbiturate therapy, and intracranial pressure monitoring on morbidity and mortality after near-drowning. Crit Care Med 14:529, 1986.

25. Conn AW, Montes JE, Barker GA, et al: Cerebral salvage in near-drowning following neurologic classification by triage. Can Anaesth Soc J 27:201, 1980.

26. Dean JM and Kaufman ND: Prognostic indicators in pediatric near-drowning. The Glasgow Coma Scale. Crit Care Med 9(7):536, 1980.

27. Frates RC: Analysis of predictive factors in the assessment of warm-water near-drowning in children. Am J Dis Child 135:1006, 1981.

28. Frewen TC, Sumabat WO, Han VK, et al: Cerebral resuscitation therapy in pediatric near-drowning. J Pediatr 106:615, 1985.

29. Jacobsen WK, Mason LJ, Briggs BA, et al: Correlation of spontaneous respiration and neurologic damage in near-drowning. Crit Care Med 11:487, 1983.

30. McComb JG: Intact survival rates in nearly-drowned comatose children. Am J Dis Child 140:504, 1986.

31. Modell JH, Graves SA, and Kuck EJ: Near-drowning: Correlation of level of consciousness and survival. Can Anaesth Soc J 27:211, 1980.

32. Nugent SK and Rogers MC: Resuscitation and intensive care monitoring following immersion hypothermia. J Trauma 20(9):814, 1980.

33. Nussbaum E: Prognostic variables in nearly-drowned comatose children. Am J Dis Child 139:1058, 1985.

34. Oakes DD, Shereck JP, Maloney JR, et al: Prognosis and management of victims of near-drowning. J Trauma 22(7):544, 1982.

35. Orlowski JP: Prognostic factors in pediatric cases of drowning and near-drowning. Ann Emerg Med 8(5):176, 1979.

36. Pearn JH, Bart RD, and Yamaoaka R: Neurologic sequelae after childhood near-drowning: A total population study from Hawaii. Pediatrics 64(2):187, 1979.

37. Peterson B: Morbidity of childhood near-drowning. Pediatrics 59:364, 1977.

38. Turner GR and Levin DL: Improvement of neurologic status after pediatric near-drowning accidents Crit Care Med 13(12):1080, 1985.

39. Weinberg HD: Prognostic variables in nearly-drowned comatose children. Am J Dis Child 140:329, 1986.

40. Reinmuth OM, Vaagene P, Abramson NS, et al: Predicting outcome after resuscitation from clinical death. Crit Care Med 16(10):1043, 1988.

41. The Compassionate Friends, Inc: National office: PO Box 3696, Oak Brook, Illinois 60522-3696 Telephone: (708) 990-0010.

42. Dollfus C, Patetta M, Siegel E, et al: Infant mortality: A practical approach to the analysis of the leading causes of death and risk factors. Pediatrics 86(2):176, 1990.

43. Grant JP: The State of the World's Children 1990. Oxford University Press. UNICEF, 3 United Nations Plaza, New York, NY 10017.

44. Lew JF, Glass RI, Gangarosa RE et al: Diarrheal Deaths in the United States, 1979 Through 1987. JAMA 265(24):3280, 1991.

45. Ho MS, Glass RI, Pinsky PF et al: Diarrheal deaths in American children: Are they preventable? JAMA 260(22):3281, 1988.

46. Wegman ME: Personal communication. June, 1991.

47. Facts for Life, A Communication Challenge. UNICEF House, DIPA H9F, 3 UN Plaza, New York, NY 10017, 1990.

48. Child Survival: A Fourth Report to Congress on the USAID Program. US Agency for International Development, Washington, DC 20523.

49. Convention of the Rights of the Child: Adopted by the General Assembly of the United Nations, November 20, 1989.

50. World Declaration on the Survival, Protection and Development of Children and Plan of Action for Implementation: World Summit for Children, United Nations, New York, September 30, 1990.

Resuscitation of the Critically Injured Child

Laurie A. Latchaw, M.D., and Burton H. Harris, M.D.

The development of pediatric trauma systems has increased the number of critically injured children who survive to reach the hospital. These children often have weak or no vital signs at the accident scene. In addition to their tissue injuries, they have neurogenic or hypovolemic shock, or both, compounded by hypoxemia. Unlike most pediatric trauma victims who do not present in profound shock, these critically injured children require advanced techniques in establishing an airway, breathing, and circulation. Recent clinical and experimental studies show that the sooner definitive resuscitation begins, the greater will be the chance of survival. The resuscitating team must be capable of expeditiously performing a wide variety of surgical and medical procedures in a limited amount of time. Thus the implementation of a pediatric trauma protocol by a trained trauma receiving unit is mandatory for the survival of these children.[1] The following information is meant to be applicable to all injured children, although because our experience is drawn predominantly from our institution, local solutions to problems are included.

RESUSCITATIVE TRAUMA TEAM

Ideally, the resuscitative trauma team consists of four physicians and three nurses. The most senior pediatric surgeon acts as the team leader. The primary responsibility of the team leader is to maintain the sequence of the defined protocol (Table 8–1), make critical decisions, and coordinate consultants. The team leader is assisted by the charge nurse, who also documents all of the team's efforts and anticipates equipment needs. An anesthesiologist, often assisted by a respiratory therapist, manages the airway and immobilizes the neck at all times. A surgeon and nurse are located on one side (usually the right) of the patient and are responsible for any surgical procedures that may be required during the resuscitation. On the opposite side of the patient, a critical care physician and nurse provide all the medical support needed.

ADVANCED TECHNIQUES USED IN RESUSCITATION OF CRITICALLY INJURED CHILDREN

Children who have no vital signs immediately after traumatic injury usually have suffered a high spinal cord or brain stem injury, complete airway obstruction, or rupture of the heart or great vessels.[2] Thus a history of cardiopulmonary resuscitation at the scene should warn the trauma team that advanced resuscitation procedures will be needed.

Airway

Airway obstruction at or below the larynx is not relieved by chin lift and suctioning secretions. Tracheal intubation is required. Nasotracheal intubation, which has been recommended to prevent hyperextension of cervical spine injuries, is difficult in children because of the anterior position of the airway in the hypopharynx. If the child's trachea accommodates at least a No. 5 endotracheal tube, flexible laryngoscopy can be used to ensure atraumatic intubation. The laryngoscope is placed through the lumen of the endotracheal tube prior to passing it through the vocal cords. The laryngoscope then acts as a guide for accurate placement of the endotracheal tube.

In children with smaller-caliber airways, direct orotracheal intubation must be attempted only by experienced operators. Similarly, emergency tracheostomy should be avoided. Poor lighting and instruments added to the chaotic environment of the trauma receiving unit renders an already difficult procedure in children nearly impossible.

In both of the preceeding situations, needle cricothyrotomy is the safest, albeit temporary, means of establishing an airway.[3] A 12- or 14-gauge catheter is "popped" through the cricothyroid membrane. This membrane is the space between the easily palpable thyroid cartilage (Adam's apple) and the cricoid cartilage (first ring-like structure of the trachea) (Fig. 8–1). Once the tracheal lumen is entered, the needle is re-

Table 8–1. RESUSCITATION PROTOCOL*

The following protocol was designed to ensure a maximal resuscitative effort for critically injured pediatric trauma patients in a 30-minute drill. Actual elapsed times will vary, especially if all advanced techniques are necessary to complete the drill and stabilize the patient. Assigned tasks with an asterisk (*) are performed only after the team leader has made an active decision to proceed.

Elapsed Time (Minutes)	Team Member	Assigned Task
0000	Team Leader (TL)	Estimate body weight and body surface area, calculate blood volume (80 × wt in kg)
	Anesthesiologist (A)	Immobilize neck—apply axial traction, place firm (Philadelphia) cervical collar
	Nurse Side 1 (N1)	Remove all clothing
	Doctor Side 1 (D1)	60-sec examination—identify life threats
	Nurse Side 2 (N2)	Apply electrocardiographic leads
	Doctor Side 2 (D2)	Perform femoral vein venipuncture at groin for complete blood count, type and crossmatch, amylase
0001	A	Airway management:
		Administer O$_2$—2–5 l/min
		Suction secretions
		Chin lift
		Ventilate with mask
	N2	Obtain vital signs
	TL	Airway decisions:
		Obstructed—orotracheal intubation versus cricothyrotomy
		Breathing decisions:
		Unequal breath sounds, shifted heart sounds, abnormal chest excursion—thoracentesis for tension pneumothorax
		Circulation decisions:
		No palpable pulse or blood pressure—begin PALS
0002	A	Orotracheal intubation*
	N1 + D1	Cricothyrotomy*
		Relieve tension pneumothorax*—thoracentesis fourth intercostal space midclavicular line
		If cardiac arrest—attempt percutaneous venous catheter once; proceed to saphenous vein cutdown at ankle
	N2	If cardiac arrest—begin chest compression
	D2	Insert percutaneous venous catheter
		If cardiac arrest—call code medications (two rounds); coordinate defibrillator
0004	A	Maintain airway and neck immobilization
	N1	Once intravenous access established—bolus (by syringe and 3-way stopcock) 25% of calculated blood volume as Ringer lactate; repeat if no response
	D1	Check for distended neck veins, pulsus paradoxus
	N2	Obtain vital signs
	TL	Circulation decisions;
		Cardiac tamponade—pericardiocentesis
0006	D1	Pericardiocentesis*—subxiphoid
	N2	Repeat vital signs after pericardiocentesis
	D2 + A	If no cardiac arrest—obtain lateral C spine
0008	TL	Consult with neurology and neurosurgery; determine C spine and airway stability; If CNS injury decide on intubation for therapeutic hyperventilation (Pco$_2$ 25–30 mm Hg)
	N1	Insert rectal temperature probe
		Place urethral catheter if no blood at meatus and no evidence of pelvic fracture
0010	N2 + D2	Insert nasogastric tube if no evidence of midfacial or base of skull fracture
		Orogastric tube can be placed in intubated patients
	TL	Suspect hemopneumothorax; confirm with portable anteroposterior chest x-ray film (semiupright if possible)
0012	N1 + D1	*Place thoracostomy tube
0015 (unstable patient)	TL	Patient hemodynamically unstable
		Consider immediate open thoracotomy for:
		penetrating heart wound
		massive intrapleural hemorrhage—cross-clamp pulmonary hilum
		massive intra-abdominal hemorrhage—cross-clamp thoracic aorta
		Consider diagnostic peritoneal lavage if abdominal injury suspected
	N1 + D1	*Perform emergency thoracotomy or *peritoneal lavage
0015 (stable patient)	D1	Perform complete examination
	N1	Dress open wounds
	N2	Leave trauma receiving unit to obtain history
	D2	Insert arterial line if needed
0018 (stable patient)	D1	Take nonemergent or post–tube thoracostomy chest x-ray film
	N2	Check laboratory results
0019 (stable patient)	D1	Calculate Glasgow Coma Score, Trauma Score, and PTS
	Consultants	Perform rapid evaluations
0020	TL	Lists positive finding
		Confer with consultants
	N1, D1, N2, D2, + A	Ready patient for transfer out of trauma receiving unit to operating room, computed tomography, intensive care unit
0025	TL	Patient unresponsive to PALS, temperature >34° C; fluid resuscitation adequate—decide to terminate resuscitation

*Modified from Harris BH, Latchaw LA, Murphy RE, et al: A protocol for pediatric trauma receiving units. J Pediatr Surg 24:419, 1989.

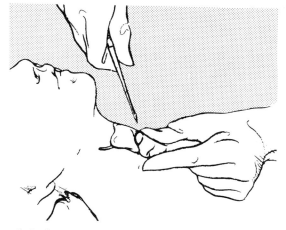

Figure 8–1. Percutaneous cricothyrotomy—a large-bore catheter-over-needle is inserted into the tracheal lumen through the cricothyroid membrane. (From Harris BH: Management of multiple trauma. Pediatr Clin North Am 32:175–181, 1985.)

moved and the cannula is connected to the adapter for a No. 3 endotracheal tube. Depending on the size of the child, satisfactory gas exchange can be maintained for about 10 minutes. This is time well spent getting organized to permanently gain access to the airway.

Breathing

Most traumatic disorders of breathing (e.g., loss of central nervous system [CNS] control, flail chest, sucking chest wounds) are amenable to airway access and positive pressure ventilation. Tension pneumothorax, massive hemothorax, or bilateral hemopneumothoraces do not, however, respond to positive pressure ventilation and may in fact be exacerbated by the increased airway pressure.

Children with unilaterally decreased breath sounds, contralaterally shifted heart sounds, or unilaterally decreased chest wall excursion who appear hypoxemic or hypotensive, or both, may benefit from needle thoracentesis to relieve a tension pneumothorax.

A confirming chest x-ray film is not necessary prior to inserting a 12-gauge catheter connected to a syringe into the suspected pleural space through the third or fourth intercostal space in the midclavicular line. Expulsion of air is usually followed by immediate improvement in oxygenation and hypotension. This improvement will be temporary if the pneumothorax is allowed to reaccumulate. Tube thoracostomy should be undertaken at the next feasible juncture of the resuscitation. Bilateral needle thoracenteses may be indicated in rare cases, but the risk of iatrogenically creating bilateral pneumothoraces using this technique must be considered.

If needle thoracentesis shows a pneumothorax or if the physical findings (flail chest, unilateral decreased breath sounds, dullness to percussion in the posterolateral portion of chest) are consistent with hemothorax, a portable anteroposterior chest x-ray film should be taken, in the semiupright position if possible. Pneumothorax alone can be treated by a small-caliber tube placed through the third intercostal space in the midclavicular line and directed in a cephalad direction. Hemothoraces and hemopneumothoraces require large-bore tubes placed through the fifth or sixth intercostal space in the midaxillary line and directed posteriorly. All tube sites require sterile technique and local 1% lidocaine anesthesia. A 1- to 1.5-cm incision is made over the rib just below the designated intercostal space. A curved clamp is used to create a tunnel over the top of the rib. The points of the clamp are then pierced through the intercostal muscles, "popped" into the pleural space, and spread open widely. The sound of rushing air or the expulsion of blood, or both, confirms that the intrapleural space has been opened. The tube is then threaded through the incision and short tunnel and into the space created by the clamp. Trocar placement of chest tubes is not recommended because the very pliable chest wall in children can be compressed so that the trocar may pierce an internal organ as it enters the pleural space. The chest tube is connected to a closed suction chest tube system, and the tube is secured to the skin with a heavy silk suture. An air-occlusive dressing is applied. The amount of air leaking and blood draining from the chest is documented as an estimate of blood loss and lower airway injury. Massive exsanguinating chest tube drainage may require emergency thoracotomy.

Circulation

The initial goal of trauma resuscitation is to reestablish adequate tissue perfusion, which is defined as the delivery of sufficient oxygen and nutrients to the cells and the removal of waste products from the cells.

The most frequent perfusion abnormality seen following traumatic injury is hemorrhagic or hypovolemic shock. In children, acute blood loss causing a loss of circulating intravascular volume is compensated by increased heart (circulating) rate and a redistribution of intravascular volume (increased peripheral vascular resistance). Experimental models suggest that children may lose up to 30% of their blood volume before decompensating (Fig. 8–2).[4] It is not unusual for children with 20 to 25% hemorrhagic blood loss to be tachycardic, combative (decreased cerebral oxygenation), and cold and clammy (increased peripheral vascular resistance) but normotensive when they present to the hospital. Immediate fluid resuscitation prevents these children from decompensating into profound and often irreversible shock.

Vascular access in the vasoconstricted child can be a challenge. Once the airway and breathing have been established, intravenous access must be obtained. Peripheral percutaneous venipuncture using the largest bore catheter possible should be attempted once. If unsuccessful, saphenous vein cutdown at the ankle should be carried out. Concerns that major intra-abdominal venous injuries would adversely affect lower extrem-

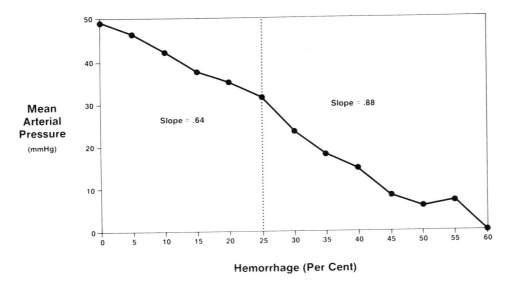

Figure 8–2. Mean response of MAP to continuous hemorrhage at 1% BV loss per minute. A break point occurs at 25% hemorrhage. (From Schwaitzberg SS, Bergman KS, and Harris BH: A pediatric trauma model of continuous hemorrhage. J Pediatr Surg 23:605–609, 1988.)

ity fluid resuscitation have not been borne out experimentally (Fig. 8–3).[5]

A standard cutdown technique is possible because of the constant position of the saphenous vein just anterior to the medial malleolus. After appropriate preparation and draping of the patient, a 1-cm skin incision is made transversely just anterior and above the medial malleolus. A curved hemostat is then placed, tips down, onto the anterior border of the medial malleolus. All structures (usually just fat, the saphenous vein, and small cutaneous nerves) are scooped onto the hemostat and brought up from the depths of the wound. Careful wiping with a gauze sponge clears away fat globules, leaving the vein exposed. Although not necessary, a proximally placed tourniquet may be applied to facilitate identification of the bluish-tinged blood-distended vein. When empty, the vein does resemble one of the small ankle tendons; however, these tendons, covered with sheaths and lying in a deeper layer, are not easy to "tent" into the wound. Once identified, the largest bore catheter possible should be used to cannulate the vein. Direct venipuncture with a catheter is preferable to distal ligation and venotomy, but both techniques are acceptable. The incision can be closed with nylon sutures or sterile adhesive strips. The catheter must be secured to the skin to prevent early dislodgment.

Intraosseous cannulation is an alternative route for emergent vascular access in children.[6] Eighteen-gauge or larger stylet needles (Seldinger needles, spinal needles, or bone marrow needles) are inserted directly into the bone marrow 1 to 2 in. below the tibial tuberosity. Fluid is infused at a pressure of 300 mm Hg. Although flow rates vary, adequate volume resuscitation is possible using this technique. Immediate complications include subcutaneous extravasation and bone, bone marrow, and fat emboli. These complications, as well as the risk of osteomyelitis, limit the use of this technique to critical situations and only until conventional access can be obtained.

Fluid resuscitation begins with calculating the patient's blood volume (80 ml × body weight in kilograms).

Crystalloid solution, most commonly lactated Ringer solution or normal saline, is given as a bolus equal to 25% of the calculated blood volume. Additional 25% aliquots are given until a normal circulating volume has been restored, as evidenced by a decreased heart rate, improved peripheral circulation, and an increase in blood pressure. Rapid infusion (by hand with a syringe) of 25% of the calculated blood volume should effect an immediate improvement in children still able to compensate for their blood loss. Children presenting with hypotension or no vital signs may require more than 25% of their calculated blood volume to effect an increase in blood pressure. Overhydration should be avoided in children with head injury, pulmonary contusions, and known pre-existing cardiac anomalies.

It is imperative that cardiac tamponade be excluded as a cause of persistent hypotension. All children not responding to fluid resuscitation should be examined specifically for distended neck veins, muffled heart

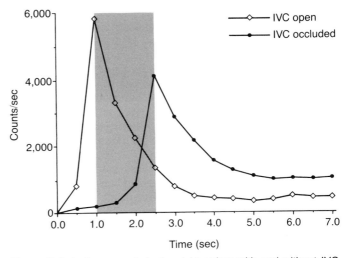

Figure 8–3. Isotope counts in the right atrium with and without IVC occlusion, showing that the isotope reaches the heart with only a 1.5-second delay despite IVC occlusion (*shaded area*).

sounds, and pulsus paradoxus. A suspicion of cardiac tamponade based upon the presence of any of these clinical findings should be followed by needle pericardiocentesis. After sterile preparation, a long, small-gauge spinal needle with stylet removed and a 20-ml syringe attached is advanced subxiphoid in line with the left midclavicle, aspirating constantly. If possible, an alligator clip electrocardiographic electrode should be attached to the metal needle near the hub so that myocardial electrical activity can be identified. This helps to differentiate pericardial blood from intracardiac blood. Since removal of even small volumes of acute pericardial fluid improves cardiac filling and increases blood pressure, aspiration of blood should be halted if no improvement is seen. Pericardial blood, its clotting factors already consumed, remains fluid in the syringe. Intracardiac blood clots.

Blood and blood products were once a routine resuscitation fluid but are now given cautiously. Adult studies show that hemoglobin levels at or even less than 7 mg/dl (hematocrit ~21%) provide adequate tissue oxygenation if the patient is not hypovolemic.[7] This level may not be adequate for the critically injured child. In addition, dilution of clotting factors and platelets by massive crystalloid infusion may result in ineffective clotting and persistent hemorrhage. The judicious use of blood and blood products remains part of the resuscitative armamentarium. Until well-conceived and well-executed studies in immature models are available, infusion of blood or blood products, or both, should commence at hemoglobin levels of 7 to 8 mg/dl (hematocrit 20 to 25%) and should be considered in children with evidence of continued bleeding at levels of 10 mg/dl (hematocrit 30 to 33%). Once the decision to give blood has been made, as much blood as tolerated from a single unit should be administered to avoid exposure to multiple blood donors.

The use of colloid in pediatric trauma resuscitation has never gained widespread use. Unpublished immature animal studies suggest that increased pulmonary edema occurs with hetastarch resuscitation compared with Ringer lactate.[8] More recently, the use of 6.5% hypertonic saline has gained some proponents, especially for use in patients with head injuries in whom increased cerebral water can result in uncontrolled intracranial hypertension. Unfortunately studies in rats have failed to show a difference in the water content of injured brain following resuscitation with hypertonic saline versus lactated Ringer fluid.[9]

Critically injured patients who have not responded to resuscitative efforts to this point have either unsalvageable CNS injury or massive uncontrolled hemorrhage. Military antishock trousers may be applied at any opportunity (hopefully at the accident scene by paramedics) but are only a temporizing measure. To work properly, they should be an appropriate size for the child.

If intra-abdominal injury is suspected but the patient is unable to have double-contrast computed tomography, diagnostic peritoneal lavage should be performed. Initially described as a percutaneous technique in traumatized adults, peritoneal lavage evolved into an open cutdown procedure in children because of iatrogenically induced intraperitoneal injuries. Using sterile technique and 1% lidocaine (Xylocaine) with epinephrine local anesthesia, a 2-cm infraumbilical incision is made in the midline and carried down until the midline fascia is identified. Stay or traction sutures are placed on either side of the fascia, which is then sharply opened. The peritoneum is identified and tented up between mosquito hemostats and then opened. (Blood is often seen through the peritoneum before opening.) A dialysis catheter is placed through the opening and directed toward the posterior cul de sac. The catheter is aspirated for blood. Gross blood is a positive finding, but when the effluent has greater than 100,000 red blood cells/mm³ quantitative lavage (600 ml of normal saline/m² body surface area) is a more reliable diagnostic technique. In the hemodynamically stable patient who must forego computed abdominal tomography because of an emergent neurosurgical or vascular procedure, lavage also provides information about intestinal or pancreatic injuries, or both, which may require surgical intervention under the same anesthetic.

If the patient remains hemodynamically unstable and massive hemorrhage is suspected, emergency thoracotomy should be considered. Indications for this procedure are (1) a penetrating heart wound confirmed by pericardiocentesis or massive chest tube hemorrhage or both; (2) massive intrapleural hemorrhage of pulmonary origin confirmed by exsanguinating chest tube drainage; and (3) massive intra-abdominal hemorrhage confirmed by a rapidly expanding abdomen or peritoneal lavage or both.[10] In each case, the goal is hemorrhage control by (1) plugging the myocardial hole, (2) cross-clamping the pulmonary hilum, or (3) cross-clamping the descending thoracic aorta. The operating room must be ready to accept the patient immediately for definitive operative repair if this ultimate resuscitative measure is performed. Under no circumstances should the chest be opened for the sole purpose of intracardiac massage, and under no circumstances should the abdomen be opened in the emergency room for hemorrhage control.

STOPPING RESUSCITATION

Knowing when to stop resuscitating the critically injured child is difficult. At the completion of the 30-minute drill, the patient should show some sign of life. The 30 minutes has allowed the medical team time to infuse two rounds of life-supporting medications while performing external cardiac massage. It has allowed the surgical team time to infuse fluid in excess of the circulating blood volume, if necessary, and correct, albeit temporarily, disorders of airway, breathing, and circulation that may prevent a response to adequate fluid resuscitation. If, at the end of the drill, the patient's temperature is more than 34° C and the patient's vital signs have remained unresponsive to pediatric advanced life support (PALS), resuscitation should be terminated.

Table 8–2. MEAN SERUM TNF ACTIVITY LEVELS†

Time	Group IA	Group IB	Group IIA	Group IIB	*Escherichia coli* Infusion
0	<1.5	<1.5	<1.5	<1.5	<1.5
30 min	<1.5	<1.5	<1.5	<1.5	5.0
60 min	<1.5	<1.5	<1.5	<1.5	126.3
90 min	<1.5	<1.5	<1.5	<1.5	136.7
120 min	<1.5	<1.5	<1.5	<1.5	106.0

*From Stylianos S, Wakabayashi G, Gelfand J, et al: Experimental hemorrhage and blunt trauma do not increase levels of circulating tumor necrosis factor. J Trauma 31:1063–1067, 1991. © by Williams & Wilkins, 1991.

†One tumor necrosis factor (TNF) activity unit is equivalent to 100 pg/ml of recombinant human TNF. Sensitivity of the TNF assay ranged from 0.8 to 1.5 activity units.

Response to hemorrhage alone (group IA), hemorrhage and resuscitation (group IB), hemorrhage with tissue trauma (group IIA), hemorrhage, tissue trauma, and resuscitation (group IIB) 30 minutes after blood loss and blunt injury. Controls were standard *E. coli* infusions.

NEW RESEARCH IN HEMORRHAGIC SHOCK

Irreversible shock despite apparent volume resuscitation and rewarming is thought to be due to the release of potent cytokine mediators in response to gastrointestinal bacterial translocation.[11] Tumor necrosis factor, which is known to be released during *Escheria coli* sepsis seems a likely culprit to initiate this shock state following hemorrhage. Immature animal studies combining hemorrhagic shock with a long bone injury failed to show any release of tumor necrosis factor (Table 8–2).[12] Undoubtedly, some other mediator will eventually be shown to influence the body's response to acute injury, at which time resuscitation will take on the additional task of suppressing or moderating these humoral influences.

References

1. Haller JA: Toward a comprehensive emergency medical system for children. *In:* Harris BH and Coran AG (eds): Pediatric Trauma, Philadelphia, JB Lippincott, 1990, pp. 1–5.
2. Bohn D, Armstrong D, Becker L, et al: Cervical spine injuries in children. J Trauma 30:463, 1990.
3. Bergman KS and Harris BH: Percutaneous transtracheal ventilation. *In:* Harris BH (ed): Progress in Pediatric Trauma, 2nd ed. Boston, Nobb Hill, 1987, p. 126.
4. Schwaitzberg SD, Bergman KS, and Harris BH: A pediatric trauma model of continuous hemorrhage. J Pediatr Surg 23:605, 1988.
5. Stylianos S, Jacir NN, Hoffman MA, et al: Optimal site for volume resuscitation in experimental hemorrhage. Submitted to J Pediatr Surg.
6. Velasco AL, Delgado-Paredes C, Templeton J, et al: Intraosseous infusion of fluids in the initial management of hypovolemic shock in young subjects. J Pediatr Surg 26:4, 1991.
7. Office of Medical Applications of Research, National Institutes of Health: Perioperative red cell transfusion. JAMA 260:1770, 1988.
8. Harris BH: Personal communication.
9. Wisner DH, Schuster L, and Quinn C: Hypertonic saline resuscitation of head injury: Effects on cerebral water content. J Trauma 30:75, 1990.
10. Eichelberger MR, Zwich HA, Pratsch GL, et al: Pediatric trauma protocol: A team approach. *In:* Eichelberger MR and Pratsch GL (eds): Pediatric Trauma Care. Rockville, MD, Aspen Publishers, 1988, pp. 11–31.
11. Baker JW, Deitch EA, Li MA, et al: Hemorrhage shock induces bacterial translocation from the gut. J Trauma 28:896, 1988.
12. Stylianos S, Wakabayashi G, Gelfand JA, et al: Experimental hemorrhage and blunt trauma do not increase circulating tumor necrosis factor. J Trauma 31:1063, 1991.

Drowning and Near-Drowning

Peter R. Holbrook, M.D., and Alan I. Fields, M.D.

Drowning is the second leading cause of accidental death in children and is also the second leading cause of years of potential life lost for all ages. As is true for other severe hypoxic ischemic injuries, the survivors are often severely damaged.

Hundreds of papers have been written on definition, pathophysiology, resuscitation, intensive care, and outcome from drowning. Sadly, no efficacious forms of therapy for the resultant hypoxic ischemic encephalopathy have emerged, and relief from the scourge of drowning must come from prevention.

EPIDEMIOLOGY

Fifteen per cent of school-aged children in the United States have experienced a life-threatening episode in the water.[1] The near ubiquitous appeal of the water in a temperate climate attracts people to pools, lakes, rivers, and oceans (also bathtubs) in prodigious numbers. Safety concerns are often ignored, because the water is synonymous with relaxation. Most persons who are prepared to swim do well, and those who swim at public supervised areas have a low risk of drowning.[2] Nonetheless, ". . . only a small proportion of the millions who swim are skilled enough to care for themselves in all the situations they are likely to encounter."[3] In addition, 55% of drowning victims had not intended to enter the water, and they often encounter water where few safety provisions have been made.[2] Sadly, it is noted that safety is less than 10 meters away in 90% of cases.[4]

Typical patterns of victims are noted. The most common example is when a toddler under adult supervision escapes for "just a few seconds" and is discovered submerged.[2] Another group of victims consists of young adults who sometimes overestimate their swimming prowess and are often under the influence of drugs or alcohol.[5, 6] An example of a third group is the infant child in a large family who is left in the bathtub under the care of an older sibling.[7-9]

Native Americans have the highest death rates from drowning. African Americans have twice the death rate of whites. Males predominate in all age groups.[10]

DEFINITIONS

Drowning is death from suffocation due to immersion in a liquid. Near-drowning implies successful resuscitation, albeit sometimes temporary, from suffocation caused by immersion. Dry drowning refers to the condition of absence of extraneous fluid in the lungs following drowning. Secondary drowning refers to fluid accumulation in the lungs following what appears to be successful recovery from a near-drowning event.[11]

ETIOLOGY

The inability to swim sufficiently well to escape the hazard presented by a body of water under the circumstances existing at the time is common to all near-drowning episodes. Although most children can be assumed to be inexperienced around all areas of water, a search for an etiology should not end with that diagnosis. All drownings should be presumed to have additional etiologic factors that may have an impact on in-hospital medical care (Table 9–1). Lack of adequate supervision and absence of barriers are routine. Some patients in this age group and many in the older population may have experienced trauma as a part of the accident. Cervical spine injuries or head trauma of sufficient degree to cause seizures or loss of consciousness may be factors, especially in children older than 8 years of age.

Drugs or alcohol are common recreational agents associated with water activities. Up to half of drownings in adults are associated with alcohol ingestion, and approximately 10% involve other drugs.[12] Hypothermia (see Chapter 83) may cause a person to drown because motor control is lost.

Table 9–1. ETIOLOGIC FACTORS IN DROWNING

Inexperience	Hypothermia
Inadequate supervision	Seizures
Absence of barriers	Hyperventilation
Trauma	Myocardial infarction
Drugs, alcohol	Exhaustion

Seizures deserve special mention. A history of seizures is found in drowning victims in a proportion that is much greater than is found in the general population.[13] Despite this, anticonvulsant levels are detected at autopsy in less than half of cases. Patients with known seizure disorders die most frequently of drowning, most commonly in their own bathtubs.[7, 14]

Hyperventilation to increase underwater endurance is common in teenage males. The artificially lowered carbon dioxide levels allow the patient to experience significant hypoxia before receiving a hypercarbic stimulus to breathe. Hypoxia may cause the patient to lose consciousness.[5, 6]

Exhaustion may cause the patient to drown even though he or she knows how to swim. Overestimation of one's swimming prowess is common. In the older patient, this may lead to myocardial infarction.

PATHOPHYSIOLOGY

Hypoxia is the fundamental pathophysiologic event in drowning and near-drowning. Initial interference with gas exchange is due to asphyxia, resulting from breath-holding, aspiration or, possibly, laryngospasm. All tissues in the body are subject to the resultant hypoxia. If the condition is not reversed, hypoxia leads to cardiovascular collapse and arrest, thus adding ischemia to the patient's problems. Each tissue in the body responds in its own pattern to the effects of hypoxia/ischemia (see Chapters 1, 13, and 19). The brain's sensitivity to hypoxia/ischemia makes it the dominant organ system dysfunction.

Oxygen demand may be altered in the patient who is submerged. Violent thrashing in an attempt to escape from the water increases demand. However, this also increases blood flow to the periphery, facilitating heat loss to the surrounding liquid. If the patient is rapidly cooled, oxygen demand may be lessened. Such protection is certainly a factor in the "miraculous" cases of good recovery of patients who have experienced prolonged submersion times.

The diving reflex, a profound redistribution of the circulation triggered by cold water in the distribution of the trigeminal nerve in the presence of breath-holding, could conceivably play a role as well in cases in which the patient recovers miraculously. The impact of this reflex in humans is unclear, because more recent data suggest that the reflex is mild and that hypothermia is the more important factor.[15]

Other pathophysiologic events occur but play a lesser role in establishing outcome in near-drowning cases. Aspiration of liquid into the lungs occurs in most patients, although in 10 to 20% of cases the patient does not aspirate (dry drowning). Aspiration of hypertonic solutions, such as salt water, induces pulmonary edema. Aspiration of hypotonic solution (fresh water) causes destruction or inactivation of surfactant. Bronchospasm, secondary to aspiration, is not uncommon. This may complicate therapy after the patient is resuscitated, but this problem is rarely the dominant one.

Swallowing large amounts of fluid is part of the pathophysiology in animal models of drowning. The potential for electrolyte abnormalities caused by absorption of hypertonic or hypotonic fluids is real.[16-19] However, electrolyte abnormalities are rarely encountered in patients who are treated in an emergency department.[20] Similarly, the effects of swallowing or aspirating large amounts of fluid on red blood cell integrity are also infrequent.

TREATMENT

Considerable effort has been expended in attempting to develop protocols that will improve the outcome in drowning patients. Unfortunately, none have shown any superiority over conventional supportive critical care.[21] Since there are no current efficacious clinical therapies for hypoxic ischemic injury other than prevention and immediate resuscitation, this result is not unexpected.

Supportive treatment of the submersion victim may be divided into prehospital and intrahospital phases. Resuscitation must be immediate. While the patient is still in the water, rescue breathing may be attempted. (Chest compressions will be fruitless.) Aggressive cardiopulmonary resuscitation (CPR) should be attempted at the scene of the accident. It is clear that effective CPR at the scene is the last time when the medical care team will be able to significantly influence the outcome for most victims of drowning.[22]

Rapid transport to an appropriate facility is essential. The patient should be neither actively warmed nor cooled during transport.

If CPR is necessary in the emergency department, the prognosis is grave unless the event was a cold water near-drowning (water temperature <5°C and the patient is hypothermic (temperature <33°C).[23] Nonetheless, CPR may be efficacious, especially if the body of water has ice in it and the child's core temperature is significantly reduced.[23, 24] Over 2 hours of CPR resulting in the return of spontaneous circulation and a good outcome has been reported.[25] Rewarming techniques include inhalation of warmed gases, peritoneal lavage or hemodialysis with warmed fluids, and cardiopulmonary bypass.

Treatment in the intensive care unit is supportive therapy of the hypoxic ischemic central nervous system injury and is directed at any underlying causes. Hypoxic ischemic injury is difficult to treat (see Chapters 13 and 19). The brain, lungs, cardiovascular system, kidneys, liver, and gastrointestinal tract may all be affected, with the dominant injury occurring in the brain. Supportive care of the brain involves ensuring adequate oxygenation and oxygen flow to the brain. Seizures are treated aggressively (see Chapter 23).

If additional lung injury is present, over and above that caused by hypoxia, aggressive therapy with various forms of mechanical ventilation and bronchodilator therapy may be necessary (see Chapters 40 and 46).

PROGNOSIS

The prognosis for the near-drowning victim is dependent on the underlying status of the patient (Was the

Table 9–2. PROGNOSTIC FACTORS IN NEAR-DROWNING

Favorable Factors	Unfavorable Factors
Age <3 yr	
Submersion (warm water) <3 min	Submersion (warm water) >9 min
Ice in water	
Core temperature <33° C	
Conscious on arrival	CPR* duration >25 min
Presence of a pulse in the emergency department	CPR needed on admission to emergency department
	ph <6.85
	Fixed and dilated pupils >6 hr after admission
	Seizures persisting >24 hr

*CPR = cardiopulmonary resuscitation.

patient exhausted, intoxicated, or hypothermic?), the circumstances of the event (Did the patient suffer a head or cervical spine injury, and what was the duration of submersion?), and, most important, how rapidly did restoration of spontaneous circulation occur? Few of these data will be available to the clinician.

Numerous attempts have been made to establish factors helpful in developing a prognosis. Some scoring systems have been developed,[23, 26] but these have not always been successful.[21, 27] Table 9–2 includes factors that have been shown to reflect favorably or unfavorably on prognosis. One should view this information with some skepticism. The exception to any of the factors may be a case report away.

OUTCOME

Outcome for survivors of near-drowning is, statistically, good[28–31]; however, these populations are not the usual ones seen in the intensive care unit, but rather usually include all patients admitted to the hospital following near-drowning. Regrettably, poor neurologic outcome is common among survivors.

References

1. Schuman SH, Rowe JR, Glazer HM, et al: Risk of drowning: An iceberg phenomenon. JACEP 6:139, 1977.
2. Rowe MI, Arango A, and Allington G: Profiles of pediatric drowning victims in a water-oriented society. J Trauma 17:587, 1977.
3. Metropolitan Life Insurance Company: Accidental drownings by age and activity. Statistical Bulletin 58:2, 1977.
4. Lamphier TA: Current status of treatment of near-drowning. Alaska Med 21:72, 1979.
5. Craig AB: Underwater swimming and loss of consciousness. JAMA 176:255, 1961.
6. Craig AB: Causes of loss of consciousness during underwater swimming. J Appl Physiol 16:583, 1961.
7. Pearn JH: Epilepsy and drowning in childhood. Br Med J 1:1510, 1977.
8. Pearn JH, Brown J III, Wong R, et al: Bathtub drownings: Report of seven cases. Pediatrics 64:68, 1979.
9. Pearn JH, Bart RD, and Yamaoka R: Neurologic sequelae after childhood near-drowning: A total population study from Hawaii. Pediatrics 64:187, 1979.
10. Center for Disease Control: Fatal injuries to children—United States, 1986. MMWR 39:442, 1990.
11. Modell JH: The Pathophysiology and Treatment of Drowning and Near-drowning. Springfield, IL, Charles C Thomas, 1971.
12. Plueckhahn VD: Alcohol and accidental drowning: A 25 year study. Med J Aust 141:22, 1984.
13. Wintemute GJ, Kraus JF, Teret SP, and Wright MA: The epidemiology of drowning in adulthood: Implications for prevention. Am J Prev Med 4:343, 1988.
14. Livingston S, Paul LL, and Pruce I: Epilepsy and drowning in childhood. Br Med J 2:515, 1977.
15. Ramey CA, Ramey DN, and Haywarb JS: Dive response of children in relation to cold-water near-drowning. J Appl Physiol 63(2):665, 1987.
16. Bennett HJ, Wagner T, and Fields A: Acute hyponatremia and seizures in an infant after a swimming lesson. Pediatrics 72:125, 1983.
17. Goldberg GN, Lightner ES, Morgan W, et al: Infantile water intoxication after a swimming lesson. Pediatrics 70:599, 1982.
18. Kropp RM and Schwartz JF: Water intoxication from swimming. J Pediatr 101:947, 1982.
19. Phillips KG: Swimming and water intoxication in infants. Can Med Assoc J 136:1147, 1987.
20. Peterson B: Morbidity of childhood near-drowning. Pediatrics 59:364, 1977.
21. Bohn DJ, Biggar WD, Smith CR, et al: Influence of hypothermia, barbiturate therapy and intracranial pressure on monitoring morbidity and mortality after near-drowning. Critical Care Med 14:529, 1986.
22. Quan L, Wentz KR, Gore EJ, et al: Outcome and predictors of outcome in pediatric submersion victims receiving prehospital care in King County, Washington. Pediatrics 86:586, 1990.
23. Orlowski JP: Drowning, near-drowning, and ice-water submersions. Pediatr Clin North Am 34:75, 1987.
24. Biggart MJ and Bohn DJ: Effect of hypothermia and cardiac arrest on outcome of near-drowning accidents in children. J Pediatr 117:179, 1990.
25. Bolt RG, Black PG, Bowers RS, et al: The use of extracorporeal rewarming in a child submerged for 66 minutes. JAMA 260:377, 1988.
26. Conn AW, Edmonda JF, and Barker GA: Cerebral resuscitation in near-drowning. Pediatr Clin North Am 26:691, 1979.
27. Bierens JJ, van der Velde EA, van Berkel M, et al: Submersion in the Netherlands: Prognostic indicators and results of resuscitation. Ann Emerg Med 19:1390, 1990.
28. Kemp AM and Sibert JR: P Outcome in children who nearly drown: a British Isles Study. Br Med J 302:931, 1991.
29. Pearn J: Survival rates after serious immersion accidents in childhood. Resuscitation 6:271, 1978.
30. Pearn J, Wong RY, Brown J III, et al: Drowning and near-drowning involving children: A five-year total population study from the city and county of Honolulu. Am J Public Health 69:450, 1979.
31. Fadel I and Bancalari E: Near-drowning in children: Clinical aspects. Pediatrics 58:573, 1976.

10

Sudden Unexpected Death

Peter R. Holbrook, M.D.

The pediatric intensive care unit (ICU) is the repository of children resuscitated from sudden death events. If the child survives, making a diagnosis of the cause of the cardiorespiratory arrest is crucial. If the child dies, a diagnosis may have implications for present or future siblings or for the parents. In addition, a correct diagnosis is an aid to relieving parental anguish. Thus, an attempt to clarify the underlying disease is imperative.

Sudden unexpected death (SUD) is a category into which almost all patients who are admitted to the pediatric ICU after cardiopulmonary resuscitation will fall. SUD may be occur in two groups of patients: (1) patients with known chronic disease, and (2) patients with either no known disease or acute, but seemingly mild disease.

The purpose of this chapter is to address the impact of SUD, review causes of SUD in patients with known chronic illness, and identify possible causes of collapse in apparently well children.

SUDDEN UNEXPECTED DEATH AS A COMPONENT OF INFANT AND CHILDHOOD MORTALITY

In the United States 2,167,999 people died in 1988.[1] Of these, 71,295 were 19 years of age or younger. The total numbers of deaths, and rates per 100,000 people, by age are in Table 10–1.

The infant mortality rate in the United States was

10.08/1,000 live births, and the rate for other nations is as low as just under 5 deaths/1,000 live births. Two thirds of U.S. infant mortality occurs in the first 28 days of life (neonatal mortality rate of 6.3 deaths/1,000 live births). In the United Kingdom almost half of infant mortality occurs after the eighth day of life (41 weeks after conception).[2] The major cause of death in the perinatal and neonatal age groups is prematurity and its complications, which are not considered here.

SUD represents a significant component of all deaths occurring in full-term infants. Even in the very young newborn group, there is a small but recognizable incidence of SUD. Polberger and Svenningsen noted an incidence in the first 4 days of life of 0.12 sudden deaths per 1,000 healthy, full-term liveborn infants.[3] In addition, based on their data, up to 0.5/1,000 may have an event that requires resuscitation.

In the postperinatal period (8 to 365 days of life) approximately half of infant deaths are unexpected,[4] and about half of these may be explained, underscoring the need to investigate all episodes of SUD.

After the first year of life, the mortality figures drop (see Table 10–1). SUD comprises about 75% of these deaths, and accidental death is the primary cause.[5] Approximately 10% of SUD is nontraumatic.[6] From another statistical approach, 20% of all nontraumatic deaths are sudden and of natural causes.[6]

SUDDEN UNEXPECTED DEATH IN PATIENTS WITH KNOWN CHRONIC DISEASE

Considering all children who experienced SUD, 6% of infants (Table 10–2) died of a known chronic disease. In the older child, 75% of mortality is caused by SUD (Table 10–3). The majority (three fourths) of these are not due to natural causes. This leaves 17% of the total mortality or 22% of all cases of SUD due to natural causes. Fifty-four per cent of children and adolescents who died of natural SUD died of a known chronic disease.[5] The breakdown by organ system of the latter group is noted in Table 10–4.

A review of the causes of death in patients under treatment for a known disease is valuable to remind the

Table 10–1. NUMBER OF DEATHS IN THE UNITED STATES—1988*

Age	No. of People	Rate (per 100,000)
All ages	2,167,999	882.0
< 19 yr of age	71,295	239.8
< 1 yr of age	38,910	1,008.3
< 1 mo	24,690	631.5
1–12 mo	14,220	383.7
1–4 yr of age	7,429	50.9
5–9 yr of age	4,357	24.2
10–14 yr of age	4,568	27.5
15–19 yr of age	16,031	88.0

*National Center for Health Statistics: Advance report of final mortality statistics—1988. Monthly Vital Statistics Report 39(7):1, 1990.

94

Table 10–2. ANALYSIS OF 115 UNEXPECTED INFANT DEATHS*

Description	No. (%)†
Pre-existing disease with a poor prognosis	7 (6)
Treatable disease	45 (39)
Minor disease	32 (28)
No disease	19 (17)
Accidental	4 (3)
Homicide†	8 (7)
Total	115 (100)

*Adapted from Taylor EM and Emery JL: Categories of preventable unexpected infant deaths. Arch Dis Child 65:535, 1990.
†Excludes deaths in which the parent or guardian was "charged with an offense."

Table 10–4. SUDDEN DEATH IN CHILDHOOD AND ADOLESCENCE*

Description	No. of Deaths
Known disease†	92
Cardiovascular	29
Respiratory	20
Neurologic	32
Diabetes	7
Miscellaneous	4
Unknown disease	77
Infection	39
Hemorrhage	13
Cardiovascular	9
Gastrointestinal	4
Diabetes	1
Unexplained	11

*Adapted from Keeling JW and Knowles SAS: Sudden death in childhood and adolescence. J Pathol 159:221–224, 1989. Reprinted by permission of John Wiley & Sons, Inc.
†Known disease includes diseases in which survival beyond 20 years is expected but which may be fatal without appropriate clinical management.

intensivist of what possibilities exist for disaster in a patient admitted to the ICU for "routine" treatment or to provide a quick differential diagnosis for a patient admitted to the ICU after a near-death event. The causes of such deterioration are the subject of other chapters in this text and lists of causes are given in Table 10–5.

SUDDEN UNEXPECTED DEATH IN PATIENTS WITH NO DISEASE OR INSIGNIFICANT DISEASE

SUD occurs in infants with no or insignificant disease at a high rate. As shown in Table 10–2, 55% of patients had no disease or minor disease at the time of death, and in an additional 39% the disease was considered to be treatable. In another study, two thirds of postperinatal infant death victims had no predisposing disease.[2]

In the older child 6.4% of all deaths, 10% of all SUD, and 46% of all SUD due to natural causes occur in patients with no disease or with insignificant disease (see Table 10–4).

The ability to establish a cause of death varies with age. In an in-hospital maternity ward (nursery) study, half of deaths could be attributed to an observed physiologic abnormality.[3] The remainder could not be explained after a clinical evaluation and an autopsy. Similarly, postneonatal infant deaths can be explained in more than 50% of cases (see Table 10–2). In the older child, the number of unexplained deaths drops but does not reach zero. Keeling and Knowles found 11 unexplained deaths among a consecutive series of 1,012

Table 10–3. ANALYSIS OF DEATHS IN CHILDHOOD AND ADOLESCENCE*

Description	No. of Deaths
Unnatural (SUD†-unnatural)	599
Natural	413
Anticipated	244
Unanticipated (SUD-natural)	169
Total	1,012

*Adapted from Keeling JW and Knowles SAS: Sudden death in childhood and adolescence. J Pathol 159:221–224, 1989. Reprinted by permission of John Wiley & Sons, Inc.
†SUD = sudden unexpected death.

deaths in children aged 2 to 20 years.[5] When only sudden, natural deaths were considered, 6.5% of deaths remained unexplained. Similarly, in a study from Sweden, only 4 of 420 SUDs (389 traumatic, 31 "natural" causes) were unexplained after a complete autopsy.[6] A complete evaluation of the cause of death in the older child usually, but not always, results in the determination of a cause.

Infections are the leading cause of death in the group with no or insignificant illness. Of 13 actual or near-miss sudden deaths in apparently healthy term infants in the first 4 days of life, four showed evidence of sepsis, which is the largest single cause.[3] Richards and McIntosh found 31% of postperinatal infant deaths at home due to infection.[2] Keeling and Knowles found that the most common cause of death in the older child with SUD (natural causes) was infection (51%), and respiratory illness was the leading cause with a frequency rate of 59%.[5] This is comparable with a Swedish study in which infections caused 52% of sudden natural death.

All other causes of death in patients with acute illness are low in frequency, except for one report of a 17% incidence of hemorrhage (90% intracranial) as a cause of death.[6]

Table 10–6 lists possible causes of sudden unexpected natural death by organ system. Several conditions merit special consideration.

The long QT syndrome has been known for 35 years. Two forms exist, the Jervell and Lange-Neilsen syndrome that combines congenital deafness, syncope, and electrocardiogram (ECG) findings of a prolongation of the QT interval, and the Romano-Ward syndrome, which is identical except for the absence of deafness. Under emotional or physical stress patients with this syndrome may develop ventricular fibrillation. ECG findings among survivors demonstrate alternation of the T wave associated with the precipitating stress. This may precede or following ventricular fibrillation. Recently, study of a kindred with the syndrome localized the gene to the short arm of chromosome 11, and strongly suggested that the disease locus is the H-ras-1 gene.[7]

Identification of patients with the syndrome allows for therapeutic trials with β-adrenergic blockade. This is effective in 75 to 80% of patients. For the remainder, good response to left cardiac sympathetic denervation has been reported.[8]

Metabolic defects causing sudden death are being increasingly recognized. The need to save a critical blood and urine sample for subsequent analysis at the time of peak malfunction is discussed in Chapter 60.

One cause of SUD, the sudden unexplained nocturnal death or lai tai, has been reported in Southeast Asian refugees and also is endemic in areas of Thailand. It is usually found in young adult males who die during sleep. The disease may be caused by a potassium deficiency that reaches its nadir during sleep. Linkage with hypokalemic periodic paralysis has been made.[9]

The sudden infant death syndrome (SIDS) is the diagnosis of exclusion for approximately half of SUD

Table 10–5. PATHOPHYSIOLOGIC CONDITIONS THAT MAY CAUSE DEATH

Known Cardiac Disease

Arrhythmias
Congestive heart failure
Pulmonary emboli
Paradoxic emboli
Hypoxia
Infundibular spasm ("tet spells")
Pulmonary artery spells
Pericardial tamponade
Inanition
Infection
Electrolyte imbalance
Intoxication

Known Cardiac Disease—Postoperative

Air emboli
Bleeding
Acute myocardial failure
Intraoperative catastrophes
  Cardioplegia
  Hypoxia
  Hemorrhage
  Electrolyte abnormalities

Known Neurologic Disease

Seizures
Herniation
Intracranial bleeding
Respiratory insufficiency
Electrolyte abnormalities
  SIADH*
  Diabetes insipidus
  Diuretic administration
Inanition
Infection

Known Pulmonary Disease

Bronchospasm
Pneumothorax
Pulmonary hemorrhage
Apnea
Hypoxia
Hypercarbia

Known Diabetes Mellitus

Hypoglycemia
Ketoacidosis
Nonketotic hyperosmolar coma
Cerebral edema

*SIADH = syndrome of inappropriate antidiuretic hormone.

Table 10–6. DIAGNOSES CAUSING SUDDEN UNEXPECTED DEATH OF NATURAL CAUSES

Central Nervous System

Intracranial Bleeding	Strokes
Arteriovenous malformation	Occlusive
Aneurysm	Sinus or venous
Bleeding disorders	Arterial
Vitamin B_1, C, and K	Embolic
deficiencies	Tumor
Hypertension	Clots
Subarachnoid hemorrhage	Seizures
Subdural hemorrhage	Infection
Bleeding into tumor	
Herniation	
Hydrocephalus	
Tumors	
Cerebral edema	

Cardiovascular

Infections	Coarctation aorta
Myocarditis	Hypertrophic cardiomyopathy
Pericarditis	Coronary artery disease
Endocarditis	Aberrant left coronary artery
Arrhythmias	Atherosclerotic disease
QT syndrome	Kawasaki disease
Wolff-Parkinson-White	Aortic rupture
syndrome	
Congenital atrioventricular	
block	

Pulmonary

Infections	Pulmonary embolus
Tonsillitis	Aspiration
Supraglottitis	Pulmonary hypertension
Laryngotracheobronchitis	
Pneumonia	

Gastrointestinal

Rupture of esophagus	Bowel obstruction
Diaphragmatic hernia	Gastroenteritis
Perforation gastrointestinal tract	Ruptured viscus
Peritonitis	Intussusception
Pancreatic necrosis	

Systemic

Sepsis	Malignant hyperthermia
Diabetic ketoacidosis	Metabolic disease

patients in infancy. Classically, this syndrome is found neither in early infancy nor beyond 1 year of age. As noted earlier, even in the newly born there are cases that remain unexplained after complete autopsy.[3] Whether these patients represent a subdivision of the basic syndrome or a unique group is unknown. Similarly, approximately 10% of SUD in older children remains unexplained.

With time the numbers of patients who fall into this group is shrinking, but only slightly. Research advances in this field have been summarized recently by Valdes-Dapena.[10]

References

1. Advance report on final mortality statistics, 1988. Monthly Vital Statistics Report, Washington, DC: National Center for Health Statistics; November 28, 1990: 39(No. 7)
2. Richards ID and McIntosh HT: Confidential inquiry into 226 consecutive infant deaths. Arch Dis Child 47:697–706, 1972.
3. Polberger S and Svenningsen NW: Early neonatal sudden infant

death and near death of full term infants in maternity wards. Acta Paediatr Scand 74:861–866, 1985.

4. Arneil GC, Brooke H, Gibson AAM, et al: Post-perinatal infant mortality in Glasgow 1979–81. Lancet ii:649, 1982.

5. Keeling JW and Knowles SAS: Sudden death in childhood and adolescence. J Pathol 159:221–224, 1989.

6. Molander N: Sudden natural death in later childhood and adolescence. Arch Dis Child 57:572–576, 1982.

7. Keating M, Atkinson A, Dunn C, et al: Linkage of a cardiac arrhythmia, the long QT syndrome, and the Harvey *ras*-1 gene. Science 252:704, 1991.

8. Schwartz PJ, Locati EH, Moss AJ, et al: Left cardiac sympathetic denervation in the therapy of congenital long QT syndrome. Circulation 84:503–511, 1991.

9. Nimmannit S, Malasit P, Chaovakul V, et al: Pathogenesis of sudden unexplained nocturnal death (lai tai) and endemic distal renal tubular acidosis. Lancet 338:930–932, 1991.

10. Valdes-Dapena M: Sudden infant death syndrome: Overview of recent research developments from a pediatric pathologist's perspective. Pediatrician 15:222–230, 1988.

III
Pansystemic Illness

11

Neonatal Sepsis

Jonathan M. Whitfield, M.B., Ch.B., F.R.C.P.(C.), F.C.C.P.,
E. Dobyns, M.D., and S. Webb, M.D.

Neonatal sepsis should be suspected in any ill-appearing neonate. The neonate with sepsis will have a predictably poor outcome unless it is treated aggressively and expeditiously with appropriate chemotherapeutic agents (antibacterial/antiviral/antifungal) as well as with intensive monitoring and supportive care. The septic neonate can present at the time of birth if the infection is acquired in utero; however, the infant may appear well initially only to present some hours to days later. Increasingly, the term newborn infant is discharged from the hospital at less than 24 hours of age and, thus, may present from home, in the physician's office, or in the emergency room with signs of sepsis. Two characteristic modes of presentation in the neonate (defined as an infant $\leq$ 28 days of age) are recognized—"early onset" less than or equal to 4 days of age, and "late onset" more than 4 days of age.[1] Late onset presentations of neonatal sepsis may have classic signs of sepsis often complicated by meningitis[2] but may also have very atypical presentations, such as cervical adenitis with stridor (Fig. 11–1).[2, 3] Interestingly, an association between early onset group B streptococcal infection and delayed right-sided diaphragmatic hernia has also been described.[4]

The clinical presentation of the septic neonate can vary from vague reports of lethargy and poor feeding to overt signs of illness, such as grunting respirations, skin mottling, or an ashen appearance with weak and rapid pulses accompanied by hypotension. Since cultures require a minimum of 12 to 24 hours to have a positive result, an infectious etiology for the septic-appearing neonate is a necessary initial presumption when the infant is first evaluated. However, it is only a presumptive diagnosis until the results of the culture are reported. It is only then that the diagnosis of sepsis becomes definitive. It is important in the interim period to thoroughly explore the differential diagnosis of the presumed septic neonate and to recognize the specific entities that masquerade as sepsis. Several of these disorders have very specific treatment interventions that can be lifesaving (Table 11–1).

EPIDEMIOLOGY

The incidence of neonatal sepsis varies widely and depends on the population of infants being studied, the gestational age, and whether an outborn or inborn population is reviewed. In one report, the 60-year experience with neonatal sepsis at the Yale New Haven Hospital was analyzed.[7] The incidence of sepsis in neonates of all weights and gestations for equal to or less than 30 days of age was 2.7 cases per 1,000 liveborn babies. The incidence for infants weighting 2,500 g or more was only 1 case per 1,000 liveborns, whereas this number increased dramatically to 86 cases per 1,000 liveborn infants in neonates weighing less than 1,000 g. The overall mortality rate for sepsis in this report was 15.9%. In addition, it was noted that prolonged lengths of stay have been associated with a significant increase in nosocomial sepsis. This had an associated 13.7% mortality rate. The microbiology of neonatal sepsis between 1979 and 1988 at Yale New Haven Hospital is shown in Table 11–2.

The continuing importance of group B streptococci (GBS) and *Escherichia coli* in neonatal sepsis is clearly shown in Table 11–2. This is the basis for combination antibiotic therapy in all neonates presenting with possible sepsis.

Early onset disease remains the predominant mode of presentation in neonatal sepsis, but it is clear that late onset and postneonatal onset beyond the first month of life is also important (Table 11–3). The organisms in late onset disease include GBS and *E. coli*, but the importance of other organisms, especially staphylococci, is clear, requiring the initiation of triple antibiotics.

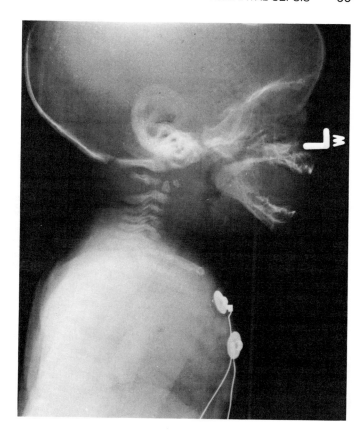

Figure 11–1. 10-week-old previous 34-week preterm male discharged from hospital 2 weeks previously who presented with a cervical mass and stridor requiring emergency intubation in the emergency room. GBS cultured. The infant responded well to intravenous antibiotics and was extubated 72 hours after admission to the hospital.

Table 11–1. MASQUERADERS OF NEONATAL SEPSIS: TIME OF ONSET AND EMERGENCY TREATMENT

Diagnosis	Typical Onset (Days)	Treatment
1. Cardiac disease:		
a. Ductal dependent structural heart disease (e.g., coarctation, interruption of aorta, hypoplastic left heart)	4–10	PGE_1 0.05–0.1 µg/kg/min
b. Paroxysmal atrial tachycardia	0–28	Synchronized DC (0.5–1 joules/kg) cardioversion IV adenosine (50–100 µg/kg)
c. Myocarditis	0–28	Supportive
d. Myocardial infarction	0–28	Supportive
2. Nonbacterial infections:		
a. Viral (e.g., HSV/varicella/RSV)	0–28	Acyclovir 10 mg/kg q 8 h VZIG 125 units IM RSVIG* 10 ml/kg IV
3. Respiratory distress (e.g., HMD, TTN)	0	Supportive
4. Endocrine/metabolic:		
a. Hypoglycemia	0–28	10% glucose IV 2 ml/kg as a bolus, then 4 ml/kg/hr
b. Lactic acidosis	0–21	
Organic acidosis	0–21	
Urea cycle defects, etc.	0–21	
Congenital adrenal hyperplasia	14–21	See ref. 5
5. Other:		
a. Gastrointestinal (e.g., NEC volvulus, appendicitis, toxic megacolon, gastroenteritis with dehydration)	Variable	May require urgent laparotomy
b. Methemoglobinemia	0–28	IV methylene blue 1–2 ml/kg
c. Drug toxicity	Variable	See ref. 6
d. Shaken infant	Variable	Supportive

*Currently in multi-institutional study.
PGEI = prostaglandin E (Prostin Upjohn Co.).
RSVIG = respiratory syncytial virus immunoglobulin.
VZIG = varicella zoster immune globulin.

NEC = necrotizing entero colitis.
HSV = herpes simplex virus.
HMD = hyaline membrane disease.
TTN = transient tachypnea of newborn.

Table 11–2. MICROBIOLOGY OF NEONATAL SEPSIS AT YALE-NEW HAVEN HOSPITAL (1979 to 1988)*

Total No. of Isolates (270)	
Organism (%)	No. of Isolates
1. Gram-positive aerobic bacteria (41%)	
β-Hemolytic streptococci group B	64
Coagulase-negative staphylococci	36
β-Hemolytic streptococci group D	
Enterococcus sp.	18
Staphylococcus aureus	14
Viridans streptococci	11
Streptococcus pneumoniae	2
Listeria monocytogenes	2
Bacillus aereus	1
2. Gram-negative aerobic bacteria (54%)	
Escherichia coli	46
Klebsiella pneumoniae	18
Haemophilus influenzae	8
Enterobacter cloacae	7
Pseudomonas aeruginosa	6
Klebsiella oxytoca	5
Serratia marcescens	3
Enterobacter agglomerans	2
Acinetobacter anitratus	2
Pseudomonas cepacia	2
Pseudomonas fluorescens	1
Arizona hinshawii	1
Morganella morgani	1
Salmonella C-2	1
Haemophilus parainfluenzae	1
3. Gram-negative anaerobic bacteria (2%)	
Bacteroides fragilis	4
Bacteroides thetaiotaomicron	1
Fusobacterium necrophorum	1
4. Fungi (3%)	
Candida albicans	10
Candida lusitaniae	1

*Modified from Gladstone IM, Ehrenkranz RA, Edberg SC, et al: A ten year review of neonatal sepsis and comparison with fifty year experience. Pediatr Infect Dis 9(11):821, 1990. © by Williams & Wilkins, 1990.

As discussed previously, the incidence of neonatal sepsis in different settings varies greatly. The actual number of suspected cases of neonatal sepsis requiring presumptive treatment with antimicrobial agents yet subsequently proven *not* to have associated bacteremia has not been well researched. Estimates suggest that up to 10% of all newborns are treated with antimicrobial agents either because of historical risk factors (e.g., prolonged rupture of membranes) or clinical suspicion of sepsis, such as temperature instability or respiratory distress. This would represent the treatment of more than 350,000 neonates per year in the United States alone. No more than 1% or 35,000 is likely to be bacteremic. This "overtreatment" results in unnecessary hospitalization. The associated increased costs have been shown to be substantially reduced with judicious use of clinical and laboratory data.[8]

RISK FACTORS

The maternal factors that are important in increasing risk of neonatal sepsis are shown in Table 11–4.

The byproducts of some of the vaginal organisms (e.g., collagenase and elastase) may weaken the intact fetal membranes prior to labor, not only exposing the fetus to ascending vaginal infective agents but also resulting in the release of mediators that can initiate labor.[9] The neonate is also at risk due to deficiencies in both cellular and noncellular components of the neonatal immune system.

Cellular Deficiencies of the Newborn

The most important phagocytic cell is the polymorphonuclear leukocyte (PMN). The neonatal PMN characteristics and how they differ from those of the adult are shown in Table 11–5. As can be seen in Table 11–6, although the intrinsic properties of the neonatal PMN are normal to increased, the response of the PMN to chemotactic signals initiated by infectious agents is poor.[10] Further, disaggregation of PMN and migration to the infected tissues that contain a focus of infection is markedly depressed. This depressed migration can result in blockage of the local microvasculature with PMN aggregates leading to tissue injury.[11] Depletion of circulating neutrophils with the exhaustion of the neutrophil storage pool in the marrow is more likely to occur because the storage pool is low (14% of the adult pool) and the turnover rate is so high.[12–14]

Noncellular Deficiences of the Newborn

Table 11–7 summarizes the known noncellular immunodeficiencies of the newborn.[15–17]

CHEMICAL MEDIATORS OF SEPSIS

The factor(s) that mediate(s) the chain of events occurring at the cellular level in neonatal septic shock are still being actively investigated. They include thromboxane, platelet-activating factor (PAF), tumor necrosis factor (TNF), leukotrienes,[18] prostaglandins, endothelial-derived relaxing factor (EDRF), free radicals, and

Table 11–3. DISTRIBUTION BY AGE OF 270 POSITIVE CULTURES AT YALE NEW HAVEN HOSPITAL (1979 TO 1988)*

	Inborn Age When Cultured Days			Outborn	Total
Number of positive cultures (% of total)	Early (0–4) 93 (35%)	Late (5–30) 54 (20%)	Postneonatal (>30) 56 (21%)	67 (25%)	270 (100%)

*Modified from Gladstone IM, Ehrenkranz RA, Edberg SC, et al: A ten year review of neonatal sepsis and comparison with fifty year experience. Pediatr Infect Dis J 9(11):821, 1990. © by Williams & Wilkins, 1990.

Table 11–4. MATERNAL RISK FACTORS FOR NEONATAL SEPSIS

Premature labor (before 37 weeks' gestation)
Prolonged rupture membranes (>12–24 hr)
Maternal fever
Chorioamnionitis
Maternal GBS carriage (up to 30% of pregnant mothers)
Maternal vaginosis

Table 11–6. OXIDATIVE METABOLIC RESPONSE OF POLYMORPHONUCLEAR LEUKOCYTES

	Normal Newborn	Stressed Newborn	Adult
Phagocytosis	Normal	Normal	Normal
Superoxide generation by PMNs	Normal to ↑	↑ ↑ ↑	Normal
Chemiluminescence response to Zymosan*	Normal	↓	Normal

*Zymosan is an oxidative stimulant, the effect of which is measured by chemical fluorescence.

interleukin-1 (IL-1). White blood cells (WBCs) release many of the proinflammatory mediators, such as lipooxygenase products, free radicals, hydrolytic enzymes, and cytokines, which act on the vascular endothelium to cause increased cellular permeability, aggregation of platelets and other blood cells, and release of additional vasoactive substances. The complex interactions and feedback cycles among these mediators contribute greatly to the hemodynamic instability and vascular leak that so commonly occur with sepsis (Fig. 11–2).

The arachidonic acid metabolite thromboxane (TxA2) appears to be a very important mediator of the pulmonary hypertensive phase of experimental GBS sepsis (GBSS)—a phase that can be blocked by cyclooxygenase inhibitors such as indomethacin[19] and the thromboxane synthetase inhibitor Dazmegrel (UK 38,485).[20] Elevations of serum thromboxane and prostacyclin have been demonstrated not only in animal models of sepsis but also in human neonates with pulmonary hypertension.[21]

Attention has focused on the inflammatory mediators PAF and TNF as having important roles in a cascade of events that result in the clinical picture of sepsis. PAF is a phospholipid that is produced by and acts on neutrophils, macrophages, monocytes, platelets, and endothelial cells and is a known inducer of microvascular permeability.[22] The extensive review article by Hosford and Braquet[22] discusses the studies that have shown that PAF infusions cause a shock state in animals often paralleling the state seen in neonatal sepsis. This mediator is also produced during shock, as noted in children with sepsis.[23] PAF is not the sole factor responsible for the circulatory changes, however, as PAF antagonists fail to reverse the pulmonary hypertension in GBSS.[24]

TNF is a powerful vasoactive cytokine produced by activated macrophages, including neonatal monocytes,[25] and is implicated as an important factor in endotoxemia and other shock-like states.[26, 27] TNF levels are elevated in humans with septic shock,[28, 29] with meningococcal

disease,[30] after endotoxin administration,[31] and in children with gram-negative septic shock.[32] Some models of experimental shock require the presence of both TNF and endotoxin.[33] Although TNF is associated with some of the vasomotor responses in sepsis, such as pulmonary hypertension and systemic hypotension,[34] it is not linked to other aspects, such as hypoxemia.[35]

Investigators suggest that overproduction of EDRF, or nitric oxide, in septic shock mediates the systemic circulatory collapse of endotoxin shock since the administration of EDRF inhibitors rapidly reversed the hypotension induced by endotoxin.[36]

Thus, it appears that no single mediator acts to cause the cardiopulmonary events seen with experimental GBSS or endotoxemia. Rather, as seen in Figure 11–2, a cascade of events occur and culminate in the clinical manifestations of sepsis and shock.

ORGAN SYSTEM RESPONSES IN NEONATAL SEPSIS

Cardiovascular Responses

Transitional Circulation

The neonate differs from the older child or adult in its cardiovascular response to many stressful stimuli, including sepsis. Some septic neonates revert to a fetal circulatory pattern. The intensivist caring for the newborn must understand both the normal fetal and transitional circulation changes as well as the abnormal perinatal circulation that is known as persistent pulmonary hypertension of the newborn (PPHN). PPHN is characterized by pulmonary hypertension and systemic arterial hypoxemia and is a consequence of extrapulmo-

Table 11–5. CHARACTERISTICS OF NEUTROPHIL IN NEWBORN COMPARED WITH ADULT

PMN Characteristics	Newborn	Adult
Neutrophil turnover rate	Extremely high	High
Neutrophil maturation storage pool (storage vs circulating pool)	2:1	14:1
Mobility after exposure to chemotactic factors	Unchanged	Enhanced
Aggregation of PMNs	Slow	Rapid
Disaggregation	Very slow to none	Rapid
Adherence	Poor	Good
Deformability	Poor	Easy

Table 11–7. NEONATAL HUMORAL DEFICITS

Specific antibody levels	↓ / ↓↓
Complement (classic)	↓
Complement (alternate)	↓↓
Fibronectin	↓
Chemotactic factors (C5a, C3a, etc.)	↓
C-reactive protein	↔ / ↑

↓ = Mild decrease.
↓↓ = Moderate to severe decrease.
↔ = Comparable to an adult.
↑ = Increased.
See Chapter 4 for further details.

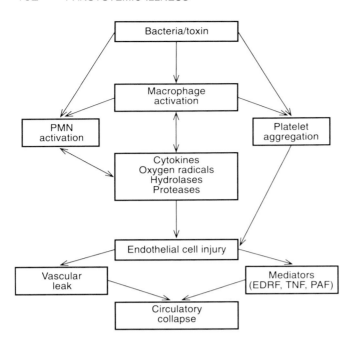

Figure 11–2. Bacteria or their toxins can trigger the release of inflammatory mediators such as tumor necrosis factor (TNF), platelet activating factor (PAF), oxygen radicals, hydrolases, and proteases from blood-borne elements. A cascade of events occurs as vascular endothelial cell injury causes subsequent increases in vascular permeability and further stimulates the release of several potent endogenous vasodilators from neutrophils, vascular endothelium, and smooth muscle cells. If not arrested, the cellular injury and continued positive feedback of circulating mediators culminates in shock and circulatory collapse.

nary right to left shunts at the foramen ovale and the ductus arteriosus (see Chapter 34 for details). These complex transitional circulation changes in the newborn are, as stated earlier, very sensitive to adverse influences. Arrest or reversal of this orderly process can tip the balance so that the neonate reverts back to a fetal circulatory pattern by reopening functionally but not yet

anatomically closed shunts and by altering the production or inhibition of vasoactive mediators.

In addition to changing flow patterns, it has become clear that structural alterations and remodeling of the existing pulmonary vascular bed can occur very rapidly in response to stress and thus potentially contribute to the perinatal circulatory abnormalities *even over short periods of time* (days). Several investigators have demonstrated that this response to injury is greater in neonatal than in adult pulmonary vasculature.[37–39] The neonatal vascular smooth muscle cell appears more metabolically reactive than the adult cell and exhibits altered responses to growth factors and inhibitors.[40] In the newborn, endothelial cell injury, smooth muscle cell and fibroblast proliferation, and increased extracellular matrix production occur more significantly after injury to the pulmonary circulation[41] than in the adult. These proliferative changes associated with pulmonary hypertension as seen in Figure 11–3 can lead to the obstruction of blood flow as well as to alterations in vasomotor responses to both endogenous and exogenous vasoactive mediators. All of these anatomic factors combine to make therapeutic intervention a challenging prospect.

Animal Models and Cardiovascular Responses to Sepsis

GBS are one of the leading causes of overwhelming neonatal sepsis, and although other organisms result in very similar clinical pictures, most investigators have used experimental animal models of GBS infections to study the pulmonary and cardiac hemodynamics of neonatal sepsis and septic shock. In addition, the clinical and pathologic features of GBSS in neonates bear marked similarity to those seen with endotoxic shock and gram-negative sepsis in adults.

Streptococcus agalactiae is the species designation for Lancefield group B β-hemolytic streptococci. Group determination is made by the group-specific antigen, in this case the group B polysaccharide antigen. This

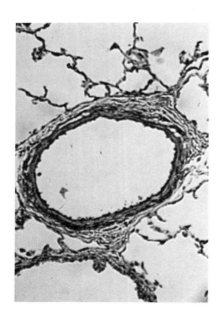

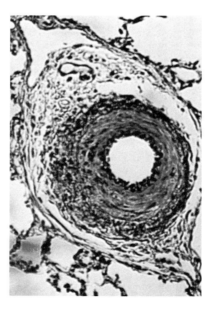

Figure 11–3. Photomicrographs showing a small pulmonary artery from a normal 15-day-old calf (left) and a 15-day-old calf after 14 days of exposure to hypobaric hypoxia (right). Pulmonary artery pressure (Ppa) in the normoxic calf was approximately 27 mm Hg, while the Ppa in the hypoxic calf was about 120 mm Hg. Note the medial and adventitial thickening in the hypertensive vessel. Original magnification 400 ×, courtesy of Kurt R. Stenmark, M.D.)

antigen contains rhamnose, galactose, and glycosamine residues. Serotyping is determined by the type-specific antigens on the GBS surface. These are primarily surface capsular polysaccharides, although some proteins are present also. The present serotype classification for the encapsulated GBS is based on polysaccharide and protein antigenic determinants and is as follows: Ia, Ib, Ia/c, II, III, IV.[42] Type III strains are the most virulent in humans. Their type-specific antigens consist of repeating units of galactose, glucose, and glycosamine with an attached sialic acid moiety. As described later, there is ongoing work to determine the nature of the active component of GBS that causes the hemodynamic instability seen with perinatal infections.

While gram-positive bacteria such as GBS do not have endotoxin, two different polysaccharide toxins have been described. An "exotoxin" consisting of a repeating unit of nine mannose residues[43] isolated from the culture media of GBS type III and another toxin[44, 45] containing capsular polysaccharide and protein each can cause the hemodynamic and gas exchange abnormalities seen with GBSS. The polysaccharide capsule may contribute to the organism's virulence via its protection from host phagocytosis, but it may not be essential to cause the thromboxane-associated pulmonary hypertension and hypoxemia seen in animal models of GBSS.[46]

Whatever the toxin is in GBS, it behaves clinically very similarly to endotoxin, which is a major initiator of the complex interactions of inflammatory mediators in gram-negative septic shock. Endotoxin has been investigated more thoroughly and is the biologically active lipopolysaccharide (LPS) component of the cell wall of gram-negative bacteria that causes a shock-like picture, including hypoxemia, pulmonary hypertension, and activation of the arachidonic acid cascade.

Experimentally, the hemodynamic effects of GBS have been studied in several animal models. The piglet's cardiovascular system is physiologically most similar to the human neonate. The hemodynamic effects of GBS infusion ($2 - 4 \times 10^{10}$ CFU/kg) in piglets is shown in Table 11–8.[47]

LV^{dp}/dt is a measure of intrinsic contractile state of the heart, and because left ventricular end-diastolic pressure (LVEDP) does not change and cardiac output (CO) decreases (even before pulmonary artery pressure [PAP] increases occurred), the primary cause of the decreased CO is considered to be a direct effect of the bacterial infusion on cardiac contractility. This is consistent with observations of adult humans suffering from endotoxic shock.[48]

Pulmonary Response to Sepsis

Most newborns with GBSS present with respiratory failure, neutropenia, and shock. Experimental GBSS has a biphasic response with initial acute pulmonary hypertension, hypoxemia, systemic hypotension, leukopenia, and increased pulmonary lymph flow followed by increased lung microvascular permeability despite a return of the pulmonary artery pressure toward baseline.[49, 50] These cardiopulmonary alterations are very

Table 11–8. HEMODYNAMIC RESPONSE OF PIGLET TO GBS INFUSION*

MAP	↓ (20–30%)
SVR	↑
CO	↓ (50% +)
LV^{dp}/dt	↓
PAP/PVR	↑
Vo$_2$	↓
H/R	↔
LVEDP	↔

*Adapted from Miller RR, et al: The effect of naloxone on the hemodynamics of the newborn piglet with septic shock. Pediatr Res 20(8):707, 1986 with permission.

CO = cardiac output.
LVdp/dt = left ventricular pressure change in unit time.
MAP = mean arterial pressure
SVR = systemic vascular resistance (MAP-CVP)/CO
PAP = pulmonary arterial pressure
PVR = pulmonary vascular resistance (PAP-LVEDP)/CO
Vo$_2$ = oxygenation consumption
(CaO$_2$-CvO$_2$ × CO)
CaO$_2$ = arterial O$_2$ content
CvO$_2$ = mixed versus O$_2$ content
H/R = heart rate (beats/min)
LVEDP = left ventricular end-diastolic pressure
↑ = increase.
↓ = decrease.
↔ = no change.

similar to septic shock from endotoxin, and the extensive review of endotoxin and lung injury by Brigham and Meyrick is recommended for a more complete description.[51]

In addition to the circulatory effects of sepsis, lung mechanics are altered (decreased dynamic compliance and increased airflow resistance) in endotoxemia,[52] TNF infusion in sheep,[53] and with GBSS in lambs.[54]

Central Nervous System Response to Sepsis

Extension of the bacteremia in neonatal sepsis to the meninges is seen 25 to 30% of the time[55] and occurs usually through susceptible portions of the blood-brain barrier (i.e., the choroid plexus or cerebral microvasculature[56]).

The pathophysiology of bacterial meningitis is extensively reviewed in an excellent article by Saez-Llorens and associates.[57] Inadequate humoral and phagocytic activity in the cerebrospinal fluid (CSF) allows organisms to reproduce rapidly. Subsequent inflammation is caused by components of the bacteria themselves and by activation of a host of inflammatory mediators. The polysaccharide capsule, found in such organisms as *E. coli, Haemophilus influenzae, Neisseria meningitidis*, and *Streptococcus pneumoniae*, is protective against host defense. As described earlier, cellular components of both gram-positive and gram-negative organisms act as potent stimulators of inflammation, shock, and ischemia.

Just as in the pulmonary condition, the presence of these components in the CSF initiate an impressive inflammatory response, a response that itself may contribute significantly to the brain damage seen with meningitis. Cytokines such as TNF[58] and IL-1[59] are produced by cells such as activated monocytes and macrophages and also by brain astrocytes and microglial cells.

These cytokines attract leukocytes for attachment to cerebral vascular endothelium and also activate phospholipases that act on membrane phopholipids to produce arachidonic acid metabolites such as prostaglandins, thromboxane, and leukotrienes. While elevated concentrations of PAF,[60] PGE$_2$, prostacyclin, IL-1, and TNF[61] have been detected in the CSF of infants with meningitis, their complex interrelationship and role in bacterial meningitis is not yet clear. Mustafa and associates[61] demonstrated that dexamethasone therapy in infants and children with bacterial meningitis resulted in a lower CSF concentration of PGE$_2$ and IL-1 after 18 to 30 hours of treatment. These proponents of dexamethasone therapy suggest that the association between anti-inflammatory treatment in meningitis and reduction in CSF inflammatory mediators results in the shorter duration of fever and lower incidence of neurologic sequelae seen in these patients. The role of other inflammatory mediators, such as complement factor C5a, IL-6, and macrophage inflammatory proteins, are being studied in meningitis.[57]

It is known that the blood-brain barrier permeability is altered in meningitis, and this is probably related to the complicated interaction among bacteria, inflammatory mediators, endothelial cells, and neutrophils.[62, 63] Once neutrophils attach to the cerebral microvasculature, transendothelial migration occurs via enzymatic digestion, paving the way for vascular leak of proteins and fluid into the CSF. The coagulation cascade is also triggered with this endothelial injury.

All of these events culminate in vasogenic edema, increased intracranial pressure, thrombosis, and reduced cerebral blood flow in the central nervous system.

Gastrointestinal Response to Sepsis

Much attention has been focused over the years on the gastrointestinal tract as a *source* for bacteremia and endotoxemia in the critically ill. Several studies have documented the adsorption or translocation of bacteria or endotoxin across gut membranes into the circulation or regional lymph nodes.[64] This was further substantiated by documenting that endotoxin was found in the portal blood but not in the systemic blood of adult patients undergoing elective abdominal surgery, thus implying that the Kupffer cells of the liver normally remove endotoxin absorbed from the gut.[65] Other investigators have studied the susceptibility of patients to the deleterious effects of endotoxemia. Caridis and associates[66] compared the existence of endotoxemia in septic and nonseptic patients and suggested that survival correlated with the integrity of the reticuloendothelial system.[66]

Although most work has focused on adults and animal models, endotoxin has been detected in the cord blood of nonseptic term and preterm infants,[67] in venous blood after feeding trials in preterm infants,[68] in nonseptic term and preterm infants with respiratory failure,[69] and in pediatric patients during and after cardiac surgery.[70] This raises the possibility that the gut may in certain circumstances be a *source* of bacteria and endotoxin in the neonate.

The potential for gut ischemia, especially in watershed areas of the bowel, is exaggerated in the neonate (the diving reflex theory). Furthermore, an overabundance of angiotensin receptors in the neonatal colon may predispose it to more vasoconstriction in low cardiac output states.[71] Whether the iatrogenic increase in α-adrenergic tone seen with the use of high-dose dopamine in the sick neonate may also compromise the splanchnic circulation sufficiently to disrupt gut integrity and permit toxin or bacterial translocation has not been proved but is certainly an intriguing possibility that requires further investigation.

Necrotizing enterocolitis (NEC) is thought to be an ischemic entity and is associated with bacteremia, sepsis, and septic shock. Studies have investigated the involvement of endotoxin and other cytokines in necrotizing enterocolitis. Although the exact pathogenesis is still being investigated,[72] it is reasonable to assume that conditions in the neonate may predispose to bacterial overgrowth of the gut, thus supplying a source for a systemic load. Several other contributing factors may coexist. Immaturity of the reticuloendothelial system in the newborn may cause failure in endotoxin clearance or the ductus venosus may remain patent in the ill neonate, permitting portal blood to bypass the liver. The immature intestinal membrane of the neonate may predispose to macromolecular passage.[73, 74] In addition, the altered carbohydrate fermentation and subsequent lower intraluminal pH in neonates may allow transepithelial passage of proinflammatory proteins across the intestinal membrane.[75] Another potential factor is the incomplete development in the neonate of gut peptides (e.g., motilin, vasoactive intestinal polypeptide, and enteroglucagon) that may alter the regulation of the intestinal response to disease states.[76]

Current research on NEC is focusing on PAF and TNF. Several investigators have shown in animals that both endotoxin and PAF can stimulate TNF production and that all three (alone or in combination) can cause bowel injury among their myriad effects.[77–79] Thus, these cytokines are implicated as mediators that act synergistically with endotoxin *to cause* bowel injury. Of note, a group of investigators has recently documented elevated TNF and PAF levels in human neonates with NEC.[80]

DIAGNOSIS AND TREATMENT

Clinical signs and symptoms of sepsis in the neonate are protean (Table 11–9).

None of the signs in the table are sufficiently specific or sensitive to distinguish sepsis from other entities, such as congenital heart disease, respiratory distress syndrome, or metabolic disease. The positive and negative predictive values of a variety of clinical and laboratory aids have been evaluated alone and in combination, and none is 100%. This is expected when the prevalence of sepsis is low. However, certain signs and symptoms seen during frequent examinations, when taken together with the perinatal history and laboratory findings, can help

Table 11–9. CLINICAL SIGNS OF NEONATAL SEPSIS

Lethargy/irritability	Tachycardia (>160/min)
Respiratory distress	Pale and/or mottled appearance
Apnea	Poor capillary refill > 3 sec
Vomiting	Hypotension (<60 mm Hg systolic)
Anorexia	Hypoglycemia (<40 mg/dl)
Abdominal distention	Hypothermia (<36.5° C)
Diarrhea	Hyperthermia (>37.8° C)
Jaundice	
Hepatosplenomegaly	
Petechiae/purpura	

the clinician to narrow the differential diagnosis and form a logical plan of treatment.

In contrast to most adults or older children, a variety of thermal responses to sepsis are seen in the neonate because temperature may be elevated, depressed, or normal. The pathophysiology of this response is poorly understood as leukocytic pyrogens such as IL-1 and IL-6 are found in neonates,[81, 82] however, hypothalamic sensitivity to such pyrogens may be depressed.[83] Retrospective studies have shown that approximately 1% of term newborns in the first week of life had a single brief episode of fever (>37.8°C), which was rarely associated

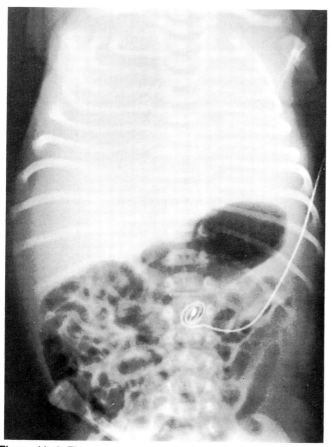

Figure 11–4. The chest roentgenogram is from a full-term neonate with severe respiratory distress. The "white out" appearance and lack of cardiac silhouette definition is apparent (see also Fig 11–5). The patient had GBSS. The patient in Figure 11–5 had HMD. Radiographs of the chest cannot distinguish these two entities.

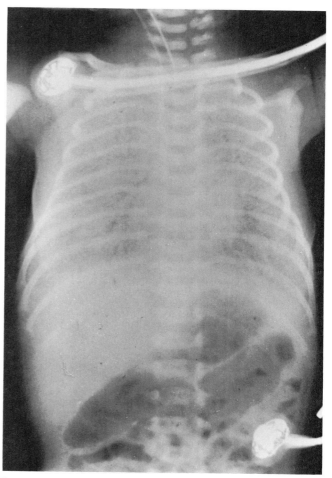

Figure 11–5. The chest roentgenogram is from a full-term neonate with severe respiratory distress. The "white out" appearance and lack of cardiac silhouette definition is apparent (see also Fig. 11–4). This patient had HMD, and the patient in Figure 11–4 had GBSS. Radiographs of the chest cannot distinguish these two entities.

with infection if no other clinical signs were present. In contrast, bacterial disease was found more frequently in infants with persistent fever or fever in conjunction with other symptoms of infection.

Respiratory distress is common in sick neonates and often is manifested by tachypnea, retractions, cyanosis, grunting, nasal flaring, or rales. Indeed, GBS pneumonia and sepsis are impossible in the earliest stages to distinguish from surfactant deficiency causing hyaline membrane disease (Figs. 11–4 and 11–5).

Apnea is an important clue in neonatal sepsis; however, it can occur late in the illness. Cardiovascular symptoms, such as tachycardia and poor capillary refill, may occur but are not specific for sepsis and frequently occur with congenital heart disease.

Jaundice occurs in about a third of the reported cases of neonatal sepsis and usually resolves after appropriate antibiotic therapy. Other skin manifestations, such as petechiae and purpura, are seen occasionally in neonatal septic shock and must be differentiated from those seen in congenital viral disease or coagulation disorders. Hepatomegaly is seen in many congenital viral infections but may also occur with congestive heart failure or metabolic diseases. Feeding difficulties (either with or without abdominal distention) can be an early sign of sepsis, and one must differentiate between an ileus secondary to sepsis from that due to NEC or anatomic abnormalities.

Meningitis is particularly difficult to diagnose or exclude in the septic neonate. There are *no* reliable symptoms to differentiate sepsis from meningitis in the neonate, such as a full fontanelle or nuchal rigidity. These signs are present in less than half of the newborns with meningitis. Both seizures, frequently focal and present in up to 75% of patients, and focal findings, such as hemiparesis and horizontal eye deviation, are often associated with neonatal meningitis.[84]

Whereas the signs and symptoms described earlier are seen in bacterial sepsis, several viruses, including herpes simplex and enteroviruses, can present with similar findings and cause significant morbidity and mortality. Disseminated neonatal herpes simplex virus (HSV) infection usually presents around 10 days of life and can adversely affect most organ systems. While the vesicular skin rash is often considered pathognomonic, it is absent in more than 20% of neonates.[85] An adage worth remembering is that a lymphocytic pleocytosis in the CSF of a neonate is HSV infection until proven otherwise. The mortality from disseminated herpes is approximately 60%, as babies usually die of complications of pneumonitis, often hemorrhagic, or disseminated intravascular coagulation (DIC). Although the morbidity is high and treatment may not halt the progression of the infection, vigorous historical and clinical investigation is warranted in these neonates to ascertain the diagnosis. Antiviral chemotherapy is relatively safe and should *not* be withheld while awaiting laboratory results.

More than 20% of infant enteroviral infections involve a sepsis-like syndrome, which again has nonspecific symptoms.[86] A high index of suspicion and knowledge of community acquired infections may be helpful in the diagnosis. Although numerous strains are documented to cause enteroviral sepsis, echovirus 11 is the most virulent and frequently leads to fulminant DIC and liver failure.[87]

In summary, there are no signs and symptoms that are 100% predictive (either positive or negative), and in the words of countless other texts on this topic, "a high degree of clinical judgment must be exercised by the prudent physician." Interestingly, studies in young infants evaluating the positive predictive value of signs and symptoms reported by caretakers (e.g., "does not look right" or "worries me") have been shown to be as reliable as a variety of other more conventional diagnostic studies. Listen to the caretakers when evaluating a neonate for possible sepsis.

INTERPRETATION OF LABORATORY DATA

Since the incidence of neonatal sepsis is so low, no laboratory test exists that is 100% predictive. The ideal

Table 11–10. INTERPRETATION OF LABORATORY TESTS

1. *Sensitivity:* When *infection* is present, the % of time the test is abnormal
2. *Specificity:* When *infection* is absent, the % of time the test is normal
3. *Positive Predictive Value:* When a *test* is abnormal, the % of time infection is truly present
4. *Negative Predictive Value:* When a *test* is normal, the % of time infection is truly absent

laboratory test would be both 100% sensitive and have a 100% negative predictive value (Table 11–10).

Most studies reviewing laboratory aids to the diagnosis of sepsis have focused on the sensitivity and specificity of tests. Sensitivity and specificity in the setting of sepsis is a *retrospective* determination, since cultures are never immediately available. The physician in the heat of clinical battle is more interested in a test's positive or negative predicative value (see definitions in Table 11–10).

Further, the presentation of the septic neonate and the rate of evolution of the disease process is very variable, and this fact must be taken into account when interpreting laboratory data. Consider the process of sepsis in the newborn analogous to a movie reel with innumerable frames that may run in slow motion (type III GBS late onset disease), regular speed (classic early onset GBS), or speeded up (in utero acquisition and presentation in the delivery room). Laboratory data may sample only one "frame" in the septic process. The sampled "frame" may *not* be representative of subsequent events (e.g., the normal white blood cell count [WBC] in the neonate that has a fulminant and fatal

Table 11–11. INTERPRETATION OF LABORATORY TESTS IN THE SEPTIC-APPEARING NEONATE

Laboratory Test	Positive Predictive Value*	Negative Predictive Value†
I/T ratio > 0.2‡	+ +	+ +
WBC < 5,000/mm³§	+ +	+ + + +
CRP + ‖	+	+ + + +
ESR > 15 mm/hr¶	+ +	+ + + +
Neutrophil morphology**	+ +	+
Platelets < 150,000/mm³	+	+
Any 2 tests or more‡**	+ +	+ + + +
Gastric aspirate	+	+
Transtracheal culture	+ +	?
Fibronectin	+ +	+ + + +
External ear aspirate	+	+
Clinical impression	+ + + +	+ + + +
Fever > 100°F	+ + +	+ + + +
CIE (or Latex agglutination)	+ + + +	+ + + +
Blood culture	+ + + +	+ + + +

*Test is positive *only* when infection is present.
†Test is negative *only* when infection is absent.
‡Immature neutrophils ÷ total neutrophil count.
§White blood cells (WBC) (see table for other causes of ↓ WBC).
‖ C-reactive protein, qualitative or quantitative.
¶Micro ESR (age in days + 2 to 3 mm/hr max. of 20 normal).
**Toxic granulations, Dohle bodies, vacuolization.
+ = 0–25%; + + = 25–50%; + + + = 50–75%; + + + + = 75–100%.

Table 11-12. FACTORS OTHER THAN SEPSIS AFFECTING POLYMORPHONUCLEAR (PMN) LEUKOCYTES IN THE NEONATE*

	Decreased Total PMNs	Increased I:T Ratio†
Maternal hypertension	+ + + +	+
Asphyxia	+	+ + +
Periventricular hemorrhage (no seizures)	+ + +	+ + + +
Hemolytic disease	+ +	+ +

*Data from Remington JS and Klein JO: Infectious Diseases of the Fetus and Newborn Infant, 3rd ed. 1990, p. 629.
†I:T = immature forms/total neutrophil count.
+ = 0–25%; + + = 25–50%; + + + = 50–75%; + + + + = 75–100%.

septic shock course in the subsequent 6 to 12 hours).[88] With these caveats in mind, Table 11–11 shows the positive and negative predictive value of commonly ordered laboratory tests.[89–107] Table 11–12 shows other conditions that affect the WBC.

When these tests are viewed from this perspective, perhaps their most useful function lies in their *negative* predictive value. Thus, laboratory tests are most helpful when done serially and when the results remain normal. If used in this way, it has been demonstrated that antibiotic treatment and duration of hospital stay can be reduced.[8]

TREATMENT

Treatment of neonatal sepsis is more likely to be successful the earlier in the septic process that therapy is initiated. From the discussion earlier, it is clear that the infecting organism initiates a series of events that can result in the release of mediators that lead to amplification of the inflammatory response with subsequent widespread organ injury. This process can continue despite adequate bacterial killing. The effectiveness of therapy is shown in Figure 11–6 in which the septic process in the neonate can be viewed as a "pyramid."

Treatment interventions targeted at the processes at the apex of the pyramid, such as antibiotics, WBC transfusions, and inotropic support, may be totally inadequate if the inflammatory process has progressed to

the base of the pyramid. Reports of neonates succumbing to sepsis yet sterile on post mortem blood cultures support this hypothesis.[108]

Standard Treatment

Antibiotics

In both early and late onset, neonatal sepsis, coverage for gram-positive and gram-negative organisms is essential, and the combination of ampicillin with an aminoglycoside or third-generation cephalosporin is appropriate. With late onset disease, the possibility of nosocomial acquisition of coagulase-negative and positive staphylococcus as well as a wide variety of gram-negative organisms such as *Pseudomonas* strains require the substitution or addition of appropriate coverage, such as vancomycin and ceftazidine, respectively. The possibility that the cause of the septic syndrome is due to herpes simplex dictates the addition of acyclovir, often empirically.

If fungal infection is considered, then amphotericin is indicated. The doses and frequency of administration of the various chemotherapeutic agents are shown in Table 11–13.

The length of treatment is not well established but is generally recommended to be 7 to 10 days for sepsis and 21 days for meningitis (after negative results have been obtained for CSF cultures).

Cessation of therapy in the infant with appropriate cultures (at least 1 ml of blood) that are negative *and* an improving clinical picture is justified at 48 to 72 hours. However, false-negative cultures are well described, and in these "septic syndromes" a full course of therapy is justified.

Cardiovascular Support

Adequate *venous access* is essential in the neonate with sepsis and septic shock. Peripheral venous access is rarely adequate in the sick neonate, and it is recommended that central access be obtained via the umbilical vein (can be cannulated up to 7 to 10 days of age) or by one of the other standard sites described elsewhere in the text. Double- and triple-lumen Silastic catheters

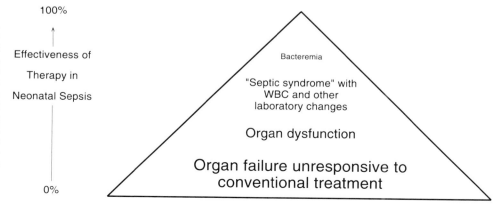

Figure 11-6. "Pyramid" of sepsis. Bacteremia represents the tip of a "pyramid" in which inflammatory cascades are initiated by the infecting organism. In the septic syndrome, the signs and symptoms and laboratory data of sepsis are apparent. After this, organ system failure occurs at the next stage. At the base of the pyramid, when organ failure has occurred, any therapy will be ineffective. The likelihood of success of therapy diminishes as the process evolves from the apex to the base of the pyramid (100% → 0%).

Table 11–13. ANTIBIOTIC DOSAGES FOR TERM NEONATES

Antibiotics	Routes of Administration	Dosages (mg/kg/day) and Intervals of Administration	
		Age 0–7 Days	Age > 7 Days
Amikacin	IM, IV	20 div q 12 hr	30 div q 8 hr
Ampicillin	IV, IM		
Meningitis		150 div q 8 hr	200 div q 6 hr
Other diseases		75 div q 8 hr	100 div q 6 hr
Aztreonam	IV, IM	90 div q 8 hr	120 div q 6 hr
Cefazolin	IV, IM	40 div q 12 hr	60 div q 8 hr
Cefotaxime	IV, IM	100 div q 12 hr	150 div q 8 hr
Ceftazidime	IV, IM	90 div q 8 hr	150 div q 8 hr
Ceftriaxone	IV, IM	50 once daily	75 once daily
Cephalothin	IV	60 div q 8 hr	80 div q 6 hr
Chloramphenicol	IV, PO	25 once daily	50 div q 12 hr
Clindamycin	IV, IM, PO	15 div q 8 hr	20 div q 6 hr
Erythromycin estolate	PO	20 div q 12 hr	30 div q 8 hr
Gentamicin	IM, IV	5 div q 12 hr	7.5 div q 8 hr
Kanamycin	IM, IV	20 div q 12 hr	30 div q 8 hr
Methicillin	IV, IM		
Meningitis		150 div q 8 hr	200 div q 6 hr
Other diseases		75 div q 8 hr	100 div q 6 hr
Metronidazole	IV, PO	15 div q 12 hr	30 div q 12 hr
Mezlocillin	IV, IM	150 div q 12 hr	225 div q 8 hr
Oxacillin	IV, IM	75 div q 8 hr	150 div q 6 hr
Nafcillin	IV	60 div q 8 hr	75 div q 6 hr
Netilmicin	IM, IV	5 div q 12 hr	7.5 div q 8 hr
Penicillin G	IV (units/kg/day)		
Meningitis		150,000 units div q 8 hr	200,000 U div q 6 hr
Other diseases		60,000 units div q 8 hr	100,000 U div q 6 hr
Penicillin G	IM (units/kg/day)		
Benzathine		50,000 units (one dose)	50,000 U (one dose)
Procaine		50,000 units once daily	50,000 U once daily
Ticarcillin	IV, IM	225 div q 8 hr	300 div q 6 hr
Tobramycin	IM, IV	4 div q 12 hr	6 div q 8 hr
Vancomycin	IV	30 div q 12 hr	30 div q 8 hr
ANTIVIRAL:			
Acyclovir	IV	30 div q 8 hr	30 div q 8 hr
ANTIFUNGAL:			
Amphotericin	IV	0.5 q day	0.5 q day (test dose required)

*Adapted from Nelson JD: 1990–1991 Pocketbook of Pediatric Antimicrobial Therapy, 9th ed. Baltimore, Williams & Wilkins, 1990. © 1990, the Williams & Wilkins Co., Baltimore.

have been used in the umbilical vein and provide excellent monitoring and infusion capability.

Maintenance fluids in the neonate: This should be D 10% with added maintenance electrolytes (3 to 4 Na$^+$ mEq/kg/day, 2 to 3 K$^+$ mEq/kg/day, 3 to 4 Cl$^-$ mEq/kg/day). Fluid infusion rates depend on postnatal age and other factors, including whether intubated (reduces insensible losses), use of radiant warmers, or phototherapy (increases insensible losses), and ranges vary from 60 to 150 + ml/kg/day.

Accurate fluid balance is essential in the sick neonate and is aided by urinary catheterization (No. 5 FG in the term neonate) and continuous weights (electronic scale), as well as judicious monitoring of serum electrolytes and uring output.

The ability to invasively monitor cardiovascular function in the newborn with shock is limited. Apart from heart rate, which is routinely monitored, blood pressure can be measured both noninvasively with the appropriate size cuffs or invasively. Percutaneous placement of arterial catheters No. 24 or 22 in the radial artery or posterior tibial artery (utilizing a transillumination technique) is safe and well tolerated. The umbilical arteries

should not be overlooked, even in the infant 7 to 10 days of age. Low placement at the L3–L4 level of the catheter tip below the renal arteries is advised. The use of femoral arteries is not recommended, and use of the temporal artery is contraindicated because ipsilateral thromboembolic complications have been documented.[109]

CVP monitoring is useful, although the limitations of this must be recognized. The fetal and newborn ventricular compliances are shifted to the left side compared with those in an older child or an adult[110] (Fig. 11–7).

The use of continuous venous oximetry in the newborn has not been systematically studied. Saturations from catheter tip placement in the right atrium must be interpreted cautiously because this is not truly mixed venous blood. However, as a trend monitor, especially when combined with systemic arterial saturations, it can be a very useful form of "dual oximetry." Placement of Swan-Ganz catheters has been reported, but the presence of extrapulmonary shunts (PDA, foramen ovale) make cardiac output calculations inaccurate, and thus they cannot be used routinely.[111]

The commonly used inotropes, vasoconstrictors, and

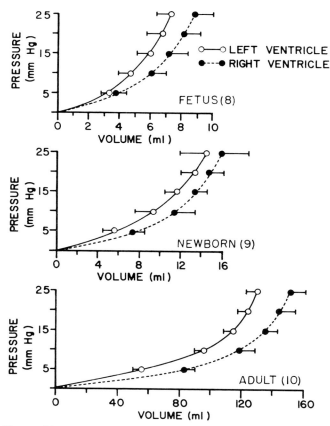

Figure 11–7. Average left and right ventricular pressure-volume curves for each age group. *Numbers in parentheses* are numbers of animals studied. Each *point* and *horizontal bars* are mean values ± SE. Note differences in the horizontal volume scale. No significant differences were observed between the two ventricles in the fetus. In the newborn, the left ventricular pressure-volume curve was significantly shifted to the left of the right ventricular curve at 15 and 20 mm Hg (P < 0.05). In the adult, significantly greater left ventricular pressures existed at every level of volume when compared with those for the right ventricle (P< 0.001). (From Romero T, Covell J, and Friedman W: A comparison of pressure-volume relations of the fetal, newborn and adult heart. Am J Physiol 222:1285, 1972.)

vasodilators used in neonatal shock are shown in Table 11–14.[112] The interactions and dose response data in the newborn are not well established. Experience has demonstrated that responses to these agents are highly variable, and recommendations for dosages must be altered on a case by case basis and carefully titrated to the desired effect. Extreme care with excessive dosages of agents with powerful α effects is advised, since the pulmonary vascular bed is well innervated with α-receptors, which when stimulated may cause vasoconstriction.[113] The septic neonate already has a propensity to vasoconstriction.

Respiratory Support

The neonate with septic shock should have mechanical respiratory support. The most commonly utilized technique includes a noncuffed orally or nasally placed ETT No. 3- to 3.5-mm I.D. in the term newborn and a continuous flow–time-cycled and pressure-limited ma-

Table 11–14. VASOACTIVE AGENTS USED IN TREATMENT OF NEONATAL SHOCK

	β₁	β₂	α₁	αB	DA₁	PDI	SMR
Dobutamine (1–20 +)	+ + +						
Dopamine (1–20 +)	+ +		+ +		+ +		
Isoproterenol (0.05–0.5)	+ +	+ +					
Epinephrine (0.05–0.5)	+ +		+ + +				
Amrinone (5–20)						+ + +	
Tolazoline (10–20)	+			+ + +			
Nitroprusside (0.5–10)							+ + +

All dosages are suggested ranges. Units used are all μg/kg/min. The effect of many drugs varies at different dosages (e.g., dopamine has α effects > 10). See Chapter 33 for further discussion.

β₁ = beta one; β₂ = beta two; α₁ = alpha one; αB = alpha blockade; DA₁ = dopamine one; PDI = phosphodiesterase inhibitor; SMR = smooth muscle relaxant.

chine utilizing an IMV mode of ventilation with positive end-expiratory pressure (PEEP). Typical initial settings are shown in Table 11–15.

Adjunctive Therapy

Immunotherapy

Adult Donor WBC Transfusion. The diminished neutrophil storage pool (NSP) and maximal proliferative state of the WBC marrow precursors and the known associated poor prognostic significance of neutropenia in the neonate with sepsis[102] has prompted attempts to modify the outcome of neonatal sepsis and accompanying neutropenia, with adult donor WBC transfusions.[114–116] Pooled data of 11 studies are shown in Table 11–16. Only six of these are controlled studies. Only four of these have shown significant benefit.

The results of WBC transfusions have been variable. For example, not all studies have established neutrophil storage pool depletion. This requires bone marrow examination. In addition, finding donors promptly and processing the WBC can result in significant time delays that may compromise the effectiveness of the therapy. Concentrates prepared by automated leukapheresis rather than from stored buffy coats seems important. The possibility that the inflammatory cascades that are central to the septic response may be accelerated by WBC transfusion is a theoretical concern also. The issue of risks of transfusion is also pertinent.

Adult Donor Fresh Whole Blood Transfusion and Exchange Transfusion. Several reports have suggested the benefit of transfusion in GBS disease.[117, 118] None

Table 11–15. RECOMMENDED INITIAL SETTINGS

Insp Flow (l/min)	i Time (sec)	PIP (cm H₂O)	PEEP (cm H₂O)	Rate (Breaths/min)
6–10	0.4–0.6	15–25	4–6	20–60

Table 11–16. COMBINED DATA FROM 11 REPORTS OF THERAPEUTIC GRANULOCYTE TRANSFUSIONS IN NEONATES*

Information Reported	Transfused	Not Transfused
No. of neonates studied	78	90
Well-documented sepsis	63	72
Blood neutrophil counts reported	47	76
Neutrophils < 1,500/μl	36	63
Neutrophils > 1,500/μl	11	13
Marrow storage pool reported	45	75
Storage pool < 7%	18	22
Storage pool > 7%	27	53
% survival	79 (62/78)	62 (56/90)

*From Strauss RG: Current status of granulocyte transfusions to treat neonatal sepsis. J Clin Apheresis 5:25–29, 1989. Copyright © 1989. Reprinted with permission of Wiley-Liss, a division of John Wiley & Sons, Inc.

have been subjected to prospective controlled randomized study. High-titer ANTI/GBS III antibody blood has been reported to be helpful in treating GBS type III sepsis, and this suggests that the specific opsonizing effects of transfused blood is the important factor. Likewise, exchange transfusions have been reported to be beneficial in treating the septic neonate.[119, 120] The benefit of this therapy is correlated with high specific antibody titers to the infecting organism, and the undoubted occasional success is likely related to high specific antibody titers in the donor blood.

Intravenous Immunoglobulin. More encouraging and well studied are the therapeutic benefits of prophylactic intravenous immunoglobulin (IVIG).[121] Studies strongly suggest that this approach to bolstering the weakened immune defenses of the newborn are beneficial.[122] Increasing the specificity of the immunoglobulin used, the precise dosages, and the appropriate timing are questions remaining to be answered in future studies. Some evidence suggests that excessive dosaging may be detrimental,[123–126] and this should be kept in mind when using IVIG in acute sepsis (Table 11–17).

Despite these potential ill effects of IVIG, more recent data support its use even acutely in the septic neonate with GBS.[126] When GBS antigen titers were more than 1:10 and neutrophils were depleted (<3,500 per mm³), benefit from this therapy was shown (i.e., the mortality rate was reduced from 58 to 17% (p<0.01)). However, this study used retrospective controls and must be interpreted with caution. This approach seems promising, and initial results are encouraging.

Newer Therapies for Neonatal Sepsis and Septic Shock

Venoarterial Extracorporeal Membrane Oxygenation (VAECMO). VAECMO is discussed in Chapter 42 as a technique for "lung rest," *and* cardiovascular support and can be a very useful form of rescue therapy for the neonate with fulminant septic shock unresponsive to the aforementioned discussed conventional treatment modalities. At the time of writing, 10 patients with septic shock have been treated at The Children's Hospital (TCH) of Denver, and 8 of these patients have survived. These numbers are small, and meaningful comparison with infants in the pre-ECMO era is, therefore, not yet possible. All of these infants met accepted mortality risk criteria (i.e., >80% risk of death) prior to initiating ECMO.

High-Frequency Ventilation (HFV) Techniques (Jet HFV or oscillator HFV). These techniques have not been studied systematically in the septic neonate. The experience at TCH with HFV suggests that in some neonates, when hypocapnic alkalosis is not attainable with conventional time-cycled, pressure-limited ventilation techniques, hypocapnia can be achieved at lower mean airway pressures with HFV and is often associated with improved oxygenation. Others have reported a decreased need for V.A. ECMO rescue therapy in patients who have received HFV trials, even when they meet accepted ECMO criteria.[127]

Surfactant Replacement. The evidence that prophylactic or rescue administration of various surfactants is beneficial in the survival of infants with primary surfactant deficiency is excellent.[128, 129]

The use of this therapy in the neonate with secondary surfactant deficiency states, as can occur in septic shock, remains to be studied.

Heparin. The use of heparin by continuous infusion (10 to 20 units/kg/hour) has been recommended as a prophylactic anticoagulant in the seriously ill neonate with sepsis and associated disseminated intravascular coagulation. Purpura fulminans can be a serious manifestation of sepsis in the newborn (Fig. 11–8). The mechanism of this devastating complication of sepsis is unknown. However, the association of homozygous protein C deficiency (a potent anticoagulant) and recurrent purpura fulminans has been described in newborns.[130] Acquired protein C deficiency can occur in disseminated intravascular coagulation.[131] Some evidence exists[132] that heparin interferes with bacterial opsonization by com-

Table 11–17. POTENTIAL ADVERSE EFFECTS OF IVIG IN THE TREATMENT OF EXPERIMENTAL BACTERIAL DISEASES*

Organism	Animal Model	Treatment	Results	Postulated Mechanisms
Group B streptococcus	Infant rat with severe GBS infection	Penicillin or ceftriaxone plus IVIG	↑ Mortality ↓ Bacterial clearance	↓ Antibiotic- and PMN-mediated killing activity
Haemophilus influenzae type B	Infant rats with Hib infection	Ceftriaxone plus IVIG or BPIG	↑ Mortality	↑ Endotoxin levels
Escherichia coli	Neutropenic mice	IVIG	↑ Susceptibility ↓ Bacterial clearance	RE blockade

*From Kim KS: High dose intravenous immune globulin impairs antibacterial activity of antibiotics. J Allergy Clin Immunol 84:579–588, 1989, with permission.
PMN = polymorphonuclear; Hib = Haemophilus influenzae type b; BPIG = bacterial polysaccharide immunoglobulin; RE = reticuloendothelial.

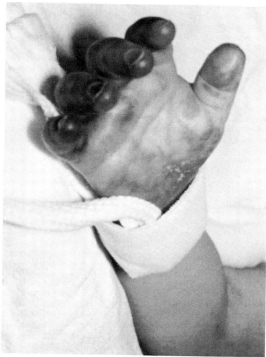

Figure 11–8. Purpura fulminans—the neonate had involvement of four extremities. The infecting organism was GBS.

plement. Heparin is often used at TCH but has not been subjected to randomized study to establish it as a form of recommended therapy in the septic newborn.

References

1. Remington JS and Klein JO: Infectious Diseases of the Fetus and Newborn Infant, 3rd ed. Philadelphia, WB Saunders, 1990.
2. Patamasucan P, Siegel JD, and McCracken GM: Streptococcal submandibular cellulitis in young infants. Pediatrics 67:378, 1981.
3. Lipson A, Vronick JB, Tewfik C, et al: Group B streptococcal supraglotittis in a 3 month old infant. Am J Dis Child 140:411, 1986.
4. Banagall RC and Watters JM: Delayed right-sided diaphragmatic hernia following group B streptococcal infection: A discussion of its pathogenesis, with a review of the literature. Hum Pathol 14:67, 1983.
5. Volpe JJ: Neurology of the Newborn, 2nd ed. Philadelphia, WB Saunders, 1987, pp. 409–433.
6. Solomon SL, Wallace EM, Ford-Jones EL, et al: Medical intelligence: Medication errors with inhalant epinephrine mimicking an epidemic of neonatal sepsis. N Engl J Med 310:166, 1984.
7. Gladstone IM, Ehrenkranz RA, Edberg SC, et al: A ten-year review of neonatal sepsis and comparison with the previous fifty-year experience. Pediatr Infect Dis J 9:819, 1990.
8. Philip AG: Decreased use of antibiotics using a neonatal sepsis screening technique. J Pediatr 98:795, 1981.
9. McGregor JA, French JI, Lawellen D, et al: Bacterial protease-induced reduction of chorioamniotic membrane strength and elasticity. Obstet Gynecol 69:167, 1987.
10. Shigeoka AL, Charette RP, Wyman MI, et al: Defective oxidative metabolic response of neutrophil from stressed neonates. J Pediatr 98:392, 1981.
11. Christensen RD, MacFarlane JL, Taylor JL, et al: Blood and marrow neutrophils during experimental group B streptococcal infection. Pediatr Res 16:549, 1982.
12. Mease AD: Tissue neutropenia: The newborn neutrophil in perspective. J Perinatol 10:55, 1990.
13. Hill HB: Biochemical structural and functional abnormalities of polymorphonuclear leukocytes in the neonate. Pediatr Res 22:375, 1987.
14. Cairo MS: Neonatal neutrophil host defense. Am J Dis Child 143:40, 1989.
15. Berger M: Complement deficiency and neutrophil dysfunction as risk factors for bacterial infection in newborns and the role of granulocyte transfusion in therapy. Rev Infect Dis 12(S-4):S401, 1990.
16. Klegman RM, Clapp DW, and Berger M: Targeted immunoglobulin therapy for the prevention of neonatal infection. Rev Infect Dis 12(S-4):S443, 1990.
17. Ferrieri P: Neonatal susceptibility and immunity to major bacterial pathogens. Rev Infect Dis 12(S-4):S394, 1990.
18. Goldberg RN, Susuihara C, Streitfeld MM, et al: Effects of a leukotriene antagonist on the early hemodynamic manifestations of group B streptococcal sepsis in piglets. Pediatr Res 20:1004, 1986.
19. Runkle B, Goldberg RN, Streitfeld MM, et al: Cardiovascular changes in group B streptococcal sepsis in the piglet: Response to indomethacin and relationship to prostacyclin and thromboxane A2. Pediatr Res 18:874, 1984.
20. Troug WE, Sorensen GK, Standaert TA, et al: Effects of the thromboxane synthetase inhibitor, dazmegrel (UK 38,485), on pulmonary gas exchange and hemodynamics in neonatal sepsis. Pediatr Res 20:481, 1986.
21. Hammerman C, Lass N, Strates E, et al: Prostanoids in neonates with persistent pulmonary hypertension. J Pediatr 110:470, 1987.
22. Hosford D and Braquet P: The potential role of platelet-activating factor in shock and ischemia. J Crit Care 5:115, 1990.
23. Bussolino F, Porcellini MG, Varese L, et al: Intravascular release of platelet-activating factor in children with sepsis. Thromb Res 48:619, 1987.
24. Pinheiro JMB, Pitt BR, and Gillis CN: Roles of platelet-activating factor and thromboxane in group B streptococcus-induced pulmonary hypertension in piglets. Pediatr Res 26:420, 1989.
25. Burckett FK, English JD, et al: Production of lymphotoxin and tumor necrosis factor by human neonatal mononuclear cells. Pediatr Res 24:717, 1988.
26. Tracey KJ, Beutler B, Lowry SF, et al: Shock and tissue injury induced by recombinant human cachectin. Science 234:470, 1986.
27. Beutler B, Milsark IW, and Cerami A: Cachectin/tumor necrosis factor: Production, distribution and metabolic fate in vivo. J Immunol 135:3972, 1985.
28. Damas P, Reuter A, Gysen P, et al: Tumor necrosis factor and interleukin-1 serum levels during severe sepsis in humans. Crit Care Med 17: 975, 1989.
29. Marks JD, Marks CB, Luce JM, et al: Plasma tumor necrosis factor in patients with septic shock: Mortality rate, incidence of ARDS, and effects of methylprednisolone administration. Am Rev Respir Dis 141:94, 1990.
30. Waage A, Halstensen A, and Espevik T: Association between tumor necrosis factor in serum and fatal outcome in patients with meningococcal disease. Lancet 1:355, 1987.
31. Michie HR, Manogue KR, Spriggs DR, et al: Detection of circulating tumor necrosis factor after endotoxin administration. N Engl J Med 318:1481, 1988.
32. Girardin E, Grau GE, Dayer JM, et al: Tumor necrosis factor and interleukin-1 in the serum of children with severe infectious purpura. N Engl J Med 319:397, 1988.
33. Neilson IR, Neilson KA, Yunis EJ, et al: Failure of tumor necrosis factor to produce hypotensive shock in the absence of endotoxin. Surgery 106:439, 1989.
34. Gibson RL, Redding GJ, and Truog WE: Tumor necrosis factor: Potential mediator of neonatal group B streptococcal sepsis. Am Rev Respir Dis 139:A439, 1989.
35. Truog WE, Gibson RL, Henderson WR, et al: Tumor necrosis factor-induced neonatal pulmonary hypertension: Effects of dazmegrel pretreatment. Pediatr Res 27:466, 1990.
36. Kilbourn RG, Jubran A, Gross SS, et al: Reversal of endotoxin mediated shock by N-methyl-L-arginine, an inhibitor of nitric oxide synthesis. Biochem Biophys Res Commun 172:1132, 1990.
37. Rabinovitch M, Gamble WJ, Miettenen OS, et al: Age and sex influence on pulmonary hypertension of chronic hypoxia and recovery. Am J Physiol 240:H62, 1981.
38. Stenmark KR, Fasules J, Hyde DM, et al: Severe pulmonary

hypertension and arterial adventitial changes in newborn calves at 4,300m. J Appl Physiol 62:821, 1987.

39. Todd L, Mullen M, Olley PM, et al: Pulmonary toxicity of monocrotaline differs at critical periods of lung development. Pediatr Res 19:731, 1985.

40. Stenmark KR and Majack RA: Response of the developing pulmonary circulation to injury. Developmental mechanisms of disease in newborns. In: Report of 101st Ross Conference on Pediatric Research, 102–110, 1991.

41. Stenmark, KR, Abman SH, and Accurso FT: Etiologic mechanisms in persistent pulmonary hypertension of the newborn. In: Weir EK and Reeves JT (eds): Pulmonary Vascular Physiology and Pathophysiology. New York, Marcel Dekker, 1989, pp. 355–402.

42. Baker CJ and Edwards MS: Group B streptococcal infections. In: Remington JS and Klein JO (eds): Infectious Diseases of the Fetus and Newborn Infant, 3rd ed. Philadelphia, WB Saunders, 1990, pp. 742–811.

43. Hellerqvist CG, Sundell H, and Gettins P: Molecular basis for group B beta-hemolytic streptococcal disease. Proc Natl Acad Sci 84:51, 1987.

44. Rojos J, Green RS, Hellerqvist CG, et al: Studies on group B beta-hemolytic streptococcus. II:Effects on pulmonary hemodynamics and vascular permeability in unanesthetized sheep. Pediatr Res 15:899, 1981.

45. Hemming VG, O'Brien WF, Fischer GW, et al: Studies of short-term pulmonary and peripheral vascular responses induced in oophorectomized sheep by the infusion of a group B streptococcal extract. Pediatr Res 18:266, 1984.

46. Gibson RL, Redding GJ, Truog WE, et al: Isogenic group B streptococci devoid of capsular polysaccharide or beta-hemolysin: Pulmonary hemodynamic and gas exchange effects during bacteremia in piglets. Pediatr Res 26:241, 1989.

47. Miller RR, Menke JA, et al: The effect of naloxone on the hemodynamics of the newborn piglet with septic shock. Pediatr Res 20(8):707, 1986.

48. Natanson C, Fink MP, Ballantyne HK, et al: Gram-negative bacteremia produces both severe systolic and diastolic cardiac dysfunction in a canine model that simulates human septic shock. J Clin Invest 78:259, 1986.

49. Rojas J, Larsson LE, Hellerqvist CG, et al: Pulmonary hemodynamic and ultrastructural changes associated with group B streptococcal toxemia in adult sheep and newborn lambs. Pediatr Res 17:1002, 1983.

50. Rojas J, Larsson LE, Oletree ML, et al: Effects of cyclooxygenase inhibition on the response to group B streptococcal toxin in sheep. Pediatr Res 17:107, 1983.

51. Brighan KL and Meyrick B: Endotoxin and lung injury. Am Rev Respir Dis 133:913, 1986.

52. Hutchinson AA, Hinson JM, Brigham KL, et al: Effect of endotoxin on airway hyperresponsiveness to aerosol histamine in sheep. J Appl Physiol 54:1463, 1983.

53. Wheeler AP, Jesmok G, and Brigham KL: Tumor necrosis factor's effects on lung mechanics, gas exchange, and airway reactivity in sheep. J Appl Physiol 68:2542, 1990.

54. Sandberg K, Engelhardt B, Hellerqvist C, et al: Pulmonary response to group B streptococcal toxin in young lambs. J Appl Physiol 63:2023, 1987.

55. Siegel JD and McCracken GH: Sepsis neonatorum. N Engl J Med 304:642, 1981.

56. Moxon ER and Ostrow PT: H. influenzae meningitis in infant rats: Role of bacteremia in pathogenesis of age-dependent inflammatory responses in cerebrospinal fluid. J Infect Dis 135:303, 1977.

57. Saez-Llorens X, Ramil O, Mustafa MM, et al: Molecular pathophysiology of bacterial meningitis: Current concepts and therapeutic implications. J Pediatr 116:671, 1990.

58. Tracey KJ, Vlassara J, and Cerami A: Cachectin/tumor necrosis factor. Lancet 1:1112, 1989.

59. Dinarello CA: Interleukin-1. Rev Infect Dis 6:51, 1984.

60. Arditi M, Caplan M, and Yogev R: Platelet-activating factor levels in CSF of children with H. influenzae. Presented to the 29th ICAAC, Abstract 1113, Houston, 1989.

61. Mustafa MM, Familo O, Saez-Llorens X, et al: Cerebrospinal fluid prostaglandins, interleukin-1, and tumor necrosis factor in bacterial meningitis. Am J Dis Child 144:883, 1990.

62. Mustafa MM, Familo O, Olsen KD, et al: Tumor necrosis factor in mediating experimental H. influenzae type B meningitis. J Clin Invest 84:1253, 1989.

63. Scheld WM, Quagliarello VJ, and Wispelwey B: The potential role of host cytokines in H. influenzae lipopolysaccharide-induced blood-brain barrier permeability. Pediatr Infect Dis J 8:910, 1989.

64. Deitch EA, Berg R, and Specian R: Endotoxin promotes the translocation of bacteria from the gut. Arch Surg 122:185, 1985.

65. Jacob AL, Goldberg PK, Bloom N, et al: Endotoxin and bacteria in portal blood. Gastroenterol 72:1268, 1977.

66. Caridis DT, Reinhold RB, Woodruff PWH, et al: Endotoxaemia in man. Lancet 1:1381, 1972.

67. Scheifele DW, Fussell S, and Olsen E: Bacterial endotoxins in umbilical cord blood of neonates. Biol Neonate 45:119, 1984.

68. Scheifele DW, Olsen E, Fussell S, et al: Spontaneous endotoxemia in premature infants: Correlations with oral feeding and bowel dysfunction. J Pediatr Gastroenterol Nutr 4:67, 1985.

69. Whitfield JM, Kotzer A, Gillespie M, et al: Aseptic spontaneous endotoxemia, respiratory failure and shock in the newborn. Crit Care Med 16:S379, 1988.

70. Hauser GJ, Casey W, Hannallah R, et al: Circulating endotoxin and tumor necrosis factor during pediatric cardiac surgery. Crit Care Med 17:S129, 1989.

71. Nowocki P: Intestinal ischemia and necrotizing enterocolitis. J Pediatr 117:S14, 1990.

72. Kosloske AM: A unifying hypothesis for pathogenesis and prevention of necrotizing enterocolitis. J Pediatr 117:S68, 1990.

73. Chu S, and Walker W: Development of the gastrointestinal mucosal barrier: Changes in phospholipid head groups and fatty acid composition of intestinal microvillus membranes from newborn and adult rats. Pediatr Res 23:439, 1988.

74. Udall JN: Gastrointestinal host defense and necrotizing enterocolitis. J Pediatr 117:S33, 1990.

75. Clark D and Miller M: Intraluminal pathogenesis of necrotizing enterocolitis. J Pediatr 117:S64, 1990.

76. Aynsley-Green A, Lucas A, Lawson G, et al: Gut hormones and regulatory peptides in relation to enteral feeding, gastroenteritis, and necrotizing enterocolitis in infancy. J Pediatr 117:S24, 1990.

77. Gonzalez-Crussi F and Hsueh W: Experimental model of ischemic bowel necrosis: The role of platelet activating factor and endotoxin. Am J Pathol 112:127, 1983.

78. Sun X-M and Hwueh W: Bowel necrosis induced by tumor necrosis factor in rats is mediated by platelet activating factor. J Clin Invest 81:1328, 1988.

79. Hsueh W, Gonzalez-Crussi F, and Arroyave JL: Platelet-activating factor: An endogenous mediator for bowel necrosis in endotoxemia. FASEB J 1:403, 1987.

80. Caplan M, Sun X, Hsueh W, et al: Role of platelet activating factor and tumor necrosis factor-alpha in neonatal necrotizing enterocolitis. J Pediatr 116:960, 1990.

81. Dinarello CA, Shparber M, and Kent EF: Production of leukocytic pyrogen from phagocytes of neonates. J Infect Dis 144:337, 1981.

82. Yachie A, Takano N, Yokoi T, et al: The capability of neonatal leukocytes to produce IL-6 on stimulation assessed by whole blood culture. Pediatr Res 27:233, 1990.

83. Blatteis C: Comparison of endotoxin and leukocytic pyrogen pyrogenicity in newborn guinea pigs. J Appl Physiol 42:3656, 1977.

84. Volpe JJ: Neurology of the Newborn, 2nd ed. Philadelphia, WB Saunders, 1987.

85. Whitley RJ, Corey L, Arvin A, et al: Changing presentation of neonatal herpes simplex virus infection. J Infect Dis 158:109, 1988.

86. Morens DM: Enteroviral disease in early infancy. J Pediatr 92:374, 1978.

87. Halfen N and Spector SA: Fatal echovirus 11 infections. Am J Dis Child 135:1017, 1981.

88. Christensen RD, Rothstein G, Hill H, et al: Fatal early onset group B streptococcal sepsis with normal leukocyte counts. Pediatr Infect Dis 4:242, 1985.

89. Philip AGS: Acute-phase proteins in neonatal infection. J Pediatr 105:940, 1984.

90. Benuck I and David, RJ: Sensitivity of published neutrophil

indexes in identifying newborn infants with sepsis. J Pediatr 103:961, 1983.

91. Liu CH, Lehan C, Speer ME, et al: Degenerative changes in neutrophils: An indicator of bacterial infection. Pediatrics 74:823, 1984.

92. Sherman MP, Chance KH, and Goetzman BW: Gram strains of tracheal secretions predict neonatal bacteremia. Am J Dis Child 138:848, 1984.

93. Philip AGS and Hewitt JR: Early diagnosis of neonatal sepsis. Pediatrics 65:1036, 1980.

94. Rodwell RL, Leslie AL, and Tudehope DI: Early diagnosis of neonatal sepsis using a hematologic scoring system. J Pediatr 112:761, 1988.

95. Koenig JM, Patterson LER, Rench MA, et al: Role of fibronectin in diagnosing bacterial infection in infancy. Am J Dis Child 142:884, 1988.

96. Manroe BL, Weinberg AG, Rosenfeld CR, et al: The neonatal blood count in health and disease. I: Reference values for neutrophilic cells. J Pediatr 95:89, 1979.

97. Sanchez PJ, Siegel JD, Cushion NB, et al: Significance of a positive urine group B streptococcal latex agglutination test in neonates. J Pediatr 116:601, 1990.

98. Harris MC, Deuber C, Polin RA, et al: Investigation of apparent false-positive urine latex particle agglutination tests for the detection of group B streptococcus antigen. J Clin Microbiol 27:2214, 1989.

99. Evans ME, Schaffner W, Federspiel C, et al: Sensitivity, specificity, and predictive value of body surface cultures in a neonatal intensive care unit. JAMA 259:249, 1988.

100. Misra PK, Kumar R, Malik GK, et al: Simple hematological tests for diagnosis of neonatal sepsis. Indian Pediatr 26:156, 1989.

101. Crain EF and Gershel, JC: Which febrile infants younger than two weeks of age are likely to have sepsis? A pilot study. Pediatr Infect Dis J 7:561, 1988.

102. Fulginiti VA, and Ray CG: Body surface cultures in the newborn infant. Am J Dis Child 142:19, 1988.

103. Okolo AA, Scott-Emuakpor AB, and Omene JA: The diagnostic value of leukocyte indices and microerythrocyte sedimentation rate in neonatal infections. Trop Georg Med 40:304, 1988.

104. Evans ME, Schaffner W, Federspiel CF, et al: Sensitivity, specificity, and predictive value of body surface cultures in a neonatal intensive care unit. JAMA 259:248, 1988.

105. Slagle TA, Bifano EM, Wolf JW, et al: Routine endotracheal cultures for the prediction of sepsis in ventilated babies. Arch Dis Child 64:34, 1989.

106. Rozycki HJ, Stahl GE, and Baumgart S: Impaired sensitivity of a single early leukocyte count in screening for neonatal sepsis. Pediatr Infect Dis J 6:440, 1987.

107. Pole JRG and McAllister TA: Gastric aspirate analysis in the newborn. Acta Paediatr Scand 64:109, 1975.

108. Squire E, Favara B, and Todd J: Diagnosis of neonatal bacterial infection: Hematologic and pathologic findings in fatal and non-fatal cases. Pediatrics 64:60, 1979.

109. Prian GW, Wright GB, Rumack CM, et al: Apparent cerebral embolization after temporal artery catheterization. J Pediatr 93:115, 1978.

110. Romero T, Covell J, and Friedman W: A comparison of pressure volume relations of the fetal, newborn and adult heart. Am J Physiol 222:1285, 1972.

111. Todres ID, Crone RK, Rogers MC, et al: Swan-Ganz catheterization in the critically ill newborn. Crit Care Med 7:330, 1979.

112. Perkins RM and Levin DL: Shock in the pediatric patient. II:Therapy. J Pediatr 101:319, 1982.

113. Haworth SG: Pulmonary vascular development. In: Long WA (ed): Fetal and Neonatal Cardiology. Philadelphia, WB Saunders, 1990.

114. Strauss RG: Current status of granulocyte transfusions to treat neonatal sepsis. J Clin Apheresis 5:25, 1989.

115. Berger M: Complement deficiency and neutrophil dysfunction as risk factors for bacterial infection in newborns and the role of granulocyte transfusion in therapy. Rev Infect Dis 12:S401, 1990.

116. Joffe A: Granulocyte transfusions in neonates with presumed sepsis. Pediatrics 80:738, 1987.

117. Courtney SE, Hall RT, and Harris DJ: Effect of blood transfusions on mortality in early-onset group B streptococcal septicaemia. Lancet 11:462–463, 1979.

118. Shigloka AO, Hall RT, and Hill HR: Blood transfusions in group B streptococcal sepsis. Lancet 636-638, 1978.

119. De Curtis M, Vetrano G, Romano G, et al: Improvement of phagocytosis and nitroblue tetrazolium reduction after exchange transfusions in two preterm infants with severe septicemia. Pediatrics 70:829–830, 1982.

120. Vain NE, Mazimuian, JR, Swarner OW, et al: Role of exchange transfusion in the treatment of severe septicemia. Pediatrics 66:693, 1980.

121. Muralt GV and Sidiropoulos D: Prenatal and postnatal prophylaxis of infections in preterm neonates. Pediatr Infect Dis J 7:S72, 1988.

122. Fischer GW: Immunoglobulin therapy of neonatal group B streptococcal infections: An overview. Pediatr Infect Dis J 7:S13, 1988.

123. Kim KS: High-dose intravenous immune globulin impairs antibacterial activity of antibiotics. J Allergy Clin Immunol 84:579, 1989.

124. Weisman LE and Lorenzetti PM: High intravenous doses of human immune globulin suppress neonatal group B streptococcal immunity in rats. J Pediatr 115:445, 1989.

125. Noya FJD and Baker CJ: Intravenously administered immune globulin for premature infants: A time to wait. J Pediatr 115:969, 1989.

126. Friedman CA, Wender DF, Temple DM, et al: Intravenous gamma globulin as adjunct therapy for severe group B streptococcal disease in the newborn. Am J Perinatol 7:1, 1990.

127. Carter MJ, Gerstmann DR, Clark MR, et al: High-frequency oscillatory ventilation and extracorporeal membrane oxygenation for the treatment of acute neonatal respiratory failure. Pediatrics 85:159–162, 1990.

128. Kendig JW, Notter RH, Cox C, et al: A comparison of surfactant as immediate prophylaxis and as rescue therapy in newborns of less than 30 weeks' gestation. N Engl J Med 324:865–871, 1991.

129. Bose C, Corbet A, Bose G, et al: Improved outcome at 28 days of age for very low birth weight infants treated with a single dose of a synthetic surfactant. J Pediatr 117:947–953, 1990.

130. Griffin JH: Clinical studies of protein C. Semin Thromb Hemost 10:162, 1984.

131. Takahashi H, Takakuwa E, Yoshino N, et al: Protein C levels in disseminated intravascular coagulation and thrombotic thrombocytopenic purpura: Its correlation with other coagulation parameters. Thromb Haemost 54:445, 1985.

132. Edwards MS, Buffone GJ, Rench MA, et al: Effect of continuous heparin infusion on bactericidal activity for group B streptococci in neonatal sera. J Pediatr 103:787, 1983.

12

Management of Pediatric Septic Shock

Joseph A. Carcillo, M.D.

In 1969, an analysis of gram-negative sepsis showed a 98% mortality rate in children in whom a shock syndrome developed.[1] Twenty years later, with the advent of pediatric intensive care, mortality in children with septic shock has been decreased to as little as 40% in the most critically ill patients. This dramatic improvement in outcome has been attained through a better understanding of the physiology of shock. The application of technologic advances in respiratory, cardiovascular, renal, and nutritional support, as well as improved antibacterial, antiviral, and antifungal therapy, has resulted in improved survival in children with septic shock and resultant multiple system organ failure.

The sepsis syndrome occurs in less than 25% of children with documented bacteremia, and blood culture results can be negative in 40% of cases.[2] These observations are compatible with current theories of pathogenesis in sepsis, which hold that invading microorganisms mediate effects primarily through release of critical levels of toxins, with secondary overactivation of the host's immune response. The most studied toxin in sepsis is endotoxin. This bacterial cell wall component can elicit myriad processes, including complement activation; platelet aggregation; Hageman factor and coagulation factor consumption; prostaglandin, thromboxane, and leukotriene production; and the release of inflammatory mediators. This latter process occurs through the activation of macrophages, lymphocytes, and polymorphonuclear leukocytes, which release monokines, lymphokines, oxygen radicals, hydrolases, and proteases. These mediators contribute to perturbation of physiologic homeostasis.

Positive feedback mechanisms between mediators and biochemical cascades can contribute to increasing cellular abnormalities and organ dysfunction. For example, endotoxin appears to mediate mortality in part through stimulation of macrophages to produce the monokine tumor necrosis factor (TNF). Michalik and colleagues[3] demonstrated that lipopolysaccharide (LPS)-resistant mouse strains exhibit macrophages incapable of releasing TNF. When these mice underwent bone marrow constitution with macrophages capable of TNF secretion, the mice became sensitive to the effects of LPS. When TNF was injected into normal rats, it caused hemoconcentration, lactic acidosis, a transient phase of hyperglycemia followed by hypoglycemia, hypotension, and death. Autopsy results showed widespread tissue necrosis in multiple organs.[4] A combination of low doses of TNF and a second LPS-induced monokine interleukin-1 (IL-1) induced thrombocytopenia, leukopenia, and a profound shock-like state in rabbits. All three effects were prevented by pretreatment with ibuprofen, suggesting that the process was mediated by prostaglandins.[5] These effects were not attainable with low levels of TNF or IL-1 alone but resulted from synergism and positive feedback mechanisms. Under normal conditions, TNF and IL-1 have important physiologic functions. These models have been used to support the concept that overactivation of physiologic immune responses and biochemical cascades can lead to pathophysiologic consequences in sepsis. Processes similar to these are proposed to occur repeatedly, with multiple mediators leading to dysfunction in multiple organ systems.[6]

The most commonly recognized and prominent clinical consequence of sepsis in children is septic shock. This failure of the cardiovascular system to maintain physiologic homeostasis is most frequently recognized in the form of hypotension. The second most common consequence is the respiratory distress syndrome, which results in hypoxia. The combination of hypoxia and hypotension causes end organ dysfunction and damage. The ability of the child with sepsis to survive depends on three requirements: (1) removal of the source of infection and restoration of normal physiologic processes, (2) reversal of shock so that continued ischemia is prevented, and (3) prevention or reversal of hypoxia so that anoxia is prevented. Children who present with overwhelming ischemia or anoxia, leading to significant end organ damage before therapy can be instituted, will have greater difficulty surviving these initial insults. Similarly, children in whom the nidus of infection cannot be removed and in whom the continued pathophysiologic processes cannot be stopped will have difficulty surviving the ongoing insult. Children in whom therapy is initiated in a timely fashion with an eradicable source of infection will benefit significantly. Before discussing the management of sepsis and septic shock in children, it is necessary to have a common insight into the evolving clinical definition of the pathophysiologic process we call shock.

CLINICAL DEFINITION AND PARAMETERS OF SHOCK

Perception of the definition and pathophysiology of septic shock and its therapy are evolving as technology expands. Initially, shock was defined as that point when the sphygmomanometer allowed recognition of a consumptive process in which decreasing blood pressure was associated with inexorable death. It was reasoned that the vital organs required a pumping pressure to maintain a perfused state. This opinion remained the consensus until the 1950s when cardiologists, armed with the vasoactive catecholamine norepinephrine, were excited by the ability to regain normal blood pressure but dismayed by the inability to meaningfully affect survival. Perfection of the indocyanine green technique for measuring cardiac output allowed more sophisticated analysis. The physical equation, flow = pressure/resistance or (Q = P/R), was used to derive the clinical equation, cardiac output = mean arterial pressure − central venous pressure/systemic vascular resistance. With further derivation, this equation (CO = MAP − CVP/ SVR) was transformed into the physiologic equation MAP − CVP = CO × SVR (Table 12–1). It was found that many patients with mean arterial pressures maintained by vasoactive therapy died with metabolic acidosis, low cardiac output, and elevated systemic vascular resistance. With these new observations, shock was perceived as a process in which the inability of the cardiovascular system to maintain cardiac output or perfusion pressure, or both, led to organ dysfunction and death.

The surgical literature soon reported a curious phenomenon in postoperative patients who died of shock associated with septicemia. These patients had low systemic vascular resistance and in some cases normal or even elevated cardiac output. Numerous reports differed on the incidence of hypodynamic or hyperdynamic states during bacteremia, but systemic vascular resistance was predominantly low when compared with that in previously reported patients with shock. This observation led to the concept that altered vascular tone might also contribute to the pathophysiologic process of shock.

The development of the bedside pulmonary artery catheter made it possible to attain information on the role of oxygen metabolism in shock. Referring to the equation $CaO_2 = 1.36 \times Hb \times O_2$ sat % + 0.003 × PaO_2, radial artery samples provide the arterial O_2 content and pulmonary artery samples yield the mixed venous O_2 content. Subtraction of mixed venous O_2 content from arterial O_2 content yields the arteriovenous difference $AVDO_2 = CaO_2 − CmvO_2$. This measure and the thermodilution catheter–derived cardiac output can be used to ascertain the patient's oxygen consumption, oxygen extraction, and oxygen delivery. Arterial O_2 content × cardiac output = oxygen delivery (CaO_2 × CO = DO_2). The product of cardiac output × the arteriovenous O_2 difference = oxygen consumption (CO × $AVDO_2 = \dot{V}O_2$). Oxygen consumption can also be calculated by subtracting the product of cardiac output × mixed venous O_2 content from the product of cardiac output × arterial O_2 content (CaO_2 × CO) − ($CmvO_2$ × CO) = $\dot{V}O_2$. Oxygen extraction can be derived as oxygen consumption ÷ oxygen delivered (O_2 ext = $\dot{V}O_2/DO_2$) (see Table 12–1).

Siegel and associates separated surgical patients into three groups: (1) those with hypovolemic shock, (2) those with cardiogenic shock, and (3) those with septic shock. They reported decreased systemic vascular resistance for a given cardiac output, as well as decreased oxygen consumption for a given oxygen delivery, in the population with septic shock. On the basis of this observation, they proposed that altered vascular tone-flow relationships and oxygen metabolism could contribute to the pathophysiologic process.[7] Since oxygen consumption was diminished, these investigators and others proposed that diminished systemic vascular resistance in sepsis might lead to a process of shunting in which oxygen extraction is adversely affected. Others proposed that this alteration in oxygen metabolism could in fact be due to an abnormality in mitochondrial oxygen metabolism that was independent of vascular tone. The concept evolved that shock could occur as a result of alterations in perfusion pressure, cardiac output, vascular tone, or oxygen metabolism.

Shoemaker and others soon characterized oxygen metabolism in surgical patients with septic shock who had high cardiac output and oxygen delivery and found that oxygen consumption was actually high in this population.[8] This high oxygen consumption state was reasoned to be a consequence of the hypermetabolic processes of sepsis. A phenomenon known as flow-dependent oxygen consumption was described in some of these patients (Fig. 12–1). In normal, healthy humans, oxygen extraction varies with changes in oxygen delivery. For example, in the face of increased oxygen delivery in the healthy subject, oxygen extraction will decrease, and oxygen consumption will be maintained at a steady state level at which oxygen metabolic needs are presumably met. In the flow-dependent state, oxy-

Table 12–1. CARDIOVASCULAR AND OXYGEN UTILIZATION VARIABLES

$$SVRI = \frac{MAP − CVP}{CI} \times 80$$

$$PVRI = \frac{MPAP − PAOP}{CI} \times 80$$

$$CaO_2 = 1.36 \times Hb \times \% \ O_2 \ sat + 0.003 \times PaO_2$$

$$AVDO_2 = CaO_2 − CmvO_2$$

$$DO_2 = CaO_2 \times CO \times 10$$

$$\dot{V}O_2 = AVDO_2 \times CO \times 10$$

$$O_2 \ ext = \dot{V}O_2/DO_2$$

SVRI = systemic vascular resistance index; PVRI = pulmonary vascular resistance index; CaO_2 = arterial oxygen content; $AVDO_2$ = arteriovenous oxygen content difference; DO_2 = oxygen delivery; $\dot{V}O_2$ = oxygen consumption; O_2 = oxygen extraction; MAP = mean arterial pressure; CVP = central venous pressure; CI = cardiac index; MPAP = mean pulmonary artery pressure; PAOP = pulmonary artery occlusion pressure; Hb = hemoglobin; CO = cardiac output; PaO_2 = partial pressure arterial oxygen.

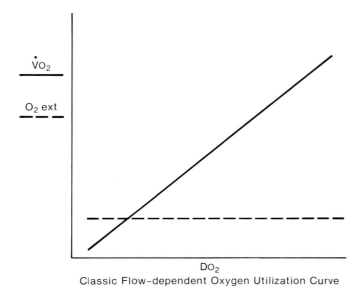

Classic Flow–dependent Oxygen Utilization Curve

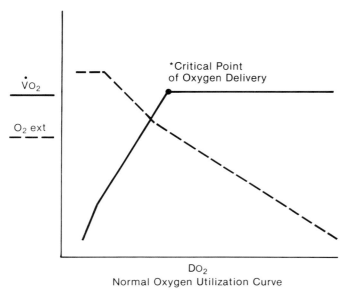

*Critical Point
of Oxygen Delivery

Normal Oxygen Utilization Curve

Figure 12–1. Oxygen utilization function curves in the normal and flow-dependent states.

gen extraction does not vary. Therefore, the hyperdynamic high oxygen delivery state yields high oxygen consumption, whereas the hypodynamic low oxygen delivery state yields low oxygen consumption. At the low end, this inability to increase oxygen extraction with decreasing oxygen delivery was interpreted as further evidence of an abnormality in oxygen utilization in sepsis. At the high end, however, the unaltered oxygen extraction, and therefore the lack of a plateau in oxygen consumption, was interpreted as evidence for a high metabolic oxygen need that was not being met by adequate delivery or extraction. This led to the consideration of whether shock could be a state in which end organ dysfunction and death could occur when increased oxygen metabolic needs were not met. Insight was provided by the observation of Bihari and coworkers.[9] Twenty-seven critically ill patients received a 30-minute infusion of prostacyclin, with significant increases in oxygen delivery. The 13 patients who showed flow-dependent increases in oxygen consumption did not survive, whereas the 12 patients who showed little increase in oxygen consumption and decreased oxygen extraction did survive. One explanation was that unrecognized and unmet oxygen requirements were associated with nonsurvival. Shoemaker's reports have provided the most direct and convincing evidence for the potential significance of treating oxygen debt during hypermetabolic states.[10] He studied critically ill patients postoperatively and used inotropic agents to maintain one random subset of patients with greater than normal oxygen delivery while allowing the remaining subset to intrinsically maintain baseline and normal oxygen delivery. The subset with pharmacologically induced increased oxygen delivery showed not only increased oxygen consumption but also clinically significant decreased mortality and morbidity. Thus, the perception of shock, and its clinically important parameters, has evolved significantly. Alterations in mean arterial pressure, cardiac output, systemic vascular resistance, oxygen delivery, and oxygen extraction may all affect oxygen consumption, organ function, and outcome.

MANAGEMENT OF SEPSIS AND SEPTIC SHOCK IN CHILDREN

Prevention

The management of sepsis and septic shock begins with prevention (Table 12–2). Children may experience life-threatening sepsis as an extension of seemingly innocuous infections, such as otitis media, sinusitis, and pneumonia, or as a consequence of occult bacteremia. Relative immunodeficiency plays a role in the tendency to acquire sepsis, with the majority of cases occurring in a bimodal distribution in children less than 2 years of age and in the neonatal period—two milestones in the development of immunocompetence. Access to, and the successful accomplishment of, prenatal care and frequent well child visits during the first years of life may allow the physician to prevent and treat infections before sepsis occurs. Children with chronic illness frequently are more immunocompromised and therefore are at greater risk for sepsis. Specific recommendations apply for specific chronic diseases (e.g., sickle cell disease, childhood cancer), but frequent access to care and immunizations remains paramount.

Nosocomial infection remains a significant contribu-

Table 12–2. STRATEGY FOR PREVENTION OF NOSOCOMIAL SEPSIS

Daily physical examination for sites of infection
Good nutrition
Tympanocentesis for otitis media in intubated children with catheters
Minimal duration for any and all indwelling lines and catheters
One team for care of chronic central catheters
Gown and glove isolation for all children after 3 days in pediatric intensive care unit

tion to sepsis in children. Hospitalized children may be at risk because of immunodeficiency, malnutrition, chronic disease, surgical wounds, invasive lines, immunosuppressive drugs, extensive antibiotic therapy, and exposure to virulent organisms. Klein and associates showed that isolation with wound, skin, and secretion precautions significantly decreased the incidence of nosocomial infection in pediatric patients in the intensive care unit (ICU) after 7 days of intensive care.[11] In addition to isolation, daily examination for localized sites of nosocomial infection may prevent extension to sepsis. For example, Persico and colleagues showed that organisms isolated by tympanocentesis in intubated children were the same organisms later isolated in blood culture specimens from these same patients during sepsis.[12] Aggressive monitoring of otitis with culture-specific antibiotics could potentially prevent the initiation of sepsis. Occult sinusitis is a particular problem in up to 10% of patients who are nasally intubated. Transition to oral intubation and appropriate antibiotics may facilitate drainage and prevent further extension. Close attention to changes in respiratory secretions will allow early management of tracheitis and pneumonia. The use of a double-lumen plugged catheter has been useful in children to assure isolation of lower respiratory organisms versus instrument contaminants.[13] All invasive lines should be examined for evidence of phlebitis or wound infection and replaced immediately if they are present. Surgical, traumatic, and burn wounds should be carefully monitored. Necrotic tissue should be débrided and wounds physically cleansed and treated with topical agents as appropriate. Careful examination may uncover other occult sources of infection (e.g., skin decubitus) or foreign bodies (e.g., vaginal tampons).

The use of surveillance cultures and prophylactic antibiotics to prevent sepsis has not been extensively studied in pediatric intensive care. However, the adult and neonatal literature have suggested its utility. Mycostatin use in patients with positive results on throat cultures for *Candida* colonization may prevent progression to candidemia and *Candida* sepsis. Nasopharyngeal cultures may also identify colonization with bacteria such as *Staphylococcus aureus,* which could be treated with rifampin to prevent dissemination. Skin cultures in burn patients with fevers have been promoted in various centers to predict sepsis when bacterial counts were greater than $100,000/cm^2$. Similarly, in culture specimens from central venous and arterial tips, bacterial counts greater than $10,000/cm^2$ have been associated with line sepsis and predicted the need for therapy when associated with positive blood culture results.

Relatively scant literature exists on the role of invasive line care in the development of sepsis in pediatric intensive care. Infection and thrombosis rates go up significantly in patients with arterial catheters after 48 hours, in patients with central venous catheters after 72 hours, and in patients with pulmonary artery catheters after 48 hours. Adult studies have suggested removal and rotating replacement of these lines at these critical times. However, the utility of this approach has not been objectively evaluated versus the risk of (1) the inability to establish access or (2) line placement com-

plications in the pediatric patient. The adult literature has suggested an alternative approach in which changing of catheters over a wire can be substituted on alternate line changes. This approach again will require investigation in pediatrics. Infection rates in chronic catheterization have been shown to be reduced when one team changes all dressings daily, an approach that would have no adverse effects in the pediatric intensive care setting. Other forms of instrumentation similarly lead to nosocomial infection. For example, patients with continuous indwelling urinary catheters show a significantly increased risk of infection after 24 hours. This can be minimized by using in-and-out catheterization in all children except those in whom strict hourly outputs are required.

Recognition

Early recognition of sepsis is a difficult clinical challenge in children because septic shock occurs as a progression of the normal inflammatory response to localized or systemic infection (Table 12–3). Release of IL-1 and other inflammatory mediators from polymorphonuclear leukocytes and the reticuloendothelial system contributes to a characteristic clinical picture of fever, tachycardia, and vasodilatation with warm, flushed skin in children with infection. This triad occurs in children with relatively innocuous viral and bacterial infections, as well as in that minority of children in whom infection progresses to sepsis. In addition, children with pneumonitis or pneumonia may also display tachypnea as a prominent symptom. Therefore, children may present with fever, tachycardia, warm skin, and tachypnea as a response to infection. The early stages of warm septic shock are heralded by signs of hypoperfusion. Clinical experience identifies a change in mental status as the earliest clinical sign of hypoperfusion and septic shock. Children may show somnolence or decreased interaction with the parent and examiner. This clinical sign, in combination with fever, tachypnea, tachycardia, and bounding pulses, presages early warm septic shock. Cardiovascular monitoring during this period characteristically shows a widened pulse pressure with an increase in cardiac index and a decrease in systemic vascular resistance, presumably secondary to increased levels of IL-1, catecholamines, and other vasoactive mediators. Pulmonary hypertension may also be noted, possibly secondary to thromboxane release. Decreased perfusion may be further evidenced by decreasing urine output. It is during this stage of sepsis, before significant ischemia or anoxia, or both, has occurred, that therapeutic intervention is theorized to be most beneficial.

Table 12–3. EARLY RECOGNITION OF SEPTIC SHOCK

Inflammatory Triad		Signs of Hypoperfusion
Fever Tachycardia Vasodilatation	+	Altered mental status, decreased urinary output, diminished capillary refill, or mottled extremities

Table 12–4. INITIAL RESUSCITATION IN WARM SEPTIC SHOCK

Presentation	Therapy	Outcome
Fever Tachycardia Bounding pulses Altered mental status Widened pulse pressure Diminished perfusion ↓ UO* ↓ ↑ Capillary refill ± Mottled extremities	Frequently requires oxygen administration alone Vigorous volume administration until signs of diminished perfusion resolve Inotropic support frequently necessary Intravascular monitoring if unacceptable diastolic pressures and vasoactive support required	If the nidus of infection can be eradicated, minimal support may suffice; continued infection may lead to multiple system organ failure

*UO = urine output.

As the untreated pathophysiologic process progresses, less subtle signs of decreased perfusion are evident, including capillary refill time longer than 2 seconds, mottled skin, and cool extremities. This occurs as blood volume is decreased secondary to a significant capillary leak. Children who are being monitored invasively may exhibit decreasing central venous or pulmonary arterial opening pressures and increasing systemic vascular resistance. Hypotension ensues, as the increase in vascular tone is not sufficient to maintain homeostasis and the patient enters into classic cold septic shock. During this final stage, the child exhibits a narrow pulse pressure, cold and clammy extremities, tachycardia, tachypnea, cyanotic nail beds, and lethargy. Monitoring reveals a decreasing cardiac index, normal or mildly elevated systemic vascular resistance, hypoxia, and metabolic acidosis. This is the clinical picture of profound hypovolemic and cardiogenic shock, with an inadequate vasoconstrictive response leading to ischemia, anoxia, and lactic acidosis.

Recognition of sepsis early in this progression, and successful rapid therapeutic intervention to either prevent or abbreviate this process, can minimize the initial anoxic and ischemic effects of septic shock. With this task accomplished, removal of the nidus of infection and support of the child allows for optimal survival and minimal morbidity. This is the goal of the pediatric intensive care team in the management of sepsis and septic shock.

Therapy

Initial Resuscitation

Initiation of therapy in septic shock requires immediate assessment of the airway, breathing, and circulation (Table 12–4). When sepsis is not recognized until late in cold septic shock, an airway may have to be established and mechanical ventilation used (Table 12–5). When sepsis is recognized during early warm septic shock, the patient frequently requires only supplemental oxygen during the initial hour of resuscitation. Establishment of venous access is the keystone of early therapy and should be attained according to Advanced Pediatric Life Support Guidelines in emergency access in children. With oxygenation and ventilation controlled, the patient should immediately receive volume resuscitation, antibiotic therapy, and vasoactive agents as necessary. Initiation of these therapies should not be delayed for the results of laboratory tests. Initial resuscitation in pediatric septic shock is based on clinical examination and noninvasive cardiovascular monitoring information.

Volume Resuscitation

Volume resuscitation is paramount to the initial therapy of septic shock. Until recently, the approach to pediatric shock was based on the physiology of the child with diarrhea and dehydration-induced hypovolemia. This called for a 10- to 20-ml/kg fluid bolus over 20 minutes. This calculation was based on the observation that children with dehydration show hypotension and decreased perfusion when there is a 10 to 20% loss in total body water. The tenet of administering a bolus slowly was founded in an era when pediatric ventilators and positive end-expiratory pressure (PEEP) were not available to treat the child with pulmonary edema. In addition, the pulmonary artery catheter was not available to assess intravascular status. Consequently, children with low filling pressures and noncardiogenic pulmonary edema (adult respiratory distress syndrome [ARDS]) could be erroneously evaluated as being hy-

Table 12–5. INITIAL RESUSCITATION IN COLD SEPTIC SHOCK

Presentation	Therapy	Outcome
Fever or hypothermia Tachycardia Poor pulses Altered mental status Narrowed pulse pressure Diminished perfusion ↓ Urine output ↓ Capillary refill Mottled extremities	Patient frequently requires ventilation for acidosis and cardiac support Vigorous volume administration is required but signs of diminished perfusion may persist Inotropic and vasoactive support are always required Intravascular monitoring for severe cardiac dysfunction	These children uniformly require sophisticated support

poxic as a result of too much volume administration. This lack of diagnostic and therapeutic sophistication led to cautious volume administration in children. This principle was further emphasized in sepsis because of preoccupation with the risk of the syndrome of inappropriate antidiuretic hormone (SIADH) in children with meningitis. Adherence to the "first do no harm" principle was the basis for the principle of administering a 20-ml/kg bolus in the first hour of pediatric shock in the early textbooks.

Modern investigation and technology revealed the pathophysiology of septic shock to be distinct from that of isolated hypovolemic shock. In addition to volume loss induced by vomiting, diarrhea, and decreased intake in the child with sepsis, effective intravascular volume is dramatically decreased by leakage across capillary membranes, as well as by venous and arteriolar pooling. The rate of extravascular transit of albumin is increased threefold in adult patients with septic shock.[14] The effect of hypovolemia can be further exacerbated by the response of the cardiovascular system during sepsis. Left ventricular end-diastolic volume has been shown to increase in adults, whereas systemic vascular resistance decreases. This is in contrast to nonseptic hypovolemia, in which left end-diastolic volume is maintained and systemic vascular resistance is markedly increased.[15] The volume required to adequately resuscitate the cardiovascular system during sepsis can be dramatic.

Inadequate volume resuscitation was the basis for failure in attaining hyperdynamic sepsis in animal models for approximately a decade. It was not until Carroll and Snyder showed that as much as 60 ml/kg of crystalloid solution was required during the first hour to produce hyperdynamic sepsis in cynomolgus monkeys that the mystery was solved.[16] Since then, these findings have been confirmed in dog and pig models. Furthermore, increased oxygen delivery and oxygen consumption have been shown to be dependent on adequate volume resuscitation in these models. Clinical investigators have now shown that volume resuscitation increases cardiac index, oxygen delivery, and oxygen consumption in patients with septic shock, as well as in patients with hypovolemic shock.[17] Hussain and associates investigated the role of volume resuscitation versus norepinephrine infusions in a canine model of endotoxin shock. In this model, norepinephrine infusion between 0.5 μg/kg/min and 1.9 μg/kg/min maintained blood pressure and increased blood flow to resting muscle (gastrocnemius) but did not improve flow to vital organs, whereas volume resuscitation up to 60 ml/kg/hr increased flow toward control levels in heart, brain, resting muscle, kidney, and gut, suggesting that volume resuscitation may be preferable to vasopressor therapy during endotoxin shock.[18]

Based on these and other observations, the American Heart Association Committee on Pediatric Life Support suggested that the clinician give a 20 ml/kg fluid bolus during volume resuscitation in septic shock and then reassess the patient's perfusion, repeating boluses to a total of 60 ml/kg in the first hour until perfusion is improved. A recent pediatric study presented data to suggest this approach can be safely accomplished with

clinical judgment and technical support.[19] In this study, 34 children with culture- or tissue-positive septic shock and a functioning pulmonary artery catheter at 6 hours following initial resuscitation were evaluated for volume requirements, cardiopulmonary characteristics, and outcome. Children at this hospital received from 5 to 120 ml/kg of volume during the first hour of resuscitation. Survivors received significantly more volume than did nonsurvivors. In addition, patients who received greater than 40 ml/kg in the first hour showed markedly increased survival as compared with those who received less than 20 ml/kg or 20 to 40 ml/kg during the first hour of resuscitation. The suspected morbidity of increased volume resuscitation was not evident in this population. There was no increased incidence in noncardiogenic pulmonary edema (ARDS) in the first 24 hours in the hyperresuscitation group. Furthermore, the incidence of cardiogenic pulmonary edema was neither clinically nor statistically significantly increased. Although new studies with greater numbers of patients will be necessary to confirm these observations, no patient with cardiogenic pulmonary edema died as a result of this process. In fact, the patients showed improved survival; however, two survivors, one who received less than 20 ml/kg in the first hour and one who received greater than 40 ml/kg in the first hour required PEEP, peritoneal dialysis, and hemofiltration within 6 hours of admission. Both of these patients were anuric on presentation. Hypovolemia at 6 hours defined by pulmonary artery occlusion pressure (PAOP) less than or equal to 8 mm Hg with a urine output less than 1 ml/kg/hr, and a blood pressure reading 2 standard deviations less than the mean were associated with significant mortality in this study. This supported the assertion that prolonged hypovolemia and subsequent ischemia during sepsis and septic shock are deleterious. Since no patient in the hyperresuscitation group met these three criteria at 6 hours, it is possible that prolonged hypovolemia may be averted with volume resuscitation. Marcier and colleagues similarly reported that hypovolemia and cardiac failure were significant contributing factors to mortality in 18 children with meningococcal septic shock, and these authors suggested aggressive resuscitation.[20] It appears that aggressive, controlled volume resuscitation may be required in some patients to avoid prolonged hypovolemia and septic shock.

Based on these observations and the recommendations of the American Heart Association Committee on Advanced Pediatric Life Support, volume in the first hour should be administered with the end point of improved perfusion as evidenced by capillary refill time of less than 2 seconds; warm, flushed extremities; strong pulses; improved mental status; diminished tachycardia; restoration of normal blood pressure; and increased urine output. The clinician may administer fluid as an intravenous push or a 20-minute bolus if it is clinically effective. The total volume required may in some cases be 20 ml/kg but can commonly be in excess of 60 ml/kg in the first hour.

Antibiotic Therapy

While volume is being given via bolus administration, antibiotics can be administered by intravenous push.

For the most part, this is done empirically and, at least initially, all patients are presumed to have bacterial septic shock (Table 12–6). As recommended by the American Academy of Pediatrics Committee on Infectious Disease, patients in the first 2 months of life may receive a combination of ampicillin and gentamicin or ampicillin and cefotaxime or ceftriaxone to cover community-acquired as well as maternally-derived vaginal flora. Children older than 2 months of age may be treated with cefotaxime or ceftriaxone alone or with a combination of ampicillin and chloramphenicol. Ampicillin may be added to the preceding cephalosporins, but it is not clearly necessary because *Listeria* and *Enterococcus* are unusual organisms in community-acquired pediatric sepsis. Nosocomial sepsis requires antibiotic therapy that is specific to hospital and ICU antibiotic susceptibility reports. *Staphylococcus* and gram-negative organisms are more common in nosocomial sepsis; therefore, a regimen of vancomycin and an aminoglycoside will usually suffice. In some circumstances, a semisynthetic penicillin such as oxacillin will suffice if *S. epidermidis* is not a pathogen. However, hospitals with significant methicillin-resistant *S. aureus* should always consider vancomycin as a first-line drug in nosocomial sepsis. Similarly, when treating sepsis and septic shock in hospitals with gentamicin-resistant *Pseudomonas* or *Klebsiella*, consideration should be given to the first-line use of an antibiotic to which these strains have shown sensitivity.

Blood culture specimens should be obtained before antibiotics are administered, if possible; however, in cases of poor access, antibiotics can be administered prior to the accomplishment of this task. Lumbar puncture is rarely indicated during septic shock. Cardiopulmonary compromise is a relative contraindication to lumbar puncture. When this procedure is felt to be necessary, consideration should be given to establishment of an airway. Studies have shown that apnea can cause significant morbidity during this procedure. The lack of diagnostic cerebrospinal fluid is not critical because blood culture results are positive in 80% of children with bacteremia-positive meningitis. If patients with sepsis are treated with antibiotic regimens appropriate for presumed meningitis, morbidity or mortality as a result of inaccessible cerebrospinal fluid culture

should be minimized. A theoretic objection to the lack of an accurate diagnosis of meningitis is the inability to enact volume restriction as prophylaxis for SIADH. During the study of 36 patients with culture-proven sepsis, no cases of SIADH occurred despite vigorous resuscitation.[19] Furthermore, the immense volume requirements of sepsis rendered volume restriction a moot alternative.

Vasoactive Agents

While volume and antibiotics are being administered via bolus, a second intravenous line should be established according to APLS guidelines. Central venous access is preferred for optimal results. If volume boluses alone restore normal perfusion, vasoactive agents are not necessary. If signs of decreased perfusion persist, however, the use of a mixed β- and α-adrenergic agent such as dopamine should be initiated. As previously discussed, individuals can respond uniquely to pharmacotherapeutic agents. However, an initial dose of 5 μg/kg/min of dopamine or dobutamine classically affects β-adrenergic stimulation. A subset of children with septic shock, particularly those recognized during warm septic shock, will respond nicely to volume resuscitation and this degree of inotropic support with 100% survival and no mortality. However, a substantial number of children will still have decreased perfusion pressure or decreased diastolic pressure and will require increased vasoactive support. This can be attained by increasing dopamine to α-adrenergic concentrations of 10 μg/kg/min or higher, or by switching to myriad vasoactive drug combinations. These children frequently require pulmonary artery catheterization to correctly manage the more profound cardiovascular dysfunction, as well as multiple technologies to support the tendency toward multiple organ system failure.

MANAGEMENT IN THE EARLY AND MIDDLE STAGES OF SEPTIC SHOCK

Prognostic Indices and Therapeutic Goals

Pollack and associates[21] evaluated 42 critically ill pediatric patients with septic shock who despite volume resuscitation required more than 5 μg/kg/min of dopamine for cardiovascular support. After pulmonary artery catheterization, all cardiopulmonary variables were obtained during active blood pressure support. The percentage of survival was significantly increased in patients with greater than normal values of oxygen consumption, arteriovenous O_2 content difference, oxygen extraction, pH, and core temperature. In addition, there were significantly more nonsurvivors with wedge pressure, pulmonary shunt, and pH values less than the survivor medians. Therapeutic goals based on the distribution of these eight variables isolated patient groups with survival rates of 59 to 75%, compared with overall survival rates of 43%.[21] This same group of investigators further examined cardiopulmonary variables sequentially in 32

Table 12–6. ANTIBIOTIC THERAPY IN SEPTIC SHOCK

Empirical therapy	
Outpatient sepsis:	Ampicillin and chloramphenicol OR
>2 mo	Third-generation cephalosporin
<2 mo	Ampicillin and gentamicin OR
	Ampicillin and cephalosporin
Nosocomial sepsis:	Staphylococcal and gram-negative coverage; consult hospital susceptibility data
Nosocomial sepsis: After 7 days on antibiotic with or without low absolute neutrophil count	Consult infectious disease specialist to rule out candidemia
Herpes or varicella sepsis	Acyclovir

children with septic shock with similar indications for pulmonary artery catheterization. According to therapeutic efforts to control blood pressure, variables were recorded during resuscitation, after resuscitation, and in the middle stages of shock. Cardiovascular support with vasoactive agents and volume therapy maintained mean arterial pressure, cardiac index, systemic vascular resistance, wedge pressure, left cardiac work index, and pulmonary circulation variables (including mean pulmonary artery pressure, pulmonary vascular resistance, central venous pressure, and right cardiac work index) similarly in survivors and nonsurvivors. However, despite similar cardiac index and oxygen delivery, nonsurvivors showed decreased oxygen utilization variables (oxygen consumption, arteriovenous O_2 content difference, O_2 extraction index, and core temperatures) during the resuscitation and postresuscitation stages when compared with survivors.[22] In these two studies, maintenance of blood pressure, systemic vascular resistance, and cardiac output with mixed α- and β-adrenergic support improved outcome from a presumed 100% mortality rate to a 43% survival rate. However, the most intriguing finding was that increased oxygen utilization was associated with as much as a 70% survival rate. Since increased oxygen extraction was similarly associated with increased survival, several questions arose about the potential of oxygen debt as a contributing factor to mortality. If oxygen delivery and oxygen requirements were the same in the survivors and nonsurvivors, children with increased oxygen extraction would have increased oxygen consumption and presumably less oxygen debt. These studies did not ascertain whether children with decreased oxygen consumption and extraction could attain therapeutically induced increased oxygen delivery or extraction with subsequently increased oxygen consumption and whether this increase in consumption would directly translate into decrease in oxygen debt and improved survival.

A rationale for future studies to answer these questions may be founded upon a recent comparison of cardiopulmonary and oxygen utilization variables during the early and middle stages of septic and cardiogenic shock in children.[23] As previously noted, altered vascular tone and flow–oxygen utilization relationships are considered a hallmark of sepsis. In contrast, this study showed that during the early and middle stages of shock in children who received inotropes, vasopressors, and in some cases vasodilators to maintain normal blood pressure, altered relationships did not exist when the septic child was compared with the child who had pure cardiogenic shock. For a given cardiac index, the septic child had the same systemic vascular resistance as did the child with cardiogenic shock. In addition, for any given oxygen delivery rate, the child with septic shock had the same if not higher oxygen consumption and extraction than did the child with cardiogenic shock. Two explanations are offered for this observation: (1) Children in the early and middle stages of septic shock had not yet reached a pathophysiologic stage of circulatory shock in which these relationships were altered or (2) the use of vasoactive agents to maintain cardiac index, systemic vascular resistance, and mean arterial pressure modified

the previously altered vascular tone and flow–oxygen utilization relationship in children so that it was similar to that observed in cardiogenic shock. In both of these populations, increased oxygen consumption and decreased oxygen extraction was associated with increasing oxygen delivery. Oxygen delivery, therefore, and not oxygen extraction was the major population determinant of increased oxygen consumption during the early and middle stages of cardiogenic and septic shock when altered vascular tone and flow–oxygen utilization relationships did not exist. On the basis of these three studies, it appears that a regimen that uses mixed α- and β-adrenergic support can restore a normal mean arterial pressure and systemic vascular resistance in child populations during the early and middle stages of septic shock. When this is accomplished, there appears to be no significant inability in children with septic shock to consume oxygen when compared with children with cardiogenic shock alone. Increased oxygen consumption appears dependent on increased oxygen delivery in this scenario.

PATTERNS OF SURVIVAL AND NONSURVIVAL AND THE FORMULATION OF A THERAPEUTIC APPROACH

Nonsurvival in sepsis and septic shock follows a continuous pattern of pathologic alterations in cardiopulmonary and oxygen utilization variables. In order to meaningfully discuss these pathophysiologic processes, we will describe several patients who show common alterations with predominant perturbation of one or the other measurable parameters. Figure 12–2A represents a patient who exhibits vascular unresponsiveness and flow-dependent oxygen utilization. The graph begins with high oxygen consumption, which is maintained primarily as a result of increased oxygen delivery from a hyperdynamic state. Although oxygen extraction is low, its significance is unknown, as oxygen consumption is at a supranormal range. Systemic vascular resistance is low but within a normal range and consistent with the hyperdynamic state. When using the variable MAP − CVP as a determinant of perfusion pressure, we find that this patient exhibits normal perfusion pressure during this early stage of shock. At this time point, the abnormal serum pH value might be an indicator of inadequate metabolism. At the next time point, systemic vascular resistance drops to less than the normal range. Although cardiac index increases, it is not enough to maintain normal perfusion pressures, and the MAP − CVP becomes abnormal. An unresponsive systemic vasculature precedes the subsequent decrease in cardiac index at the next time point. This may be due to inadequate perfusion of the heart during diastole or perhaps secondary to direct cardiac unresponsiveness. This is accompanied by a further decrease in systemic vascular resistance and perfusion pressure. As cardiac index and oxygen delivery decrease, so does oxygen consumption. In fact, oxygen extraction remains significantly unchanged throughout the course. Oxygen con-

Text continued on page 126

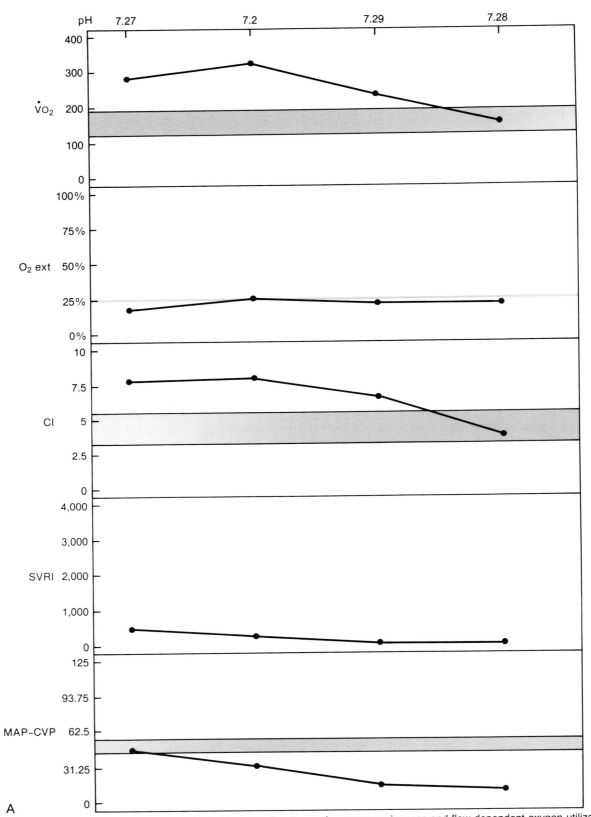

Figure 12–2. *A,* Pattern of nonsurvival in a child with predominant vascular unresponsiveness and flow-dependent oxygen utilization.

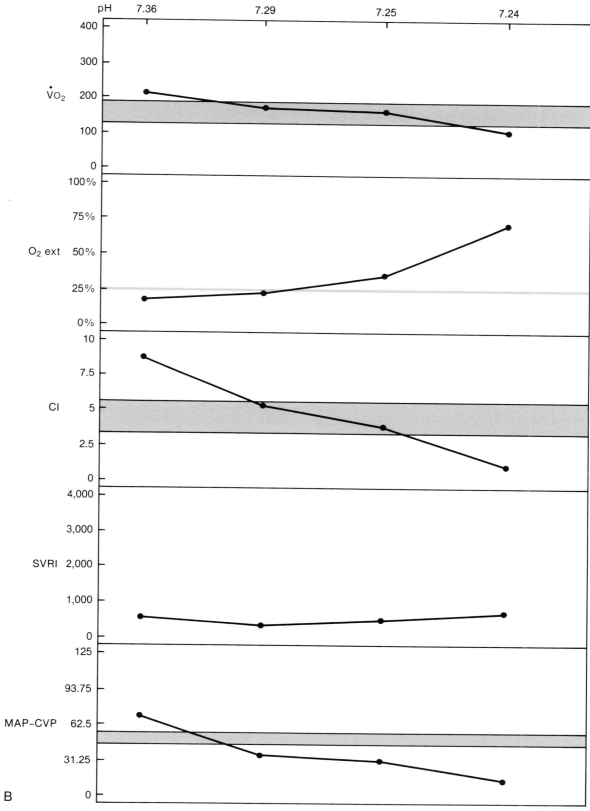

Figure 12–2 *Continued B,* Pattern of nonsurvival in a child with predominant cardiac failure.

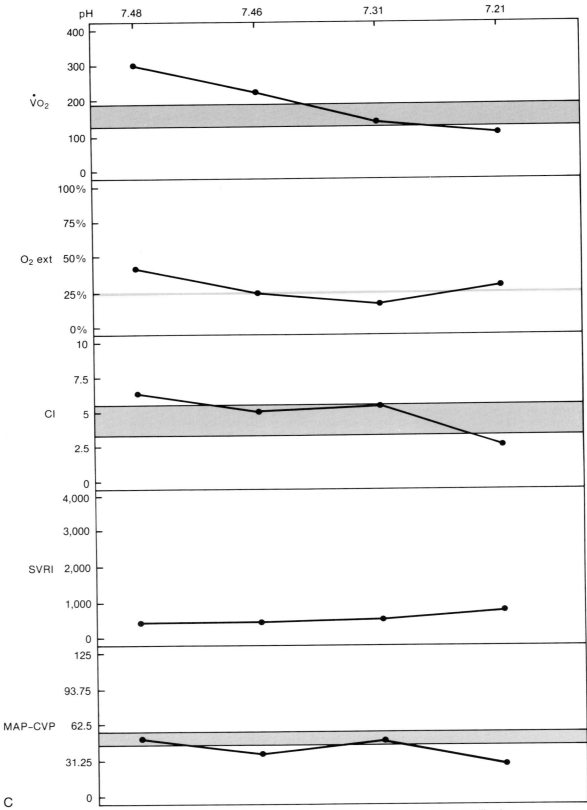

Figure 12–2 *Continued C,* Pattern of nonsurvival in a child with inadequate oxygen utilization.

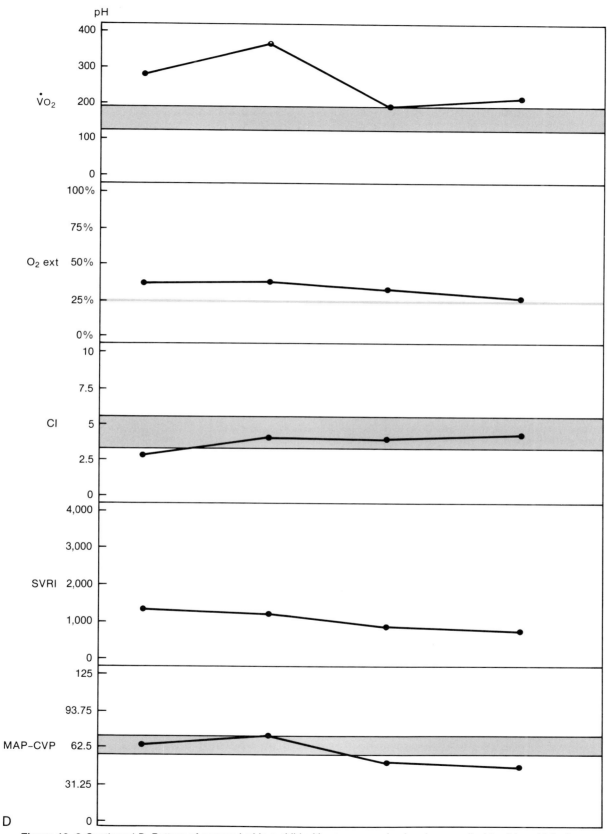

Figure 12–2 *Continued D,* Pattern of nonsurvival in a child with an unrecognized and noneradicable nidus of infection.

sumption is completely flow-dependent. At the last time point before the child's demise, oxygen consumption, oxygen extraction, and cardiac index remain within what are considered normal limits. However, this is misleading. The severe decrease in systemic vascular resistance would require a greater than normal cardiac index to maintain perfusion pressure. The heart is relatively dysfunctional and unable to accomplish this, which subsequently results in systemic perfusion pressure that is inadequate to sustain life. It is also possible that the patient still requires supranormal oxygen delivery and consumption to fulfill her O_2 requirement. The inability to increase extraction presumably contributes to a continued oxygen debt.

Figure 12–2B is representative of a child in whom cardiac failure with decreased cardiac output and oxygen delivery significantly contributes to mortality. This child, in a fashion similar to the first patient, begins early septic shock with supranormal oxygen consumption that is maintained by an increased cardiac index and oxygen delivery. The perfusion pressure and cardiac index–systemic vascular resistance relationship is within normal limits, and though oxygen extraction is low, there is no overt evidence of oxygen debt. The next time point reveals a progressive pattern of decreasing cardiac output. This is accompanied by a notable lack of systemic vascular response, leading to a subnormal perfusion pressure and altered cardiac index–systemic vascular resistance relationship. Unlike the child in Figure 12–2A, oxygen extraction is increased in response to decreased delivery in a decidedly non–flow-dependent manner. Significantly, acidemia ensues, suggesting oxygen debt. The third time point reveals progressively decreased yet normal cardiac indices with more markedly increased oxygen extraction to maintain a high normal oxygen consumption. However, metabolic acidosis and decreased perfusion pressure continue as the vascular response to decrease in cardiac output remains conspicuously lacking. The last time point reveals severe cardiac failure with a low-normal systemic vascular resistance index and inadequate perfusion pressure. Despite an increase in oxygen extraction to 70%, oxygen consumption drops to subnormal levels, metabolic acidosis continues, and death ensues. In contrast to our first patient, this child shows no evidence of an inability to extract oxygen. Furthermore, the predominant cardiovascular dysfunction in this patient is diminished cardiac output. Vascular unresponsiveness does, however, significantly contribute to the child's inability to maintain adequate perfusion pressure. The onset of metabolic acidosis at the time point of decreased perfusion pressure and decreasing oxygen consumption further suggests that oxygen debt was a contributing factor.

Figure 12–2C represents a patient in whom inadequate oxygen utilization is the predominant contributor to mortality. This child begins in the early stage of septic shock with a hyperoxygen utilization that is attained through increased oxygen extraction as well as increased delivery—two prognostically favorable variables. This occurs during a hyperdynamic state with normal perfusion pressure and cardiac index–systemic vascular resis-

tance relationships. Over time, however, oxygen extraction decreases with a resultant decrease in oxygen consumption—first to normal levels and then to low-normal levels. This is accompanied by a decreasing serum pH value. Cardiac index, systemic vascular resistance index, and perfusion pressure remain relatively unchanged during this period. At the final time point, the child becomes hypodynamic with a moderate but inadequate systemic vascular response, leading to decreased perfusion pressure. This is accompanied by subnormal oxygen consumption, normal rather than increased oxygen extraction, and increasing metabolic acidosis, suggesting progressive oxygen debt. Again we see elements of vascular unresponsiveness and cardiac dysfunction, but in this child abnormal oxygen utilization appears to be the predominant perturbation.

Figure 12–2D represents a child who survived the initial period of observation but eventually succumbed to unrecognized *Candida* sepsis and multiple organ system failure. Initially this child presented in a hypodynamic state, with increased systemic vascular resistance and normal perfusion pressure. The increased oxygen consumption state was maintained through increased oxygen extraction, which continued to the second time point when an increased cardiac index further increased oxygen utilization. The systemic vascular response was sufficient to maintain normal perfusion as well. Over a 3-day period, this child maintained a high oxygen utilization state with normal perfusion pressures. However, the continued nidus of infection led to multiple organ system failure and eventual mortality.

The first three children illustrate scenarios in which alterations in the cardiac index–systemic vascular resistance relationship led to decreased perfusion, and the oxygen consumption and oxygen delivery relationship led to oxygen debt, contributing to metabolic acidosis, shock, and death. The fourth patient illustrates the fundamental tenet that without eradication of the source of infection, eventual multiple organ system failure and death will ensue.

Survivors respond to therapeutic maneuvers without development of refractory cardiac, vascular, or oxygen consumption dysfunction. On the basis of these observations, the goal, but not the guarantee, of therapy is to treat such alterations in the hope that refractoriness will not occur. It is proposed that the response will depend upon the degree to which the presence of mediators or the persistent effect of ischemia has affected the intrinsic function of the child's multiple cardiovascular and oxygen utilization systems.

Based on these observations, Figure 12–3 graphically illustrates a therapeutic approach to management during septic shock. The shaded area represents the accepted boundaries of normal perfusion pressure, or MAP − CVP. The curve represents increasing oxygen consumption as a parameter of increasing oxygen delivery. Maintaining normal perfusion pressure, the physician can then increase oxygen delivery to the point of maximal oxygen consumption. This is represented as the intersection of these two curves. Once maximal oxygen consumption has been attained, there is no need to further increase oxygen delivery. Perfusion pressure can

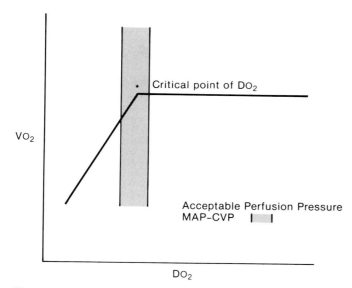

Figure 12–3. This illustration represents a therapeutic approach to shock. Therapy is directed at an acceptable perfusion pressure and the oxygen delivery that accomplishes the highest oxygen consumption (critical point of oxygen delivery).

be maintained by increasing cardiac index or systemic vascular resistance, or both, as long as this point of intersection occurs.

CARDIOVASCULAR MANAGEMENT DURING THE EARLY AND MIDDLE STAGES OF SEPTIC SHOCK

Cardiac and vascular functions are compromised in sepsis. Myocardial depression has been shown in vitro, in vivo, and in clinical studies. Endotoxin and plasma from septic patients have been shown to decrease contractility in both cell culture and isolated cardiac muscle preparations. Clinical studies in adults have shown that dysfunction begins within hours of sepsis and peaks in 1½ to 2 days, with survivors returning to normal function over a 7- to 10-day period. Parrillo's group has proposed that a hyperdynamic state is maintained by the dilatation of the ventricles during sepsis.[15] In this manner, high cardiac output can be produced despite a decreased ejection fraction. According to these investigators, survivors can be anticipated on the basis of their ability to accomplish this cardiac response. In a smaller group of patients, these investigators also measured coronary artery blood flow and concluded that dysfunction is not the result of inadequate perfusion. They proposed that dysfunction is the result of a myocardial depressant factor, which has been isolated but neither purified nor sequenced.[15]

Equivalent studies in children are thus far unavailable. Cardiac output in children is classically thought to be more rate- than stroke-volume–dependent. Thus, it remains to be seen to what extent ventricular dilatation plays a significant role in the maintenance of the hyperdynamic state in children. Interestingly, hyperdynamic sepsis is not the rule in children during blood pressure support with vasoactive agents during the early and middle stages of sepsis. In fact, the mean cardiac index in 56 children with septic shock was 4.05 ± 0.25 l/min/m² (a eudynamic state) compared with the 34 children with pure cardiogenic shock who showed a mean cardiac index of 2.5 ± 0.6 l/min/m² (a hypodynamic state).[23] Marcier has further documented a clinically significant incidence of hypodynamic sepsis in meningococcal shock in children.[20]

Vascular dysfunction in sepsis is clinically evidenced as lower than normal systemic vascular resistance and diminished vascular response to vasoactive agents or decreased cardiac output, or both. Animal models have shown a diminished dose response curve of mean arterial pressure to adrenergic stimulation during sepsis. Aortic rings from these models have similarly shown the same responsiveness in an isolated organ bath. Since this dysfunction remains when LPS or mediators are lacking, it is postulated that there are intrinsic alterations in the contractile response, which remain even after removal of the nidus of infection. This intrinsic change has been documented on multiple biochemical levels.[24] Although TNF and IL-1 have been shown to decrease responsiveness of vascular tissue to α-adrenergic stimulation in vitro, effects at the biochemical level have not yet been investigated.[25] The clinical significance of vascular tissue dysfunction has been emphasized by the findings of Lucking and coworkers[26] in adults and of Pollack and coworkers[21] in children. They have shown that low systemic vascular resistance is associated with decreased survival. Clearly, vascular dysfunction in the face of cardiac failure is deleterious.

CLINICAL PRINCIPLES OF CARDIOVASCULAR MANAGEMENT

Clinical management of cardiac index is based on several principles. The first is the Starling law, which is the basis for cardiac volume resuscitation in sepsis. As illustrated in Figure 12–4A, this law states that cardiac output or ventricular muscle shortening velocity increases with increasing left ventricular end-diastolic volume or muscle fiber length. When the heart muscle is dysfunctional, as is frequently the case in sepsis, the Starling curve is diminished such that less cardiac output is evident for a given left ventricular end-diastolic volume. Inotropic agents may be used to improve contractility and hence elevate the dysfunctional cardiac curve toward normal parameters. Inotropic agents thus have an important role in improving cardiac function in sepsis.

The second principle is the observation that increasing aortic impedance or afterload decreases cardiac output. This is illustrated in Figure 12–4B. According to this curve, cardiac output remains optimal at a given aortic impedance but then drops disproportionately with increasing resistance. Once again the curve representing a patient with cardiac dysfunction, as is frequent in the case of sepsis, shows decreased cardiac output for any given aortic impedance. This is the basis for the use of afterload reducing agents in patients with cardiogenic shock and elevated systemic vascular resistance or aortic

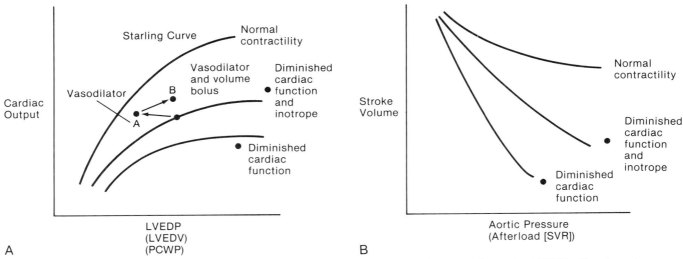

Figure 12–4. Two important principles of cardiac performance. *A,* The Starling curve shows that increasing LVEDV with volume increases cardiac output. In the dysfunctional heart, the curve can be improved with inotropic therapy. (Afterload reduction improves cardiac output (A) with the use of a vasodilatory agent. The addition of volume to attain optimal cardiac output (B). *B,* Stroke volume is inversely proportional to afterload. The function curve in the dysfunctional heart can be improved with inotropy.

impedance. In these patients, minimal reductions of aortic impedance result in marked improvement in cardiac output. This physiologic principle contributes in part to the increased cardiac output frequently observed in early warm sepsis. In the patient with sepsis and adequate volume loading, cardiac output may be increased in part because aortic impedance or systemic vascular resistance is low. This allows the dysfunctional heart in sepsis to perform in a eudynamic or perhaps even hyperdynamic state. The corollary of this observation is that any therapeutic maneuver that increases systemic vascular resistance or aortic impedance in a dysfunctional heart, as may be the case in sepsis, will significantly decrease cardiac index and lower the Starling curve. Therefore, therapeutic approaches that aim to improve systemic vascular resistance through the use of α-adrenergic agents in sepsis will require the simultaneous use of β-adrenergic agents to improve cardiac function or will result in decreased cardiac output.

The third principle on which therapy can be based is the tenet that two thirds of coronary artery perfusion occurs during diastole. Aortic diastolic pressure and duration of diastole are two main determinants of cardiac perfusion and ultimate performance. At some level, low systemic vascular resistance and tachycardia may contribute to progressive cardiac dysfunction. As a result, optimal cardiac function may require some degree of α-adrenergic stimulation and increased systemic vascular resistance for proper perfusion. This increased systemic vascular resistance may also control tachycardia to some degree if cardiac filling is improved on the basis of improved venous return.

Figure 12–5 shows the proposed cardiac index–systemic vascular resistance relationship of a healthy child and the hypothesized abnormal tone-flow relationship of a child with sepsis in which vascular tone is diminished for any given cardiac index. In order to establish the normal relationship and adequate perfusion pressure,

the physician can manipulate cardiac index (β-adrenergic stimulation) or systemic vascular resistance (α-adrenergic stimulation), or both. This illustration assumes optimal volume loading and proposes that with β-adrenergic stimulation, cardiac index improves along the same curve, whereas systemic vascular resistance decreases, and with pure α-stimulation, cardiac index decreases along the same curve, whereas systemic vascular resistance increases. However, mixed α and β

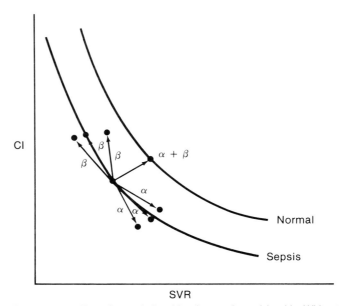

Figure 12–5. Tone-flow relationships in sepsis and health. Without inotropic or vasoactive support an abnormal tone-flow relationship exists in which SVR is low for any given CI. The use of a pure β-agonist increases CI and may decrease SVR. The use of a pure α-agonist increases SVR but may decrease CI. The use of β- and α-agonists may restore "normal" tone-flow relationships with an acceptable SVR for any given CI.

Table 12–7. CALCULATED SYSTEMIC VASCULAR RESISTANCE INDEX FOR GIVEN PERFUSION PRESSURES AND CARDIAC INDICES

	12 Yr			6 Mo	
CI*	SVRI†	MAP − CVP‡		SVRI	MAP − CVP
3.5	1371	60		1211	53
4.5	1067	60		942	53
5.5	873	60		771	53
6.5	738(873)	60 (71)		652(771)	53(63)
7.5	640(873)	60 (82)		565(771)	53(73)
8.5	565(873)	60 (93)		499(771)	53(82)

*CI = cardiac index.
†SVRI = systemic vascular resistance index.
‡MAP − CVP = mean arterial pressure minus central venous pressure.

In attaining an acceptable SVRI several considerations may be made. Age and CI are important determinants. Also minimal SVRI requirements may necessitate increased pharmacotherapeutically induced MAP. This is represented by parentheses. The clinician may use a given MAP − CVP or a minimal (SVRI) in these calculations according to interpretation of the literature.

stimulation allows the child to experience a different curve or tone-flow relationship. It is proposed that at each level of α-adrenergic stimulation, a new curve is generated when accompanied by β-adrenergic stimulation. This theoretic manipulation of tone-flow relationships is offered as a possible explanation for the observed lack of decreased systemic vascular resistance for any given cardiac index in early pediatric septic shock when mixed adrenergic agents were used to maintain normal mean arterial pressure.[23] In theory, maintenance of normal perfusion pressure or mean arterial pressure minus central venous pressure with mixed α- and β-adrenergic agents rather than α or β agents alone can have greater utility. For example, use of a pure α-adrenergic agonist might increase systemic vascular resistance but decrease cardiac index, whereas pure β-adrenergic agents might increase cardiac index but neither maintain systemic vascular resistance nor prevent an increase in tachycardia. The use of both agents could produce an increased cardiac index, systemic vascular resistance, and mean arterial pressure minus central venous pressure, and prevent unnecessary tachycardia.

Using varied combinations, the physician can manipulate perfusion through systemic vascular resistance or cardiac index. Determination of therapeutic goals can begin with the equation SVR = (MAP − CVP/cardiac index) × 80 and the accepted perfusion pressure for age. For example, in children older than 12 years of age, a mean arterial pressure of 65 mm Hg, a central venous pressure of 5 mm Hg, and an accepted cardiac index range from 3.5 to 5.5 l/min/m² gives a perfusion pressure of 60 mm Hg and a range of acceptable systemic vascular resistance indices of 872 to 1,371 dyne·sec/cm⁵·m². In children who are 6 months old, a mean arterial pressure of 53 mm Hg, central venous pressure of 5 mm Hg, and an accepted cardiac index range of 3.5 to 5.5 l/min/m² gives a perfusion pressure of 48 mm Hg and a range of acceptable systemic vascular resistance indices from 689 to 1,097 dyne·sec/cm⁵·m². Maintenance of normal perfusion pressure with a systemic vascular resistance index within these ranges would suffice unless the cardiac index was greater than 5.5 l/min/m². Since the systemic vascular resistance index is calculated, maintenance of these same parameters of

systemic vascular resistance in a hyperdynamic state with a cardiac output greater than 5.5 l/min/m² would require increased perfusion pressure or mean arterial pressure. Some have suggested, but it is not currently known, that decreased systemic vascular resistance is deleterious even when it occurs in the presence of normal perfusion pressure. Table 12–7 shows the calculated systemic vascular resistance indices for various cardiac indices with maintained perfusion pressure. At this time, the physician should at the very least maintain these minimal systemic vascular resistance indices for each cardiac index. When high output and higher systemic vascular resistance indices are determined to be prudent, increased mean arterial pressure must be accepted.

As discussed, since cardiac dysfunction exists, maintenance of an acceptable perfusion pressure and systemic vascular resistance index with pure α-adrenergic support can decrease cardiac index in the hyperdynamic patient with a lower than expected systemic vascular resistance index and perfusion pressure. The addition of inotropic agents will increase cardiac output. It remains to be seen to what degree this should be implemented. If the cardiac index in a patient is 6.5 and decreases to 4 with restoration of normal systemic vascular resistance and perfusion pressure by α-adrenergic support, should the physician be satisfied with a cardiac index of 4 l/min/m², or should further inotropic support be used to increase the cardiac index to 6.5 l/min/m²? Should the physician attempt an even greater level of support to maintain a more hyperdynamic state? At present, this decision may be based on the effects that these levels of oxygen delivery, as dictated by cardiac output, have on oxygen consumption. For example, if oxygen consumption remains the same at a cardiac index of 4 l/min/m² as it does at 6.5 l/min/m², the cardiac index of 4 l/min/m² is considered sufficient. If oxygen consumption instead decreases, consideration may be given to the use of an inotrope to increase oxygen delivery and oxygen consumption.

CLINICAL PRINCIPLES OF OXYGEN UTILIZATION

Clinical manipulation of oxygen utilization as targeted in Figure 12–3 is based on several principles. First, oxygen consumption and oxygen extraction are dependent on oxygen delivery. Oxygen delivery has three components: (1) hemoglobin concentration, (2) percentage of hemoglobin oxygen saturation and to a much lesser extent dissolved plasma oxygen, and (3) cardiac output. This is evident in the equation, $D_{O_2} = CO \times (1.36 \times \% \, Hb \times \% \, O_2 \, sat + Pa_{O_2} \times 0.0003)$. Oxygenation is made optimal in the patient through the use of supplemental oxygen as well as mechanical ventilation and PEEP. The well-known hemoglobin O_2 association-dissociation saturation curve illustrates that saturation is dependent on P_{O_2} in a nonlinear fashion. This relationship is under the control of the Bohr effect, which states that temperature, pH, and 2,3-diphosphoglycerate levels all affect the level of P_{O_2} at which oxygen associates and dissociates with hemoglobin. In the critically ill child, measured oxygen saturation is necessary for accurate evaluation of oxygen content. As a therapeutic goal, oxygen saturation rather than P_{O_2} should be targeted. A saturation of 95% or higher should be attained if clinically reasonable. Hemoglobin concentration has become an important topic in medicine with more sophisticated understanding of blood-borne viruses. The recent National Institutes of Health consensus conference suggested that hemoglobin concentrations of less than 10 g/dl are acceptable in patients without cardiopulmonary compromise. Two groups have recently investigated the role of hemoglobin transfusion in children with septic shock, with conflicting results. One group found that packed red blood cell transfusions increased hemoglobin, oxygen delivery, and oxygen consumption.[26] The other group demonstrated no increase in oxygen consumption in their population.[27] However, this latter population was not tested to determine whether other maneuvers that increased oxygen delivery, such as administration of inotropic agents, increased oxygen consumption. Therefore, it is unknown whether the oxygen requirement had already been met in these children. Until further data are available, hemoglobin concentration may be maintained at the level considered acceptable in cardiopulmonary compromise, which according to most opinions is 10 g/dl or higher. After attaining these O_2 content goals, cardiac output becomes the primary determinant of oxygen delivery.

The relationship between oxygen consumption and oxygen delivery is illustrated in Figure 12-1. Oxygen consumption at very low levels of oxygen delivery is maintained with maximal extraction. This is limited by the fact that when the oxygen saturation of hemoglobin is 20%, no further oxygen can be extracted by the mitochondrial apparatus. Therefore, maximum extraction is in the range of somewhat less than 80%. As delivery is increased, consumption increases with decreasing O_2 extraction until a "critical point" of oxygen delivery is attained. It is assumed that this represents the delivery at which the patient's oxygen requirements are satisfied. At oxygen delivery greater than this level, oxygen consumption is unchanged and oxygen extraction decreases proportionately. It has been proposed that hypermetabolism, mitochondrial dysfunction, and vasomotor shunting alter this relationship in sepsis. Depending on the degree of perturbation, the patient may have

mild effects manifested as an inability to maximally extract up to 80% oxygen during the low-flow state and an increased critical point of oxygen delivery, or more severe effects may be present, manifested as a flow-dependent state in which increased oxygen extraction is unattainable to any meaningful degree and the predicted critical point of oxygen delivery is beyond attainability within meaningful clinical parameters (Fig. 12-6).

When one clinically manipulates oxygen utilization variables, it is important that increased oxygen consumption is indicative of a satisfaction of oxygen debt rather than a satisfaction of artifactually elevated oxygen requirements. For example, fever, tachycardia, and catecholamines can all increase oxygen consumption in animals and normal humans. In addition, as previously described, increased oxygen consumption may occur in skeletal muscle rather than in vital organs, depending on the therapeutic modality. In adult studies, serum lactate levels and metabolic acidosis have been correlated with oxygen debt, which has been corrected when therapy has increased oxygen delivery and consumption.[28, 29] A similar study remains to be done in children. However, the previously mentioned correlation of serum pH to outcome suggests that these parameters are useful until more sophisticated measures of tissue oxygen debt are devised. At present, three factors can be most reliable in guiding the physician to a rational use of therapies that increase oxygen delivery: (1) identification of the critical oxygen delivery point, (2) elimination of metabolic acidosis, and (3) prevention of pharmacologically induced clinically significant tachycardia. This approach provides the physician some guidelines for rational therapy in cardiovascular and oxygen utilization management during pediatric septic shock.

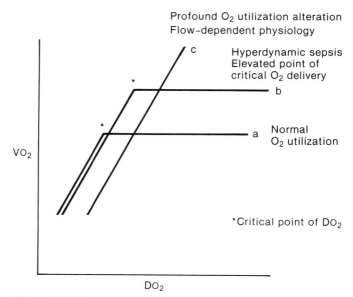

Figure 12-6. Degrees of abnormal O_2 utilization in sepsis. Graphic representation of alterations in oxygen utilization physiology. Depending on stage of pathophysiology, sepsis may result in a hyperutilization state (b) with increased oxygen utilization and intact O_2 extraction, or in the pathologic flow-dependent state in which increased extraction is nonexistent (c).

INOTROPES, VASODILATORS, AND VASOPRESSORS FOR MANIPULATION OF CARDIOVASCULAR AND OXYGEN UTILIZATION PARAMETERS DURING EARLY SEPSIS AND SEPTIC SHOCK

At present, there is no consensus on which particular inotropes, vasopressors, or vasodilators are most useful in attaining therapeutic goals during sepsis. Table 12–8 illustrates some of the more commonly used agents. Phenylephrine and norepinephrine are classically used for their predominant α-adrenergic effects, whereas dobutamine and isoproterenol may be used as predominant β-adrenergic agonists. Mixed agents, including dopamine and epinephrine, both of which are predominant β-agonists at lower doses and α-agonists at higher doses, may have expanded utility. Afterload reducing agents such as nitroprusside, nitroglycerin, and phentolamine are also available. Nitroprusside, a predominant systemic arterial vasodilator, and nitroglycerin, a predominant pulmonary artery vasodilator, can be used in combination to reduce vascular resistance in sepsis during predominant cardiac dysfunction and increased vascular tone.

These pharmacotherapeutic agents may be used in combination for varied effects. For example, phentolamine or low-dose dopamine has been advocated in combination with norepinephrine. Through α-adrenergic blockade, the former regimen allows the β-adrenergic component of norepinephrine to become predominant and transforms its function from a potent vasopressor to a potent inotrope. The latter regimen allows predominant α-agonist–mediated systemic vasoconstriction to occur while promoting renal artery dilatation and protection of renal function through dopaminergic-receptor stimulation. Nitroprusside can similarly be used in combination with norepinephrine, epinephrine, or dopamine, offsetting α-adrenergic–mediated arterial vasoconstriction with nitrate-mediated dilatation. This allows the direct contractile effect of epinephrine or dopamine to promote cardiac output without significantly increased afterload. Other goals may be attained with a combination of predominant β-agonists and phenylephrine. Dobutamine and isoproter-

enol have mild systemic vasodilating effects, isoproterenol through β_2-adrenergic stimulation and dobutamine as a result of its α_2-racemate. Phenylephrine may be titrated to allow these cardiotonic drugs to improve cardiac output without decreasing systemic vascular resistance. The corollary of this approach is the addition of dobutamine or isoproterenol to provide inotropic support and improve cardiac function when pure α agents are being used. For example, when systemic vascular resistance is being maintained with phenylephrine, a β-adrenergic agent can be added to improve cardiac output.

The use of vasopressors, inotropes, and vasodilating agents to manipulate cardiac index, systemic vascular resistance, and oxygen delivery and to attain normal perfusion pressure and oxygen consumption is illustrated in Figure 12–7 in children in early and middle stages of septic shock. Figure 12–7A shows three patients in whom increased α-adrenergic agonist stimulation was employed to increase systemic vascular resistance. This led to a disproportionate decrease in cardiac index in all three children, as predicted by Figure 12–4B. The decrease in oxygen delivery was so significant that despite increased oxygen extraction in the second patient, oxygen consumption was decreased in all three patients. Furthermore, this adverse effect on cardiac function was such that perfusion pressure actually decreased in the second patient despite increased systemic vascular resistance. The corollary to this phenomenon is seen in Figure 12–7B. In these children, α-agonist stimulation was removed and replaced with β-agonist stimulation, causing a significant increase in cardiac index but a concomitant decrease in systemic vascular resistance. This resulted in a marked increase in oxygen delivery and oxygen consumption.

Figure 12–7C represents two patients in whom the use of combined α- and β-adrenergic stimulation led to an increase in cardiac index and maintenance of systemic vascular resistance. This resulted in increased perfusion pressure. Since oxygen delivery was similarly increased, the first patient had increased oxygen consumption as well. The second patient had decreased oxygen extraction and showed no increase in oxygen consumption despite increased oxygen delivery. This patient, it appears, had already reached the point of critical oxygen

Table 12–8. PHARMACOTHERAPEUTIC AGENTS COMMONLY USED TO MODERATE CARDIAC INDEX, SYSTEMIC VASCULAR RESISTANCE INDEX, MEAN ARTERIAL PRESSURE, OXYGEN CONSUMPTION, AND OXYGEN DELIVERY

Dopamine	Excellent first-line choice, 0–3 μg/kg/min dopaminergic, 3–10 μg/kg/min β, >10 μg/kg/min α
Epinephrine	Excellent choice in patients who are unresponsive to dopamine at 0.01–0.05 μg/kg/min β, >0.05 μg/kg/min increasing α effect
Dobutamine	Excellent β-agonist with minimal tachycardia; may widen pulse pressure at concentration >10 μg/kg/min
Isoproterenol	Excellent β_1- and β_2-agonist; helpful during pulmonary hypertension; may increase pulmonary shunting; use 0.01–1 μg/kg/min
Norepinephrine	Excellent α-agonist with β-agonist activity that is frequently inapparent; use 0.05–1 μg/kg/min
Phenylephrine	Partial α-agonist; excellent combination agent with β-agonists
Norepinephrine and Phentolamine	This combination allows β-agonist activity to be manifested through α-blockade; begin phentolamine at 1 μg/kg/min in advance according to outcome variable
Nitroglycerin	Excellent vasodilator; 1–3 μg/kg/min pulmonary vasodilator, >3 μg/kg/min systemic vasodilator
Nitroprusside	Premiere afterload reducing agent; frequently requires simultaneous administration of volume bolus; long-term use may be associated with cyanide toxicity

Higher concentrations of all agents may be used according to measured variables.

Text continued on page 136

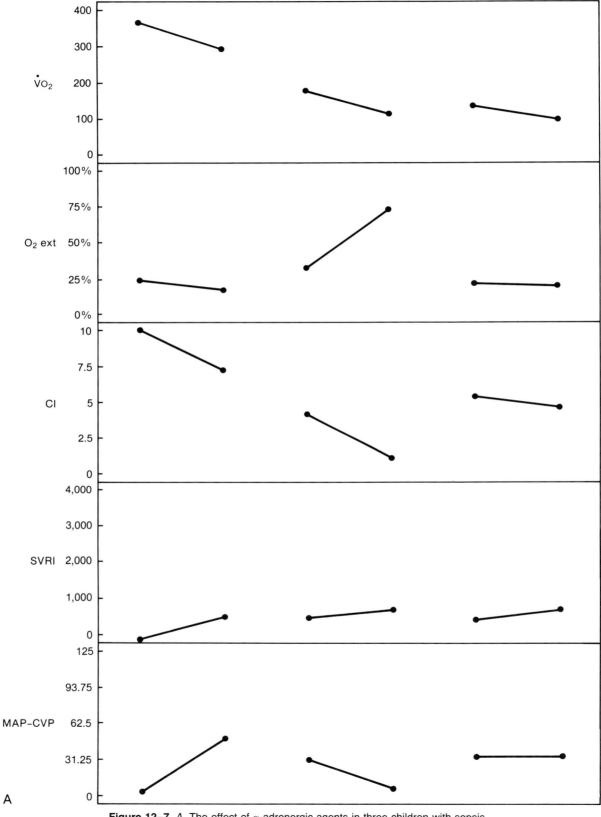

Figure 12–7. *A,* The effect of α-adrenergic agents in three children with sepsis.

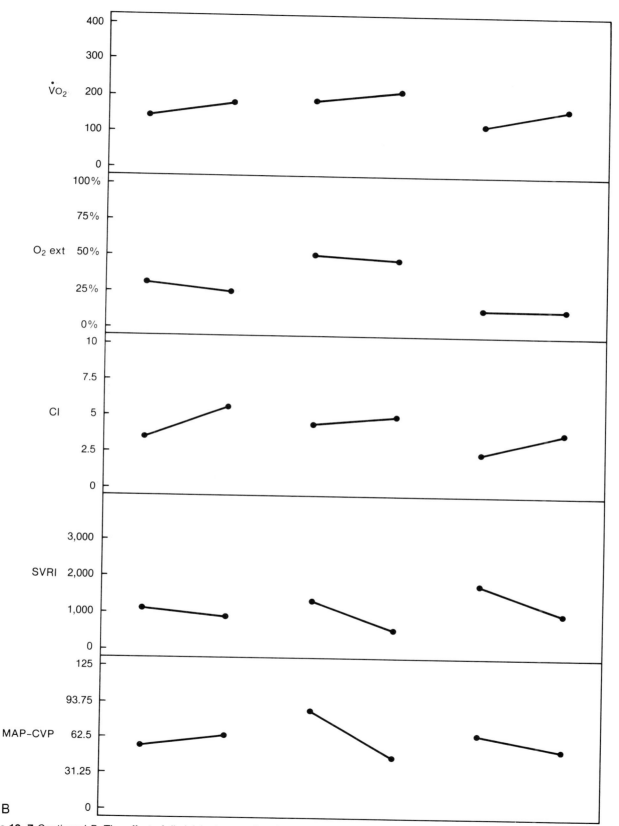

Figure 12–7 *Continued B,* The effect of diminished α-agonist stimulation and increased β-agonist stimulation in three children with sepsis.

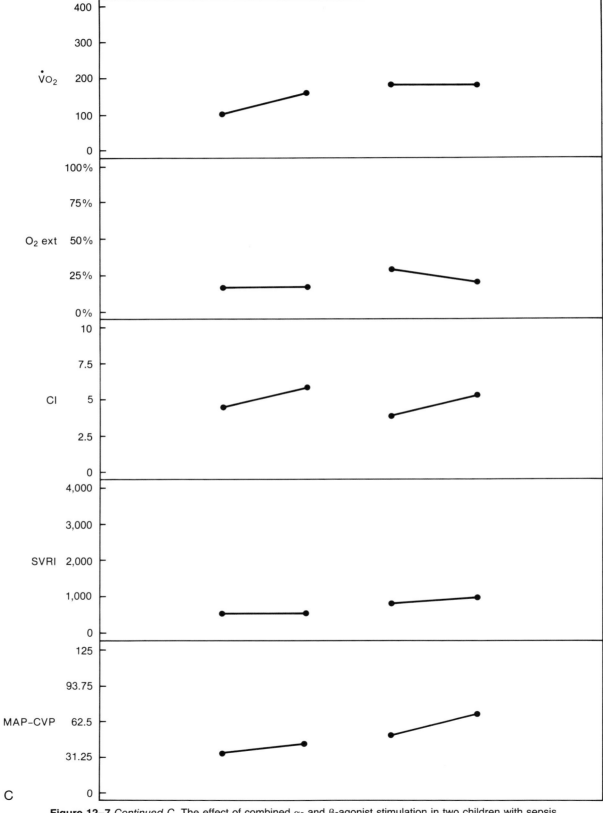

Figure 12–7 *Continued C,* The effect of combined α- and β-agonist stimulation in two children with sepsis.

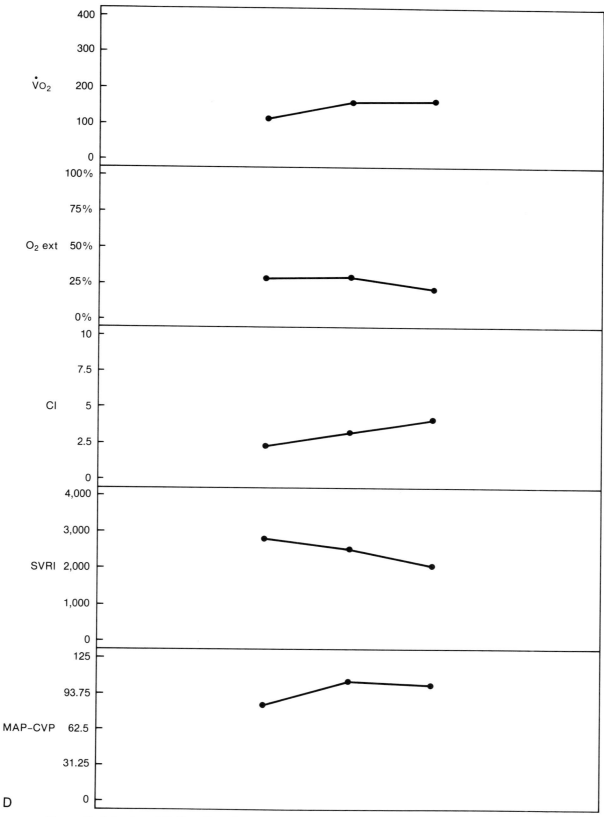

Figure 12–7 *Continued D,* The effect of β-agonist stimulation and afterload reduction in a child with sepsis.

delivery, suggesting no further increase in cardiac index was required. This ability to reach the point of critical oxygen delivery is further illustrated by Figure 12–7D. This patient presented with cardiac dysfunction and flow dependence but elevated systemic vascular resistance. The use of β-agonists and afterload reduction in this patient resulted in increased cardiac index, decreased systemic vascular resistance, and improved perfusion pressure. With this increase in oxygen delivery, oxygen consumption increased from the subnormal to the normal range and then reached a plateau. Thus, perfusion pressure in this patient was maintained at the point of critical oxygen delivery. In the latter two cases, no further manipulation of oxygen delivery was necessary when the critical O_2 delivery point was met.

Re-evaluation of the effects of combinations of vasoactive and cardiotonic drugs on oxygen utilization and the cardiovascular state should occur at intervals throughout the early and middle stages of septic shock. Observation of decreasing α-adrenergic or β-adrenergic responsiveness presages a worsening prognosis, whereas decreasing requirements for support suggest recovery. When cardiovascular stabilization is attainable, other areas of multiple organ system failure take on increasing significance.

RESPIRATORY MANAGEMENT AND ADULT RESPIRATORY DISTRESS SYNDROME, IN THE EARLY AND MIDDLE STAGES OF SEPSIS AND SEPTIC SHOCK

As many as 80% of critically ill children with septic shock are intubated and started on mechanical ventilation within 24 hours of admission.[19] Indications include hypoxia, hypercarbia, metabolic acidosis, increased work of breathing, and the use of neuromuscular blockade for central line placement. Forty per cent of children have the criteria of ARDS, including alveolar infiltrates, a PO_2 of less than 60 mm Hg on room air, and pulmonary artery occlusion pressure less than or equal to 15 mm Hg.[30] This process is thought to be mediated in part by white blood cell–induced autoinjury, macrophage-released mediators, complement, ischemia, and endotoxin. The clinical result is increased capillary permeability with alveolar collapse, increased extravascular lung water, and decreased lung compliance. In children with heart failure, work of breathing can require as much as 25% of oxygen consumption. Extrapolating a similar effect of cardiac dysfunction and increased work of breathing to ARDS in sepsis, it has generally been recommended that early intubation and ventilation be instituted to allow for optimal oxygen metabolism in other vital organs.

The hallmark of respiratory management of ARDS during mechanical ventilation is the significant requirement for PEEP. ARDS is predominantly a disease of significantly reduced functional residual capacity (FRC). PEEP allows recruitment of alveoli, restoring FRC with beneficial cardiopulmonary effects. Increasing FRC results in improved lung compliance and work of breathing for a given minute ventilation. Increasing FRC can also have an ameliorating effect on increased pulmonary vascular resistance. This is in part due to anatomic considerations, but most significantly it is related to decreased hypoxia-mediated vasoconstriction. Since increased pulmonary vascular resistance, pulmonary hypertension, and right ventricular dysfunction are hallmarks of sepsis, the salutary cardiopulmonary effect is especially significant. Hypoxia is reversed by PEEP through alveolar effects. FRC is more crucial to oxygenation than ventilation because O_2 diffuses more slowly than CO_2. PEEP allows continued oxygen diffusion in alveoli that were previously collapsed. PEEP can therefore improve oxygenation, compliance, work of breathing, pulmonary vascular resistance, and right heart function.

Adverse cardiopulmonary interactions can also occur with PEEP. In order to increase FRC, PEEP increases intrathoracic pressure. This can decrease venous return and ventricular filling, resulting in diminished cardiac output. At higher levels of PEEP, generally in excess of 20 mm Hg in adults, it has been reported that PEEP can increase right ventricular afterload as well. This results in right ventricular dilatation, septal deviation, decreased left ventricular filling, and decreased cardiac output. Increased systemic venous pressure is required to overcome intrathoracic pressure and improve ventricular filling. This can be achieved in part through volume loading and vasoactive agents that improve vascular tone and venous return.

The therapeutic goal of PEEP in sepsis-induced ARDS is to attain optimal oxygen delivery with nontoxic oxygen administration. This goal is attained by therapeutic manipulations of oxygen content and cardiac output. Since FiO_2 concentrations greater than 60% are considered to contribute to pulmonary toxicity, the clinician increases PEEP to maintain optimal oxygen (95% saturation) when an FiO_2 greater than 0.6 is required. As PEEP levels increase to greater than 12 cm H_2O, increased intrathoracic pressure can lead to decreased cardiac output, as well as an increased risk of pneumothorax. Initially, high FiO_2 is relatively more tolerated, as irreversible lung damage has been documented after only 24 hours of 100% oxygen administration. However, over time, PEEP must be increased to allow adequate oxygenation within acceptable FiO_2 levels. If increased PEEP adversely affects oxygen delivery, additional therapeutic maneuvers must be employed.

Figure 12–8 illustrates the scenario in a child with *Candida* sepsis, ARDS, and "PEEP toxicity." In this case, the increase in PEEP from 18 to 20 cm H_2O allowed optimal oxygenation at 0.6% FiO_2 but resulted in a significant decrease in oxygen delivery, cardiac index, and oxygen consumption. Volume resuscitation to improve venous return (the best, first therapeutic maneuver) and the addition of vasoactive agents to increase cardiac output resulted in improved oxygen delivery and consumption. In the child in Figure 12–8D during the use of super-PEEP (PEEP > 20 cm H_2O), the addition of an α-adrenergic agonist, as well as continued inotropic support, led to increased oxygen

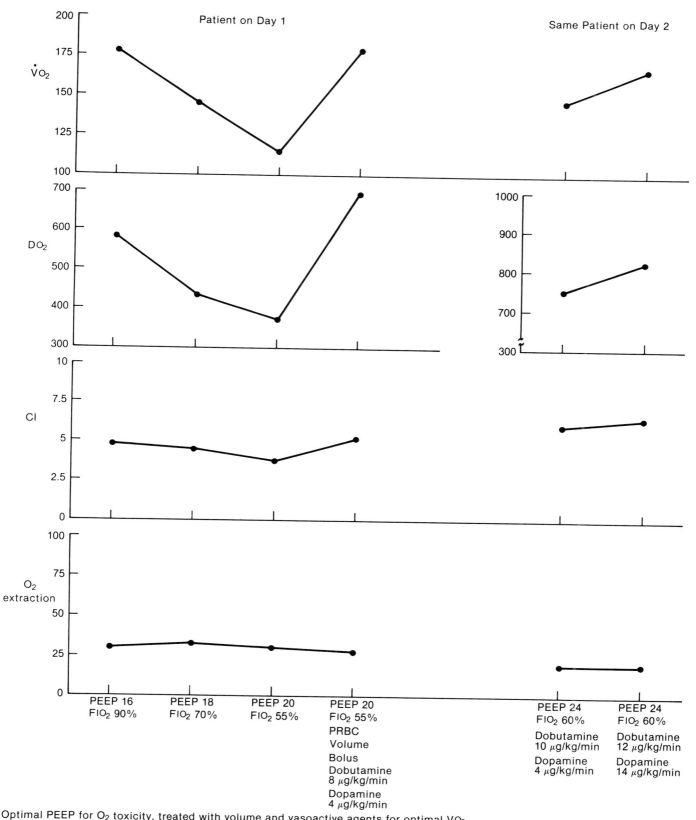

Optimal PEEP for O₂ toxicity, treated with volume and vasoactive agents for optimal VO₂
Super PEEP for O₂ toxicity requires vasopressor to improve venous return, VO₂, DO₂, and CI

Figure 12–8. PEEP and flow-dependent oxygen consumption during *Candida* ARDS.

delivery and consumption. This volume-pressor approach can be repeated periodically during the early and middle stages of sepsis.

Once adequate cardiac output is established, fluid management in children with ARDS and sepsis becomes one of delicate balance. Increased capillary permeability results in increased extra lung water for any given filling pressure. This, in turn, can lead to increased PEEP requirements. On the basis of this principle, it has been recommended that oxygen delivery be maintained at the lowest filling pressure possible. When volume is required to maintain cardiac output because of decreased systemic venous return, packed red blood cells have been theoretically advocated over crystalloid solutions because oncotic forces partially offset the hydrostatic effect of volume infusion. Other colloids such as albumin may have no long-term benefit, as eventual leaking into interstitial spaces may potentiate the pathophysiologic process. Others have proposed the use of small-volume boluses of salt-poor albumin or hyperoncotic colloid solution with furosemide. This approach has a theoretic advantage of increased filling and oncotic pressures with a minimal increase in total body water. The confounding variable in attaining minimal filling pressures while maintaining optimal oxygen delivery is the unreliability of the pulmonary artery occlusion pressure readings with the administration of PEEP. Transmitted transmural pressure may be partly distinguished from the true pulmonary artery occlusion pressure by placing an esophageal pressure transducer and subtracting its reading from the pulmonary artery occlusion pressure. However, this method assumes 100% transmission of transmural pressure, an incorrect assumption. Therefore, the physician has, at best, an estimated pulmonary artery occlusion pressure with which to determine volume status. The use of diuretics in the hemodynamically stable patient with ARDS can result in decreased PEEP requirements, increased lung compliance, and improved oxygenation. This can be attained with decreased extravascular lung water. The cardiovascular management of ARDS requires continuous attention, as capillary permeability, fluid shifts, and cardiovascular function evolve.

MANAGEMENT OF RENAL FUNCTION IN SEPTIC SHOCK

Preservation of renal function is crucial to the management of cardiopulmonary and metabolic homeostasis in the early and middle stages of septic shock. Renal function may be preserved with adequate maintenance of renal blood flow. This can be facilitated with measures that increase cardiac output as well as regional perfusion. Low-dose dopamine has been shown to increase renal blood flow and preserve renal function in studies in animals and adults when used as a primary inotrope, as well as when used as a dopaminergic agent during norepinephrine infusion. The use of furosemide and mannitol with volume expansion has similarly been proposed to prevent or attenuate renal failure when initiated before an insult secondary to shock, or when α-adrenergic–mediated vasoconstriction occurs. On the basis of these observations, low-dose dopamine with or without furosemide and mannitol may be used during the early and middle stages of septic shock to preserve urine output. More aggressive regimens are required in children in whom cardiovascular and renal resuscitation is unsuccessful in preventing oliguria or anuria. Diuretics are the first line of therapy. The loop diuretics furosemide or the more potent bumetanide may be employed to promote urine output. When unsuccessful, these therapies may be repeated 20 minutes after administering a bolus of a hyperoncotic volume expander such as salt-poor albumin or mannitol. These expanders presumably increase renal blood flow by oncotically drawing interstitial water into the intravascular space with a minimal administered volume. If this regimen is successful, attention to hyperosmolar effects of repeated mannitol administration or the eventual reverse osmotic effects of salt-poor albumin in the interstitial space, or both, must be carefully monitored and considered. The distal loop diuretic metolazone may act synergistically with furosemide or bumetanide.

Unlike in other conditions, volume restriction is not the hallmark of therapy for acute renal failure during the early and middle stages of septic shock. This strategy is unsuccessful because significant capillary leaking leads to worsening intravascular hypovolemia and decreased renal blood flow. In addition, worsening total body fluid overload does not present as hypertension but rather as overwhelming interstitial edema and third spacing. This results in increased PEEP requirements that eventually lead to decreased cardiac output and renal blood flow. For these reasons, indications for dialysis or filtration in children with sepsis and the capillary leak syndrome should include not only hyperkalemia, a blood urea nitrogen value greater than 100 mg/dl, and refractory metabolic acidosis but also anuria or significant oliguria that is unresponsive to diuretic therapy.

Peritoneal dialysis provides therapy rapidly and safely. In one study, it was reported that two children underwent bedside placement of a Tenckhoff peritoneal dialysis catheter for anuria and increased PEEP requirements within 8 hours of admission for septic shock.[19] Both children survived, with return of spontaneous renal function within 72 hours. Peritoneal dialysis cannot be used when an adequate peritoneal space or intact bowel is lacking. Continuous arteriovenous hemofiltration or dialysis provides a rapid and safe bedside technique for removing volume or correcting acidosis during anuria or significant oliguria. In this method, functioning intraarterial and intravenous catheters are connected in line with a filter and a bedside pump. The only disadvantage to this technique is the potential lack of adequate vascular access during septic shock. This approach, however, may prevent the need for hemodialysis with its known cardiovascular side effects.

MANAGEMENT OF METABOLIC DERANGEMENTS IN THE EARLY AND MIDDLE STAGES OF SEPTIC SHOCK

Disseminated Intravascular Coagulation

Alteration of the coagulation cascade is common in children during septic shock. It is believed that LPS activates the Hageman factor as well as various proteases, leading to hypofibrinogenemia, thrombocytopenia, reduced concentrations of Factors II, V, and VIII, and resultant prothrombin time and partial thromboplastin time prolongation. In addition, thrombocytopenia has been reported in 57 to 77% of children during septicemia.[31] Studies in pediatrics have suggested that restoration of perfusion can improve these parameters.[32] However, component replacement remains the hallmark of therapy during sepsis and septic shock. During the consumptive process, maintenance of normal prothrombin time and partial thromboplastin time, fibrinogen levels, and a platelet count between 40,000 and 100,000/mm^3 are the goals.

Fresh frozen plasma (FFP) can be most beneficial during the early stages of septic shock. It not only allows correction of deficient factor levels but also provides an ideal volume resuscitation fluid. One may consider transfusing a unit of cryoprecipitate for every 2 to 3 units of FFP given. This blood product is rich in fibrinogen and Factor VIII. An additional potential benefit is its high content of fibronectin. This α_2-glycoprotein, an opsonin that can increase phagocytosis in the reticuloendothelial system, is markedly decreased in adult sepsis. Replacement with cryoprecipitate has been shown to correlate with an increased survival of 77 versus 42% during sepsis in adult studies.[33] Platelet transfusions may be given with or without FFP as necessary.

Electrolyte Abnormalities

Hypocalcemia, hypophosphatemia, and metabolic acidosis are all common during septic shock. Since hypocalcemia has been correlated with decreased cardiac output in adults, it is generally recommended that low ionized serum calcium levels be corrected. Hypophosphatemia is similarly important, as phosphate is crucial to cardiac, diaphragmatic, and mitochondrial function. According to new American Heart Association APLS guidelines, metabolic acidosis should be treated initially with respiratory alkalosis induced by hyperventilation, as the primary use of sodium bicarbonate may correct metabolic acidosis but actually decrease tissue pH. Once adequate ventilation is assured, bicarbonate may be used according to clinical judgment. When acidosis is due to renal failure or serum bicarbonate levels less than 12 mEq/l, the use of sodium bicarbonate remains the treatment of choice.

Hyperglycemia and Hypoglycemia

Hyperglycemia or hypoglycemia may be present in children during early sepsis. Hyperglycemia is thought to be in part the result of glycogenolysis and gluconeogenesis secondary to elevated levels of hormones, including catecholamines and glucagon. This hyperglycemic state is also accompanied by insulin resistance. In a study of septic adults, Weisul and colleagues identified a group of patients whose presenting state was hypodynamic in which insulin levels were diminished when compared with those of patients in a normodynamic state. Using a glucose, insulin, and potassium infusion, these authors were able to demonstrate improved cardiac output in this hypodynamic group of patients.[34] This remains the only study to suggest a potential efficacy for the treatment of hyperglycemia. When hyperglycemia is associated with glycosuria, metabolic acidosis, or decreased cardiac output, the physician may consider the use of insulin. Hypoglycemia may result from the depletion of glycogen stores, decreased muscle mass, or inhibition of hepatic gluconeogenesis. Hypoglycemia always requires immediate correction. For this reason, many clinicians suggest the use of 10% glucose solution with appropriate electrolytes for maintenance of fluids in sepsis.

Nutrition

Surprisingly little work has been done on the important subject of nutrition in children during sepsis. In addition to the previously mentioned alterations in glucose utilization, lipid and protein metabolism is also altered. Catecholamines and glucagon-induced lipolysis lead to triglyceridemia, as well as increased fatty acid production. Fatty acid utilization is impaired by cachectin (TNF)-induced inhibition of lipoprotein lipase. The lack of energy substrates is complemented by hyperutilization of branched-chain amino acids from skeletal muscle. The significance of this process in children, who have little muscle mass, is not known, but it has been shown that adults who survive sepsis have a higher level of branched-chain amino acids than do nonsurvivors.

In the early stages of sepsis, it is prudent to monitor closely for hypoglycemia. Once resuscitation has been attained and maintenance fluids have been established, it is reasonable to provide proper energy substrates, including carbohydrates, lipids, and proteins. Until studies are performed, it is reasonable to use maintenance calories for growth in children, assuring the presence of branched-chain amino acids in the protein source. This number of calories is in excess of that required for basal metabolic rates and presumably will be sufficient to meet the hypermetabolic needs in sepsis. While administering nutrition, careful monitoring of glucose and triglyceride levels should continue.

MANAGEMENT OF THE THROMBOTIC COMPLICATIONS OF SEPTIC SHOCK

During the middle stage of sepsis, children may exhibit decreased perfusion and early autoinfarction of the peripheral extremities. This is noted particularly in children with purpura fulminans. It is thought to be secondary to decreased perfusion during shock, as well as to thrombosis. Girardin and associates recently showed that high levels of TNF occur in children with purpura fulminans.[35] This monokine is known to elicit endothelial damage, as well as increased thrombosis. Several reports have used heparin to treat the malady with varied success.[36, 37] At present, there are no reports of the use of local thrombolytic or vasodilating agents. Unfortunately, this malady can result in above-the-knee and above-the-elbow amputations.

ALTERNATIVE THERAPIES

Alternative therapies in sepsis and septic shock have been directed at interrupting the pathophysiologic process and have evolved as the biochemical understanding of the host's response to systemic infection has increased. Corticosteroids have been the most commonly used therapy in intensive care. Steroids are thought to mediate several potentially beneficial effects, including cell membrane and lysosomal stabilization, inhibition of the phospholipase A_2–mediated arachidonic acid cascade, inhibition of complement-activated granulocyte aggregation and oxygen radical release, and macrophage-released TNF production. Clinical studies showed that 30 mg/kg of methylprednisone significantly decreased alveolocapillary permeability when given early in adult septic shock.[38] Furthermore, in another adult study, the use of 30 mg/kg of methylprednisone or 3 mg/kg of dexamethasone early in septic shock resulted in a 10.4% (9 of 86 patients) mortality rate versus a 38.4% (33 of 86 patients) mortality rate in saline-matched controls with a P value of less than 0.001.[39, 40] Since this time, two adult clinical studies have shown no beneficial effect when steroids were used.[41, 42] The most recent study, in fact, has shown deleterious effects, including increased risk of secondary infection. At this high dose, steroids are not indicated in adult septic shock. The pertinence of these findings to pediatric intensive care remains unclear. For example, children, particularly those with purpura fulminans, frequently experience adrenal necrosis. Unfortunately, few data are available as to the role of adrenal function and cortisol levels in pediatric septic shock. At present, the use or nonuse of steroids in children remains a clinical judgment until pediatric studies are completed. Various other agents that inhibit biochemical cascades include prostaglandin synthetase inhibitors, phospholipase A_2 inhibitors, opiate antagonists, and oxygen free radical scavengers. All of these agents have been shown to have some efficacy in animal models but their efficacy has yet to be corroborated in the clinical setting.

Another approach to sepsis is the use of antibody technology. Ziegler and colleagues studied core LPS–lipid A complex human antiserum and showed efficacy in adult clinical trials. Therapy with J-5 antiserum decreased mortality during profound shock from 76% (26 of 34 patients) to 46% (17 of 37 patients) with a P value equal to 0.009.[43] More recently, investigations have shown that the HA-1A human monoclonal IgM antibody, which binds to the lipid A portion of endotoxin, accomplished similar results during gram-negative bacteremia and shock in adults. In this study, there were 27 deaths among the 47 recipients of placebo (57%) and 18 deaths among the 54 patients who received antibody (33%) with a P value equal to 0.0017. Trials in children are ongoing.[44] The use of C5A and TNF antibodies has shown dramatic improvement in survival in pretreated animal models of endotoxin-mediated shock.[45, 46] Since this technology has its greatest potential benefit before infection begins with bacteremia and endotoxemia, it may be most beneficial as a prophylactic therapy in children at risk for nosocomial sepsis. A final approach has been the use of extracorporeal filtration, pheresis, and perfusion technology. The collaborative adult studies of extracorporeal membrane oxygenation in sepsis have not been promising. However, analysis of neonatal data from extracorporeal membrane oxygenation studies has not compared outcome in sepsis with and without this therapy. The use of hemofiltration to remove circulating myocardial depressant factors, TNF, and proteases (all of which have a kilodalton less than the filter pore size of the hemofilter) has been considered on the basis of a canine study, which showed improved cardiovascular function with hemofiltration during sepsis.[47] Similarly, animal studies using charcoal hemoperfusion to absorb LPS or remove complement have shown benefit, and its use has also been reported in adults and children. The use of whole blood exchange has efficacy in neonates.[48] However, studies took place before the discovery of the human immunodeficiency virus and therefore have not been repeated in children. At present, these potentially promising methods have not undergone clinical evaluation.

CONCLUSION

Outcome in pediatric septic shock has improved dramatically with advanced pediatric life support techniques and intensive care. This remarkable accomplishment remains shadowed by the prevalence of the process in critically ill children. The incidence is high enough to be a significant contributor to morbidity and mortality in the pediatric intensive care arena but too low for any one university to study in an effective manner over a reasonable period. A similar dilemma prompted pediatric oncologists to develop the highly productive Children's Cancer Study Group in the 1970s. National or multinational collaborative group studies will be necessary to allow the advances of biochemical and molecular technologies to contribute to the advance of intensive care technology.

The biases of this chapter are that among children with sepsis and septic shock, there may be subgroups that require identification in order to ascertain expected mortalities and optimal therapies. The classification of these groups might be dependent on the degree of immunocompromise, ability to eradicate infection, baseline organ function or dysfunction, and period of ischemia before resuscitation.[49] The time-honored approach of applying adult studies to pediatric therapy is not optimal.

With a uniform approach to prevention, early recognition, and therapeutic goals in a large cohort of pediatric patients, it will be possible to assess the remaining important questions: (1) To what degree can prevention with prophylactic measures decrease the incidence of septic shock in patients at risk for nosocomial infection? (2) To what degree can early recognition and aggressive resuscitation prevent morbidity and mortality in outpatient sepsis? and (3) To what degree can new therapies affect outcome once septic shock has occurred? Until this time, using the principles outlined in this chapter, we can be excited by our ability to dramatically improve survival in this previously uniformly fatal disease process.

References

1. Dupont HL and Spink WW: Infections due to gram-negative organisms: An analysis of 860 patients with bacteremia at the University of Minnesota Medical Center, 1958–1966. Medicine 48:507, 1969.
2. Naqvi JH, Chundu KR, and Friedman AD: Shock in children with gram negative bacillary sepsis and *Haemophilus influenzae* type B sepsis. Pediatr Infect Dis 5(5):512, 1986.
3. Michalik JM, Moore RN, McGhee JR, et al: The primary role of lymphoreticular cells in the mediation of host responses to bacterial endotoxin. J Infect Dis 141:55, 1980.
4. Tracey WJ, Beutler B, Lowry SF, et al: Shock and tissue injury induced by recombinant human cachectin. Science 23:470, 1986.
5. Dinarello CA, Okusawa S, and Gelfand JA: IL-1 induces a shock like state in rabbits. *In:* Roth BL, Nielsen TB, and McKee AE (eds): Progress in Clinical and Biological Research, Vol 286. Molecular and Cellular Mechanisms of Septic Shock. New York, Alan R Liss, 1988, pp 243–263.
6. Zimmerman JJ and Dietrich KA: Current prospectives on septic shock. *In:* Orlowski JP (ed): Pediatric Clinics of North America, Vol 34, No 1. Philadelphia, WB Saunders, 1987 pp. 131–163.
7. Siegel JH, Greenspan M, and Del Guercio LRM: Abnormal vascular tone, defective oxygen transport, and myocardial failure in human septic shock. Ann Surg 165:504, 1967.
8. Shoemaker WC: Circulatory mechanisms of shock and their mediators. Crit Care Med 15:787, 1987.
9. Bihari MA, Smithics M, Gimson A, et al: The effects of vasodilation with prostacyclin on oxygen delivery and uptake in critically ill patients. N Engl J Med 317:399, 1987.
10. Shoemaker WC: Shock states: Pathophysiology, monitoring, outcome prediction, and therapy. *In:* Shoemaker WC, Ayres S, Grenvik A, et al (eds): Textbook of Critical Care, 2nd ed. Philadelphia, WB Saunders, 1989, pp. 977–993.
11. Klein BS, Perloff WH, and Maki DG: Reduction of nosocomial infection during pediatric intensive care by protective isolation. N Engl J Med 320:171, 1989.
12. Persico M, Barker GA, and Mitchell DP: Purulent otitis media—a "silent" source of sepsis in the pediatric intensive care unit. Otolaryngol Head Neck Surg 93:330, 1985.
13. Zucker A, Pollack M, and Katz K: Blind use of the double lumen plugged catheter for diagnosis of respiratory tract infections in critical ill children. Crit Care Med 12:867, 1984.
14. Ellman H: Capillary permeability in septic patients. Crit Care Med 12:629, 1984.
15. Parillo JE: Septic shock in humans: Clinical evaluation, pathogenesis, and therapeutic approach. *In:* Shoemaker WC, Ayres S, Grenvik A, et al (eds): Textbook of Critical Care Medicine, 2nd ed. Philadelphia, WB Saunders, 1989, pp. 1006–1024.
16. Carroll GC and Snyder JV: Hyperdynamic severe intravascular sepsis depends on fluid administration in cynomolgus monkeys. Am J Phys 243:R131, 1982.
17. Kaufman BS, Rackow FC, and Falk JC: The relationship between oxygen delivery and consumption during fluid resuscitation of hypovolemic and septic shock. Chest 85(3):336, 1984.
18. Hussain SNA, Rutledge F, Roussos C, et al: Effects of norepi-
nephrine and fluid administration on the selective blood flow distribution in endotoxic shock. JCC 3(1):32, 1988.
19. Carcillo JA, Davis AI, and Zaritsky A: Role of early fluid resuscitation in pediatric septic shock. JAMA 226:1242, 1991.
20. Marcier JC, Beaufils F, Hartmann JF, et al: Hemodynamic patterns of meningococcal septic shock in children. Crit Care Med 16(1):27, 1988.
21. Pollack MM, Fields AI, and Ruttimann UE: Distribution of cardiopulmonary variables in pediatric survivors and nonsurvivors of septic shock. Crit Care Med 13(6):454, 1985.
22. Pollack MM, Fields AI, and Ruttimann UE: Sequential cardiopulmonary variables of infants and children in septic shock. Crit Care Med 12(7):554, 1984.
23. Carcillo JA, Pollack MM, Ruttimann UE, et al: Sequential physiologic interaction in pediatric cardiogenic and septic shock. Crit Care Med 17(1):12, 1989.
24. Roth BL, Suba EA, and Carcillo JA: Alternations in hepatic and aortic phospholipase C coupled receptors and signal transduction in rat intraperitoneal sepsis. *In:* Roth BL, Nielson TB, and McKee AE (eds): Progress in Clinical and Biological Research, Vol 286. Molecular and Cellular Mechanisms of Septic Shock. New York, Alan R Liss, 1988, p. 41.
25. McKenna TM and Titius WAW: Role of monokines in altering receptor and non-receptor mediated vascular contraction in sepsis. *In:* Roth BL, Nielson TB, and McKee AE: Progress in Clinical and Biologic Research, Vol 286. Molecular and Cellular Mechanisms of Septic Shock. New York, Alan R Liss, 1989, p. 279.
26. Lucking SE, Williams TM, and Chaden FC, et al: Oxygen consumption in pediatric septic shock with initial low O_2 extraction. Crit Care Med 17:S141, 1989.
27. Mink RB and Pollack MM: Effect of blood transfusion on oxygen consumption in pediatric septic shock. Crit Care Med 18:1087, 1990.
28. Astiz ME, Rackow EC, Kaufman I, et al: Relationship of oxygen delivery and mixed venous oxygenation to lactic acidosis. Crit Care Med 16:655, 1988.
29. Astiz ME, Rackow EC, Falk JC, et al: Oxygen delivery and consumption in patients with hyperdynamic sepsis. Crit Care Med 15:26, 1987.
30. Holbrook PR, Taylor G, Pollack MM, et al: Adult respiratory distress syndrome in children. Pediatr Clin North Am 27:677, 1930.
31. Corrigan JJ: Thrombocytopenia: A laboratory sign of septicemia in infants and children. J Pediatr 85:219, 1974.
32. Corrigan JJ: Disseminated intravascular coagulopathy. Pediatrics 64:37, 1978.
33. Steven LE, Clemmer TP, Lamb M, et al: Fibronectin in severe sepsis. Surg Gynecol Obstet 162:222, 1986.
34. Weisul JP, O'Donnell TF, Stone MA, et al: Myocardial performance in clinical septic shock: Effects of isoproterenol and glucose potassium insulin. J Surg Res 18:357, 1975.
35. Girardin MD, Grau GB, Dayer JM, et al: Tumor necrosis factor and IL in the serum of children with severe infectious purpura. N Engl J Med 319(7):397, 1988.
36. Corrigan JJ and Jordan CM: Heparin therapy in septicemia with disseminated intravascular coagulation. N Engl J Med 283(15):778, 1978.
37. LeCoultre C and Halperin D: Treatment of skin necrosis in fulminant meningococcemia. Z Kinderchir 41(3):174, 1986.
38. Sibbald WJ, Anderson RR, Reid B, et al: Alveolocapillary permeability in human ARDS. Chest 79:133, 1981.
39. Schumer W: Steroids in the treatment of clinical septic shock. Ann Surg 184:333, 1976.
40. Sprung CL, Coralis PV, Marcial E, et al: The effect of high dose corticosteroids in patients with septic shock. N Engl J Med 311(13):1137, 1984.
41. Bone RC, Fisher CJ, Clemmer TP, et al: A controlled clinical trial of high dose methyl prednisolone in the treatment of severe sepsis and septic shock. N Engl J Med 317:653, 1987.
42. Veterans Administration Systemic Sepsis Cooperative Study Group: Effect of high-dose glucocorticoid therapy on mortality in patients with clinical signs of sepsis. N Engl J Med 317:659, 1987.
43. Ziegler EJ, McCutchan JA, Fierer J, et al: Treatment of gram-negative bacteremia and shock with human antiserum to a mutant *E. coli.* N Engl J Med 307:1225, 1982.
44. Ziegler EJ, Fisher CJ, Sprung CL, et al: Treatment of gram-

negative bacteremia and septic shock with HA-1A human mono-clonal antibody against endotoxin. N Engl J Med 324:429, 1991.

45. Calandra T, Glausner MP, Schollekens J, et al: Treatment of gram-negative septic shock with human IgG antibody to *E. coli* J5. J Infect Dis 153(2):312, 1988.

46. Tracey KJ, Fong Y, Hesse DG, et al: Anticachectin/TNF mono-clonal antibodies prevent septic shock during lethal bacteremia. Nature 330(6149):662, 1987.

47. Gomez A, Wang R, Unruh H, et al: Hemofiltration reverses left ventricular dysfunction during sepsis in dogs. Anesthesiology 73(4):671, 1990.

48. Hagisawa M, Ogins T, Goto R, et al: Endotoxin clearance by exchange blood transfusion in septic shock neonates. Acta Pae-diatr Scand 72(1):87, 1983.

49. Parker MM, Shelhammer JH, Natanson C, et al: Prognostic hemodynamic parameters in septic shock in humans. Clin Res 33:294A, 1985.

13

Hypoxic-Ischemic Injuries

Richard B. Mink, M.D.

Tissue oxygen delivery depends on several factors, including blood flow, hemoglobin content, hemoglobin oxygen saturation, and dissolved oxygen in the blood. An uncompensated change in any one of these components will alter tissue oxygen delivery. Hypoxia results when the partial pressure of oxygen in the blood is severely lowered; both oxygen saturation and dissolved oxygen are reduced. Oxygen delivery also may be decreased by a reduction or complete cessation of blood flow (ischemia) (see also Chapter 1).

Hypoxic injuries, as opposed to ischemic injuries, are more likely to occur in infants and children, because respiratory disease is more prevalent than cardiac disease in this population. Generally, hypoxia results in less permanent tissue damage than does ischemia. When severe, however, hypoxia can lead to cardiac arrest and a combined hypoxic-ischemic injury. Nonetheless, correction of severe hypoxia prior to the complete cessation of blood flow generally results in a more favorable outcome.

Specific organ damage after a hypoxic-ischemic insult varies. This variability is due to several factors. First, blood flow may be preferentially shunted to the heart and the brain in an attempt to minimize injury to these vital organs, resulting in blood flow being shunted away from other organs. Second, the metabolic needs of organs differ. For example, the metabolic demands of the heart and brain are significantly greater than that of peripheral, resting skeletal muscle. Tissue damage results when the oxygen supplied is insufficient to meet the metabolic demands of the tissue. Third, specific critical regions within a particular organ may be very susceptible to hypoxia-ischemia, and damage to these areas may compromise whole organ function.

EFFECT OF HYPOXIA-ISCHEMIA ON SPECIFIC ORGANS

Brain

The brain accounts for 20 to 25% of total oxygen consumption. To meet this high metabolic demand, the brain receives approximately one fifth of the total cardiac output. Although it is assumed that the brain can tolerate only 3 or 4 minutes of ischemia without serious damage, animal investigations suggest that this time may be as long as 60 minutes.[1] Since the outcome from hypoxia-ischemia is frequently determined by the extent of cerebral recovery, research has focused on understanding the pathophysiology of cerebral hypoxia-ischemia with the hope of improving neurologic recovery by providing specific therapies to reduce brain damage.

A significant portion of the damage incurred from hypoxia-ischemia is believed to occur during the reperfusion period when oxygen is provided and other blood components are available. Multiple mechanisms have been implicated, but no one dominant hypothesis has emerged. It is likely that more than one mechanism is important in reperfusion injury and that therapies directed at several pathways will be necessary.[2]

Current therapy is supportive and involves providing adequate ventilation, oxygenation, and blood flow. Although "brain resuscitation" protocols are a useful guide to therapy, there is no evidence that they improve central nervous system outcome. Intracranial pressure monitoring has also not diminished morbidity (see also Chapter 19).

Heart

The heart is of critical importance in the pathophysiology of most hypoxic-ischemic injuries. It may play a primary role, as in cardiogenic shock secondary to a cardiomyopathy, or its role may be participatory, such as in cardiac arrest caused by severe hypoxia from respiratory failure.

Myocardial oxygen consumption is predominantly influenced by three factors: heart rate, systolic wall tension (afterload), and myocardial contractility. Under normal circumstances, oxygen supply and oxygen consumption are closely linked. In the resting state, myocardial oxygen extraction is near maximal, with the heart using about 70% of the oxygen supplied. With increased demands, metabolic needs are met by an increase in coronary blood flow, which increases myocardial oxygen delivery. In periods of hypotension, coronary vessels are maximally dilatated, and since coronary perfusion pressure is reduced, coronary blood flow is diminished.[3] As a result, oxygen delivery is insufficient to meet metabolic demands, and myocardial function is impaired. Cardiac output may be further compromised by dysrhythmias caused by hypoxemia and acidemia. Acute ischemia also decreases left ventricular compliance, presumably by inhibiting ventricular relaxation. Blood flow to the endocardium is particularly compromised, since systole inhibits blood flow in the layers near the endocardium more than in epicardial layers.[4]

Pathologic lesions may be observed if the hypoxic-ischemic insult is severe and prolonged. Hemorrhages and necrosis may be seen first in the subendocardial region and then, if the ischemia is prolonged, in the subepicardium. The area of necrosis may be small and limited to a few myofibers, or it may involve a large area and constitute a myocardial infarct.

Therapy is directed at maintaining adequate cardiac output and coronary blood flow so as to reduce further ischemia to the heart and other organs. The circulation should be supported while minimizing increases in myocardial oxygen consumption, particularly if the heart is the primary cause for the hypoxic-ischemic event. Afterload reduction can frequently be used to improve blood flow without increasing myocardial oxygen demands.

Lungs

Unless severe, the lungs are generally resistant to hypoxia-ischemia, as hypoperfusion per se does not usually result in significant lung injury. This probably relates to the lungs having three sources of oxygen supply: the pulmonary arteries, the bronchial arteries, and the airways. However, gas exchange may be compromised by pulmonary edema from left ventricular failure. In a severe hypoxic-ischemic injury, which occurs with cardiac arrest, the lung itself may be damaged, resulting in severe abnormalities in gas exchange. The pathophysiology of this alveolar-capillary injury is similar to that from other causes, and this condition is referred to as the adult respiratory distress syndrome (ARDS).

ARDS is a clinical syndrome of noncardiac origin that occurs in patients with previously normal lungs. It is defined by criteria that include hypoxemia refractory to supplemental oxygen, increased intrapulmonary shunting, reduced lung compliance, and radiographic evidence of bilateral pulmonary infiltrates.[5] ARDS appears to be a final common pathway of lung injury, since a similar morphologic appearance is observed following pulmonary injury from different causes.

The pathophysiology of ARDS involves damage to the alveolar-capillary membrane, which results in extravasation of fluid of high protein concentration (75 to 95% of plasma protein concentration) into the alveolar spaces. This is associated with surfactant deficiency through inactivation of surfactant from protein in the pulmonary edema fluid or a decrease in surfactant synthesis, or both.[6] Many mediators have been implicated in the pathogenesis of ARDS,[7] and it is likely that more than one is involved (Table 13–1). The activated neutrophil probably plays an important role, though this

Table 13–1. POSSIBLE MEDIATORS IN ADULT RESPIRATORY DISTRESS SYNDROME

Complement
Bradykinin
Prostaglandins
Leukotrienes
Oxygen-free radicals
Neutrophil proteases
Platelet-activating factor
Cytokines

is still somewhat controversial, since ARDS has been observed in neutropenic patients.[8]

There is no specific treatment for ARDS; management is therefore supportive. The goal is to maintain adequate tissue oxygen delivery while minimizing pulmonary barotrauma and oxygen toxicity.[9] To reduce the contribution of hydrostatic forces to pulmonary edema, left ventricular filling pressures should be as low as possible without compromising cardiac output. Corticosteroids are of no proven benefit. Clinical trials to evaluate surfactant as a therapeutic agent are in progress. Since mortality from ARDS is related to associated organ failure, often from sepsis, care should be taken to reduce the risk of nosocomial infection[5] (see also Chapter 47).

Kidneys

Compared with other organs, the kidney has a very high resting oxygen delivery and a low oxygen extraction ratio (Table 13–2). Theoretically, then, the kidney would be expected to be an organ relatively resistant to hypoperfusion, since renal oxygen supply is in much greater excess than is oxygen demand. This is contrary to what is observed, however, as the kidney is usually the organ most susceptible to ischemic injury. Hypotheses for the pathophysiology of renal failure following ischemia have only recently attempted to explain this vulnerability. The actual levels of renal blood flow and oxygen delivery below which renal failure occurs are unknown.

Acute renal failure is the sudden deterioration of renal function to a level insufficient to maintain homeostasis—specifically, to maintain fluid and electrolyte balance, acid-base status, and blood pressure control.[10] The pathogenesis of renal failure resulting from hypoperfusion remains poorly understood. This is due to, at least in part, conflicting data in differing animal models of renal failure, all of which have limited application to acute renal failure in humans. Frequently, the pathology seen in animal models contrasts with that seen in human acute renal failure.[11]

Although a decrease in renal blood flow may be responsible for *initiating* renal failure, it is not clear that renal blood flow is of importance in the *maintenance* of renal failure.[12] Restoration of renal blood flow to normal levels after ischemia does not correlate with recovery of renal function, implicating other mechanisms for the maintenance of renal failure. The explanations for this

Table 13–2. COMPARISON OF WHOLE ORGAN OXYGEN DELIVERY, OXYGEN CONSUMPTION, AND OXYGEN EXTRACTION*

Region or Organ	O₂ Delivery (ml/min/100 g)	Blood Flow Rate (ml/min/100 g)	O₂ Consumption (ml/min/100 g)	O₂ Consumption/ O₂ Delivery (%)
Hepatoportal	11.6	58	2.2	18
Kidney	84.0	420	6.8	8
Brain	10.8	54	3.7	34
Skin	2.6	13	0.38	15
Skeletal muscle	0.5	2.7	0.18	34
Heart	16.8	84	11.0	65

*Modified from Brezis M, Rosen S, Silva P, et al: Renal ischemia: A new perspective. Kidney Int 26:376, 1984. All measurements are for humans.

disparity of renal blood flow and glomerular filtration rate (GFR) have focused predominately on two mechanisms: tubular and vascular (Fig. 13–1). Tubular mechanisms include (1) tubule obstruction from casts, cellular debris, or swelling of injured epithelium and (2) tubule backleak in which there is increased reabsorption of luminal fluid through the damaged tubule epithelium. Vascular mechanisms are thought to decrease the GFR by altering the filtration coefficient or through afferent arteriolar constriction and efferent arteriolar vasodilatation via still-undefined mediators. It is likely that multiple factors are responsible for the decrease in the GFR and that these factors may be important at different times and in different nephrons.[13] The predominance of a vascular or tubular mechanism in a particular patient may explain the variability observed in response to different therapies for oliguria.

Tubular and vascular mechanisms may serve to explain the maintenance of acute renal failure, but they do not explain why the kidney is unusually susceptible to hypoperfusion. Although oxygen delivery to the kidney as a whole is high, recent data have shown that oxygen delivery and blood flow within the kidney are inhomogeneous.[14, 15] The PaO₂ in the medullary region of the dog and rat kidney is approximately 10 mm Hg, presumably because of countercurrent exchange (Fig. 13–2). Brezis and associates[11] have proposed that the initial injury following renal hypoperfusion occurs in the medullary thick ascending loop of Henle. Since the cells

of the medullary thick ascending loop of Henle have a high metabolic rate that is related to active chloride reabsorption, and since oxygen delivery is near the critical value, these cells would be expected to be very susceptible to hypoxia-ischemia. Although whole organ blood flow may be restored to normal after ischemia, medullary blood flow remains depressed. The depressed GFR seen after normalization of renal blood flow may serve as a compensatory mechanism to reduce the metabolic requirements of the medullary thick ascending loop of Henle cells and thus prevent additional damage. With more severe injury, tubule factors may play an additional role in depressing the GFR. Acute renal failure is therefore hypothesized to be a spectrum of injury ranging from medullary thick ascending loop of Henle ischemia to the widespread focal necrosis seen in animal models. Cited in support of this hypothesis are the observations that a renal concentrating defect is often the first sign of acute renal failure and that agents given to reduce medullary thick ascending loop of Henle metabolism (e.g., loop diuretics) increase resistance to ischemic injury.[11]

Following ischemia, therapy is directed at the restoration of renal perfusion, since usually it is not possible to know whether renal failure is in the maintenance phase. Once renal failure is established, treatment is supportive. Adequate intake of protein and carbohydrate is important to avoid the catabolic state. The

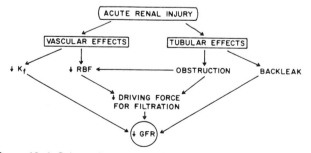

Figure 13–1. Schematic representation of the mechanisms implicated in the maintenance of acute renal failure. Different animal models of injury have been shown to have various preferential effects. GFR = glomerular filtration rate; RBF = renal blood flow. (From Brezis M, Rosen S, Epstein F, et al: Acute renal failure. *In:* Brenner BM and Rector FC Jr [eds]: The Kidney, 3rd ed. Philadelphia, WB Saunders, 1986, p 748.)

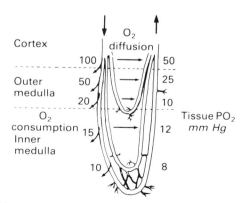

Figure 13–2. The countercurrent exchange of oxygen in the vasa recta. Diffusion of oxygen from arterial to venous limbs leads to a lower tissue PO₂ in the medulla. (Modified from Brezis M, Rosen S, Silva P, et al: Renal ischemia: A new perspective. Kidney Int 26:377, 1984.)

possible benefits of mannitol, loop diuretics, or dopamine in established acute renal failure are controversial, reflecting the lack of controlled studies.[13] Unlike the brain, the kidney has the capacity for both functional and morphologic recovery after ischemia, even if the insult is severe. Functional recovery typically occurs 1 to 2 weeks after the initial insult (see also Chapter 53).

Liver

The liver is somewhat resistant to reductions in oxygen delivery, as it compensates for decreases in oxygen supply by increasing oxygen extraction, thereby maintaining oxygen consumption. The liver receives a dual blood supply through the hepatic artery and the portal vein, partially protecting it from hemodynamic disturbances. Although the traditionally described pathologic unit of the liver is the lobule (composed of a central vein and outlined by six portal spaces), the hepatic acinus is the microvascular unit of the hepatic parenchyma (Fig. 13–3). Blood flows from the terminal portal venule and the terminal hepatic arteriole, through the acinar sinusoids, and exits via the terminal hepatic venules (central veins). Thus all hepatocytes in one acinus receive their blood supply from a common source. It is hypothesized that there is a steep oxygen gradient

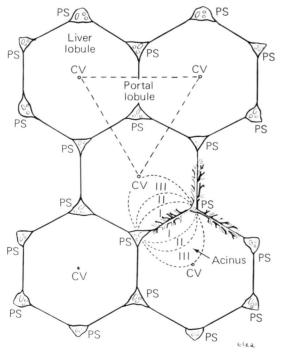

Figure 13–3. Schematic illustrating the classic liver lobules, hepatic acini, and portal lobules. The classic lobule has a central vein (CV) and is outlined by lines that connect the portal spaces (PS). The portal lobules have their center in the portal space and are outlined by lines that connect the central veins. The hepatic acinus, the microvascular unit of the liver parenchyma, consists of the region supplied by the terminal portal venule and terminal hepatic arteriole. Blood enters the acinar sinusoid in zone I and flows sequentially into zones II and III, where it leaves through the central vein. (From Junquera LC and Carneiro J: Basic Histology, 3rd ed., Los Altos, CA, Lange Medical, 1980, p 349.)

between hepatocytes in acinar zone I and those in zone III, with the oxygen tension in the latter zone close to the critical level, making these cells more susceptible to ischemia.[16]

Hepatic hypoperfusion can result in liver injury with biochemical changes similar to those seen in acute hepatitis. This clinical syndrome, known as ischemic hepatitis, is characterized by sudden elevations of serum glutamic-oxalacetic transaminase and serum glutamic-pyruvic transaminase levels of up to 100 times normal (Fig. 13–4).[17, 18] The levels typically peak at 24 to 48 hours after adequate perfusion is re-established and resolve to near normal values within 7 to 10 days. Serum lactic dehydrogenase levels are also increased and follow a similar pattern. Bilirubin levels are transiently elevated but are usually not more than four times the normal value. Cholestasis is not a feature of this syndrome, as the alkaline phosphatase level is rarely increased more than twice that of normal. Some patients may have a prolonged prothrombin time and partial thromboplastin time, though it may be difficult to determine the cause of the coagulopathy if disseminated intravascular coagulation coexists. Liver biopsy shows a "centrilobular" (acinar zone III) focal necrosis, with focal collapse of the reticulin infrastructure but preservation of overall acinar architecture. Inflammation is scant, in contrast to viral hepatitis. Gibson and Dudley have proposed that ischemic hepatitis can be differentiated from viral hepatitis on clinical and biochemical criteria alone.[18] These criteria include (1) an appropriate clinical setting with evidence of hypoperfusion; (2) elevation of serum transaminase and lactate dehydrogenase levels, the latter of which is not significantly increased in viral hepatitis; and (3) an appropriate time course of transaminase elevation with peak levels at 24 to 48 hours.

Although ischemic hepatitis is frequently associated with congestive heart failure, hepatic passive congestion appears to play a minor, if any, role, in its pathogenesis. Passive congestion without a significant reduction in cardiac output results in only minimal elevation of transaminase levels.[19] Furthermore, liver biopsy in passive congestion reveals sinusoidal congestion and hemorrhage, as opposed to the zone III focal necrosis seen with left ventricular failure.[20] Since it is thought that the oxygen tension in acinar zone III is near the critical level, focal necrosis in zone III supports the theory that ischemic hepatitis results predominantly from hepatic perfusion failure.

Mortality associated with ischemic hepatitis in children is reportedly as high as 40%.[17] However, mortality is related to the underlying disease and not to hepatic dysfunction. There is usually little evidence of overt hepatic failure, and the pathologic lesions usually resolve without fibrosis. If the liver had been previously damaged or if the period of hypoperfusion is particularly severe and long (greater than 24 hours), significant hepatic dysfunction may follow. The absolute level of transaminase elevation does not correlate with mortality; however, patients with ischemic hepatitis who fail to demonstrate a reduction in transaminase levels have a high incidence of mortality, which is likely related to persistent hypoperfusion.[21] Therapy is directed at im-

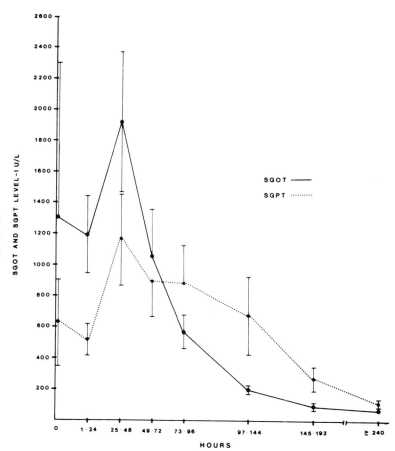

Figure 13–4. The time course of serum transaminase levels after a hypoxic-ischemic injury. (From Garland JS, Werlin SL, and Rice TB: Ischemic hepatitis in children: Diagnosis and clinical course. Crit Care Med 16:1211, 1988. © by Williams & Wilkins, 1988.)

proving perfusion and treating the underlying cause, as ischemic hepatitis requires no specific therapy (see also Chapter 56).

Gastrointestinal Tract

Information regarding ischemic injury to the gut in children is sparse, and extrapolating the adult experience to the infant and child is complicated by atherosclerotic narrowing of blood vessels in the adult. Nonetheless, there are similarities between cases of necrotizing enterocolitis in the newborn and the adult counterpart of acute intestinal necrosis, suggesting a common ischemic pathogenesis for both entities.

Pathologic changes can be observed after only 5 to 10 minutes of intestinal ischemia.[22] The lesions are usually restricted to the mucosa, but with increasing severity or duration of ischemia, or both, deeper layers may be involved. The injury tends to be patchy and segmental, and the distribution of damage does not seem to conform to an area supplied by any one major blood vessel. Based on a compilation of autopsy specimen results, the small bowel is the most sensitive to injury from hypoperfusion (Table 13–3).[23]

Within 30 to 60 minutes of ischemia, the luminal portion of the small intestinal villi are denuded of epithelium. Capillary permeability and capillary integrity are altered, leading to hemorrhage and edematous thickening of the mucosa and submucosa. Depending on the extent of injury, an inflammatory infiltrate may appear 12 to 24 hours following injury. Since the intestinal mucosa has an extremely rapid turnover rate, complete resolution is often possible within 48 to 72 hours after injury but only if the superficial mucosa is damaged. The critical factor seems to be whether there is injury to the intestinal crypts.[24] Damage to the deeper muscularis layer may lead to varying degrees of inflam-

Table 13–3. PREVALENCE OF LESIONS (PERCENT) AT AUTOPSY IN REGIONS OF THE GASTROINTESTINAL TRACT FOLLOWING HYPOPERFUSION OF DIFFERING ETIOLOGIES*

Primary Etiology	Stomach	Duodenum	Small Bowel	Colon
Heart failure	20.0	23.2	92.1	57.2
Postoperative hypotension	5.2	8.5	73.5	45.8
Hemorrhage	9.1	9.1	90.9	27.3

*Modified from Bounous G: Acute necrosis of the intestinal mucosa. Gastroenterology 82:1458, 1982.

matory fibrosis and stricture formation. If the injury is severe and involves the entire intestinal wall, bowel rupture may result. Generally, perforation resulting from full-thickness necrosis is rare beyond the neonatal period. In the colon, luminal bacteria may influence recovery by causing infection or producing toxins.

The pathophysiology of intestinal ischemic injury may be different from that of other organs in view of the unique contents of the intestinal lumen. Various mechanisms have been proposed to explain the susceptibility of the intestinal villus to ischemia, including a counter-current exchange mechanism in the villi similar to that in the kidney medulla, selective constriction of the mesenteric vascular bed, portal hypertension leading to intravascular pooling of blood in the villus, and free radicals derived from xanthine oxidase.[23] A current hypothesis favors a role for pancreatic proteases.[25] In the initial phase of injury, pancreatic elastase and bile salts located within the intestinal lumen lead to the loss of the brush border proteins, since ischemia prevents the regeneration of the protective glycoproteins on the brush border. As ischemia is prolonged, the brush border disappears, and the underlying structures are then accessible to the digestive action of the pancreatic endopeptidases trypsin and chymotrypsin.

Therapy requires only the maintenance of perfusion and the replacement of lost fluid and electrolytes. Ileus often accompanies the injury, resulting in the accumulation of fluid within the intestinal lumen. In the majority of cases, there is complete resolution of bowel function (see also Chapter 57).

Pancreas

Ischemia as a cause of pancreatitis has been largely ignored in both children and adults. This is from, in part, the difficulty in making the diagnosis of pancreatitis, especially in the pediatric patient.[26] No single laboratory test is of high enough specificity, so the diagnosis is made by a combination of clinical signs and symptoms, biochemical abnormalities, and the finding of pancreatic inflammation through imaging techniques.

Pancreatitis results from the autodigestion of the pancreas as a consequence of inappropriate activation of pancreatic zymogens to active enzymes within the pancreatic parenchyma. The pancreas normally has an array of safeguards designed to prevent autodigestion; the sequence of events needed to trigger activation is unknown. Inflammation can range from mild edema to generalized necrosis with or without hemorrhage. Histologic severity correlates with the clinical course, which ranges from a mild, self-limited disease to one that is fulminant.[27]

Clinical symptoms may be lacking in pancreatitis resulting from ischemia. In an adult study of patients with pancreatitis in shock, 75% had no clinical symptoms. All of these patients had complete resolution of the disease. In another study of patients with cardiogenic shock, pancreatitis found at autopsy was rarely suspected antemortem.[28] Although pancreatitis is infre-

quent in infants and children, it is likely that many cases are undetected.

Diagnosis requires a high index of suspicion. Signs that may be present in critically ill patients include excessive nasogastric drainage, left pleural effusion, and abdominal ascites.[29] Hyperamylasemia has traditionally been used to indicate pancreatic inflammation, but the amylase can be elevated in other disorders, and pancreatitis has been observed in the presence of normal levels. Other assays, such as serum trypsinogen and pancreatic isoamylase, may improve specificity. Edema of the pancreas may be visualized by sonography, and gland enlargement can be seen with computerized tomography.[27]

Since "third-space" losses may be significant, treatment is directed at maintaining intravascular volume by replacing fluid and electrolytes. Severe cases may result in hypocalcemia or hyperglycemia. Enteral feeding should be avoided to "rest" the pancreas in an attempt to reduce pancreatic secretions and thereby reduce the intensity of inflammation. If narcotic analgesics are used, meperidine is preferred to morphine, because morphine increases contraction of the sphincter of Oddi.

References

1. Hossmann KA and Kleihues P: Reversibility of ischemic brain damage. Arch Neurol 29:375, 1973.
2. Bircher NG: Brain resuscitation. Resuscitation 18(Suppl):S1, 1989.
3. Mosher P, Ross J Jr, McFate A, et al: Control of coronary blood flow by an autoregulatory mechanism. Circ Res 24:250, 1964.
4. Factor SM and Kirk ES: Pathophysiology of myocardial ischemia. In: Hurst JW (ed): The Heart, 6th ed. New York, McGraw Hill, 1986, p 856.
5. Wiener-Kronish JP, Gropper MA, and Matthay MA: The adult respiratory distress syndrome: Definition and prognosis, pathogenesis and treatment. Br J Anaesth 65:107, 1990.
6. Petty TL: Acute respiratory distress syndrome (ARDS). Dis Mon 36:1, 1990.
7. Demling RH: Current concepts on the adult respiratory distress syndrome. Circ Shock 30:297, 1990.
8. Maunder RJ, Hackman RC, Riff E, et al: Occurrence of the adult respiratory distress syndrome in neutropenic patients. Am Rev Respir Dis 133:313, 1986.
9. Pfenninger J, Gerber A, Tschappeler H, et al: Adult respiratory distress syndrome in children. J Pediatr 101:352, 1982.
10. Ellis D, Gartner JC, and Galvis AG: Acute renal failure in infants and children: Diagnosis, complications and treatment. Crit Care Med 9:607, 1981.
11. Brezis M, Rosen S, Silva P, et al: Renal ischemia: A new perspective. Kidney Int 26:375, 1984.
12. Conger JD and Schrier RW: Renal hemodynamics in acute renal failure. Ann Rev Physiol 42:603, 1980.
13. Brezis M, Rosen S, and Epstein F: Acute renal failure. In: Brenner BM and Rector FC Jr (eds): The Kidney, 3rd ed. Philadelphia, WB Saunders, 1986, p 748.
14. Ratcliffe PJ, Endre ZH, Tange JD, et al: Ischaemic acute renal failure: Why does it occur? Nephron 52:1, 1989.
15. Epstein FH and Brown RS: Acute renal failure: A collection of paradoxes. Hosp Pract (Off) 23:171, 1988.
16. Gumucio JJ and Miller DL: Functional implications of liver cell heterogeneity. Gastroenterology 80:393, 1981.
17. Garland JS, Werlin SL, and Rice TB: Ischemic hepatitis in children: Diagnosis and clinical course. Crit Care Med 16:1209, 1988.
18. Gibson PR and Dudley FJ: Ischemic hepatitis: Clinical features, diagnosis and prognosis. Aust NZ J Med 14:822, 1984.

19. Mace S, Borkat G, and Liebman J: Hepatic dysfunction and cardiovascular abnormalities. Am J Dis Child 139:60, 1985.
20. Arcidi JM Jr, Moore GW, and Hutchins GM: Hepatic morphology in cardiac dysfunction. Am J Pathol 104:159, 1981.
21. Hickman PE and Potter JM: Mortality associated with ischaemic hepatitis. Aust NZ J Med 20:32, 1990.
22. Robinson JWL, Mirkovitch V, Winistörfer B, et al: Response of the intestinal mucosa to ischaemia. Gut 22:512, 1981.
23. Bounous G: Acute necrosis of the intestinal mucosa. Gastroenterology 82:1457, 1982.
24. Whitehead R: The pathology of ischemia of the intestines. Pathol Annu 11:1, 1976.
25. Bounous G, Menard D, and DeMedicis E: Role of pancreatic proteases in the pathogenesis of ischemic enteropathy. Gastroenterology 73:102, 1977.
26. Tam PKH, Saing H, Irving IM, et al: Acute pancreatitis in children. J Pediatr Surg 20:58, 1985.
27. Geokas MC, Baltaxe HA, Banks PA, et al: Acute pancreatitis. Ann Intern Med 103:86, 1985.
28. Warshaw AL, and O'Hara PJ: Susceptibility of the pancreas to ischemic injury in shock. Ann Surg 188:197, 1978.
29. Nguyen T, Abramowsky C, Ashenburg C, et al: Clinicopathologic studies in childhood pancreatitis. Hum Pathol 19:343, 1988.

Nutritional Failure and Therapy

Catherine A. Musemeche, M.D., and
Richard J. Andrassy, M.D.

The effective management of nutritional failure in the critically ill child is essential for recovery. Such nutritional intervention can increase resistance to infection, improve wound healing, prevent organ failure, and reduce mortality. An aggressive nutritional plan must be instituted early in the course of severe illness and updated as the child's clinical status evolves to accompany changes in metabolic requirements and routes of support. It has been well documented that major nutritional deficiencies develop within 48 hours of admission to the pediatric intensive care unit in 16 to 20% of patients.[1]

As recently as 15 years ago, many ill and injured children died from a sequence of malnutrition, sepsis, and multiple organ system failure because nutritional support was inadequate. Today these patients may receive nutritional support because of (1) the development of techniques for central venous cannulation and infusion of hypertonic nutrient solutions, (2) the development of specific enteral formula diets that can be provided orally or by feeding catheter, and (3) the development of fat emulsions for safe intravenous administration.[2]

Multiple organ system failure can develop after trauma, severe aspiration, or prolonged sepsis. It is accompanied by a sustained phase of hypermetabolism. During this time, energy expenditure may exceed two times basal requirements.[3] Total body protein catabolism is markedly increased, and lean body mass can be depleted in 7 days. Within skeletal muscle, branched chain amino acids (leucine, isoleucine, valine) are predominantly oxidized for energy production. It is important to guard against excess total calories, and specifically excess glucose calories, because of the side effects of fatty liver syndrome, hyperosmolar states, and excess carbon dioxide production. There is little doubt that effective nutritional support can help reduce morbidity and mortality when multiple organ system failure occurs.

NUTRITIONAL REQUIREMENTS AND ASSESSMENT

An understanding of the alterations in metabolic regulation that occur in severe illness has improved the nutritional management of critically ill children. The calorie and protein requirement for these patients usually increases substantially with the hypercatabolic response associated with stress. Catecholamines stimulate tissue metabolism thereby increasing energy expenditure and necessitating an increased oxygen consumption.[4] The metabolic rate is increased up to 100% from burns, by 50% from sepsis, and by 20% from long bone fractures.[5]

There are also physiologic differences between children and adults that leave children at a significant nutritional disadvantage in times of stress. In addition to increased caloric demands, there is usually a decrease in caloric intake during times of severe illness. Nutritional stores in the pediatric patient younger than 1 year of age are considerably less than in adults because of a decreased percentage of body fat and protein. In a premature baby, fat makes up approximately 1% of body weight, whereas in a 1-year-old child, 20% of the body weight may be fat. This compares with 21% in adults. Children also have an increased need for calories, compared with adults, because of a higher basal metabolic rate (55 versus 35 kcal/m²/hr).[5] Children have increased requirements because they are growing and because metabolic organs compose a greater percentage of their body weight.

Determining energy requirements begins with a knowledge of the basal metabolic rate (BMR) for infants and children. The BMR is derived from a measurement of heat production in a resting fasting state. Maintenance requirements are 120 to 150% of the BMR. Growth requirements are an additional 5 kcal/g of weight gained. An approximation of energy needs during critical illness is 150 to 200% of the BMR (Table 14–1).

Protein requirements are also age-dependent and are as follows: infants less than 6 months, 2 to 3 g/kg/day; and adults, 0.5 to 2.0 g/kg/day.[5] Critically ill children require protein intake in greater amounts to achieve a positive nitrogen balance. No more than 30% of calories should be provided in the form of protein.[6] The amount of protein required depends on its essential amino acid content. Essential amino acids should compose 40% of

Table 14–1. ENERGY REQUIREMENTS (Kcal/kg/24 hr) FOR VARIOUS AGES AT BASAL, MAINTENANCE, GROWTH, AND ILLNESS LEVELS*

	1 Yr	5 Yr	10 Yr	16 Yr
Basal	55	45	38	27
Maintenance	83	75	56	42
Growth	89	77	78	43
Illness	95	78	66	45

*Modified from Briglia FA and Pollak MM: Fluid and nutritional therapy in the critically ill child. Indian J Pediatr 54:819, 1987.

an infant's protein intake, 30% of a child's protein intake, and 20% of an adult's protein intake.[6]

Essential fatty acid requirements (linoleic acid) may be met by supplying 4 to 8% of the daily caloric requirements with fat,[7] but on the average, fat is used to provide 30% of total caloric requirements. In the past, up to 60% of nonprotein calories have been supplied by fat. This should not be exceeded, especially in light of recent evidence that high levels of polyunsaturated fatty acids have an immunosuppressive effect in burn patients.[8] Because of an impairment in the utilization of fat during severe sepsis, not more than 10% of energy requirements should be provided by fat.

Complete nutritional support requires adequate amounts of vitamins, minerals, and trace elements. Vitamins are especially important in wound healing and immunity. Thiamine, riboflavin, niacin, and vitamin B_6 are components of enzymes and coenzymes used to metabolize carbohydrate, fat, and protein. Animal studies suggest that deficiencies in vitamins A and D, ascorbic acid, thiamine, folic acid, and others may reduce host resistance to infection.[9] The strength of vitamin supplements depends on preinjury nutritional status, and for children not previously deficient it is approximately two to three times the minimum daily requirement.[10] Excesses of fat-soluble vitamins (A, D, and E) can be toxic in large quantities and should be limited to recommended allowances.

Calcium and phosphorus supplementation are especially important in infants and children because of the increased requirements for bone growth (Table 14–2). Hypophosphatemia can cause red blood cell and leukocyte dysfunction, encephalopathy, and myopathy.[11] Hypomagnesemia can cause nausea, anorexia, neuromuscular irritability, and encephalopathy. Magnesium requirements are 1 to 2 mEq/kg/day for infants less than 6 months of age and 0.5 mEq/kg/day for older infants and children.

The nutritional assessment provides a baseline of the patient's nutritional state and aids in decisions regarding timing and route of support. It begins with the dietary history, which defines the chronicity of the nutritional deficiencies (weight change, previous illness) and documents gastrointestinal complaints (i.e., vomiting or diarrhea or food intolerance). Objective data include anthropometric measurements and biochemical testing. The triceps skinfold thickness provides an estimate of body fat stores, because 50% of body fat is situated in subcutaneous sites.[12] Protein stores are determined by estimating skeletal muscle mass from midarm muscle circumference. The excretion of creatinine, a by-product

of creatine (muscle protein), can also be used to estimate total body muscle mass. Normal daily creatinine excretion (mg/kg/day) is equal to 15 plus ½ the patient's age in years.[10] Visceral protein mass can be assessed indirectly from albumin and transferrin levels. Albumin has a half-life of 20 days so that there is a delay in the measured decrease with protein malnutrition. It is therefore more indicative of chronic changes in nutrition. An albumin level less than 3 g/l is indicative of either protein malnutrition or liver dysfunction. Transferrin (normal = 150 mg/dl), in contrast, has a shorter half-life of 9 days and is a more reliable indicator of recent protein depletion.

ENTERAL FEEDINGS

There are definite physiologic and economic advantages to enteral feedings, and they are preferred if the gastrointestinal tract is functioning. A knowledge of the effects of critical illness on the gastrointestinal tract can aid in determining when enteral feedings can be tolerated.

There are alterations in gastrointestinal enzymes and the structure of intestinal villi in critically ill children. Animal studies have shown that this gastrointestinal dysfunction is most likely to occur with parenteral nutrition and after burn injury over a large portion of the body.[13-16] Ileus in critically ill patients can result from many different causes, including abdominal surgery, intra-abdominal sepsis, head or spinal injury, and metabolic disturbances. Postoperative ileus does not affect the entire gastrointestinal tract uniformly. The stomach may be nonfunctional for 2 to 3 days. The motility of the small bowel, however, usually returns within 24 hours.[17] Colonic function may take 3 to 5 days to return to normal.[18]

Enteral nutrition has been shown to be superior to parenteral nutrition in maintaining gastrointestinal integrity and gut hormonal balance. Food ingestion stimulates growth and replication of enterocytes and secre-

Table 14–2. CALCIUM AND PHOSPHOROUS REQUIREMENTS IN INFANTS AND CHILDREN

Age	Calcium	Phosphorous
<6 mo	80 mg/kg/day	1–2 mM/kg/day
6 mo–2 yr	40 mg/kg/day	1 mM/kg/day
2 yr–10 yr	400 mg/day	10–30 mM/day
>10 yr	600 mg/day	15–20 mM/day

Table 14–3. COMPOSITION OF ENTERAL FORMULAS

	Calories (cal/ml)	Osmolality (mOsm/l)	Carbohydrate (g/l)	Fat (g/l)	Protein (g/l)
Normal digestion					
Ensure	1	450	145	37	37
Isocal	1	300	132	44	34
Pregestimil	0.67	350	90	27	18
Citrotein	0.71	495	130	1.7	44
Elemental					
Vivonex	1	550	231	1	22
Criticare HN	1	650	222	3	38
Modular components					
Polycose	2	850	500		
MCT Oil	7.7	N/A		933	

tion of mucus.[19] In studying the nutritional requirements of the gut itself, glutamine has been found to be a major energy source and nutrient. The gut uptake of glutamine exceeds that of any other amino acid. After severe injury, the glutamine concentration in blood and skeletal muscle decreases, and the intestinal glutamine uptake increases. Current parenteral solutions contain no glutamine, and this may partly explain the villous atrophy in patients on long-term total parenteral nutrition (TPN). Preserving the gut mucosal barrier through enteral nutrition may also affect the incidence of bacterial translocation from the gut to the systemic circulation. This can be of major concern in critically ill patients with compromised immune systems.

Enteral nutrition preserves the normal physiologic sequence of nutrient absorption and metabolism. Enteral feeding stimulates secretion of bile salts, and there is decreased cholestasis.

The safety of enteral nutrition over parenteral nutrition has been debated. Clearly, the complications that can occur from central line insertion, such as pneumothorax, hydrothorax, hemothorax, and catheter embolus, are avoided with enteral nutrition. There are inherent risks to enteral alimentation as well, however, such as vomiting, aspiration, and diarrhea.

Enteral feeding can be instituted orally if the patient is awake and cooperative, but in critically ill individuals this is not usually an alternative. A nasoenteric tube is a traditional option. To avoid the hazards of reflux and aspiration, the tip of the tube should be positioned in the duodenum. A Dobhoff tube (weighted with mercury) is designed to be passed through the pylorus. Nasogastric or gastrostomy tube feedings, if tolerated without reflux, allow one to choose the option of bolus feedings at some point. Children who require laparotomy for trauma, or other operative interventions, are candidates for placement of a needle catheter jejunostomy at the time of the operation.[20] Intestinal feedings should be given by continuous infusion, beginning with small volumes (1 ml/kg/hr) of half-strength formula.[12] If this is well tolerated during the first 24 hours, the volume can be increased by 0.5/ml/kg/hr until the desired volume is being delivered. Once the required volume has been achieved, the concentration can be increased. If the enteral feedings are delivered into the stomach, bolus feedings can be initiated by delivering 2 ml of formula/kg

of body weight every 3 to 4 hours, starting with half-strength formula on the first day. If gastric residuals are not substantial, the volume can be gradually increased. The strength of the formula can be increased after the first day if diarrhea does not ensue. If stool output becomes unmanageable at any point in the tube feeding regimen, both the strength and volume of formula can be decreased until tolerated.

The formula chosen for enteral feeds depends on the child's digestive activity, as well as on individual metabolic restrictions. These formulas can be thought of in three broad categories: formulas requiring normal digestion, elemental diets, and caloric additive or "modular" formulas (Table 14–3). Normal digestion formulas are composed of protein hydrolysates, glucose polymers, and long chain fatty acids. They require intact lipolytic and proteolytic activity for digestion.

If the child has limited digestive ability, elemental diets are available. These are solutions of short chain peptides or amino acids and simple sugars. They are usually low in fat. Elemental diets provide the advantage of easy and complete absorption in the upper small intestine and minimal residue. They are hyperosmolar, and gradual introduction is necessary to minimize osmotic diarrhea. Elemental diets are particularly useful in the management of gastrointestinal fistulas, inflammatory bowel disease, short bowel syndrome, and for early postoperative feeding via jejunostomy.

Caloric additive diets are designed to provide extra calories or supplement a specific nutrient. They also allow possible mixing of separate sources—that is, "modules" for protein, carbohydrate, and fat.

TOTAL PARENTERAL NUTRITION

When use of the gastrointestinal tract is precluded because of severe acute illness and intestinal dysfunction, TPN can be instituted. Since 1968, when Dudrick demonstrated that central venous alimentation was life-sustaining, this technique has been particularly valuable in infants and children in whom nutritional reserves are limited.[21]

TPN can be implemented by either a peripheral or a central route. Peripheral TPN offers the advantage of a lower incidence of catheter-related complications; however, it is difficult to achieve full nutritional support through the peripheral route. Peripheral infusion of glucose in concentrations greater than 10 to 12% damages the intima of veins, which can result in phlebitis and sclerosis. The peripheral administration of fat emulsions greatly augments the caloric value of peripheral nutrition. However, lipid intake (3 to 4 g/kg/day) is on average limited to 30% of total caloric requirements. In addition to caloric restraints, peripheral TPN prevents the use of hyperconcentrated glucose and amino acids, which are valuable when fluid restriction is indicated. Peripheral TPN may serve its greatest role as a supplement to an enteral diet in the child who will not or cannot eat enough to meet caloric needs.

Critical illness frequently precludes enteral feeding, and central TPN then becomes the best option for complete nutritional support. This is particularly appropriate when prolonged support is anticipated and peripheral venous access is limited. The technique of central venous cannulation varies, depending on the size of the child, previous sites of insertion, and patient injuries. In infants and young children, the apex of the lung is high and the subclavian and jugular veins are small. Central venous lines in these patients are usually inserted in the operating room by cutdown on the external or internal jugular vein. Older children, or those weighing more than 10 kg, can generally safely undergo percutaneous subclavian catheter placement.

Although parenteral nutrition in children has been used for about 20 years, very little data exist on what the specific intravenous nutrient requirements are. There are large variations in TPN solution formulations.

Dextrose is the predominant carbohydrate source in parenteral solutions. In infants and children, a final solution containing 20 to 25% dextrose is usually sufficient if intralipid is also used. This hyperosmolar solution must be infused centrally, at which point it is rapidly diluted.

All of the amino acid solutions contain the eight known essential amino acids plus histidine, which is considered essential in children.[22] There is much variability in the provision of "nonessential" amino acids. Some feel that all 20 amino acids used in protein synthesis should be provided in these formulations; however, they are not, usually for technical reasons.[23] Of the total amino acids provided, 40 to 50% are essential amino acids. The amino acid form is made up of 50% free amino acids and 50% polypeptides. The utilization of polypeptides is not fully understood, though it is probably not as energy-efficient as using free amino acids. Amino acids are available in 3 to 10% solutions. Metabolism in infants is more sensitive to varying mixtures of amino acids, and the content of methionine, cysteine, phenylalanine, tyrosine, and glycine are of particular concern.

The high caloric density of lipid (9 kcal/g) has made it an excellent caloric supplementation. It is available in 10 or 20% solutions, either of which may be infused centrally or peripherally. As previously mentioned, fat generally composes approximately 30% of total caloric intake and should not exceed 60% or 4 g/kg/day. Intravenous fat solutions should be initiated at a slow rate in

children and gradually increased if the patient is having no reaction and if the serum triglyceride level does not exceed 150 mg/dl. At levels greater than this, the lipoprotein lipase enzyme system that metabolizes fat emulsions is saturated. The total daily amount of fat should be infused over at least 8 hours, and bolus infusion should be avoided. Fat emulsions are now stable in hypertonic glucose solutions, and it is possible to infuse the two simultaneously.

The addition of electrolytes and minerals to the TPN solutions depends on the maintenance needs and ongoing losses of the patient. Calcium (see Table 14–2), in the form of gluconate or chloride, and phosphorous, as sodium or potassium phosphate and magnesium sulfate, should be added. Trace elements (zinc, copper, manganese, and chromium) are routinely provided on a daily basis but are actually not required for several weeks after TPN is instituted.

Difficulty in maintaining intravenous access in infants and children may necessitate the concomitant administration of medications while the TPN solution is infusing. The list of drugs compatible with TPN includes ampicillin, cefazolin, clindamycin, cloxacillin, gentamicin, tobramycin, cimetidine, furosemide, heparin, hydrocortisone, regular insulin, and phenobarbital.[24] When drugs are administered, intravenous lipid should be discontinued because it is unstable when in contact with most additives.[22]

COMPLICATIONS OF TOTAL PARENTERAL NUTRITION

Complications of TPN can be divided into technical complications from catheter insertion, infectious complications, and metabolic complications. Most complications of central line insertion are related to the percutaneous approach to the subclavian vein, and this should be avoided in children who weigh less than 10 kg. Pneumothorax, hemothorax, chylothorax, and brachial plexus injury can occur upon insertion of a subclavian line.

Late complications of a central venous catheter include venous thrombosis in up to 20% of patients, thromboemboli from the catheter tip, air embolism, and catheter erosion. Central line infections are usually a result of contamination during blood withdrawal or medication infusion. If possible, the catheter should be limited to TPN infusion only to minimize the risk of infection.

There are many potential metabolic complications of TPN. One of the most common is hyperglycemia secondary to overinfusion of glucose. This may be an acute concern in patients with diabetes, sepsis, or stress-related insulin resistance. Hypoglycemia can accompany a rapid cessation of TPN therapy, especially in neonates and infants. It is therefore important to wean TPN gradually if possible.

A wide variety of fluid, electrolyte, and mineral abnormalities can also result from TPN administration. Hypernatremia, especially in young infants, can result from dehydration and the inefficient urine concentration capacity of the kidney. Hyponatremia, in contrast, is likely to result from water retention secondary to an impaired ability to excrete free water. Serum potassium levels may decrease, depending on gastrointestinal and renal losses and should be replaced as necessary. Hyperkalemia is a possible danger in patients with severe catabolism or acidosis or after extensive muscle injury.

Intrahepatic cholestasis is a well-documented complication of prolonged TPN administration in infants. Jaundice and an elevation in liver enzymes are typically seen. This is a condition that may be alleviated or prevented by cycling the TPN intermittently throughout the day. Severe cases have progressed to cirrhosis and liver failure.

Hypertriglyceridemia secondary to excessive intravenous fat administration is to be avoided. Recent data in neonates have shown that intravenous fat infusion can inhibit polymorphonuclear leukocyte and platelet function.[25]

MONITORING THERAPY

Monitoring of TPN therapy has a two-fold purpose. The first is to ensure safe and accurate therapy by biochemical measurements, which fluctuate acutely. The second is to measure the success or failure of therapy by assessing weight gain, muscle mass, and fat stores.

Biochemical parameters are measured more frequently at the beginning of therapy. Initially, a complete baseline determination of blood count and blood chemistries is obtained. During the first 1 to 2 weeks, serum electrolytes, blood urea nitrogen, creatinine, and glucose determinations are obtained daily. The urine is checked at each shift to assess glucose levels. A complete blood count, prothrombin time, partial thromboplastin time, liver function studies, and calcium, phosphorous, and magnesium determinations are obtained two to three times a week. After therapy has been adjusted to the patient's metabolic needs and no further acute changes in formulations are expected, laboratory studies, including determinations of serum electrolytes, glucose, and creatinine, as well as liver function tests and a complete blood count are performed once or twice a week. Blood for cultures is drawn only if there is a clinical suspicion of infection and not on a routine basis.

References

1. Pollack MM, Wiley JS, and Holbrook PR: Early nutritional depletion in critically ill children. Crit Care Med 9:580, 1981.
2. Hauser GJ and Holbrook PR: Immune dysfunction in the critically ill infant and child. Crit Care Clin 4:711, 1988.
3. Cerra FB: Hypermetabolism-organ failure syndrome: A metabolic response to injury. Crit Care Clin 5:289, 1989.
4. Wilmore DW, Long JM, Mason AD, et al: Catecholamines: Mediator of the hypermetabolic response to thermal injury. Ann Surg 180:653, 1974.
5. Briglia FA and Pollack MM: Fluid and nutritional therapy in the critically ill child. Indian J Pediatr 54:819, 1987.
6. Dominioni L, Trocki O, Fang C, et al: Enteral feeding in burn hypermetabolism: Nutritional and metabolic effects of different levels of caloric and protein intake. JPEN 9:269, 1985.
7. Reimer SL, Michener WM, and Steiger E: Nutritional support of the critically ill child. Pediatr Clin North Am 27:647, 1980.
8. Alexander JW: Nutrition and infection: New perspectives for an old problem. Arch Surg 121:966, 1986.
9. Andrassy RJ, Nirgiotis JG, and Hennessey PJ: Preserving the gut and enhancing the immune response: The role of enteral nutrition in decreasing sepsis. J Jpn Soc Pediatr Surg 26:1057, 1990.
10. Alexander SJW: Nutrition and surgical infection. Manual of Surgical Nutrition. American College of Surgeons Committee on Pre- and Postoperative Care, Philadelphia, WB Saunders, 1975, p 393.
11. Krochel JP: The pathophysiology and clinical characteristics of severe hypophosphatemia. Arch Intern Med 137:203, 1977.
12. Siegler RL: Nutritional support. In: Mayer TA (ed): Emergency Management of Pediatric Trauma, 1st ed. Philadelphia, WB Saunders, 1985, pp 125–138.
13. Eastwood GL: Small bowel morphology and epithelial proliferation in intravenously alimented rabbits. Surgery 82:613, 1977.
14. Johnson LR, Copeland EM, Dudrick SJ, et al: Structural and hormonal alterations in the gastrointestinal tract of parenterally fed rats. Gastroenterology 68:1177, 1975.
15. Levine GM, Dren JJ, Steiger ET, et al: Role of oral intake in maintenance of gut mass and disaccharide activity. Gastroenterology 67:975, 1974.
16. Mochizuki H, Trocki O, Dominioni L, et al: Mechanism of prevention of postburn hypermetabolism and catabolism by early enteral feeding. Ann Surg 200:297, 1984.
17. Wells C, Tinkler L, Rawlinson K, et al: Postoperative gastrointestinal motility. Lancet 1:4, 1964.
18. Woods JH, Erickson LW, Condon RE, et al: Postoperative ileus: A colonic problem. Surgery 84:527, 1978.
19. Alverdy J, Chi HS, and Sheldon GF: The effect of parenteral nutrition on gastrointestinal immunity: The importance of enteral stimulation. Ann Surg 202:681, 1985.
20. Page CP, Carlton PK, Andrassy RJ, et al: Safe, cost-effective postoperative nutrition. Defined formula diet via needle-catheter jejunostomy. Am J Surg 138:939, 1979.
21. Wilmore DW and Dudrick SJ: Growth and development of an infant receiving all nutrients exclusively by vein. JAMA 203:860, 1968.
22. Zlotkin SH, Stallings VA, and Pencharz PB: Total parenteral nutrition in children. Pediatr Clin North Am 32:381, 1985.
23. Jackson AA: Amino acids: Essential and nonessential? Lancet 6(8332):1034, 1983.
24. Fargo S: Compatibility of antibiotics and other drugs in total parenteral nutrition solutions. Can J Hosp Pharm 34:43, 1983.
25. Herson VC, Block C, Eisenfeld L, et al: Effects of intravenous fat infusion on neonatal neutrophil and platelet function. JPEN 6:620, 1989.

15

Multiple Organ System Failure

Vinay M. Nadkarni, M.D.

BACKGROUND

Multiple organ system failure (MOSF) is broadly defined as the progressive concurrent failure of two or more organ systems. It is a nonspecific expression of critical illness resulting from the amplification of a systemic inflammatory process. The insult leads to dead or injured tissue, infection, or severe sepsis ("sepsis syndrome"), or a combination of these conditions. Perfusion deficit or shock leads to a series of events involving the central nervous system (CNS), endocrine system, and cell to cell communications systems, which cascades to amplify the inflammatory response, resulting in hypermetabolism and progressive organ failure.[1-12]

MOSF was initially identified in critically ill adult patients who had been recently resuscitated from severe trauma, hemorrhage, major surgery, sepsis, or myocardial infarction. By the mid-1970s, a specific syndrome of sequential organ failure following well-defined inciting injuries, the multiple organ failure syndrome, was described in the adult literature.[1, 2, 13-17] MOSF has become a leading cause of death in the critical care setting. Critically ill adults with MOSF have an associated mortality rate of 60 to 90%.[1, 2, 5, 13, 17-22]

MOSF is less well recognized in children. In large pediatric centers, approximately one quarter of patients acquire MOSF, and only approximately half of these patients survive.[23, 24] The tight association of sepsis and sepsis syndrome with MOSF in adults does not appear to be true in the pediatric age group,[7, 8, 23, 24-30] although the common histologic and clinical features of tissue hypoperfusion and shock, leading to MOSF via mechanisms that produce tissue necrosis, vascular congestion, microthromboembolism, and tissue inflammation are believed to pertain to children. Twenty-six to 88% of pediatric patients with MOSF succumb.[23, 24, 31, 32]

Although technology and supportive care techniques are rapidly advancing, the incidence and prevalence of MOSF does not appear to be declining. As our ability to resuscitate patients from sepsis, shock, and severe trauma improves, we may expect an increased incidence of MOSF.

The objective of this chapter is to provide an overview of MOSF in pediatric critical care, define the multiple organ failure syndrome, relate the pathophysiology of MOSF to mechanisms of disease presented in Chapters 1 to 3, review diagnostic criteria for pediatric organ-specific system failure, and review present and possible future therapeutic interventions and goals. It is anticipated that as our understanding of the pathophysiologic mechanisms leading to MOSF evolves, we may be able to further subdivide patients with MOSF into entities with distinct metabolic pathologic features and therapeutic goals.

MULTIPLE ORGAN FAILURE SYNDROME

The classic adult progression of MOSF is the sequential failure of the lungs (first 2 to 3 days), liver (7 to 10 days), and kidneys (14 to 21 days)[8, 13] following a defined traumatic inciting event. This clinical constellation is termed the *multiple organ failure syndrome* or *multiple organ dysfunction syndrome*. This particular complex of injury, pulmonary dysfunction, and hypermetabolism leads to sequential organ failure over a 14- to 21-day time course and ultimately results in death.[1, 2, 8, 13-15, 33-35] As the syndrome progresses from single to multiorgan involvement, the risk of mortality increases from 25 to 80%.[5, 17, 22-24] The multiple organ failure syndrome has not been well characterized in the pediatric population partly because fewer numbers of patients with multiorgan involvement are identified and partly because the resiliency of organ systems among pediatric patients complicates the definition of true age-specific organ system failure.

PATHOPHYSIOLOGY OVERVIEW

The development of MOSF results from dysfunctional compensatory pathophysiologic processes, as well as amplification of inflammatory and immune cascades. As MOSF progresses, maldistribution of circulating volume occurs, resulting in imbalance of tissue oxygen supply and demand. Metabolic derangements become prominent. The maldistribution of circulating volume may evolve as the hyperdynamic phase of disease progresses and cellular energy stores become exhausted.[1, 3, 6, 8, 36–40] When the kidneys fail, volume overload may ensue, and inadequate cardiac output may induce systemic vasoconstriction. Sustained sympathetic nervous system activation or infusion of vasopressors may further exacerbate this problem, and specific mediators (e.g., thromboxane A_2, platelet-activating factor) may further induce pulmonary artery hypertension and right ventricular failure. Decreased cardiac output and reserve may result from the production of myocardial depressant factor,[41] ischemic myocardium, acidosis, and the use of positive end-expiratory pressure. Capillary leak often develops as endothelium is damaged by thrombosis, disseminated intravascular coagulopathy, and prothrombotic mediators.[2, 7, 33, 42–47] An imbalance in oxygen supply and demand results. When the failing circulatory system is unable to supply adequate oxygen to the tissues, the tissue metabolic needs are not met. It has been proposed that tissue metabolism may be altered and unable to use available substrates in a normal manner.[34, 36–38, 40, 48] Metabolic derangements then result as energy depletion occurs. Cellular damage becomes permanent. Cell death may evolve from lack of substrate, resistance to exogenous administration of substrates, or failure of peripheral metabolism secondary to exhaustion of intracellular energy stores. With cellular death, there is the potential for release of encephalopathic mediators in the peripheral nervous system and the CNS.

The contributions of the inflammatory and immune responses are key in the pathophysiology of MOSF. Multiple organ failure syndrome exemplifies the presumed course of events resulting from a local traumatic or inflammatory event triggering a cascade of platelet activation, endothelial injury, and tissue necrosis, which induces the release of inflammatory mediators, creating a systemic response. As the immune and inflammatory responses are amplified, the patient becomes hypermetabolic and the cell-to-cell interactive components perpetuate the local and systemic responses.[2, 7, 8, 12, 26, 33, 42, 43, 49, 50] Once the cascade has progressed to the point of MOSF, the risk of mortality is extremely high.

The amplification of the systemic response to local injury involves both cellular and protein component function. The critical target cell is the neutrophil, which plays a key role in the inflammatory response, undergoing a respiratory burst during the process of phagocytosis and releasing mediators that propagate the immune response. These mediators include oxygen free radicals, prostaglandins, leukotrienes, interleukins, platelet-activating factors, tissue thromboplastin, and proteases.[2, 7, 8, 25, 29, 43, 44, 47] In the tissue, the macrophage is the first line of defense and the major source of mediator release.[26, 42] Specific tissue macrophages assume different roles based on their location: The alveolar macrophage in the lung functions differently from the Kupffer cells in the liver. Specific macrophages exist for the lung, liver, bone, CNS, subcutaneous tissue, lymph nodes, and spleen. Mediators released by macrophages include tumor necrosis factor, interleukins, prostaglandins, complement, coagulation factors, plasminogen activators, and oxygen free radicals. The lymphocytes are the major cellular component of the lymph nodes and spleen. They are the most important cellular agent in mediating the immune response and amplifying the regulator, stimulator, and suppressor functions of the cellular immune response. T cells may amplify MOSF by direct cytotoxicity, enhancement of B cell activity, activation or suppression of cytoxic cells, or release of mediators that affect the metabolic response of tissues. B cells have an active role in antibody production. Platelets are circulating cellular components that function in both coagulation and regulation of the immune response, which amplifies MOSF. Thrombosis enhances granulocyte aggregation and cytotoxicity and may result in the release of inflammatory mediators, including thromboxane, serotonin, chemotactic factors, and complement activators.

Protein systems are likewise activated. Complement triggers a complex cascade of events that further amplifies the immune response. Small peptides (anaphylatoxins) that result from this amplification may exacerbate multiple organ failure as neutrophil chemotaxis and aggregation are enhanced, production of oxygen free radicals is increased, and proinflammatory products are released.[2, 7, 8, 25, 29, 43, 44, 47] The kallikrein and kinin systems further enhance the immune response and regulate microvascular perfusion. Often the coagulation and fibrinolytic pathways are triggered. Biochemical components that are described in Chapters 2 and 4, including tumor necrosis factor, interleukin-1, arachidonic acid metabolites, and histamine, play immunoregulatory roles that lead to the systemic changes seen in MOSF. MOSF, then, appears to be independent of the cause of the initial trauma or septic episode but instead represents amplification of the inflammatory response with a resultant dysfunctional outcome.

CONTRASTS: ADULT VERSUS PEDIATRIC MULTIPLE ORGAN SYSTEM FAILURE

Pathophysiologic elements that lead to MOSF in children and adults may be similar, but there are some clear differences. Ontologic changes occur in organ systems with age. In infants, the immature immune response and magnitude of immune mediator amplification may be affected by maternal antibody transmission, activity of the lymphatic organs, and developing enzymatic systems. In addition, organs in infants and children may have a "resiliency" attributable to number, type, or composition of cellular components and regenerative capability. Although children with sepsis and MOSF exhibit a systemic mediator response that is similar to that of their adult counterparts,[7, 19, 28, 42–44, 47] it remains to be demonstrated that the local activity and effects of these systemic mediators are similar in pediatric and adult populations.

The prognosis of MOSF in adults with sepsis syndrome and disseminated intravascular coagulation appears closely linked.[5, 8, 17, 18] In children, however, the mortality associated with MOSF and sepsis appears less clearly related.[23, 24] One study of pediatric MOSF showed a 26% mortality rate when two organ systems failed, a 62% mortality rate when three organ systems failed, and an 88% mortality rate when four or more organ systems failed.[4] Although 47% of those patients with MOSF had associated sepsis syndrome, sepsis did not significantly increase mortality rates in the groups with organ system failure. Although sepsis is a major risk factor for MOSF,[5, 9, 17] even in adults, a nonspecific host response to critical illness contributes to the syndrome in at least 35% of patients.[20, 22]

ORGAN INVOLVEMENT—DIAGNOSTIC CRITERIA

Lungs

The lungs present a large surface area of pulmonary endothelium, and cellular damage rapidly leads to vasoconstriction and increased capillary permeability with development of pulmonary edema. Adult respiratory distress syndrome often follows, with characteristic hypoxemia, loss of alveolar integrity, atelectasis, and decreased pulmonary compliance. The ensuing refractory hypoxemia compromises oxygen delivery and offers a seeding ground for pulmonary infection. Damaged pulmonary endothelium activates the previously described cascade of cellular protein and biochemical mediators (Table 15–1).

Liver

The liver has assumed a central role in the study of MOSF. The liver metabolizes carbohydrates, proteins, lipids, vitamins, and iron and detoxifies or modifies numerous drugs, hormones, and toxins. The liver performs circulatory and immune functions in the storage and filtration of blood, in lymph production and processing, in phagocytosis of translocated intestinal bacteria in the portal circulation, and in production of coagulation factors in acute phase reactions. The liver functions in a secretory and excretory role in the production of bile and the metabolism of bilirubin. Because of the liver's diverse functions, diverse blood supply, and proximity to the gastrointestinal tract and lungs, it is perceived to play a central role in the evolution of MOSF.[2, 13, 27, 30, 40, 51, 52] No consensus exists as to whether it is the ischemia, hypoxia, or direct cellular damage by toxins that causes the evolution of MOSF. The specifics of liver metabolic function are presented elsewhere (see Chapter 56). Alterations in the metabolic function of the liver that herald MOSF include alterations of carbohydrate metabolism, glycogen storage, gluconeogenesis, and blood glucose homeostasis.[2, 13, 27, 30, 40, 51, 52] Impaired deamination of amino acids for energy production or conversion of carbohydrate or lipid to energy sources may occur. Ureagenesis to remove ammonia may be impaired, and plasma protein synthesis may decrease. The rate of oxidation of fatty acids for adenosine triphosphate (ATP) production may lead to formation of ketones, and the detoxification capacity of the liver for secretion of drugs, hormones, and toxins may be impaired (see Table 15–1).

Kidneys

The development of renal failure in MOSF is often a late phenomenon that is increasingly attributed to the acute renal tubular dysfunction caused by hypoperfusion, immune mediators, antibiotics, vasopressor therapy, and immune complex deposition. Failure of renal function includes alterations in the following: hematopoiesis, acid-base regulation, urea clearance, electrolyte balance, and chemical detoxification. Although renal function is vitally important and renal failure complicates the management of the critically ill pediatric patient, children do not die primarily of renal disease.

Table 15–1. CRITERIA FOR FAILURE OF SPECIFIC PEDIATRIC ORGAN SYSTEMS*

Organ System	Criteria
Cardiovascular	MAP† <40 mm Hg (infants <12 mo)
	MAP <50 mm Hg (children ≥12 mo)
	HR‡ <50 beats/min (infants <12 mo)
	HR <40 beats/min (children ≥12 mo)
	Cardiac arrest
	Continuous vasoactive drug infusion for hemodynamic support
Respiratory	§RR >90/min (infants < 12mo)
	RR >70 /min (children ≥12 mo)
	PaO_2 <40 mm Hg (in absence of cyanotic heart disease)
	$PaCO_2$ >65 mm Hg
	PaO_2/FiO_2 <250 mm Hg
	Mechanical ventilation (>24 hr if postoperative)
	Tracheal intubation for airway obstruction or acute respiratory failure
Neurologic	Glasgow Coma Scale <5
	Fixed, dilated pupils
	Persistent (>20 min) intracranial pressure >20 mm Hg or requiring therapeutic intervention
Hematologic	Hemoglobin <5 g/dl
	WBC <3,000 cells/mm³
	Platelets <20,000/mm³
	Disseminated intravascular coagulopathy (PT‖ >20 sec or aPTT** >60 sec in presence of positive FSP†† assay)
Renal	BUN >100 mg/dl
	Serum creatinine >2 mg/dl
	Dialysis
Gastrointestinal	Blood transfusions >20 ml/kg in 24 hr because of GI hemorrhage (endoscopic confirmation optional)
Hepatic	Total bilirubin >5 mg/dl and SGOT‡‡ or LDH§§ more than twice normal value (without evidence of hemolysis)
	Hepatic encephalopathy ≥ grade II

*From Wilkinson JD, Pollack MM, Glass NL, et al: Mortality associated with multiple organ system failure and sepsis in pediatric intensive care unit. J Pediatr 111:324, 1987.
†MAP = mean arterial pressure.
‡HR = heart rate.
§RR = respiratory rate.
‖PT = prothrombin time.
**aPTT = activated partial thromboplastin time.
††FSP = fibrin split products.
‡‡SGOT = serum glutamate-oxalate transaminase
§§LDH = lactic dehydrogenase.

Renal replacement therapy in the modern intensive care unit setting can adequately replace the metabolic and excretory functions of the kidneys. The failure of the renal organ system often simply reflects the severity of the underlying disease (see Table 15–1).

Cardiovascular System

A perfusion deficit from cardiovascular failure is discussed in detail elsewhere (see Chapters 30 and 31). Whether primary cardiovascular failure leads to organ damage or whether cardiovascular failure is a reflection of ongoing regional organ damage already occurring in the periphery is controversial. The myocardium itself is sensitive to specific mediators of ischemia, depressant factors, and acidosis. Dysfunctional compensation for inadequate cardiac output with intractable vasoconstriction can lead to a progressive low cardiac output state.

Infants and children rarely present with clinical evidence of cardiac failure by the adult criteria of ventricular tachycardia or fibrillation, a cardiac index of less than 2 l/min/m^2, or increased cardiac isoenzyme levels. Cardiovascular pressor support must be based on receptor ontogeny, as the density and affinity of inotrope receptors and amounts of neurotransmitter stores vary with age (see Table 15–1).

Central Nervous System

MOSF affecting the CNS usually involves a decrease in both the cerebral blood flow[53] and the effects of mediators on CNS endothelium. Damage may result directly from ischemia or from the indirect release of toxic mediators, such as false neurotransmitters, endogenous opioids, oxygen free radicals, or arachidonic acid metabolites.[3, 8] Hepatic failure may contribute to this process. Children with MOSF involving the CNS frequently exhibit temperature instability, alterations in vascular tone, and vagal fluctuations in blood pressure and heart rate. Vagal influence in infants and children appears more prominent than in older patients. Criteria for CNS failure based on clinical scoring systems are less well defined in children (and certainly in neonates) than in adults (see Table 15–1).

Gastrointestinal Tract

The gastrointestinal tract is very sensitive to ischemic injury and sustains a high metabolic rate. As the mucosal integrity of the gut is damaged during ischemia, ulceration and necrosis of the bowel wall occur.[2, 13, 27, 30, 40, 51, 52] Gastrointestinal bleeding may exacerbate this process, and treatment with antibiotics may allow overgrowth of certain pathogenic bacterial species. It has been proposed that bacterial translocation through an injured gut wall may play an integral role in the induction of sepsis and the association with MOSF.[2, 10, 30] Both endocrine and exocrine organs of the gastrointestinal system, including the pancreas, may be severely affected.[41] Endocrine hormones, such as insulin and glucogen, that affect metabolism and cardiovascular function may be altered. Release of lysosomal enzymes may cause extensive local tissue damage. As organs such as the pancreas are damaged, the precise feedback control mechanisms for carbohydrate regulation and intestinal function may be lost. Numerous factors that may play a role in the development of multisystem involvement, including myocardial depressant factor, may be released. Characteristic changes in serum amino acid profiles occur over time, and hypertriglyceridemia becomes prominent.[8, 36, 40] Criteria for failure of the gastrointestinal tract are nonspecific in the pediatric age group (see Table 15–1).

Hematologic-Immune System

The hematologic and immune systems are affected in both decreased production of cellular components in the bone marrow and spleen and increased consumption by sustained immune stimulation (disseminated intravascular coagulopathy is often a prominent feature). The hematologic system also serves as a vehicle for soluble factors and mediators of MOSF to be distributed to distant tissue and organ beds. Pediatric hematologic-immune system failure criteria do not differ significantly from the adult criteria (see Table 15–1).

THERAPEUTIC INTERVENTIONS AND GOALS: SUPPORT, MONITORING, AND SPECIFIC THERAPEUTIC INTERVENTION

MOSF appears to result from dysfunctional cellular interactions among organs perpetuated by inflammatory cascades that create imbalances in substrate delivery and utilization. Early identification and supportive care of those patients at risk for MOSF and intervention to block the progression of single-organ system failure to MOSF remain the principal precepts of caring for the critically ill patient. Therapeutic management of MOSF hinges on the same goals as those for severe sepsis and septic shock in the pediatric age group (see also Chapter 12). Supportive care with close attention to the prevention of nosocomial infections and adequate oxygen delivery to meet tissue oxygen demand is critical. As MOSF progresses, hemodynamic monitoring, including oxygen delivery and utilization data, is often helpful to ensure that oxygen delivery is meeting metabolic demands.[21, 26, 34, 54–57] Unfortunately, state of the art monitoring gives only a gross measure of total body oxygen delivery and consumption, and much current work focuses on more organ-specific and tissue-specific metabolic energy markers. The value of continuous metabolic monitoring, meaningful organ-specific lactate analysis, serum amino acid analysis, and analysis of mediator levels is not clear, but these measures are increasingly employed in many institutions. The limitations of most monitoring systems are (1) the information is sporadic as opposed to continuous, (2) measures are generally those of serum or plasma as opposed to tissue levels, and (3) measurements lack standards, particularly in the pediatric age group.

Methods of resuscitation and restoration of the balance of oxygen supply and demand are currently the focus of therapeutic intervention. Increasing oxygen supply until the global oxygen demand plateaus and systemic assays of cellular utilization improve is the principle applied. Nutritional and metabolic support is fastidiously provided, which becomes increasingly complicated as liver failure becomes more prominent.[36, 37, 40] Reversal of acidosis and a supply of energy-rich substrates to reduce autocannibalism are used. To date, manipulation of the amino acid composition of hyperalimentation formulas (most notably branched chain amino acids) has great theoretical potential but has not demonstrated significant decreases in MOSF mortality. Supplementation with alternative sources of fatty acids is being explored (see also Chapter 14).

THERAPEUTIC TRENDS FOR THE FUTURE

Immune Modulation

Immune and inflammatory response modulation by the infusion of protective cytokines or monoclonal antibodies to destructive cytokines is under study. Modulation of both specific and nonspecific arachidonic acid metabolite levels by infusion of prostaglandins, platelet-activating factors, and nutritional immunomodulation offer areas for future research. Efforts at gastrointestinal decontamination to decrease the likelihood of bacterial translocation through the gastrointestinal tract also hold promise.[7, 27, 30] Extracorporeal therapy aimed at filtration or adsorption of toxic and systemic mediators of MOSF may similarly alter systemic levels of these "toxins."[31, 58] Infusion of opsonins[59] (e.g., fibronectin) may also have a global effect. Clearly the explosion of information on mediators of sepsis in recent years and the characterization of many of the mediators that appear to play a role in the translation of local inflammatory responses to systemic inflammatory responses will play a prominent role in therapeutic trends for MOSF in the future.

Flow Distribution

Optimizing blood flow distribution theoretically decreases the incidence of multiorgan system involvement by decreasing the amount of tissue hypoxia and ischemia. Proposed modalities include hyperosmolar-hyperoncotic solutions, in which hypertonic solutions might minimize interstitial and intracellular edema by drawing fluid into the extracellular spaces of the vasculature.[60] Artificial hemoglobins might similarly provide improved oxygen-carrying capacity and systemic oxygen delivery to meet increased metabolic demands. Selective nutritional energy sources that would minimize autocannibalism, amino acid flux, and ureagenesis may further improve flow distribution. β-Endorphin antagonists (nal-

oxone) and steroids may experimentally improve the peripheral response to adrenergic stimulation.[51, 50] Further experimental studies and clinical trials are evolving along these lines. New cardiovascular agents, inotropes, vasodilators, and combinations of these agents may not only improve cardiovascular function but may also improve microvascular tissue blood flow. Pharmacologic agents such as pentoxifylline[61] may serve to decrease the blood viscosity, improving microvascular flow and altering adherence of activated white blood cells to vascular endothelium in order to block release of toxic mediators of MOSF.[54, 62, 63] In the future, improved monitoring and assessment techniques for assaying microvascular blood flow (e.g., laser Doppler velocimetry, tissue PO_2 and pH assays, continuous magnetic resonance imaging of organ beds) may improve our ability to assay oxygen delivery and consumption needs. Improved mechanisms of delivering substrates to tissue when single organ systems fail (extracorporeal methods, including extracorporeal membrane oxygenation [ECMO] and intravenous oxygenation [IVOX] and extracorporeal CO_2 removal [ECCOR]) may in the future be used at an earlier time.[8, 54, 56, 58, 63]

Improvement of Tissue Energy Metabolism

Another focus of future studies will be the infusion of substrates aimed at improving cellular energy production. Following shock, ischemia, and reperfusion, decreases in cellular ATP stores, tissue and mitochondrial magnesium levels, and impaired mitochondrial function have been documented experimentally.[6, 8, 51] The administration of the substrate $ATP-MgCl_2$ complex may improve microcirculatory blood flow, tissue and mitochondrial magnesium levels, tissue ATP stores, and cellular metabolic function.[51] Oxygen free radical scavengers, such as xanthine oxidase inhibitors, mannitol, and vitamin E, may block or prevent cellular damage from hypoxia.[8] Calcium flux alteration using calcium channel blockers or G protein genetic modulation may emerge as a viable option. New buffers of acidosis (e.g., dichloroacetate) that may improve tissue perfusion without generating paradoxic intracellular acidosis may be increasingly used.[64] Hormonal modulation (e.g., granulocyte-monocyte colony stimulating factors, growth hormone, thyrotropin-releasing factor) may be utilized to stimulate and improve wound healing and alter metabolic responses to multiple organ failure.

It is important to realize that each of these therapeutic modalities has theoretical benefit for halting the progression of MOSF but that each is in the early developmental stages and has *not* been shown to alter the course of MOSF once initiated. It is increasingly evident that no single treatment modality will serve to treat or prevent all forms of MOSF but that a combination of modalities will need to be employed in order to have significant impact on the outcome of MOSF.

SUMMARY

In summary, MOSF in pediatric critical care remains a condition associated with extremely high morbidity and mortality. MOSF is currently a marker for the severity of the underlying illness and reflects a condition in which multiple organ systems contribute to inadequate substrate perfusion of vitally important organs, and unmet metabolic demands perpetuate a vicious cycle, which frequently leads to death. As our understanding of MOSF progresses and our ability to define the metabolic and hormonal mediator patterns that control cellular metabolism at the cellular and subcellular levels increases, we are likely to categorize the MOSF syndromes into a series of subgroupings and develop successful specific therapeutic interventions.

References

1. Borzatta A and Polk H: Multiple system organ failure. Surg Clin North Am 63(2):315, 1983.
2. Cerra FB and Bihari D: Multiple organ failure: Critical care, state of the art. Soc Crit Care Med 3:1–397, 1989.
3. Astiz M, Rackow EC, Weil MH, et al: Early impairment of oxidative metabolism and energy production in severe sepsis. Circ Shock 26(3):311, 1988.
4. Bersten A and Sibbald WJ: Circulatory disturbances in multiple systems organ failure. Crit Care Clin 5(2):233, 1989.
5. Knaus WA, Draper EA, Wagner DP, et al: Prognosis in acute organ-system failure. Ann Surg 202(6):685, 1985.
6. Cerra FB: Hypermetabolism-organ failure syndrome: A metabolic response to injury. Crit Care Clin 5(2):289, 1989.
7. Demling RH: Wound inflammatory mediators and multisystem organ failure. Prog Clin Biol Res 236A:525, 1987.
8. Huddleston VB: Multisystem organ failure: A pathophysiologic approach. Presentation, Barbara Clark Mims Associates, 1989.
9. Lehmkuhl P, Schultz A, and Gebert J: Risk factors of the multiple organ failure syndrome. Prog Clin Biol Res 308:643, 1989.
10. Nuytinck JK and Goris RJ: Pathophysiology of the adult respiratory distress syndrome and multiple organ failure—a hypothesis. Neth J Surg 37(5):131, 1985.
11. Pinsky MR: Multiple systems organ failure: Malignant intravascular inflammation. Crit Care Clin 5(2):195, 1989.
12. Pinsky MR and Matuschak GM: Multiple systems organ failure: Failure of host defense homeostasis. Crit Care Clin 5(2):199, 1989.
13. Barton R and Cerra F: The hypermetabolism-multiple organ failure syndrome. Chest 96(5):1153, 1989.
14. Fry DE: Multiple system organ failure. Surg Clin North Am 68(1):107, 1988.
15. Schuster HP: Multisystem organ failure. Prog Clin Biol Res 236A:459, 1989.
16. Shen PF and Zhang SC: Acute renal failure and multiple organ system failure. Arch Surg 122(100):1131, 1987.
17. Knaus WA and Wagner DP: Multiple systems organ failure: Epidemiology and prognosis. Crit Care Clin 5(2):221, 1989.
18. Balk RA and Bone RC: The Septic syndrome: Definition and clinical implications. Crit Care Clin 15(1):1, 1989.
19. Brandtzaeg P, Kierulf P, Gaustad P, et al: Plasma endotoxin as a predictor of multiple organ failure and death in systemic meningococcal disease. J Infect Dis 159(2):195, 1989.
20. Darling GE, Duff JH, Mustard RA, et al: Multiorgan failure in critically ill patients. Can J Surg 31(3):172, 1988.
21. Russell JA, Ronco JJ, Lockhat D, et al: Oxygen delivery and consumption and ventricular preload are greater in survivors than in nonsurvivors in the adult respiratory distress syndrome. Am Rev Respir Dis 141(3):659, 1990.
22. Tran DD, Groeneveld AB, van der Meulen J, et al: Age, chronic disease, sepsis, organ system failure, and mortality in a medical intensive care unit. Crit Care Med 18(5):474, 1990.
23. Wilkinson JD, Pollack MM, Glass NL, et al: Mortality associated with multiple organ system failure and sepsis in a pediatric intensive care unit. J Pediatr 111(3):324, 1987.
24. Wilkinson JD, Pollack MM, Ruttimann UE, et al: Outcome of pediatric patients with multiple organ system failure. Crit Care Med 14(4):271, 1986.
25. Border JR: Hypothesis: Sepsis, multiple systems organ failure, and the macrophage. Arch Surg 123(3):285, 1988.
26. Parker MM, Parillo JE. Septic Shock: Hemodynamics and pathogenesis. JAMA 250(24):3324, 1983.
27. Marshall JC, Christou NV, Horn R, et al: The microbiology of multiple organ failure. The proximal gastrointestinal tract as an occult reservoir of pathogens. Arch Surg 123(3):309, 1988.
28. Hervas JA, Lopez P, de la Fuente A, et al: Multiple organ system failure in an infant with *Legionella* infection. Pediatr Infect Dis J 7(9):671, 1988.
29. Heideman M and Hugli TE: Anaphylatoxin generation in multisystem organ failure. J Trauma 24(12):1038, 1984.
30. Border JR, Hassett J, LaDuca J, et al: The gut origin septic states in blunt multiple trauma in the ICU. Ann Surg 206(4):427, 1987.
31. Zobel G, Trop M, Ring E, et al: Arteriovenous hemofiltration in children with multiple organ system failure. Int J Artif Organ 10(4):233, 1987.
32. Price HL and Matthew DJ: Evaluation of pediatric intensive care scoring systems. Intensive Care Med 15(2):79, 1989.
33. Hyers TM, Gee M, and Andreadis NA: Cellular interactions in the multiple organ injury syndrome. Am Rev Respir Dis 135(4):952, 1987.
34. Siegel JH: Cardiorespiratory manifestations of metabolic failure in sepsis and the multiple organ failure syndrome. Surg Clin North Am 63:379, 1983.
35. Barlett RH, Morris AH, Fairley HB, et al: A prospective study of acute hypoxic respiratory failure. Chest 78(5):684, 1986.
36. Cerra FB: Hypermetabolism, organ failure, and metabolic support. Surgery 101(1):1, 1987.
37. Gutierrez G, Lund N, and Bryan-Brown CW: Cellular oxygen utilization during multiple organ failure. Crit Care Clin 5(2):271, 1989.
38. Ozawa K, Aoyama H, Yasuda K, et al: Metabolic abnormalities associated with postoperative organ failure: A redox theory. Arch Surg 118(110):1245, 1983.
39. Ozawa K: Biological significance of mitochondrial redox potential in shock and multiple organ failure—redox theory. Prog Clin Biol Res 111:39, 1983.
40. Pittiruti M, Siegel JH, Sanga G, et al: Increased dependence of leucine in posttraumatic sepsis: Leucine/tyrosine clearance ratio as an indicator of hepatic impairment in septic multiple organ failure syndrome. Surgery 98(3):378, 1985.
41. Lefer AM: Role of a myocardial depressant factor in the pathogenesis of circulatory shock. Fed Proc Am Phys Soc 29:1836, 1970.
42. Vedder NB, Winn RK, Rice CL, et al: Neutrophil-mediated vascular injury in shock and multiple organ failure. Prog Clin Biol Res 16(2):111, 1989.
43. Petrak RA, Balk RA, and Bone RC: Prostaglandins, cyclooxygenase inhibitors, and thromboxane synthetase inhibitors in the pathogenesis of multiple systems organ failure. Crit Care Clin 5(2):302, 1989.
44. Beutler B: Cachectin in tissue injury, shock, and related states. Crit Care Clin 5(2):353, 1989.
45. Bihari DJ and Tinker J: The therapeutic value of vasodilator prostaglandins in multiple organ failure associated with sepsis. Intensive Care Med 15(1):2, 1988.
46. Sprague RS, Stephenson AH, Dahms TE, et al: Proposed role for leukotrienes in the pathophysiology of multiple systems organ failure. Crit Care Clin 5(2):315, 1989.
47. Tracey KJ and Cerami A: Cachectin/tumor necrosis factor and other cytokines in infectious disease. Curr Opin Immunol 1(3):454, 1989.
48. Nasraway SA, Rackow EC, Astiz ME, et al: Inotropic response to digoxin and dopamine in patients with severe sepsis, cardiac failure, and systemic hypoperfusion. Chest 95(3):612, 1989.
49. Roth BL, Nielson TB, and McKee AE (eds): Molecular and Cellular Mechanisms of Septic Shock. New York, John Wiley, 1988.
50. Cerra FB, West M, Keller G, et al: Hypermetabolism/organ failure: The role of the activated macrophage as a metabolic regulator. Prog Clin Biol Res 264:27, 1988.
51. Chaudry IH: ATP-MgCl₂ and liver blood flow following shock and ischemia. Prog Clin Biol Res 299:19, 1989.

52. Schwartz DB, Bone RC, Balk RA, et al: Hepatic dysfunction in the adult respiratory distress syndrome. Chest 95(4):871, 1989.
53. Bowton JL, Bertels NH, Prough DS, et al: Cerebral blood flow is reduced in patients with sepsis syndrome. Crit Care Med 17(5):399, 1989.
54. Macho JR and Luce JM: Rational approach of the management of multiple systems organ failure. Crit Care Clin 5(2):379, 1989.
55. Papile LA: The management of hypoxic-ischemic encephalopathy. Pediatr Ann 17(8):524, 1988.
56. Sheagren JN: Mechanism-oriented therapy for multiple systems organ failure. Crit Care Clin 5(2):393, 1989.
57. Vincent J and De Backer D: Initial management of circulatory shock as prevention of MSOF. Crit Care Clin 5(2):369, 1989.
58. DiCarlo JV, Dudley TE, Sherbotie JR, et al: Continuous arterio-venous hemofiltration improves pulmonary gas exchange in children with multiple organ failure. Crit Care Med 18:822, 1990.
59. Grossman JE: Clinical use of fibronectin in critically ill patients. Prog Clin Biol Res 299:157, 1989.
60. Kramer GC, English TP, Gunther RA, et al: Physiologic mechanisms of fluid resuscitation with hyperosmotic/hyperoncotic solutions. Prog Clin Biol Res 299:311, 1989.
61. Schonharting MM and Schade UF: The effect of pentoxifylline in septic shock—new pharmacologic aspects of an established drug. J Med 20(1):97, 1989.
62. Machiedo GW, Powell RJ, Rush BF, et al: The incidence of decreased red blood cell deformability in sepsis and the association with oxygen free radical damage and multiple-system organ failure. Arch Surg 124(12):1386, 1989.
63. Borelli M, Kolobow T, Spatola R, et al: Severe acute respiratory failure managed with continuous positive airway pressure and partial extracorporeal carbon dioxide removal by an artificial membrane lung. Am Rev Respir Dis 138(6):1480, 1988.
64. Stacpoole PW, Harman EM, Curry SH, et al: Treatment of lactic acidosis with dichloroacetate. N Engl J Med 309(7):390, 1983.

IV Organ System Failure

Central Nervous System

16

Central Nervous System Evaluation and Monitoring

Ido Yatsiv, M.D.

Several groups of patients present to pediatric critical care units with pathologic conditions of the central nervous system (CNS). These individuals require evaluation and monitoring. These groups include patients with (1) head trauma, (2) multiple trauma with head or spine involvement, (3) infections of the CNS, and (4) hypoxic-ischemic and metabolic encephalopathies, as well as (5) postoperative neurosurgical patients. Commonly, these patients are acutely ill, have unstable physiologic parameters, and need continuous monitoring both at the cardiopulmonary level and at a more specific neurologic level.

Effective monitoring of patients with CNS illness or injuries dictates a certain setting and equipment, as well as specifically trained medical personnel.

This chapter reviews the clinical approach to the pediatric patient with CNS involvement who presents to the intensive care unit (ICU), with an emphasis on the approach to patients with altered mental status. This will be followed by a review of various monitoring devices, including intracranial pressure (ICP) monitoring systems and electrophysiologic monitoring.

EVALUATION OF THE PEDIATRIC NEUROSURGICAL PATIENT

The initial evaluation of the pediatric patient in the ICU begins with a complete history. Patients admitted following planned surgery and some patients who arrive through the emergency department have a reliable and useful history. Relevant points in the history include exact timing of events, estimated velocity in the case of car accidents, immediate neurologic response, seizure activity, and a review of the transport. However, many patients arrive with altered mental status and without a known medical background, posing a special diagnostic problem. In this section, we delineate the approach to the child with altered mental status and follow that with a discussion of neurologic scoring systems.

Physical Examination of the Child with Altered Mental State

An altered mental state can originate from a pathologic process in one of two neuroanatomic structures: (1) a lesion involving *both* cerebral hemispheres, such as hypoxic-ischemic encephalopathy (HIE), an acute intoxication, or a metabolic disorder or (2) a lesion involving the reticular formation, which is a brain stem structure involved in the preservation of consciousness. In order to define a change in mental status and localize its origin to one of these two areas, five features of the physical examination need to be assessed: (1) degree of altered mental status, (2) pattern of respirations, (3) pupillary response, (4) extraocular movements (caloric testing, doll's eye reflex), and (5) the motor examination.[1]

Degree of Altered Mental Status

In order to use common terminology and enable comparisons among studies, the following terms are accepted:

1. An *awake* person is alert without needing any external stimuli; however, the patient can be either coherent or demented.
2. A *lethargic* patient seems to be asleep but can be aroused to an awake state with verbal or mild physical stimuli. When awakened, he or she inter-

acts in some way with the examiner, but when left alone he or she quickly drifts back to the original sleep state.

3. A *stuporous* patient does not become fully awake even in the face of strong stimuli; however such a patient does respond, either by withdrawing from pain or by moaning.

4. The truly *comatose* patient does not have any purposeful movements in response to stimulation of any magnitude.

Respiratory Pattern

An assessment of the respiratory pattern can help localize the region accountable for the change in consciousness.

1. *Cheyne-Stokes respiration:* A bilateral hemispheric involvement (such as drug ingestion, hypoxia, or a metabolic factor) can result in Cheyne-Stokes breathing. In this disturbance, the breathing rate gradually increases and deepens to a peak of hyperventilation followed by a gradual decrease all the way to a short apneic period.

2. *Central neurogenic hyperventilation:* This pattern, which results from a lesion in the midbrain, is characterized by a rapid rate unexplained by a basic metabolic derangement. This diagnosis depends on the exclusion of any metabolic cause for acidosis.

3. *Apneustic breathing:* This pattern results from a pontine lesion and is manifested by a very long inspiratory phase followed by a short exhalation.

4. *Cluster breathing:* Low pontine and high medullary lesions sometimes result in this pattern, in which clusters of breaths may follow each other with irregular intervals between them.

5. *Ataxic breathing:* Lesions in the medulla result in this breathing pattern, which is completely irregular. It is frequently insufficient for adequate oxygenation and is reason to perform intubation and artificial ventilation (Fig. 16–1).

Pupillary Response

Although many of the metabolic diseases cause a mental change through their influence on both cortical hemispheres, they do not induce a pupillary effect. However, many drug ingestions do, and a short list has been composed by James (Table 16–1).[2]

Midbrain lesions typically present with pupillary dilatation, usually via pressure on the third cranial nerve or its nucleus. This explains the pupillary manifestations of cerebral herniation following increased ICP, resulting in dilated, nonresponsive pupils.

Pontine lesions result in very constricted ("pinpoint") pupils. The exact neuroanatomic reason for this remains unclear. Medullary lesions seldom manifest any change in pupillary size or function (Fig. 16–2).

Extraocular Movements

In order to have appropriate conjugate eye movements in response to vestibular stimulation, large seg-

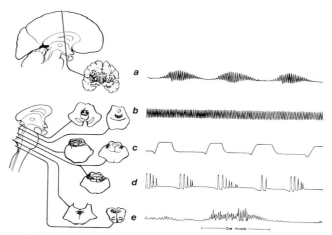

Figure 16–1. Abnormal respiratory patterns associated with pathologic lesions (*shaded areas*) at various levels of the brain. Tracings by chest-abdomen pneumograph inspiration read up. *a,* Cheyne-Stokes respiration. *b,* Central neurogenic hyperventilation. *c,* Apneusis. *d,* Cluster breathing. *e,* Ataxic breathing. (From Plum F and Posner JB: The Diagnosis of Stupor and Coma, 3rd ed. Philadelphia, FA Davis, 1980.)

ments of the brain stem—that is, midbrain, pons, and medulla—must be intact. Stimulation of the vestibular system involves the eighth cranial nerve (medulla), which is connected to the paramedian pontine reticular formation. The latter is the part of the reticular formation responsible for the coordination of lateral conjugated gaze and is located in the pons by the sixth nerve nucleus. The synchronized symmetric movement of the eyes also requires a connection between the third and sixth nuclei, a link accomplished by the medial longitudinal fasciculus, which is a tract running from the pons to the midbrain.

In order to elicit the *vestibulo-ocular reflex* (caloric reflex), ice water is injected into one of the ear canals, thus inactivating the vestibular system on that side. Since the contralateral vestibular system remains active, this maneuver results in driving the eyes *toward* the side that has had the ice water injection. A normal caloric reflex implies an essentially intact and well-functioning brain stem.

Since the reticular formation is a brain stem component that is crucial to intact consciousness, a lesion there

Table 16–1. INTOXICATIONS AND PUPILLARY EXAMINATION IN COMA*

Mydriasis	Miosis
Amphetamines	Barbiturates
Antihistamines	Opiates
Atropine	Propoxyphene
Cocaine	Meperidine
Ephedrine	Methadone
Ethyl alcohol	Carbon monoxide
Glutethimide	Organophosphates
	Thallium

*From James HE: Therapy-directed diagnosis in coma. *In*: James HE, Anas NG, and Perkin RM (eds): Brain Insults in Infants and Children: Pathophysiology and Management. Orlando, Grune & Stratton, 1985, p. 170.

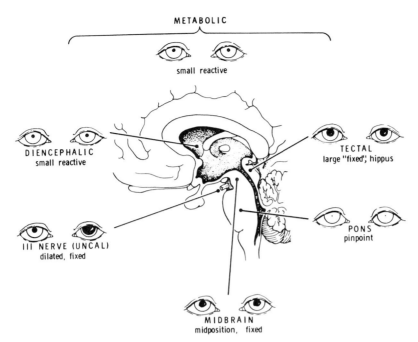

Figure 16–2. Pupils in comatose patients. (From Plum F, Posner JB: The Diagnosis of Stupor and Coma, 3rd ed. Philadelphia, FA Davis, 1980.)

would cause impaired consciousness, as well as an abnormal caloric response.

Another reflex that depends on the same neural tracts is the *oculocephalic reflex,* also known as the *doll's eye reflex.* This should be assessed *only* after the cervical spine has been deemed intact. This reflex produces a typical eye response to head movements in a comatose patient with an intact brain stem. In order to invoke this reflex, the head has to be moved either horizontally or vertically while the eyes are kept open. When the reflex is normal, the eyes move contralaterally to the head's direction, as if fixated on a constant point in space. A normal reflex implies that the brain stem is *not* the cause of impaired consciousness. Brain stem involvement results in an abnormal reflex, leaving the eyes "fixed" in the orbits and moving concomitantly with the head (Fig. 16–3).

Motor Examination

The motor examination reflects the function of the motor cortex, the pyramidal tracts, and some thalamic nuclei. It is not related to consciousness but can contribute to localization of the lesion in two aspects: focalization and posturing.

A focal lesion along the pyramidal tracts can be localized by observing asymmetric spontaneous or invoked movements and abnormal (hyperactive or diminished) deep tendon reflexes.

Stuporous patients can respond to noxious stimuli with a stereotyped motor response, which is defined as posturing. The relevant types of posturing in the critical care context are *decorticate* and *decerebrate.*

Decorticate posturing is typified by *extension* of the legs and *flexion* of all the joints in the arms in response to pain. This response points to a lesion above the red nucleus (the middle part of the midbrain).

Decerebrate posturing is characterized by *extension* of the legs as well, but the arms *extend and rotate internally.* Such a response to pain is a result of a lesion in the lower brain stem, below the red nucleus down to the top of the medulla (Fig. 16–4).

Glasgow Coma Score

Neurologic scoring systems were developed soon after the evolution of intensive care units. Scoring systems quantify injuries or disease states according to a certain scale, with the goal of being able to compare the degree of disease acuity, indicate thresholds for treatments and monitoring decisions, and predict outcome.

The most commonly used scoring scale is the Glasgow Coma Score (GCS).[3] The scale was developed from data collected from adult patients with head injuries and consists of ascribing points to certain patient behaviors in three fields: (1) eye opening, (2) verbal response, and (3) motor response to stimuli (Table 16–2).

The GCS is simple to employ and does not require an extensive knowledge of physical examination or neurologic procedures. This causes it to be remarkably reproducible, it can be used by nonphysicians, and it is very practical in the acute setting, both in the field and in the emergency room. Most critical care units use it as an addition to charting of vital signs in the appropriate patients, thus adding another component to monitoring the neurologic status.

Although it was developed from observations in adults with head injuries, the GCS has been widely used in pediatrics. Some adjustments have been made in infants and toddlers to cope with differences in verbal responses, and thus under the verbal response part of the GCS, "oriented" is exchanged for "cooing or babbling" and "confused" is exchanged for "irritable cries."[4] Other

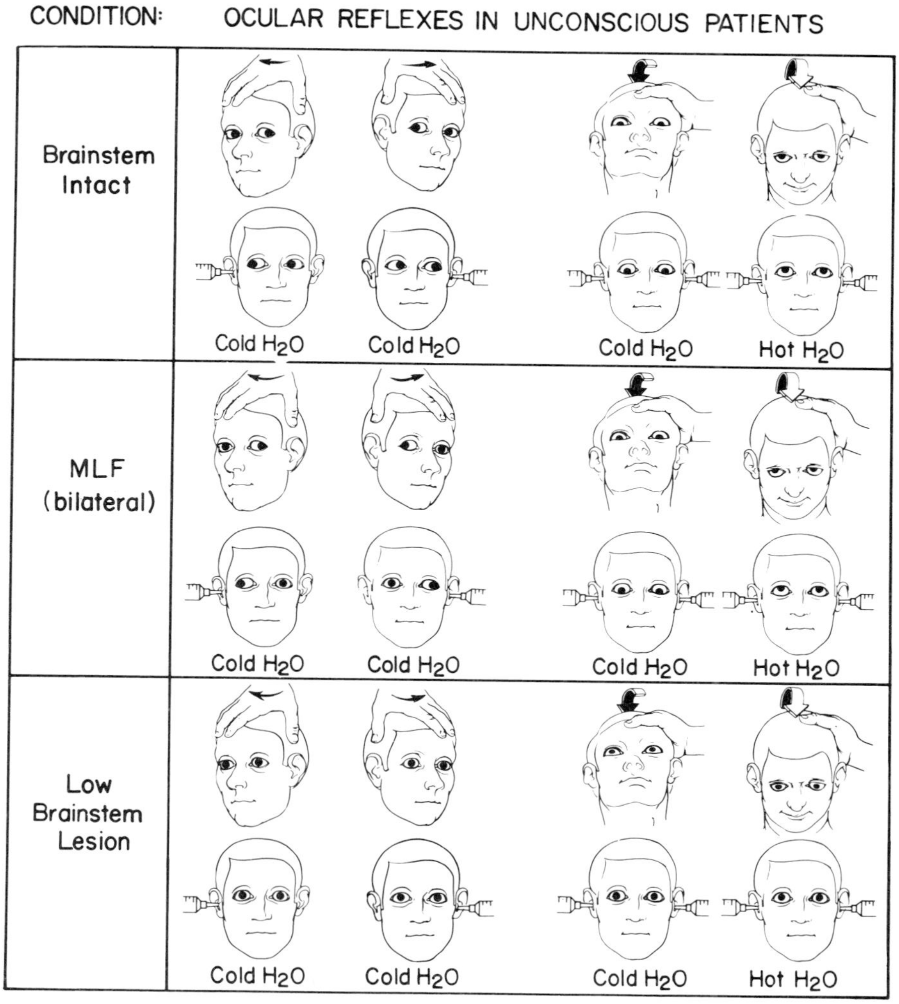

CONDITION: OCULAR REFLEXES IN UNCONSCIOUS PATIENTS

Figure 16–3. Ocular reflexes in unconscious patients. The top row in each compartment illustrates the oculocephalic reflex, and the lower row shows the oculovestibular reflex. The upper compartment reflects the responses when the brain stem tracts are intact. The middle compartment corresponds with bilateral MLF lesions, and the lower compartment exhibits the effects of a low brain stem lesion (see text). (From Plum F and Posner JB: The Diagnosis of Stupor and Coma, 3rd ed. Philadelphia, FA Davis, 1980.)

neurologic scoring systems have been developed, but they are not as widely used and commonly accepted as the GCS.

MONITORING OF INCREASED INTRACRANIAL PRESSURE

Increased ICP is the common denominator in many pediatric patients with CNS involvement in the ICU. Increased ICP and the resultant drop in cerebral blood flow are thought to be major factors in morbidity and mortality in these patients. Therefore measurement, recording, and aggressive treatment of elevated ICP are the cornerstones of neurologic critical care.

At the beginning of the 19th century, Monro and Kellie proposed the fundamental concept of the skull as a closed cavity containing three minimally compressible compartments: (1) neural tissue composing 80 to 90% of the intracranial volume, (2) circulating cerebrospinal fluid (CSF) composing 5 to 10% of the intracranial volume, and the cerebral vascular bed composing 5 to 10% of this volume. Addition of volume to the intracranial space results in an immediate increase in the ICP unless a parallel decrease in one of the compartments

can be achieved. Since neural tissue is not able to contract under normal (nonedematous) conditions, reduction in the CSF volume or a drop in the cerebral blood volume is the only way to maintain normal ICP, as is discussed in detail in Chapter 17.

Table 16–2. Glasgow Coma Score*

Activity	Best Response	Score
Eye opening	Spontaneous	4
	To verbal stimuli	3
	To pain	2
	None	1
Verbal	Oriented	5
	Confused	4
	Inappropriate words	3
	Nonspecific sounds	2
	None	1
Motor	Follows commands	6
	Localizes pain	5
	Withdraws in response to pain	4
	Flexion in response to pain	3
	Extension in response to pain	2
	None	1

*From Teasdale G and Jennett B: Assessment of coma and impaired consciousness: A practical side. Lancet 2:81, 1974.

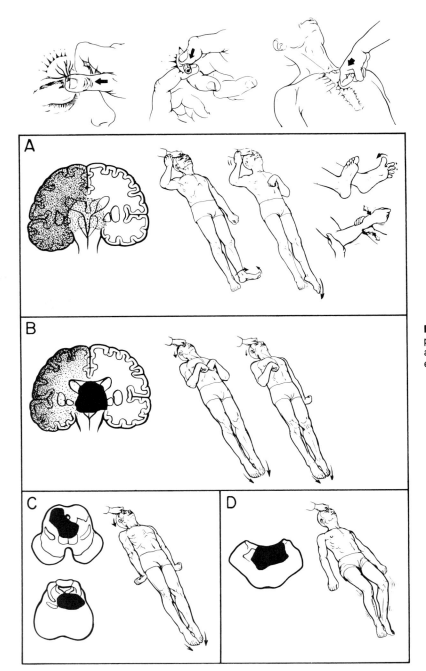

Figure 16–4. Motor responses to noxious stimulation in patients with acute cerebral dysfunction. (From Plum F and Posner JB: The Diagnosis of Stupor and Coma, 3rd ed. Philadelphia, FA Davis, 1980.)

Methods Used in the Assessment of Intracranial Pressure

Physical Examination

The physical and neurologic examinations can suggest that the ICP is elevated. Increased ICP is known to increase blood pressure, cause bradycardia, and change the breathing pattern (Cushing's triad); impair the level of consciousness; and cause bulging of the fontanelles and sutures in infants and papilledema in children and adults.

Unfortunately, these well-documented findings rarely correlate with more precise and sophisticated methods, such as direct intraventricular pressure measurement (the gold standard of ICP measurement), and can never replace invasive ICP monitoring techniques.

ICP Monitoring Devices

Various CNS compartments can be transduced for pressure monitoring, with the assumption that there is an equal transmission of pressure within the cranium. The ventricular pressure can be measured by ventriculostomy, the brain parenchyma can be measured by a fiberoptic pressure transducer, and the subarachnoid and subdural spaces can be measured by specially designed catheters or the "bolt" (Fig. 16–5).

Spinal Catheter. The oldest method of ICP measurement is the lumbar puncture (LP). Through the needle, a low-compliance catheter is placed in the lumbar subarachnoid space and is connected to a manometer. Measuring ICP this way has several disadvantages:

1. Patients with noncommunicating hydrocephalus do not have a continuous fluid column of CSF and consequently have two compartments with different pressures. This means that the measured pressure does not reflect the ICP proximal to the occlusion.
2. Introducing a needle and *removing* fluid via an LP is sometimes dangerous and can cause fluid shifts, leading to rostrocaudal herniation in patients with increased ICP.

Intraventricular Catheter—Ventriculostomy. In 1960, Lundberg[5] described a simple technique for the direct measurement of intraventricular pressure by a fluid-filled catheter system inserted straight into the ventricle (ventriculostomy). This device is still commonly used and remains the gold standard by which other techniques are evaluated.

The ventriculostomy avoids the drawbacks of the LP catheter and remains the only ICP monitoring method that enables the therapeutic drainage of CSF under certain circumstances. The procedure is simple and can be done in an ICU setting. It also enables the measurement of intracranial compliance.

Risk factors associated with ventriculostomy include infection and hemorrhage. An infection rate of 6 to 21% has been reported in several studies, and prophylactic treatment is often instituted.[6,7] Intracerebral hemorrhage occurs infrequently (in 1 to 2% of cases[6]) and rarely becomes clinically significant. Raftopoulos and colleagues[8] studied patients shortly after they underwent a ventricular catheterization. Computed tomography

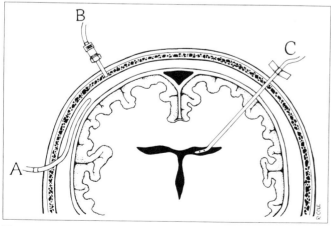

Figure 16–5. Placement of intracranial pressure monitoring devices: *A*, subdural cap catheter; *B*, subarachnoid screw; and *C*, ventriculostomy catheter. (From Aucoin JP, Kotilainen HR, Gantz NM, et al: Intracranial pressure monitors: Epidemiologic study of risk factors and infection. Am J Med 80:369–376, 1986.)

(CT) scans were compared with magnetic resonance imaging (MRI) scans in order to evaluate radiologic changes around the catheter. The study found a significant MRI signal in all patients, corresponding to brain edema around the catheter, which in some cases lasted days after the catheter was removed.

One of the drawbacks of intraventricular catheters is that they cannot be inserted when the ventricular system has collapsed, a situation frequently occurring in severe brain edema.

Fiberoptic pressure transducers can be inserted into patients' ventricles when drainage is not necessary. This method has the advantage of being a closed system without any flow and therefore presumably with a reduced potential for infectious complications.

Subarachnoid Pressure Monitoring Devices. When CSF drainage is not necessary or when there are contraindications to an intraventricular catheter, a subarachnoid pressure monitoring apparatus can be inserted. The more common device is the subarachnoid screw (bolt), which was invented by Vries and colleagues[9] in 1973. In this method, a burr hole is drilled in the skull after the appropriate shaving, cleansing, and preparation. Once the hole is complete, the dura (and sometimes the arachnoid) is cut under direct vision. The bolt, which has the same diameter as the burr hole, is screwed in place and is connected to a closed fluid-filled pressure-transducing system.

The bolt has gained wide acceptance in pediatric critical care practice and was the main ICP monitoring device until the invention of the fiberoptic monitor. The bolt has the advantage of not involving major penetration of brain parenchyma, thus reducing edema, scar formation, infection, and hemorrhage. Its limitations include underestimation of "true" pressure when that is determined by an intraventricular catheter as the reference point,[10] dampening of the pressure waveform when use is prolonged because of partial obliteration of the system, and an inability to drain a substantial amount of CSF fluid as a therapeutic measure. Insertion in infants is also limited by skull thickness—that is, in order to be appropriately mounted, the skull needs to be rigid and thick enough, which usually excludes infants younger than 6 months of age.

Fiberoptic Intracranial Pressure Monitors. The most recent development in ICP monitoring devices are the fiberoptic intracranial pressure monitors. These devices use a monitor that senses changes in the amount of light reflected off of a pressure-sensitive diaphragm located at the tip of a fiberoptic catheter. The mean pressure is then displayed digitally on the monitor and can also be presented on a multichannel monitor. Since the device is a catheter-tipped transducer, it is effective in the subdural, intraparenchymal, and intraventricular compartments. Its advantages, in addition to being applicable in different compartments, include a no-flow closed system (low infection rates), no need for recalibration following the initial insertion, continuous reading, and avoidance of complications resulting from occlusion.

Crutchfield[11] evaluated fiberoptic intracranial pressure monitors of the Camino type (digital pressure monitor, Model 420, Camino Laboratories, San Diego, CA), both as to their in vitro accuracy and drift in time and as compared with other modes of ICP monitoring in a canine model. The monitor was found to be accurate (± 3 mm Hg at greater than the 0 to 30 mm Hg range) with a low drift (average daily drift ± 0.6 mm Hg) and correlated well with measurements from the intraventricular and subarachnoid compartments. Chambers and coworkers[12] compared the same device in humans. It was placed either in the subdural compartment or in the ventricle with a fluid-filled ventricular system. These investigators found an excellent correlation between the methods. A drawback of the device is the inability to withdraw CSF and thus alleviate increased ICP in selected cases.

Indications and Benefits of Intracranial Pressure Monitoring

All currently available ICP monitors require access to the intracranial space. Patients who have not undergone a craniectomy for their initial problem are subject to an invasive procedure for the placement of the device. Consequently, it is relevant to define the indications for ICP monitoring.

ICP monitoring is indicated when there is reason to believe that the ICP is increased or will be increased in the ensuing hours *and* that treatment of the elevated ICP improves outcome.

In reviewing head trauma series both in adults and in children, it becomes evident that there are no axioms regarding the placement of an ICP monitor. Eisenberg and colleagues[13] prospectively studied head trauma patients who were older than 15 years and had a GCS less than or equal to 7 and found an elevated ICP in more than 90% of them. Narayan and colleagues[7] analyzed ICP retrospectively in regard to various parameters and found an *abnormal CT scan* (the presence of a high-density or low-density lesion) to be a strong predictor of elevated ICP. In patients with a normal CT scan, three features were related to elevated ICP: age greater than 40 years, systolic blood pressure less than 90 mm Hg, and unilateral or bilateral motor posturing. In children with head injuries, Muizelaar and associates[14] studied a group of 32 pediatric head trauma patients who all had a GCS less than or equal to 7 and found 72% of them to have ICP greater than 20 mm Hg in the first 6 hours following injury.

As to the benefit of ICP treatment in pediatric head trauma, recent studies[15-17] strongly suggest that effective control of ICP significantly improves outcome. Similar findings are found in the adult literature.

Other disease entities in which control of ICP seems to be beneficial include metabolic encephalopathies and infectious processes. The clinical outcome of patients with Reye's syndrome, in which brain edema and increased ICP are common and often lethal findings, has been apparently improved with the application of aggressive ICP control.[18] The recommended threshold for inserting an ICP monitor is when the patient's disease is in stage IV or V.[15]

It is well established that elevated ICP may develop in meningitis, especially the bacterial form. ICP monitoring in these patients is mentioned in various series. Goitein and colleagues[19] studied 14 infants with CNS infections. Their indication for placement of an ICP monitor included clinical signs of increased ICP, a modified (for nonverbal response) GCS less than 7, and an abnormal CT scan. In this group, successful control of ICP correlated with a favorable outcome, as compared with the outcome of patients in which ICP did not respond to treatment. Le Roux and coworkers[15] also reported four pediatric patients with bacterial meningitis who responded favorably to ICP reducing treatment.

HIE is another disease entity in which ICP often increases. A decade ago, it was common to vigorously treat raised ICP in these patients. However, studies evaluating the outcome of these patients are disappointing, pointing to a failure to alter morbidity despite control of increased ICP[15, 19-21] (see also Chapter 17). It seems that in HIE, the increased ICP reflects the initial acute injury sustained by the brain; therefore, treating the elevated ICP is futile.

ELECTROPHYSIOLOGIC MONITORING

The information derived from ICP monitoring, though useful in acute management and prognostically valuable to a certain degree, does not directly reflect changes in cerebral function. Additional information regarding cerebral function may be obtained by electrophysiologic testing, including electroencephalography and evoked potentials.

Electroencephalography

Electroencephalography provides information about the severity and distribution of the altered CNS function and the presence of electrical seizure activity. It may also point to a cause. In several studies, it was found to correlate with outcome.[22]

Tasker and coworkers[22] reported 48 nontrauma pediatric patients who were admitted to an ICU and had ICP monitoring. All patients had an electroencephalogram (EEG) within 36 hours of admission, and the majority had two or more studies. The EEG tracings were graded in order of severity into one of four categories, and both the initial and the worst studies were correlated with the eventual outcome. It was found that patients who had low-grade activity on the EEG (isoelectric or generalized low-voltage activity) had a poor outcome (p less than 0.001). The study emphasizes that EEG studies may contribute to the prediction of prognosis in nontraumatic coma.[22]

Stone[23] reviewed studies evaluating electroencephalography in head trauma. There is a consistent sequence of EEG changes that correlates with the degree of injury. In some cases, injury of specific anatomic areas of the CNS produces distinct EEG patterns. Other studies find significant correlations between changes in the EEG and eventual outcome in head trauma patients.[23] In patients with head trauma and altered consciousness who are admitted to the ICU, it may be beneficial to obtain an EEG even without the presence of clinical seizures.

Electroencephalography also has a role in monitoring therapeutic barbiturate-induced coma. This technique depends on continuous or frequent EEG monitoring, since the goal is to titrate therapy to reach burst suppression.

The place of the EEG in brain death determination is discussed in Chapter 93.

Evoked Responses

Evoked responses represent the brain's electrical response to external stimuli. These techniques entail repeated stimulation and the use of computed signal averaging in order to extract the signal from the background EEG activity. This group of studies includes visual evoked responses (VER), brain stem auditory evoked responses, (BAER), and somatosensory evoked potentials (SER).

Several studies have looked at BAER or SER in critically ill patients.[24, 25] Judson and colleagues[24] evaluated SER in 100 head trauma patients (a mixed pediatric and adult group). SER was divided into three categories (from normal and symmetric central conduction time to lack of the cortical waveform). When SER was compared with outcome for each patient, a significant association (p less than 0.0001) was found, and the test was highly specific and sensitive. SER is considered to be unaffected by sedation or paralysis and therefore has distinct advantages in the ICU setting. At present, SER is mainly an investigational tool but may eventually find its place as an adjunct to standard monitoring in certain patients. Narayan and associates[25] studied patients with severe head injury, analyzing the predictive value of various parameters in relation to outcome and found that a battery of evoked response tests (including those mentioned previously) was a strong predictor of outcome.

References

1. Plum F and Posner JB: The diagnosis of Stupor and Coma, 3rd ed. Philadelphia, FA Davis, 1980.
2. James HE: Therapy-directed diagnosis in coma. *In:* James HE, Anas NG, and Perkin RM (eds): Brain Insults in Infants and Children: Pathophysiology and Management. Orlando, Grune & Stratton, 1985, p 170.
3. Teasdale G and Jennett B: Assessment of coma and impaired consciousness. A practical scale. Lancet 2:81, 1974.
4. James HE and Trauner DA: The Glasgow Coma Scale. *In:* James HE, Anas NG, and Perkin RM (eds): Brain Insults in Infants and Children: Pathophysiology and Management. Orlando, Grune & Stratton, 1985, 179.
5. Lundberg N: Continuous recording and control of ventricular fluid pressure in neurosurgical practice. Acta Psychiatr Neurol Scand 36 (Suppl) 149:1, 1960.
6. Aucoin JP, Kotilainen HR, Gantz NM, et al: Intracranial pressure monitors. Epidemiologic study of risk factors and infection. Am J Med 80:369, 1986.
7. Narayan RK, Kishore RSP, Becker DP, et al: Intracranial pressure: To monitor or not to monitor? A review of our experience with severe head injury. J Neurosurg 56:650, 1982.
8. Raftopoulos C, Baleriaux D, Brotchi J, et al: The traumatic aspect of ventricular catheterization demonstrated by magnetic resonance imaging. Clin Neurol Neurosurg 90:47, 1988.
9. Vries JK, Becker DP, and Young HF: A subarachnoid screw for monitoring intracranial pressure. J Neurosurg 39:419, 1973.
10. Lehman LB: Intracranial pressure monitoring and treatment: A contemporary view. Ann Emerg Med 19:295, 1990.
11. Crutchfield JS, Narayan RK, Robertson CS, et al: Evaluation of a fiberoptic intracranial pressure monitor. J Neurosurg 72:482, 1990.
12. Chambers IR, Mendelow AD, Sinar EJ, et al: A clinical evaluation of the Camino subdural screw and ventricular monitoring kits. Neurosurgery 26:421, 1990.
13. Eisenberg HM, Frankowski RF, Contant CF, et al: High-dose barbiturate control of elevated intracranial pressure in patients with severe head injury. J Neurosurg 69:15, 1988.
14. Muizelaar JP, Marmarou A, and DeSalles AA: Cerebral blood flow and metabolism in severely head-injured children. Part 1: Relationship with GCS score, outcome, ICP and PVI. J Neurosurg 71:63, 1989.
15. Le Roux PD, Jardine DS, Kanev PM, et al: Pediatric intracranial pressure in hypoxic and nonhypoxic brain injury. Child Nerv Syst 7:34, 1991.
16. Bruce DA, Alavi A, and Bilanuik L: Diffuse cerebral swelling following head injuries in children: The syndrome of "malignant brain edema." J Neurosurg 54:170, 1981.
17. Cordobes F, LeBato RP, and Rivas JS: Post-traumatic diffuse brain swelling, isolated or associated with cerebral axonal injury. Child Nerv Syst 3:235, 1987.
18. Shaywitz BA, Rothstein P, and Venes JL: Monitoring and management of increased intracranial pressure in Reye syndrome: Results in 29 children. Pediatrics 66:198, 1980.
19. Goitein KJ, Amit Y, and Musaffi H: Intracranial pressure in central nervous system infections and cerebral ischaemia of infancy. Arch Dis Child 58:184, 1983.
20. Bohn DJ, Biggar WD, Smith CR, et al: Influence of hypothermia, barbiturate therapy, and intracranial pressure monitoring on morbidity and mortality after near-drowning. Crit Care Med 14:529, 1986.
21. Frewen TC, Somabot WO, and Han UK: Cerebral resuscitation therapy in pediatric near drowning. J Pediatr 106:615, 1985.
22. Tasker RC, Boyd S, Harden A, et al: Monitoring in nontraumatic coma. Part II: Electroencephalography. Arch Dis Child 63:895, 1988.
23. Stone JL, Ghaly RF, and Hughes JR: Electroencephalography in acute head injury. J Clin Neurophysiol 5(2):125, 1988.
24. Judson JA, Cant BR, and Shaw NA: Early prediction of outcome from cerebral trauma by somatosensory evoked potentials. Crit Care Med 18:363, 1990.
25. Narayan RK, Greenberg RP, Miller JD, et al: Improved confidence of outcome prediction in severe head injury. A comparative analysis of the clinical examination, multimodality evoked potentials, CT scanning, and intracranial pressure. J Neurosurg 54:751, 1981.

17

Central Nervous System Support Techniques

Ido Yatsiv, M.D.

Support of central nervous system (CNS) function and integrity is in essence the primary goal of critical care medicine. The diseased CNS poses a unique problem because of three distinctive characteristics:

1. It is located in a closed cavity with a constant volume, resulting in a delicate balance between the volumes of the various compartments. Alterations of any volume can lead to problems of intracranial pressure (ICP) control (see Chapter 16).
2. Neural tissue is extremely susceptible to hypoxia and ischemia.
3. CNS damage is largely irreversible, since neuronal tissue cannot regenerate itself.

This chapter discusses the general supportive approach to patients with CNS insult and follows with an evaluation of specific treatment modalities aimed at reducing ICP and thus protecting brain function.

THE APPROACH TO THE PATIENT WITH AN ACUTE CENTRAL NERVOUS SYSTEM INSULT

The application of life support measures, such as maintaining a patent airway, controlling breathing, and sustaining adequate blood pressure and circulation constitutes an important aspect in the treatment of acute CNS injury.

Airway Management and Ventilation

The patient with a CNS insult who requires critical care observation and treatment must always have a patent airway. An endotracheal tube is often necessary. There are three reasons for intubation of the trachea that are unique to the child with severe CNS injury:

1. Most of these patients have depressed consciousness and bulbar reflexes and cannot protect the airway from aspiration.
2. These patients often present with breathing irregularities caused by brain stem involvement.

3. Increased ICP necessitating hyperventilation is a major and common complication.

Head trauma patients require *oral* intubation because it is difficult to exclude a basal skull fracture, and a nasally inserted tube can find its way into the cranial cavity. Cervical spine injury occurs concomitantly in 5 to 10% of head trauma patients; therefore, it is essential to obtain radiologic clearance or stabilization in a neck collar prior to intubation.

When intubating these patients, the physician must consider the high likelihood of increased ICP. Further increase of ICP induced by the intubation technique can result in further ischemic damage secondary to low cerebral perfusion pressure (CPP) and in extreme cases can cause herniation. Intubation requires two classes of drugs: a sedative and a muscle relaxant. As a sedative, a short-acting barbiturate (thiopental, 2 to 7 mg/kg) has the advantage of short-term sedation and lowering of the ICP; however, it is a cardiodepressant and may cause hypotension. Alternatively, narcotics (fentanyl, 1 to 5 µg/kg) or benzodiazepines (midazolam, 0.1 to 0.2 mg/kg) can be used, the former having the benefit of a short duration of action and reversibility. Lidocaine (1 to 1.5 mg/kg) is effective for blunting laryngeal reflexes that cause ICP to increase during intubation. The muscle relaxant of choice for rapid sequence intubation is succinylcholine (1 to 2 mg/kg) because it induces paralysis within seconds. However, succinylcholine may increase ICP either by increasing cerebral blood flow[1] or by increasing central venous pressure (CVP) because of fasciculations. The latter can usually be overcome by a priming dose of a nonpolarizing agent. Vecuronium (0.1 to 0.2 mg/kg) is probably the best alternative to succinylcholine because it is a nondepolarizing agent, it has minimal cerebro- and cardiovascular effects, and its onset of action, albeit longer than succinylcholine's, can be shortened if a higher dose is given.

In adults, some authors advocate awake intubation if the patient seems to be capable of cooperating. This approach has a limited role, if any, in pediatrics.

Once the patient is intubated, adequate ventilation and oxygenation is the goal. Hyperventilation (which will be discussed later at length) is aimed at lowering

Pa_{CO_2} to 25 to 30 mm Hg, a level that reduces cerebral blood flow (CBF) and is one of the mainstays in the treatment of elevated ICP. Hypoxia is also an important consideration, since a Pa_{O_2} less than 60 mm Hg invokes cerebral vasodilatation and increases CBF. The patient should therefore receive supplemental oxygen so that the Pa_{O_2} is greater than 90 mm Hg.

Patients with increased ICP often have concomitant respiratory problems, including aspiration pneumonia, neurogenic pulmonary edema,[2] and chest trauma. Positive end-expiratory pressure (PEEP) is used to increase functional residual capacity (see Chapter 40) and is a cornerstone in the treatment of these conditions. PEEP may increase ICP by increasing CVP and impeding cerebrovascular drainage, or it may reduce ICP by decreasing cardiac output and blood pressure through its effect on venous return and the pulmonary vascular bed. The net effect of PEEP on the hypertensive brain remains controversial, but it seems beneficial to monitor ICP in these patients, especially if high levels of PEEP (>15 mm Hg) are being employed.

Circulation

One of the primary goals in the treatment of the brain-injured patient is maintenance of CPP at greater than a certain limit. CPP is an artificial number derived from subtracting the ICP from the mean arterial pressure (MAP); CPP reflects the driving pressure along the cerebrovascular bed. In adult studies, the minimal adequate CPP is considered to be 50 mm Hg; data in children are lacking, but most practitioners of intensive care medicine consider the critical CPP to be 35 to 45 mm Hg, depending on age. It is therefore clear that in addition to preserving low ICP, the other important factor is to keep the MAP sufficiently high.

The patient with a head insult often has noncranial injuries that result in hypovolemia and hypotension. These injuries must be treated and adequate blood volume restored. It has been well documented that even without extracranial injuries, head trauma can produce cardiac depression. This is thought to be a result of massive sympathetic discharge, systemic and pulmonary artery hypertension, and acute right and left heart strain and may require placement of a pulmonary artery catheter to measure cardiac output and assist in monitoring fluid and vasopressor therapy.

Head Positioning

Proper positioning of the head is another way of facilitating cerebral venous drainage and lowering ICP. This is achieved by creating a hydrostatic pressure gradient between the intracranial sinuses that drain the CNS and the right atrium.[3] Theoretically, a 90-degree angle would provide the highest gradient; however, at this level it is difficult to avoid a degree of neck flexion, leading to obstruction and engorgement of the jugular veins, which results in increased cerebral blood volume (CBV) and ICP. In addition, at angles greater than 45 degrees, orthostatic hypotension may become significant, resulting in a decline of cranial MAP and failure to maintain CPP.[4, 5] It is therefore recommended that the head of the bed should be elevated to *15 to 30 degrees*.

In addition to elevation, the head must also be kept at a midline position because rotation tends to partially obstruct flow in the ipsilateral jugular vein, resulting in increased CBV and ICP.

Fluid Management

The common denominator of most brain insults is brain edema. Consequently, dehydration of the brain causes decreased brain edema and a decline in ICP. Fluid management in patients with brain edema is complex and has to take into consideration the goal of brain dehydration, as well the need to prevent systemic hypotension and shock in patients who often suffer extracranial trauma and blood loss and are treated with diuretics and osmotherapy. In order to manage these patients closely, continuous monitoring of blood pressure and fluid status is needed. This is achieved by the placement of an indwelling arterial line, a urethral catheter, and a central line, preferably a pulmonary artery catheter. Fluid is administered at an initial rate of 40 to 60% of calculated maintenance, but careful adjustments are made according to urine output (aiming at 0.5 to 1 ml/kg/hr), serum electrolytes and osmolarity, blood pressure, and atrial filling pressures. Adequate cardiac function must be preserved constantly, and frequently a vasopressor agent such as dopamine is needed.

Recently, attention has been given to the type of fluid being delivered. Nonelectrolyte solutions should be avoided because the sugar is utilized and the remaining "free water" contributes to brain edema.[6] Tranmer and associates[7] have compared crystalloid and colloid solutions (hetastarch) in a canine brain edema model and found that the use of the latter resulted in lower ICP values and less pathologic electroencephalogram (EEG) tracings. At present, there are no clinical studies of this issue in humans.

Sedation and Paralysis

Painful and stressful stimulation is unfortunately unavoidable during the management of patients in the intensive care unit. The need to control ventilation and the inability of critically ill neurologic patients (especially children) to breathe synchronously with the ventilator often dictate the need for continuous paralysis. In addition, it is well documented that routine treatments such as endotracheal suctioning, dressing changes, and repositioning of the patient cause an increase in ICP. Consequently, these patients need to undergo continuous paralysis and sedation with muscle relaxants and sedatives, and special attention has to be given to adequate prophylactic sedation and analgesia prior to invasive procedures, suctioning, and other painful or irritating stimuli.

The ideal sedative in these circumstances has minimal side effects and a short duration of action or is reversible in order to enable clinical evaluation (an option essentially lost during paralysis and sedation). Barbiturates (thiopental, 5 mg/kg), benzodiazepines (midazolam, 0.1 to 0.2 mg/kg), or narcotics (fentanyl, 1 to 4 µg/kg) are being used either in repeated boluses or as continuous drips. It should be mentioned that if pain is anticipated, narcotics should probably be used, since only they provide analgesia. Narcotics are also the only agents readily reversible.

The choice of a muscle relaxant is also dictated by side effects and length of action. Pancuronium, which was the drug of choice for years, has been largely abandoned because of its adverse cardiovascular effects. It has largely been replaced by vecuronium (0.1 to 0.2 mg/kg), which is also a nondepolarizing agent that has almost no side effects and can be administered by boluses or continuous infusion.

Seizure Control

Seizures are a serious complication of CNS insult, especially when ICP is elevated. Seizures augment brain damage by raising the cerebral metabolic rate ($CMRO_2$), increasing O_2 demand, and consequently raising CBF and ICP.

Data regarding the prevalence of seizures in different pediatric CNS insults are scarce. The largest segment of CNS disease that requires critical care is head trauma. Hahn and colleagues[8] studied 937 children hospitalized for head trauma. They found a 9.8% rate of post-traumatic seizures; 94.5% of these seizures developed within 24 hours of the insult. The risk groups included patients with cerebral edema, acute subdural hematoma, open depressed skull fractures, and severe head injury. Based on these observations, they recommend prophylactic use of anticonvulsants in high-risk patients.

Phenytoin (10 mg/kg loading dose followed by 5 mg/kg/day, aiming at a level of 10 to 15 mg/l) is the initial recommended drug, since it lacks cardiodepressant side effects and does not alter mental status.[9] It is important to remember that paralyzed patients can have electrical seizure activity that is undetectable clinically but is nevertheless just as deleterious. Consequently, in these patients there should be a low threshold for prophylactic anticonvulsive treatment as well as for *continuous* monitoring by multichannel or single electrode EEG tracings.

Temperature Control

Body temperature has a linear correlation with cerebral metabolism as reflected by $CMRO_2$. Between 25 and 37° C, $CMRO_2$ increases by 9 to 19% for every degree centigrade increase.[10-12] Based on theoretic reasons and data from animal models, hypothermia has been advocated as another mode of reducing ICP. Hypothermia lowers CBF and decreases cerebral metabolism and thus has been thought to have a protective effect on the brain. Hypothermia was studied in patients with brain ischemia,[13] neurosurgical operations,[14] severe head injury,[15] and in near-drowning.[16] Despite initial enthusiasm, hypothermia does not seem to add significantly to ICP control when other methods are used and has not been demonstrated to improve neurologic outcome in any of these conditions. Conversely, it was found to have detrimental effects on neutrophil function and clearance by the reticuloendothelial system and was found to be arrythmogenic (at a body temperature less than 28° C) as well.

In the last decade, hypothermia has been largely abandoned in critical care but continues to have limited use in neuroanesthesia. It should be emphasized, however, that clinically controlled studies of the effect of hypothermia on clinical outcome in patients with neuroaxial trauma have never been published.[17]

Along the same line of reasoning, it is clear that *fever* in these patients is harmful and should be rapidly reduced to a normothermic range of 35 to 36° C. This is accomplished by using antipyretics as well as cooling devices (cooling blankets, cooling mattresses). Cooling often produces shivering, which may result in an increase in CVP and ICP and should be promptly stopped using muscle relaxants or a phenothiazine.

As fever is detrimental, temperature should be closely monitored and measured centrally by devices such as rectal or esophageal probes or a pulmonary artery catheter.

SPECIFIC MEASURES OF INTRACRANIAL PRESSURE CONTROL

In addition to the general considerations and treatment modes discussed so far, more specific modalities have been developed. These include hyperventilation and the induction of hypocapnia, hyperosmolar therapy, barbiturates, and steroids.

Hyperventilation and Hypocapnia

The cerebrovascular vasculature is exceptionally sensitive to the pH of the interstitial fluid surrounding those vessels as mediated by changes in CO_2,[18, 19] causing them to constrict at an alkaline pH and to dilate at an acidic pH. This physiologic response has been attributed to the action of adenosine[20] or prostaglandins[21] on vascular smooth muscle. Since CO_2 rapidly crosses the blood-brain barrier (BBB), changes in $PaCO_2$ are the sole way to induce rapid changes in cerebral interstitial pH and thus changes in cerebrovascular resistance, flow, and volume. Measurements of CBF changes in response to changes in $PaCO_2$—that is, *CO_2 reactivity*—indicate that in a normal brain at a $PaCO_2$ between 38 and 45 mm Hg, a change of 1 mm Hg in $PaCO_2$ leads to a 4% change in CBF. CO_2 reactivity alters with $PaCO_2$, decreasing to 2% at the 22 to 38 mm Hg range and increasing to 6% when $PaCO_2$ is greater than 45 mm HG.[22]

In the normal brain, compensatory mechanisms respond to artificially increased pH, resulting in adaptation and return to baseline pH values within 24 to 48 hours. This adaptation may explain the fact that prolonged hyperventilation ceases to reduce ICP in some patients, and further reduction of $PaCO_2$ is needed. In some head trauma patients, however, this adaptive mechanism does not seem to occur, and hyperventilation may be efficacious for a long period.[23]

In a small segment of patients with severe head injuries, the cerebrovascular response to CO_2 changes is lacking or significantly diminished. In this group of patients, the response to barbiturates is also significantly reduced, and the overall outcome has been shown to be extremely poor.[23, 24]

In addition to the well-studied cerebrovascular responses to pH changes, prolonged hypocapnia has been found to decrease the rate of cerebrospinal fluid production.[25, 26] The clinical significance of this observation is not clear.

In the clinical setting, hypocapnia is the most rapid method of alleviating increased ICP. When there is reason to suspect high ICP, hyperventilation should be started as soon as possible, justifying intubation and control of ventilation. As to the desired $PaCO_2$, some authors recommend aiming at an initial level of 32 to 36 mm Hg, claiming that it may be enough for ICP reduction and it leaves room for increased hyperventilation if adaptation develops,[9] whereas others set a $PaCO_2$ of 24 to 28 mm Hg as a treatment goal.

It seems that the most logical approach is to adjust the desired $PaCO_2$ to the measured ICP and CPP, since these are the only readily measurable neurophysiologic parameters that can be monitored in the clinical setting.

It has been argued that hypocapnia less than a $PaCO_2$ of 20 mm Hg can create ischemia by vasoconstriction. In cats, hypocapnia at a $PaCO_2$ of 20 mm Hg generated an increase in lactate concentration in cerebral tissue and cerebrospinal fluid.[27] Canine studies of brain tissue during extreme hypocapnia-induced alkalosis also demonstrate ischemia.[28] These studies and glucose metabolism studies in humans subjected to hypocapnia[29] support the view that excessive hyperventilation might result in brain ischemia. It is therefore not recommended to hyperventilate patients at a $PaCO_2$ of less than 20 mm Hg.

Osmotherapy and Diuretics

Osmotic agents such as glycerol, urea, and mannitol are known to decrease ICP and have been used clinically since the early 1960s.[30] Glycerol and urea have been largely abandoned because of vein irritation and a higher BBB permeability, leaving mannitol as the most commonly used agent in clinical practice.

Mannitol, administered as a bolus or a rapid infusion, decreases ICP in 10 to 15 minutes, a drop that is normally maintained for several hours.[31] This immediate decrease in ICP occurs about 15 minutes before the onset of diuresis and is observed in nephrectomized animals as well.

Mannitol's exact mode of action remains controver-

sial. The more widely accepted mechanism entails an increase of the osmotic pressure in the intravascular compartment, resulting in an osmotic gradient along the BBB, decrease of brain tissue water content, and a parallel decrease in ICP.[32, 33] The effect of mannitol on cerebral tissue water content in head trauma patients was investigated by Nath and Galbraith.[33] They measured white matter specific gravity before and after mannitol infusion and documented a significant decrease in brain water content from 80.9 to 75.3%.

Another proposed mechanism centers on the drop in hematocrit and blood viscosity following mannitol infusion. It is thought that this drop improves oxygen transport to the brain, leading to an autoregulatory response of vasoconstriction and decrease in CBV and ICP.[34] In accordance with this theory, patients who lose cerebral autoregulation following a head insult do not experience vasoconstriction after the treatment, and its effect is diminished. One way of approaching this issue has been the use of the cranial window technique. In this research method, a "cranial window" is made and sealed with cover glass. A special microscope-video system enables the continuous measurement of pial vessels, thus making investigation of cerebral vascular changes feasible. Using this technique, Muizelaar and coworkers[35] have found vasoconstriction of pial vessels in response to mannitol. Conflicting data, despite the use of a similar technique, were reported by Auer and Haselsberger,[36] who did not observe such a response.

When the time sequence of ICP response to mannitol is studied, an initial *increase* in ICP lasting several minutes is detected in patients with normal ICP. This elevation is attributed to an initial increase of CBF and CBV. When patients with an initial state of elevated ICP were studied, a further increase in ICP was not found.[37] The latter observation may serve to support the safety of rapid infusion of mannitol in patients suspected of having high ICP. Another approach in that circumstance is to administer a loop diuretic first, thus obtunding that initial ICP peak.

Mannitol has some detrimental effects. It produces transient intravascular hypervolemia, which may be harmful to patients with cardiovascular instability. It may also generate a rebound increase in ICP following prolonged use. The presumption is that in patients with disrupted BBB, the normally slow penetration of the BBB by mannitol may be accelerated, leading to local retention of water in that part of the brain. This consideration may point to a drawback in prolonged treatment with mannitol; however, there are no clinical studies clarifying this issue.

Initially, recommended doses of mannitol based on experience with urea and glycerol were 1 to 4 gr/kg. Since then studies have indicated that much smaller doses result in similar effects, and it is now customary to use doses in the 0.25 to 1 gr/kg range.

Treatment with mannitol requires electrolyte and osmolarity monitoring, since serum osmolarity is expected to increase, and hyponatremia often develops. Serum osmolarity should be in the 300 to 310 mOsm range and should *not* exceed 320 mOsm, since beyond that level renal and neurologic dysfunction may occur.

Loop diuretics (furosemide, ethacrynic acid) are also being used in patients with elevated ICP. These agents act nonspecifically, causing water depletion, and have the advantage of not causing the initial increase in ICP. In addition, they do not have the rebound phenomenon. It contrast, they are nonspecific and tend to cause more electrolyte abnormalities. The combined use of diuretics and mannitol is an effective treatment mode and is often used.

In addition to osmotic and diuretic therapy, it should again be emphasized that strict and judicious fluid management is an important aspect in the treatment of these patients.

Barbiturates

In 1966 Ishii[38] first proposed that high-dose barbiturates might be useful in the control of increased ICP. In the late 1970s, the first clinical reports of the use of barbiturates in Reye syndrome[39] and in head trauma[40] were published. In Reye syndrome, aggressive ICP control including barbiturate coma appeared to reverse the natural history of the disease, resulting in 100% survival in seven children. In the head injury series, ICP reduction occurred in 75% of the patients who were refractory to intensive treatment with hyperventilation and mannitol. Since then, barbiturates have been added to the list of drugs effective in decreasing ICP.

Barbiturates induce a dose-dependent decrease in cerebral metabolism (as measured by the cerebral metabolic rate of oxygen [$CMRO_2$]). Since cerebral metabolism is coupled with CBF, a parallel reduction in CBF occurs, and CBV and ICP decrease as well.[41] At barbiturate levels sufficient to produce burst suppression on the EEG, the CBF decreases to one third of normal and the $CMRO_2$ decreases to 45% of normal. Since barbiturates affect only electrical activity–related metabolism, once an isoelectric EEG is achieved, there is a maximal trough in oxygen consumption; hence, a further increase in the barbiturate level will result in *no* further change in $CMRO_2$ or CBF and would *not* contribute to a further decrease in ICP.[42, 43]

There are conflicting results from clinical trials designed to examine the role of barbiturates as an adjuvant to ICP therapy. Eisenberg and associates[44] reported a five center study comparing treatment for increased ICP in which half of the patients whose ICP did not respond adequately to intensive conventional treatment received high-dose pentobarbital. In this group of extremely sick patients, barbiturates were found to reduce ICP in 32% of patients, a significant difference compared with controls. Conversely, when relative efficacy or outcome was compared, barbiturates did not prove superior to other treatment modalities. Schwartz and colleagues[45] compared mannitol treatment to pentobarbital and Ward and associates[46] examined outcome following prophylactic pentobarbital therapy, both in severe head trauma patients. Both studies failed to demonstrate an advantage in using barbiturates.

Despite the conflicting reports, when ICP control is warranted, barbiturates should be used if other means

fail. One commonly used regimen is pentobarbital infusion, in which a loading dose of 10 to 20 mg/kg over 1 to 2 hours is administered, followed by a 1 to 2 mg/kg/hr continuous infusion.[47] The therapeutic goal is control of ICP, but repeated EEG tracings are necessary in order to detect burst suppression. When burst suppression is achieved, a further increase in barbiturate level is useless. Satisfactory control of ICP is usually reached at pentobarbital levels of 20 to 25 mg/l.

Barbiturates are known to produce cardiac depression and hypotension; consequently, when high-dose barbiturate therapy is started, placement of a pulmonary artery catheter and repeated determinations of cardiac function are mandatory.

Steroid Therapy

The role of steroids in the treatment of increased ICP has been a matter of controversy throughout the years. Steroids have been shown to decrease ICP in several animal head trauma models. Conversely, most of the human head trauma studies fail to prove either an ICP reducing effect or improved outcome,[48] and therefore their use in head injury has been largely abandoned. Braughler and Hall[49] have addressed the inconsistency between animal and human studies, arguing that human studies employed an insufficient dosage that was often administered too late. The recent proof that megadoses of steroids improve outcome in *spinal* injury[50] may support their reasoning. However, steroids do have an undebatable role in the treatment of increased ICP as a result of vasogenic edema around masses such as tumors, abscesses, and organized subdural hematomas.[51]

References

1. Lanier WL, Milde JH, and Michenfelder JD: Cerebral stimulation following succinylcholine in dogs. Anesthesiology 64:551, 1986.
2. Milley JR, Nugent SK, and Rogers MC: Neurogenic pulmonary edema in childhood. J Pediatr 94:706, 1979.
3. Cowan F and Thoresen M: Changes in superior sinus blood velocities due to postural alterations and pressure on the head of the newborn infant. Pediatrics 75:1038, 1985.
4. Durward QJ, Amacher AL, Del Maestro RF, et al: Cerebral and cardiovascular responses to changes in head elevation in patients with intracranial hypertension. J Neurosurg 59:938, 1983.
5. Trost HA: The cerebral perfusion pressure. Problems of measurement and treatment after head injury. Neurosurg Rev 12 (Suppl) 1:382, 1989.
6. Lehman LB: Intracranial pressure monitoring and treatment: A contemporary view. Ann Emerg Med 19:295, 1990.
7. Tranmer BI, Iacobacci RI, and Kindt GW: Effects of crystalloid and colloid infusions on intracranial pressure and computerized electroencephalographic data in dogs with vasogenic brain edema. Neurosurgery 25:173, 1989.
8. Hahn YS, Fuchs S, Flannery AM, et al: Factors influencing posttraumatic seizures in children. Neurosurgery 22:864, 1988.
9. Pascucci RC: Head trauma in the child. Intensive Care Med 14:185, 1988.
10. Astrup J, Sorensen PM, and Sorensen HR: Inhibition of oxygen and glucose consumption in the dog by hypothermia, pentobarbital, and lidocaine. Anesthesiology 55:263, 1981.
11. Adams JE, Elliot H, Sutherland VC, et al: Cerebral metabolic studies of hypothermia in the human. Surg Forum 7:535, 1957.
12. Tabaddor K, Gardner TJ, and Walker AE: Cerebral circulation

and metabolism at deep hypothermia. Neurology (Minneapolis) 22:1065, 1972.

13. Cohen PJ: To dream the impossible dream (editorial view). Anesthesiology 55:491, 1981.

14. White RJ, Albin MS, Verdura J, et al: Differential extracorporal hypothermic perfusion of and circulatory arrest to the human brain. Med Res Engineer 6:18, 1967.

15. Shapiro HM, Wyte SR, and Loeser J: Barbiturate-augmented hypothermia for reduction of persistent intracranial hypertension. J Neurosurg 40:90, 1974.

16. Bohn DJ, Biggar WD, Smith CR, et al: Influence of hypothermia, barbiturate therapy, and intracranial pressure monitoring on morbidity and mortality after near-drowning. Crit Care Med 14:529, 1986.

17. Cold GE: Cerebral blood flow in acute head injury. The regulation of cerebral blood flow and metabolism during the acute phase of head injury, and its significance for therapy. Acta Neurochir (Wien) (Suppl) 49:1, 1990.

18. Cotev S and Severinghous JW: Role of cerebrospinal fluid pH in management of respiratory problems. Anesth Analg 48:42, 1969.

19. Plum F and Siesjo BK: Recent advances in CSF physiology. Anesthesiology 42:708, 1975.

20. Phillis JW and De Long RE: An involvement of adenosine in cerebral blood flow regulation during hypercapnia. Gen Pharmacol 18:133, 1987.

21. Dahlgren W, Nilsson B, Sakabe T, et al: The effect of indomethacin on cerebral blood flow and oxygen consumption in the rat in normal and increased carbon dioxide tensions. Acta Physiol Scand 111:475, 1981.

22. Olesen J: Contralateral focal increase of cerebral blood flow in man during arm work. Brain 94:635, 1971.

23. Cold GE, Jensen FT, and Malmros R: The cerebrovascular CO_2 reactivity during the acute phase of brain injury. Acta Anaesthesiol Scand 21:222, 1977.

24. Messeter K, Nordstrom C-H, Sundbarg G, et al: Cerebral hemodynamics in patients with severe head trauma. J Neurosurg 64:231, 1986.

25. Hochwald GM, Wald A, and Malhan C: The sink action of cerebrospinal fluid volume flow. Arch Neurol 33:339, 1976.

26. Martins AN, Doyle TF, and Newby N: PCO_2 and rate of formation of cerebrospinal fluid in monkey. Am J Physiol 231:127, 1976.

27. Granholm L and Siesjo BK: The effects of hypercapnia and hypocapnia upon the cerebrospinal fluid lactate and pyruvate concentrations and upon the lactate, pyruvate, ATP, ADP, phosphocreatine and creatine concentrations of the cat brain. Acta Physiol Scand 75:257, 1969.

28. Hilberman M, Nioka S, Subramanian H, et al: Brain pH during respiratory acidosis and alkalosis, a 31P NMR study. Anesthesiology 61:A317, 1984.

29. Alexander SC, Smith TC, Strobel G, et al: Cerebral carbohydrate metabolism of man during respiratory and metabolic alkalosis. J Appl Physiol 24:66, 1968.

30. Wise BL and Chater N: The value of hypertonic mannitol solution in decreasing brain mass and lowering cerebrospinal-fluid pressure. J Neurosurg 19:1038, 1962.

31. James HE: Methodology for the control of intracranial pressure with hypertonic mannitol. Acta Neurochir (Wien) 51:161, 1980.

32. Marshall LF, Smith RW, Rauscher LA, et al: Mannitol dose requirements in brain injured patients. J Neurosurg 48:169, 1978.

33. Nath F and Galbraith S: The effect of mannitol on cerebral white matter water content. J Neurosurg 65:41, 1986.

34. Muizelaar JP, Lutz HA, and Becker DP: Effect of mannitol on ICP and CBF and correlation with pressure autoregulation in severely head-injured patients. J Neurosurg 61:700, 1984.

35. Muizelaar JP, Wei EP, Kontos HA, et al: Mannitol causes compensatory cerebral vasoconstriction and vasodilation in response to blood viscosity changes. J Neurosurg 59:822, 1983.

36. Auer LM and Haselsberger K: Effect of intravenous mannitol on cat pial arteries and veins during normal and elevated intracranial pressure. Neurosurgery 21:142, 1987.

37. Ravussin P, Abou-Madi M, Archer D, et al: Changes in CSF pressure after mannitol in patients with and without elevated CSF pressure. J Neurosurg 69:869, 1988.

38. Ishii S: Brain swelling. Studies of structural, physiologic and biochemical alterations. In: Caveness WF and Walker AE (eds): Head Injury. Conference Proceedings. Philadelphia, JB Lippincott, 1966, p 276.

39. Marshall LF, Shapiro HM, Rauscher A, et al: Pentobarbital therapy for intracranial hypertension in metabolic coma: Reye syndrome. Crit Care Med 6:1, 1978.

40. Marshall LF, Smith RW, and Shapiro HM: The outcome with aggressive treatment in severe head injuries. Part 2: Acute and chronic barbiturate administration in the management of head injury. J Neurosurg 50:26, 1979.

41. Nillson L and Siesjo BK: The effect of phenobarbitone anesthesia on blood flow and oxygen consumption in the rat brain. Acta Anaesth Scand (Suppl) 57:18, 1975.

42. Donegan JH, Traystman RJ, Koehler RC, et al: Cerebrovascular hypoxic and autoregulatory responses during reduced brain metabolism. Am J Physiol 249:H421, 1985.

43. Trauner DA: Barbiturate therapy in acute brain injury. J Pediatr 109:742, 1986.

44. Eisenberg HM, Frankowski RF, Contant CF, et al: High-dose barbiturate control of elevated intracranial pressure in patients with severe head injury. J Neurosurg 69:15, 1988.

45. Schwartz ML, Tator CH, Rowed DW, et al: The University of Toronto Head Injury Treatment Study: A prospective, randomized comparison of pentobarbital and mannitol. Can J Neurol Sci 11:434, 1984.

46. Ward JD, Becker DP, Miller JD, et al: Failure of prophylactic barbiturate coma in the treatment of severe head injury. J Neurosurg 62:383, 1985.

47. Swedlow DB and Schreiner MS: Management of Reye syndrome. Crit Care Clin 1:285, 1985.

48. Cooper PR, Moody S, Clark WK, et al: Dexamethasone and severe head injury: A prospective double-blind study. J Neurosurg 51:307, 1979.

49. Braughler JM and Hall ED: Current application of "high dose" steroid therapy for CNS injury. J Neurosurg 62:806, 1985.

50. Bracken MB, Shepard MJ, Collins WF, et al: A randomized control trial of methylprednisolone or naloxone in the treatment of acute spinal-cord injury. Results of the Second National Acute Spinal Cord Injury Study. N Engl J Med 322:1405, 1990.

51. Brock M, Weingand H, Zillig C, et al: The effect of dexamethasone on intracranial pressure in patients with supratentorial tumors. In: Pappius HM and Fiendel W (eds): Dynamics of Brain Edema. New York, Springer Verlag, 1976, p 330.

Hypoxic-Ischemic Cerebral Injury in the Newborn

Alan Hill, M.D., Ph.D., and Joseph J. Volpe, M.D.

Despite major advances in obstetric and neonatal care, approximately 2% of all pregnancies are complicated by perinatal asphyxia with consequent mortality or long-term neurologic sequelae.[1] Improved techniques for assessment of fetal well-being have focused greater attention on hypoxic-ischemic insults that occur during the antepartum period. Nevertheless, the precise incidence and significance of antepartum asphyxia is difficult to ascertain because affected infants may be asymptomatic during the neonatal period. In contrast, term newborns who sustain intrapartum hypoxic-ischemic cerebral injury of sufficient magnitude to result in long-term neurologic abnormalities invariably have clinical features of encephalopathy during the first days of life. In fact, the lack of an acute recognizable neonatal encephalopathy argues strongly against significant intrapartum hypoxic-ischemic cerebral injury in the term newborn. In any event, it is critical that a diagnosis of hypoxic-ischemic cerebral injury be made cautiously and only after careful consideration of historical details and laboratory investigations. This caution is warranted because the clinical features are nonspecific and may occur in the context of numerous other insults to the nervous system (e.g., infection, metabolic derangements, cerebral dysgenesis), some of which require specific treatments. This chapter will review the pathogenesis, diagnosis, and management of acute intrapartum hypoxic-ischemic cerebral injury in the term newborn.

PATHOGENESIS

The extent of hypoxic-ischemic cerebral injury is determined both by the maturity of the central nervous system of the affected newborn at the time of the insult and by the severity and duration of the hypoxic-ischemic insult.[2] The latter is often difficult to quantify in the human newborn. However, studies of asphyxiated near-term fetal rhesus monkeys have established clearly that there is a critical duration of hypoxic-ischemic insult necessary to cause irreversible cerebral injury.[3] In most instances, cerebral injury results from a combination of hypoxia (decreased blood oxygen content) and ischemia (decreased cerebral perfusion), which increases anaerobic cerebral metabolism with decreased production of high-energy phosphate compounds and the accumulation of potentially toxic metabolites (e.g., lactate, intracellular calcium, extracellular potassium, excitatory neurotransmitters, and free radicals). Recent studies suggest that these toxic substances may mediate the major portion of the cerebral injury.

The neuropathologic patterns of hypoxic-ischemic cerebral injury differ considerably between premature and term infants, principally because of the difference in the extent of maturation of the cerebral vasculature. Thus in the term newborn, the watershed zones of arterial supply of the brain are located principally in parasagittal cortical regions between territories supplied by the anterior, middle, and posterior cerebral arteries. In contrast, in the premature infant, the watershed zone is located in the periventricular white matter.[2] Of course, it must be recognized that there is variation in the rate of maturation of cerebral vasculature, which further determines the spectrum of injury. Thus in some instances, there may be a pattern of injury in the term newborn resembling that observed more commonly in an infant of younger gestational age—for example, injury involving predominantly periventricular white matter. The major features of the newborn brain that govern, in part, the extent of hypoxic-ischemic cerebral injury are listed in Table 18–1.

The major neuropathologic patterns of hypoxic-ischemic cerebral injury and their clinical correlates are summarized in Table 18–2. The localization of cerebral injury in the human newborn may be achieved by the use of radiologic imaging techniques, which are discussed further on.

DIAGNOSIS

Because approximately 90% of hypoxic-ischemic cerebral injury originates during the prenatal and intrapartum period,[2] accurate diagnosis depends on a detailed history of complications of pregnancy, labor, and delivery.

Table 18–1. FEATURES OF THE NEWBORN BRAIN THAT DETERMINE EXTENT AND TOPOGRAPHY OF HYPOXIC-ISCHEMIC INJURY

Impaired cerebrovascular autoregulation
Degree of maturation of the cerebral vascular supply:
  Watershed zones of arterial supply, presence of germinal matrix
Water content of cerebral tissue
Pre-existing chronic intrauterine hypoxic-ischemic insult or
  undernutrition

History

Clinical features that may be useful for the diagnosis of significant hypoxic-ischemic insult include electronic fetal heart rate monitoring, acid-base status of the fetus determined by scalp and cord blood sampling, delayed Apgar scores after 5 minutes of age, the presence of thick meconium in the amniotic fluid, and placental pathologic features. Although each of these parameters has been used to define hypoxic-ischemic cerebral insult, it must be recognized that no *single* clinical factor correlates closely with poor neurologic outcome.[4–6] Improved techniques for assessment of fetal well-being permit more accurate timing of insult.[7, 8] Furthermore, historical details are essential in infants who may have sustained hypoxic-ischemic cerebral injury earlier in gestation and who will not necessarily display clinical abnormalities during the newborn period. Finally, attention must be directed toward the exclusion of other potential causes of encephalopathy, such as cerebral dysgenesis, infection, a metabolic disorder, and so on.

Physical Examination

A detailed examination is essential for the diagnosis of hypoxic-ischemic cerebral injury in the term newborn.

Clinical abnormalities may be more difficult to ascertain in the premature newborn or in term newborns who have received muscle-paralyzing agents (e.g., pancuronium) to facilitate mechanical ventilation. In general, term newborns who sustain acute intrapartum hypoxic-ischemic insult of sufficient severity to result in long-term neurologic sequelae will demonstrate a recognizable clinical encephalopathy during the first week of life.[9] Both the severity and duration of acute hypoxic-ischemic encephalopathy have prognostic value. Although there exists a continuum of severity of hypoxic-ischemic encephalopathy, distinct categories of severity may be defined that correlate closely with outcome[10, 11] (Table 18–3). Table 18–4 outlines the evolution of severe encephalopathy that results almost invariably in death or severe neurologic sequelae (e.g., microcephaly, seizures, cerebral palsy).

Several aspects of this clinical syndrome warrant further elaboration. Although some dysfunction of cranial nerves occurs commonly, a specific pattern of hypoxic-ischemic cerebral injury with disproportionate involvement of brain stem nuclei and the thalamus and relative preservation of cortex and subcortical white matter may occur occasionally following acute, apparently total, asphyxia. This pattern of cerebral injury may originate before birth and is manifested by persistent severe cranial nerve abnormalities (e.g., facial diplegia, tongue fasciculations, skew deviation of the eyes).[12] This pattern of injury may be incompatible with long-term survival.[13]

Seizures occur in approximately 50% of asphyxiated term newborns. They usually begin before 24 hours of age. During the acute phase, the seizures may be difficult to control despite high doses of multiple anticonvulsants. Repeated electroencephalographic (EEG) recordings or continuous monitoring, when available, may be indicated in infants who have been given paralyzing drugs to facilitate mechanical ventilation. It has not been

Table 18–2. CLINICAL AND RADIOLOGIC DIAGNOSIS OF MAJOR NEUROPATHOLOGIC PATTERNS OF HYPOXIC-ISCHEMIC CEREBRAL INJURY

Neuropathologic Pattern of Injury	Clinical Features in Newborn	Long-term Neurologic Sequelae	Radiologic Techniques for Diagnosis			
			CT*	US†	MRI‡	Radio-nuclide
Selective neuronal necrosis (cerebral cortex, cerebellum, thalamus, brain stem)	Seizures, hypotonia, decreased level of consciousness, cranial nerve dysfunction	Intellectual impairment, seizures, cerebral palsy, attention deficit disorders	+ §	+	+	
Status marmoratus of basal ganglia, thalamus, cortex	Unknown	Intellectual impairment, choreoathetotic cerebral palsy	±	– ‖	?	+
Parasagittal	Hypotonia-weakness of proximal limbs	Spastic quadriparesis, visual-spatial dysfunction	+	–	?	+
Focal-multifocal	Focal seizures, hemiparesis (upper limb weakness > lower limb weakness)	Hemiparesis, quadriparesis, seizures, intellectual impairment	+	+	+	+
Periventricular leukomalacia	?Weakness of lower extremities	Spastic diplegia	±	+	+	±

*CT = computed tomography.
†US = ultrasonography.
‡MRI = magnetic resonance imaging.
§ + = useful.
‖ – = not useful.

Table 18–3. CORRELATION OF SEVERITY AND DURATION OF HYPOXIC-ISCHEMIC ENCEPHALOPATHY WITH OUTCOME IN THE TERM NEWBORN

Severity of Encephalopathy	Clinical Features	Duration	% with Neurologic Sequelae*
Mild	Hyperalertness, uninhibited Moro and stretch reflexes, sympathetic overactivity	<24 hr	0
Moderate	Lethargy-stupor, hypotonia, suppressed primitive reflexes, seizures	<1 wk ≥1 wk	0 20–40
Severe	Stupor-coma, flaccidity, suppressed brain stem and autonomic activities, increased intracranial pressure, seizures	>1 wk	100 (i.e., cerebral palsy, seizures, mental retardation)

*Modified from Robertson C and Finer N: Term infants with hypoxic-ischemic encephalopathy: Outcome at 3.5 years. Dev Med Child Neurol 27:473, 1985.

clarified whether electrographic seizures are harmful to the newborn human brain as long as systemic cardiovascular and metabolic homeostasis is maintained.[14] Recent EEG-video recordings of infants with apparent "subtle" seizures (e.g., abnormal eye movements, repetitive sucking) have not been consistently associated with electrical discharges on EEG recordings. This inconsistency raises the possibility that some of these movements may represent brain stem release phenomena rather than seizures originating in cortical regions.[15, 16] However, it is also possible that these seizures originate in limbic structures and thus may be undetectable by surface EEG. Infants with diffuse neuronal injury usually experience multifocal clonic seizures. Focal seizures may be indicative of focal ischemia-infarction, most commonly in the territory of the middle cerebral artery.[2, 17, 18] It is important to distinguish between jitteriness (i.e., stimulus-sensitive tremor that ceases with passive flexion of the affected limb) and actual seizures, which are often associated with abnormal eye movements and usually are not affected directly by environmental factors. This distinction may have important prognostic value because jitteriness may be a feature of mild encephalopathy and does not necessarily imply a poor outcome.

Most infants who sustain significant hypoxic-ischemic cerebral injury are initially hypotonic. Specific patterns of motor weakness correlate with specific anatomic distribution of injury—for example, in the term newborn, disproportionate weakness of the shoulder girdle signifies parasagittal injury in watershed zones of arterial supply of anterior, middle, and posterior cerebral arteries. Unilateral weakness may indicate focal cerebral injury. Clinical suspicion of specific neuropathologic patterns of injury may be confirmed by neuroimaging techniques (see further on).

Cerebral edema that is detectable clinically occurs relatively infrequently in the asphyxiated newborn. It is not a feature of hypoxic-ischemic cerebral injury in the premature newborn, perhaps because of the normal high water content of the immature brain. Even in the term newborn, raised intracranial pressure (ICP) occurs only in severely asphyxiated infants. Estimation of ICP may be performed clinically by palpation of the anterior fontanelle or may be quantified by measurement with a Ladd ICP monitor or subarachnoid screw. We have documented the temporal profile of increased ICP by performing serial ICP measurements in 32 asphyxiated term newborns using a Ladd ICP monitor. In all cases, the ICP was normal initially (less than 10 mm Hg) and rose subsequently to a maximal level between 24 and 72 hours of age. Only seven infants experienced an elevated ICP. All of them either died (three infants) or experienced severe neurologic sequelae (four infants). The temporal profile of increased ICP is most consistent with extensive cerebral necrosis as a cause of the cerebral edema. Thus, elevated ICP in the term newborn should be considered a consequence rather than a cause of ischemic cerebral injury.[19] Similar results have been obtained using a more invasive subarachnoid bolt to measure ICP.[20]

Adjunctive Investigations

Although detailed history and physical examinations are of paramount importance in all instances of sus-

Table 18–4. EVOLUTION OF SEVERE HYPOXIC-ISCHEMIC ENCEPHALOPATHY IN TERM NEWBORNS

Clinical Features	Age after Birth (hr)			
	0–12	12–24	24–72	>72
Level of consciousness	Stupor-coma	"Apparent" alertness	Stupor-coma → death	Persistent, diminishing stupor
Respiratory pattern	Periodic breathing	Apnea	Possible respiratory arrest	± Persistent apneic spells
Other brain stem function	Intact pupillary light response and extraocular movements	Impaired visual fixation	Pupillary-oculomotor abnormalities	Bulbar dysfunction (e.g., abnormal gag, sucking)
Seizures	Present (50%)	Worsening seizures, jitteriness	Tonic posturing (?seizures)	± Seizures
Motor examination	Severe hypotonia	Specific patterns of weakness	Flaccidity	Hypotonia evolving into hypertonia
Intracranial pressure	Normal	Gradual increase	Maximum increase	Gradual decrease

pected hypoxic-ischemic cerebral injury, adjunctive electrodiagnostic and radiologic procedures may provide important confirmatory information, particularly in infants who require complex life support apparatus or those who have been given paralyzing drugs to facilitate mechanical ventilation.

Electroencephalography

Following severe hypoxic-ischemic cerebral insult, there is a characteristic evolution of EEG abnormalities. Initially there is generalized slowing of activity with suppression of amplitude. After 24 to 48 hours, a discontinuous "burst-suppression" pattern may appear, which consists of intermittent high-voltage sharp and slow waves with periods of marked voltage suppression. This ominous pattern must be distinguished from the normal trace alternant pattern of quiet sleep seen in the normal term newborn. After approximately 3 days, the periodicity may deteriorate to an isoelectric recording. As discussed previously, continuous EEG monitoring is useful for diagnosis of seizure activity in paralyzed infants. Rapid resolution of EEG abnormalities is associated with a good prognosis.[11]

Evoked Responses

Both brain stem auditory evoked responses and visual evoked responses are of value for assessment of the integrity of brain stem structures or visual pathways.[21-23]

Radiologic Techniques

A variety of radiologic techniques are of proven value for assessment of severity and anatomic location of hypoxic-ischemic cerebral injury in the term newborn.

Computed Tomography. In the term newborn, visualization of decreased brain tissue attenuation on computed tomography (CT) scans permits accurate assessment of both the severity and extent of hypoxic-ischemic cerebral injury, provided that an appropriate imaging technique is used. Thus, CT images of the newborn brain should be viewed and documented using a narrow window width of 60 to 80 Hounsfield units. The correct window level is between 25 and 30 Hounsfield units. The numeric value of brain attenuation (in Hounsfield units) must be determined for accurate assessment. The optimal timing of CT studies to demonstrate the maximal extent of parenchymal injury (hypodensities) in the acute period is 2 to 4 days following the insult. This corresponds to the timing of maximal ICP following injury. Thus the presence of decreased tissue attenuation on CT correlates with the presence of brain swelling or edema.[19] CT scans performed later in infancy may demonstrate the signs of tissue loss or dissolution—that is, generalized cerebral atrophy or multicystic encephalomalacia (Fig. 18-1).

In addition to the severity of injury, CT scanning may permit identification of the precise distribution of hypoxic-ischemic cerebral injury. Patterns of hypoxic-ischemic cerebral injury recognizable on CT include dif-

fuse neuronal necrosis,[19] parasagittal injury[24] (Fig. 18-2), focal infarction,[25] and thalamic and brain stem injury.[12]

The diagnostic value of CT for the assessment of hypoxic-ischemic cerebral injury in the premature newborn in the acute period is limited because of the high water content of the immature brain, which results in normally low tissue attenuation. In this age group, CT scanning is best for the identification of acute hemorrhagic cerebral infarction. Subsequently, CT is useful to demonstrate long-term sequelae of hypoxic-ischemic brain injury, that is, ventriculomegaly caused by loss of white matter or multicystic leukomalacia.

Cranial Ultrasonography. Cranial ultrasonography is the method of choice for the diagnosis of hypoxic-ischemic and hemorrhagic injury in the premature newborn. In contrast, this technique is of somewhat more limited value in the term newborn. Hypoxic-ischemic injury may be suspected on the basis of increased echogenicity.[26] Thus generalized increased echogenicity on ultrasonographic scans may reflect diffuse cerebral necrosis. Furthermore, focal areas of increased echodensity may correspond to focal cerebral infarction.[27] The major limitations of cranial ultrasound technique relate to its inability to distinguish between hemorrhagic and nonhemorrhagic hypoxic-ischemic cerebral injury (both of which may appear as areas of increased echogenicity), as well as the subjective nature of interpretation of apparent increased echogenicity.

Magnetic Resonance Imaging. Preliminary studies of hypoxic-ischemic cerebral injury in term newborns suggest that the deep gray matter structures and cerebral cortex are most susceptible to injury. Delayed myelination has been documented in asphyxiated infants.[28-31] To date, the precise role of magnetic resonance imaging for diagnosis of perinatal hypoxic-ischemic injury has not been defined clearly.

Monitoring of Intracranial Pressure

As discussed previously, the presence of a clinically recognizable elevated ICP indicates extensive cerebral necrosis and poor prognosis in the context of the asphyxiated term newborn. Among the techniques available for noninvasive measurement of ICP, palpation of the anterior fontanelle is probably adequate for routine clinical management, whereas instruments such as the Ladd ICP monitor may provide more quantitative data.[19] Unfortunately, there is no convincing evidence that treatment of elevated ICP improves outcome.

Measurement of Cerebral Blood Flow and Cerebral Blood Flow Velocity

Alterations in cerebral perfusion (both increased and decreased cerebral blood flow) have been documented in the asphyxiated newborn. Thus a "pressure-passive" relationship between systemic blood pressure and cerebral perfusion has been documented even following mild hypoxic-ischemic cerebral injury.[32, 33] Subsequently following asphyxia, there may be a decrease in cardiac output with systemic hypotension and decreased cere-

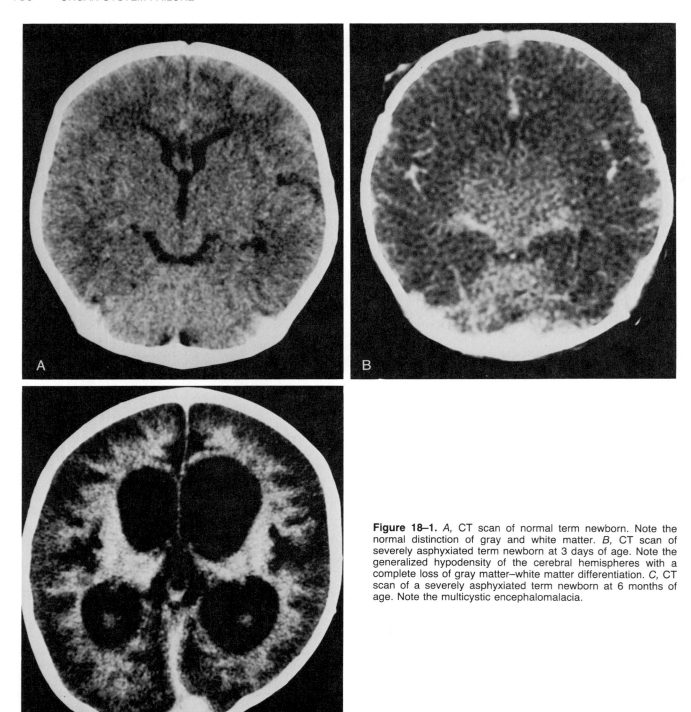

Figure 18–1. *A,* CT scan of normal term newborn. Note the normal distinction of gray and white matter. *B,* CT scan of severely asphyxiated term newborn at 3 days of age. Note the generalized hypodensity of the cerebral hemispheres with a complete loss of gray matter–white matter differentiation. *C,* CT scan of a severely asphyxiated term newborn at 6 months of age. Note the multicystic encephalomalacia.

bral perfusion. A variety of techniques are available for estimation of cerebral perfusion. Doppler ultrasound methodology permits measurement of cerebral blood flow velocity, which is an indicator of actual cerebral blood flow if the caliber of the insonated vessel remains constant. Regional cerebral blood flow may be assessed by positron emission tomography, which is not available currently for routine clinical evaluation. However, re-

search studies indicate clearly the potential of this technique for delineation of the anatomic location of injury.[34]

Biochemical Markers

A variety of biochemical disturbances may be associated with hypoxic-ischemic insult and can contribute to the clinical abnormalities (e.g., hypoglycemia, hypocal-

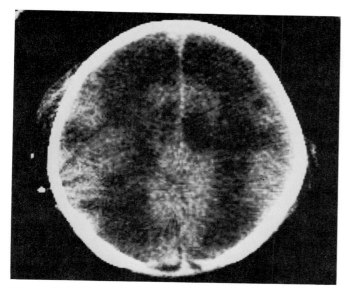

Figure 18–2. CT scan of parasagittal hypoxic-ischemic injury. Note the low-density changes in the parasagittal regions.

cemia, hyponatremia, hyperammonemia, and lactic acidosis). Such metabolic derangements should be investigated and the abnormalities corrected. Other metabolic derangements produce identifiable enzymes or metabolites (e.g., creatine kinase, hypoxanthine), which may serve as "markers" of the presence and severity of hypoxic-ischemic injury.[2]

MANAGEMENT OF HYPOXIC-ISCHEMIC ENCEPHALOPATHY

At present, there is no standardized protocol for the management of acute perinatal hypoxic-ischemic encephalopathy.[14, 35] Clearly, infants who sustain severe cerebral hypoxic-ischemic injury often, though not invariably, experience dysfunction of other organ systems (e.g., cardiac, pulmonary, hepatic, or renal, see Chapter 13). Although the management of these systemic complications is of critical importance, the discussion in this chapter will be limited to cerebral complications.

Prevention

Because hypoxic-ischemic insult occurs during the intrauterine period, early recognition of adverse maternal factors and close monitoring of the high-risk fetus are of paramount importance for prevention of severe insult.[2, 5–8] However, it should be recognized that many infants with signs of "distress" during labor have no neonatal neurologic abnormalities or subsequent deficits.

Maintenance of Adequate Ventilation and Perfusion

The importance of maintaining adequate ventilation and perfusion cannot be overemphasized. Thus hyper-

capnia may result in impaired autoregulation, cerebral acidosis, or focal ischemia related to "intracranial steal."[2] Impairment of cerebrovascular autoregulation with a "pressure-passive" relationship between systemic blood pressure and cerebral perfusion, which has been documented following even mild hypoxic-ischemic cerebral injury, underscores the importance of avoiding systemic hypotension. Other complications (e.g., polycythemia) have been associated with reduced cerebral perfusion and cerebral infarction.[36]

Maintenance of Adequate Blood Glucose Levels

The optimal level of blood glucose needed to prevent brain injury at the time of hypoxic-ischemic insult has not been defined precisely. During the period following the insult, hypoglycemia should be avoided.

Control of Seizures

Moderate or severe hypoxic-ischemic encephalopathy may be the single most important cause of neonatal seizures. In this context, seizures usually begin during the first 24 hours following the insult and may be difficult to control initially, despite high doses of numerous anticonvulsants. Seizure types include subtle, focal or multifocal clonic, tonic, or myoclonic. They may be difficult to recognize in infants who require complex life support apparatus or in those who have been given paralyzing drugs to facilitate mechanical ventilation. In these instances, EEG monitoring may be helpful. Although to date there is no conclusive clinical evidence that seizures per se are harmful to the newborn brain without associated cardiovascular or metabolic disturbances, it is recommended that persistent seizures be treated aggressively. When there are no treatable metabolic disturbances (e.g., hypoglycemia), anticonvulsant treatment should begin with a loading dose of phenobarbital (20 mg/kg) administered intravenously. If seizures persist, additional aliquots of 5 mg/kg may be given every 5 minutes up to a total dose of 40 mg/kg while monitoring cardiorespiratory function carefully. With this regimen, it has been reported that seizures may be controlled adequately in 88% of infants.[37, 38] When seizures persist, 20 mg/kg of phenytoin may be given slowly by an intravenous route with monitoring of cardiac function.[2] Rarely, it may be necessary to give intermittent doses of paraldehyde or diazepam.[39]

Control of Brain Swelling

In the asphyxiated term newborn, it is appropriate to avoid fluid overload and maintain careful surveillance of serum electrolyte levels, osmolality, urine output, and body weight. Although elevated ICP may be normalized by certain interventions (e.g., hyperventilation, administration of glucocorticosteroids or osmotic diuretics, and hypothermia), there is no convincing evidence that neurologic morbidity is reduced by these maneuvers.[14] In fact, mortality in experimental animals treated with high-dose dexamethasone was higher than in saline-treated controls, suggesting that steroid therapy should probably be avoided in this context.[40]

Experimental Pharmacologic Intervention

Oxygen-free Radical Inhibitors and Scavengers

Oxygen-free radicals (e.g., O_2^- or OH^-) are produced following hypoxic-ischemic insult either as by-products in the metabolism of prostaglandins or hypoxanthine or within mitochondria when cytochrome oxidase is not fully oxygenated. Oxygen-free radicals may attack the fatty acid components of cellular membranes and cause membrane fragmentation and additional cerebral injury.[41-43] It may be speculated that drugs that inhibit formation or rapidly destroy free radicals—for example, inhibitors of prostaglandin synthesis, indomethacin (a cyclooxygenase inhibitor), phospholipase A_2 inhibitors, and xanthine oxidase inhibitors (allopurinol)—may minimize the extent of hypoxic-ischemic brain injury. Thus asphyxiated immature rats that were pretreated with allopurinol experienced less severe cerebral edema and fewer long-term neurologic abnormalities than did controls[44] (see Chapters 1 and 19).

Excitatory Amino Acid Antagonists

Experimental studies suggest that excitatory amino acids, especially glutamate, may produce neuronal injury identical to that observed following hypoxia-ischemia.[45] It appears that excessive stimulation of cell surface receptors by glutamate released from axons during hypoxia-ischemia promotes neuronal death.[46] Experimental evidence in developing rats indicates that antagonists of the glutamate receptor channel complex, such as phencyclidine, dextromethorphan, ketamine, and MK-801, are capable of reducing the severity of hypoxic-ischemic brain injury.[14, 47, 48] It has been reported that pretreatment of animals (including immature animals) with MK-801 may prevent occurrence of tissue injury. Moreover, treatment administered shortly after the insult has been shown to be effective in some experimental models (see Chapter 22).

Calcium Channel Blockers

An increase in cytosolic calcium concentrations results in activation of lipases, proteases, and endonucleases, which disrupt cell membranes and may result in neuronal death.[49] At the present time, several calcium channel blockers (e.g., flunarizine, nimodipine) are under active investigation for protection against hypoxic-ischemic cerebral injury.[14]

At present, there is not sufficient experimental evidence for the new pharmacologic agents to warrant their recommendation for routine clinical use.

Table 18–5. USEFUL PROGNOSTIC FACTORS FOR HYPOXIC-ISCHEMIC CEREBRAL INJURY

Data from electronic fetal heart rate monitoring and fetal blood gas sampling

Presence of thick meconium

Apgar scores: "extended" scores after 5 minutes of age

Neonatal neurologic syndrome:
  Duration: longer than 1–2 weeks[11]
  Severity: moderate or severe[11]
  Presence of seizures: 30–75% sequelae
  Presence of cerebral edema

Radiologic imaging data:
  Cranial ultrasonography
  Computed tomography
  Magnetic resonance imaging

Neurophysiologic techniques:
  Electroencephalography
  Brain stem auditory evoked potentials
  Visual evoked potentials

Biochemical markers
  Creatine kinase
  Hypoxanthine

OUTCOME

The accurate prediction in the neonatal period of outcome following perinatal hypoxic-ischemic injury is difficult because of the frequent inability to delineate the severity of insult and location of injury. Major prognostic factors, which have already been discussed, are summarized in Table 18–5. The outcome following asphyxia sustained earlier in utero and not necessarily associated with clinical abnormalities during the newborn period has not been established.

REFERENCES

1. Low JA: Fetal asphyxia in the antepartum and intrapartum period. *In*: Perinatal asphyxia. Its role in developmental deficits in children. Can Med Assoc J (Suppl):49, 1989.
2. Volpe JJ: Neurology of the Newborn, 2nd ed. Philadelphia, WB Saunders, 1987.
3. Myers RE: Experimental models of perinatal brain damage: Relevance to human pathology. *In*: Intrauterine Asphyxia and the Developing Fetal Brain. Chicago, Year Book Medical Publishers, 1977, pp 37–97.
4. Nelson KB and Ellenburg JH: Antecedents of cerebral palsy: Multivariante analysis of risk. N Engl J Med 315:81, 1986.
5. Freeman JM and Nelson KB: Intrapartum asphyxia and cerebral palsy. Pediatrics 82:240, 1988.
6. Nelson KB: Perspective on the role of perinatal asphyxia in neurologic outcome. *In*: Perinatal asphyxia. Its role in developmental deficits in children. Can Med Assoc J (Suppl) 1989, pp 3–10.
7. Hill A and Volpe JJ: Fetal Neurology. New York, Raven Press, 1989.
8. Hill A: Assessment of the fetus: Relevance to brain injury. Clin Perinatol 16:413, 1989.
9. Hill A: Clinical assessment of perinatal asphyxia in the newborn. *In*: Perinatal asphyxia. Its role in developmental deficits in children. Can Med Assoc J (Suppl):53, 1989.
10. Robertson C and Finer N: Term infants with hypoxic-ischemic encephalopathy: Outcome at 3.5 years. Dev Med Child Neurol 27:473, 1985.
11. Sarnat HB and Sarnat MS: Neonatal encephalopathy following

fetal distress: A clinical and electroencephalographic study. Arch Neurol 33:695, 1976.

12. Roland EH, Norman MG, MacNab A, et al: Selective brainstem injury in an asphyxiated newborn: Correlation of clinical, radiological and neuropathological features. Ann Neurol 23:89, 1988.

13. Norman MG: Antenatal neuronal loss and gliosis of the reticular formatin, thalamus and hypothalamus. Neurology 22:910, 1972.

14. Vannuci RC: Current and potentially new management strategies for perinatal hypoxic-ischemic encephalopathy. Pediatrics 85:961, 1990.

15. Mizrahi EM and Kellaway P: Characterization and classification of neonatal seizures. Neurology 37:1837, 1987.

16. Volpe JJ: Neonatal seizures: Current concepts and revised classification. Pediatrics 84:422, 1989.

17. Mannino FL and Trauner D: Stroke in neonates. J Pediatr 102:605, 1983.

18. Ment LR, Duncan CC, and Ehrenkranz RA: Perinatal cerebral infarction. Ann Neurol 16:559, 1984.

19. Lupton BA, Hill A, Roland EH, et al: Brain swelling in the asphyxiated term newborn: Pathogenesis and outcome. Pediatrics 82:139, 1988.

20. Clancy R, Legido A, Newell R, et al: Continuous intracranial pressure monitoring and serial electroencephalographic recordings in severely asphyxiated term newborns. Am J Dis Child 142:740, 1988.

21. Hakamada S, Watanabe K, Hara K, et al: The evolution of visual and auditory evoked potentials in infants with perinatal disorder. Brain Dev 3:339, 1981.

22. Hecox KE and Cone B: Prognostic importance of brainstem auditory evoked responses after asphyxia. Neurology 31:1429, 1981.

23. Whyte HE, Taylor MS, Menzies R, et al: Prognostic utility of visual evoked potentials in term asphyxiated neonates. Pediatr Neurol 2:220, 1986.

24. Pasternak JF: Parasagittal infarction in neonatal asphyxia. Ann Neurol 21:202, 1987.

25. Clancy R, Malin S, Larague D, et al: Focal motor seizures heralding stroke in neonates and infants. Am J Dis Child 139:601, 1985.

26. Siegel MJ, Shackelford GD, Perlman JM, et al: Hypoxic-ischemic encephalopathy in term infants: Diagnosis and prognosis evaluated by ultrasound. Radiology 152:395, 1984.

27. Martin DJ, Hill A, Daneman AR, et al: Hypoxic-ischemic cerebral injury in the neonatal brain: A report of sonographic features with computed tomographic correlation. J Pediatr Radiol 13:307, 1983.

28. Johnson MA, Pennock JM, Bydder GM, et al: Serial MR imaging in neonatal cerebral injury. AJNR 8:89, 1987.

29. McArdle CB, Richardson CJ, Hayden CK, et al: Abnormalities of the neonatal brain in MR imaging, Part II. Hypoxic-ischemic brain injury. Radiology 163:395, 1987.

30. Barkovich JA and Truwit CL: Brain damage from perinatal asphyxia: Correlation of MR findings with gestational age. AJNR 11:1087, 1990.

31. Byrne P, Welch R, Johnson MA, et al: Serial magnetic resonance imaging in neonatal hypoxic-ischemic encephalopathy. J Pediatr 117:694, 1990.

32. Lou HC, Lassen NA, and Friis-Hansen B: Impaired autoregulation of cerebral blood flow in the distressed newborn. J Pediatr 94:119, 1979.

33. Lou HC, Lassen NA, Tweed WA, et al: Pressure-passive cerebral blood flow and breakdown of the blood-brain barrier in experimental fetal asphyxia. Acta Pediatr Scand 68:35, 1979.

34. Volpe JJ, Herscovitch P, Perlman JM, et al: Positron emission tomography in the asphyxiated term newborn: Parasagittal impairment of cerebral blood flow. Ann Neurol 17:287, 1985.

35. Donn SM, Goldstein GW, and Schork A: Asphyxia neonatorum: A national survey of management practices. Pediatr Res 20:461A, 1986.

36. Black VD, Lubchenco LO, Koops BL, et al: Neonatal hyperviscosity: Randomized study of effect of partial plasma exchange transfusion on long-term outcome. Pediatrics 75:1048, 1985.

37. Gal P, Toback J, Boer H, et al: Efficacy of phenobarbital monotherapy in treatment on neonatal seizures: Relationships to blood levels. Neurology 32:1401, 1982.

38. Gilman JT, Gal P, Duchowny MS, et al: Rapid sequential phenobarbital treatment of neonatal seizures. Pediatrics 83:674, 1989.

39. Koren G, Butt W, Rajchgot P, et al: Intravenous paraldehyde for seizure control in newborn infants. Neurology 36:108, 1986.

40. Altman DI, Young RSK, and Yagel SK: Effects of dexamethasone in hypoxic-ischemic brain injury in the neonatal rat. Biol Neonate 46:149, 1984.

41. Siesjo BK: Cell damage in the brain: A speculative synthesis. J Cereb Blood Flow Metab 1:155, 1981.

42. Raichle ME: The pathophysiology of brain ischemia. Ann Neurol 13:2, 1983.

43. McCord JM: Oxygen-derived free radicals in postischemic tissue injury. N Engl J Med 312:159, 1985.

44. Palmer C, Vannucci RC, and Towfighi J: Reduction of perinatal hypoxic-ischemic brain damage with allopurinol. Pediatr Res 10:227, 1990.

45. Coyle JT, Bird SJ, Evans RH, et al: Excitatory amino acid neurotoxins: Selectivity, specificity and mechanism of action. Neurosci Res Prog Bull 19:329, 1981.

46. Rothman SM and Olney JW: Glutamate and the pathophysiology of hypoxic-ischemic brain damage. Ann Neurol 19:105, 1986.

47. McDonald JW, Silverstein FS, and Johnston MW: Neuroprotective effects of MK-801, TCP, PCP and CPP against N-methyl-D-aspartate induced neurotoxicity in an in vivo perinatal rat model. Brain Res 490:33, 1989.

48. Hattori H, Morin AM, Schwartz PH, et al: Posthypoxic treatment with MK-801 reduces hypoxic-ischemic damage in the neonatal rat. Neurology 39:713, 1989.

49. Siesjo BK and Bengtsson F: Calcium fluxes, calcium antagonists and calcium-related pathology in brain ischemia, hypoglycemia and spreading depression: A unifying hypothesis. J Cereb Blood Flow Metab 9:127, 1989.

19

Hypoxic-Ischemic Encephalopathy in the Child

Richard B. Mink, M.D.

Cerebral metabolism accounts for approximately 25% of oxygen consumption in humans, with the majority of cerebral energy supplied through aerobic metabolism. Glucose is virtually the sole source of energy, as the brain respiratory quotient (CO_2 produced/O_2 consumed) is near unity. To supply the required oxygen and glucose, the brain receives approximately one fifth of the total body cardiac output. Hence the brain is highly susceptible to injury when either blood flow or blood oxygen content is significantly reduced.

DEFINITIONS

Hypoxia refers to a reduced partial pressure of oxygen in the blood, whereas *anoxia* is used to indicate the complete lack of oxygen in the circulation. The cessation of blood flow is designated *ischemia*, and oligemia implies a reduction in blood flow. Decreased brain oxygen utilization *(brain hypoxia)* can result from an abnormality of blood flow *(stagnant hypoxia)*, a reduction in the arterial partial pressure of oxygen *(hypoxic hypoxia)*, or from insufficient hemoglobin to bind and transport oxygen *(anemic hypoxia)*. Brain hypoxia also can result from the metabolic blockade of the respiratory chain *(histotoxic hypoxia)*, as occurs in cyanide poisoning. Although these terms are of value for classifying experimental situations, they are less useful clinically, as the net effect in all is to deprive the brain of its critical oxygen supply. Furthermore, in the majority of cases, brain injury is the result of more than one category, giving rise to the term *hypoxic-ischemic* encephalopathy. This results in a *global* injury—that is, one that affects the entire brain.

ETIOLOGY

Hypoxic-ischemic encephalopathy is the most common neurologic syndrome encountered in the pediatric intensive care unit. Although the understanding of the pathophysiologic events that occur with brain hypoxia has increased immensely, there is still high morbidity and mortality associated with this entity. It is a common sequela of pediatric out-of-hospital cardiac arrests. Several studies have shown a mortality rate approaching 90%, and hospital survivors are frequently severely impaired neurologically.[1, 2]

Hypoxic-ischemic encephalopathy represents a collection of clinical entities that have in common a reduction of oxygen delivery to the brain. No study has identified the most common causes of this syndrome, though they are likely similar to the causes of pediatric respiratory and cardiac arrests. Sudden infant death syndrome and near drowning are cited as the most common causes of out-of-hospital pediatric arrests. Other causes of hypoxic-ischemic encephalopathy are listed in Table 19–1. Although the primary cause may be respiratory in nature, most often the hypoxic environment also impairs circulatory function, leading to a combined hypoxic-ischemic insult.

PATHOPHYSIOLOGY

Physiologic Determinants

Normal cerebral gray matter blood flow ranges from 80 to 100 ml/100 g tissue/min. In adults studied during carotid artery occlusion, interruption of cerebral blood flow (CBF) results in loss of consciousness within 10

Table 19–1. SOME CAUSES OF HYPOXIC-ISCHEMIC ENCEPHALOPATHY IN THE PEDIATRIC INTENSIVE CARE UNIT

Respiratory Causes	Circulatory Causes	Miscellaneous Causes
Sudden infant death syndrome	Cardiac dysrhythmia	Carbon monoxide intoxication
Near drowning	Congenital heart disease	Cyanide intoxication
Neuromuscular dysfunction	Cardiopulmonary bypass	Hemorrhage
Airway obstruction	Heart failure	
Pneumonia	Septic shock	
	Hypovolemic shock	

seconds, and the electroencephalogram (EEG) is abolished after 15 to 20 seconds when blood flow is decreased to less than 18 ml/100 g tissue/min. However, somatosensory evoked potentials are still elicited until gray matter blood flow is decreased to less than 12 ml/100 g tissue/min. White matter blood flow is lower than that in the cortical gray matter (20 to 40 ml/100 g tissue/min), but the thresholds for conduction failure are as yet undefined.

Blood flow through the brain is dependent upon three factors: cardiac output, the pressure difference between the arteries and the veins in the brain, and the vascular resistance of the intervening vessels. Cerebral perfusion pressure (CPP) is usually denoted as the mean arterial pressure minus the intracranial pressure. This assumes that intracranial pressure is higher than cerebral venous pressure, as is the usual clinical circumstance. In the event that cerebral venous pressure is greater than intracranial pressure, the CPP is more appropriately designated as mean arterial pressure minus cerebral venous pressure (Fig. 19–1). The cerebral vascular resistance is influenced by several factors, including the tone of the smooth muscle in the vessel walls and the viscosity of blood flowing through the vessels. When brain oxygen delivery is impaired, compensatory responses include an increase in CBF and an increase in oxygen extraction.

The relationship between CPP and CBF is complex and is governed by the principle of autoregulation. This is the tendency of the brain to maintain a relatively constant blood flow in the face of variations in CPP. The range of blood pressures through which the brain autoregulates CBF is well defined in the adult. At less than the lower limit (approximately 60 mm Hg), cerebral vessels are maximally dilatated and further reduction of the CPP lowers CBF. At the upper limit (approximately 160 mm Hg), vessels are maximally constricted, and elevation of the CPP results in an increase in CBF. Autoregulation in the neonate and infant is not well studied but probably differs somewhat from that in the adult. Nonetheless, in the injured brain, cerebral vessels lose their ability to autoregulate and are maximally dilatated. In this situation, CBF varies directly with the CPP. Since it is difficult to measure CBF in the clinical circumstance, the CPP is used as an index of blood flow. Experimental evidence suggests that a CPP of at least 50 mm Hg is needed to provide adequate CBF.

Biochemical Determinants

Although the general perception is that the brain can tolerate only 3 to 4 minutes of ischemia, there is evidence that neurons may be able to withstand much

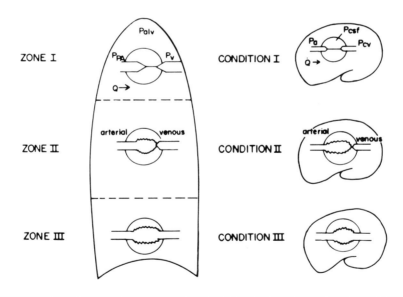

Zone/Condition	Lung		Brain	
	Pressures	Flow gradient	Pressures	Flow gradient
I	$P_{alv} > P_{PA} > P_v$	No flow	$P_{csf} > P_a > P_{cv}$	No flow
II	$P_{PA} > P_{alv} > P_v$	$P_{PA} - P_{alv}$	$P_a > P_{csf} > P_{cv}$	$P_a - P_{csf}$
III	$P_{PA} > P_v > P_{alv}$	$P_{PA} - P_v$	$P_a > P_{cv} > P_{csf}$	$P_a - P_{cv}$

Figure 19–1. Schematic diagram showing the different pressure gradients that regulate blood flow in the lung and brain. Cerebral perfusion pressure is usually represented by *condition II*, analogous to West's *zone II* of the lung. However, when $P_{cv} > P_{csf}$, the pressure gradient governing blood flow is $P_a - P_{cv}$ (*condition III*). P_{alv} = alveolar pressure; P_{PA} = pulmonary artery pressure; P_v = pulmonary venous pressure; P_{csf} = CSF pressure; P_a = arterial blood pressure; P_{cv} = cerebral venous pressure; Q = blood flow. (From Traystman RJ: Microcirculation of the brain. *In:* Mortillaro NA [ed]: Physiology and Pharmacology of the Microcirculation, Vol. 1. New York, Academic Press, 1983.)

longer periods of oxygen deprivation. Dogs subjected to 25 minutes of global ischemia had complete neurologic recovery when evaluated several days after the insult,[3] and there was significant neurophysiologic recovery in primates subjected to 60 minutes of global ischemia.[4] Studies in other species with different models of ischemia have yielded similar results. It is now believed that neurologic recovery is related not only to the circumstances surrounding the ischemic event, such as brain temperature, serum glucose levels, and the duration of ischemia, but also to events that occur when blood flow is restored, the reperfusion phase. If it is of sufficient magnitude, the hypoxic-ischemic period sets into motion a cascade of events that cause brain injury during this reperfusion period. Research has focused on understanding these events with the hope of improving neurologic outcome by providing specific therapies to prevent this added injury (see also Chapter 1).

Multiple mechanisms that may contribute to hypoxic-ischemic brain injury have been investigated. Although each pathway is discussed individually, it is important to recognize that these events are occurring simultaneously (Fig. 19–2). It is also likely that more than one mechanism is important in reperfusion injury, and therapies directed at several pathways will be necessary.

Interest in calcium as a mediator of hypoxic-ischemic injury was stimulated by studies of Schanne and colleagues, which suggested that calcium influx was the final common pathway of cell death.[5] The cell normally maintains an intracellular to extracellular calcium ratio of approximately 1:10,000 through energy-requiring processes. During ischemia when energy (adenosine triphosphate [ATP]) supplies are depleted, this gradient cannot be maintained, and calcium infuses into the cell. Calcium influx results in the activation of phospholipases, leading to the formation of free fatty acids and additional vasoactive and toxic products. Proteases are also activated by the calcium influx, leading to the breakdown of neurofilaments. Finally, calcium causes an uncoupling of mitochondrial oxidative phosphorylation. The energy provided by the reduction of oxygen is usually coupled to the production of ATP. With the increased intracellular calcium concentration, this energy is now used to sequester calcium in the mitochondria. The net effect is to deprive the cell of ATP production at a time of energy shortage.

Free radicals are highly reactive species that have an unpaired electron. They are a by-product of many "normal" cellular reactions, and as a consequence there are both nonenzymatic (e.g., ascorbic acid, tocopherol) and enzymatic (e.g., superoxide dismutase) scavenging systems that protect the cell from intrinsic damage. In reperfusion injury, it is thought that free radicals are produced at a rate that overwhelms these scavenging systems, causing damage to the lipid membrane, transport proteins, and possibly deoxyribonucleic acid (DNA). The primary oxygen-derived free radical formed, superoxide anion, is thought to be converted to the more highly reactive hydroxyl radical through reactions catalyzed by iron. Several sources of free radicals have been suggested, including the synthesis of prostaglandins, oxidation of hypoxanthine by xanthine oxidase, a mitochondrial "leak" during electron transport and through the leukocyte-associated reduced form of nicotinamide-adenine dinucleotide phosphate (NADPH) oxidase. Demonstration of a pathologic role for free radicals has been complicated by their extremely short half-life. Injury attributable to free radicals is often inferred from indirect techniques, such as an improved neurologic recovery after administration of free radical scavengers prior to reperfusion.

The accumulation of free fatty acids during ischemia also leads to the accumulation of arachidonic acid. When oxygen becomes available during reperfusion, arachidonic acid may be further metabolized by the enzyme cyclooxygenase to unstable prostaglandin intermediates. In the endothelial cell, these intermediates are converted to prostacyclin, a potent vasodilator and inhibitor of platelet aggregation, whereas in the platelet and macrophage, they are converted to the potent vasoconstrictor and platelet aggregator, thromboxane A$_2$. During reperfusion, the thromboxane-prostacyclin balance may shift, favoring vasoconstriction and thrombosis and contributing to the altered blood flow observed following ischemia. In addition, metabolism of arachidonic acid by lipooxygenase produces the hydroxyeicosatetraenoic (HETE) compounds, which are powerful vasoconstrictors and chemotactants.

Recent experimental evidence suggests that excitatory neurotransmitter amino acids, specifically L-glutamate and L-aspartate, may contribute to brain injury after ischemia. It is thought that following ischemia, these amino acids are released, leading to neuronal depolarization at a time of energy depletion. The net result is additional neurologic injury. Support for this hypothesis is gained from experiments in which interruption of excitatory pathways protects against neuronal damage,[6] and when a glutamate receptor antagonist is adminis-

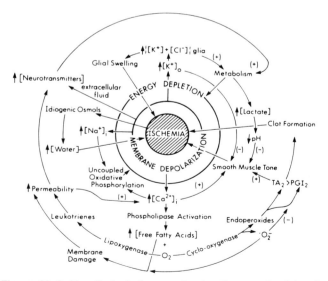

Figure 19–2. Hypothetical diagram showing the complex interrelationships between biochemical events promoting tissue injury in brain ischemia-reperfusion. $(+)$ = stimulatory effect; $(-)$ = inhibitory effect; TA$_2$ = thromboxane A$_2$; PGI$_2$ = prostacyclin; $\cdot$O$_2^-$ = superoxide anion. (From Raichle ME: The pathophysiology of brain ischemia. Ann Neurol 13:3, 1983.)

tered prior to ischemia, brain injury is reduced[7] (see also Chapter 23).

Since the brain is highly dependent upon the oxidation of glucose as a source of energy, interest has focused on altering the brain glucose supply to reduce brain injury. Contrary to what was expected, Myers and Yamaguchi found that the administration of glucose to primates prior to ischemia worsened neurologic outcome.[8] Furthermore, recovery was significantly worse in those primates who had incomplete ischemia (trickle flow) when compared with those subjected to complete ischemia (no flow). This apparent paradox is explained as follows. Brain tissue lactate levels have been shown to be inversely correlated with tissue damage. In incomplete ischemia, oxygen delivery is inadequate, and energy production shifts to anaerobic pathways. However, because there is a small amount of blood flow, glucose is continuously supplied and lactate accumulates. In complete ischemia, lactate accumulation is limited, since substrate is not continuously supplied. In a few clinical investigations, hyperglycemia following resuscitation has been associated with reduced neurologic recovery.

Morphologic Determinants

Reperfusion of a previously ischemic area results in a heterogeneous pattern of microcirculatory blood flow, with areas of very low flow juxtaposed with areas of high flow. Presumably these areas of hypoperfusion do not receive adequate oxygen and glucose for continued neuronal survival, leading to additional tissue injury. Various mechanisms have been proposed to explain postischemic hypoperfusion, including blockage of vessels by swollen astrocytes, obstruction by aggregated platelets and leukocytes, intravascular coagulation, and vascular spasm. An improvement in postischemic blood flow has been associated with improved neuronal recovery.

Two pathologic patterns may be observed following cerebral hypoxia-ischemia. Injury may involve neurons in specific regions of the brain that are particularly sensitive to ischemia. These so-called selectively vulnerable areas include the CA1 and CA4 areas of the hippocampus, the parahippocampal gyrus, parts of the cortical layers, the Purkinje cells, and specific areas in the brain stem. Brain stem damage in the infant and child is particularly more extensive than that seen in the adult. Brain injury also may involve damage to neurons in the arterial boundary (or "watershed") zones, though this pattern is usually seen after severe hypotension, an unusual cause of hypoxic-ischemic encephalopathy in children. If blood flow is completely interrupted for a long enough time and, supportive care is subsequently provided for a sufficient time, the brain will undergo a process of in vivo autolysis, resulting in liquefaction necrosis of all tissue elements, the "respirator brain."

CLINICAL MANAGEMENT

Although the body of information concerning the pathophysiology of hypoxic-ischemic encephalopathy

has increased immensely in the past few years, no single therapeutic agent has emerged that will prevent the neurologic damage that occurs after a severe hypoxic-ischemic episode. Current treatment is thus supportive, with the goal of care to minimize further neurologic injury. Supportive care must encompass all organ systems, since other organs have also sustained a hypoxic-ischemic insult (see also Chapter 13).

General Principles

Since the initial pathophysiologic event is one of brain oxygen deprivation, foremost in care should be the maintenance of adequate ventilation, oxygenation, and circulation. In most cases of severe hypoxia-ischemia, tracheal intubation is necessary, not only for mechanical ventilation but also for airway protection. Oxygenation should be maintained in the normal range. In order to minimize the toxic effects of a high FIO_2, positive end-expiratory pressure should be used as necessary. Although there is little clinical data to document that hyperventilation will improve outcome, it is prudent to maintain PCO_2 at 30 to 35 mm Hg to compensate for cerebral tissue acidosis. Muscle relaxants may be used, but they should be periodically discontinued to allow assessment of the neurologic status.

Because global brain injury leads to alterations in microcirculatory blood flow and loss of vessel autoregulation, support of the circulation following ischemia is critical. Hypotension should be aggressively treated with either inotropes or fluid boluses, but care should be exercised to avoid overhydration. Severe hypertension should also be avoided, because this has been demonstrated to augment neurologic damage.[9] If cardiac function is severely compromised and blood pressure is difficult to maintain, consideration may be given to placement of a pulmonary artery catheter to aid in assessing fluid status and to measure cardiac output. However, in the usual case, cardiac function that has been this severely compromised by hypoxia-ischemia usually portends a very poor neurologic outcome.

Serum glucose concentration should be monitored, and hypoglycemia should be treated without delay. There is controversy as to whether hyperglycemia during the reperfusion phase is detrimental to neurologic recovery; however, it seems prudent to avoid it.

Central Nervous System Management

Serial neurologic examinations are of critical importance in the management of the patient with hypoxic-ischemic encephalopathy. Repetitive examinations are necessary to assess the extent of injury, rule out seizure activity, evaluate treatment, and eventually ascertain prognosis. If sedatives, analgesics, or muscle relaxants are required, short-acting agents should be administered. This will allow intermittent emergence and an accurate neurologic assessment. A computed tomographic scan of the brain is not essential for management, though it may be required to exclude mass lesions, especially if head trauma is part of the differential diagnosis.

Seizures are not infrequent after a cerebral hypoxic-ischemic insult. In adult studies, 20 to 30% of patients have seizures following cardiopulmonary arrest[10, 11]; the incidence is unknown in children. Detection of seizure activity may be difficult and require EEG confirmation. Patients with seizures who are receiving muscle relaxants should have continuous EEG monitoring to eliminate the possibility of undiagnosed seizure activity. Seizures should be treated aggressively, because they increase cerebral metabolism at a time of diminished oxygen delivery. Treatment with anticonvulsants such as phenobarbital or benzodiazepines may interfere with an accurate neurologic assessment. Many advocate the use of phenytoin because of its lesser sedating properties. Seizure prophylaxis has not been demonstrated to be of any benefit in altering neurologic outcome.

There is controversy surrounding the use of intracranial pressure monitoring in hypoxic-ischemic brain injury in children. Although cerebral edema is a prominent feature of focal cerebral ischemia and contributes to intracranial compartment shifts, the role of cerebral swelling and increased intracranial pressure in hypoxic-ischemic encephalopathy is unclear. In experimental models of global ischemia, brain water content increases after reperfusion, and may progress for several days before it subsides. Intracranial pressure is moderately elevated after the ischemic episode but then normalizes. In some studies, an increase in intracranial pressure is seen at 48 to 72 hours in association with poor neurologic recovery.[12] Results from clinical studies of hypoxic-ischemic encephalopathy have been inconsistent, with some studies reporting increased intracranial pressure and others reporting normal pressure.[13, 14] Therapies directed at maintaining normal intracranial pressure have failed to alter neurologic outcome, although an elevated intracranial pressure may be prognostic. Studies by Black and colleagues[15] and Nussbaum and Galant[16] in pediatric near-drowning found that an intracranial pressure greater than 20 mm Hg was associated with a poor outcome. Evidence suggests that increased intracranial pressure is more a manifestation of severe brain injury and that treatments directed at control of intracranial pressure will be ineffective. As a consequence, many centers have now abandoned the practice of monitoring intracranial pressure in hypoxic-ischemic encephalopathy.

Hypothermia prior to an ischemic insult is efficacious in preventing neurologic damage, as it reduces cellular metabolism, thereby decreasing substrate requirements. It is routinely used for cerebral protection for surgical repair of congenital heart disease. In addition, many children who have experienced prolonged cold water submersion had full neurologic recovery. When used as a therapy after an ischemic insult, hypothermia has not been demonstrated to be of benefit, and its use is associated with an increase in septic complications.[17] It also may be detrimental by increasing blood viscosity and thereby lowering blood flow. At present, this therapy cannot be recommended.

The role of glucocorticoids in the treatment of hy-poxic-ischemic encephalopathy is controversial, but their use appears to be of little benefit. Recent studies evaluating steroid treatment following cardiac arrest in adults have not shown improvement in neurologic recovery.[18] Furthermore, an animal study suggests that neurologic injury is potentiated by steroid treatment following global cerebral ischemia.[19]

Barbiturates have been intensively investigated as drugs that may ameliorate damage from global ischemia. Among their many effects, barbiturates have been shown to lower cerebral metabolism and CBF, reduce intracranial pressure, reduce free fatty acid generation during ischemia, and scavenge free radicals. Favorable results examining barbiturate therapy in animal models of cerebral ischemia in the early 1970s led to a large, prospective, randomized study of thiopental after cardiac arrest in adults.[20] In this study of comatose patients, thiopental administered within 1 hour of resuscitation failed to improve neurologic outcome. Another barbiturate, pentobarbital, also did not improve neurologic outcome in nearly drowned children.[21] More recent animal studies have not confirmed the efficacy of barbiturates observed in the earlier investigations. Furthermore, large doses of these drugs frequently produce hypotension, compromising cerebral perfusion. Barbiturates should not be used routinely in the management of hypoxic-ischemic encephalopathy, though they may be administered to treat seizures or, if so desired, to reduce intracranial pressure.

Future Therapeutic Modalities

The increased understanding of the pathophysiologic events that contribute to neurologic injury after cerebral ischemia has led to several promising therapeutic strategies (Table 19–2). These therapies require additional evaluation before they can be advocated for "brain resuscitation." It is likely that successful treatment of cerebral ischemia will encompass multiple modalities.

Calcium antagonists have been investigated in animal models with the intent of preventing the postischemic intracellular accumulation of calcium associated with neuronal cell death. Of the many agents evaluated, nimodipine has shown the most promise, as it seems to selectively increase CBF. Although many studies have shown some benefit of nimodipine, even when administered after ischemia, neurologic recovery has been

Table 19–2. FUTURE THERAPEUTIC AGENTS

Pathophysiologic Goal	Proposed Agents
Decrease intracellular calcium accumulation	Calcium channel blockers
Decrease free radical damage	Free radical scavengers Allopurinol
Inhibit excitatory neurotransmitters	Excitatory amino acid blockers
Improve tissue oxygen delivery	
1. Decrease blood viscosity	Hemodilution
2. Increase blood oxygen-carrying capacity	Perfluorocarbons Hyperbaric oxygen

variable. Since calcium antagonists block only voltage-regulated channels, additional agents may be necessary to inhibit receptor-mediated channels to prevent intracellular calcium accumulation.

Free radical scavengers present an exciting but challenging area of therapeutic intervention. To be effective, free radical scavengers must be administered during the early stages of reperfusion, and they must be able to cross the blood-brain barrier. The administration of superoxide dismutase and catalase prior to reperfusion has improved neurologic recovery in some models of global ischemia. Pretreatment with the xanthine oxidase inhibitor allopurinol has also shown some value, possibly by preventing the formation of xanthine oxidase–derived free radicals. Other scavengers, such as ascorbate, α-tocopherol, and mannitol, have been of variable benefit. The effectiveness of free radical scavengers in the clinical realm remains to be determined.

The development of excitatory amino acid inhibitors that cross the blood-brain barrier has stimulated interest in these drugs as potential therapeutic agents. One such agent, MK-801, an antagonist to the N-methyl-D-aspartate (NMDA) receptor, showed early promise in ameliorating neurologic injury, even when given after ischemia. Newer agents are currently under investigation, but it is unlikely that these drugs will be available clinically for several years (see also Chapter 23).

Several therapeutic strategies have been proposed to improve postischemic oxygen delivery. These methods attempt to increase oxygen delivery to neurons located in marginally or hypoperfused regions. One such method is hemodilution. Since blood flow is inversely related to blood viscosity, it is hypothesized that lowering viscosity will improve microcirculatory blood flow. Clinical studies have failed to show a significant benefit of this therapy in patients who have had a stroke; however, these studies have been criticized for initiating therapy too long after the event, lowering the hematocrit too slowly, and not lowering it enough.[22] Clinical studies of hemodilution following global cerebral ischemia are lacking.

A second approach to increasing oxygen delivery is through the administration of perfluorocarbons. These chemicals have been advocated as blood substitutes because of their high affinity for O_2 and CO_2. Furthermore, their small particle size could increase oxygen-carrying capacity without a corresponding increase in blood viscosity. Animal studies with early perfluorocarbon preparations showed only a small benefit, but newer preparations carry significantly more oxygen and are currently under evaluation.

Hyperbaric oxygen is another method to increase tissue oxygen delivery (see Chapter 43). Normally, oxygen in the blood is transported bound to erythrocytes; dissolved oxygen accounts for less than 2% of the total oxygen carried. However, hyperbaric oxygen can significantly increase the contribution of dissolved oxygen to total oxygen delivery. For example, when breathing 100% O_2 at 2.8 atm absolute, and assuming a hemoglobin of 12 g/dl, dissolved oxygen provides about 25% of total oxygen delivery. This is equivalent to the oxygen transported by 4.8 g/dl of fully saturated hemoglobin.

Hyperbaric oxygen has been shown to improve mortality in models of focal ischemia (i.e., stroke), and evidence suggests that it does not increase free radical production. Only one study has evaluated hyperbaric oxygen therapy after global cerebral ischemia.[23] In this investigation, cats who were subjected to 5 minutes of circulatory arrest had improved EEG recovery and decreased cerebrospinal fluid lactate accumulation when treated with hyperbaric oxygen. Although more work needs to be done, hyperbaric oxygen is a promising adjunctive therapy in the treatment of hypoxic-ischemic encephalopathy.

PROGNOSIS

The prognosis following cerebral hypoxia-ischemia depends upon several factors, foremost of which is the duration of time that the brain is deprived of oxygen. Other factors, such as core (or more appropriately brain) temperature at the time of the event, also must be taken into account. Generally, any incident that does not lead to complete loss of consciousness rarely, if ever, causes permanent neurologic injury.

Prediction of the neurologic outcome of the child in coma is based on the clinical examination. Therefore, care must be taken to address those factors that interfere with an accurate neurologic assessment. The child should be normotensive and normothermic, and medications that preclude an accurate clinical examination (i.e., sedatives, muscle relaxants) should be discontinued. A metabolic cause for coma should be excluded, since prognostic data derived from studies of hypoxic-ischemic encephalopathy are not applicable to this situation. Furthermore, one must be cautious in interpreting the neurologic examination of the postictal patient.

Only a few studies have evaluated prognostic factors in hypoxic-ischemic encephalopathy in children. Most investigations have been in near-drowning and have focused on the early neurologic examination, predominantly using the Glasgow Coma Score. One study of children experiencing cardiopulmonary arrest after nearly drowning found that an early (2 to 6 hours after resuscitation) Glasgow Coma Score of 3 was predictive of a poor neurologic outcome.[24] Furthermore, patients with unreactive pupils at the time of admission to the intensive care unit either died or had severe brain damage. The applicability of these data to other causes of hypoxic-ischemic encephalopathy is unknown. Studies by Snyder and associates[25, 26] and by Levy and colleagues[11] of adults in hypoxic-ischemic coma have identified neurologic findings of prognostic significance; however, caution is advised when extrapolating these findings to children, especially very young children. In these studies, the level of consciousness was associated with neurologic recovery. Most adults who became fully alert did so within the first 72 hours after resuscitation; a deepening coma within the first 48 hours was associated with a poor outcome. Neurologic findings within 6 hours of resuscitation were of lesser prognostic significance; however, abnormalities after this period were predictive. Specifically, the lack of the pupillary light reflex or of the corneal reflex after 6 hours indicated an extremely poor prognosis. Although the lack of brain stem reflexes was of prognostic significance, the presence of intact brain stem reflexes was not predictive of good recovery. After 3 days, the motor response was a good predictor; no better than a flexor response indicated a poor recovery. The presence of seizures following resuscitation was not correlated with neurologic recovery.

The use of the EEG as a prognostic tool has had variable success. Overall, it is of limited benefit, except when the abnormality is mild or extremely severe. Some studies suggest that continuous EEG monitoring with frequency analysis methods (e.g., compressed spectral array) improves the predictive capability. Somatosensory evoked potentials have shown some prognostic value in adults with coma of various causes. It remains to be seen whether these methods will augment the clinical examination and improve outcome prediction in hypoxic-ischemic encephalopathy.

References

1. Lewis JK, Minter MG, and Eshelman SJ: Outcome of pediatric resuscitation. Ann Emerg Med 12:5, 1983.
2. Zaritsky A, Nadkarni V, Getson P, et al: CPR in children. Ann Emerg Med 16:10, 1987.
3. Neely WA and Youmans JR: Anoxia of canine brain without damage. JAMA 183:1085, 1963.
4. Hossmann KA and Kleihues P: Reversibility of ischemic brain damage. Arch Neurol 29:375, 1973.
5. Schanne FAX, Kane AB, Young EE, et al: Calcium dependence of toxic cell death: A final common pathway. Science 206:700, 1979.
6. Pulsinelli WA: Deafferentation of the hippocampus protects CA1 pyramidal neurons against ischemic injury. Stroke 16:144, 1985.
7. Kochlar A, Zivin JA, and Lyden PD: Glutamate antagonist therapy reduces neurologic deficits produced by focal central nervous system ischemia. Arch Neurol 45:148, 1988.
8. Myers RE and Yamaguchi M: Effects of serum glucose concentration on brain response to circulatory arrest. J Neuropathol Exp Neurol 35:301, 1976.
9. Kontos HA: Oxygen radicals in cerebral vascular injury. Circ Res 57:508, 1985.
10. Snyder BA, Hauser WA, Loewenson RB, et al: Neurologic prognosis after cardiopulmonary arrest. III: Seizure activity. Neurology 30:1292, 1980.
11. Levy DE, Caronna JJ, Singer BH, et al: Predicting outcome from hypoxic-ischemic coma. JAMA 253:1420, 1985.
12. Snyder JV, Nemoto EM, Carroll RG, et al: Global ischemia in dogs: Intracranial pressures, brain blood flow and metabolism. Stroke 6:21, 1975.
13. Senter HJ, Wolf A, and Wagner FC: Intracranial pressure in nontraumatic ischemic and hypoxic cerebral insults. J Neurosurg 54:489, 1981.
14. Snyder BD and Tabbaa MA: Assessment and treatment of neurological dysfunction after cardiac arrest. Curr Concepts Cardiovasc Dis (Stroke) 12:1, 1987.
15. Black PR, Van Devanter S, and Cohn LH: Effect of hypothermia on systemic and organ system metabolism and function. J Surg Res 20:49, 1976.
16. Nussbaum E and Galant SP: Intracranial pressure monitoring as a guide to prognosis in the nearly drowned, severely comatose child. J Pediatr 102:215, 1983.
17. Bohn DJ, Biggar WD, Smith CR, et al: Influence of hypothermia, barbiturate therapy, and intracranial pressure monitoring on morbidity and mortality after near-drowning. Crit Care Med 14:529, 1986.
18. Jastremski M, Sutton-Tyrell K, Vaagenes P, et al: Glucocorticoid treatment does not improve neurological recovery following cardiac arrest. JAMA 262:3427, 1989.
19. Sapolsky RM and Pulsinelli WA: Glucocorticoids potentiate ischemic injury to neurons: Therapeutic implications. Science 229:1397, 1985.
20. Brain Resuscitation Clinical Trial I Study Group: Randomized clinical study of thiopental loading in comatose survivors of cardiac arrest. N Engl J Med 314:397, 1986.
21. Nussbaum E and Maggi JC: Pentobarbital therapy does not improve neurologic outcome in nearly drowned, flaccid-comatose children. Pediatrics 81:630, 1988.
22. Heros RC and Korosue K: Hemodilution for acute stroke. Stroke 20:423, 1989.
23. Kapp JP, Phillips M, Markov A, et al: Hyperbaric oxygen after circulatory arrest: Modification of postischemic encephalopathy. Neurosurgery 11:496, 1982.
24. Allman FD, Nelson WB, Pacentine GA, et al: Outcome following cardiopulmonary resuscitation in severe pediatric near-drowning. Am J Dis Child 140:571, 1986.
25. Snyder BD, Gumnit RJ, Leppik IE, et al: Neurologic prognosis after cardiopulmonary arrest. IV: Brain stem reflexes. Neurology 31:1092, 1981.
26. Snyder BD, Loewenson RB, Gumnit RJ, et al: Neurologic prognosis after cardiopulmonary arrest. II: Level of consciousness. Neurology 30:52, 1980.

General References

Bircher NG: Brain resuscitation. Resuscitation 18(Suppl):S1, 1989.
Brierley JB and Graham DI: Hypoxia and vascular disorders of the central nervous system. In: Adams JHM, Corsellis JAN, and Duchen LW (eds): Greenfield's Neuropathology, 4th ed. New York, John Wiley & Sons, 1984, pp 125–156.
Kochanek PM: Novel pharmacologic approaches to brain resuscitation after cardiorespiratory arrest in the pediatric patient. Crit Care Clin 4:661, 1988.
Rogers MC and Kirsch JR: Current concepts in brain resuscitation. JAMA 261:3143, 1989.
Siesjö BK: Cell damage in the brain: A speculative synthesis. J Cereb Blood Flow Metab 1:155, 1981.
Snyder BD (ed): Anoxic and ischemic encephalopathies. In: Bradley W, Daroff R, Fenichel G, et al (eds): Neurology in Clinical Practice. Stoneham, MA, Butterworths, in press.

20

Intracranial Infections

Barbara A. Jantausch, M.D.

Central nervous system infections are a significant cause of morbidity and mortality in the pediatric population. The serious neurologic consequences of these infections as well as secondary failure of other organ systems mandates the management of severely affected patients to critical care specialists. This chapter outlines the presentation, diagnostic evaluation, and management of pediatric patients with encephalitis, meningitis, brain abscess, subdural empyema, and epidural abscess.

ENCEPHALITIS

Encephalitis is an inflammation of the brain, often including the meninges, resulting in meningoencephalitis. Patients who present with clinical signs of encephalitis but lack signs of inflammation have an encephalopathy. Encephalitis can result from direct involvement of the brain by a pathogen such as rabies or herpes simplex virus (HSV) or from indirect effects mediated by a toxin or vasculitis, such as that which occurs in Rocky Mountain spotted fever. Pathogens can reach the brain through hematogenous spread or along neuronal pathways. In most cases of encephalitis, no etiologic agent is identified.[1]

Fever, headache, altered mental status, abnormal behavior, focal neurologic signs, and seizures characterize encephalitis.

PATHOGENS

Etiologic agents for infectious encephalitis are listed in Table 20–1. Viruses are a common cause of encephalitis in children.

Enteroviruses

Enteroviral encephalitis is caused by coxsackieviruses A and B, echoviruses, and enterovirus 71. These agents are present during late summer and early fall. The outcome following enteroviral encephalitis is generally good; however, death may occur. Disease in immunocompromised patients can be very severe.

Arboviruses

Arthropod-borne viruses (arboviruses) are ribonucleic acid (RNA) viruses transmitted by ticks and mosquitoes during the summer and early fall. Disease may occur in isolated cases or in epidemics and is caused primarily by California encephalitis (CE) virus, St. Louis encephalitis (SLE) virus, eastern equine encephalitis (EEE) virus and western equine encephalitis (WEE) virus in the

Table 20–1. ETIOLOGIC AGENTS IN ENCEPHALITIS

Viruses:	Enteroviruses	Parainfluenza I, II, and III
	Arboviruses	Influenza
	Herpes simplex I and II	Epstein-Barr virus
	Varicella	Adenovirus
	Mumps	Cytomegalovirus
	Measles	Rubella
	Rabies	
	Herpesvirus simiae (herpes B)	
	Lymphocytic choriomeningitis	
Bacteria:	*Haemophilus influenzae*	
	Streptococcus pneumoniae	
	Neisseria meningitidis	
	Mycobacteria	
Rickettsiae:	Rocky Mountain spotted fever	
	Typhus	
Spirochetes:	*Leptospira*	
	Borrelia burgdorferi	
	Treponema pallidum	
Fungi:	*Blastomyces dermatidis*	
	Coccidioides immitis	
	Cryptococcus neoformans	
	Histoplasma capsulatum	
	Nocardia asteroides	
Parasites:	*Plasmodium falciparum* malaria	
	Naegleria, Acanthamoeba	
	Toxoplasmosis	
	Schistosomiasis, trichinosis, *Strongyloides stercoralis*	
Other:	*Mycoplasma pneumoniae, M. hominis*	
	Cat-scratch disease	

United States.[2] Japanese B encephalitis virus is common in China and southeast Asia.[3]

Herpes Simplex

HSV is responsible for 10% of encephalitis cases in the United States; the annual incidence is 1/250,000 to 1/500,000 people per year. One third of the cases of HSV encephalitis occur within the pediatric population (individuals younger than 20 years of age).[3] Neonatal HSV encephalitis can be caused by either HSV type 1 or HSV type 2; HSV encephalitis in older children is usually secondary to HSV type 1.

Other Viruses

Varicella encephalitis occurs in 0.3/1,000 patients with chickenpox and has a fatality rate of 17%. With the advent of measles, mumps, and rubella vaccine (MMR), mumps and measles are less common causes of encephalitis but still occur. Encephalitis occurs in 3/1,000 patients with mumps and 0.74/1,000 patients with measles and has fatality rates of 1.4% and 14%, respectively.[1] Cytomegalovirus, toxoplasmosis, and rubella encephalitis can be seen in association with congenital infection. *Herpesvirus simiae* (herpes B) can be transmitted by a bite from a monkey.[3]

Other Pathogens

Common pediatric bacterial meningitis pathogens can produce meningoencephalitis. Encephalitis secondary to *Spirochetes*,[4, 5] *Rickettsia*,[6] *Mycoplasma*,[7] and cat-scratch disease[8] can occur in normal children, whereas fungal infections such as *Blastomyces dermatitidis*, *Coccidiodes immitis*, and *Cryptococcus neoformans* are most often seen in immunocompromised hosts.[6] Parasitic species such as *Plasmodium falciparum* malaria[9] and schistosomiasis are suspected if the patient has travelled to an endemic area. History of swimming in a freshwater lake suggests the possibility of amebic encephalitis with *Naegleria* and *Acanthamoeba*[10]; history of ingestion of raw meat or contact with cat litter boxes suggests toxoplasmosis.[6]

DIAGNOSTIC EVALUATION

Diagnostic evaluation of a patient with clinical signs and symptoms of encephalitis includes a careful history to (1) exclude other causes of pathology, including toxin ingestion or exposure and head trauma and (2) gain information that may help to identify the etiologic agent. This history should include exposure to persons who are ill, especially individuals with rashes or who have travelled to outside areas or foreign countries, or exposure to animals (especially horses) and to any mosquito, tick, or animal bites. A physical examination of the patient should include a detailed neurologic examination and

an evaluation for signs of increased intracranial pressure (ICP), impending herniation, and focal neurologic signs.

The presence of cutaneous HSV lesions in a neonate is an indication for acyclovir therapy. In the older child, HSV skin lesions can occur with other diagnoses and are present in only a few patients with HSV encephalitis. The neonate may present with focal seizures that progress to generalized seizures having little response to anticonvulsant therapy; infants may develop abnormal breathing patterns and apnea.[11]

Patients who present with fever, altered mental status, or other signs of encephalitis should have a lumbar puncture (LP) unless contraindicated by increased ICP, a computed tomography (CT) scan of the head with and without contrast, and an electroencephalogram (EEG) as part of the initial diagnostic evaluation. Most patients with encephalitis have a cerebrospinal fluid (CSF) pleocytosis on LP, elevated protein, and usually normal glucose. If done early in the course of illness, the initial LP may be normal and become abnormal later in the course of disease. A few patients may have persistently normal CSF examinations in encephalitis. A CT scan of the head (including contrast) should be done to rule out other diagnostic possibilities, such as brain abscess, tumor, or hemorrhage, and to look for evidence of focal involvement in an encephalitic process. Brain scan or magnetic resonance imaging (MRI) may localize lesions that are not present on a CT scan.[12] In many cases of encephalitis, the EEG shows diffuse slowing with no focality; focality on an EEG in encephalitis suggests HSV disease.

Depending on the season of the year and outbreaks in the community, the diagnostic evaluation outlined in Table 20–2 should be appropriately modified and pursued. All patients should have viral and bacterial cultures taken. A sample of serum should be frozen and saved for a comparison of acute and convalescent sera.

A definitive diagnosis in encephalitis cannot be made unless the etiologic agent is recovered from brain tissue by culture or identified by histopathology or by special staining (i.e., immunofluorescence). Presumptive diagnosis in the case of encephalitis is often made by identification of an organism from another focus in the body, by positive serology finding,[1] and retrospectively by use of acute and convalescent titers.

Herpes simplex is the only viral agent for which effective chemotherapy has been documented to improve outcome; therefore, it is essential that the diagnosis of HSV encephalitis is recognized so that antiviral therapy may be instituted as early as possible. Acute febrile encephalitis with focal signs suggests the diagnosis of HSV encephalitis.[13] Focal seizures or localizing findings on neurologic examination may clinically suggest focality as may the diagnostic studies listed in Table 20–3.

A brain biopsy is the most sensitive and specific test for the diagnosis of HSV encephalitis and can diagnose other conditions for which alternate therapy is available. HSV has been isolated from 33 to 45% of brain biopsy specimens from patients with presumptive HSV encephalitis.[14, 15] Other authors contend that a brain biopsy is an invasive diagnostic modality, which rarely

Table 20–2. DIAGNOSTIC EVALUATION IN
ENCEPHALITIS

Baseline evaluation
Cerebrospinal fluid (unless contraindicated by increased ICP)
   Cell count, protein
   Chemistry
   HSV I and II titers
Electroencephalogram
CT* scan (with and without contrast)

Cultures
Viral:
Nose, throat, conjunctiva, rectum, spinal fluid, blood, urine, genital
   swab from the mother (when the patient is a neonate)
Bacterial:
Spinal fluid, blood urine, stool

Serology
Viral
Arbovirus; measles; mumps; varicella; adenovirus; parainfluenza I,
   II, and III; influenza; Epstein-Barr virus; TORCH
Other Pathogens
Mycoplasma (CF), RPR, Rocky Mountain spotted fever, leptospira,
   Lyme, fungal

Imaging
MRI
Brain scan

Miscellaneous
Chest x-ray
Slit-lamp examination (for chorioretinitis in CMV, toxoplasmosis)
PPD, anergy panel
CSF for AFB smear, culture, and fungal culture

AFB = acid-fast bacteria; CMV = cytomegalovirus; CT = computed
tomography; HSV = herpes simplex virus; ICP = intracranial pressure; MRI
= magnetic resonance imaging; PPD = purified protein derivative; RPR =
rapid plasma-reagin; TORCH = toxoplasmosis, rubella, cytomegalovirus, and
herpes simplex.

yields information on alternate diagnoses that cannot be obtained from noninvasive testing.[16] Currently, brain biopsy in cases of suspected HSV encephalitis is recommended for patients who do not respond to acyclovir therapy within 72 hours and who have a focal abnormality on a CT scan, MRI, or brain scan. HSV antigen

Table 20–3. DIAGNOSTIC EVALUATION OF A PATIENT
WITH HERPES SIMPLEX ENCEPHALITIS

Test	Result	Onset Positivity
EEG*	Periodic lateralized epileptiform discharges	1 day
MRI†	Focal lesion, temporal lobe most common, also frontal and parietal lobes	3 days
Brain scan	Focal lesion	3 days
CT‡ scan (contrast)	Focal lesion	5–7 days
HSV§ antigen (CSF‖)	Positive	3–7 days
HSV antibody	Fourfold increase in titer (of retrospective use only)	2–3 weeks

*EEG = electroencephalogram.
†MRI = magnetic resonance imaging.
‡CT = computed tomography.
§HSV = herpes simplex virus.
‖CSF = cerebrospinal fluid.

testing from CSF, although not commercially available, has a sensitivity of 62% and a specificity of 82% on samples obtained within the first week of onset of symptoms. These values reach 100% sensitivity and 89% specificity in patients who are symptomatic for 8 to 14 days.[17]

A brain biopsy should be performed in immunocompromised patients who have a focal lesion present on imaging studies and in whom the diagnosis is unknown. The pathology and clinical microbiology laboratories should be notified in advance when a brain biopsy is to be performed so that a pathologist, neuropathology technician, and microbiology technician are available to process the specimen and to inoculate cultures. A piece of tissue should be sent to pathology for histopathology, routine staining, and special staining, including immunofluorescence for HSV; a second piece should be sent to the microbiology laboratory for Gram stain, routine culture, anaerobic culture, fungal culture, acid-fast bacteria (AFB) smear and culture, and viral cultures.

MANAGEMENT

The underlying disease process should be treated once an agent is identified. Patients in whom bacteriologic disease is not ruled out should receive empiric antibiotic therapy for 10 to 14 days if no agent is identified. Acyclovir therapy should be considered in patients with varicella encephalitis.[18] The patient with encephalitis should be monitored closely for the development of cerebral edema and increased ICP and monitored for signs of early herniation (see Chapters 19 and 20). Use of dexamethasone may not be appropriate in cases of acute viral encephalitis in which it may enhance the viral process. Seizures should be treated with dilantin preferably, so as not to alter neurologic status.

Fluids and electrolytes should be monitored closely, because these patients are likely to develop syndrome of inappropriate antidiuretic hormone secretion (SIADH). All medications should be given parenterally. Hyperalimentation may be required if symptoms persist and adequate intake is not established. Patients may experience deterioration in respiratory function or sudden cardiorespiratory arrest from a central origin. Gastrointestinal bleeding and disseminated intravascular coagulation (DIC) can also occur.[1]

Untreated HSV encephalitis has a mortality of 70%. Patients treated with acyclovir with Glasgow coma scores of 6 or less have an overall mortality of 25%, whereas those with scores above 6 and above 10 have mortality rates of 17% and 0%, respectively. The overall mortality rate for acyclovir-treated patients younger than 30 years of age is 6%.[14]

Patients with HSV encephalitis should receive a 10- to 14-day course of antiviral chemotherapy with intravenous acyclovir, 30 mg/kg/day divided every 8 hours. Neonates with HSV encephalitis should receive a 14-day course of acyclovir to minimize the risk of a recurrence. Patients with HSV encephalitis with ocular infection should be treated with topical antiviral therapy in addition to systemic therapy.

The few viral isolates examined from patients who had a relapse have retained sensitivity to acyclovir; higher doses of acyclovir 45 mg/kg/day divided every 8 hours for a longer duration (21 days) and in combination with vidarabine have been used for some patients who have had a relapse. A brain biopsy should be considered in the case of a suspected relapse. Postinfectious encephalomyelitis with demyelination has been described after cases of HSV encephalitis.[3, 19]

MENINGITIS

Meningitis is an inflammation of the meninges. Infection can be caused by bacteria, viruses, fungi, and other agents, including spirochetes.

PATHOGENESIS

Infection of the meninges most commonly occurs through hematogenous spread and rarely from the contiguous spread of organisms from the sinuses, middle ear, or mastoids. Organisms commonly progress from the nasopharynx to the blood stream, then to the meninges. Meningitis can occur after head trauma, and *S. pneumoniae* or *H. influenzae* may be isolated following breaks in the cribiform plate or fractures of the sinuses. Meningitis can develop as a complication of neurosurgical procedures and from direct inoculation of organisms into the CSF from meningomyeloceles or dermoid sinus tracts.[20, 21]

PRESENTATION

The clinical presentation of patients with meningitis varies according to the age of the patient. Neonates with meningitis usually present with nonlocalizing signs and symptoms, such as lethargy, irritability, vomiting, dehydration, and possibly fever, and rarely with a bulging fontanelle, seizures, or nuchal rigidity. The older child and adolescent typically present with altered consciousness, headache, nuchal rigidity, fever, and photophobia. Cranial nerve palsies may also be present. Skin lesions progressing from maculopapular lesions to petechiae and purpura also occur. Outside the neonatal period it may be possible to elicit a positive Kernig or Brudzinski sign. Patients with meningitis may present with an insidious course or with one marked by an abrupt onset with rapid deterioration in which the risk of herniation and death is pronounced.

Focal signs, including hemiparesis, facial nerve palsy, and endophthalmitis occur in 15% of patients with meningitis and may be the result of cortical vessel thrombosis. The presence of focal neurologic signs or papilledema is an indication for a CT scan.[20]

DIAGNOSIS

The definitive diagnosis of meningitis is made by analysis of CSF. An LP should be performed on patients suspected of having meningitis unless contraindicated by: (1) cardiorespiratory instability; (2) increased ICP; and (3) local infection overlying the site of LP.[21] Thrombocytopenia may delay performance of an LP until platelet levels are adequate. Patients suspected of having meningitis in whom LP is contraindicated or delayed should be presumptively treated for meningitis.

In meningitis, the CSF usually reveals a pleocytosis; however, 30% of infants with group B streptococcus meningitis may have a normal cell count. A differential cell count of CSF in most cases reveals a predominance of neutrophils; this finding is usually indicative of a bacterial process, although it can be seen early in viral infections. Later in the course of disease, lymphocytes predominate in the CSF. The CSF protein is usually elevated, and CSF glucose is decreased to less than half of the serum glucose. It is rare for all CSF parameters to be normal in a patient with meningitis.

A Gram stain of the CSF can be used as a method to make an early diagnosis and to broaden the spectrum of antibiotic therapy. CSF should be sent for routine bacterial culture; fungal culture; and AFB smear and culture, and viral culture may be indicated in some patients. Countercurrent immunoelectrophoresis (CIE) and latex particle agglutination (LPA) are a rapid means of antigen detection in the CSF. They are useful in the management of patients previously treated with antibiotics in whom culture results may not be reliable; false-negative results can occur with CIE and LPA.

NEONATAL MENINGITIS

Neonatal meningitis has a mortality rate of 15 to 20%. The most common pathogens are group B streptococcus, *Escherichia coli*, and *Listeria monocytogenes*. *Enterobacter*, *Klebsiella*, *Citrobacter diversus*, *Salmonella*, *Streptococcus pneumoniae*, and other organisms listed as meningitis pathogens in the older child can cause neonatal meningitis. Neonatal meningitis pathogens are listed with their initial empiric therapy in Table 20–4.

Therapy

Ampicillin and cefotaxime have replaced ampicillin and gentamicin as initial broad-spectrum therapy for the neonate with meningitis at many institutions, especially when gram-negative organisms are present on Gram stain. Cefotaxime affords better CSF penetration and effectiveness against organisms that may be resistant to aminoglycosides without the ototoxicity and the need to monitor aminoglycoside levels.[22] Empiric therapy with cefotaxime is recommended for *E. coli*, other gram-negative enteric organisms, and *H. influenzae* type B until sensitivity results are available. The combination of cefotaxime plus an aminoglycoside is used in the initial management of patients with gram-negative meningitis other than *Pseudomonas* and when resistance to cephalosporins is suspected. Therapy for *Pseudomonas* meningitis requires ceftazidime plus an aminoglycoside.

Table 20–4. INITIAL THERAPY OF MENINGITIS*

Organism	Antibiotic Coverage	Duration of Therapy
Common Neonatal Pathogens		
Group B streptococcus	Penicillin G + aminoglycoside or ampicillin + aminoglycoside	3 weeks
Escherichia coli	Cefotaxime + aminoglycoside	3 weeks†
Listeria monocytogenes	Ampicillin + aminoglycoside	2–3 weeks
Gram-negative agents‡	Cefotaxime + aminoglycoside	3 weeks†
Enterococci§	Ampicillin + aminoglycoside	2 weeks
Haemophilus influenzae	Cefotaxime	10–14 days
Anaerobes	Metronidazole‖	
Common Childhood Pathogens		
Haemophilus influenzae	Cefotaxime	10–14 days
Streptococcus pneumoniae	Cefotaxime	10–14 days
Neisseria meningitidis	Cefotaxime	7 days

*Definitive and final therapy is determined by susceptibility test results.
†May require longer duration of therapy.
‡In the case of *Pseudomonas*, ceftazidime and an aminoglycoside should be used.
§5% of enterococci are resistant to ampicillin and require vancomycin with an aminoglycoside.
‖May require additional agent for gram-positive anaerobic coverage.

Definitive therapy is determined by susceptibility test results.

Antibiotic dosages in neonates less than 1 week old and weighing more than 2,000 grams are the following: ampicillin, 50 mg/kg every 8 hours; gentamicin, 2.5 mg/kg every 12 hours; cefotaxime, 50 mg/kg every 12 hours; penicillin G, 50,000 units/kg every 8 hours; metronidazole, 7.5 mg/kg every 12 hours; and vancomycin, 15 mg/kg every 12 hours.[23]

Patients with tolerant group B streptococcus organisms (minimum bactericidal concentration (MBC) greater than fivefold minimum inhibitory concentration (MIC)) should receive combined therapy with penicillin and an aminoglycoside for 2 weeks and with penicillin alone the third week of therapy. Patients with nontolerant organisms need receive combined antibiotic therapy for only 1 week, with penicillin administered alone the last 14 days of therapy. Aminoglycoside levels should be obtained after the third to fifth dose of antibiotic and followed weekly thereafter with complete blood count (CBC), blood urea nitrogen (BUN), creatinine, and urinalysis. Gentamicin trough levels should be below 2 µg/ml, and peak levels should be between 5 and 10 µg/ml. Hearing evaluation by brain stem auditory evoked response (BAER) should be performed as a baseline and weekly thereafter in patients who are to receive 2 weeks or longer of aminoglycoside therapy.

Management

Patients with gram-negative meninigitis should have repeat LPs on a daily basis until CSF is sterile. Patients with a positive finding on repeat cultures should have a CT scan of the head to rule out subdural fluid collection or an abscess. Complications of neonatal meningitis include ventriculitis, which occurs in 70% of infants with gram-negative meningitis. Brain abscess is usually rare but occurs in 77% of patients with *C. diversus* meningitis.[24, 25] Patients with *C. diversus* meningitis should routinely have a CT evaluation of the head at an early stage since clinical signs and symptoms of intracranial pathology are often not apparent (Fig. 20–1 *A* and *B*). Subdural effusions commonly accompany meningitis in the young infant and generally do not require tapping. Hydrocephalus frequently accompanies neonatal meningitis; therefore, daily transillumination and head circumference measurement should be performed. A CT

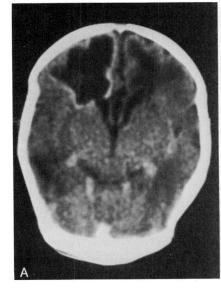
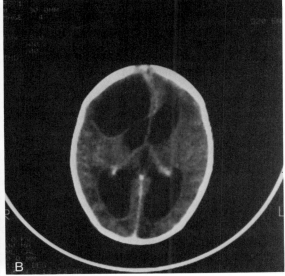

Figure 20–1. *A*, Neonate with *Citrobacter diversus* meningitis and cerebritis. *B*, The follow-up CT scan reveals posterior infarcts with hydrocephalus.

scan should be ordered to evaluate increasing head size. Further management recommendations are outlined in the following section.

MENINGITIS IN THE OLDER CHILD

H. influenzae type B meningitis has an incidence of 32 to 71/100,000 U.S. children below the age of 5 years and is the most common cause of bacterial meningitis in the older infant and child in the United States.[20] *Streptococcus pneumoniae* and *Neisseria meningitidis* are also common pathogens (see Table 20–4). Children between the age of 3 to 8 months are at greatest risk for having meningitis.[21] The mortality rate following meningitis is 5 to 10%, with 25 to 50% of survivors having some sequelae.[26]

Therapy

Antibiotic Therapy

Antibiotic therapy for the older infant and for the child with meningitis should be effective against the common encapsulated organisms—*H. influenzae* type B, *S. pneumoniae*, and *N. meningitidis*—that cause most infections in this age group. Cefotaxime 200 mg/kg/day divided into four daily doses given intravenously every 6 hours to treat β-lactamase–producing or otherwise ampicillin-resistant *H. influenzae* type B strains is the mainstay of therapy in this group. Ampicillin 400 mg/kg/day divided into six daily doses given every 4 hours is effective therapy for *H. influenzae* strains with documented ampicillin sensitivity. The incidence of ampicillin-resistant *H. influenzae* type B varies geographically and has reached 50% in some areas. Sporadic cases of ampicillin and chloramphenicol-resistant *H. influenzae* type B have been reported in the United States. Use of cefuroxime (225 mg/kg/day divided into three daily doses) has been associated with delayed sterilization of the CSF[27] and should not be used. Other third-generation cephalosporins, ceftriaxone 100 mg/kg/day in two divided daily doses given every 12 hours, and ceftazidime (150 mg/kg/day divided into three daily doses given 8 hours apart) have also been used in the child with meningitis. All patients with meningitis should be treated with parenteral antibiotics. Optimally, the patient should be afebrile for 5 days prior to the discontinuation of antibiotics, but other than for group B streptococcus and gram-negative meningitis, rarely does one treat a patient without other complications for more than 14 days.

S. pneumoniae usually has an MIC to penicillin of less than 0.1 μg/ml; isolates with MICs of 0.1 to 1.0 μg/ml are relatively resistant to penicillin and in the case of meningitis mandate the use of alternate therapy. (*S. pneumoniae* organisms with MICs to penicillin greater than 1.0 μg/ml are resistant and also indicate the need for alternate therapy.) Empirically, vancomycin (60 mg/kg/day divided into four daily doses given every 6 hours) or chloramphenicol should be used in cases of

suspected penicillin-resistant pneumococci; these organisms can be sensitive to the cephalosporins such as cefotaxime, but one must obtain sensitivity results before using cephalosporins as alternate therapy. General durations of therapy are listed in Tables 20–1 to 20–4. Antibiotic levels as well as a hearing evaluation need to be obtained when vancomycin is administered.

Steroid Therapy

Dexamethasone (0.6 mg/kg/day given in four divided doses 6 hours apart intravenously for 4 days at the start of parenteral antibiotic therapy) has been shown to have a beneficial effect in decreasing the hearing loss in children with bacterial meningitis.[28] However, its use in patients with meningitis is still controversial.[29, 30] The bulk of the data has been acquired in patients with *H. influenzae* type B meningitis. The use of dexamethasone may be considered in patients with bacterial meningitis over the age of 2 months.[30] Gastrointestinal bleeding has been reported following the use of dexamethasone, therefore careful monitoring of hemoglobin concentration and stool occult blood is necessary when this drug is used.

Rifampin Prophylaxis

Patients with *H. influenzae* type B and *N. meningitidis* meningitis and their close contacts[31, 32] should receive oral rifampin to eradicate these organisms from the nasopharynx in order to prevent secondary cases of meningitis. The prophylactic dose of rifampin for *H. influenzae* type B disease is 20 mg/kg/day (maximum and adult daily dose is 600 mg), given once a day for 4 days. The dosage of rifampin for *N. meningitidis* disease is 10 mg/kg in two daily doses given 12 hours apart for 2 days; the adult and maximum dose is 600 mg given twice a day for 2 days. A liquid suspension of rifampin can be prepared. Some authorities recommend giving infants less than 1 month old half the aforementioned dose—10 mg/kg per dose daily for 4 days, and 5 mg/kg per dose every 12 hours for 2 days for *H. influenzae* and *N. meningitidis*, respectively. The effect of rifampin on the fetus is not known; pregnant women should consult their obstetricians regarding the use of rifampin. Prophylaxis should be given as soon as possible to people in the same household and other close contacts, optimally within 24 hours after the diagnosis of the index case. The physician should promptly notify the infection control officer of the hospital and the local health department of cases of meningitis.

Management

Vital signs, including blood pressure, should be monitored every 15 minutes until the patient is stable, then at 1- to 2-hour intervals during the first 24 hours. Shock occurs in 4% of patients with meningococcal disease and in 5.5% of patients with *H. influenzae* type B disease.[20] The patient should be given sufficient fluids to maintain adequate blood pressure, urine output, and cerebral perfusion. The use of pressor agents, such as dopamine, may be necessary. The patient should be given nothing by mouth (NPO) for the first 24 hours and should be kept NPO until he or she is able to tolerate oral feedings. Fluid and electrolyte monitoring including strict input and output measurements, with urine specific gravity calibrations on each voiding, and daily weights should be performed to monitor for SIADH. Patients who are not dehydrated, hypotensive, or exhibiting poor perfusion should initially have restrictions on fluid intake to one-half to three-fourths maintenance with serum sodium and serum osmolality measured every 12 hours for the first 48 hours. If sodium and osmolality measurements remain within normal limits, fluids may then be liberalized. Patients who are hyponatremic or have other manifestations of SIADH are best managed with fluid restriction. The patient with meningitis should have a complete physical examination daily, and attention should be paid to the character of heart sounds, joints, and spontaneous movement of extremities. The neurologic examination should be performed several times a day until the patient is stable, then twice daily; transillumination (in patients younger than 18 months of age) and head circumference measurement should be performed daily. Patients with systemic meningococcal disease may have an underlying complement deficiency; therefore, a CH50 screening test should be obtained on these patients.[33]

Neurologic Complications

Neurologic complications of meningitis include increased ICP, cortical vascular thrombosis with infarction, and rarely, brain abscess.

ICP can be managed as discussed for encephalitis, with the exception that ICP monitors and barbiturate coma are usually not used in the management of patients with meningitis.

Seizures occur in 30% of patients with bacterial meningitis; in 20% of patients prior to arrival at the hospital; and in 26% within the first 2 days of hospitalization. Nonpersistent generalized seizures are not associated with a poor prognosis; however, focal seizures at any time in the course of illness or generalized seizures after the fourth day of hospitalization are generally associated with a poorer outcome. Seizures late in the course of meningitis can be the result of ICF collections, thrombosis, or abscess. EEG is usually not indicated for self-limited seizures but may be helpful in the evaluation of focal seizures, seizures persisting longer than 72 hours, seizures occurring after the third or fourth day, and in patients with an altered mental status.[20] Seizures can usually be managed with phenytoin and phenobarbital but may require the administration of Valium for status epilepticus. Anticonvulsant therapy usually does not need to be continued after hospital discharge in patients whose seizures abate within 48 hours and in whom no focal signs are present on discharge.

A CT scan is indicated in children with focal seizures, focal findings on neurologic examination, increasing head circumference, or signs of increased ICP.

Prolonged Fever

Fever can persist for 7 days in 20% of patients with meningitis and for as long as 10 days in 13% of patients.[34] Causes of persistent fever include subdural effusions, other foci of infection such as pneumonia, arthritis, or osteomyelitis, and drug fever, which is primarily a diagnosis of exclusion. Recurrent fever is usually secondary to nosocomial infection, such as phlebitis from intravenous catheters or nosocomial respiratory and gastrointestinal infections. A physical examination should be performed in the case of these patients; patients with focal findings on examination should have a CT scan. The decision to repeat the LP should be made on an individual basis.

Other Complications

Other complications of meningitis include the development of arthritis[35, 36] or osteomyelitis, endophthalmitis, and pericarditis.[36]

Sequelae

Patients with meningitis may develop the following sequelae: significant hearing loss (10 to 11%), vision defects (2 to 4%), motor deficits (3 to 7%), seizures requiring long-term anticonvulsants (2 to 8%), and mental retardation (10 to 11%).[37] Hearing deficits were noted in 31% of patients following meningitis with S. pneumoniae, 10.5% after N. meningitidis, and 6% after H. influenzae.[38] A hearing evaluation should be obtained in all patients with meningitis prior to discharge by conventional methods or by BAER, and at 3 to 6 months post discharge. Developmental evaluation and careful follow-up is essential for meningitis patients post discharge.

Tuberculous Meningitis

Tuberculous meningitis most commonly occurs in children less than 6 years of age. Tubercle bacilli enter the subarachnoid space from caseated lesions in the brain or meninges. Disease occurs in three stages: (1) systemic symptoms of fever, malaise, and irritability; (2) vomiting, signs of increased ICP, nuchal rigidity, seizures, and cranial nerve palsies; and (3) coma and cardiorespiratory irregularity.[39, 40] Disease is fatal in 3 to 4 weeks without therapy. Virtually all patients who present in the initial stage survive, whereas those presenting in stages two and three have mortality rates of 15% and 50%, respectively.[40]

A CSF examination usually reveals a pleocytosis with less than 500 cells, with an initial predominance of neutrophils that progresses to a lymphocytosis. CSF protein is usually elevated, and glucose is decreased; however, each of these values may be normal on an initial CSF examination. AFB may not be seen on smear in a significant number of patients, and cultures may have a positive result in only 45 to 90% of patients with actual disease.[41] Repeat CSF examination with additional specimens submitted for AFB smear and culture may help to document the diagnosis. Most children have an abnormal chest x-ray and a positive PPD.

Three early morning gastric aspirates should be sent for AFB smear and culture. All patients should have a CT scan of the brain to look for tuberculomas and hydrocephalus. Therapy should consist of at least three antituberculous drugs initially, isoniazid plus rifampin with either pyrazinamide or streptomycin. Steroid therapy for a minimum of 1 month is recommended for patients with increased ICP.[39, 40] Sequelae of disease include visual and auditory deficits, mental retardation, seizures, motor abnormalities, diabetes insipidus, and other endocrinopathies.

Fungal Meningitis

Fungal meningitis can be caused by *Candida* species and by the same pathogens that cause encephalitis. Presentation may be insidious in the normal host and may be more pronounced in the immunocompromised patient. While one should attempt to isolate the organism from the CSF by repeated culture, organisms such as *Coccidiodes* and *Cryptococcus* can be identified more efficiently by serology on CSF and serum. India ink stain and cryptococcal antigen testing performed on CSF are useful in the identification of cryptococcal meningitis; the India ink smear requires an experienced reader for accurate interpretation. Standard therapy for fungal meningitis consists of the combination of amphotericin B and flucytosine.[42] Promising therapeutic agents include the triazoles, particularly fluconazole.[43]

Partially Treated Meningitis

Partially treated meningitis occurs in children who have received antibiotic therapy that alters the signs and symptoms of meningitis and potentially the recovery of the causal organism from spinal fluid but that was insufficient to adequately treat the patient for meningitis. Antigen detection tests on the CSF often identify the organism in the case of negative cultures. If no pathogen is identified, these children are treated empirically with broad-spectrum antibiotic therapy, such as cefotaxime for 10 days in the older child and ampicillin and cefotaxime for 14 days in the neonate, to eradicate the likely pathogens for the particular age group.

Viral Meningitis

Viral meningitis secondary to enteroviruses commonly presents in the summer. CSF pleocytosis does not usually exceed 2,000 cells/mm³. CSF protein is usually elevated; mumps and coxsackie viruses can cause hypoglycorrhachia. Viruses in many cases can be grown from CSF, but this usually requires several days. The illness is self-limited in the normal host. Infants under 1 year of age should have BAER testing, because hearing defects may occur in this age group.

BRAIN ABSCESS

Brain abscess can develop in the presence of ischemia and necrosis in the brain. Microorganisms reach the brain via hematogenous dissemination, spread from contiguous structures such as the middle ear, orbit, mastoid, and face, as a complication of neurosurgery and through penetrating head trauma.[44] Four stages correlating CT scan findings with histologic appearance have been described in the evolution of brain abscess: (1) early cerebritis on days 1 to 3 characterized by the presence of inflammatory cells, a developing necrotic center, and surrounding cerebral edema; (2) late cerebritis on days 4 to 9, characterized by an enlarging necrotic center and the presence of fibroblasts; (3) early capsule formation on days 10 to 13, with increased number of fibroblasts, presence of mature collagen, and diminishing cerebritis; and (4) late capsule formation on day 14 and later, coinciding with completion of the encapsulation process (Fig. 20–2).[45] Brain abscess is commonly associated with ear, nose, and throat infections and cyanotic congenital heart disease and is rare following meningitis. Prior to the advent of CT scanning in 1974, the mortality from brain abscess was 40%; the current mortality is 5 to 10%. Morbidity is still high, and 29 to 52% of children have sequelae.

Children with brain abscess commonly present with headache, malaise, vomiting, and seizures; fever is present in less than 50%. Papilledema and focal neurologic signs may also be present during the initial examination. LP is contraindicated because of the risk of herniation from increased ICP. CSF analysis may reveal a pleocytosis but is usually not helpful in the evaluation of these patients.[46] A CT scan with and without contrast should be performed.

CSF and blood cultures usually have negative results, except in the presence of endocarditis when the blood culture may have a positive finding. Culture of the abscess with material submitted for Gram stain, routine, anaerobic, fungal, AFB smear and cultures and pathol-

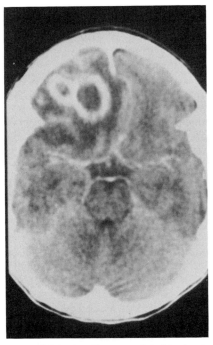

Figure 20–2. Bilobed well-encapsulated brain abscess.

ogy is necessary for identification of the causative organisms. Streptococci are the most common organisms present in these infections; a significant number also contain anaerobes. Other organisms, such as gram-negative agents, *H. influenzae*, *S. pneumoniae*, and *N. meningitidis*, from ear and sinus infections, may also be present. Microbial flora vary with the etiology. Initial antibiotic coverage has consisted of the combination of penicillin 300,000 units/kg/day divided into six doses given every 4 hours and chloramphenicol. Metronidazole affords excellent anaerobic coverage; however, its usage has not been clearly established in pediatric brain abscess. If *S. aureus* is suspected, a semisynthetic penicillin such as oxacillin should be added to the treatment regimen; vancomycin is an alternative in patients who are allergic to penicillin. Antibiotic therapy should be administered intravenously and should be continued for 6 to 8 weeks. The use of steroids in these patients is controversial. They are used in patients with increased ICP with clinical deterioration but may impair antibiotic penetration into the abscess and host immune defenses. The patient's progress should be monitored on the basis of a physical examination and serial CT scans.

All patients with brain abscess should have a consultation regarding neurosurgery. The standard therapy of brain abscess has included surgical drainage by excision or by repeat aspiration and prolonged antibiotic therapy.[47-49] Selected cases have responded to medical management, that is, antibiotic therapy alone.[50-52]

SUBDURAL EMPYEMA

Subdural empyema is an accumulation of pus between the dura and arachnoid membranes. It arises most commonly from contiguous spread of infection from nearby structures, such as the middle ear and paranasal sinuses by transport of infectious material through the valveless emissary veins, and from penetrating trauma or neurosurgery. Current mortality from subdural empyema is 10 to 20%.

Patients commonly present with headache, alterations in consciousness, vomiting, papilledema, and focal neurologic deficits. Patients may present with fever and nuchal rigidity, simulating meningitis; focal signs such as hemiparesis may aid in the differentiation of these patients.[53, 54] A CT scan commonly reveals a hypodense area below the cranial vault or adjacent to the falx; false-negative CT scans do occur. In some patients, subdural empyema is more readily detected by coronal CT cuts (Fig. 20–3). Clinical suspicion should dictate the management of the patient; a repeat CT scan within 24 hours may delineate a developing lesion.

Streptococci, staphylococci, and anaerobes are frequent pathogens. Initial antibiotic therapy should consist of penicillin, a semisynthetic penicillin, and chloramphenicol pending culture results. Surgical drainage is mandatory in these patients.[53] Intravenous antibiotic therapy should be continued for 6 weeks. The patient should be followed clinically and with repeat CT scans.

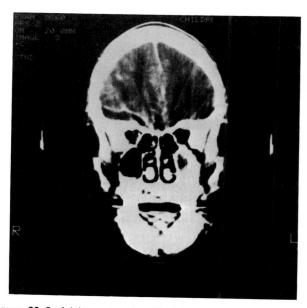

Figure 20–3. Adolescent male with right frontal sinusitis; subdural fluid collection is visible beneath the right frontal lobe on the coronal cut.

EPIDURAL ABSCESS

Epidural abscess is a collection of pus located between the dura mater and overlying cranium. The pathogenesis and microbiology of these infections are similar to those of subdural empyema.[53] Patients commonly present with headache and fever and rarely focal findings until the subdural space is involved. Osteomyelitis of the overlying bone may also be present. Meningitis and other intracranial infections may develop as complications of epidural abscess. Diagnosis is often delayed.[54] A CT scan with contrast is used to delineate the lesion. Emergent neurosurgical drainage is mandatory, coupled with appropriate long-term intravenous antimicrobial therapy.

References

1. Cherry JD and Shields WD: Encephalitis and meningoencephalitis. *In:* Feigin RD and Cherry JD (eds): Textbook of Pediatric Infectious Diseases, 2nd ed. Philadelphia, WB Saunders, 1987, pp. 484–496.
2. Ho DD and Hirsch MS: Acute viral encephalitis. Med Clin North Am 69:415, 1985.
3. Whitley RJ: Viral encephalitis. N Engl J Med 323:242, 1990.
4. Feder HM, Zalneraitis EL, and Reik L: Lyme disease: Acute focal meningoencephalitis in a child. Pediatrics 82:931, 1988.
5. Dattwyler RJ, Halperin JJ, Pass H, and Luft BJ: Ceftriaxone as effective therapy in refractory Lyme disease. J Infect Dis 155:1322, 1987.
6. Meloff KL: Fungal, rickettsial, and parasitic diseases of the nervous system. *In:* Swaiman KF (ed): Pediatric Neurology: Principles and Practice, Vol. 1. Baltimore, CV Mosby, 1989, pp. 517–540.
7. Lehtokoski-Lehtiniemi E and Koskiniemi M-L: *Mycoplasma pneumoniae* encephalitis: A severe entity in children. Pediatr Infect Dis J 8:651, 1989.
8. Lewis DW and Tucker SH: Central nervous system involvement in cat-scratch disease. Pediatrics 77:714, 1986.

9. Miller KD, Greenberg AE, and Campbell CC: Treatment of severe malaria in the United States with a continuous infusion of quinidine gluconate and exchange transfusion. N Engl J Med 321:65, 1989.

10. Seidel JS, Harmatz P, Visvesvara GS, et al: Successful treatment of primary amebic meningoencephalitis. N Engl J Med 306:346, 1982.

11. Arvin AM, Johnson RT, Whitley RT, et al: Consensus: Management of the patient with herpes simplex encephalitis. Pediatr Infect Dis J 6:2, 1987.

12. Schroth G, Gawehn J, and Thron A: Early diagnosis of herpes simplex encephalitis by MRI. Neurology 37:179, 1987.

13. Kohl S: Herpes simplex virus encephalitis in children. Pediatr Clin North Am 35:465, 1988.

14. Whitley RJ, Alford CA, Hirsch MS, et al: Vidarabine versus acyclovir therapy in herpes simplex encephalitis. N Engl J Med 314:144, 1986.

15. Whitley RJ, Cobbs CG, Alford CA, et al: Diseases that mimic herpes simplex encephalitis: Diagnosis, presentation and outcome. JAMA 262:234, 1989.

16. Wasiewski WW and Fishman MA: Herpes simplex encephalitis: The brain biopsy controversy. J Pediatr 113:575, 1988.

17. Lakeman FD, Koga J, and Whitley RJ: Detection of antigen to herpes simplex virus in cerebrospinal fluid from patients with herpes simplex encephalitis. J Infect Dis 155:1172, 1987.

18. Maguire JF and Meissner HC: Onset of encephalitis early in the course of varicella infection. Pediatr Infect Dis 4:699, 1985.

19. Johnson RT, Griffin DE, and Gendelman HE: Postinfectious encephalomyelitis. Semin Neurol 5:180, 1985.

20. Feigin RD: Bacterial meningitis beyond the neonatal period. In: Feigin RD and Cherry JD (eds): Textbook of Pediatric Infectious Diseases. Philadelphia, WB Saunders, 1987, pp. 439–465.

21. Klein JO, Feigin RD, and McCracken GH: Report of the task force on diagnosis and management of meningitis. Pediatrics 78 (Suppl):959, 1986.

22. McCracken GH: Current management of bacterial meningitis. Pediatr Infect Dis J 8:919, 1989.

23. Nelson JD: Table of antibiotic dosages for neonates. In: Nelson JD (ed): 1989–1990 Pocketbook of Pediatric Antimicrobial Therapy. Baltimore, Williams & Wilkins, 1989, pp. 20–21.

24. McCracken GH and Freij BJ: Perinatal bacterial diseases. In: Feigin RD and Cherry JD (eds): Textbook of Pediatric Infectious Diseases. Philadelphia, WB Saunders, 1987, pp. 940–966.

25. Graham DR and Band JD: Citrobacter diversus brain abscess and meningitis in neonates. JAMA 245:1923, 1981.

26. McCracken GH, Nelson JD, Kaplan SL, et al: Consensus report: Antimicrobial therapy for bacterial meningitis in infants and children. Pediatr Infect Dis J 6:501, 1987.

27. Marks WA, Stutman HR, Marks MI, et al: Cefuroxime versus ampicillin plus chloramphenicol in childhood bacterial meningitis: A multicenter randomized controlled trial. J Pediatr 109:123, 1986.

28. Lebel MH, Freij BJ, Syrogiannopoulos GA, et al: Dexamethasone therapy for bacterial meningitis: Results of two double-blind, placebo-controlled trials. N Engl J Med 319:964, 1988.

29. Kaplan SL: Dexamethasone for children with bacterial meningitis: Should it be routine therapy (Editorial)? Am J Dis Child 143:290, 1989.

30. McCracken GH and Lebel MH: Dexamethasone therapy for bacterial meningitis in infants and children (Editorial). Am J Dis Child 143:287, 1989.

31. Committee on Infectious Diseases, American Academy of Pediatrics: Haemophilus influenzae infections. In: Report of the Committee on Infectious Diseases. 1988 Redbook, 21st ed. Elk Grove Village, IL, American Academy of Pediatrics, pp. 204–210.

32. Committee on Infectious Diseases, American Academy of Pediatrics: Meningococcal infections. In: Report of the Committee on Infectious Diseases. 1988 Redbook, 21st ed. Elk Grove Village, IL, American Academy of Pediatrics, pp. 289–292.

33. Leggiadro RJ: Prevalence of complement deficiencies in children with systemic meningococcal infections. Pediatr Infect Dis J 6:75, 1987.

34. Lin T-Y, Nelson JD, and McCracken GH: Fever during treatment for bacterial meningitis. Pediatr Infect Dis 3:319, 1984.

35. Rush PJ, Shore A, Inman R, et al: Arthritis associated with Haemophilus influenzae meningitis: Septic or reactive? J Pediatr 109:412, 1986.

36. Edwards MS and Baker CJ: Complications and sequelae of meningococcal infections in children. J Pediatr 99:540, 1981.

37. Sell SH: Long-term sequelae of bacterial meningitis in children. Pediatr Infect Dis 2:90, 1983.

38. Dodge PR, Davis H, Feigin RD, et al: Prospective evaluation of hearing impairment as a sequela of acute bacterial meningitis. N Engl J Med 311:871 1984.

39. Smith MH and Marquis JR: Tuberculosis and other mycobacterial infections. In: Feigin RD and Cherry JD (eds): Textbook of Pediatric Infectious Diseases. Philadelphia, WB Saunders, 1987, pp. 1342–1387.

40. Idriss ZH, Sinno AA, and Kronfol NB: Tuberculous meningitis in childhood. Am J Dis Child 130:364, 1976.

41. Molavi A and LeFrock JL: Tuberculous meningitis. Med Clin North Am 69:315, 1985.

42. Diamond RD: Fungal meningitis. In: Feigin RD and Cherry JD (eds): Textbook of Pediatric Infectious Diseases. Philadelphia, WB Saunders, 1987, pp. 467–475.

43. Sugar AM, Stern JJ, and Dupont B: Overview: Treatment of cryptococcal meningitis. Rev Infect Dis 12:S338, 1990.

44. Dodge PR: Parameningeal infections (including brain abscess, epidural abscess, subdural empyema). In: Feigin RD and Cherry JD (eds): Textbook of Pediatric Infectious Diseases, 2nd ed. Philadelphia, WB Saunders, 1987, pp. 496–505.

45. Britt RH, Enzmann DR, and Yeager AS: Neuropathological and computerized tomographic findings in experimental brain abscess. J Neurosurg 55:590, 1981.

46. Patrick CC and Kaplan SL: Current concepts in the pathogenesis and management of brain abscess in children. Pediatr Clin North Am 35:625, 1988.

47. Johnson DL, Markle BM, Wiedermann BL, and Hanahan, L: Treatment of intracranial abscesses associated with sinusitis in children and adolescents. J Pediatr 113:15, 1988.

48. Jadavji T, Humphreys RP, and Prober CG: Brain abscesses in infants and children. Pediatr Infect Dis J 4:394, 1985.

49. Young RF and Frazee J: Gas within intracranial abscess cavities: An indication for surgical excision. Ann Neurol 16:35, 1984.

50. Keren G and Tyrrell DL: Nonsurgical treatment of brain abscesses: Report of two cases. Pediatr Infect Dis 3:331, 1984.

51. Rennels MB, Woodward CL, Robinson WL, et al: Medical cure of apparent brain abscesses. Pediatrics 72:220, 1983.

52. Rosenblum ML, Hoff JT, Norman D, et al: Nonoperative treatment of brain abscesses in selected high-risk patients. J Neurosurg 52:217, 1980.

53. Silverberg AL and DiNubile MJ: Subdural empyema and cranial epidural abscess. Med Clin North Am 69:361, 1985.

54. Smith HP and Hendrick EB: Subdural empyema and epidural abscess in children. J Neurosurg 58:392, 1983.

21

Head Trauma

Hector E. James, M.D.

INTRACRANIAL DYNAMICS

Anatomy

The intracranial contents are divided into partial compartments by various structures that limit to some degree the movement of the brain and the cerebellum. The falx cerebri incompletely separates the left cerebral hemisphere from the right cerebral hemisphere, and the tentorium cerebelli divides the cerebellum in the infratentorial compartment from the cerebrum in the supratentorial compartment. These compartments communicate with each another by the various cerebrospinal fluid (CSF)-containing cisterns. Communication between the supratentorial and infratentorial compartments exists within the brain stem by the sylvian aqueduct and around the brain stem, by the cisterns at the level of the opening of the tentorium cerebelli, the tentorial incisura. The intracranial compartment communicates by the spinal subarachnoid space in the foramen magnum. Under normal conditions, all these spaces communicate freely. However, in pathologic conditions, shifts of structures may separate these spaces and give rise to complete isolation and compartmentalization. Usually the more rapid the change, the less well it is tolerated. This is because the faster the separation from one compartment to the other, the less time will be available for adaptation and accommodation of the surrounding structures. What then follows is a more sudden and massive displacement of the neural elements.

In infancy, the intracranial volume increases rapidly and the brain attains 75% of its adult size by 18 months of age. The final volume is made up of approximately 80% brain parenchyma, 10% blood, and 10% CSF.[1]

Physiology

Cerebrospinal Fluid

The production, circulation, and reabsorption of CSF is a very dynamic phenomenon. The production rate is 0.33 ± 0.2 ml/min.[2, 3] Consequently, the same amount needs to be reabsorbed so that a build-up of CSF in the cisterns and ventricles does not ensue. The primary sites of reabsorption are in the arachnoid villi. These sites are located at the level of venous sinuses. The villi are microscopic valves that open at an approximate pressure of 5 mm Hg. Reabsorption does increase in the face of elevations of ICP.[4–6]

Vascular

Most of the intracranial blood volume is in the venous sinuses and the pial veins; however, there is very rapid flow through the cerebrovascular system. Cerebral blood flow (CBF) is 75 ml to 80 ml/100g/min in the gray matter and 25 ml/100g/min in the white matter. In infants, the global CBF is 40 ml/100g/min; in children, it can range from 75 to 110 ml/100g/min; and in adolescents, it is 50 ml/100 mg/min. From the standpoint of the vascular properties, CBF seems to follow Poiseuille's law. In most conditions, the length of the blood vessels and the viscosity can be considered constant, and in order to maintain a constant blood flow, only the radius of the arteries and pressure gradient across the brain can be varied. CBF is maintained at a constant rate over a large range of perfusion pressures. The ability of the cerebral arteriolar bed to maintain a constant flow in the face of changing perfusion pressure is believed to be a myogenic response of the muscular walls to changes in transmural pressure.[7] This ability is called cerebrovascular autoregulation. If the blood pressure drops, the transmural pressure is decreased, arterioles dilate, flow resistance is lowered, and blood flow is maintained even in the face of a reduction in blood pressure.[8] In the absence of trauma or a significant brain insult, the normal range of cerebral autoregulation seems to be 45 to 150 mm Hg of mean arterial pressure (MAP).[8] At a mean blood pressure of approximately 45 mm Hg, autoregulation fails and CBF decreases.[8] At mean blood pressure values over 150 mm Hg, there can be a disruption of the blood-brain barrier owing to the head of pressure being so elevated at meta-arteriolar level that vasogenic brain edema may ensue.[9] Above and below the range of good autoregulation, CBF is passively dependent on the perfusion pressure.[8] The effective perfusion pressure for the cerebral circulation is approximated by measuring the difference between the MAP and the mean intracranial pressure (ICP).

The most important factors controlling intracranial

201

circulation are the partial pressure of arterial carbon dioxide (Pa_{CO_2}) and the local metabolic requirements of the brain (metabolic autoregulation).[10, 11] Increases in Pa_{CO_2} lead to vasodilatation and an increase in CBF and consequently in the cerebral blood volume.[11, 12] This control and influence of the CO_2 seems to be closely related to the local metabolism through tissue pH. Thus, increases in local metabolism as may be seen with seizure activity are accompanied by increased CBF.

Concepts on Intracranial Volume and Pressure

Normally there is an interaction between the CSF, cerebral blood volume, and the water of the brain parenchyma that allows for a constant overall volume of the intracranial contents to be maintained. The Monro-Kellie hypothesis states that the sum of the volumes of brain-blood, CSF, and other components should remain constant.[13] Consequently, ICP stays constant, with little variation. When additional volume is added, a progressive increase in ICP is noted.[14] The initial lack of elevation of ICP when a mass expands in the cranium due to a reduction in the CSF volume is because of the compression of the ventricles and the subarachnoid spaces. As further expansion of the mass occurs and no further compensation can occur due to the reduction of the CSF and brain water, the additional volume results in a visible and progressive elevation of ICP. This creates mechanical distortion of the neural structures, seen as shift and displacements, and a reduction of CBF, owing to intracranial hypertension and an impairment of cerebral perfusion. These changes of ICP with increasing intracranial volume constitute the volume-pressure curve.[15] The importance of this concept is that as ICP is elevated, small changes in intracranial volume may bring about very dramatic further changes in ICP.[15] This situation is commonly seen in clinical practice and, if unrecognized, may result in irreversible cerebral ischemic damage.

When ICP is recorded under normal conditions, the tracing displays vascular and respiratory oscillations and the pulse pressure is readily visualized.[16] The normal ICP in the adult and the child is under 15 mm Hg (204 mm H_2O), and in the infant it is under 8 to 10 mm Hg.[16, 17] ICP does not remain at a given value, and it fluctuates constantly. Brief elevations in ICP are seen in the normal situations of coughing and straining.[15]

Pathology

Mass effects may occur intracranially as a result of intracranial hemorrhage and hematoma formation, or from cerebrovascular engorgement due to an impairment of cerebral autoregulation and increased blood volume. In the more severe head injuries, it may be a combination of these factors. As a consequence, a shift of intracranial structures may follow.

Transtentorial herniation is the most commonly described syndrome due to mass effect and displacements. Clinically, it is characterized by a progressive impair-

ment of consciousness, pupillary dilatation ipsilateral to the expanding mass, and contralateral or ipsilateral hemiparesis. This constellation is the result of the expansion of a supratentorial mass causing displacement of the medial aspect of the ipsilateral temporal lobe into the tentorial hiatus, which results in obliteration of the cisterna ambiens. This leads to an obstruction of the communication between the infratentorial and supratentorial compartments. Pressure on the brain stem creates mechanical distortion and local ischemia. Consequently the reticular activating system dysfunctions, and impairment of consciousness follows. Since the third cranial nerve travels through the tentorial incisura from the infratentorial compartment to the supratentorial one, it is trapped between the herniating mesial temporal lobe, the brain stem, and the hard edge of the dura of the tentorial incisura. That is why the ipsilateral pupil to the mass effect dilates; the third cranial nerve is parasympathetic and is responsible for miosis, and its dysfunction leaves a dominant sympathetic (mydriatic) innervation.[18] If the herniation progresses, it can manifest bilateral signs, caudal brain stem deterioration with unresponsiveness, Cheyne-Stokes respiration, central neurogenic hyperventilation, decerebration, apnea, and death.[19]

Tonsillar or *foramen magnum herniation* occurs owing to intracranial hypertension, with caudal gradients of pressure displacing the brain stem and cerebellar tonsils into the foramen magnum. The progressive pressure on the lower brain stem creates impairment of consciousness, hypertension, bradycardia and respiratory irregularities, and finally apnea. The bradycardia, hypertension, and respiratory irregularities are commonly known as the cushing triad.[19] *Upward tentorial herniation* occurs when the infratentorial hypertension is associated with a lower supratentorial compartment pressure. This gradient moves the high cerebellar vermis into the incisura, causing brain stem pressure with consequent alterations of consciousness, respiratory irregularities and, owing to compression of the posterior cerebral arteries, occipital lobe ischemia (cortical blindness). *Cingulate* or *subfalcine herniation* occurs as a result of supratentorial herniation from one compartment to the other, underneath the falx cerebri. Compression of the anterior cerebral artery may ensue with damage to the ipsilateral mesial motor cortex. The patient then manifests a loss of motor control of the contralateral lower extremity and may have urinary sphincter incontinence.

Brain swelling due to cerebrovascular engorgement is the most common neuropathologic finding in severe pediatric head injuries. This is seen at autopsy as swollen and distended cerebral circumvolutions with distended cortical blood vessels.[20] On a cranial computed tomography (CT) scan, there are crowded subarachnoid spaces and small ventricles with or without midline displacement. Increased brain density on a CT scan, seen in children shortly after head trauma, is associated with increased cerebral blood volume measurements.[21] Brain edema is an abnormal increase in brain water. This is less commonly part of the acute head injury unless there has been a severe hypoxic-ischemic event at the time or during the resuscitation.[21] It may occur in the subsequent course of the disease, and it becomes obvious as a low-density finding on follow-up CT studies. Focal edema may be seen as part of cerebral "cortical" contusions on the initial CT scan. This is seen as a hemorrhagic area within the brain parenchyma, surrounded by the low-density edematous regions. It signals significant focal cerebral disruption.[22]

Note that common usage has led to the incorrect interchanging of the terms brain swelling and cerebral edema.

PATHOPHYSIOLOGY OF HEAD TRAUMA

Following head injury cerebral autoregulation may be impaired, and it may be intact in some areas of a hemisphere at the same time that it is altered in others.[18] In more severe injuries the impact itself creates a transient apneic spell that, if sufficiently prolonged, leads to severe hypoxic insult prior to any resuscitation measures. This is commonly accompanied by a brief, significant hypotensive spell that can aggravate neuronal damage by superimposing an ischemic injury. The combination and magnitude of the mechanical impact, hypoxic-ischemic event, and timeliness of resuscitation determine the outcome prior to the patient's arriving at the hospital. In nonfulminant injuries cerebral swelling is the most common finding. This is due to the increased blood volume and CBF because of the impaired autoregulation.[21, 22] Associating and potentially aggravating factors are cortical contusions in which the disruption of neural tissue and blood vessels can in themselves generate further change to the surrounding areas. The breakdown of membranes can release into the extracellular spaces products of cellular metabolism such as glutamate, free fatty acids, and vasoactive compounds that bring about a series of secondary changes.[23] These changes include further impairment of autoregulation, interference of neuronal and glial metabolism, and further tissue breakdown.[23] Local and generalized ischemic hypoxia creates metabolic derangement and tissue acidosis. Local acidosis enhances further metabolic disarray and magnifies the cycle of impairment of regional and generalized cerebrovascular autoregulation. Cerebral perfusion pressure can maintain a normal CBF when it is over 40 mm Hg. Under this value, the cerebral arteriovenous O_2 difference increases rapidly.[9] When CBF is reduced below 40% of its normal value, the electroencephalogram (EEG) tracing becomes flat, anaerobic metabolism is magnified, and the cerebral levels of adenosine triphosphate (ATP) fall.[24] When CBF is less than 20 ml/100g/min, there are no longer cortical responses on the somatosensory evoked stimuli.[25] Ischemic hypoxia may be made worse by seizures due to the increased metabolic demand that the seizure creates on the neurons. This further mismatches the CBF-metabolism coupling, enhances local acidosis, and further interferes with autoregulation. Hypercarbia and hypoxia follow.

INJURIES TO THE SKULL AND ITS COVERINGS

Scalp Injuries

Collections under the scalp following traumatic injuries are most commonly subgaleal hematomas. These are hemorrhages between the galea and the underlying pericranium. They can be extensive, and in the smaller child they may create a significant reduction in the hematocrit. They do not require treatment, and they will most commonly tamponade and then reabsorb over several days. They may be present due to bleeding from an underlying linear fracture, particularly in infants.

Scalp abrasions require thorough cleansing and an assessment of tetanus prophylaxis. Daily care with an application of topical antibiotic ointment is the extent of what is required in most cases. Scalp lacerations require prompt and immediate attention by the first physician who comes into contact with the child. The smaller child and the infant may exsanguinate from such injuries. Prompt and effective cleansing should be immediately followed by a tight closure by suturing in order to stop the blood loss. This may be readily performed with a vertical mattress suture to incorporate skin and galea in the same layer. Tetanus prophylaxis should be always assessed.

Neuroimaging of Cranial Trauma

Skull x-rays may reveal a fracture in approximately 11% of children who have a head injury.[26] However, plain x-rays do not indicate the lack or presence of underlying brain disease. Intracranial hematomas may be present in the absence of skull fractures.[27] On the other hand, the association of skull fracture on x-rays and neurologic signs or symptoms should mandate an assessment by cranial CT, owing to the higher incidence of intracranial hematomas.[26]

CT scanning is the most important diagnostic tool for the management of an acute head injury. This is due to the rapidity of the neuroimaging assessment as well as its noninvasiveness. Magnetic resonance imaging is used for the less acute stage of the disease process due to the limitations imposed on life support and resuscitation systems that go with the acutely injured child.[28] The most common CT finding in the child with a significant head injury is the presence of subarachnoid blood. This finding is noted in approximately 79% of patients.[21, 22] It is noted as a sheet-like high-density image on the falx cerebri and the tentorium.[22] In approximately 50% of significant pediatric head injuries, diffuse brain swelling is present.[22] This is seen as crowded and small ventricles and obliterated subarachnoid spaces. The white matter images may be more prominent than normal, indicating cerebral vasocongestion.[22] Areas of low density surrounding high-density areas that represent edema around small focal hemorrhages may be seen in approximately 10% of significant head injuries, and they represent cerebral contusions.

In severe injuries the acceleration-deceleration forces

may produce such movements of the brain on itself and the brain stem that tears are created in the white matter of the centrally placed structures (shear injuries). They present on a CT scan as areas of pinpoint or patchy hemorrhages in the corpus callosum, surrounding white matter, and brain stem (Fig. 21–1).[22]

Intracranial hematomas from head injury are less frequent in the pediatric population than in the adult population (26% versus 46%).[29] However, their significance is no less important owing to the fact that they indicate an adverse prognosis. Although the overall mortality from significant head injury is lower in children than in adults, when children with surgical mass lesions were compared with those of the adult population with mass lesions, the outcome in both groups was similar.[29] Therefore, prompt diagnosis and management of intracranial hematomas are of utmost importance.[21, 29]

Acute subdural hematomas are seen as high-density lesions of varying sizes, usually over the convexity of the hemispheres unilaterally or bilaterally (Fig. 21–2). They may be interhemispheric. Hematomas that are more difficult to locate on a CT scan may be those that are subfrontal or infratemporal and those in the posterior fossa.[22] Acute epidural hematomas are also high-density lesions, characteristically over the temporoparietal regions, with an hour-glass shape that is commonly associated with a fracture of the temporal bone, dural laceration, and a tear of the middle meningeal artery (Fig. 21–3). They vary in size. Acute intracerebral hematomas are usually associated with severe head injuries and shear injuries. They present as high-density lesions in the white matter or basal ganglia.[22, 28] They may follow penetrating injuries.

Skull Fractures

Linear Skull Fractures

Linear skull fractures may present with or without external evidence of trauma. In the infant with a subgaleal collection, they should always be suspected. For the most part these occur as a consequence of a fall, but child abuse should always be considered (see also Chapter 86). In the otherwise intact infant or child, they do not require treatment. In the child with an impairment of consciousness, hospitalization and observation is needed. It is recommended for the child under 2 years of age with a linear fracture that a follow-up anteroposterior and lateral skull film be obtained 7 to 8 weeks following the injury. This is done to detect the potential presence of a leptomeningeal cyst (growing skull fracture), which may occur as a result of the fracture opening in the face of a rapidly growing brain.[30]

Compound and Comminuted Skull Fractures

Compound skull fractures may have a significant laceration over the site or may be present as a small pinpoint opening of the scalp. The underlying fracture needs to be confirmed. In these situations the area needs to be urgently débrided and thoroughly cleansed, and

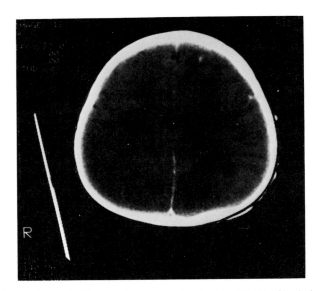

Figure 21–1. A CT scan is shown of a 5-year-old girl after being injured in a severe motor vehicle accident and arrest at the scene. Note the loss of normal differentiation between gray and white matter, with a central haziness in the white matter ventricle interface and, in the left hemisphere, the punctate areas of high density in the frontal region, indicative of hemorrhagic contusions and shear injuries.

the scalp should be repaired. If these steps are not done, the child is at subsequent risk of presenting with intracranial infections.[31] In the presence of a comminuted fracture or a depressed fracture, this is even more important owing to the potential laceration and communication with the CSF pathways.[31] These are explored by the neurosurgeon in the operating room to ensure maximal cleansing and dural repair.[31] Tetanus prophylaxis should always be assessed.

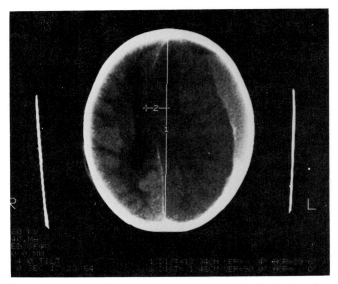

Figure 21–2. The CT scan illustrates a high-density image of an acute subdural hematoma on the left side in a 2-year-old girl after a motor vehicle accident. A significant shift to the midline is pointed out by the cursor, of 2 cm. Note the complete obliteration of the left ventricle by the displacement and mass effect.

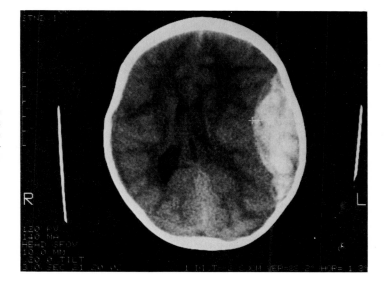

Figure 21–3. A CT scan is shown of a high-density lesion on the left side, characteristic of an acute epidural hematoma. This occurred in a 2-year-old girl after a fall. Note the particular shape of the high-density lesion, compared with the lesion in Figure 21–2. A significant midline shift and effacement of the ipsilateral ventricle are also present.

Depressed Skull Fractures

These fractures may vary in extent and severity and may or may not create dural tears and laceration of vessels, such as the middle meningeal artery or venous sinuses. Therefore, they should be assessed thoroughly, and the patient's neurologic status should be monitored carefully. The neuroimaging that yields the most information is the CT scan (bone windows).[22] The less significant ones do not require operative treatment, unless they are part of a compound fracture. The more significant ones require surgical exploration and correction to determine that the dura has not been involved, as well as for the correction of the deformity.

Basilar Skull Fractures

These fractures may present in the acute state with otorrhea, hemotympanum or vertigo (fracture in the middle cranial fossa), or rhinorrhea (fracture in the frontal fossa) with or without pneumocephalus (fracture involving sinus mucosa or mastoid cell). The diagnosis is made during the clinical examination, since apart from pneumocephalus the neuroimaging studies are often not revealing due to the thickness of the bones of the cranial base. The major concern about basilar skull fractures is that of infection. The management is bed rest till the CSF fistula ceases to leak. Antibiotic prophylaxis is not recommended, because this may lead to subsequent meningitis with antibiotic-resistant bacterial strains.[32] If fever does occur, a lumbar puncture should follow and the patient should be then promptly initiated on intravenous (IV) broad-spectrum antibiotic coverage.[32] Antibiotic adjustments can then be performed when the organism's sensitivities become available.

INTRACRANIAL HEMATOMAS

Extradural Hematomas

Extradural or epidural hematomas in children occur in approximately 6% of significant head injuries.[33] Most patients have sustained a blow to the temporoparietal region and usually have transient unconsciousness. They then improve neurologically before they deteriorate once more. This is called the lucid interval. However, most patients do not return to a true normal state during the lucid interval, and it is important to note that contrary to what occurs in adults, the subsequent neurologic deterioration occurs 24 to 72 hours after the trauma.[27] Therefore, if a child fails to improve neurologically or keeps complaining of a headache 2 to 3 days after the injury, he or she should be reassessed by a CT scan. Epidural hematomas are of varying size, and minimal collections do not need operative intervention. More important is the need to assess the neurologic state of the child and the presence of associated changes on the CT scan, such as diffuse brain swelling. If the patient has a significant epidural hematoma, prompt surgical evacuation is mandatory prior to the patient's manifesting the signs and symptoms of transtentorial herniation. Obliteration of the perimesencephalic cistern on the CT scan is a finding that may indicate the anatomic shift of structures, and it should be given the necessary clinical consideration.

With prompt diagnosis and early surgical intervention, patients with an epidural hematoma and no other significant injury should have a zero mortality rate.[33]

Subdural Hematomas

Acute subdural hematomas are usually bilateral, and they tend to occur more commonly after 1 year of age. In the infant, they may present with a bulging and tense fontanelle and split cranial sutures in a very irritable child, who then develops progressive obtundation. The older child presents with the usual signs and symptoms of intracranial hypertension and then progresses if untreated to obtundation. The most common finding in the child admitted to the hospital after a motor vehicle accident or a significant fall is evidence of trauma to other parts of the body. This mandates a thorough examination of the child to detect the presence of internal hemorrhage in other locations, as well as intracranially. The severity of the associated brain injury, together with the rapidity of expansion of the subdural hematoma(s), determines the gravity of the clinical state.

In an infant with a deteriorating level of consciousness, accompanied by a bulging and tense fontanelle and split cranial sutures, emergent bilateral subdural taps are indicated. This is performed under aseptic technique with 22-gauge subdural or spinal needles. Once the pressure is relieved, a CT scan of the head is mandatory. This determines the extent of the residual subdurals, but more important the presence or absence of other injuries as well as the extent of the brain swelling and shift of structures. Surgical intervention may then follow to obliterate the point of hemorrhage or to place an intracranial pressure monitor, if brain swelling is significant.[34] In the older child surgical drainage of the subdural collection is done by open craniotomy as an emergency, in the face of clinical deterioration and significant mass effect. In patients with a good clinical status and small subdural hematomas, surgical intervention is not needed. It is important to note that close monitoring and repeated CT scans may be required in these children, because subsequent enlargement of the subdural collections may follow initial stabilization.[33]

Intracerebral Hematomas

As previously stated, intracerebral hematomas are indicative of a significant acceleration-deceleration force applied to the child's cranium, with subsequent shear injury of the deeper white matter tracts, lacerations of deep veins, and hemorrhage. The hemorrhagic points may be small but can be asymmetric and large, with low-density areas around them indicating focal edema.[28] In most cases, surgical intervention is unwarranted because they usually do not expand further; however, ICP monitoring and maintenance of cerebral perfusion pressure and ventilation is mandatory. The patient with intracerebral hemorrhage needs to be monitored closely. Poorly controlled ICP should mandate a repeat CT scan, because subsequent expansion of the pre-existing clot may lead to further mass effect.[35] In some cases, if ICP does not respond to medical management, consideration should be given to surgical removal of the clot. The combination of a severe head injury and intracerebral hemorrhage is usually indicative of a poor neurologic outcome with significant neurologic handicaps.[29, 35, 36]

BRAIN INJURIES SECONDARY TO CHILD ABUSE

In the presence of a comatose child or severely obtunded infant who has a history that does not seem to concur with the clinical findings, child abuse should be a serious concern. It should be remembered that the child may have suffered more than one cerebral insult in the past and that the child may have been brought to the hospital only after being ill for a prolonged time. It should be presumed therefore that seizures or hypoxic-ischemic insults have been ongoing for an undetermined period, prior to the current emergency. This explains the poor clinical outcome in many of these children.

Visible External Cranial Evidence of Trauma

The presence of scalp contusions accompanied or not by subgaleal collections needs to be correlated with the history obtained in reference to the mechanism of injury. Periorbital ecchymosis immediately following an impact indicates a direct traumatic injury to the orbit(s). This should be differentiated from the findings of fractures in the anterior skull base that present as crescentic hemorrhagic accumulation at the conicoconjunctival junction. This is caused by retro-orbital bleeding that seeps forward by gravity to the lateral orbital canthus under the conjunctiva and then become visible. This process takes hours to 1 day to develop[37] and therefore may indicate a different history from the one given for the child in the current emergency. A similar statement can be said for a blue discoloration behind the ear, over the mastoid (Battle sign). The mechanism here is that of a fracture in the skull base at the level of the middle cranial fossa, with subsequent seepage of blood that later presents in the dermis and subcutaneous tissues of that region.[37]

Nonvisible External Cranial Trauma and Shaking Injuries

If the infant is taken by the shoulders and shaken violently, no clear external impact sites may be visible; however, the child may have had significant acceleration-deceleration brain injuries. The child may then present with obtundation, coma, apneic spells, a bulging and tense fontanelle, varying degrees of motor deficits or flaccidity, and retinal and preretinal hemorrhages on funduscopic examination.[38] The CT scan may reveal the presence of subarachnoid blood, primarily in the interhemispheric cistern and tentorium, and a swollen brain. Closer inspection may reveal areas of atrophic focal changes (from old cerebral contusions) and the presence of some fresh subcortical-cortical bleeding and edema (from fresh contusions).[28]

The outcome of these children may be poor owing to the magnitude and repetitiveness of previous injuries, the associated delay in seeking medical attention, and the hypoxic-ischemic insults that may or may not be accompanied by seizures. Unfortunately, if these children survive hospitalization, the outcome is compounded by the subsequent possible medical and social complicating factors (see also Chapter 86).[39]

ACUTE MANAGEMENT AND MULTIDISCIPLINARY CARE

Priorities and Acute Management Strategies

The specific aspects of resuscitation from trauma are addressed in another section (see Chapter 8). Priorities relate to ensuring airway control and venous access, as the cervical spine and remainder of the spine, if indicated, are assessed radiologically. An overall physical examination determines other management priorities. The level of consciousness mandates the next therapeutic steps. Patients with Glasgow Coma Scale scores of 8 or less, infants with coma, and patients who are convulsing should be promptly intubated and taken to the CT suite for neuroimaging studies. Intracranial hematomas should be promptly evacuated if their size and location indicate this step. If the impairment of consciousness is due to brain swelling, an ICP monitor should be promptly placed to assist in the critical care management.

Recognition and Management of Post-Traumatic Seizures

Seizures lead to secondary brain insults due to blood flow-metabolism mismatch, local lactic acidosis, and elevation of ICP secondary to all of these effects. Historical facts suggesting seizures should be sought. Seizures may be of a focal motor type and may or may not develop into full generalized seizures. In the patient with head injury and seizures, airway control is of utmost importance in order to prevent the secondary brain damage that may occur with the seizure and ventilatory embarrassment. If the impairment of consciousness is related to the seizures, once they are controlled, the patient's alertness may improve and extubation may follow. Electroencephalography is helpful in clinically equivocal cases.

Operative Priorities

Patients with expanding intracranial hematomas may deteriorate very rapidly according to the rapidity of the accumulation of the blood. This deterioration may be worsened by poor airway control and brain swelling. The importance of prompt detection of the underlying pathology by CT scanning is reiterated. The location, mass, and extent of intracranial disease direct the necessary neurosurgical intervention(s) and minimize the effects of intracranial hypertension and impairment of cerebral perfusion pressure (CPP). Subsequent postoperative management is tailored to the individual needs of the patient, related to the presence or absence of significant trauma to other organs, the presence of associated brain swelling, and respiratory status. The patients with a significant shift and brain swelling are best managed with ICP and systemic monitoring and airway control.

Maintaining Neuronal and Glial Function

The postoperative patient after removal of an intracranial hematoma and significant head injury is still at high risk. Therapy to support CPP, control ICP, and maintain oxygenation and hypocarbia should be continued. The neurons and glia have been subjected to an insult that may not allow them to readily recover. Falls in CPP, repeated elevations of ICP, or respiratory difficulties add secondary brain insults that can create further dysfunction. Seizures should be watched for, and if anticonvulsant therapy was not already initiated, this therapy should be promptly and effectively started. As the clinical parameters improve, then invasive monitoring and aggressive therapy are gradually withdrawn.

References

1. Kuhl DE, Reivich M, Alvai M, et al: Local cerebral blood volume determined by three-dimensional reconstruction of radionuclide scan data. Circ Res 36:610, 1975.
2. Milhorat TH: Hydrocephalus and the Cerebrospinal Fluid. Baltimore, Williams & Wilkins, 1972.
3. Sato O and Bering EA: Extra ventricular formation of cerebrospinal fluid. Brain Nerve 19:883, 1967.
4. Gomez DG, Potts TG, and Deonarine V: Arachnoid granulations of the sheep: Structural and ultrastructural changes with varying pressure differences. Arch Neurol 30:169, 1974.
5. Welch K and Friedman V: The cerebrospinal fluid valves. Brain 83:454, 1961.
6. Welch K and Pollay M: Perfusion of particles through arachnoid villi of the monkey. Am J Physiol 210:651, 1961.
7. Bayliss WM: On the local reaction of the arterial wall to changes of internal pressure. J Physiol 28:220, 1902.
8. Lassen NA: Control of cerebral circulation in health and disease. Circ Res 34:749, 1970.
9. Haggendal E, Loffgren J, and Nillson NJ: Effect of varied CSF pressure of cerebral blood flow in dogs. Acta Physiol Scand 79:262, 1970.
10. Cohen PJ, Alexander SC, Smith TF, et al: Effects of hypoxia and normocarbia on cerebral blood flow in conscious man. J Appl Physiol 23:183, 1967.
11. Reivich N: Arterial pCO_2 and cerebral hemodynamics. Am J Physiol 206:25, 1964.
12. Phelps ME, Grubb RL, and Terpogossian MM: Correlation between $pACO_2$ and regional blood volume by x-ray fluorescence. J Appl Physiol 34:741, 1973.
13. Monro A: Observations on the Structure and Function of the Nervous System. Edinburgh, Creech & Johnson, 1783.
14. Langfitt TW: Increased intracranial pressure. Clin Neurosurg 16:436, 1969.
15. Langfitt TW, Weinstein JD, and Kassell NF: Cerebral vasomotor paralysis produced by intracranial hypertension. Neurology 15:622, 1965.
16. Lundberg N: Continuous recording and control of ventricular fluid pressure in neurosurgical practice. Acta Psychiatr Neurol Scand 36(Suppl. 149):1, 1960.
17. Donn SM and Phillip AGS: Early increase in intracranial pressure in pre-term infants. Pediatrics 61:904, 1978.
18. Jefferson G: The tentorial pressure cone. Arch Neurol Psychiatr 40:857, 1938.
19. Plum F and Posner JB: Diagnosis of Stupor and Coma. Philadelphia, FA Davis, 1980.
20. Lindenberg R, Fisher RS, Durlacher S, et al: Pathology of the Brain in Blunt Head Injuries of Infants and Children. In: International Congress of Neuropathology Proceedings. Amsterdam, Excerpta Medica, 1955, pp. 477–479.
21. Bruce DA, Raphaely RC, Goldberg AI, et al: Pathophysiology, treatment and outcome following severe head injury in children. Child's Brain 5:174, 1979.

22. Zimmerman RA, Bilaniuk LT, Bruce DA, et al: Computed tomography of pediatric head trauma: Acute general cerebral swelling. J Radiol 126:403, 1978.
23. Unterberg A and Baethmann A: Secondary changes in brain biochemistry with brain edema. *In* Brain Insults in Infants and Children. Orlando, Grune & Stratton, 1985, pp. 61–73.
24. McKenzie EI, McGeorge AP, Graham DI, et al: Breakthrough of cerebral autoregulation in the sympathetic nervous system. *In*: Ingvar DH and Lassen NA (eds): Cerebral Function: Metabolism and Circulation. Copenhagen, Munksgaard, 1977, pp. 48–49.
25. Astrup J, Symon L, Branstorn NN, et al: Cortical evoked potential and extracellular potassium and hydrogen at critical levels of brain ischemia. Stroke 8:51, 1977.
26. Rosenthal BW and Bergman I: Intracranial injury after moderate head trauma in children. J Pediatr 115:346, 1989.
27. Galbraith S and Smith J: Acute traumatic intracranial hematomas without skull fracture. Lancet 1:501, 1973.
28. Zimmerman RA, Bilaniuk LT, Hackney DB, et al: Head injury: Early results of comparing CT and high field MR. AJNR 7:757, 1986.
29. Alberico AM, Ward JD, Marmarou A, et al: Outcome after severe head injury: Relationship to mass lesions, diffuse injury, and ICP course in pediatric and adult patients. J Neurosurg 67:648, 1987.
30. Sato O, Tsugane R, and Kageyama N: Growing skull fractures of childhood. Child's Brain 1:148, 1975.
31. Jennett WP and Miller JD: Infections after depressed fracture of the skull. J Neurosurg 36:333, 1972.
32. Ignelzi RJ and VanderArk GD: Analysis of treatment of basilar skull fractures with and without antibiotics. J Neurosurg 43:721, 1975.
33. Bruce DA, Schut L, Bruno LA, et al: Outcome following severe head injuries in children. J Neurosurg 48:679, 1978.
34. James HE: Analysis of therapeutic modalities for head injured children. Child's Brain 5:263, 1979.
35. Atluru V, Epstein LG, and Zilka A: Delayed traumatic intracerebral hemorrhage in children. Pediatr Neurol 2:297, 1986.
36. Luerssen TG, Klauber MR, and Marshall LF: Outcome from head injury related to patient's age: A longitudinal prospective study of adult and pediatric head injury. J Neurosurg 68:409, 1988.
37. Lewin W: The Management of Head Injuries. Baltimore, Williams & Wilkins, 1966.
38. Caffey J: The whiplash-shaken infant syndrome: Manual shaking by the extremities with whiplash-induced intracranial and intraocular bleedings, linked with residual permanent brain damage and mental retardation. Pediatrics 54:396, 1974.
39. James HE and Schut L: The neurosurgeon and the battered child. Surg Neurol 2:415, 1974.

22

Spinal Cord Injury in Children

Dennis L. Johnson, M.D.

Every year more than 1,000 children sustain paralyzing spinal cord injuries in the United States.[1] The tragedy and costs of acute and continuing care of a paralyzed child are staggering. Since the cord does not repair itself and the primary injury is not "curable," treatment is designed to prevent secondary injury. Although the primary focus of this chapter is on the diagnosis and acute care of pediatric spinal cord injuries, prevention deserves highest priority: primary prevention in our homes and schools, secondary prevention at the scene of the accident, and tertiary prevention when the injured child first enters the health care system.

The fundamental differences between pediatric and adult trauma victims are self-evident and provide the framework for this chapter. The typical child is neither cooperative nor able to articulate neurologic symptoms. Radiographic examination is complicated by technical problems associated with the small uncooperative patient: overpenetrated films, motion artifacts, and imperfect alignment. Interpretation of the x-rays is confounded by the immature skeleton and ligaments as well as by congenital abnormalities. Moreover, since spinal cord injury can occur without radiographic abnormality, the integrity of the spine in children can never be ensured by x-ray alone. Falls and accidents related to motor vehicles are characteristic mechanisms of injury seen in children. The patterns of injury are determined by the child's unique anatomic vulnerability. Management of pediatric spine injuries differs from adult injuries in that immobilization plays a much greater role than traction, and the indications for surgical fusion are more stringent. Finally, although children are expected to achieve more than adults, the outcome for children may be worse.

DEVELOPMENT OF THE SPINE

Recognition of normal variants and correct interpretation of congenitally abnormal spines depend on a knowledge of the development and maturation of the spine. All vertebral bodies are shaped by ossification centers. Most vertebrae are composed of an anterior or ventral ossification center (OC) and two posterior or lateral ossification centers. The anterior center forms the body of the vertebra, and the lateral centers extend dorsally or posteriorly to encircle the spinal cord and to form the pedicles, transverse processes, neural arches, and the spinous processes. The atlas and axis are the only vertebrae that do not conform to this pattern of development. The atlas has the usual three OCs, but part of the anterior OC migrates caudally to form the odontoid process, which is the most cephalad portion of the axis. The odontoid process lies anteriorly within the ring of the atlas to provide a pivot joint where the head joins the neck to convey tremendous rotatory capability. The odontoid peg or process has two OCs that take the shape of two pillars positioned side by side and capped by a third OC, the os terminale (Fig. 22–1A and B). The growth and fusion of OCs vary by vertebral level, but the OCs of the upper most cervical vertebrae are the last to appear.[2, 3]

The development of the spine can be chronicled radiographically (Table 22–1). The ventral OC that forms the anterior arch of the atlas is visible at birth in only 20% of normal children, but by 1 year of age the anterior arch of the atlas becomes visible.[3, 11] At 2 years of age the os terminale is seen. By 4 years of age the lateral OCs have fused posteriorly to complete the neural arch around the spinal cord.[4] The neurosynchondrosis at the base of the odontoid begins to close by 6 years of age but may remain visible up to 11 years of age.[5, 6] By 8 years of age, the lateral OCs have fused with the anterior OCs and the child's spine begins to assume its adult configuration. Not only does the flattened, wedged appearance of the body become more rectangular but the ligamentous laxity, which is best illustrated by pseudosubluxation of C2–C3, also disappears. The point of maximal flexion shifts from C2–C3 to C4–C5 and C5–C6 by the end of the first decade. By the age of 12, the os terminale has fused to the remainder of the odontoid.[6] At 15 or 16 years of age, secondary ossification centers develop at the tips of the transverse processes and inferior articulations as well as the spinous processes.[2, 3] Several normal radiographic variants are based on these developmental guidelines.

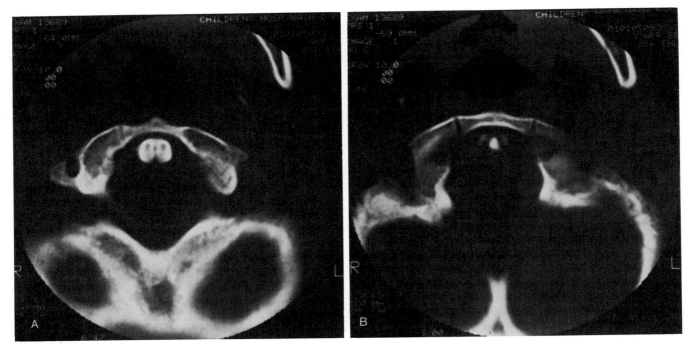

Figure 22–1. *A,* Axial CT scan through the base of the skull, including the atlas and odontoid process: Two ossification centers form the body of the odontoid process. *B,* Axial CT scan imaged in a slightly more cephalad plane to show all three ossification centers, including os terminale.

NORMAL VARIANTS

In children less than 1 year old the anterior arch of C1 may not be visible. "Fractures" of the anterior arch may also occur where the anterior OC of the atlas joins the lateral OCs. Up to 2 years of age the odontoid process appears foreshortened and may be overridden by the anterior ring of the atlas when the child's head and neck are in extension.

Prior to 8 years of age, pseudosubluxation of C2 on C3 or C3 on C4 is common. Up to 4 mm is seen in 37% of routine lateral cervical spine x-rays done for trauma. Pseudosubluxation is always anterior and is most pronounced in flexion. It disappears in extension and can be further differentiated from fracture-dislocation by tracing Swishchuck line, the posterior aspect of the spinal canal (Fig. 22–2A and B).[7]

The radiographic gap between the ossification centers

of the odontoid process and the body of the axis corresponds to a cartilaginous plate known as the basilar odontoid synchondrosis. In the high-risk age group of 6 to 9 years fractures of the axis occur through this synchondrosis, and to the inexperienced eye the normal synchondrosis can simulate a fracture. By the age of 12 the basilar odontoid synchondrosis has ossified.[6] Fractures in this older age group are through the base of the odontoid and not through the synchondrosis. On the anteroposterior view of the x-ray film the normal is below the base of the odontoid at the level of the superior articulating facets.[8]

Finally, large secondary ossification centers in the spinous processes of adolescents may mimic fractures such as clay-shoveler's fracture of the spinous process of C7. True fractures of the spinous process are very painful and can be easily differentiated from this normal variation.

Table 22–1. DEVELOPMENTAL EVENTS

Age (Yr)	Radiographic Feature
0	Anterior mass of the atlas may be absent
1	Anterior mass of the atlas present; dens short with overriding atlas; os terminale not seen; vertebrae wedge-shaped; ligamentous laxity (pseudosubluxation) evident
2	Os terminale appears
4	Neural arches fuse posteriorly
6	Odontoid synchondrosis of axis begins to disappear
8	Pseudosubluxation disappears; adult configuration (rectangular instead of wedge-shaped) of the vertebral body
12	Os terminale fuses to the remainder of the dens
16	Secondary ossification centers may be seen at the tips of the spinous processes

ABNORMAL VARIANTS

Anomalies of the spine are rare but pertinent to interpretation of the injured spine. Most anomalies are discovered when the child develops persistent neck pain or torticollis after a trivial injury. The best known anomaly is the atlantoaxial instability of Down syndrome that has been brought to public attention by the Special Olympics. Seventeen per cent of these special children have excessive motion of the odontoid within the ring of the atlas.[9] Participation in the high jump and pole vault places these children at risk for a hyperflexion injury and possible quadriplegia. Rotatory subluxation is not uncommon in Down syndrome and can be differ-

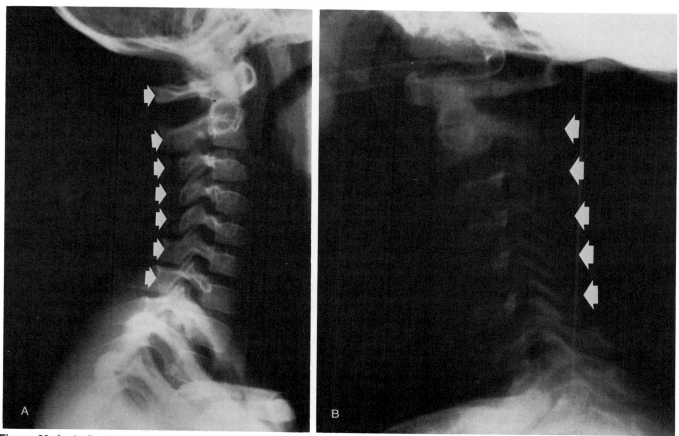

Figure 22–2. *A*, Routine lateral cervical spine with arrows marking Swischuck's line. *B*, Pseudosubluxation. Swishchuck's line remains unbroken.

entiated from acute torticollis by computed tomography (CT) or plain tomography. Occipitoatlantoaxial ligamentous instability is seen in juvenile rheumatoid arthritis, Reiter syndrome, Larsen syndrome, Hurler syndrome, and Morquio syndrome.[10] Achondroplastic dwarfs may also present with severe spinal cord injury after trivial trauma because of associated craniovertebral anomalies and spinal stenosis.

Klippel-Feil syndrome is characterized by a short, immobile neck and a low hairline. Radiographically, fusion of adjacent segments of both the anterior and posterior elements is apparent, and occasionally vertebrae are absent. The spine is particularly vulnerable to injury at levels adjacent to the fused segments. Uncommonly, fusion of the scapulae with the posterior arches of the lower cervical vertebrae is seen. Odontoid hypoplasia and absence of the posterior arch of C1 are common.[3, 11]

Odontoid hypoplasia is also seen in Morquio syndrome, the most common of the mucopolysaccharidoses.[12] Flattening of the vertebrae or platyspondilia in this syndrome produces such a short neck that the head appears to be attached directly to the shoulders. Fortunately, extension of the head is usually checked by the kyphotic chest, and flexion is limited by a sternal kyphos. However, by sudden forward flexion of the head and neck, the spinal cord can be garrotted by the anterior arch of C1 as the hypoplastic odontoid process slips forward under the arch.

Os odontoideum is peculiar to childhood but is probably not a congenital abnormality. It is most commonly confused with os terminale, which is a normal feature of the cervical spine in children under the age of 12. The os terminale is the third ossification center of the odontoid process and is firmly morticed to the rest of the odontoid by cartilage. It moves as a unit in flexion and extension of the neck and does not cause symptoms (Figs. 22–3 and 22–4). In contrast, os odontoideum becomes apparent after a minor injury because of persistent discomfort or torticollis. The bony apical fragment is clearly separated from the rest of the odontoid and remains fixed to the anterior arch of the atlas by the transverse ligament during flexion and extension (Fig. 22–5). The rest of the odontoid moves unchecked posteriorly in flexion and impinges on the spinal cord. Trauma in early childhood is the most probable cause of os odontoideum. Several cases of a normal odontoid process replaced by an "os" following trauma have been documented radiographically, but there have been no documented cases of a post-traumatic os beyond 3 years of age.[13, 14] The argument against a traumatic etiology is that the abnormal articulation of the os is cephalad and well removed from the basilar synchondrosis, which is the site of odontoid fractures in young children. The cephalad position of the os is due to impaired development caused by disruption of the blood supply.

Central vascularization of the odontoid process, which is normally reduced through the cartilaginous synchon-

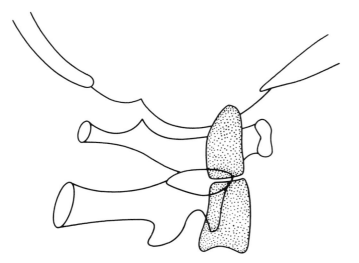

Figure 22–3. Craniovertebral junction: normal relation of posterior lip of foramen magnum, tip of clivus, atlas, body of the axis, odontoid, and basilar synchondrosis. Fractures usually occur through the synchondrosis.

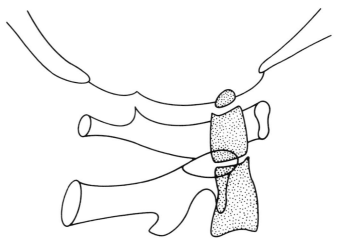

Figure 22–5. Os terminale: the terminal ossification center has not yet fused to the remainder of axis but a firm cartilaginous framework ensures that it moves together with the rest of the axis in flexion and extension, in contrast to os odontoideum.

drosis, is interrupted or severely impaired by the fracture. Thus the vascularization necessary for fracture healing must come from the vascular arcade that encircles the tip of the odontoid and the anastomotic collar around its base.[15] The distal tip of the odontoid has the most fragile blood supply and is more likely to undergo resorption than the base. The base of the odontoid continues to develop but much of the apex resorbs and becomes separated from the main body of the odontoid. The os articulation thus comes to lie superior to the synchondrosis and the original site of the injury.

BIOMECHANICS OF SPINAL INJURIES

Extension, flexion, rotation, and axial compression, singularly or in combination, are the moments of force

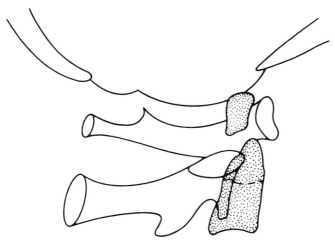

Figure 22–4. Os odontoideum: top of odontoid is separated from remainder of axis and moves with atlas in flexion/extension because it is secured by the transverse ligament. The remainder of the axis extends above the C1–C2 facet joints, in contrast to a fracture through the basilar synchondrosis that is at or just below the articulating surfaces.

that result in spinal cord injury. The mechanism of injury provides insight into the severity of injury, the integrity of the anterior and posterior elements of the spine, and stability.

Spine injuries in children are most common in the upper three cervical segments. This is due in part to the disproportionately large head, the horizontal orientation of the facets of the upper three vertebrae, ligamentous laxity, hypoplastic occipital condyles, and poorly developed uncinate processes. The relatively large and ponderous skull is attached to the cervical spine by the anterior and posterior atlanto-occipital membranes, the ligamentum nuchae, the apical and alar ligaments of the odontoid, and the tectorial membrane. The mobility of the head on the neck is also dependent on this same ligamentous complex.

Atlanto-occipital dislocation (AOD) was previously thought to be a fatal injury, but because of prompt transport and sophisticated prehospital care, children with this injury are surviving to reach medical attention.[16] AOD has been conventionally classified by the radiographic direction of dislocation, but this classification scheme does not have prognostic value nor does it guide treatment.[17] Distraction is the primary radiographic finding, and the degree to which the ligamentous complex is disrupted depends on the direction of force. Hyperflexion is less likely to be fatal since the anterior displacement of the head is checked by the chin on the chest and also by all atlanto-occipital ligaments except the anterior atlanto-occipital membrane. The potential arc of movement of the atlanto-occipital joint and the risk of injury to the upper spinal cord and lower brain stem are much greater in hyperextension. Pedestrians are particularly vulnerable to AOD and often present comatose with a moderately severe head injury, an occipital skull fracture, and a long bone fracture. The impact is so great that the skull and long bones are fractured. As the child is "run over," the distracting force is sufficient to detach the ligaments and stretch lower cranial nerves.

Upper cervical cord injuries are also seen in fatal child abuse presumably due to violent shaking of the relatively heavy head on a poorly muscled neck.[18] Spinal cord injuries (SCI) may be overlooked if attention is focused solely on the management of acute subdural hematomas. Spinal cord injury without radiographic abnormality (SCIWORA) is common, and the clinical picture is often clouded by hypoxia, seizures, and severe brain injury.[19–23]

Jefferson fractures or burst fractures of the atlas are uncommon in children and are often confused with normal developmental variants (synchondroses between anterior and lateral OCs). They usually result from a blow to the vertex of the skull.

Fractures of the odontoid are one of the most common in children. In children less than 8 years of age the fracture occurs at the point of least resistance, which is the basilar odontoid synchondrosis (Fig. 22–6).[24] Fracture and separation can best be defined on fluoroscopically controlled flexion-extension views of the cervical spine. Remnants of the odontoid synchondrosis may simulate fractures in children up to 12 years of age. In contrast to fractures of the base of the odontoid, the synchondrosis lies below the level of the superior articular facets because the odontoid is recessed into the body of the axis as a tenon in a mortise.

Atlantoaxial rotatory fixation (AARF) presents as acute torticollis associated with a wrestling or football injury. AARF is not uncommon in Down syndrome. If the rotatory excursion of the atlas exceeds 40 degrees, the alar or "check" ligaments are torn and the superior articulating facet of the atlas becomes perched on the occipital condyle. The child presents with acute torticollis and occasionally with a "cocked robin" appearance (head tilted and flexed to one side and then rotated to the opposite side). Acute torticollis in childhood is more often spontaneous or associated with upper respiratory infection, cervical adenitis, tonsillitis, minor trauma, or even after cleft palate surgery.[25] In contrast to AARF, acute torticollis is characterized by spasm of the shorter sternocleidomastoid muscle (SCM). The longer SCM is in spasm in AARF. Unless the transverse ligament is torn and the anterior arch of the atlas is displaced forward of the odontoid, these injuries can be managed with tong or halter traction to reduce the subluxation. Immobilization will be necessary to maintain alignment.

Most motor vehicle injuries occur because the occupant is not restrained. Hangman fractures (bipedicular fracture of C2) are seen in high-speed accidents when the unrestrained child is thrown from the vehicle and sustains a hyperextension injury. Unless there is an associated C2–C3 spondylolisthesis, these injuries are stable and only require a Philadelphia collar for support.

Restraint devices can contribute to injury if they are not applied and secured correctly (e.g., an infant restraint device should face backward rather than forward). A three-point restraint system holds the chest adequately but allows the head and neck to snap forward. Sufficient force can cause injury to the spinal cord at the cervicothoracic junction or the atlantoaxial junction. These injuries can be missed, especially if there is no radiographic abnormality or when attention is diverted to life-threatening chest injuries. The initial survey must include a careful neurologic examination.

Rear seat lap belts are another significant source of spinal cord injury.[26] In children, the lap belt easily slips up over the immature anterior superior iliac spines and bands the abdomen tightly just above the umbilicus. Tremendous bending forces are exerted on the upper lumbar spine to cause compression and fracture of the vertebral body. The interspinous ligament is disrupted, and the laminae and articulating facets are distracted. Rarely, a Chance fracture is seen that extends horizontally through the body, pedicles, laminae, and spinous process. In addition to a spinal cord injury, many of these children also have a duodenal injury, and tears in the mesentery and mesenteric vessels, pancreas, liver, and spleen. A significant head injury often complicates their care. These fractures are unstable and require surgical reduction and fusion.

Beyond the age of 8 years the spine assumes its adult configuration, and the point of maximal flexion shifts from the upper cervical spine to the low and midcervical spine. Football, wrestling, diving, and motorcycle injuries are confined to the older adolescents. The pattern of injury is more characteristic of the mature skeleton and adult injuries: low to midcervical fracture dislocation.

Even with modern radiographic techniques, SCIWORA is encountered in at least 35% of pediatric injuries.[25] SCIWORA is seen most commonly in children younger than 8 years of age and is usually associated with severe spinal cord injury.

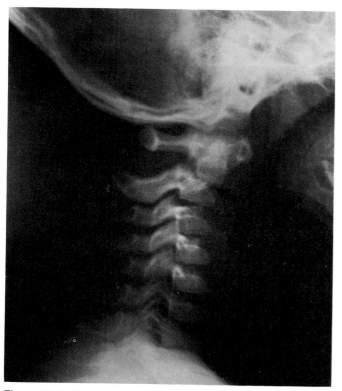

Figure 22–6. Odontoid fracture-subluxation through basilar odontoid synchondrosis.

SCIWORA may also be delayed in onset. In most of the cases reported by Osenbach and Menezes, premonitory complaints of weakness, paresthesias, or numbness could be elicited. Recurrent SCIWORA with previous mild spinal cord injury has also been described.[27] The ligamentous laxity and hypermobility of the spine provide the basis for SCIWORA.[28] The neonatal spine can be stretched a full 2 inches before disruption, but the neonatal spinal cord can only be stretched one quarter of an inch.[29]

Cervical straightening, kyphosis, or prevertebral swelling on the lateral cervical spine x-ray are not reliable clues to SCI in children. Cervical kyphosis is common in younger children, perhaps because when the proportionately larger head rests on the examining table the neck is straightened or slightly flexed. Loss of cervical lordosis is evident in 30% of routine "normal" lateral cervical spine x-rays for trauma. Moreover, during forced expiration associated with crying, the hypopharynx enlarges to give the appearance of prevertebral swelling.

Careful plain film radiographs and CT scanning will not replace a detailed history and physical examination. Children should remain immobilized until a thorough neurologic examination has been done.

NEUROLOGIC EXAMINATION

The neurologic examination is an integral part of assessing every trauma patient. The neurologic examination is usually directed by symptomatology, but the injured child cannot always articulate pain, paresthesias, or anesthesia. A careful evaluation of the mental status is followed by a quick survey of the cranial nerves. In addition to pupillary reactions and symmetry, eye movements are also assessed. An inability to look lateral may be a manifestation of sixth cranial nerve palsy and correlate with atlanto-occipital distraction. Facial asymmetry and tongue deviation may be important signs of significant concomitant head injury or reflect lower brain stem injury associated with upper cervical spine trauma.

Gross motor function may be apparent as the child is wheeled into the trauma bay struggling and screaming. Guarding or torticollis may be important clues to cervical spine injury. The child must be treated for an SCI until an adequate examination and radiographic survey have been completed, especially if the child is intubated. Right-left symmetry and an assessment of upper versus lower extremity function is particularly valuable. The lack of motor function helps to localize the anatomic level of the injury. Muscle strength or power can be graded, but it is more meaningful to ascribe function. Describing a marginal function that the child can barely perform provides a basis for serial evaluation (e.g., "child is able to move fingers but unable to hold tennis ball"). The sensory level is much more difficult to assess in children: they may be frightened, noncommunicative, comatose, or simply uncooperative. Nevertheless the response to touch or pinprick may not only establish the anatomic level of injury but also predict how badly the cord is damaged. Complete loss of motor and sensory function below the anatomic or radiologic level of injury precludes recovery. The extent of recovery is directly correlated with the degree of motor and sensory preservation below the level of the injury. If perineal sensation is present or "spared" in an otherwise paralyzed patient, some hope for recovery can be garnered. Reflexes are not particularly helpful in the assessment of the cord-injured patient. Reflexes are often absent; both extensor and flexor plantar responses can be transiently observed following complete cord transection. Priapism and a bulbocavernosus reflex carry a particularly poor prognosis for recovery. An intact anal sphincter reflex may be a sign of sacral sparing.

Traumatic lesions seldom manifest with neurologic precision, but certain patterns of neurologic dysfunction provide an anatomic signature for the injury: central cord syndrome, anterior cord syndrome, Brown-Sequard syndrome, and cruciate paralysis of Bell.

The central cord syndrome is characterized by paresis of the arms with relative sparing of the legs.[30] The long tracts are somatotopically organized in the cord such that the fibers supplying the arms are located centrally, whereas the legs are represented more peripherally. This pattern of injury is usually seen in older children and in adults after extension injuries and is attributed to occlusion of penetrating vessels; it can also be associated with hematomyelia.

The anterior cord syndrome is attributed to hyperflexion or axial compression injuries and presents with analgesia and paresis below the level of the lesion with preservation of proprioception, light touch, and vibration.[31] This syndrome can be caused by ruptured disc or fracture fragments pushing posteriorly against the anterior or ventral surface of the cord.

The Brown-Sequard syndrome is characterized by ipsilateral motor paralysis and loss of touch and proprioception combined with contralateral loss of pain and temperature. The anatomic injury is to the side of the cord.[32, 33] Stabbing is the usual mechanism of injury.

Cruciate paralysis of Bell is characteristic of injuries at the level of the foramen magnum, such as odontoid fractures.[34] The motor tracts supplying the arms decussate at the level of the foramen magnum and the motor fibers to the legs decussate at C1–C2. If the injury is midline and centered at the foramen magnum, a cruciate paralysis manifests predominantly as arm paralysis; a lower injury at the C1–C2 level will present with more leg than arm paralysis. If the injury is off to the side, motor fibers to the ipsilateral arm (which have not yet crossed) will be injured with decussating leg fibers from the contralateral side. The neurologic result is a crossed (cruciate) paralysis—an arm and the contralateral leg.

These patterns of neurologic dysfunction are incomplete injuries of the spinal cord and have the potential for recovery. They deserve careful radiographic investigation. CT scanning provides excellent detail of the bone structure and can be done expeditiously (3 minutes with current software) in the course of the initial trauma work-up. Magnetic resonance imaging (MRI) produces the invaluable sagittal image and better neuroanatomic detail but requires more time (minimum of 20 minutes) and does not image bone well. Moreover, because of the magnetic fields, an MRI cannot be performed on patients who are supported on ventilators with metallic parts. Spinal traction must be applied by hand, which contributes to movement artifact.

MANAGEMENT

Nearly all trauma victims are immobilized in the field and transported on a board with a collar around the neck or with sand bags supporting each side of the head. In the emergency department the primary concerns are alignment and stability. Pain is the first clue to a significant injury, and persistent pain or an abnormal posture imply that the spine is not anatomically aligned. If a ligamentous or bone injury significantly alters alignment, then stability is also compromised. Malalignment and instability can then be corroborated radiographically. More commonly, this clinical sequence is reversed in the emergency department: the routine lateral cervical spine x-ray exposes an abnormality that must be further investigated radiographically and corroborated by physical examination. Normal and abnormal variants must be recognized, and the radiographic abnormality must be brought into perspective. Alignment can be assessed by Swishchuck line, and stability must be ensured by fluoroscopically controlled flexion-extension views of the lateral cervical spine. Flexion-extension dynamic views (FEDS) should not be done on obvious subluxations or on the very uncooperative child. Good judgment mandates immobilization until the child's condition has stabilized and until the child has been fully assessed radiographically and neurologically. Care should be taken when studies are equivocal or when pain persists despite normal FEDS. Continued immobilization and repeat studies may be in order.

In the acute care of children with spine injuries, immobilization takes precedence over axial traction. However, axial traction may be necessary to achieve alignment and to ensure temporary immobilization of the spine. Since most fractures are in the upper cervical spine, traction is used with caution. Alignment is usually achieved with little (< 5 lb) or no traction. For traction, Gardner-Wells skull tongs are easy to insert (in the parietal bones 2 finger-breadths above the ear in line with the external auditory meatus) and are usually more readily available than the alternative, a halo ring. The advantage of the halo ring is that with a single procedure alignment can be restored and external fixation secured by attaching it to a jacket. Since in the supine position the cervical spine is flexed into slight kyphosis by the child's relatively large head, bolsters should be placed under the shoulders to achieve a neutral position. The same effect can be achieved with a mattress split cephalad from the shoulders. The occiput or the back of the halo ring must be suspended so that the force of the traction is not absorbed in friction on the mattress. Cervical kyphosis cannot be reversed by simple extension of the head, because most of that movement takes place at the atlanto-occipital joint. Adjustable halo rings, which accommodate any head size, are available, and some halo devices also have cranial tongs built into

the halo to hasten use. Application of the halo requires two pairs of hands and a ring-spacing device (either pin spacers or the Hershey "spoon"). Adequate analgesia can be achieved with a combination of local anesthesia, fentanyl, and midazolam. The four pins are torqued to 4 or 5 foot-pounds. In children less than 2 years of age 6 to 8 pins can be torqued to 3 or 4 foot-pounds.

The extent of immobilization should be guided by the degree of instability. Relatively stable fractures include isolated fractures of the posterior ring of the atlas or axis and nondisplaced fractures of the thoracic spine. Anterior compression fractures of the middle and lower cervical spine that are not associated with subluxation either on static x-rays or FEDS should be immobilized with a two- or four-posted brace to prevent any change in the natural configuration of the spine. Atlanto-occipital distraction, atlantoaxial subluxation, and fractures of the odontoid including the basilar odontoid synchondrosis are best immobilized in a halo jacket for 3 months, followed by a stiff Philadelphia collar for 6 weeks, then a soft collar for another 4 to 6 weeks. This sequence should be monitored radiographically at each anticipated change of the fixation device or orthosis.

If the bone injury is associated with spinal cord injury, intravenous methylprednisolone (a 30 mg/kg push followed by 5.4 mg/kg/hr for 23 hours) is administered. One multicenter trial has shown that this high-dose regimen improves neurologic recovery in adults if given within 8 hours.[35]

The only indication for immediate surgery is an incomplete injury with progressive loss of neurologic function. Urgent surgery is indicated for thoracic and lumbar spine subluxations that compromise 50% or more of the spinal canal. Harrington rod distraction and fixation are preferable to laminectomy or costotransversectomy in reducing these fractures. Severe head injury or major chest injury are relative contraindications to early surgical reduction and fusion. Facet subluxations may be reduced by traction, but bilateral facet fracture/subluxations are inherently unstable and must be fused. The continuing care of these children can be best directed by a pediatrician who can coordinate multidisciplinary care involving a neurosurgeon, urologist, orthopedic surgeon, and physiatrist.

OUTCOME

Prognosis in pediatric spinal cord injury has not been studied extensively. Although probably not substantially different from adult injuries, the outcome may, indeed, be worse. Children who are immediately and completely paralyzed are not likely to recover useful function below the level of the injury. Those with an incomplete injury have a good chance of recovering sufficient neurologic function to walk and to live independently. Children with an anterior cord syndrome seldom recover function below the level of the lesion.

Future direction for management of SCI should concentrate on exploring mechanisms of injury that would open new possibilities for prevention.

CONCLUSION

Since most injuries can be prevented, it is appropriate that we should conclude this chapter as we began it. Primary prevention of cervical spine injuries involves teaching young people and their parents how to prevent neck injuries. There are laws in many states mandating the use of seat belts, but the devices must be attached properly to the seat and the infant or child positioned properly for restraint. The biomechanics of each SCI should be studied in minute detail to provide input into the manufacture of safety restraint devices and to provide a basis for rule changes in contact sports to make participation safer. The dangers of diving should be publicized. Parents should know the ramifications of shaking a child in anger and the risk of an open staircase to a child in a walker. Moreover, cervical spine radiographs should be mandatory for amateur wrestlers and participants in Special Olympics.

Secondary prevention mandates that the neck of every child at the scene of an accident be immobilized and protected from further injury that might be caused by rescue. Each child is assumed to have a neck injury until they can be thoroughly evaluated.

Tertiary prevention dictates a lateral spine x-ray and a thorough neurologic evaluation on every pediatric trauma victim. SCIWORA is surprisingly common and greatly complicates the care of the injured child. The integrity of the spine cannot be ensured by x-ray alone.

Knowledge of the development of the spine allows recognition of normal variants such as pseudosubluxation, pseudofractures of the basilar odontoid synchondrosis, and os terminale. These variants disappear between the ages of 8 and 12 as the pediatric spine assumes its adult configuration. Abnormal variants such as os odontoideum are an extension of our knowledge of normal variants.

Diagnostic tests must be undertaken cautiously and under the supervision of a neurosurgeon. Myelography and MRI have little value in the treatment of the acutely ill child with a complete injury. MRI is the test of choice for incomplete lesions once the child is beyond the acute phase.

Immobilization and external fixation are the first priorities of treatment. If a neurologic deficit is evident, steroids should be given for 24 hours. Surgery is reserved for deterioration of a partially paralyzed patient. Dislocations that cannot be reduced by traction and bilateral facet dislocation should also be operated early before the injury becomes fixed by the healing process.

The severity of the neurologic deficit at the initial examination is the best predictor of outcome. The child who is completely paralyzed and insensate below the level of the injury will not recover function. The majority of children with incomplete lesions recover sufficient function to walk. Children with central cord and Brown-Sequard syndromes recover much of their deficit and are ambulatory; in contrast, those with anterior cord syndrome seldom recover motor function.

The child with an SCI is a national tragedy. Public awareness, commitment, and investment will hopefully prevent most injuries. A responsive, well-informed health care system will temper the personal tragedy of lifelong paralysis.

References

1. Kewalramini LS and Tori JA: Spinal cord trauma in children: Neurologic patterns, radiologic features, and pathomechanics of injury. Spine 5:11, 1980.
2. Parke WW: Development of the spine. In: Rothman RH and Simeone FA (eds): The Spine. Philadelphia, WB Saunders, 1975, pp. 1–17.
3. Harwood-Nash DC and Fitz CR: Neuroradiology in Infants and Children. St. Louis, CV Mosby, 1976, p. 1059.
4. Allen BL and Ferguson RL: Cervical spine trauma in children. In: Bradford D and Hensinger R (eds): The Pediatric Spine. New York, Thieme Inc, 1985, pp. 89–104.
5. Bailey DK: The normal cervical spine in infants and children. Radiology 59:712, 1952.
6. Cattel HS and Filtzer DL: Pseudosubluxation and other normal variations in the cervical spine in children. J Bone Joint Surg 47(A):1295, 1965.
7. Swishchuck LE: Anterior displacement of C2 in children: Physiologic or pathologic? Radiology 122:759, 1977.
8. Stauffer ES and Mazur JM: Cervical spine injuries in children. Pediatr Ann 11:502, 1982.
9. Pueschel SM: Atlanto-axial subluxation in Down's syndrome. Lancet i:980, 1983.
10. Hensinger RN and MacEwen GD: Congenital anomalies of the spine. In: Rothman RH and Simeone FA (eds): The Spine. Philadelphia, WB Saunders, 1975, pp. 157–200.
11. Harwood-Nash DC and Fitz CR: Neuroradiology in Infants and Children. St. Louis, CV Mosby, 1976, p. 1003.
12. Tolo VT: Spinal deformity in dwarfs. In: Bradford DS and Hensinger RN (eds): The Pediatric Spine. New York, Thieme Inc, 1985, pp. 338–349.
13. Hawkins RJ, Fielding JO, and Thompson W: Os odontoideum: Congenital or acquired. J Bone Joint Surg 58(A):413, 1976.
14. Fielding JW, Hensinger RN, and Hawkins RJ: Os odontoideum. J Bone Joint Surg 62(A):376, 1980.
15. Schiff DCM and Parke WW: The arterial supply of the odontoid process. J Bone Joint Surg 55(A):1450, 1973.
16. Pang D and Wilberger JE: Traumatic atlanto-occipital dislocation with survival: Case report and review. Neurosurgery 7:503, 1980.
17. Fielding JW and Hawkins RJ: Atlanto-axial rotatory fixation. J Bone Joint Surg 59(A):37, 1977.
18. Duhaime AC, Gennarelli TA, Thibault LE, et al: The shaken baby syndrome: A clinical pathological and biomechanical study. J Neurosurg 66:409–415, 1987.
19. Burke DC: Spinal cord trauma in children. Paraplegia 11:268, 1974.
20. Osenbach RK and Menezes AH: Spinal cord injury without radiographic abnormality in children. Pediatr Neurosci 15:168, 1990.
21. Pang D and Wilberger JE Jr: Spinal cord injury without radiographic abnormalities in children. J Neurosurg 57:114, 1982.
22. Walsh JW, Stevens DB, and Young AB: Traumatic paraplegia in children without contiguous spinal fracture or dislocation. Neurosurgery 12:439, 1983.
23. Hill SA, Miller CA, Kosnik EJ, and Hunt WE: Pediatric neck injuries. J Neurosurg 60:700, 1984.
24. Sherk HH, Nicholson JT, and Chung SMK: Fractures of the odontoid process in young children. J Bone Joint Surg 60(A):921, 1978.
25. Menezes AH, Godersky JC, and Smoker WRK: Spinal cord injury. In: McLaurin RL, Schut L, Venes JL, and Epstein F (eds): Pediatric Neurosurgery. Philadelphia, WB Saunders, 1989, pp. 298–317.
26. Johnson DL: Head injury. In: Eichelberger M (ed): Pediatric Trauma Care. Rockville, MD, Aspen Publishers, 1988, pp. 87–99.
27. Pollack IF, Pang D, and Sclabassi R: Recurrent spinal cord injury without radiographic abnormality in children. J Neursurg 69:177, 1988.

28. Townsend EH Jr and Rowe ML: Mobility of the upper cervical spine in health and disease. Pediatrics 10:567, 1952.
29. Levanthal HR: Birth injuries of the spinal cord. J Pediatr 56:447, 1960.
30. Schneider RC, Cherry G, and Pantek H: The syndrome of acute central cervical spine injury with special references to the mechanism involved in hyperextension injuries of the cervical spine. J Neurosurg 11:546, 1954.
31. Schneider RC: The syndrome of acute anterior spinal cord injury. J Neurosurg 12:95, 1955.
32. Brown-Sequard M: Del la transmission des impressions sensitives par la moelle épinière. Compt Rend Soc Biol 1:192, 1849.
33. Chilton J and Dagi TF: Acute cervical spinal cord injury. Am J Emerg Med 3:340, 1985.
34. Bell HS: Paralysis of both arms from injury of the upper portion of the pyramidal decussation: "Cruciate paralysis." J Neurosurg 33:376, 1970.
35. Bracken MB, Shepard MJ, Collins WF, et al: A randomized, controlled trial of methylprednisolone or naloxone in the treatment of acute spinal cord injury. N Engl J Med 322:1405, 1990.

Neuroexcitatory Syndromes

Michael V. Johnston, M.D.

Hyperexcitability is one of the most common nonspecific signs of brain dysfunction seen in patients in the intensive care unit. Seizures, status epilepticus, and myoclonus occur frequently in individuals with a wide range of brain disorders associated with congenital heart disease, metabolic disorders, hypoxia-ischemia, trauma, infections, and neoplasms. This chapter reviews the major mechanisms that control excitability in the nervous system and describes the phenomena that are observed when the brain is overexcited. The diagnosis and management of individual neuroexcitatory syndromes are then discussed.

BASIC MECHANISMS FOR HYPEREXCITABILITY AND BRAIN INJURY

Control of Excitability in the Central Nervous System

Normal functioning of the brain depends upon controlled electrical firing of networks of thousands of individual neurons. Excessive uncontrolled neuroexcitation requires at least two physiologic abnormalities: excessive excitation of individual neurons and synchronization of large networks of neurons.[1] Many of the details that underlie seizures and other excitatory syndromes remain elusive. However, a major factor controlling neuroexcitability is the pathologic interaction between excitatory and inhibitory neurotransmitters that synapse on individual neurons (Fig. 23–1). In brain structures that are capable of initiating and sustaining seizure activity, predominantly the cerebral cortex and hippocampus, excitatory and inhibitory neurons synapse on principal neurons in a fairly consistent fashion. Excitatory neurons tend to form synapses on the network of dendrites that collects large arrays of excitatory inputs to the neuron. Inhibitory neurons tend to synapse on the cell body or the proximal axon that emerges from the neuron.[2] The arrangement of excitatory inputs on the dendritic arbor tends to summate and amplify excitatory inputs from diverse regions, and the synapses from inhibitory neurons are arranged so as to gate or dampen the final output of summated excitatory activity. The

major excitatory neurotransmitter in the brain appears to be the amino acid L-glutamate, and the primary inhibitory neurotransmitter is γ-aminobutyric acid (GABA). Together glutamate and GABA are used at more than half the synapses in the brain.

The physiologic interactions between glutamate and GABA on a typical principal output neuron in the human cerebral cortex are shown in Figure 23–2. The

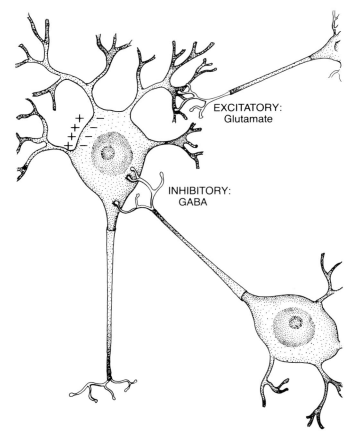

Figure 23–1. Schematic drawing of a principal neuron in the cerebral cortex or hippocampus. Excitatory neuronal axons synapse predominantly on dendrites, but inhibitory neurons synapse primarily on the neuronal cell body or proximal axon. The major excitatory neurotransmitter is glutamate, and the major inhibitory neurotransmitter is GABA. The rows of (+) and (−) indicate a resting membrane potential (−90 mV) that is negative inside. GABA = γ-aminobutyric acid.

218

cerebral cortex and the hippocampus, located in the medial temporal lobe, receive strong excitatory inputs. The neuronal circuits that connect excitatory and inhibitory neurons in the cerebral cortex and hippocampus create a physiologic "checks and balances" system to control neuronal excitability. When receptors for the excitatory amino acid neurotransmitters are stimulated by glutamate, or are stimulated electrically in an experimental setting, a single, large depolarizing spike is produced.[3, 4] However, the excitatory depolarization is usually followed immediately by a smaller hyperpolarizing current caused by synaptic release of the inhibitory transmitter GABA and stimulation of inhibitory receptors. The importance of the counteracting release of GABA is shown in Figure 23–2. If the GABA receptor is blocked by a drug, stimulation of the cerebral cortex leads to a more prolonged excitatory depolarizing current. This prolonged depolarization is one of the components that may lead to initiation of a seizure. The combination of reduced inhibition and excessive stimulation of excitatory neurotransmitter receptors appears to play an important role in the generation of hyperexcitable neurons.

Effects of Neurotransmitters on Neuronal Membranes

The interplay between excitatory and inhibitory neurotransmitters is expressed through alterations in *effector* molecules within neuronal membranes.[5] These effector molecules are either membrane channels that control passage of ions through the membrane or membrane-bound enzymes. Both membrane channels and enzymes control the neuron's membrane potential and intracellular metabolism. They control the opening of ionic channels and the production of intracellular second messengers (Fig. 23–3). Changes in ionic gradients across the neuronal membrane have the most immediate and dramatic effects on brain excitability. The most prominent effect of excitatory neurotransmitters is to open channels that allow sodium and calcium ions to travel into neurons and depolarize them. In contrast, the most prominent effect of the major inhibitory transmitter, GABA, is to increase the entry of chloride ions into neurons. Entry of chloride ions increases the negative membrane potential inside the neuron, compared with the outside, and this hyperpolarization makes the neuron more refractory to excitation (see also Chapter 3).

Effects of Metabolism on Neuronal Excitability

Because of the critical importance of ionic gradients and changes in membrane potential in normal brain function, neurons have developed an extensive metabolic machinery to control them (see Fig. 23–3). A large share of the energy requirements of neurons is expended to power membrane pumps that stabilize ion gradients and membrane potentials. In pathologic situations in

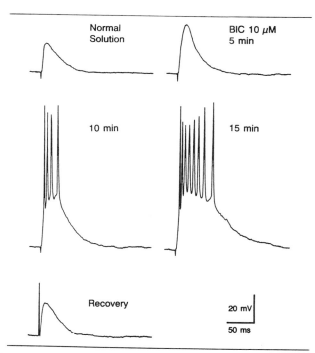

Figure 23–2. An intracellular neuronal recording from neocortex removed during surgery for epilepsy from a 4-year-old child. The response is a postsynaptic potential elicited by electrical stimulation of the neuron. The excitatory postsynaptic potential *(top left)* became larger when a GABA-receptor antagonist bicuculline was added to the incubation bath (*BIC*, 10 μM; *top right* and *middle left*). After 15 minutes of GABA-receptor blockade the excitatory bursting became prolonged into an epileptiform burst *(middle right)*. The bursting was reversible when bicuculline was removed from the bath. (From Wuarin J-P, Kim YI; Cepeda C, et al: Synaptic transmission in human neocortex removed for treatment of intractable epilepsy in children. Ann Neurol 28:507, 1990.)

which stores of energy are reduced, reduced pump activity and membrane depolarization predispose the brain to hyperexcitability and seizures.

Control of calcium ion homeostasis appears to be particularly important for the control of neuronal excitability, as well as the overall health of neurons.[6] Under normal resting conditions, the concentration of calcium is 10,000 times greater in the extracellular fluid than within neurons (Fig. 23–4). Two types of membrane channels allow calcium to enter neurons. Neurotransmitter-operated calcium channels are triggered by glutamate to open in response to stimulation from adjacent excitatory neurons. In contrast, voltage-sensitive calcium channels, resembling those found in the heart, open passively as the neuronal membrane is depolarized. These two types of channels modulate major changes in intracellular calcium levels by controlling the strong tendency of calcium to flow into the neurons. Receptor-operated second messenger systems (e.g., products of phosphoinositide turnover) also help to control intracellular calcium levels. These mechanisms for controlling calcium have a major impact on neuronal excitability and also help to regulate a diverse group of metabolic processes within neurons.

When receptor-operated ion channels allow large amounts of calcium to flow into neurons, raising the

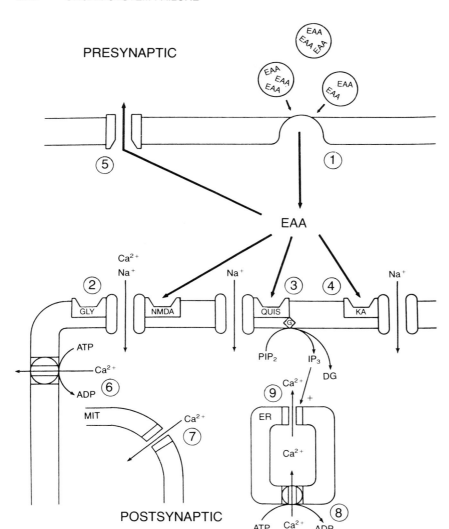

PRESYNAPTIC

EAA

POSTSYNAPTIC

Figure 23–3. This schematic diagram outlines the synaptic components that contribute to excitatory amino acid *(EAA)*-mediated synaptic transmission, second-messenger generation, and calcium homeostasis. *1,* EAAs such as glutamate are released from presynaptic terminals in a calcium-dependent process by presynaptic depolarization. *2–4,* Glutamate in the synaptic cleft can depolarize the postsynaptic membrane by binding to at least three subsets of EAA receptors. Activation of *(2)* the NMDA receptor-channel complex, *(3)* quisqualate (QUIS) receptors, or *(4)* kainate (KA) receptors produces calcium (Ca^{2+}) and sodium (Na^+) entry through receptor-associated ionophores. Furthermore, activation of a subset of quisqualate receptors that are linked to phospholipase C produces phosphoinositol *(PIP₂)* hydrolysis and generation of the second messengers inositol triphosphate *(IP₃)* and diacylglycerol *(DG)*. *5,* The excitatory action of synaptically released EAA is terminated by a presynaptic high-affinity, energy-dependent, transport process. ADP = adenosine diphosphate; ATP = adenosine triphosphate; ER = evoked response; MIT = monoiodotyrosine. (From Johnston MV and McDonald JW: Metabolic and pharmacologic consequences of seizures. *In:* Dodson WE and Pellock JM [eds]: Epilepsy in Childhood. New York, Demos Publications, 1991.)

intracellular calcium concentration, several events are triggered that attempt to restore normal ion gradients. Energy-requiring chemical pumps extrude calcium from the cytoplasm outward across the cell membrane. Calcium is also sequestered by the endoplasmic reticulum and within mitochondria. A variety of cytoplasmic proteins also serve to "buffer" free calcium. Mitochondria are particularly important because they act as high-capacity "sponges" for calcium. Inherited disorders of mitochondria can cause inadequate calcium buffering, as well as a shortage of energy substrates that are needed to power the membrane pumps. Normally functioning energy-dependent mechanisms that restore cellular ionic homeostasis are essential for maintaining normal neuronal excitability.

Relationship Between Hyperexcitability and Brain Injury

The relationship between neuronal hyperexcitability and brain injury is complex.[7, 8] In most situations, self-limited seizures are harmless because of the numerous mechanisms present in the brain to correct rapid alterations in neurotransmitters, ionic gradients, and metabolism. However, several experimental observations in animals suggest that excessive excitation from prolonged seizures can cause brain damage even when the systemic metabolic state is normal (Fig. 23–5). In subhuman primates, seizures produced by kainic acid, an analogue of glutamate, can produce status epilepticus and brain damage resembling the pattern found in humans.[9] This excitotoxin causes damage by two mechanisms: a direct injury at the site of injection and indirect injury that is caused by the spread of seizures from the primary site. In another experimental model, repetitive firing of an excitatory pathway that enters the hippocampus can produce brain damage resembling that seen in humans with status epilepticus.[10] In a third experimental model, damage can be produced by application to the cerebral cortex of a substance that blocks the effects of the inhibitory transmitter GABA.[11] The damage occurs in the thalamus, an area to which the rapidly firing cortical neurons project. These experimental results indicate that prolonged intense neuronal firing may lead to brain damage. Seizures can also enhance brain damage by

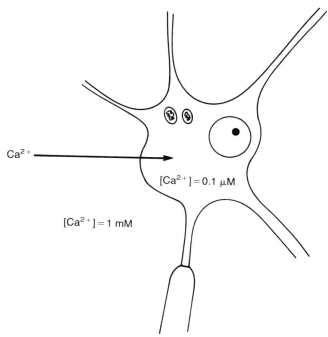

Figure 23–4. Schematic diagram of calcium gradient across the neuronal membrane in resting state. Usually there is a 10,000 times higher concentration of calcium outside the cell than inside the cell.

Ca^{2+}

$[Ca^{2+}] = 0.1\ \mu M$

$[Ca^{2+}] = 1\ mM$

increasing cerebral blood flow and intracranial pressure in certain critically ill patients.

A proposal that links the mechanism of neuronal injury from prolonged seizures to injury from other causes (e.g., hypoxia-ischemia, hypoglycemia, and head injury) is the *calcium overload hypothesis* (Fig. 23–6). This hypothesis states that the final common pathway that causes neuronal injury from these diverse causes is the inability of neurons to withstand flooding by calcium.[7, 12, 13] According to this hypothesis, the differences in the neuropathologic and the characteristic incidence

of seizures among these disorders depend upon the variation in pathogenetic mechanisms that result in the calcium overload. Calcium overload can kill neurons through a variety of mechanisms (Fig. 23–6). The **calcium overload hypothesis** is compatible with the observation that seizures may be a harmless sign in certain situations (e.g., acute head injury, acute hypoxia) or may act synergistically with other disorders to cause further damage.

CLINICAL NEUROEXCITATORY SYNDROMES

Virtually all of the neuroexcitatory syndromes encountered in clinical practice can be classified as seizures or related epileptic phenomena. An exception is the infectious disorder tetanus, which produces segmental hyperexcitability in the brain stem and spinal cord through inactivation of inhibitory neurons by the tetanus toxin. The clinical presentation and pathophysiologic characteristics of this disorder can be understood in terms of the model of inhibitory and excitatory neuronal interactions presented earlier. The clinical presentation and management of the disorder is considered elsewhere (see Chapters 24, 51, and 72).

Classification of Seizures

A seizure is the clinical manifestation of a sudden, massive, and synchronized electrical discharge of central nervous system (CNS) neurons.[1] Seizures may occur as isolated manifestations of nervous system dysfunction or as part of a chronic epileptic disorder in which the recurrence of seizures is predictable. Seizures are usually self-limited, probably because the brain's compensatory inhibitory mechanisms act to restore normal electrical function. Seizures that last longer than 30 minutes are

Figure 23–5. This diagram illustrates the possible role of EAA neurotoxicity in acute brain injury. EAA neurotoxicity may be a common mechanism in neuronal injury resulting from sustained seizures, hypoxia-ischemia, and physical brain trauma. All these conditions tend to elevate the extracellular concentration of EAAs via different mechanisms. EAA = excitatory amino acid. (From McDonald JW and Johnston MV: Physiological and pathophysiological roles of excitatory amino acids during central nervous system development. Brain Res Rev 15:41, 1990. Modified from Choi DW: Glutamate neurotoxicity and diseases of the nervous system. Neuron 1:623, 1988.)

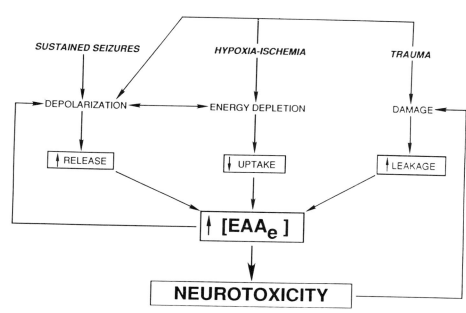

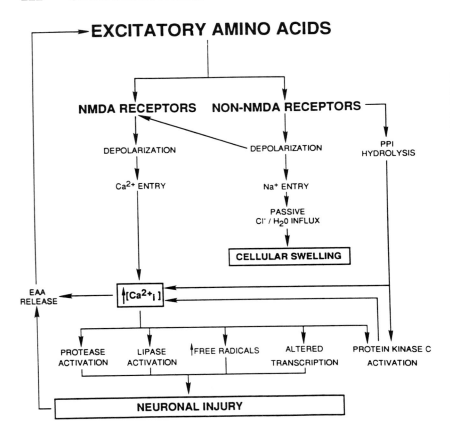

EXCITATORY AMINO ACIDS

Figure 23–6. This schematic diagram summarizes some of the mechanisms that may contribute to EAA neurotoxicity. In vitro experiments suggest that EAA neurotoxicity may have two components. The first component, mediated by excessive activation of non-NMDA receptors, is characterized by influx of Na^+ followed by passive influx of Cl^- and H_2O, which may produce osmotic neuronal swelling. These acute events occur within hours of exposure to EAA agonists. The second, more prominent component is produced by overactivation of NMDA receptors, which leads to an intracellular CA^{2+} that may trigger a biochemical cascade of events that lead to neuronal injury and death. Furthermore, activation of a subset of non-NMDA receptors coupled to polyphosphoinositide *(PPI)* hydrolysis may also elevate intracellular CA^{2+}. EAAs released from synaptic terminals would further propagate neuronal injury. NMDA = *n*-methyl-D-aspartate; EEA = excitatory amino acid. (From McDonald JW and Johnston MV: Physiological and pathophysiological roles of excitatory amino acids during central nervous system development. Brain Res Rev 15:41, 1990. Modified from Choi DW: Glutamate neurotoxicity and diseases of the nervous system. Neuron 1:623, 1988.)

generally considered to have crossed over into the condition known as status epilepticus (see further on). Another condition, myoclonus, is closely related to motor seizures but is distinctive. Myoclonus is composed of very brief shock-like jerks of a muscle or group of muscles. It is different from other seizure manifestations because the shock-like jerks occur as relatively isolated or widely spaced events. In contrast to the massive discharges of neurons in the brain that produce seizures, myoclonus can originate at any level in the nervous system, such as the spinal cord, brain stem, or an isolated part of the cerebral cortex. Myoclonus is particularly likely to occur in a nervous system injured by hypoxia-ischemia or other metabolic disorders encountered in the pediatric intensive care unit. Myoclonus also occurs as part of certain genetic or sporadic epileptic syndromes.

Clinical presentations of neuroexcitatory phenomena are often confusing, and it has been useful in practice to assign two somewhat separate classifications of these disorders. The first classification, the International Classification of epileptic seizures is useful for organizing observations made from patients and for creating a differential diagnosis[14] (Table 23–1). A second classification of epileptic syndromes is also useful diagnostically and is helpful for thinking about the pathophysiology of seizures.

International Classification of Seizures

The International Classification of seizures was based on a worldwide consensus, though there are continuing efforts to revise it. The terms it uses to describe seizures are the ones currently accepted by most neurologists. This classification separates seizures into two major categories: partial and generalized seizures. Partial sei-

Table 23–1. INTERNATIONAL CLASSIFICATION OF EPILEPTIC SEIZURES*

Partial (Focal, Local) Seizures
A. Simple partial seizures
  1. With motor signs
  2. With somatosensory or special sensory symptoms
  3. With autonomic symptoms or signs
  4. With psychic symptoms
B. Complex partial seizures
  1. Simple partial onset followed by impairment of consciousness
  2. With impairment of consciousness at onset
C. Partial seizures evolving to secondarily generalized seizures
  1. Simple partial seizures evolving to generalized seizures
  2. Complex partial seizures evolving to generalized seizures
  3. Simple partial seizures evolving to complex partial seizures evolving to generalized seizures

Generalized Seizures (Convulsive or Nonconvulsive)
A. Absence seizures
  1. Typical absences
  2. Atypical absences
B. Myoclonic seizures
C. Clonic seizures
D. Tonic seizures
E. Tonic-clonic seizures
F. Atonic seizures (astatic seizures)

Unclassified epileptic seizures

*From Commission on Classification and Terminology of the International League Against Epilepsy: Proposal for revised clinical and electroencephalographic classification of epileptic seizures. Epilepsia 22:489, 1981.

Table 23–2. PHARMACOKINETIC PROPERTIES OF ANTICONVULSANT DRUGS*

Drug Use	Daily Dosage (mg/kg)	Rx Plasma Conc (μg/ml)	Plasma half-life (hr)	Peak Time (hr)	Time to Steady State (days)	Protein bound (%)
Phenytoin GTCS,† CPS,‡ SPS§	4–7	10–20	14 ± 12	4–8	5–10	90
Carbamazepine GTCS, CPS, SPS	10–20	4–12	12 ± 3	2–6	2–4	80
Sodium valproate Absence, GTCS, CPS, MCS ‖	20–60	50–100	12 ± 6	1–4	2–4	90
Primidone GTCS, CPS, SPS	10–15	5–15	12 ± 6	2–4	4–7	0–20
Phenobarbital GTCS, CPS, SPS	2–3	10–30	96 ± 12	4–8	14–21	40–50
Clonazepam Absence, MCS, CPS, SPS	0.1–0.2	0.02–0.08	20 ± 50	1–4	6	87
Ethosuximide Absence	20–60	40–100	30 ± 6	1–4	5–8	0

*From Macdonald RL: Antiepileptic drug therapy. *In*: Johnston MV, Macdonald RL, and Young AB (eds): Principles of Drug Therapy in Neurology. Philadelphia, FA Davis, 1992.
†GTCS = generalized tonic-clonic seizures.
‡CPS = complex partial seizures.
§SPS = simple partial seizures.
‖ MCS = myoclonic seizures.

zures, which begin or remain in one part of the brain, can be expressed as either *simple partial* seizures if their manifestation is relatively focal and discrete or *complex partial* if they are expressed as complex states of impaired consciousness. A third category of *partial seizures with secondary generalization,* is related to the spread of seizures from one part of the brain to another. In contrast to partial seizures, generalized seizures involve virtually all parts of the brain simultaneously. Generalized seizures may be either convulsive, such as the common clonic or tonic-clonic motor seizures, or nonconvulsive and characterized by staring and unresponsiveness with few motor movements.

In most cases, observation is sufficient to classify seizure types according to the International Classification. At times, however, electrical monitoring of seizures using electroencephalography is needed to classify them correctly. For example, absence seizures, a form of generalized epilepsy, may produce staring episodes that superficially resemble the episodes of unconsciousness produced by complex partial seizures. Electrical monitoring during the seizure would, most likely, distinguish between these two types. Monitoring during a generalized absence seizure would most likely show generalized three/second spike and wave activity, whereas monitoring during a partial complex seizure would most likely show more localized, less frequent spike activity over the temporal or frontal region.

Clinical classification of seizure types is useful for making a determination about the site of origin in the brain and the cause of the seizure. Although generalized metabolic or toxic brain disorders can produce all types of seizures, partial seizures are more likely to indicate a focal process. For example, new onset of a simple partial seizure, a partial seizure with secondary generalization, or a complex partial seizure in a confused febrile patient

admitted to the intensive care unit would be strong evidence for a focal infectious process such as a focal encephalitis or abscess. The electroencephalogram (EEG) and neuroradiologic imaging studies (computed tomography and magnetic resonance imaging) are important tools for supplementing careful clinical observations in critical care patients.

The International Classification of seizures is also useful for planning drug therapy. The most widely used anticonvulsants, such as phenytoin, phenobarbital, and carbamazepine, are useful for all kinds of partial seizures and generalized motor or convulsive seizures but not for absence seizures[15, 16] (Table 23–2). Prescription of one of these major anticonvulsants for absence seizures often causes them to worsen. In contrast, the drug ethosuximide is useful for generalized absence seizures but not for other generalized or partial seizures. Valproic acid has the widest spectrum of all anticonvulsant drugs. It is useful for both partial seizures and all kinds of generalized seizures. Carbamazepine is favored by many clinicians for partial complex seizures and other types of partial seizures, but phenytoin may be equally effective. Barbiturate anticonvulsants such as phenobarbital are effective for all types of partial and convulsive generalized seizures and are useful drugs for refractory seizures. However, their use in patients with chronic epilepsy is diminishing because of the cognitive side effects.

Classification of Neonatal Seizures

The neonatal period and infancy are probably the most seizure-prone periods of life. Experience with neonates indicates that a special classification is needed to encompass the variety of neuroexcitatory events that are observed.[17] Recently, the classification of these events has been improved by the use of simultaneous video and EEG observation of infants (Table 23–3). These observations distinguished seizure-like motor events that are correlated with EEG activity from those that are not. These observations suggest that some of the seizure-like events observed in young infants may not have an epileptic origin. In particular, the generalized tonic extensor movements observed in infants after an hypoxic-ischemic insult may reflect disinhibition of lower brain stem centers rather than an epileptic discharge. This suggests that these infants could be spared vigorous anticonvulsant treatment if there is no EEG confirmation of seizures. Conversely, certain behavioral patterns appear to be closely associated with epileptic EEG activity despite relatively subtle behavioral changes. These patterns include focal clonic seizures, myoclonic jerks, focal tonic seizures, and eye deviation. These events probably should be treated with anticonvulsant medication.

Epileptic Syndromes Commonly Encountered in the Intensive Care Unit

A number of relatively specific combinations of seizures and patient characteristics compose "syndromes"

Table 23–3. CLASSIFICATION OF CLINICAL NEONATAL SEIZURES AND RELATIONSHIP TO EEG SEIZURE DISCHARGES*

Seizures with Close Association to EEG Seizure Discharges
A. Focal clonic
  1. Unifocal
  2. Multifocal
    a. Alternating
    b. Migrating
  3. Hemiconvulsive
  4. Axial
B. Myoclonic
  1. Generalized
  2. Focal
C. Focal tonic
  1. Asymmetric truncal
  2. Eye deviation
D. Apnea

Seizures with an Inconsistent or No Relationship to EEG Seizure Discharges
A. Motor automatisms
  1. Oral-buccal-lingual movements
  2. Ocular signs
  3. Progression movements
    a. Pedaling
    b. Stepping
    c. Rotary arm movements
  4. Complex purposeless movements
B. Generalized tonic
  1. Extensor
  2. Flexor
  3. Mixed extensor-flexor
C. Myoclonic
  1. Generalized
  2. Focal
  3. Fragmentary

Infantile Spasms

EEG Seizures without Clinical Seizures

*From Mizrahi EM and Kellaway P: Characterization and classification of neonatal seizures. Neurology 37:1837, 1987.

Table 23–4. SYNDROMES ASSOCIATED WITH SEIZURES AND EPILEPSY IN CHILDREN*

Secondary or Symptomatic Syndromes
Febrile convulsions
Reactive seizures (e.g., breath-holding)
Metabolic and systemic disorders (see Table 23–6)
Drugs and toxins (see Table 23–7)
Hypoxic-ischemic encephalopathy
Traumatic brain injury
Brain malformations
Temporal lobe epilepsy
Infantile spasms
Lennox-Gastaut syndrome
Rasmussen's syndrome

Primary or Idiopathic syndromes
Benign neonatal convulsions
Benign rolandic epilepsy
Childhood and juvenile absence epilepsy (petit mal)
Generalized tonic-clonic seizures
Juvenile myoclonic epilepsy
Severe and benign myoclonic epilepsy of infancy
Myoclonic astatic epilepsy

*Data from Engel J: Seizures and Epilepsy. Philadelphia, FA Davis, 1989.

that are seen fairly commonly in critical care pediatric practice[1] (Table 23–4). In neurologic practice, an attempt has been made to distinguish primary or idiopathic epileptic syndromes and secondary or symptomatic syndromes.

The secondary or symptomatic syndromes are the ones most commonly encountered in the intensive care unit. Seizures or status epilepticus from high fever, traumatic brain injury, meningitis and other infections, hypoxic-ischemic encephalopathy, drug ingestion, and metabolic and systemic disorders are very common. Seizures from rare disorders such as the Lennox-Gastaut syndrome and chronic temporal lobe epilepsy are rarer but may be seen more frequently at specialized centers that care for these patients.

Febrile Convulsions and Reactive Seizures

Febrile convulsions and reactive seizures represent an extreme of normal CNS excitability in response to physiologic stress, such as a high fever, breath-holding, or a brief hypoxic episode. As shown in Table 23–5, the peak age for febrile convulsions is between 18 and 22

Table 23–5. FEBRILE CONVULSIONS

Characteristics of Complex Febrile Convulsions
Duration longer than 15 minutes
Partial features or focal seizures
Multiple seizures in 1 day
Family history of nonfebrile seizures
Neurologic deficits or developmental delay

Characteristics of Benign or Simple Febrile Convulsions
Age—3 months to 5 years (peak 18–22 months)
Generalized tonic-clonic seizures
Duration less than 15 minutes
Occurs on first day of illness with high fever
Family history of febrile convulsions common

months, and they are usually restricted to children between the ages of 3 months and 5 years.[1] Febrile seizures may occur in approximately 6% of normal infants. Large follow-up studies indicate that febrile convulsions with certain characteristics are benign.[18] These so-called simple febrile convulsions appear to have no impact on later CNS development. The characteristics of simple febrile convulsions are shown in Table 23–5. In contrast to simple febrile convulsions, complex febrile convulsions may indicate patients with a higher risk for experiencing epilepsy at a later time. Even in this group, however, the risk of developing nonfebrile seizures at a later time is only approximately 13%.

In a critical care setting, any seizure is cause for concern, and a detailed assessment should be made of the patient's condition to determine the cause. If the patient is febrile, a lumbar puncture is essential to detect meningitis. A radiologic imaging study such as a computed tomographic scan of the brain may be useful if there is a suspicion of a focal pathologic condition such as an abcess or hemorrhage or evidence of increased intracranial pressure.

If the diagnostic work-up suggests that the seizure is "febrile" or reactive, the plan of therapy should take into account its generally benign nature. Prolonged febrile convulsions can be treated effectively with diazepam, 0.3 mg/kg, or phenobarbital, 10 mg/kg, intramuscularly or intravenously. This dose may be repeated in 10 to 15 minutes if necessary. If higher doses are needed, the protocol for status epilepticus (see further on) can be used. Prophylactic treatment with phenobarbital is not recommended for most children with febrile convulsions, though patients with very prolonged or otherwise complex febrile convulsions may be treated.[19] Phenobarbital, 3 to 5 mg/kg/day, to achieve a serum drug level of greater than 15 µg/ml is usually effective, but phenytoin is not. Primidone and valproic acid may also be effective. Prophylactic treatment with phenobarbital is being used less frequently because of potential effects on learning and memory and also because parents often do not comply with recommendations for long-term treatment. Use of rectal or oral diazepam is being investigated for prevention of febrile seizures.[20]

Metabolic and Systemic Disorders

A variety of temporary and chronic systemic disorders and diseases may cause seizures in critically ill children (Table 23–6). Patients whose seizures occur in the intensive care unit or those who have seizures severe enough to prompt admission to the intensive care unit should be screened carefully for acute disorders of glucose, water and electrolyte metabolism, and infections. Patients cared for in the intensive care unit may also have a variety of rarer disorders that should be considered in the differential diagnosis. Among infants with prolonged seizures, aminoacidopathies, organic acidurias, urea cycle defects, and pyridoxine deficiency should be considered.[21, 22] Several rare genetic abnormalities of mitochondria may produce seizures and

Table 23–6. SYSTEMIC DISORDERS THAT CAUSE SEIZURES

Electrolyte disturbances	*Circulatory-cardiovascular disorders*
Water intoxication	Congenital heart disease
Hyponatremia	Hypoxic-ischemic
Hypocalcemia	encephalopathy
Hypomagnesemia	Hypertensive encephalopathy
Metabolic-endocrine disorders	Hypertension
Hypoglycemia	Stroke
Uremia	Subarachnoid hemorrhage
Liver failure	Venous sinus thrombosis
Adrenoleukodystrophy	*Hematologic disorders*
Aminoacidopathies,	Sickle cell anemia
hyperglycinemia	Henoch-Schönlein and
Homocystinuria	thrombotic
Ceroid lipofuscinosis	thrombocytopenic purpura
Gaucher disease	*Infections*
Leigh disease	Viral (e.g., encephalitis)
Pyridoxine deficiency	Rickettsia
Organic acidurias	Bacterial (meningitis, abcess,
Zellweger disease	empyema)
Reye syndrome	Spirochetal
Mitochondrial disorders	Fungal
	Toxoplasmosis
	Cysticercosis, *Echinococcus*
	Genetic-neurocutaneous disorders
	Tuberous sclerosis
	Sturge-Weber syndrome
	Incontinentia pigmenti

stroke in infants. One disorder referred to as mitochondrial encephalopathy and stroke-like episodes may produce seizures through combinations of strokes and energy failure.[23] Another disorder called medium chain acyl-CoA-dehydrogense deficiency may produce seizures and an illness that resembles Reye's syndrome[24] (see Chapter 60). Several genetic neurocutaneous disorders should also be considered, especially in young infants. Tuberous sclerosis, Zellweger's syndrome, and other inherited disorders of peroxisomes may produce refractory seizures in infants.[21, 25] Seizures are also seen in patients with a variety of unusual chronic infectious disorders. Parasites are a common cause of seizures in certain parts of the United States and in other countries.[26]

Hypoxic-Ischemic Disorders and Stroke

Seizures are a virtually constant sign of hypoxic-ischemic encephalopathy that is severe enough to damage the brain. This is especially true in infants and younger children.[27] Seizures also occur frequently with other vascular disorders, such as stroke associated with congenital heart disease, venous sinus thrombosis, sickle cell cerebrovascular disease, and intracranial hemorrhage. As described earlier, seizures are first and foremost a sign of brain dysfunction produced by the metabolic, membranous, and structural disorders triggered by hypoxia-ischemia. However, continued intense seizure activity can worsen metabolic abnormalities that may enhance injury.

A variety of seizure types are encountered in patients

with hypoxic-ischemic encephalopathy. Frequently these seizures are intermixed with focal or multifocal myoclonic jerks. The metabolic consequences of focal or segmental myoclonus are probably less serious than those for generalized motor seizures. Although seizures or myoclonus occurring in the context of hypoxia-ischemia are often refractory to treatment, it seems worthwhile to attempt to treat them as outlined further on for status epilepticus. Myoclonic jerks often respond better to benzodiazepines, such as clonazepam, than to other anticonvulsants (see Table 23–2). Focal myoclonus coming from the spinal cord may continue even when there is no cerebral function.

Drugs and Toxins

Various drugs, usually in toxic doses, produce seizures or status epilepticus[28] (Table 23–7). Among commonly ingested toxins, anticholinergic organophosphates are a potent cause of seizures. Increasingly, accidental cocaine ingestion is a cause of severe seizures in children.[29] Seizures related to ingestion of methylxanthine drugs prescribed for asthma and tricyclic antidepressants are also seen with some frequency in patients hospitalized in the critical care unit.

Traumatic Brain Injury

Severe head injury is an important cause of seizures in the first week after injury and may also cause epilepsy that is delayed for many months. It has been estimated that approximately 5% of children with severe head injury experience seizures within the first week after injury, though the incidence increases with the severity of the trauma.[30] If there is an open brain injury, the incidence may rise to 25%. Seizures from head injury probably originate from a combination of primary traumatic injury and secondary hypoxic-ischemic injury.

Leakage of blood into the brain substance may also play a role in the development of post-traumatic epilepsy.

Antiepileptic drugs are commonly prescribed in the immediate period following injury to prevent the onset of seizures, and some clinicians continue them for months later. Recent studies suggest that phenytoin loading prevents seizures in the early period following trauma but does not prevent the onset of delayed epilepsy. One study examined a large group of adults with severe head injury (prolonged unconsciousness or intracranial bleeding, or both) and found that phenytoin loading exerted a beneficial effect by reducing seizures within the first week after severe head injury from 14.2% in patients assigned to placebo to 3.6% in patients assigned to phenytoin.[31] However, the incidence of late seizures over 2 years was 21.5% in the phenytoin group and 15.7% in the placebo group. Although this evidence suggests that early phenytoin loading may be useful in preventing early seizures, it is not clear whether preventing the early seizures has any impact on the outcome of injury. In patients with severe head injuries and with increased intracranial pressure, as well as rare secondary syndromes, prevention of seizures would have potential benefit.

Primary or Idiopathic Epileptic Syndromes

Several important idiopathic epilepsy syndromes that may come to the attention of the physician in the intensive care unit have been defined over the last few years[1] (see Table 23–4). They are not common causes for admission to most intensive care units, but they are occasionally encountered and it is important to understand them in the context of neuroexcitatory phenomena or syndromes. Benign familial neonatal convulsions are important to recognize because they have a strong genetic component and appear to be harmless.[32] Rec-

Table 23–7. DRUGS REPORTED TO CAUSE CONVULSIONS*

Aqueous iodinated contrast agents	Mefenamic acid
Anticholinesterase agents (organophosphates, physostigmine)	Methylxanthines
Antihistamines	Metronidazol
Antidepressants	Misonidazole
Antipsychotics	Nalidixic acid
Baclofen	Narcotic analgesics (fentanyl, meperidine, pentazocine, propoxyphene)
β-Blockers (propranolol, oxprenolol)	
Camphor	Oxytocin (secondary to water intoxication)
Chlorambucil	Penicillins
Cocaine	Phencyclidine
Cycloserine	Phenytoin
Cyclosporin A	Prednisone (with hypocalcemia)
Ergonovine	Sympathomimetics (amphetamines, ephedrine, phenylpropanolamine, terbutaline)
Folic acid	
General anesthetics (ketamine, halothane, althesin, enflurane, propanidid)	Tricyclic antidepressants
	Vitamin K oxide
Hyperbaric oxygen	
Hypoglycemic agents	
Hypo-osmolar parenteral solutions	
Isoniazid	
Local anesthetics (bupivacaine, lidocaine, procaine, etidocaine)	

*From Messing RO, Closson RG, and Simon RP: Drug-induced seizures: A 10-year experience. Neurology 34:1582, 1984.

ognition of this entity in a family may reduce the apprehension and extensive work-up that is often required to define neonatal seizures in other patients. The disorder is also important because it indicates that there is a strong genetic component for certain types of epilepsy. Several other genetic types of epilepsy have been defined recently. They include childhood and juvenile absence epilepsy, certain types of generalized tonic-clonic seizures, and several myoclonic syndromes.[1] In several of the myoclonic syndromes, generalized tonic-clonic seizures occur independently of myoclonus. Another important disorder is benign rolandic epilepsy. This disorder typically occurs in school-aged children and begins with focal movements that involve the tongue and the mouth and may involve drooling. The EEG typically shows spikes over the midsylvian region. The seizures may generalize secondarily into tonic-clonic seizures. The importance of recognizing them is that they generally have a good prognosis and typically disappear after puberty.

When complications develop or epilepsy surgery is performed, rare "secondary" syndromes are occasionally encountered in the intensive care unit and include the Lennox-Gastaut syndrome and Rasmussen syndrome.[1] Both of these disorders produce refractory seizure disorders with multiple seizure types. The Lennox-Gastaut syndrome is usually associated with mental retardation and a slow (less than three/second) spike and wave pattern on the EEG. It may occur in children with a variety of pre-existing conditions, such as infantile spasms, hypoxic brain injury, and tuberous sclerosis. Rasmussen syndrome is a form of refractory partial motor epilepsy. Resection of the seizure focus in the brain shows a chronic inflammatory infiltrate. Rasmussen syndrome may present as epilepsia partialis continua, or focal continuous jerking of one part of the body lasting months or years.

Status Epilepticus

Status epilepticus, or a seizure lasting longer than 30 minutes, is an extremely serious and potentially lethal disorder. Status epilepticus may be idiopathic or may be initiated by any of the primary or secondary epileptic syndromes already described. Several forms of status epilepticus have been identified[33] (Table 23–8). Convulsive, major motor, generalized status epilepticus is probably the most dangerous. However, the impact of partial status epilepticus and generalized absence status epilepticus has not been well defined. A number of systemic disorders may complicate major motor status epilepticus[1] (Table 23–9). In the presence of increased intracranial pressure, even nonconvulsive status epilepticus may be dangerous.

Although modern intensive care has reduced the morbidity and mortality from status epilepticus in children, one study of 193 children with this condition demonstrated that neurologic sequelae occurred in 29% of infants younger than 1 year of age, in 11% of children 1 to 3 years of age, and in 6% of children older than 3 years of age.[34] Of the 125 children with no prior history of unprovoked seizures, 30% had subsequent unprovoked seizures. Another study found that the occurrence of febrile status epilepticus in a neurologically impaired child is a risk factor for subsequent febrile, as well as afebrile, seizures.[35] These clinical studies indicate that status epilepticus is an important risk factor for the development of subsequent neurologic disability in patients who are critically ill. However, the incidence of later neurologic sequelae appeared to correlate better with the severity of the underlying brain disorder than with the severity of the status epilepticus. It is difficult to determine how much of the subsequent brain injury is contributed by excessive neuronal excitability alone as opposed to direct effects of the underlying condition. It is possible that an underlying condition, such as encephalitis, may be the predominant cause of injury. Conversely, these studies could also be interpreted to mean that status epilepticus is more damaging in the presence of an underlying brain disorder. This interpretation is supported by the information presented earlier about the potential synergism of mechanisms that enhance neuronal excitability and produce brain injury.[36–38] Status epilepticus may also produce dangerous increases in intracranial pressure in critically ill patients whose intracranial pressure is already elevated. Therefore, this disorder should be regarded as a serious medical emergency.

Therapy for status epilepticus should attempt to terminate the seizure while avoiding potentially serious morbidity for the patient.[39] Adverse effects of parenteral anticonvulsant treatment can be minimized in the critical care unit, because of the respiratory support and cardiovascular monitoring that is readily at hand. The clinical

Table 23–8. CLASSIFICATION OF STATUS EPILEPTICUS*

Generalized status epilepticus
  Convulsive
  Absence

Partial status epilepticus
  Simple partial ("epilepsia partialis continua"
    when prolonged over days to months)
  Complex partial

*Data from Gaustaut H: Classification of status epilepticus. Adv Neurol 34:15, 1983.

Table 23–9. SYSTEMIC COMPLICATIONS OF MAJOR MOTOR STATUS EPILEPTICUS

Respiratory failure
Lactic acidosis
Hyperkalemia
Hypoglycemia
Hypertension
Cardiovascular collapse
Cardiac arrhythmias
Congestive heart failure
Pulmonary edema
Aspiration pneumonia
Acute tubular necrosis and myoglobinuria
  secondary to rhabdomyolysis
Hyperuricemia
Fever
Dehydration

Table 23-10. PROTOCOL FOR TREATMENT OF STATUS EPILEPTICUS IN CHILDREN

Time	Procedure
0-5 min	Assessment
	Airway, breathing management
	Blood withdrawal: drug levels, glucose level, toxic screen, BUN,* electrolytes
5-10 min	Start IV† infusion
	Administer: Glucose (25%, 1 ml/kg)
10-30 min	Lorazepam: 0.03-0.05 mg/kg/dose IV in repeated doses every 5-10 min (usual maximum three doses) OR
	Diazepam: 0.2-0.5 mg/kg IV in repeated doses every 5-10 min (usual maximum three doses)
	Phenytoin: 20 mg/kg IV in <5 mg/ml solution in normal saline, rate of <1 mg/kg/min with cardiac and blood pressure monitoring
30-60 min	If seizures persist: Phenobarbital
	15-25 mg/kg IV at <30 mg/min, may repeat with secure airway
	Aim for maximum blood level of 50 μg/ml (however, higher levels have been used safely in children)[44]
>1 hr	Consider pentobarbital coma, general anesthesia
	Also consider pyridoxine, 100 mg IV with EEG‡ monitoring

*BUN = blood urea nitrogen.
†IV = intravenous.
‡EEG = electroencephalogram.

research data reviewed earlier suggest that status epilepticus in children without underlying brain disorders has a relatively good prognosis. However, in individual clinical situations, especially in the intensive care unit, it may be impossible to distinguish immediately between patients with and those without an underlying brain disorder. Therefore, a similar protocol is suggested for all patients with status epilepticus. Neuromuscular paralysis is not adequate therapy for status epilepticus because prolonged seizures can damage the brain even without motor convulsions. Patients given paralyzing drugs should be monitored carefully to detect status epilepticus.

The standard drugs used to treat status epilepticus are combinations of benzodiazepines, phenytoin, and barbiturates (Table 23-10). Most standard protocols recommend the use of general anesthesia or barbiturate coma for status epilepticus lasting longer that 1 hour.[39-42] The side effects of this protocol include respiratory and cardiovascular depression at very high doses of barbiturates (Table 23-11). Benzodiazepines have also been administered successfully by the rectal route for status epilepticus.[39, 43] Several new parenteral preparations of these and other drugs are under development.

Table 23-11. PROTOCOL FOR PENTOBARBITAL COMA IN REFRACTORY STATUS EPILEPTICUS

Preparation:	Intubate and mechanically ventilate in intensive care unit, cardiovascular and EEG* monitoring
Loading dose:	5-8 mg/kg IV† bolus supplement with 25-50 mg every 5 minutes to produce EEG burst suppression or nearly flat for 2 to 4 hr
	Taper and observe for seizures and repeat induction if seizures reemerge
Maintenance:	1-6 mg/kg/hr, as needed to maintain burst suppression pattern
Plasma therapeutic concentrations:	25-50 μg/ml

*EEG = electroencephalogram.
†IV = intravenous.

The anticonvulsants that are used to treat status epilepticus appear to work by a combination of stabilizing the membrane potential and increasing the inhibition produced by GABAergic neurons.[15] At present, there are no clinically available drugs that work primarily by diminishing excitatory neurotransmission.

SUMMARY AND CONCLUSION

Neuroexcitatory disorders encountered in the intensive care unit are produced by a variety of conditions. The most common syndromes are prolonged seizures and status epilepticus produced by a variety of brain disorders. Seizures are produced by a sudden massive discharge of neurons in the brain, whereas more discrete neuronal firing anywhere in the central nervous system may produce myoclonus. Excessive neuroexcitation is caused by combinations of reduced inhibition and uncontrolled or excessive excitation in the nervous system. The most prominent mechanisms that control excitability are the synaptic interactions between excitatory and inhibitory neurons to control neuronal membrane potential. The most serious neuroexcitatory disorder, status epilepticus, has a good prognosis in most children if adequate treatment is provided. The morbidity from status epilepticus appears to relate to the severity of the underlying brain disorder that produces it. Nevertheless, status epilepticus itself is capable of damaging the brain by a direct neuroexcitatory mechanism, and vigorous therapy is warranted especially in the setting of primary brain disorder such as encephalitis or hypoxia-ischemia.

REFERENCES

1. Engel J: Seizures and Epilepsy. Philadelphia, FA Davis, 1989.
2. Cooper JR, Bloom FE, and Roth RN: The Biochemical Basis of Neuropharmacology, 2nd ed. New York, Macmillan, 1980.
3. Cotman CW and Iverson LL: Excitatory amino acids in the brain—focus on NMDA receptors. Trends Neurosci 10:263, 1987.
4. Wuarin J-P, Kim YI, Cepeda C, et al: Synaptic transmission in human neocortex removed for treatment of intractable epilepsy in children. Ann Neurol 28:503, 1990.

5. McDonald JW and Johnston MV: Physiological and pathophysiological roles of excitatory amino acids during central nervous system development. Brain Res Rev 15:41, 1990.
6. Siesjo BK: Cell damage in the brain: A speculative synthesis. J Cereb Blood Flow Metab 1:155, 1981.
7. Johnston MV and McDonald JW: Metabolic and pharmacologic consequences of seizures. In: Dodson WE and Pellock JM (eds): Epilepsy in Childhood. New York, Demos Publications, 1991.
8. Choi DW: Glutamate neurotoxicity and diseases of the nervous system. Neuron 1:623, 1988.
9. Meldrum BS and Brierly JB: Prolonged epileptic seizures in primates. Ischemic cell change and its relationship to ictal physiological events. Arch Neurol 28:10, 1973.
10. Sloviter RS: Epileptic brain damage in rats induced by sustained electrical stimulation of perforant cells. I. Acute electrophysiological and light microscope studies. Brain Res Bull 10:675, 1983.
11. Collins RC and Olney JW: Focal cortical seizures cause distant thalamic lesions. Science 218:177, 1982.
12. Rothman SV and Olney JW: Glutamate and pathophysiology of hypoxic-ischemic brain damage. Ann Neurol 19:105, 1986.
13. Auer RN and Siesjo BK: Biological differences between ischemia, hypoglycemia and epilepsy. Ann Neurol 24:699, 1988.
14. Commission on Classification and Terminology of the International League Against Epilepsy: Proposal for revised clinical and electroencephalographic classification of epileptic seizures. Epilepsia 22:489, 1981.
15. Macdonald RL: Antiepileptic drug therapy. In: Johnston MV, Macdonald RL, and Young AB (eds): Principles of Drug Therapy in Neurology. Philadelphia, FA Davis, 1992.
16. Woodbury SM, Penry JK, and Pippenger CE: Anticonvulsant Drugs, 2nd ed. New York, Raven Press, 1982.
17. Mizrahi EM and Kellaway P: Characterization and classification of neonatal seizures. Neurology 37:1837, 1987.
18. Nelson KB and Ellenberg JH: Prognosis in children with febrile seizures. Pediatrics 61:720, 1978.
19. Nelson, KB and Ellenberg JH (eds): Febrile Seizures. New York, Raven Press, 1981.
20. Knudsen FU: Frequent febrile episodes and recurrent febrile convulsions. Acta Neurol Scand 78:414, 1988.
21. Adams RD and Lyon G: Neurology of Hereditary Metabolic Diseases in Children. New York, Hemisphere, 1982.
22. McDonald JW and Johnston MV: Non-ketotic hyperglycinemia: Possible pathophysiological role of NMDA type excitatory amino acid receptors. Ann Neurol 27:449, 1990.
23. DiMauro S, Bonilla E, Zeviani M, et al: Mitochondrial myopathies. Ann Neurol 17:521, 1985.
24. Vianey-Liaud C, Divry P, Gregersen N, et al: The inborn errors of mitochondrial fatty acid oxidation. J Inher Metab Dis 10 (Suppl 1):159, 1987.
25. Lazarow PB and Moser HW: Disorders of peroxisome biogenesis. In: Scriber CR, Beaudet AL, Sly WS, et al (eds): The Metabolic Bases of Inherited Disease, 6th ed. New York, McGraw-Hill, 1989.
26. Mitchell WG and Crawford TO: Seizures in children with intraparenchymal cerebral cysticercosis. Epilepsia 28:627, 1987.
27. Johnston MV: Intracranial hemorrhage, periventricular leukomalacia and hypoxicischemic encephalopathy in the neonate. In: Johnson RT (ed): Current Therapy In Neurologic Disease—3. Philadelphia, BC Decker, 1990.
28. Messing RO, Closson RG, and Simon RP: Drug-induced seizures: A 10-year experience. Neurology 34:1582, 1984.
29. Rivkin M and Gilmore HE: Generalized seizures in an infant due to environmentally acquired cocaine. Pediatrics 84:1100, 1989.
30. Rosman NP and Oppenheimer EY: Post-traumatic epilepsy. Pediatr Rev 3:221, 1982.
31. Temkin NR, Dikmen SS, Wilensky J, et al: A randomized double blind study of phenytoin for the prevention of post-traumatic seizures. N Engl J Med 323:497, 1990.
32. Leppert M, Anderson VE, Quattlebaum T, et al: Benign familial neonatal convulsions linked to genetic markers on chromosome 20. Nature 337:647, 1989.
33. Gastaut H: Classification of status epilepticus. Adv Neurol 34:15, 1983.
34. Maytal J, Shinnar S, Moshe SL, et al: Low morbidity and mortality of status epilepticus in children. Pediatrics 83:323, 1989.
35. Maytal J and Shinnar S: Febrile status epilepticus. Pediatrics 86:611, 1990.
36. Aicardi J and Chevrie J-J: Status epilepticus. Pediatrics 84:939, 1989.
37. Aicardi J and Chevrie J-J: Convulsive status epilepticus in infants and children: A study of 239 cases. Epilepsia 11:167, 1970.
38. Meldrum BS: Physiological changes during prolonged seizures and epileptic brain damage. Neuropediatrie 9:203, 1978.
39. Lockman LA: Treatment of status epilepticus in children. Neurology 40 (Suppl 2):43, 1990.
40. Delgado-Escueta AV, Wasterlain C, Treiman DM, et al: Management of status epilepticus. N Engl J Med 306:1337, 1982.
41. DeLorenzo RJ: Status epilepticus. In: Johnson RT (ed): Current Therapy in Neurologic Disease—3. Philadelphia, BC Decker, 1990, p 47.
42. Rowe PC: The Harriet Lane Handbook, 11th ed. Chicago, Year Book Medical Publishers, 1987, p. 269.
43. Albano A, Raisdorff EJ, and Weigenstein JG: Rectal diazepam in pediatric status epilepticus. Am J Emerg Med 7:168, 1989.
44. Crawford TO, Mitchell WG, Fishman LS, et al: Very high dose phenobarbital for refractory status epilepticus in children. Neurology 38:1035, 1988.

Respiratory Failure and Other Complications of Neuromuscular Disease

Thomas O. Crawford, M.D.

PERIPHERAL NEUROMUSCULAR DISEASE

Severe neuromuscular disease is unusual in children, but in most major pediatric critical care centers, such disease underlies a significant number of long-term admissions for associated respiratory insufficiency. Such children often present to the intensive care unit (ICU) with complex and interwoven issues of respiratory, nutritional, and neuromuscular management, with results measured over weeks or months rather than shifts or days. Successful outcome may often depend on the appreciation of many subtle nursing and medical responsibilities.

Appropriate intensive care for children with neuromuscular disease depends not only on a correct diagnosis but also on an understanding of a number of basic issues underlying the physiology of the motor unit as well as the functioning and vulnerabilities of each of its parts. This involves identifying both the anatomic location and the pathophysiology of the disease. This chapter is divided into two sections: the first section considers normal anatomy and physiology of the motor unit, and the second section contains issues that are specific to individual diseases.

MOTOR UNIT

The motor unit is defined as a motor neuron and all of the individual muscle fibers that it innervates. Functionally, the motor unit consists of several distinct parts. The neuron cell body, or perikaryon, resides in the anterior horn of the spinal cord or motor nuclei of the brain stem. It gives rise to a single axon that is myelinated within the spinal cord by oligodendrocytes and within the roots and peripheral nerves by Schwann cells. After penetrating the target muscle, the axon has numerous branches that innervate widely scattered muscle fibers. The number of muscle fibers innervated by one

motor neuron varies widely, from as low as 10 in the extraocular muscles to as high as 2,000 in large muscles of the leg. The point of contact between the axon and the muscle is a specialized cholinergic synapse called the neuromuscular junction.

The motor neuron is perhaps the most extraordinary cell in the body for its size and complexity. The perikaryon is large, with an average diameter of 50 μM, yet the total volume of its axon may exceed the perikaryon by 1,000 fold. To support the axon, the perikaryon is highly active metabolically, synthesizing and transporting into the axon the equivalent of 25% of its volume daily. Another unique feature of the motor neuron—for central nervous system (CNS) neurons at least—is that the terminal portion of its axon is unprotected by the blood-brain or blood-nerve barrier. This specialization of the vascular endothelium has many functions, significant among them the barrier to multiple environmental agents such as drugs, toxins, or viruses. Exposure of the terminal motor axon to the systemic interstitial environment thus provides a "back-door" entrance through which pathogenic agents can gain access to the cell and can be transported by active axonal transport systems back to the perikaryon. These unique features may explain, in part, the special vulnerability of the motor neuron to disease.

In the anterior horn of the spinal cord motor neuron perikarya are arranged in groups defined by basic mechanical function. Neurons innervating a single muscle are pooled, but to a great extent these pools overlap with those of neurons innervating other functionally related muscles. Motor neurons receive synaptic input from a variety of different sources, both segmental (e.g., interneurons) and suprasegmental (e.g., the corticospinal tract). A common misunderstanding, possibly arising from the simplification necessary to make a diagram of neuronal pathways, is that a single corticospinal tract neuron innervates one motor neuron. Instead, both suprasegmental and intersegmental axons are themselves branched (like motor axons within the muscle), innervating multiple different motor neurons within a single muscle pool and functionally related pools, as well as antagonistic muscle pools acting through inhibitory interneurons. The effect of all this richly redundant branched innervation is to undermine the importance of any one or few neurons.

In addition to being robust, however, this system of organization modulates muscle tension in an exquisitely sensitive manner. The net amount of excitatory influence on a pool of motor neurons is carefully matched by corresponding tension in the innervated muscle. According to the Henneman size principle,[1] motor neurons within a pool are graded by size in their responsiveness to excitatory stimulus. The smallest motor neurons are the first recruited to discharge. Corresponding to the size of the perikarya are a number of other important physiologic features, including the size of the motor unit, velocity of axonal conduction, and the type of innervated muscle fiber (with the associated features of twitch speed, force of contraction, and fatigue resistance). This progression allows precision of movement and high exercise tolerance at low levels of excitation of the motor unit pool, with a reserve of high power but imprecise and fatiguable muscle tension available on demand.

An action potential is initiated by the axon hillock, which acts as an integrator of all excitatory and inhibitory influences before then reaching the firing threshold. Once initiated, the impulse may propagate toward the muscle at speeds up to 100 m/sec in large healthy nerve fibers. The conduction velocity is determined by several factors, one of which is axonal caliber, with larger axons conducting impulses more rapidly. Another factor, often disrupted by disease, is the myelin sheath. In human peripheral nerve, individual myelin segments may be as long as 1 mm. With acute demyelinating disease myelin segments may be lost, thus significantly slowing conduction. If several adjacent segments are lost, the action potential rapidly diminishes in this region, blocking axonal conduction, despite an anatomically normal nerve fiber distal to the block. Over time, Schwann cells divide and migrate to the exposed portion of axon, investing it with a new myelin sheath. The new myelin segments are smaller with thinner myelin, however, causing a chronic slowing of conduction.

The neuromuscular junction is an especially extensive and complex cholinergic synapse that virtually ensures one-to-one transmission of action potential to depolarizing muscle fiber potential. At the presynaptic terminal, the arrival of an action potential changes the transmembrane voltage, which opens specialized voltage-sensitive Ca^{2+} channels. The local influx of Ca^{2+} is necessary for release of vesicles containing acetylcholine into the synaptic cleft. On the postsynaptic side of the neuromuscular junction, the quantal release of acetylcholine produces a small depolarization of the membrane. Each action potential of the motor neuron normally releases enough quanta of acetylcholine that the small depolarizations sum together easily to surpass the threshold for a muscle fiber action potential, which then propagates along the length of the muscle fiber.

Muscle fibers are generally divided into two groups, types I and II, based on myosin type, twitch characteristics, metabolic source of energy, fatiguability, and other characteristics. Type I fibers are relatively slow to generate twitch tension, are supplied adenosine triphosphate (ATP) from aerobic metabolism in richly abundant mitochondria, and are resistant to fatigue. Type II fibers are the opposite: fast to generate twitch tension, supplied ATP chiefly by anaerobic glycolytic metabolism (with resultant lactate build-up with exercise), and relative fatiguability. The fiber type is determined by the innervating neuron, with type I motor units recruited first (in accordance with the Henneman size principle). In most human skeletal muscles, type I and type II fibers are nearly equal in abundance and are distributed in an apparent random fashion throughout the muscle.

Each muscle fiber is a syncytium, representing the fusion of up to 10,000 myoblasts (in large muscles) during development. In healthy mature muscle the nuclei occupy a peripheral location, just under the cell membrane. The bulk of the cytoplasm is filled with the contractile apparatus, organized into bundles called myofibrils. The myofibril consists of numerous repeated sarcomeres (the basic contractile unit) arranged end to end in series. The sarcomere represents one set of myosin and actin molecules that slide over one another to produce contractile force. Also prominent throughout the muscle cytoplasm is an extensive membrane network, the T tubule system, which is intimately related to the contractile apparatus. The T tubules are continuous with the muscle fiber surface and distribute the electrostatic and ionic effects of a depolarizing action potential throughout the cytoplasm of this very large cell. This leads to the local release of Ca^{2+} from the adjacent sarcoplasmic reticulum, which is the molecular signal for the production of contractile force. The Ca^{2+} is quickly cleared, requiring successive action potentials to maintain tetanic contraction.

Muscle contraction is mediated by the interaction of myosin and actin through cross-bridges that form, break, and re-form as the two fibrous proteins slide over one another. The actual movement is generated by a conformational change in the cross-bridge itself, sliding the fibers 7 nm for each molecule of ATP. The resultant force varies with the number of sites available for crossbridging, which in turn is related to the length of the muscle. The length by which maximum force is generated is called L_O: available force drops off quickly at either longer or shorter lengths (Fig. 24–1).

Another important aspect of the length-force relationship is the amount of tension generated by passive stretch. This passive tension also varies with length and is a function of two factors. The first, the contractile apparatus itself, resists stretch because it requires the breaking of formed cross-bridges between actin and myosin. This component of passive tension is not easily manifest since these cross-bridges are usually quickly recycled to preserve mobility. In some pathologic states with muscle ischemia, or after death, the release of Ca^{2+} into muscle fixes myosin/actin cross-bridges and leads to rigor. The other factor in passive tension is the combined resistance to stretch of all the other elements of muscle. Within the functional range of motion of normal skeletal muscles, passive tension to stretch is not apparent. As

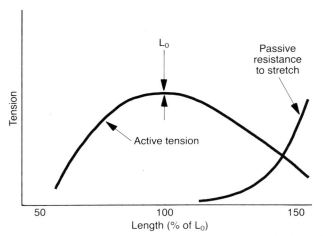

Figure 24–1. The relationship between length and tension in skeletal muscle.

seen in many muscular dystrophies, however, muscle fibrosis can become a significant factor in limiting passive stretch, resulting in joint contractures.

Response of the Motor Unit to Stress and Injury

With the exception of injury to the motor neuron perikaryon itself, the motor unit is capable of repair and regeneration to a degree that is extraordinary for the nervous system. Moreover, in response to unusual demands—as with the loss of adjacent motor units or other extremes of use—the motor unit is very plastic. Some of the responses are immediate, such as the increased firing frequency of remaining motor units, whereas others may take months or years to become manifest, such as the regrowth of axons to a remote muscle after axonal injury.

When a peripheral nerve is severed or crushed, the portion of nerve distal to the injury undergoes wallerian degeneration. Axonal dissolution is accompanied by break-up of myelin into clumps. Macrophages enter the nerve to digest the debris, while Schwann cells proliferate. The one remaining unaltered feature is the basal lamina that originally ensheathed the myelin-containing Schwann cell. With time, the basal lamina tubes contain a solid core of Schwann cells and are called Bunger bands. These bands are a favored substrate for the growth of axon sprouts, directing regeneration toward the original target. In these circumstances regeneration can proceed as fast as 1 mm/day. Without the support of the distal stump, extension of axonal sprouts is slow and directionless and may eventually cease in a painful, tangled neuroma.

Muscle fibers that have been "orphaned" by denervation respond with a sequence of reactions. The first reaction is to diminish the resting membrane potential to a value close to the threshold for generation of an action potential. Acetylcholine receptors spread from the site of the original neuromuscular junction over the surface of the fiber, increasing the sensitivity to exoge-

nous acetylcholine. The denervated muscle fiber thus fires spontaneously and randomly in fibrillations. These are too small to be seen clinically but can easily be discerned by electromyography. Following these membrane changes, the muscle fiber begins to lose volume as contractile proteins are lost.

The orphaned muscle fiber is hypothesized to produce a diffusible factor that directs the growth of sprouts from adjacent healthy nerve fibers in the region to "rescue" it. An important consequence of this process is that the size of each motor unit expands as the number of motor units decreases. Total muscle power and endurance are relatively preserved at the expense of fine control. Rescued muscle fibers eventually take on the type of the innervating neuron, so that the chronically denervated/reinnervated muscle eventually evolves from a random distribution of fiber types to manifest large clumps of fibers of a single type. There is a limit to the total number of muscle fibers that any one neuron can support however, after which the remaining orphaned muscle fibers atrophy and are eventually lost.

The setting of the ICU is one in which extremes of muscle use and disuse are probable. With disuse, type II muscle fibers atrophy. Although type I muscle fibers generally appear unchanged, disuse is associated with earlier fatigue. Increased use usually involves conditions favoring increases in strength or increases in endurance. Recurrent high-load weight-bearing is necessary to increase strength, which is accomplished by the addition of more contractile proteins within hypertrophied muscle fibers, chiefly type II. The physiology of this hypertrophy is complex, however, because increased tension loads alone are sufficient to enlarge denervated muscle fibers in some special experimental conditions. Persistent low-load work is necessary to increase exercise tolerance and oxygen utilization. Changes in the muscle anatomy are more subtle but involve an increase in muscle mitochondria and the density of capillaries.

SPECIFIC NEUROMUSCULAR DISEASES

Diagnosis

Beyond the concerns of general care for all children with neuromuscular disease, certain issues are affected by the specific neuromuscular diagnosis or at least by an understanding of the location of the lesion within the motor unit. Many children with chronic weakness will have had a thorough diagnostic evaluation prior to the intercurrent illness that precipitates ICU care. Thus the question of diagnosis in the ICU is confined mainly to causes of acute weakness in previously normal children. The full diagnostic evaluation of such children is beyond the scope of this chapter, but a listing of commonly considered causes of acute weakness is presented in Table 24–1. In general, the most important clues to diagnosis are available from the history and physical examination, as well as from the demographic variables of age and gender. Diseases that are linked specifically to the newborn period are listed in Table 24–2.

Table 24–1. CAUSES OF ACUTE AND SUBACUTE WEAKNESS

Central nervous system
  Spinal cord injury, infarct or hemorrhage with spinal shock
  Acute transverse myelitis

Motor neuron
  Poliomyelitis
  Enteroviral polio syndromes

Motor nerve
  Guillain-Barré syndrome
  Acute intermittent porphyria
  Toxic neuropathy
    Heavy metals
    Organic solvents
    Drugs, especially chemotherapeutic agents
  Diphtheria

Neuromuscular junction
  Myasthenia gravis
  Botulism (infantile or adult forms)
  Organophosphate poisoning

Muscle
  Metabolic myopathy (especially disorders of energy metabolism)
  Dermatomyositis/polymyositis

Unknown
  Tick paralysis

Table 24–2. NEUROMUSCULAR DISEASES OF THE NEWBORN

Spinal muscular atrophy (Werdnig-Hoffmann disease)
Myotonic dystrophy
Neonatal myasthenia gravis
Congenital myopathy
Congenital muscular dystrophy
Tetanus
Disorders mimicking motor-unit disease
  Central nervous system disorders (e.g., hypotonic cerebral palsy)
  Metabolic disease
  Genetic disease (e.g., Prader-Willi syndrome)
  Connective tissue disorders (e.g., Ehlers-Danlos syndrome)

Table 24–3. CHILDHOOD NEUROMUSCULAR DISEASES THAT MAY PREDOMINATELY AFFECT RESPIRATORY MUSCLE FUNCTION

Myasthenia gravis
Guillain-Barré syndrome
Polymyositis and dermatomyositis

It should be possible to answer several important questions after performing the physical examination: (1) is the weakness regional (arms, legs, or face; proximal or distal) or generalized? Diseases that exclusively affect one or more limbs are more likely to be either in the CNS or due to local disease or injury such as a mononeuropathy. With few exceptions, generalized myopathies affect proximal muscle function more than distal muscle function, and neuropathies affect distal muscle functions more than proximal ones. Neuromuscular diseases that affect the respiratory muscles out of proportion to other muscles are listed in Table 24–3. (2) Is weakness a consequence of diminished effort? If so, consider CNS dysfunction or incomplete cooperation as a cause. (3) Is passive tone affected as much as active strength? Is there any evidence of regional spasticity? Neuromuscular diseases diminish both tone and strength. In contrast, floppiness caused by CNS disease often affects tone more than strength. Further, CNS disease often affects tone in a regional manner, with some movements, such as thumb adduction/abduction or wrist supination/pronation, demonstrating increased

tone. (4) Is the muscle strength highly variable, suggesting fatigue as a factor? If so, consider myasthenia gravis. (5) Is there evidence for other neurologic dysfunction? Seizures or altered mental status implicate the CNS but do not exclude disease of the motor unit as well. Ataxia out of proportion to weakness suggests either cerebellar dysfunction or possible sensory involvement either in the peripheral nerves or dorsal columns of the spinal cord.

Disorders of the Motor Neuron and Nerve

Spinal Muscular Atrophy

Childhood spinal muscular atrophy (SMA) is the second most common recessive genetic disease that is lethal. At any age a child or adult may be affected, but two broad groups have been distinguished by age of onset, the first group including children with an onset of weakness between birth and 6 months of age (Werdnig-Hoffmann disease or acute childhood SMA), and the second group including those with a later age of onset (chronic childhood SMA). These groups are important chiefly for genetic counseling but also because age of onset correlates somewhat with the degree of weakness and predicted life span. Affected children typically are thought to be normal prior to a subacute period of advancing weakness, followed by a long period of relatively stable weakness. There is a classic distribution of weakness and strength (especially in younger patients), with the trunkal and proximal limb muscles most affected while the diaphragm, extraocular muscles, upper facial muscles, extreme distal fingers and toes, and anal sphincter are relatively spared (although weak on an absolute scale). The relative preservation of the strength of the diaphragm despite chest and abdominal weakness leads to the collapse of the chest and to protrusion of the abdomen on inspiration, a pattern called paradoxic breathing.

Weakness is associated with paucity of motor neurons in the spinal cord. The remaining motor units are often very large, with each neuron innervating many times the usual number of muscle fibers. In turn, many of the remaining viable muscle fibers are massively hypertrophied while the residual bulk of muscle is atrophic or replaced with fat. The functional consequence of this mixture of hypertrophy and atrophy is that baseline muscle strength is especially subject to loss with disuse.

Children with SMA are especially vulnerable to respiratory crises with otherwise minor upper respiratory illnesses. Treatment of such respiratory crises is especially difficult, because of rapidly developing disuse atrophy of respiratory muscles on the ventilator. Every effort should be made to avoid assisted ventilation, but once initiated, attempts should be made to clear the airway and, as soon as respiratory muscle fatigue is relieved, reinstitute respiratory muscle work as quickly as possible. These children are often quite sensitive to postural adjustments and prefer to lie prone or on one side rather than supine.

One of the most difficult issues is the determination of appropriate resuscitation status for children with SMA. If young infants with SMA require, and are provided with, maximum ventilatory support, they may be sustained possibly for an extended time. With virtually no movement, however, the quality of life on the ventilator is very poor. On the other hand, older children may remain functional for many years with assistive devices. The need for ventilatory assistance is not necessarily associated with a "locked-in" state. The issue of code status for young infants with SMA should be discussed carefully before the onset of respiratory crisis. Pediatric hospice service may be very helpful to the family if available.

Experience suggests that many children and adolescents with SMA benefit from night-time ventilatory assistance (either by mask or with a tracheostomy), with improved daytime alertness, strength, and endurance.[2] By regularly relieving respiratory muscle fatigue, there may be long-term beneficial effects as well.

Guillain-Barré Syndrome

The acute polyneuropathy of Guillain-Barré syndrome (GBS) is an inflammatory disorder of presumably autoimmune origin. It is a relatively common disorder, with highest incidence in persons over 60 years of age; nonetheless, 0.8 children (under 18 years) per 100,000 are affected annually,[3] and rare cases are reported in infants. Because it is often a rapidly advancing disorder with numerous life-threatening but treatable complications, early recognition and treatment are critical.

The clinical presentation of GBS is highly variable, especially at the outset. Research criteria for the definition of GBS have been established, although necessarily these attempt only to define the core syndrome.[4] The onset of weakness is often preceded, usually by 2 to 4 weeks, by a diverse number of "triggers." Most often this is a viral infection, either with upper respiratory or gastrointestinal symptoms. Apart from its course, acute GBS is clinically similar to chronic inflammatory demyelinating polyneuropathy, which is slower in onset and persists for years. On occasion the chronic form presents with an acute onset that is indistinguishable from GBS.

The initial symptoms of GBS in older children are often sensory, and complaints (but not findings) of tingling paresthesias, distal limb pain, and back pain predominate. Younger children refuse, or are unable, to walk. Much attention has been focused on the "ascending" nature of weakness, from legs to arms to bulbar muscles. This may in fact represent the nature of symptoms found with progressive diffuse weakness, with deficiencies in running, stair-climbing, and walking

noted prior to loss of maximum arm strength functions. Regional areas of weakness may predominate in any one patient, although loss is relatively symmetric. Patients with rapidly progressive weakness almost always have some loss of vital capacity by the time of admission to an ICU. Depression of deep tendon reflexes in general correlates with weakness.

The early diagnosis of GBS is based on clinical suspicion and consideration of the other causes of acute weakness listed in Table 24–2. In some centers, early electrophysiologic studies may be highly suggestive. The classic features of demyelination (i.e., slowed conduction velocity and conduction block) may take days or weeks to develop or may never be manifest. A large decrease in the compound muscle action potential generated by stimulation of the distal nerve has been shown to be the best prognostic feature for recovery in adults.[5] After 7 to 10 days, characteristic elevations of the cerebrospinal fluid (CSF) protein without corresponding elevations of the cell count are almost always present.

The level of appropriate care is related to the duration and severity of weakness. The immediate concern for any new patient is the status of respiratory and airway function. The total vital capacity, a simple but reliable measure of respiratory muscle reserve, should be followed closely. Younger, uncooperative patients are a special problem and must be evaluated frequently for respiratory rate, quality of cough, and handling of secretions. These patients are also vulnerable because they are frequently sedated for diagnostic procedures, a practice that may precipitate "silent" respiratory failure. Patients with rapidly declining respiratory indices, or those with slower decline to marginal respiratory status, should be intubated early: There is no advantage in waiting for respiratory failure. Although most patients recover sufficiently quickly to avoid tracheostomy, occasionally patients lacking significant improvement require tracheostomy to avoid long-term complications of the endotracheal tube.

Other than respiratory failure, the chief complications of severely affected patients are disorders of autonomic function. These may be an excess or deficit of either sympathetic or parasympathetic tone. The most common finding, sinus tachycardia, is usually well tolerated and does not require treatment. Other features include bradycardia, T wave changes, hypertension, hypotension, and urinary sphincteric disturbance. Occasionally severe vasomotor collapse, presumably from diminished sympathetic-mediated vascular tone, requires large increases in circulating volume and continuous measurement of central venous pressure (CVP). Agents acting directly on the autonomic system should be avoided because of the potential for wide and unpredictable responses. Depolarizing muscle relaxants (e.g., succinylcholine) should be avoided for the same reason. However, almost any anesthetic or sedative can have unexpected consequences and should be monitored carefully.

Other complications include syndrome of inappropriate antidiuretic hormone (SIADH), acquired infection of lungs or urinary tract, pulmonary emboli, and decubitus ulcers. Patients sometimes have severe back pain that may require opiate analgesics acutely or tricyclic antidepressant agents chronically for management. In very weak patients, the possibility of pain should be explored carefully because it may manifest only as otherwise overlooked autonomic symptoms. Careful attention to nutritional status, either with gavage feedings or intravenous alimentation, is important. Passive range of motion of all joints, especially the hips and ankles, is necessary to prevent contractures in long-term patients.

The possibility of quickly altering humoral immunity with plasmapheresis has introduced a specific therapy for GBS. In a large cooperative trial of plasmapheresis versus control in adults, plasmapheresis was shown to be effective.[6] Patients receiving plasmapheresis spent less time on a ventilator, walked sooner, and were less likely to have residual neurologic involvement at 6 months. The plasmapheresis protocol varied, but generally 40 to 50 ml of plasma per kilogram of body weight were exchanged with plasmanate every other day for three to five sessions. A study of plasmapheresis in children with GBS, comparing a retrospective control group with a group of serial patients receiving pheresis, suggests that the benefit can be extended to children.[7] Nevertheless, plasmapheresis for younger children with GBS may not have the same favorable balance of risks and benefits. Plasmapheresis is more difficult in smaller children, both because of vascular access problems and because of proportionally greater shifts of fluids and electrolytes. The balance of these risks and benefits clearly requires individual judgments considering age, size, severity of disease, technical issues, and institutional experience.

Anecdotal reports suggest that intravenous immunoglobulin (400 mg/kg/day for 5 days) may be beneficial.[8] The mechanism of action is unknown, although benefit in other acute, presumably autoimmune, diseases is well documented.[9] Whether or not intravenous immunoglobulin is equal to plasmapheresis in benefit, and thus probably superior overall because of expected fewer complications, awaits a controlled trial.

Diseases of the Neuromuscular Junction

Myasthenia Gravis

Myasthenia gravis (MG) is a chronic autoimmune disorder of the neuromuscular junction associated with antibodies directed against the postsynaptic acetylcholine receptor. The clinical hallmark of MG is excessive fatiguability of muscles, but weakness independent of fatigue is apparent in more severe cases. Because the symptoms may appear to be both protean and variable, the diagnosis (especially in mild cases) can be very difficult. In patients who are admitted to the ICU for crisis management, however, the diagnosis is often more straightforward.

MG often affects the ocular, bulbar, and respiratory muscles disproportionately to other muscles. Common manifestations include (any combination of) ptosis, paralysis of extraocular movements, fatigue of the jaw with chewing, and palatal weakness characterized by a weak, nasal dysarthria after prolonged speaking or by nasal regurgitation of ingested liquids. In the limbs proximal muscles are typically more affected than distal muscles. The disease usually develops insidiously over weeks or months, but in some cases more rapid progression may precipitate an initial diagnosis in the ICU.

The diagnosis of MG rests on the clinical demonstration of excessive muscle fatigue and a on number of ancillary tests. The first of these is the rapid recovery of strength following intravenous edrophonium (0.2 mg/kg). This test is useful only in patients who have easily appreciable weakness at the time of infusion (excluding long-standing ophthalmoplegia, which usually does not respond). Because of cholinergic side effects, edrophonium should only be given in a controlled setting with adequate resuscitation equipment available (including atropine). Certain electrophysiologic features are also helpful to confirm the diagnosis. The best known is a characteristic decremental response to rapid nerve stimulation. Finally, many (but not all) patients with MG have elevated antiacetylcholine receptor antibody titers. The level of antibody titer does not correlate with the severity of disease, although in any one patient changes in antibody concentration may manifest clinically.

Therapy for autoimmune MG is based on two broad principles: first, direct improvement of the security of transmission through the neuromuscular junction with cholinergic drugs; and second, suppression of the immune system. The mainstay of cholinergic treatments is pyridostigmine, an anticholinesterase agent that prolongs the synaptic half-life of released acetylcholine. The peak of activity occurs about 2 hours after an oral dose. The dose and dosing interval must be individualized; starting doses of 60 mg in adults, 30 mg in children, and 6 mg in infants every 4 hours are typical. The chief side effect of a dose that is too high is diarrhea and abdominal cramping, although in some cases excessive anticholinergics can exacerbate weakness. Another agent of occasional benefit as a supplement is ephedrine. The usual starting dose is 25 mg for adults and 10 mg in children, given two or three times a day. The effects are usually not dramatic and must be balanced against the side effects of anxiety and sleep disruption.

Weakness leading to functional impairment of respiratory or bulbar muscles can be life-threatening and is termed a myasthenic crisis. Any patient complaining of new dyspnea or dysphagia is at risk and should be evaluated carefully and probably hospitalized. Because fatigue is highly variable, evaluation of vital capacity and swallowing competence must be made at frequent intervals over time. Any patient with progressive dyspnea, increasing respiratory rate, falling vital capacity, or poor handling of secretions should be intubated. There is no advantage in waiting for respiratory failure. Ventilatory support should be maintained on intermittent mandatory ventilation (IMV) mode with occasional sighs to minimize atelectasis. Because the fatigue of MG is at the level of the neuromuscular junction and not the energy production or contractile apparatus of the muscle itself, no improvement is likely with conditioning regimes. In fact, incentive spirometry may needlessly exhaust marginally fatigued muscle. In IMV mode, disuse atrophy should be minimal.

Infection or other metabolic stress is a frequent precipitant of myasthenic crisis and should be sought assiduously. If the patient is taking immunosuppressive agents, antibiotic therapy should be initiated empirically after appropriate cultures are obtained. Rarely patients in crisis have overdosed on anticholinesterase inhibitors and may benefit from withdrawal. These patients often have other problems, however, and may require more than just a drug "holiday."

After securing ventilation and treating any infection or pulmonary disease, the mainstay of treatment for myasthenic crisis is treatment of the underlying disease. Anticholinesterase drugs should be continued, if necessary intravenously (1 mg of neostigmine intravenously is equivalent to 60 mg of pyridostigmine orally). Measures that quickly modify immune function should be initiated as soon as possible. Alternate-day plasmapheresis for five sessions is often associated with rapid improvement that may last up to 28 days. This can "buy time" until other immunosuppressive agents have taken effect. If plasmapheresis is not logistically or technically possible, some authorities recommend the use of intravenous immunoglobulin, in doses of 400 mg/kg/day for 5 days. In the absence of bacterial infection (or after several days of specific therapy), high-dose corticosteroids can be introduced. Concern about transient worsening of the respiratory muscle function, sometimes seen with the initiation of steroids, is moot when the patient is intubated. In many cases of myasthenic crisis, initial high doses of corticosteroids are necessary to recover strength sufficient for weaning from the ventilator.

Many children, school age and older, with autoimmune MG benefit from thymectomy[10] with an increase in spontaneous remission rate or diminished need for immunosuppressive agents. Because this is an elective procedure, it should be performed only in institutions with experience, and then only with very careful preoperative preparation. Corticosteroids and other immunosuppressive agents should be avoided, if possible, with strength optimized by anticholinesterase drugs and plasmapheresis when necessary. Postoperatively, the equivalent intravenous dose of neostigmine may be slightly high; some authorities start with three fourths of the equivalent dose and administer it by constant infusion pump.

Patients with myasthenia require careful attention during surgery for other indications. All patients with active disease should be considered in potential myasthenic crisis postoperatively and should be managed accordingly. Curare-like agents should be avoided because of the possibility of prolonged paralysis (in some very unusual situations, extreme curare sensitivity has been used as a provocative diagnostic test). Certain drugs used in the ICU, including the aminoglycoside antibiotics, β-blockers, quinidine or quinine, and lithium, may be associated with an unmasking of nascent MG or exacerbation of known MG.[11, 12] Other than D-penicillamine, however, no drug should be considered absolutely contraindicated if equivalent substitutes are not available.

Fifteen per cent of babies born to mothers with MG have a transient neonatal form. Affected neonates present within the first minutes to days after birth with a feeble cry and suck, and floppy tone with potential respiratory failure. There is little correlation of risk with maternal severity or antibody titer—on occasion neonatal MG directs attention to previously unsuspected maternal disease. Expectant mothers with MG should be encouraged to deliver in hospitals equipped to care for such infants. The treatment is initially supportive, with assisted ventilation and gavage feeds as necessary. When stable, cautious therapy with anticholinergic agents (4 to 10 mg of pyridostigmine orally or 0.05 to 0.1 mg intravenously of neostigmine) can be advanced. In these infants, weakness usually resolves within the first month, because titers of circulating maternal antibody drop with age.

Congenital myasthenic syndrome, caused by a genetic defect of some portion of the neuromuscular junction, often presents in childhood or infancy.[13] Diagnosis depends on electrophysiologic testing. Some patients respond to anticholinesterase agents. There is generally no role for immunosuppressive therapy.

Infant Botulism

Botulism affects infants generally in the first 6 months of life. Infants most often present having been constipated for a few days with progressively declining feeding. They are often admitted and (appropriately) placed on antibiotics as part of a "rule out sepsis" protocol. The pattern of weakness is characteristic, with features of autonomic failure (constipation and sluggish pupillary response to light), followed by restricted extraocular movements, bulbar weakness, and weakness of the limbs. The limb muscles may be relatively spared, obscuring the severity of chest and bulbar weakness from casual observation. Early recognition is very important; respiratory failure is most likely to occur with the stress of admission to the hospital. Respiratory failure may be due to either a direct effect on respiratory muscles, upper airway collapse as the pharyngeal muscles become flaccid, or with aspiration. The diagnosis can be confirmed by characteristic incremental responses of the muscle to rapid nerve stimulation or by isolation of toxin from the stool.

Infant botulism has an unusual epidemiology, and most recognized cases in the United States occur in distinct regions around southern California, Utah, and southeastern Pennsylvania. Many infants are breast-fed. There is a low but relatively increased incidence of dietary exposure to honey. Around Philadelphia, most patients are from middle and upper socioeconomic groups; in southern California hospitals serving lower socioeconomic groups have a high incidence of cases.

The botulinum toxin is extremely potent, lethal in nanogram quantities. The toxin enters the motor axon terminus through specific uptake sites, then binds covalently to the inner face of the axonal synaptic membrane and prevents fusion and exocytosis of vesicles containing acetylcholine.[14] Recovery of function is prolonged, requiring the production of new membrane proteins. Affected axons can be observed with new sprouts growing outward, presumably to re-establish new connections with muscle. Infant botulism differs from conventional adult poisoning by the route of intoxication. In infants the toxin is produced by the *Clostridium botulinum* organism colonizing the intestinal lumen, whereas conventional botulism occurs after the ingestion of preformed toxin produced by spores growing in anaerobic conditions in canned food.

Treatment is largely supportive. Antibiotics have not shortened the morbidity, as infants spontaneously clear the clostridia. Most hospitalized patients require intubation and mechanical ventilation for several weeks or more. This is usually well tolerated.[15] Relatively loose-fitting endotracheal tubes are sufficient because of minimal air leak—a consequence of laryngeal flaccidity and low peak inspiratory pressure (PIP) requirements. This and the paucity of movement combine to lower the risk of subglottic stenosis (in the absence of trauma during endotracheal tube insertion) despite prolonged intubation. Most patients do not require a tracheostomy. Perhaps the greatest risk to affected infants is loss of vigilance and impatience. One should not rely too much on external monitors and alarms, because these infants cannot signal distress when the airway is plugged or disconnected. Because recovery of limb strength often precedes respiratory muscle and bulbar function, increased movement is not sufficient to predict successful weaning. Once extubated, affected children should be watched very carefully for aspiration of secretions. There is a small but significant risk of relapse.[16] Because of this risk, discharge from the hospital should probably be delayed until independent feeding is established.

Diseases of Muscle

Duchenne Muscular Dystrophy

Duchenne muscular dystrophy (DMD) is the most common, best understood, and among the most severe forms of muscular dystrophy. A deficiency in the protein dystrophin, coded by the X chromosome, is responsible. Characteristic features include proximal weakness, calf pseudohypertrophy, ankle and hip contractures, and extreme elevations of the serum creatine kinase (CK). The average age of confinement to a wheelchair is 11 years;[17] boys who are affected usually survive until the late teens or early twenties.

Boys with DMD are generally in the ICU either for postoperative care or in the terminal stage of the disease. They frequently require major orthopedic surgery for scoliosis to preserve good pulmonary function and diminish the need for painful bracing and support. The timing of this operation is critical; too late and the diminished respiratory strength can significantly increase postoperative risk for prolonged ventilation. If done too soon, the indication for surgery may not be clear. We try to follow the scoliosis and vital capacity carefully in the first years after the patient is confined to a wheelchair

to determine the proper temporal window for lowest risk. Surgery before the vital capacity drops below 35% of predicted value is advisable: postoperative complications increase when the vital capacity drops below 30% of predicted value.[18] Inspiratory resistive training to improve respiratory muscle function may be especially useful 6 to 12 weeks preoperatively.[19]

Most institutions have for many years discouraged intervention with mechanical ventilation in the terminal phase of the disease. More recently the availability of better portable ventilators, better assistive devices, and early aggressive medical and orthopedic care have improved the quality of life such that assisted ventilation is being reconsidered on an individual basis.[20] With this help, a few patients have survived into the fourth decade. The decision is obviously complex and most difficult. Support services offered by the Muscular Dystrophy Association can play a pivotal role in informed choice. It is very important, however, for medical as well as social reasons, that the decision be made prior to a respiratory crisis in terminal care. Patients with DMD are particularly susceptible to nocturnal hypoventilation. Treatment with night-time nasal mask-assisted ventilation can improve both night and daytime respiratory function. Thus, patients who benefit most from mechanical ventilation progress through a number of stages of assistance, from night-time nasal mask-assisted ventilation through tracheostomy with night-time IMV to full-time controlled ventilation.[21]

Chronically ventilated patients (and some boys much earlier) have a high risk for symptomatic cardiac insufficiency. The severity of cardiac involvement in DMD does not correlate with respiratory muscle strength. Thus, cardiac status (in many patients best evaluated by gated radionuclide ventriculography) is an important factor when long-term assisted ventilation is being considered.[22]

Other Myopathies

A wide range of both inherited and acquired inflammatory, metabolic, or toxic disorders diminish muscle function. Most myopathies are apparent more in the loss of strength of proximal muscles of the arm and leg than in the loss of more distal functions. Because a number of myopathies improve with specific treatment, a thorough diagnostic evaluation is most important. Diagnosis depends on an evaluation of information from many sources. Muscle biopsy should be done only in centers experienced in the histochemical evaluation of frozen tissue sections: Improper freezing or transport prior to freezing often introduces artifacts that render the specimen useless.

In the ICU, the treatment of children with myopathies follows the general guidelines suggested for all forms of weakness. Two points are often neglected. First, nutritional status should be assessed carefully and frequently (see also Chapter 16). Weak children may not be able to eat a full caloric load. Because they are often frail secondary to the underlying disease, standard anthropometric measures of nutritional status may not apply, and greater reliance on biochemical markers becomes necessary. A carefully monitored trial (checking for excessive fat gain or metabolic intolerance) of supplemental nutrition can be rewarded with useful strength and weight gain. Second, the role of disuse in myopathic weakness is easy to underestimate. In general, weak patients should have regular exercise to fatigue, followed by sufficient rest to recover muscle function fully. Unfortunately, the design of a proper training program for weak patients, with optimal workload and timing, falls short of the present sophisticated approach to sports training programs.

Malignant hyperthermia is a clinically silent or subtle myopathy that is only expressed in response to severe metabolic stress or certain anesthetic agents. The presenting signs of tachycardia, dysrhythmias, fever, and rigidity despite neuromuscular blockade strongly suggest the diagnosis. Untreated, the course may be fatal, with hyperpyrexia, ventilatory failure, myoglobinuria, and acute renal failure. The agents most commonly associated with malignant hyperthermic reactions are the inhaled anesthetics and depolarizing neuromuscular blockers, especially succinylcholine. Early treatment with dantrolene sodium (Dantrium) can abort or minimize complications (see also Chapters 80 and 86).

Acknowledgments. I would like to thank John L. Carroll, Pamela Talalay, and Miriam L. Freimer for critical review of the manuscript.

References

1. Henneman E: Recruitment of motoneurons: The size principle. *In*: Desmedt JE (ed): Motor unit types, recruitment and plasticity in health and disease. Prog Clin Neurophysiol 9:26–60, 1981.
2. Gilgoff IS, Kahlstrom E, MacLaughlin E, and Keens TG: Long term ventilatory support in spinal muscular atrophy. J Pediatr 115:904–909, 1989.
3. Beghi E, Kurland LT, Mulder DW, and Wiederhold WC: Guillain-Barré syndrome: Clinicoepidemiologic features and effect of influenza vaccine. Arch Neurol 42:1053–1057, 1985.
4. Asbury AK: Guillain-Barré syndrome: Historical aspects. Ann Neurol 27(Suppl):s2–s6, 1990.
5. Cornblath DR, Mellits ED, Griffin JW, et al: Motor conduction studies in Guillain-Barré syndrome: Description and prognostic value. Ann Neurol 23:354–359, 1988.
6. Guillain-Barré Syndrome Study Group: Plasmapheresis and acute Guillain-Barré syndrome. Neurology 35:1096–1104, 1985.
7. Epstein MA and Sladky JT: The role of plasmapheresis in childhood Guillain-Barré syndrome. Ann Neurol 28:65–69, 1990.
8. Kleyweg RP, van der Meche FGA, and Meulstee J: Treatment of Guillain-Barré syndrome with high dose gammaglobulin. Neurology 38:1639–1641, 1988.
9. Steele RW, Burks AW, and Williams LW: Intravenous immunoglobulin: New clinical applications. Ann Allergy 60:89–94, 1988.
10. Rodriguez M, Gomez MR, Howard FM, and Taylor WF: Myasthenia gravis in children: Long-term follow up. Ann Neurol 13:504–510, 1983.
11. Argov Z and Mastaglia FL: Disorders of neuromuscular transmission caused by drugs. N Engl J Med 301:409–413, 1979.
12. Howard JF: Adverse drug effects of neuromuscular transmission. Semin Neurol 10:89–102, 1990.
13. Engel AG: Congenital disorders of neuromuscular transmission. Semin Neurol 10:12–26, 1990.
14. Simpson LL: Molecular pharmacology of botulinum toxin and tetanus toxin. Ann Rev Pharmacol Toxicol 26:427–453, 1986.
15. Schreiner MS, Field E, and Ruddy R: Infant botulism: A review of 12 years' experience at the Children's Hospital of Philadelphia. Pediatrics 87:159–165, 1991.
16. Glauser TA, Maguire HC, and Sladky JT: Relapse of infant botulism. Ann Neurol 28:187–189, 1990.
17. Brooke MH, Fenichel GM, Griggs RC, et al: Clinical investigation in Duchenne dystrophy. 2: Determination of the "power" of therapeutic trials based on the natural history. Muscle Nerve 6:91–103, 1983.
18. Jenkins JG, Bohn D, Edmonds JF, et al: Evaluation of pulmonary function in muscular dystrophy patients requiring spinal surgery. Crit Care Med 10:645–649, 1982.
19. Dimarco AF, Kelling JS, DiMarco MS, et al: The effects of inspiratory resistive training on respiratory muscle function in patients with muscular dystrophy. Muscle Nerve 8:284–290, 1985.
20. Gilgoff I, Prentice RN, and Baydur A: Patient and family participation in the management of respiratory failure in Duchenne's muscular dystrophy. Chest 95:519–524, 1989.
21. Baydur A, Gilgoff I, Prentice W, et al: Decline in respiratory function and experience with long-term assisted ventilation in advanced Duchenne's muscular dystrophy. Chest 97:884–889, 1990.
22. Stewart CA, Gilgoff I, Baydur A, et al: Gated radionuclide ventriculography in the evaluation of cardiac function in Duchenne's muscular dystrophy. Chest 94:1245–1248, 1986.

25

Postoperative Neurosurgical Management

Ido Yatsiv, M.D.

Most neurosurgical patients who require intensive care monitoring are head-trauma patients at risk of developing increased intracranial pressure (ICP) and of having decreased mental status. These patients require basic life support including airway control, mechanical ventilation, and treatment aimed at normalizing ICP. These aspects of patient management have been discussed in Chapters 16 and 17.

There are several additional groups of pediatric neurosurgical patients that require postoperative monitoring in the intensive care unit (ICU). This monitoring is directed at early detection of anticipated complications (Table 25–1). Bleeding, seizures, and intracranial pressure control are discussed in Chapters 16, 17, 23, and 64. The remaining fluid and electrolyte complications are discussed here and are related to specific disease entities.

DISORDERS OF WATER AND ELECTROLYTES

The central nervous system (CNS) regulates water metabolism by way of secretion of antidiuretic hormone (ADH). ADH is produced by neurons in the supraoptic and paraventricular nuclei of the hypothalamus and is delivered by a hypothalamoneurohypophyseal tract to the posterior hypophysis, where it is stored. Secretion of ADH from the neurohypophysis is regulated by

intravascular osmolality and its effect on hypothalamic osmoreceptors and also by volume receptors in the left atrial wall and carotid sinus. The hormone binds to cells in the distal renal tubule and the collecting duct and activates adenylate cyclase with a resultant increase in intracellular cyclic adenosinemonophosphate (cAMP). The elevated cAMP increases the luminal cell membrane permeability to water, thus allowing water reabsorption and hypersthenuria.

In postoperative neurosurgical patients, either undersecretion (central diabetes insipidus [CDI]) or oversecretion of ADH (syndrome of inappropriate ADH secretion [SIADH]) may occur.

DIABETES INSIPIDUS

CDI is well recognized both as a primary symptom of various diseases such as brain tumors (craniopharyngioma, dysgerminoma, supraoptic glioma, and astrocytoma), histiocytosis, brain cysts, and granulomas and as a frequent result of suprasellar surgery.[1, 2] It also occurs in severe head trauma[3] and in brain death.[4, 5] In a large series of pediatric patients presenting with CDI, the principal etiologies were intracranial tumors (47%), intracranial anatomic defects (15.0%), postinfectious disease (11%), and histiocytosis (8.2%).[1] Most (80%) tumor-related CDI developed *after* surgery, and almost all of these patients had craniopharyngioma.

Various studies define slightly different clinical and laboratory criteria for CDI,[5, 6] some of which are listed in Table 25–2.

The intensivist should be aware of the likelihood that CDI might develop and make an early diagnosis so that

Table 25–1. PEDIATRIC NEUROSURGICAL PROCEDURES AND ASSOCIATED COMPLICATIONS

Operation	Complication
Craniotomy/tumor resection	Cerebral edema
	Bleeding
	Diabetes insipidus
	SIADH*
	Seizures
AVM† resection	Bleeding
Ventriculoperitoneal shunt	Shunt malfunction

*SIADH = syndrome of inappropriate antidiuretic hormone.
†AVM = arteriovenous malformation.

Table 25–2. LABORATORY FEATURES OF DIABETES INSIPIDUS

Polyuria: urine output >30 ml/kg/day
Hypernatremia: Na >145–150 mEq/l
Elevated serum osmolality: >310 mOsm
Decreased urine osmolality: <300 mOsm
Low urine specific gravity: <1.005

239

appropriate treatment can be administered. In the immediate postoperative period, the clinical picture might be obscured by other causes of increased urine output, such as mobilization of fluids administered during surgery, mannitol or radiographic contrast material leading to osmotic diuresis, and treatment with corticosteroids that magnifies urinary water loss by increasing the glomerular filtration rate. Use of the criteria mentioned earlier will usually help to confirm the diagnosis. If, however, the diagnosis remains in doubt, no harm will result from a brief fluid restriction and the documentation of a negative fluid balance. Postoperative CDI can sometimes remain chronic and require chronic maintenance therapy; however, in most cases in which surgery involved only the hypophysis, CDI reverses within 2 to 3 days and therapy can then be discontinued.

Treatment

Patients who slowly develop CDI rely initially on thirst for adequate fluid intake. Since the typical postoperative patient cannot drink freely, fluid replacement should begin promptly once the diagnosis of CDI has been made. Fluid replacement in these patients is monitored by accurate urine output measurements as well as by blood and urine electrolyte determinations. The recommended solutions contain one fourth to one half normal saline with 2.5 to 5% dextrose, to avoid excessive sodium or glucose overload.

The mainstay of treatment of CDI are the synthetic ADH analogues. There are four types of analogues: aqueous pitressin, pitressin tannate in oil, lysine vasopressin nasal spray, and desmopressin acetate nasal drops. The drug of choice in this category is desmopressin acetate (1-deamino-8-D-arginine vasopressin [DDAVP]), which was first synthesized in 1968.[7] DDAVP is delivered by intranasal insufflation. There is a wide variation in dose that does not seem to correlate with the age or the size of the patient. The usual starting dose is 2.5 mg, and the duration of action may last from 8 to 20 hours, thus making individualized dosing necessary. Several reports of *continuous* intravenous treatment with aqueous vasopressin in critically ill pediatric patients have been published.[6, 8-9] The advantage of this mode of therapy lies in the short duration of action of aqueous vasopressin (2 to 8 hours), which enables an accurate control of dosage in the immediate postoperative situation. The doses reported ranged between 1 to 15 mU/kg/hr of aqueous vasopressin.

In selected mild cases drugs that potentiate the effects of ADH (e.g., chlorpropamide, carbamazepine, and clofibrate) can support the water balance. These drugs, however, do not have a role in critically ill patients.

SYNDROME OF INAPPROPRIATE SECRETION OF ANTIDIURETIC HORMONE

SIADH secretion is frequently seen in neurosurgical patients as well as in other critically ill patients. The syndrome consists of *continuous* secretion of ADH, despite a hypo-osmolar state with an expanded extracellular volume. The secretion is "inappropriate" because under normal conditions, once the osmolality is lower than 280 mOsm ADH, secretion essentially shuts off. The syndrome is also associated with hyponatremia and natriuresis secondary both to low aldosterone and to an increase in the filtered load of sodium.

The laboratory criteria for the diagnosis of SIADH are listed in Table 25-3.

The variety of clinical situations associated with SIADH in children can be grouped into four broad categories: CNS disorders, intrathoracic disorders, neoplasia, and drug-related SIADH.[10] CNS disorders associated with SIADH include CNS tumors, blocked ventriculoperitoneal (VP) shunts, head trauma, and CNS infections.

In the clinical setting, SIADH is diagnosed by the clinical and laboratory criteria mentioned earlier; however, studies have measured elevated plasma and urine vasopressin levels in pediatric patients with SIADH following head trauma,[3] bacterial meningitis,[11] and postasphyxia.[12] The intensivist should anticipate and diagnose SIADH in time in the postoperative neurosurgical patient so that treatment is not delayed.

Treatment

Effective treatment of SIADH consists of the correction of the primary disorder, strict fluid restriction, and in some cases the use of hypertonic (3%) saline. Postoperative pediatric patients with conditions that are likely to cause SIADH should have their serum and urine electrolytes checked frequently and should have an accurate fluid balance. Unless there is a contraindication, it is probably advisable to put these patients on a fluid restriction regimen of 40 to 60% maintenance or 800 to 1,000 ml/m²/day. If the hyponatremia is severe and symptomatic (seizure activity, extreme lethargy, or altered mental status), it needs to be reversed rapidly by use of hypertonic saline. The dose of 3% saline is calculated to replace the deficit, and the goal is a serum sodium of 125 to 128 mEq/l. This solution is hypertonic and should be administered through a large intravenous catheter.

Lithium and demeclocycline have a potential role in the pharmacologic treatment of SIADH, because both impair the kidney's ability to concentrate urine; however, the pediatric experience with them is limited since there is seldom a need for more than fluid restriction.

Table 25-3. LABORATORY FEATURES OF SIADH*

Serum Na <135 mEq/l
Urinary Na >25 mEq/l
Serum osmolality <280 mOsm/kg
Urinary osmolality >serum osmolality
No renal, adrenal, or thyroid disease
No dehydration

*SIADH = syndrome of inappropriate antidiuretic hormone.

References

1. Greger NG, Kirkland RT, Clayton GW, et al: Central diabetes insipidus—22 years' experience. Am J Dis Child 140:551–554, 1986.
2. Baskin DS and Wilson CB: Surgical management of craniopharyngiomas: A review of 74 cases. J Neurosurg 65:22, 1986.
3. Padilla G, Leake JA, Castro R, et al: Vasopressin levels and pediatric head trauma. Pediatrics 83:700–705, 1989.
4. Outwater KM and Rockoff MA: Diabetes insipidus accompanying brain death in children. Neurology (Cleveland) 34:1243–1246, 1984.
5. Fiser DH, Jimenez JF, Wrape V, et al: Diabetes insipidus in children with brain death. Crit Care Med 15:551–553, 1987.
6. Chanson P, Jedynak CP, Dabrowski G, et al: Ultralow doses of vasopressin in the management of diabetes insipidus. Crit Care Med 15:44–46, 1987.
7. Vavra I, Machova A, Holeck V, et al: Effect of a synthetic analogue of vasopressin in animals and in patients with diabetes insipidus. Lancet 1:948–952, 1968.
8. Ralston C and Warwick B: Continuous vasopressin replacement in diabetes insipidus. Arch Dis Child 65:896–897, 1990.
9. McDonald JA, Martha PM, Kerrigan J, et al: Treatment of the young child with postoperative central diabetes insipidus. Am J Dis Child 143:201–204, 1989.
10. Kaplan SL and Feigin RD: Syndromes of inappropriate secretion of antidiuretic hormone in children. Adv Pediatr 27:247–274, 1980.
11. Kaplan SL and Feigin RD: The syndrome of inappropriate secretion of antidiuretic hormone in children with bacterial meningitis. J Pediatr 92:758–761, 1978.
12. Kaplan SL and Feigin RD: Inappropriate secretion of antidiuretic hormone complicating neonatal hypoxic-ischemic encephalopathy. J Pediatr 92:431–433, 1978.

26

Development and Maturation of the Cardiovascular System

Roger N. Ruckman, M.D.

FUNCTIONAL DEVELOPMENT OF THE HEART

The embryonic heart progresses from a straight tube to a beating, septated heart through a series of cellular changes and hemodynamic events. Important developmental stages in the human embryo occur between 21 and 24 days' gestation. The initial cell migration, torsion, and flexion of the tube allow the establishment of a pump with a regular heart rhythm. Modelling of the heart then proceeds through cell shape change, cell death, and tissue proliferation. By day 22, major progress in development proceeds through the contractile activity of the heart. Forward blood flow is achieved, and important aspects of the heart that are flow-dependent are shaped. Circulating blood volume begins to rapidly increase, and changes in stroke volume and blood pressure occur. Further hemodynamic molding of the heart is defined. During these developmental stages, the cardiac jelly participates by augmenting the contractile force transmitted to intracardiac structures, by enhancing primitive valve action, and by preserving ventricular shape. This is important especially during these stages with sparse myocyte development. The endocardium takes on a heaped-up appearance that aids the initiation of septation as well as allowing better contractile force and uniform blood flow. By 24 days, the regulation of heart rate, vascular tone, and cardiac output is established through innervation and the action of circulating catecholamines.[1]

Bulbus Cordis

At 25 days' gestation, the straight tube has flexed into a loop in which the bulbus cordis lies to the right (D-loop) of the primitive ventricle (left ventricle) (Fig. 26–242

1A and B). Growth of the proximal one third of the bulbus cordis gives rise to the right ventricle. The midportion of the bulbus cordis, referred to as the conus cordis, gives rise to the outflow portions of both ventricles. The distal one third of the bulbus cordis, the truncus arteriosus, divides into the aortic and pulmonary roots.[2]

Septation of the Heart

The ventricles are initially enlargements of adjacent portions of the cardiac tube, connected by a narrowed portion of the tube, the primary interventricular foramen (see Fig. 26–1). At these early stages, the developing atrioventricular (AV) canal is connected only to the left ventricle. The only pathway for flow into the developing right ventricle is the primary interventricular foramen. As the ventricles enlarge, the muscular septum is formed. The primary interventricular foramen also enlarges and serves as a pathway to the outflow portion of the heart (conus cordis). In the early embryo, the aorta is rightward and receives the flow from the primitive left ventricle via the primary interventricular foramen. The endocardial cushions, which appear initially as heaped up masses of endocardium, define the AV canal that is aligned with the primitive left ventricle. At 30 days' gestation, the well-developed superior and inferior cushions are noted to grow toward each other. With contributions from the bulbar ridges, lateral cushions, and a shift of the AV canal to the right, the fusion process gives rise to two AV valve orifices, each aligned to one ventricle. There also remains a communication between the ventricles that is called the secondary interventricular foramen (Fig. 26–2). This communication goes on to close by 6 weeks' gestation.

The first partition to form in the atrial cavity is the

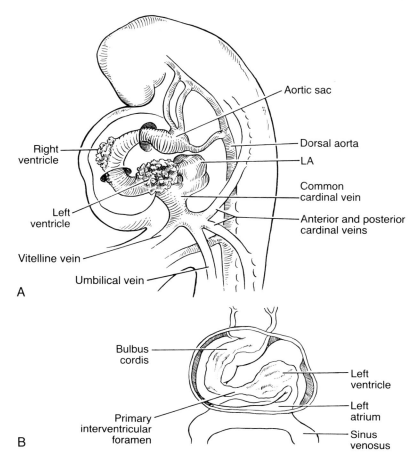

Figure 26–1. *A* and *B,* The early embryonic heart. The straight tube has looped; the ventricle is left and posterior; and the bulbus cordis is right and anterior. The definitive right ventricle is noted to bud out of the bulbus cordis. The earliest connection between the primitive (left) ventricle and the evolving right ventricle is the primary interventricular foramen (bulboventricular foramen).

septum primum, and the first communication defined by this wall is the ostium primum. As septum primum joins the AV septal portion of the AV canal, perforations of septum primum join to give rise to ostium secundum. Growth of the septum secundum to the right of ostium secundum gradually leads to fusion and obliteration of any communication except for the foramen ovale, which is covered by a portion of septum primum.

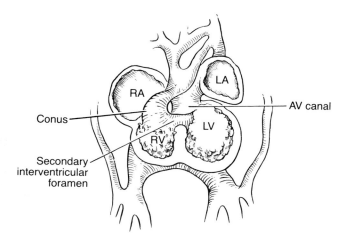

Figure 26–2. Septation of the ventricles. The two ventricles are well formed and are connected by the secondary interventricular foramen. The outflow region of the heart is defined by the conus.

The truncus arteriosus is ultimately separated into an aortic and a pulmonary trunk through, in part, growth of truncal ridges distally and bulbar ridges proximally. As described earlier, the bulbar ridges also contribute to ventricular septation. Individual pulmonary arteries also depend on contributions from the sixth arches. The pulmonary arteries can remain a part of the common trunk if aorticopulmonary septation fails to occur. Such a failure of septation implies a deficiency of the conal septum. Accordingly, persistent truncus arteriosus tends to have an associated large ventricular septal defect. In cases in which the common trunk is divided but with unequal partitioning, either the aorta or the pulmonary trunk can end up small. In addition, the aorticopulmonary septum fails to align with the interventricular septum and a ventricular septal defect is noted with the larger vessel overriding the defect.[2]

Conus

The midportion of the developing bulbus cordis is referred to as the conus cordis and is important in the development of the right ventricle, particularly the right ventricular outflow tract (see Fig. 26–2). The distal portions of the conus cushions participate in the partitioning of the truncus. The posteromedial portion of the conus enlarges into the primary interventricular foramen, thus establishing a channel under the aorta. As

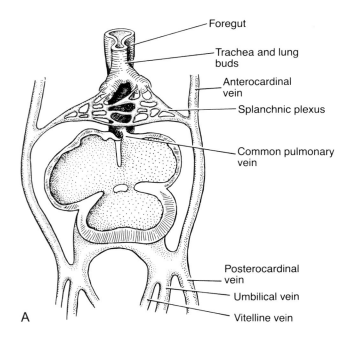

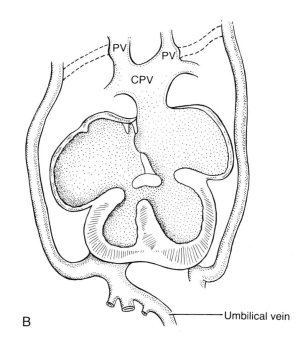

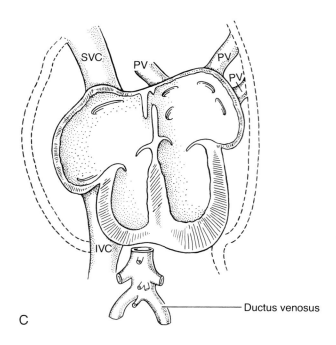

Figure 26–3. *A,* Development of systemic and pulmonary veins. The splanchnic plexus allows interconnection of the cardinal system and the common pulmonary vein noted to emerge from the back wall of the left atrium. The trachea and lung buds, which relate to the splanchnic plexus, are derived from the foregut. *B,* Development of the common pulmonary vein. As the individual pulmonary veins are defined, connections to the systemic veins are lost. During this time, ventricular and atrial septation are proceeding. *C,* Connection of the pulmonary veins. The common pulmonary vein becomes incorporated into the back of the left atrium, allowing connection of four individual veins. Septation is complete, and the cardinal system has atrophied.

this subaortic infundibulum is progressively effaced, the aorta shifts to the left, and definitive continuity between the left ventricle and the aorta is established. The small remaining secondary interventricular foramen is then closed by 6 weeks' gestation through contributions from muscular septum, endocardial cushion tissue, and conus septum.[2]

Pulmonary and Systemic Veins

As atrial septation is proceeding, the common pulmonary vein grows out from the posterior atrial wall and forms connections with the splanchnic vascular bed, which is associated with the developing lungs (Fig. 26–3A). The expansion of the common pulmonary vein with four channels of drainage from the lungs leads to enlargement of the left atrium and incorporation of the pulmonary veins into the left atrium (see Fig. 26–3B). In normal development, the systemic veins that connect into the splanchnic plexus become separated such that all pulmonary drainage from the splanchnic plexus proceeds to the left atrium via the pulmonary veins (see Fig. 26–3C).

The proximal end of the heart tube is the sinus venosus. Its two ends are called the sinus horns. The right sinus horn assumes a vertical orientation adjacent to the right atrium, ultimately forming the superior vena cava (SVC). The proximal portions of the left sinus horn and the connection of the two sinus horns develop into the coronary sinus. Veins that normally involute by the end of the sixth week include the left common cardinal vein and the distal portion of the left sinus horn. A pathway of the right common cardinal system may persist as the azygos vein. The left innominate vein is derived from the left common cardinal system.[2]

Atrioventricular Valves

The mitral and tricuspid valves are derived mainly from the ventricles with small contributions to the anterior leaflets from the mesenchymal tissue that surrounds the developing AV valve orifices. Through a process of undermining of the ventricular muscle, thick, fleshy sheets of tissue are formed along with a trabecular network. The mitral valve originates as a quadricuspid skirt of tissue. Each component has its own tensor apparatus. With subsequent development, adjacent cusps and papillary muscles fuse to create the definitive anterior and posterior leaflets with the supporting anterolateral and posteromedial papillary muscles. The anterior leaflet of the mitral valve receives an important contribution from the superior endocardial cushion whereas the tricuspid valve is derived mostly from the right ventricle. For each AV valve, the anterior leaflet forms first. The mitral valve development is completed before the tricuspid valve, the latter proceeding into 12 weeks of gestation.[2]

Semilunar Valves

By 33 days' gestation, the truncus arteriosus has been partitioned into the aorta and pulmonary trunk. Paired swellings of truncus cushion tissue fuse with a third small cushion to form the primitive valves. With blood flow through the valves, a process of excavation and migration of the valves proceeds through 55 days' gestation. The finished valves are thus located more proximally than in early embryonic development.[2]

FETAL CIRCULATION

The Pathways

Certain patterns of blood flow are noted in the fetus, which allow efficient delivery of maternal placental flow to developing organ systems (Fig. 26–4). The most oxygen-rich blood passes up to the fetal IVC from the umbilical vein. In turn, blood from the inferior vena cava (IVC) preferentially streams across the foramen ovale to the left atrium and on to left ventricle, aortic arch, and the developing heart (coronary circulation) and brain. Flow from the SVC, which is less rich in oxygen, proceeds to the right ventricle, into the pulmonary artery, and across the ductus arteriosus to the descending aorta. The majority of flow to the fetal heart is through the IVC. Consequently, the hepatic and

ductus venosus channels are important as regulators of total venous return to the heart. Umbilical venous flow is directed to the ductus venosus which, at times of fetal stress or hypoxia, can dilate to preserve delivery of oxygenated blood. At the same time, less blood is directed through the hepatic veins. In addition, a greater percentage of SVC flow streams across the foramen ovale rather than emptying almost exclusively into the right ventricle. The streaming patterns of blood not only allow more efficient oxygen delivery but also substrate (e.g., glucose) distribution.[3–5]

Cardiac Output

Work done in fetal sheep has shown that 60 to 65% of combined ventricular output is supplied by the right ventricle, and the remainder is supplied by the left ventricle. Of that 60 to 65%, all but 7 to 8% is shunted through the ductus to the descending aorta. Of the 35 to 40% supplied by the left ventricle, 20% goes to the head and upper body, 3% to the heart, and 15% to the descending aorta. The proportionate flows provided by each ventricle relate to the resistances seen downstream rather than differences in size, muscle mass, or filling pressures. The aortic isthmus serves as an important point of resistance for left ventricular (LV) output. Changes in cardiac output are regulated through similar mechanisms as in the mature heart. However, responsiveness to regulatory mechanisms is different in the fetus. The heart rate response is especially important since the capacity for change of stroke volume is limited in the fetus. Similarly, although the Frank-Starling relation holds, the fetal heart is near the top of the curve, and changes in filling pressure or volume cause little change in cardiac output. The reduced distensibility of fetal myocardium contributes to this reduced response. The fetal heart is affected particularly by changes in afterload. Cardiac output can be augmented by afterload reduction but, even more striking, is the fall in cardiac output when afterload increases. Fundamental contractility of the heart shows limited capacity for increase in early fetal life owing to limited numbers of myofibrils and to less efficient calcium mobilization.[3]

Ventricular Growth and Mechanics

Even though the right ventricle contributes a larger percentage of flow to combined ventricular output, the right ventricle is not "dominant" in terms of size. Studies of spontaneously aborted human fetuses have shown that total heart weight, right ventricular (RV) wall weight, and LV wall weight all increase linearly with body weight from 8 weeks to term. Wall thickness and surface area measurements confirm similarity of RV and LV. Other studies in fetal sheep have confirmed similar behavior in terms of pressure-volume and wall tension-radius relationships.[6]

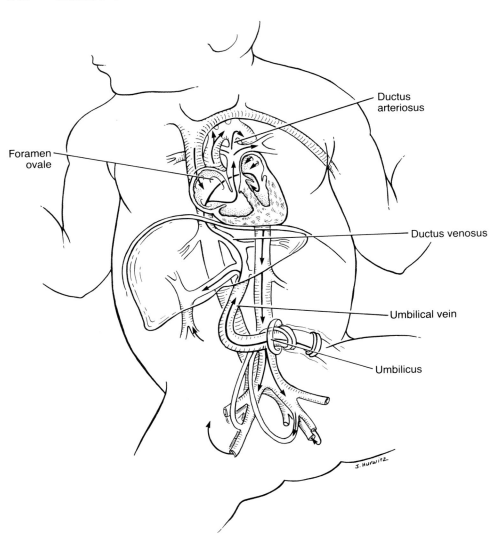

Figure 26—4. The fetal circulation. Flow from the placenta is directed into the umbilical vein, through the liver via the ductus venosus, and into the right atrium. Streaming, aided by venous valves, carries the oxygenated blood through the foramen ovale to the systemic circulation. Smaller flows proceed through the right heart and ductus arteriosus to the descending aorta.

Stress Responses

A major stress to the fetal heart is hypoxia. The responses are very different from those of the adult heart in which neurohumoral and local vascular responses contribute to hypertension, tachycardia, increase in cardiac output, and redistribution of flows to preserve the brain and myocardium. Fetal studies show that peripheral chemoreceptors and a baroreflex response to hypertension lead to bradycardia rather than tachycardia after hypoxic stress. Both vagal action and direct hypoxic depression of myocardium are involved in the bradycardia that is observed. Because hypoxia causes a hypertensive response and an associated increase in afterload, both LV and RV outputs decrease. However, the major cause for decreased cardiac output is the fall in heart rate. Circulation in the liver is important because of regional differences in oxygen saturation. The hepatic veins drain to the IVC, where flow preferentially streams across the foramen ovale to the left atrium. In the fetal lamb, the oxygen saturation in the right hepatic veins is 55%, while that in the left hepatic veins is 70%. This reflects preferential distribution of lower saturation portal venous blood to the right

lobe of the liver. After hypoxic stress, flow into the liver, as opposed to flow through the ductus venosus, is decreased. Flow is decreased more to the right lobe than to the left lobe. Consequently, aggregate flow into the IVC, after hypoxic stress, is made up of streams of blood that are most highly oxygenated. Of those streams, that from the ductus venosus and left hepatic veins show more direct flow across the foramen ovale. Venous valves in the high IVC-low right atrium further facilitate streaming effects. Accordingly, delivery of oxygen to vital organs is maintained.[7]

Pulmonary Circulation

The ductus arteriosus diverts blood away from the pulmonary circuit in fetal life. This right-to-left shunt may persist for the first 3 days in a normal newborn, reflecting nearly equal pulmonary artery and aortic pressures. More commonly, the pulmonary artery pressure shows a rapid fall such that right-to-left shunting is only observed for about 6 hours followed by left-to-right shunting for an additional 9 hours. At about 15 hours after birth, the ductus shows physiologic closure. Anatomic closure then takes several more days, and the ductus may open and close physiologically during this time.[8]

In early fetal life, prostacyclin is undetectable. After the onset of spontaneous respiration, there is active prostacyclin synthesis. This synthesis coupled with the pulmonary vasodilatory effects of increased PO_2 leads to an associated fall in pulmonary vascular resistance within 15 minutes. At the same time, the ductus arteriosus begins to close, also partly in response to increased PO_2. Prostacyclin synthesis decreases significantly by 5 hours of life. Accordingly, other factors are important in maintaining low pulmonary artery pressure after the initial fall in pressure. Direct inhibition of prostacyclin synthesis by agents such as indomethacin will stimulate ductal closure, a useful clinical effect in cases of persistent patency of the ductus.[9, 10]

Metabolic Changes at Birth

From work in fetal sheep, it has been demonstrated that the process of delivery and cutting of the umbilical cord leads to a significant increase in catecholamine production and release. The presence of acidosis also triggers release of catecholamines. At the same time free fatty acids are mobilized, the liver increases its production of glucose, and chemical thermogenesis is stimulated. The other key metabolic change at the time of birth is the regulation of thyroid hormone. Current evidence suggests that the build-up of plasma thyroid concentrations in the 2 to 3 weeks prior to delivery is important for appropriate cardiac performance after delivery. Experiments with fetal lambs subjected to thyroidectomy near term versus a similar group with thyroidectomy done during delivery before cord cutting show that the fetal thyroidectomy group has no measurable plasma T3. In addition, that group, unlike controls or those operated during delivery, shows depression of left ventricular function, heart rate, blood pressure, and systemic blood flow. Oxygen consumption is also reduced. All groups showed similar flows into the lung, demonstrating that ductal shunting is not different in the three groups of animals. The normal newborn lamb should show a two- to three-fold increase in LV output. This change is noted by 1 hour after delivery, and the determining factors for this increase in output may be developing just before birth. One of the determining factors appears to be thyroid-stimulated new cardiac myosin with actin-activated ATPase activity. Other possible mechanisms of thyroid effect on cardiac contractility include enhanced sodium-potassium ATPase activity and augmented energy conservation in mitochondria. Thyroid hormone may affect the appearance of β-adrenergic receptors in the heart, but the hormone does not appear to directly affect the observed changes in circulating catecholamines. Thyroid hormone may play some role in the hypertrophy of cardiac muscle that is observed after birth, but the major stimulus for hypertrophy is the sudden increase in systemic vascular resistance and closure of fetal shunts with the associated increase in cardiac work.[11, 12]

VENTRICULAR SEPTAL DEFECT

Development of the Interventricular Septum

As discussed in the section on septation of the heart, the interventricular septum receives contributions from several sources of embryonic tissue. In terms of the mature heart, the smooth septum is derived from growth of the margins of the interventricular foramen. The trabecular septum is defined by expansion of the two ventricles. The crista supraventricularis, or conus septum, develops from conus ridges. The conus septum is important as a boundary between the pulmonary and aortic outflows as well as a contributor to closure of the interventricular foramen. The interventricular foramen, in turn, initially develops as a communication between the primitive (left) ventricle and the bulbus cordis (see Fig. 26–1). With looping and development of the right ventricle, the interventricular foramen becomes the communication between the developing left and right ventricles. This bulboventricular foramen, and the ridge adjacent to it, shifts to the left and allows the aorta to align with the left ventricle. With further development of the AV cushions, the communication between the ventricles takes on the appearance of a membranous ventricular septal defect. The muscular ventricular septum has three developmental portions as viewed from the left ventricle: the posterior smooth septum that is the superior one third to one half of the septum; the posterior trabecular septum that is the apical one half to two thirds of the septum; and the anterior septum that lies between the membranous septum and the anterior wall of the left ventricle. Important anatomic details of the septum as viewed from the right ventricle are the pars interventriculare, which is that part of the membranous septum under the septal leaflet of the tricuspid valve, and the pars atrioventriculare, which lies just above the septal leaflet of the tricuspid valve and forms part of the floor of the right atrium. Accordingly, this part of the septum divides the left ventricle from the right atrium. On the right ventricular side of the septum, the papillary muscle of the conus serves as the boundary between the body of the right ventricle and its outflow tract or infundibulum.

On closer study of the development of the membranous septum, there is some evidence to suggest that the pars atrioventriculare is the only portion present for much of fetal life. In later fetal life, undermining of tricuspid leaflet tissue allows the pars interventriculare to form. This process of undermining occurs after the secondary interventricular foramen has closed. A perimembranous ventricular septal defect can involve any combination of deficiency of pars atrioventriculare or pars interventriculare. Part of the anomalous development may include some degree of malalignment of the aorta with the left ventricle. The additional feature required in cases of LV to right atrial shunting is a wide anteroseptal commissure of the tricuspid valve.[13, 14]

Timing of Closure

The normal embryology of the ventricular septum leads to closure by 6 weeks in the human fetus. It appears that most of the development of the ventricular septum occurs during the fourth and fifth weeks of pregnancy. This is the time of proliferation of the right and left bulbar ridges, growth of the endocardial cushions, and expansion of the muscular septum. However, clinical data suggest that development of these tissues may continue through fetal life and on into infancy, thus explaining the significant percentage of ventricular septal defects that show spontaneous closure.[15]

Conal Ventricular Septal Defect

A variety of terms have been used to describe the ventricular septal defect that occurs above the lower border of the crista supraventicularis (Fig. 26–5). This defect is important because of its location just below the pulmonary valve (subpulmonary ventricular septal defect) and the frequent clinical association with a prolapsed aortic cusp, particularly the right coronary cusp. Aortic insufficiency, which develops after birth, is more common in conal (either intracristal or supracristal) ventricular septal defects than in subcristal defects. It is also more common to see conal defects in Asian populations. The particular etiologic factors for this observed distribution of defects are not understood.[16]

Displacement of the Atrioventricular Canal

The common AV canal initially relates to the primitive (left) ventricle. The communication to the bulbus cordis, which gives rise to the right ventricle, is the bulboventricular foramen. With further development, the AV canal shows movement towards the bulbus cordis to

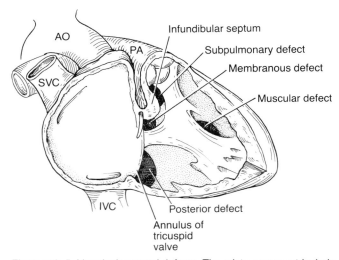

Figure 26–5. Ventricular septal defects. The crista supraventricularis, which forms a "Y" through its septal and parietal bands, helps to define the location of the defects. Note the supracristal location of the subpulmonary defect (conal ventricular septal defect). A shift in the infundibular septum would add the feature of malalignment. The posterior defect, in the inlet portion, is also called "canal type" VSD. The perimembranous defect is close to the tricuspid annulus.

allow connection of the canal into the developing right ventricle. The AV canal then undergoes division into two separate orifices. If the shift of the AV canal fails to occur, the result is a single (left) ventricle with a rudimentary outlet chamber. The single ventricle has a double inlet configuration. In cases of partial shift of the AV canal, straddling of the tricuspid valve may be seen. If, on the other hand, an exaggerated shift of the AV canal occurs, a single right ventricle with double inlet and double outlet configuration is noted. In these cases of "single" right ventricle, careful examination will define at least a remnant (slit) of left ventricular cavity. The region bordered by the two descending coronary arteries corresponds to the remnant of left ventricle. An intermediate shift of the AV canal gives rise to the situation of "unbalanced" ventricles. For example, an exaggerated shift to the right leads to the formation of a small tricuspid valve and right ventricle with a correspondingly larger mitral valve and left ventricle. In cases of only partial shift, a small or atretic mitral valve, small left ventricle, and double-outlet right ventricle arrangement is noted. When one considers all segments of the heart, the arrangement of the great arteries in most of these cases tends to involve a D-loop ventricle with D-malposition or transposition of the great arteries. However, the single left ventricle with persistent bulboventricular foramen to an outlet chamber, tends to have an L-loop arrangement. If the AV canal remains undivided, these hearts would be classified as complete AV canal rather than ventricular septal defect or single ventricle.[17]

Straddling and Overriding of Atrioventricular Valves

As noted earlier, a persistent ventricular septal defect or AV canal can be associated with malalignment of the AV valve orifices. Further examination of the anatomic details of such hearts reveals that the support structure for the valves is also variable. A distinction should be made between overriding of an orifice and straddling of the tension apparatus (Fig. 26–6). In general, when there is overriding, there is also straddling, but one can occur without the other. The terms concordance or discordance are introduced to describe hearts in which the right-sided AV valve empties into a right-sided anatomic right ventricle (concordance) or the right-sided AV valve empties into a right-sided anatomic left ventricle (discordance). Cases with more than 50% override are generally classified as double-inlet single ventricles. Straddling is of particular importance because of the impact on the approach to surgical repair. When a mitral papillary muscle with its associated chordae tendineae is found in the anatomic right ventricle or a tricuspid papillary muscle is found in the anatomic left ventricle, then straddling is present. This is true for both concordant and discordant AV valves. The orientation of the ventricular septum is important in these hearts. The septum may or may not extend to the crux of the heart. In cases with a straddling tricuspid valve, the tensor apparatus extends across the posterior part of the sep-

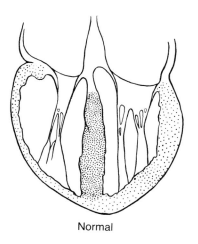
Normal

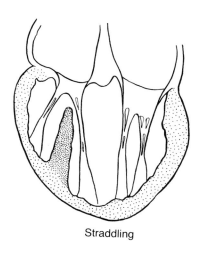
Straddling

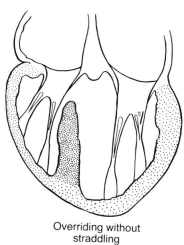
Overriding without straddling

Figure 26–6. Straddling and overriding atrioventricular (AV) valves. The normally related AV valve is committed to its ventricle and papillary muscle support on one side of the ventricular septum. An AV valve shows straddling when one of its papillary muscle supports is attached to the opposite ventricle through a ventricular septal defect. Overriding occurs when the AV valve annulus is shifted over the crest of the septum.

tum and the septum fails to extend to the crux. In contrast, straddling mitral valves show chordae crossing the anterior part of the septum and the septum does extend to the crux. When there is straddling of the mitral valve into a small right-sided anatomic left ventricle, a unique physiologic arrangement occurs. Flow from right atrium proceeds across to the left-sided anatomic right ventricle while flow from the left atrium is directed into the right-sided anatomic left ventricle. This is called a criss-cross heart. These hearts tend to have only one outlet, the aorta, from the primary (anatomic right) ventricle, and the pulmonary artery is atretic. Even with this abnormal rotation of the left ventricle, the septum is noted to extend to the crux. In cases of straddling common AV valves, the hearts are univentricular in type and the major distinction from hearts already described is that the common valve drains both atria to the ventricular mass. The most unusual variation of straddling is the rare heart that has a mitral papillary muscle in the anatomic right ventricle and a tricuspid papillary muscle in the anatomic left ventricle. These cases represent a greater risk for block at the time of operation. Also uncommon are hearts with overriding of the valve annulus but all tensor apparatus in the appropriate anatomic ventricle. Consequently, the four most common arrangements are straddling right AV valve with either concordance or discordance or straddling left AV valve with either concordance or discordance.[18]

Double-Inlet Left Ventricle

When the embryonic heart is developing, one of the normal stages of development involves a left ventricle with the AV canal committed to it and a separate bulboventricular foramen that allows connection of the left ventricle to the developing right ventricle. The two great arteries at this stage are noted to arise from the bulbus cordis (developing right ventricle) with the aorta to the right, elevated anterior and superior above a

conus. The cephalic portion of the outflow tract is derived from the conus. The aorta, which starts out elevated above conus tissue, should migrate to a definitive connection with the left ventricle as the conoventricular flange is effaced. These findings at about 30 days of pregnancy also include drainage of both atria into the left ventricle. Accordingly, it is understandable that a developmental error at this stage could lead to the typical arrangement of double inlet left ventricle with D-malposition of the great arteries. If the bulboventricular foramen is small, the pathway to the right-sided aorta is restricted and functional subaortic stenosis results. The anatomy may be complicated further by ventricular inversion, giving an overall segmental arrangement of S,L,L. Studies in the chick embryo have shown that the anatomic right ventricle, derived from the bulbus cordis, is small until the migration of the AV canal allows the right atrium to establish connection to the right ventricle. In essence, embryonic flow to the right heart is provided by the left ventricle and is directed to the outflow tracts. Growth of the inflow and body of the right ventricle is dependent on the establishment of contact from right atrium to right ventricle. Cases of double-inlet left ventricle (DILV) will show a right ventricular infundibulum since that portion of the right ventricle is derived from the conus portion of the bulbus cordis. The orientation of the ventricular septum is abnormal in these hearts due to the lack of development of RV sinus. If the truncus arteriosus fails to partition equally, there may be pulmonary stenosis. In addition, unequal partitioning of the AV canal leads to the appearance of mitral stenosis.[19]

Rudimentary Outlet Chamber

In order to understand DILV versus single ventricle with a rudimentary outlet chamber, it is important to remember that the development of DILV relates to the failure of the two atria, which are initially both connected to the left ventricle, to establish, through shift of the AV canal, communications with both ventricles. The rudimentary outlet chamber is made up of the infundibulum of the right ventricle, the embryonic bulbus cordis. The anatomy of this chamber is smooth. By contrast, the small right ventricle in DILV has an inflow portion with its characteristic rough trabecular pattern. There is also a moderator band. The ventricular septal defect in DILV tends to be large and involves the posterior and midportions of the septum.[20]

Transition at Birth

At birth, as circulation is established to the lungs, the presence of a ventricular septal defect becomes manifest. In the first few hours after birth, pulmonary vascular resistance is high and pressures in the pulmonary and systemic beds are equal. Consequently, there may be little shunting initially. This left-to-right shunt is a dependent shunt since the flow depends on the fall in pulmonary vascular resistance. The drop in pulmonary vascular resistance over time is exponential, and, by 6 weeks of age, resistance values fall to levels close to the normal adult range. Accordingly, some of the clinical manifestations of the left-to-right shunt may be delayed to the first month of age. At that point, increasing flow into the pulmonary bed stimulates receptors that mediate the tachypnea which, along with the heart murmur, provides early evidence of the defect. If the shunt flow is large, the full picture of congestive heart failure may develop.

Surgical Implications

The location of the ventricular septal defect is particularly important to the surgeon from the standpoint of accessibility and relation to the conduction system. The most common defects are located in the perimembranous region. Malalignment defects are adjacent to the "Y" of the crista supraventricularis. These defects have in common the ability to be visualized from a transatrial surgical approach. The supracristal and apical muscular defects are harder to visualize by this approach. In all of these defects, whether approached from the atrium or by a ventriculotomy, attention has to be directed to preservation of the conduction system, since conduction fibers skirt along the rim of the defect. Other important issues for the surgeon in terms of increasing the risk of the procedure include multiple ventricular septal defects, associated mitral valve disease, and the straddling tricuspid valve. This latter condition poses two problems. The valve may be insufficient, necessitating repair or replacement, and the AV node may be anomalously positioned, increasing the possibility of heart block.[21]

TETRALOGY OF FALLOT

Embryologic Development

Experimental work in the chick has shown that abnormal development of the conus is central to the subsequent appearance of the complex of tetralogy of Fallot. Placement of a ligature in the conus region of the chick in early development alters the hemodynamics in that region and interferes with the ability of the conus to achieve its normal position. The result in half of the chicks is a ventricular septal defect, an overriding aorta, and an obstructed right ventricular outflow tract. The obstructive component is found in 85% of cases. Timing of the ligature placement is critical to the appearance of these anomalies. The embryologic insult must occur at the point when the conotruncal cushions are just beginning to develop. This corresponds to a developmental stage in which septation has not yet occurred and the aorta has not migrated to its definitive position. The conoventricular groove is disturbed by the ligature such that the components of the septum are not properly assembled and the aorta remains partially committed to the right ventricle. The fourth component of tetralogy of Fallot, hypertrophy of the right ventricle, is a secondary change developing in response to the pulmonary stenosis. From the embryologic standpoint, as has been described by Van Praagh, this complex of anomalies is actually a "monology," all features relating to the underdevelopment of the subpulmonary infundibulum (conus). The conus is defined by the crista supraventricularis, which extends as the parietal band to the right ventricular free wall. During development, the crista must show movement and expansile growth in a posterior, inferior, and rightward direction to achieve proper closure of the ventricular septal defect and allow an unobstructed right ventricular outflow tract (Fig. 26–7A). The crista should ultimately fill the "Y" created by the arms of the septal band that extends up from the body of the ventricle. Failure of this embryologic step leads to the appearance of a malalignment type of ventricular septal defect that is characteristic of tetralogy of Fallot (see Fig. 26–7B). In addition, the underdeveloped infundibulum, through a process of hypertrophy, causes the obstruction of the right ventricular outflow tract. Overriding of the aorta, as seen in tetralogy of Fallot, is an expression of a normal developmental stage. The aorta is often dilated in reciprocal proportion to the underdevelopment of the pulmonary artery, reflecting altered flows in the embryo due to the primary developmental abnormality of the conus. In addition, the degree of overriding tends to be related to the degree of underdevelopment of the pulmonary artery. This leads to an alteration in the degree of mitral-aortic fibrous continuity. Specifically, the contact with the noncoronary aortic leaflet is not seen. There is contact with the left coronary leaflet. By contrast, in double-outlet right ventricle there is loss of continuity to both leaflets. In cases of tetralogy of Fallot with significant override, the aorta ends up in an abnormally anterior, superior, and rightward location. Since the coronary arteries, as they grow up from the ventricles, seek attachments to the closest coronary ostium, one may find the left anterior descending coronary artery attached to the abnormally anterior facing right coronary ostium.[22, 23]

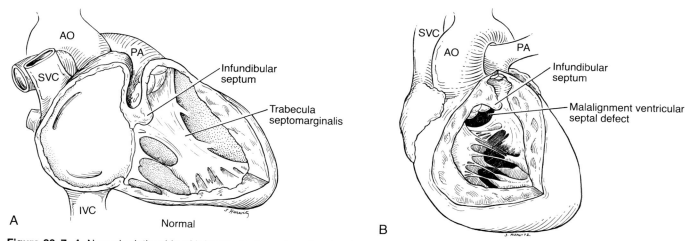

Figure 26–7. *A,* Normal relationship of infundibular (conus) septum to crista supraventricularis. The infundibular septum is noted to fill the "Y" of parietal and septal bands. *B,* Tetralogy of Fallot. The infundibular septum has shifted anterior, superior, and to the left. A malalignment ventricular septal defect and obstruction of the right ventricular outflow tract result. There is resultant right ventricular hypertrophy. The aorta overrides the large defect and is often enlarged.

Subpulmonary Ventricular Septal Defect

The usual ventricular septal defect in tetralogy of Fallot is located beneath the commissure between the right and noncoronary cusp. In addition, the aorta is located posterior and to the right of the pulmonary valve. A variation of these usual findings is the presence of a subpulmonary (doubly committed subarterial) ventricular septal defect. This defect is either immediately adjacent to the pulmonary valve or separated by a thin fibrous ridge. The pulmonary valve is noted to be in a more side-by-side relationship to the aortic valve. The parietal and septal bands that normally join are found to be separate, displaced, and contributing to the obstruction in the right ventricular outflow tract (RVOT). However, the RVOT tends to be less obstructed than in the usual tetralogy. In addition, the main and branch pulmonary arteries tend to be better developed. These cases represent an absence (in most cases) or hypoplasia of the infundibular (conus) septum.[24]

Variations of Anatomy

The main variations of anatomy in tetralogy of Fallot involve the location of the ventricular septal defect, the degree of overriding of the aorta, the amount of infundibular obstruction, the degree of obstruction presented by the pulmonary valve or its annulus, the size of the pulmonary arteries, the nature of the coronary distribution, and the location of the conduction tissue pathways. The usual ventricular septal defect is a malalignment type of defect in a perimembranous location (infracristal). One variation, as described earlier, is the subpulmonary (intracristal or supracristal) defect (see Fig. 26–5). The other type, which may coexist, is the muscular ventricular septal defect, defined by a rim of muscle all the way around the defect. Such a defect may still be in an infundibular location if the posterior limb of septal band is fused with the ventriculoinfundibular fold. Conduction tissue is closest to the defect, in the

usual tetralogy, in which the aortic, mitral, and tricuspid valves come together. In the muscular type defects in the infundibulum and in canal-type defects, the conduction fibers are further away from the rim. The association of tetralogy of Fallot with an AV septal defect is discussed later.

The degree of overriding of the aorta varies from 85% commitment to the left ventricle to 95% commitment to the right ventricle. The latter group is distinguished from double-outlet right ventricle by the presence of mitral-aortic fibrous continuity. Most cases of tetralogy of Fallot have less than half of the aorta overriding the right ventricle.

Obstruction of the pathway to the pulmonary bed can occur at several levels, but the major obstruction in most cases is related to the failure of the crista to grow posterior, inferior, and rightward. The resultant anterior deviation of the crista places muscle directly in the flow pathway through the right ventricular outflow tract. Hypertrophy of adjacent muscle bundles in the anterior ventricular wall adds to the obstruction. In the cases with subpulmonary ventricular septal defect, the obstruction is related to the deviation of arterial septum tissue that separates the two great arteries. Such deviation, in conjunction with muscle bundle hypertrophy, compromises the flow pathway to the pulmonary artery. Additional sources of obstruction in classic tetralogy of Fallot are hypertrophy of the septal band or other muscle bundles, fibrous rings, abnormal position of the moderator band or apical muscle growth leading, in the extreme, to double-chamber right ventricle, and abnormalities of the pulmonary valve leaflets or annulus. The pulmonary arteries may be sufficiently small that "complete" repair may not be possible due to the extensive distal obstruction that persists after relief of infundibular or valvular stenosis.[25]

Complete Atrioventricular Canal

The combination of AV canal (AV septal defect) with tetralogy of Fallot is uncommon. As with classic tetralogy of Fallot, there is a large, nonrestrictive ventricular septal defect and severe outflow tract obstruction with anterosuperior displacement of the infundibular septum and normal pressures in the pulmonary artery distally. The other features that are typically present include primum atrial septal defect, apically displaced AV valve leaflet tissue, and anterior leaflet tissue that at least partially bridges the ventricular septal defect. The ventricular septal defect has features of both tetralogy of Fallot and AV canal in that it involves portions of the perimembranous region and the inlet septum. There is some subaortic extension of the defect in contrast to the AV canal with simple valvular pulmonary stenosis in which the defect is in the inlet portion of the septum.[26]

Double-Outlet Right Ventricle and Tetralogy of Fallot

These two conditions may have considerable overlap. If one notes that the conus muscle that constitutes the infundibular septum serves to define the boundary between the two outflow tracts, then it follows that overriding will have associated malalignment of the conus and, therefore, malalignment of the superior rim of the ventricular septal defect with the inferior border of the ventricular septum. A helpful feature that is characteristic of tetralogy of Fallot is a malalignment ventricular septal defect that includes insertion of the infundibular septum anterosuperior to the superior limb of septal band (see Fig. 26–7B). There is an abnormal insertion of the infundibular septum in double-outlet right ventricle but the point of insertion varies, allowing the ventricular septal defect to be subaortic, subpulmonary, or doubly committed (Fig. 26–8). The defect in tetralogy of Fallot tends to be more extensive, involving both the perimembranous region and the infundibular area, such that the superior rim of the defect is bounded by the aortic cusps. Loss of continuity between the mitral valve and aortic valve is not necessarily a requirement for the

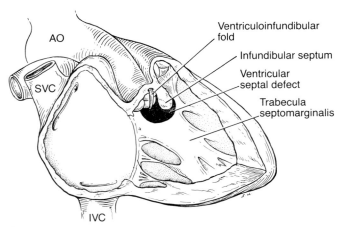

Figure 26–8. Double-outlet right ventricle. There is a large ventricular septal defect which, depending on the position of the infundibular septum, can be subaortic, subpulmonary, or doubly committed. The degree of outflow obstruction is variable. At least 50% of the aorta is noted to override the crest of the septum.

diagnosis of double-outlet right ventricle. A simpler definition is the origin of at least 50% of both great arteries from the right ventricle. This definition would include cases with malposition of the aorta. A further distinction of double-outlet right ventricle is the variability of the pulmonary stenosis that may or may not be due to the anterosuperior insertion of the superior limb of septal band.[27]

Aortopulmonary Collateral Arteries

Cases of tetralogy of Fallot can have aortopulmonary collateral arteries but not to the extent of pulmonary atresia with ventricular septal defect (tetralogy-pulmonary atresia). In cases of tetralogy of Fallot, the central pulmonary arteries are developed and all the bronchopulmonary segments are connected to them. Collaterals, when present, are fewer in number than cases with pulmonary atresia. The presence of collaterals does not necessarily correlate with the severity of the tetralogy of Fallot. The severity of obstruction, which is complete in cases with pulmonary atresia, does appear to contribute to the embryologic sequence that allows multiple collaterals to be present. One view of tetralogy of Fallot with pulmonary atresia is that there is an error in partitioning the distal bulbus cordis and the truncus arteriosus. Consequently, the flow from both ventricles is into the developing fourth arch at the expense of the sixth arch. Impaired development of the sixth arch can lead to absent ductus, small or absent pulmonary artery branches, and persistence of the more primitive intersegmental arteries that link the developing pulmonary vascular bed with the descending aorta.[28, 29]

Surgical Implications

The classic tetralogy of Fallot with severe obstruction will present in infancy and require a shunt or corrective procedure. By contrast, those cases with subpulmonary ventricular septal defect tend to have less obstruction both at the infundibular level and in the main pulmonary artery and branches. Such infants are seldom cyanotic and rarely require operation in infancy. However, when surgery is done, the act of closing the ventricular septal defect increases the severity of the outflow obstruction such that a majority end up needing patch graft enlargement of the RV outflow tract. The cases with tetralogy and AV canal are a major surgical challenge. The ventricular septal defect, because of its extent and multiplanar arrangement, represents a more complex repair. In addition, the patch has to be tailored to avoid subaortic obstruction. In cases of AV canal in which the aortic overriding is more consistent with double-outlet right ventricle, and the ventricular septal defect is doubly committed, successful direct repair is difficult, necessitating a Rastelli procedure or modified Fontan type of palliation. In patients with tetralogy of Fallot with collaterals, particularly when the central or intrapulmonary arteries are small, the goal of surgery is to promote growth of those arteries. Accordingly, a shunt to increase pulmonary blood flow may be a necessary first step before complete repair. The steps of balloon angioplasty and embolization, frequently required in cases with pulmonary atresia, are less often needed in classic tetralogy of Fallot. An interesting anatomic variation in severe tetralogy of Fallot is the origin of a pulmonary artery, usually the left, from the ductus arteriosus. In some cases with bilateral ducti, both the left and right pulmonary arteries can have a ductal origin. These can be confusing when the ductus closes after birth, suggesting that the involved pulmonary artery is absent when, in fact, it is present but isolated and not able to be filled on an angiogram in the main pulmonary artery. Prostaglandin can be used to achieve ductal patency, allow antegrade filling of the involved pulmonary artery, and clarify the surgical approach.[24-30]

ATRIOVENTRICULAR CANAL

Embryologic Development

As the interventricular foramen is realigned to allow communication between the developing left ventricle and the aorta, the AV canal undergoes medial shifting to allow the right atrium to communicate with the developing right ventricle. Two separate AV valve orifices begin to be defined when the superior and inferior cushions fuse. The point of fusion takes on the shape of an arch, the rightward portion contributing to the septal leaflet of tricuspid valve and the left portion contributing to the anterior leaflet of the mitral valve. Septum primum normally fuses with the top of this "arch" of cushion tissue to close the ostium primum. The right side of the "arch" fuses with the muscular septum to close the interventricular foramen. This point of fusion is to the right of the point of atrial fusion, thus leaving an area, the AV septum, where, if deficient, left ventricle to right atrium shunting can occur. In cases with complete AV canal, there is failure of fusion of the endocardial cushions and deficiency of the "arch." Consequently, septum primum has no point of fusion, and a primum atrial septal defect is noted. This communication is different than ostium primum that occurs at an earlier developmental stage. The AV septum is absent, and the AV valves are noted to develop in an apically displaced location. This failure of "arch" development also contributes to a failure of proper seating of the aortic valve. Accordingly, the high position of the aortic valve and the low position of the left AV valve defines a long, narrow LVOT, described as a "gooseneck" deformity. When partial fusion of endocardial cushions occur, a cleft in the involved AV valve is noted. When no endocardial cushion fusion occurs, each cushion gives rise to an AV valve leaflet which, in the most extreme form, spans the ventricular septal defect and lacks chordal attachments to the ventricle.

Variations in the shift of the AV canal help to account for certain forms of univentricular heart. These hearts have a common ventricular chamber with the internal morphology of either a right ventricle (excessive shift of AV canal) or left ventricle (inadequate shift of AV

canal). The more common form is a single left ventricle that gives rise to the aorta (transposed) through an outlet chamber. Since the AV canal failed to shift to the right to allow right atrial to RV communication, the only access to the developing right ventricle is through the interventricular foramen. Since development of the right ventricle is arrested, flow from the left ventricle is into the bulbus cordis. Consequently, the persistent communication is called a bulboventricular foramen. The outlet chamber represents the persisting remnant of bulbus cordis. In cases in which the pulmonary artery relates to the outlet chamber, the condition is referred to as a Holmes' heart. It is often noted that the bulbo-ventricular foramen has a horizontal orientation to the outlet chamber. This finding is related to failure of the aorta and the interventricular foramen to align toward the left ventricle.

The AV valves receive some contributions from the endocardial cushions, but most of the leaflet tissue, the supporting chordal apparatus, and the papillary muscles are derived from a process of diverticulation and undermining of the ventricle. The leaflets themselves therefore start out as muscular structures and evolve to fibrous cusps. The presence of an anterior papillary muscle and a moderator band in the right ventricle depends on a partial shift of the AV canal towards the right ventricle. If no shift occurs, the anterior papillary muscle and moderator band will be absent. If one considers the developing mitral valve in more detail, it is noted that this left AV valve is receiving contributions from two main endocardial cushions and two left lateral cushions. Accordingly, one developmental stage of the valve consists of four leaflets and four papillary muscles. Normally two of the leaflets are quite small and are situated at the commissures of the main leaflets. In addition, the anterior two papillary muscles move toward each other and fuse. A similar process occurs with the posterior papillary muscles. Variations in these developmental steps or in fundamental gene expression account for the range of left AV valve morphology seen in complete atrioventricular canal. The right AV valve has similar embryology except that there are also contributions to the valve from the conus septum, further complicating the potential arrangement of the anterior and septal leaflets of the tricuspid valve. A unique variation of development of the mitral valve occurs when one of the endocardial cushions partly fuses with one of the lateral cushions. The orifice of the mitral valve ends up divided, a condition referred to as double-orifice mitral valve.[31-33]

Classification of Atrioventricular Canal Defects

The term AV septal defect has been applied to this group of anomalies, because the one consistent feature of all of them is deficiency of the AV septum. Other variations have been described, using the terms endocardial cushion defect (any combination of primum atrial septal defect, canal type ventricular septal defect, or cleft AV valve), partial AV canal (primum atrial septal defect with cleft AV valve), and transitional AV canal (primum atrial septal defect and ventricular septal defect occluded by abnormal chordae/leaflet tissue). The term unbalanced AV canal is used when one of the ventricles fails to develop to normal size. This latter condition is a major concern for the surgeon, particularly when the left ventricle is small. Better understanding of this spectrum of anomalies, particularly as relates to surgical repair, is achieved by defining the character of the AV valve leaflet tissue. In cases with either a common AV valve orifice or two separate orifices, there will be at least five recognizable AV valve leaflets. Of particular interest are the two leaflets that are common to both ventricles: the superior (anterior) and inferior (posterior) leaflets. These leaflets tend to bridge the crest of the ventricular septum to varying degrees. The other three leaflets are confined to one ventricle: mural leaflet in the left ventricle; mural and anterosuperior leaflets in the right ventricle. The nature of the bridging leaflets and their papillary muscle support is central to the Rastelli classification of the AV canal. As viewed from the right ventricle, a papillary muscle is noted at the base of the septal band. It supports the commissure between the mural leaflet and the inferior bridging leaflet. When a medial papillary muscle is noted to support the commissure between the superior bridging leaflet and the anterosuperior leaflet, the pattern fits the classification of Rastelli, type A. With extreme bridging of the superior leaflet, an anterior papillary muscle serves the dual role of supporting both commissures. The anterosuperior leaflet is small in these cases. Such an anatomic arrangement fits the classification of Rastelli, type C. An intermediate form, Rastelli, type B, has an intermediate papillary muscle, part way down the septal band, which supports the commissure between the superior bridging leaflet and the anterosuperior leaflet. This intermediate papillary muscle is sometimes immediately adjacent to the anterior papillary muscle, giving a B/C configuration. An examination of the left ventricle reveals the anterolateral and posteromedial papillary muscles, but they are more lateral than usual in cases of AV septal defect. They serve to support the commissures between the bridging leaflets and the mural leaflet. The latter is smaller than in normal hearts. In cases with dual orifice mitral valve, there are abnormal connections to the more inferior papillary muscle. Some hearts may show a single papillary muscle that is associated with a parachute deformity of the valve.

The relationship between the superior and inferior bridging leaflets is important in the context of ventricular level shunting. In cases with two separate AV valve orifices, the leaflets tend to be fused and connected to the crest of the ventricular septum, preventing any ventricular level shunt. By contrast, those with a common AV valve orifice often have interchordal shunting under the bridging leaflets. More direct shunting is noted in those at the type C end of the spectrum and more interchordal shunting at the type A end of the spectrum.

Independent of the Rastelli type of configuration, there are certain associations of anomalies with AV septal defects that are important. Those with common AV orifice often have associated complex malforma-tions, such as double-outlet right ventricle, tetralogy of Fallot, pulmonary atresia, or total anomalous pulmonary venous return (TAPVR). Those with separate AV valve orifices are more likely to show left heart hypoplasia or obstruction. Coarctation of the aorta can be seen in both types. The association of Down syndrome is four times more likely in those with common AV orifice (41%) than in those with separate orifices (11%). The incomplete types of AV canal are less commonly associated with Down syndrome. Splenic anomalies are seen more in complex, complete AV canal anomalies.[34, 35]

Surgical Implications

If one thinks of AV canal anomalies in terms of the degree of bridging of the superior leaflet, a more accurate Rastelli classification can be achieved. Type B may not always be recognized, however, since it depends on identification of the anomalous papillary muscle that supports the commissure between the superior bridging and anterosuperior leaflet. Cases with unbalanced ventricular development are a major surgical challenge. In cases with a dominant right ventricle, the leaflets on the left tend to be smaller than usual and the right leaflets larger than normal. In cases with a dominant left ventricle, there is a small amount of bridging leaflet tissue attached to the anterolateral papillary muscle with the remainder of the valve attached in the left ventricle. Some of these cases do not lend themselves to standard canal repair. Those with dominant right ventricle and underdevelopment of the left ventricle are further complicated by obstructions in the left ventricular outflow tract (LVOT) and in the arch. The LVOT obstruction is due to a combination of medial attachment of the anterior leaflet, hypertrophy of septal muscle, presence of accessory endocardial cushion tissue, and/or leftward deviation of the conal septum. In the extreme form, the subaortic area may be atretic. Such cases, all related to excessive displacement of the embryologic AV canal toward the bulbus cordis, tend to preclude standard surgical intervention and may require transplantation.[36]

COARCTATION/INTERRUPTION OF THE AORTIC ARCH

Embryologic Development

In early development, the aortic isthmus is uniquely affected by changes in flow since it is positioned between relatively low antegrade flow in the distal arch and variable ductal shunting to the descending aorta. Obstructions to flow across the LVOT reduce flow to the isthmus and narrowing or interruption tends to result. By contrast, cases of aortic atresia have flow by retrograde filling from the ductus, and the isthmus tends to be normal in size. The isthmus tends to be larger than normal in cases of pulmonary atresia since more of the fetal cardiac output is directed into the ascending aorta. Cases of interruption usually have a large ventricular septal defect and associated complex anomalies such as double-outlet right ventricle or transposition. The interruption appears to reflect events during cardiogenesis. Coarctation may occur as an isolated anomaly, suggesting that the hemodynamic events contributing to its appearance may occur after embryologic development of the heart is complete. In fact, some cases of coarctation may be related to the postnatal event of ductal closure. Coarctation usually involves a shelf of tissue that extends in the aortic wall around its circumference skipping the lower portion of the wall in which the ductus inserts. There is debate about the role of ductal tissue as a participant in this shelf. Some have suggested that the observed alteration in the media is derived from thickening of the rim of the orifice of the left subclavian artery. This, in turn, is felt to be related to the embryologic event of migration of dorsal intersegmental arteries. Rolling in of the fourth aortic arch towards the future ascending aorta leads to a medial pull on the left subclavian artery (derived from the sixth cervical intersegmental artery), thus creating a shelf. Similar shelves can be associated with the orifices of the other arch vessels. When a shelf is present, a newborn may show no evidence for obstruction during the first week or two but then show loss of femoral pulses as the ductus closes. Histologic study of cases of coarctation and tubular hypoplasia of the aorta has shown that the isthmus has normal histology compared with the rest of the aorta, showing regularly spaced elastic lamellae. The ductus has a more muscular makeup. This ductal tissue can be found to form a sling around the distal orifice of the aortic isthmus, contributing to obstruction in cases of tubular hypoplasia and coarctation. The presence of this tissue is felt to be derived from the sixth arch rather than an ectopic spread of ductal tissue into the aorta. Specifically, the left sixth arch gives rise in its proximal portion to the pulmonary artery and in its distal portion to the ductus. The distal left sixth arch fuses with the left fourth aortic arch and descending aorta. This junction, just opposite the ductus, is the site of obstruction in coarctation. Accordingly, there may be a dynamic component to coarctation obstruction related to ductal closure and an associated "lasso" constriction of the circumference of the aorta (Fig. 26–9).

The development of interruption of the aortic arch may be affected not only by changes in flow in the embryo but also by altered migration of neural crest cells. Such cells contribute to the development of the aortic arch and the conotruncal region of the heart. In addition, neural crest cells are important in the development of the thymus. Consequently, the association of DiGeorge syndrome and interruption of the aortic arch may be related to neural crest abnormalities.[37-43]

Associated Intracardiac Anomalies

Certain intracardiac anomalies contribute to diminished aortic blood flow that may contribute to arch obstruction. The malalignment type of ventricular septal defect in which there is a deviation of the conus septum into the LVOT causes obstruction to the outflow tract. The pathology of hearts with this type of ventricular septal defect invariably includes coarctation, tubular hypoplasia, or interruption of the aorta. By contrast, the "Eisenmenger" type of ventricular septal defect, in which there is anterior deviation of the conus septum into the RVOT, is associated with a normal aortic arch. In a significant number of hearts, there is noted an anterolateral muscle bundle adjacent to the LVOT, lying between the left coronary cusp and the anterior leaflet of the mitral valve. This muscle bundle is derived from the fold of tissue in the embryo that helps to define the ostium between the developing (left) ventricle and the bulbus cordis. If there is abnormal myocardial growth in this bulboventricular region, a prominent anterolateral muscle bundle results. Additional abnormal trabeculae may result in the LVOT, contributing to obstruction. In addition, since the anterior leaflet of the mitral valve is partly derived from the bulboventricular fold, there can be associated mitral valve disease. The aortic arch obstructions in cases with prominent anterolateral muscle bundle tend to be less severe with fewer interruptions than cases with deviated conal septum in which the obstruction to the LVOT tends to be greater. An error in the process of septation can give rise to an additional source of LVOT obstruction, a posteromedial muscle bundle, which sits in the groove where membranous septum, mitral valve, and aortic valve come together.

In hearts with a restrictive bulboventricular foramen, there can be diminished flow to a malposed or transposed aorta with associated arch obstruction. It is apparent that the sixth week of embryologic development is a critical time since the processes of arch formation, ductal development, and septation are all proceeding simultaneously. A structural abnormality or even a transient flow disturbance at this stage can contribute to arch malformations.[44-46]

Aortic Valve

Obstruction of the aortic arch is commonly associated with an abnormality of the aortic valve. A bicuspid aortic valve will be found in many cases of coarctation of the aorta. The valve may show a band at the base of the undivided cusp instead of a normal commissure

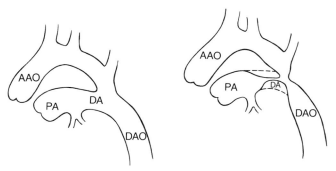

Figure 26–9. Coarctation of the aorta. Some cases of coarctation have a well-developed "shelf" that obstructs flow. Other cases, as shown here, develop an obstruction as ductal tissue "lassos" the aortic wall postnatally.

between the right and left coronary cusps. Actual aortic stenosis tends to be less common, less than 10% of cases in an autopsy series. However, the presence of a bicuspid aortic valve can lead to stenosis and/or regurgitation over time. These processes can be further complicated by calcification or infection.[47]

Mitral Valve

A range of abnormalities of the mitral valve can be found on examination of cases of coarctation of the aorta. If diminished flow occurs in the embryo during the period of undermining and diverticulation of the left ventricle, two possible developmental errors of the mitral valve may occur: the leaflet tissue may be deficient, creating a small valve, or the papillary muscles may form abnormally, showing adherence to each other or lack of separation from the ventricular wall. Independent of changes of flow, primary developmental errors in formation of ventricular myocardium may contribute to the observed abnormalities. Cases with a single papillary muscle, the parachute mitral valve, may fall into this category. The mitral valve may also show restricted movement of the free margin of the leaflets due to alteration of chordal length and space between chordae tendineae. Variations in papillary muscle separation and in chordal length can lead to either stenosis or regurgitation of the valve. Both types of abnormalities have been noted in association with coarctation of the aorta.[48]

Surgical Implications

Identification of coarctation of the aorta should lead to investigation of the size of the left ventricle, the nature of the mitral and aortic valves, the status of the LVOT, and the association of intracardiac shunts. The specific type of any associated ventricular septal defect should be determined. Surgical correction of the coarctation may not significantly benefit the patient if more proximal obstructions or intracardiac shunts are left unrepaired. In many cases, an initial coarctation repair from a left thoracotomy can be followed later by a median sternotomy approach to intracardiac repair. Cases with multiple ventricular septal defects often require pulmonary artery banding at the time of coarctation repair. Some with severe but correctible intracardiac anomalies require a one-stage approach. Such an approach is now used in most cases with interruption of the aortic arch. In such cases, the ventricular septal defect is large and there is a leftward shift of the conus septum that obstructs the LVOT. Reconstruction of the arch in these cases is more easily accomplished in type A (interruption distal to the left subclavian artery) since the left fourth arch has been incorporated in development giving more arch tissue. Failure of arch incorporation is noted in type B (interruption between the left common carotid and left subclavian arteries), and reconstruction of the arch is more difficult. Some cases may require a tube graft to reconstitute the arch, and banding of the pulmonary arteries may be required.

Infants with interrupted aortic arch, particularly type B, undergoing surgical repair should receive only irradiated blood due to the common association with DiGeorge syndrome and the related risk of graft versus host disease. Type C interruption (between the right common carotid and left common carotid arteries) is rare and represents a major surgical risk due to the high association of severe intracardiac defects.[43–49]

TOTAL ANOMALOUS PULMONARY VENOUS RETURN

Embryologic Development

The vascular system of the developing lung initially relates to the foregut through the splanchnic plexus (see Fig. 26–3A). Connections to the primitive systemic veins are also noted at this time. The cardinal venous system ultimately gives rise to the left superior vena cava, the coronary sinus, and the left innominate vein. The omphalomesenteric (umbilicovitelline) system becomes the portal vein and ductus venosus. Initially, there is no connection of the developing pulmonary veins to the heart. This connection depends on the outgrowth, from the sinoatrial portion of the heart, of the common pulmonary vein (see Fig. 26–3B). The common pulmonary vein becomes incorporated into the back wall of the left atrium, allowing definitive pulmonary venous connection (see Fig. 26–3C). These events proceed during the fourth week of intrauterine development, a time when the embryonic heart is establishing an active heart beat.[50–54]

Anomalies of pulmonary venous return and obstructions of flow to the left heart can occur through several embryologic errors. If the common pulmonary vein becomes obliterated early in development, the developing pulmonary venous drainage will proceed through the splanchnic plexus to one or more of the systemic venous systems. Connection to the cardinal system leads to total anomalous pulmonary venous return of the supracardiac type (to the left innominate vein or left superior vena cava), intracardiac type (to the coronary sinus), or mixed types. Persistent connection to the umbilicovitelline system leads to infradiaphragmatic TAPVR. Since the ductus venosus constricts after birth, this form of TAPVR is usually obstructed. If the connection between the common pulmonary vein and the left atrium is narrowed but not obliterated, the resultant developmental steps lead to cor triatriatum. If the stenosis is severe, the connections to the primitive venous systems are maintained, and both cor triatriatum and total anomalous pulmonary venous return are noted. Occasional cases of TAPVD are noted in which the common pulmonary vein persists as an atretic strand. An additional factor influencing the pattern of anomalous venous return is the point of connection of the common pulmonary vein to the left atrium. A shift in its position to either side can lead to connection to either the right horn of sinus venosus, which drains the right common cardinal system, or the left horn of sinus venosus, which drains the left common cardinal system.

The right cardinal system ultimately gives rise to the azygos vein and superior vena cava while the left cardinal system gives rise to the coronary sinus. Cases of partial anomalous pulmonary venous return occur if some of the lung buds maintain persistent communication with the primitive systemic venous system despite appropriate development of the common pulmonary vein. If the right lung bud itself develops abnormally, the pattern of scimitar syndrome can be seen. This syndrome includes anomalous venous drainage of all lobes of the right lung, systemic arterial supply to one lobe (usually right lower lobe) of the right lung, and appropriate connection of the right lung to the right bronchus. Since the embryologic error occurs at an earlier stage, the lung itself is underdeveloped. The right lung pulmonary veins connect to the inferior vena cava, which is nearly always right sided, thus explaining the lack of cases of left-sided scimitar syndrome.[55]

Transition at Birth

Anomalous pulmonary venous return, when obstructed, presents early as pulmonary edema. Specifically, there is pulmonary venous hypertension that leads to increased pulmonary capillary pressure and leak of fluid into alveoli. Several mechanisms may come into play to minimize pulmonary edema. The pulmonary arteriolar bed may show constriction as a reflex, thus reducing flow into the pulmonary vascular bed. In addition, bronchopulmonary veins may be recruited to allow a path from the lungs to the systemic venous bed. In turn, the lymphatic system can provide some alternative drainage. Finally, over time, there may be some alteration of the permeability in the pulmonary capillary walls themselves.[51] Once the obstruction is relieved, reflex pulmonary arteriolar hypertension, even that associated with changes in the media histologically, should resolve in infants. Protection of the pulmonary bed by isolated pulmonary stenosis is an uncommon association in TAVR. On the other hand, a broad range of complex associated heart disease has been found, particularly in cases of asplenia and polysplenia.[56]

Surgical Implications

Patients with total anomalous pulmonary venous disease (TAPVD) may be noted to have pulmonary artery pressure equal to or greater than systemic pressure at preoperative cardiac catheterization, but not all such cases are obstructed (about three quarters of such patients are obstructed). Similarly, patients with pulmonary artery pressure less than systemic pressure are usually (87%) unobstructed.[54]

Successful surgery depends on the presence of a connecting vein that runs behind the back wall of the left atrium, thus allowing a natural site for anastomosis. Certain cases, such as TAPVD to the right atrium may lack such a vein, necessitating a "tunnel" procedure from the right atrium to the left atrium via an atrial communication. A similar lack of a convenient vein for anastomosis may be seen in cases with drainage to the coronary sinus. Such cases may require creation of a partially unroofed coronary sinus to allow communication into the left atrium.[54] Innovative approaches are needed for mixed types of TAPVD, and staged procedures may be required in cases with anomalous pulmonary venous return and associated complex heart disease.

References

1. Ruckman RN: Functional development of the heart: Hemodynamics. In: Meisami E and Timiras PS (eds): Handbook of Human Growth and Developmental Biology, Vol. 3. Boca Raton, CRC Press, 1990, pp. 69–83.
2. Van Mierop LHS: Morphological development of the heart. In: Berne RM, Sperelakis N, and Geiger SR (eds): Handbook of Physiology, Section 2. Bethesda, American Physiological Society, 1979, pp. 1–28.
3. Rudolph AM: Distribution and regulation of blood flow in the fetal lamb. Circ Res 57(6):811, 1985.
4. Anderson DA, Faber JJ, Morton MJ, et al: Flow through the foramen ovale of the fetal and newborn lamb. J Physiol 365:29, 1985.
5. Edelstone DI: Regulation of blood flow through the ductus venosus. J Dev Physiol 2:219, 1980.
6. St. John Sutton MG, Raichlen JS, Reichek N, et al: Quantitative assessment of right and left ventricular growth in the human fetal heart: A pathoanatomic study. Circulation 70(6):935, 1984.
7. Rudolph AM: The fetal circulation and its response to stress. J Dev Physiol 6:11, 1984.
8. Moss AJ, Emmanouilides G, and Duffie ER: Closure of the ductus arteriosus in the newborn infant. Pediatrics 32:25, 1963.
9. Leffler CW, Hessler JR, and Green RS: The onset of breathing at birth stimulates pulmonary vascular prostacyclin synthesis. Pediatr Res 18(10):938, 1984.
10. Heymann MA, Rudolph AM, and Silverman NH: Closure of the ductus arteriosus in premature infants by inhibition of prostaglandin synthesis. N Engl J Med 295(10):530, 1976.
11. Padbury JF, Diakomanolis ES, Hobel CJ, et al: Neonatal adaptation: Sympatho-adrenal response to neonatal cord cutting. Pediatr Res 15:1483, 1981.
12. Breall JA, Rudolph AM, and Heymann MA: Role of thyroid hormone in postnatal circulatory and metabolic adjustments. J Clin Invest 73:1418, 1984.
13. Goor DA, Edwards JE, and Lillehei W: The development of the interventricular septum of the human heart. Chest 58(5):453, 1970.
14. Allwork SP and Anderson RH: Developmental anatomy of the membranous part of the ventricular septum in the human heart. Br Heart J 41:275, 1979.
15. Mitchell SC, Berendes HW, and Clark WM: The normal closure of the ventricular septum. Am Heart J 73(3):334, 1967.
16. Tatsuno K, Ando M, Takao A, et al: Diagnostic importance of aortography in conal ventricular septal defect. Am Heart J 89(2):171, 1975.
17. Jimenez MQ, Martinez VMP, Azcarate MJM, et al: Exaggerated displacement of the atrioventricular canal towards the bulbus cordis (rightward displacement of the mitral valve). Br Heart J 35:65, 1973.
18. Milo S, Ho SY, Macartney FJ, et al: Straddling and overriding atrioventricular valves: Morphology and classification. Am J Cardiol 44:1122, 1979.
19. De La Cruz MV and Miller BL: Double inlet left ventricle: Two pathological specimens with comments on the embryology and on its relation to single ventricle. Circulation 37:249, 1968.
20. Mehrizi A, McMurphy DM, Ottesen OE, et al: Syndrome of double inlet left ventricle: Angiocardiographic differentiation from single ventricle with rudimentary outlet chamber. Bull Johns Hopkins Hosp 119:255, 1966.
21. Lincoln C, Jamieson S, Joseph M, et al: Transatrial repair of

ventricular septal defects with reference to their anatomic classification. J Thorac Cardiovasc Surg 74(2):183, 1977.

22. Aranega A, Egea J, Alvarez L, et al: Tetralogy of Fallot produced in chick embryos by mechanical interference with cardiogenesis. Anat Rec 213:560, 1985.

23. Van Praagh RV, Van Praagh S, Nebesar RA, et al: Tetralogy of Fallot: Underdevelopment of the pulmonary infundibulum and its sequelae. Am J Cardiol 26:25, 1970.

24. Neirotti R, Galindez E, Kreutzer G, et al: Tetralogy of Fallot with subpulmonary ventricular septal defect. Ann Thorac Surg 25(1):51, 1978.

25. Anderson RH, Allwork SP, Ho SY, et al: Surgical anatomy of tetralogy of Fallot. J Thorac Cardiovasc Surg 81:887, 1981.

26. Uretzky G, Puga FJ, Danielson GK, et al: Complete atrioventricular canal associated with tetralogy of Fallot: Morphologic and surgical considerations. J Thorac Cardiovasc Surg 87:756, 1984.

27. Edwards WD: Double outlet right ventricle and tetralogy of Fallot: Two distinct but not mutually exclusive entities. J Thorac Cardiovasc Surg 82:418, 1981.

28. Ramsay JM, Macartney FJ, and Haworth SG: Tetralogy of Fallot with major aortopulmonary collateral arteries. Br Heart J 53:167, 1985.

29. Thiene G, Frescura C, Bortolotti U, et al: The systemic pulmonary circulation in pulmonary atresia with ventricular septal defect: Concept of reciprocal development of the fourth and sixth aortic arches. Am Heart J 101(3):339, 1981.

30. Jedeikin R, Rheuban KS, Carpenter MA, et al: Ductal origin of the left pulmonary artery in severe tetralogy of Fallot: Problems in management. Pediatr Cardiol 5:323, 1984.

31. Van Mierop LHS: Embryology of the atrioventricular canal region and pathogenesis of endocardial cushion defects. In: Feldt RH (ed): Atrioventricular Canal Defects. Philadelphia, WB Saunders Company, 1976, pp. 1–12.

32. Van Mierop LHS: Embryology of the univentricular heart. Herz 4(2):78, 1979.

33. Van Mierop LHS, Alley RD, Kausel HW, et al: The anatomy and embryology of endocardial cushion defects. J Thorac Cardiovasc Surg 43:71, 1962.

34. Penkoske PA, Neches WH, Anderson RH, et al: Further observations on the morphology of atrioventricular septal defects. J Thorac Cardiovasc Surg 90:611, 1985.

35. Bharati S and Lev M: The spectrum of common atrioventricular orifice (canal). Am Heart J 86(4):553, 1973.

36. Freedom RM, Bini M, and Rowe RD: Endocardial cushion defect and significant hypoplasia of the left ventricle: A distinct clinical and pathological entity. Eur J Cardiol 7:263, 1978.

37. Rudolph AM, Heymann MA, and Spitznas U: Hemodynamic considerations in the development of narrowing of the aorta. Am J Cardiol 30:514, 1972.

38. Talner NS and Berman MA: Postnatal development of obstruction in coarctation of the aorta: Role of the ductus arteriosus. Pediatrics 56(4):562, 1975.

39. Moffat DB: Pre- and post-natal changes in the left subclavian artery and their possible relationship to coarctation of the aorta. Acta Anat 43:346, 1960.

40. Ho SY and Anderson RH: Coarctation, tubular hypoplasia, and the ductus arteriosus: Histological study of 35 specimens. Br Heart J 41:268, 1979.

41. Rosenberg HS: Coarctation of the aorta: Morphology and pathogenetic considerations. Perspec Pediatr Pathol 1:339, 1973.

42. Kirby ML and Bockman DE: Neural crest and normal development: A new perspective. Anat Rec 209:1, 1984.

43. Van Mierop LHS and Kutsche LM: Cardiovascular anomalies in DiGeorge syndrome and importance of neural crest as a possible pathogenetic factor. Am J Cardiol 58:133, 1986.

44. Moulaert AJ, Bruins CC, and Oppenheimer-Dekker A: Anomalies of the aortic arch and ventricular septal defects. Circulation 53(6):1011, 1976.

45. Moene RJ, Oppenheimer-Dekker A, and Wenink ACG: Relation between aortic arch hypoplasia of variable severity and central muscular ventricular septal defects: Emphasis on associated left ventricular abnormalities. Am J Cardiol 48:111, 1981.

46. Moene RJ, Oppenheimer-Dekker A, Moulaert AJ, et al: The concurrence of dimensional aortic arch anomalies and abnormal left ventricular muscle bundles. Pediatr Cardiol 2(2):107, 1982.

47. Tawes RL, Berry CL, and Aberdeen E: Congenital bicuspid aortic valves associated with coarctation of the aorta in children. Br Heart J 31:127, 1969.

48. Rosenquist GC: Congenital mitral valve disease associated with coarctation of the aorta: A spectrum that includes parachute deformity of the mitral valve. Circulation 49:985, 1974.

49. Van Praagh R, Bernhard WF, Rosenthal A, et al: Interrupted aortic arch: Surgical treatment. Am J Cardiol 27:203, 1971.

50. Lucas RV, Woolfrey BF, Anderson RC, et al: Atresia of the common pulmonary vein. Pediatrics 29:729, 1962.

51. Lucas RV, Anderson RC, Amplatz K, et al: Congenital causes of pulmonary venous obstruction. Pediatr Clin North Am 10:781, 1963.

52. Hickie JB, Gimlette TMD, and Bacon APC: Anomalous pulmonary venous drainage. Br Heart J 18:365, 1956.

53. Neill CA: Development of the pulmonary veins with reference to the embryology of anomalies of pulmonary venous return. Pediatrics 18:880, 1956.

54. Delisle G, Ando M, Calder AL, et al: Total anomalous pulmonary venous connection: Report of 93 autopsied cases with emphasis on diagnostic and surgical considerations. Am Heart J 91:99, 1976.

55. Neill C, Ferencz C, Sabiston DC, et al: Familial occurrence of hypoplastic right lung with systemic arterial supply and venous drainage "scimitar syndrome." Bull Johns Hopkins Hosp 107:1, 1960.

56. Bharati S and Lev M: Congenital anomalies of the pulmonary veins. Cardiovasc Clin 5:23, 1973.

Cardiovascular Monitoring and Evaluation

Gerard R. Martin, M.D., and
Deidre G. Holley, M.B., B.S.

Knowledge of cardiovascular monitoring and evaluation is important for all personnel involved in pediatric critical care medicine. The primary function of the cardiovascular system is the transport of oxygen and other nutrients and the removal of metabolic waste products.[1] This is achieved by the pumping action of the heart and the propulsion of blood through the vascular tree. Maintenance of a normal cardiac output is dependent on normal systolic function of the heart. The four major determinants of systolic function are heart rate, preload, afterload, and contractility. There are important interactions among these determinants that have an impact on systolic function of the heart.[2]

Heart function may also be affected by alterations in filling properties (diastolic function), respiratory function, and pulmonary arterial pressure and resistance. This chapter focuses on noninvasive and invasive methods of cardiovascular monitoring in the pediatric critical care patient (Table 27–1) and shows how to separate the four determinants of cardiac function using both of these methods of cardiovascular monitoring.

NONINVASIVE EVALUATION

Physical Examination

Cardiac structural abnormalities can be detected by physical examination. This type of evaluation also aids in the assessment of cardiac function because of its

ability to detect patients with low cardiac output states. The physical findings of low cardiac output are weak peripheral pulses, cool extremities, pallor, decreased capillary refill, tachycardia, and hypotension. Detection of low cardiac output by physical examination has been noted to have particular significance in the prognosis of postoperative cardiac surgical patients.[3] Surgical mortality is increased when low cardiac output is detected in the early postoperative period. However, the accuracy of physical examination in predicting cardiac output has been a subject of controversy.[4, 5] In controlled studies, estimates of cardiac output based on physical examination have lacked both sensitivity and specificity when compared with cardiac output measurements made by thermodilution technique. Physical examination appears to be better suited for identifying relative changes in cardiac output rather than isolated cardiac output measurements in time.

Tachycardia and weak peripheral pulses are signs of low cardiac output that should be readily apparent on physical examination. Heart rate abnormalities, which cause low cardiac output states, should also be readily apparent on physical examination. Ascertaining whether tachycardia is a sign or the cause of the low cardiac output may, however, be difficult. Bradycardia, caused by complete heart block, should be easily detected by physical examination. Heart rates less than 60 beats per minute (bpm) in association with other signs of congestive heart failure should immediately lead to the suspicion of heart block, and a electrocardiogram should be obtained. Abnormalities of preload, afterload, and contractility are less well defined by physical examination and require further evaluation.

Laboratory Evaluation

The evaluation of cardiac function can be helped by laboratory tests. Determination of electrolyte, acid-base, and substrate abnormalities is important because of their direct effects on cardiac function. Also, abnor-

Table 27–1. NONINVASIVE AND INVASIVE CARDIOVASCULAR MONITORING

Noninvasive	Invasive
Physical examination	Intra-arterial pressure
Laboratory evaluation	Central venous pressure
Electrocardiography	Pulmonary wedge pressure
Oximetry-capnography	Cardiac output
Echocardiography	Cardiac catheterization
Roentgenography	

malities in electrolytes, acid-base balance, and substrates may occur because of low cardiac output, thus compounding the decreased cardiac function. Serum electrolyte, blood urea nitrogen, creatinine, calcium, and blood glucose levels, as well as arterial blood gases, should be measured at baseline and then periodically during the period of suspected low cardiac output.

Electrocardiography

Both primary and secondary cardiac abnormalities can be detected by electrocardiography. When cardiac function is abnormal or when structural heart disease is suspected, a 12-lead electrocardiogram should be obtained. Interpretation of electrocardiograms in children is different than it is in adults, and appropriate references should be used.[6, 7] Rate, rhythm, axis, electrical intervals (PR, QRS, QTc), and chamber size should be determined, and injury patterns (ischemia) should be identified. A full discussion of electrocardiographic abnormalities is beyond the scope of this chapter, but a few monitoring aspects deserve special mention (see also Chapter 36).

Difficulties may arise in determining whether tachycardia results from a sinus mechanism (sinus tachycardia) or from paroxysmal atrial tachycardia. The heart rate may provide clues to the diagnosis. The heart rate in sinus tachycardia rarely exceeds 200 bpm, and in paroxysmal atrial tachycardia it is usually greater than 200 bpm unless there is associated 2:1 atrioventricular block. Signs of atrial depolarization (p waves) are usually present on the electrocardiogram in sinus tachycardia, but they may be lacking or retrograde in many cases of paroxysmal atrial tachycardia. The QRS interval is most often narrow in both instances, but it can be widened if there is a rate-dependent bundle branch block in sinus tachycardia or aberration in paroxysmal atrial tachycardia. If previous electrocardiograms are available, it is useful to compare the QRS vectors during tachycardia and sinus rhythm.

During the early postoperative period following a cardiothoracic procedure, p waves may be difficult to visualize on surface electrocardiography. Temporary atrial pacemaker wires can be used to record an atrial electrocardiogram.[8] These leads are more likely to allow definitive diagnosis of atrial tachycardia (Fig. 27–1). If atrial pacemaker wires are not available, an esophageal electrode may be placed to obtain a similar atrial tracing.[9]

When paroxysmal atrial tachycardia is diagnosed, rhythm strips should be obtained during therapeutic trials. Many drugs that are used in the treatment of tachycardia have significant rhythm abnormalities as side effects. Adenosine has become a frequently used drug for the treatment of paroxysmal atrial tachycardia, which results from a re-entry mechanism that usually involves the atrioventricular node. Adenosine causes a transient, complete heart block that interrupts the re-entry cycle, and thus it medically converts the rhythm to a sinus mechanism (Fig. 27–2). In atrial ectopic tachycardia, there is no re-entry cycle to interrupt. Adenosine still

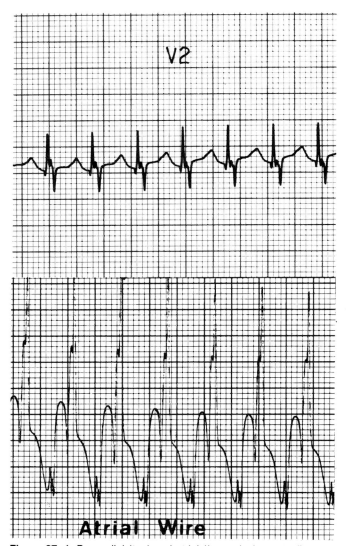

Figure 27–1. Precordial (*top*) and atrial (*bottom*) electrocardiograms in a cardiac patient postoperatively. Precordial lead shows rapid, narrow QRS rhythm. Atrial lead shows atrial depolarizations preceding each ventricular depolarization, confirming sinus tachycardia.

causes transient, complete heart block in atrial ectopic tachycardia, but rapid atrial depolarizations continue to be present on the rhythm strip.

Correct diagnosis of rhythm abnormalities often requires that rhythm strips be recorded from multiple leads, since rhythm strips from only one lead may lead to an incorrect diagnosis or fail to clearly delineate a rhythm abnormality (Fig. 27–3). Obtaining rhythm strips from other leads may make the diagnosis of premature ventricular contractions obvious (Fig. 27–4). A complete 12-lead electrocardiogram can be informative when trying to ascertain if there are any electrolyte abnormalities, ischemia, or hypertrophy associated with the rhythm abnormality. All pediatric intensive care patients should receive continuous electrocardiographic monitoring. Tachycardia or bradycardia or other arrhythmias may be the first sign of a change in the patient's status, and thus further evaluation can be performed in a timely fashion.

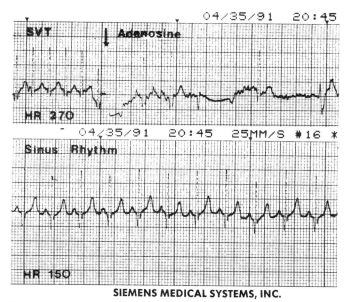

Figure 27–2. Treatment of supraventricular tachycardia (*SVT*) with Adenosine. Adenosine converted SVT to normal sinus rhythm. Short period of complete heart block is present before conversion to sinus rhythm. HR = heart rate.

Atrial enlargement or ventricular hypertrophy is often first suspected after examination of a 12-lead electrocardiogram. The sensitivity and specificity of electrocardiography are good, but errors do occur and confirmatory studies should be obtained.

Respiratory Evaluation

Noninvasive respiratory monitoring has become quite sophisticated. Respiratory rate, oxygenation, and ventilation can all be evaluated noninvasively. Oxygenation can be determined by either transcutaneous oxygen

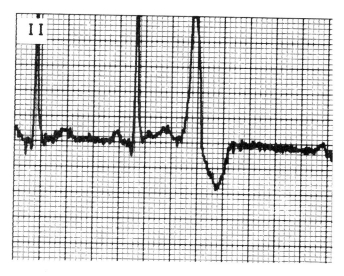

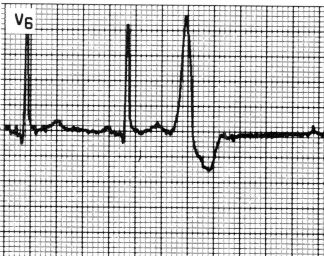

Figure 27–4. Rhythm strip from patient in Figure 27–3 obtained from two other leads. There is more significant aberration of the QRS and T waves, indicating that this ectopic beat is a premature ventricular contraction.

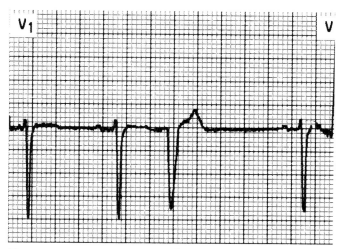

Figure 27–3. Rhythm strip from a single precordial lead shows premature beat. There is only minimal aberration of the QRS shown by this lead.

monitoring (Po_2) or by pulse oximetry (O_2 saturation).[10] Transcutaneous oxygen monitoring has become routine in neonatal intensive care units. Transient periods of high or low oxygen tension can be detected, decreasing the likelihood of oxygen toxicity or hypoxic damage. Pulse oximetry is the simplest means of oxygen saturation monitoring, and it has excellent correlation with measured arterial saturation between values of 60 and 100%. Correlation between pulse oximetry and calculated oxygen saturation may vary significantly. Continuous oxygen saturation monitoring has led to important observations about some disease processes. For instance, pulmonary hypertensive crisis has been shown to be initiated by an abrupt decrease in oxygen saturation. This decrease is usually in response to a painful procedure, a decrease in sedation, or inadequate ventilation. Following the decrease in oxygen saturation, heart rate increases, pulmonary arterial pressure increases, systemic arterial pressure decreases, and metabolic acidosis follows. End-tidal CO_2 measurements are a reliable method of monitoring ventilation.[11] When arterial access is limited, end-tidal gas measurements can be used in the weaning of ventilatory assistance. End-tidal CO_2 measurements should be correlated periodically with arterial P_{CO_2} measurements.

Echocardiography

The most complete noninvasive assessment of cardiac structure and function is provided by echocardiography. Accurate delineation of normal and abnormal cardiac structure is obtained primarily by two-dimensional echocardiographic imaging.[12-15] Atrial and ventricular septal defects can be identified by two-dimensional echocardiography (Fig. 27–5). It also provides information about the size and position of septal defects. Atrial septal defects that have well-defined margins and are safely away from the pulmonary veins and mitral valve may be closed during an interventional cardiac catheterization using a double clamshell device.[16] Echocardiography has proved to be a useful adjunct in the proper placement of the clamshell device[17] (Fig. 27–6).

Knowledge of the size and position of ventricular septal defects in children allows the proper timing of invasive testing and intervention. Nonrestrictive ventricular septal defects have a diameter similar to the outflow tract of the aorta. Nonrestrictive defects result in equalization of pressures between the right and left ventricles. These defects are less likely to close spontaneously and are more likely to cause pulmonary vascular obstructive disease if they are left uncorrected.

Two-dimensional echocardiography not only visualizes the cardiac defect but also, in combination with pulsed Doppler echocardiography, can determine the presence, timing, and direction of shunting, as well as the pressure difference between chambers (Fig. 27–7).

In a patent ductus arteriosus, Doppler echocardiography detects turbulence during both systole and diastole in the pulmonary artery. The Doppler signal also identifies the direction of shunting. Signals displayed above the baseline represent flow that is directed toward the transducer, and signals displayed beneath the baseline represent flow away from the transducer. Thus in the patient in Figure 27–7, flow is identified as traveling from the aorta to the pulmonary artery during both diastole and systole. The velocity of flow between two chambers is related to the pressure difference between the chambers. Using the Bernoulli principle, pulmonary arterial pressure or right ventricular pressure can be predicted in patients with patent ductus arteriosus or ventricular septal defect.[18, 19]

Pulsed Doppler echocardiography can determine the magnitude of the shunt. Calculations of systemic and pulmonary blood flow are made by measuring the cross-sectional areas and mean blood flow velocities of the pulmonary and systemic outflow tracts.[20] The pulmonary:systemic blood flow ratio is a measure of the hemodynamic significance of a septal defect, and the ratio of these measures compares favorably with those that are made at cardiac catheterization.[21] Errors can occur in this measurement, especially in the calculation of the cross-sectional area of the outflow tracts.

Echocardiography has had a dramatic effect on the need for invasive evaluation of congenital heart disease. Although physical examination may not always be able to exclude structural heart disease, echocardiography has been shown to accurately detect and guide the care of infants with heart disease.[22-24] Tetralogy of Fallot is the most common form of cyanotic congenital heart disease (Fig. 27–8). Two-dimensional echocardiography clearly shows the anatomic features of tetralogy of Fallot: large ventricular septal defect, overriding aorta, right ventricular outflow tract stenosis, and right ventricular hypertrophy.

Echocardiography may also be helpful in the thera-

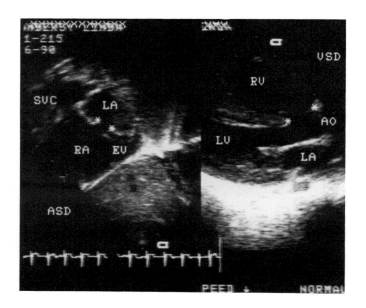

Figure 27–5. Two-dimensional echocardiogram of an atrial septal defect (ASD) (*left*); and a ventricular septal defect (*right; VSD*). Secundum atrial septal defect (*asterisks on left*) is shown from the subcostal short axis view of the heart. Ventricular septal defect (*asterisks on right*) is shown from the parasternal long axis view of the heart. AO = aorta; EV = eustachian valve, LA = left atrium, LV = left ventricle, RA = right atrium, RV = right ventricle, SVC = superior vena cava.

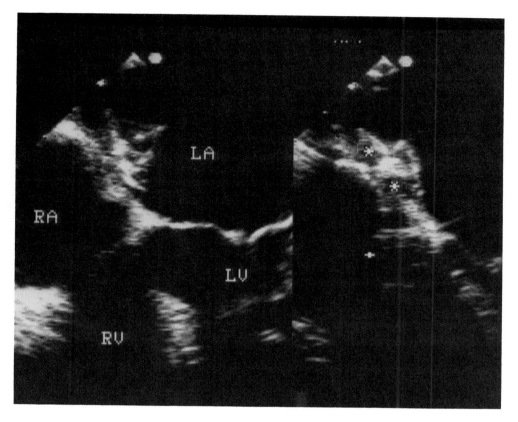

Figure 27–6. Transesophageal echocardiogram during an interventional catheterization. Clamshell device is opened in the left atrium and positioned in the midportion of the atrial septal defect (*left*). The right atrial arms of the device are then opened after confirming the location of the edges (*asterisks*) of the defect (*right*). LA = left atrium; LV = left ventricle; RA = right atrium; RV = right ventricle.

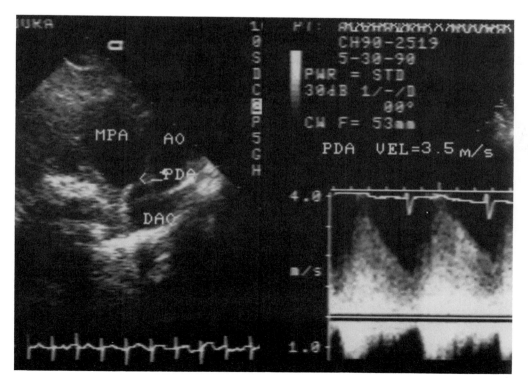

Figure 21–7. Two-dimensional echocardiogram of a patent ductus arteriosus (*left; PDA*) The arrow shows the pulmonary arterial end of the ductus arteriosus. Continuous wave Doppler signal from a patent ductus arteriosus (*right*) shows a peak velocity (VEL) of 3.5 m/sec, which is consistent with a pressure difference of 50 mm Hg between the aorta and pulmonary artery. AO = aorta; MPA = main pulmonary artery; DAO = descending aorta.

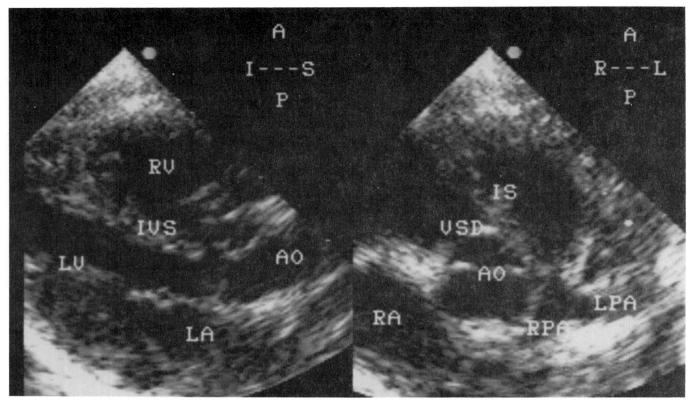

Figure 27–8. Two-dimensional echocardiogram in a patient with tetralogy of Fallot. Ascending aorta straddles the ventricular septum (*IVS*) just above the ventricular septal defect (*left*). Infundibular septum (IS) is deviated anteriorly, narrowing the right ventricular outflow tract (*right*). A = anterior; P = posterior; I = inferior; S = superior; AO = aorta; LPA = left pulmonary artery; LA = left atrium; LV = left ventricle; RV = right ventricle; RA = right atrium; VSD = ventricular septal defect; RPA = right pulmonary artery.

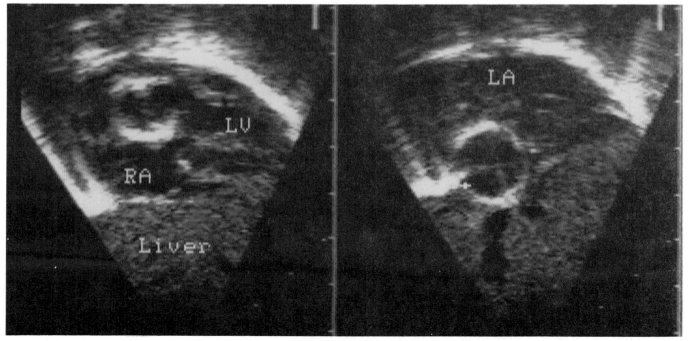

Figure 27–9. Two-dimensional echocardiogram during balloon atrial septostomy. The septostomy catheter is positioned and inflated in the left atrium (*left*) and then pulled across the atrial septum to the right atrium (*right*). LV = left ventricle; RA = right atrium; LA = left atrium.

peutic management of some diseases—for example, it has been helpful in documenting the position of septostomy catheters during cardiac catheterization in infants with d-transposition of the great arteries.[25] In some situations, balloon septostomy is performed in the intensive care unit without fluoroscopic guidance (Fig. 27–9). In the postoperative cardiac patient, pericardial effusion is a potentially life-threatening condition. Echocardiography can make the diagnosis, guide the positioning of the pericardiocentesis needle, and confirm the final position of the needle prior to removing fluid (Fig. 27–10). Saline contrast may be used to aid in the identification of needle position.

Occasionally transthoracic echocardiography does not provide adequate images for definitive diagnosis. Transesophageal echocardiography can be performed in the intensive care unit and provides images when there are inadequate transthoracic windows (Fig. 27–11). Obesity, prior cardiac surgery, ventilator therapy, and chest wall deformities can all impede adequate transthoracic imaging. The diagnosis of intracardiac vegetations, small cardiac tumors or thrombi, valvular disease, aortic dissection, and atrial septal defects, and the timely assessment of cardiac repairs intraoperatively and postoperatively have been improved by transesophageal imaging (Fig. 27–12).[26, 27]

Many useful measures of systolic cardiac function can be made by echocardiography; however, only ejection phase indexes have gained wide clinical acceptance.[28] The simplest measures of cardiac performance are diameters of the cardiac chambers at end diastole (left ventricular end diastole [LVED]) and end systole (left ventricular end systole [LVES]) (Fig. 27–13). End-diastolic measures are a gross measure of the volume status of a patient. Left ventricular shortening fraction (LVED-LVES/LVED, %) is a predictor of the systolic function of the heart. Ejection fraction is similar to shortening fraction but has the advantage of being able to estimate cardiac stroke volume. The velocity of ventricular shortening and left ventricular systolic time intervals have also been noted to be good predictors of ventricular performance. Shortening fraction, ejection fraction, velocity of shortening, and systolic time intervals are simple to measure, readily repeatable, and reliably separate ventricles that perform normally from those that do not, and thus they are appealing to physicians. Ventricular shortening fraction can quickly differentiate the patient with normal systolic function (see Fig. 27–13) from the patient with abnormal systolic function (Fig. 27–14).

Conditions such as hypertrophic cardiomyopathy are associated with increased systolic cardiac function. Hypertrophic cardiomyopathy is readily diagnosed by two-dimensional echocardiography (Fig. 27–15), and Doppler echocardiography is able to detect the presence of any associated left ventricular outflow tract obstruction. The two-dimensional echocardiogram shows the highlights of this condition: thickened cardiac walls, disproportionate septal thickening, decreased left ventricular end-systolic dimension, and increased percentage shortening fraction.

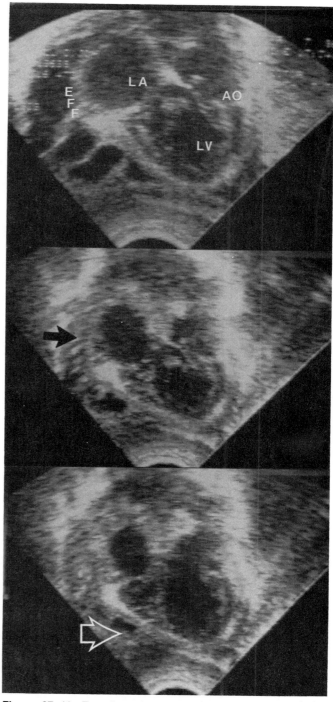

Figure 27–10. Two-dimensional echocardiogram shows a large, loculated pericardial effusion (*top*). After inserting the needle into the pericardium, contrast is injected into and visualized (*black arrow*) in the pericardial space (*middle*). Contrast has filled the pericardial space (*bottom*) except in loculated areas (*open arrow*). AO = aorta; EFF = effusion; LA = left atrium; LV = left ventricle.

The ejection phase indexes of systolic cardiac function measure the global performance of the heart.[29] Performance, however, is determined by heart rate, loading conditions, and contractility of the heart. Heart rate influences systolic function by changes in calcium me-

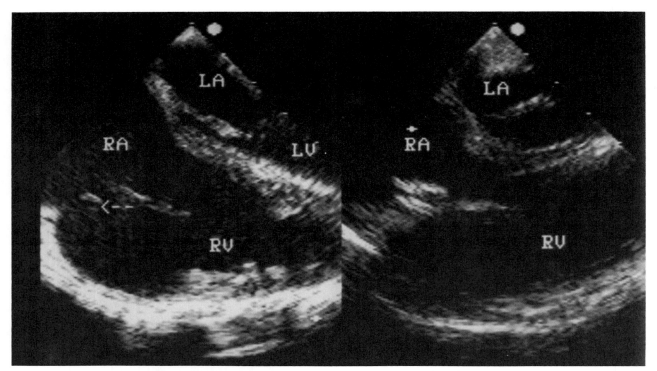

Figure 27–11. Transesophageal echocardiogram in a patient following blunt chest trauma shows a ruptured tricuspid annulus (*left*). Intraoperative transesophageal echocardiogram shows repaired tricuspid annulus (*right*). LA = left atrium; RA = right atrium; LV = left ventricle; RV = right ventricle. Arrow = annulus ruptured.

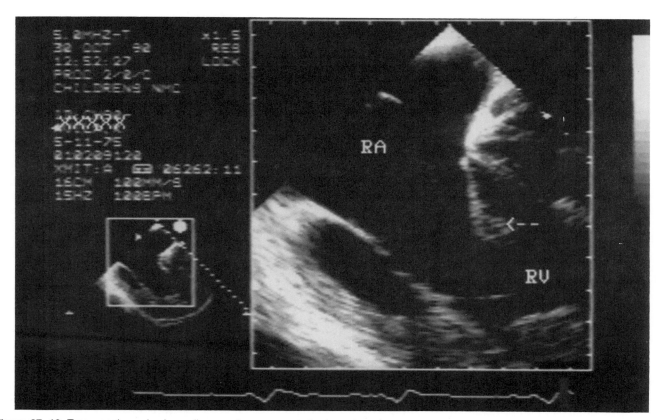

Figure 27–12. Transesophageal echocardiogram shows a vegetation(*arrow*) on the septal leaflet of the tricuspid valve. RA = right atrium; RV = right ventricle.

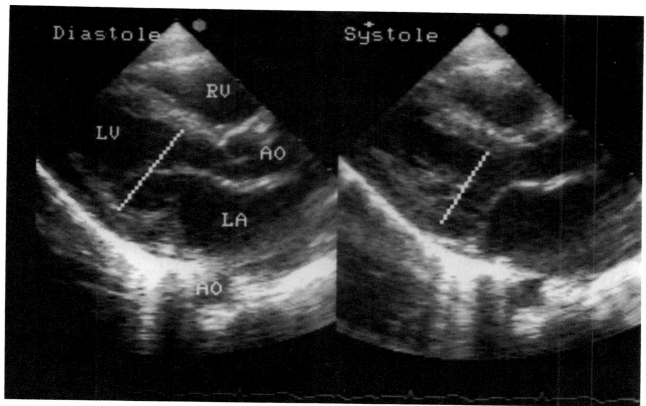

Figure 27–13. Parasternal long axis view of a normal left ventricle shows end-diastolic dimension of 2.5 cm (*left*) and end-systolic dimension of 1.7 cm (*right*). The calculated shortening fraction is 32%. AO = aorta; LA = left atrium; LV = left ventricle; RV = right ventricle.

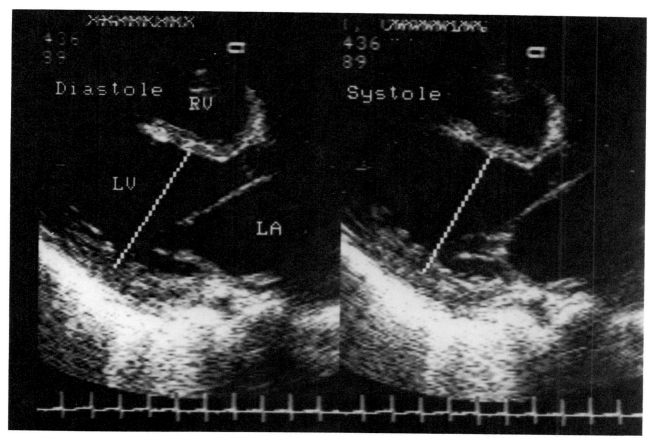

Figure 27–14. Parasternal long axis view of a dilated left ventricle shows an increased left ventricular end-diastolic dimension of 4.0 cm (*left*) and an increased end-systolic dimension of 3.7 cm (*right*). The calculated shortening fraction is 7%. LA = left ventricle; LV = left ventricle: RV = right ventricle.

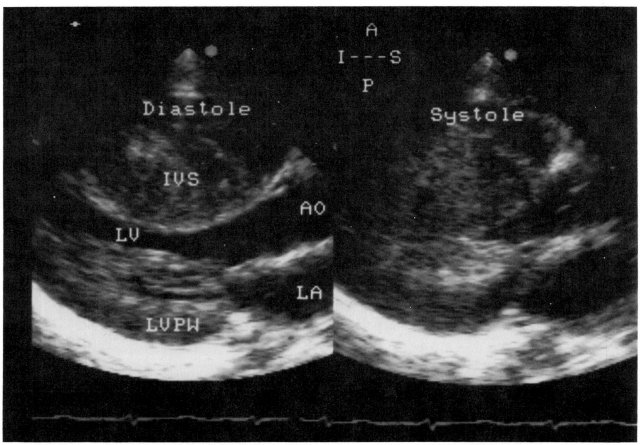

Figure 27–15. Parasternal long axis view of an echocardiogram performed on a child with hypertrophic cardiomyopathy. There is tremendous septal hypertrophy, diminished end-diastolic dimensions (*left*) and cavitary obliteration during systole (*right*). A = anterior; P = posterior; I = inferior; S = superior; AO = aorta; LA = left atrium; LV = left ventricle; IVS = interventricular septum; LVPW = left ventricular posterior wall.

tabolism. Increases in heart rate result in decreased time for uptake of calcium out of the cell and cause an increase in calcium available to the contractile apparatus. The loading conditions of the heart are preload and afterload. Preload is the load felt by the heart muscle before the heart begins to contract. The Frank-Starling phenomenon states that the greater the length of the muscle before the contraction, the greater the development of force. Afterload is the load opposing the muscle once ventricular shortening has begun. The greater the afterload, the less the shortening of muscle that will occur. Echocardiography is able to estimate both preload and afterload. Preload is estimated by the end-diastolic dimensions of the ventricular chambers. Afterload is estimated by ventricular wall stress.

The major determinants of ventricular wall stress are systolic blood pressure, left ventricular chamber diameter, and wall thickness. The relationship between ejection phase indexes of left ventricular performance and wall stress has been studied in children.[29] It has been shown that there is an inverse relationship between left ventricular shortening and wall stress that is independent of preload. For any given patient, there is a range of normal shortening for any given afterload. We routinely perform measures of end-systolic wall stress and velocity of circumferential fiber shortening in all patients in whom cardiac function is in question.

Measurements of diastolic function are being performed with increasing frequency. Many cardiac and noncardiac diseases have been shown to result in altered filling patterns that may be of clinical importance. It is important to note that there are important maturational changes that take place in the filling patterns of the ventricles and that these patterns are also affected by the loading conditions of the heart. The normal and abnormal filling patterns of the heart have recently been reviewed.[30, 31] There are two phases of filling: early or rapid filling and late or slow filling. The normal pattern of filling has a predominance of early or rapid filling. In fetal life, infancy, and old age, and in diseases with decreased diastolic function, the slow filling phase predominates.

Echocardiography has been used to estimate pulmonary arterial pressure. Many different methods derived from M-mode, two-dimensional, and Doppler echocardiography have been used to estimate pulmonary artery pressure.[32-34] These measures of pulmonary arterial pressure are particularly important in evaluating the child with known congenital heart disease because many decisions regarding therapy are based on the pulmonary arterial pressure or pulmonary vascular resistance, or both. Doppler velocimetry of tricuspid regurgitant jets is perhaps the most reliable and useful method for predicting pulmonary arterial pressure. Tricuspid regurgitation is found in the majority of normal adults (80%) and in a large number of children, particularly if there are associated pulmonary problems. The maximal velocity of the tricuspid regurgitant jet is measured by Doppler technique, and using the Bernoulli equation, the pressure difference between the right ventricle and the atrium is calculated (pressure difference = 4 × velocity^2). Right ventricular pressure is then estimated by the formula

RV pressure = RA pressure + pressure difference.

When no pulmonary stenosis is present, right ventricular pressure is equal to pulmonary arterial pressure (Fig. 27–16).

Cardiac output measurements can also be made by Doppler echocardiography.[20] Doppler cardiac output measurements are based on the principle that blood flow in a tube is proportional to the cross-sectional area of the tube and the velocity of blood in the tube. Measurements of cardiac output by Doppler echocardiography have been shown to correlate well with other measures of cardiac output, and there is a small amount of error in the estimate. Errors in cardiac output measurements come predominantly from inaccuracies in the measurement of cross-sectional area of the outflow tracts. Small inaccuracies in diameter of the outflow tracts are magnified when the diameters are squared to calculate cross-sectional area. Despite this limitation, Doppler measures of cardiac output are particularly useful when following trends in a patient. Thus the error in measurement of cross-sectional area is cancelled out, and relative changes in cardiac output can be followed.

Radiographic Evaluation

A vital role has always been played by radiography in intensive care units. Most intensive care patients have a chest x-ray film taken daily. Important information is obtained about lung fluid, lung expansion, heart size, and catheter and endotracheal tube position. Pediatric roentgenographic texts are available for a full discussion of cardiac evaluation.[35] However, we would mention two particularly useful radiographic evaluations: Magnetic resonance imaging has added much to the evaluation of both intracardiac and great vessel delineation. The magnetic resonance image is particularly useful in the older child with suspected coarctation of the aorta

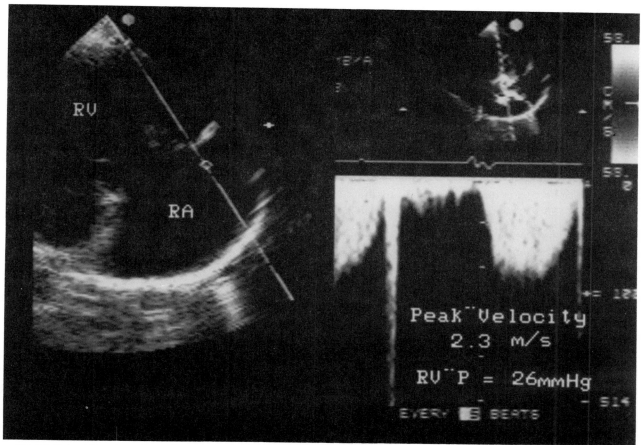

Figure 27–16. Pulsed Doppler echocardiogram in patient with tricuspid regurgitation. The sample volume of the pulsed Doppler is placed near the tricuspid valve in the right atrium (*left*). Doppler recording shows peak velocity of 2.3 m/sec, indicating a pressure difference of 21 mm Hg between the right ventricle and the atrium (*right*). The estimated right ventricular pressure is 26 mm Hg. RA = right atrium; RV = right ventricle.

or postoperative coarctation of the aorta (Fig. 27–17). Barium swallow esophagrams have long been used in the detection of atrial enlargement. Currently echocardiography has replaced the barium swallow for this indication; however, the barium swallow remains a useful method of detecting infants and children with airway and esophageal symptoms due to vascular rings (Fig. 27–18).

INVASIVE EVALUATION

Invasive evaluation of cardiac performance has become commonplace in pediatric intensive care units. The two most common parameters followed in the intensive care unit setting are intra-arterial pressure and central venous pressure. *Intra-arterial* access is usually obtained from the radial artery by either percutaneous technique or arterial cutdown. Posterior tibial or dorsalis pedis arteries are also readily available. In some situations, femoral arterial or axillary arterial access can be obtained by percutaneous technique. Although not confirmed by clinical studies, it would seem prudent to attempt to avoid central arteries such as the axillary or femoral artery because of the risk of arterial damage and subsequent ischemic limb damage. Umbilical arterial access is routine in the neonatal period, and its risks have been well described.[36] Excellent reviews are available for more information on arterial access procedures and their risks.[37]

The most common uses of intra-arterial lines are for observation of blood pressure trends and for blood withdrawal. The contours of the arterial pulse pressure tracing can be very useful in the evaluation of cardiac function. The normal arterial pulse contour has a sharp upstroke during the rapid ejection phase (Fig. 27–19). This phase is followed by slow ejection, which results in a plateau phase and a subsequent decrease in arterial pressure. The dicrotic notch notes the end of ejection and the closure of the aortic valve. The subsequent decrease in arterial pressure during diastole is attributed to normal aortic run-off into the systemic arterial bed. The normal decline in pressure can be increased in patients with accentuated run-off, as occurs in severe aortic insufficiency. There is also an increased stroke volume in patients with aortic insufficiency and, as such, there is an increase in blood pressure in the rapid phase of ejection. The plateau phase of ejection is lost, and there is an exaggerated decline in aortic pressure during diastole resulting from run-off into the left ventricular cavity. This type of tracing can be seen with other types of aortic run-off, such as patent ductus arteriosus, arteriovenous malformations, truncus arteriosus, or an aortopulmonary window. Fever with marked vasodilatation and anemia may also result in a widened arterial pulse pressure.

Estimates of cardiac output can be made by the quality of arterial pulse contours. One can compare the normal pulse contour with the pulse contour seen in patients with low cardiac output. The patient in Figure 27–20 has idiopathic dilatated cardiomyopathy and low cardiac

output syndrome. There is a slow rapid ejection phase and narrow pulse pressure. The area under the curve can be integrated to estimate cardiac output. A note of caution is necessary, however, as dampened arterial wave forms may falsely mislead one to the diagnosis of hypotension or low cardiac output. Arterial blood pressure measurements should be confirmed routinely by standard cuff blood pressure measurements.

Central venous pressure is the most common measure of preload. It is useful in assessing preload in a given patient over a short period; however, central venous

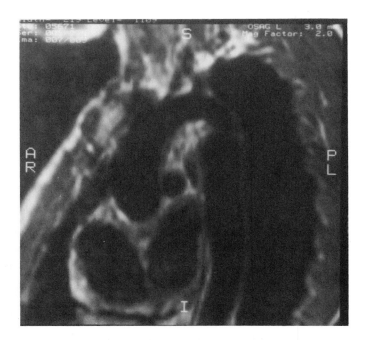

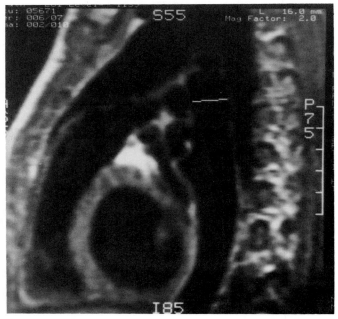

Figure 27–17. Magnetic resonance image of a patient after correction of coarctation of the aorta. There is a residual narrowing (*bottom*) between the transverse and descending aorta.

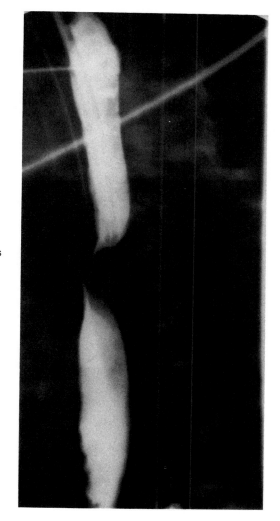

Figure 27–18. Barium swallow performed in an infant with double aortic arch shows severe compression of the esophagus.

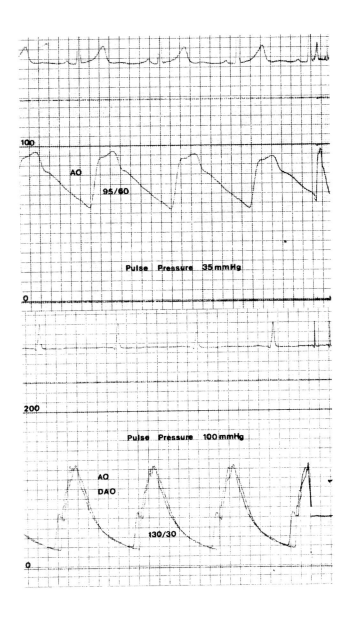

AO

95/60

Pulse Pressure 35 mmHg

100

0

200

Pulse Pressure 100 mmHg

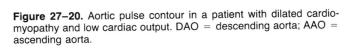

AO
DAO

130/30

0

Figure 27–19. Aortic pulse contours in a normal patient (*top*) and in a patient with severe aortic insuficiency (*bottom*). AO = aorta; DA = descending aorta.

Figure 27–20. Aortic pulse contour in a patient with dilated cardiomyopathy and low cardiac output. DAO = descending aorta; AAO = ascending aorta.

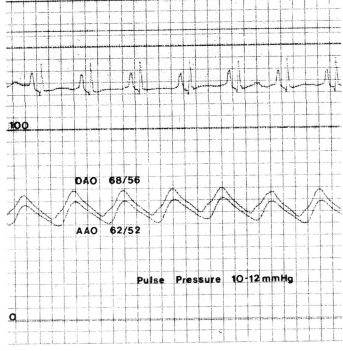

100

DAO 68/56

AAO 62/52

Pulse Pressure 10-12 mmHg

0

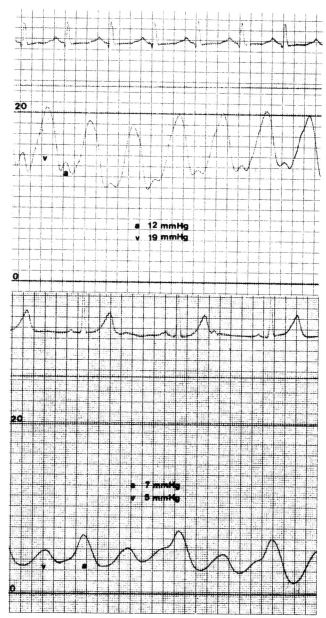

Figure 27-21. Right atrial pressure tracing in a normal patient (*bottom*) and in a patient with severe tricuspid regurgitation (*top*). In the normal patient, there is a dominant a wave, and in the patient with tricuspid regurgitation there is a dominant v wave.

pressure is difficult to assess chronically or to compare between patients. Ventricular hypertrophy may result in less filling of the heart in diastole for any given central venous pressure. These measurements are best obtained with a catheter positioned in the caval-atrial junction. In this position, there is less motion of the catheter with respect to the heart and less of a chance of arrhythmias or thrombus formation. Excellent reviews of central venous catheterization are available.[38]

The normal right atrial pressure tracing is characterized by two waveforms (Fig. 27-21, *bottom*). There is a dominant "a" wave following atrial contraction and a lesser "v" wave following ventricular contraction. A "c"

wave can often be seen during the period of isovolumetric contraction. Ventricular hypertrophy or dysfunction and tricuspid stenosis result in an increase in right atrial pressure and marked elevation of the "a" wave. Severe tricuspid regurgitation results in an increase in right atrial pressure. Unlike the previously mentioned conditions, in this case there is a marked increase in the right atrial v wave (see Fig. 27-21, *top*). Timing the onset of the atrial waveforms with the electrocardiogram is crucial for a correct diagnosis.

Central venous lines may be useful in the estimation of cardiac output or in the detection of intracardiac shunts. In the setting of normal oxygen consumption and normal arterial oxygen saturation, mixed venous

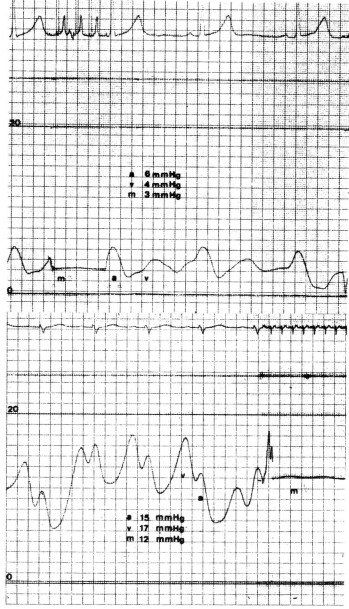

Figure 27-22. Comparison of normal right atrial (*top*) and left atrial (*bottom*) pressure tracings. The left atrial tracing has a dominant v wave and higher mean pressure (*m*).

oxygen saturation reflects cardiac output. Right atrial oxygen saturation can be used as the mixed venous measure only when there is no atrial left-to-right shunting. Pulmonary arterial oxygen saturation should be similar to right atrial saturation unless there is an intracardiac left-to-right shunt. Comparison of the pulmonary and central venous oxygen saturations can be used to quantify the left-to-right shunt.[2] This is particularly useful in the postoperative assessment of children following septal defect closure.

The *left atrial* pressure tracing is easily recognized in comparison with the right atrial tracing (Fig. 27–22). The left atrial pressure tracing is "v" wave–dominant and has a higher mean pressure than does the right atrium. This higher pressure reflects the need for a higher filling pressure because the left ventricle is thicker and less compliant.

In most circumstances, it is impractical to have a catheter in the left atrium or ventricle for measurements of pressure. A balloon-tipped flow-directed catheter can be inserted into the *pulmonary artery* for monitoring pulmonary arterial or pulmonary capillary wedge pressures.[39] Pulmonary capillary wedge pressure has been found to be an excellent measure of left-sided filling pressures (Fig. 27–23).[40] There is a time delay in the wedge pressure waveform such that the "a" wave does not closely follow the p wave on the electrocardiogram. In some patients, it is difficult to wedge the balloon catheter consistently. In these cases, pulmonary arterial diastolic pressure can be substituted for wedge pressure

as the estimate of left ventricular filling pressure (Fig. 27–24). There are circumstances when pressures from the wedge catheter can be misleading.[41]

Most pulmonary artery catheters are equipped with a thermistor for measurements of cardiac output by the thermodilution technique.[42] Thus pulmonary arterial catheters are able to measure cardiac output, right atrial pressure, pulmonary arterial pressure, and pulmonary and capillary wedge pressures. These measurements can be used to calculate systemic vascular resistance, pulmonary vascular resistance, stroke volume index, and cardiac index.[43] Normal values are shown in Table 27–2. Serial measures allow detection of trends in the course of an illness and objective measures of the responses to therapy.

Another use for pulmonary arterial catheters is in patients with pulmonary arterial hypertension. In the postoperative patient with congenital heart disease, pulmonary arterial hypertensive crisis can be lethal. Monitoring pulmonary arterial pressure can guide therapy in this difficult situation. Primary pulmonary arterial hypertension is an uncommon disease in childhood; however, when it is present it is difficult to manage. We have placed pulmonary arterial pressure lines in these patients for drug studies in the intensive care unit. The child in Figure 27–25 had nearly systemic levels of pulmonary arterial pressure and did not respond to oxygen, calcium channel blockers, or other vasodilators.

Intensive care units should now include monitoring units that provide capabilities for monitoring the elec-

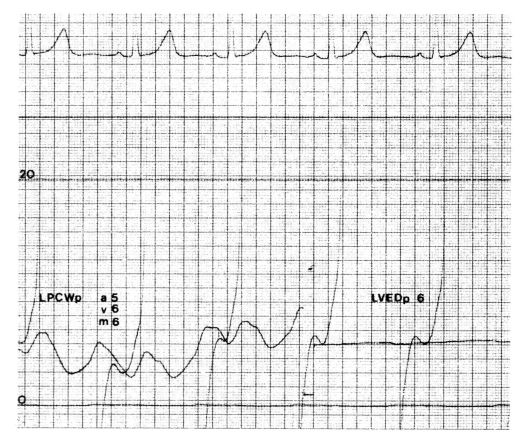

Figure 27–23. Comparison of L pulmonary capillary wedge pressure (LPCWp) and left ventricular end-diastolic pressure (LVED$_P$). There is good correlation between the wedge pressure at end-expiration and the mean wedge pressure with left ventricular end-diastolic pressure.

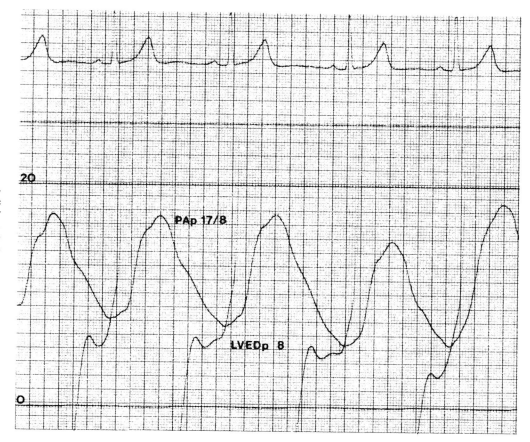

Figure 27–24. Comparison between pulmonary arterial diastolic pressure (PAp) and left ventricular end-diastolic pressure (LVEDp). When wedge pressure cannot be obtained, PA diastolic pressure is a good approximation of LVEDp.

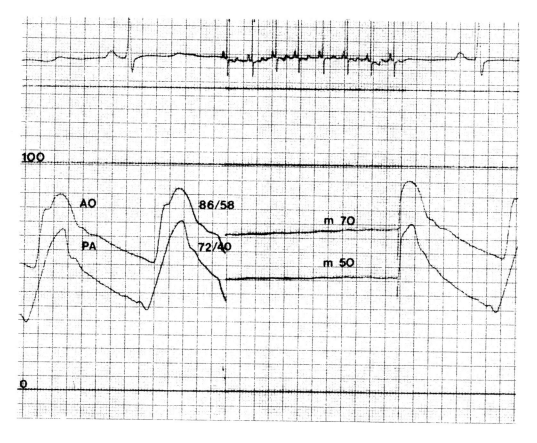

Figure 27–25. Pulmonary and aortic pressure tracings in a patient with idiopathic primary pulmonary artery hypertension. AO = aorta; PA = pulmonary artery.

Table 27–2. NORMAL VALUES FOR HEMODYNAMIC MEASUREMENTS

Pressures	Value
Right atrium (mm Hg)	"a" wave: 2–10; "v" wave 2–10; mean: 2–8
Pulmonary artery (mm Hg)	Systolic peak: 15–30; mean 9–18
Left atrium (mm Hg)	"a" wave: 3–15; "v" wave 3–15; mean: 2–10
Oxygen Saturation	
Mixed venous (%)	65–80
Left atrial (%)	96–100
Calculated Values	
Stroke volume index (ml/beat/m²)	30–65
Cardiac index (l/min/m²)	2.6–4.2
Systemic vascular resistance (dynes/sec/cm⁻⁵)	700–1600
Pulmonary vascular resistance (dynes/sec/cm⁻⁵)	20–130

trocardiogram, respiratory rate, arterial pressure waveform, and at least two other waveforms. The patient in Figure 27–26 had recently undergone a repair of a complete atrioventricular canal defect. Normal sinus rhythm was present, and blood pressure was adequate

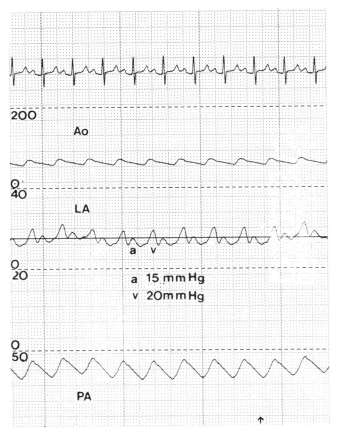

Figure 27–26. Monitor print-out in a patient following surgery for complete atrioventricular canal defect. Electrocardiogram (*top*), aortic and left atrial pressure (*middle*), and pulmonary artery pressure (*bottom*) all presented on a single monitor allows complete assessment of hemodynamic status following surgical correction. A = aorta; LA = left atrium; PA = pulmonary artery.

on inotropic support. Two important points are present on the left atrial and pulmonary arterial pressure waveforms. Left atrial pressure is increased, and there is a "v" wave of 20 mm Hg, indicating mitral regurgitation. In chronic mitral regurgitation, elevated atrial mean and "v" wave pressures indicate severe mitral regurgitation. When mitral regurgitation is acute, as in the early postoperative period following atrioventricular canal correction, an elevated v wave may occur with only mild regurgitation because the left atrium is relatively noncompliant. Severe mitral regurgitation is associated with secondary pulmonary arterial hypertension. In the patient shown in Figure 27–26, pulmonary arterial pressure is only mildly increased, and thus we have secondary information that the mitral regurgitation is not severe. Afterload reduction was begun, and over the ensuing 48 hours left atrial pressure decreased to normal values, and the patient was successfully extubated.

The use of intravascular catheters has greatly improved the care of patients in the intensive care setting. However, it is important to note that there have been significant complications associated with the use of these catheters (Table 27–3). Infection is one complication that can be reduced if precautions are taken during the insertion and management of the catheter and the dressing after insertion.[44] Like any other manipulation involving patient care, there must be an analysis of the risk:benefit ratio before employing invasive monitoring.

Cardiac catheterization provides the most complete hemodynamic evaluation of the pediatric intensive care patient. This invasive procedure can be performed safely with relatively few complications.[45] Hemodynamic measures obtained in the laboratory include oxygen consumption, cardiac output (Fick method or thermodilution), shunt detection and quantification, intracardiac and great vessel pressure measurements, vascular resistances, pressure differences across obstructions (Fig. 27–27), and valve area. Angiography is used to provide anatomic information to aid in the diagnosis of cardiac disease. Despite the use of noninvasive techniques for many of the measurements provided by cardiac catheterization, the number of catheterizations performed has not dramatically decreased. This is because of an increasing number of interventional procedures now being performed in the cardiac catheterization laboratory.[46]

Table 27–3. COMPLICATIONS OF CENTRAL VENOUS AND ARTERIAL ACCESS

Arterial	Central Venous	Pulmonary Artery
Thrombosis	Thrombosis	Vessel injury
Infection	Infection	Pneumothorax
Embolism	Embolism	Arrhythmia
Nerve injury	Pneumothorax	Pulmonary infarction
Skin necrosis	Arrhythmia	Embolism
Hematoma	Phrenic nerve injury	Cardiac rupture
AV* fistula	Thoracic duct injury	PA† rupture
	Hemorrhage	Catheter knotting
		Infection
		Valvular injury

*AV = arteriovenous.
†PA = pulmonary artery.

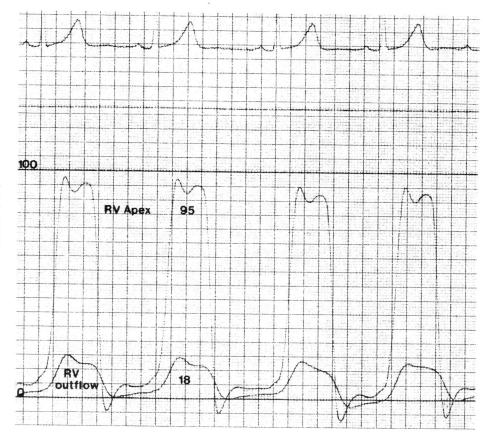

Figure 27–27. Pressure tracings from a patient with double-chamber right ventricle. There is increased pressure in the body (*Apex*) of the right ventricle and normal pressure in the right ventricular outflow tract, confirming that the obstruction is at the ventricular level. RV = right ventricle.

References

1. Katz AM: Physiology of the Heart, 4th ed. New York, Raven Press, 1983, pp 1–24.
2. Grossman W: Cardiac Catheterization and Angiography, 3rd ed. Philadelphia, Lea & Febiger, 1986, pp 301–319.
3. Kirklin JK, Blackstone EH, Kirklin JW, et al: Intracardiac surgery in infants under age 3 months: Predictors of postoperative in-hospital cardiac death. Am J Cardiol 48:507, 1981.
4. Eisenberg PR, Jaffe AS, and Schuster DP: Clinical evaluation compared to pulmonary artery catheterization in the hemodynamic assessment of critically ill patients. Crit Care Med 12:549, 1984.
5. Connors AF, McCaffree DR, and Gray BA: Evaluation of right heart catheterization in the critically ill patient without acute infarction. N Engl J Med 308:263, 1983.
6. Garson A: The Electrocardiogram in Infants and Children: A Systematic Approach. Philadelphia, Lea & Febiger, 1983.
7. Gillette PC and Garson A: Pediatric Arrhythmias: Electrophysiology and Pacing. Philadelphia, WB Saunders, 1990.
8. Humes RA, Porter CJ, Puga FJ, et al: Utility of temporary atrial epicardial electrodes in postoperative pediatric cardiac patients. Mayo Clin Proc 64:516, 1989.
9. Benson DW, Dunnigan A, Sterba R, et al: Atrial pacing from the esophagus in the diagnosis and management of tachycardia and palpitations. J Pediatr 102:40, 1983.
10. Brown M and Vender JS: Noninvasive oxygen monitoring. Crit Care Clin 4:493, 1988.
11. Morley TF: Capnography in the intensive care unit. J Intensive Care Med 5:209, 1990.
12. Silverman NH and Snider AR: Two-dimensional Echocardiography in Congenital Heart Disease. E. Norwalk, Appleton-Century-Crofts, 1982.
13. Williams RG, Bierman FZ, and Sanders SP: Echocardiographic Diagnosis of Cardiac Malformations. Boston, Little, Brown, 1986.
14. Seward JB, Tajik AJ, Edwards WD, et al: Two-dimensional

Echocardiographic Atlas. Vol 1: Congenital Heart Disease. New York, Springer-Verlag, 1987.
15. Snider AR and Serwer GA: Echocardiography in Pediatric Heart Disease. Chicago, Year Book Medical Publishers, 1990.
16. Rome JJ, Keane JF, Perry SB, et al: Double umbrella closure of atrial defects: Initial clinical applications. Circulation 82:751, 1990.
17. Hellenbrand WE, Fahey JT, McGowan FX, et al: Transesophageal echocardiographic guidance of transcatheter closure of atrial septal defect. Am J Cardiol 66:207, 1990.
18. Musewe NN, Smallhorn JF, Benson LN, et al: Validation of Doppler-derived pulmonary arterial pressure in patients with ductus arteriosus under different hemodynamic states. Circulation 76:1081, 1987.
19. Murphy DJ, Ludomirsky A, and Huhta JC: Continuous wave Doppler in children with ventricular septal defect: Noninvasive estimation of interventricular pressure gradient. Am J Cardiol 57:428, 1986.
20. Alverson DC, Eldridge M, Dillon T, et al: Noninvasive pulsed Doppler determination of cardiac output in neonates and children. J Pediatr 101:46, 1982.
21. Sanders SP, Yeager S, and Williams RG: Measurements of systemic and pulmonary blood flow and QP/QS ratio using Doppler and two-dimensional echocardiography. Am J Cardiol 51:952, 1983.
22. Alboliras ET, Seward JB, Hagler DJ, et al: Impact of two-dimensional and Doppler echocardiography on care of children aged two years and younger. Am J Cardiol 61:166, 1988.
23. Gutgesell HP, Huhta JC, Latson LA, et al: Accuracy of two-dimensional echocardiography in the diagnosis of congenital heart disease. Am J Cardiol 55:514, 1985.
24. Krabill KA, Ring S, Foker JE, et al: Echocardiographic versus cardiac catheterization diagnosis of infants with congenital heart disease requiring cardiac surgery. Am J Cardiol 60:351, 1987.
25. Perry LW, Ruckman RN, Galioto FM, et al: Echocardiographically assisted balloon atrial septostomy. Pediatrics 70:403, 1982.
26. Seward JB, Khandheria BK, Oh JK, et al: Transesophageal

echocardiography: Technique, anatomic correlations, implementation and clinical applications. Mayo Clin Proc 63:649, 1988.

27. Matsuzaki M, Toma Y, and Kusukawa R: Clinical applications of transesophageal echocardiography. Circulation 82:709, 1990.

28. Feigenbaum H: Echocardiography, 4th ed. Philadelphia, Lea & Febiger, 1986, pp 12–188.

29. Colan SD, Borow KM, and Neumann A: Left ventricular end-systolic wall stress-velocity of fiber shortening relation: A load independent index of myocardial contractility. J Am Coll Cardiol 4:715, 1984.

30. Nishimura RA, Housmans PR, Hatle LK, et al: Assessment of diastolic function of the heart: Background and current applications of Doppler echocardiography. Part I: Physiology and pathophysiologic features. Mayo Clin Proc 64:71, 1989.

31. Nishimura RA, Abel MD, Hatle LK, et al: Assessment of diastolic function of the heart: Background and current applications of Doppler echocardiography. Part II: Clinical studies. Mayo Clin Proc 64:181, 1989.

32. Robinson PJ, Macartney FJ, and Wyse RKH: Non-invasive diagnosis of pulmonary hypertension. Int J Cardiol 11:253, 1986.

33. Yock PG and Popp RL: Noninvasive estimation of right ventricular systolic pressure by Doppler ultrasound in patients with tricuspid regurgitation. Circulation 70:657, 1984.

34. Chan KL, Currie PJ, Seward JB, et al: Comparison of three Doppler ultrasound methods in the prediction of pulmonary artery pressure. J Am Coll Cardiol 9:549, 1987.

35. Kirks DR: Practical Pediatric Imaging: Diagnostic Radiology of Infants and Children. Boston, Little, Brown, 1984.

36. Kitterman JA, Phibbs RH, and Tooley WH: Catheterization of umbilical vessels in newborn infants. Pediatr Clin North Am 17:895, 1972.

37. MacDonald MG and Eichelberger MR: Peripheral arterial cannulation. In: Fletcher MA, MacDonald MG, and Avery GB (eds): Atlas of Procedures in Neonatology. Philadelphia, JB Lippincott, 1983, pp 154–165.

38. Seneff MG: Central venous catheterizations: A comprehensive review. Part I. J Intensive Care Med 2:163, 1987.

39. Grossman W: Cardiac Catheterization and Angiography, 3rd ed. Philadelphia, Lea & Febiger, 1986, pp 88–97.

40. Voyce SJ and Rippe JM: Pulmonary artery catheters: An update. J Intensive Care Med 5:175, 1990.

41. Raper R and Sibbald WJ: Misled by the wedge? The Swan-Ganz catheter and left ventricular preload. Chest 89:427, 1986.

42. Grossman W: Cardiac Catheterization and Angiography, 3rd ed. Philadelphia, Lea & Febiger, 1986, pp 101–117.

43. Grossman W: Cardiac Catheterization and Angiography, 3rd ed. Philadelphia, Lea & Febiger, 1986, pp 135–142.

44. Corona ML, Peters SG, Narr BJ, et al: Infections related to central venous catheters. Mayo Clin Proc 65:979, 1990.

45. Cohn HE, Freed MD, Hellenbrand WF, et al: Complications and mortality associated with cardiac catheterization in infants under one year: A prospective study. Pediatr Cardiol 6:123, 1985.

46. Lock JE, Keane JF, and Fellows KE: Diagnostic and Interventional Catheterization in Congenital Heart Disease. Boston, Martinus Nijhoff, 1987.

Cardiovascular Support—Mechanical

Stephen A. Klem, M.D.

Although contemporary management of cardiovascular failure is primarily drug-oriented, circumstances may arise when mechanical adjuncts to circulation can improve perfusion and corresponding survival. These modalities will likely never replace the initial approach of volume expansion and appropriate use of various inotropic, afterload reducing, or diuretic medications. The mechanical manipulation of pressures around or within the cardiovascular system, however, can be effective in assisting or even replacing autologous cardiac function. Many of the techniques discussed in this chapter are routinely applied in pediatric critical care—for example, mechanical ventilation or closed-chest compression. Other techniques, such as intra-aortic balloon pumping (IABP), are used with greater frequency in critical care of adult patients and are available in only a few pediatric centers. Still others, such as ventricular assist devices (VADs) or artificial hearts, remain intriguing research tools undergoing further evaluation and refinement.

The purpose of this chapter is to outline the underlying physiology, benefits or relative advantages, and risks or complications of several examples of indirect or noninvasive mechanical therapies that are currently available to treat children with cardiovascular failure. In addition, research about invasive mechanical supports that promises wider clinical application in the next decade is briefly discussed, along with a consideration of the ethical and economic implications of these therapies.

ROLE AND INDICATIONS IN PEDIATRICS

The definition, differential diagnosis, and pharmacologic management of cardiovascular failure in pediatrics are discussed elsewhere (see Chapters 29 to 31). Due to the risks of invasive support, many present mechanical modalities are reserved for compassionate use in cases of cardiogenic shock refractory to conventional treatments. Supportive modalities with well-established utilization criteria and benefits, such as mechanical ventilation, are integral parts of conventional therapy,

however. Just as cardiopulmonary resuscitation (CPR) has resulted in successful resuscitation of children arresting from a variety of otherwise fatal causes, the severity and acuity of circulatory failure are stronger criteria for deciding when to institute mechanical support than is etiology.

Medical Congestive Heart Failure

Therapeutic benefit from various mechanical circulatory adjuncts has been established for pediatric patients with congestive heart failure (CHF) from a variety of medical causes, such as posthypoxia or ischemic shock, myocarditis or cardiomyopathy, congenital or inflammatory coronary abnormalities, or ventricular hypertrophy associated with congenital heart diseases.

Postoperative Congestive Heart Failure

Benefit has also been noted in acute postoperative patients with deterioration after cardiac surgery and bypass. Myocardial "stunning" has been observed in the absence of significant myocardial necrosis in patients with severely depressed cardiac function after bypass.[1] The skills of cardiovascular surgeons and the convenience of ready access to the same circulatory support modalities used intraoperatively for chest surgery lends itself to extracorporeal pump assist.

Bridge to Transplantation

Other groups have found great success in supporting patients with end-stage myocardial failure from many causes with mechanical circulation assist until a matching donor organ can be transplanted.[2, 3]

INDIRECT/SUPPORTIVE

The initial approach to imminent or actual circulatory failure should include assessment and possible diagnosis, adequate volume expansion, and appropriate use of inotropic infusions. At the same time, the critically important interdependence between the respiratory and circulatory systems (see Chapter 41) needs to be addressed through aggressive respiratory support.

Positive-Pressure Ventilation

Although obviously indicated for imminent respiratory failure, mechanical ventilation can have several beneficial functions for patients with heart failure, even in the absence of significant carbon dioxide retention or hypoxemia. In the progression of cardiogenic shock, respiratory arrest occurs prior to cardiac arrest.[4]

Work of Breathing

Up to 80% of total oxygen delivery may flow to respiratory muscles in patients with increased elastic or resistive work loads.[5] A patient in heart failure with adequate hemoglobin and cardiac output may still develop increased lactic acidosis that responds to mechanical ventilation.[6] Mechanical ventilation can improve hemodynamics by decreasing blood flow to the diaphragm and intercostal muscles.[7] Due to the relatively high oxygen consumption of the respiratory muscles of dyspneic patients, oxygen delivery to other organs with less replaceable function (e.g., brain, heart, liver) can be increased by decreasing the metabolic demand of chest expansion.

Positive End-Expiratory Pressure

The appropriate use of positive end-expiratory pressure (PEEP) may have several benefits in treating circulatory dysfunction (Table 28–1). PEEP's effect in alveolar recruitment reduces intrapulmonary shunting and therefore improves arterial oxygenation.[8] Depending on pulmonary condition, PEEP may restore lung volume to functional reserve capacity (FRC) and decrease pulmonary vascular resistance (PVR), or increase PVR if inflation exceeds FRC.[9] Increasing intrathoracic pressure (ITP) can improve cardiac function by reducing left-ventricular (LV) wall stress and therefore by decreasing afterload.[10] Most often, however, the increases in ITP from positive-pressure ventilation and PEEP decrease cardiac output by decreasing the transmural right atrial pressure gradient for systemic venous return.[11] Cardiac index and oxygen delivery can be decreased even by PEEP in the 5 to 10 cm H_2O range in adult respiratory distress syndrome (ARDS).[12] If LV end-diastolic volume can be maintained by administration of fluids, however, LV performance is not adversely affected by increases in ITP.[13] PEEP's effects in decreasing LV afterload may in fact improve performance when contractility is limited.[14] The net effect is usually to increase myocardial and systemic oxygen delivery when optimal PEEP levels are chosen and supplemental volume expansion is provided.

Synchronized Ventilation

The principle that ITP can generate flow of blood even without cardiac compression ("the thoracic pump", see later) was originally proposed as "the lungs as a pump" concept in 1963.[21] In animal studies, elevations of ITP applied in synchrony with the cardiac cycle in closed-chest dogs had little hemodynamic effect unless the thorax and abdomen were enclosed in binders, even when pulmonary hypertension was induced by microembolization.[22] Synchronizing binding pulses to early diastole decreased LV filling pressure and LV stroke volume. With propranolol-induced acute LV failure, the pulses improved LV performance by increasing LV stroke volume, despite decreases in LV filling pressure.

Table 28–1. VENTILATOR STRATEGIES BY MEDICAL AND SURGICAL CONDITION

Condition	Ventilator Strategy	Rationale	References
Apnea, hypoventilation	Intubation and PPV	Prevent respiratory acidosis	
Neuromuscular disease	Pressure support, or negative-pressure ventilation	Decrease work of breathing	
Restrictive lung disease (e.g., scoliosis, pulmonary hypoplasia)	Prolonged T_{insp} or inspiratory plateau	Allow gas distribution	
Upper airway obstruction	Artificial airway, usually with IMV	Maintain patent airway	
Small airways disease (asthma, bronchiolitis, BPD)	Bronchodilation, prolonging T_{exp}	Diminish air trapping	15
Alveolar disease; atelectasis; pulmonary edema	PEEP, inverse ratio ventilation	See text	
Flail chest	Moderate PEEP	Stabilize chest wall	
Bronchopleural fistula	Minimum necessary PIP, PEEP, and T_{insp}	Minimize air leak	
Low-output state; cardiogenic shock	PPV with minimal PEEP necessary	Avert acidosis, decrease PVR	
Pulmonary hypertension; elevated PVR	Elevated PO_2, hyperventilation	Pulmonary vasodilation	16, 17
Left-to-right shunt—pulmonary hyperemia	Minimize FiO_2, moderate-high PEEP; avoid hyperventilation	Increase PVR, reduce pulmonary blood flow	
Fontan physiology (right atrium to pulmonary artery)	Low PIP and PEEP, early extubation	Minimize PVR	18
Pulmonary or pericardial hemorrhage	High PEEP	Tamponade bleeding	19, 20

PEEP = positive end-expiratory pressure; PPV = positive pressure ventilation; T_{insp} = inspiratory phase time; IMV = intermittent mandatory ventilation; BPD = bronchopulmonary dysplasia; T_{exp} = expiratory phase time; PVR = pulmonary vascular resistance.

The effect was more pronounced when the pulses were timed to occur with systole.[23] The only published human data, gathered from patients undergoing extracorporeal shock wave lithotripsy and given QRS-synchronized high-frequency jet ventilation, did not show significant hemodynamic changes.[24]

Fluid Management and Removal

Although most pediatric patients acutely in shock benefit from expansion of intravascular volume, patients with cardiogenic shock or following prolonged fluid resuscitation may benefit from volume unloading. If intrinsic renal function or supplementation with a loop diuretic such as furosemide or bumetanide fails to result in diuresis, extrarenal removal of fluid may be necessary. Support with peritoneal dialysis, hemodialysis, continuous arteriovenous hemofiltration (CAVH), or CAVH with dialysis (CAVH-D) may be indicated (see Chapter 53). Ultrafiltration can reduce fluid overload with few detrimental hemodynamic effects.[25] Hemodialysis has been emergently initiated for cardiac arrest due to hyperkalemia in an adult, with subsequent successful resuscitation and recovery.[26]

NONINVASIVE ASSIST—EXTERNAL BODY COMPRESSION

Static—MAST/PASG

The military antishock trouser (MAST) garment was first used in 1903 by Crile as a means of controlling intra-abdominal hemorrhage.[27]

Mechanism of Action

At least four mechanisms are considered to be involved in its effect on reversing shock[28]:

1. Increase in peripheral resistance in the lower body
2. Selective perfusion of the upper body
3. Initial increase of venous return (preload) from the lower body
4. Tamponade of bleeding in the lower body

It is important to distinguish between the pneumatic antishock garment's (PASG) capability to redistribute blood *flow* versus redistribution of blood *volume*.[29] An early explanation for the mechanism of action of the compression garment was "autotransfusion"—shift of blood volume from the lower body. Some estimated this volume to be as much as 1,000 ml in adult trauma patients, based on the amount of volume required to maintain blood pressure during garment deflation.[30] An earlier study, however, measured a shift of 250 ml being displaced to the thorax based on the shift in center of gravity during MAST device inflation.[31] Further, the use of volume expansion to elevate central venous pressure in normal humans to the same level seen with MAST garment inflation causes no change in mean arterial pressure (MAP), compared with the significant elevation in MAP measured with the lower body compressed.[32] Instead, the likely mechanism is redistribution of blood flow—increases in carotid and coronary flow have been measured with coincident decreases in femoral flow during MAST garment inflation.[33]

Benefits and Efficacy

Among the MAST garment's greatest advantages are the ease and speed with which it can be applied or reversed, should adverse results occur. In a retrospective study of PASG use in 1,120 adults with hypotension and poor tissue perfusion or tachycardia in the field or emergency room, 84% showed significant elevation in blood pressure, a decreased heart rate, or clinically improved perfusion.[34] Despite these changes, PASG use may not increase long-term survival for patients with prehospital injuries—one prospective study of 911 patients found 31% mortality in the MAST group compared with 25% in the group in whom MAST was not used.[35] There are no studies published to date on the efficacy of the PASG therapy in children, other than case reports following trauma[36-39] and after Fontan surgery (see later).

Indications, Hazards, and Contraindications

The PASG device has been recommended for use in patients incurring clinical shock or hypotension, especially if associated with pelvic or femur fracture or intra-abdominal hemorrhage. This device has also been reported to increase blood pressure in patients with cardiogenic shock but causes an acute increase in LV afterload.[40] Pulmonary edema is the only absolute contraindication. Inflation of the leg compartments only is recommended during pregnancy. Despite small increases in intracranial pressure, use of PASG increases cerebral perfusion pressure and thus is not contraindicated in patients with increased intracranial pressure. Lower extremity ischemia and lactate accumulation have been reported in a small number of adults.

Dynamic/Intermittent

Chest Compression

The physiologic explanation for how blood flow is generated during closed-chest compression varies based on species of study, depth and duration of compression, age of subject, and duration of resuscitation. Although blood flow was originally considered to be generated from direct compression of the heart and intact valve function, in many situations changes in ITP (the "thoracic pump" mechanism) better explain how CPR works.[41] The reader is referred to Chapter 5 and other fine reviews[42] for a thorough discussion of this concept.

Based on the observation that voluntary coughing generated sufficient blood flow to maintain consciousness during ventricular fibrillation,[43] the role of manipulating ITP to augment cardiac output has been studied.

Simultaneous chest compression and ventilation CPR increased blood flow to the brain and to a lesser degree to the heart and kidneys than did nonsimultaneous CPR in a dog[44] and in infant pigs.[45] Another group found that the addition of abdominal binding to simultaneous compression with lung inflation improved cerebral blood flow to 32% of prearrest flow, compared with 3% for conventional CPR.[46]

Abdominal Compression

When the abdomen is compressed 400 ms prior to each thoracic compression (phased compression) in dogs, carotid flow index is increased by 77% (to 23% of prearrest flow) and cardiac output index is increased by 65% (to 12.5% of prearrest).[47] A human study, however, found that simultaneous chest and abdominal compression provided the largest increase in aortic pressures compared with standard CPR.[48] In actual practice interposed abdominal and chest compression showed no improvement in prehospital resuscitation rate over standard CPR but was associated with improved survival to discharge for adults in a randomized inpatient study.[49]

Lower Body and Abdomen Phasic Compression

Via cyclic pressure waves properly timed to the cardiac cycle, hemodynamic energy can be transmitted noninvasively to assist the circulation.[50] Cyclic pressure waves to the lower body require that the high pressure occur during diastole in order to augment cardiac output or coronary flow. In contrast, chest compression should be timed to fall at the onset of ventricular systole to optimally augment cardiac output.[51] A cooperative study of external pressure circulatory assist, timed to occur during diastole, decreased mortality of randomized adult patients with acute myocardial infarction from 17.5% to 8.3%.[52] In the process of augmenting diastolic pressure, however, venous return (preload) and risk of pulmonary edema are increased. If maximal vasoconstriction is present peripherally or LV function is severely compromised, external compression may have minimal benefit.

Phasic external lower body compression (below the costal margin, to 45 to 50 mm Hg × 45 sec/min) increased right atrial pressure by 44% (mean of 7 mm Hg) and systolic arterial pressure by 30% (mean of 20 mm Hg) in nine postoperative Fontan patients, the youngest patient being 9 years of age.[53] More recently, two younger 10- to 18-kg post-Fontan patients were reported as benefitting from cyclic inflation of a MAST suit to 25 mm Hg 45 sec/min. As the use of a MAST suit can decrease vital capacity, its use was discontinued prior to extubation. The authors ascribed the improvement to increased venous return leading to increased pulmonary blood flow, left-sided filling pressures, and cardiac output.[54] Unlike present pharmacologic means of manipulating vascular tone, this mechanical therapy may provide a specific means of affecting systemic vascular resistance independent from PVR. This would allow the clinician to titrate systemic (Q_s) against pulmonary (Q_p) blood flow in patients with bidirectional intracardiac shunts.

INVASIVE ASSIST

Temporary

Cardiopulmonary Bypass Pump

Intraoperative cardiopulmonary bypass (CPB) using an extracorporeal pump and an oxygenator is standard therapy for most cardiac surgery. It is a natural extension to resume this support for patients who deteriorate during or shortly following weaning from CPB. Spencer and colleagues first reported the successful treatment of postcardiotomy cardiogenic shock in an adult patient with prolonged LV bypass.[55] Similar to extracorporeal membrane oxygenation (ECMO) (see later), however, survival for pediatric patients placed on bypass due to circulatory failure is poor.

Emergency Bypass as Part of Resuscitation. CPB has been studied in the treatment of cardiac arrest of nonoperative patients. In one study, five of five adult patients with mean of 25 minutes of advanced life support placed on femorofemoral CPB in an emergency department had return of spontaneous circulation.[56] None survived more than 28 hours, however, most commonly due to subacute pulmonary or neurologic sequelae.

One of 29 patients who were placed on CPB within a mean of 9.5 minutes after telephone request survived to hospital discharge in another study of adult hospital inpatients.[57] The Hemopump (see later) has been placed after 3 hours of "mechanical resuscitation" and succeeded in maintaining life for another 20 hours.[58] Although emergency CPB is still an exciting avenue of research in adult resuscitation, the technical difficulties of cannulation and of obtaining adequate flow will probably prevent the use of this technology in children.

Extracorporeal Membrane Oxygenation

Based on a growing body of experience, ECMO may be the mode of extracorporeal circulatory assist that is best suited to small patients. Although its popularity has been based on success in treating neonatal respiratory failure, it has also been used for respiratory failure in older children.[59] This subject is addressed in Chapter 42. Children with circulatory failure following cardiac surgery have been treated with ECMO, although only 20 of 48 patients survived and were discharged from hospital.[60–62a] The inclusion of a membrane oxygenator may be beneficial compared with LV assist alone, especially when postoperative biventricular or primary right ventricular (RV) failure is present. Bleeding, infection, and vascular injury are potential major complications.

Intra-Aortic Balloon

Physiology. The concept of IABP was first demonstrated in 1961,[63] but was not utilized clinically until

1968.[64] A catheter is positioned with a distal-end polyurethane balloon located in the descending thoracic aorta. The balloon is rapidly inflated with CO_2 or helium during diastole (beginning with aortic valve closure) and serves to displace blood more proximally and distally in the aorta. This acts to increase blood flow and oxygen delivery to the coronary and peripheral circulation. Balloon deflation occurs just before systole and creates a negative aortic pressure to facilitate ventricular ejection. The latter serves to decrease LV afterload and consequent myocardial oxygen consumption. Additionally, pulmonary artery wedge pressure and pulmonary vascular resistance are reduced. The reader is referred to an excellent review of the mechanical, hemodynamic, and metabolic effects of IABP.[65] Although it is common to see a fall in a IABP patient's end-diastolic pressure (Fig. 28–1), balloon timing that minimizes aortic end-diastolic pressure will not always maximize oxygen delivery or minimize oxygen consumption.[66] IABP can be considered only as a circulatory assist device rather than as cardiac replacement, because it depends on a minimum adequate stroke volume ejected from the left ventricle for effect.

Indications. IABP has become a common technique in adult patients with cardiogenic shock owing to acute myocardial infarction, unstable angina refractory to medical management, and for postoperative LV dysfunction.[67] For conditions other than acute, reversible LV failure, however, IABP has been less effective. Although sepsis is known to produce LV dysfunction (see Chapter 12), IABP therapy in adults with sepsis has been disappointing.[68] Owing to relative ease of placement and availability, it is frequently used in transplant centers as a temporizing measure before cardiac transplantation. With some risk, patients can even be transported while undergoing IABP, making referral to

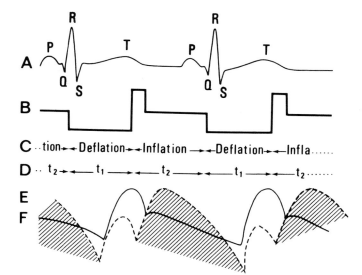

Figure 28–1. Inflation and deflation timing diagram for intra-aortic balloon pumping. A, ECG tracing. B, Balloon pump timing trace. C, Inflation and deflation intervals. D, timing of inflation and deflation depicted as t_1 and t_2. E and F, Assisted and unassisted arterial pressure trace indicating the point of balloon inflation and deflation. (From Bolooki H: Clinical Application of Intra-aortic Balloon Pump, 2nd ed. Mt. Kisco, NY, Futura Publishing Co., 1984, p. 38.)

specialty centers or movement between the catherization laboratory, operating room, and intensive care unit (ICU) possible.[69]

Pediatric Use. Problems specific to IABP use in children include[70]: (1) small size of the aorta, severely limiting the size of balloon that can be placed—most adult-sized balloons would extend to below the diaphragm. (2) The high elasticity of a child's aorta (more so under 5 years of age), combined with large collateral bronchial flow in cyanotic heart disease, may preclude effective balloon pumping by dissipating kinetic energy. (3) Pediatric patients with severe LV failure may produce insufficient stroke volume to permit balloon augmentation. In addition, the rapid heart rates of smaller children preclude pump support for each beat. Owing to time delays in balloon inflation/deflation, heart rates above 110 beats/min cannot be matched at a 1:1 rate.

Balloon catheters best suited for pediatric use should be (1) large enough to adequately increase aortic diastolic pressure and lower aortic end-diastolic and peak systolic pressure, (2) small enough to avoid aortic wall injury and also not impair renal and mesenteric circulation by extending below the diaphragm, (3) be rapidly inflated and deflated to match rapid heart rates on children, and (4) have a narrow catheter to minimize distal ischemia of the lower extremity.[71] Commercially available IABP sizes now include No. 5 and 7 French catheters with 5- to 20-ml balloons.

IABP has been applied to pediatric patients after open-heart surgery. In one series, 6 of 14 patients survived, although none were under 5 years of age.[72] In another study of pediatric patients with postoperative cardiogenic shock, four of eight patients were successfully weaned from IABP, and two (the youngest patients—6 weeks and 6 months) of eight patients were discharged from the hospital.[73] A larger study looked at children who could not be weaned from CPB after cardiac surgery.[74] Of 41 patients, 19 survived, most of them older than 5 years of age. No patient had suprasystolic augmentation of diastolic blood pressure. Of patients in whom augmentation could be achieved, 63% survived. Renal failure developed in more than half of the patients. Reversible thrombocytopenia and liver failure occurred in almost every patient, as did decreased pulse in the target limb. Of 41 patients, five had residual severe limb ischemia.

Pulmonary Artery Balloon Pumping (PABP). Many patients with transient perioperative RV failure can be managed with longer CPB time. Some benefit from IABP. There have been case reports of PABP with long-term survival in adults.[75] PABP has several theoretic advantages for pediatric patients undergoing correction of congenital heart defects with RV hypertrophy and risk of RV failure after ventriculotomy (e.g., tetralogy of Fallot), although this finding has only been reported in an animal model.[76]

Long-Term

The aforementioned techniques, which all work in *series* with the left ventricle to deliver flow output to the aorta, each have disadvantages precluding their long-term use. Inability to supply more than 20 to 40% of cardiac output (except for CPB and ECMO), risk of infection, need for systemic anticoagulation, and problems with hemolysis are all limiting factors. Techniques for long-term circulatory assist take the strategies of ventricular assistance in *parallel* circuits or of heart replacement.[77]

Ventricular Assist Device

VADs work in parallel with the ventricles to draw blood flow from the atrium or ventricle and return it to the aorta or pulmonary artery. The advantages of VAD support include allowing the natural heart to remain in place (with recovery potential), the capability of providing almost all cardiac output on a short-term basis, and consequently sustaining life in patients with a high risk of mortality from LV failure until recovery or transplantation takes place. Their disadvantages include the risk of infection and disconnection of percutaneous access, need for anticoagulation (in most cases), dangers of device dependence (device failure or myocardial atrophy), and limits to duration of use. Similar to IABP, their present role is short-term (several hours to 1 to 2 weeks) support for patients with cardiac failure that is reversible or treatable (e.g., transplantation). Failure to wean from CPB or IABP, acute viral myocarditis, transplant rejection, or end-stage cardiomyopathy prior to cardiac transplantation have all led to the development and use of VAD.

Generally accepted indications for pursuing circulatory assist over IABP were developed by Norman.[78] Current criteria include: (1) cardiac index < 2.0 l/min/m^2, (2) systemic vascular resistance (SVR) $> 2,100$ dynes/sec/cm^5, (3) atrial pressure > 20 mm Hg, and (4) urine output < 20 ml/hr, along with additional requirements of optimal preload, maximal drug therapy, corrected metabolism, and IABP already in use. Patients to be excluded are those with perioperative myocardial infarction or organ system failure: renal, hepatic, central nervous system, or multiple, or those with extensive bleeding.[79] Between 1.5 to 10% of adult patients undergo IABP after CPB in major centers, and only 0.2 to 1% receive a left ventricular assist device (LVAD) or a partial artificial heart.[80]

A variety of designs and types of devices are undergoing an evaluation in animal studies and in adult patients. Their relative advantages and disadvantages are reviewed elsewhere.[81–83] A pediatric VAD could reduce the risks of bleeding and infection that form the major complications during ECMO.[84] One pediatric VAD has been developed, with proportionately smaller stroke volumes (20 and 40 ml) and higher rates (up to 200/min).[85] When applied to three patients with "profound heart failure," circulation could be maintained adequately for 3 to 5 days.[86] Another device that could conceivably benefit pediatric patients is the Hemopump, which is a 7-mm diameter axial flow pump that can be placed in the aorta, similar to IABP, to draw blood from the left ventricle into the aorta.[87]

Muscle Grafts, Dynamic Aortic Patch

Skeletal muscle ventricles constructed from latissimus dorsi in dogs were capable of performing the work of the right heart with near-physiologic filling pressures.[88] There has been some work in humans with using skeletal muscle flaps to "patch" areas of ventricular aneurysm.[89]

Artificial Ventricle/Heart

Although the goal of much research on assisted circulation is the development of an implantable artificial heart, the major bioengineering hurdles of compatible materials design, power supply, hemolysis and complement activation, adequate output, and durability are significant. Due to thromboembolic complications, the famous Jarvik-7 device, which was first implanted in Barney Clark for 112 days and 12,912,499 beats, is no longer being used as a permanent cardiac replacement. It has been successful as an intermediate-term (2 to 35 days) bridge to eventual orthotopic heart transplantation.[90] The implantation of artificial hearts or VADs significantly increases the risk of infection, especially if used as a bridge to transplantation.[91] One reason for this may be a decrease in T lymphocyte function observed after VAD insertion, although this has been attributed to underlying severity of illness rather than to the presence of the device itself.[92] The fully implantable permanent total artificial heart is probably a distant hope as an alternative to transplantation.[93]

CONSIDERATIONS

Economics

It has been estimated that totally implantable VADs have the potential for helping 17,000 to 35,000 patients annually at an estimated cost to society of $2.5 to $5 billion per annum.[94] Compared with other therapies presently available in pediatric ICUs, assisted circulation by ECMO or IABP is the most labor- and resource-intensive. The essential requirements of a high degree of skill, experience, and commitment to this technology on the part of cardiothoracic surgeons, operating room and perfusion staff, critical care physicians, and nursing staff will restrict its use to a small number of patients in a small number of centers. The development of such extremely expensive technology poses major socioeconomic and ethical questions for society.

Ethics

Therapeutic versus Sustaining Treatment

In evaluating any therapy that results in a cure, the potential years of good-quality life gained are greater for a pediatric patient than for an adult. For children with reversible cardiac failure or for those who go on to cardiac transplantation, assisted circulation can serve as a lifesaving temporizing measure. Although hospital mortality is high for patients requiring VADs (72%), 28% of adult patients who would have otherwise died were "long-term" survivors.[95] In another study, those who did survive ventricular assist pumping had a good chance of resuming active lives. The risk of residual cardiac or noncardiac disability was small.[96]

Some of the ethical issues involved in experimental studies of VADs are discussed by Parker and associates.[97] The issues raised include assessing a therapy that is not believed to be as safe or as effective as cardiac transplantation (or even hold promise of such within a patient's lifetime) but which may still have a role due to the short supply of donor organs. In choosing to enroll randomized end-stage cardiac patients 60 years or older, the authors believed that they had identified a patient population for whom admittedly inferior experimental therapy was comparable with the patients' other therapeutic options. Extrapolation to the pediatric setting would permit the enrollment only of moribund patients and would therefore minimize the opportunity to establish efficacy or beneficial long-term outcome.

Although many support research into *temporary* artificial hearts,[98] Annas argues that "as long as there is a shortage of transplantable human hearts, temporary artificial hearts cannot increase the total numbers of human heart transplants; they can only change the identity of the individuals who receive them."[99]

Role of Assisted Circulation in Pediatric Critical Care

Presently, there is no safe means of assisting circulation on a long-term basis for pediatric patients. Several current technologies have a role for short-term use, however. The most important mechanical device for assisting the failing heart is a ventilator. Early intubation and aggressive support with positive-pressure ventilation and PEEP are key therapies for shock while fluid and inotropic management is initiated. There is great promise in the development of external compression garments with or without cardiac synchronization, although only limited human data have been published. For invasive support, ECMO is the modality with the largest volume of pediatric experience at this time, particularly for smaller patients. IABP may have a role in supporting the larger child with transient cardiogenic shock. VADs and implantable artificial hearts are not likely to benefit pediatric patients for many years to come.

References

1. Braunwald E and Kloner RA: The stunned myocardium: Prolonged, postischemic ventricular dysfunction. Circulation 66:1146, 1982.
2. Kanter KR, McBride LR, Pennington DG, et al: Bridging to cardiac transplantation with pulsatile ventricular assist devices. Ann Thorac Surg 46:134, 1988.
3. Joyce LD, Emery RW, Eales F, et al: Mechanical circulatory support as a bridge to transplantation. J Thorac Cardiovasc Surg 98:935, 1989.
4. Aubier M, Trippenbach T, and Roussos C: Respiratory muscle fatigue in cardiogenic shock. J Appl Physiol 51:499, 1981.
5. Roussos C and Macklem PT: The respiratory muscles. N Engl J Med 307:786, 1982.
6. Aubier M, Viires N, Syllic G, et al: Respiratory muscle contribution to lactic acidosis in low cardiac output. Am Rev Respir Dis 126:648, 1982.
7. Viires N, Sillye G, Aubier M, et al: Regional blood flow distribution in dog during induced hypotension and low cardiac output: Spontaneous breathing versus artificial ventilation. J Clin Invest 72:935, 1983.
8. Kumar A, Falke KI, Geffin B, et al: Continuous positive pressure plateau: Effects on hemodynamics and lung function. N Engl J Med 238:1430, 1970.
9. Canada E, Benumof JL, and Tousdale FR: Pulmonary vascular resistance correlated in intact normal and abnormal canine lungs. Crit Care Med 10:719, 1982.
10. Pinsky MR, Summer WR, Wise RA, et al: Augmentation of cardiac function by elevation of intrathoracic pressure. J Appl Physiol: Respirat Environ Exercise Physiol 54:950, 1983.
11. Pinsky MR: Hemodynamic effects of artificial ventilation. In: Shoemaker WC, Ayres S, Grenvik A, et al (eds): Textbook of Critical Care, 2nd ed. Philadelphia, WB Saunders, 1989, p. 679.
12. Brear SG, Edwards JD, and Nightingale P: Optimal cardiorespiratory patterns: Implications for positive and expiratory pressure (PEEP) therapy. Thorax 43:827P, 1988.
13. Qvist J, Pontoppidian H, Wilson HS, et al: Hemodynamic response to mechanical ventilation with PEEP: The effect of hypervolemia. Anesthesiology 42:45, 1975.
14. Pinsky MR and Summer WR: Cardiac augmentation by phasic high intrathoracic pressure support in man. Chest 84:370, 1983.
15. Hubmayr RD, Abel MD, and Rehder K: Physiological approach to mechanical ventilation. Crit Care Med 18:103, 1990.
16. Rudolph AM and Yuan S: Response of the pulmonary vasculature to hypoxia and H+ ion concentration changes. J Clin Invest 45:399, 1966.
17. Bell TJ: Postoperative care. In: Garson AG Jr, Bricker JT, and McNamara DG (eds): The Science and Practice of Pediatric Cardiology, Vol. III. Philadelphia, Lea & Febiger, 1990, p. 2264.
18. Behrendt DM and Austen WG: Patient Care in Cardiac Surgery, 4th ed. Boston, Little, Brown, 1985, pp. 106–107.
19. Ilabaca PA, Ochsner JL, and Mills NL: Positive end-expiratory pressure in the management of the patient with a postoperative bleeding heart. Ann Thorac Surg 30:282, 1980.
20. Hoffman WS, Tomasello DN, and MacVaugh H. Control of postcardiotomy bleeding with PEEP. Ann Thorac Surg 34:71, 1982.
21. Bertwell WC, Soroff HS, Sachs BF, et al: The use of the lungs as a pump: A method for assisting pulmonary blood flow by varying airway pressure synchronously with EKG. Trans Am Soc Artif Intern Organs 9:192–201, 1963.
22. Naeije R, Maarek JM, and Chang HK: Pulmonary vascular impedance in microembolic pulmonary hypertension: Effects of synchronous high-frequency jet ventilation. Respir Physiol 79:205–217, 1990.
23. Pinsky MR, Matuschak GM, Bernardi L, et al: Hemodynamic effects of cardiac cycle-specific increases in intrathoracic pressure. J Appl Physiol 60:604, 1986.
24. Jansson L, Bengtsson M, and Carlsson C: Heart-synchronized ventilation during general anesthesia for extracorporeal shock wave lithotripsy. Anesth Analg 67:706, 1988.
25. L'Abbate A, Emdin M, Piacenti M, et al: Ultrafiltration: A rational treatment for heart failure. Cardiology 76:384, 1989.
26. Lin JL and Huang CC: Successful initiation of hemodialysis during cardiopulmonary resuscitation due to lethal hyperkalemia. Crit Care Med 18:342, 1990.
27. Crile GW: The resuscitation of the apparently dead and demonstration of the pneumatic blood pressure. Trans South Surg Gynecol Assoc 16:361, 1904.
28. McSwain NE Jr: Pneumatic anti-shock garment: State of the art 1988. Ann Emerg Med 17:506, 1988.
29. Freeman S: Adjunctive techniques for cardiopulmonary resuscitation. In: Tintinalli JE, Rothstein RJ, and Krome RL (eds): Emergency Medicine: A comprehensive Study Guide. N York, McGraw-Hill, 1985, pp. 10–13.
30. Kaplan BC, Civetta JM, Nasel EL, et al: The military anti-shock trouser in civilian pre-hospital emergency care. J Trauma 13:843, 1973.
31. Tenney SM and Honig CR: The effect of the anti-G suit on the ballistocardiogram. J Aviation Med 26:194, 1955.

32. Goldsmith SR: Comparative hemodynamic effects of antishock suit and volume expansion in normal human beings. Ann Emerg Med 12:348, 1983.
33. Wangensteen SL, Ludewig RM, and Eddy DM: The effect of external counterpressure on the intact circulation. Surg Gynecol Obstet 125:253, 1968.
34. Wayne MA and MacDonald SC: Clinical evaluation of the antishock trouser: Retrospective analysis of five years of experience. Ann Emerg Med 12:342, 1983.
35. Mattox KL, Bickell W, Pepe PE, et al: Prospective MAST study in 911 patients. J Trauma 29:1104, 1989.
36. Garcia V, Eichelberger M, Ziegler M, et al: Use of military antishock trousers in a child. J Pediatr Surg 16:544, 1981.
37. Concannon JR, Matre WM, and Verhagen AD: Antishock trousers in pediatrics—a case management report. Clin Pediatr 23:78, 1984.
38. Brunette DD, Fifield G, and Ruiz E: Use of pneumatic antishock trousers in the management of pediatric pelvic hemorrhage. Pediatr Emerg Care 3:86, 1987.
39. Walker LA 3rd, MacMath TL, Chipman H, et al: MAST application in the treatment of paroxysmal supraventricular tachycardia in a child. Ann Emerg Med 17:529, 1988.
40. Rubal BJ, Geer MR, and Bickell WH: Effects of pneumatic antishock garment inflation in normovolemic subjects. J Appl Physiol 67:339, 1989.
41. Rudikoff MT, Maughan WL, Effron M, et al: Mechanisms of blood flow during cardiopulmonary resuscitation. Circulation 61:345, 1980.
42. Weisfeldt ML and Halperin HR: Cardiopulmonary resuscitation: Beyond cardiac massage. Circulation 74:443, 1986.
43. Criley J, Blaufass A, and Kissel G: Cough induced cardiac compression: Self-administered form of cardiopulmonary resuscitation. JAMA 136:1246, 1976.
44. Luce JM, Ross BK, O'Quin RJ, et al: Regional blood flow during cardiopulmonary resuscitation in dogs using simultaneous and nonsimultaneous compression and ventilation. Circulation 67:259, 1983.
45. Berkowitz ID, Chantarojanasiri T, Koehler RC, et al: Blood flow during cardiopulmonary resuscitation with simultaneous compression and ventilation in infant pigs. Pediatr Res 26:558, 1989.
46. Koehler RC, Chandra N, Guerci AD, et al: Augmentation of cerebral perfusion by simultaneous chest compression and lung inflation with abdominal binding after cardiac arrest in dogs. Circulation 67:266, 1983.
47. Kimmel E, Beyar R, Dinnar U, et al: Augmentation of cardiac output and carotid blood flow by chest and abdomen phased compression cardiopulmonary resuscitation. Cardiovasc Res 20:574, 1986.
48. Barranco F, Lesmes A, Irles JA, et al: Cardiopulmonary resuscitation with simultaneous chest and abdominal compression: Comparative study in humans. Resuscitation 20:67, 1990.
49. Mateer JR, Stueven HA, Thompson BM, et al: Interposed abdominal compression CPR versus standard CPR in prehospital cardiopulmonary arrest. Ann Emerg Med 13:764, 1984.
49a. Sack JB, Kesselbrenner MB, and Bergman D: Survival from in-hospital cardiac arrest with interposed abdominal counterpulsation during cardiopulmonary resuscitation. JAMA 267:379, 1992.
50. Mueller H, Ayres M, Grace W, et al: External counterpulsation: A noninvasive method to protect ischemic myocardium in man. Circulation 45, 46 (Suppl. 2): II-195, 1972.
51. Beyar R, Halperin HR, Chandra NC, et al: Manipulation of external pressure as a method to assist the failing heart. IEEE Trans Biomed Eng 37:197, 1990.
52. Amsterdam EA, Banas J, Criley JM, et al: Clinical assessment of external pressure circulatory assistance in acute myocardial infarction: Report of a cooperative clinical trial. Am J Cardiol 45:349, 1980.
53. Heck HA Jr and Doty DB: Assisted circulation by phasic external lower body compression. Circulation 64:II–118, 1981.
54. Tobias JD, Schleien CL, and Reitz BA: Use of the MAST suit in the postoperative care of patients after the Fontan procedure. Crit Care Med 18:781, 1990.
55. Spencer FC, Eiseman B, Trinkle JK, et al: Assisted circulation for cardiac failure following intracardiac surgery with cardiopulmonary bypass. J Thorac Cardiovasc Surg 49:56, 1965.
56. Martin GB, Paradis NA, Rivers EP, et al: Cardiopulmonary bypass in the treatment of cardiac arrest in humans. Crit Care Med 18:S247, 1990.
57. Hartz R, LoCicero L III, Sanders, Jr JH, et al: Clinical experience with portable cardiopulmonary bypass in cardiac arrest patients. Ann Thorac Surg 50:437, 1990.
58. Scholz KH, Tebbe U, Chomnitius M, et al: Transfemoral placement of the left ventricular assist device "Hemopump" during mechanical resuscitation. Thorac Cardiovasc Surg 38:69, 1990.
59. Redmond CR, Graves ED, Falterman KW, et al: Extracorporeal membrane oxygenation for respiratory and cardiac failure in infants and children. J Thorac Cardiovasc Surg 93:199, 1987.
60. Kanter KR, Pennington DG, Weber TR, et al: Extracorporeal membrane oxygenation for postoperative cardiac support in children. J Thorac Cardiovasc Surg 93:27, 1987.
61. Kanter KR, Ruzevich SA, Pennington DG, et al: Follow-up of survivors of mechanical circulatory support. J Thorac Cardiovasc Surg 96:72, 1988.
62. Reedy JE, Swartz MT, Raithel SC, et al: Mechanical cardiopulmonary support for refractory cardiogenic shock. Heart Lung 19:514, 1990.
62a. Dalton HJ, Siewers RD, Fuhrman BP, et al: Extracorporeal membrane oxygenation for cardiac rescue in children with severe myocardial dysfunction. Crit Care Med (in press).
63. Moulopoulos SD, Topaz S, and Kolff WJ: Diastolic balloon pumping (with carbon dioxide) in aorta: Mechanical assistance to failing circulation. Am Heart J 66:669, 1962.
64. Kantrowitz A, Tjonneland S, Freed PS, et al: Initial clinical experience with intraaortic balloon pumping in cardiogenic shock. JAMA 203:113, 1968.
65. Bolooki H: Clinical Application of Intra-aortic Balloon Pump, 2nd ed. Mt. Kisco, NY, Futura Publishing Co., 1984, pp. 57–90.
66. Barnea O, Moore TW, Dubin SE, et al: Cardiac energy considerations during intraaortic balloon pumping. IEEE Trans Biomed Eng 37:170, 1990.
67. Reemtsma K, Bregman D, Cohen SS, et al: Mechanical circulatory support—advances in intra-aortic balloon pumping. In: Shoemaker WC, Ayres SA, Grenvik A, et al (eds): Textbook of Critical Care, 2nd ed. Philadelphia, WB Saunders, 1989, pp. 420–428.
68. Berger RL, Saini VK, Long W, et al: The use of diastolic augmentation with the intra-aortic balloon in human septic shock with associated coronary artery disease. Surgery 74:601, 1973.
69. LoCicero L III, Hartz RS, Sanders JH Jr, et al: Interhospital transport of patients with ongoing intraaortic balloon pumping. Am J Cardiol 56:59, 1985.
70. Bolooki H: Clinical Application of Intra-aortic Balloon Pump, 2nd ed. Mt. Kisco, NY, Futura Publishing Co., 1984, pp. 408–409.
71. Veasy LG, Blaylock RC, Daitoh N, et al: Preclinical evaluation of intra-aortic balloon pumping for pediatric use. Trans Am Soc Artif Intern Organs 27:490, 1981.
72. Pollock JC, Charlton MC, Williams WG, et al: Intraaortic balloon pumping in children. Ann Thorac Surg 29:522, 1980.
73. Veasy LG, Blalock RC, Orth JL, et al: Intra-aortic balloon pumping in infants and children. Circulation 68:1095, 1983.
74. Al Mofada S, Edmonds J, Vobecky S, et al: Intra-aortic balloon pumping (IABP) in children. Crit Care Med 18:S230, 1990.
75. Moran J, Opravil M, Gorman A, et al: Pulmonary artery balloon counterpulsation for right ventricular failure. II: Clinical experiences. Ann Thorac Surg 38:254, 1984.
76. Jett GK, Siwek LG, Picone AL, et al: Pulmonary artery balloon counterpulsation for right ventricular failure—an experimental evaluation. J Thorac Cardiovasc Surg 86:364, 1983.
77. Ghosh PK: Precedents and perspectives. In: Unger F (ed): Assisted Circulation, Vol. 3. Berlin, Springer-Verlag, 1989, pp. 8–45.
78. Norman JC, Cooley DA, Igo SR, et al: Prognostic indices for survival during postcardiotomy intra-aortic balloon pumping: Methods of scoring and classification, with implications for left ventricular assist device utilization. J Thorac Cardiovasc Surg 74:709, 1977.
79. Pennington DG (moderator), Joyce LD, Pae WE Jr, and Burkholder JA: Panel—patient selection. Ann Thorac Surg 47:77, 1989.
80. McGee MG, Zillgitt SL, Trono R, et al: Retrospective analyses of the need for mechanical circulatory support (intra-aortic balloon

pump/abdominal left ventricular assist device or partial artificial heart) after cardiopulmonary bypass: A 44 month study of 14,168 patients. Am J Cardiol 46:135, 1980.

81. Graham TR and Chalmers AC: Temporary mechanical ventricular support, Part 1. Br J Hosp Med 41:420, 1989.
82. Graham TR and Chalmers AC: Temporary mechanical ventricular support, Part 2. Br J Hosp Med 41:520, 1989.
83. Macoviak JA, Dasse KA, and Poirier VL: Mechanical cardiac assistance and replacement. Cardiol Clin 8:39, 1990.
84. Pennington DG and Swartz MT: Management—by circulatory assist devices. Cardiol Clin 7:195, 1989.
85. Taeneka Y, Takano H, Nakatani T, et al: Ventricular assist device (VAD) for children: In vitro and in vivo evaluation. Trans Am Soc Artif Intern Organs 30:155, 1984.
86. Taenaka Y, Takano H, Noda H, et al: A pediatric ventricular assist device: Its development and experimental evaluation of hemodynamic effects on postoperative heart failure of congenital heart diseases. Artif Organs 14:49, 1990.
87. Butler KC, Moise JC, and Wampler RK: The Hemopump®—a new cardiac prosthesis device. IEEE Trans Biomed Eng 37:193, 1990.
88. Bridges CR, Jr, Hammond RL, Dimeo F, et al: Functional right-heart replacement with skeletal muscle ventricles. Circulation 80:III–183, 1989.
89. Chachques JC, Grandjean PA, Bourgeois I, et al: Dynamic cardiomyoplasty to improve ventricular function. In: Unger F

(ed): Assisted Circulation 3. Berlin, Springer-Verlag, 1989, pp. 525–541.
90. Griffith BP, Hardesty RL, Kormos RL, et al: Temporary use of the Jarvik-7 total artificial heart prior to transplantation. N Engl J Med 316:130, 1987.
91. Griffith BP, Kormos RL, Hardesty RL, et al: The artificial heart: Infection-related morbidity and its effect on transplantation. Ann Thorac Surg 45:409, 1988.
92. Termuhlen DF, Pennington DG, Roodman ST, et al: T cells in ventricular assist device patients. Circulation 80:III–174, 1989.
93. Wolner E, Portner PM, Pierce WS, et al: Cardiovascular support versus total artificial heart. Artif Organs 12:242, 1988.
94. Firth BG: Replacement of the failing heart. Am J Med Sci 293:50, 1987.
95. Adamson RM, Dembitsky WP, Reichman RT, et al: Mechanical support: assist or nemesis? J Thorac Cardiovasc Surg 98:915, 1989.
96. Pae WE, Jr, Pierce WS, Pennock JL, et al: Long-term results of ventricular assist pumping in postcardiotomy shock. J Thorac Cardiovasc Surg 93:434, 1987.
97. Parker LS, Arnold RM, Meisel A, et al: Ethical factors in the allocation of experimental medical therapies: The chronic left ventricular assist system. Clin Res 38:537, 1990.
98. Relman AS: Artificial hearts—permanent and temporary. N Engl J Med 314:644, 1986.
99. Annas GJ: No cheers for temporary artificial hearts. Hastings Cent Rep 15:27, 1985.

Cardiovascular Support— Pharmacologic

Daniel A. Notterman, M.D.

Support of the failing circulation is one of the major responsibilities of pediatric critical care. This task is multifaceted, often requiring (1) treatment of abnormal peripheral vascular capacitance and resistance, (2) correction of impaired contractility, (3) suppression of abnormal cardiac rate or rhythm, and (4) restoration of intravascular volume. The focus in this chapter will be on pharmacotherapy that is designed to improve peripheral vascular function or to enhance the inotropic, or contractile, state of the myocardium. The clinical pharmacology of the five catecholamines employed in pediatric critical care will be reviewed, along with that of a newer class, the bipyridines (amrinone, milrinone), and the cardiac glycosides. Nitroprusside and nitroglycerine are presented as examples of vasodilators. Receptor pharmacology is reviewed in Chapter 75, and the treatment of dysrhythmia is presented in Chapter 36.

HISTORY

Cardiac glycosides have been used for medicinal and hunting purposes for millennia. For example, squill is mentioned in the Ebers Papyrus of 1500 B.C;[1] this plant is rich in the glycoside scillaren A and was also used by the Romans to treat heart failure. Early descriptions of foxglove appeared in writings of Welsh physicians, and the plant was given its modern name, *digitalis purpurea,* by Fuchsius in 1542. Withering[2] in his 1785 classic, *An Account of the Foxglove and some of its Medicinal Uses: With Practical Remarks on Dropsy and Other Diseases,* was the first to present a scientific description of the uses and adverse effects of the "foxglove" plant. The importance of this work is not vitiated by the fact that Withering incorrectly attributed the effectiveness of digitoxin in treating edema to a specific renal effect. Ferrier, in 1799, was the first to correctly attribute the mode of action to a direct effect on the heart. In this century, digitalis was used mainly to treat atrial fibrillation; later, it was agreed that glycosides also improve congestive heart failure (CHF) by enhancing contractility.[3]

Catecholamines have also been used for centuries: For example, the skin of dried toad, employed by Chinese physicians for toothache and bleeding gums and by English physicians for dropsy, contains epinephrine and cardiac glycosides.[1] The pressor effect of the catecholamines was demonstrated by Oliver and Schäfer[4] in 1895, who produced hypertension by intravenous injection of extracts of adrenal medulla. Epinephrine was synthesized by Stolz in 1904,[5] who also reported the synthesis of norepinephrine in the same year. Barger and Dale[6] introduced the term *sympathomimetic* in the course of their survey of structure-activity relationships, applying the term to all amines that have, "An action simulating that of the true sympathetic nervous system. . . ."

The era of receptor pharmacology was introduced by Alquist's understanding that the different responses elicited by norepinephrine, epinephrine, and isoproterenol in various tissues could be explained by positing two types of receptors: α and β.[7] Work by Lands and associates led to differentiating β_1 (chiefly cardiac) from β_2 (airway, vascular smooth muscle, glandular tissue) receptors.[8, 9] Subsequently, Langer proposed that α-receptors are also heterogenous and suggested that postsynaptic α-receptors be termed α_1 and that presynaptic α-receptors be termed α_2.[10] Elliot had described the pharmacologic activity of epinephrine by 1905.[11, 12] However, the integration of catecholamines into the treatment of shock was delayed. Thus, in the first edition of Goodman and Gilman's *The Pharmacologic Basis of Therapeutics,* the authors wrote, "Epinephrine has little place in the therapy of shock because the arterioles are already constricted maximally. . . ." Much safer and more effective measures are available for the management of shock than the use of vasopressor drugs.[1]

With a better understanding of the interdependence of preload, contractility, and afterload upon cardiovascular performance, the role of epinephrine and the other endogenous catecholamines has expanded.[13, 14] With this expansion came the desire to develop synthetic catecholamines. Isoproterenol was the first synthetic catecholamine that enjoyed wide clinical use. It was described by Konzett in 1940 and was employed as vasodilator and bronchodilator.[15] Isoproterenol was used to treat shock during the 1960s but was largely abandoned in adult critical care when dopamine was introduced. Norepinephrine, too, was employed extensively during this interval. However, inappropriate use without attention to either cardiac filling pressures or systemic vascular resistance (SVR) produced poor results, and the agent was nearly abandoned until recently. Dopamine, an endogenous neurotransmitter, was introduced for the treatment of shock and other hemodynamic disturbances in the early 1970s by Goldberg.[16] The fifth clinically used catecholamine, dobutamine, was synthesized in 1973 and was soon released to the clinical market in the United States. The newest catecholamine, dopexamine, is a strong β_2-agonist with weaker agonist activity at β_1- and dopaminergic (D_1- and D_2-) receptors. Dopexamine reduces afterload and improves contractility. Preliminary results in treating acute reductions in contractility in adults are encouraging, but information in children is still not available.[17]

MECHANISMS OF RESPONSE

Adrenergic Receptors

Alquist understood that sympathomimetics modify cellular physiology by interacting with a cell surface receptor. Chapter 3 discusses signal transduction, and Chapter 75 describes the physiology of adrenergic receptors in detail; the present chapter offers only such detail as is necessary to explicate the clinical pharmacology of the catecholamines. A clinically useful classification of adrenergic receptors is indicated in Table 29–1.

Adrenergic receptors are members of a family of structurally and genetically related glycoproteins. By extending between the external and the internal surface of the cell membrane, they transduce information. Except for the α_1-receptor, adrenergic receptors affect cell function by altering the intracellular concentration of cyclic adenosine monophosphate (cAMP). When an adrenergic receptor is engaged by an appropriate ligand, the *receptor recognition unit* located on the external

surface of the cell membrane interacts with a *nucleoside regulatory protein,* termed G_s (stimulatory) or G_i (inhibitory). Under appropriate circumstances, the resulting *receptor-G binary complex* associates with the catalytic unit, adenylate cyclase. When G_s is involved, the activity of adenylate cyclase increases. The intracellular concentration of cAMP rises. When the regulatory protein is G_i, this interaction leads to a decrease in the activity of adenylate cyclase, and the intracellular concentration of cAMP falls.[18, 19] This decrease in cAMP is facilitated by the enzyme *phosphodiesterase* (PDE), which degrades cAMP.

Typically, an increase in the concentration of cAMP leads to activation of a cAMP-dependent protein kinase.[20] This kinase, in turn, phosphorylates and activates other structures and enzymes. The ultimate effect is an increase in either the fraction of membrane calcium channels that are open or the time that they are open to calcium.[14, 21] Another process, involving phosphorylation of phospholamban, leads to translocation of calcium from the cytosol into the endoplasmic reticulum. This promotes diastolic relaxation of the myocardium and enhances sarcoplasmic reticulum storage of calcium. Contractility during the subsequent systole is further augmented.[22] Thus, β_1-adrenergic stimulation accentuates both contraction and relaxation.[23] Stimulating myocardial β_1-receptors also produces chronotropic effects. Automaticity is enhanced because diastolic (phase 4) depolarization of the sinoatrial node occurs more rapidly. The refractory period of the atrioventricular (AV) node is shortened. There is evidence that β-adrenergic stimulation increases the degree of heterogeneity between the refractory periods of different areas of the ventricular myocardium and that this may promote myocardial irritability.[24]

In vascular and bronchiolar smooth muscle, activation of β_2-receptors also enhances formation of cAMP; the resulting activation of cAMP-dependent protein kinase in that cell, however, leads to removal of calcium from the cytosol. Smooth muscle relaxes and the blood vessel or bronchiole dilates.

As indicated in Table 29–1, D_1- and D_2-receptors also

Table 29–1. ADRENERGIC RECEPTORS: PHYSIOLOGIC RESPONSES, AGONIST POTENCY, AND REPRESENTATIVE ANTAGONISTS*

Receptor	G Protein	Physiologic Response	Agonist	Antagonist
α_1	G_x†	Increase InsP$_3$, 1,2DG, and intracellular Ca^{2+}, muscle contraction; vasoconstriction; inhibit insulin secretion	E‡>NE§>D‖	Prazosin
α_2	G_i	Decrease cAMP; inhibit NE release; vasodilation; negative chronotropy	E>NE	Yohimbine
β_1	G_s	Increase cAMP; inotropy, chronotropy; enhance renin secretion	I[19]>E≥D≥NE	Propranolol Metoprolol
β_2	G_s	Increase cAMP; smooth muscle relaxation; vasodilatation; bronchodilation; enhance glucagon secretion; hypokalemia	I≥E>D>NE	Propranolol
D_1	G_s	Increase cAMP; smooth muscle relaxation	D	Haloperidol Metoclopramide
D_2	G_i	Decrease cAMP; inhibit prolactin and β-endorphin	D	Domperidone

*Modified from Notterman DA: Pharmacologic support of the failing circulation: An approach for infants and children. Probl Anesth 3:288, 1989.
†Hypothetical.
‡E = epinephrine.
§NE = norepinephrine.
‖D = dopamine.
¶ = isoproterenol.

modify adenylate cyclase. D_1 is associated with G_s and produces stimulation of adenylate cyclase, whereas D_2 is associated with G_i and inhibits adenylate cyclase.

Many nonadrenergic compounds also increase intracellular levels of cAMP. Some, such as prostaglandin E and glucagon, do so through separate, distinct membrane receptors that are also coupled to G_s, whereas others, such as forskolin, stimulate adenylate cyclase directly without the intermediate step of receptor interaction. The *methylxanthines* (theophylline) and the *bipyridines* (amrinone, milrinone) increase cAMP levels by inhibiting PDE. Whether the mechanism is receptor-mediated or not and whether the increase in cAMP is produced by more rapid synthesis or less rapid destruction, the result of a rise in concentration of cAMP in myocytes is enhanced contractility.[18, 19]

The α_1-receptor is an exception to the receptor–G protein–adenylate cyclase model. Signal transduction across this receptor also involves a G protein but not G_s or G_i. When activated, this system causes an enzyme called *phospholipase C* to generate hydrolytic products that enhance extracellular and sarcoplasmic calcium movement into the cytosol.[18, 19, 25]

Changes in the responsiveness of adrenergic receptors to stimulation have been extensively documented. Some of these changes are important to the critical care physician. The best documented is agonist-mediated receptor desensitization. Exposure of receptors to agonists reduces the sensitivity of the target cell to that agonist family (*homologous desensitization*) or to other agonist families (*heterologous desensitization*).[26]

It is known that this process of regulation involves several different mechanisms.[27] Stimuli other than receptor agonists have been implicated in desensitization. These stimuli include endotoxin,[28] tumor necrosis factor,[29, 30] and CHF.[31]

Phosphodiesterase Inhibition

Modification of PDE activity has recently assumed greater importance to the critical care specialist, because the *bipyridines,* a relatively new family of inotropic agents, appear to function through direct inhibition of phosphodiesterase III (PDE III).[32–35] As explained earlier, inhibition of this enzyme is expected to increase cAMP concentration. The concentration of cyclic guanosine monophosphate (cGMP) is not affected by selective inhibition of PDE III.[34, 36] In contrast, methylxanthines, such as theophylline, inhibit all phosphodiesterases (PDE I, PDE II, PDE III). These other PDEs affect the concentration of cGMP as well as that of cAMP. Therefore, broad spectrum PDE inhibitors such as theophylline cause levels of both cGMP and cAMP to increase. It has been argued that the balanced increase in both cAMP and cGMP explains the limited inotropic and marked chronotropic activity of theophylline,[37, 38] though other explanations remain to be considered.[39]

Adenosine Triphosphatase Inhibition

The discussion has thus far emphasized stimuli that enhance production or retard destruction of cAMP. The glycosides act through a different mechanism, though the final common pathway, increased cytosolic calcium, is similar. The target of digitalis is membrane-bound sodium, potassium-adenosine triphosphatase (Na,K-ATPase). This enzyme extrudes sodium from the cell and incorporates potassium into the cell. Inhibition of this pump by the digitalis glycosides produces an increase in intracellular sodium concentration.[40] Secondary exchange of extracellular sodium for intracellular calcium is thereby impeded, and the concentration of intracellular calcium rises. Contractility is enhanced.

Development Issues

The immature heart and vascular system may respond differently to inotropic agents than do adult organs. For example, the inotropic response to dopamine and isoproterenol increases with increasing puppy age.[41, 42] In developing swine, Gootman and associates[43] found that the peripheral vascular response to several adrenergic agonists developed at different rates and that complete reflex integration was not present at birth. These studies are complemented by receptor binding studies that indicate that there are developmental differences in the adrenergic receptor content of a variety of organs,[44] though more recent work indicates that lymphocyte β-adrenergic receptors are fully mature and functional at birth.[45]

Also of potential importance are structural and ultrastructural differences in the hearts of infants, children, and adults. These differences include reduced ventricular compliance, greater ventricular interdependence, and a reduction in the ratio of myocardial contractile:noncontractile protein in the immature heart. For these reasons, the infant's heart neither responds to nor tolerates volume loading as well as the adult heart does, thus limiting this mode of therapy.

The twin limitations of restricted response to augmentation of preload and reduced sensitivity of the heart and peripheral vasculature to adrenergic agents has been taken to imply that the response of the immature organism to infusion of inotropic and vasopressor agents differs from the pattern noted in adults.[46, 47] However, the practical consequences of these differences have not yet been experimentally or clinically established in critically ill children, and an age-based paradigm for therapy with these drugs is still not possible.

CATECHOLAMINES

With very few exceptions, catecholamines are the only sympathomimetic amines employed in Western countries to treat acute disease of the cardiovascular system; the noncatecholamine phenylephrine is occasionally employed as a pressor. This chapter discusses the endogenous catecholamines epinephrine, norepinephrine, and dopamine and the synthetic products isoproterenol and dobutamine. The new agent, dopexamine has not been evaluated in children. Catecholamines are based upon the catechol structure: 3,4 phenylethylamine (Fig.

29–1). Structure-activity relationships are complex and have been recently reviewed.[13] It is possible to generalize by noting that increasing size of the substituent on the amino group enhances β-adrenergic activity, whereas decreasing size of that substituent is associated with α-adrenergic selectivity.

Although it is a simplification of clinical practice, it is useful to categorize catecholamines (and other sympathomimetics) as either *inotropes* or *vasopressors*. An inotrope improves contractility, augmenting stroke work at a given preload and afterload. These agents activate β₁-adrenergic receptors; in so doing, they also increase heart rate, unless this increase is attenuated by other properties of the drug or by reflex activity. As with any treatment that improves cardiac function, improvement in cardiac output may also be accompanied by a desirable reflex relaxation of vascular tone. Inotropic agents that also activate β₂-receptors directly produce peripheral vasodilatation. One result is reflex tachycardia; another can be diversion of blood from vital organs. Vasopressors interact with α₁-adrenergic receptors, increase peripheral vascular tone, and elevate SVR and blood pressure. *In theory, vasopressors treat peripheral vascular failure, whereas inotropic agents treat impaired cardiac contractility.* In practice, most available agents display a blend of inotropic, chronotropic, and vasopressor activity. Norepinephrine and phenylephrine have considerable specificity for the α-adrenergic receptor. Isoproterenol and dobutamine have little α-adrenergic agonist activity but retain considerable activity at the β-receptor. Epinephrine and dopamine are Janus-like. At relatively low infusion rates, they enhance myocardial function, produce vasodilatation, and increase heart rate (β₁ and β₂). At higher rates, pressor activity (α₁) becomes manifested.

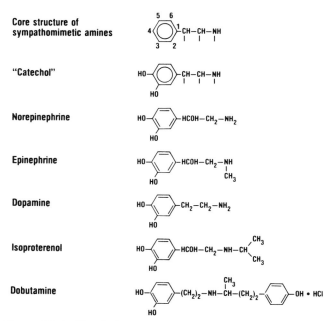

Figure 29–1. Chemical structure of the catecholamines. (Reprinted with permission from Chernow B, Rainey T, and Lake R: Endogenous and exogenous catecholamines in critical care medicine. Crit Care Med 10:6, 1982. © by Williams & Wilkins, 1982.)

Table 29–2. SUMMARY OF INTERACTIONS BETWEEN TRICYCLIC ANTIDEPRESSANTS, MONOAMINE OXIDASE (MAO) INHIBITORS, AND SYMPATHOMIMETICS*

Amplified by MAO Inhibitors
Dopamine
Levodopa
Ephedrine
Phenylephrine
Pseudoephedrine

Amplified by Tricyclics
Dopamine
Epinephrine
Norepinephrine

*Some compounds not discussed in the text are included.

Termination of activity occurs through a variety of different processes, including excretion of unchanged drug in the urine, O-methylation by catechol-O-methyltransferase (COMT), deamination by monoamine oxidase (MAO), sulfoconjugation by phenolsulfotransferase, glucuronidation, and neuronal and extraneuronal uptake. Elimination pathways vary among catecholamines; in addition, for the same substance, methods of elimination depend upon whether the drug is secreted endogenously or administered in pharmacologic doses. The mechanism by which the pharmacologic effect is terminated may be important, because it is likely that processes, or drugs that disturb these processes, will affect dosage requirements. For example, with liver dysfunction, and probably with renal dysfunction, the clearance of dopamine is reduced,[48] implying a need to reduce dosage. Very little is known regarding the effect of coadministered drugs upon catecholamine clearance or duration of action, and there is meager literature regarding pharmacokinetic interactions among the catecholamines themselves. Tricyclic antidepressants such as imipramine and nortriptyline inhibit reuptake of norepinephrine in the synaptic terminal.[13] This may result in an exaggerated pressor response and an increased frequency of dysrhythmias during epinephrine or norepinephrine infusion. It is prudent to begin therapy with these drugs at a starting dose much lower than usual.[49] MAO is not necessary for ending the pharmacologic response to infused epinephrine or norepinephrine; this can be accomplished by COMT. Therefore, it is not obligatory to adjust norepinephrine or epinephrine dosage in patients receiving MAO inhibitors, though the physician should be alert to the possibility of some enhancement of epinephrine's activity. Generally the response to compounds that act *directly* at the nerve terminal (epinephrine, norepinephrine) is *relatively* unaffected by MAO inhibition but is affected by tricyclic antidepressants. The response of compounds that act indirectly, by promoting synaptic release of norepinephrine (tyramine, metaraminol, dopamine), is profoundly amplified by MAO inhibition but is relatively insensitive to tricyclic antidepressants (Table 29–2). Dopamine is both an indirect- and direct-acting compound. With dopamine, caution is needed if a patient is receiving either a tricyclic antidepressant or an MAO inhibitor. In this regard, critical care physicians should recall that

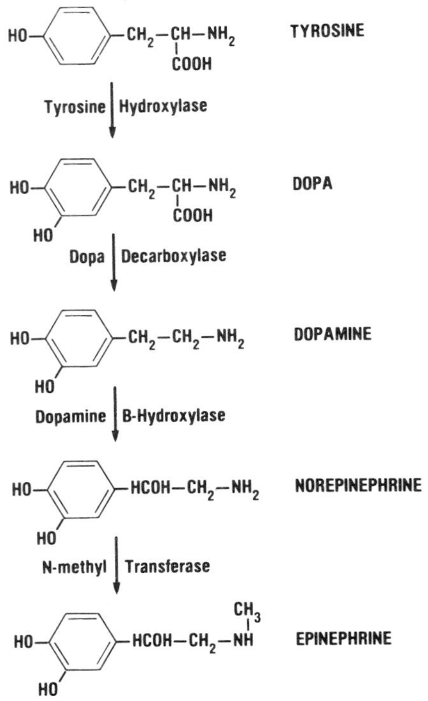

Figure 29–2. Biosynthetic pathway of the endogenous catecholamines. (Reprinted with permission from Chernow B, Rainey T, and Lake R: Endogenous and exogenous catecholamines in critical care medicine. Crit Care Med 10:6, 1982. © by Williams & Wilkins, 1982.)

imipramine is frequently prescribed to young children for treatment of enuresis.

DOPAMINE

Decarboxylation transforms L-DOPA to dopamine (Fig. 29–2). Dopamine is a central neurotransmitter and is also found in sympathetic nerve terminals and in the adrenal medulla, in which it is the immediate precursor of norepinephrine. In healthy individuals, plasma levels of dopamine are in the range of 50 to 100 pg/ml.

Clinical Pharmacology

Dopamine simulates dopamine (D_1 and D_2) receptors located in the brain and in vascular beds in the kidney, mesentery, and coronary arteries (Table 29–3). As the plasma dopamine concentration increases, β-receptors and then α-receptors are activated. In addition to these direct sympathomimetic effects, dopamine also acts as an indirect sympathomimetic, causing release of norepinephrine from sympathetic nerve terminals.

D_1-receptors are coupled (through G_s) to adenylate cyclase (see Table 29–1). The rise in cAMP produced by their activation evokes *vasodilatation*, increasing blood flow to the kidney, gut, and coronary arterial bed. Renal solute and water excretion increases. Dopamine also inhibits release of thyrotropin, aldosterone, and prolactin (D_2-receptors), facilitating renal solute clearance.[14, 50]

Response to infusion of dopamine has been examined in both healthy adult volunteers and critically ill patients. In healthy volunteers, infusion rates between 1 and 10 μg/kg/min increase stroke volume and cardiac output without major effect upon heart rate or blood pressure. These infusion rates are associated with concentrations of 50 to 100 ng/ml. Low infusion rates augment renal sodium excretion, intermediate rates produce chronotropic and inotropic effects, and still higher infusion rates increase vascular resistance.[51–53] These effects are expected from knowledge of the affinity for dopamine of the various classes of adrenergic receptor. Although dopamine produces less tachycardia than does isoproterenol, in healthy adults receiving a relatively low infusion rate of 400 μg/min (5 to 6 μg/kg/min), there is significant augmentation of heart rate and blood pressure.[54] Renal blood flow (RBF), glomerular filtration rate (GFR), and sodium excretion are maintained or even increased during dopamine infusion in patients with poor cardiac output.

There is some information that infants display reduced sensitivity to dopamine; however, the evidence for this view is not strong. In support of reduced sensitivity, one group[55] found that in critically ill neonates, infusion rates of 50 μg/kg/min did not cause clinically evident impairment of cutaneous or renal perfusion. There is

Table 29–3. MAJOR HEMODYNAMIC EFFECTS OF ADRENERGIC RECEPTOR ACTIVATION BY CATECHOLAMINES*

Agent	Receptor			
	α_1	β_1	β_2	D_1†
Dopamine‡	Vasoconstriction, ↑ SVR§, PVR‖	Inotropy, chronotropy	Vasodilatation	Vasodilatation (renal)
Norepinephrine	Vasoconstriction, ↑ SVR, PVR	Inotropy (minor)	—	—
Epinephrine**	Vasoconstriction, ↑ SVR, PVR	Inotropy, chronotropy	Vasodilatation	—
Isoproterenol	—	Inotropy, chronotropy	Vasodilatation	—
Dobutamine	See text	Inotropy	—	—
Amrinone	Nonreceptor-mediated inotropy and vasodilatation			

*Adapted from Notterman DA: Pharmacologic support of the failing circulation: An approach for infants and children. Probl Anesth 3:288, 1989.
†D_1 = dopamine receptor.
‡Dose-related. At low infusion rates, D_1-receptor effects predominate; at intermediate rates, β_1- and β_2-receptor effects predominate; and at high rates, α-receptor effects predominate.
§SVR = systemic vascular resistance.
‖PVR = pulmonary vascular resistance.
**Dose-related. At low infusion rates, β_1- and β_2-receptor effects predominate; at high rates, α-receptor effects predominate.

also some experimental evidence for diminished sensitivity to dopamine in infants; however, this is limited to studies in immature animals.[41, 42] Padbury and associates[56] measured cardiac output in a group of infants and found that mean blood pressure increased at doses of 0.5 to 1.0 μg/kg/min, whereas heart rate increased at doses greater than 2 to 3 μg/kg/min. Cardiac output (and stroke volume) increased before heart rate, and SVR did not change within the range of dopamine infusion rates (0.5 to 8 μg/kg/min).

In contrast to the situation in adults, infused dopamine crosses the blood-brain barrier in preterm neonates. The fact that dopamine crosses the blood-brain barrier should mitigate against use of this drug for trivial indications in preterm infants.

Low infusion rates of dopamine are frequently employed to augment renal function during critical illness.[57–59] This may promote salt excretion and renal plasma flow; however, it is unlikely that the incidence of renal failure due to poor perfusion is thereby modified.

Pharmacokinetics

Plasma dopamine clearance ranges from 60 to 80 ml/kg/min in normal adults.[54] The half-life has not been reliably determined but probably is in the range of 2 to 4 minutes. As mentioned before, clearance is lower in patients with renal or hepatic disease.[48, 60] Clearance in children younger than 2 years of age is approximately twice as rapid as it is in older children (82 versus 46 ml/kg/min).[48] This pharmacokinetic difference, rather than a difference in receptors or myocardial sensitivity, may account for the observations that infants require and tolerate higher infusion rates. Dopamine crosses the human placenta, but the effect on the fetus is not known.

Role in Therapy

There is little systematically collected information concerning the use of dopamine in children; however, dopamine is very widely employed in pediatric critical care. This important role is due to its blend of inotropic and vasopressor properties and its potential enhancement of renal function. Dopamine is less likely than either epinephrine or isoproterenol to evoke tachycardia or dysrhythmias at modest infusion rates. One group[61] employed dopamine in 24 children (newborn to 18 years of age). In 20 of 24 of these children, CHF was the cause of shock or cardiovascular insufficiency. More than half of the subjects displayed at least a 15% increase in blood pressure at an average rate of 8.3 μg/kg/min. Tachycardia was not a limiting problem. Dopamine has also been effective in infants with a variety of conditions associated with circulatory failure, including hyaline membrane disease, asphyxia, sepsis syndrome, and cyanotic CHF.[62, 63]

After ensuring an adequate circulating volume, dopamine is administered to treat moderately severe degrees of distributive shock. In this context, it is valuable when mean blood pressure is normal or when there are modest degrees of hypotension. However, in septic shock, dopamine is *not* the agent of choice when hemodynamic measurements reveal an elevated cardiac output in the context of a markedly reduced SVR and profound hypotension. This pattern is best treated by judicious use of a vasopressor such as norepinephrine. Dopamine is also not the drug of choice to treat severe hypotension associated with major reductions in cardiac index (e.g., <2 to 2.5 l/min/m²), regardless of the primary cause of shock. Epinephrine is more appropriate. When contractility and blood pressure are only moderately depressed, dopamine may be effective.

Abnormal contractility that is not complicated by frank hypotension is better treated with a purely inotropic agent such as dobutamine or amrinone. This is because the infusion rates of dopamine needed to ameliorate severe myocardial dysfunction may be associated with troublesome tachycardia, dysrhythmia, hypertension, and probably untoward increases in myocardial oxygen consumption.

Following cardiac surgery, dopamine is extensively employed to provide hemodynamic support. There are surprisingly few data with which to evaluate this practice in children.[64]

Therapy is initiated with an infusion rate of 5 to 10 μg/kg/min (Table 29–4). The rate of infusion is increased in steps of 2 to 5 μg/kg/min, guided by evidence of improved blood flow (skin temperature, capillary refill, sensorium, urine output) and restoration of blood pressure appropriate for age. Infusion rates greater than 25 to 30 μg/kg/min of dopamine are not customary, even if "normal" blood pressure is maintained. At infusion rates of this magnitude, the effect upon blood pressure is likely to represent an increase in SVR (α-adrenergic activation) rather than cardiac output. A requirement for a dopamine infusion of this magnitude suggests reevaluation of the physiologic diagnosis or changing to a different agent such as epinephrine or norepinephrine. A comparison of dopamine with other agents described in this chapter is presented in Table 29–5.

Adverse Effects

Central Nervous System

Nausea and vomiting are relatively common during infusion of dopamine and may reflect stimulation of

Table 29–4. SUGGESTED INFUSION RATES (μg/kg⁻¹/ min⁻¹) FOR CATECHOLAMINES AND AMRINONE

Agent	Saluretic	Inotropic	Pressor
Dopamine	0.5–2	2–15	>15 (25)*
Norepinephrine	—	—	0.05–1(2)
Epinephrine	—	0.05–0.5	0.1–1(3)
Isoproterenol	—	0.05–1†	—
Dobutamine	—	5.0–20(40)	—
Amrinone	—	5–10‡	—

*Number in parentheses indicated suggested maximum infusion rate.
†For inotropy or chronotropy.
‡Loading dose required (see text).

Table 29–5. SELECTING INOTROPIC AND VASOPRESSOR AGENTS FOR SPECIFIC HEMODYNAMIC DISTURBANCES IN CHILDREN*†

Hemodynamic Pattern	Blood Pressure or SVR		
	Normal	Decreased	Elevated
Septic shock			
Stroke index ↑ ↔	None or dopamine‡	Norepinephrine	None
Stroke index ↓	Dobutamine or dopamine	Dopamine or epinephrine or dobutamine + norepinephrine	Dobutamine + nitroprusside
Cardiogenic shock§	Dobutamine or amrinone or dopamine	Epinephrine or dopamine	—
Myocardial dysfunction (complicating critical illness)‖	Dobutamine or dopamine or amrinone	Epinephrine or dobutamine + norepinephrine	Dobutamine + nitroprusside
CHF	Dobutamine or dopamine or amrinone	—	Dobutamine + nitroprusside
Bradycardia	None	Isoproterenol or epinephrine	None

*Adapted from Notterman DA: Pharmacologic support of the failing circulation: An approach for infants and children. Probl Anesth 3:288, 1989.
†Combinations of drugs are denoted by " + ". Alternatives are denoted by "or."
‡0.5–2 μg/kg/min.
§Isoproterenol may be effective following open heart surgery in infants.
‖For example, ARDS, anthracycline therapy, and so on.

dopamine receptors located in the fourth ventricle of the brain.

Dopamine depresses the ventilatory response to both hypoxemia and hypercarbia.[65] In patients who were already hypoxemic, an infusion of dopamine (3 μg/kg/min) reduced minute ventilation by 60%.[66] The potential effect of dopamine infusion upon apnea testing for brain death determination has not been examined.

Heart

As a class, the catecholamines produce qualitatively similar adverse cardiac effects. Increased oxygen consumption and induction of atrial and ventricular dysrhythmias are the two most important potential problems. Neither has been adequately defined in the pediatric age group.

All inotropes, with the possible exception of amrinone, increase myocardial oxygen consumption. This is because the ultimate effect of increasing myocardial contractility is to increase myocardial work. Increasing myocardial work is not necessarily desirable, and chronic CHF is frequently better treated by improving cardiac performance through modification of afterload and preload.[67] This may not be possible in the critical care setting, and it is often necessary to increase cardiac output by directly stimulating ventricular performance. If the resulting increase in oxygen utilization is balanced by improved coronary blood flow, the net effect upon oxygen balance is salutary. In shock caused or complicated by myocardial failure, an inotrope may lead to reduced ventricular size and wall tension, a decrease in preload and afterload, an increase in coronary artery perfusion pressure and, if heart rate decreases, prolongation of diastolic coronary flow. The result is a net improvement in oxygen balance. The same agent, producing the same increment in contractility in a person who is not experiencing heart failure, may merely increase cardiac work and oxygen utilization without a concomitant increase in myocardial oxygen delivery. Drugs evoking significant tachycardia (isoproterenol,

epinephrine) are more likely to be associated with an unfavorable net effect upon oxygen balance than those associated with less tachycardia, such as dobutamine.

Although the effect upon myocardial oxygen balance is probably more favorable during dopamine infusion than it is during infusion of isoproterenol[68] or epinephrine, it is less favorable than during infusion of dobutamine[69] or amrinone.[70] Compared with other agents now available to treat CHF, such as dobutamine and amrinone, dopamine is more likely to evoke tachycardia and dysrhythmias.[71]

Vascular System

As the dosage increases, α_1-adrenergic activation becomes important, and vasoconstriction replaces vasodilatation. Taken to an extreme, tissue perfusion is embarrassed, and delivery of oxygen and other nutrients is impaired.

Skin

Dopamine has been frequently involved in limb ischemia, gangrene of distal parts and entire extremities, and extensive loss of skin. This has occurred with infusion rates as low as 1.5 μg/kg/min.[72-74] Pre-existing vascular disease and prior frostbite increase the chance of this occurring. The presence of an arterial catheter also increases the possibility of limb ischemia. Because dopamine promotes release of norepinephrine from synaptic terminals (and is also converted to norepinephrine in vivo[75]), it is more often associated with limb ischemia than are other adrenergic compounds. Extravasation of dopamine should be treated immediately by local infiltration with a solution of phentolamine (Regitine) (5 to 10 mg in 15 ml of normal saline) administered with a fine hypodermic needle.[76]

Respiratory System

Several catecholamines decrease PaO_2 by perturbing ventilation perfusion ($\dot{V}/\dot{Q}$) matching.[77] Mechanisms include pulmonary vascular recruitment and attenuation of hypoxic vasoconstriction. This phenomenon is not observed (and can be reversed) with α-agonists such as phenylephrine and norepinephrine. It is best described following administration of dopamine, isoproterenol, or dobutamine. In one study, dopamine increased shunt in patients with adult respiratory distress syndrome (ARDS) from 27 to 40%.[78]

Drug Interactions

The interaction with MAO inhibitors has been described. Reports indicate that coadministration of dopamine with ergot alkaloids increases the risk of distal limb ischemia and gangrene.[79]

Although dopamine receptor antagonists, such as metoclopramide and haloperidol, could plausibly be expected to affect the response to infused dopamine, convincing evidence that this occurs is not available.

Preparation and Administration

To avoid the risk of skin injury from extravasation, dopamine is administered by central vein. It may be administered through an intraosseous needle for limited periods.[80] Tables 29–6 and 29–7 provide information regarding compatibility and preparation of infusions. At the low infusion volumes often employed in infants and children, available infusion pumps produce cyclic variations in fluid delivery rate. These may be of sufficient magnitude to cause oscillations in hemodynamic response.[81] Therefore when treating infants and small children, it is good practice to administer dopamine (and other vasoactive compounds) by a syringe-type pump.

Clinical Summary

Dopamine is employed in the setting of moderately severe cardiogenic or distributive shock associated with modest hypotension. When there is no hypotension, acute severe cardiac failure is treated with dobutamine or amrinone. When septic or cardiogenic shock is complicated by severe hypotension, norepinephrine or epinephrine is preferred, depending upon hemodynamic measurements (see Table 29–5).

Table 29–6. A METHOD FOR PREPARING CATECHOLAMINE INFUSIONS IN PEDIATRIC PATIENTS*

Drug	Preparation	Infusion Rate
Isoproterenol Epinephrine Norepinephrine	0.6 mg × body weight (kg) added to diluent to make 100 ml	1 ml/hour delivers 0.1 μg/kg/min
Dopamine Dobutamine Amrinone†	6 mg × body weight (kg) added to diluent to make 100 ml	1 ml/hour delivers 1 μg/kg/min

*Adapted from Zaritsky A and Chernow B: Use of catecholamines in pediatrics. J Pediatr 105:341, 1984.
†Avoid dextrose-containing solutions.

Table 29–7. INTRAVENOUS FLUIDS AND DRUGS COMPATIBLE WITH CATECHOLAMINE INFUSION*†

Intravenous Fluids
Dextrose (5–20%) in water or normal saline
Dextran 40,000
Mannitol 20%
Normal saline
Protein hydrolysate 5% in dextrose 5%
Ringer's lactate
TPN‡ solution
Drugs
Aminophylline
Other catecholamines
Heparin
Lidocaine
Methylprednisolone
Nitroglycerin
Potassium chloride

*Adapted from Notterman DA: Pharmacologic support of the failing circulation: An approach for infants and children. Probl Anesth 3:288, 1989.
†Consult manufacturer for more specific information.
‡TPN = total parenteral nutrition.

NOREPINEPHRINE

Hydroxylation of dopamine at the β carbon yields norepinephrine, the principal neurotransmitter of the sympathetic nervous system (see Figs. 29–1 and 29–2). Because a substituent on the N (amino)-terminus is lacking, it is a moderately potent α- and β₁-agonist.

Clinical Pharmacology

Administration to normal subjects sharply elevates SVR because α-adrenergic stimulation is not opposed by β₂-adrenergic stimulation (Fig. 29–3). Reflex vagal activity slows the rate of sinus node discharge. Renal, splanchnic, and hepatic blood flow decreases. Coronary blood flow may increase because of the rise in diastolic blood pressure and because of vasodilator α-adrenergic receptors located in the coronary arteries. Improved coronary blood flow is more likely to occur in patients who are hypotensive. Similarly, in hypotensive patients, norepinephrine may produce an increase in urine output.[82]

Pharmacokinetics

In the healthy supine adult, plasma levels of norepinephrine are much higher than those of epinephrine (250 to 500 versus 20 to 60 pg/ml). The minimum concentration at which norepinephrine produces detectable hemodynamic activity is at least 1,500 to 2,000 pg/ml.[83] The clearance of norepinephrine in healthy adults is 24 to 40 ml/kg/min.

Role in Therapy

Norepinephrine is employed to improve perfusion to vital organs in children with low blood pressure and

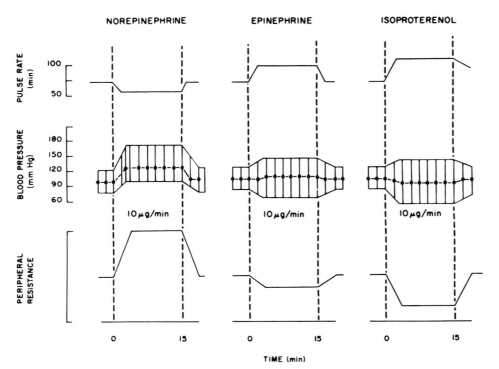

Figure 29–3. The effects of intravenous infusion of norepinephrine, epinephrine, and isoproterenol in humans. (Reprinted with permission from Allwood MJ, Cobbold AF, and Ginsberg J: Peripheral vascular effects of noradrenaline, isopropylnoradrenaline and dopamine. Br Med Bull 19:132, 1963.)

normal or elevated cardiac index. This virtually limits its use in pediatric practice to the treatment of septic shock. Even in this setting, norepinephrine is administered only after intravascular volume repletion and is best guided by knowledge of cardiac output and SVR. Published experience with norepinephrine used to treat children is limited. Recent publications concerning adult patients have supported its use in the clinical context in which hypotension is unresponsive to volume repletion and infusion of dopamine.[84–87] In these individuals, norepinephrine has produced increases in SVR, arterial blood pressure, and urine flow. If successful, treatment with norepinephrine (starting infusion rate: 0.1 μg/kg/min) should elevate perfusion pressure so that vital organ function is maintained. Practically speaking, this means employing the lowest infusion rate that improves perfusion, as judged by skin color and temperature, mental status, and urine flow. Although invasive monitoring, including pulmonary artery catheterization, is desirable for safe use, specific values of SVR or blood pressure are not appropriate end points for therapy.

Adverse Effects

Heart

The net effect of norepinephrine infusion upon oxygen balance is difficult to predict. The increase in afterload that it produces would be expected to increase myocardial oxygen consumption; however, norepinephrine also decreases heart rate, a factor that should reduce oxygen consumption and improve diastolic coronary perfusion.[88] Norepinephrine will not promote or exacerbate tachy-dysrhythmias, which is a major advantage.

Vascular System

Injudicious use of norepinephrine will lead to compromised organ blood flow. In some patients, norepinephrine infusion elevates blood pressure but does not improve clinical indices of perfusion. A poor clinical response of this type is usually associated with an abnormally low cardiac index, stroke volume, left ventricular stroke work index, and an elevated pulmonary capillary wedge pressure (PCWP).[85, 86] Employing excessive dosages, or using norepinephrine in circumstances in which it elevates blood pressure without improving perfusion, may lead to ischemic injury to extremities, widespread organ system failure, and death.

Infusion of norepinephrine constricts pulmonary as well as systemic arterial vessels, and increases pulmonary vascular resistance (PVR).

Drug Interactions

The interaction between tricyclic antidepressents and norepinephrine has been described. Guanethidine, an antihypertensive agent, potentiates the pressor effect of norepinephrine.[89] Clearance of lidocaine is reduced by norepinephrine.[90]

Preparation and Administration

Norepinephrine is administered only by central venous catheter, except in emergency. Extravasation of norepinephrine will result in injury to skin and deeper tissues. Extravasation is treated by infiltrating phentolamine, as described for dopamine. The practice of adding small amounts of phentolamine to norepinephrine infusate is irrational and should be abandoned.

Clinical Summary

Norepinephrine is an excellent choice when the principal hemodynamic disturbance involves hypotension with abnormally low SVR and normal or high cardiac output (see Table 29–5). The best described indication is septic shock, and in this condition the compound is effective and well tolerated.

EPINEPHRINE

Unlike norepinephrine, synthesis of epinephrine is confined to a single site, the adrenal medulla. There, it is formed from norepinephrine by the addition of a methyl group to the N-terminus (see Fig. 29–2). Epinephrine is a hormone, and endogenous levels change with the physiologic state of the organism. The metabolic and hemodynamic effects of this hormone of stress have been extensively reviewed.[13]

Clinical Pharmacology

Epinephrine activates receptors of the α, β_1, and β_2 types. β_1-receptors are affected by very low concentrations of epinephrine; consequently, one of the early effects of epinephrine infusion is activation of β_1-receptors in the myocardium and conducting systems (infusion rates 0.05 to 0.2 μg/kg/min). Heart rate increases, and systolic time intervals are shortened. Contractility is augmented: The force of contraction and rate of rise of pressure increase. Stimulation of peripheral β_2-receptors relaxes resistance arterioles; SVR decreases and diastolic blood pressure falls (see Fig. 29–3). As SVR falls, reflex tachycardia is superimposed on the direct chronotropic effect of epinephrine. Higher plasma concentrations (infusion rates 0.5 to 2 μg/kg/min) are associated with activation of vascular α-receptors, and SVR increases.

The relationship between plasma epinephrine concentration and response was determined by Cryer.[83] Basal levels are around 40 pg/ml. In a group of critically ill children not receiving catecholamines, epinephrine levels were between 0 and 1,378 pg/ml at admission (mean 508 pg/ml).[91] In healthy individuals, heart rate accelerates at levels between 50 and 100 pg/ml; changes in blood pressure (systolic blood pressure increases, diastolic blood pressure decreases) occur at levels between 75 and 100 pg/ml. Hepatic and splanchnic blood flow increase, whereas RBF may be reduced. A variety of metabolic effects (hyperglycemia, hyperlactemia, ketogenesis, and glycolysis) occur at levels between 150 and 200 pg/ml. Insulinopenia occurs at 400 pg/ml. Concentrations of this magnitude are achieved during therapeutic infusion of the drug, accounting for the hyperglycemia that is frequently encountered. Other metabolic effects include hypophosphatemia and hypokalemia. Desensitization to elevated levels of epinephrine occurs rapidly and may be present prior to administration of exogenous catecholamines in the intensive care unit.

Pharmacokinetics

The pharmacokinetics of infused epinephrine have not been determined in the pediatric age group, and factors affecting kinetics in critically ill patients have not been examined.

Role in Therapy

Epinephrine is employed to treat shock associated with myocardial dysfunction. The setting is usually one in which dopamine or dobutamine has not produced an adequate improvement in perfusion. In this setting, epinephrine is employed whether myocardial dysfunction is primary (e.g., cardiomyopathy or following open heart surgery[92]) or secondary (e.g., septic shock).

Epinephrine is most likely to be useful when hypotension exists in the context of a low stroke index. In treating *septic shock*, epinephrine is indicated for the subset of patients in whom significant myocardial dysfunction coexists with abnormal regulation of vascular tone. In treating *cardiogenic shock*, epinephrine is considered when contractility is so poor that it embarrasses perfusion even after administration of other inotropic agents. Epinephrine by infusion is also the agent of choice for hypotension or shock following successful treatment of cardiac arrest. Shock following an episode of hypoxemia or ischemia is usually cardiogenic[93] and may respond to epinephrine infusion.

Bolus injections of epinephrine are used to treat asystole and other nonperfusing rhythms. The recommended dosage is 0.01 mg/kg (10 μg/kg or 0.1 ml/kg of the 1:10,000 solution), though recently some have suggested that "high-dose epinephrine" is more likely to be associated with successful resuscitation. Proponents of higher doses have employed 0.2 mg/kg for treatment of pediatric cardiac arrest.[94, 95] More work is needed to define the optimal dosage of epinephrine in this setting. Epinephrine may be given by endotracheal tube; acquisition of a high plasma epinephrine concentration has been demonstrated, though the dosage required for endotracheal administration has not been settled. It seems appropriate to double the usual dosage (i.e., administer 0.02 mg/kg) diluted in 1 ml of saline to ensure delivery to the distal airway. Intraosseous administration is useful for both bolus and continuous infusion (for short periods) when direct vascular access is difficult,[80] and is preferred to endotracheal administration.

Adverse Effects

Central Nervous System

Epinephrine produces unpleasant subjective symptoms of central nervous system excitation, including anxiety, dread, vascular-type headaches, weakness, nausea, emesis, and dyspnea. Although these sensations may be disturbing, they rarely interfere with therapy.

Heart

Adverse cardiac effects associated with epinephrine are qualitatively similar to those noted during infusion of dopamine, but they are of greater magnitude. Although myocardial oxygen balance is surely affected by administration of epinephrine, there is no data from children to assist the practitioner in predicting circumstances in which the effect will be favorable or unfavorable. The best that can be said, given the paucity of objective data, is that the lowest dose that increases global systemic perfusion should be employed. Extreme tachycardia carries a substantial oxygen penalty, as does hypertension. Acute, severe mismatching of myocardial oxygen delivery to oxygen consumption may be recognized by characteristic electrocardiographic changes of ischemia or by chest pain. More subtle, however, is the effect of a subischemic, but persistently unfavorable, ratio of oxygen delivery:consumption. This subject has not been adequately examined in the setting of critical illness in children.

Epinephrine always produces tachycardia. Increases in infusion rate lead to successively more serious events, including atrial and ventricular extrasystoles, atrial ventricular tachycardia, and, ultimately, ventricular fibrillation and death. In preadolescent children, epinephrine infusion is frequently associated with heart rates as high as 150 to 180 bpm. It appears to be well tolerated. Ventricular dysrhythmias in this age group are not frequent, but they can be evoked by the presence of another risk factor, such as myocarditis, hypokalemia, or hypoxemia. Induction of dysrhythmias is traditionally ascribed to stimulation of β_1 adrenergic receptors; however, recent evidence indicates that ischemia (or hypoxia) is associated with an increase in the number of myocardial α_1 adrenergic receptors.[24] These receptors elicit responses that are proarrhythmogenic. It is possible that these receptors are involved in catecholamine-induced dysrhythmias.

Epinephrine overdosage is serious. Toxicity developed in neonates because similar labeling of bottles containing DL (racemic)-epinephrine and vitamin E led to oral administration of huge amounts of epinephrine. The syndrome mimicked an epidemic of neonatal sepsis with shock and metabolic acidosis.[96] Intra-aortic injection in infants (via umbilical artery) produces tachycardia, hypertension, and renal failure.[97] Intravenous overdosage of epinephrine is immediately life-threatening. In adults, myocardial infarction, ventricular tachycardia, extreme hypertension (up to 400/300), cerebral hemorrhage, seizures, renal failure, and pulmonary edema have occurred. Bradycardia has also been observed.[98]

Manifestations of acute overdosage are treated symptomatically. β-Receptor antagonists such as propranolol are avoided (see further on). Hypertension is treated symptomatically with short-acting antihypertensive agents (i.e., nitroprusside). Nitroglycerin has been employed to ameliorate myocardial ischemia.[99]

Vascular System

In the critical care setting, excessive infusion rates of epinephrine (and other catecholamines) will be heralded by a decreasing urine output and clinical signs of poor cutaneous perfusion (distal coolness and cyanosis, poor capillary refill, narrow pulse volume). Ultimately there is evidence of widespread tissue ischemia with metabolic acidosis and multiple organ system failure.

Respiratory System

Epinephrine variably increases PVR. Central venous and pulmonary arterial and venous pressures increase because of redistribution of blood from the systemic to the pulmonary arterial system. In overdosage, this effect is accentuated, and pulmonary edema occurs.[100]

Metabolic Effects

Hypokalemia is frequently encountered during epinephrine infusion and has been attributed to activation of β_2-adrenergic receptors, which are linked to Na,K-ATPase located in skeletal muscle. In normal volunteers, infusion of 0.1 µg/kg/min lowered serum potassium levels by 0.8 mEq/l.[101] Hyperglycemia results from α-adrenergic–mediated suppression of insulin release; usually this effect is undesirable and may compel use of exogenous insulin. Epinephrine also accelerates glucose metabolism by activating glycogen phosphorylase, and it decreases production of glycogen by inhibiting glycogen synthetase. Gluconeogenesis is accelerated. In infants, this effect is occasionally exploited to treat refractory hypoglycemia. Accelerated glycogenolysis in muscle ultimately leads to production of lactate, and lacticacidemia results.[102] Therefore, on occasion it may be incorrect to attribute increasing plasma lactate levels during catecholamine infusion to worsening tissue perfusion. Another effect is activation of lipase, which elevates free fatty acid concentration and increases concentrations of cholesterol and low-density lipoprotein.

Infusion of epinephrine in normal volunteers increases global oxygen consumption by 20 to 30%.[13] The importance of this response in critically ill children is unknown.

Skin

Epinephrine is an α_1-adrenergic agonist, and infiltration into local tissues or intra-arterial injection can produce severe vasospasm and tissue injury; however, activation of β_2-receptors by epinephrine limits vasospasm, and local injury to tissue is less frequent than with either norepinephrine or dopamine.

Drug Interactions

The need to avoid epinephrine in children who are receiving tricyclic antidepressants has been mentioned. Administration of epinephrine to patients receiving a nonselective β-adrenergic antagonist, such as propranolol, permits unopposed α_1-receptor stimulation and produces hypertension and reflex bradycardia. These events have terminated in cardiac arrest or hypertensive stroke.[49, 103] Cardioselective antagonists such as metoprolol, atenolol, or acebutolol may be safer in this context than nonselective β-blockers. *Halogenated anesthetics,* particularly halothane, have been implicated in sensitizing the myocardium to the arrhythmogenic effects of epinephrine.[104–106] This is less likely to be a problem in children and is more likely in the context of hypoxemia or hypercarbia. Enflurane and isoflurane produce fewer dysrhythmias when used in patients who require catecholamine infusion. Chloral hydrate, a sedative hypnotic, has also been associated with induction of arrhythmias and should be avoided, if possible, in children receiving epinephrine.[107, 108]

Preparation and Administration

Epinephrine should be infused by a syringe-type pump into a central vein. Consult Tables 29–6 and 29–7 for compatibility and dilution information.

Clinical Summary

Epinephrine is useful in treating shock associated with myocardial dysfunction and hypotension when other agents have not been successful. Appropriate settings for epinephrine infusion are (1) cardiogenic shock, (2) septic shock associated with reduced stroke volume, and (3) shock following severe hypoxemia-ischemia (see Table 29–5).

ISOPROTERENOL

Isoproterenol is structurally related to norepinephrine (see Fig. 29–1). The isopropyl N-terminal substituent confers β (β$_1$ and β$_2$)-receptor specificity; the compound does not affect the α-adrenergic receptor. Its cardiovascular activities thus relate to its inotropic, chronotropic, and vasodilator effects.

Clinical Pharmacology

Isoproterenol enhances cardiac contractility and cardiac rate. Peripheral vasodilatation produces a fall in SVR, which augments the direct chronotropic action of the drug. Systolic blood pressure increases, whereas mean and diastolic pressures fall. Tachycardia may be extreme (see Fig. 29–3). If the patient is normal prior to infusion of isoproterenol, mesenteric and renal perfusion fall; however, if the subject is in shock prior to administration, the increase in cardiac output associated with isoproterenol may result in an increase in blood flow to these tissues.[13] When the intravascular compartment is depleted, hypotension complicates initiation of isoproterenol infusion.

Isoproterenol has few important metabolic effects. Hyperglycemia is not usually observed, though the drug does promote release of free fatty acids.

Pharmacokinetics

Isoproterenol is metabolized by COMT. The half-life of elimination is about 2 minutes. Information about therapeutic isoproterenol concentrations is not available in critically ill patients. In healthy volunteers, tachycardia and increases in stroke volume were observed at 50 pg/ml.[109]

Role in Therapy

Stimulation of pulmonary bronchial and vascular bed β$_2$ adrenergic receptors produces bronchodilatation. The principle indication for continuous intravenous infusion of isoproterenol is in children with refractory or rapidly worsening status asthmaticus.[110] Formerly, isoproterenol was used to treat a variety of problems, including septic shock and cardiogenic shock associated with myocardial infarction; however, newer agents such as dopamine and dobutamine, together with a better understanding of the pathophysiology of shock, have made isoproterenol largely obsolete as therapy for shock.

Isoproterenol is still employed to treat hemodynamically significant bradycardia. This indication is narrow: When bradycardia results from heart block, atropine is the initial form of drug therapy, and placement of a pacemaker is definitive treatment. Isoproterenol is used when bradycardia is resistant to atropine, or when there is a delay in placing a pacing device. Many physicians prefer to use epinephrine infusion for this purpose. Of course, bradycardia caused by anoxia is treated by administering oxygen and improving gas exchange.

Some clinicians prefer isoproterenol as a first-line agent for infants following cardiac surgery. Although this indication is not well explored in the literature, it appears rational, because, as discussed, it may be difficult to obtain inotropic augmentation in young infants.[46] The remaining method to increase cardiac output may be to increase heart rate. A second advantage is that isoproterenol causes vasodilatation. In one report, isoproterenol provided a greater improvement in cardiac output than did either atrial pacing or atrial pacing combined with dobutamine,[111] and other physicians have found isoproterenol useful following a Senning repair of transposition of the great vessels.[112]

Adverse Effects

Heart

Isoproterenol causes intense tachycardia. During infusion in children for treatment of status asthmaticus, sinus rates of 180 to 190 bpm are anticipated. It is not surprising that the full range of ventricular and atrial tachydysrhythmias has been encountered during infusion of isoproterenol.

Isoproterenol imposes a substantial increase in myocardial oxygen demand. Myocardial oxygen delivery *decreases* because of shortened diastole and a decrease in diastolic blood pressure.[68] Oxygen balance is so adversely affected that it is possible to induce myocardial infarction when there is no coronary artery disease. Myocardial ischemia, myocardial infarction, and fatal myocardial necrosis have occurred in teen-aged children who received the drug by infusion for status asthmaticus.[113–115]

Drug Interactions

Isoproterenol infusion increases clearance of theophylline[116, 117] and lidocaine,[90] decreasing the blood concentration of these compounds. The interaction with theophylline is clinically important, since the two compounds are frequently coadministered. MAO inhibitors and tricyclic antidepressants do not affect the response to isoproterenol. Propranolol attenuates the cardiovascular and bronchodilator effects of isoproterenol and other catecholamines.[118] This needs to be considered following cardiac surgery in the child who has received propranolol preoperatively.

Preparation and Administration

Isoproterenol administration requires very careful cardiovascular monitoring. Continuous electrocardiographic monitoring is important, with attention to evidence of myocardial ischemia. Chest pain or other symptoms of ischemia should prompt immediate reduction in the dosage. Daily determination of cardiac enzyme levels is appropriate.

Relative intolerance to sustained tachycardia and the possibility of coronary artery disease suggest that isoproterenol should not be employed to treat refractory status asthmaticus in individuals older than 18 to 20 years of age. Isoproterenol can be safely administered by peripheral vein because extravasation does not produce skin necrosis.

Clinical Summary

Isoproterenol is effective adjunctive therapy for respiratory failure associated with status asthmaticus. In the infant recovering from open heart surgery, it may be employed as the primary agent for increasing cardiac output and peripheral perfusion. A pronounced effect on myocardial oxygen balance should limit its use in older children and adolescents.

DOBUTAMINE

Dobutamine is unique in that it is synthesized to contain a large aromatic substituent on the N-terminus (see Fig. 29–1). It is administered as a racemate. (+) Dobutamine is a strong β-agonist and an α-antagonist; (−) dobutamine is an α-agonist and a weak β-agonist.[119] Partly because of this combination of receptor activities, dobutamine provides significant inotropic benefit with limited chronotropic and vasopressor activity.[120]

Clinical Pharmacology

Infusion of dobutamine produces prompt improvement in cardiac performance. Adults with CHF record a 50 to 80% increase in cardiac output, which is almost entirely due to greater stroke volume. With improved contractility follows a decrease in left atrial pressure and SVR. Tachycardia usually does not occur. Use of dobutamine is associated with a decrease in PVR.[121] Renal function and urine output should improve.

Pharmacokinetics

The half-life is about 2.4 minutes in adults, and the volume of distribution is 0.2 l/kg. Published data in children are still quite limited. Within the therapeutic dobutamine concentration range of 40 to 190 ng/ml, there is a linear relationship between improvement in stroke volume and plasma dobutamine concentration. Tachycardia occurs beyond this range. Dobutamine is metabolized by glucuronide conjugation and 3-O-methylation.

Role in Therapy

Work in adults has established that dobutamine improves cardiac function in settings such as cardiomyopathy, atherosclerotic heart disease, and acute myocardial infarction.[122–124] It has been effective following surgery for myocardial revascularization, cardiac transplantation, and other procedures associated with postoperative myocardial dysfunction, though undesirable chronotropic effects have been recorded when used after cardiac surgery.[125–127]

In one study,[128] dobutamine was effective in treating children with cardiogenic or septic shock, (2.5 to 10 μg/kg/min). In these children, as in adults, cardiac index and stroke index increased, with a concomitant decrease in SVR. Dobutamine was less effective in patients with septic shock than in those with cardiogenic shock. Another group[129] also documented a positive inotropic effect with little increase in heart rate in 12 children with shock of various causes, including trauma, septic shock, and ARDS. Mean cardiac output increased from 2.4 to 3.2 l/min. Both SVR and PVR decreased. When children with congenital heart disease were treated with 2 and 7.5 μg/kg/min, they displayed an increase in stroke volume.[130] In newborns with "heart failure" of various causes, left ventricular systolic time intervals improved during infusion of dobutamine.[131]

Results in children following cardiac surgery with cardiopulmonary bypass have been uneven. One group[132] found that dobutamine enhanced cardiac output only by increasing heart rate, and tachycardia led to termination of the infusion in several patients. The expected fall in SVR was not observed, and the authors of this study were not impressed by any benefit over isoproterenol or dopamine. This finding may be related to the fact that significant impairment of contractility is not characteristic of the disease process affecting children who undergo repair of congenital heart disease. It is also plausible that dissimilar lesions may respond differently to inotropic support. For example, one author[133] found that children undergoing operation for mitral valve disease responded to dobutamine with an increase in stroke volume; children having repair of tetralogy of Fallot did not, and their cardiac output increased only through a faster heart rate.

Although the practice appears to be a frequent one, it is not clear that septic shock or ARDS are appropriate settings for the use of dobutamine, unless the primary disturbance is complicated by myocardial dysfunction. In that context, dobutamine alone or in combination with dopamine has produced an increase in cardiac output, left ventricular stroke work, and blood pressure.[134] A frequently encountered problem in pediatric critical care is the child with septic shock who has severely degraded contractility in conjunction with an inappropriately low SVR. An example is the child who has received a cardiotoxic agent to treat cancer and has subsequently experienced septic shock. In this setting, dobutamine may be effective when combined with norepinephrine. It is unusual for dobutamine to be useful as a single agent to treat hemodynamic compromise associated with sepsis, ARDS, or shock following an episode of severe hypoxia-ischemia unless clinical signs or hemodynamic data document an isolated problem with contractility.

Typical indications in which dobutamine is useful include viral myocarditis, cardiomyopathy associated with the use of anthracyclines and cyclophosphamide, or with hemochromatosis (related to hypertransfusion therapy) or myocardial infarction (Kawasaki disease). Patients with CHF who have normal or slightly low blood pressure may benefit by combining inotropic support using dobutamine with a left ventricular afterload reducing agent such as nitroprusside. The subsequent decrease in afterload further improves stroke volume, augmenting cardiac output at a lower cost of oxygen consumption than does an inotropic agent alone. In addition, use of a balanced arterial and venous dilator such as nitroprusside may improve pulmonary function in the setting of left ventricular failure.[135, 136]

Therapy is initiated at a rate of 5 μg/kg/min (see Table 29–4) and is titrated to effect. It is unlikely that infusion rates greater than approximately 40 μg/kg/min will be useful. However, a definitive statement in this regard awaits pharmacokinetic and pharmacodynamic data in children.

Preparation and Administration

Tables 29–6 and 29–7 provide information regarding dilution and compatibility.

Adverse Effects

Heart

In adults, dobutamine usually increases myocardial oxygen demand. In subjects with myocardial dysfunction

but patent coronary arteries, coronary blood flow and oxygen supply increase to keep pace with or exceed demand. Myocardial oxygen balance is favorably affected.[137] It is likely that this is also true in children with depressed contractility. However, when dobutamine is employed in a setting in which contractility is normal, the effect upon oxygen balance will be unfavorable—a good reason to avoid this practice. Positive chronotropy is another limiting factor: When dobutamine increases heart rate, oxygen balance is unfavorably affected because tachycardia increases oxygen consumption and decreases diastolic time for coronary artery perfusion.[120, 138] An advantage relative to other catecholamines is that dobutamine is usually associated with a modest chronotropic effect—an increase on the order of 10 to 20% is observed at infusion rates between 7.5 and 10 μg/kg/min.[121, 139, 140] In a small number of patients (7.5 to 10%), even these rates produce marked tachycardia or hypertension.

Although dobutamine is less likely than other catecholamines to induce serious atrial and ventricular dysrhythmias, these conditions do occur in patients receiving this agent, particularly in the context of myocarditis, electrolyte imbalance, or high infusion rates. Dobutamine and other inotropes should be administered cautiously to patients with dynamic left ventricular outflow obstruction (hypertrophic aortic stenosis).

Hematologic Effects

Dobutamine inhibits platelet function; the mechanism is probably inhibition of the secondary wave of adenosine diphosphate–induced aggregation. Although generally of no consequence, petechial bleeding was described in one report.[141] In the critically ill child with thrombocytopenia, the physician may wish to limit the use of dobutamine for this reason.

Clinical Summary

Dobutamine is a positive inotropic agent that should be reserved to treat poor myocardial contractility. Dobutamine is used with varying success following cardiac surgery, when contractility is abnormal. Similarly, in septic shock and other acute hemodynamic disturbances, dobutamine is useful when the primary problem is complicated by poor myocardial function. In this setting, combination therapy with a vasopressor such as norepinephrine may be appropriate, particularly in children who have been subjected to cancer chemotherapy.

BIPYRIDINES (AMRINONE)

Amrinone (Fig. 29–4) is a noncatecholamine inotropic agent. Milrinone, enoximone, and piroximone are other members of the same class, the *bipyridines*. Amrinone is the only bipyridine generally available in the United States. Recall that the pharmacologic effects of amrinone are ascribed to inhibition of phosphodiesterase III rather than to adrenergic receptor activation.[32] In addi-

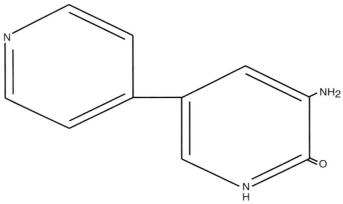

Figure 29–4. Structure of amrinone.

tion to having a positive inotropic effect in in vitro models of isolated ventricular tissue, these agents also have the advantageous property of inducing relaxation of vascular smooth muscle.[142]

Clinical Pharmacology

When administered to subjects with CHF, amrinone increases stroke volume in association with a reduction of SVR, central venous pressure (CVP), and PCWP. Tachycardia is not observed.[143] Therapeutically effective concentrations are in the range of 2 to 7 μg/ml, and there is a strong correlation between plasma amrinone concentration and improvement in hemodynamic function.[38, 144, 145] Clinical and laboratory observations suggest that the improvement in stroke volume is due to the combination of a positive inotropic effect and relaxation of SVR.[32, 142, 146] Amrinone may also be a direct pulmonary vasodilator.[147] The improvement in contractility and stroke volume means that blood pressure is usually well maintained, even as the SVR falls. However, this is not always so, and when amrinone is administered to patients whose intravascular volume is depleted or in whom the expected improvement in cardiac output does not occur, hypotension may result.[148]

Amrinone differs from previously described inotropic agents in that its use is associated with a *decrease* in myocardial oxygen consumption. Reductions of 50% or greater have been observed.[149–151] Even in the context of coronary artery disease and coexistent CHF, amrinone improves contractility without increasing myocardial energy consumption.[70] Although not examined in children, it is likely that the effect of amrinone on oxygen delivery and consumption by the myocardium is also favorable, at least when the drug is used in the appropriate setting of impaired contractility.

Pharmacokinetics

Amrinone is metabolized by *N*-acetyl transferase, the same system involved in biotransformation of isoniazid; thus, like isoniazid, the rate of metabolism depends upon acetylator status. In healthy adults, the half-life of

amrinone in slow acetylators is 4.4 hours, and in fast acetylators it is 2 hours.[152] It is not known whether this difference is clinically important. Protein binding is not important. Amrinone and its metabolites are eliminated by the kidney. The rate of elimination appears to be reduced in CHF.[153] There is little information available regarding the use of amrinone in children. One study of children younger than 1 year of age who were given amrinone following cardiopulmonary bypass found that the half-life was prolonged in those younger than 4 weeks of age (22.8 hours in infants less than 4 weeks of age and 6.8 hours in infants older than 4 weeks of age) and that the mean volume of distribution (1.6 to 1.8 l/kg) was threefold greater than others have reported in adults.[38, 145] No information is available in children with multiple organ system failure.

Role in Therapy

Amrinone is safe and effective in adults with CHF, and its role in short-term management of patients with impaired contractility is established.[142] Although studies in children are limited, it is likely that the bipyridines will also be useful in management of children and adolescents who require short-term treatment of impaired contractility. Amrinone provides both inotropic support and afterload reduction and may be an alternative to coadministration of dobutamine and an afterload-reducing agent (see Table 29–5). Since dysrhythmias are uncommon as a result of amrinone, it may be a first-line agent in the setting of myocardial irritability. Prime examples include the child with myocarditis or a postoperative dysrhythmia.

It is premature to assign amrinone a major role in the management of critically ill children in whom the primary disturbance is other than myocardial failure. In patients with septic shock or ARDS, for example, it is prudent to reserve amrinone for the child with impaired myocardial contractility who has not responded adequately to (or does not tolerate) other agents such as dobutamine or dopamine. The concern is that the relatively long half-life, coupled with the observation that clearance is depressed in patients with cardiac or hepatic dysfunction,[143] may lead to drug accumulation and dose-related toxicity. In the future, more extensive pharmacokinetic data, and even availability of therapeutic drug monitoring, may make one more sanguine regarding the use of this drug in children with multisystem illness.

More information regarding the effect of age upon potential pharmacodynamic differences among infants, children, and adults is also needed. For instance, it has been noted that application of low concentrations of amrinone on neonatal myocardium has a *negative inotropic* effect, but it is not known whether this translates to critically ill infants.[154]

Adverse Effects

Cardiovascular Effects

Hypotension is the principle concern. In one study, mean blood pressure fell from an average of 82 to 68 mm Hg in 36 of 40 patients (chronic CHF, NYHA grades 2 to 4) who received 1.5 to 2 mg/kg of amrinone intravenously.[148] In five of these patients, albumin infusion was necessary to correct the fall in blood pressure. The high rate of hypotension in this study may have been related to very rapid injection of amrinone. In addition, hypotension is more likely to occur in a subject with low cardiac filling pressures.[142] Hypotension is best avoided by administering the loading dose slowly and by assuring adequate intravascular volume status. Supraventricular and ventricular dysrhythmias have occurred during infusion of amrinone but may have been related to the underlying condition of the patient.

Hematologic Effects

Thrombocytopenia is probably the most common adverse effect of amrinone.[155, 156] In the trials of oral amrinone, 10 to 20% of patients had platelet counts less than 100,000/ml. The frequency and magnitude of thrombocytopenia is related to both the dose and duration of therapy. The incidence of thrombocytopenia during *intravenous* administration of amrinone is much lower. In one large study, only 2.4% of patients had platelet counts less than 100,000/ml.[157] However, recent experience indicates a higher frequency in acutely ill children.

Thrombocytopenia is due to increased peripheral destruction of platelets, with decreased platelet survival. The bone marrow is normal. There is no solid evidence of an immunologic process. Although bleeding as a result of amrinone-induced thrombocytopenia has not been documented, it is wise to determine the platelet count prior to beginning therapy with this drug. Mild thrombocytopenia (>50,000 platelets/ml) prior to treatment probably does *not* contraindicate short-term use of intravenous amrinone. Similarly, the development of mild thrombocytopenia in patients receiving amrinone does not necessarily require discontinuation of the drug.[156] Coexisting diseases that impair platelet function, or a coagulopathy, mitigate in favor of discontinuation of amrinone even in the setting of mild thrombocytopenia. Renal disease, which increases plasma levels of the drug, may increase the incidence and severity of thrombocytopenia.

Once amrinone is discontinued, platelet counts return toward normal within several days.

Hypersensitivity

Patients receiving oral amrinone have experienced a syndrome characterized by an elevated erythrocyte sedimentation rate, pericarditis, pleuritis, ascites, myositis, and vasculitis with nodular pulmonary densities, hypoxemia, and jaundice.[148] There are not sufficient data to know if this occurs in children.

Drug Interactions

Clinically significant interactions have not been substantiated.

Preparation and Administration

In adults, the manufacturer recommends a loading dose of 0.75 mg/kg, which may be repeated once. This is followed by a continuous infusion of 5 to 10 μg/kg/min. Adjustments for age and development have not been established. A study suggests a much higher loading dose (children younger than 1 year of age—initial intravenous amrinone bolus of 3 to 4.5 mg/kg in divided doses followed by a continuous infusion of 10 μg/kg/min; neonates—a similar bolus followed by a continuous infusion of 3 to 5 μg/kg/min).[38] These recommendations are based on a small number of patients in a single clinical context; the reader should be cautious in their application.

Amrinone may be prepared for intravenous administration as indicated in Table 29-6. It should not be diluted in solutions that contain dextrose.

Clinical Summary

Amrinone is the first bipyridine to be widely used in the United States. It is effective in short-term management of the older child, adolescent, and adult with impaired myocardial contractility. Amrinone is usually not the first-line inotrope for use in the patient whose primary disease does not involve the heart, though the virtual lack of induced arrhythmias may outweigh other concerns in the setting of myocardial irritability. The clinical pharmacology of amrinone still must be evaluated in infants and children. Questions regarding amrinone's pharmacokinetic properties in the child with multiple organ system disease need to be addressed.

DIGITALIS GLYCOSIDES

Physicians are hesitant to prescribe digitalis glycosides in the intensive care unit for several valid reasons, including a narrow therapeutic range, slow onset of action, and the relatively frequent occurrence of significant and even life-threatening adverse effects. However, glycosides are frequently employed for control of supraventricular dysrhythmias and as adjunctive support for poor myocardial contractility that is expected to persist beyond several days or weeks.

Cardiac glycosides consist of a steroid moiety (the *aglycone* or *genin*) with 1 to 4 sugar molecules attached.[40] For digoxin, there are three molecules of a 2,6-dideoxyribose, digitoxose. All digitalis glycosides have similar pharmacodynamic properties, the number and composition of sugars affecting only the pharmacokinetics.

Glycosides bind to and inhibit Na,K-ATPase, thereby increasing intracellular calcium. Binding of digoxin to ATPase is affected by serum potassium. Hyperkalemia depresses digoxin binding, whereas hypokalemia has the opposite effect,[158] accounting in part for potentiation of digoxin-induced arrhythmias during hypokalemia.

Clinical Pharmacology

Digoxin increases contractility in normal and diseased hearts. When CHF is present, digoxin leads to increased stroke volume and reduction of elevated filling pressures. A recent study[159] of 10 adults patients with acute myocardial failure indicated that a single dose of digoxin, 10 μg/kg, produced a 69% increase in left ventricular stroke work index, a 25% reduction in PCWP, a 16 to 28% increase in cardiac index, and a 25% increase in stroke index within 2 hours of infusion. Many of these changes were present within 60 minutes. When administered to infants, digoxin has been shown to increase contractility as judged by echocardiography, though invasive hemodynamic measurements have not been made in infants or children.[160–162] When CHF results from obstructive lesions or left-to-right shunts, it is more difficult to demonstrate benefit than when CHF is caused by poor contractility.

Administration of digoxin reduces the elevated heart rate associated with CHF. Digoxin both permits reduction in compensatory sympathetic activity and enhances vagal tone by increasing baroceptor sensitivity and by directly stimulating central vagal centers.[158, 163] This property underlies the effectiveness of digoxin in treating and preventing supraventricular rhythm disturbances such as supraventricular tachycardia, atrial flutter, or atrial fibrillation. This aspect of digitalis pharmacology is reviewed in Chapter 36.

Pharmacokinetics

Children and infants require higher dosages than do adults in order to achieve a therapeutically effective plasma concentration of 1 to 2 ng/ml.[161] Infants are not less sensitive to digoxin; the dosage discrepancy is pharmacokinetic in origin, since infants and young children eliminate digoxin more rapidly and have larger volumes of distribution for the drug. Digoxin is eliminated by the kidney through glomerular filtration and renal tubular secretion. Elimination is strongly affected by renal dysfunction, complicating the use of the agent in the critically ill child.

Dosage

The dosage of digoxin depends upon the age of the patient, the indication for therapy, the route of administration, and the presumed sensitivity of the myocardium to toxicity. Dosage must be individualized. Table 29–8 indicates *intravenous* dosages of digoxin that are appropriate in patients with normal electrolytes and renal function and without evidence of myocardial irritability. These dosages must be reduced and the pace of digitalization slowed if these conditions are present.

Digitalis Toxicity

The frequency and severity of digitalis toxicity is the major limiting factor in treating critically ill patients.

Table 29–8. RECOMMENDED INTRAVENOUS DIGOXIN DOSAGE FOR CONGESTIVE HEART FAILURE*

	Digitalizing Dose (μg/kg)	Maintenance Dose (μg/kg/day)
Premature infant	15	3–4
Term neonate	20	6–7.5
Children <2 year	30–35	7.5–9
Children >2 year	25–30	6–7.5

*Adapted from Park MK: Use of digoxin in infants and children, with specific emphasis on dosage. J Pediatr 108:871, 1986.

The most frequent side effects are gastrointestinal; the most serious are disturbances in cardiac rhythm. The intensive care practitioner encounters digitalis toxicity in the following two distinct patterns.

1. *Iatrogenic Digitalis Intoxication* occurs in as many as 30% of hospitalized adults;[164] the frequency in children has never been established. Toxicity during treatment reflects one of three general conditions: (1) dosage error, (2) a change in the pharmacokinetics of digoxin (drug interaction, increase in bioavailability, decreased renal clearance), or (3) a change in sensitivity to digoxin causing an alteration in the response of the heart to a stable plasma digoxin concentration.[165] Although digoxin is not frequently prescribed in the pediatric intensive care unit, many patients entering an intensive care unit have previously received the drug. Thus the primary illness may be complicated by the emergence of digitalis toxicity.

2. *Acute massive ingestion,* whether deliberate (suicide) or accidental (pediatric) is very dangerous. In one series, deliberate digoxin overdose was fatal in half the cases.[166]

Cardiac Effects of Toxicity

Conduction and automaticity are both affected by toxicity. Almost every rhythm disturbance known has been recorded.[167, 168] Table 29–9 provides a summary of these dysrhythmias. Most frequent are ventricular premature systole, supraventricular tachycardia, and coupled ventricular beats. One may also observe ventricular tachycardia and fibrillation.

Digoxin produces sinus bradycardia by suppressing sinus node discharge. All degrees of AV block occur and may be associated with ectopic atrial beats and junctional ectopic tachycardia. Digitalis toxicity is strongly implied by AV block occurring in conjunction with ventricular irritability.

Infants and children are more likely to experience bradycardia and AV conduction disturbances than ectopic activity or tachydysrhythmia. In children, AV block may be the first evidence of toxicity. This difference reflects higher underlying vagal tone and the lack of myocardial damage related to coronary artery occlusion. Although specific manifestations may differ, the myocardium of the child or infant is no less sensitive to digoxin than is that of the older patient, and serum digoxin levels that produce toxicity in older patients will do so in infants, as well.[161]

Table 29–9. DYSRHYTHMIAS ASSOCIATED WITH DIGITALIS TOXICITY*

Due to Conduction Delay
Sinus bradycardia
SA block or arrest
1st, 2nd, 3rd degree AV block
Bundle branch block

Due to Abnormal Excitability
Atrial premature beats
Supraventricular tachycardia
Junctional tachycardia
Accelerated junctional rhythm
Ventricular premature beats
Ventricular and atrial fibrillation

Due to Abnormal Excitability with Conduction Delay
Atrial tachycardia with block
Sinus bradycardia with junctional or ventricular tachycardia
AV dissociation

*Adapted from Goodman L: Digitalis. *In:* Haddad LM and Winchester JF (eds): Clinical Management of Poisoning. Philadelphia, WB Saunders, 1983, p. 813.
AV = atrioventricular.

Knowledge of digoxin concentration is helpful in determining whether a particular electrocardiographic finding represents digoxin toxicity, though interpretation of this measurement may be complicated by the presence of endogenous digoxin-like substance in infants and in patients with organ system dysfunction.[169, 170] It is pertinent to note that amrinone has also been reported to interfere with measurement of digoxin.[171] Ideally, the concentration of digoxin should be determined at least 6 hours after the ingestion or injection of the drug. Digitalis toxicity is unlikely to be involved when the level is less than 1.5 ng/ml and is quite likely to be involved when the concentration is relatively great (i.e.,>3 ng/ml).[165]

Hypokalemia, hypomagnesemia, hypoxemia, myocarditis, hypothyroidism, and coadministration of a catecholamine or calcium salt all exacerbate digitalis toxicity. These risk factors may provoke serious toxicity even when the drug's concentration is within the usual therapeutic range. For this reason, as cardiac disease progresses or new electrolyte or metabolic disturbances occur, digitalis toxicity can develop in the patient receiving a constant dosage and having stable digitalis levels.

Treatment of acute massive intoxication is discussed in depth in Chapter 80. Briefly, it presents with severe disturbances in cardiac rhythm, which range from resistant ventricular tachycardia to AV block and asystole. In acute massive ingestions *hyperkalemia* is often present. Hyperkalemia exacerbates AV block and depresses automaticity. Mild hyperkalemia does not require specific therapy, but when it is severe and associated with characteristic electrocardiographic changes (elevation and peaking of T waves, ST segment depression, widened QRS complex), specific treatment is required. Therapy for digitalis-induced hyperkalemia is similar to treatment of hyperkalemia from other causes, except that rapid infusion of calcium salts has a great likelihood of inducing ventricular fibrillation and is *absolutely contraindicated.*

Drug Interactions

Digoxin and digitoxin interact with a large number of other drugs. These interactions can be of major significance and have been recently reviewed.[49, 172] Cotreatment with quinidine produces a dose-dependent increase in digoxin levels,[173] which can lead to serious toxicity. In addition to these pharmacokinetic interactions, several drugs affect the sensitivity of the myocardium to glycosides. The interaction may be indirect, as when furosemide or amphotericin induce potassium and magnesium depletion, or they may be direct, as when calcium or β-adrenergic agonists potentiate the prodysrhythmic effect of digitalis.

Clinical Summary

As an inotropic agent in the intensive care unit, digoxin offers two advantages: (1) It does not induce β-adrenergic receptor desensitization, remaining effective even when myocardial β-receptor desensitization is presumed to have occurred and (2) it does not increase heart rate. These properties make digoxin useful for treatment of primary disturbances in myocardial function, such as those associated with cardiomyopathy, myocardial infarction, and myocarditis or for treatment following cardiopulmonary bypass. Unfortunately, each of these conditions is associated with enhanced susceptibility to digitalis toxicity. Thus, digoxin is much more often employed in the period of convalescence and recovery than during the acute illness. At that time its administration may substantially reduce heart rate and permit withdrawal of other inotropic support.

VASODILATOR THERAPY

In the setting of markedly reduced stroke volume and systemic vasoconstriction, inotropic support alone may be ineffective in adequately increasing cardiac output and may exact a significant penalty in increased myocardial oxygen consumption. For these reasons, *vasodilator* therapy is frequently employed to alter either venous capacitance or arterial resistance.

Vasodilators have been classified on the basis of their principal circulatory action (Table 29–10). *Venous* dilators decrease venous tone, thereby increasing venous capacitance and reducing elevated central and ventricular filling pressures. This results in a decrease in pre-

Table 29–10. CLASSIFICATION OF VASODILATORS BASED ON PRINCIPAL HEMODYNAMIC EFFECT*

Venous	Arteriolar	Balanced
Nitroglycerin	Diazoxide	Nitroprusside
	Nifedipine	Phentolamine
	Tolazoline	Captopril
	Hydralazine	Enalapril
		Prazosin

*Data from Steward DJ: Afterload: Nonsurgical manipulation of the failing circulation. *In:* Swedlow DB and Raphaely RC (eds): Cardiovascular Problems in Pediatric Critical Care, Chapter 6. New York, Churchill Livingstone, 1986.

load. *Arterial* dilators decrease arterial vascular tone and resistance, thereby contributing to a decrease in arterial impedance. The result is a decrease in ventricular afterload, the tension in the ventricular wall during systole.[174] As aortic impedance falls, stroke volume increases and organ blood flow improves. *Balanced* vasodilators affect both venous and arterial vessels in approximately equal proportion.[175] These agents reduce both afterload and preload. This classification is a useful oversimplification; all vasodilators have some effect upon both venous and arterial systems.

Table 29–11 provides a summary of the hemodynamic effects of various vasodilator drugs. Many of these compounds are discussed elsewhere in the text. This section will review the two drugs that, historically, have been most frequently employed in the pediatric critical care unit and remain quite useful: nitroprusside and nitroglycerin.

NITROPRUSSIDE

Sodium nitroprusside is a *balanced* vasodilator, producing arterial and venous dilatation in approximately equal proportion.[176–178] Treatment of acute severe hypertension is the principal critical care indication in children. Other important indications are adjunctive therapy of CHF, cardiogenic shock, and myocardial ischemia. The drug is also employed to improve cardiac output and perfusion in the period following cardiac surgery. Less well defined indications include therapy for pulmonary hypertension and instances of distributive (e.g., septic) shock complicated by inappropriate elevation of peripheral vascular tone.

Clinical Pharmacology

Nitroprusside is an iron-containing inorganic nitrate. Like other nitrovasodilators, its mechanism of action involves release of nitric oxide (NO).[179] Nitroprusside reacts with oxyhemoglobin to produce NO, cyanomethemoglobin, and cyanide.[180] NO subsequently activates soluble guanylate cyclase, resulting in an increase in production of cyclic $3'5'$ guanosine monophosphate (cGMP). Ultimately, formation of cGMP leads to dephosphorylation of myosin light chain and smooth muscle relaxation in vascular beds as well as the trachea and gut.[176, 179]

Infusion of nitroprusside evokes rapid, profound, and widespread vasodilatation affecting both the arterial and venous systems. The effect upon hemodynamic function depends upon the underlying circulatory status. In normotensive and hypertensive patients with normal cardiac function, the decrease in central pressures and preload produces a modest decrease in stroke volume and cardiac index. As SVR decreases, systolic and diastolic blood pressures are reduced. The reduction is amplified by a vertical position. Heart rate increases reflexively and generally modestly, but sometimes profoundly. Contractility is not directly affected. In patients with depressed contractility and CHF, the reduction in SVR and left ventricular afterload outweighs the effect of venous pooling, and stroke volume increases. Blood pressure is usually well maintained because the decrease in SVR is matched by the improved cardiac output. Limb blood flow and RBF usually increase. Heart rate generally decreases and the skin becomes warm and well perfused. These effects are examined in the context of the Starling relationship shown in Figure 29–5.

Developmental effects upon nitroprusside have not been extensively investigated. It is known that the elderly are more sensitive to the drug than are younger adults.[181] One study in guinea pig aorta suggests that smooth muscle sensitivity to nitroprusside increases from fetal to adult life;[182] work in lambs suggests that there may be developmental differences in the response of

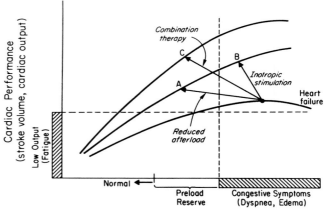

Figure 29–5. Response to treatment with inotropic drugs or afterload reduction. Afterload reduction alone (line A) or inotropic stimulation alone (line B) provide some improvement in cardiac performance, from the low to the intermediate curve. Through combining inotropic and afterload reducing agents (line C), greater improvement is achieved than with either agent alone. If *preload* is not maintained at an adequate level, however, cardiac function will follow the intermediate curve downward to the low output area; there will be no improvement in performance. (From Friedman WF, and George BL: New concepts and drugs for heart failure. Pediatr Clin North Am 31:1197—1227, 1984.)

Table 29–11. HEMODYNAMIC EFFECTS OF VASODILATOR DRUGS*

	Cardiac Output	Heart Rate	PAP†	RAP‡	SVR§	PVR‖	BP**
Tolazoline	↑	↑	0–↓	?	0–↓	0–↓	0–↓
Phentolamine	↑	↑	0–↓	?	0–↓	0–↓	0–↓
Isoproterenol	↑↑	↑↑	0–↑	↓	↓↓	0–↓	0–↓
Diazoxide	↑	↑	0	0	↓↓	↓	↓
Hydralazine	↑	↑	0	0	↓↓	↓	↓
Nifedipine	0–↑	0–↑	↓↓	↑	↓↓	↓	↓↓
Nitroglycerin	0–↑	0	↓↓	↓	0–↓	↓↓	↓
Nitroprusside	0–↑↑	↑	↓	↓	↓↓	↓↓	0–↓↓
Captopril	0	0	0	0	↓↓	0–↓	↓

*Adapted from Packer M: Vasodilator therapy for primary pulmonary hypertension: Limitations and hazards. Ann Intern Med 103:258, 1985.
†PAP = pulmonary artery pressure.
‡RAP = right atrial pressure.
§SVR = systemic vascular resistance.
‖PVR = pulmonary vascular resistance.
**BP = blood pressure.

the pulmonary arterial bed to nitroprusside.[183] Whether these observations translate into clinical effect is unknown.

The effects upon RBF and GFR are variable. In patients with poor cardiac function, nitroprusside causes a decrease in renal vascular resistance. Renal blood flow increases, but GFR is not affected.[178] In individuals treated for hypertension, rather than CHF, RBF may decrease from reduced perfusion pressure.

Pharmacokinetics

Nitroprusside undergoes intravascular decomposition to both nitric oxide, which is responsible for the therapeutic effect, and cyanide. Cyanide is rapidly metabolized by hepatic rhodanase (in a reaction that employs thiosulfate as a cofactor) to thiocyanate, which is then excreted by the kidney. Although it is not possible to specifically measure the blood concentration of nitroprusside, the half-life of nitroprusside must be extremely short, since peak effects are noted within 2 minutes of altering the infusion rate, and the pharmacologic effect dissipates within 3 minutes of stopping an infusion. The half-life of thiocyanate is about 3 days in patients with normal renal function, but it is greatly prolonged in those with renal disease.

Role in Therapy

Hypertension

Although several other agents are now available to treat hypertensive emergencies, nitroprusside remains the mainstay of treatment in children because of its consistent efficacy, ease of titration, and relatively low incidence of toxicity. In children, the starting dosage is 0.5 μg/kg/min, and most children respond to an infusion rate of 1.5 to 2 μg/kg/min. In an early study, an average infusion rate of 1.4 μg/kg/min produced adequate blood pressure control within 20 minutes.[184] Occasionally, dosages to 10 μg/kg/min may be required. Need for higher dosages may represent so-called nitroprusside resistance (see further on) or simply compensatory tachycardia and fluid retention. The dosage needed to reduce a normal blood pressure (i.e., as in hypotensive anesthesia) is much higher (i.e., 6 to 8 μg/kg/min)[185] than that required to treat hypertension.

In children who experience an excessive or dangerous increase in cardiac rate during infusion of nitroprusside, adjunctive use of a β-blocking agent (propranolol, esmolol, labetalol) may be considered if cardiac contractility is not a concern. Indeed, under some circumstances a β-blocking agent is preferred as the sole therapy for hypertension. For example, compared with nitroprusside, esmolol produces a lower cardiac index and heart rate but does not affect SVR; thus, pulse pressure is reduced rather than amplified. Esmolol has been advocated in the patient with a vascular anastomosis, in whom a hyperdynamic circulation may be dangerous.[186] Nitroprusside, but not esmolol, reduces PaO_2. As practitioners gain experience with esmolol in children, it is likely that it will displace some of the indications for nitroprusside use.

Other factors that reduce efficacy of nitroprusside include compensatory fluid retention, which can be counteracted by judicious use of a diuretic, and reflexive increases in norepinephrine and renin secretion, which are counteracted by an increase in dosage or addition of a β-adrenergic blocking agent.

Once a desirable reduction in blood pressure is achieved, therapy is gradually changed to a more chronic form. This is discussed in Chapter 54.

Nitroprusside is extensively employed to control the hypertension that occurs postoperatively following coarctation repair, though esmolol may become the agent of choice.

Congestive Heart Failure

Nitroprusside is effective in treating CHF caused by either diminished myocardial contractility or certain specific structural lesions, such as mitral or aortic regurgitation.

Poor Myocardial Contractility. In adult patients with CHF (with or without associated acute myocardial infarction) nitroprusside decreases CVP and PCWP. End-diastolic pressure and ventricular radius fall in both the right and left ventricle. As PVR and SVR fall, stroke volume increases in proportion to the decrease in SVR. Wall tension (the product of chamber radius and pressure) is reduced, and ventricular compliance is increased. Subendocardial blood flow is augmented, even in the presence of a fixed coronary artery obstruction, because ventricular diastolic pressure is lower. Stroke work decreases. Thus, oxygen requirements tend to decrease as oxygen supply increases—a desirable effect.[186–189] Pulmonary function may improve with the fall in left atrial pressure.

A study by Beekman[190] showed that in children with either cardiomyopathy or mitral regurgitation, nitroprusside (2 μg/kg/min) produced a 30% increase in cardiac index and stroke index. PCWP decreased by 28% and SVR decreased by nearly 40%. Other studies support the efficacy of nitroprusside in children.[191]

Several reports indicate that nitroprusside is also effective for adjunctive treatment of *impaired ventricular function* in the immediate postoperative period.[175, 192, 193] Benzing and coworkers[194] employed nitroprusside alone and in combination with epinephrine to augment hemodynamic performance following open heart surgery in a group of children in whom the cardiac index was less than 2 l/min/m². There was substantial improvement in cardiac output, and SVR decreased. Stephenson and associates[195] found that a combination of dopamine and nitroprusside produced a greater increase in cardiac index (13%) than did either agent alone, though there was an important increase in heart rate. With the combination, SVR and PVR each decreased about 20%.

As suggested by Figure 29–5, maximizing stroke volume and preventing hypotension require that the physician administer sufficient fluid to maintain an adequate preload (CVP and PCWP or left arterial pressure) during infusion of nitroprusside.

Amrinone, discussed earlier in this chapter, is now frequently employed as a single agent to produce both vasodilatation and inotropic support. In many patients, it may be preferable to the combination of dobutamine and nitroprusside. However, a remaining advantage of the nitroprusside and dobutamine combination is the short half-life of both agents, thus permitting very rapid titration.

Cardiogenic Shock. Nitroprusside is employed to treat adult patients with cardiogenic shock. Unfortunately, there are no systematically collected data in children. In adults (most often following acute myocardial infarction), nitroprusside is used in combination with an inotropic agent, such as dobutamine, and occasionally with mechanical afterload reduction, such as aortic balloon counterpulsation.[188, 196]

In treating CHF or cardiogenic shock, initiation and titration of nitroprusside are done cautiously to avoid inducing hypotension. In practice, children are initially treated with dobutamine or epinephrine. Once an acceptable blood pressure has been restored, nitroprusside is considered if SVR remains elevated, stroke volume is inadequate, and PCWP is still elevated or normal. In this setting, nitroprusside is started at 0.10 to 0.25 μg/kg/min. Subsequent decreases in blood pressure or perfusion are treated with cautious fluid administration and adjustment of inotropic support; it is most important to maintain filling pressures that are adequate to support the stroke volume. If tolerated, nitroprusside is increased until cutaneous perfusion is improved (warm to midcalf) and until further increases in infusion rate do not evoke an increase in stroke volume.

Structural Heart Disease

Nitroprusside ameliorates symptoms of CHF caused by mitral and aortic regurgitation. It is less consistently effective for ventricular septal defect (VSD).

Treatment with pure arterial dilators such as hydralazine[175, 190, 197] or phentolamine may reduce interventricular shunt flow in infants with VSD, improving CHF. In contrast, nitroprusside appears to produce undesirable hemodynamic effects in this setting. In one study, five infants with CHF secondary to VSD experienced a 35% increase in the pulmonary:systemic flow ratio because of a marked decrease in systemic blood flow and enhanced shunt across the VSD.[198] This is attributed to a decrease in venous return that impairs right ventricular filling, facilitating the left-to-right shunt.

In individuals with left-sided regurgitant lesions, reducing aortic impedance facilitates forward (i.e., nonregurgitant) flow. Several studies document that nitroprusside effectively increases forward flow and decreases regurgitation in mitral and aortic insufficiency. The improvement in forward stroke volume may be quite large (50%) and may occur even without the presence of impaired contractility.[188, 190, 199]

Pulmonary Hypertension

Nitroprusside has been examined for treatment of nonsurgical pulmonary hypertension in newborns[200] and adults.[201] To the extent that vasoconstriction contributes to elevated PVR, infusion of a vasodilator may be helpful. Unfortunately, no selective pulmonary vasodilator of any class has yet been identified. Treatment of pulmonary hypertension by vasodilators is often complicated by systemic hypotension and tachycardia.[202] Additionally, hypoxemia is exacerbated by ablation of protective regional pulmonary vasoconstriction.

Nonetheless, there is support for use of a vasodilator, usually nitroprusside, in the setting of pulmonary hypertension that follows surgery, such as repair of VSD or truncus arteriosus.[174, 195, 203] Even in this limited setting, systemic hypotension may be a prohibitive penalty. For this reason, other adjustments that are known to reduce PVR, such as elevating FiO_2, hyperventilation, correction of metabolic acidosis, adequate postoperative anesthesia, and ventilation with relatively low mean airway pressure, are probably more effective in controlling postoperative pulmonary hypertension than are currently available vasodilator drugs. A trial of nitroprusside (or nitroglycerin) is warranted, however, when these other techniques fail to correct or prevent life-threatening, postoperative pulmonary hypertension.[204]

Beyond use in the postoperative setting, vasodilator therapy of pulmonary hypertension is empirical, and guidelines for patient selection, specific drug, and clinical context have not been established. (See also Chapter 34).

Although employed occasionally to treat neonatal hyaline membrane disease,[200] this practice is limited. Nitroprusside is not likely to be effective in treating the pulmonary hypertension associated with ARDS, and it is not recommended in this disease except in conjunction with an approved experimental protocol.

Septic Shock

A dominant hemodynamic manifestation of septic shock is disturbed vasomotor regulation. The most frequent pattern is associated with inappropriate vasodilatation and is often associated with mild to severe impairment of contractility.[188, 205] An inappropriately low SVR characterizes septic shock in children as well as in adults, even when the shock state is far advanced or preterminal. Obviously, the use of a vasodilator is not appropriate in this context. Occasionally, a picture develops in children that is characterized by hypotension, excessive vasoconstriction, sharply reduced cardiac output and stroke index, and very poor peripheral perfusion. Measurements also reveal elevated central filling pressures. This hemodynamic picture is encountered, for example, in children who have received cardiotoxic drugs to treat a malignancy and who subsequently experience septic shock. It is actually a blend of cardiogenic and distributive shock. In this context, nitroprusside may be effective in improving stroke volume and distribution of blood flow. However, unless elevated SVR is documented by hemodynamic measurements, there is no rationale for vasodilator treatment.

If selected, vasodilator therapy is initiated very cautiously, as described previously for cardiogenic shock, and should follow restoration of adequate blood pressure by use of fluid infusion and inotropic support. Pulmonary artery catheterization is necessary. Frequently, contractility is so severely impaired that treatment with a vasodilator is complicated by hypotension. An unacceptable decrease in blood pressure may be corrected by infusion of fluid, added inotropic support, or a reduction in the nitroprusside dosage. Successful therapy is marked by an increase in cardiac output and a perceptible improvement in perfusion of the extremities and in urine output.

Toxicity and Adverse Effects

Hypotension is the major dose-related toxicity of all vasodilators. An important advantage of both nitroprusside and nitroglycerin is that this complication is rapidly corrected by a reduction in dosage. As described for β-adrenergic agonists, nitroprusside and nitroglycerin may worsen hypoxemia by ablating regional hypoxia-induced pulmonary vasoconstriction.

Accumulation of thiocyanate may occur in the patient with poor renal function. Neuroexcitatory signs and symptoms such as confusion, delirium, and convulsions have been attributed to thiocyanate when the concentration exceeds 10 mg/dl.[178] Thiocyanate also inhibits the iodide-concentrating capacity of the thyroid gland, reportedly producing hypothyroidism.[206] Blood thiocyanate concentration should be determined in patients with poor renal function or in those who receive nitroprusside for longer than 72 hours. Thiocyanate is removed during hemodialysis and peritoneal dialysis. There is little evidence that thiocyanate accumulation occurs during short-term use (3 to 4 days) in children who do not have renal failure, and routine monitoring of thiocyanate is not indicated.

Administration of nitroprusside causes cyanide to be released into the circulation and, in animal models, cyanide poisoning is the cause of death following massive doses of nitroprusside.[180] Although cyanide toxicity has been reported occasionally in humans,[177] and coadministration of thiosulfate or cyanocobalamine has been advised as a precaution, the relevance of this concern is probably overstated. Cyanide accumulation has been suggested as a potential cause of nitroprusside resistance.[207, 208] Since an early sign of cyanide intoxication is lactic acidosis, it is prudent to monitor blood lactate levels in children receiving prolonged or high-dosage infusions of nitroprusside. However, a normal lactate level does not exclude the possibility of cyanide toxicity. Measurement of thiocyanate concentration does not have relevance to detecting cyanide toxicity. Methemoglobin levels should also be determined during prolonged infusion, since methemoglobin is an intermediate product of nitroprusside metabolism.

Preparation and Administration

Nitroprusside is light-sensitive. Only fresh solutions in 5% dextrose should be employed and the administration container wrapped in an opaque cover. Syringe-type infusion devices should be employed. Infusion rates greater than 10 μg/kg/min are rarely necessary and may enhance the possibility of cyanide intoxication.

Clinical Summary

Nitroprusside is a balanced vasodilator with an extremely rapid onset and short duration of action. These properties make it nearly ideal for treating critically ill children. Important indications include hypertensive emergency, CHF, cardiogenic shock, and valvular regurgitation. Nitroprusside is also of adjunctive value in the setting of hypertension and pulmonary hypertension following cardiac surgery.

NITROGLYCERIN

Nitroglycerin is a venous dilator. Its major indication is myocardial ischemia that is caused by coronary artery disease. Therefore, though extensively employed in the critical care of adult patients, it has a limited role in the treatment of children. Occasional indications in the pediatric age group are CHF, pulmonary edema, and pulmonary hypertension. Nitroglycerin is occasionally employed in adults (in combination with vasopressin) to acutely ameliorate portal hypertension.

Clinical Pharmacology

Nitroglycerin (or glyceryl trinitrate) relaxes vascular smooth muscle by activating guanylate cyclase. This reaction involves intermediate formation of S-nitrosothiols.[209] Venous dilatation predominates over arteriolar dilatation, but at higher dosages SVR does decrease. CVP, left atrial pressure, and ventricular end-diastolic pressure decrease. Pulmonary arterial pressure falls, mainly from the increase in venous capacitance rather than direct pulmonary vasodilatation. In normal subjects, cardiac output may decrease because of venous pooling. However, in patients with CHF, cardiac output and stroke volume increase during nitroglycerin infusion, though the increase is more profound following infusion of nitroprusside.[189] Nitroglycerin and nitroprusside evoke similar reductions in PCWP and pulmonary arterial pressures.

Pharmacokinetics

The half-life of nitroglycerin is approximately 2 minutes. Nitroglycerin (and other organic nitrates) are hydrolyzed by hepatic glutathione–organic nitrate reductase. The resulting dinitrates have some vasodilator activity; their half-lives are 30 to 60 minutes. Developmental aspects of nitrate metabolism have not been examined. Tolerance to nitroglycerin develops over several days of continuous infusion; it can be reversed by infusion of acetylcysteine or by temporary cessation of the infusion.

Role in Therapy

Myocardial Ischemia

Nitroglycerin is rapidly effective in relief of anginal pain; its routine use in patients with acute myocardial infarction remains controversial. Although there is insufficient experience in children with myocardial ischemia and coronary artery disease to merit a specific recommendation, critical care management of this process should be comparable to adults. Vasodilators have been employed for myocardial infarction in the setting of Kawasaki's disease.[210]

Congestive Heart Failure

In adults who have CHF, infusion of nitroglycerin rapidly reduces CVP, PCWP, and pulmonary artery pressure.[189] At lower dosages, the major effect is upon preload and ventricular end-diastolic pressure. Signs and symptoms of pulmonary edema improve rapidly. At higher dosages, nitroglycerin begins to induce arteriolar dilatation, SVR falls, and the cardiac output increases proportionately.

Published experience in children is scanty, but reports by Ilbawi and colleagues[211] and Benson and associates[212] suggest that the hemodynamic response is comparable to that observed in adults. Both groups employed nitroglycerin following hypothermic cardiac arrest for open heart surgery.

A few tentative generalizations are possible. Compared with nitroprusside, nitroglycerin is more likely to effect a reduction in CPV and PCWP without inducing systemic arterial hypotension. This suggests that nitroglycerin is the preferred agent when treating the child with acute CHF, pulmonary edema, and marginal blood pressure. In contrast, when blood pressure is well preserved, the preferred vasodilator is nitroprusside, because this drug will produce a greater increase in cardiac output. Nitroprusside is also the preferred agent when the dominant manifestation of CHF is poor peripheral perfusion rather than pulmonary edema or when CHF results from mitral or aortic regurgitation.

Pulmonary Hypertension

Infusion of nitroglycerin reduces pulmonary arterial pressure. This is secondary in part to increased venous capacitance, but at higher rates of infusion there is also a true decrease in PVR. Notwithstanding favorable evaluations in adults,[213] there is little reason to believe that nitroglycerin will be of significant benefit to most children who experience primary or idiopathic pulmonary hypertension. Indeed, Rudinsky and coworkers[214] recently confirmed that neither nitroprusside nor nitroglycerin selectively reduced pulmonary resistance in sepsis-induced hypertension in piglets. However, circumstances may be different in the setting of pulmonary hypertension following surgery to repair left-to-right shunts. Ilbawi and colleagues[211] administered 1 to 6 µg/kg/min to children following open heart surgery. Several children had elevated PVR prior to surgery. At low infusion rates (<3 µg/kg/min), the principal effect was upon preload. As the dosage was increased, SVR and left ventricular stroke work decreased with a reciprocal increase in cardiac output. All patients experienced a decrease in PVR as dosage was increased. This decrease was much more pronounced in children with *preoperative* pulmonary hypertension. In some children, the decrease in PVR was much greater than the associated decrease in SVR. Interestingly, this group of children enjoyed the greatest improvement in cardiac output. This single study suggests that nitroglycerin may be the preferred vasodilator in children with pulmonary hypertension following cardiac surgery. The reader should be aware, however, that the dosages employed in this study were much higher, by comparison, than those used when initiating therapy in adults (about 0.1 µg/kg/min). This may have resulted, in part, from adsorption of nitroglycerin by the plastic employed in the infusion sets.

There is a case report[215] in which nitroglycerin was transiently effective in reducing pulmonary artery pressure in a child with pulmonary hemosiderosis.

Adverse Effects

The principal adverse effect is hypotension. As is true for nitroprusside, nitroglycerin regularly reduces PaO_2 in children with pulmonary disease; on occasion this may be clinically significant. Nitroglycerin has been documented to increase intracranial pressure.[216, 217] This suggests that nitroglycerin (and nitroprusside) should be used cautiously in the patient in whom this may be a potential problem. Ethanol toxicity has occurred in several patients who received very high (more than 2,000 µg/min) dosages of nitroglycerin.[218] The ethanol employed as a diluent is responsible (about 0.1 ml ethanol/mg nitroglycerin).

Preparation and Administration

Nitroglycerin migrates into many plastics, resulting in substantial loss of potency when conventional polyvinyl chloride (PVC) intravenous sets are employed. This phenomenon is more pronounced at low infusion rates, such as are employed for children. Loss of drug is minimized when polyolefin or another non-PVC infusion set is employed. Thus, the dosage prescribed must be lower when the non-PVC infusion set is employed. *Available studies in children do not indicate whether a special infusion set was employed.* It is possible that infusion rates indicated in these studies (as high as 20 µg/kg/min)[213] would be much too high when using the appropriate non-PVC infusion set. Thus, these reported infusion rates should be considered illustrative rather than prescriptive. Data in adults suggest that it is reasonable to begin with a dosage of 0.1 µg/kg/min, increasing by 0.1 to 0.2 µg/kg/min until the desired effect is achieved. In order to minimize variation in dosage and the possibility of error, it is recommended that nitroglycerin be administered only with a specifically designed infusion set.

Clinical Summary

Nitroglycerin is primarily a venous dilator. Its rapid onset and short duration of action make it an excellent choice for critical care applications. In the child with marginal systemic blood pressure and pulmonary edema, nitroglycerin may be preferable to nitroprusside.

References

1. Goodman L and Gilman A: The Pharmacologic Basic of Therapeutics. New York, MacMillan, 1940.
2. Withering W: An Account of the Foxglove and Some of its Medicinal Uses: With Practical Remarks on Dropsy and other Diseases. London, 1785.
3. Braunwald E, Bloodwell RD, Goldberg LI, et al: Studies on digitalis. IV. Observations in man on the effects of digitalis preparations on the contractility of the nonfailing heart and on total vascular resistance. J Clin Invest 40:52, 1961.
4. Oliver G and Schäfer EA: The physiological effect of extracts of the suprarenal capsules. J Physiol 18:230, 1895.
5. Stolz F: Uber Adrenalin und Alkylaminoacetobrenzcatechin. Ber Deutsch chem Ges 37:4149, 1904.
6. Barger G and Dale HH: Chemical structure and sympathomimetic action of amines. J Physiol 126:237, 1932.
7. Alquist RP: A study of adrenotropic receptors. Am J Physiol 153:586, 1948.
8. Lands AM, Arnold A, McAuliff JP, et al: Differentiation of receptors systems activated by sympathomimetic amines. Nature 214:597, 1967.
9. Lands AM, Luduena FP, and Buzzo HJ: Differentiation of receptors responsive to isoproterenol. Life Sci 6:2241, 1967.
10. Langer SZ: Presynaptic regulation of catecholamine release. Br J Pharmacol 60:481, 1974.
11. Eliot R: The action of adrenaline. J Physiol (Lond) 32:401, 1905.
12. Farah AE: Historical perspectives on inotropic agents. Circulation 73 (Suppl III):III-4, 1986.
13. Weiner N: Norepinephrine, epinephrine, and the sympathomimetic amines. In: Gilman AG, Goodman LS, Rall TW, et al (eds): The Pharmacologic Basis of Therapeutics, 7th ed, Chapter 8. New York, MacMillan, 1985.
14. Chernow B, Rainey T, and Lake R: Endogenous and exogenous catecholamines in critical care medicine. Crit Care Med 10:6, 1982.
15. Lands AM and Brown TG: Sympathomimetic (adrenergic) stimulants. In: Burger A (ed): Drugs Affecting the Peripheral Nervous System, Chapter 8. New York, Marcel Dekker, 1967.
16. Goldberg LI: Cardiovascular and renal actions of dopamine: Potential clinical applications. Pharmacol Rev 24:1, 1972.
17. Fitton A and Benfield P: Dopexamine hydrochloride. A review of its pharmacodynamic and pharmacokinetic properties and therapeutic potential in acute cardiac insufficiency. Drugs 39:308, 1990.
18. Michell RH: Post-receptor signalling pathways. Lancet 1:765, 1989.
19. Insel P: Adrenergic receptors. Am J Hypertens 2:112S, 1989.
20. Evans DB: Modulation of cAMP: Mechanism for positive inotropic action. J Cardiovasc Pharmacol (Suppl) 9:522, 1986.
21. Sperelakis N: Cyclic AMP and phosphorylation in regulation of Ca+2 influx into myocardial cells and blockade by calcium antagonist drugs. Am Heart J 107:347, 1984.
22. Tada M and Katz A: Phosphorylation of the sarcoplasmic reticulum and sarcolemma. Ann Rev Physiol 44:401, 1982.
23. Carcillo J: Signal transduction: How the cell processes information. Crit Care Clin 4:679, 1988.
24. Corr PB: Mechanisms contributing to the arrhythmogenic influ-

ences of α_1 adrenergic stimulation of the ischemic heart. Am J Med (Suppl 2A) 87:19S, 1989.
25. Minneman KP: α_1-Adrenergic receptor subtypes, inositol phosphates, and sources of cell Ca^{2+}. Pharmacol Rev 40:87, 1988.
26. Lefkowitz RJ, Caron MG, and Stiles GL: Mechanisms of membrane-receptor regulation. Biochemical, physiological, and clinical insights derived from studies of the adrenergic receptors. N Engl J Med 310:1570, 1984.
27. Sibley DR and Lefkowitz RJ: Molecular mechanisms of receptor desensitization using the β-adrenergic receptor-coupled adenylate cyclase system as a model. Nature 317:124, 1985.
28. Shepherd RE, Lang CH, and McDonough KH: Myocardial adrenergic responsiveness after lethal and nonlethal doses of endotoxin. Am J Physiol 252:H410, 1987.
29. Notterman DA, Hardman R, and Moldawer LL: Human recombinant tumor necrosis factor desensitizes the lymphocyte β-adrenergic complex. Pediatr Res 25:42A, 1989.
30. Notterman DA, Steinberg C, Metakis L, et al: Tumor necrosis factor produces homologous desensitization of the β adrenergic receptor complex. Crit Care Med 19:S74, 1991.
31. Bristow MR, Ginsburg R, and Minobe W: Decreased catecholamine sensitivity and β-adrenergic-receptor density in failing human hearts. N Engl J Med 307:205, 1982.
32. Schlepper M, Thormann J, Kremer P, et al: Present use of positive inotropic drugs in heart failure. J Cardiovasc Pharmacol (Suppl 1) 14:S9, 1989.
33. Farah AE and Frangakis CJ: Studies on the mechanism of action of the bipyridine milrinone on the heart. Basic Res Cardiol (Suppl 1) 84:85, 1989.
34. Weishaar RE, Quade MM, Schenden JA, et al: Relationship between inhibition of cardiac muscle phosphodiesterases, changes in cyclic nucleotide levels, and contractile response for CI-914 and other novel cardiotonics. J Cyclic Nucleotide Protein Phosphor Res 10:551, 1985.
35. Weishaar RE, Burrows SD, Kobylarz DC, at al: Multiple molecular forms of cyclic nucleotide phosphodiesterase in cardiac smooth muscle and in platelets. Biochem Pharmacol 35:787, 1986.
36. Endoh M, Yamashita S, and Taira N: Positive inotropic effect of amrinone in relation to cyclic nucleotide metabolism in the canine ventricular muscle. J Pharmacol Exp Ther 221:775, 1982.
37. Goldberg ND, Haddox MK, Nicol SE, et al: Bioregulation through opposing influences of cyclic GMP and cyclic AMP: The Yin Yang hypothesis. Adv Cyclic Nucleotide Res 5:307, 1975.
38. Lawless S, Burckart G, Diven W, et al: Amrinone in neonates and infants after cardiac surgery. Crit Care Med 17:751, 1989.
39. Chatterjee K: New oral inotropic agents: Phosphodiesterase inhibitors. Crit Care Med (Suppl 1) 18:S34, 1990.
40. Hoffman BF and Bigger JT Jr: Digitalis and allied cardiac glycosides. In: Goodman A, Gillman LS, Rall T, et al (eds): The Pharmacological Basis of Therapeutics, 7th ed, Chapter 30. New York, MacMillan, 1985.
41. Rockson SG, Homcy CJ, Quinn P, et al: Cellular mechanisms of impaired adrenergic responsiveness in neonatal dogs. J Clin Invest 67:319, 1981.
42. Driscoll DJ, Gillette PC, Ezrailson EG, et al: Inotropic response of the neonatal canine myocardium to dopamine. Pediatr Res 12:42, 1978.
43. Gootman N, Gootman PM, Buckley BJ, et al: Cardiovascular effects of catecholamine infusions in developing swine. In: Tumbleson ME (ed): Swine in Biomedical Research. New York, Plenum, 1986, p 1615.
44. Whitsett JA, Noguchi A, and Moore JJ: Developmental aspects of alpha and beta-adrenergic receptors. Semin Perinatol 6:125, 1982.
45. Boreus LO, Hjemdahl P, and Lagercrantz H: β-Adrenoceptor function in white blood cells from newborn infants: No relation to plasma catecholamine levels. Pediatr Res 20:1152, 1986.
46. Perloff WH: Physiology of the heart and circulation. Cardiovascular Problems in Pediatric Critical Care. In: Swedlow DB and Raphaely RC (eds): New York, Churchill Livingston, 1986.
47. Friedman WF and George BL: New concepts and drugs in the treatment of congestive heart failure. Pediatr Clin North Am 31:1197, 1984.
48. Notterman DA, Greenwald B, Moran F, et al: Dopamine clearance in critically ill infants and children: Effect of age and organ system dysfunction. Clin Pharmacol Ther 48:138, 1990.

49. Hansten PD, and Horn JR: Drug Interactions, 6th ed. Philadelphia, Lea & Febiger, 1989.

50. Seri I, Tulassay T, and Kiszel J: Effect of low dose dopamine infusion on prolactin and thyrotropin secretion in preterm infants with hyaline membrane disease. Biol Neonate 47:317, 1985.

51. Beregovich J, Bianchi C, and Rubler S: Dose-related hemodynamic and renal effects of dopamine in congestive heart failure. Am Heart J 87:550, 1974.

52. Goldberg LI: Dopamine-clinical use of an endogenous catecholamine. N Engl J Med 291:707, 1974.

53. Wilson RF, Sibbald WJ, and Jaanimagi JL: Hemodynamic effects of dopamine in critically ill septic patients. J Surg Res 20:163, 1976.

54. Gundert-Remy U, Penzien J, Hildebrandt R, et al: Correlation between the pharmacokinetics and pharmacodynamics of dopamine in healthy subjects. Eur J Clin Pharmacol 26:163, 1984.

55. Perez CA, Reimer JM, Schreiber MD, et al: Effect of high dose dopamine on urine output in newborn infants. Crit Care Med 14:1045, 1986.

56. Padbury JF, Agata Y, Baylen BG, et al: Dopamine pharmacokinetics in critically ill newborn infants. J Pediatr 110:2, 1987.

57. Girardin E, Berner M, Rouge JC, et al: Effect of low dose dopamine on hemodynamic and renal function in children. Pediatr Res 26:200, 1989.

58. Tulassay T, Rascher W, and Scharer K: Effect of low dose dopamine on kidney function and vasoactive hormones in pediatric patients with advanced renal failure. Clin Nephrol 28:22, 1987.

59. Schaer GL, Fink MP, and Parillo JE: Norepinephrine alone vs. norepinephrine plus low dose dopamine: Enhanced renal blood flow with combination pressor therapy. Crit Care Med 13:492, 1985.

60. Zaritsky A, Lotze A, and Stull R: Steady state dopamine clearance in critically ill infants and children. Crit Care Med 16:3, 1988.

61. Driscoll DJ, Gillette PC, and McNamara DG: The use of dopamine in children. J Pediatr 92:309, 1978.

62. Zaritsky A and Chernow B: Use of catecholamines in pediatrics. J Pediatr 105:341, 1984.

63. Seri I, Tulassay T, Kiszel J, et al: Cardiovascular response to dopamine in hypotensive preterm neonates with severe hyaline membrane disease. Eur J Pediatr 142:3, 1984.

64. Lang P, Williams RG, Norwood WI, et al: Hemodynamic effects of dopamine in infants after corrective cardiac surgery. J Pediatr 96:630, 1980.

65. Sabol SJ and Ward DS: Effect of dopamine on hypoxic-hypercapnic interaction in humans. Anesth Analg 66:19, 1987.

66. Ward DS and Bellville JW: Reduction of hypoxic ventilatory drive by dopamine. Anesth Analg 61:333, 1982.

67. LeJemtel T and Sonnenblick EH: Should the failing heart be stimulated? N Engl J Med 21:1384, 1984.

68. Mueller H, Ayres SM, Gregory JJ, et al: Hemodynamics, coronary blood flow, and myocardial metabolism in coronary shock; Response to 1-norepinephrine and isoproterenol. J Clin Invest 49:1885, 1970.

69. Fowler MB, Alderman EL, Oesterk SN, et al: Dobutamine and dopamine after cardiac surgery: Greater augmentation of myocardial blood flow with dobutamine. Circulation 70(Suppl I):103, 1984.

70. Benotti JR, Grossman W, Braunwald E, et al: Effects of amrinone on myocardial energy metabolism and hemodynamics in patients with severe congestive heart failure due to coronary artery disease. Circulation 62:28, 1980.

71. Benotti JR, McCue JE, and Alpert JS: Comparative vasoactive therapy for heart failure. Am J Cardiol 56:19B, 1985.

72. Golbranson FL, Lurie L, Vance RM, et al: Multiple extremity amputations in hypotensive patients treated with dopamine. JAMA 243:1145, 1980.

73. Alexander C, Sako Y, and Mikulic E: Pedal gangrene associated with use of dopamine. N Engl J Med 293:591, 1975.

74. Greene SI and Smith JW: Dopamine gangrene. N Engl J Med 294:114, 1976.

75. Dutz W: Drugs affecting autonomic functions of the extrapyramidal system. In: Dukes MNG (ed): Meyler's Side Effects of Drugs, 11th ed, Chapter 14. Amsterdam, Elsevier, 1988, p. 258.

76. Product Information: Inotropin®, dopamine. Du Pont Pharmaceuticals, Wilmington, 1989.

77. Rennotte MT, Reynaert M, Clerbaux T, et al: Effects of two inotropic drugs, dopamine and dobutamine, on pulmonary gas exchange in artificially ventilated patients. Intensive Care Med 15:160, 1989.

78. Lemaire F: Effect of catecholamines on pulmonary right-to-left shunt. Int Anesthesiol Clin 21:43, 1983.

79. Buchanan N, Cane RD, Miller M: Symmetrical gangrene of the extremities associated with the use of dopamine subsequent to ergometrine administration. Intensive Care Med 3:55, 1977.

80. Orlowski JP, Porembka DT, and Gallagher JM: Comparison study of intraosseous, central intravenous, and peripheral intravenous infusions of emergency drugs. Am J Dis Child 144:112, 1990.

81. Schulze KF, Graff M, Schimmel MS, et al: Physiologic oscillations produced by an infusion pump. J Pediatr 103:5, 1986.

82. Desjars P, Pinaud M, Potel G, et al: A reappraisal of norepinephrine therapy in human septic shock. Crit Care Med 15:2, 1987.

83. Cryer PE: Physiology and pathophysiology of the human sympathoadrenal neuroendocrine system. New Engl J Med 303:8, 1980.

84. Marin C, Eon B, Saux P, et al: Renal effects of norepinephrine used to treat septic shock patient. Crit Care Med 18:282, 1990.

85. Fukuoka T, Nishimura M, Imanaka H, et al: Effects of norepinephrine on renal function in septic patients with normal and elevated serum lactate levels. Crit Care Med 17:1104, 1989.

86. Desjars P, Pinaud M, Bugnon D, et al: Norepinephrine therapy has no deleterious renal effects in human septic shock. Crit Care Med 17:426, 1989.

87. Hesselvik JF and Brodin B: Low dose norepinephrine in patients with septic shock and oliguria: Effects on afterload, urine flow, and oxygen transport. Crit Care Med 17:179, 1989.

88. Mueller H, Ayres SM, Gregory JJ, et al: Hemodynamics, coronary blood flow, and myocardial metabolism in coronary shock; response to 1-norepinephrine and isoproterenol. J Clin Invest 49:1885, 1970.

89. Dollery CT: Physiological and pharmacological interactions of antihypertensive drugs. Proc R Soc Med 58:983, 1965.

90. Benowitz N, Forsyth RP, Melmon KL, et al: Lidocaine disposition kinetics in monkey and man. Effects of hemorrhage and sympathomimetic drug administration. Clin Pharmacol Ther 16:99, 1974.

91. Notterman DA, DeBruin W, and Metakis L: Plasma catecholamine concentrations in critically ill children—evidence of early β-adrenergic receptor desensitization. Pediatr Res 25:42A, 1989.

92. Benzig G III, Helmsworth JA, Schreiber JT, et al: Nitroprusside and epinephrine for treatment of low output in children after open-heart surgery. Ann Thorac Surg 27:523, 1979.

93. Lucking SE, Pollack MM, and Fields AI: Shock following generalized hypoxic ischemic injury in previously healthy infants and children. J Pediatr 108:359, 1986.

94. Goetting MG and Paradis NA: High dose epinephrine improves outcome from pediatric cardiac arrest. Ann Emerg Med 20:P22, 1991.

95. Brown CG and Kelen GD: High dose epinephrine in pediatric cardiac arrest [editorial]. Ann Emerg Med 20:104, 1991.

96. Solomon SL, Wallace EM, Ford-Jones EL, et al: Medication errors with inhalant epinephrine mimicking an epidemic of neonatal sepsis. N Engl J Med 310:166, 1984.

97. Levine DH, Levkoff AH, Pappu LD, et al: Renal failure and other serious sequelae of epinephrine toxicity in neonates. South Med J 78:874, 1985.

98. Kurachek SC and Rockoff MA: Inadvertent intravenous administration of racemic epinephrine. JAMA 253:1441, 1985.

99. Horak A, Raine R, Opie LH, et al: Severe ischaemia induced by intravenous adrenaline. Br Med J (Clin Res) 286:519, 1983.

100. Carter BT, Westfall UK, Heironimus TW, et al: Severe reaction to accidental subcutaneous administration of large doses of epinephrine. Anesth Analg 50:175, 1971.

101. Brown MJ, Brown DC, and Murphy MB: Hypokalemia from beta$_2$-receptor stimulation by circulating epinephrine. N Engl J Med 309:1414, 1983.

102. Weiner N and Taylor P: Neurohumoral transmission: The autonomic and somatic motor nervous system. In: Gilman AG, Goodman LS, Rall TW, et al (eds): The Pharmacologic Basis of Therapeutics, 7th ed, Chapter 4. New York, MacMillan, 1985.

103. Houben H, Thien T, De Boo T, et al: Influence of selective and non-selective beta-adrenoreceptor blockade on the haemodynamic effect of adrenaline during combined antihypertensive drug therapy. Clin Sci 57:397s, 1979.

104. Snow JC, Shamsai J, and Sakarya I: Effects of epinephrine during halothane anesthesia in mastoidotympanoplastic surgery. Anesth Analg 47:252, 1968.

105. Johnston RR, Eger EI II, and Wilson C: A comparative interaction of epinephrine with enflurane, isoflurane and halothane in man. Anesth Analg 55:709, 1976.

106. Lippmann M and Reisner LS: Epinephrine injection with enflurane anesthesia: Incidence of cardiac arrhythmias. Anesth Analg 53:886, 1974.

107. Nordenberg A, Delisle G, and Izukawa T: Cardiac arrhythmia in a child due to chloral hydrate ingestion. Pediatrics 47:134, 1971.

108. Bowyer K and Glasser SP: Chloral hydrate overdose and cardiac arrhythmias. Chest 77:232, 1980.

109. Goldstein DS, Zimlichman R, Stull R, et al: Plasma catecholamine and hemodynamic responses during isoproterenol infusions in humans. Clin Pharmacol Ther 40:2, 1986.

110. Downes J, Wood DW, and Harwood I: Intravenous isoproterenol infusion in children with severe hypercapnia due to status asthmaticus. Crit Care Med 1:63, 1973.

111. Berner M, Oberhansli I, Rouge JC, et al: Chronotropic and inotropic supports are both required to increase cardiac output early after corrective operations for tetralogy of Fallot. J Thorac Cardiovasc Surg 97:297, 1989.

112. Steinberg, C: Personal communication, 1990.

113. Page R, Gay W, Friday G, et al: Isoproterenol-associated myocardial dysfunction during status asthmaticus. Ann Allergy 57:402, 429, 1986.

114. Kurland G, Williams J, and Lewiston NJ: Fatal myocardial toxicity during continuous infusion intravenous isoproterenol therapy of asthma. J Allergy Clin Immunol 63:407, 1979.

115. Matson JR, Loughlin GM, and Strunk RC: Myocardial ischemia complicating the use of isoproterenol in asthmatic children. J Pediatr 92:776, 1978.

116. Hamstreet MP, Miles MV, and Rutland, RO: Effect of intravenous isoproterenol on theophylline kinetics. J Allergy Clin Immunol 69:360, 1982.

117. O'Rourke PP and Crone RK: Effect of isoproterenol on measured theophylline levels. Crit Care Med 12:373, 1974.

118. Barrazzone C, Jaccard C, Berner M, et al: Propranolol treatment in children with tetralogy of Fallot alters the response to isoprenaline after surgical repair. Br Heart J 60:2, 1988.

119. Ruffolo RR, Spradlin D, Pollock D, et al: Alpha and beta adrenergic effects of the stereoisomers of dobutamine. J Pharm Exp Ther 219:447, 1981.

120. Leier CV and Unverferth DV: Dobutamine. Ann Intern Med 99:4, 1983.

121. Leier CV, Unverferth DV, and Kates RE: The relationship between plasma dobutamine concentrations and cardiovascular responses in cardiac failure. Am J Med 66:238, 1979.

122. MacCannell KL, Giraud GD, Hamilton Pl, et al: Hemodynamic responses to dopamine and dobutamine infusions as a function of duration of infusion. Pharmacology 26:29, 1983.

123. Leier CV, Heban PT, Huss P, et al: Comparative systemic and regional hemodynamic effects of dopamine and dobutamine in patients with cardiomyopathic heart failure. Circulation 58:466, 1978.

124. Stoner JD III, Bolen JL, and Harrison DC: Comparison of dobutamine and dopamine in treatment of severe heart failure. Br Heart J 39:536, 1977.

125. Steen PA, Tinker JH, Pluth JR, et al: Efficacy of dopamine, dobutamine, and epinephrine during emergence from cardiopulmonary bypass in man. Circulation 57:378, 1978.

126. Majerus TC, Dasta JF, Bauman JL, et al: Dobutamine: Ten years later. Pharmacotherapy 9:245, 1989.

127. Sakamoto T and Yamada T: Hemodynamic effects of dobutamine in patients following open heart surgery. Circulation 55:525, 1977.

128. Perkin RM, Levin DL, and Webb R: Dobutamine: A hemodynamic evaluation in children with shock. J Pediatr 100:977, 1982.

129. Schrantz D, Stopfkuchen H, Jungst BK, et al: Hemodynamic effects of dobutamine in children with cardiovascular failure. Eur J Pediatr 139:4, 1982.

130. Driscoll DJ and Gillette PC: Hemodynamic effects of dobutamine in children. Am J Cardiol 43:581, 1979.

131. Stopfkuchen H, Schranz D, Huth R, et al: Effects of dobutamine on left ventricular performance in newborns as determined by systolic time intervals. Eur J Pediatr 146:135, 1987.

132. Bohn DJ, Poirier CS, and Edmonds JF: Hemodynamic effects of dobutamine after cardiopulmonary bypass in children. Crit Care Med 8:367, 1980.

133. Berner M, Rouge JC, and Friedli B: The hemodynamic effect of phentolamine and dobutamine after open-heart operations in children: Influence of the underlying heart defect. Ann Thorac Surg 35:643, 1983.

134. Schremmer B and Dhainaut JF: Heart failure in septic shock: effects of inotropic support. Crit Care Med (Suppl 1) 18:S49, 1990.

135. Berkowitz C, McKeever L, Crike RP, et al: Comparative responses to dobutamine and nitroprusside in patients with chronic low output cardiac failure. Circulation 56:918, 1977.

136. Franciosa JA, Guiha NH, Limas C, et al: Improved left ventricular function during nitroprusside infusion in acute myocardial infarction. Lancet 1:650, 1972.

137. Magorien RD, Unverferth DV, Brown GP, et al: Dobutamine and hydralazine: Comparative influences of positive inotropy and vasodilation on coronary blood flow and myocardial energetics in nonischemic congestive heart failure. J Am Coll Cardiol 1:499, 1983.

138. Kupper W, Waller D, Hanrath P, et al: Hemodynamic and cardiac metabolic effects of inotropic stimulation with dobutamine in patients with coronary artery disease. Eur Heart J 3:29, 1982.

139. Tinker JH, Tarkan S, and White RD: Dobutamine for inotropic support during emergence from cardiopulmonary bypass. Anesthesiology 44:281, 1976.

140. Loeb H, Bredakis J, Gunner, RM, et al: Superiority of dobutamine over dopamine for augmentation of cardiac output in patients with cardiac failure. Circulation 55:375–378, 1977.

141. Smith RE, Briggs B, Unverferth DV, et al: Dobutamine-induced inhibition of platelet function. Int J Clin Pharmacol Res 2:89, 1982.

142. Colucci W, Wright R, and Braunwald E: New positive inotropic agents in the treatment of congestive heart failure. N Engl J Med 314:291 (Part 1) and 349 (Part 2), 1986.

143. Bottorff MB, Rutledge DR, and Pieper JA: Evaluation of intravenous amrinone: The first of a new class of positive inotropic agents with vasodilator properties. Pharmacotherapy 5:227, 1985.

144. Benotti JR, Lesko LJ, and McCue JE: Acute pharmacodynamics and pharmacokinetics of oral amrinone. J Clin Pharmacol 22:425, 1982.

145. Edelson J, Stroshane R, Benziger DP, et al: Pharmacokinetics of the bipyridines amrinone and milrinone. Circulation 73:III, 145, 1986.

146. Chatterjee K: Phosphodiesterase inhibitors: Alterations in systemic and coronary hemodynamics. Basic Res Cardiol 84 (Suppl 1): 213, 1989.

147. Mammel MC, Einzig S, Kulik TJ, et al: Pulmonary vascular effects of amrinone in conscious lambs. Pediatr Res 17:720, 1983.

148. Wilsmhurst PT and Webb-Peploe MM: Side effects of amrinone therapy. Br Heart J 49:447, 1983.

149. Benotti JR, Grossman W, Braunwald E, et al: Hemodynamic assessment of amrinone: A new inotropic agent. N Engl J Med 299:1373, 1978.

150. Ward A, Brogden RN, Heel RC, et al: Amrinone—a preliminary review of it pharmacological properties and therapeutic use. Drugs 26:468, 1983.

151. Weber KT, Andrews V, Janicki JS, et al: Amrinone and exercise performance in patients with chronic heart failure. Am J Cardiol 48:164, 1981.

152. Hamilton RA, Kowalsky SF, Wright EM, et al: Effect of the acetylator phenotype on amrinone pharmacokinetics. Clin Pharmacol Ther 40:615, 1986.

153. Rocci ML Jr and Wilson H: The pharmacokinetics and pharmacodynamics of newer inotropic agents. Clin Pharmacokinet 13:91, 1987.

154. Klitzner TS, Shapir Y, Ravin R, et al: The biphasic effect of amrinone on tension development in newborn mammalian myocardium. Pediatr Res 27:144, 1990.

155. Wilmshurst PT and Webb-Peploe MM: The effects of amrinone on platelet count, survival and function in patients with congestive heart failure. Br J Clin Pharmacol 17:317, 1984.

156. Ansell J, Tiarks C, McCue J, et al: Amrinone-induced thrombocytopenia. Arch Intern Med 144:949, 1984.

157. Treadway G: Clinical safety of intravenous amrinone—a review. Am J Cardiol 56:39, 1985.

158. Lewis RP: Digitalis: A drug that refuses to die. Crit Care Med 18:S5, 1990.

159. Rackow EC, Packman MI, and Weil MH: Hemodynamic effects of digoxin during acute cardiac failure: A comparison in patients with and without acute myocardial infarction. Crit Care Med 12:1001, 1987.

160. Berman W, Yabek SM, Dillon T, et al: Effects of digoxin in infants with a congested circulatory state due to a ventricular septal defect. N Engl J Med 308:363, 1983.

161. Park MK: Use of digoxin in infants and children, with specific emphasis on dosage. J Pediatr 108:871, 1986.

162. Sandor GGS, Bloom KR, Izukawa T, et al: Noninvasive assessment of left ventricular function related to serum digoxin levels in neonates. Pediatrics 65:541, 1980.

163. Ferrari A, Gregorini L, Ferrari MC, et al: Digitalis and baroceptor reflexes in man. Circulation 63:279, 1981.

164. Beller GA, Smith TW, Abelmann WH, et al: Digitalis intoxication: A prospective clinical study with serum level correlations. N Engl J Med 284:989, 1971.

165. Aronson JK: Positive inotropic drugs and drugs used in dysrhythmias, Chapter 18. In: Dukes MNG (ed): Meyler's Side Effects of Drugs, 11th ed. Amsterdam, Elsevier, 1988, p. 333.

166. Ordog GI and Beneron S: Serum digoxin levels and mortality in 5,100 patients. Ann Emerg Med 16:32, 1987.

167. Lathers CM and Roberts J: Minireview: Digitalis cardiotoxicity revisited. Life Sci 27:1713, 1980.

168. Chung EK: Digitalis Intoxication. Amsterdam, Excerpta Medica, 1969.

169. Vlasses PH, Besarab A, Lottes SR, et al: False-positive digoxin measurements due to conjugated metabolite accumulation in combined renal and hepatic dysfunction. Am J Nephrol 7:355, 1987.

170. Witherspoon L, Shuler S, Alyea K, et al: Digoxin-like substance in term pregnancy, newborns, and renal failure. J Nucl Med 27:1418, 1986.

171. Perkins SL and Ooi DS: Inocor (amrinone lactate) interferences with TDX digoxin measurements. Clin Chem 33:1944, 1987.

172. Rodin SM and Johnson BF: Pharmacokinetic interactions with digoxin. Clin Pharmacokinet 15:227, 1988.

173. Bigger JT and Leahey EB: Quinidine and digoxin: An important interaction. Drugs 24:229, 1982.

174. Steward DJ: Afterload: Nonsurgical manipulation of the failing circulation. In: Swedlow DB and Raphaely RC (eds): Cardiovascular Problems in Pediatric Critical Care, Chapter 6. New York, Churchill Livingstone, 1986.

175. Artman M and Graham TP Jr: Guidelines for vasodilator therapy of congestive heart failure in infants and children. Am Heart J 113:994, 1987.

176. Murad F: Drugs used for the treatment of angina: Organic nitrates, calcium-channel blockers, and β adrenergic antagonists. In: Gilman AG, Rall TW, Nies AS, et al (eds): The Pharmacologic Basis of Therapeutics, 8th ed, Chapter 32. New York, Pergamon Press, 1990.

177. Cohn JN and Burke LP: Nitroprusside. Ann Intern Med 91:752, 1979.

178. Palmer RF and Lasseter KC: Sodium nitroprusside. N Engl J Med 292:294, 1975.

179. Murad F: Cyclic guanosine monophosphate as a mediator of vasodilation. J Clin Invest 78:1, 1986.

180. Smith RP and Kruszyna H: Toxicology of some inorganic antihypertensive anions. Fed Proc 35:69, 1976.

181. Wood M, Hyman S, and Wood AJJ: A clinical study of sensitivity to sodium nitroprusside during controlled hypotensive anesthesia in young and elderly patients. Anesth Analg 66:132, 1987.

182. Balaraman V, Kullama LK, Easa D, et al: Developmental changes in sodium nitroprusside and atrial natriuretic factor mediated relaxation in the guinea pig aorta. Pediatr Res 27:392, 1990.

183. Getman CE, Goetzman BW, and Bennett S: Age-dependent effects of sodium nitroprusside and dopamine in lambs. Pediatr Res 29:329, 1991.

184. Gordillo-Paniagua G, Velasquez-Jones L, Martini R, et al: Sodium nitroprusside treatment of severe arterial hypertension in children. J Pediatr 87:799, 1975.

185. Yaster M, Simmons RS, Tolo VT, et al: A comparison of nitroglycerin and nitroprusside for inducing hypotension in children: A double-blind study. Anesthesiology 65:175, 1986.

186. Gray RJ, Bateman TM, Czer LSC, et al: Use of esmolol in hypertension after cardiac surgery. Am J Cardiol 56:49F, 1985.

187. Miller RR, Vismara LA, and Williams DO: Pharmacological mechanism for left ventricular unloading in clinical congestive heart failure. Circ Res 39:127, 1976.

188. Parillo J: Vasodilator therapy. In: Chernow B, (ed): The Pharmacologic Approach to the Critically Ill Patient, 2nd ed, Chapter 19. Baltimore, Williams & Wilkins, 1988.

189. Leir CV, Bambach D, and Thompson MJ: Central and regional effects of intravenous isosorbide dinitrate, nitroglycerin and nitroprusside in patients with congestive heart failure. Am J Cardiol 48:1115, 1981.

190. Beekman RH, Rocchini AP, Macdonald D II, et al: Vasodilator therapy in children: Acute and chronic effects in children with left ventricular dysfunction or mitral regurgitation. Pediatrics 73:43, 1984.

191. Dillon TR, Janos CG, Meyer RA, et al: Vasodilator therapy for congestive heart failure. J Pediatr 96:623, 1980.

192. Appelbaum A, Blackstone EH, Kouchoukos NT, et al: Afterload reduction and cardiac output in infants early after cardiac surgery. Am J Cardiol 39:445, 1977.

193. Appelbaum A, Bitran D, Merin G, et al: Afterload reduction and cardiac output in patients after mitral valve surgery. Thorac Cardiovasc Surg 28:414, 1980.

194. Benzing G, Helmsworth JA, Schrieber, et al: Nitroprusside after open heart surgery. Circulation 54:467, 1976.

195. Stephenson LW, Edmunds LH Jr, and Raphealy R: Effects of nitroprusside and dopamine on pulmonary arterial vasculature in children after cardiac surgery. Circulation 60:104, 1979.

196. Rude RE: Pharmacologic support in cardiogenic shock. Adv Shock Res 10:35, 1983.

197. Nakazawa M, Takao A, and Shimizu T: Afterload reduction for large ventricular septal defects. Br Heart J:49:461, 1983.

198. Beekman RH, Rocchini AP, and Rosenthal A: Hemodynamic effects of nitroprusside in infants with a large ventricular septal defect. Circulation 64:553, 1981.

199. Nakano H, Ueda K, and Saito A: Acute hemodynamic effects of nitroprusside in children with isolated mitral regurgitation. Am J Cardiol 56:351, 1985.

200. Benitz WE, Malachowski N, Cohen RS, et al: Use of sodium nitroprusside in neonates: Efficacy and safety. J Pediatr 106:102, 1985.

201. Knapp E and Gmeiner R: Reduction of pulmonary hypertension by nitroprusside. Int J Clin Pharm 15:75, 1977.

202. Packer M: Vasodilator therapy for primary pulmonary hypertension: Limitations and hazards. Ann Intern Med 103:258, 1985.

203. Rubis LJ, Stephenson LW, and Jonston MR: Comparison of effects of prostaglandin E1 and nitroprusside on pulmonary vascular resistance in children after open-heart surgery. Ann Thorac Surg 32:563, 1981.

204. Mayer JE Jr, Walsh E, and Castanada AR: Intensive care management of pediatric cardiac surgical patients. In: Fuhrman BP and Shoemaker WC (eds): Critical Care: State of the Art, Vol 10, Chapter 10. Fullerton, CA, The Society of Critical Care Medicine, 1989.

205. Pollack MM, Fields AI, and Ruttimann UE: Sequential cardiopulmonary variables of infants and children in septic shock. Crit Care Med 12:554, 1984.

206. Nourok DS, Glassock RJ, Solomon DH, et al: Hypothyroidism following prolonged sodium nitroprusside therapy. Am J Med Sci 248:129, 1964.

207. Cottrell JE, Casthely P, Brodie JD, et al: Prevention of nitroprusside-induced cyanide toxicity with hydroxocobalamin. N Engl J Med 298:809, 1978.

208. Cottrell JE, Patel K, Casthely P, et al: Nitroprusside tachyphylaxis without acidosis. Anesthesiology 49:141, 1978.

209. May DC, Popma JJ, Black WH, et al: In vivo induction and reversal of nitroglycerin tolerance in human coronary arteries. N Engl J Med 317:805, 1987.

210. Nakano H, Saito A, and Ueda K: Clinical characteristics of myocardial infarction following Kawasaki disease. J Pediatr 108:198, 1986.
211. Ilbawi MN, Idriss FS, DeLeon SY, et al: Hemodynamic effects of intravenous nitroglycerine in pediatric patients after heart surgery. Circulation 72 (Part 2): II 101, 1985.
212. Benson LN, Bohn D, and Edmods JF: Nitroglycerine therapy in children with low cardiac index after heart surgery. Cardiovasc Med 4:207, 1979.
213. Pearl RG, Rosenthal MH, Schroeder JS, et al: Acute hemodynamic effects of nitroglycerin in pulmonary hypertension. Ann Intern Med 99:9, 1983.
214. Rudinsky BF, Komar KJ, Strates E, et al: Neither nitroglycerin nor nitroprusside selectively reduces sepsis-induced pulmonary hypertension in piglets. Crit Care Med 15:1127, 1987.
215. Frankel LR, Smith DW, and Pearl RG: Nitroglycerin-responsive pulmonary hypertension in idiopathic pulmonary hemosiderosis. Am Rev Respir Dis 133:170, 1987.
216. Dohi S, Matsumoto N, and Tahahashi T: The effects of nitroglycerin on cerebrospinal fluid pressure in awake and anesthetized humans. Anesthesiology 54:511, 1981.
217. Ghani GA, Sung YF, Weinstein MS, et al: Effects of intravenous nitroglycerin on the intracranial pressure and volume pressure response. J Neurosurg 58:562, 1983.
218. Shook TL, Kirshenbaum JM, Hundley RF, et al: Ethanol intoxication complicating intravenous nitroglycerin therapy. Ann Intern Med 101:498, 1984.

30

Congestive Heart Failure

Theresa A. Hantsch, M.D., and Scott J. Soifer, M.D.

Congestive heart failure (CHF) is the pathophysiologic condition in which the heart is unable to provide adequate cardiac output or regional blood flow to meet the circulatory and metabolic requirements of the body. There is, in effect, an "exhaustion of the reserve force of the heart muscle."[1] This condition may result from structural abnormalities that place pressure or volume loads on the heart's pumping mechanism or from intrinsic myocardial dysfunction. CHF is a frequent disorder in children, particularly in infants. The clinical presentation of CHF in infants and children differs from that in adults. In fact, the age at presentation is often a guide to the likely cause of CHF (Fig. 30–1). In particular, congenital heart disease more commonly causes CHF in newborns, infants, and younger children, whereas acquired heart disease more commonly causes CHF in older children. Complex interactions among neurohormonal agents mediate the predominant effects of CHF on the cardiovascular, pulmonary, and renal systems. These effects of CHF are compensated for by the therapy for CHF.

ETIOLOGY

There are many causes of CHF in newborns, infants, children, and adolescents. Most cases occur in infancy, and in general the age at onset of CHF places a patient in a category of likely causes, particularly for congenital heart disease.[2, 3] The majority of causes of CHF are cardiac processes, either congenital or acquired; however, there are also a number of noncardiac causes of CHF (Table 30–1).

Congenital Cardiac Conditions (see also Chapter 33)

Defects producing left-sided obstruction produce CHF in the first few days to the first 2 weeks of life. Newborns with the hypoplastic left heart syndrome present in the first days of life with the acute onset of tachypnea, tachycardia, decreased perfusion, and weak pulses. These symptoms develop when the ductus arteriosus closes after birth. Newborns with severe coarctation of the aorta or interrupted aortic arch may similarly present

in the first days of life in cardiogenic shock, but presentation may be delayed. These infants may then present at 7 to 14 days of age with signs of CHF and a discrepancy between upper and lower body pulse quality and blood pressure. CHF results from the constriction of the aortic end of the ductus arteriosus, causing an increase in left ventricular afterload and a decrease in blood flow distal to the constriction. Infants with severe aortic stenosis present in the first few days of life with severe CHF. Physical examination reveals decreased upper and lower body pulse quality and a systolic murmur at the upper right sternal border. The electrocardiogram (ECG) shows left ventricular hypertrophy with strain. Newborns with total anomalous pulmonary venous return (TAPVR) with obstruction typically present in the first few days of life with tachypnea, cyanosis, and mild hypercarbia. The chest x-ray film reveals a small- or normal-sized heart and pulmonary venous congestion. It is difficult to distinguish patients with TAPVR from those with pulmonary disease. Echocardiography and frequently cardiac catheterization are necessary for diagnosis. Cor triatriatum is similar to TAPVR but is more difficult to diagnose without cardiac catheterization.

Defects with left-to-right shunting of blood at the atrial, ventricular, or great vessel level can produce CHF. In the premature infant, a patent ductus arteriosus may produce CHF in the first week of life, most often as the infant is recovering from the respiratory distress syndrome. The peripheral pulses are bounding, the precordium is hyperdynamic, and a continuous to-and-fro murmur is present, though occasionally only a systolic murmur is heard. In the premature infant, the pulmonary arteries are less able to constrict, and the immature myocardium is less distensible and thus less tolerant of a volume load than in the term infant. When a left-to-right shunt is present in the term infant, the left ventricle is not subjected to a volume load until 1 to 2 months of age when the normal fall in pulmonary vascular resistance occurs, allowing pulmonary blood flow to increase. Thus the term infant with a patent ductus arteriosus, ventricular septal defect (VSD), or atrioventricular septal defect (AVSD) without mitral insufficiency presents with CHF at 1 to 2 months, though there is often a history of tachypnea, sweating, or poor feeding. Newborns with AVSD with mitral insufficiency, however,

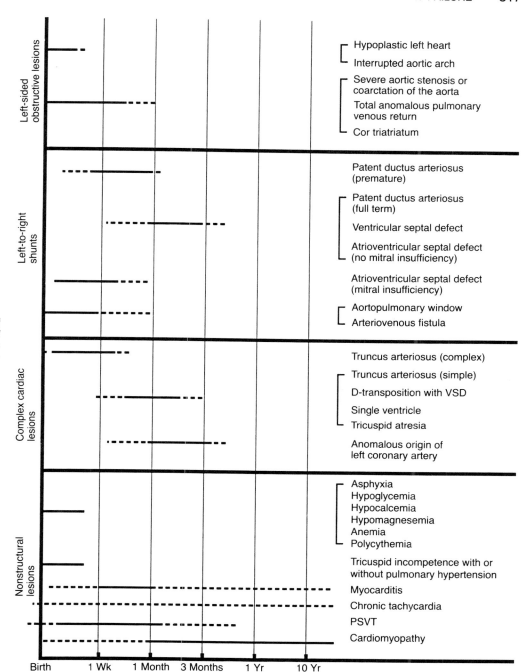

Figure 30–1. The age of onset of congestive heart failure (*solid lines* = more frequent occurrence; *dashed lines* = less frequent occurrence).

usually present in the first 2 weeks of life because of the associated pulmonary venous congestion in addition to the large left-to-right shunt. Similarly, with aortopulmonary window, newborns present in the first 2 weeks of life, since shunting is not limited by pulmonary vascular resistance and is consequently massive. Shunting at the atrial level, as in an atrial septal defect, is an infrequent cause of CHF. An atrial septal defect is usually diagnosed in a child with a murmur due to relative pulmonary stenosis and cardiomegaly. Nonobstructed TAPVR is a rarer disorder with a large atrial level shunt that usually produces CHF in the first few months of life.

Complex congenital cardiac defects, including truncus arteriosus, d-transposition of the great arteries (d-TGA) with VSD, tricuspid atresia, or single ventricle cause CHF. Infants with these defects usually experience CHF by 1 month of age. Since all these defects have both left-to-right and right-to-left shunting of blood and increased pulmonary blood flow, these infants also demonstrate a variable degree of desaturation, which may or may not be clinically apparent, depending on the type of defect and the infant's hemoglobin value. Infants with truncus arteriosus have a single second heart sound, mild desaturation (80 to 90%), and if truncal insufficiency is present, a see-saw murmur. Infants with

Table 30–1. CAUSES OF CONGESTIVE HEART FAILURE

Cardiac	Noncardiac
Congenital	**Systemic**
Left-sided obstructive defects	Asphyxia
Hypoplastic left-sided heart	Hypoglycemia
syndrome	Hypocalcemia
Interrupted aortic arch	Hypomagnesemia
Coarctation of the aorta	Sepsis
Aortic stenosis	Kawasaki disease
Total anomalous pulmonary	Diffuse vasculitis
venous return (obstructed)	Neuromuscular degenerative
Cor triatriatum	disorders
Left-to-right shunting defects	**Pulmonary**
Patent ductus arteriosus	Upper airway obstruction
Ventricular septal defect	(tonsillar hypertrophy,
Atrioventricular septal defect	subglottic stenosis)
Aortopulmonary window	Bronchopulmonary dysplasia
Atrial septal defect	Persistent primary pulmonary
Total anomalous pulmonary	hypertension
venous return	Cystic fibrosis
Complex congenital defects	**Hematologic**
Truncus arteriosus	Anemia
d-transposition of the great	Polycythemia
arteries with ventricular	**Renal**
septal defect	Failure
Tricuspid atresia	Intravascular volume overload
Single ventricle	Hypertension (renovascular)
Other	**Endocrine**
Anomalous origin of left	Hyperthyroidism
coronary artery	Hypothyroidism
Pulmonary insufficiency	Adrenal insufficiency
Tricuspid insufficiency	**Vascular**
Pulmonary stenosis	Systemic arteriovenous fistula
Tetralogy of Fallot, absent	Multiple cutaneous
pulmonary valve variant	hemangiomas
Postoperative	Large vascular tumor
Myocardial ischemia	
Inadequate repair	
Ventricular dysfunction	
Acquired	
Dysrhythmia	
Complete heart block	
Supraventricular tachycardia	
Chronic tachycardia	
Other tachyarrhythmia	
Cardiomyopathy	
Myocarditis	
Endocardial fibroelastosis	
Anthracycline-induced	
Human immunodeficiency	
virus	
Hypertrophic	
Hypertensive	
Familial	
Storage disease	
Idiopathic	
Valvular dysfunction	
Rheumatic	
Acute bacterial endocarditis	

d-TGA with VSD are usually the most cyanotic, depending on the size of the VSD. Single ventricle is an echocardiographic diagnosis, but the ECG characteristically reveals that Q waves are lacking.

Several other congenital cardiac defects may also produce CHF. Infants with anomalous origin of the left coronary artery present in the first few months of life with CHF due to anterolateral myocardial ischemia or infarction. The newborn with elevated pulmonary vascular resistance may experience transient tricuspid and pulmonary insufficiency and may have accompanying CHF, which is usually self-limited. Newborns with pulmonary stenosis may experience right-sided CHF and a right-to-left atrial shunt resulting in cyanosis; a murmur is heard at the upper left sternal border. In the absent pulmonary valve variant of tetralogy of Fallot, severe pulmonary insufficiency, in addition to the left-to-right ventricular shunt, increases pulmonary blood flow and causes enlargement of the pulmonary arteries and bronchial compression. Tricuspid insufficiency and systemic venous congestion are usually associated. This syndrome can present shortly after birth.

Other patients with congenital heart defects experience CHF in late infancy and childhood. In these patients, the onset of CHF is usually coincident with the occurrence or worsening of valvular insufficiency or the development of an arrhythmia. CHF occurs in patients with Ebstein's anomaly from the neonatal period to late childhood when the degree of tricuspid insufficiency becomes severe. Right-sided CHF also occurs in older children and young adults with Eisenmenger syndrome (irreversible pulmonary vascular disease due to a long-standing left-to-right shunt) with the development of atrial fibrillation. Left-sided CHF occurs in older children and young adults who experience aortic insufficiency secondary to either the progressive prolapse of an aortic valve cusp through a VSD or the development of acute bacterial endocarditis on a structurally abnormal aortic valve. Insufficiency of the systemic atrioventricular valve commonly occurs in patients with AVSD, congenitally corrected transposition of the great arteries, or single ventricle with common atrioventricular valve, and may also lead to left-sided CHF, which is often severe and difficult to treat. In all these cases, the most effective therapy is generally repair of the dysfunctional valve or treatment of the tachyarrhythmia that precipitated CHF.

Patients with congenital heart disease may experience CHF in the *postoperative* period, usually for one of three reasons: (1) myocardial ischemia secondary to cardiopulmonary bypass, (2) inadequate surgical repair, or (3) ventricular dysfunction secondary to ventriculotomy or coronary artery injury. Cardiopulmonary bypass may result in a diffuse ischemic injury to the myocardium, which impairs the intrinsic contractile function of the myocardium. This generally leads to CHF in the immediate postoperative period, which resolves slowly, if at all, over several weeks to months. In patients who had CHF preoperatively, the condition may persist following inadequate surgical repair of defects such as a VSD that is incompletely closed. CHF may also develop following surgical repair when prosthetic valves or shunts become obstructed or dysfunctional. This complication may occur at any point in the postoperative period and usually resolves after further surgical intervention. In some patients in whom an aortopulmonary shunt is placed to increase pulmonary flow, CHF may develop from excessive volume loading of the left ventricle; these patients may require either banding or snaring of the shunt to decrease pulmonary blood flow. Ventriculotomy and isolated coronary artery injury may compromise both the compliance and the contractility of the ventricle, which results in ventricular dysfunction and, consequently, CHF. This is particularly common after tetralogy of Fallot repair in which a right ventriculotomy is performed to attain access to the pulmonary outflow tract. Occasionally, in either tetralogy of Fallot repair or the arterial switch procedure for d-TGA, a coronary artery is injured, resulting in significant ventricular dysfunction and CHF. After the Fontan procedure, patients frequently have signs of severe right ventricular failure resulting from a lack of a pumping chamber between the systemic venous atrium and the pulmonary circulation. These patients typically have pleural effusions, hepatomegaly, ascites, and anasarca. In all patients with postoperative ventricular dysfunction, CHF is present in the immediate postoperative period and resolves very gradually, usually over a period of months.

Acquired Cardiac Conditions (see also Chapter 35)

Dysrhythmias are an important cause of CHF, though the patient often presents initially with symptoms related to the rhythm disturbance—for example, palpitations, chest pain, or syncope. Newborns and infants with very slow heart rates, as in congenital heart block, or very fast heart rates, as in paroxysmal supraventricular tachycardia, may initially present with symptoms of CHF or may experience these symptoms if treatment is delayed or unsuccessful. Asymptomatic chronic tachycardia may remain undiagnosed until the patient manifests symptoms of CHF. Other tachyarrhythmias not associated with congenital cardiac defects may arise at any age and remain clinically inapparent until CHF occurs.

Cardiomyopathy is a disease process of the heart muscle usually involving inflammation or fibrosis, which results from a variety of disorders. These changes in the myocardium impair the contractility of the heart and compromise ventricular compliance. Children present with CHF during either the early or late phases of the illness. A common cause of cardiomyopathy in childhood is myocarditis, which is defined as a round cell infiltration of the myocardium.[4] Myocarditis is a nonspecific inflammatory response to a variety of agents, most commonly viral infections. Although there are many subclinical cases of myocarditis, those patients with clinical findings typically have a history of an antecedent viral illness and present with fever, dyspnea, and progressive findings of CHF. Myocarditis may occur at any age but is most common in newborns and infants, in whom the course is frequently fulminant, and in older children and adolescents, in whom the course is usually more insidious.[5] The toxic myocarditis of diphtheria is characterized by the development of arrhythmias, including atrioventricular block and bundle branch block. In viral myocarditis, the ECG frequently shows only mild ST-T wave abnormalities, low QRS voltages without evidence of ischemia or ventricular hypertrophy, and arrhythmias, usually tachycardias.

Another cause of cardiomyopathy is endocardial fibroelastosis (EFE), which usually produces CHF in infancy or early childhood. The ECG reveals left ventricular hypertrophy, with increased QRS voltages, large Q waves in the lateral precordial leads, and deep inverted T waves.[6] Whether EFE is a separate entity or a pathologic stage in the progression of other cardiomyopathies remains controversial; however, the clinical course of EFE is of severe CHF that deteriorates steadily and usually ends in death.

The use of anthracyclines such as doxorubicin (Adriamycin) in the treatment of childhood cancer has a direct, dose-related irreversible cardiotoxic effect that produces CHF in about 5% of patients receiving total cumulative doses of 400 to 500 mg/m^2 and in 30% of those receiving doses greater than 550 mg/m^2.[7] Pathologic changes are noninflammatory and include myocytic injury of two types: myofibrillar loss and vacuolar degeneration.[8] Interstitial fibrosis may also be present. The severity of the pathologic changes correlates with both increasing total dose and degree of myocardial dysfunction.[9] Both the pathologic findings and the clinical condition may be worse in patients who have received radiation therapy.[8, 10] There has been an increasing number of reports of the delayed onset of CHF in children, suggesting an inability of myocardial growth to match somatic growth following anthracycline administration.[11] The treatment of CHF induced by anthracyclines consists of discontinuation of anthracycline therapy and administration of digoxin, diuretics, and afterload reducing agents; this treatment has had mixed reports of success.[12, 13]

An increasingly important cause of cardiomyopathy in children is the acquired immunodeficiency syndrome (AIDS). The pathogenesis of this cardiomyopathy may be a direct effect of human immunodeficiency virus infection or may reflect other factors such as secondary infection, immunologic abnormalities, anemia, or nutritional deficiencies, which may also depress myocardial function. Pathologic findings are predominantly myopathic in some series[14] and inflammatory in others.[15] AIDS is associated with a dilated cardiomyopathy, which may be difficult to diagnose because many of the signs and symptoms of CHF may already be present in patients with AIDS; however, medical therapy appears to improve cardiac function in these patients.[16]

Several other types of cardiomyopathy may also produce CHF. Infants of diabetic mothers may have neonatal hypertrophic cardiomyopathy that generally resolves but may be significant enough to require treatment of CHF. Hypertrophic cardiomyopathy may be identified in infants who are initially thought to have structural heart disease, usually caused by cyanosis or CHF. The occurrence of CHF despite increased ventricular function with hypertrophic cardiomyopathy in infancy is a poor prognostic sign.[17] Following infancy, hypertrophic cardiomyopathy does not usually cause CHF until late adolescence or adulthood. Hypertensive cardiomyopathy is extremely rare in childhood, as is familial cardiomyopathy. Pompe disease, a glycogen storage disorder, may present with a cardiomyopathy very similar to that in EFE. Infants with Pompe disease may be distinguished by their generalized hypotonia, a very thick-walled left ventricle, and a short PR interval on the ECG. Idiopathic cardiomyopathy may also present with CHF.

Valvular dysfunction from rheumatic heart disease or from acute bacterial endocarditis may cause CHF. Although the incidence of acute rheumatic fever has decreased, it is again increasing in the United States and remains common in many other countries. Mitral insufficiency, and less frequently aortic insufficiency, coupled with myocarditis cause CHF in rheumatic heart disease.[18] Acute bacterial endocarditis may cause the destruction of valvular tissue in otherwise asymptomatic patients with bicuspid aortic valves or mitral valve prolapse, and the resultant insufficiency may produce CHF.[19]

Noncardiac Conditions

CHF may develop during many *systemic* diseases. Cardiac muscle dysfunction may result from asphyxia, hypoglycemia, hypocalcemia, hypomagnesemia, or sepsis. Myocarditis or coronary artery abnormalities that occur in Kawasaki disease can result in CHF. Similarly, the diffuse vasculitis of collagen-vascular diseases may cause a myocarditis that can cause CHF. Severe cardiomyopathy may also be a component of degenerative neuromuscular disorders such as Duchenne muscular dystrophy and Friedreich ataxia. Several chronic *pulmonary* conditions may lead to the development of right-sided CHF and cor pulmonale. These conditions include upper airway obstruction such as tonsillar hypertrophy or subglottic stenosis, bronchopulmonary dysplasia, persistent primary pulmonary hypertension, and cystic fibrosis. *Hematologic* disorders such as severe anemia and polycythemia may cause CHF. In severe anemia in neonates, infants, and younger children, the myocardium may be incapable of increasing cardiac output sufficiently to compensate for the decreased oxygen-carrying capacity. In polycythemia, the hyperviscosity of the blood results in elevation of vascular resistances, which may decrease coronary blood flow, produce myocardial ischemia, and decrease cardiac output. *Renal* disorders such as acute renal failure may result in CHF from fluid overload. Similarly, iatrogenic fluid administration or maternal-fetal or twin-twin transfusion may produce intravascular volume overload and CHF. Hypertension secondary to renal vascular disease may cause a cardiomyopathy and CHF. *Endocrine* disorders such as hyperthyroidism may produce high-output CHF, whereas hypothyroidism and adrenal insufficiency may produce low-output CHF. *Vascular* abnormalities such as a large systemic arteriovenous malformation, multiple cutaneous hemangiomas, and large vascular tumors may cause high-output CHF.

DIAGNOSIS—SYMPTOMS AND SIGNS (PATHOGENESIS)

Cardiac output is determined by four components: preload, afterload, contractility, and heart rate.[20, 21] Preload, which is the diastolic loading state of the heart, relates to venous return and ventricular compliance and determines the end-diastolic volume and pressure of the ventricle. Increased ventricular volume increases both the force of contraction and the extent of fiber shortening, which correspond to systolic wall force and stroke volume, respectively, thus increasing cardiac output. Preload corresponds to ventricular end-diastolic pressure and clinically to right and left atrial pressures for the right and left ventricles, respectively. Afterload, the systolic loading state of the heart, relates to vascular resistance or the total force opposing ventricular ejection. Increased afterload decreases stroke volume and cardiac output, whereas decreased afterload increases stroke volume and cardiac output. The effects of these changes in preload or afterload are purely mechanical and do not relate to the contractile function of the myocardium. Contractility is the intrinsic ability of the myocardium to generate force. The intensity of the contractile force is determined by the availability of cytoplasmic calcium ions to the contractile proteins actin and myosin. The intracellular concentration of calcium ions depends on the release of calcium ions from the sarcoplasmic reticulum into the cytoplasm. This release, in turn, depends on the entry of extracellular calcium ions via calcium channels that are regulated by cyclic adenosine monophosphate (cAMP).[21] Changes in contractility, or the inotropic state of the heart, are independent of preload and afterload. Heart rate, or the frequency of cardiac contraction, affects the amount of work/unit time and the amount of time available for diastolic filling.

The ability of the heart to maintain adequate cardiac output during CHF is due to the cardiac reserve, which is much more limited in newborns and infants than in older children and adults for a number of reasons.[20, 21] First, the newborn heart functions at a higher diastolic volume (preload), so there is less ability to increase cardiac output from a given increase in preload. Second, the newborn heart has a decreased ability to develop tension in response to increased afterload. Third, the newborn heart has a greater proportion of noncontractile elements and generates less tension during contraction than does the adult heart. Finally, the newborn heart has an intrinsically higher heart rate; therefore, the ability of further increases in heart rate to augment cardiac output is limited and may be outweighed by decreased diastolic filling time and increased myocardial oxygen demand. Thus newborns and infants have less cardiac reserve than do older children and adults. As cardiac reserve is exceeded, signs and symptoms of CHF become manifested in response to physiologic stimuli (e.g., exercise and feeding) and pathophysiologic stimuli (e.g., fever), and eventually at rest.[23]

The clinical presentation of CHF is primarily the result of the side effects from the compensatory mechanisms that strive to maintain adequate cardiac output in the setting of extrinsic pressure or volume loads on the heart or intrinsic myocardial dysfunction. Because the failing ventricle (left or right or both) is unable to eject a normal stroke volume, it dilates to increase end-diastolic volume, thus maintaining cardiac output via the Frank-Starling mechanism (Fig. 30–2). This requires increased wall tension and increased myocardial oxygen demand. The ventricle may also dilate as a result of large volume loads. Ventricular dilatation causes elevation of ventric-

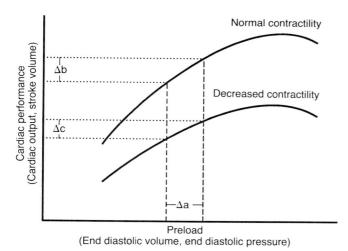

Figure 30–2. Cardiac performance (measured as cardiac output or stroke volume) is related to preload (measured as end-diastolic volume or pressure). The cardiac performance is depressed at all preloads when contractility is decreased. The same absolute increase in preload (Δa) yields a significantly smaller increase in cardiac performance than normal (Δb) when contractility is decreased (Δc).

ular end-diastolic pressure and, in turn, the corresponding atrial and venous pressures rise, leading to congestion of the venous bed.

In CHF of either the left or right ventricle, the resultant atrial and venous distention stimulates stretch receptors; low aortic blood pressure and pulse pressure stimulate aortic and carotid sinus baroreceptors. Stimulation of the stretch receptors and the baroreceptors causes an increase in sympathetic tone, which, in turn, stimulates α- and β-adrenergic and cholinergic receptors. α-Adrenergic receptor stimulation causes constriction of the vascular beds of the gastrointestinal tract, kidneys, muscles, and skin. As a result, urine output is decreased, and the extremities are usually cool and pale with decreased pulses. β-Adrenergic receptor stimulation causes tachycardia, increased contractility, bronchodilatation, and, possibly, increased secretion of bronchial mucus. Cholinergic receptor stimulation causes sweating, which is usually generalized but may be more marked on the scalp. Sweating is more prominent during exertion or feeding. Malaise, fatigue, anorexia (due to reduced blood flow and venous congestion of the gastrointestinal tract), and feeding difficulty (due to tachypnea) are often present. Irritability may also be present in infants. Impaired growth results from chronic CHF.

In left-sided CHF, the elevation of left atrial and pulmonary venous pressures results in an increase in pulmonary blood volume and an increase in lung interstitial water secondary to transudation of fluid. Consequently, the lungs become less compliant. As a result, the patient experiences many symptoms and signs, including tachypnea (rapid, shallow breaths) and dyspnea on exertion. As ventilatory requirements increase with exertion, a maximal respiratory rate is reached, and larger tidal volumes are required to achieve the necessary minute ventilation. To achieve these tidal volumes, markedly negative thoracic pressures must be generated, and retractions of the soft portions of the thorax result.

In addition, there are fine rales secondary to increased alveolar edema from the increased interstitial water, wheezing from the mucosal edema of small airways, and rhonchi due to increased mucus secretion in the larger airways.

In right-sided CHF, right atrial and systemic venous pressures are elevated from fluid retention. In older children and young adults, this produces dependent pitting edema, jugular venous distention, and hepatomegaly. In infants, however, pitting edema is unusual unless there is hypoalbuminemia, a history of excessive salt intake, associated renal dysfunction, or advanced CHF. If present, peripheral edema is best seen in the periorbital region. In infants, jugular venous distention is also unreliable because the veins are difficult to visualize and the venous pressure may not be elevated. In fact, systemic venous pressures may remain normal in infants until CHF is severe because the venous bed is very compliant. The liver is particularly distensible, and hepatomegaly is always present in infants with CHF. Right-sided CHF is usually present in conjunction with left-sided CHF.

CHF is diagnosed on the basis of the history and physical examination, with supportive information from laboratory test results and imaging studies. In the infant, a history of feeding difficulties, poor weight gain, tachypnea, noisy breathing, dyspnea, weak cry, and sweating can be obtained. In older children, the history is similar to that in adults, with symptoms of fatigue, dyspnea on exertion, cough, and anorexia. The physical examination may reveal signs of pulmonary venous congestion (tachypnea, rales, wheezing, and rhonchi) or systemic venous congestion (peripheral edema, hepatomegaly, and jugular venous distention). Tachycardia and cool extremities with delayed capillary refill resulting from enhanced sympathetic tone are often present. Examination of the heart may show a third heart sound and pulsus alternans secondary to ventricular dilatation and a fourth heart sound from atrial dilatation. In patients with congenital heart defects, the corresponding murmurs are also heard.

A number of laboratory tests and imaging studies may be useful in supporting the clinical diagnosis of CHF. An arterial blood gas determination may demonstrate mild respiratory alkalosis from tachypnea or mild respiratory acidosis from pulmonary edema. The arterial blood gas determination may also demonstrate hypoxemia secondary to a ventilation-perfusion mismatch from pulmonary edema or an underlying cyanotic congenital cardiac defect, or a combination of both. Metabolic acidosis is often present in severe CHF secondary to anaerobic metabolism. Although total body sodium and chloride levels are increased, electrolytes may reveal dilutional hyponatremia and hypochloremia. Hemoglobin determination may reveal polycythemia (which may develop in patients with cyanotic congenital cardiac defects) or severe anemia. The chest x-ray film shows cardiomegaly and possibly pulmonary venous congestion or increased pulmonary arterial vascular markings, or both, depending on the cause and severity of the condition. Except in dysrhythmias, the ECG is not diagnostic, but it may be helpful in identifying specific chamber enlargement or hypertrophy and ischemic changes, which may suggest a particular cause or correlate with the compromise of cardiac function. The echocardiogram (M-mode, two-dimensional imaging, and Doppler) can be very useful in identifying congenital cardiac defects, other structural abnormalities, chamber enlargement or hypertrophy, and associated findings (e.g., pericardial effusion, valvular insufficiency). It is also particularly helpful in providing noninvasive, objective measures of cardiac function such as shortening fraction (normal, 0.35 ± 0.06),[24] ejection fraction (normal, 0.66 ± 0.08),[24] and pre-ejection period:ejection period ratio (normal, 0.31 ± 0.06).[25] Ejection fractions may also be measured by radionuclide studies.

IMPACT ON ORGAN SYSTEMS (PATHOPHYSIOLOGY)

The pathophysiology of CHF primarily alters cardiovascular, pulmonary, and renal physiology. Complex interactions among a number of neurohormonal agents (including norepinephrine, the renin-angiotensin-aldosterone system, vasopressin, atrial natriuretic factor [ANF], dopamine, and a number of paracrine agents that exert their effects on local vascular beds) affect vascular tone, myocardial function, sodium balance, and free water balance.[26, 27] Blood flow is redistributed via the vasoconstricting and vasodilating effects of these neurohormonal agents. The extracellular fluid volume expands because of increased renal reabsorption of sodium and retention of free water, both of which are mediated by these neurohormonal agents. The exact nature of the interactions among these neurohormonal agents, in terms of which are primary and which are secondary, and the feedback mechanisms among them are complex and not well defined (Fig. 30–3).

Increased sympathetic tone increases renal vascular resistance, causing a decrease in renal blood flow, which, in turn, decreases the glomerular filtration rate. However, vasoconstriction of the efferent arteriole increases the filtration fraction. This increased filtration fraction lowers the postglomerular capillary hydrostatic pressure and increases its oncotic pressure, which promotes peritubular capillary uptake of proximal tubular fluid. Thus the amount of sodium reabsorbed in the proximal nephron increases.

Although norepinephrine is a neurotransmitter, it may have systemic effects much like a hormone in CHF because the excessive stimulation of the sympathetic nervous system results in marked elevation of plasma concentrations. These elevated concentrations, which correlate directly with the severity of hemodynamic compromise in children,[28] are a result of decreased clearance as well as increased synthesis of norepinephrine.[26] The most significant effect of norepinephrine is to redistribute blood flow to maintain perfusion of the heart and central nervous system at the expense of the kidneys, liver, and skin. However, the persistent stimulation of the sympathetic nervous system in CHF may cause autonomic abnormalities. In particular, patients with CHF demonstrate blunted baroreceptor responsiveness, β-adrenergic receptor down-regulation, and blunted end-organ responsiveness.[29–32] Nevertheless, there is potential for therapeutic benefit from inotropic agents that promote sympathetic activity by increasing cyclic adenosine monophosphate (cAMP) production via the β-receptor–mediated stimulation of adenylate cyclase.[33] This causes increased contractility and heart rate in the myocardium and vasodilatation in the vascular smooth muscle.

The renin-angiotensin-aldosterone system is a major contributor to the pathophysiologic mechanisms involved in sodium and fluid retention in CHF. Several factors stimulate the release of renin from the juxtaglomerular cells surrounding the renal afferent arterioles. Reduced renal blood flow and perfusion pressure and a reduced sodium load to the macula densa are important stimuli of renin production. Sympathetic nervous system activation via β-adrenergic receptor stimulation is also an important stimulus of renin production, though its contribution may be less significant in patients with CHF because end-organ responsiveness is blunted. In addition, the use of diuretic therapy and dietary sodium restriction in the treatment of CHF is a potent stimulus for renin production. In contrast, digoxin, the most commonly used pharmacologic agent in the treatment of CHF, suppresses renin production. Renin converts angiotensinogen to angiotensin I, which is then converted to angiotensin II by an enzyme present on endothelial cells. Thus angiotensin II, the most potent endogenous vasoconstrictor known, is produced in excess in CHF. It is indirectly responsible for sodium retention via renal vasoconstriction and the subsequent reduction in glomerular filtration rate; it is directly responsible for aldosterone secretion via stimulation of adrenal cortical receptors. Aldosterone not only is produced in excess in CHF but because it is metabolized primarily by the liver and because hepatic blood flow is reduced in CHF, its half-life may also be markedly prolonged. The resultant increase in the serum concentration of aldosterone increases sodium transport from the lumen of the distal convoluted tubules and the collecting ducts to the blood, and therefore this is a major cause of sodium retention in CHF. Aldosterone also causes water retention, which produces dilutional hyponatremia.

The excessive production of vasopressin in CHF is an important hormonal mediator of dilutional hyponatremia. The regulation of vasopressin release is complex under normal conditions, but it is further complicated by CHF and its pharmacologic therapy. Although osmolar mechanisms of regulation appear preserved, the serum vasopressin concentration is moderately elevated in CHF, most likely because of the stimulation of vasopressin release by angiotensin II. In addition to its role in free water retention, which may be attenuated by uncontrolled free water intake, vasopressin in pharmacologic doses causes potent vasoconstriction, and in pathophysiologic doses it causes both vasoconstriction and reduced cardiac output. Although the degree of vasoconstriction produced by vasopressin is not of the same magnitude as that produced by angiotensin II or even that produced by norepinephrine, it is such that it may be of clinical significance in patients with CHF.

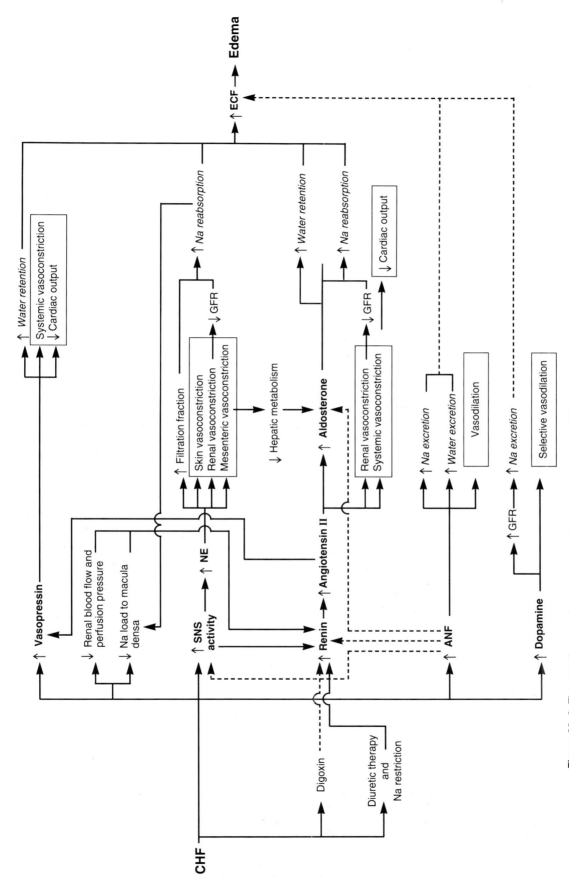

Figure 30–3. The complex neurohormonal interactions in congestive heart failure. Underlined items are end-organ responses that mediate the expansion in extracellular fluid volume. *Boxed* items are end-organ responses that mediate the redistribution of blood flow. *Solid lines* = stimulating effects; *dashed lines* = inhibiting effects; CHF = congestive heart failure; SNS = sympathetic nervous system; NE = norepinephrine; GFR = glomerular filtration rate; ECF = extracellular fluid; ANF = atrial natriuretic factor.

323

An important balancing component to the neurohormonal vasoconstrictors in CHF is ANF, which is a peptide hormone produced by atrial myocytes that is released in response to increases in atrial pressure and wall tension. It induces marked natriuresis and diuresis and is a potent vasodilator. Additionally, ANF suppresses both renin secretion, presumably through increased sodium delivery to the distal tubule and macula densa, and aldosterone secretion. It appears that the natriuretic and diuretic effects of ANF are blunted in patients with CHF. However, there is controversy regarding the vasodilating effects of ANF in patients with CHF. Blunting of ANF-mediated vasodilatation has been reported[34] as has augmentation of this vasodilatation.[35] The latter reports suggest that ANF has a balanced vasodilator effect, with reduction in both preload and afterload in patients with CHF. ANF also appears to have inhibitory effects on the sympathetic nervous system, which may facilitate its natriuretic and vasodilating effects, which sympathetic nervous activity would normally counteract. The plasma concentrations of ANF in patients with CHF are moderately elevated, which may explain the controversy regarding ANF's vasodilating effects, since higher levels may be necessary to induce these effects in patients with CHF. Thus ANF probably serves an important role in counterregulation of the effects of the sympathetic nervous and renin-angiotensin-aldosterone systems in CHF. However, therapeutic benefit from the administration of ANF to patients in CHF is unlikely, since it does not demonstrate effects superior to those of existing diuretic and vasodilating agents.

Another counterregulator of vascular tone and sodium excretion is dopamine. In pharmacologic doses, dopamine produces vasodilatation of selected vascular beds, including the renal, coronary, mesenteric, and cerebral circulations via the stimulation of dopamine$_1$ receptors located in these vascular beds and the stimulation of dopamine$_2$ receptors located in autonomic ganglia and sympathetic nerve tracts. In the kidney, dopamine increases the glomerular filtration rate, decreases proximal tubular reabsorption of sodium, and redistributes intrarenal blood flow toward the cortical region. These changes increase sodium excretion. Dopamine concentrations are increased mildly in CHF, and less specific α- and β-adrenergic stimulation may produce vasoconstriction at these higher concentrations.

There are several agents that exert their effects locally on vascular tissue. These paracrine agents may be very important in regional blood flow regulation and may also exert a systemic effect indirectly by dilating or constricting the resistance vessels, thereby changing the total cross-sectional area of the vascular bed. Thromboxane A$_2$, serotonin, and endothelin are paracrine vasoconstrictors. Thromboxane A$_2$ is produced in platelets from arachidonic acid and is likely involved in local vasoconstriction. Serotonin has both inotropic and vasoconstrictor effects that are likely mediated by the release of norepinephrine from sympathetic nerve endings.[36] Endothelin is a recently discovered peptide that has been found to exert a profound vasoconstrictor effect.[37] Prostaglandins E$_2$ and I$_2$, bradykinin, and endothelium-derived relaxing factor (EDRF) are paracrine vasodilators. The vasodilating effects of prostaglandins E$_2$ and I$_2$ are greatest in regional beds like the renal and coronary circulations. In fact, the production of prostaglandin E$_2$ by the renal vasculature is stimulated in CHF by the elevated concentrations of angiotensin II and norepinephrine. This may help maintain renal blood flow.[38] Prostaglandin I$_2$ is preferentially produced by vascular endothelial cells in which its role as a local vasodilator is probably quite significant.[39] Bradykinin is also predominantly a local vasodilator; its effects may be promoted by angiotensin-converting enzyme (ACE) inhibitors (which are frequently used in the therapy of CHF), since the enzyme responsible for the degradation of bradykinin is very similar to ACE.[26] EDRF has recently been identified as nitric oxide,[40] though other compounds that are also endothelium-derived vasodilators may exist. EDRF is the local mediator of the vasodilating effects of many pharmacologic agents, but its role in systemic regulation of vascular tone remains to be defined. The precise role of these paracrine vasoregulators and the interaction between them in the patient with CHF remains under investigation.

Although the major impact of CHF is on the heart, lungs, and kidneys, several other effects are worthy of note. The redistribution of blood flow in CHF, though protective for the heart and brain, may result in impaired function of the gastrointestinal system. Hepatic metabolism of carbohydrates and proteins may become markedly abnormal. Protein loss across the gastrointestinal tract and fat malabsorption also occur. The increased work of breathing and the elevated plasma concentration and activity of catecholamines generate increased caloric needs; the adverse cardiopulmonary effects of CHF often limit caloric intake. The combination of increased caloric needs and decreased caloric intake frequently results in malnutrition and growth failure. Oxygen delivery, despite a 2,3-diphosphoglycerate–mediated increase in tissue delivery (via a right shift of the oxyhemoglobin dissociation curve)[21] reaches a maximal level that may be exceeded by oxygen consumption, further promoting growth failure. Finally, insulin production is reduced in CHF, either as a result of diminished pancreatic blood flow or by direct α-adrenergic–mediated suppression, resulting in a catabolic state that further compounds the problem of growth.[41]

TREATMENT

The methods of treatment of CHF range from simple, supportive, and symptomatic measures to pharmacologic therapy to complex invasive mechanical methods and surgery. The severity of the patient's condition dictates the amount of supportive, symptomatic, and pharmacologic intervention needed. Mechanical methods of treatment are generally reserved for the most critically compromised patients and are primarily employed in the postoperative period. Although surgical repair may ultimately be required for definitive treatment of CHF resulting from congenital heart defects, it is preferable to optimize the patient's condition with medical therapy prior to surgery.

Supportive measures address the issues of oxygen requirements and salt and water balance. Oxygen requirements may be improved by increasing the oxygen supply or by decreasing the oxygen demand. Oxygen supply can be increased by administration of supplemental oxygen, patient positioning to increase tidal volume (semi-Fowler position), and bronchodilator administration if significant wheezing is present. Oxygen demand can be decreased by maintenance of normothermia, reduction in activity, digoxin therapy, sedation, and, if necessary, mechanical ventilation following muscle relaxation and intubation. Positive pressure mechanical ventilation will also decrease the alveolar component of pulmonary edema. Salt and water balance may be maintained by decreasing intake via salt and fluid restriction and by increasing output with diuretic therapy. Symptomatic measures of treatment address the correction of metabolic and hematologic derangements that have adversely altered myocardial function. This may involve the administration of glucose, calcium, or magnesium; the correction of endocrine abnormalities with the appropriate hormonal therapy; or the management of illnesses such as sepsis, collagen-vascular disease, and Kawasaki syndrome with antibiotics, steroids, and aspirin and gamma globulin, respectively, as indicated. Anemia may require transfusion to augment oxygen-carrying capacity, which will allow a decrease in cardiac output and consequently a decrease in myocardial oxygen consumption. Polycythemia may require phlebotomy or partial exchange transfusion to lower the hematocrit value to an acceptable range.

The premise of pharmacologic therapy, other than the administration of diuretics, is to alter the principal determinants of cardiac output: preload, afterload, contractility, and heart rate (see also Chapter 29). Vasodilating agents affect preload and afterload; inotropic agents primarily affect contractility but also affect other determinants of cardiac output to varying degrees. There are three types of vasodilators: venous dilators (nitroglycerin), which reduce preload; arteriolar dilators (hydralazine, nifedipine), which reduce afterload; and mixed dilators (nitroprusside, phentolamine, captopril, enalapril, prazosin), which reduce both. Similarly, there are three types of inotropic agents: digitalis glycosides, catecholamines, and the phosphodiesterase inhibitors. Digitalis glycosides are the traditional, standard therapy for CHF. A significant advantage is their availability in oral form for chronic usage; significant disadvantages include a low toxic:therapeutic ratio, increased myocardial oxygen demand, and increased arrhythmogenicity.[20] The catecholamines (norepinephrine, epinephrine, isoproterenol, dopamine, and dobutamine) exert their inotropic effect via stimulation of β-adrenergic receptors.[20, 42] They differ in their systemic cardiovascular effects on the basis of their varying degrees of β_1 and β_2 stimulation, and in several, on the basis of their α stimulation. Side effects include tachycardia, arrhythmogenicity, and vasoconstriction or vasodilation. These compounds must all be administered by continuous intravenous infusion. A useful technique is the combination of two of these agents, usually low-dose dopamine (renal effective range) and either dobutamine or epinephrine. The third category of inotropic agents, the phosphodiesterase inhibitors, are also peripheral vasodilators.[43] Amrinone is the most commonly used of these drugs. The mechanism of action of these compounds has not been fully described, but the inotropic effect is thought to be mediated by inhibition of the cAMP-specific cardiac phosphodiesterase; this results in increased intracellular cAMP concentration and increased activity of cAMP-dependent protein kinases.[44] These protein kinases activate proteins that cause increased intracellular calcium ion concentrations, which, in turn, increases myocardial contractility.[45] The advantage of these agents in the therapy of CHF is that they have both a positive inotropic effect, which is nonadrenergically mediated, and an afterload reducing effect. The disadvantages are that there are numerous toxicities and that benefits appear to be short term only.[45]

Surgical intervention is indicated when the cause of CHF is directly related to a correctable congenital cardiac defect, and even then surgery is usually undertaken only after the patient's condition has been optimized with medical management. Mechanical interventions such as intra-aortic balloon pumps and extracorporeal membrane oxygenation are generally treatment modalities of last resort in patients with CHF and cardiogenic shock (see Chapter 28).

SUMMARY

Congestive heart failure is a common disease process in children, particularly infants. CHF compromises infants and younger children more than older children and adults because the cardiac reserve of the former is more limited. Cardiac processes, in particular congenital structural defects but also cardiomyopathies and dysrhythmias, are the predominant causes of CHF. However, a number of noncardiac processes may also cause CHF. The symptoms and signs of CHF are manifestations of the body's compensatory mechanisms for this process. These compensatory mechanisms include the responses to systemic and pulmonary venous congestion and the role of sympathetic nervous system activation. Although these manifestations are primarily of a cardiovascular or pulmonary nature, CHF has systemic effects that are largely the result of complex interactions among a variety of neurohormonal agents that affect vascular tone, myocardial function, and sodium and free water balance. The goal of treatment of CHF is to restore sodium and free water balance and to optimize vascular tone (preload and afterload) and myocardial function (contractility and heart rate). Thus cardiac output is improved and the circulatory and metabolic requirements of the body can be met.

References

1. Mackenzie J: Diseases of the Heart. London, Oxford Medical Publications, 1908.

2. Artman M and Graham TP: Congestive heart failure in infancy: Recognition and management. Am Heart J 103:1040, 1982.
3. Artman M, Parrish MD, and Graham, TP: Congestive heart failure in childhood and adolescence: Recognition and management. Am Heart J 105:471, 1983.
4. Noren GR, Staley NA, and Kaplan EL: Nonrheumatic inflammatory diseases. *In*: Adams FH, Emmanouilides GC, and Riemenschneider TA (eds): Moss' Heart Disease in Infants, Children and Adolescents, 4th ed. Baltimore, Williams & Wilkins, 1989, pp 730–748.
5. Hohn AR and Stanton RE: Myocarditis in children. Pediatr Rev 9:83, 1987.
6. Maron BJ: Cardiomyopathies. *In*: Adams FH, Emmanouilides GC, and Riemenschneider TA (eds): Moss' Heart Disease in Infants, Children and Adolescents, 4th ed. Baltimore, Williams & Wilkins, 1989, pp 940–964.
7. Von Hoff DD, Layard MW, Basa P, et al: Risk factors for doxorubicin-induced congestive heart failure. Ann Intern Med 91:710, 1979.
8. Billingham ME, Mason JW, Bristow MR, et al: Anthracycline cardiomyopathy monitored by morphologic changes. Cancer Treat Rep 62:865, 1978.
9. Mason JW, Bristow MR, Billingham ME, et al: Invasive and noninvasive methods of assessing adriamycin cardiotoxic effects in man: Superiority of histopathologic assessment using endomyocardial biopsy. Cancer Treat Rep 62:857, 1978.
10. Gilladoga AC, Manuel C, Tan CT, et al: The cardiotoxicity of adriamycin and daunomycin in children. Cancer 37:1070, 1976.
11. Goorin AM, Chauvenet AR, Perez-Atayde AR, et al: Initial congestive heart failure, six to ten years after doxorubicin chemotherapy for childhood cancer. J Pediatr 116:144, 1990.
12. Biancaniello T, Meyer RA, Wong KY, et al: Doxorubicin cardiotoxicity in children. J Pediatr 97:45, 1980.
13. Goorin AM, Borow KM, Goldman A, et al: Congestive heart failure due to adriamycin cardiotoxicity: Its natural history in children. Cancer 47:2810, 1981.
14. Joshi VV, Gadol C, Connor E, et al: Dilated cardiomyopathy in children with acquired immunodeficiency syndrome: a pathologic study of five cases. Hum Pathol 19:69, 1988.
15. Lipshultz SE, Chanock S, Sanders SP, et al: Cardiovascular manifestations of human immunodeficiency virus infection in infants and children. Am J Cardiol 63:1489, 1989.
16. Stewart JM, Kaul A, Gromisch DS, et al: Symptomatic cardiac dysfunction in children with human immunodeficiency virus infection. Am Heart J 117:140, 1989.
17. Maron BJ, Tajik AJ, and Ruttenberg HD: Hypertrophic cardiomyopathy in infants: Clinical features and natural history. Circulation 65:7, 1982.
18. Kaplan S: Chronic rheumatic heart disease. *In*: Adams FH, Emmanouilides GC, and Riemenschneider TA (eds): Moss' Heart Disease in Infants, Children and Adolescents, 4th ed. Baltimore, MD, Williams & Wilkins, 1989, pp 705–718.
19. Kaplan EL and Shulman ST: Endocarditis. *In*: Adams FH, Emmanouilides GC, and Riemenschneider TA (eds): Moss' Heart Disease in Infants, Children and Adolescents, 4th ed. Baltimore, Williams & Wilkins, 1989, pp 718–730.
20. Friedman WF and George BL: New concepts and drugs in the treatment of congestive heart failure. Pediatr Clin North Am 31:1197, 1984.
21. Talner NS: Heart failure. *In*: Adams FH, Emmanouilides GC, and Riemenschneider TA (eds): Moss' Heart Disease in Infants, Children and Adolescents, 4th ed. Baltimore, Williams & Wilkins, 1989, pp 890–911.
22. Weber KT and Janicki JS: Pathogenesis of heart failure. Cardiol Clin 7:11, 1989.
23. McElroy PA, Shroff SG, and Weber KT: Pathophysiology of the failing heart. Cardiol Clin 7:25, 1989.
24. Franklin RG, Wyse RK, Graham TP, et al: Normal values for noninvasive estimation of left ventricular contractile state and afterload in children. Am J Cardiol 65:505, 1990.
25. Gutgesell HP and Paquet M: Atlas of Pediatric Echocardiography. Hagerstown, MD, Harper & Row, 1978, p 205.
26. Cody RJ: Neurohormonal influences in the pathogenesis of congestive heart failure. Cardiol Clin 7:73, 1989.
27. Cannon PJ: The kidney in heart failure. N Engl J Med 296:26, 1977.
28. Ross RD, Daniels SR, Schwartz DC, et al: Plasma norepinephrine levels in infants and children with congestive heart failure. Am J Cardiol 59:911, 1987.
29. Bristow MR, Ginsburg R, Minobe W, et al: Decreased catecholamine sensitivity and β-adrenergic-receptor density in failing human hearts. N Engl J Med 307:205, 1982.
30. Fowler MG, Laser JA, and Hopkins GL, et al: Assessment of the beta-adrenergic receptor pathway in the intact failing human heart: Progressive receptor down-regulation and subsensitivity to agonist response. Circulation 74:1290, 1986.
31. Kubo SH and Cody RJ: Circulatory autoregulation in chronic congestive heart failure: Responses to head-up tilt in 41 patients. Am J Cardiol 52:512, 1983.
32. Zucker IH and Gilmore JP: Aspects of cardiovascular reflexes in pathologic states. Fed Proc 44:2400, 1985.
33. Wit AL, Hoffman BF, and Rosen MR: Electrophysiology and pharmacology of cardiac arrhythmias IX. Cardiac electrophysiologic effects of beta adrenergic receptor stimulation and blockade. Part A. Am Heart J 90:521, 1975.
34. Cody RJ, Kubo SH, Atlas SA, et al: Direct demonstration of the vasodilator properties of atrial natriuretic factor in normal man and heart failure patients. Clin Res 34:476A, 1986.
35. Kubo SH: Neurohormonal activity in congestive heart failure. Crit Care Med 18:S39, 1990.
36. Majid PA and Sole MJ: Effect of 5-hydroxytryptamine blockade with ketanserin on myocardial uptake of epinephrine and norepinephrine in patients with congestive heart failure. J Clin Pharmacol 27:661, 1987.
37. Yanagisawa M, Kurihara H, Kimura S, et al: A novel potent vasoconstrictor peptide produced by vascular endothelial cells. Nature 332:411, 1988.
38. Oliver JA, Sciacca RR, Pinto J, et al: Participation of the prostaglandins in the control of renal blood flow during acute reduction of cardiac output in the dog. J Clin Invest 67:229, 1981.
39. Needleman P, Bronson SD, Wyche A, et al: Cardiac and renal prostaglandin I_2: Biosynthesis and biological effects in isolated perfused rabbit tissues. J Clin Invest 61:839, 1978.
40. Palmer RM, Ferrige AG, and Moncada S: Nitric oxide release accounts for the biological activity of endothelium-derived relaxing factor. Nature 327:524, 1987.
41. Hait G, Gruskin AB, and Paulsen EP: Insulin suppression in children with congestive heart failure. Pediatrics 50:451, 1972.
42. Notterman DA: Pharmacologic support of the failing circulation: An approach for infants and children. Prob Anesth 3:288, 1989.
43. Ward A, Brogden RN, Heel RC, et al: Amrinone: A preliminary review of its pharmacological properties and therapeutic use. Drugs 26:468, 1983.
44. Colucci WS, Wright RF, and Braunwald E: New positive inotropic agents in the treatment of congestive heart failure: Mechanisms of action and recent clinical developments (second of two parts). N Engl J Med 314:349, 1986.
45. Chatterjee K: Newer oral inotropic agents: Phosphodiesterase inhibitors. Crit Care Med 18:S34, 1990.

31

Cardiogenic Shock

Margaret M. Parker, M.D.

Severe heart failure in infants and children may progress to cardiogenic shock, a state in which the forward output of blood from the left ventricle is inadequate to meet the body's metabolic needs. The diagnosis and management of cardiogenic shock present a difficult challenge for intensivists caring for children.

ETIOLOGY

Heart failure in children presents most commonly within the first year of life and is usually the result of congenital mechanical defects (see also Chapter 30).[1] Structural defects in the heart produce volume or pressure overload on the ventricles, which, if severe enough, may overcome the heart's ability to compensate and lead to cardiogenic shock. Heart failure may also develop as a complication of surgery to correct congenital defects. See Chapter 33 for a detailed discussion of congenital heart disease.

After the first year of life, heart failure may result from high-output states such as anemia or hyperthyroidism. Rheumatic heart disease, endocarditis, or nutritional deficiencies may also lead to the development of heart failure in children.[1] In children with chronic illnesses, heart failure may be a complication of the therapy for that illness, such as hemochromatosis in children with transfusion-dependent anemia or anthracycline cardiomyopathy in children with malignancies. Idiopathic cardiomyopathy may follow a viral illness, presumably as a result of acute viral myocarditis. Symptomatic cardiac dysfunction has been reported in children with human immunodeficiency virus infection and could potentially lead to cardiogenic shock.[2] Severe dysrhythmias may also compromise cardiac output enough to produce circulatory failure. Less common causes of heart failure include Kawasaki disease, glycogen storage diseases, mucopolysaccharide disorders, Friedreich ataxia, muscular dystrophy, and cardiac tumors. Heart failure may also be produced iatrogenically by overly aggressive administration of intravenous fluids, although this rarely results in cardiogenic shock. Heart failure of any etiology may progress to cardiogenic shock if the heart is no longer able to produce enough forward flow of blood to meet the metabolic needs of the tissues.

PATHOPHYSIOLOGY OF HEART FAILURE

As described in Chapter 30, there are four major determinants of ventricular function: contractility, heart rate, preload, and afterload.[3] The Frank-Starling relationship is the family of curves of preload versus ventricular function (Fig. 31–1). Different contractile states are described by different curves. Increases in contractility (e.g., in inotropic therapy) will shift the ventricular function curve upward and to the left. In the failing heart, the curve is shifted downward and to the right. Changes in contractility directly alter stroke volume and secondarily alter cardiac output if the heart rate does not change. The relative inability of the young child to increase stroke volume makes the cardiac output heart rate–dependent. According to the Frank-Starling relationship of preload to ventricular function, increases in preload will increase the cardiac output (if all else stays the same), up to the point at which the myocardial cells are stretched to their maximum efficiency (see Fig. 31–1).[1, 3] Increased afterload generally has the effect of decreasing the cardiac output in a structurally normal heart. Each of these four factors is important in determining cardiac output. Isolated changes in one factor without affecting the others is unusual. Thus the net effect on cardiac function from altering contractility, heart rate, preload, or afterload, and hence the patient's response to a therapeutic intervention, depends on the state of the myocardium and on the interactions of these factors in the individual patient.

In addition to the four primary determinants of ventricular function, there is an interaction between the right and left ventricles in vivo that may be enhanced by the constraining effect of the pericardium (see also Chapter 45).[4] The contribution of the pericardium in enhancing ventricular interdependence varies and may depend on the patient population studied. The clinical importance of this phenomenon remains to be determined.

The heart has a number of compensatory mechanisms that can help to maintain perfusion to the tissues in heart failure. When these are overwhelmed, cardiogenic shock ensues. When there is volume overload, the increased stretch on the myocytes enables them to

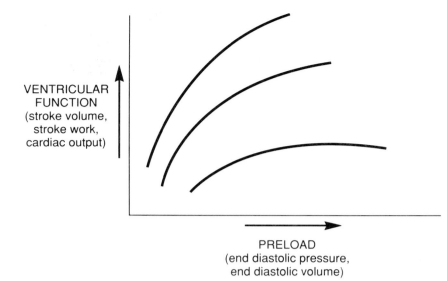

Figure 31–1. Frank-Starling relationship of preload versus ventricular function. In the normal heart, increased preload produces improved ventricular function. In the failing heart, the curve is shifted downward and to the right. Inotropic therapy shifts the curve upward and to the left.

increase the force of contraction.[1, 3, 5] The Frank-Starling relationship of preload to ventricular function describes the increase in stroke work or other measure of ventricular function that follows an increase in preload. The curve levels off as preload increases to very high levels and the myocytes are stretched beyond their ability to generate increased force by increasing cross-bridges between actin and myosin.[5]

The response to pressure overload, in contrast to volume overload, is one of hypertrophy.[3] Table 31–1 shows the short-term and long-term effects of the adaptive responses to impaired cardiac performance. The overall cardiac mass increases over a period of prolonged pressure overload, with the individual myocytes becoming larger and adding new sarcomeres. There is a decrease in contractility of each individual sarcomere, but the increase in overall mass allows the heart to maintain stroke volume and cardiac output with a decrease in energy required. There is not an increase in blood supply, however; thus in the long term energy starvation may develop, and cellular hypertrophy may contribute in the future to the deterioration and death of cardiac cells and to the transition from cardiac failure to cardiogenic shock. There is an increase in collagen as well in the hypertrophied heart, which may serve on a short-

term basis to reduce dilation but in the long term will impair relaxation and produce diastolic dysfunction.[6, 7]

Many changes take place at the cellular and subcellular level in response to decreased cardiac performance. Intracellular calcium shifts are the major determinants of contractility. An influx of calcium into the myocardial cell initiates contraction by binding to troponin and by allowing the interaction of actin and myosin. In the presence of adenosine triphosphate (ATP), actin and myosin form cross-bridges that cause the myocardial cell to shorten or develop force.[8] Active pumping of calcium out of the cell allows relaxation of the myocardial cell in diastole. Intracellular calcium handling has been shown to be abnormal in the failing human heart, leading to systolic and diastolic dysfunction manifested by delayed contraction and relaxation. The inability to maintain intracellular calcium homeostasis may cause an abnormality of contractility.[9] In addition, systolic function and some measures of diastolic function have been shown to correlate with high-energy phosphate content in myocardial cells.[10]

Changes in gene expression have been shown in the failing heart. Regulation of cardiac myocyte growth in the development of hypertrophy results from the action of proto-oncogene products such as growth factors,

Table 31–1. SHORT-TERM AND LONG-TERM RESPONSES TO IMPAIRED CARDIAC PERFORMANCE*

Response	Short-Term Effects†	Long-Term Effects‡
Hypertrophy	Unloads individual muscle fibers	Leads to deterioration and death of cardiac cells; cardiomyopathy of overload
Increased collagen	May reduce dilatation	Leads to energy starvation Impairs relaxation
Salt and water retention	Augments preload	Causes pulmonary congestion, anasarca
Vasoconstriction	Maintains blood pressure for perfusion of vital organs (brain, heart)	Exacerbates pump dysfunction (afterload mismatch); increases cardiac energy expenditure
Sympathetic stimulation	Increases heart rate and ejection	Increases energy expenditure
Sympathetic desensitization	—	Spares energy

*Adapted from Katz AM: Cardiomyopathy of overload. N Engl J Med 322:100–110, 1990. Reprinted by permission of The New England Journal of Medicine.
†Short-term effects are mainly adaptive and occur after hemorrhage and in acute heart failure.
‡Long-term effects are mainly deleterious and occur in chronic heart failure.

receptors, intracellular signaling proteins, and transcription factors.[11, 12] Guanine nucleotide-binding regulatory proteins have been shown to be increased in failing human hearts, compared with normal hearts.[13] The increase in these proteins may serve as a marker for heart failure. They may also account partially for the decrease in responsiveness to β-adrenergic agonists seen in heart failure. Pressure overload leads to changes in the protein content of myocytes as an indication of altered gene expression. Within a few hours of acute pressure overload in the rat's heart, there is an accumulation of α-skeletal actin, and within a few days there is an increase in β-myosin, indicating that there are at least two different regulatory mechanisms of myocyte protein content.[14]

In addition to the compensatory responses of the heart, there are adaptive mechanisms of the body as a whole that initially serve to maintain peripheral perfusion. Many of these responses have beneficial short-term effects, but over the long term they may be deleterious and produce further progression of heart failure (see Table 31–1).[7] Production of renin from relatively hypoperfused renal juxtaglomerular cells leads to increased angiotensin II and increased production of aldosterone. The effect on the kidney is to retain salt and water. In the short term, this increases preload and cardiac function by the Frank-Starling effect. On a long-term basis, salt and water retention cause pulmonary and peripheral edema.[15, 16] The beneficial effect seen with the use of angiotensin-converting enzyme inhibitors suggests that activation of the renin/angiotensin/aldosterone system may contribute to the pathogenesis of progressive heart failure.[17]

Activation of the sympathetic nervous system, with release of endogenous catecholamines, is an early response to heart failure.[18, 19] An immediate increase in cardiac output is produced by the increase in heart rate caused by adrenergic stimulation. There is an increase in the velocity of ejection and in the rate of tension developed. Endogenous catecholamines also increase vasoconstriction. This effect helps to maintain the blood pressure and perfusion to the tissues, but a long-term increase in afterload will reduce cardiac output, increase the workload on the heart, and may contribute to progressive myocyte death. Long-term vasoconstriction potentially alters regional blood flow, thus contributing to further organ dysfunction.[20] Chronic adaptation to decreased organ blood flow may partly explain why the early hemodynamic improvement seen with vasodilator therapy may not be followed by an immediate improvement in symptoms, although chronic vasodilator therapy may produce a beneficial clinical effect.[20] The reduced local vasodilation that is seen in chronic heart failure with a low-flow state may be caused by the inability of the endothelial cells to produce adequate quantities of endothelial-derived relaxing factor.[20] Another result of chronic endogenous catecholamine release is the downregulation of β-adrenergic receptors, with decreasing cardiac responsiveness to sympathetic stimulation.[21] This phenomenon has led some investigators and clinicians to use β-blocker therapy in some patients with chronic heart failure.[22, 23] Additionally, sympathetic stimulation may contribute to arrhythmias, which are commonly seen in heart failure.

DIAGNOSIS OF CARDIOGENIC SHOCK

The clinical syndrome of cardiogenic shock is one of failure of organ perfusion. Lethargy or mental status changes, oliguria, hypotension, and cool, clammy extremities may be seen in shock of a variety of etiologies. Signs or symptoms of forward heart failure and the adaptive responses to it include tachycardia, an S3 gallop, cardiomegaly, growth failure, irritability, and sweating. Signs of backward failure are those of pulmonary congestion/edema: tachypnea, wheezing, rales, cyanosis, dyspnea manifest as slow or poor feeding, and cough. In the patient with right heart failure as a major component of the process, hepatomegaly, jugular venous distention (which is often difficult to assess in infants), and peripheral edema (uncommon in infants) may be seen.[1, 3]

Chest roentgenography in the child with cardiogenic shock usually shows cardiomegaly. Pulmonary congestion may also be present, as may pleural effusions, if backward failure is present.[1] Electrocardiographic findings are not specific for cardiogenic shock but depend more on the underlying heart disease that has produced heart failure. Echocardiography is extremely useful in the evaluation of the child with cardiogenic shock. The type of congenital abnormality present (if any) can be diagnosed, and systolic function and valvular structure can be assessed. Systolic time intervals can also be measured to estimate ventricular function. Radionuclide ventriculography may be helpful in quantifying ventricular systolic function as well as in providing structural information in the case of patients with congenital heart disease.[24] All of these studies are useful in assessing the clinical state of the child, although they do not specifically diagnose cardiogenic shock.[1]

Laboratory studies are also helpful in evaluating the child's clinical state. Arterial blood gases show hypoxia and possibly a respiratory acidosis if there is significant pulmonary congestion. Respiratory alkalosis may be present in less severe cases of heart failure. Metabolic acidosis is present in most cases of true cardiogenic shock with failure of adequate forward flow. As tissue perfusion becomes increasingly compromised, anaerobic metabolism ensues, and lactate accumulates.[1] Hyponatremia with hypochloremia and an increase in bicarbonate are common in patients who have received diuretics chronically. Hyperkalemia suggests a marked compromise of renal function and possibly cell death in severe cases of cardiogenic shock. Hypoglycemia may be seen, because children with severe heart failure may develop a depletion of hepatic glucogen stores. In this case, therapy with glucose may result in clinical improvement of the heart failure.[5] In the patient with hypocalcemia (particularly common in infants of diabetic mothers), therapy with calcium may improve cardiac function.[1] A laboratory evaluation of renal and hepatic function is also helpful in evaluating the clinical state of the critically ill child and in assessing the prognosis, with failure of multiple organs due to inadequate perfusion being of obviously poor prognosis.

The diagnosis of cardiogenic shock itself is based on the clinical presentation of shock (see earlier) and on the hemodynamic differentiation from other types of shock.[26] In the newborn with congenital heart disease, hemodynamic assessment other than vital signs and the assessment of peripheral perfusion are difficult, as is differentiating respiratory distress from cardiac disease versus pulmonary disease.

Echocardiography is very useful in defining the cardiac abnormality and in establishing the diagnosis as possibly one of cardiogenic shock. In the larger child, a pulmonary artery catheter may be placed to measure right heart pressure and cardiac output and also to evaluate shunts. In cardiogenic shock the cardiac output is low, and the systemic vascular resistance and pulmonary artery wedge pressure are high. Hypovolemic shock is characterized by a low-cardiac output and high systemic vascular resistance, but with a low pulmonary artery wedge pressure. In extracardiac obstructive shock, such as pericardial tamponade, the right heart pressures are all elevated and equilibrated within 5 mm Hg of each other. Here again, the cardiac output is low and the systemic vascular resistance is high. In adults and larger children, septic shock is contrasted to cardiogenic shock by a high-cardiac output and low systemic vascular resistance. It is not clear that this hemodynamic profile is seen in smaller children. In any case, septic shock may progress to produce a cardiogenic shock-like state, with a low-cardiac output and high systemic vascular resistance, which is managed clinically in the same way as cardiogenic shock.

MANAGEMENT

The principles of therapy in cardiogenic shock are to increase cardiac function by reducing the workload and by improving the efficiency of the heart. Therapeutic interventions may be directed at correcting the primary cause of heart failure or at altering the adaptive responses that may have become deleterious. In children with congenital heart disease, surgery may be the most important intervention. Inotropic therapy is an important part of supportive therapy in cardiogenic shock, with the intent of improving contractility and thus cardiac output and tissue perfusion. However, downregulation of β-adrenergic receptors may make the heart less responsive to catecholamines, and the use of these agents may increase the energy demands of the failing heart, further exacerbating the problem.[8, 27] Inotropic agents may also be arrhythmogenic, and careful monitoring is required when using these agents. As noted earlier, β-blocker therapy may be beneficial in some patients with chronic heart failure.[22, 23] In the setting of cardiogenic shock, only very short-acting β-blockers should be used if they are used at all, because the negative inotropic effect may produce further decompensation of the cardiac output.

Afterload reduction with vasodilators or angiotensin-converting enzyme inhibitors may have a marked effect in decreasing the workload of the heart and thus improving cardiac output.[28–31] In the patient with cardiogenic shock and hypotension, these agents must be used with great care to avoid increasing hypotension. Intravenous agents with a short half-life are the most easy to titrate in the critically ill child. Preload reduction with diuretics or vasodilators may also improve ventricular function and is particularly useful in patients with backward failure who have pulmonary congestion and a high pulmonary artery wedge pressure. Treatment of arrhythmias with appropriate anti-arrhythmic therapy is also essential to restoring and maintaining hemodynamic stability.

References

1. Talner NS: Heart failure. *In:* Adams FH and Emmanouilides GC (eds), Heart Disease in Infants, Children, and Adolescents, 3rd ed. Baltimore, Williams & Wilkins, 1983, pp. 708–725.
2. Stewart JM, Kaul A, Gromisch DS, et al: Symptomatic cardiac dysfunction in children with human immunodeficiency virus infection. Am Heart J 117:140–144, 1989.
3. Moller JH and Neal WA: Specific cardiopulmonary problems of the neonate and their management. *In:* Moller JH and Neal WA: Heart Disease in Infancy. East Norwalk, CT, Appleton-Century-Crofts, 1981, pp. 463–483.
4. Janicki JS: Influence of the pericardium and ventricular interdependence on left ventricular diastolic and systolic function in patients with heart failure. Circulation 81:III-15–III-20, 1990.
5. Braunwald E, Ross J, and Sonnenblick EH: Mechanisms of contraction of the normal and failing heart. N Engl J Med 277:853–863, 1967.
6. Wexler LF, Lorell BH, Momomura S, et al: Enhanced sensitivity to hypoxia-induced diastolic dysfunction in pressure-overload left ventricular hypertrophy in the rat: Role of high-energy phosphate depletion. Circ Res 62:766–775, 1988.
7. Katz AM: Cardiomyopathy of overload. N Engl J Med 322:100–110, 1990.
8. Colucci WS, Wright RF, and Braunwald E: New positive inotropic agents in the treatment of congestive heart failure (First of two parts). N Engl J Med 314:290–299, 1986.
9. Gwathmey JK, Copelas L, MacKinnon R, et al: Abnormal intracellular calcium handling in myocardium from patients with end-stage heart failure. Circ Res 61:70–76, 1987.
10. Bashore TM, Magorien D, Letterio J, et al: Histologic and biochemical correlates of left ventricular chamber dynamics in man. J Am Coll Cardiol 9:734–742, 1987.
11. Simpson PC: Proto-oncogenes and cardiac hypertrophy. Annu Rev Physiol 51:189–202, 1988.
12. Izumo S, Nadal-Ginard B, and Mahdavi V: Proto-oncogene induction and reprogramming of cardiac gene expression produced by pressure overload. Prog Nat Acad Sci 85:339–343, 1988.
13. Feldman AM, Cates AE, Veazey WB, et al: Increase of the 40,000-mol wt pertussis toxin substrate (G protein) in the failing human heart. J Clin Invest 82:189–197, 1988.
14. Schiaffino S, Samuel JL, Sassoon D, et al: Nonsynchronous accumulation of alpha-skeletal actin and beta-myosin heavy chain mRNAs during early stages of pressure-overload-induced cardiac hypertrophy demonstrated by in situ hybridization. Circ Res 64:937–948, 1989.
15. Cannon PJ: The kidney in heart failure. N Engl J Med 296:26–32, 1977.
16. Baylen BG, Johnson G, Tsang R, et al: The occurrence of hyperaldosteronism in infants with congestive heart failure. Am J Cardiol 45:305–310, 1980.
17. Francis GS, Goldsmith SR, Levine TB, et al: The neurohumoral axis in congestive heart failure. Ann Intern Med 101:370–377, 1984.
18. Levine TB, Francis GS, Goldsmith SR, et al: Activity of the sympathetic nervous system and renin-angiotensin system assessed by plasma hormone levels and their relation to hemodynamic

abnormalities in congestive heart failure. Am J Cardiol 49:1659–1666, 1982.

19. Lees MH: Catecholamine metabolite excretion of infants with heart failure. J Pediatr 69:259–265, 1966.

20. Zelis R, Sinoway LI, Musch TI, et al: Regional blood flow in congestive heart failure: Concept of compensatory mechanisms with short and long time constants. Am J Cardiol 62:2E–8E, 1988.

21. Bristow MR, Ginsburg R, Minobe W, et al: Decreased catecholamine sensitivity and beta-adrenergic-receptor density in failing human hearts. N Engl J Med 307:205–211, 1982.

22. Engelmeier RS, O'Connell JB, Walsh R, et al: Improvement in symptoms and exercise tolerance by metoprolol in patients with dilated cardiomyopathy: A double-blind, randomized, placebo-controlled trial. Circulation 72:536–546, 1985.

23. Waagstein F, Caidahl K, Wallentin I, et al: Long-term beta-blockade in dilated cardiomyopathy. Circulation 80:551–563, 1989.

24. Treves S, Fogle R, and Lang P: Radionuclide angiography in congenital heart disease. Am J Cardiol 46:1247–1255, 1980.

25. Benzing G, Schubert W, Hug G, and Kaplan S: Simultaneous hypoglycemia and acute congestive heart failure. Circulation 40:209–216, 1969.

26. Weil MH and Shubin H: Diagnosis and Treatment of Shock. Baltimore, Williams & Wilkins, 1967, p. 10.

27. Colucci WS, Wright RF, and Braunwald E: New positive inotropic agents in the treatment of congestive heart failure (Second of two parts). N Engl J Med 314:349–358, 1986.

28. Fried R, Steinherz LJ, Levin AR, et al: Use of hydralazine for intractable cardiac failure in childhood. J Pediatr 97:1009–1011, 1980.

29. Cohn JN, Archibald DG, Ziesche S, et al: Effect of vasodilator therapy on mortality in chronic congestive heart failure: Results of a Veterans Administration Cooperative Study. N Engl J Med 314:1547–1552, 1986.

30. Massie BM, Packer M, Hanlon JT, and Combs DT: Hemodynamic responses to combined therapy with captopril and hydralazine in patients with severe heart failure. J Am Coll Cardiol 2:338–344, 1983.

31. Captopril Multicenter Research Group: A placebo controlled trial of captopril in refractory chronic congestive heart failure. J Am Coll Cardiol 2:755–763, 1983.

Cardiac Transplantation

Marshall L. Jacobs, M.D., Barbara B. Sands, R.N., and
William I. Norwood, M.D., Ph.D.

The concept of treating infants and children with lethal heart disease by means of heart replacement is not a new one. Shortly after the first successful heart transplant in a human adult had been accomplished, Kantrowitz and associates in 1967 attempted to treat a 3-month-old baby with tricuspid atresia by heart transplantation using an anencephalic infant as the donor.[1] The following year, Cooley and associates treated an infant with a complete common atrioventricular canal defect by combined heart and lung transplantation.[2] These early attempts demonstrated the technical feasibility of thoracic organ transplantation in small children, but neither of the recipients survived for more than a few hours. For the most part, heart transplantation between the late 1960s and the early 1980s was performed at a small number of centers, and most recipients were young adults. The Registry of the International Society for Heart Transplantation recorded fewer than five pediatric heart transplants per year prior to 1980. The major resurgence of activity in the field of heart transplantation that took place in the early 1980s was accompanied by an increased level of enthusiasm for pediatric heart transplantation as well. In 1984, the Registry recorded 37 pediatric heart transplants at 15 reporting centers.[3] In 1984 to 1988 there were 205 heart transplants in patients under 10 years of age, and there were 377 heart transplants in patients between 10 and 19 years of age. The latter half of the 1980s was marked also by a major resurgence of interest and level of activity in heart transplantation as a means of treating newborns and infants with lethal heart disease. Those who are engaged in this exciting and rapidly growing field owe considerable knowledge to the vastly larger experience in the field of adult heart transplantation. At the same time, the success and practicality of heart transplantation in children depends on special considerations with regard to the availability of appropriate infant and pediatric donors, the growth and long-term function of transplanted organs, and the implications of lifelong immunosuppressive therapy in very young patients.

PATIENT SELECTION

Heart transplantation is indicated for infants and children who have a cardiac lesion or disease that is associated with a worse prognosis and natural history than the current results of heart transplantation. In general, this implies that heart transplantation is offered to infants and children with a prognosis of surviving only several months to 1 year with any other form of therapy. This includes children with certain cardiomyopathies (viral, familial, metabolic, hypertrophic, drug-induced, or idiopathic), congenital structural cardiac lesions (palliated or unoperated), ischemic heart disease, life-threatening arrhythmias resistant to conventional therapy, and graft failure following previous transplantation. Relative contraindications to heart transplantation include the presence of uncontrolled neoplastic or infectious processes, recent or unresolved pulmonary infarction, and severe irreversible dysfunction of other vital organs. High pulmonary vascular resistance and anatomic distortion of the pulmonary arteries can certainly increase the challenge of heart transplantation but should not be considered absolute contraindications.

A stable family support system is important to the successful long-term outcome of pediatric heart transplantation. When heart transplantation is considered as a mode of therapy for an infant or child, an evaluation of the patient and the family is undertaken by a team consisting of transplant surgeons, pediatric cardiologists, transplant physicians, a transplant nurse clinician, and social worker. Neurology, psychiatry, and dentistry consultations are occasionally helpful.

The potential heart transplant recipient is characterized as to ABO blood type and HLA phenotype, and the patient's blood is tested against a panel of donor sera to detect the presence of preformed circulating antibodies. For patients who are highly sensitized (high levels of circulating preformed antibodies), a prospective lymphocytotoxic cross-match is advisable at the time of transplantation. Pulmonary function may be assessed by standard objective measures. Heart catheterization is performed to assess hemodynamics and measure the pulmonary vascular resistance. An assessment of renal function is accomplished by means of serum determinations of urea nitrogen and creatinine and by measurement of creatinine clearance. Liver function and other metabolic parameters are assessed with standard blood chemistry tests. A prospective transplant recipient is screened for the presence or absence of antibodies to the hepatitis viruses, human immunodeficiency virus, herpes simplex virus, cytomegalovirus (CMV), and varicella virus, as well as tuberculosis. A complete and accurate history of prior immunizations must be obtained. When the possibility of transplantation is anticipated at some point beyond the immediate future, it is desirable to update the patient's immunizations, with the important exclusion of live-attenuated virus vaccines.

While some children may await heart transplantation at home in the care of their family, it has been our experience that most pediatric patients referred for heart transplantation are sufficiently ill as to require management in the hospital, and frequently in an intensive care unit setting. This includes neonates whose pulmonary or systemic circulation depends on the patency of the ductus arteriosus and who therefore require a continuous intravenous infusion of prostaglandin to maintain satisfactory hemodynamics and oxygenation. Some but not all of these infants also require mechanical ventilatory support. Unfortunately, many additional pediatric patients are not referred for heart transplantation until their condition has deteriorated to a point requiring a significant level of support in the hospital, often with intravenous inotropic agents or vasodilators and occasionally with mechanical circulatory support.

Markedly elevated pulmonary vascular resistance has been considered by some to be an absolute contraindication to heart transplantation. It has been our experience, however, that the pulmonary vasculature of many children with heart failure is still very dynamic and may in fact be extremely responsive to alterations in the arterial blood gases, to reduction of the left atrial pressure (and thus the pulmonary venous pressure), and to vasodilator therapy. An example is the case of a 1-year-old child who was born with transposition of the great arteries (S, D, D) and underwent an arterial switch procedure in the newborn period. This was complicated by a major ischemic insult to the left ventricle and resulted in chronic ventricular dysfunction, congestive heart failure, and failure to thrive. When the child was first evaluated by us at 1 year of age, cardiac catheterization demonstrated pulmonary artery pressure that was equal to systemic arterial pressure, a transpulmonary gradient of 49 mm Hg, and a pulmonary vascular resistance of 26 Wood units/m^2/body surface area. This physiology might be considered by many to preclude successful heart transplantation. The child was treated with administration of intravenous amrinone at a dose of 10 μg/kg/min. After 3 weeks of inotropic and vasodilator therapy, hemodynamics were assessed by repeat cardiac catheterization. The pulmonary artery pressure was then found to be approximately one half of the systemic arterial pressure; the transpulmonary gradient was 16 mm Hg; and the calculated pulmonary vascular resistance was 8.2 Wood units/m^2/body surface area. Furthermore, it was demonstrated that the pulmonary artery pressure and resistance were responsive to increasing the oxygen content of inspired gases and to hyperventilation with a reduction of the level of arterial P_{CO_2}. The child subsequently underwent orthotopic heart transplantation with a very benign postoperative course, and pulmonary artery pressure at subsequent catheterization is in the normal range.

DONOR SELECTION AND MANAGEMENT

As for all heart transplantation, ABO compatability between the donor and the recipient is a requirement. HLA compatability has not been demonstrated to have an important impact on the outcome, and at the present time is not a criterion for donor selection. For heart transplantation in adults, it is conventional to try to match donor and recipient body mass. The scarcity of pediatric donors has necessitated considerably greater flexibility in donor-recipient size matching than is generally considered acceptable for adults. Bailey and associates[4] have emphasized the flexibility with regard to size matching that is possible in an infant heart transplant program, and Mavroudis and colleagues[5] have stated that satisfactory heart size matching can be achieved with body size variation of more than 60%. Our experience has in fact extended well beyond such variances. We have achieved satisfactory results with donor-recipient body mass mismatches of more than 300%. For example, the heart of a 20-month-old donor weighing 11.0 kg was transplanted successfully into a 6-week-old infant weighing 2.8 kg. Most of the neonates that we treat by heart transplantation at the Children's Hospital of Philadelphia have cardiac lesions that are associated with significant cardiomegaly. Neonatal heart donors are very scarce, but it is technically feasible to transplant the hearts of considerably older and larger babies into these newborns. Accordingly, the average donor weight for neonatal heart transplant recipients at our center is 8.6 kg, and the mean weight of the newborn recipients is 3.6 kg (Table 32–1).

Maintenance of adequate intravascular volume is essential to the preservation of satisfactory hemodynamics in potential cardiac donors. Vasopressor support should be minimized, and cardiac anatomy and function should be assessed by echocardiography whenever possible. There have been many cases of successful pediatric heart transplantation with extremely long graft ischemic times. Whenever possible, we make efforts to stay within limits of approximately 4 hours of cold ischemia, and in particular, we try to minimize graft ischemic time (as well as maximizing graft size) if the recipient has significantly elevated pulmonary vascular resistance. Others have emphasized the usefulness of donor transport to the transplant center for neonatal heart transplantation.[5, 6] With the current prevalence of multiple organ harvesting from each donor, this is rarely a practical possibility. It is also worth noting that a history of cardiac arrest with prompt and successful resuscitation is not an absolute contraindication to cardiac donation.

Donor serology with regard to human immunodeficiency virus, CMV, and the hepatitis viruses must be available prior to transplantation. It is likely that the incidence and severity of CMV infection following transplantation may be greatest if an organ from a CMV-seropositive donor is transplanted into a seronegative recipient. Some centers routinely avoid such a scenario by declining the offer of a CMV-positive donor for a CMV-negative recipient. Others routinely administer human immunoglobulins to CMV-mismatched recipi-

Table 32–1. HEART TRANSPLANTS (JUNE 1990 TO JUNE 1991) AT THE CHILDREN'S HOSPITAL OF PHILADELPHIA

		Patient Age	Donor Age	Patient Weight (Kg)	Donor Weight (Kg)	Ischemic Time (min)	COD*
1.	DM	15 mo	31 mo	7.0	13.0	196	MVA†
2.	CT	4 wk	3 mo	3.5	5.7	290	SIDS‡
3.	JH	5 wk	3 mo	4.4	5.6	64	SIDS
4.	AM	6 wk	2 yr	4.0	11.4	120	Fall
5.	SO	6 wk	20 mo	2.8	11.0	68	Fall
6.	AB	3 mo	13 mo	4.0	10.0	135	MVA
7.	AB	3 mo	3 yr	4.0	11.4	175	Sepsis
8.	MT	11 yr	10 yr	26.0	39.0	90	MVA
9.	MW	6 yr	6 yr	19.0	16.0	153	Blocked shunt
10.	TH	5 wk	14 mo	3.0	8.0	43	Child abuse
11.	TM	1 yr	6 mo	8.5	9.0	152	MVA
12.	JC	19 yr	14 yr	52.0	45.0	168	GSW§
13.	MN	2 wk	7 mo	3.9	9.7	53	Head trauma
14.	WM	2 yr	3 yr	12.4	19.5	191	Moya-Moya

*COD = cause of death (donor).
†MVA = motor vehicle accident.
‡SIDS = sudden infant death syndrome.
§GSW = gun shot wound.

ents. There is some preliminary experience (as yet unpublished) that suggests that the routine administration of gancyclovir may reduce the frequency and severity of CMV infections in these circumstances.

OPERATIVE TECHNIQUE

Donor cardiectomy is accomplished with inflow occlusion and aortic cross-clamping. Myocardial protection is achieved with topical hypothermia and with cold crystalloid cardioplegia that is infused into the coronary arteries via the ascending aorta. In cases in which the recipient has undergone previous heart surgery or in which there are anatomic abnormalities such as malposition of the great vessels, anomalous systemic or pulmonary venous connections, or stenosis or hypoplasia of the pulmonary arteries or systemic arteries, it is important to obtain as much donor tissue as possible including significant length of the donor great vessels. This generally involves removal of the graft with the confluence and branch pulmonary arteries intact, with some or all of the aortic arch, and with all of the superior vena cava and left innominate vein.

The recipient operation begins with the establishment of cardiopulmonary bypass in a conventional fashion. Transplantation may be performed either with deep hypothermia and circulatory arrest or with moderate hypothermia and continuous perfusion. For virtually all babies, and for many older children who have undergone previous reconstructive procedures or who have anomalies of the great vessels or systemic or pulmonary veins, the use of deep hypothermia and circulatory arrest significantly facilitates the accomplishment of the operative procedure. In most cases, satisfactory reconstruction can be accomplished at the time of orthotopic transplantation using autologous tissue from the donor and the recipient. This is exemplified by the use of the donor aortic arch in orthotopic heart transplantation of neonates with lesions that include hypoplasia of the aortic arch or coarctation of the thoracic aorta, or both,

as described by Bailey and associates.[7] In that instance, the donor aortic arch is used to augment the hypoplastic recipient aortic arch and to accomplish an aortoplasty of the region of juxtaductal coarctation of the thoracic aorta (Fig. 32–1). After implantation of the graft, perfusion may be accomplished by cannulation of the brachiocephalic trunk of the graft (Fig. 32–2).

Heterotopic heart transplantation in children has been

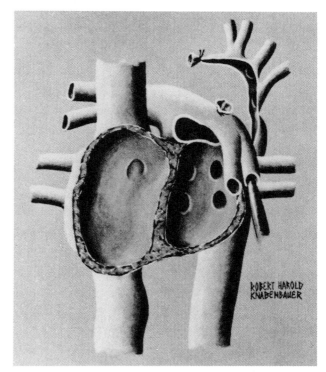

Figure 32–1. Artist's rendering of the appearance of the atria and great vessels of an infant with hypoplastic left heart syndrome following excision of the ventricular mass and valves. The tiny ascending aorta has been ligated proximal to the brachiocephalic trunk. (From Bailey L, Concepcion W, Shattuck H, et al: Method of heart transplantation for treatment of hypoplastic left heart syndrome. J Thorac Cardiovasc Surg 92:1–5, 1986.)

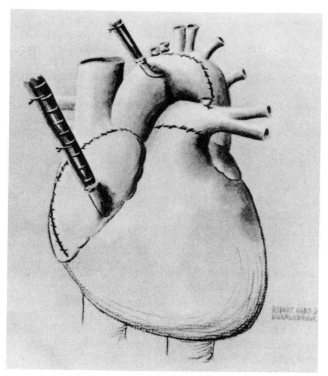

Figure 32–2. Artist's rendering of the appearance of the completed graft implantation with insertion of the arterial perfusion cannula via the donor brachiocephalic trunk. (From Bailey L, Concepcion W, Shattuck H, et al: Method of heart transplantation for treatment of hypoplastic left heart syndrome. J Thorac Cardiovasc Surg 92:1–5, 1986.)

undertaken less commonly than orthotopic transplantation. The predominant indication has been elevated pulmonary vascular resistance in the recipient rather than insufficient graft size. It is not clear how the long-term natural history of heterotopic transplantation compares with that of combined heart and lung transplantation.

PERIOPERATIVE MANAGEMENT

Each institution, of course, has individual preferences with regard to the management of pediatric heart transplantation recipients. At the Children's Hospital of Philadelphia, we currently use a triple-drug regimen consisting of cyclosporine, azathioprine, and steroids for the induction and maintenance of immunosuppression in most patients. When a potential donor is identified, the prospective recipient is given an oral dose of cyclosprine A of 6 to 10 mg/kg depending on the adequacy of the recipient's renal function. Following the completion of the implantation operation and after separation from cardiopulmonary bypass, azathioprine 5 mg/kg and methylprednisolone 10 mg/kg are administered by vein. Postoperatively, cyclosporine is given orally or by nasogastric tube at intervals of every 8 or every 12 hours. The dose may range from a typical adult dose of 8 to 10 mg/kg/day to as high as 45 mg/kg/day in infants and children. Infants and children may require and tolerate

both higher doses and higher blood levels of cyclosporine than adults in order to achieve adequate immunosuppression. A variety of assays are used for the measurement of blood and serum levels of cyclosporine and its metabolites. Accordingly, there is no such thing as a uniformly desirable therapeutic level. Even within a given institution, therapeutic and toxic effects of the drug may be observed at widely varying levels from one patient to another. We generally begin by administering 10 mg/kg/day of cyclosporine A and by steadily increasing the dose until a slight rise in the serum creatinine is observed, or other manifestations of toxicity such as hypertension or irritability occur. Steroids are administered as methyprednisolone 2 mg/kg/every 8 hours for six doses, and then as prednisone, which is given by mouth every 12 hours. The steroid dose is tapered gradually from 2 mg/kg/day of prednisone 48 hours postoperatively to 0.3 mg/kg/day by 6 weeks. In the absence of rejection, it has been our practice to leave the steroid dose at the level that is achieved approximately 6 weeks after transplantation, rather than increasing it with respect to body mass as the child grows. We have not, however, weaned our patients from steroids entirely, as has been the practice at some other centers. After the initial intravenous loading dose in the operating room, azathioprine is administered once a day at a usual dose of 2 to 3 mg/kg, which is reduced or deleted if the total white blood cell count falls below 4,000 or if significant thrombocytopenia occurs.

In patients who have important but potentially reversible renal dysfunction at the time of transplantation, we have selectively used OKT-3 for the first 10 to 14 days of immunosuppression and we have postponed the administration of cyclosporine until approximately the fifth day after transplantation or until adequate renal function and urine output are observed. Starnes and associates[8] at Stanford University reported excellent results in pediatric patients using a triple-drug regimen but with the routine addition of OKT-3 for the first 14 days of immunosuppression. Fricker[9] at the University of Pittsburgh utilized triple-drug therapy with the addition of antithymocyte globulin for the first week. Bailey and associates[4] at Loma Linda University have been extremely successful in utilizing an immunosuppressive drug regimen consisting of cyclosporine and azathioprine following neonatal heart transplantation. They reserve the use of steroids for the treatment of clinically evident episodes of acute rejection.

Intravenous catecholamines are frequently used during the early postoperative period following cardiac transplantation. Approximately one half of our patients receive infusions of low doses of either dopamine or isoproterenol, or both. If a sinus mechanism is not present in the early postoperative period, atrial or sequential atrioventricular pacing may be utilized. The potential for right ventricular dysfunction of the graft in the setting of either elevated recipient pulmonary vascular resistance or prolonged graft ischemic time is one of the most important challenges in the postoperative management of heart transplant recipients. In such circumstances, adjustment of ventilatory parameters to achieve a low arterial P_{CO_2} is often sufficient to reduce the pulmonary vascular resistance. In some cases, the addition of adrenergic inotropic agents to improve ventricular contractility and vasodilators such as sodium nitroprusside or prostaglandin E_1 to reduce pulmonary vascular resistance (or a combination of these two types of agents) may be beneficial. When hemodynamics are satisfactory, every attempt is made to wean mechanical ventilatory support when the child is fully awake, but infants and children who have been severely compromised prior to transplantation may require several days of endotracheal intubation and mechanical ventilation. Handwashing and other fundamental measures to prevent cross-contamination from other patients are important. Our heart transplant recipients are managed in the same cardiac surgical intensive care unit environment as all of the other infants and children undergoing heart surgery. Some institutions still adhere to practices of full reverse isolation.

In older children, endomyocardial biopsies are easily performed using the femoral vein or jugular vein approach. Clinical signs suggestive of acute rejection include unexplained fever, tachycardia, arrhythmias, hypotension, weakness, lethargy, and fluid retention. The presence of these signs may be an indication for emergent myocardial biopsy. Clearly, the pediatric transplant patient would benefit from the development of a noninvasive technique of assessing rejection with the same sensitivity and specificity as the endomyocardial biopsy. The utility of echocardiography as a screening tool for acute rejection in heart transplant recipients has been the subject of considerable debate. In our experience, the two-dimensional echocardiogram has reliably detected decrements in systolic function (left ventricular ejection fraction and fractional shortening), changes in ventricular wall thickness and compliance, and the presence of new pericardial effusions, which have correlated with biopsy proven acute rejection in the absence of overt clinical signs. The Stanford group has reported a high degree of correlation between two Doppler-derived indices (the isovolumetric relaxation time and the pressure half-time of the maximal velocity of blood flow decline across the mitral valve opening) and the histologic results of endomyocardial biopsies.[8] Our heart transplant recipients undergo weekly echocardiographic evaluation in the early post-transplant period. Bailey and associates at Loma Linda University do not routinely perform endomyocardial biopsies on neonatal heart transplant recipients until 1 year after transplantation.[6] They diagnose and treat episodes of rejection on the basis of clinical observation of changes in the infant's vital signs, behavior, and appetite, as well as noninvasive analysis including electrocardiogram, chest radiography, echocardiogram, and laboratory assays including cytoimmunologic monitoring. There is, however, extensive experience elsewhere with endomyocardial biopsies in children and infants. Bhargava and associates reported no serious complications with 71 consecutive biopsy procedures in infants and children.[10] Our practice is to reserve endomyocardial biopsies in infants and small children for circumstances in which the differentiation between acute rejection or some other process such as viral infection, for example, is not evident on a clinical basis alone. Otherwise, the diagnosis of acute rejection is made on the basis of clinical signs, and treatment is undertaken without histologic confirmation.

When an episode of acute rejection has hemodynamic consequences, or when the endomyocardial biopsy demonstrates myocyte necrosis of any degree, we initiate high-dose steroid therapy. In the early post-transplant period (the first 6 to 8 weeks after surgery), this generally consists of methylprednisolone 15 mg/kg/day by vein for 3 days. More than 2 months after transplantation, or in the absence of any signs of hemodynamic compromise, a significant increase in the dose of oral steroids may be substituted for the intravenous regimen. A steroid-resistant rejection, or any episode of acute rejection accompanied by major hemodynamic compromise, is treated with specific anti-T cell preparations. The results of such therapy can be dramatic and lifesaving. We have managed an episode of steroid-resistant rejection 4 months following transplantation in an 11-year-old girl that was associated with cardiogenic shock and multiple cardiac arrests. The profound low cardiac output state was reversed successfully by day 5 of a 14-day course of OKT-3. Several months later the patient's cardiac function was normal.

Toxic effects of the immunosuppressive drugs are observed occasionally in the early post-transplant period. Hypertension related to the administration of cyclosporine is generally responsive to some combination of diuretics and to either central vasodilators or calcium channel blockers. Neurologic manifestations of cyclosporine toxicity include irritability, tremors, seizures, and transient cortical blindness. The maintenance of adequate levels of anticonvulsant agents is of particular importance in cyclosporine-treated patients with a past history of seizures. Oliguria and renal dysfunction related to cyclosporine toxicity are almost always reversible with temporary discontinuation of the drug. On rare occasions, dialysis may be required for a period of up to several days. The administration of azathioprine may be associated with leukopenia or thrombocytopenia. In these cases, the drug should be discontinued until blood counts begin to rise. In the setting of profound granulocytopenia, broad-spectrum antibiotic therapy may be indicated.

RESULTS OF PEDIATRIC HEART TRANSPLANTATION

In 1989, the Stanford group[8] reported an actuarial survival of 75% at 1 year and at 5 years for a group of 17 patients, aged 5 months to 14 years, who had undergone transplantation since 1981 (Fig. 32–3). All deaths occurred in the first 6-month period following transplantation. In 1987, the Columbia University transplant group[11] reported the results of 15 pediatric heart transplants, with one operative death and three early deaths. One year later, these authors reviewed the effect of preoperative pulmonary hypertension and severe hemodynamic deterioration on the outcome of transplantation.[12] They found that all of the early deaths were

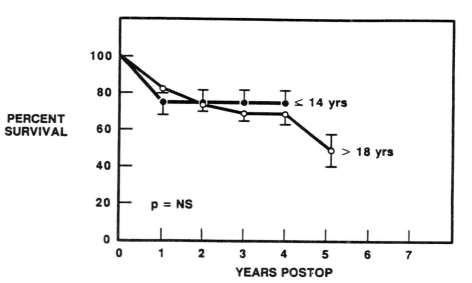

PERCENT SURVIVAL

Figure 32–3. Actuarial survival after heart transplantation by patient age. (From Starnes VA, Bernstein D, Oyer PE, et al: Heart transplantation in children. J Heart Transplant 8:20–26, 1989.)

due to right ventricular failure in the setting of pulmonary hypertension. These authors argued that pediatric cardiac patients with poor prognosis for long-term survival should be referred for transplantation prior to the development of severe pulmonary artery hypertension or hemodynamic deterioration.

In 1988, Bailey and associates[4] from Loma Linda University presented their early results of infant heart transplantation. Of 14 transplant recipients, 11 had survived. Three recipients had required perioperative peritoneal dialysis. All but one had demonstrated evidence of at least one episode of acute rejection. Also in 1988, Mavroudis[5] reported the early results of the University of Louisville heart transplant program. They reported five transplants including four neonates with hypoplastic left heart syndrome and one infant with previously undiagnosed anomalous origin of the left coronary artery. There was one early death from graft dysfunction. Three of the four survivors had sustained major complications, including renal failure requiring dialysis (one patient), and tamponade requiring delayed sternal closure (two patients).

The reported incidence of acute rejection following pediatric heart transplantation varies considerably from one center to another and importantly according to the criteria and methods utilized to make the diagnosis of rejection. The Stanford University group[13] reported no statistically significant differences between pediatric and adult heart transplant patients with regard to the incidence and linearized rates of rejection episodes (Fig. 32–4). Fricker and associates[14] at the University of Pittsburgh reported a higher incidence and a greater frequency of morbidity and mortality from rejection in children compared with adults. Among their pediatric patients, all of the short-term survivors had at least one treated rejection episode in the first 2 months. Three of the 12 children who survived the perioperative period died of chronic rejection. With the possible exception of neonates (whom Bailey[6] believes manifest a less virulent response to the allograft), pediatric heart transplant patients as a group seem to manifest rejection with comparable or greater frequency than adults.

As noted earlier, hypertension and renal dysfunction are among the major toxic side effects of cyclosporine.

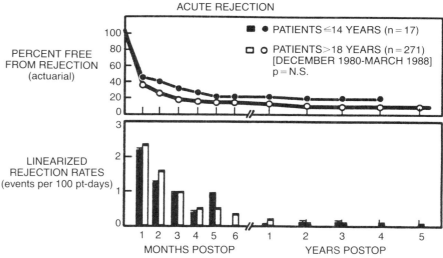

Figure 32–4. Actuarial incidence *(top)* and linearized rate *(bottom)* of acute rejection following transplantation. (From Starnes VA, Bernstein D, Oyer PE, et al: Heart transplantation in children. J Heart Transplant 8:20–26, 1989.)

Chartrand and associates[15] at the University of Montreal reported normal blood pressure in all seven of their pediatric patients 2 months to 4 years after transplantation. Dunn and associates[16] observed hypertension in two of seven long-term survivors using a triple-drug regimen. Pahl and associates[17] at the University of Pittsburgh observed significant hypertension in more than half of their long-term survivors. Some had increased ventricular wall thickness by echo and increased left ventricular end-diastolic pressure, but all had normal left ventricular ejection fractions. Starnes and the Stanford University group[13] observed hypertension in 96% of their pediatric heart transplant patients. We have observed systemic hypertension in almost all of the infants who have undergone heart transplantation at the Children's Hospital of Philadelphia, but the use of antihypertensive agents has been transient, with virtually none of these infants requiring blood pressure therapy for more than 2 months after transplantation. Pahl and associates[18] at the University of Pittsburgh reported that urea nitrogen and creatinine levels were normal in all of their patients who were followed for more than 1 year. Our experience has been similar, with essentially normal renal function in all long-term survivors.

CONCLUSION

Pediatric heart transplantation is an exciting and rapidly evolving field. Experience over the past decade has clearly demonstrated that gratifying results can be achieved in terms of short- and medium-term survival and rehabilitation. Principles of intensive care management of the heart transplant recipient continue to evolve with a major emphasis on the techniques of management of pulmonary hypertension and elevated pulmonary vascular resistance, aimed at prevention and amelioration of graft dysfunction that persists as a major cause of morbidity and early mortality. Time, scrupulous observation, and careful reporting will undoubtedly shed new light on important questions regarding long-term survival, quality of life, and the effects of years and decades of immunosuppressive therapy. In the meantime, while it is clear that most infants and children with structural heart disease are well served by reconstructive surgical procedures, patients whose myocardial dysfunction is associated with an unfavorable long-term prognosis may be best served by heart transplantation.

References

1. Kantrowitz A, Haller SD, Joos H, et al: Transplantation of the heart in an infant and an adult. Am J Cardiol 22:782, 1968.
2. Cooley DA, Bloodwell RD, Hallman GL, et al: Organ transplantation for advanced cardiopulmonary disease. Ann Thorac Surg 8:30, 1969.
3. Pennington DG, Sarafian J, and Swartz M: Heart transplantation in children. J Heart Transplant 4:441–445, 1985.
4. Bailey LL, Assaad AN, Trimm RF, et al: Orthotopic transplantation during early infancy as therapy for incurable congenital heart disease. Ann Surg 208:279–286, 1988.
5. Mavroudis C, Harrison H, Klein JB, et al: Infant orthotopic cardiac transplantation. J Thorac Cardiovasc Surg 96:912–924, 1988.
6. Bailey LL, Nehlsen-Cannarella SL, Doroshow RW, et al: Cardiac allotransplantation in newborns as therapy for hypoplastic left heart syndrome. N Engl J Med 315:949–951, 1986.
7. Bailey L, Concepcion W, Shattuck H, et al: Method of heart transplantation for treatment of hypoplastic left heart syndrome. J Thorac Cardiovasc Surg 92:1–5, 1986.
8. Starnes VA, Bernstein D, Oyer PE, et al: Heart transplantation in children. J Heart Transplant 8:20–26, 1989.
9. Fricker FJ, Griffith BP, Hardesty RL, et al: Experience with heart transplantation in children. Pediatrics 79:138–146, 1987.
10. Bhargava H, Donner RM, Sanchez G, et al: Endomyocardial biopsy after heart transplantation in children. J Heart Transplant 6:298–302, 1987.
11. Addonizio LJ and Rose EA: Cardiac transplantation in children and adolescents. J Pediatr 111:1034–1038, 1987.
12. Rose EA, Addonizio LJ, and Smith CR: Optimal timing of pediatric heart transplantation. Circulation 78(Suppl. II)II-278, 1988.
13. Starnes VA, Stinson EB, Oyer PE, et al: Cardiac transplantation in children and adolescents. Circulation 76(Suppl. V):43–47, 1987.
14. Fricker F, Beerman L, Trento A, et al: Cardiac allograft rejection is more frequent in children than in adults. Am J Cardiol 60:642, 1987.
15. Chartrand C, Dumont L, and Stanley P: Pediatric cardiac transplantation. Transplant Proc 21:3349–3350, 1989.
16. Dunn JM, Cavarocchi NC, Balsara RK, et al: Pediatric heart transplantation at St. Christopher's Hospital for Children. J Heart Transplant 6:334–342, 1987.
17. Pahl E, Fricker F, Trento A, et al: Long-term follow-up of children following heart/heart-lung transplantation. Circulation 76(Suppl. IV):IV-24, 1987.
18. Pahl E, Fricker FJ, Trento A, et al: Late follow-up of children after heart transplantation. Transplant Proc 20:743–746, 1988.

Bibliography

Guidelines for the Determination of Death: Report of the medical consultants on the diagnosis of death to the President's Commission for the Study of Ethical Problems in Medicine and Biomedical and Behavioral Research. JAMA 246:2184–2186, 1981.

Guidelines for the Determination of Brain Death in Children. Pediatrics 80:298–300, 1987.

Heck CF, Shumway SJ, and Kaye MP: The registry of the International Society for Heart Transplantation: Six official reports—1989. J Heart Transplant 8:271–276, 1989.

Kanakrieyeh MS, Pai RG, Bansal RC, et al: Systolic and diastolic function in the non-rejecting transplanted heart in infants. Circulation 78(Suppl II):II–395, 1988.

Lawrence KS and Fricker FJ: Pediatric heart transplantation: Quality of life. J Heart Transplant 6:329–333, 1987.

Pahl E, Fricker FJ, Trento A, et al: Coronary artery disease after pediatric heart transplantation: Limitation of long term allograft survival. Circulation 78(Suppl II):II–278, 1988.

Radley-Smith R and Yacoub MH: Heart and heart-lung transplantation in children. Circulation 76(Suppl. IV):IV–24, 1987.

Shewmon DA, Capron AM, Peacock WJ, et al: The use of anencephalic infants as organ sources. JAMA 261:1773–1781, 1989.

Uzark K, Crowley D, Callow L, et al: Linear growth after pediatric heart transplantation. Circulation 78(Suppl. II):II–492, 1988.

Wray J, Potts-Moes C, Banner N, et al: Mental and psychological development of children after heart and heart-lung transplantation. Circulation 78(Suppl. II)II–86, 1988.

Congenital Heart Disease

Roberta G. Williams, M.D., and Ronald Day, M.D.

The advances in cardiac diagnosis and surgical techniques have had a remarkable impact on the problems encountered in the perioperative management of children with congenital heart disease. Accurate and complete fetal and neonatal diagnosis using echocardiography has paved the way for improved management of the very young patient. Early diagnosis not only provides an improved surgical candidate in most cases but also permits the survival of marginally viable individuals. As a result, perioperative management is much simplified for the less severe lesions but remains a challenge for the high-risk surgical patient. Complete surgical repair is accomplished in the neonatal period in lesions such as transposition of the great arteries. Increasingly, early repair is favored in order to reduce secondary disability in other lesions, such as tetralogy of Fallot and truncus arteriosus. Since the immature heart differs significantly in structural, mechanical, and biochemical characteristics, perioperative management must be customized for the infant. Advancements in the surgical management of patients with a single functioning ventricular chamber have required improved strategies for hemodynamic and pulmonary management. The interactions among diagnosis, surgery, and medical management are closely intertwined as advances in one area both change the requirements and permit the success of the others. This chapter will outline the major congenital cardiac defects, their surgical repair, and perioperative management.

LEFT-TO-RIGHT SHUNT LESIONS

Atrial Septal Defect

Anatomy

Several types of atrial septal defect (ASD) are illustrated in Figure 33–1. Secundum ASD, the most common type of atrial defect, is caused by a defect in the septum primum, the flap valve of the foramen ovale.[1] This centrally located communication may result from a large defect in this structure, fenestrations of the septum primum, or a gap between a well-formed septum primum and the superior limbic band. The latter is called a patent foramen ovale and may be the route of significant atrial shunting in the presence of abnormal loading conditions of the right or left ventricle. Defects in the more rightward portion of the interatrial septum, sinus venosus defects, are commonly located at the orifice of the superior vena cava (superior type) or less commonly near the inferior vena cava (inferior type).[2] They may be associated with anomalies of pulmonary venous drainage, particularly anomalous return of the right upper and middle pulmonary veins. Primum-type ASD is found in the leftward portion of the interatrial septum and is associated with a trileaflet or cleft left atrioventricular (AV) valve. This lesion is described in the family of lesions known as atrioventricular septal defects (ASVDs). A rare cause of shunting at the atrial level is a defect in the roof of the coronary sinus known as a sinoseptal defect.[3]

Physiology

The magnitude and direction of shunting at the atrial level is determined by the compliance and loading conditions of the right and left ventricles. As right ventricular hypertrophy normally regresses during infancy, predominant left-to-right shunting will occur across an ASD, though minimal right-to-left shunting is usually present during atrial contraction when right atrial pressure transiently exceeds left atrial pressure. Left-to-right shunting sufficient to produce a Qp:Qs ratio of 2:1 is usually associated with measurable right ventricular enlargement on the electrocardiogram and the echocardiogram. Symptoms of right ventricular failure and pulmonary congestion are rare unless associated with left ventricular obstruction or mitral regurgitation.

Surgical Repair

An atrial defect is repaired by suture or patch closure on cardiopulmonary bypass. Catheter device closure of small and medium-sized secundum defects in early clinical trials show great promise.[4] Sinus venosus defects with anomalous pulmonary venous return will require placement of the patch in a manner that baffles the anomalous pulmonary vein into the left atrium. Occasionally the right upper pulmonary vein may enter high on the superior vena cava and must be left with the systemic venous return in order to prevent pulmonary vascular obstruction. This does not usually cause a

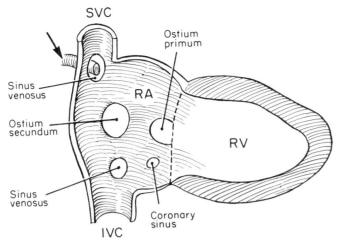

Figure 33–1. The locations of ostium secundum and ostium primum atrial septal defects, sinus venosus defects of the superior vena caval (*SVC*) and inferior vena caval (*IVC*) types, and of a coronary sinus defect. Unmarked arrow identifies the right superior pulmonary vein. RV = right ventricle. (From Perloff JK: The Clinical Recognition of Congenital Heart Disease, 3rd ed. Philadelphia, WB Saunders, 1987, p, 273.)

significant residual shunt. The repair of primum-type ASD will be discussed further on.

Perioperative Management

ASDs are closed with a very low rate of resultant morbidity and mortality, and the postoperative course is generally benign. Atrial tachyarrhythmias and brady-arrhythmias occur rarely in all types of ASD but are more common in sinus venosus ASD. Some patients with ASD have an underlying propensity for arrhythmia, and postoperative rhythm disturbances represent only an exacerbation of a pre-existing problem; therefore, a preoperative history of arrhythmia should be sought and appropriate monitoring obtained in this situation.

Air embolism is a disastrous but fortunately rare complication of ASD closure and should be suspected if seizures or other neurologic signs appear following surgery.

The most frequent complication of ASD repair is postpericardiotomy syndrome. This problem appears insidiously 2 days to several weeks postoperatively and may cause considerable hemodynamic compromise before it is recognized.[5] Low-grade fever and abdominal pain are frequent complaints. Tachycardia is a sensitive indicator of tamponade unless there is an underlying arrhythmia. A paradoxical pulse may be difficult to recognize in a young child. Distention of the neck and hepatic veins is a late finding. Patients should be routinely screened for cardiomegaly by chest radiograph or for pericardial effusion by echocardiography at discharge and 1 to 2 weeks after repair.

An indication for urgent pericardiocentesis is tamponade, which can be confirmed by the echocardiographic findings of right atrial wall indentation and variable ventricular inflow or outflow velocities. Smaller accumulations of pericardial fluid without tamponade are

treated with anti-inflammatory doses of aspirin, indomethacin or, more rarely, steroids for a period of several weeks. Recurrent pericardial effusion is occasionally seen.

Ventricular Septal Defects

Anatomy

As illustrated in Figure 33–2, defects may occur in the perimembraneous, inlet, trabecular muscular, or outlet portions of the interventricular septum. Various terminologies are used, to the confusion of some.[6–9] The perimembraneous defect is found at the superior corner of the tricuspid valve septal leaflet near the rightward border of the aortic annulus, and it may be partially covered by accessory AV valve tissue, sometimes referred to as an aneurysm of the membranous septum. Inlet defects refer to either (1) a defect in the AV septum that extends to the AV valve annulus or (2) a posterior muscular ventricular septal defect (VSD). Muscular defects may also occur in the middle, apical, or anterior (extreme leftward) septum. Outlet defects may be caused by malalignment of the outlet septum (infundibular or conal septum), as in tetralogy of Fallot, or by deficiency in the outlet septum (known as doubly committed subarterial or subpulmonary VSD). This defect may be associated with prolapse of one or more of the aortic cusps and progressive aortic insufficiency.[10]

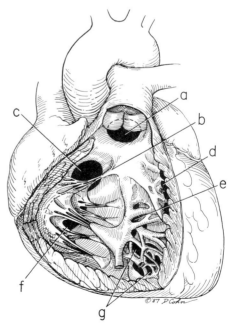

Figure 33–2. Anatomic positions of ventricular septal defects. (*a*) Subarterial defect, (*b*) papillary muscle of the conus, (*c*) perimembranous defect, (*d*) anterior muscular defects, (*e*) central muscular defects, (*f*) inlet defect, and (*g*) apical muscular defects. (From Adams FH, Emmanouilides GC, and Riemenschneider TA [eds]: Moss' Heart Disease in Infants, Children, and Adolescents, 4th ed, p. 191. © 1989, the Williams & Wilkins Co., Baltimore.

Physiology

Left-to-right shunting occurs across a VSD as pulmonary vascular resistance drops to less than systemic levels.[11] The magnitude of the shunt is determined by defect size, the balance between pulmonary and systemic resistances, and the presence of associated anomalies. Significant left-to-right shunting through the defect results in pulmonary overcirculation with left atrial and left ventricular enlargement. In response to elevated pulmonary arterial blood flow and pressure, the pulmonary vascular resistance may rise because of progressive intimal proliferation and medial hypertrophy leading to obliteration of small pulmonary arteries.[12]

Surgical Repair

VSDs are usually repaired by patch closure, though primary closure of slit-like defects or perimembranous defects with a well-formed aneurysm of the pars membranacea septi is possible. Perimembranous VSDs that extend into the inlet septum may require detachment of the septal tricuspid leaflet in order to close the posterior extent of the defect. Most defects may be closed via the tricuspid valve, but apical defects may require an approach via the left ventricular apex, and subpulmonary defects may require a right ventriculotomy or pulmonary artery approach for closure of the upper defect margin.[7, 13, 14] Subpulmonary defects with aortic valve prolapse may require aortic annuloplasty to reduce aortic insufficiency.[15] The term *Swiss cheese* interventricular septum refers to a single large defect that is overlaid by right ventricular trabeculations and appears as multiple muscular defects when viewed from the right side. This defect may require closure via the left ventricular apex.[16, 17] Preoperative assessment by echocardiography or angiography, or both, should include careful search for additional muscular defects.

Perioperative Management

Preoperative patients with increased pulmonary vascular resistance should be assessed by cardiac catheterization to determine the response of the pulmonary vascular bed to alveolar hyperoxia or pharmacologic vasodilatation, or both. A patient with a large septal defect, elevated pulmonary vascular resistance, and only slight left-to-right shunting in room air may benefit from several days of supplemental oxygen before surgical repair. Placement of a pulmonary artery line at the time of surgical repair facilitates postoperative management in patients with high pulmonary vascular resistance. In general, these patients should be well sedated during the postoperative period and managed with alveolar hyperoxia, mild hyperventilation, and vasodilatory agents such as prostaglandin E_1, prostacyclin, or nitroglycerin.[18, 19] Ventilatory support should be cautiously weaned, and the patient should continue to receive supplemental oxygen until signs of right ventricular failure and pulmonary hypertension resolve. Some patients may survive surgery but continue to have moderate pulmonary vascular disease and limited exercise tolerance.

Residual or recurrent VSD in the early postoperative state may present as respiratory failure or a low output state. Increasing heart size and pulmonary vascularity are suggestive findings. There may or may not be a loud systolic murmur, depending upon the cardiac output and pulmonary arterial pressure. Echocardiography with Doppler examination should be able to establish the presence and nature of the left-to-right shunt. Intraoperative echocardiography has also proved useful in detecting additional defects prior to repair and in assessing the integrity of VSD closure after repair.[20] Complete heart block is an uncommon complication that is more likely to occur in inlet or AVSDs. Early postoperative pacing is accomplished with temporary epicardial ventricular wires that are routinely placed after intracardiac repair. The sensitivity and threshold of the wire must be checked at least daily to predict and avoid the consequences of pacing failure when the patient is dependent on a pacemaker. Permanent surgical heart block is considered an indication for permanent pacing because the escape rhythm is generally distal to the bundle of His and is considered unreliable. Fortunately, most heart block after VSD repair is only temporary, caused by edema in the area of the conduction tissue. After recovery of conduction, the patient must be evaluated for residual bifascicular block or transient high-grade heart block.

Atrioventricular Septal Defects

Anatomy

The family of AVSDs, also known as AV canal defects, is characterized by a large central defect with a common AV valve annulus as shown in Figure 33–3.[21, 22] In the case of a primum ASD, the defect lies entirely above the AV valve, which has a common annulus but separate orifices that extend into the right and left ventricles. The left AV valve is trileaflet (cleft mitral valve). The valve may be deficient or densely bound to the interventricular septum, in which case it is usually regurgitant. In the typical form of complete AVSD, the common valve lies in the middle of the large central defect, associated with both the interatrial and interventricular communications. The separate ASD and VSD components may be large or small. The common AV valve may have a central sail-like portion of the superior leaflet or a divided superior leaflet that is attached to the crest of the interventricular septum by chordae tendineae. The length of the mural (true posterior) leaflet and the distance between its chordal attachments to left ventricular papillary muscles has implications for surgical palliation. Both a very wide and a very narrow mural leaflet have been related to postoperative valve dysfunction, characterized by stenosis with a narrow mural leaflet or regurgitation with an unusually broad mural leaflet.

The common AV valve may not straddle the interventricular septum symmetrically but may be aligned more over the right or left ventricle, causing hypoplasia of the contralateral ventricle. Careful assessment of

Figure 33–3. Embryology of atrio-ventricular canal and spectrum of atrioventricular canal defects. *Center panel,* In the embryologic atrioventricular canal, the superior (*SEC*) and inferior (*IEC*) endocardial cushions fuse, thereby forming two orifices. Lateral endocardial cushion (*LEC*) on left forms posterior (*P*) mitral leaflet, *LEC* on right forms posterior tricuspid leaflet, and *LEC* on the right and dextrodorsal conus cushion (*DDCC*) form anterior tricuspid leaflet (*A*). *Top panel,* Fused superior and inferior endocardial cushions form anterior mitral and septal (*S*) tricuspid leaflets in normal heart. In partial form of atrioventricular canal, anterior mitral leaflet is cleft, and medial tricuspid commissure is widened. In intermediate form, anterior (*AB*) and posterior (*PB*) bridging leaflets are fused in midline. *Bottom panel,* Complete forms of atrioventricular canal. With progression of type A to type C, anterior bridging leaflet becomes larger, anterior tricuspid leaflet becomes smaller, and medial tricuspid papillary muscle migrates from ventricular septum to moderator band to anterior tricuspid papillary muscle. Anterior bridging leaflet is attached by chordae tendineae to ventricular septal summit in type A but not in type B or C (so-called free-floating leaflet). (From Adams FH, Emmanouilides GC, and Riemenschneider TA [eds]: Moss' Heart Disease in Infants, Children, and Adolescents, 4th ed, p. 176. © 1989, the Williams & Wilkins Co., Baltimore.

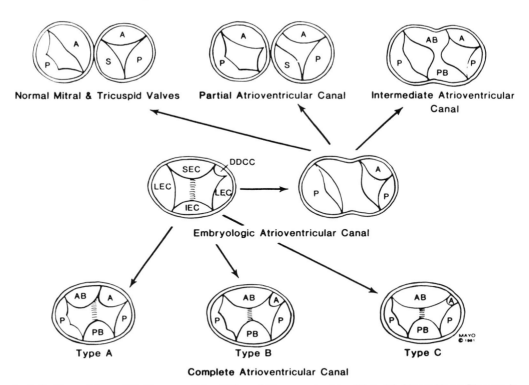

CONGENITAL DEFECTS

ATRIAL SEPTAL DEFECTS AND ATRIOVENTRICULAR CANAL

Normal Mitral & Tricuspid Valves — Partial Atrioventricular Canal — Intermediate Atrioventricular Canal

Embryologic Atrioventricular Canal

Type A — Type B — Type C

Complete Atrioventricular Canal

Physiology

Shunting may occur from left atrium to right atrium, from left ventricle to right ventricle, or from left ventricle to right atrium. Right and left AV valve insufficiency may be present and may range from mild to severe. Thus varying degrees of volume overload in the left and right ventricles may result from the level of shunting and valve function. As in simple VSD, the degree of shunting at the ventricular level depends upon the size of the interventricular communication and the balance between pulmonary and systemic vascular resistances. In patients with Down's syndrome, hypoventilation or mild airway obstruction may elevate pulmonary vascular resistance, limit the left-to-right shunt, and mask the findings of a septal defect.

Surgical Repair

The central defect is repaired by a single-or two-patch technique, dividing the common AV valve into two portions and anchoring the medial halves to the central patch or patches.[23-25] When chordae tendineae are foreshortened and limit valve excursion, extensive recon-struction of the subvalvar elements may be required to provide successful coaptation of the three components of the left AV valve. In some cases, the superior and inferior leaflet portions of the valve are sutured together, but this maneuver is subject to great variation, dictated by surgical choice and individual morphologic characteristics. Occasionally, a prosthetic valve is required to assure valve competence.

Perioperative Management

Intraoperative echocardiography has been used to assess the adequacy of AV valve repair.[26,27] The accuracy of this assessment is limited by variable systemic resistance, cardiac output, and ventricular loading conditions. Echocardiography may be more useful several hours after surgery when these variables have stabilized. As in VSD, postoperative complications may include pulmonary artery hypertension and complete heart block. In patients with severe preoperative congestive heart failure, poor nutrition and left ventricular failure may result in the need for inotropic support and prolonged ventilatory management. Patients with a low output state or respiratory failure should be studied aggressively for residual AV valve insufficiency or acquired stenosis.

Patent Ductus Arteriosus

A patent ductus arteriosus is usually a short, broad structure in a premature infant but is often a long and tortuous channel in the older infant and child. The degree of left-to-right shunting is determined by the resistance at the ductal vessel and in the pulmonary vascular bed. Left-to-right shunting usually occurs throughout the cardiac cycle. The resulting aortic run-off produces bounding pulses and widened pulse pressure. Left atrial and left ventricular enlargement with pulmonary overcirculation is seen. The patent ductus arteriosus may be closed by a transcatheter device in some centers or ligated via left thoracotomy.[28, 29] The complication rate of either procedure is low. Embolization and significant residual shunting are unusual occurrences after transcatheter closure. Residual shunting and chylothorax are rare complications following surgical ligation.

RIGHT VENTRICULAR OBSTRUCTIVE LESIONS

Valvular Pulmonary Stenosis, Critical Pulmonary Stenosis, and Pulmonary Atresia with Intact Interventricular Septum

Anatomy

Since balloon valvuloplasty has become the strategy of choice for the management of simple valvular pulmonary stenosis, patients undergoing surgical valvotomy will be limited to those with severely dysplastic pulmonary valves in which the pulmonary valve is formed by thick, myxomatous ridges.[30, 31] Critical pulmonary stenosis is seen in the newborn patient and is associated with varying degrees of hypoplasia of the right ventricle and pulmonary annulus. In pulmonary atresia with interventricular septum (PA:IVS), the pulmonary valve is usually an imperforate membrane. The pulmonary arteries are usually normal in size or only mildly hypoplastic. The right ventricle and tricuspid valve are usually, but not invariably, hypoplastic with variable representation of the inflow, apical trabecular, and outflow ventricular portions.[32] There may be connections of the right ventricular cavity and distal coronary arteries. Occasionally, this is also associated with interruption of the proximal coronary arteries.[33]

Physiology

Right ventricular hypertension is a universal finding in these forms of outflow obstruction. In critical pulmonary stenosis and PA:IVS, tricuspid valve incompetence may lower right ventricular pressure from suprasystemic levels. In both lesions, ductal patency must be maintained to provide pulmonary blood flow. Patients with suprasystemic right ventricular pressure and ventriculocoronary arterial connections may have right-to-left shunting into the coronary arteries. When there are coexisting obstructions within the coronary arteries, myocardial perfusion may be dependent on flow from a suprasystemic right ventricle.[34] In critical pulmonary stenosis and PA:IVS, when the right ventricle cannot deliver the full systemic venous return to the pulmonary artery, the balance flows across the interatrial septum to the left ventricle. Pulmonary blood flow is dependent on left-to-right shunting via the ductus arteriosus.

Surgery

The surgical approach to dysplastic pulmonary valves is often removal of the entire valve. Occasionally, the right ventricular outflow tract must be resected or enlarged by a patch to correct associated infundibular obstruction. In critical pulmonary stenosis and PA:IVS with mild to moderate right ventricular hypoplasia, open or closed pulmonary valvotomy may be performed with or without a right ventricular outflow tract patch.[35-37] In many cases, the patent ductus arteriosus is closed, and a small GoreTex shunt from either the ascending aorta or a subclavian artery to the pulmonary artery may be placed to provide pulmonary blood flow until right ventricular filling and ejection improve. In patients with PA:IVS with moderate to severe right ventricular hypoplasia, large fistulous ventriculocoronary arterial connections, or right ventricle–dependent coronary perfusion, a left subclavian to pulmonary artery shunt is placed without decompression of the right ventricle.

As illustrated in Figure 33–4, the second stage of surgical management of critical pulmonary stenosis or PA:IVS is also dependent on the degree of right ventricular hypoplasia and the characteristics of the ventriculocoronary arterial connections. If the right ventricle appears large enough to sustain the cardiac output, the shunt is ligated, residual right ventricular outflow obstruction is alleviated by resection or patch augmentation, and the ASD is closed. Alternatively, an adjustable snare can be used to gradually close the ASD as right ventricular function and volume increase.

In some cases of mild to moderate right ventricular hypoplasia, a partial biventricular repair is performed by a bidirectional cavopulmonary shunt that diverts blood from the superior vena cava directly to the pulmonary vascular bed. The ASD is snared or completely closed, and blood from the inferior vena cava is pumped by the right ventricle to the pulmonary artery.[38]

When right ventricular hypoplasia or ventriculocoronary arterial connections preclude biventricular repair, a Fontan operation is performed. A lateral tunnel is created in the right atrium, which diverts systemic venous return to the proximal right pulmonary artery. Thus the systemic and pulmonary circulations are distinct, and saturated blood supplies all myocardial regions. Sudden death occurs in some patients with PA:IVS and right ventricular hypertension or ventriculocoronary arterial connections. Thus heart transplantation is an alternative approach to the surgical management of the severe form of this lesion.

Perioperative Management

The postoperative course of severe pulmonary stenosis with dysplastic pulmonary valve is usually benign,

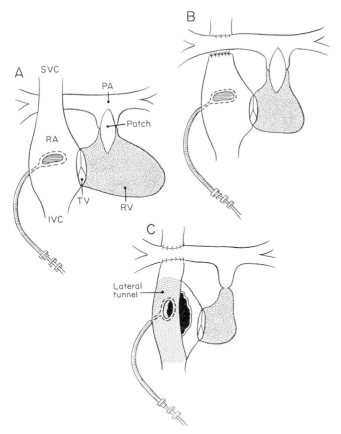

Figure 33–4. Surgical approach to pulmonary atresia with intact ventricular septum and varying degrees of right ventricular hypoplasia following neonatal palliation. A, Following successful alleviation of right ventricular outflow obstruction, the ASD is closed or is left with an adjustable snare for subsequent closure. B, A partial biventricular repair is performed by excision of residual right ventricular outflow obstruction, a bidirectional cavopulmonary shunt, and an ASD snare or closure to divert inferior caval return to the right ventricle. C, When biventricular repair is not possible, the ASD is enlarged, and a lateral tunnel Fontan operation is performed to separate systemic and pulmonary circulation and allow saturated blood to perfuse right ventricle–dependent ventriculocoronary arterial connections. SVC = superior vena cava; RA = right atrium; IVC = inferior vena cava; TV = tricuspid valve; RV = right ventricle; PA = pulmonary artery.

with only mild findings of elevated right ventricular filling pressures secondary to poor right ventricular compliance that is temporarily worsened by mild to moderate pulmonary insufficiency. Rarely, the combination of severe right ventricular hypertrophy and a sudden drop in right ventricular afterload may produce severe dynamic infundibular obstruction, the so-called suicidal right ventricle. This may be treated with β-adrenergic blockade and volume infusion.

Patients will have varying degrees of right ventricular failure after surgery for critical pulmonary stenosis and PA:IVS. Until right ventricular compliance improves, a residual right-to-left shunt across the interatrial septum will persist.

PA:IVS may present unique postoperative problems because of associated coronary abnormalities. Although careful preoperative assessment of the coronary circulation by selective coronary or aortic root angiography

and right ventricular angiography is helpful, there is still an unpredictable incidence of myocardial ischemia, left ventricular failure, and sudden death that may occur during the early or late postoperative period. Management includes close monitoring of left ventricular filling pressures, the electrocardiogram, and cardiac output. If left ventricular failure is present, afterload reduction may be of benefit, but care must be taken to maintain adequate aortic diastolic pressure in order to perfuse the myocardial bed.

Left Ventricular Obstructive Lesions

Aortic Stenosis, Subaortic Stenosis, and Supravalvular Aortic Stenosis

The stenotic aortic valve many be unicuspid, bicuspid, or tricuspid.[39–42] The valve cusps may be thin and pliable with commissural fusion, thick and dysplastic without commissural fusion, or all gradations in between. In the former, the cusps dome in systole as seen on echocardiography or angiography. This type of valve is more favorable for surgical or balloon valvuloplasty.[43] A unicommissural valve is most often seen when aortic stenosis causes heart failure in the neonate. The valve is commonly dysplastic and is associated with hypoplasia of the left ventricle, aortic annulus and ascending aorta. In the most severe form, the systemic circulation cannot be supported by left ventricular output and is dependent on right-to-left shunting at the ductus arteriosus.

Valvular aortic stenosis is a progressive disorder—for example, a bicuspid aortic valve may cause no gradient during infancy yet may result in severe stenosis later in life because of progressive thickening and calcification of the valve. The timing of intervention is dependent on the gradient, associated symptoms, ventricular function, and the presence of concurrent aortic insufficiency.

Subvalvular aortic stenosis may take several forms, from a discrete membrane across the left ventricular outflow tract to a long, tunnel-like narrowing beneath the aortic valve.[41, 44–46] A membrane with a fibromuscular base attaching as a ring to the anterior mitral leaflet occurs most commonly. There may be secondary abnormalities of the aortic valve cusps due to turbulence from subaortic obstruction. Hypertrophic cardiomyopathy with dynamic left ventricular outflow obstruction will not be included in this category (see Chapter 35).

Supravalvular aortic stenosis is seen in children with hypercalcemia of infancy (Williams syndrome) or as an isolated familial form and consists of a tubular "waist" that generally lies above the aortic sinuses but sometimes includes the orifice of the coronary arteries.[47, 48]

Surgical Management

Increasingly, balloon valvuloplasty is employed for palliation of valvular aortic stenosis.[49–51] Surgical valvotomy is more commonly performed on patients with a dysplastic aortic valve.[52–55] Incision of the commissures is carefully undertaken in order not to undermine the commissural support of the aortic cusps in diastole.

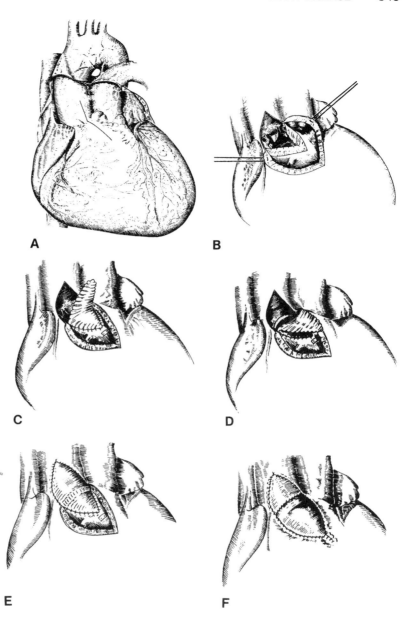

Figure 33–5. Operative technique of aortoventriculo-plasty (Konno-Rastan procedure). *A,* Direction of incision on the aorta and right ventricular outflow tract. *B,* Opening of the aorta, right ventricle, and interventricular septum. *C,* Widening of the subaortic area and the aortic ring by patching of the septal incision. *D,* Excision and replacement of the aortic valve. *E,* Closure of the aortic incision by the remainder of the same patch. *F,* Closure of the right ventricular outflow tract incision by a second Dacron patch, which is sutured to the inner patch over the aorta. (From Baue AE, Geha AS, Hammond GL, et al [eds]: Glenn's Thoracic and Cardiovascular Surgery, 5th ed. E. Norwalk, Appleton and Lange, 1991, p. 1708.)

However, it is often impossible to relieve the obstruction without a concomitant increase in aortic insufficiency. Valvotomy in patients with valvular aortic stenosis is only palliative. Recurrence of significant obstruction is common.[56, 57] Prosthetic aortic valve replacement is eventually required in many patients because of either progressive aortic stenosis or aortic insufficiency.

In neonates with critical aortic stenosis, partial relief of obstruction by open or closed aortic valvotomy is a realistic objective. Balloon valvuloplasty is employed in some centers as an investigational procedure. When critical aortic stenosis in the neonate is associated with left ventricular hypoplasia, and a significant proportion of systemic blood flow is provided by the right ventricle, cardiac transplantation or a palliative strategy such as a Norwood procedure may be preferred.[58, 59] In any case, this severe subset of aortic stenosis is associated with high mortality and morbidity, whether approached by balloon or surgical palliation, Norwood procedure, or cardiac transplantation.

Surgical relief of subaortic obstruction involves resection of the entire ring of subaortic tissue, together with myectomy at the base of the obstruction along the left septal surface, taking care not to injure the mitral valve or conduction tissue.[60, 61]

The Konno-Rastan procedure is used to alleviate a long segment of subaortic obstruction.[63–66] As illustrated in Figure 33–5, an anterior approach is used by performing a right ventriculotomy beneath the pulmonary valve to expose the ventricular septum beneath the aortic valve. The stenotic portion of the left ventricular outflow septum is resected. If necessary, the aortic valve is also replaced with a homograft or a prosthetic valve. The interventricular septum is then closed with a patch, and the right ventriculotomy is also closed with a patch to provide unobstructed outflow for each ventricle.

Supravalvular aortic stenosis is repaired by a patch over the affected area.[67–71] Occasionally, the distal tips of the coronary cusps are attached to a supravalvular ridge, requiring aortic valvuloplasty to avoid valvular insufficiency after resection of the obstruction.

Perioperative Management

The infant with critical aortic stenosis will often present with shock or a low output state. Stabilization with prostaglandin E_1 infusion, to maintain ductal patency, and inotropic support is sometimes necessary for several days while monitoring improvement in the renal and neurologic status. When possible, surgical intervention should be delayed until other organ system damage has been at least partly reversed. Postoperative management involves careful manipulation of intravascular volume, inotropic support, afterload reduction, and prolonged ventilatory support.

Intraoperative echo Doppler offers some advantage in the immediate evaluation of aortic valvotomy and subaortic resection. Care must be taken to interpret Doppler assessment of residual gradient and valvular insufficiency in light of changing cardiac output, ventricular filling, and aortic pressures. In the early postoperative period, left ventricular volume should be adjusted to accommodate left ventricular stiffness and the usual requirement for a slight increase in filling pressures. Widened aortic pulse pressure may be the only clinical indication of significant aortic insufficiency because a diastolic murmur may be difficult to discern in the early postoperative period. This finding indicates a need to monitor for ischemia and diminished left ventricular function by electrocardiogram and echocardiography. The combination of lowered aortic diastolic pressure and elevated left ventricular filling pressure greatly diminished coronary perfusion of the hypertrophied left ventricle. Following subaortic resection, one should survey carefully for signs of heart block, mitral insufficiency, and aortic insufficiency.

The postoperative care of patients with supravalvular aortic stenosis is usually benign, but the patient must be assessed for signs of impaired coronary perfusion and aortic insufficiency.

Coarctation of the Aorta, Interrupted Aortic Arch

Anatomy

Coarctation of the aorta is usually caused by a ledge along the outer curvature of the distal aortic arch opposite the position of the ductus arteriosus or ligamentum.[72, 73] This is usually associated with some hypoplasia of the distal transverse arch in neonates and is especially severe when associated with VSD and left ventricular outflow obstruction.

The most common form of aortic arch interruption occurs between the left carotid and left subclavian arteries (type B). Less commonly, interruption may occur distal to the left subclavian artery (type A) or between the innominate and the left carotid arteries (type C).[74–77]

Physiology

In the neonate with coarctation of the aorta and interrupted aortic arch, blood flow distal to the site of obstruction becomes compromised when the ductus arteriosus closes.[78] In some patients, this causes immediate systemic collapse because the left ventricle cannot adapt to the demands of excessive pressure overload. The ensuing acidosis often causes the ductus arteriosus to reopen transiently. The effect of this dynamic interaction is the waxing and waning of pulses in the lower extremities.

Differential cyanosis may occur when upper body blood is supplied by the left ventricle and lower body blood is supplied by the right ventricle. Since the left ventricle of the neonate is not capable of suddenly generating high pressure, systolic blood pressure usually is not increased in the upper extremities, however, it is decreased or not detectable in the lower extremities. The young child with coarctation of the aorta is compensated by appropriate ventricular hypertrophy and can generate high pressures in the proximal aorta. In such patients, blood pressure is usually elevated in the upper extremities and nearly normal in the lower extremities. With age, collateral vessels develop between the upper and lower segments, thus bypassing the obstruction and lowering the upper segment hypertension. However, hypertension may persist because of activation of the renin-angiotensin system.

Surgical Repair

Coarctation of the aorta is repaired by resection of the narrow segment with end-to-end anastomosis or by the subclavian flap technique as illustrated in Figures 33–6 and 33–7.[79–83] Balloon angioplasty of native aortic coarctation warrants further investigation.[84–87] Aortic hypoplasia or interruption often requires placement of an interposition graft to alleviate obstruction.[88–90]

Perioperative Management

In the neonate, prostaglandin E_1 is usually effective at maintaining ductal patency and establishing adequate lower body perfusion until surgery is performed.[91] The risk of aortic cross-clamping is decreased when collateral flow has been established in older children. Intraoperative evaluation of somatosensory evoked potentials may be used to monitor spinal function during aortic cross-clamping and thus avoid neurologic injury.[92] Early postoperative hypertension is frequently encountered and usually responds to nitroprusside or β-blockade, or both. β-Adrenergic antagonists and angiotensin-converting enzyme inhibitors may be used to treat persistent hypertension. Mesenteric arteritis may occur, and splanchnic function may require time to recover following coarctation repair.[93] Initial feedings should be delayed and advanced cautiously once bowel activity returns.

CYANOTIC HEART DISEASE

Transposition of the Great Arteries

Anatomy

In the common form of transposition of the great arteries (TGA), the atria and ventricles are in a normal position, but the great arteries are transposed, the aorta arising from the right ventricle and the pulmonary artery arising from the left ventricle.[94, 95] The ventricular septum is most often intact in this lesion. The VSD, if present, is commonly associated with posterior deviation of the outflow (infundibular) septum. This defect is subpulmonary in location. The associated deviation of the outflow septum is accompanied by variable degrees of subpulmonary obstruction and hypoplasia of the pulmonary annulus and the main pulmonary artery and its branches. Defects may also be found in the AV and muscular trabecular septum.

Some variations of coronary anatomy in TGA are illustrated in Figure 33–8. The most common pattern consists of the left coronary (anterior descending and circumflex) originating from the left aortic sinus and the right coronary originating from the posterior sinus. Although techniques have been developed to perform the arterial switch operation for all variations of coronary anatomy, there may be increased risk of early or late coronary ischemia for some patterns.[96, 97]

Subpulmonary stenosis may be found in TGA with intact ventricular septum (IVS) or a VSD. In patients with TGA and IVS, dynamic subpulmonary stenosis may occur in time as the IVS bulges leftward when pulmonary vascular resistance and left ventricular pressure fall.

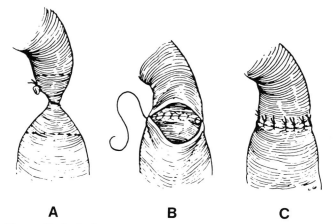

Figure 33–6. *A,* Coarctation repair using end-to-end anastomosis. The ductus arteriosus has been ligated and transected. The proposed sites of aortic transection and the extent of coarctectomy are depicted. The adequate but conservative margins of resection reflect the need to negotiate competing interests: to maximize the luminal diameter at the site of eventual anastomosis without producing excessive anastomotic tension. *B,* The coarctectomy has been accomplished. The "back" wall of the anastomosis has been performed with a continuous suture technique. *C,* The end-to-end anastomosis has been completed. Note the interrupted suture technique utilized in the "front" wall. (From Long WA: Fetal and Neonatal Cardiology. Philadelphia, WB Saunders, 1990, p. 765.)

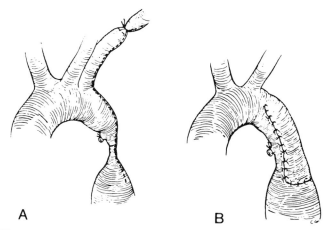

Figure 33–7. *A,* Juxtaductal coarctation of the aorta. The ductus arteriosus has been ligated and transected; the left subclavian artery has been ligated proximal to the origin of the vertebral artery. The proposed location and extent of incision in the proximal subclavian artery and aorta are depicted. *B,* Subclavian flap coarctation repair. The proximal subclavian artery has been transected. After excision of any intimal shelf at the coarctation site, the incised subclavian stump has been fashioned into a turned-down flap and has been interposed within the longitudinal defect created by the aortic incision. (From Long WA: Fetal and Neonatal Cardiology. Philadelphia, WB Saunders, 1990, p. 763.)

Physiology

TGA creates separate and parallel systemic and pulmonary circulations. Deoxygenated blood from systemic veins is directed through the right atrium and right ventricle to the aorta, whereas oxygen-rich blood travels from pulmonary veins through the left ventricle to the pulmonary arteries. Extrauterine survival depends on a communication between these circuits—commonly, a patent foramen ovale or a patent ductus arteriosus, or both. Shunting from the systemic to the pulmonary circulation must be accompanied by an equal and opposite shunt from the pulmonary to the systemic circulation. Thus when blood flows via a patent ductus arteriosus to the pulmonary artery, an equal amount of blood will shunt via an ASD from the left atrium to the right atrium. If communication is available at one site only, bidirectional shunting must occur.

As pulmonary vascular resistance falls during the transitional period, pulmonary blood flow increases, systemic saturation improves, and the change in left ventricular pressure leads to a fall in left ventricular mass.

Surgical Repair

A switch at either the atrial or the great artery level will convert the pulmonary and systemic circulations in TGA from a parallel to a serial relationship. Two variations of interatrial baffle repair, the Mustard and Senning procedures, divert systemic venous blood to the left ventricle and hence to the pulmonary artery.[98, 99] Pulmonary venous return is directed to the right ventricle and aorta. The long-term complications of this approach are arrhythmias, venous obstruction, and failure of the morphologic right ventricle to perform as a

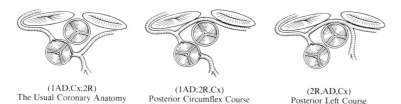

(1AD,Cx;2R)
The Usual Coronary Anatomy

(1AD;2R,Cx)
Posterior Circumflex Course

(2R,AD,Cx)
Posterior Left Course

(1AD,Cx;2R)
Commissural Origins
Between the Great Arteries

(2R;2AD,Cx)
Intramural Coronary Course
Between the Great Arteries

(1R;2AD,Cx)
Anterior Right Course
Posterior Left Course

(1R,AD;2Cx)
Anterior Right Course
Posterior Circumflex Course

Figure 33–8. Some of the variations of coronary anatomy in d-transposition of the great arteries. The Leiden classification is used to identify the sinus of origin for each major coronary branch. 1 = the left aortic sinus; 2 = the posterior aortic sinus; R = right coronary artery; AD = anterior descending artery; CX = circumflex artery. Eccentric origins (commissural and intramural) and coronary segments passing anterior to, between, or posterior to the great arteries are descriptively stated.

systemic ventricle.[100–106] The atrial switch is usually performed in the first 6 months of life; therefore, balloon atrial septostomy must be performed during the neonatal period in order to provide adequate mixing to maintain systemic oxygenation when the ductus arteriosus closes.

The arterial switch repair involves transection of the aorta and pulmonary artery above the sinuses of Valsalva. As shown in Figure 33–9, the coronary ostia and a button of surrounding tissue are transposed to the native main pulmonary artery root. The numerous variations in coronary anatomy require modifications of the technique according to individual surgical choice.[96, 97, 107–110]

Complex TGA is managed with a variety of techniques, depending on the type of associated anomalies. The association of TGA with large subarterial VSD and subpulmonary stenosis is suited for the Rastelli approach, which entails patching the anterior aorta into the left ventricle by means of an interventricular tunnel,

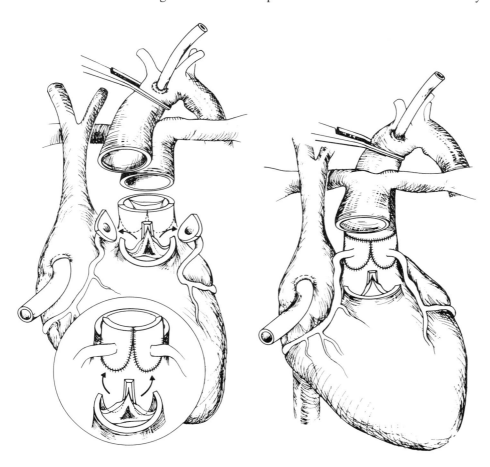

Figure 33–9. The arterial switch operation. *A*, On cardiopulmonary bypass, the ductus arteriosus is divided, and both great arteries are transected approximately 1 cm above the valve commissures. The coronary arteries are excised with a generous patch of aortic wall. The coronary artery buttons are reimplanted on the proximal pulmonary trunk or the neoaorta. *B*, The pulmonary artery confluence and branches are mobilized and brought anterior to the ascending aorta (LeCompte maneuver). End-to-end anastomosis of the great arteries is performed. A pericardial patch is used to augment the neopulmonary artery anastomosis. (Modified from Long WA: Fetal and Neonatal Cardiology. Philadelphia, WB Saunders, 1990.)

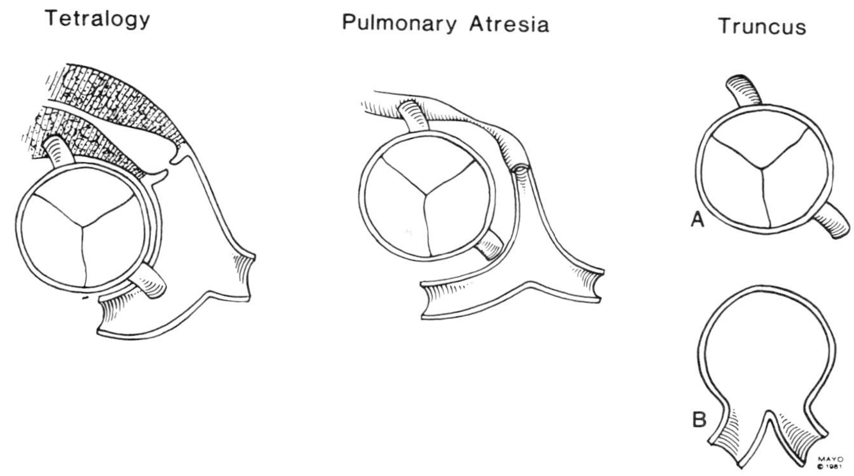

Tetralogy   Pulmonary Atresia   Truncus

Figure 33–10. Cross-sectional views of the cardiac base in tetralogy of Fallot *(left)* and tetralogy with pulmonary atresia *(center)* show the relationship of the right ventricular outflow tract to the aorta (marked by the coronary arteries). Views from the aortic root *(A)* and higher in the great artery trunk *(B)* in a patient with truncus arteriosus shows the complete absence of the right ventricular outflow tract. (From Moller JH and Neal WA [eds]: Fetal, Neonatal and Infant Cardiac Disease. E. Norwalk, Appleton and Lange, 1990, p. 649.)

dividing the main pulmonary artery, and establishing continuity between the right ventricle and distal main pulmonary artery via an external conduit and valved homograft.[111, 112]

Perioperative Management

The newborn with simple TGA presents with severe systemic desaturation and perhaps acidosis without respiratory distress. Initial stabilization is carried out with prostaglandin E_1 infusion. When transport to a tertiary center is required, prophylactic intubation and positive pressure ventilation are advisable. Echocardiographic diagnosis confirms the anatomic diagnosis and defines proximal coronary anatomy, the nature of the interatrial communication, patency of the ductus arteriosus, and a rough estimation of left ventricular pressure. Cardiac catheterization and angiography may be performed to further delineate coronary anatomy and associated anomalies when uncertainty exists. Balloon atrial septostomy can be performed by echocardiographic or fluoroscopic guidance to establish optimal mixing until an atrial or arterial switch procedure is performed.[113] Care must be taken to maintain adequate central volume and a hematocrit value greater than 45%. Falling arterial saturation and acidosis should be treated with immediate volume expansion. Blood losses should be aggressively replaced. Ideally, transfusion with whole blood or packed red blood cells and albumin will serve to provide volume expansion and will also substitute mature hemoglobin for fetal hemoglobin and improve oxygen delivery to the peripheral tissues.

Following the neonatal arterial switch repair of simple TGA, peripheral and central edema is a prominent finding. This appears to be due to a tendency to extravasate fluid during cardiopulmonary bypass, which is perhaps accentuated by previous prostaglandin E_1 infusion or volume expansion, or both. This does not compromise stability but requires a significant negative fluid balance through diuresis and free water restriction before extubation is attempted. Significant inotropic support is not usually needed, but a combination of low-dose dopamine and dobutamine (3 to 5 µg/kg/min each)

with mild afterload reduction (e.g., with nitroglycerin) promotes adequate diuresis and maintains optimal cardiac output during the initial postoperative period. Monitoring the 12-lead electrocardiogram and wall motion by echocardiogram is recommended during the first postoperative days. Evidence of myocardial ischemia or wall motion abnormalities should prompt early postoperative angiography.

Following interatrial baffle repair, stabilization with mild inotropic support and diuresis and free water restriction speed the clearance of mild pulmonary and peripheral edema. Sinus node dysfunction and atrial tachyarrhythmias are infrequent early complications of this surgical approach, but they are seen with increasing frequency in later years. Postoperatively, the physical examination, chest radiograph, and echocardiogram are useful to exclude obstruction of pulmonary and systemic venous return.

Tetralogy of Fallot and Truncus Arteriosus

Anatomy

Tetralogy of Fallot, with or without pulmonary atresia, and truncus arteriosus are selected lesions among the family of conotruncal abnormalities. Tetralogy of Fallot results from a rotational abnormality of the most distal part of the embryonic cardiac tube and the proximal truncus arteriosus.[114–118] The infundibular septum, which separates the right and left ventricular outflow obstruction, is shifted anteriorly, superiorly, and leftward, creating subpulmonary stenosis and a large subaortic interventricular communication. An associated abnormality in truncal division results in a large aortic root overriding the ventricular septum and hypoplasia of the pulmonary annulus, main pulmonary artery, and distal pulmonary branches.

As shown in Figure 33–10, tetralogy of Fallot with pulmonary atresia is associated with more severe hypoplasia of the pulmonary arteries. Moreover, the pulmonary artery anatomy is often complex and variable in these patients.[119, 120] The native pulmonary arteries frequently are not confluent, and several lung regions may be supplied by systemic collaterals.

Three types of truncus arteriosus are illustrated in Figure 33–11. In type I, a single main pulmonary artery arises from the left posterolateral aspect of the truncus and bifurcates into left and right pulmonary branches.[121] The pulmonary branches originate separately in truncus arteriosus, types II and III. Varying degrees of branch pulmonary stenosis have been observed in all types of truncus arteriosus. The number of truncal valve leaflets is variable, and truncal valve stenosis or insufficiency may occur.[122]

Physiology

In tetralogy of Fallot, the right ventricular outflow obstruction takes place at the infundibular, pulmonary valvular, and pulmonary arterial level. Infundibular obstruction is often dynamic, whereas more distal obstruction is fixed. As shown in Figure 33–12, shunting across the VSD depends upon the balance between systemic arteriolar and combined pulmonary outflow resistance. Episodes of severe cyanosis may result from systemic vasodilatation or increased dynamic outflow tract obstruction. These "hypercyanotic spells" may initially be treated with sedation, oxygen, volume expansion, β-adrenergic antagonists, and agents or maneuvers to increase systemic vascular resistance. Occasionally, such an episode is fatal; thus early palliation with a systemic to pulmonary shunt or complete repair is often indicated.

In contrast to tetralogy of Fallot, pulmonary pressures and blood flow are markedly increased in truncus arteriosus. Pulmonary overcirculation results in minimal cyanosis and congestive heart failure with a risk of early pulmonary vascular disease.

Surgical Repair

Surgical management of tetralogy of Fallot is influenced in part by the size of the pulmonary valve annulus and the morphologic features of the pulmonary artery.[121–131] The VSD is patched via a right atrial approach. When there is predominant infundibular obstruction, the muscle may often be resected through the tricuspid valve as well. When there is significant hypo-

plasia of the right ventricular infundibulum, pulmonary annulus, or main pulmonary artery, an outflow patch is required in the affected area. Placing a patch across the pulmonary annulus produces pulmonary insufficiency, which is not usually severe unless there is distal arterial obstruction. When a transannular patch is required and the distal pulmonary arteries are hypoplastic or stenotic, a prosthetic pulmonary valve is needed to prevent severe pulmonary insufficiency. When the pulmonary annulus and main pulmonary artery are atretic, a conduit between the right ventricle and pulmonary arteries may be required. In many cases, a homograft or a conduit containing a valve is used. Severe hypoplasia of the main and branch pulmonary arteries requires a staged approach, promoting branch pulmonary artery growth by selective shunt placement or bringing true pulmonary artery and collateral vessels into a single system through lateral thoracotomies, followed by a more definitive procedure via midline sternotomy.[132–134]

Definitive repair for truncus arteriosus is usually performed during the early months of life.[135] Banding the branch pulmonary arteries has a high rate of mortality, may distort the pulmonary branches, and may not adequately reduce pulmonary blood flow or prevent pulmonary vascular disease.[136] As shown in Figure 33–13, truncus arteriosus, types I and II, are repaired by VSD closure, detachment of the pulmonary artery or arteries, patch reconstruction of the truncal root, and placement of a conduit composed of a distal aortic valve homograft and a proximal polyester (Dacron) tube between the right ventricle and pulmonary artery confluence.[137] Truncus arteriosus, type III, may require a staged approach to establish branch pulmonary continuity prior to repair. Subsequently, the conduit from the right ventricle to the pulmonary artery is replaced as the child grows.

Postoperative Care

Right ventricular failure is a variable feature following repair of tetralogy of Fallot, being more prevalent in patients with a large ventriculotomy, severe pulmonary insufficiency, or residual outflow obstruction. This is managed by correction of residual obstruction and placement of a prosthetic pulmonary valve if there is an important residual hemodynamic abnormality. Other supportive maneuvers include moderate inotropic sup-

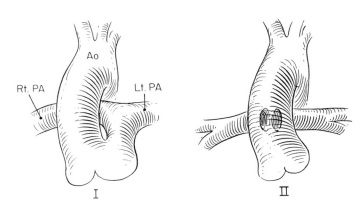
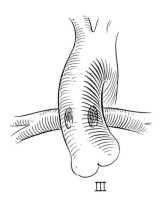

Figure 33–11. Truncus arteriosus. In type (*I*), a single main pulmonary artery usually arises from the truncal root and bifurcates after a short course into right and left branch pulmonary arteries. In type (*II*), the right and left pulmonary arteries originate side by side from the truncal root with separate orifices. In type (*III*), the right and left pulmonary arteries are widely separated and originate from the posterolateral aspects of the truncal root. Rt. PA = right pulmonary artery; Ao = aorta; Lt. PA = left pulmonary artery.)

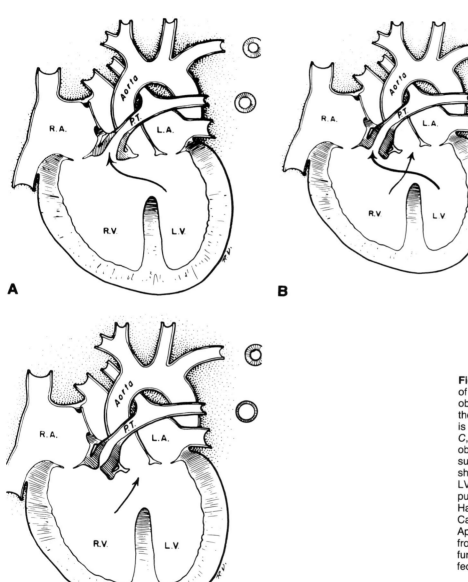

Figure 33–12. The spectrum seen in tetralogy of Fallot. *A*, The right ventricular outflow tract obstruction is mild, and the shunt indicated by the arrow is from left to right. *B*, The obstruction is moderate and the shunting is bidirectional. *C*, The usual situation, with severe outflow tract obstruction and right-to-left shunting, which results in cyanosis. The overriding aorta is well shown. RA = right atrium; RV = right ventricle; LV = left ventricle; LA = left atrium; PT = pulmonary trunk. (From Baue AE, Geha AS, Hammond GL, et al [eds]: Glenn's Thoracic and Cardiovascular Surgery, 5th ed. E. Norwalk, Appleton and Lange, 1991, p 1183. Modified from Edwards JE: Recent concepts on the functional pathology in ventricular septal defects. Wisc Med J 56:484, 1957.)

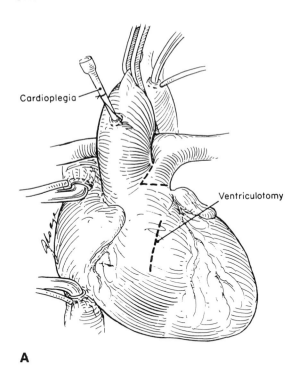

A

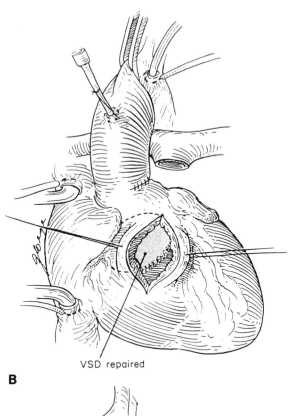

B

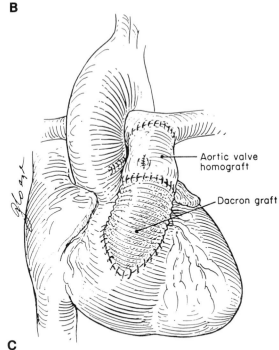

C

Figure 33–13. Complete intracardiac repair of truncus arteriosus, type I. *A*, Surgical anatomy and incision for detachment of main pulmonary artery from the truncus and right ventriculotomy. *B*, After pulmonary artery detachment, reconstruction of the ascending aorta and patch closure of the VSD. *C*, Completed repair with the conduit composed of cryopreserved aortic valve homograft with proximal albumin-pretreated Dacron graft in place. (From Baue AE, Geha AS, Hammond GL, et al: Glenn's Thoracic and Cardiovascular Surgery, 5th ed. E. Norwalk, Appleton and Lange, 1991, p. 1084.)

port and volume replacement to maintain adequate left ventricular filling. Left ventricular failure is a rare occurrence that should prompt a search for left-to-right shunting through a residual VSD. However, some degree of right or left ventricular failure is a common finding during the early postoperative period and responds to low-dose inotropic support with dopamine and dobutamine, followed by digoxin and moderate diuretics for a few weeks. The postoperative management of patients following repair of truncus arteriosus

is similar to that in other lesions with a risk of increased pulmonary vascular resistance.

Tricuspid Atresia and Single Ventricle (Univentricular Heart)

Because of a commonality of management issues, tricuspid atresia and single ventricle are discussed together.

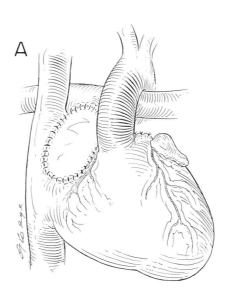
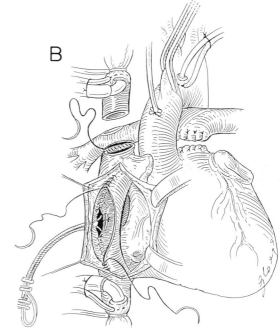

Figure 33–14. Modifications of the Fontan operation. *A,* The pulmonary artery is mobilized posterior to the aorta and is anastomosed directly with the right atrium. *B,* A synthetic patch is used to create a lateral tunnel within the atrium. The superior atrial margins of this tunnel and the SVC are anastomosed to the proximal right pulmonary artery. A fenestration or an adjustable ASD may be left to allow a residual right-to-left shunt during the early postoperative period.

Anatomy

Tricuspid atresia usually involves the total lack of an atrial–right ventricular connection.[138, 139] The left ventricle and mitral valve are usually normal. A diminutive right ventricle communicates with the left ventricle via a VSD. The right ventricle lacks a significant inflow portion and consists of an outflow chamber with a underdeveloped trabecular portion. There may be muscular obstruction of the right ventricular outflow tract. The great arteries are usually normally related but may be transposed.

There are many forms of single ventricle (univentricular heart).[140–142] They have one feature in common—that is, only one ventricular chamber of a size to accommodate systemic blood flow. There may be two AV valves, a common valve, or a solitary tricuspid or mitral valve. Ventricular morphologic features and great artery relations may be variable, and either pulmonary or systemic outflow may be obstructed. Patients with subaortic obstruction often have associated coarctation of the aorta or interrupted aortic arch.

Physiology

In tricuspid atresia, systemic venous return must exit the right atrium via a patent foramen ovale or an ASD. Systemic and pulmonary venous blood is mixed in the left atrium and is delivered to the left ventricle at which point output is distributed to the aorta and pulmonary artery according to the balance between total pulmonary and systemic outflow resistance. With normally related great arteries, obstruction to pulmonary flow may occur at the VSD or the right ventricular infundibulum. Depending on these features, the patient may present with variable degrees of cyanosis or congestive heart failure.

The many forms of single ventricle have diverse physiologic features, but they have in common with tricuspid atresia complete mixing of pulmonary and systemic venous return and distribution of pulmonary and systemic arterial flow, according to their relative total resistance to outflow. The variables that influence outcome and management are pulmonary vascular resistance and morphologic characteristics, obstruction to systemic or pulmonary venous return, AV valve insufficiency, ventricular mass, compliance and systolic function, and obstruction to pulmonary or systemic outflow.

Surgical Repair

Early surgical management of this diverse group of lesions is directed toward providing a limited but reliable source of pulmonary arterial flow, ensuring unobstructed systemic and pulmonary venous return and eliminating subaortic and aortic obstruction.[143–145]

The object is to preserve normal pulmonary vascular resistance, allow good growth of the branch pulmonary arteries, and preserve ventricular function. These are the features required for a successful outcome from a Fontan operation.[146] This procedure connects systemic venous return directly to the pulmonary arteries.[147, 148] Two of the several modifications of the Fontan procedure are illustrated in Figure 33–14. Venous pressure is the driving force across the pulmonary vascular bed. Pulmonary venous return is directed to the single ventricular chamber to supply the systemic output.[149, 150]

Postoperative Management

The object of postoperative management following a Fontan procedure is to maintain optimal cardiac output at the lowest systemic venous pressure. Because flow across the pulmonary vascular bed is passive, systemic venous pressure is directly related to pulmonary vascular resistance and ventricular diastolic pressure (assuming no mechanical obstruction at the anastomosis site, the pulmonary veins, or within the pulmonary venous atrium). For this reason, it is important to support the ventricle with inotropic agents and to maintain effective afterload reduction. Since ventricular afterload is directly related to filling pressure, it not only promotes systemic output but also lowers left atrial and, hence, systemic venous pressure. The efficacy of early management can be monitored by trends in the mixed venous oxygen saturation and the patient's toe temperature. It is also important to keep pulmonary vascular resistance at a minimum. This is promoted by alveolar hyperoxia, aggressive maintenance of acid-base balance, and prevention of lung compression or collapse. Since positive pressure ventilation may impede systemic venous return, ventilatory pressures are kept at a minimum, and early extubation is encouraged. Pleural and pericardial effusions must be aggressively removed because they increase systemic venous pressure. Elevated systemic venous pressure, in turn, leads to further accumulation of pleural and pericardial effusion.

Recently, several institutions found that systemic output can be preserved at the expense of variable degrees of cyanosis by leaving a residual ASD or fenestration in the atrial tunnel of the Fontan procedure.[38, 151] As pulmonary vascular resistance and ventricular function improves, the residual defect can be closed. Some institutions close this fenestration transvenously with a catheter closure device.[151] We have had good results using an adjustable snare that provides the flexibility of closing the fenestration gradually, partially, or completely at the patient's bedside. This approach has the advantage of being reversible if elevated systemic venous pressures ensue. A modified bidirectional cavopulmonary anastomosis is an alternative method of managing patients with single ventricle and less than ideal hemodynamics.[152] As shown in Figure 33-15, superior vena caval return is diverted to the lungs. Since systemic oxygen saturation is improved, other sources of pulmonary flow can be restricted to protect the pulmonary vascular bed and decrease the volume load on the ventricle. Thus the hemodynamics and ventricular function may be made more favorable for a subsequent Fontan procedure.

Following the initial postoperative day, the management of the patient who has undergone a Fontan procedure changes considerably. During the earliest postoperative period, it is important to maintain inotropic support and adequate central volume. This involves sustaining a central venous pressure that is high enough to maintain adequate cardiac output without raising central venous pressure to the point of encouraging extravasation of fluid. In the uncomplicated course, weaning and extubation may be accomplished after several hours of stabilization. Over the next several days, fluid restriction to one half of normal maintenance and vigorous diuresis are necessary to discourage pleural effusion. Continued afterload reduction may be of benefit in most patients, since some degree of ventricular dysfunction is common. In patients with chylous pleural effusion, dietary fat restriction is important. Fluid restriction, diuretics, and afterload reduction may be required for months, or even years, postoperatively.

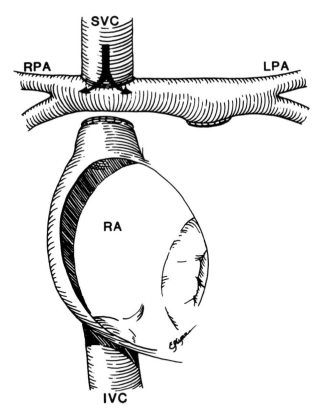

Figure 33–15. Schematic of bidirectional cavopulmonary anastomosis showing end-to-side anastomosis of the superior vena cava (*SVC*) to the ipsilateral pulmonary artery (*RPA*), with the junction of the SVC and the right atrium (*RA*) oversewn. Pulmonary arteries are in continuity. RPA = right pulmonary artery; IVC = inferior vena cava. (From Bridges ND, Jonas RA, Mayer JE, et al: Bidirectional cavopulmonary anastomosis as interim palliation for high-risk Fontan candidates. Circulation 82 [Suppl IV]:IV–170, 1990. By permission of the American Heart Association, Inc.)

Total Anomalous Pulmonary Venous Return

Anatomy

Anomalous pulmonary veins may connect with the right side of the heart through a variety of channels as shown in Figure 33–16.[153–156] Supracardiac-type total anomalous pulmonary venous return may connect with the innominate vein via a vertical vein in the mediastinum, the coronary sinus, the right superior vena cava, or directly to the back wall of the right atrium. The infradiaphragmatic type of anomalous pulmonary venous return connects by means of a vertical vein to either the portal system or the inferior vena cava. Pulmonary venous connections may be mixed—for example, when left pulmonary veins ascend via a vertical vein to the innominate vein, and right pulmonary veins enter the right superior vena cava. There is complete mixing of pulmonary and systemic return at the right atrial level. The right ventricle is dilated as a result of excessive pulmonary blood flow unless there is severe obstruction within the pulmonary venous system. Venous return to the left ventricle must pass through a patent foramen ovale or ASD. Left ventricular volumes are usually at the lower limits of normal.

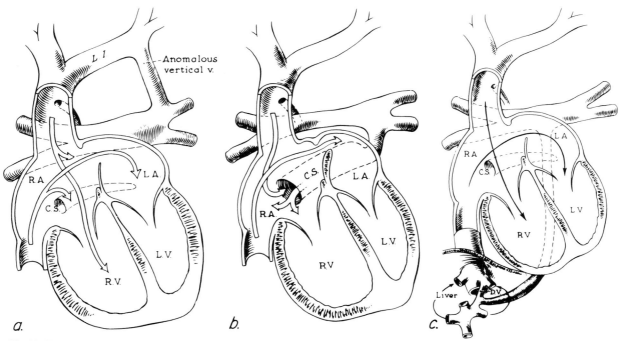

Figure 33–16. Three common types of total anomalous pulmonary venous connection. In each instance blood from the lungs is ultimately delivered to the right atrium, whence it transverses an interatrial communication for delivery to the left atrium (*LA*). *a*, Total anomalous pulmonary venous connection to the left brachiocephalic (innominate) vein (*LI*). *b*, Total anomalous pulmonary venous connection to the coronary sinus (*CS*). *c*, Total anomalous pulmonary venous connection of the infradiaphragmatic type. In the details shown, the anomalous pulmonary vein inserts into the ductus venosus (*DV*). In other instances such an anomalous pulmonary vein may connect with the portal vein or with the left gastric vein. (From Hurst JW, Schlant RC, Rackley CE, et al [eds]. The Heart, 7th ed. New York, McGraw-Hill Information Services, 1990, p. 752. Reproduced with permission of McGraw-Hill, Inc.)

Physiology

Unobstructed pulmonary venous return to the right ventricle is usually associated with excessive pulmonary blood flow and signs of congestive heart failure. Although there is complete mixing of systemic and pulmonary venous return, systemic saturation is only mildly lowered because of the large pulmonary:systemic flow ratio. Oxygen saturation in all cardiac chambers and great arteries will be approximately the same. Obstruction of the pulmonary venous pathway occurs commonly in the infradiaphragmatic type of anomalous pulmonary venous return. This obstruction may be at the point at which the vertical vein crosses the diaphragm at the ductus venosus or elsewhere in the venous system. The supracardiac type of anomalous venous return may also be involved with obstruction, particularly when there is a long, tortuous course of venous return via a vertical vein that may be caught between the left mainstem bronchus and other vascular structures such as the left pulmonary artery. When pulmonary venous obstruction is severe, the patient will usually present in the first days of life with pulmonary edema and severe cyanosis. In such patients, pulmonary arterial flow is not increased and there is little right ventricular enlargement.

Surgical Repair

Since the anatomy is quite varied in this condition, diverse surgical techniques are required to baffle pulmonary venous return into the left atrium.[157–159] Usually, a common pulmonary vein lies behind the atrial cavity, facilitating a side-to-side anastomosis between this venous structure and the left atrial posterior wall. Pulmonary venous return to the coronary sinus is approached by unroofing the coronary sinus and closing the right atrial orifice, thereby diverting both pulmonary venous and coronary sinus flow to the left atrium. In the infradiaphragmatic type of total anomalous pulmonary venous return, there may be some distance between the entry of upper and lower pulmonary veins into the long vertical vein. This may require a more complex anastomosis between the vertical vein and the left atrium. In addition to establishing communication between the pulmonary veins and the left atrium, it is important to eliminate the previous connection with the systemic venous return by ligating the common pulmonary vein beyond the area of anastomosis.

Postoperative Support

Many patients, particularly those with preoperative pulmonary venous obstruction, require prolonged ventilatory support and vigorous diuresis to clear pulmonary edema. Left atrial pressures are often elevated during the initial postoperative period. Whether this is due to decreased left ventricular compliance, left ventricular dysfunction, or small left atrial volume is a matter of debate. Occasionally, there is evidence of continued pulmonary venous hypertension. In some cases, this results from long segment obstruction of pulmonary veins. This is a particularly devastating association because there is no successful surgical or catheter intervention for this type of obstruction. Whether this obstruction is due to primary pulmonary venous hypoplasia or a sclerosing type of mediastinitis is unclear. Some patients with repair of total anomalous pulmonary venous return have successful recovery despite a prolonged period of mechanical ventilation and supportive therapy.

Aortic Atresia with Hypoplastic Left-sided Heart Syndrome

Anatomy

In aortic atresia with hypoplastic left-sided heart syndrome, there is severe hypoplasia of the left ventricle. The mitral valve may be atretic or stenotic. The left ventricle is smaller than normal and may be represented by a slit-like cavity in the back of the heart. The aortic valve is atretic, and the size of the ascending aorta is variable but is usually only several millimeters in diameter. Since the ascending aorta serves to carry blood between the aortic arch and the coronary arteries, the structure is usually approximately the size of the combined coronary arteries. A ductus arteriosus is present in surviving patients. Pulmonary veins return most commonly to the left atrium. Since egress from the left atrium through the mitral valve is blocked, pulmonary venous return must egress via the patent foramen ovale, which is often obstructed.[160-162]

Physiology

Ductal patency is required to maintain systemic blood flow. The right ventricle delivers blood directly to the pulmonary arteries and to the aorta by way of the ductus arteriosus. The balance between the pulmonary flow and the systemic flow depends upon the degree of pulmonary vascular resistance and obstruction to aortic flow at the ductus arteriosus. Pulmonary venous hypertension caused by an obstructed foramen ovale also increases pulmonary arterial resistance. For this reason, though the pulmonary arteries are unobstructed, pulmonary flow may be limited by pulmonary vasoconstriction, promoting perfusion of the systemic vascular bed. In patients with an unobstructed interatrial septum that may result from balloon atrial septostomy, a protective degree of pulmonary vasoconstriction may not occur, and a low systemic output state may ensue. Closure of the ductus arteriosus is also a cause for a sudden drop in systemic perfusion. Classically, the ductus arteriosus may constrict several times before finally closing, leading to a waxing and waning of the low output state.

Surgical Approach

A series of palliative procedures versus neonatal cardiac transplantation are the two currently available surgical approaches for the management of this disorder. Neonatal cardiac transplantation will not be described here (see Chapter 32). The palliative approach involves an initial Norwood procedure in which the pulmonary

blood flow is restricted and a large and reliable connection is created between the main pulmonary artery and the aorta.[58, 163] As illustrated in Figure 33–17, this is done by transecting the main pulmonary artery, anastomosing the proximal portion to the ascending aorta, and patching the inferior aspect of the aortic arch and proximal descending aorta in order to ensure an unlimited pathway for aortic flow. The distal pulmonary arteries are perfused by a Gore-Tex shunt. The proximal pulmonary arteries are patched to avoid distortion. Following the initial procedure, the patient with ideal hemodynamics will progress to a Fontan repair, whereas those with pulmonary artery distortion, elevated pulmonary arterial resistance, or poor ventricular function may be candidates for a bidirectional cavopulmonary shunt (anastomosis between the superior vena cava and pulmonary artery) or cardiac transplantation.

Postoperative Management

Successful transition to a Norwood procedure requires careful preoperative management. This includes maintenance of ductal patency with prostaglandin E_1 infusion and promotion of pulmonary vasoconstriction. This may be accomplished by hypoventilation and mild hypercarbia and avoidance of balloon atrial septostomy. The postoperative period is often stormy because these patients are recovering from a major open heart procedure

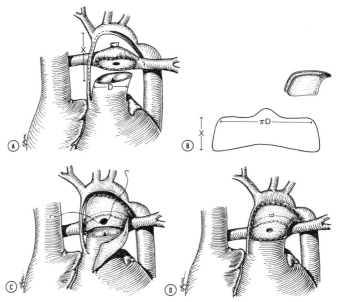

Figure 33–17. First-staged palliation of hypoplastic left heart syndrome. *A,* The main pulmonary artery is transected, and the ductus arteriosus is divided. A long incision is made in the thoracic aorta as shown by the dashed line. *B, C,* A patch of polytetrafluoroethylene (PTFE) or a portion of adult pulmonary artery homograft is used to close the distal pulmonary artery confluence and create a new ascending aortic segment that is anastomosed to the proximal pulmonary arterial trunk. *C, D,* A hole in the PTFE or a separate PTFE tube is used to provide a shunt from the neoaorta to the pulmonary artery confluence. (From Jonas RA, Lang P, Hansen D, et al: First-stage palliation of hypoplastic left heart syndrome. J Thorac Cardiovasc Surg 92:6–13, 1986.)

and have the abnormal physiologic state of a mixed circulation and a systemic right ventricle. Moreover, this occurs during a period of physiologic change as pulmonary vascular resistance is dropping. Balancing the pulmonary and systemic circulations is difficult and requires frequent adjustments in management. Significant cyanosis must be tolerated during the early postoperative period. This should abate as pulmonary vascular resistance decreases. If pulmonary blood flow is optimal during the early postoperative period, it may become excessive and produce severe ventricular failure as pulmonary vascular resistance decreases. Afterload reduction may have an unpredictable effect on the balance between pulmonary and systemic vascular resistances, but a trial may be indicated in patients with low output state. Substantial inotropic support is usually indicated. Postoperative evaluation with cardiac catheterization is advised in order to ascertain whether any substantial hemodynamic abnormalities are present that would compromise the patient's candidacy for later Fontan repair.

References

1. Bedford DE: The anatomical type of atrial septal defects, their incidence and clinical diagnosis. Am J Cardiol 37:805, 1968.
2. Edwards JE: Malformations of the atrial septal complex. In: Gould SE (ed): Pathology of the Heart and Blood Vessels, 3rd ed. Springfield, IL, Charles C Thomas, 1968, pp 262–274.
3. Raghib G, Ruttenberg HD, Anderson RC, et al: Termination of left superior vena cava in left atrium, atrial septal defect and absence of coronary sinus. A developmental complex. Circulation 31:906, 1965.
4. Rome JJ, Keane JF, Perry SB, et al: Double-umbrella closure of atrial defects: Initial clinical applications. Circulation 82:751, 1990.
5. Engle MA, Klein AA, and Hepner S: The post-pericardiotomy and similar syndromes. Cardiovasc Clin 7:211, 1976.
6. Moulaert AJ: Anatomy of ventricular septal defect. In: Anderson RH and Shinebourne EA (eds): Pediatric Cardiology 1977. Edinburgh, Churchill Livingstone, 1978, pp 113–124.
7. Lincoln C, Jamieson S, Joseph M, et al: Transatrial repair of ventricular septal defects with reference to their anatomic classification. J Thorac Cardiovasc Surg 74:183, 1977.
8. Soto B, Ceballas R, and Kirklin JW: Ventricular septal defects: A surgical view point. J Am Coll Cardiol 14(5):12:91, 1989.
9. Van Praagh R, Geva T, and Kreutzer J: Ventricular septal defects: How shall we describe, name and classify them (editorial comment). J Am Coll Cardiol 14(5)12:98, 1989.
10. Schmidt KG, Cassidy SC, Silverman NH, et al: Doubly committed subarterial ventricular septal defects: Echocardiographic features and surgical implications. J Am Coll Cardiol 12:38, 1988.
11. Hoffman JIE and Rudolph AM: The natural history of ventricular septal defects in infancy. Am J Cardiol 16:634, 1965.
12. Hislop A and Reid L: Pulmonary artery development during childhood: Branching pattern and structure. Thorax 28:129, 1973.
13. Rein JG, Freed MD, Norwood WI, et al: Early and late results of closure of ventricular septal defect in infancy. Ann Thorac Surg 24:19, 1977.
14. Blackstone EH, Kirklin JW, Bradley EL, et al: Optimal age and results in repair of large ventricular septal defects. J Thorac Cardiovasc Surg 72:661, 1976.
15. Moreno-Cabral JR, Mamiya RT, Nakamura FF, et al: Ventricular septal defect and aortic insufficiency. Surgical treatment. J Thorac Cardiovasc Surg 73:358, 1977.
16. Zavanella C, Matsuda H, Jara F, et al: Left ventricular approach to multiple ventricular septal defects. Ann Thorac Surg 24:537, 1977.
17. Kirklin JK, Castaneda AR, Keane JF, et al: Surgical management of multiple ventricular septal defects. J Thorac Cardiovasc Surg 80:485, 1980.
18. Wheller J, George BL, Mulder DG, et al: Diagnosis and management of postoperative pulmonary hypertensive crisis. Circulation 60:164, 1979.
19. Bush A, Busst C, Booth K, et al: Does prostacyclin enhance the selective pulmonary vasodilator effect of oxygen in children with congenital heart disease? Circulation 74:135, 1986.
20. Ungerleider RM, Greeley WJ, Sheiki KH, et al: The use of intraoperative echo with Doppler color flow imaging to predict outcome after repair of congenital heart defects. Ann Surg 210:526, 1989.
21. Goor DA and Lillehei CW: Atrioventricular canal malformations. In: Goor DA and Lillehei CW (eds): Congenital Malformations of the Heart. New York, Grune & Stratton, 1975, pp 132–153.
22. Piccoli GP, Gerlis LM, Wilkinson JL, et al: Morphology and classification of atrioventricular defects. Br Heart J 42:621, 1979.
23. Danielson GK: The "classic" (one-patch) operative approach. In: Moulton AL (ed): Congenital Heart Surgery—Current Techniques and Controversies. Pasadena, Appleton-Davies, 1984, pp 136–150.
24. Moreno-Cabral RJ and Shumway NE: Double-patch technique for correction of complete atrioventricular canal. Ann Thorac Surg 33:88, 1982.
25. Bove EL, Sondheimer HM, Kavey REW, et al: Results with the two-patch technique for repair of complete atrioventricular septal defect. Ann Thorac Surg 38(2):158, 1984.
26. Hagler DJ, Tajik AJ, Seward JB, et al: Intraoperative two-dimensional Doppler echocardiography. Thorac Cardiovasc Surg 95:516, 1988.
27. Ungerleider RM, Kisslo JA, Greeley WJ, et al: Intraoperative pre-bypass and post-bypass epicardial color flow imaging in the repair of atrioventricular septal defects. J Thorac Cardiovasc Surg 98:90, 1989.
28. Rashkind WJ, Mullins CE, Hellenbrand WE, et al: Non-surgical closure of patent ductus arteriosus: Clinical application of the Rashkind PDA occluder system. Circulation 75:583, 1987.
29. Gross RE and Hubbard JP: Surgical ligation of a patent ductus arteriosus. JAMA 112:729, 1939.
30. Koretzky ED, Moller JS, Dorns MD, et al: Congenital pulmonary stenosis resulting from dysplasia of the valve. Circulation 40:43, 1969.
31. Schneeweiss A, Blieden LC, Shem-Tov A, et al: Diagnostic angiocardiographic criteria in dysplastic stenotic pulmonic valve. Am Heart J 106:761, 1983.
32. deLeval MR, Bull C, Stark J, et al: Pulmonary atresia and intact ventricular septum: Surgical management based on a revised classification. Circulation 66:272, 1982.
33. Gittenberger-deGroot AC, Sauer U, Bindl L, et al: Competition of coronary arteries and ventriculo-coronary arterial communications in pulmonary atresia with intact ventricular septum. Int J Cardiol 18:243, 1988.
34. Freedom RM: Pulmonary valve stenosis with intact ventricular septum and congenital pulmonary valve regurgitation. In: Freedom RM (ed): Angiocardiography of Congenital Heart Disease. New York, MacMillan, 1984, pp 222–230.
35. Coles JG, Freedom RM, Olley PM, et al: Surgical management of critical pulmonary stenosis in the neonate. Am Thorac Surg 38:458, 1984.
36. Weldon CS, Hartmann AF Jr, and McNight RC: Surgical management of hypoplastic right ventricle with pulmonary atresia or critical pulmonary stenosis and intact ventricular septum. Am Thorac Surg 37:12, 1984.
37. Merrill WH, Shuman TA, Graham TP Jr, et al: Surgical intervention in neonates with critical pulmonary stenosis. Ann Surg 205:712, 1987.
38. Billingsley AM, Laks H, Boyce SW, et al: Definitive repair in patients with pulmonary atresia and intact ventricular septum. J Thorac Cardiovasc Surg 97:746, 1989.
39. Spencer FC, Neill CA, Sank L, et al: Anatomical variations in 46 patients with congenital aortic stenosis. Am Surg 26:294, 1960.
40. Braunwald E, Goldblatt A, Aygen MM, et al: Congenital aortic stenosis. I: Clinical and hemodynamic findings in 100 patients. II: Surgical treatment and the results of operation. Circulation 27:426, 1963.
41. Roberts WC: Valvular, subvalvular, and supravalvular aortic stenosis: Morphologic features. Cardiovasc Clin 5:126, 1973.

42. Roberts WC: The congenitally bicuspid aortic valve. A study of 85 autopsy cases. Am J Cardiol 26:72, 1970.
43. Sholler GF, Keane JF, Perry SB, et al: Balloon dilation of congenital aortic valve stenosis. Results and influence of technical and morphological features on outcome. Circulation 78:351, 1988.
44. Newfeld EA, Muster AJ, Paul MH, et al: Discrete subvalvular aortic stenosis in childhood. Study of 51 patients. Am J Cardiol 38:53, 1976.
45. Moses RD, Barnhart GR, and Jones M: The late prognosis after localized resection for fixed (discrete and tunnel) left ventricular outflow tract obstruction. J Thorac Cardiovasc Surg 87:410, 1984.
46. Maron BJ, Redwood DR, Roberts WC, et al: Tunnel subaortic stenosis: Left ventricular outflow tract obstruction produced by fibromuscular tubular narrowing. Circulation 54:404, 1976.
47. Williams JC, Barratt-Boyes BG, and Lowe JB: Supravalvular aortic stenosis. Circulation 24:1311, 1961.
48. Beuren AJ, Schulze C, Eberle P, et al: The syndrome of supravalvular aortic stenosis, peripheral pulmonary stenosis, mental retardation and similar facial appearance. Am J Cardiol 13:471, 1964.
49. Lababidi Z, Wu JR, and Walls JT: Percutaneous balloon aortic valvuloplasty: Results in 23 patients. Am J Cardiol 53:194, 1984.
50. Choy M, Beekman RH, Rocchini AP, et al: Percutaneous balloon valvuloplasty for valvar aortic stenosis in infants and children. Am J Cardiol 59:1010, 1987.
51. Kasten-Sportes CH, Piechard JF, Sidi D, et al: Percutaneous balloon valvuloplasty in neonates with critical aortic stenosis. J Am Coll Cardiol 13(5):1101, 1989.
52. McGoon DC, Geha AS, Scofield EL, et al: Surgical treatment of congenital aortic stenosis. Dis Chest 55:388, 1969.
53. Reid JM, Coleman EN, and Stevenson JG: Management of congenital aortic stenosis. Arch Dis Child 45:201, 1970.
54. Cheitlin MD, Fenoglio JJ Jr, McAllister HA Jr, et al: Congenital aortic stenosis secondary to dysplasia of congenital bicuspid aortic valves without commissural fusion. Am J Cardiol 42:102, 1978.
55. Kugler JD, Campbell E, Vargo TA, et al: Results of aortic valvotomy in infants with isolated aortic valvular stenosis. J Thorac Cardiovasc Surg 78:553, 1979.
56. Lawson RM, Bonchek LI, Menashe V, et al: Late results of surgery for left ventricular outflow tract obstruction in children. J Thorac Cardiovasc Surg 71:334, 1976.
57. Wagner HR, Ellison RC, Keane JF, et al: Clinical course in aortic stenosis. Report from the Joint Study on the Natural History of Congenital Heart Defects. Circulation 56(Suppl I):I-47–I-56, 1976.
58. Norwood WI, Lang P, and Hansen DD: Physiologic repair of aortic atresia-hypoplastic left heart syndrome. N Engl J Med 308:23, 1983.
59. Bailey L, Concepcion W, Shattuck H, et al: Method of heart transplantation for treatment of hypoplastic left heart syndrome. J Thorac Cardiovasc Surg 92:1, 1986.
60. Binet JP, Losay J, Demontous S, et al: Subvalvular aortic stenosis: Long-term surgical results. Thorac Cardiovasc Surg 31:96, 1983.
61. Cain T, Campbell D, Patron B, et al: Operation for discrete subvalvular aortic stenosis. J Thorac Cardiovasc Surg 87:366, 1984.
62. Brown J, Stevens L, Lynch L, et al: Surgery for discrete subvalvular aortic stenosis: Actuarial survival, hemodynamic results, and acquired aortic regurgitation. Ann Thorac Surg 40:151, 1985.
63. Konno S, Imai Y, Iida Y, et al: A new method for prosthetic valve replacement in congenital aortic stenosis associated with hypoplasia of the aortic valve ring. J Thorac Cardiovasc Surg 70:909, 1975.
64. Bjornstad PG, Rastan H, Keutel J, et al: Aortoventriculoplasty for tunnel subaortic stenosis and other obstructions of the left ventricular outflow tract. Clinical and hemodynamic results. Circulation 60:59, 1979.
65. Misbach GA, Turley K, Ullyot DJ, et al: Left ventricular outflow enlargement by the Konno procedure. J Thorac Cardiovasc Surg 84:696, 1982.
66. Vouhe PR, Poulain H, Bloch G, et al: Aortoseptal approach for optimal resection of diffuse subvalvular aortic stenosis. J Thorac Cardiovasc Surg 87:887, 1984.
67. Rastelli GC, McGoon DC, Ongley PA, et al: Surgical treatment of supravalvular aortic stenosis. Report of 16 cases and review of literature. J Thorac Cardiovasc Surg 51:873, 1966.
68. Keane JF, Fellows KE, LaFarge CG, et al: The surgical management of discrete and diffuse supravalvar aortic stenosis. Circulation 54:112, 1976.
69. Weisz D, Hartmann AF Jr, and Weldon CS: Results of surgery for congenital supravalvular aortic stenosis. Am J Cardiol 37:73, 1976.
70. Doty DB, Polansky DB, and Jenson CB: Supravalvular aortic stenosis. Repair by extended aortoplasty. J Thorac Cardiovasc Surg 74:362, 1977.
71. Flaker G, Teske D, Kilman J, et al: Supravalvular aortic stenosis. A 20 year clinical perspective and experience with patch aortoplasty. Am J Cardiol 51:256, 1983.
72. Edwards JE, Christensen NA, Clagett OT, et al: Pathologic considerations in coarctation of the aorta. Mayo Clin Proc 23:324, 1948.
73. Ho SY and Anderson RH: Coarctation tubular hypoplasia and the ductus arteriosus: Histological study of 35 specimens. Br Heart J 41:268, 1979.
74. Moller JH and Edward JE: Interruption of aortic arch. Anatomic patterns and associated cardiac malformations. AJR 95:557, 1965.
75. Van Praagh R, Bernhard WF, Rosenthal A, et al: Interrupted aortic arch: Surgical treatment. Am J Cardiol 27:200, 1971.
76. Jaffe RB: Complete interruption of the aortic arch. 1. Characteristic radiographic findings in 21 patients. Circulation 52:714, 1975.
77. Neye-Bock S and Fellows KE: Aortic arch interruption in infancy: Radio- and angiographic features. AJR 135:1005, 1980.
78. Collins-Nakai RL, Dick M, Parisi-Buckley L, et al: Interrupted aortic arch in infancy. J Pediatr 88:959, 1976.
79. Gersony WM: Coarctation of the aorta. In: Adams FH and Emmanouilides GC (eds): Moss' Heart Disease in Infants, Children and Adolescents, 3rd ed. Baltimore, Williams & Wilkins, 1983, pp 188–199.
80. Harlan JL, Doty DB, Brandt B, et al: Coarctation of the aorta in infants. J Thorac Cardiovasc Surg 88:1012, 1984.
81. Kirklin JW, Burchell HB, Pugh DG, et al: Surgical treatment of coarctation of the aorta in a ten-week old infant: Report of a case. Circulation 6:411, 1952.
82. Thibault WN, Sperling DR, and Gazzaniga AB: Subclavian artery patch angioplasty. Treatment of infants and young children with aorta coarctation. Arch Surg 110:1095, 1975.
83. Hamilton DI, DiEusanio G, Sandrasagra FA, et al: Early and late results of aortoplasty with a left subclavian flap for coarctation of the aorta in infancy. J Thorac Cardiovas Surg 75:699, 1978.
84. Lock JE, Bass JL, Amplaz K, et al: Balloon dilatation angioplasty of aortic coarctation in infants and children. Circulation 68:109, 1983.
85. Finley JB, Beaulieu RG, Nanton MA, et al: Balloon catheter dilatation of coarctation of the aorta in young infants. Br Heart J 50:411, 1983.
86. Lababidi ZA, Daskapoulos DA, and Stoechkle H Jr: Transluminal balloon coarctation angioplasty: Experience with 27 patients. Am J Cardiol 54:1288, 1984.
87. Wren C, Pearl I, Bain H, et al: Balloon dilatation of unoperated aortic coarctation: Immediate results and one year follow-up. Br Heart J 58:369, 1984.
88. Zahka KG, Roland JM, Cutilletta AF, et al: Management of aortic arch interruption with prostaglandin E_1 infusion and microporous expanded polytetrafluoroethylene grafts. Am J Cardiol 46:1001, 1980.
89. Tyson KR, Harris LC, and Ngiem QX: Repair of aortic arch interruption in the neonate. Surgery 67:1006, 1970.
90. Fishman NH, Bronstein MH, Berman W Jr, et al: Surgical management of severe aortic coarctation and interrupted aortic arch in neonates. J Thorac Cardiovasc Surg 71:35, 1976.
91. Freed MD, Heymann MA, Lewis AB, et al: Prostaglandin E_1 in infants with ductus arteriosus–dependent congenital heart disease. Circulation 64:899, 1981.
92. Kreiger KH and Spencer FC: Is paraplegia after repair of coarctation of the aorta due principally to distal hypotension during aortic cross-clamping? Surgery 97:2, 1985.

93. Ho ECK and Moss AJ: The syndrome of mesenteric arteritis following surgical repair of aortic coarctation. Pediatrics 49:40, 1972.

94. Van Praagh R and Van Praagh S: Isolated ventricular inversion. A consideration on the morphogenesis, definition and diagnosis of nontransposed and transposed great arteries. Am J Cardiol 17:395, 1966.

95. Van Praagh R, Weinberg PM, Matsuora R, et al: Malpositions of the heart. In: Adams FH and Emmanouilides CG (eds): Heart Disease in Infants, Children and Adolescents. Baltimore, Williams & Wilkins, 1983, p 422.

96. Planche C, Bruniaux J, Lacour-Gayet F, et al: Switch operation for transposition of the great arteries in neonates. J Thorac Cardiovasc Surg 96:354, 1988.

97. Mayer JE, Sanders SP, Jonas RA, et al: Coronary artery pattern and outcome of arterial switch operation for transposition of the great arteries. Circulation 82(Suppl IV):IV-139, 1990.

98. Senning A: Surgical correction of transposition of the great vessels. Surgery 45:966, 1959.

99. Mustard WT: Successful two-stage correction of transposition of the great vessels. Surgery 55:469, 1964.

100. Marx GR, Hougen TI, Norwood WI, et al: Transposition of the great arteries with intact ventricular septum: Results of Mustard and Senning operations in 123 consecutive patients. J Am Coll Cardiol 1:476, 1983.

101. George BL, Laks H, Klitzner TS, et al: Results of the Senning procedure in infants with simple and complex transposition of the great arteries. Am J Cardiol 59:426, 1987.

102. Goodman MR, Friedli B, Pasternac A, et al: Hemodynamic studies in children four to ten years after the Mustard operation for transposition of the great arteries. Circulation 53:532, 1976.

103. Borrow KM, Keane JF, Castaneda AR, et al: Systemic ventricular function in patients with tetralogy of Fallot, ventricular septal defect and transposition of the great arteries repaired during infancy. Circulation 64:878, 1981.

104. Mee RB: Severe right ventricular failure after Mustard or Senning operation. Two-stage repair: Pulmonary artery banding and switch. J Thorac Cardiovasc Surg 92:385, 1986.

105. Martin TC, Smith L, Hernandez A, et al: Dysrhythmias following the Senning operation for dextro-transposition of the great arteries. J Thorac Cardiovasc Surg 85:928, 1983.

106. Gillette PC, Kugler JD, Garson A Jr, et al: Mechanisms of cardiac arrhythmias after Mustard operation for transposition of the great arteries. Am J Cardiol 45:1225, 1980.

107. Jatene AD, Fontes VF, Paulista PP, et al: Anatomic correction of transposition of the great vessels. J Thorac Cardiovasc Surg 72:364, 1976.

108. Castaneda AR, Norwood WI, Jonas RA, et al: Transposition of the great arteries and intact ventricular septum: Anatomical repair of the neonate. Ann Thorac Surg 38:438, 1984.

109. Quaegebeur JM, Rohmer J, Ottenkamp J, et al: The arterial switch operation. An eight year experience. J Thorac Cardiovasc Surg 92:361, 1986.

110. Yacoub MH and Radley-Smith R: Anatomy of the coronary arteries transposition of the great arteries and methods for their transfer in anatomical correction. Thorax 33:418, 1978.

111. Rastelli GC, McGoon DC, and Wallace RB: Anatomic correction of transposition of the great arteries with ventricular septal defect and subpulmonary stenosis. J Thorac Cardiovasc Surg 58:545, 1969.

112. McGoon DC, Danielson GK, Puga FJ, et al: Late results after extracardiac conduit repair for congenital cardiac defects. Am J Cardiol 49:1741, 1982.

113. Rashkind WJ and Miller WW: Creation of an atrial septal defect without thoracotomy. A palliative approach to complete transposition of the great arteries. JAMA 196:991, 1966.

114. Lev M, Rimoldi JA, and Rowlatt UF: The quantitative anatomy of cyanotic tetralogy of Fallot. Circulation 30:531, 1964.

115. Becker AE, Connor M, and Anderson RH: Tetralogy of Fallot: A morphometric and geometric study. Am J Cardiol 35:402, 1975.

116. Anderson RH, Allwork SP, Ho SY, et al: Surgical anatomy of tetralogy of Fallot. J Thorac Cardiovasc Surg 81:887, 1981.

117. Edwards WD: Double-outlet right ventricle and tetralogy of Fallot. Two distinct but not mutually exclusive entities. J Thorac Cardiovasc Surg 82:418, 1981.

118. Van Praagh R, Van Praagh S, Nebesar RA, et al: Tetralogy of Fallot: Underdevelopment of the pulmonary infundibulum and its sequelae. Am J Cardiol 26:25, 1970.

119. Bharati S, Paul MH, Idriss FS, et al: The surgical anatomy of pulmonary atresia with ventricular septal defect: Pseudotruncus. J Thorac Cardiovasc Surg 69:713, 1975.

120. Haworth SG and Macartney FJ: Growth and development of pulmonary circulation in pulmonary atresia with ventricular septal defect and major aortopulmonary collateral arteries. Br Heart J 44:12, 1980.

121. Collett RW and Edwards JE: Persistent truncus arteriosus: A classification according to anatomic types. Surg Clin North Am 29:1256, 1949.

122. Calder L, Van Praagh R, Van Praagh S, et al: Truncus arteriosus communis. Clinical, angiographic and pathologic findings in 100 patients. Am Heart J 92:23, 1976.

123. Blackstone EH, Kirklin JW, and Pacifico AD: Decision-making in repair of tetralogy of Fallot based upon intraoperative measurements of pulmonary arterial outflow tract. J Thorac Cardiovasc Surg 77:526, 1979.

124. Zhao H, Miller DC, Reitz BA, et al: Surgical repair of tetralogy of Fallot. J Thorac Cardiovasc Surg 89:204, 1985.

125. Sanchez HE, Cornish EM, Shih FC, et al: The surgical treatment of tetralogy of Fallot. Ann Thorac Surg 37:431, 1984.

126. Finck SJ, Puga FJ, and Danielson GK: Pulmonary valve insertion during reoperation for tetralogy of Fallot. Ann Thorac Surg 45:610, 1988.

127. Blackstone EH, Kirklin JW, and Pacifico AD: Decision-making in repair of tetralogy of Fallot based on intraoperative measurements of pulmonary arterial outflow tract. J Thorac Cardiovasc Surg 77:526, 1979.

128. Kurosawa H, Imai Y, Nakazawa M, et al: Conotruncal repair of tetralogy of Fallot. Ann Thorac Surg 45:661, 1988.

129. Coles JG, Kirklin JW, Pacifico AD, et al: The relief of pulmonary stenosis by a transatrial versus a transventricular approach to the repair of tetralogy of Fallot. Ann Thorac Surg 45:7, 1988.

130. Castaneda AR and Norwood WI: Fallot's tetralogy. In: Stark J and de Leval M (eds): Surgery for Congenital Heart Defects. London, Grune & Stratton, 1983, pp 321–329.

131. Laks H, Hellenbrand WE, Kleinman CS, et al: Patch reconstruction of the right ventricular outflow tract with pulmonary valve insertion. Circulation 64:154, 1981.

132. Kirklin JW, Bargeron LM, and Pacifico AD: The enlargement of small pulmonary arteries by preliminary palliative operations. Circulation 56:612, 1977.

133. Kirklin JW, Blackstone EH, Smmazaki Y, et al: Survival, functional status, and reoperations after repair of tetralogy of Fallot with pulmonary atresia. J Thorac Cardiovasc Surg 96:102, 1988.

134. Millikan JS, Puga FJ, Danielson GK, et al: Staged surgical repair of pulmonary atresia, ventricular septal defect, and hypoplastic confluent pulmonary arteries. J Thorac Cardiovasc Surg 91:818, 1986.

135. Ebert PA, Turley K, Stanger P, et al: Surgical treatment of truncus arteriosus in the first six months of life. Ann Surg 200:451, 1984.

136. Singh AK, de val MR, Pincott JR, et al: Pulmonary artery banding for truncus arteriosus in the first year of life. Circulation 54(Suppl 3):17, 1976.

137. Milgalter E and Laks H: Truncus arteriosus. In: Baue AE, Geha AS, Hammond GL, et al (eds): Glenn's Thoracic and Cardiovascular Surgery, 5th ed. Norwalk, Appleton & Lange, 1991, pp 1079–1087.

138. Rosenthal A and Dick M: Tricuspid atresia. In: Adams FH and Emmanouilides GC (eds): Moss' Heart Disease in Infants, Children and Adolescents, 4th ed. Baltimore, Williams & Wilkins, 1990, pp 348–361.

139. Weinberg PM: Anatomy of tricuspid atresia and its relevance to current forms of surgical therapy. Ann Thorac Surg 29:306, 1980.

140. Van Praagh R, Ongley PA, and Swan HJC: Anatomic types of single or common ventricle in man. Morphologic and geometric aspect of 60 necropsied cases. Am J Cardiol 13:367, 1964.

141. Anderson RH, Macartney FJ, Tynan M, et al: Univentricular atrioventricular connection: The single ventricle trap unsprung. Pediatr Cardiol 4:273, 1983.

142. Anderson RH, Lenox CC, Zuberbuhler JR, et al: Double-inlet left ventricle with rudimentary right ventricle and ventriculoarterial concordance. Am J Cardiol 52:573, 1983.

143. Freedom RM, Sondheimer H, Dische R, et al: Development of "subaortic stenosis" after pulmonary arterial banding for common ventricle. Am J Cardiol 39:78, 1977.

144. Park SC, Siewers RD, Neches WH, et al: Surgical management of univentricular heart with subaortic obstruction. Ann Thorac Surg 37:417, 1984.

145. Girod DA, Lima RC, Anderson RH, et al: Double-inlet ventricle: Morphologic analysis and surgical implications in 32 cases. J Thorac Cardiovasc Surg 88:590, 1984.

146. Choussat A, Fontan F, Bosse P, et al: Selection criteria for Fontan's procedure. *In*: Anderson RH and Shinebourne EA (eds): Pediatric Cardiology. Edinburgh, Churchill Livingstone, 1978, pp 559–566.

147. Gale AW, Danielson GK, McGoon DC, et al: Fontan procedure for tricuspid atresia. Circulation 62:91, 1980.

148. Fontan F and Baudet E: Surgical repair of tricuspid atresia. Thorax 26:240, 1971.

149. Kreutzer G, Galindez E, Bono H, et al: An operation for the correction of tricuspid atresia. J Thorac Cardiovasc Surg 66:613, 1973.

150. Humes RA, Porter CJ, Mair DD, et al: Intermediate follow-up and predicted survival after the modified Fontan procedure for tricuspid atresia and double-inlet ventricle. Circulation 76(Suppl III):III-67, 1987.

151. Bridges AD, Lock JE, and Castaneda AR: Baffle fenestration with subsequent transcatheter closure: Modification of the Fontan operation for patients at increased risk. Circulation 82:1681, 1990.

152. Bridges AD, Jonas RA, Mayer JE, et al: Bidirectional cavopulmonary anastomosis as interim palliation for high-risk Fontan candidates: Early results. Circulation 82(Suppl IV):IV-170, 1990.

153. Neill CA: Development of the pulmonary veins with reference to the embryology of anomalies of pulmonary venous return. Pediatrics 18:880, 1956.

154. Lucas RV Jr, Lock JE, Tandon R, et al: Gross and histological anatomy of total anomalous pulmonary venous connection. Am J Cardiol 62:292, 1988.

155. Burroughs JT and Edwards JE: Total anomalous pulmonary venous connection. Am Heart J 59:913, 1960.

156. Delisle G, Ando M, Calder AL, et al: Total anomalous pulmonary venous connection. Report of 93 autopsied cases with emphasis on diagnostic and surgical considerations. Am Heart J 91:99, 1976.

157. Norwood WI, Hougen TJ, and Castaneda AR: Total anomalous pulmonary venous connection: Surgical considerations. Cardiovasc Clin 11:353, 1981.

158. Yee ES, Turley K, Hsieh W, et al: Infant total anomalous pulmonary venous connection: Factors influencing timing of presentation and operative outcome. Circulation 76(Suppl III):III-83, 1987.

159. Galloway AC, Campbell DN, and Clarke DR: The value of early repair for total anomalous pulmonary venous drainage. Pediatr Cardiol 6:77, 1985.

160. Lev M: Pathologic anatomy and interrelationship of hypoplasia of the aortic tract complexes. Lab Invest 1:61, 1952.

161. Noonan JA and Nadas AS: The hypoplastic left heart syndrome: An analysis of 101 cases. Pediatr Clin North Am 5:1029, 1958.

162. Mahowald JM, Lucas RV Jr, and Edwards JE: Aortic valvular atresia. Associated cardiovascular anomalies. Pediatr Cardiol 2:99, 1982.

34

Chest Vasculature

Linda M. Bradley, M.D.

Abnormalities in either the structure or function of the chest vasculature are a source of morbidity and mortality in the pediatric intensive care unit (ICU). This chapter first reviews anomalies in vascular development commonly encountered in the ICU. These lesions include abnormalities of lung bud development and arteriovenous malformations. Vascular rings and malformations of the aortic arch are reviewed elsewhere (see Chapters 37 and 49).

Because the response of the pulmonary circulation to a wide variety of conditions and disease states can influence clinical outcome in critically ill children, this chapter focuses on the pathogenesis and management of pulmonary hypertension in infancy and childhood. Research concerning the cell biology of the vessel wall, endothelial-smooth muscle interactions, and endogenous regulators of vascular tone are discussed in detail.

PULMONARY HYPOPLASIA SYNDROMES

Pulmonary Hypoplasia

Hypoplasia of the lung may be primary or secondary to reduced intrathoracic volume, which occurs with congenital diaphragmatic hernia. In the primary disorders, the pulmonary artery is small and hypoplasia may result from failure of bronchial branching. The signs and symptoms of a hypoplastic lung may be minimal. The involved hemithorax tends to be smaller than the contralateral side. Breath sounds may be normal or diminished. Recurrent pulmonary infections may be frequent. The main clinical complication of this disorder is airway compression. In patients with agenesis or severe hypoplasia of the right lung, the aorta is deviated to the right and compresses the trachea.[1] Radiographic manifestations include mediastinal shift, elevation of the hemidiaphragm, closer rib approximation, and sparse-appearing pulmonary vessels. Ventilation and perfusion radionuclide lung imaging provides a valuable noninvasive technique for detecting this disorder, but definitive diagnosis is by pulmonary angiography and bronchography.

Pulmonary Hypoplasia with Abnormal Vascular Connections (Scimitar Syndrome)

The scimitar syndrome consists of hypoplastic right lung that has a systemic arterial supply, an anomalous right pulmonary vein, and dextroposition of the heart (Fig. 34–1). The arterial supply to the hypoplastic lung varies, but the venous drainage is almost always by a single vein coursing the right atrium and returning to the inferior vena cava just below the diaphragm. Associated lesions include atrial septal defect, eventration of the diaphragm, and accessory diaphragm. Some studies suggest that this disorder may be inherited as an autosomal dominant trait.[2]

The child may be asymptomatic but more often suffers from chronic, recurrent respiratory infections. Physical findings include diminished right-sided breath sounds, a systolic ejection murmur along the right sternal border, and a widely split second heart sound. The anomalous "scimitar" vein is best seen on lateral or right anterior oblique radiographic projection and can be confirmed angiographically when other cardiac anomalies are suspected (Fig. 34–1).

Horseshoe Lung

Horseshoe lung is an unusual malformation in which the right and left lungs are joined behind the pericardial sac. Salient features include right lung hypoplasia, partial anomalous pulmonary venous drainage (right lung to inferior vena cava), and aberrant systemic arterial supply to all or most of the right lung. Like those with scimitar syndrome, patients with horseshoe lung frequently have recurrent pneumonia.

PULMONARY SEQUESTRATION

A sequestration consists of embryonic lung tissue that does not function and derives its blood supply from anomalous systemic arteries. Intralobar sequestrations are located within the normal visceral pleura, whereas extralobar sequestrations have a separate pleura.

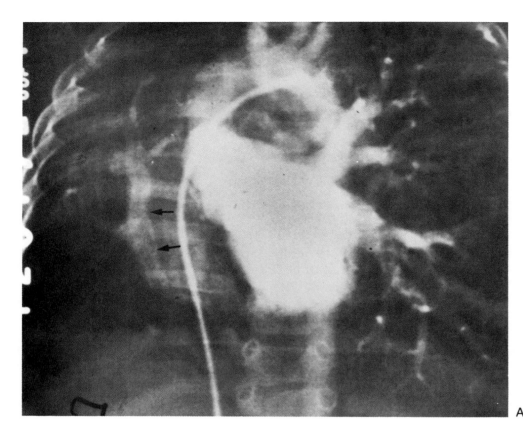

Figure 34–1. Scimitar syndrome. *A,* The right lung is hypoplastic, and the heart occupies a considerable portion of the right hemithorax. A curvilinear density (*arrow*) represents an anomalous pulmonary vein.

A

Intralobar sequestrations usually occur in the posterior basilar segments. Two thirds are left sided. Their blood supply usually comes from a single, large artery off the aorta; venous drainage is via the pulmonary veins. Communications with the gastrointestinal tract are rare. Extralobar sequestrations are just above or below the diaphragm. Ninety per cent are left sided. Their arterial supply is usually from small anomalous branches of the pulmonary artery, and venous drainage is to a systemic (azygous or portal) vein. Gastrointestinal communications are common as are other associated anomalies including bronchial agenesis, duplication of the colon, vertebral anomalies, and diaphragmatic defects. Most extralobar sequestrations are diagnosed in the neonatal period.

Patients usually present with some form of respiratory difficulty. Occasionally, they present with cardiac failure as a result of a large left-to-right shunt through the sequestration. Differential diagnosis includes pneumonia, empyema, lung abscess, bronchiectasis, adenomatoid malformation, Bochdalek hernia, and intrathoracic kidney.

The chest x-ray is almost always abnormal, but findings are nonspecific. Radionuclide scanning can be useful to demonstrate late filling in the vessels of the sequestration compared with the rest of the lung. Aortography is helpful to identify anomalous vessels if surgery is needed for relief of symptoms.

PULMONARY FISTULAS

Pulmonary arteriovenous fistulas are almost always congenital, although they can be acquired due to schistosomiasis, juvenile hepatic cirrhosis, metastatic carcinoma of the thyroid, or trauma. When congenital, its origin appears to be abnormal development of pulmonary arteries and veins in a common vascular network.

Approximately 60% of patients with pulmonary arteriovenous fistulas have Rendu-Osler-Weber syndrome.[3] Other associated anomalies include malformations of the bronchial tree, absent right lower lobe, and congenital heart disease.

The central physiologic disturbance is the shunting of venous blood from the pulmonary arteries to the pulmonary veins, causing systemic arterial oxygen saturation to range from 50 to 85%. Since ventilation is unaffected, arterial P_{CO_2} is normal. Rapid pulmonary circulation time can be seen by contrast echocardiography and radioisotope studies. Pulmonary flow and pressure are normal. Polycythemia develops in response to arterial hypoxemia. The lack of capillary filter in the affected lung predisposes to the development of brain abscesses.

Clinically, symptoms related to cyanosis are common (e.g., exercise intolerance, dyspnea on exertion). One fourth of the patients present with neurologic complaints (e.g., speech disorders, diplopia, transitory numbness). These symptoms are thought to be due to a combination of factors—hypoxemia, polycythemia, small-vessel thrombosis, and repeated hemorrhage in telangiectatic brain lesions. Physical signs vary and may include digital clubbing, cyanosis, or a faint ($\leq$ grade II/VI) continuous murmur that increases with inspiration. Radiographically, the size of the heart is usually normal. In 50% of cases, x-ray films reveal one or more rounded opacities in one or both lung fields. Angiographically, injection

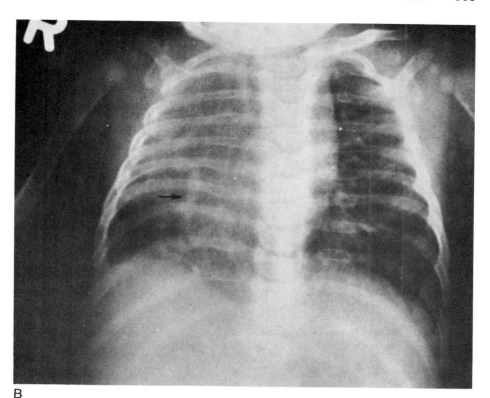

Figure 34–1 *Continued B*, Hypoplasia of the right pulmonary artery is seen on pulmonary angiography. *C*, Levophase shows the aberrant pulmonary vein (*arrows*) carrying contrast to the right atrium. Aberrant systemic arterial supply to the right lower lobe was visible on other films. (From Felman AH: Abnormal lung bud development. *In*: Felman AH [ed]: The Pediatric Chest, 1st ed. Springfield, IL, 1983, pp. 38–39. Courtesy of Charles C Thomas, Publisher, Springfield, Illinois.)

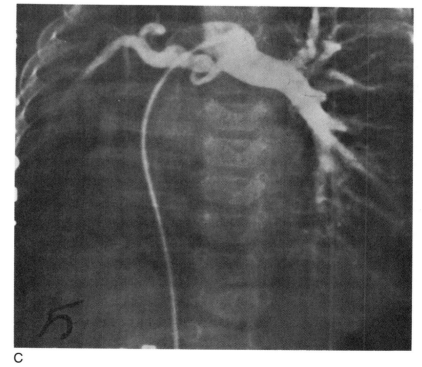

B

C

of contrast into the affected pulmonary artery will show dilated, tortuous afferent and efferent vessels, early opacification of the left atrium, and scarce opacification of the uninvolved lung.

Most patients with pulmonary arteriovenous fistulas require treatment due to the frequency of fatal complications such as aneurysm rupture, massive hemorrhage, endocarditis, and brain abscess.[4] Until recently, treatment has been surgical—the goal being to remove the lesions and preserve as much healthy lung as possible. A new technique, detachable balloon embolization, is now available and provides nonsurgical closure of aberrant vessels.[5] Partially inflated balloons are floated to the desired position, fully inflated, and then detached

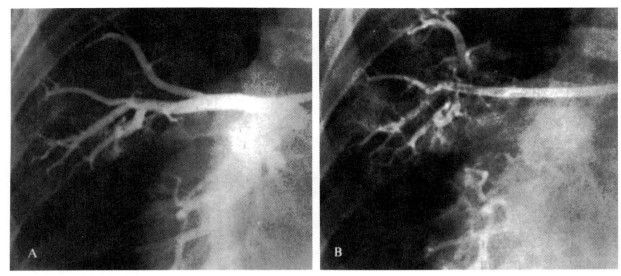

Figure 34–2. Eisenmenger syndrome with ventricular septal defect in a 9-year-old patient. Pulmonary artery pressure = 110/70 (mean pressure 85 mm Hg), PVR = 46.4 Wood units/m². *A,* Midarterial and *B,* flush phases demonstrate severe pruning of the upper lobe vessels and very few supernumerary vessels. Sparse capillary filling produces little background haze. (From Nihill MR and McNamara DG: Magnification pulmonary wedge angiography in the evaluation of children with congenital heart disease and pulmonary hypertension. Circulation 58:1094, 1978. By permission of the American Heart Association, Inc.)

from the catheter. Initially, the balloons cause occlusion by obstructing the vascular lumen; within days, thrombus forms to provide a permanent occlusion.

PULMONARY HYPERTENSION

Natural history studies document that the frequency and severity of pulmonary hypertension varies considerably among the different congenital heart defects. Severity of pulmonary hypertension is determined by the absolute level of the pulmonary vascular resistance (PVR), its rate of rise, and its reversibility in response to various vasodilators. This topic has been thoroughly reviewed by Rabinovitch.[6]

Of babies with large ventricular septal defects, 15% develop increased PVR in early childhood. If surgical repair is performed in the first 2 years, the increased PVR generally reverses. Delays in surgical correction can result in permanent elevation in PVR. Patients with a large patent ductus arteriosus have a comparable incidence of pulmonary hypertension.[7] Severe pulmonary hypertension occurs in 8% of patients with transposition of the great arteries and intact ventricular septum versus 40% in those with an accompanying ventricular septal defect or patent ductus arteriosus.[8] Almost all patients with common atrioventricular canal have pulmonary hypertension. Pulmonary vascular obstructive disease has been reported in the first year of life. The extent and progression of increased PVR in children with Down syndrome and a complete atrioventricular canal defect remain controversial. Histologic studies have failed to disclose any differences between patients with Down syndrome and age-matched controls with atrioventricular canal defect.[9] Others have documented an increased incidence of pulmonary hypoplasia in children with Down syndrome.[10]

Infants with truncus arteriosus and unrestricted pulmonary blood flow have a similar incidence and progression of pulmonary hypertension, as do those with an atrioventricular defect canal.[11]

Hemodynamic criteria have been suggested to identify patients at high risk for persistent postoperative severe elevation in PVR—a calculated PVR of greater than or equal to 10 Wood units/m². PVR values from 8 to 10 Wood units/m² are considered borderline; postoperative prognosis improves if PVR decreases to 6 Wood units/m² with inhalation of 100% oxygen. Unfortunately, PVR measurements reflect only one point in time and are influenced by hypoxemia, polycythemia, and sedation.[12, 13] Supplementation of the hemodynamic assessment with a structural evaluation of the pulmonary vascular bed can be useful in complex cases.

One method of quantitating changes in the pulmonary vascular bed is by wedge angiography (Fig. 34–2).[14, 15] A balloon catheter is placed at the origin of a lower lobe pulmonary artery; contrast is injected; and the angiogram is filmed on biplane cine. The three features of each wedge study that are of particular importance are the rate of vessel tapering, the background filling, and the pulmonary circulation time. Abrupt tapering, lack of background filling, and prolonged circulation time correlate with advanced changes on a lung biopsy.[14, 15]

A major challenge in the pediatric ICU is postoperative control of the reactive pulmonary circulation. The cause of the "pulmonary hypertensive crisis" is unclear. It is thought to result from interaction of vascular endothelial cells with platelets and leukocytes that have been activated by hypothermia and cardiopulmonary bypass.[16–18] Platelets release potent vasoconstrictor thromboxanes[19]; activated leukocytes produce leukotrienes[20] and platelet-activating factor.[21] Elaboration of these substances produces profound pulmonary hypertension (Figs. 34–3 and 34–4).[22–24] Endothelin, an endothelial cell-derived peptide, may also be important, because its effects can be vasoconstrictor or vasodilator depending on concentration (Figs. 34–5 and 34–6).[25–27]

These vasoactive mediators may play a role either in causing or perpetuating the pulmonary hypertensive state. Pilot studies have suggested that pulmonary endothelial cell function is affected in infants and children after cardiopulmonary bypass; postoperative patients with congenital heart disease display decreased acetylcholine-induced vasodilation compared with controls (T. Giglia, personal communication). It is possible that the hypertensive pulmonary vascular bed, having been subjected to prolonged stretching and shearing forces, may have diminished production and responsiveness to endogenous vasodilators such as endothelium-derived relaxing factor (EDRF).[28–32] There is a substantial body of evidence from experiments in animals that EDRF deficiency contributes to the pathogenesis of hypertension in the systemic and pulmonary circulations. Interestingly, EDRF also has both antiproliferative and antiplatelet action; defective production or release of EDRF

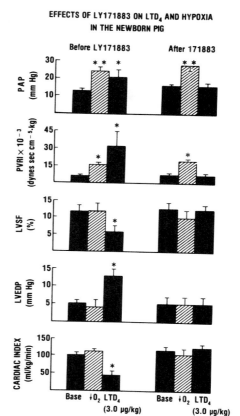

EFFECTS OF LY171883 ON LTD₄ AND HYPOXIA IN THE NEWBORN PIG

*p < 0.05 vs base; **p < 0.01 vs base

Figure 34–4. Effects of leukotriene D₄ on the newborn pulmonary circulation. Baseline values were calculated before the administration of 12% O_2, 88% N_2, and LTD_4 before and 60 minutes after injection of the leukotriene D_4 receptor antagonist, LY 171883. Values for ↓ O_2 were calculated after a 3-minute exposure to 12% O_2 and 88% N_2; values for LTD_4 were determined 1 minute after injection. Results are expressed as absolute values. * p < 0.05 versus baseline, ** = p < 0.01 versus baseline. (From Bradley LM, Feuerstein GF, and Goldstein RE: Leukotriene D_4 and Hypoxia: Differential effects on the pulmonary and systemic circulations in newborn piglets. Eicosanoids 2:15, 1989.)

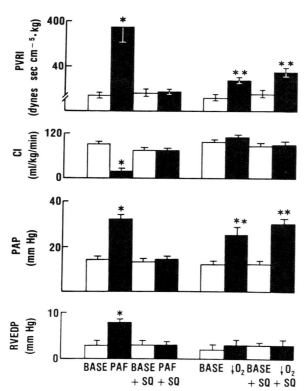

Figure 34–3. Influence of TxA₂ receptor antagonism on pulmonary vasoconstrictor responses to PAF-acether and hypoxia. Both PAF-acether 0.1 nmol/kg and hypoxia caused significant uses in pulmonary artery pressure (PAP) and PVRI when compared with baseline; PAF also caused RVEDP to increase and CI to decrease. TxA₂ receptor antagonism with SQ 29, 548 completely blocked PAF-induced pulmonary vasoconstriction; hypoxic pulmonary vasoconstrictor responses remained intact. Results are expressed as absolute values ± SEM. PVRI data are shown on a logarithmic scale × 10⁻³. *p < 0.05 versus BASE; ** p < 0.01 versus BASE + SQ. (From Bradley LM, Stambouly JJ, and Goldstein RE: Influence of thromboxane A₂ receptor antagonism on pulmonary vasoconstrictor responses. Pediatr Res 26:175, 1989.)

favors abnormal muscularization of small arteries as well as platelet deposition.

To optimize postoperative care in patients with increased pulmonary vascular reactivity, prolonged anesthesia with fentanyl and hyperventilation are useful.[33, 34] Continuous monitoring of both pulmonary arterial and left atrial pressure aids management. Hyperventilation, (Pco_2 25 to 30 mm Hg) adjusted to maintain pulmonary artery pressure equal to or less than half of systemic pressure, can be continued for several days. Ventilatory weaning is best done gradually to avoid the wide swings in airway pressure that can exacerbate increased PVR.[35] The use of intravenous prostacyclin is controversial, and its availability is quite limited.[36]

What constitutes optimal medical management of persistent pulmonary hypertension secondary to congenital heart disease remains unclear. The use of antiplatelet agents is clearly beneficial for patients with primary pulmonary hypertension.[37] Chronic prostacyclin therapy and calcium channel blockade may also prolong survival.[38, 39] Heart-lung transplantation may ultimately

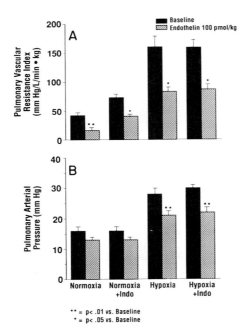

Figure 34–5. Effects of endothelin on mean pulmonary arterial pressure (PAP, B) and pulmonary vascular resistance index (PVRI, A) during nomoxia and hypoxia in control (n = 8) and indomethacin-pretreated (n = 6) piglets. Results are expressed as peak percent change from baseline. Low-dose endothelin (100 pmol/kg) caused mild decreases in PAP in both groups. High-dose endothelin (1,000 pmol/kg) produced a substantial rise in PAP in controls, an effect blocked by indomethacin pre-treatment. Low-dose endothelin also significantly decreased PVRI in both groups during nomoxia and hypoxia. Values are means ± SE. (From Bradley LM, Czaja JF, and Goldstein RE: Circulatory effects of endothelin in newborn piglets. Am J Physiol [Heart Circ Physiol] 28:H1613, 1990.)

be the treatment of choice for irreversible pulmonary hypertension.[40]

The mechanisms of pulmonary vascular changes are the subject of considerable research. Rabinovitch and associates have shown that the hypertensive endothelium is coarse and ridged compared with the normotensive endothelium (Fig. 34–7).[41] In addition to these ultrastructural changes, hypertensive pulmonary arteries have been found to produce abnormal von Willebrand factor and increased amounts of connective tissue proteins.[42] Whether or not hypertensive pulmonary arteries produce decreased amounts of EDRF or increased amounts of endothelin is unknown.

Congenital Heart Disease—Lesions with Decreased Pulmonary Blood Flow

Congenital heart lesions with diminished pulmonary blood flow may demonstrate increased PVR even after correction.[43] Pulmonary hypertension is seen in patients with pulmonary atresia with large systemic to pulmonary artery collaterals.[44] An assessment of the extent of pulmonary hypertension in these patients is often difficult to make. In such patients, the pulmonary arterial musculature is hypoplastic and the axial arteries are abnormally few and narrow.[45, 46]

The degree of elevation of PVR becomes important

particularly in the postoperative course of patients undergoing the Fontan operation. In this procedure, systemic venous blood is diverted directly into the pulmonary arteries without a ventricular pump. While the operative mortality rate remains low (<7%) for patients with tricuspid atresia, patients with complex congenital heart disease and a functional single ventricle carry higher operative risk.[47]

To maximize survival in these high-risk patients, the Fontan operation has been revised in several ways. Modifications of the operation include the use of a direct cavopulmonary connection and placement of a fenestration between the systemic and pulmonary venous chambers. The fenestration results in an atrial right-to-left shunt that can be hemodynamically advantageous in several ways: It allows cardiac output to be maintained (at the cost of oxygenation) in the presence of increased PVR; it increases left ventricular preload; and it prevents excessively high right atrial pressure. The fenestration can then be closed at a later date, either surgically or at cardiac catheterization with a clamshell double umbrella.

Hypoxic Pulmonary Vasoconstriction

The rise in PVR that occurs in response to acute hypoxia is frequently mild and rapidly reversible. An elegant study by Raj and Chen has demonstrated that both small arteries and veins are involved in the constrictor response to hypoxia.[48] In humans, PVR increases by approximately 50% when alveolar P_{O_2} falls to 50 mm Hg. As yet, no single vasoactive mediator has been

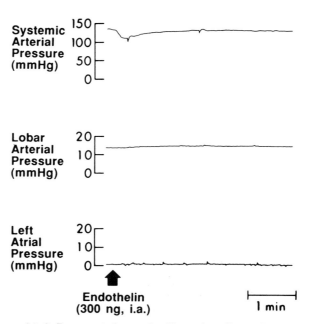

Figure 34–6. Representative tracing illustrating effects of endothelin on systemic arterial, lobar arterial, and left atrial pressures under conditions of resting pulmonary vasomotor tone in cats. Endothelin was injected as bolus into the left lobar artery. (From Lippton HL, Nauth TA, Summer WR, et al: Endothelin produces pulmonary vasoconstriction and systemic vasodilation. J Appl Physiol 66[2]:1008, 1989. With permission from the American Physiological Society.)

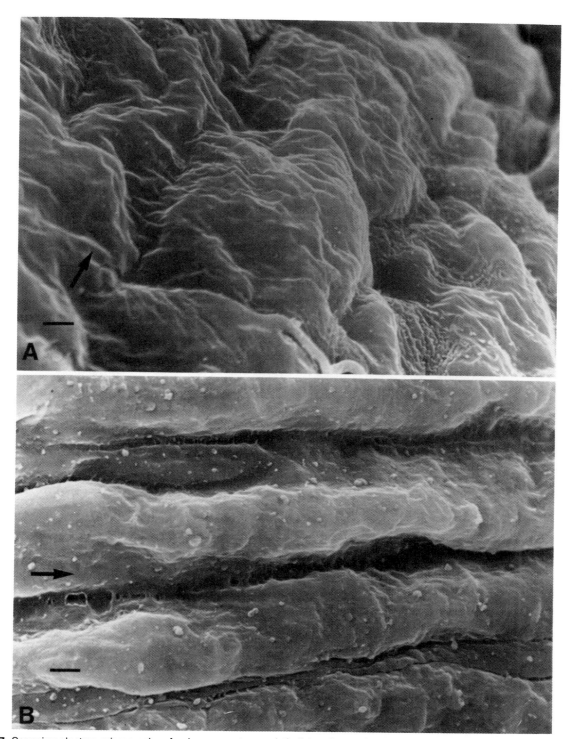

Figure 34–7. Scanning electron micrographs of pulmonary artery endothelial surfaces. *A*, Normal pulmonary artery shows "corduroy pattern," closely aligned ridges. *B*, Hypertensive pulmonary artery shows "cable" pattern, deep knotted ridges and numerous microvilli (mv). (Magnification × 810.) (From Rabinovitch M, Bothwell T, Hayakawa BN, et al: Pulmonary artery endothelial abnormalities in patients with congenital heart defects and pulmonary hypertension: A correlation of light with scanning electron microscopy and transmission electron microscopy. Lab Invest 55:632, 1986. © by the U.S. and Canadian Academy of Pathology, Inc.)

proved responsible for acute hypoxic vasoconstriction. Histamine, serotonin, norepinephrine, and the vasoconstrictor prostaglandins do not mediate the hypoxia-induced rise in PVR. The role of leukotrienes remains controversial.[50–52]

Thromboembolic Pulmonary Hypertension

The accurate diagnosis of thromboembolic disease depends on the clinician's index of suspicion. It is important to be aware of the disorders that predispose patients to develop pulmonary thromboemboli. Such diseases include sickle cell anemia,[53] hydrocephalus with ventriculoatrial shunts,[54] sepsis and right-sided endocarditis,[55] and portal or renal vein thrombosis. Fat emboli may occur in the setting of trauma as well as in patients with collagen vascular disease.[56] Tumor emboli from the abdominal organs as well as from the right heart are also occasional sources of pulmonary emboli.[57]

Acute pulmonary embolism can produce circulatory failure through a variety of mechanisms. Mechanical blockage of the pulmonary artery abruptly increases right ventricular afterload, resulting in right ventricular failure, diminished left ventricular preload, and shock. Massive release of inflammatory mediators from activated leukocytes and platelets serves to maintain profound pulmonary vasoconstriction.

All pulmonary emboli are associated with low-output states, hypoxia, and hypercarbia. If an indwelling pulmonary artery catheter is present, aspiration may demonstrate air or fat. The diagnosis of pulmonary embolism is best established with a lung perfusion scan. Therapy is directed toward hemodynamic and ventilatory support, prevention of further embolization, and removal of emboli. Optimal treatment depends on the underlying disease and on the localization and distribution of emboli. Standard medical management involves systemic anticoagulation for 5 to 7 days. Patients are loaded with heparin (50 units/kg intravenous bolus) and placed on a maintenance infusion of heparin (10 to 25 units/kg/hr), adjusting the dose to give a clotting time of 20 to 30 minutes or a partial thromboplastin of 1½ to two times the control value. Oral anticoagulants are generally started within 48 hours of diagnosis of pulmonary emboli. Chronic therapy is recommended for 3 to 6 months. In patients with relative contraindications to anticoagulation (i.e., intracranial hemorrhage), prevention of recurrent embolization can be accomplished with the placement of filters in the inferior vena cava. In patients for whom there is no clear predisposing etiology, a hematologic work-up for hypercoagulable states (e.g., protein C, protein S) should be conducted 3 to 6 months after the acute illness.

Collagen Vascular Disease

Pulmonary hypertension can occur in almost all forms of collagen vascular disease.[58] Systemic lupus erythematosus, juvenile rheumatoid arthritis, scleroderma, dermatomyositis, and Takayasu arteritis are all associated with the development of pulmonary hypertension. The etiology of elevated PVR in collagen vascular disease is variable: Some patients have advanced interstitial lung disease with secondary reduction in pulmonary vascular cross-sectional area, whereas others have little parenchymal disease but advanced vasculitis.

Primary Pulmonary Hypertension

Idiopathic or primary pulmonary hypertension always involves a structural abnormality in either the arteries or veins. There are three pathologically distinct types of primary pulmonary hypertension: plexogenic pulmonary arteriopathy, recurrent thromboembolism, and pulmonary veno-occlusive disease. Primary pulmonary hypertension can occur in families. In childhood, males and females are equally affected. The diagnosis is usually made in the first year of life.

The disease progresses rapidly and is generally fatal. Different series report a mean PVR ranging from 15 to 21 Wood units/m² at the time of diagnosis. Treatment has been uniformly disappointing.[59] Patients in whom intravenous prostacyclin produces a decrease in pulmonary artery pressure may benefit from oral prostacyclin.[60] Other treatments that have been useful for selected patients include oxygen administered at home, hydralazine, and calcium channel blockers.[61, 62]

References

1. Felman AH: Abnormal lung bud development. In: Felman AH (ed): The Pediatric Chest, 1st ed. Springfield, Charles C Thomas, 1983, pp. 32–52.
2. Morgan JR and Forker AD: Syndrome of hypoplasia of the right lung and dextroposition of the heart; "scimitar sign." Circulation 43:27, 1971.
3. Moyer JH, Glantz G, and Brest AN: Pulmonary arteriovenous fistulas. Am J Med 32:417, 1962.
4. Jimenez MQ and Guillen FA: Arteriovenous fistulas. In: Moss AJ and Adams FH (eds): Heart Disease in Infants, Children, and Adolescents, 4th ed. Baltimore, Williams & Wilkins, 1989.
5. Barth KH, White RI, and Kaufman SL: Embolotherapy of pulmonary arteriovenous malformations with detachable balloons. Radiology 142:599, 1982.
6. Rabinovitch M: Pulmonary hypertension. In: Moss AJ and Adams FH (eds): Heart Disease in Infants, Children, and Adolescents, 3rd ed. Baltimore, Williams & Wilkins, 1983, pp. 669–692.
7. Hoffman JIE, Rudolph AM, and Heymann MA: Pulmonary vascular disease with congenital heart lesions: Pathologic features and causes. Circulation 64:873, 1981.
8. Newfeld EA, Paul MH, and Muster AJ: Pulmonary vascular disease in complete transposition of the great arteries: A study of 200 patients. Am J Cardiol 34:75, 1974.
9. Newfeld EA, Sher M, and Paul MH: Pulmonary vascular disease in complete atrioventricular canal defect. Am J Cardiol 39:721, 1977.
10. Cooney TP and Thurlbeck WM: Pulmonary hypoplasia in Down syndrome. N Engl J Med 307:1170, 1982.
11. Juneda E and Haworth SG: Pulmonary vascular disease in children with truncus arteriosus. Br Heart J 52:1314, 1984.
12. Vogel JHK, McNamara DC, and Blount SG Jr: Role of hypoxia in determining pulmonary vascular resistance in infants with ventricular septal defect. Am J Cardiol 20:346, 1967.
13. Rosenthal AM, Nathan DJ, and Marty AT: Acute hemodynamic

effects of red cell volume reduction in polycythemia of cyanotic congenital heart disease. Circulation 42:297, 1970.

14. Nihill MR and McNamara DG: Magnification pulmonary wedge angiography in the evaluation of children with congenital heart disease and pulmonary hypertension. Circulation 58:1094, 1978.

15. Rabinovitch M, Keane JF, and Fellows KE: Quantitative analysis of the pulmonary wedge angiogram in congenital heart defects: Correlation of hemodynamic data and morphometric findings in lung biopsy tissue. Circulation 63:152, 1981.

16. Biggar WD, Bohn DJ, and Kent G: Neutrophil migration in vitro and in vivo during hypothermia. Infect Immun 46:857, 1984.

17. Faymonville ME, Debry-Dupont G, and Larbuisson R: Prostaglandin E_2, prostacyclin, and thromboxane changes during nonpulsatile cardiopulmonary bypass. J Thorac Cardiovasc Surg 91:858, 1986.

18. Fleming WH, Sarafian LB, and Leuschen MP: Serum concentrations of thromboxane and prostacyclin in children before, during, and after cardiopulmonary bypass. J Thorac Cardiovasc Surg 92:73, 1986.

19. Oates JA: The 1982 Nobel Prize in Physiology on Medicine. Science 218:765, 1982.

20. Yokochi K, Olley PM, and Sideris E: Leukotriene D_4: A potent vasoconstrictor of the pulmonary and systemic circulation in the newborn lamb. In: Samuelsson B (ed): Leukotrienes and other Lipoxygenase Products, 1st ed. New York, Raven Press, 1982, pp. 214–221.

21. Bradley LM, Goldstein RE, and Feuerstein G: Circulatory effects of PAF-acether in newborn piglets. Am J Physiol 256 (Heart Circ Physiol 25):H202, 1989.

22. Bradley LM, Stambouly JJ, and Czaja JF: Influence of thromboxane A_2 receptor antagonism on pulmonary vasoconstrictor responses. Pediatr Res 26:175, 1989.

23. Voelkel NF, Worthen S, and Reeves JT: Non-immunological production of leukotrienes by platelet activating factor. Science 218:286, 1982.

24. Caplan MS, Sun X, and Hageman JR: Platelet activating factor is elevated in persistent pulmonary hypertension of the newborn. Pediatr Res 25:305A, 1989.

25. Vane JR, Anggard EE, and Botting RM: Regulatory functions of the vascular endothelium. N Engl J Med 323:27, 1990.

26. Lippton HL, Hauth TA, and Summer WR: Endothelia produces pulmonary vasoconstriction and systemic vasodilation. J Appl Physiol 66(2):1008, 1989.

27. Bradley LM, Czaja JF, and Goldstein RE: Circulatory effects of endothelin in newborn piglets. Am J Physiol 259 (Heart Circ Physiol 28):H1613, 1990.

28. Panza JA, Quyyum AA, and Brush JE: Abnormal endothelium dependent vascular relation in patients with hypertension. N Engl J Med 323:22, 1990.

29. Moore P, Velmis H, and Heymann MA: The effects of EDRF inhibition on resting pulmonary vascular tone in fetal lambs. Pediatr Res 29:245A, 1991.

30. Cornfield DN, Chatfield BA, McMurtry IF, and Abman SH: Effects of EDRF inhibition on the fetal pulmonary vascular response to partial compression of the ductus arteriosus. Pediatr Res 29:311A, 1991.

31. Furchgott RF: Role of endothelium in vascular responses of smooth muscle. Circ Res 53:557, 1983.

32. Vanhoutte PM, Rubyanyi GM, and Miller VM: Modulation of vascular smooth muscle contraction by the endothelium. Ann Rev Physiol 48:962, 1986.

33. Hickey PR, Hansen DD, and Wessel DL: Pulmonary and systemic hemodynamic responses to fentanyl in infants. Anesth Analg 64:483, 1985.

34. Hickey PR, Hansen DD, and Wessel DL: Blunting of stress responses in the pulmonary circulation in infants with fentanyl. Anesth Analg 64:1137, 1985.

35. Fuhrman BP, Smith-Wright DL, and Kulik TJ: Effects of static and fluctuating airway pressure on intact pulmonary circulation. J Appl Physiol 60:114, 1986.

36. Friedman WF: Proceedings of National Heart, Lung and Blood Institute Pediatric Cardiology Workshop: Pulmonary Hypertension. Pediatr Res 20:811, 1986.

37. Fuster V, Steele PM, and Edwards WD: Primary pulmonary hypertension natural history and the importance of thrombosis. Circulation 70:580, 1984.

38. Brownlee JR, Beckman RH, and Rosenthal A: Acute hemodynamic effects of nifedipine in infants with pulmonary hypertension. Pediatr Res 24:186, 1988.

39. Higgenbottam T: The place of prostacyclin in the clinical management of primary pulmonary hypertension. Am Rev Respir Dis 136:782, 1987.

40. Fricker FJ, Griffith BP, and Hardesty RL: Experience with heart transplantation in children. Pediatrics 79:138, 1987.

41. Rabinovitch M, Bothwell T, and Hayakawa BN: Pulmonary artery endothelial abnormalities in patients with congenital heart defects and pulmonary hypertension: A correlation of light with scanning electron microscopy and transmission electron microscopy. Lab Invest 55:632, 1986.

42. Rabinovitch M, Andrew M, and Thom H: Abnormal endothelial factor VIII associated with pulmonary hypertension and congenital heart defects. Circulation 76:1043, 1987.

43. Pulmonary arterial hypertension after repair of tetralogy of Fallot. J Thorac Cardiovasc Surg 67:110, 1974.

44. Haworth SG, Rees PG, and Taylor JF: Pulmonary atresia with ventricular septal defect and major aortopulmonary collaterals. Br Heart J 45:133, 1981.

45. Rabinovitch M, Herrera-DeLeon V, and Castaneda AR: Growth and development of the pulmonary vascular bed in patients with tetralogy of Fallot with or without pulmonary atresia. Circulation 64:1234, 1978.

46. Haworth SG and Macartney FJ: Growth and development of the pulmonary circulation in pulmonary atresia. Br Heart J 44:14, 1980.

47. Gale AW, Danielson GK, and McGoon DC: Fontan procedure for tricuspid atresia. Circulation 62:91, 1980.

48. Raj UJ and Chen P: Role of eicosanoids in hypoxia vasoconstriction in isolated lamb lungs. Am J Physiol 253:H626, 1987.

49. Tucker A, Weir EK, and Reeves JT: Failure of histamine antagonists to prevent hypoxic pulmonary vasoconstriction in dogs. J Appl Physiol 40:496, 1976.

50. Morganroth ML, Reeves JT, and Murphy RC: Leukotriene synthesis and receptor blockers block hypoxic pulmonary vasoconstriction. J Appl Physiol 56:1340, 1984.

51. Bradley LM, Feuerstein G, and Goldstein RE: Leukotriene D_4 and hypoxia: Differential effects in the pulmonary and systemic circulations in newborn piglets. Eicosanoids 2:15, 1989.

52. Voelkel NF, Worthen S, and Reeves JT: Non-immunological production of leukotrienes induced by platelet activating factor. Science 218:286, 1982.

53. Moser KM and Shea JG: The relationship between pulmonary infarction, cor pulmonale, and sickle cell states. Am J Med 22:561, 1957.

54. Noonan JA and Ehmke DA: Complications of ventriculoatrial shunts for control of hydrocephalus: Report of 3 cases with thromboembolism to the lung. N Engl J Med 269:70, 1963.

55. Newburger JW and Nadas AS: Infective endocarditis. Pediatr Rev 3:226, 1982.

56. Nair SS, Askart AD, and Popelka CG: Pulmonary hypertension and systemic lupus erythematosus. Arch Intern Med 140:109, 1980.

57. Fyke FE, Seward JB, and Edwards WD: Primary cardiac tumors: Experience with 30 consecutive patients since the introduction of 2-dimensional echocardiography. J Am Coll Cardiol 5:1465, 1985.

58. Ammann AJ and Wara DW: Collagen vascular diseases. In: Rudolph Am (ed): Pediatrics, 17th ed. E. Norwalk, CT, Appleton-Century-Crofts, 1982, pp. 431–439.

59. Haworth SG: Primary pulmonary hypertension. Br Heart J 49:517, 1983.

60. Barst RJ: Pharmacologically induced pulmonary vasodilation in children and young adults with primary pulmonary hypertension. Chest 89:497, 1986.

61. Rich S and Brundage BH: High dose calcium channel-blocking therapy for primary pulmonary hypertension: Evidence for long term reduction in pulmonary arterial pressure and regression of right ventricular hypertrophy. Circulation 76:135, 1987.

62. Rich S, Dantzker DR, and Ayers SM: Primary pulmonary hypertension: A national prospective study. Ann Intern Med 107:216, 1987.

Acquired Heart Disease

Philip Moore, M.D., and Scott J. Soifer, M.D.

Acquired heart disease is much less common in children than is congenital heart disease. Cardiac dysfunction resulting from infection, autoimmune-mediated injury, systemic illnesses, or infiltrative processes can lead to significant morbidity and mortality. This chapter focuses on the common acquired heart diseases of children (Kawasaki disease, myocarditis, infectious endocarditis, pericarditis, acute rheumatic fever, and cardiomyopathy), which frequently necessitate diagnosis and treatment in the pediatric intensive care unit.

KAWASAKI DISEASE

Kawasaki disease, an acute febrile exanthematous illness with multisystem organ involvement, was first described in Japan in 1967.[1, 2] Although the extent of cardiac involvement is variable, it remains the leading cause of acquired ischemic heart disease in children, causing significant morbidity and mortality.

Epidemiology. Kawasaki disease affects infants and children, with a peak incidence at 9 to 12 months of age in Japan and 3 years of age in the United States.[3, 4] There appears to be no definite seasonal pattern and no predisposing factors.

Pathophysiology. Kawasaki disease causes an acute vasculitis of medium-sized arteries, small arterioles, and venules throughout the body, with a predilection for the coronary vessels.[5] Initially, there is acute inflammation of the arterioles and venules, which peaks within 10 days of illness and resolves within 25 days, causing no permanent damage. The vasculitis of the coronary arteries peaks at 12 to 20 days after the onset of illness and may cause aneurysm formation, severe stenosis from granulating thrombi, or scar formation with calcification. The myocardium shows involvement in approximately 40 to 60% of cases, with myocellular hypertrophy, degeneration of myocytes, and endocardial changes that lead to myocarditis and decreased cardiac function.[6]

There are three clinical stages of Kawasaki disease. The first stage is an acute febrile period of 5 to 14 days; the second stage is a subacute period of 2 to 6 weeks, during which there may be further multisystem involvement; and the third stage is a convalescent phase, during which recovery occurs (Table 35–1).[7] During these stages, cardiac manifestations include mild to moderate

congestive heart failure from either myocarditis or ischemia, left ventricular dilatation with mitral insufficiency, and pericardial effusion. Arrhythmias may occur, including first- or second-degree atrioventricular (AV) block, a prolonged QT interval, abnormal ST-T segments, and low R wave amplitude. Late cardiac manifestations include coronary artery aneurysms, coronary artery stenosis, and myocardial ischemia or infarction. The incidence of coronary artery aneurysm varies between 20 and 50%. Aneurysms usually form after 2 weeks, with the majority resolving by 6 to 12 months. Eight per cent of patients with coronary aneurysms experience coronary stenosis. Right coronary artery stenosis is relatively benign compared with left coronary artery stenosis, which has a high incidence of producing myocardial infarction and death.[8] Two to 4% of patients with Kawasaki disease die of cardiac involvement. Most deaths occur between the 10th and 29th days of illness. Early deaths result from myocarditis or arrhythmias, whereas late deaths are caused by ischemia from coronary artery involvement.

Diagnosis. The diagnosis of Kawasaki disease is based on the presence of certain clinical criteria, but it remains a diagnosis of exclusion (Table 35–2). The presence of prolonged fever plus four of the remaining five criteria listed in the table, without evidence of another known disease, is required to establish the diagnosis. Typical laboratory findings include an elevated erythrocyte sedimentation rate, leukocytosis, thrombocytosis, a mild normochromic and normocytic anemia, and proteinuria. An echocardiogram is the standard for evaluating coronary artery involvement and cardiac function and should be performed by day 7 or earlier if clinically indicated. Serial echocardiograms should be performed every 6 months until (1) there has been no evidence of coronary artery involvement for 2 years or (2) the coronary artery aneurysms are stable, showing no regression (Fig. 35–1).

Treatment. Because of insufficient knowledge about the cause and pathogenesis of Kawasaki disease, treatment remains nonspecific and controversial. Antibiotic therapy has not been shown to shorten the acute febrile period or to prevent long-term complications. Similarly, neither has low-dose aspirin or steroids. However, high-dose aspirin (100 mg/kg/day) during the acute febrile phase has been shown to decrease the duration of fever,

Table 35–1. THE INCIDENCE OF COMMON SYMPTOMS AND ORGAN SYSTEM INVOLVEMENT DURING THE ACUTE STAGES OF KAWASAKI DISEASE

Symptom	Incidence (%)
Carditis	50
Coronary involvement	50 (no treatment)
	20 (treatment)
Conduction system abnormalities	30–50
Diarrhea	40
Arthritis	30
Aseptic meningitis	25
Urethritis	25
Hepatitis	Rare
Hydrops of the gallbladder	Rare

improve comfort, and decrease the formation of coronary artery aneurysms.[10]

High-dose intravenous gamma globulin, 400 mg/kg/day for 4 consecutive days, given during the acute febrile phase reduces fever and laboratory signs of inflammation, and decreases the incidence of coronary artery aneurysm formation.[11] The optimal dose and duration of treatment remain unclear and are currently under study.

Aspirin (3 to 5 mg/kg/day) and other antiplatelet aggregating drugs, such as dipyridamole (5 mg/kg/day), are used to prevent coronary artery thrombosis and myocardial infarction in patients with Kawasaki disease. Patients without coronary artery abnormalities should be treated for 2 years, whereas patients with coronary artery abnormalities should be treated for life. In patients with giant aneurysms, both aspirin and dipyridamole are used (Table 35–3).

Treatment of severe complications of Kawasaki disease remains supportive. Congestive heart failure is treated with diuretics, inotropic support and, if severe, positive pressure ventilation. Symptomatic ventricular arrhythmias are treated with lidocaine. Evidence of acute myocardial ischemia or infarction or echocardiographic findings of coronary thrombosis warrant further evaluation with selective coronary artery angiography and treatment with thrombolytic agents. The latter consists of the intravenous infusion of tissue plasminogen activator (1.25 mg/kg over 30 minutes) or streptokinase (21,000 units/kg over 1 hour) followed by an infusion of heparin to keep the partial thromboplastin time one and one-half to two times the control value. If angiography shows evidence of left main coronary artery stenosis or high-grade stenosis in two or more major coronary arteries, coronary artery bypass surgery should be considered.

Table 35–2. CLINICAL CRITERIA FOR THE DIAGNOSIS OF KAWASAKI DISEASE

Fever, >5 days' duration (spiking 101–104° F)
Rash, generalized erythematous
Edema-erythema, of hands and feet, with periungual desquamation
Conjunctivitis, bilateral
Stomatitis, typically fissuring of lips or strawberry tongue
Lymphadenitis, nonsuppurative cervical node >1.5 cm

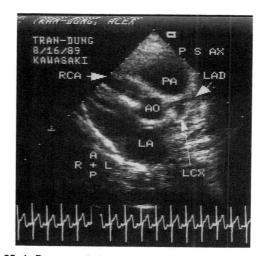

Figure 35–1. Parasternal short-axis echocardiogram of a 3-year-old child with Kawasaki disease. Note the size of the proximal right coronary artery aneurysm as compared with the left main coronary artery. AO = aorta; LA = left atrium; LAD = left anterior descending coronary artery; LCX = left circumflex coronary artery; PA = pulmonary artery; RCA = right coronary artery.

MYOCARDITIS

Myocarditis is an inflammation of the heart that may produce decreased cardiac performance and, if severe, congestive heart failure and death. Myocarditis is usually caused by a viral infection, but it may be secondary to systemic illness (Table 35–4). Because of the high incidence of life-threatening sequelae, many children with myocarditis will require treatment in the pediatric intensive care unit.

Viral Myocarditis

Epidemiology. Myocarditis is a common disease that has been documented in 4% of autopsies in adults and

Table 35–3. TREATMENT REGIMEN FOR KAWASAKI DISEASE

Acute Phase	
Aspirin	100 mg/kg/day PO* × 7–14 days
Gamma globulin	400 mg/kg/day IV† × 4 days
Antiplatelet	
Aspirin	5 mg/kg/day PO (begin following high dose)
Dipyridamole	5 mg/kg PO divided bid‡
Thrombolytic	
Tissue plasminogen activator (r-TPA)	1.25 mg/kg IV over 30 minutes
OR	
streptokinase	21,000 units/kg IV over 1 hour (premedicate with hydrocortisone and diphenhydramine)
AND	
heparin	50 units/kg IV load followed by 12–25 units/kg/hr, maintaining PTT§ 1.5–2 × control

*PO = by mouth.
†IV = intravenously.
‡bid = twice daily.
§PTT = partial thromboplastin time.

Table 35–4. CAUSES OF MYOCARDITIS

Infections	Toxin
Coxsackie virus B and A	Scorpion bites
Influenza A and B	
Echovirus	**Drugs**
Mumps	Sulfonamides
Rubella	Phenylbutazone
Varicella zoster	Cyclophosphamide
Herpes	Acetozolamide
Diphtheria	Amphotericin B
	Indomethacin
Systemic Illnesses	Tetracycline
Rheumatoid arthritis	Isoniazid
Systemic lupus erythematosus	Methyldopa
Rheumatic fever	Phenytoin
Ulcerative colitis	Penicillin
Scleroderma	
Polymyositis	
Dermatomyositis	
Sarcoidosis	

7% of autopsies in children.[12] In autopsy studies, the incidence of acute or previous myocarditis is 25%.[13, 14] However, only 0.3% of all patients seen by pediatric cardiologists have clinical evidence of myocarditis. This discrepancy between the clinical findings and the autopsy findings is due to a large percentage of asymptomatic or subclinical cases.

There are a wide variety of infectious agents that cause myocarditis, with coxsackievirus B serotypes 1 to 6 being the most common. Of 228 cases of suspected myocarditis, 41% were caused by coxsackievirus B.[15] Between 5 and 12% of children infected with either coxsackievirus B or influenza viruses will acquire clinical myocarditis.[16, 17] Myocarditis will develop in 20% of neonates with congenital rubella,[18] 6% of children with varicella zoster,[19] and 40% of children with infectious mononucleosis. The incidence of myocarditis is highest in children less than 1 year of age.

Pathophysiology. The mechanism of tissue injury in myocarditis has been studied in humans and in animal models. Tissue injury results from direct destruction of myofibers by the virus, cytotoxic T cell destruction of myocytes, and possibly antibody complement–mediated destruction of noninfected cells.

The gross pathologic findings are nonspecific. The heart is pale and flabby with mild to moderate dilatation of the left ventricle and petechial hemorrhages on the epicardial surface. Microscopically, there is a patchy focal or diffuse interstitial infiltrate of lymphocytes, plasma cells, and eosinophils, occasionally extending to the perivascular areas. In severe cases, edema and necrosis of the myocardium are seen.

These inflammatory and necrotic changes in the myocardium decrease cardiac function. Cardiac dilatation leads to increased left ventricular end-diastolic volume and mitral insufficiency. This results in increased left ventricular end-diastolic pressure, which is transmitted through the left atrium to the pulmonary veins, causing elevated pulmonary venous pressure and pulmonary edema. In autopsy cases of children with myocarditis, 33% had clinical evidence of pulmonary edema and congestive heart failure.[12] The inflammatory changes of the heart also involve the conducting system, producing arrhythmias and conduction abnormalities. Paroxysmal atrial tachycardia, complete AV block, premature ventricular contractions, and ventricular tachycardia occur and contribute to the 15% incidence of sudden death in children with myocarditis[12] (see also Chapter 36). Mortality rates vary from 75% of newborns to 10 to 25% of older children with coxsackievirus B myocarditis.[20]

As healing occurs, necrotic myocytes are replaced with scar tissue, decreasing cardiac elasticity and causing permanent impairment of ventricular function. This, together with ongoing immunologically mediated myocardial injury, may produce idiopathic dilated cardiomyopathy.[21, 22] Persistent congestive heart failure may occur.

Diagnosis. The clinical presentation of patients with myocarditis varies from those who are asymptomatic to those who progress to fulminant congestive heart failure and death. Typically, newborns and young infants are more critically ill than are older children. In newborns, the onset of symptoms is sudden.[20] Lethargy, fever, tachycardia out of proportion to the fever, respiratory distress, cyanosis, and vomiting may be present. In older children, the symptoms are less severe and include fever, malaise, myalgia, gastroenteritis, pleurodynia, pharyngitis, and meningitis. The cardiac examination typically shows tachycardia and a thready pulse. The heart sounds are soft if a pericardial effusion is present. In severe cases, a gallop rhythm is heard. Frequently, a high-frequency blowing pansystolic murmur is present; this murmur is loudest at the apex and is caused by mitral regurgitation.

Various laboratory studies should be performed to confirm the diagnosis of myocarditis. Typical laboratory findings include an elevated white blood cell count without leftward shift, an elevated erythrocyte sedimentation rate, abnormal liver function tests, elevated levels of lactate dehydrogenase isoenzyme 1, and an elevated creatine phosphokinase MB fraction. A blood culture specimen should be obtained to rule out bacterial infection. Nasopharyngeal and stool cultures for viral isolation should also be performed. The classic electrocardiographic findings of myocarditis include low QRS voltages, low or inverted T waves, and decreased or absent Q waves in leads V_5 and V_6. More importantly, the electrocardiogram (ECG) can detect life-threatening arrhythmias. An echocardiogram is useful in myocarditis to evaluate cardiac function and to detect pericardial effusions. Typically the left ventricle is mildly dilated, with increased left ventricular end-systolic and end-diastolic dimensions.[23] The left ventricular free wall may have asymmetric motion or there may be global myocardial depression.

Endomyocardial biopsy is the "gold standard" for the diagnosis of myocarditis. Three or more samples are taken from the right ventricular apex and septum, using a myocardial bioptome introduced into the internal jugular or femoral veins. The specimens are examined by both light and electron microscopy and recently by in situ hybridization of complementary nucleotide sequences to viral ribonucleic acid (RNA).[24] Because of the patchy nature of the inflammation, however, a normal biopsy result does not exclude the diagnosis. In fact, up to 30% of patients with clinical evidence of myocarditis have normal biopsy results.[25, 26] Recently, ^{67}Ga nuclear medicine imaging has been used to detect active inflammation in the heart. This may be useful in directing the location for biopsy.[27]

Treatment. Treatment of children with myocarditis remains supportive (Table 35–5). Animal studies have shown that exercise during the acute phase of myocarditis increases intramyocardial viral replication and worsens outcome.[28] Supplemental oxygen to maintain adequate oxygen delivery in the face of congestive heart failure with pulmonary edema is essential. Diuretic therapy, inotropic support, and afterload reduction may all be necessary (see Chapter 29). During the acute inflammatory stage, the heart may be overly sensitive to digoxin-induced arrhythmias; therefore, careful monitoring is essential.

Because arrhythmias can be life-threatening, they should be treated aggressively. Supraventricular tachycardia should be treated with digoxin, whereas ventricular arrhythmias should be treated with lidocaine. Second- or third-degree AV block should be treated with a temporary pacemaker, which should be converted to a permanent pacemaker electively if the AV block persists longer than 2 weeks.

Nonsteroidal anti-inflammatory agents have been shown to increase mortality in animals with myocarditis and are, therefore, contraindicated. The use of more powerful anti-inflammatory agents, such as prednisone or cyclosporine, is more controversial. Animal studies have shown either worsening myocardial necrosis or no effect with these agents.[29–31] However, several nonrandomized human studies have suggested a benefit. These studies are difficult to interpret. First, 45 to 50% of the patients with myocarditis improve spontaneously.[32] Second, though 60% of patients with biopsy-proven myocarditis treated with steroids improved,[21] only 1 of 21 patients with rapidly progressive myocarditis improved,

whereas 21 of 22 patients with low-grade inflammation improved. There is an ongoing multicenter randomized trial evaluating the efficacy of conventional therapy versus conventional therapy plus cyclosporine and prednisone. Currently there are not enough data to support the use of steroids or cyclosporine in children with myocarditis. Several experimental treatments, including the use of interferon[33] and FLM 5011, an inhibitor of the 5′-lipoxygenase pathway of the arachidonic acid cascade, are showing promise.[34]

Noninfectious Causes of Myocarditis

Myocarditis also occurs in a number of systemic diseases (including systemic lupus erythematosus and juvenile rheumatoid arthritis) and after exposure to toxins and drugs (see Table 35–4).

Systemic Lupus Erythematosus

Although 40 to 50% of patients with systemic lupus erythematosus (SLE) acquire symptoms of cardiac disease, most commonly pericarditis, only 8% experience clinical signs of myocarditis, and 20% show microscopic evidence at autopsy.[35] Even in asymptomatic patients, SLE causes abnormalities in ventricular function, including elevated right and left ventricular end-diastolic pressures, elevated left ventricular end-systolic volume, and decreased ejection fraction.[36]

The mechanism of tissue injury is unknown.[37] It has been proposed that either antiheart antibodies or immune complex deposition leading to complement activation causes small coronary vessel vasculitis, focal inflammation and, eventually, myocardial necrosis.[37, 38]

There are many symptoms specific to SLE.[39, 40] However, the signs and symptoms and the ECG and echocardiographic findings of SLE myocarditis are nonspecific, similar to those described for viral myocarditis. In addition to these symptoms, a blowing apical pansystolic murmur of mitral regurgitation may be heard; however, it is most often due to valvular vegetations (Libman-Sacks endocarditis). Laboratory findings include low C3 and C4 complement levels. Treatment includes the use of diuretics, inotropic agents, and steroid therapy (if viral myocarditis can be excluded).

Juvenile Rheumatoid Arthritis

As with SLE, pericarditis is the most common manifestation of juvenile rheumatoid arthritis (JRA). However, myocarditis occurs in approximately 10% of patients.[41] The cause is unknown, but it is presumed to involve the deposition of immune complexes in the small coronary vessels. Even patients with JRA without cardiac symptoms demonstrate abnormalities on the echocardiogram, suggesting depressed myocardial function.[41] The signs and symptoms of JRA myocarditis are similar to those in viral myocarditis, and the diagnosis can be made only by their association with an exacerbation of JRA. Therapy includes vigorous diuresis and the use of

---

Table 35–5. CURRENT TREATMENT REGIMEN FOR MYOCARDITIS

Bed rest during the acute phase (7–14 days)
  O₂ supplementation to maintain normal arterial oxygen saturation
  Supportive treatment of mild congestive heart failure
    Diuresis with furosemide 1 mg/kg/dose PO* bid† to qid‖
    Add spironolactone 1 mg/kg/dose PO bid, if furosemide given three or more times daily
    Digoxin 30 μg/kg load given in three doses every 8 hr, followed by 10 μg/kg/day PO divided bid
  Supportive treatment for severe congestive heart failure
    If hypotensive and poor perfusion: 5–10 ml/kg IV‡ bolus of 5% albumin or packed red blood cells
    Furosemide 1 mg/kg/dose IV tid§ to qid
    Dopamine 5–15 μg/kg/min IV
    If more inotropic support required: dobutamine 10–20 μg/kg/min IV with reduction in dopamine dose
    If adequate systemic blood pressure: nitroprusside 0.5–5 μg/kg/min IV

*PO = by mouth.
†bid = twice daily.
‡IV = intravenous.
§tid = three times daily.
‖qid = four times daily.

high-dose steroids. The clinical response to steroids occurs within 12 to 48 hours.[42]

INFECTIOUS ENDOCARDITIS

Infectious endocarditis is an inflammatory process of a cardiac valve, mural endocardium, or vascular endothelium resulting from infection with bacteria, viruses, or fungi. Because of the high rate of severe sequelae and an increasing incidence within the pediatric population, it has become a common cause for admission to the pediatric intensive care unit.

Epidemiology. The overall incidence of infectious endocarditis in adults has decreased over the last decade, but it has increased in children.[43–45] This is secondary to the increased survival and life expectancy of children after cardiac surgery. More than 50% of cases occur in children older than 10 years of age. There has also been a marked increase in the incidence of infectious endocarditis in neonates secondary to the increased use of indwelling catheters for nutritional and pharmacologic support.[46]

Risk factors for infectious endocarditis include congenital heart disease, with the exception of a secundum atrial septal defect; rheumatic heart disease; previous cardiac surgery, especially if a prosthetic valve, synthetic shunt, or patch material was used; and intravenous drug use. The most common congenital defects associated with infectious endocarditis are tetralogy of Fallot, ventricular septal defect, aortic stenosis, patent ductus arteriosus, and pulmonary stenosis. The lifetime risk for infectious endocarditis has been estimated to be 10% for patients with ventricular septal defect, 1.4% for patients with aortic stenosis, and 0.9% for patients with pulmonary stenosis. Approximately 17 to 23% of patients who acquire infectious endocarditis will have no risk factors.[45, 47]

Pathophysiology. Two conditions lead to infectious endocarditis in most cases. The first is bacteremia, which is most commonly associated with dental or surgical procedures (Table 35–6). The second is the presence of a defect of the heart or great vessels associated with turbulent blood flow that produces endothelial damage and initiates platelet and fibrin deposition, causing the formation of a nonbacterial thrombotic vegetation. During transient bacteremia, microorganisms become trapped within the platelet, fibrin, and thrombus meshwork, leading to colonization and eventually infection of the vegetation.

In the subacute form of infectious endocarditis, caused by *Streptococcus viridans*, large colonies of bacteria grow, with constant seeding of the blood stream. The bacteria become encased in an organizing mass of fibrin, cellular debris, and leukocytes, which may protect the bacteria from invasion by phagocytic leukocytes and circulating antimicrobial agents, making sterilization difficult. Large vegetations may cause obstruction of heart valves or great vessels, whereas friable vegetations may embolize, causing myocardial infarction or injury to distant organs. In addition, there is an immunologic reaction, with an elevated rheumatoid factor and circu-

Table 35–6. PROCEDURES ASSOCIATED WITH BACTEREMIA

Procedure	Organism	% Positive Blood Cultures
Dental extraction	S. viridans, diphtheroids	30–65
Brushing teeth	S. viridans	0–26
Tonsillectomy	S. viridans, Haemophilus influenzae, diphtheroids	28–38
Bronchoscopy (rigid)	S. viridans, Staphylococcus epidermidis	15
Bronchoscopy (flexible)		0
Intubation (nasal)	S. viridans, gram-negative rods	16
Intubation (oral)		0
Endoscopy	S. viridans, Neisseria meningitidis, S. epidermidis, diphtheroids	8–12
Colonoscopy	Enterococci, gram-negative rods	0–10
Percutaneous liver biopsy	Pneumococci, gram-negative rods, S. aureus	3–14
Urethral catheter	Not stated	8

lating immune complexes and antibodies, which contributes to both the cardiac and extracardiac manifestations of infectious endocarditis.[48] The overall mortality rate in children with the subacute form of infectious endocarditis is 8 to 12%.

In the acute form of infectious endocarditis caused by *Staphylococcus aureus*, large vegetations do not form; however, there is direct extension from the infected vegetation to surrounding cardiac tissue, causing endocardial abscesses, ventricular aneurysms, fistula formation with development of pericardial empyema-tamponade, valvular ring abscesses, valvular perforation, or chordae tendineae rupture. These conditions cause acute congestive heart failure by direct myocardial injury or by the sudden onset of valvular regurgitation. Congestive heart failure occurs in approximately 40% of patients with the acute form of infectious endocarditis, producing an overall mortality rate in children of 14 to 26%.[45, 49]

Microbiologic Features. Ninety per cent of all cases of infectious endocarditis are caused by gram-positive cocci. *S. viridans* is the most common organism (35%). The increasing frequency of infectious endocarditis caused by *S. aureus* (33%), *S. epidermidis* (5%), gram-negative organisms (5%), and fungi (3%) is due to their association with infections in patients who have undergone cardiac surgery, in patients who are immunocompromised, in patients who have indwelling catheters, or in those who are intravenous drug users. Cultures are negative in 14 to 20% of pathologically proven cases of infectious endocarditis.

Diagnosis. The diagnosis of infectious endocarditis is often difficult to make. Therefore, it must be considered in any child with known cardiac disease who presents with positive blood cultures or persistent fever. Presenting symptoms vary from malaise or other nonspecific symptoms in the subacute form to septic shock in the acute form (Table 35–7).

Table 35–7. CLINICAL SYMPTOMS AND LABORATORY FINDINGS IN PATIENTS WITH INFECTIOUS ENDOCARDITIS

Symptoms		Laboratory Findings
Common	Fever New or changing heart murmur	Positive blood culture Elevated ESR,* C-reactive protein
Usually present	Myalgia Arthralgia Headache Malaise	Anemia Leukemia Leukocytosis Hematuria
Occasional	Petechiae Splenomegaly Pneumonia Splinter hemorrhages	Positive rheumatoid factor Positive circulating immune complexes
Rare	Janeway lesions Osler nodes	

*ESR = erythrocyte sedimentation rate.

Congestive heart failure occurs in 25 to 30% of patients secondary to acute valvular insufficiency from chordae tendineae rupture or valvular ulceration, acute valvular stenosis from a large vegetation, decreased myocardial contractility from a myocardial abscess, purulent pericarditis with cardiac tamponade, or coronary artery emboli with concomitant myocardial infarction. Congestive heart failure is the most important prognostic factor for overall outcome. Other factors include the underlying cardiac defect, the presence of prosthetic material, the infecting organism, and the duration of illness prior to initiation of treatment. Currently, the overall mortality rate in children with infectious endocarditis is 20 to 30%.

A blood culture is the single most important diagnostic test. Blood cultures are positive in 92% of autopsy-proven cases of bacterial endocarditis and in 50% of cases of fungal endocarditis. The bacteremia of infectious endocarditis is continuous; therefore, the timing and site of collection of blood culture specimens does not affect their yield. Multiple blood cultures do increase yield; 66% for one specimen, 90% for two specimens, and 97% for three blood culture specimens.[50] Current recommendations are for three blood culture specimens to be obtained within the first 24 hours of evaluation. The blood volume of each should be as large as possible for the patient's size. Blood cultures from patients pretreated with antibiotics must be placed in a special culture medium that absorbs or inactivates the antibiotics present.

Echocardiography is a useful adjunct to the evaluation of a patient suspected of having infectious endocarditis. It should be performed immediately in patients with congestive heart failure or in those with evidence of acute valvular insufficiency to evaluate myocardial and valvular function. All patients suspected of infectious endocarditis should have an elective echocardiogram to look for vegetations, which are present in 66% of children. Although echocardiography has an 83% sensitivity for detecting vegetations,[51] it cannot visualize vegetations smaller than 2 to 3 mm in diameter and,

therefore, the lack of vegetations on an echocardiogram does not rule out infectious endocarditis. Serial echocardiograms are not useful to assess the efficacy of treatment; however, new vegetations or enlargement of existing vegetations with persistent bacteremia indicates treatment failure or the need for surgical intervention, or both.

Treatment. It is necessary to diagnose the causative agent before starting antibiotic therapy in order to prevent (1) prolonged hospitalization, (2) nosocomial infection, (3) the drug toxicity risks of empiric therapy, or (4) inadequate treatment of infectious endocarditis. Antibiotic therapy should be initiated empirically, after obtaining blood cultures, in cases of fulminant infections only. Antibiotics should be given parenterally for 4 to 6 weeks. Bactericidal agents are preferred over bacteriostatic drugs, and synergism between agents may increase efficacy (Table 35–8). Daily blood culture specimens should be drawn until they are consistently negative. Positive blood cultures while the patient is receiving therapy warrant evaluating the adequacy of antibiotic treatment by measuring the minimal bactericidal concentration of the patient's serum (Schlichter test) and altering therapy if there is less than a 1:8 dilution. Repeat blood cultures during the first few weeks following the completed course of antibiotics should be performed to investigate relapse during this vulnerable period.

Surgical treatment of infectious endocarditis includes removal of large vegetations and replacement of insufficient native or infected synthetic valves, conduits, or patches. Indications for surgery include valve obstruction or regurgitation causing congestive heart failure, fungal infection with large vegetations, recurrent emboli, or persistent positive blood cultures following 2 weeks of appropriate antibiotic therapy. Early surgical replacement of infected prosthetic valves reduces mortality.[52, 53]

Prophylaxis is an attempt to prevent infectious endocarditis by reducing high-risk patients' exposure to circulating bacteria with the use of antibiotics in instances in which bacteremia is likely to occur. Common procedures performed in the pediatric intensive care unit, such as bladder catheterization, nasotracheal intubation, rigid bronchoscopy, and endoscopy, put children with congenital heart disease at risk for the development of infectious endocarditis (Table 35–9). All children with congenital heart disease, except those with isolated secundum atrial septal defect, require antibiotics for prophylaxis during procedures involving the oral mucosa and upper respiratory tract (against *S. viridans*) and genitourinary or gastrointestinal tract (against enterococci). Patients undergoing cardiac surgery should have perioperative prophylaxis against *S. aureus*.

PERICARDITIS

Pericarditis is the inflammation of the sac surrounding the heart, which causes fluid accumulation. The causes of pericarditis include infections, systemic inflammatory illnesses, and neoplasms, among others (Table 35–10).

Table 35–8. TREATMENT REGIMEN

Infecting Organism	Treatment	Duration (wk)
Streptococcus viridans	Penicillin G* plus gentamicin†	4 (gentamicin × 2)
penicillin-allergic	Vancomycin‡ plus gentamicin†	4 (gentamicin × 2)
Enterococci	Same	Same
Staphylococcus aureus	Nafcillin§ plus gentamicin†	6 (gentamicin × 2)
methicillin-resistant	Vancomycin‡	6
penicillin-allergic	Same	Same
S. epidermidis	Vancomycin‡ plus or minus rifampin‖	6
prosthetic valve	Vancomycin‡ plus rifampin‖ plus gentamicin†	8
Enteric bacilli	Ampicillin** plus gentamicin†	6
Pseudomonas spp.	Ticarcillin†† plus gentamicin†	6
Haemophilus spp.	Ampicillin** plus or minus gentamicin†	4 (gentamicin × 2)
Culture-negative		
nonoperative	Nafcillin§ plus gentamicin† plus penicillin G*	6
postoperative	Vancomycin‡ plus gentamicin†	6
Fungus	Amphotericin B‡‡	8

*Aqueous penicillin G, 250,000 units/kg/day divided every 4 hr
†Gentamicin, 7 mg/kg/day divided every 8 hr
‡Vancomycin, 60 mg/kg/day divided every 6 hr
§Nafcillin, 200 mg/kg/day divided every 6 hr
‖Rifampin, 30 mg/kg/day divided every 12 hr
**Ampicillin, 300 mg/kg/day divided every 6 hr
††Ticarcillin, 400 mg/kg/day divided every 6 hr
‡‡Amphotericin B, 1 mg/kg/day over 6–12 hr

Patients with pericarditis, regardless of the cause, may experience a pericardial effusion and cardiac tamponade and therefore require rapid diagnosis and treatment provided by the pediatric intensive care unit team.

Pathophysiology. The pericardium is made up of two layers, a visceral layer of mesothelial tissue adhering to the epicardium and a parietal layer of collagen interlaced with elastic fibers. They form a sac enveloping the heart, proximal great vessels, and cardiac junction of the systemic and pulmonary veins. The pericardial sac of an adult usually contains less than 50 ml of clear serous fluid.

Acute inflammation, effusion with or without tampon-ade, or fibrosis with or without constriction may develop in response to acute injury to the pericardium. Initially, fine fibrin strands are deposited within the pericardial space, followed by fluid accumulation. The rate of fluid accumulation determines the severity of symptoms. Rapid accumulation of fluid does not allow time for expansion of the parietal pericardium, which leads to dramatic increases in pericardial pressure, causing car-

Table 35–9. PROPHYLAXIS AGAINST INFECTIOUS ENDOCARDITIS

Oral and Upper Respiratory Tract Procedures
Standard
  Amoxicillin, 50 mg/kg PO* 1 hr before, 25 mg/kg IV† 6 hr after
  Ampicillin, 50 mg/kg IV 1 hr before, 25 mg/kg IV 6 hr after

High risk
  Add gentamicin, 2 mg/kg IV 30 min before and 6 hr after to IV ampicillin

Penicillin-allergic
  Erythromycin ES, 20 mg/kg PO 2 hr before, 10 mg/kg 6 hr after
  Clindamycin, 10 mg/kg IV 30 min before, 5 mg/kg IV 6 hr after

Genitourinary and Gastrointestinal Procedures
Low risk
  Amoxicillin, 50 mg/kg PO 1 hr before, 25 mg/kg PO 6 hr after

Standard
  Ampicillin, 50 mg/kg IV plus gentamicin, 2 mg/kg IV 30 min before and 8 hr after

Penicillin-allergic
  Vancomycin, 20 mg/kg IV plus gentamicin 2 mg/kg IV 1 hr before and 8 hr after

*PO = by mouth.
†IV = intravenous.

Table 35–10. CAUSES OF PERICARDITIS

Infectious
Bacterial
  Staphylococcus aureus, Haemophilus influenzae, Streptococcus pneumoniae, β-hemolytic streptococci, *Neisseria meningitidis,* gonococci, *Pseudomonas aeruginosa, Salmonella, Mycoplasma pneumoniae, Mycobacterium tuberculosis*

Viral
  Coxsackievirus B, influenza types A and B, adenovirus, echovirus, mumps, mononucleosis, measles, hepatitis, cytomegalovirus, varicella zoster
Fungal
  Candida, Aspergillus

Other
  Syphilis, leptospirosis, psittacosis, typhus, Q fever, *Entamoeba histolytica, Echinococcus, Toxoplasma gondii*

Systemic Illness
  Systemic lupus erythematosus
  Juvenile rheumatoid arthritis
  Rheumatic fever
  Chronic renal failure–uremia
  Ulcerative colitis

Neoplasm
  Leukemia, lymphoma
  Metastatic

Other
  Postpericardiotomy syndrome
  Postirradiation syndrome
  Trauma
  Hypersensitivity: drugs, serum sickness, Stevens-Johnson syndrome

diac tamponade. As little as 100 ml of pericardial fluid may cause tamponade in a small child if it accumulates rapidly, whereas 3 l of pericardial fluid may cause no symptoms in an older child if it accumulates slowly. There is little change in pressure as the volume of fluid in the pericardial sac increases until a critical point is reached, after which pressure rises rapidly, causing tamponade.[54] Increased pericardial sac pressure decreases diastolic filling of the heart by increasing both the right and left ventricular end-diastolic pressures. The decreased diastolic filling reduces stroke volume and cardiac output, whereas the increased end-diastolic pressure decreases coronary blood flow, which decreases myocardial contractility, further reducing cardiac function.

Infectious Pericarditis

In children, pericarditis with effusion is most often associated with systemic illness or cardiac surgery; however, purulent pericarditis causes the majority of deaths, especially in children younger than 2 years of age.[55, 56] In more than 90% of cases, there is another site of infection that seeds the pericardium, either by direct extension or hematogenous spread.[57] *S. aureus* is the most common organism producing pericarditis[57] and is responsible for 73% of all deaths from purulent pericarditis[58] and 50% of deaths from purulent pericarditis in children 1 to 4 years of age.[57]

Haemophilus influenzae is the second most common organism causing purulent pericarditis in children, accounting for 22% of cases.[57] It is generally associated with meningitis or pneumonia. Twenty per cent of children with *H. influenzae* meningitis have an associated pericardial effusion.[59] *S. pneumoniae* pericarditis occurs in association with pneumonia or empyema. Pericarditis is a late complication of other serious infections. Other infectious agents, including viruses, cause pericarditis; however, in 20% of cases no infectious agent can be identified.[60]

Diagnosis. The most common symptoms of purulent pericarditis are fever, tachypnea, and tachycardia. There is often precordial pain that is made worse with inspiration or supine positioning. The heart sounds are muffled, and a pericardial friction rub is present. As the pericardial pressure rises, jugular venous distention, hepatomegaly, pulsus paradoxus, and hypotension with a narrow pulse pressure develop. Pulsus paradoxus is an exaggerated fall in systolic blood pressure during inspiration (greater than 10 mm Hg). It is calculated by subtracting the peak systolic blood pressure during inspiration from that during expiration.[61]

Laboratory tests are performed to document infection and to isolate the organism from pericardial fluid, blood, or urine. The complete blood count will be elevated with a leftward shift. Blood culture specimens must be obtained prior to initiating treatment; the cultures are positive in 80% of cases. A urinalysis may show hematuria, or urine culture may identify the organism, as may a urine sample for latex agglutination tests. If a viral cause is suspected, nasopharyngeal and stool swabs for viral culture, as well as serum for acute and convalescent antibody titers, should be obtained. A purified protein derivative patch (PPD) should be placed to evaluate for infection with *Mycobacterium tuberculosis*.

A chest x-ray film shows cardiomegaly without congestive heart failure, unless there is an associated myocarditis. The ECG findings include low QRS voltages and ST segment elevation in leads I, II V5, and V6, with or without T wave inversion.[62] Electrical alternans (alternation in the electrical amplitude of QRS and T waves with each cardiac cycle) may be seen.

Echocardiography is useful for diagnosing pericardial effusion and quantitating the amount of fluid present. Echocardiographic signs of tamponade include compression of the atrial free walls or right ventricular outflow tract and a decreased ejection fraction (Fig. 35-2).

Examination of the pericardial fluid is the most specific aid in diagnosing purulent pericarditis. Pericardial fluid samples should be obtained for a cell count; cytologic studies; glucose, protein, and LDH determinations; Gram staining and acid fast staining ; cultures for bacteria, fungi, viruses, and tuberculosis; and latex agglutination studies.

Treatment. The treatment of purulent pericarditis with specific antibiotic therapy and surgical drainage has reduced the overall mortality rate to less than 20%.[63] Prior to identification of an organism, antibiotic coverage must be broad, including a penicillinase-resistant penicillin (methicillin or nafcillin, 200 mg/kg/day) to cover *S. aureus* and ampicillin (300 mg/kg/day), or a third-generation cephalosporin (ceftriaxone, 100 mg/kg/day) to cover *S. pneumoniae*, meningococcus, and *H. influenzae*. An aminoglycoside (gentamicin, 7.5 mg/kg/day) should be added if purulent pericarditis is associated with a genitourinary infection or postoperative cardiac surgery or is present in an immunocompro-

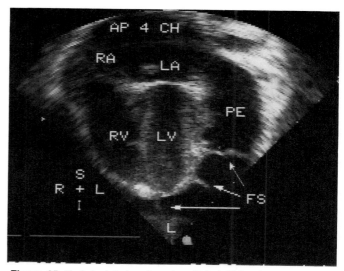

Figure 35-2. Apical 4-chamber view (*AP 4 CH*) echocardiogram of a 1-year-old child with a pericardial effusion (*PE*). Note the PE extends completely around the heart. There are fibrous strands (*FS*) visualized. S = superior; R + L = right and left; I = inferior; RA = right atrium; LA = left atrium; RV = right ventricle; LV = left ventricle; L = liver.

mised patient. The total length of treatment is 4 to 6 weeks, with the agents given parenterally in the initial 3 to 4 weeks. Lifesaving supportive measures must be instituted immediately if the patient shows evidence of cardiac tamponade. These measures include pericardiocentesis (needle aspiration or catheter placement), volume expansion with 10 to 15 ml/kg normal saline or 5% albumin, and inotropic support.

Pericardiocentesis is most safely and easily performed using echocardiographic guidance in the pediatric intensive care unit. The patient should be adequately sedated and monitored with a 12-lead ECG. The head of the bed should be elevated 30 degrees to allow the pericardial fluid to collect on the diaphragmatic surface. After the chest and abdomen are prepared and draped in sterile fashion, the skin and subcutaneous tissue immediately inferior to the xyphoid process are infiltrated with lidocaine. Through a small stab wound in the skin immediately below the xyphoid process, an 18-gauge needle with a plastic catheter is advanced toward the left scapula at a 30-degree angle. Using a syringe, constant suction is applied to the needle while it is being advanced. Once fluid is encountered or a dysrhythmia is noted, the advancement is stopped. Using a sterile alligator clip, an ECG chest lead can record and monitor the ECG directly from the needle to increase the sensitivity for detecting injury current. If grossly bloody fluid is obtained, it should be sent for measurement of hematocrit, and another sample should be allowed to stand for 5 minutes. If the hematocrit value is the same as that for venous blood or the sample clots, it was probably obtained from the right ventricle. If location of the needle is still uncertain, 2 to 3 ml of agitated sterile saline is injected through the needle while an echocardiogram is obtained. If the needle is in the heart, the right ventricular chamber will fill with microbubbles. If it is in the pericardial space, microbubbles will fill the pericardial space and outline the heart. Once it is certain that the needle is in the pericardial space, the catheter is advanced over the needle and the needle is withdrawn. If a catheter is to be left in the pericardial space to drain an effusion, we recommend inserting a No. 5 French 30-cm pigtail catheter over a 0.0028-in. flexible J wire. The catheter should be sutured in place and connected in a sterile manner to a closed gravity drainage system. Surgical drainage, either by a subxyphoid pericardial window or an anterior pericardiotomy, should be performed as soon as the diagnosis is certain.

Treatment of viral pericarditis is supportive, including bed rest until evidence of acute inflammation is gone and the use of nonsteroidal anti-inflammatory agents for pain. Cardiac tamponade is less common than in bacterial pericarditis. Tuberculous pericarditis is treated with isoniazid (20 mg/kg/day), pyrazinamide (15 to 30 mg/kg/day), rifampin (20 mg/kg/day) and, if needed, streptomycin (40 mg/kg/day). Prednisone (2 mg/kg/day) is recommended during the first several weeks of tuberculous pericarditis to decrease inflammation and speed resorption of pericardial fluid. Fungal pericarditis is treated with amphotericin B.

There are many noninfectious causes of pericarditis (see Table 35–10). Although more common than purulent or constrictive pericarditis, these causes have a much lower incidence of associated morbidity and mortality. One of the most common causes is postpericardiotomy syndrome, a febrile illness with pericardial and pleural reaction that occurs after cardiac surgery in which the pericardium was opened. It occurs in 25 to 30% of children undergoing open heart surgery for congenital heart disease. It is uncommon in children less than 2 years of age.[64] The pathogenesis is likely caused by an autoimmune response to an associated viral infection.[65] The illness is generally self-limited, lasting 2 to 3 weeks, but occasionally cardiac tamponade develops. Therefore, careful monitoring is warranted. Symptoms are similar to those for infectious pericarditis. Treatment is with nonsteroidal anti-inflammatory agents (aspirin 100 mg/kg/day) for 5 to 7 days. If symptoms are severe, steroids (prednisone 1 to 2 mg/kg/day for 3 to 5 days) cause a more prompt response. Catheter or surgical drainage may be necessary.

Malignancy may cause pericarditis by direct extension or hematogenous spread of the tumor. Mediastinal radiation causes pericarditis in 2% of patients treated for Hodgkin disease.[66] Conservative medical management with nonsteroidal anti-inflammatory agents or short-course steroids is adequate, though catheter or surgical drainage may be necessary.

Constrictive Pericarditis

In constrictive pericarditis, a thickened, fibrotic, calcified, inelastic pericardial sac impairs the diastolic filling of the heart, leading to a decrease in stroke volume. The thickening and fibrosis of the pericardium are due to chronic infection.[55, 56] In more than 50% of cases, however, no cause is found.

Typical symptoms include jugular venous distention and hepatomegaly. There may be signs of decreased cardiac output. A chest x-ray film shows a normal heart size; however, calcification of the pericardium may be seen. Magnetic resonance imaging is useful to look for pericardial thickening and evidence of fibrosis. Echocardiography should be used to rule out an associated pericardial effusion and to evaluate cardiac function.

ACUTE RHEUMATIC FEVER

Acute rheumatic fever (ARF) is an inflammatory process affecting the heart, skin, joints, and brain. It is mediated by an immunologic reaction to streptococcal infections. ARF is the leading cause of acquired heart disease in children in the United States. Many of these children experience valvular heart disease, congestive heart failure, or pericarditis, necessitating admission to the pediatric intensive care unit.

Epidemiology. ARF is directly caused by group A β-hemolytic streptococcal pharyngitis. Approximately 3% of patients with streptococcal pharyngitis will acquire ARF;[67] however, 33% of children with ARF will have no history of pharyngitis. The peak incidence is in the spring and winter. The incidence of ARF has increased dramatically over the past years.[68, 69]

Pathophysiology. The pathophysiology of ARF is an immune-mediated reaction to a streptococcal infection producing vasculitis of the skin, which leads to erythema marginatum, arthritis of large joints, vasculitis in the basal ganglia and cerebellum, causing Sydenham chorea, and cardiac involvement, including valvular endocarditis, myocarditis, and pericarditis. The incidence of cardiac involvement in ARF is approximately 70% when diagnosed clinically and 90% when diagnosed by color Doppler echocardiography.[70] The most common cardiac finding is valvular endocarditis, with the mitral valve affected most often, followed by the aortic valve and the tricuspid valve. The pulmonary valve is only very rarely affected. Congestive heart failure occurs in 7% of patients and is the most common reason for admission to the pediatric intensive care unit. The mortality rate from ARF is 3%, with approximately one half of those deaths occurring several years later from chronic congestive heart failure.[71]

The histologic findings of acute rheumatic carditis are nonspecific. There is edema and cellular infiltrates of lymphocytes, plasma cells, and fibrinoid (an eosinophilic granular substance) scattered throughout the myocardium.[72] The valvular tissue and chordae tendineae also show edema, with cellular infiltration eventually leading to hyaline degeneration, fibrosis, and calcification. Pericarditis is often present.

Diagnosis. Because there is no specific test for ARF, the diagnosis is based on the presence of clinical criteria initially established by Jones in 1944 and later modified.[73, 74] The modified Jones criteria, which include major and minor clinical manifestations of the disease, are used to indicate a high probability of ARF. However, these criteria are not specific for ARF, and overdiagnosis is common. To make the diagnosis of ARF, the patient must demonstrate two of the major criteria or one major and two minor criteria if supported by evidence of a preceding group A β-hemolytic streptococcal infection (Table 35–11).

The diagnosis of carditis is made clinically but is aided by the ECG and the echocardiogram. The onset of a

Table 35–11. MODIFIED JONES' CRITERIA TO DIAGNOSE ACUTE RHEUMATIC FEVER

Major	Minor
Carditis (70%)	Previous episode of ARF* (25%)
Polyarthritis (70%)	Arthralgia
Chorea (15%)	Fever (60%)
Erythema marginatum (5%)	Prolonged PR interval (40%)
Subcutaneous nodules (<5%)	Elevated ESR† (95%)
	Leukocytosis
	Elevated C-reactive protein

Supporting Evidence of Streptococcal Infection
Increased titer of antistreptococcal antibodies: ASO, anti-DNAse B, streptozyme
Recent scarlet fever
Positive throat culture for group A β-hemolytic streptococci

(_____) = % of patients with specific criteria
*ARF = acute rheumatic fever.
†ESR = erythrocyte sedimentation rate.

Table 35–12. TREATMENT REGIMENS FOR ACUTE RHEUMATIC FEVER

Eradication of Group A β-Hemolytic Streptococci
Benzathine penicillin IM,* 600,000 to 1.2 million units
Penicillin V, 125–250 mg PO† qid‡ × 10 days
Erythromycin, 40 mg/kg/day PO tid§ × 10 days

Arthritis plus Mild Carditis
ASA,‖ 100 mg/kg/day PO q4h** × 2–6 wk
Follow with ASA taper over 3 wk to 25 mg/kg/day

Carditis, Moderate to Severe
Prednisone, 2 mg/kg/day PO or IV × 2 wk
Follow with prednisone taper over 3 wk to 10 mg/day
During second week of taper, begin ASA as above

Secondary Prophylaxis
Benzathine penicillin, 600,000 to 1.2 million units IM q4wk
Penicillin VK, 125–250 mg PO bid††
Erythromycin, 250 mg PO bid

*IM = intramuscular.
†PO = by mouth.
‡qid = four times daily.
§tid = three times daily.
‖ASA = acetylsalicylic acid.
**q4h = every 4 hours.
††bid = twice daily.

new heart murmur occurs in 65% of patients with ARF. A murmur of mitral insufficiency is the most common manifestation of carditis, whereas aortic insufficiency will present as a short, high-frequency decrescendo diastolic murmur that is loudest at the left-mid sternal border. A gallop rhythm is heard in 30% of patients who have associated congestive heart failure. Conduction abnormalities occur frequently. Forty per cent of patients have prolongation of the PR interval, 30% have resting bradycardia, and 30% experience second- or third-degree heart block.[75] An echocardiogram will show a dilated left atrium with mitral insufficiency and can be used to assess the severity of the regurgitation. With aortic insufficiency, dilatation of the left ventricle may be present.

There are no specific laboratory tests to diagnose ARF. Elevation of the acute phase reactants are nonspecific indicators of inflammation, but they can be used to monitor ongoing activity of ARF; however, they do not correlate with severity. A throat culture is positive in only one third of patients with ARF. Assays for antibodies (antistreptolyson-O [ASO], antideoxyribonuclease B [anti–DNAse-B], and the streptozyme test, an agglutination test to several antigens) to group A β-hemolytic streptococcal antigens must be performed to document previous streptococcal infection.

Treatment. Therapy for ARF has several goals, including eradication of the streptococcal infection to prevent immediate recurrence (regardless of the period from the initial infection or throat culture result at the time of presentation), symptomatic treatment of the major manifestations and acute complications, rest to allow adequate cardiac recovery, and prophylaxis against recurrent episodes (Table 35–12). Whether aspirin or steroids are more effective for the treatment of carditis is controversial. The two large multicenter prospective studies have shown no significant difference in the drugs' efficacy for reducing the acute inflammation of carditis, although prednisone may be more effective at improving the symptoms of severe carditis.[71, 76–78] However, these drugs have no effect on reducing or preventing chronic valvular heart disease or mortality. Plasmapheresis has been used to treat three patients, with resultant improvement in the symptoms of carditis and arthritis.[79] Because of the high risk of recurrence in patients who have had ARF, prophylaxis against streptococcal infection is essential and should be continued for life.

CARDIOMYOPATHY

Cardiomyopathy refers to any structural or functional abnormality of the ventricular myocardium. It may be primary or secondary to other cardiovascular or systemic diseases (Table 35–13). Cardiomyopathies are either dilated, hypertrophic, or restrictive, depending on the characteristic structural and functional abnormalities. Because of the frequent sequelae of congestive heart failure, arrhythmias, and sudden death, diagnosis and treatment in the pediatric intensive care unit is often required.

Dilated Cardiomyopathy

Dilated cardiomyopathy is the most common cardiomyopathy in infants and children. The two most com-

Table 35–13. CAUSES OF CARDIOMYOPATHY

Infectious
    Myocarditis-endocarditis

Metabolic
    Thyrotoxicosis
    Hypothyroidism
    Diabetic cardiomyopathy
    Infant of a diabetic mother
    Carnitine deficiency

Storage disease
    Glycogen types II–VI
    Mucopolysaccharidoses (all)
    Sphingolipidoses (all)

Systemic diseases
    SLE*
    JRA†
    Kawasaki disease
    Mitochondrial cytopathy
    Osteogenesis imperfecta
    Noonan syndrome

Genetic disorders
    Muscular dystrophy (Duchenne, Steinert, Erb)
    Myopathy (nemaline, myotubular)
    Friedreich ataxia

Nutritional deficiency
    Protein (kwashiorkor)
    Thiamine (beriberi)
    Vitamine E and selenium

Drugs
    Anthracyclines
    Iron
    Chloramphenicol

*SLE = systemic lupus erythematosus.
†JRA = juvenile rheumatoid arthritis.

mon types are idiopathic dilated cardiomyopathy and endocardial fibroelastosis.

The cause of idiopathic dilated cardiomyopathy remains unknown. In adults, it occurs after viral myocarditis, whereas in children there is a genetic predisposition. The heart shows diffuse chamber dilatation, mild ventricular hypertrophy, and patchy scarring of the subendocardium or papillary muscles. Microscopically, there is chronic inflammation, interstitial fibrosis, and myofibril hypertrophy, degeneration, or necrosis. There is decreased contractility, which may produce congestive heart failure. The poor contractility allow stasis of blood in the ventricular apex, with resultant thrombus formation in up to 75% of patients.

Most pediatric patients typically present by 2 years of age with signs of respiratory distress, congestive heart failure, or isolated cardiac enlargement.[80] The physical examination reveals pulmonary congestion, a quiet precordium, distant heart sounds, a prominent S3 gallop, and hepatomegaly. A chest x-ray film shows marked cardiomegaly and pulmonary edema. An ECG shows nonspecific ST-T wave abnormalities. Because of the risk of ventricular arrhythmias, ECG monitoring is indicated. An echocardiogram shows marked dilatation of all cardiac chambers, decreased shortening and ejection fractions and, occasionally, regional wall motion abnormalities. In these patients, cardiac catheterization carries a significant risk of producing ventricular arrhythmias or worsening congestive heart failure and should be performed only if there is a high suspicion of an anomalous origin of the left coronary artery, if a biopsy is needed to rule out acute myocarditis or glycogen storage disease, or to prepare the patient for cardiac transplantation.

The overall prognosis for patients with idiopathic dilated cardiomyopathy is poor, with a 65% survival at 1 year and a 33% survival at 5 years.[81] Intractable congestive heart failure is the most common cause of death, followed by arrhythmias. Of the survivors, 50% will have residual myocardial dysfunction.

Initial management includes reduction in activity, fluid restriction, diuretic therapy, and the use of inotropic and afterload reducing agents if symptoms are more severe (see Table 35–5). Supplemental O_2, intubation, and mechanical ventilation may be necessary. If the patient is unresponsive to medical management or if the disease is rapidly progressive, cardiac transplantation should be considered.

Endocardial fibroelastosis is a dilated cardiomyopathy with marked left ventricular endocardial thickening. It occurs in 1/6,000 live births,[82] with more than 75% of patients presenting by 1 year of age. Viral myocarditis, carnitine deficiency, and left-sided obstructive lesions may produce endocardial fibroelastosis secondarily. The common pathophysiologic mechanism appears to be increased left ventricular wall tension, leading to endocardial injury. This causes an overproduction and deposition of collagen and elastin in the endocardium.[83] The heart is markedly enlarged. The left ventricular walls are normal to slightly increased in size, with a diffusely thickened, opaque, glistening endocardium that may extend onto the surface of the left atrium and mitral and aortic valves.

Diagnosis. Most patients present within the first year of life with signs and symptoms of congestive heart failure. The physical examination shows lateral displacement of the apical impulse, normal to muffled heart sounds, a gallop rhythm, and an apical holosystolic murmur of mitral insufficiency. An ECG shows left or right atrial enlargement or both, and left ventricular hypertrophy. Dysrhythmias are common and include both tachycardias and heart block. A chest x-ray film shows cardiomegaly with or without pulmonary venous congestion. An echocardiogram shows a markedly dilated left atrium and ventricle and a decreased ejection fraction. A bright, thickened endocardium can be seen. Cardiac catheterization shows elevated atrial and ventricular end-diastolic pressures. Catheterization should be performed only if endomyocardial biopsy is required for definitive diagnosis.

Treatment. The treatment of endocardial fibroelastosis is supportive and is directed toward relief of congestive heart failure symptoms (see Table 35–5). The overall prognosis for patients with endocardial fibroelastosis is poor, with the majority of patients dying within the first year of life. The onset of congestive heart failure as a newborn or recurrent episodes of congestive heart failure despite adequate treatment are poor prognostic indicators. Those patients who survive have persistent left ventricular dysfunction.

Hypertrophic Cardiomyopathy

In hypertrophic cardiomyopathy, there is hypertrophy of the left ventricle leading to abnormal relaxation, which can result in congestive heart failure, arrhythmias, and sudden death.[84] In 60% of cases, there is an autosomal-dominant mode of transmission with variable penetrance.[85]

The underlying pathologic mechanism appears to be myofibril disarray, leading to increased wall stress and resultant hypertrophy. The heart shows hypertrophy of the intraventricular septum and left ventricular free wall, with a small left ventricular cavity. Histologically, the myocardial cells are hypertrophied and are oriented in a disorganized fashion.[86]

These pathologic changes lead to impaired diastolic function, with decreased compliance and filling of the left ventricle. The elevated left ventricular end-diastolic pressure leads eventually to pulmonary venous congestion and signs of congestive heart failure. Severe left ventricular outflow tract obstruction results from systolic anterior motion of the anterior mitral leaflet as it comes in contact with the hypertrophied intraventricular septum. This may produce congestive heart failure, chest pain, arrhythmias, and sudden death.

Infants with hypertrophic cardiomyopathy typically present with a systolic murmur and signs of congestive heart failure and, occasionally, cyanosis. Congestive heart failure is rare in older children, who more frequently present with symptoms of dyspnea, exercise intolerance, chest pain, palpitations, or syncope. The physical examination may be normal in 25% of patients. The first heart sound is normal; however, the second heart sound may be paradoxically split. In many patients, S3 and S4 gallops are heard. A systolic ejection murmur at the left lower sternal border will be heard due to left ventricular outflow tract obstruction. This can be accentuated by maneuvers that increase contractility or decrease systemic vascular resistance, such as exercise, the Valsalva maneuver, standing, or the administration of amyl nitrate. A chest x-ray film shows cardiomegaly with normal pulmonary vascularity. ECG abnormalities occur in 90% of patients and include left atrial enlargement, left ventricular hypertrophy, ST-T segment changes, and abnormal Q waves.[87] Dysrhythmias, including premature ventricular contractions, may occur. An echocardiogram shows asymmetric left ventricular hypertrophy, with the intraventricular septum affected most severely. There is systolic anterior motion of the anterior leaflet of the mitral valve, with or without mitral regurgitation, which correlates with the degree of left ventricular outflow tract obstruction. Because of the sensitivity of the echocardiogram, cardiac catheterization is no longer needed unless surgical treatment is required. A thallium perfusion scan for detecting regional myocardial perfusion abnormalities may be useful in patients suspected of having subendocardial ischemia.

In infants, the differential diagnosis of hypertrophic cardiomyopathy includes congenital heart disease causing left-sided hypertrophy and cardiomyopathy in infants of diabetic mothers. Although rare, Pompe disease and Friedreich ataxia must be considered in older children.

The clinical course of hypertrophic cardiomyopathy in infants and children is variable, ranging from stable without symptoms to rapidly progressive. The prognosis for infants presenting with congestive heart failure is poor, with most dying by 1 year of age, whereas asymptomatic infants have a 50% survival rate at 1 year.[88] Of the infants who survive, 40% will die, 40% will improve, and 20% will have severe residual disease. Patients who present after 1 year of age do not typically experience severe congestive heart failure; however, 3 to 7%/year die suddenly.[89] There is an increase in left ventricular hypertrophy, especially with somatic growth; however, this does not correlate well with symptoms. The cause of sudden death is unknown but is presumed to be secondary to arrhythmias. The risk factors for sudden death include age 12 to 35 years, exercise, and evidence of ventricular tachycardia on a Holter monitor.

Treatment. The goal of treatment in hypertrophic cardiomyopathy is to decrease symptoms by improving diastolic function and relieving left ventricular outflow tract obstruction. However, no therapy has been successful at reversing ventricular hypertrophy or preventing sudden death. Calcium channel blockers such as verapamil (2 to 5 mg/kg/dose PO tid) or nifedipine (0.25 to 0.5 mg/kg/dose PO tid) are effective for relieving symptoms in more than 60% of patients. They improve left ventricular diastolic relaxation and filling, decrease myocardial oxygen consumption by decreasing heart rate and afterload, and may decrease systolic anterior motion of the anterior leaflet of the mitral valve, thereby reducing left ventricular outflow obstruction.[90] Their full effect may not occur until several weeks of therapy. Propranolol (2 mg/kg/day, maximum 320 mg/day) relieves symptoms in 30 to 50% of patients.[91] The exact mechanism of action is unknown; however, it may decrease the left ventricular outflow tract gradient during sympathetic stimulation or decrease myocardial oxygen consumption through its effect on heart rate. Diuretics should be used sparingly to decrease pulmonary edema, because overdiuresis may result in decreased left ventricular filling and worsening obstructive symptoms. Patients with marked pulmonary edema and left ventricular outflow tract obstruction may require oxygen supplementation, mechanical ventilation, and aggressive afterload reduction with intravenous nitroprusside. Careful observation for arrhythmias and myocardial ischemia is warranted. Both atrial and ventricular arrhythmias should be treated aggressively.

Surgical treatment should be considered in patients with severe symptoms that are unresponsive to medical treatment and a left ventricular outflow tract gradient of greater than or equal to 150 mm Hg. As with medical treatment, surgery does not reverse the left ventricular hypertrophy or decrease the incidence of sudden death; however, it does improve symptoms. A transaortic ventricular septal myotomy-myomectomy is performed.[92] The perioperative mortality rate is 8%, and relief of symptoms occurs in 70% of patients.

Restrictive Cardiomyopathy

Restrictive cardiomyopathy is characterized by markedly reduced ventricular compliance, normal left ventricular end-diastolic volume, mild symmetric ventricular wall thickening, and a mildly decreased ejection fraction. Restrictive cardiomyopathy is very rare in children.

References

1. Kawasaki T, Kosaki F, Okawa S, et al: A new infantile acute febrile mucocutaneous lymph node syndrome (MLNS) prevailing in Japan. Pediatrics 54:271, 1974.
2. Kawasaki T: MCLS—clinical observation of 50 cases (Japanese). Jpn J Allerg 16:178, 1967.
3. Yanagihara R and Todd J: Acute febrile mucocutaneous lymph node syndrome. Am J Dis Child 134:603, 1980.
4. Morens DM and O'Brien RJ: Kawasaki disease in the United States. J Infect Dis 137:91, 1978.
5. Fujiwara H and Hamashima Y: Pathology of the heart in Kawasaki disease. Pediatrics 61:100, 1978.
6. Yonesaka S, Nakada T, Sunagawa Y, et al: Histopathologic studies of endomyocardial biopsy on the children with Kawasaki disease (Japanese). Kokyu To Junkan 37:429, 1989.
7. Hiraishi S, Yashiro K, Oguchi K, et al: Clinical course of cardiovascular involvement in the mucocutaneous lymph node syndrome. Am J Cardiol 47:323, 1981.
8. Nakanishi T, Takao A, Nakazawa M, et al: Mucocutaneous lymph node syndrome: Clinical, hemodynamic and angiographic features of coronary obstructive disease. Am J Cardiol 55:662, 1985.
9. Kato H, Hoike S, and Yokohama T: Kawasaki disease: Effect of treatment in coronary artery involvement. Pediatrics 63:175, 1979.
10. Koren G, Rose V, Lavi S, et al: Probable efficacy of high dose salicylates in reducing coronary involvement in Kawasaki disease. JAMA 254:767, 1985.
11. Newburger JW, Takahashi M, Burns J, et al: The treatment of Kawasaki syndrome with intravenous gamma globulin. N Engl J Med 315:341, 1986.
12. Sophir D, Simon W, and Reingold M: Myocarditis in children. Am J Dis Child 67:294, 1944.
13. Koren G, Staley N, Bendt C, et al: Occurrence of myocarditis in sudden death in children. J Forensic Sci 22:188, 1978.
14. Burch GE, Sun S, Chu K, et al: Interstitial and coxsackie B myocarditis in infants and children: A comparative histologic and immunofluorescent study of 50 autopsied hearts. JAMA 203:1, 1968.
15. Woodruff J: Viral myocarditis: A review. Am J Pathol 101:425, 1980.
16. Helin M, Savola J, and Lapinleimu K: Cardiac manifestations during a coxsackie B$_5$ epidemic. Br Med J 3:97, 1968.
17. Karjalainen J, Nieminen M, and Heikkila J: Influenza A$_1$ myocarditis in conscripts. Acta Med Scand 207:27, 1980.
18. Ainger L, Lawger N, and Fitch C: Neonatal rubella myocarditis. Br Heart J 28:691, 1966.
19. Osama S, Krishnamurti S, and Gupta D: Incidence of myocarditis in varicella. Indian Heart J 31:315, 1979.
20. Kibrick S and Benirschke K: Severe generalized (encephalohepatomyocarditis) occurring in the newborn period due to infection with coxsackie group B: Evidence of intrauterine infection with the agent. Pediatrics 22:857, 1958.
21. Kereiakes D and Parmley W: Myocarditis and cardiomyopathy. Am Heart J 108:1318, 1984.
22. Kitaura Y and Morita H: Secondary myocardial virus myocarditis and cardiomyopathy. Jpn Circ J 43:1017, 1979.
23. Goldberg S, Valdes-Cruz L, Sahn D, et al: Two-dimensional echocardiographic evaluation of dilated cardiomyopathy in children. Am J Cardiol 52:1244, 1983.
24. Bowles N, Richardson P, Olsen E, et al: Detection of coxsackie B-virus specific RNA sequences in myocardial biopsy samples from patients with myocarditis and dilated cardiomyopathy. Lancet 1:1120, 1986.
25. Cassling R, Linder J, Sears TD, et al: Quantitative evaluation of inflammation in biopsy specimens from idiopathically failing or irritable hearts: Experience in 80 pediatric and adult patients. Am Heart J 110:713, 1985.
26. Dec G, Palacios IF, Fallon JT, et al: Acute myocarditis in the spectrum of acute dilated cardiomyopathy. N Engl J Med 312:885, 1985.
27. O'Connell J, Henkin RE, Robinson JA, et al: Gallium-67 imaging in patients with dilated cardiomyopathy and biopsy proven myocarditis. Circulation 70:58, 1984.
28. Cabinian AE, Kiel RJ, Smith F, et al: Modification of exercise-aggravated coxsackievirus B3 murine myocarditis by T lymphocyte suppression in an inbred model. J Lab Clin Med 115:454, 1990.
29. Estrin M, Smith C, and Huber S: Coxsackievirus B-3 myocarditis: T-cell autoimmunity to heart antigens is resistant to cyclosporin-A treatment. Am J Pathol 125:244, 1986.
30. Kishimoto C and Abelmann WH: Absence of effects of cyclosporine on myocardial lymphocyte subsets in coxsackievirus B3 myocarditis in the aviremic stage. Circ Res 65:934, 1989.
31. Matsumori A, Tomioka N, and Kawai C: Viral myocarditis: Immunopathogenesis and the effect of immunosuppressive treatment in a murine model. Jpn Circ J 53:58, 1989.
32. Schieken R and Myers M: Complete heart block in viral myocarditis. J Pediatr 87:831, 1975.
33. Matsumori A, Tomioka N, and Kawai C: Protective effect of recombinant alpha interferon on coxsackievirus B3 myocarditis in mice. Am Heart J 115:1229, 1988.
34. Geissler W, Forster A, Schewe T, et al: Antiinflammatory effect of a lipoxygenase inhibitor (FLM 5011) in severe active myocarditis. Biomed Biochim Acta 47:S311, 1988.
35. Bulkey BH and Roberts WC: The heart in systemic lupus erythematosus and the changes induced in it by corticosteroid therapy. Am J Med 58:243, 1975.
36. Strauer BE, Brune I, Schenk H, et al: Lupus cardiomyopathy: Cardiac mechanics, hemodynamics, and coronary blood flow in uncomplicated systemic lupus erythematosus. Am Heart J 92:715, 1976.
37. Das SL and Cassidy JT: Antiheart antibodies in patients with SLE. Am J Med Sci 265:275, 1973.
38. Doherty NE and Siegal RJ: Cardiovascular manifestations of systemic lupus erythematosus. Am Heart J 110:1257, 1985.
39. Dubois EL and Wallace DT: Clinical and laboratory manifestations of systemic lupus. In: Dubois EL (ed): Lupus Erythematosus, 3rd ed. Philadelphia, Lea & Febiger, 1987, pp 317–450.

40. Tan EM, Cohen AS, Fries JF, et al: The 1982 revised criteria for the classification of systemic lupus erythematosus. Arthritis Rheum 25:1271, 1982.
41. Bernstein B, Takahashi M, and Hansen V: Cardiac involvement in juvenile rheumatoid arthritis. J Pediatr 85:313, 1974.
42. Miller JJ and French J: Myocarditis in juvenile rheumatoid arthritis. Am J Dis Child 131:205, 1977.
43. Zakrzewski T and Kieth JD: Bacterial endocarditis in infants and children. J Pediatr 67:1179, 1965.
44. Johnson D, Rosenthal A, and Nadas A: A forty-year review of bacterial endocarditis in infancy and childhood. Circulation 51:581, 1975.
45. Van Hare G, Ben-Shachar G, Liebman J, et al: Infective endocarditis in infants and children during the past 10 years: A decade of change. Am Heart J 107:1235, 1984.
46. McGuinness G, Schieken R, and Maguire G: Endocarditis in the newborn. Am J Dis Child 134:577, 1980.
47. Kaplan EL, Rich H, Gersony W, et al: A collaborative study of infective endocarditis in the 1970's: Emphasis on patients who have undergone cardiovascular surgery. Circulation 59:327, 1979.
48. Maisch B, Eichstadt H, and Kochsiek K: Immunologic reactions in infective endocarditis. I: Clinical data and diagnostic relevance of antimyocardial antibodies. Am Heart J 106:329, 1983.
49. Parras F, Bouza E, Romero J, et al: Infectious endocarditis in children. Pediatr Cardiol 11:77, 1990.
50. Washington JA II: Blood cultures: Principles and techniques. Mayo Clin Proc 50:91, 1975.
51. Becher H, Hanrath P, Bleifeld W, et al: Correlation of echocardiographic and surgical findings in acute bacterial endocarditis. Eur Heart J 5(Suppl C):67, 1984.
52. Prager RL, Maples MD, Hammon JW, et al: Early operative intervention in aortic bacterial endocarditis. Am Thorac Surg 32:347, 1981.
53. Nihoyannopoulos P, Oakley CM, Exadactylos N, et al: Duration of symptoms and the effects of a more aggressive surgical policy: Two factors affecting prognosis of infective endocarditis. Eur Heart J 6:380, 1985.
54. Shabetai R, Fowler N, and Guntheroth W: The hemodynamics of cardiac tamponade and constrictive pericarditis. Am J Cardiol 26:480, 1970.
55. Boyle J, Pearce M, and Gaze L: Purulent pericarditis: Review of literature and report of 11 cases. Medicine 40:119, 1961.
56. Strouss AW, Santa-Maria M, and Goldring D: Constrictive pericarditis in children. Am J Dis Child 129:822, 1975.
57. Feldman WE: Bacterial etiology and mortality of purulent pericarditis in pediatric patients: Review of 162 cases. Am J Dis Child 133:641, 1979.
58. Gersony WM and McCracken GM: Purulent pericarditis in infancy. Pediatrics 40:224, 1967.
50. Laird WP, Nelson JD, and Huffines FD: The frequency of pericardial effusion in bacterial meningitis. Pediatrics 63:764, 1979.
60. Fowler NO and Monitsas G: Infectious pericarditis. Prog Cardiovasc Dis 16:323, 1973.
61. Fowler NO: Physiology of cardiac tamponade and pulsus paradoxus. Mod Conc Cardiovasc Dis 47:109, 1978.
62. Gurzton LE and Laks M: The differential diagnosis of acute pericarditis from the normal variant: New electrocardiographic criteria. Circulation 65:1004, 1982.
63. Fyfe DA, Hagler DJ, Puga FJ, et al: Clinical and therapeutic aspects of *Haemophilus influenzae* pericarditis in pediatric patients. Mayo Clin Proc 59:415, 1984.
64. Engle MA, Zabriskie JB, Senderfit LB, et al: Viral illness and the postpericardiotomy syndrome: A prospective study in children. Circulation 62:1151, 1980.
65. Engle MA, Zabriskie JB, Senderfit LB, et al: Immunologic and virologic studies in postpericardiotomy syndrome. J Pediatr 87:1103, 1975.
66. Tarbell N, Thompson L, and Mouch P: Thoracic irradiation in Hodgkin's disease: Disease control and long term complications. Int J Radiat Oncol Biol Phys 18:275, 1980.
67. Rammelkamp CH Jr, Denny FW Jr, and Wannamaker LW: Studies on the epidemiology of rheumatic fever in the armed services. *In*: Thomas L (ed): Rheumatic Fever. Minneapolis, University of Minnesota Press, 1952, pp 72–89.
68. Gordis L: The virtual disappearance of rheumatic fever in the United States: Lessons in the rise and fall of a disease. Circulation 72:1155, 1985.
69. Lennon D, Martin D, Wong E, et al: Longitudinal study of poststreptococcal disease in Auckland; rheumatic fever, glomerulonephritis, epidemiology and M typing 1981–1986. N Zealand Med J 8:396, 1988.
70. Veasey LG, Wiedmeier SE, Orsmond GS, et al: Resurgence of acute rheumatic fever in the intermountain area of the United Stated. N Engl J Med 316:421, 1987.
71. Cooperative Rheumatic Fever Study: The treatment of acute rheumatic fever in children. A cooperative clinical trial of ACTH, cortisone and aspirin. Circulation 22:503, 1960.
72. Murphy GE: Nature of rheumatic heart disease with special reference to myocardial disease and heart failure. Medicine 39:289, 1960.
73. Jones TD: The diagnosis of rheumatic fever. JAMA 126:481, 1944.
74. Committee on Rheumatic Fever and Infectious Endocarditis of the Council on Cardiovascular Disease in the Young, American Heart Association: Jones' criteria (revised) for guidance in the diagnosis of rheumatic fever. Circulation 60:204A, 1984.
75. Clarke M and Keith J: Atrioventricular conduction in acute rheumatic fever. Br Heart J 34:472, 1972.
76. Cooperative Rheumatic Fever Study: The treatment of acute rheumatic fever in children: A cooperative clinical trial of ACTH, cortisone and aspirin. Circulation 11:343, 1955.
77. Combined Rheumatic Fever Study Group (1960): A comparison of the effect of prednisone and acetylsalicylic acid therapy on the incidence of residual rheumatic heart disease. N Engl J Med 262:895, 1960.
78. Combined Rheumatic Fever Study Group (1965): A comparison of short term intensive prednisone and acetylsalicylic acid therapy in the treatment of acute rheumatic fever. N Engl J Med 272:63, 1965.
79. Shiokawa Y and Yamagata J: Plasmapheresis in the treatment of rheumatic fever. Jpn Circ J 44:797, 1980.
80. Schmaltz AA, Apitz J, and Hort W: Dilated cardiomyopathy in childhood: Problems of diagnosis and long term follow-up. Eur Heart J 8:100, 1987.
81. Griffin ML, Hernandez A, Martin TC, et al: Dilated cardiomyopathy in infants and children. J Am Coll Cardiol 11:139, 1988.
82. Mitchell HC, Froehlich LA, Bones JS, et al: An epidemiologic assessment of primary endocardial fibroelastosis. Am J Cardiol 18:859, 1966.
83. Fishbein MC, Ferrans VJ, and Roberts WC: Histologic and ultrastructural features of primary and secondary endocardial fibroelastosis. Arch Pathol Lab Med 101:49, 1977.
84. Teare D: Asymetrical hypertrophy of the heart in young patients. Br Heart J 20:1, 1958.
85. Maron BJ, Nichols PF, Pickle LW, et al: Patterns of inheritance in hypertrophic cardiomyopathy: Assessment by M-mode and two-dimensional echocardiography. Am J Cardiol 53:1087, 1984.
86. Ferrans VJ, Morrow AG, and Roberts WC: Myocardial ultrastructure in idiopathic hypertrophic subaortic stenosis: A study of operatively excised left ventricular outflow tract muscle in 14 patients. Circulation 45:769, 1972.
87. Maron BJ, Wolfson JR, Ciro E, et al: Relation of electrocardiographic abnormalities and patterns of left ventricular hypertrophy identified by two-dimensional echocardiography in patients with hypertrophic cardiomyopathy. Am J Cardiol 51:189, 1983.
88. Greenwood RD, Nadas AS, and Fyler DC: The clinical course of primary myocardial disease in infants and children. Am Heart J 92:549, 1976.
89. Maron BJ, Roberts WC, and Epstein SE: Sudden death in HCM: A profile of 78 patients. Circulation 65:1388, 1982.
90. Spicer RL, Rocchini AP, Crowley DC, et al: Hemodynamic effects of verapamil in children and adolescents with hypertrophic cardiomyopathy. Circulation 67:413, 1983.
91. Gillum RF: Idiopathic cardiomyopathy in the United States, 1970–1982. Am Heart J 111:752, 1986.
92. Maron BJ, Epstein SE, and Morrow AG: Symptomatic status and prognosis of patients after operation of hypertrophic obstructive cardiomyopathy: Efficacy of ventricular septal myotomy and myectomy. Eur Heart J 4(Suppl F):175, 1983.

36

Arrhythmias

Victoria L. Vetter, M.D.

ANATOMY

The specialized conduction system of the heart consists of the sinus node, the atrioventricular (AV) node, the His bundle, the bundle branches, and the peripheral Purkinje fibers. The sinus node is the primary pacemaker of the heart, having a faster rate of discharge than any other structure of the heart. It is the remnant of the right horn of the sinus venosus and is located on the anterolateral margin of the superior vena caval–right atrial junction just under the epicardial surface. The sinus node artery arises from the right coronary artery in 60% and from the left circumflex artery in 40% of individuals. The sinus node consists of three types of cells: P cells, T cells, and working atrial myocardial cells. The P cells, or nodal cells, are thought to be responsible for impulse formation in the sinus node. They are connected to the myocardial cells by the T, or transitional, cells. The sinus node is richly innervated with postganglionic adrenergic and cholinergic nerve terminals.[1, 2]

Although specific anatomic tracts have not been confirmed, it is generally agreed that impulses travel from the sinus node to the AV node along preferential pathways of atrial myocardium. These pathways have been designated anterior, middle, and posterior internodal tracts.

The AV node is located between the opening of the coronary sinus and the posterior border of the membranous interventricular septum, just below the right atrial endocardium and above the insertion of the tricuspid valve. The AV node is composed of three or four different types of cells whose structural and functional characteristics remain the subject of investigation. The AV node functions to direct the electrical impulse into the ventricle after a slight delay, during which time the ventricle fills. It also serves as a gate to prevent rapid electrical impulses from stimulating the ventricle. It is the major secondary pacemaker of the heart. The blood supply is from the posterior descending coronary artery.[3]

The His bundle is in direct continuity with the AV node, becoming the penetrating bundle (His bundle) as it traverses the central fibrous body and runs along the upper margin of the muscular interventricular septum. The left bundle branch leaves the branching bundle and cascades down the left ventricular septal surface, possi-

bly in a trifascicular rather than a bifascicular form. The right bundle branch continues from the branching bundle running intramyocardially. It is a cord-like structure in a fibrous sheath that subdivides into three portions and is distributed throughout the right ventricle.

Accessory pathways associated with the Wolff-Parkinson-White (WPW) syndrome are muscular connections of atrial and ventricular myocardium outside the normal area of the specialized conduction system. These pathways can exist at any point around the AV junction where atrial and ventricular myocardium is adjacent. They may occur around the tricuspid valve ring, mitral valve ring, or septal area and are designated right-sided, left-sided, or septal. Tracts exist that are designated atriofascicular, nodoventricular, or fasciculoventricular, according to their connections. Accessory pathways are composed of working atrial or ventricular myocardium, but they may consist of specialized conduction tissue similar to AV nodal cells.[4]

PHYSIOLOGY

Cardiac Action Potential

The cardiac action potential (Fig. 36–1) has five phases: phase 0, the upstroke or rapid depolarization; phase 1, early rapid repolarization; phase 2, plateau; phase 3, final rapid repolarization; and phase 4, resting membrane potential and diastolic depolarization. The phases result from passive fluxes of ions through specific channels and are regulated by their individual electrochemical gradients, resulting from active ion pumps and exchange mechanisms. Each ion has its own specific channel. Sodium and calcium channels provide the depolarizing currents and potassium channels provide the repolarizing currents. Sodium channels are referred to as fast channels and calcium channels are referred to as slow channels, although the rapidity relates to the increased number of sodium channels.[3, 5, 6]

A typical atrial or ventricular cardiac myocardial cell has a resting membrane potential of -90 mV with respect to the outside of the cell, resulting from the high permeability of K^+, which is the major ion that determines the resting potential. Sodium is pumped out of the cell and K^+ is pumped into the cell by the Na, K

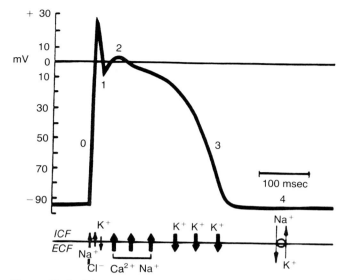

Figure 36–1. Schematic diagram of action potential of ventricular myocardium indicating ionic fluxes and phases of depolarization and repolarization. See text for details.

pump against their electrochemical gradients, allowing intracellular K^+ to remain high and intracellular Na^+ to remain low. In diastole, the cell membrane is permeable to K^+ and is relatively impermeable to Na^+, Cl^-, and Ca^{2+}. The rapid Na^+ current is responsible for activation of the atrial and ventricular myocardial cells. The slow Ca^{2+} current is responsible for activation in depolarized cells exhibiting the slow response and for activation in sinus and AV nodal cells.[7, 8]

Phase 0: Upstroke or Depolarization

The rapid upstroke in atrial and ventricular muscle and His-Purkinje fibers of the action potential is caused by a sudden increase in the membrane conductance to Na^+, generating a fast sodium current. The increase in Na^+ conductance results from the opening of voltage-gated Na^+ channels, with rapid depolarization opening the channels while maintained depolarization inactivates them. The steady state availability of Na^+ channels is regulated by resting potential such that at -90 mV, more than 80% of Na^+ channels are available for activation, whereas at -60 mV (a level present in ischemic myocardium), only 10 to 20% of Na^+ channels are available for activation. Larger Na^+ currents that produce rapid upstroke velocity, resulting in more rapidly propagating waveforms, are seen in myocardium with high (-90 mV) resting potential. Tissue with lower resting potential, such as the sinus and AV nodes and ischemic tissue, have slower velocity and propagating waveforms. During phase 0, when the membrane is depolarized to potentials positive to -40 mV, a slower inward current is activated, which is carried by the opening of Ca^{2+} channels.

Phase 1: Early Rapid Repolarization

Rapid repolarization of the membrane to 0 mV occurs with partial inactivation of the rapid inward Na^+ current

and activation of a transient outward K^+ current and possibly a Cl^- current at potentials positive to 0 mV. A slow inward Ca^{2+} current is activated at membrane potentials positive to -40 mV mediated by highly selective Ca^{2+} channels that inactivate slowly, maintaining the plateau. Phases 0 and 1 occur during inscription of the QRS complex of the electrocardiogram (ECG).

Phase 2: Plateau

The plateau phase lasts several hundred milliseconds, during which time conductance of the membrane to all ions is low. The primary inward current supporting the plateau is the Ca^{2+} current. Compared with the resting state, Na^+ and Ca^{2+} conductance is significantly enhanced, and K^+ permeability is markedly diminished during the plateau phase. The Ca^{2+} current provides the trigger for the release of Ca^{2+} from the sarcoplasmic reticulum, resulting in activation of myofilaments that provide the link between excitation and contraction. At the end of phase 2, when a sufficient number of Na^+ and Ca^{2+} channels are inactivated, the cell becomes inexcitable, and the absolute or effective refractory period occurs. As the membrane becomes partially repolarized and more Na^+ channels become available, a phase known as the relative refractory period occurs. Although an action potential may be initiated during this interval, its rate of rise and propagation velocity is slow, and the action potential duration is shorter. This results in slow aberrant conduction or block. Phase 2 occurs during the ST segment of the ECG.

Phase 3: Final Rapid Repolarization

Repolarization occurs with inactivation of the inward Ca^{2+} current and activation of an outward K^+ current (delayed rectifier), resulting in a net efflux of positive charges shifting the membrane toward a more negative potential. This results in the activation of inwardly rectifying K^+ current, which is the dominant current of the resting membrane.

Phase 4: Resting Membrane Potential and Diastolic Depolarization

In atrial and ventricular muscle cells, the resting membrane potential remains stable throughout diastole, controlled by the inwardly rectifying K^+ channel. In pacemaker cells, the membrane potential gradually depolarizes, resulting in a spontaneous action potential when the threshold level is reached. The slow diastolic depolarization, or phase 4 depolarization, is affected by a number of factors. The slope of diastolic depolarization determines the rate of pacemaker firing. For example, sympathetic stimulation (catecholamines) increases the slope of phase 4 or diastolic depolarization, whereas parasympathetic stimulation (acetylcholine) decreases the slope. A number of ionic currents controls the pacemaker potential.

Antiarrhythmic agents affect resting membrane potential, threshold potential, and phase 4 depolarization.[9]

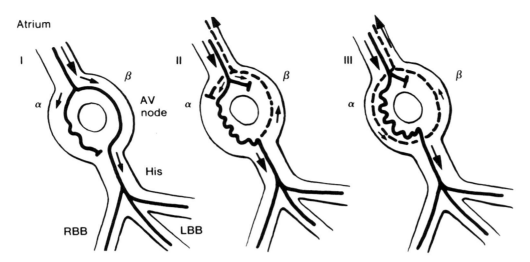

Figure 36–2. Diagram of dual AV nodal pathways showing normal conduction *(I)*, atrial echo *(II)*, and AV re-entrant tachycardia *(III)*. RBB = right bundle branch; LBB = left bundle branch.

Electrophysiologic Mechanisms of Arrhythmias

Cardiac arrhythmias are the result of abnormal impulse formation or abnormal impulse conduction, or a combination of both.[5, 10, 11]

All cardiac fibers are excitable. Certain cells in the specialized conducting system in the sinus and AV nodes depolarize spontaneously during phase 4 until threshold potential is attained and an action potential is initiated. This ability to spontaneously depolarize is called automaticity. In automatic fibers, the outward potassium current may decrease or an inward sodium current may increase with time, resulting in gradual depolarization. The rate at which normally automatic cells fire is controlled primarily by the activity of the autonomic nervous system and secondarily by changes in the local environment, including K^+ concentration, pH, PO_2, and extracellular calcium concentration.

Abnormal automaticity occurs when the function of the normal sinus pacemaker is depressed or when ectopic pacemakers compete with the sinus node. Depression of sinus node automaticity by an increase in vagal activity may shift the site of origin of the cardiac impulse to other automatic cells proximal to the AV node or to cells in the His-Purkinje system, which are not strongly influenced by vagal activity. Similarly, there may be an increase in automaticity at an ectopic site because of a local increase in sympathetic efferent activity or some local change in the condition of the cells that decreases membrane potential, such as that caused by ischemia or stretch. Enhanced phase 4 depolarization is seen in digoxin toxicity and low K^+ states. The presence of sympathetic stimulation or catecholamine excess may result in ectopic impulse initiation that competes with a normal sinus node. Triggered activity results from a second depolarization that occurs during repolarization and is referred to as an early afterdepolarization, or it occurs after repolarization has been completed and is referred to as a delayed afterdepolarization. With delayed afterdepolarizations, the slope of phase 4 is increased as the rate of stimulus is increased. This mechanism is felt to be responsible for digoxin toxic rhythms.[12]

Abnormal impulse conduction is another mechanism responsible for arrhythmias. Conduction velocity of the cardiac impulse is determined by the level of resting membrane potential and the amplitude and upstroke velocity of the action potential and by the so-called passive or cable properties of the fibers themselves.[13] Abnormal conduction occurs when conduction proceeds along abnormal pathways as in pre-excitation (the WPW syndrome) or other re-entrant pathways or when normal conduction is blocked as in sinoatrial block or AV conduction block.

Three conditions are required for re-entry to occur, and include (1) a closed circuit of conduction, (2) unidirectional block in the circuit, and (3) slow conduction. A closed circuit may exist in the atrium, AV node, or Purkinje fibers of the ventricle. Re-entry within the AV node illustrates this concept. Mines first described AV nodal re-entry in 1913,[14] and Moe described the presence of dual AV nodal pathways in 1956.[15] By convention, dual pathways have been labeled α and β. The α pathway is slower conducting but has a shorter refractory period than the faster conducting β pathway. The application of this concept to human supraventricular tachycardia (SVT) is shown in Figure 36–2. During sinus rhythm (Fig. 36–2*I*), the atrial impulse traverses the faster conducting β pathway to produce a single QRS complex. The impulse simultaneously travels down the α (slow) pathway, reaching the His bundle shortly after it has been depolarized and rendered refractory by the impulse that was conducted down the β pathway. In response to an atrial premature depolarization (Fig. 36–2*II*), the impulse is blocked in the β pathway as a result of its longer refractory period and proceeds slowly down the α pathway. If conduction down the α pathway is slow enough to allow the previously refractory β pathway time to recover, an atrial echo results. If the α pathway does not recover in time to permit subsequent antegrade conduction, only a single atrial echo results. In Figure 36–2*II*, an earlier atrial premature depolarization also blocks in the β pathway but conducts more slowly down the α pathway and arrives later to exit retrogradely from the β pathway and produce an atrial echo. However, because of the longer antegrade conduction time, the α pathway has sufficient time to recover, and a sustained AV nodal re-entrant tachycardia results. If conduction delay and refractoriness in both pathways are appropriate, a continuously circulating wave front of electrical activity ensues, resulting in a re-entrant tachycardia. The condition for re-entry may be found in the sinus node, atrium, AV node and accessory pathways, and the Purkinje fibers of the ventricle.

Simultaneous abnormalities of impulse generation and conduction result in abnormal rhythms such as parasystole.[16]

ELECTROPHARMACOLOGY OF ANTIARRHYTHMIC AGENTS

General Principles

Determination of the site of origin and the electrophysiologic mechanism of an arrhythmia allows one to select pharmacologic therapy. The selection is based on knowledge of the types of tissue affected by the agent and its ability to interfere with the specific underlying mechanism of the arrhythmia. Antiarrhythmic agents also may be grouped according to their mechanisms of action and electrophysiologic properties, as shown in Table 36–1, or by the types of arrhythmias they are used to treat. In the 1960s, Vaughan-Williams developed a classification of antiarrhythmic drugs based on electrophysiologic properties.[17, 18] Although many drugs have multiple actions, this scheme is helpful for understanding drug actions and selecting drugs that may be effective in the treatment of specific arrhythmias. Antiarrhythmic agents are grouped by their blocking actions on sodium, potassium, or calcium channels or by their ability to block adrenoreceptors. The actions of these drugs on a

Table 36–1. CLASSIFICATION OF ANTIARRHYTHMIC AGENTS

Class I	A	Procainamide
		Quinidine
		Disopyramide
	B	Lidocaine
		Phenytoin
		Mexiletine
		Tocainide
	C	Flecainide
		Encainide
		Propafenone
Class II		β-Adrenergic blockers
		Propranolol
		Nadolol
		Atenolol
		Acebutolol
		Esmolol
Class III		Amiodarone
		Bretylium
Class IV		Calcium channel blockers
		Verapamil
Other		Digoxin
		Adenosine

normal fiber will differ somewhat from their actions on damaged fibers or fibers exposed to variable external factors, such as hypoxia, acid-base or electrolyte imbalance, or variable heart rates.[9] It is important to keep in mind the effects of the various agents on cardiovascular function and interactions with the autonomic nervous system and other major organ systems. It should be noted that many drugs have metabolites that may behave differently from the parent compound.

Class I agents block the fast sodium channel.[19] Further subclassifications are based primarily on effects on action potential duration.[9] Class IA agents decrease the maximum rate of rise of phase 0 ($\dot{V}_{max}$), which prolongs refractoriness and slows conduction. Class IB agents do not reduce $\dot{V}_{max}$ but shorten the action potential duration and effective refractory period. Class IC agents reduce $\dot{V}_{max}$ and slow conduction to a greater extent than prolongation of refractoriness. Class II agents block adrenoreceptors.[20] Class III agents block potassium channels and prolong repolarization.[21] Class IV agents block the slow calcium channel.[22]

Antiarrhythmic drugs are thought to interact with receptors in the membrane channels when these channels are in the rested, activated, or inactivated states.[23] When the drug is bound to the receptor, the channel cannot conduct. These interactions vary in relation to the rate of association and dissociation of the drug. These interactions may be voltage- or time-dependent.

In general, most drug levels are trough levels and should be obtained just prior to the next dose. Digoxin levels are steady state and should be obtained 6 to 12 hours after a dose is administered. Levels should not absolutely direct therapy, but in some instances they may be an adjunct to help guide therapy and evaluate possible toxicities.

A few of the more commonly used antiarrhythmics will be discussed as representative examples.

Class I Antiarrhythmic Agents

Quinidine and Procainamide

Class IA agents act on the Na^+ channel, interfering with reactivation of this channel and prolonging the action potential duration and effective refractory period in atrial, ventricular, and Purkinje cells.[19] They also decrease membrane responsiveness and conduction velocity without changing resting membrane potential. These drugs decrease automaticity by decreasing the slope of phase 4 depolarization except at high concentrations when phase 4 depolarization is increased and automaticity is enhanced.[24] These drugs also have a vagolytic action, with a resultant increase in sinus rate and AV conduction. In patients with sinus node dysfunction, sinus node automaticity may be depressed. AV nodal and His-Purkinje conduction times may be prolonged. Because of a property referred to as use dependence, more channels are blocked at faster rates. These drugs are effective in treating AV re-entrant tachycardias related to accessory pathways because they prolong refractoriness and slow conduction in the accessory pathway. When class IA agents are used to treat atrial tachycardias, such as atrial flutter or fibrillation, previous administration of digoxin or propranolol should be used to block AV nodal conduction. Slowing of the atrial flutter rate in combination with improved AV nodal conduction (secondary vagolytic effects of class IA agents) may actually increase the ventricular response and result in hemodynamic deterioration if AV nodal blockade is not present. Class IA agents affect the ECG by prolongation of the PR interval, QRS duration, and QTc interval. Because of their ability to suppress abnormal automaticity, they may be effective in treating automatic atrial or junctional ectopic tachycardias and ventricular tachycardia.

Procainamide. The major metabolite of procainamide, N-acetylprocainamide (NAPA), is an active antiarrhythmic agent but differs from procainamide in that it does not suppress the rate of phase 4 depolarization and does not alter resting membrane potential, action potential, or the rate of rise of phase 0.[25] It does prolong action potential duration. Compared with quinidine and disopyramide, procainamide has less vagolytic effect but greater local anesthetic effect.

Side Effects. Side effects include a lupus-like syndrome that is generally reversible; gastrointestinal symptoms, especially diarrhea; confusion; disorientation and depression; blood dyscrasias; decreased myocardial function; and hypotension. Cardiac side effects include significant QTc prolongation, which is associated with proarrhythmic events (occurrence of a new arrhythmia or production of an incessant existing arrhythmia), especially a torsades de pointes type of polymorphic ventricular tachycardia.[26] This type of proarrhythmia occurs less frequently in children than in adults and less commonly with procainamide than with quinidine. An increase in the QTc interval of more than 30% or more than 0.5 second should be considered a harbinger of possible proarrhythmia, and the class IA agent should be stopped or the dosage reduced appropriately. In addition to ventricular arrhythmias, AV block may occur.

Other. Young children may require high doses to maintain adequate blood levels. Dosages up to 150 mg/kg/day may be given to infants, with careful monitoring of blood levels and side effects. Consistent levels are obtained by the intravenous route, but the infusion must be continuous, as the intravenous half-life is quite short. The best oral absorption in children too young to take the capsule or tablets is from use of the intravenous form orally. In our experience, absorption from a suspension of the oral powder (from the capsule) has been erratic, and levels have been difficult to maintain. Levels should be obtained after five doses (half-lives) and the dosage adjusted appropriately to obtain a therapeutic response with as little toxicity as possible.

Quinidine. This agent exerts α-adrenoreceptor blocking effects that decrease peripheral vascular resistance and cause hypotension. Because these effects are pronounced when given intravenously, the parenteral route is generally not used. Therefore, quinidine is rarely used in pediatrics in emergent situations. Its oral dosage formulation also limits its use somewhat in smaller children.

Side Effects. The most common side effects of quinidine use are gastrointestinal, consisting of abdominal pain, diarrhea, and anorexia. Central nervous system toxicity includes visual disturbances, hearing loss, confusion, and delirium referred to as cinchonism. ECG effects are similar to those of procainamide, though quinidine seems to have a higher incidence of proarrhythmia and QTc prolongation in children than does procainamide, especially in patients who have undergone surgery for congenital heart defects.[27]

Quinidine-induced syncope is associated with the development of polymorphic ventricular tachycardia or torsades de pointes.[28] Quinidine- or procainamide-induced torsades de pointes is treated by increasing the heart rate by pacing, usually atrial pacing.[29] If pacing cannot be achieved, isoproterenol may be used cautiously.[30] Intravenous magnesium has also been used.[31]

Class IB Antiarrhythmic Agents

Lidocaine. This agent is the most commonly used class IB agent employed in the critical care setting. It is the most effective agent used to treat ventricular arrhythmias. Lidocaine suppresses normal and abnormal automaticity in Purkinje fibers, including early and late afterdepolarizations.[32] It shortens action potential duration to a greater extent than it shortens the effective refractory period. Its effect is greater in association with acidosis, high K^+ levels, and decreased membrane potential, which are seen in ischemic states.

Side Effects. Major side effects involve the gastrointestinal tract and central nervous system. When used as a constant infusion, levels should be monitored, as they correlate well with side effects. With high levels, drowsiness, agitation, slurred speech, tinnitus, disorientation, seizures, coma, and paresthesias may occur.

Mexiletine. This agent is similar to lidocaine and may be given orally; therefore it may be used as a maintenance therapy in patients in whom lidocaine has been effective but who need long-term oral therapy. Mexiletine depresses the rate of rise of phase 0 of the action potential and depresses Purkinje fiber automaticity.[33] Mexiletine has been effective in treating ventricular arrhythmias seen after repair of tetralogy of Fallot and in association with β-blockers in the congenital long QT syndrome.[34]

Side Effects. The major side effects are gastrointestinal and consist of nausea and abdominal pain. Many of these side effects may be avoided by giving the drug after a meal. Central nervous system effects are primarily dizziness, headache, visual disturbance, tremor, and convulsions. Blood dyscrasias and hepatic toxicity may occur. Cardiac effects are infrequent but may be manifested as bradycardia.

Tocainide. This agent is similar to mexiletine. It may need to be given four times daily in children because of more rapid metabolism.

Side Effects. The side effects are similar to mexiletine; however, blood dyscrasias and pulmonary fibrosis have been noted to occur in adults.

Phenytoin. This agent has electrophysiologic actions similar to those of lidocaine and mexiletine. It may increase phase 0 upstroke velocity, may be effective in the presence of digoxin toxicity in suppressing afterdepolarizations, and may be effective in treating digoxin-related ventricular arrhythmias.[35] It has also been noted to be effective in the congenital long QT syndrome and after repair of tetralogy of Fallot.[36]

Side Effects. The side effects include myocardial depression with rapid intravenous infusion. Allergic reactions manifested by a rash are relatively common. Central nervous system effects include ataxia, nystagmus, drowsiness, and coma.

Class IC Antiarrhythmic Agents

Flecainide. Flecainide is the most commonly used class IC agent. Its role is that of maintenance therapy after acute treatment of SVT or ventricular tachycardia. In pediatrics, it has been used with greatest efficacy in the treatment of SVT associated with accessory pathways, especially permanent junctional reciprocating tachycardia.[37, 38] In this setting, it appears to be relatively safe in the treatment of re-entrant SVT, as shown by a collaborative pediatric study.[39] Nevertheless, its use must be carefully monitored, as its potential to cause proarrhythmia, torsades de pointes types of polymorphic ventricular tachycardia, and sudden death has been noted in adults treated for ventricular arrhythmias after myocardial infarction. Concerns have also been raised in pediatric patients with congenital heart defects and atrial flutter.

Flecainide blocks the rapid Na channel, decreasing V_{max}. Purkinje fiber action potential durations are decreased, whereas those of ventricular myocardium are increased. Conduction is reduced in all tissues.

Side Effects. The previously discussed proarrhythmic effects are the most serious side effects, and careful ECG monitoring must be employed for several days in the hospital when this drug is first used.

Flecainide is a negative ionotrope and should be used cautiously and only after careful consideration in patients with depressed ventricular function.

Because of its effect on conduction, patients with AV conduction system delays or damage may experience heart block using this drug. Central nervous system effects include blurred vision, dizziness, and headache.

Class II Antiarrhythmic Agents

β-Blocking Agents. The β-adrenoreceptor–blocking agents most commonly used to treat arrhythmias in children include propranolol, nadolol, and atenolol.[40] β-Blockers act by competitive inhibition of catecholamine binding at β-receptor sites. Higher concentrations exert a local anesthetic effect that depresses the inward Na current and membrane responsiveness in Purkinje fibers. Propranolol slows automaticity in fibers, especially automaticity that occurs in response to adrenergic stimulation. β-Blockers slow sinus rate and prolong the PR interval by slowing AV nodal conduction.

Side Effects. β-Blockers are negative inotropes and may decrease ventricular function, resulting in a worsening of congestive heart failure in some patients. This

effect may be seen particularly when propranolol is given intravenously. It should be noted that the intravenous dose is one tenth of the oral dose.

Other side effects include hypoglycemia, gastrointestinal symptoms of abdominal pain, diarrhea, anorexia, and bronchospasm. AV block and sinus bradycardia may occur.

Class III Antiarrhythmic Agents

Amiodarone. This agent prolongs action potential duration by blocking K channels and prolonging repolarization.[41, 42] At faster rates, V_{max} is reduced. These effects result in prolonged refractoriness and slowed conduction. Amiodarone blocks inactivated Na^+ channels, decreases automaticity, and blocks α and β receptors. Amiodarone is generally given orally, as its effects on conduction and refractoriness are less when the intravenous route is used. This may be related to the 15 to 50 times concentration of amiodarone in the myocardium compared with its concentration in plasma after chronic use. Thus its onset after oral administration is 2 to 3 days at the earliest and may be 1 to 3 weeks. Elimination is extremely slow after stopping therapy, with a mean of 53 days required.

Amiodarone is effective in children in suppressing refractory arrhythmias, especially ventricular tachycardia, atrial flutter, and junctional ectopic tachycardia.[43]

Side Effects. Although side effects are less likely to occur in children than in adults, significant side effects do exist and this drug should be used cautiously. The most significant side effect in adults, pulmonary fibrosis, has not been reported in children. Liver function abnormalities, photosensitivity, bluish gray skin discoloration, corneal deposits, and thyroid dysfunction (both hypo- and hyperthyroidism) are among the more commonly noted side effects. Because amiodarone inhibits the conversion of T_4 (thyroxine) to T_3 (triiodothyroxine), reverse T_3 is elevated. Levels of reverse T_3 greater than 90 ng/dl have correlated with a greater likelihood of toxicities developing.

Cardiac side effects of significance include marked sinus bradycardia, AV block, and polymorphic ventricular tachycardia. Patients with sinus node dysfunction or AV nodal disease may need a pacemaker when amiodarone is introduced because of its profound effects on all areas of the conduction system. Electrocardiographic effects include PR, QRS, and QTc prolongation. Because of all of these significant side effects, it is recommended that amiodarone be used in treatment of refractory life-threatening arrhythmias.

Bretylium. This agent is concentrated in sympathetic ganglia and postganglionic adrenergic nerve terminals. Initially, it causes norepinephrine release but subsequently prevents this release.[44, 45] Initial norepinephrine release may aggravate some arrhythmias. Prolonged administration prolongs action potential duration and refractoriness. Bretylium increases ventricular fibrillation thresholds, thus exerting an antifibrillatory effect. Bretylium is generally used in cases of recurrent ventricular fibrillation or ventricular tachycardia after lidocaine, procainamide, and β-blockers have failed.

Side Effects. Hypotension may occur because the efferent limb of the baroreceptor reflex is blocked. Gastrointestinal side effects are also noted and include nausea and vomiting.

Class IV Antiarrhythmic Agents

Verapamil. The calcium channel blocker used most commonly to treat arrhythmias is verapamil. Its electrophysiologic effect is to block the slow inward calcium current. It is most effective in decreasing the slope of diastolic depolarization in sinus node cells and reducing the rate of rise of phase 0, maximum diastolic potential, and action potential amplitude in sinus and AV nodal cells.[46] Therefore, it slows AV nodal conduction and prolongs AV nodal refractoriness. Verapamil also suppresses early and late afterdepolarizations. Verapamil is most effective in treating AV nodal SVT or AV reentrant SVT. One form of exercise-related ventricular tachycardia is responsive to verapamil.[47]

Side Effects. Verapamil, by virtue of its calcium channel blockade, interferes with excitation-contraction coupling and depresses myocardial function. This effect is especially pronounced in the young child and infant, in whom cardiovascular collapse and death have been reported.[48] Verapamil is not recommended for use in children less than 1 year of age or in those with impaired ventricular function. Pretreatment with calcium does not prevent this depression of cardiac function. In patients with atrial flutter or fibrillation and the WPW syndrome, verapamil may result in an increased ventricular response over the accessory pathway and should be avoided in this setting.[49] Bradycardia and AV block may occur.

Agents for Treatment of Supraventricular Tachycardia

Adenosine. This agent is a naturally occurring purine nucleoside. Adenosine decreases automaticity and slows conduction in the sinus and AV nodes.[50] It terminates AV re-entrant tachycardia by blocking the impulse in the AV node.[51] Its extremely short half-life (<10 seconds) makes it a very attractive drug for use in pediatrics, as side effects are short-lived and repetitive doses may be given starting at 50 to 100 μg/kg and increasing the dose by 50 μg/kg at 2-minute intervals until an effect has occurred, to a maximum dose of 350 μg/kg or 12 mg. The dose is given by rapid intravenous bolus followed by a saline flush.

Side Effects. The side effects include transient shortness of breath, bronchospasm, hypotension, flushing, and irritability. AV block or marked sinus bradycardia may occur. Although these effects are generally transient, administrators of this drug must be prepared to support the patient's circulation and ventilation, if necessary, until a normal rhythm resumes.

Digitalis. This agent is a cardiac glycoside, with digoxin being the most commonly used form. Digoxin has a direct effect on myocardial cells and indirect effects mediated by the parasympathetic nervous system.[52, 53] Digoxin administration results in slowing of the sinus rate by both a direct and an indirect effect. The AV nodal effects result in slowing of conduction and prolongation of the effective refractory period. The direct effects on the AV node are to decrease maximum diastolic potential, action potential amplitude, and the rate of rise of phase 0. The slope of phase 4 depolarization is increased, resulting in ectopic rhythms in toxic states.[54]

Digoxin is most effective in the treatment of AV nodal re-entrant SVT or AV re-entrant SVT, using a concealed accessory pathway. It should be avoided in patients with manifested accessory pathways (as in the WPW syndrome) because it may decrease the refractory period of the accessory pathway, increasing the ventricular response to atrial fibrillation.[55, 56] In patients with the syndrome in whom digoxin is used, usually for the treatment of congestive heart failure associated with acquired or congenital heart disease, the effect of digoxin on the refractory period of the accessory pathway should be evaluated by electrophysiologic study.

Both amiodarone and quinidine increase digoxin levels. Digoxin doses must be decreased and levels followed during concomitant use of these drugs.

Side Effects. Cardiac side effects include sinus bradycardia or sinus arrest, junctional rhythm, AV block, and ventricular arrhythmias. Gastrointestinal side effects include anorexia, nausea, vomiting, diarrhea, and abdominal pain. Central nervous system side effects include headaches, confusion, visual changes, lethargy, and irritability.

SYSTEMIC CONDITIONS ASSOCIATED WITH ARRHYTHMIAS

Collagen Vascular Diseases

Although myocardial involvement is not uncommon in children with collagen vascular diseases such as systemic lupus erythematosus, scleroderma, or polymyositis, arrhythmias are relatively uncommon. When they occur, one generally sees abnormalities of AV conduction with heart block or ventricular arrhythmias, including premature ventricular contractions or ventricular tachycardia.[57] These arrhythmias may be secondary to myocarditis or myocardial fibrosis, coronary artery involvement, systemic or pulmonary hypertension with secondary effects on the heart, or central nervous system involvement. Complete heart block has been reported in both neonatal and childhood systemic lupus erythematosus.[58, 59] Myocardial infarction from coronary artery vasculitis has also been reported and may lead to significant arrhythmias. Scleroderma and dermatomyositis produce extensive myocardial fibrosis and have been associated with AV block; ventricular arrhythmias, including ventricular tachycardia; atrial fibrillation; multifocal atrial tachycardia; and sudden death.[60]

Infection

Infection may precipitate arrhythmias in children in whom there is an underlying tendency toward arrhythmia. This is most commonly seen in patients with accessory pathways who have episodes of re-entrant SVT in the presence of an infection. This is presumed to be related to stress of the underlying infection with intrinsic changes in the sympathetic nervous system and circulating catecholamines. Treatment of even mild respiratory infections with drugs that contain sympathomimetic amines may also be a contributing factor.

More serious infections may cause arrhythmias by direct effects on the heart or other organs such as the brain or kidneys, which then affect the heart secondarily.[61] With sepsis or toxic shock syndrome, toxins directly affect myocardial function. The precise effects on conduction tissue are unknown, but these patients are known to experience delays in AV conduction, including heart block and ventricular arrhythmias, especially in the presence of diminished cardiac function.

Renal Diseases

Arrhythmias are produced in renal disease by the secondary effects of hypertension with myocardial depression or by interference with normal electrolyte balance, especially sodium, potassium, or calcium.[62] Uremic myocarditis may occur in patients with renal failure and elevated blood urea nitrogen levels. In patients taking digoxin, renal failure may precipitate digoxin toxic rhythms.

Oncologic Diseases

Primary cardiac tumors may result in life-threatening ventricular arrhythmias, including ventricular tachycardia. This has been noted with cardiac rhabdomyomas, fibromas, and oncocytic transformation of the myocardium.[63] The WPW syndrome in conjunction with SVT has been noted in association with cardiac rhabdomyomas.[64] A refractory form of ventricular tachycardia secondary to Purkinje cell tumors has been reported and has been treated surgically.[65]

Children with extracardiac tumors may acquire arrhythmias by two different mechanisms: (1) Metastases to the heart may result in ectopic rhythms[66] or (2) chemotherapeutic agents, especially anthracycline, or radiation, or both may induce cardiac arrhythmias, most commonly ventricular.[67] A number of arrhythmias, including premature atrial and ventricular beats, atrial fibrillation, SVT, ventricular tachycardia, and AV block have been noted in patients with acute leukemia.

Neuromuscular Disorders

Cardiac involvement is most commonly seen in the progressive muscular dystrophies (Duchenne), myotonic muscular dystrophy, and Friedreich ataxia[68] (see also Chapter 57).

Duchenne muscular dystrophy is a sex-linked recessive disorder with cardiac involvement most commonly manifested in the teenaged years when the patient is wheelchair-bound and often experiencing respiratory difficulties. Even prior to this time, a common ECG pattern with deep Q waves in the lateral leads (I and aV_L and V_4 to V_6) and a prominence of right-sided forces in the precordial leads is often seen. This is felt to be due to myocardial fibrosis in the posterobasal and lateral ventricular walls of the heart.[69] A short PR interval has been noted, but SVT is seldom seen. Sinus tachycardia is the most common abnormality in cardiac rhythm that is seen, but atrial flutter has been reported in patients who are in the late stage of disease and may precipitate congestive heart failure. Patients at this stage have been reported to have ventricular arrhythmias, including single or coupled premature ventricular contractions and ventricular tachycardia. Sudden death without respiratory involvement may be related to these arrhythmias. Right bundle branch block and left anterior hemiblock have been reported. Complete heart block is more commonly noted in the more slowly progressive muscular dystrophies.[70] Atrial standstill has been reported in association with facioscapulohumeral and humeroperoneal dystrophy.[71]

Myotonic dystrophy is an autosomal dominant disorder with multisystem involvement. The conduction tissues of the heart are commonly involved, especially the area of the His-Purkinje system. First-degree AV block, right bundle branch block, and left anterior hemiblock have been seen. Progression to complete heart block may result in syncope or sudden death. Other reported arrhythmias include atrial premature contractions, atrial flutter or fibrillation, premature ventricular contractions, and ventricular tachycardia.[72]

Friedreich ataxia is an autosomal recessive trait characterized by progressive spinocerebellar degeneration. Cardiac involvement (i.e., hypertrophic or dilated cardiomyopathy) occurs in the majority of patients. Premature atrial and ventricular contractions, atrial fibrillation, and ventricular arrhythmias have been reported.[73, 74]

The Kearns-Sayre syndrome consists of progressive external ophthalmoplegia, pigmentary retinopathy, and heart block. Progressive involvement of the infranodal conduction system occurs, with the development of right bundle branch block, left anterior hemiblock, and subsequent complete heart block resulting in syncope or sudden death.[75]

Familial periodic paralysis is associated with cardiac arrhythmias even without the presence of an abnormal potassium level. This usually consists of ventricular arrhythmias, including bidirectional ventricular tachycardia.[76]

Central Nervous System

Patients with intracerebral or subarachnoid hemorrhages, brain tumors, head trauma, infections of the central nervous system, or those who have undergone neurosurgical procedures have been reported to have arrhythmias. In the presence of increased intracranial pressure, sinus bradycardia and prolonged QT intervals are common, as are ST and T wave changes. AV block has been noted in association with intracerebral hemorrhage and cerebral abscesses. Brain tumors have been associated with ventricular tachycardia.[77]

Metabolic Disorders

Many inherited disorders of metabolism affect the heart[78] (see also Chapter 60). Enzyme deficiencies result in accumulation of abnormal substances in the myocardium or conduction system. The heart may be secondarily affected when central nervous system or autonomic nervous system deterioration occurs.

The lysosomal enzyme deficiencies resulting in mucopolysaccharidosis, such as the Hurler syndrome, can result in cardiomyopathy with mitral and aortic valve regurgitation and congestive heart failure. Coronary artery involvement and myocardial infarction may result in associated ventricular arrhythmias.[79, 80] Fabry disease, a deficiency of α-galactosidase A (a lysosomal enzyme) has been associated with atrial fibrillation and right bundle branch block.[81] Tay-Sachs, a gangliosidosis that results from a deficiency of hexosaminidase A, results in QTc prolongation. It is not known whether this is secondary to cardiac or central nervous system involvement. Pompe disease, or type II glycogen storage disease, is a deficiency in acid maltose (α-1,4-glucosidase) and results in storage of glycogen in lysosomes, cytoplasm, and other tissues. It results in a short PR interval, which has been seen in many of the storage diseases, and is felt to be related to deposition of abnormal material in the AV node, interrupting the normal conduction delay.[82, 83] Cytoplasmic disorders, such as selenium deficiency (Keshan disease), result in a congestive cardiomyopathy with associated atrial and ventricular arrhythmias.

Mitochondrial disorders, including acyl coenzyme A (CoA) dehydrogenase deficiency and the Kearns-Sayre syndrome, have been associated with the development of complete AV block and may require pacemaker implantation.[75] Refsum disease is a peroxisomal disorder in which phytanic acid accumulates. Complete AV block has been reported, requiring pacemaker implantation.

Familial hyperlipoproteinemias have been associated with myocardial infarction and sudden death, presumably from ventricular arrhythmias.[84]

Pulmonary Disorders

Most arrhythmias associated with pulmonary disorders are secondary to hypoxemia and acidosis.[85] Many of the drugs used to treat airway disease are sympathetic stimulants and secondarily affect the heart, producing arrhythmias. This is commonly seen in patients with asthma, especially when theophylline preparations or adrenergic drugs are used. Ventricular ectopy is the most common arrhythmia in this setting. An episode of SVT may be triggered in a susceptible patient. Use of selective β₂ agents is preferred when possible.

Cor pulmonale may result from chronic parenchymal lung disease or upper airway obstruction and can result

in arrhythmias, again usually secondary to hypoxia or hypercarbia, or both. These patients are especially sensitive to the toxic effects of digoxin.

Hematologic Disorders

The two most common hematologic disorders associated with cardiac arrhythmias are thalassemia major and sickle cell disease (see also Chapter 62). Thalassemia major results in cardiac hemosiderosis secondary to the necessary repetitive blood transfusions. Iron is deposited in ventricular and atrial myocardium and the conduction tissue. Although supraventricular arrhythmias are most common, ventricular tachycardia and AV block are the most serious conditions.[86] Administration of the iron chelator deferoxamine is being used successfully to prevent severe hemosiderosis or to treat patients with pre-existing hemosiderosis.[87] Sickle cell anemia results in atrial and ventricular arrhythmias, including atrial fibrillation. First-degree AV block and QTc prolongation are not uncommon.[88]

Endocrine Disorders

Cardiac arrhythmias may be seen in patients with disorders of the thyroid, adrenal, pituitary, and parathyroid glands (see Chapter 59).

Children with hyperthyroidism most commonly have sinus tachycardia but may present with atrial arrhythmias, including re-entrant SVT and atrial flutter or fibrillation.[89] When thyrotoxicosis is present, the arrhythmias may be resistant to the usual therapy, whereas propranolol may be effective. Care should be taken when congestive heart failure is present. Life-threatening arrhythmias are less common in patients with hypothyroidism and are usually manifested as sinus bradycardia, prolonged PR or QT intervals, and ST or T wave abnormalities.[90]

The adrenogenital syndrome produces arrhythmias by its associated hyperkalemia. AV block and ventricular tachycardia are the most common serious arrhythmias. Pheochromocytomas produce elevated levels of catecholamines, which lead to atrial or ventricular tachycardia or fibrillation.[91] These arrhythmias are a result of enhanced automaticity and respond to α-receptor blockade with phentolamine and to β-receptor blockers. Patients with hyperparathyroidism or hypoparathyroidism have arrhythmias associated with hypercalcemia or hypocalcemia. Pituitary tumors may result in arrhythmias associated with an elevated growth hormone level. This is especially noted when congestive heart failure ensues.[92]

Drugs, Toxins, and Anesthetic Agents

Accidental ingestions are quite common in pediatrics. Many of the agents ingested can produce arrhythmias, as shown in Table 36–2 (see also Chapter 80). The general procedures for acute poisoning are recom-

Table 36–2. DRUGS, TOXINS, AND ANESTHETIC AGENTS

Agent	Common Arrhythmias
Tricyclic antidepressants	Atrial flutter or fibrillation
	Ventricular tachycardia or fibrillation
	Atrioventricular block
	Asystole
Phenylephrine	Ventricular arrhythmia
	Bradycardia
	Supraventricular tachycardia
Sympathomimetic amines	Supraventricular tachycardia
Antihistamine-decongestant preparations	
Volatile hydrocarbons	Ventricular fibrillation
Benzene	
Cocaine-crack	Ventricular tachycardia
	Ventricular fibrillation
Anesthetic agents	Ventricular arrhythmia
Halothane	
Enflurane	
Ketamine	

mended, but specific arrhythmias must be recognized and treated appropriately. In addition to the usual antiarrhythmic agents, the anticholinesterase agent physostigmine is indicated to treat life-threatening arrhythmias, usually ventricular tachycardia, atrial flutter, or atrial fibrillation associated with tricyclic antidepressant toxicity.[93] Intravenous lidocaine and β-blockers may also be indicated.

A number of factors related to general anesthesia and surgery may result in cardiac arrhythmias.[94] These factors include abnormal blood gas concentrations or electrolyte imbalances, endotracheal intubation with exaggeration of vagal reflexes, central nervous system or sympathetic nervous system involvement or stimulation, dental surgery with autonomic nervous system stimulation, pre-existing cardiac disease, and placement of wires or catheters in the heart.

TRAUMA

Blunt Trauma

Cardiac contusion from blunt trauma to the heart is unusual in children but may occur without the presence of obvious chest wall injury. Precordial chest pain is the most common symptom. Evidence of myocardial injury may be evident on the ECG with ST-T wave changes and abnormal Q waves. Premature ventricular contractions are the most common arrhythmias seen. Other reported arrhythmias include SVT, ventricular tachycardia, AV block, or bundle branch block and ventricular fibrillation[95] (see also Chapter 85).

Electrical Trauma

Electrocution as the result of accidents in children has been known to result in ventricular fibrillation.[96] Low levels of electrical shock that may not produce ventric-

ular fibrillation may result in frequent ventricular premature complexes, ventricular tachycardia, and evidence of myocardial damage on the ECG (see also Chapter 88).

UNOPERATED CONGENITAL HEART DISEASE

Eisenmenger Syndrome and Pulmonary Vascular Obstructive Disease

Because of early recognition and repair of congenital heart defects, few new patients are now experiencing pulmonary vascular obstructive disease, although a population of patients exist who already have irreversible pulmonary hypertension. These are generally patients with complex congenital heart diseases, including single ventricles and transposition complexes. These patients are at high risk for the development of cardiac arrhythmias and sudden death, which has been reported at an incidence of 14 to 47% in patients with Eisenmenger syndrome.[97] These patients frequently experience ventricular arrhythmias due to long-standing ventricular volume and pressure overload. Many of these patients have associated severe semilunar or AV valve regurgitation. Those with AV valve regurgitation are prone to the development of atrial flutter or fibrillation.

Cyanotic Congenital Heart Disease with Pulmonary Stenosis or Atresia

A variety of arrhythmias have been reported in patients with cyanotic congenital heart disease and pulmonary stenosis or atresia, including SVT, atrial flutter, and ventricular arrhythmias. In older patients with marked polycythemia, ventricular arrhythmias are not uncommon.

Ebstein Anomaly

Up to 40 to 80% of patients with the Ebstein anomaly have arrhythmias preoperatively.[98] The arrythmia most commonly associated with this lesion is SVT, occurring in 30% of patients. The WPW syndrome occurs in 10 to 15% of these patients with associated SVT. The pathways are most commonly located in the posterior septal and right ventricular free wall sites. AV nodal reentry has been seen. Atrial flutter or fibrillation, junctional rhythms, AV block, and ventricular tachycardia and fibrillation are known to occur. Sudden death occurs in up to 20% of these patients. Arrhythmias are common during cardiac catheterization and surgery.

D-Transposition of the Great Arteries

Although infrequent supraventricular arrhythmias have been seen, including atrial flutter and premature atrial contractions and ventricular arrhythmias, preoperative arrhythmias are uncommon in patients with D-transposition of the great arteries.[99]

Corrected Transposition of the Great Arteries

The most commonly associated arrhythmias include the WPW syndrome with SVT, second- or third-degree heart block, and ventricular tachycardia or fibrillation.[100] AV block occurs in 30 to 60% of patients with complete heart block in at least 30% of cases. This may occur quite late in life and may result in sudden death.

Tricuspid Atresia

Preoperative arrhythmias, including atrial arrhythmias and ventricular ectopy, have been reported in older patients before repair. It has been suggested that some of the postoperative arrhythmias that occur may be part of the natural history of this lesion.[101]

Aortic Stenosis and Coarctation of the Aorta

Ventricular arrhythmias may occur in patients with aortic stenosis and coarctation of the aorta, particularly in the presence of a marked elevation of left ventricular pressure.[102] AV block and the WPW syndrome have been reported to be associated with coarctation of the aorta, though this is uncommon.[103]

Tetralogy of Fallot

Ventricular arrhythmias occur with increasing frequency in older patients with unoperated tetralogy of Fallot.[104] Twenty-one per cent of patients older than 16 years of age have been reported to experience ventricular tachycardia. SVT may occur in older patients as well.

Atrial Septal Defects

A number of supraventricular arrhythmias occur in patients with atrial septal defects (ASD), particularly in patients who reach an older age before diagnosis and repair. Preoperative arrhythmias occur in more than 50% of patients older than 30 years of age at the time of surgery.[105] Atrial flutter and fibrillation are the most common arrhythmias, but SVT and junctional and ectopic atrial rhythms are not uncommon. Sinus node dysfunction is seen in 18% of patients with sinus venosus ASD, compared with 4% of patients with secundum ASD.[106] AV block may be seen in primum ASD or in association with ASD syndromes such as the Holt-Oram syndrome.

Miscellaneous Conditions

Any type of unoperated congenital lesion may have associated arrhythmias. The lesions just described are those most commonly seen but do not represent an exhaustive list (see also Chapter 33).

POSTOPERATIVE ARRHYTHMIAS IN CONGENITAL HEART DISEASE

The correction of specific cardiac defects predisposes one to the development of specific types of arrhythmias.[107] The significant abnormal postoperative arrhythmias include SVT, atrial flutter, accelerated junctional rhythm, ventricular tachycardia, sick sinus syndrome, and complete heart block.[108] Supraventricular arrhythmias are more common in association with lesions requiring extensive atrial surgery or after repairs with elevated preoperative or postoperative atrial pressure. Intra-atrial repairs such as the Mustard or Senning repair for D-transposition of the great arteries[109] and the Fontan repair for complex single-ventricle lesions are associated with sick sinus syndrome and SVT, especially atrial flutter.[110] Similar arrhythmias occur after repair of ASDs or total anomalous pulmonary venous return. Supraventricular arrhythmias are associated with sudden death in 2 to 8% of these patients. More than 90% of patients who undergo the Mustard procedure will have evidence of sinus node dysfunction 10 years after the surgery, and 10 to 20% will be affected sufficiently to require pacemaker implantation. Close to 25% will require treatment for atrial flutter.[111] As these patients age, ventricular arrhythmias are reported more frequently.[112] Forty per cent of patients who undergo Fontan repair will have SVT postoperatively; sinus node dysfunction and ventricular tachycardia have also been noted.

Lesions associated with postoperative ventricular tachycardia include tetralogy of Fallot, ventricular septal defects, AV canal defects, aortic stenosis, idiopathic hypertrophic subaortic stenosis, the Ebstein anomaly, coronary artery anomalies, single-ventricle complexes after Fontan repair, and D-transposition of the great arteries.[113] Ten to 15% of these patients have ventricular tachycardia postoperatively. Sudden death occurs in 5 to 10% of patients.[114]

An interesting postoperative arrhythmia that occurs in the acute postoperative setting is the rhythm designated as accelerated junctional rhythm or junctional ectopic tachycardia.[115] In the postoperative setting, this rhythm carries a high mortality if it cannot be slowed.[116] It is seen most commonly after repair of tetralogy of Fallot or the Fontan repair. The rates often accelerate to more than 250 bpm and produce severe hemodynamic compromise.

ACQUIRED HEART DISEASE

A variety of acquired infections and inflammatory disorders are associated with arrhythmias. They include viral myocarditis,[117, 118] rheumatic fever,[119] Lyme disease,[120] and Kawasaki disease.

Viral Myocarditis

Viral myocarditis is an inflammation of the myocardium associated with a number of viral illnesses (see also Chapter 35). Myocardial damage in myocarditis is related to direct viral damage of the cell and to an immune response against cells that have been infected by the virus. Arrhythmias include premature atrial contractions, SVT, premature ventricular contractions, ventricular tachycardia, and AV conduction disturbances. Myocarditis may occur with other infectious agents, including rickettsia, bacteria, protozoa, parasites, fungi, and yeasts.

Although all areas of the conduction system may be involved with myocarditis, the most serious arrhythmias are AV block and ventricular tachycardia. AV block may be transient, but in cases in which cardiac output is limited, temporary intracardiac pacing should be performed. If normal conduction does not return after 2 weeks, permanent pacing is indicated. Because of the tendency toward development of ventricular arrhythmias, the heart rate should not be increased with adrenergic agents. Infection with diphtheria is interesting in that the diphtheria exotoxin has an affinity for conduction tissue, often with resultant complete AV block.

Ventricular arrhythmias should be treated if ventricular function is compromised by the arrhythmias or if the nature of the arrhythmia is such that deterioration to a more malignant arrhythmia is likely to occur. In the presence of depressed ventricular function, aggressive treatment of ventricular arrhythmias is indicated. Improvement of ventricular function with inotropic support and correction of metabolic and electrolyte aberrations generally improves arrhythmia control. Careful monitoring is essential, as many of the inotropic agents will be arrhythmogenic in this setting. Although individual responses vary, dobutamine is generally less arrhythmogenic than is dopamine. Rhythm responses to amrinone vary. Epinephrine and isoproterenol have the greatest arrhythmogenic potential.

Patients with myocarditis may be overly sensitive to digoxin, and digitalization should be achieved slowly with lower doses than those used for the usual patient with congestive heart failure and under careful continuous electrocardiographic monitoring.

Rheumatic Fever

Rheumatic fever is a result of an upper respiratory tract infection with group A β-hemolytic streptococci. It is an inflammatory process involving connective tissue and affecting the heart, along with joints, brain, blood vessels, and subcutaneous tissue. Cross-reacting antibodies against the streptococcus appear to interact with the cardiac cell.[121] Other abnormalities in the immune system occur, adding to the abnormal autoimmune responses seen in this illness. Cytotoxic substances play a role in the pathogenesis of this disease. These factors may be responsible for the myocarditis associated with acute rheumatic fever.

Serious arrhythmias are uncommon in acute rheumatic fever. The AV conduction system is most commonly involved, as manifested by the typical PR prolongation seen on the ECG. Complete heart block may occur. Specific lesions have not been found in the specialized conducting tissues, suggesting a transient vasculitis could be responsible. The most common arrhythmia associated with long-standing rheumatic heart disease relates to the mitral valve involvement, particularly mitral stenosis. Atrial fibrillation is a common occurrence in patients with severe mitral stenosis and may not resolve after relief of the mitral stenosis.[122]

Lyme Disease

Lyme disease is a multisystem disease involving skin, joints, nervous system, and heart. It is caused by a spirochete called *Borrelia burgdorferi* generally transmitted by the deer tick *Ixodes dammini*. Cardiac involvement occurs in 8% of individuals with Lyme disease and may consist of a mild myopericarditis. Although uncommon, AV conduction disturbances that may progress to complete AV block are the most common arrhythmias.[120] Occasional pacing may be necessary. Premature atrial contractions, SVT, premature ventricular contractions, and ventricular arrhythmias may occur. The usual antiarrhythmic agents for the specific arrhythmia may be indicated to temporarily suppress the arrhythmias. Antibiotic treatment generally results in resolution of the arrhythmia after several weeks. Steroids have been used in patients with AV block with resultant resolution of the block.

Kawasaki Disease

Kawasaki disease is an acute febrile syndrome of unknown etiology that was first reported from Japan in 1967. The most serious, acute, and long-term involvement involves the cardiovascular system. There is a 15 to 20% incidence of coronary artery aneurysms. They may be manifested early or late by acute myocardial infarction and associated ventricular arrhythmias, SVT, atrial fibrillation, or AV block.[123] Myocarditis is seen in more than 50% of patients and may be manifested by electrocardiographic changes, including PR or QTc prolongation, low QRS voltage, and ST-T wave changes. Arrhythmias are unusual and generally transient, usually consisting of premature atrial or ventricular contractions (see also Chapters 35 and 67).

ELECTROLYTE IMBALANCES

Abnormalities in electrolyte concentrations may affect heart rate, rhythm, and automaticity and lead to arrhythmias. Potassium and calcium abnormalities most commonly result in abnormal rhythms, though alterations in magnesium and acid-base balance may produce arrhythmias.[124, 125] Any patient with significant unexplained arrhythmia should undergo electrolyte testing. Electrocardiographic changes are characteristic and should lead to suspicion of a specific electrolyte abnormality.

Hyperkalemia

Electrocardiographic abnormalities may be roughly associated with serum levels.[126] Peaked T waves are seen at a serum concentration of 5 to 6 mEq/l, and the QRS widens when the concentration exceeds 6 mEq/l. When the concentration is greater than 7 mEq/l, the QT interval increases, the QRS complex widens, P wave amplitude decreases and duration increases, and the PR interval increases. When the concentration exceeds 8 to 9 mEq/l, P waves disappear, the ventricular rate becomes irregular, and severe bradycardia with sinus arrest, block, or idioventricular rhythms occurs, often with a sinusoidal wave pattern. Ventricular fibrillation or asystole occurs at serum concentrations greater than 12 to 14 mEq/l. The myocardial toxicity of hyperkalemia is enhanced by low serum calcium levels.

Hypokalemia

Potassium concentrations of less than 2.7 mEq/l produce electrocardiographic changes, including a U wave with an amplitude of more than 1 mm, and ST segment depression greater than 0.5 mm. The QT interval becomes prolonged, and the T wave becomes flattened with progressive hypokalemia. The PR interval becomes prolonged, and intraventricular conduction becomes delayed with a widened QRS complex. P wave and QRS amplitude may become increased with marked hypokalemia. Other arrhythmias have been associated with low serum potassium levels, including ectopic atrial and ventricular complexes, ectopic or automatic atrial tachycardia with block, AV dissociation, second-degree AV block, and ventricular tachycardia and fibrillation. Patients with hypokalemia who are taking digoxin are particularly susceptible to digoxin toxic arrhythmias related to the combined effects on automaticity and conduction.[127]

Hypocalcemia

The electrocardiographic changes noted correlate with ionized calcium, with the degree of QT prolongation (ST segment prolongation) being proportional to the degree of hypocalcemia. Other associated arrhythmias include SVT and second-degree and complete heart block. The effects of potassium and calcium on myocardial cells are antagonistic. Calcium should be administered cautiously to patients taking digoxin, with continuous cardiac monitoring because of the possibility of precipitating digoxin toxic rhythms.

Hypercalcemia

Calcium levels greater than 12 mg/dl result in a shortened QT interval, a shortened ST segment, and normal or prominent U waves. More marked hypercalcemia may produce PR and QRS prolongation, and second- and third-degree AV block. Elevated levels of serum calcium decrease the effect of hyperkalemia and potentiate digoxin toxicity.

Hypomagnesemia

Low magnesium levels are frequently associated with hypokalemia or hypocalcemia, with the electrocardiographic abnormalities reflecting the combined effects of all of these aberrations. Noted arrhythmias have included ectopic complexes and ventricular fibrillation.[31]

Hypermagnesemia

Magnesium levels of 3 to 5 mEq/l are associated with delays in AV and intraventricular conduction (see also Chapter 58).

SPECIFIC ARRHYTHMIAS

General Principles

Appropriate management of pediatric arrhythmias requires correct and rapid diagnosis of the specific type of arrhythmia. This section is not intended to be an exhaustive compendium of the electrocardiographic diagnosis of cardiac arrhythmias, but a few suggestions will be made that should simplify the diagnosis of arrhythmias in the intensive care setting.

When an abnormal rhythm is appreciated, a 12-lead ECG should be obtained if at all possible. The ECG should be scanned to determine if the heart rate is abnormally high or low. The next factor to be considered is whether the abnormal rhythm is of sinus origin or is originating from an abnormal mechanism. Because of the multiple stresses experienced by the patient in intensive care, sinus tachycardia is often the rule rather than the exception. The most common causes of sinus tachycardia and bradycardia in the critical care setting are shown in Table 36–3. The relationship of the P wave to the QRS complex, the P wave axis, as well as the PR interval should be considered in differentiating between a sinus and an abnormal tachycardia.

If it is determined that the rhythm is not sinus in origin, the next factor to be determined is the origin. Is it supraventricular or ventricular? Although most narrow complex tachycardias are of supraventricular origin and most wide complex tachycardias are of ventricular origin, it is well known that wide complex tachycardias include, in addition to ventricular tachycardia, antidromic SVT, atrial flutter or fibrillation with aberration, nodofascicular or nodoventricular accessory pathways

Table 36–3. COMMON CAUSES OF ARRHYTHMIAS

Sinus Tachycardia	Sinus Bradycardia
Fever, infection	Hypothermia
Anemia	Increased intracranial pressure
Myocarditis	Head trauma
Hyperthyroidism	Brain tumor
Drugs: sympathomimetic	Meningitis
Fear, anxiety	Infections
Pheochromocytoma	Typhoid fever
Hypoxia	Q fever
Dehydration, hypovolemia	Chagas disease
Hypotension	Hypothyroidism
	Drugs: digoxin, propranolol, morphine
	Anorexia

with reciprocating tachycardia, and orthodromic reciprocating tachycardia with aberration. The other confounding issue is the fact that many ventricular rhythms in infants are only 80 or 90 msec in duration, making the distinction between wide and narrow complex tachycardia difficult until the sinus rhythm is present for comparison. It should be noted that many intensive care unit patients who have had cardiac surgery will have a bundle branch block, especially of the right bundle. Sinus tachycardia, especially if associated with first-degree AV block, will be a wide QRS tachycardia with a P wave that is somewhat difficult or impossible to visualize often being on top of the T wave.

Noncritical Arrhythmias

Certain arrhythmias are critical because they produce hemodynamic instability, and others are critical because of their potential to do so. Before instituting a therapy that may complicate or worsen the patient's condition, the physician must be certain that the clinical problem warrants intervention.

Premature ventricular contractions are not an absolute indication for intervention unless they are frequent enough to interfere with cardiac output, are closely coupled or frequently fall on the T wave in a patient judged to be vulnerable to such occurrences, or occur in runs, resulting in hemodynamic instability.

Premature atrial contractions or premature junctional contractions rarely require intervention. Second-degree AV block can usually be observed without intervention unless long pauses occur or a medication is found to be responsible.

Critical Arrhythmias

As previously mentioned, arrhythmias become critical because of their hemodynamic effects. However, certain arrhythmias are likely to produce instability and are discussed in the following sections.

Supraventricular Tachycardia

Paroxysmal SVT, also known as paroxysmal atrial tachycardia, is the most common significant arrhythmia seen in children. SVT describes a group of arrhythmias with similar electrocardiographic manifestations but different mechanisms. A typical example is shown in Figure 36–3. The rate of the tachycardia in infants ranges from 220 to 320 bpm and in older children, it ranges from 150 to 250 bpm.

The incidence of SVT is estimated to be 1 in 250 to 1000 children.[128] It occurs most commonly in boys less than 4 months of age. Predisposing factors are present in more than half of cases and include infection, fever, or drug exposure (20 to 24%); the WPW syndrome (10 to 22%); and congenital heart disease (20 to 23%). Ventricular septal defects, the Ebstein anomaly of the tricuspid valve, corrected transposition of the great arteries, and cardiomyopathies are the most common unoperated lesions. The most common postoperative congenital heart lesions are D-transposition of the great arteries, ASDs, AV canal defects, and Fontan repairs. The 40 to 50% of patients without associated conditions are considered to have idiopathic SVT, but most probably there are concealed accessory pathways or AV nodal re-entry that explain their propensity to have this type of arrhythmia. Congestive heart failure occurs most commonly in infants less than 4 months of age but is unlikely to occur in children with normal hearts in the first 24 hours of the arrhythmia. Children with extremely

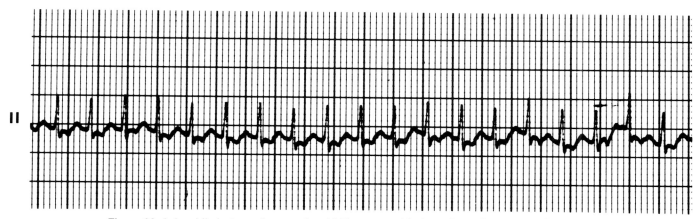

Figure 36–3. Lead II electrocardiogram of a child in supraventricular tachycardia at a rate of 270 bpm.

fast heart rates or underlying abnormalities of the heart or other systems will be less tolerant of rapid arrhythmias.

Electrophysiologic mechanisms of SVT include (1) re-entry within the sinus node, atrium, AV node, or accessory pathways or (2) enhanced automaticity of the atrial or AV junctional tissues. The most common supraventricular arrhythmias seen in children include concealed bypass tracts with SVT, the WPW syndrome with SVT, AV nodal re-entry, and atrial flutter or fibrillation.

The most common type of SVT seen in children is that associated with an accessory pathway with antegrade conduction—the WPW syndrome.[129] The WPW syndrome occurs in as many as 0.1% of children. SVT associated with this syndrome occurs most commonly in infants less than 1 month of age. A congenital heart defect is seen in approximately one fifth to one third of these patients. A positive family history has been reported. One third of the accessory tracts are located in the right ventricular free wall, one third are located in the left ventricle, and one third are located in the septal area. The WPW syndrome is diagnosed from the ECG performed when the patient is in sinus rhythm, as shown in Figure 36–4. The PR interval is short because the accessory pathway bypasses the normal delay that occurs in the AV node. There is a slurred upstroke (delta wave) at the onset of the QRS complex related to delayed conduction as the impulse traverses normal ventricular myocardium to reach the specialized conduction tissues when the rapid portion of the QRS complex is inscribed. The typical WPW complex is not seen in most episodes of SVT associated with these pathways, as the tachycardia is initiated by a premature complex that becomes blocked in the accessory pathway and is conducted antegradely through the AV node and in a retrograde fashion through the accessory pathway. A continuation of this circuit results in an orthodromic AV reciprocating SVT with a narrow complex QRS tachycardia. Thus, re-entrant SVT in the WPW syndrome is analogous to AV nodal re-entrant SVT, with the bypass tract functioning like a β pathway (fast conduction, long refractory period) and the AV node functioning like an α pathway (slow conduction, short refractory period). In approximately 10% of cases in children, the route of re-entry is reversed, and the bypass tract forms the antegrade limb, with the AV node forming the retrograde limb of the re-entrant circuit. These tachycardias are referred to as antidromic and present as a wide QRS tachycardia that may be difficult to distinguish from ventricular tachycardia. Although atrial fibrillation occurs commonly in adults with the WPW syndrome, it is less common in children and when seen occurs most often after 10 years of age. The danger of atrial fibrillation is that a pathway with a short refractory period and rapid conduction may allow rapid conduction of the impulse to the ventricle, with hemodynamic deterioration or ventricular fibrillation.[49, 55, 56]

In some patients with the WPW syndrome, the pathway is difficult to see on the surface ECG, becoming manifested only at faster heart rates or in other instances when AV conduction slows. These pathways are referred to as latent.

A concealed bypass tract, sometimes referred to as concealed WPW, indicates that the bypass tract is used only as the retrograde limb of the re-entrant circuit during SVT but is not used during normal sinus rhythm.[130] The resting ECG will show no evidence of a delta wave, as no antegrade conduction occurs over this tract. When accessory pathways form part of the re-entrant circuit, the atrium will always be depolarized after the ventricle, and the ECG during SVT will reveal a retrograde P wave in both the WPW syndrome SVT and SVT associated with a concealed accessory pathway. The P wave may be difficult to see, as it occurs during the T wave. The RP interval is usually less than the PR interval.

An unusual form of SVT known as permanent junctional reciprocating tachycardia has a slow retrograde pathway and therefore a long RP interval compared with the faster antegrade pathway as evidenced by a shorter PR interval.[131] An example is shown in Figure 36–5.

A study by Gillette in 1977 describing the location of concealed bypass tracts found 60% in the left atrium, 30% in the right atrium, and 10% in the septum.[132]

In one study, AV nodal re-entry was the second most common type of SVT in children, occurring in 24% of subjects and was the most common type in children older than 5 years of age.[133] Retrograde P waves may not be seen in this type of SVT, as atrial and ventricular activation occur almost simultaneously. If the P wave is visible, it is closely related to the preceding QRS complex. Treatment of AV nodal re-entrant SVT consists of drugs that primarily affect the AV node, such as digoxin, propranolol, and verapamil.

Sinus node re-entry is uncommon in children but may present as an unexplained sinus tachycardia. The electrocardiographic presentation is that of a sinus tachycardia, but onset and offset may be sudden. β-Blockers are the most effective treatment for this arrhythmia. If sinus node automaticity is abnormal, a pacemaker may be needed to provide an adequate heart rate.

Although the ECG during SVT may be suggestive of the mechanism, an electrophysiologic study may be needed to determine the precise mechanism of the tachycardia if it is determined that this information is necessary. The electrophysiologic study may be used to locate the site of the accessory pathway in both the WPW syndrome and concealed accessory pathway SVT.

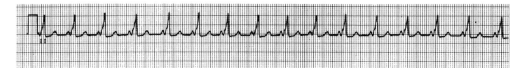

Figure 36–4. Lead II electrocardiogram of a patient with Wolff-Parkinson-White syndrome illustrating short PR interval and delta wave.

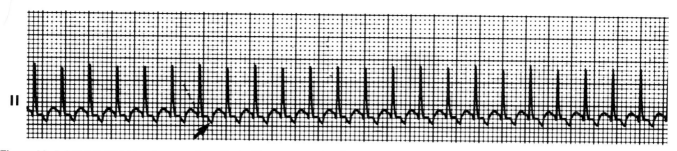

Figure 36–5. Lead II electrocardiogram of a patient with permanent junctional reciprocating tachycardia (PJRT). *Solid arrow* indicates retrograde P wave with long PR interval.

It is also used to determine the refractory period of the accessory pathway, to induce the SVT, and to determine the ventricular response to atrial fibrillation when it can be induced in patients with the WPW syndrome.[134]

Treatment. Since the mechanisms can usually be identified, treatment can be chosen for the specific forms of SVT.[135] The main principle of treatment in any cardiac arrhythmia is that the form of therapy is determined by the clinical status of the patient. Thus the type of treatment chosen for the patient in shock is different from that given to the patient who is asymptomatic and has only a fast heart rate, as shown in Table 36–4. When the SVT is caused by AV re-entry, any intervention that interrupts the critical relationship of conduction and refractoriness between the two limbs of the re-entrant circuit can interrupt the tachycardia. Carotid sinus pressure or the Valsalva maneuver is rarely successful in children but may be attempted. In children not attached to life support systems, a headstand will often successfully interrupt the tachycardia. More commonly, especially in infants, application of an ice or ice-water bag directly to the center of the infant's face will recruit the diving reflex and stop the SVT.[136]

A new rapid pharmacologic treatment now available is adenosine. It has a rapid onset, usually within 10 seconds, and a short half-life, with side effects lasting less than a minute and rarely being serious.[137] Adenosine may be used in acutely ill patients but should not delay immediate cardioversion in severely compromised patients. For those patients who become acidotic or hypotensive, synchronized DC cardioversion is advised, with a dosage of 1 to 2 watt-sec/kg. The dosage may be continually doubled until it is effective or until a level of 10 watt-sec/kg is reached. The older patient should be given a sedative or short-acting anesthetic agent, and preparation should be made for airway support and ventilation if needed. The underlying acidosis should be treated, and adequate ventilation and oxygenation of the patient provided, as cardioversion may not be successful in the presence of hypoxia and acid-base imbalance. However, cardioversion should not be delayed to make these corrections but should be performed immediately in emergent situations. The presence of digoxin in the patient should not prevent the use of cardioversion when needed. Evidence of digoxin toxicity, such as ventricular arrhythmias, may be treated with intravenous lidocaine (1 mg/kg). Once the patient's rhythm has been converted, the chosen chronic treatment should be initiated immediately.

Children with mild to moderate congestive heart failure may be treated initially with adenosine if vagal maneuvers are unsuccessful. Pharmacologic agents such as digoxin, procainamide, or propranolol may be used. Intravenous digoxin is the preferred route in the critically ill patient. The digitalizing dose intervals may be given at 2 to 4 hours as determined by the patient's status. Although digoxin toxic rhythms may not be noted as easily with this type of rapid digitalization, the need to convert the tachycardia takes precedence in this instance. If the tachycardia persists after three doses, one to two additional doses equivalent to one quarter of the total digitalizing dose may be given. The maintenance dose should be determined according to the total digitalizing dose required and is one eighth of the total digitalizing dose given twice daily.

Other pharmacologic agents that may be used acutely are shown in Table 36–5. Propranolol, which prolongs

Table 36–4. ACUTE TREATMENT OF SUPRAVENTRICULAR TACHYCARDIA

Asymptomatic
Ice, vagal maneuvers
IV* adenosine
Pharmacologic agents
  IV digoxin
  Oral procainamide
  Oral propranolol

Mild Congestive Heart Failure
Ice, vagal maneuvers
IV adenosine
Pharmacologic agents
  IV digoxin
  Oral procainamide
  Oral propranolol

Moderate Congestive Heart Failure
Ice, vagal maneuvers
IV adenosine
Pacing, esophageal or intracardiac
Pharmacologic agents
  IV digoxin
  IV procainamide
Cardioversion, synchronized

Severe Congestive Heart Failure
Cardioversion, synchronized
IV adenosine
Pacing, esophageal or intracardiac
Pharmacologic agents
  IV digoxin
  IV procainamide

*IV = intravenous.

Table 36–5. PHARMACOLOGIC AGENTS FOR ACUTE TREATMENT OF SUPRAVENTRICULAR TACHYCARDIA

Agent	Initial Treatment (IV)*
Adenosine	50–100 µg/kg; increase by 50-µg/kg increments every 2 min to 350 µg/kg or 12 mg maximal dose
Digoxin	30 µg/kg TDD†; maximum dose = 1 mg
Procainamide	5 mg/kg over 5–10 min 10–15 mg/kg over 30–45 min Infusion: 20–100 µg/kg/min
Propranolol	0.05–0.1 mg/kg over 5 min every 6 hr
Phenylephrine	100 µg/kg IV bolus Infusion: 10 µg/kg/min
Verapamil	0.15 mg/kg over 3–5 min
Amiodarone	IV: 1 mg/kg every 10 min every 12 hr for 10 doses ORAL: 10–20 mg/kg/day PO‡ bid§ × 7–14 days, then 5–10 mg/kg/day PO every day

*IV = intravenous.
†TDD = total digitalizing dose.
‡PO = by mouth.
§bid = twice daily.

AV nodal conduction and refractoriness in both α and β pathways should be used with caution in the ill child, as it may further depress cardiac function. In instances in which cardiac function is not compromised, a slow intravenous dose may be given. Some have recommended using a shorter acting β-blocker such as esmolol in this setting, but little data are available in children. Propranolol or other β-blockers may be quite effective in treating SVT associated with accessory pathways, as it slows the AV nodal limb of the circuit without affecting the accessory pathway.[138] β-Blockers are preferred over digoxin for SVT treatment in the presence of the WPW syndrome.

Phenylephrine is effective because it raises the blood pressure and thus recruits the baroreceptor-vagal reflexes. Termination usually occurs in the antegrade slow pathway.[139]

The class I agents such as procainamide may be given intravenously, and they terminate the SVT by blocking retrograde conduction in the fast (β) pathway of the AV node or in the accessory pathway when it is a part of the circuit. These agents are particularly effective for permanent junctional reciprocating tachycardia (PJRT).

Overdrive pacing may be used to convert SVT to sinus rhythm.[140] Previously, this had involved the placement of an intracardiac catheter with pacing of the atrium at a rate slightly higher than the rate of the tachycardia. Cessation of pacing often results in resumption of normal rhythm. A less invasive method of overdrive pacing involves the use of an esophageal pacing catheter, which is placed, via the nose or mouth, in the esophagus behind the heart and is used in the same manner to capture the atrial rhythm and interrupt the re-entrant circuit.[141] It is effective in most instances of AV reciprocating tachycardia and in more than half of the cases of atrial flutter. In postoperative cardiac surgery patients, epicardial wires may be present and may be used for pacing to terminate the tachycardia.

Although verapamil has been an effective treatment of SVT in adults, serious problems have occurred with its use in pediatric patients. This is a particular problem in patients less than 1 year of age and in those with severe congestive heart failure. The use of verapamil in this patient population has resulted in cardiovascular collapse and death.[48, 142] Pretreatment with calcium does not prevent this complication in all patients. For these reasons, we generally avoid verapamil in patients less than 3 years of age. Even in older patients, we would use other regimens first before giving verapamil. Adenosine is more rapid in its action, has a much lower risk, and is preferred.

As soon as there is conversion from the SVT, an ECG in sinus rhythm should be obtained. This will allow the physician to determine the presence of the WPW syndrome or other abnormalities that will affect the choice of chronic therapy. In general, digoxin is not advised in the presence of the WPW syndrome unless one knows that the accessory pathway refractory period is relatively long and is unaffected by the digoxin. Often, digoxin (and verapamil) have been shown to shorten the refractory period of an accessory pathway, facilitating conduction of electrical impulses to the ventricle, especially in the presence of atrial fibrillation.[49, 55, 56] In patients with congestive heart failure secondary to the arrhythmias, digoxin may be used under careful electrocardiographic monitoring. If the congestive heart failure resolves after conversion to sinus rhythm, the treatment may be changed to another antiarrhythmic agent. If digoxin is continued, an assessment of its effect on the accessory pathway should be made. Once the SVT has been successfully converted, one of the chronic treatment regimens shown in Table 36–6 should be instituted to prevent recurrence of the arrhythmia.

The preferred medical treatment of AV nodal SVT or SVT using a concealed bypass tract is digoxin.[143] It is effective by prolonging AV nodal conduction and refractoriness in both the fast (β) and slow (α) pathways. When refractoriness of the fast pathway is prolonged more than conduction down the slow pathway, SVT cannot be initiated. Class I antiarrhythmic agents may be more effective in some patients with the WPW syndrome, as these agents affect the accessory pathway in addition to the AV node.[144] A combination of accessory pathway and AV nodal effects may be necessary in some refractory tachycardias.

Atrial Flutter

Atrial flutter is defined by its characteristic electrocardiographic manifestations, which consist of a sawtooth flutter wave best seen in leads II, III, aVF, and V₁. At times, the flutter waves are less distinct, and the ECG must be carefully scrutinized. An example is shown in Figure 36–6. Atrial flutter consists of rapid, regular atrial excitation at rates of 280 to 480 bpm. The ventricular response is related to AV nodal conduction, which may allow 1:1, 2:1, or 3 to 4:1 or greater conduction. In pediatrics, atrial flutter is seen in three distinct groups, including fetal or neonatal patients,[145] in patients with acquired heart disease or unoperated congenital heart disease, and in patients with postoperative congenital heart disease.[111, 146] When noted in utero, hydrops fetalis may be present. Infants with atrial flutter usually

Table 36–6. CHRONIC ANTIARRHYTHMIC AGENTS FOR SUPRAVENTRICULAR AND VENTRICULAR TACHYCARDIA

Arrhythmia	Agent	Dose	Level
SVT*	Digoxin	40–60 μg/kg TDD† oral (IV‡ 3/4 PO§) Maintenance: 10–15 μg/kg/day every 12 hr	1–2.5 ng/ml
SVT or VT	Verapamil	2–7 mg/kg/day tid**	
	Propranolol	0.5–2 mg/kg/dose every 6 hr	100–300 ng/ml
	Nadolol	0.5–1 mg/kg/dose every 12 hr	50–100 μg/l
	Atenolol	0.5–1 mg/kg/day every day	0.03–0.13 μg/ml
	Procainamide	20–100 mg/kg/day every 4–6 hr	4–10 mg/l NAPA†† = 4-8 mg/l
	Quinidine	20–60 mg/kg/day every 6–8 hr	2–5 mg/l
	Disopyramide	1–3 mg/kg/day every 6 hr	2–4 μg/ml
	Flecainide	50–200 mg/m²/day every 12 hr	0.2–1.0 mg/l
	Ethmosine	200–600 mg/m²/day every 8 hr	Not established
	Amiodarone	Loading dose: 5–10 mg/kg/dose bid‡‡ × 7–14 days Maintenance: 5–10 mg/kg/dose every day	Not established
VT	Phenytoin	Loading dose: 10–20 mg/kg/day every 12 hr × 2 days Maintenance: 2–4 mg/kg/dose every 12 hr	10–20 μg/ml
	Mexiletine	2–5 mg/kg/dose every 8 hr	0.5–2.0 μg/ml
	Tocainide	2–5 mg/kg/dose every 8 hr	3–10 μg/ml

*SVT = supraventricular tachycardia.
†VT = ventricular tachycardia.
‡IV = intravenous.
§PO = by mouth.
∥ TDD = total digitalizing dose.
**tid = three times daily.
††NAPA = *n*-acetylprocainamide.
‡‡bid = twice daily.

have normal hearts. Those who respond initially to medical management usually have a good prognosis, whereas those requiring multiple drugs and emergency delivery may do poorly even after birth, especially in the presence of associated congenital heart defects.

Treatment. The initial medical treatment should be digitalization of the infant or of the mother and the fetus. The initial effect is to increase AV block, which slows the heart rate and improves cardiac function, but conversion to sinus rhythm may occur. A number of other agents, including procainamide, quinidine, propranolol, and amiodarone have been used to treat the fetus in atrial flutter.

Atrial flutter is most commonly seen postoperatively in patients who have had intra-atrial repair of D-transposition of the great arteries, repair of ASDs, or the Fontan repair. It is also common in lesions with associated AV valve regurgitation. As with other arrhythmias, the mode of therapy is determined by the patient's status. Immediate synchronous cardioversion should be performed in the infant or child with severe congestive heart failure. Digoxin should be used to maintain sinus rhythm. If digoxin is not effective in maintaining sinus rhythm, cardioversion should be performed and a second drug added if adequate digoxin has been given. In children, especially in acute situations, intravenous procainamide is recommended. Infants frequently require higher than expected doses of procainamide to obtain therapeutic levels. Drug levels are quite helpful in determining the appropriate dose of this drug. Once the rhythm is converted, the patient may be switched to the oral formulation. If the child is too young to take the capsule or sustained-release tablet, the intravenous form may be used orally. A suspension made from the powder

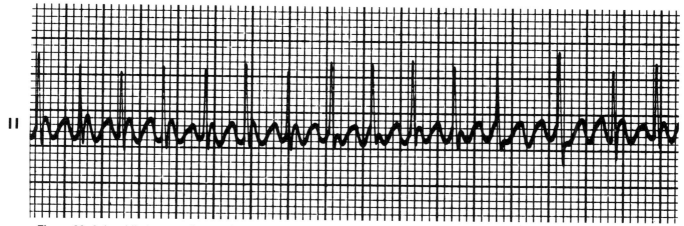

Figure 36–6. Lead II electrocardiogram from a patient with atrial flutter with an atrial rate of 500 bpm and 2 to 3:1 AV conduction.

contained in the capsule often results in erratic absorption and failure to maintain adequate levels. Other class I agents have been successful in treating atrial flutter but should not be used unless an AV nodal blocking agent is used concomitantly. Chronic intractable cases may require amiodarone. If amiodarone is used in a patient with sinus node dysfunction or marked AV nodal dysfunction, a pacemaker should be in place to provide an adequate escape rhythm.[147]

Adenosine may be helpful in confirming the diagnosis of atrial flutter, if there is a question, by increasing the degree of AV block and clarifying the flutter waves, but conversion to sinus rhythm is not to be expected.

Atrial pacing techniques, either esophageal or intracardiac, may be used. Esophageal pacing is effective in only 50% of patients. Intracardiac pacing is usually effective but may result in conversion from atrial flutter to atrial fibrillation, which then requires elective cardioversion. New antitachycardia pacemakers are a helpful adjunct in selective patients as a chronic therapy for refractory atrial flutter.[148]

Atrial Fibrillation

Atrial fibrillation is less common than atrial flutter in pediatric patients.[149] The atrial rate is rapid and irregular, from 400 to 700 bpm. The ventricular rhythm is irregular secondary to variable AV block. Atrial fibrillation is seen in association with rheumatic heart disease, congenital heart defects such as the Ebstein anomaly of the tricuspid valve, tricuspid atresia, ASDs, AV valve regurgitation, and acquired heart disease, including cardiomyopathies.[150] Atrial fibrillation is associated with the WPW syndrome and may be life-threatening because of rapid conduction to the ventricle, resulting in a rapid ventricular response and possible ventricular fibrillation.[151]

Treatment. Digoxin should be avoided in the presence of the WPW syndrome with atrial fibrillation because of its potential to further shorten the refractory period of the accessory pathway.[55, 56] β-Blockers may be used in combination with class I agents such as procainamide or quinidine. It should be noted that esophageal or intracardiac pacing is not effective in these patients, and synchronized electrical cardioversion may be required.

Automatic Atrial Tachycardia

Automatic atrial tachycardia or ectopic atrial tachycardia is a tachycardia arising from a site in the atrium other than the sinus node. The P wave axis and morphologic characteristics and the PR interval are different from those present during sinus rhythm. Ectopic foci may occur anywhere but are most commonly seen in the area of the atrial appendages (the right atrium more than the left atrium). Tachycardias from the automatic ectopic focus tend to be chronic and incessant. Congestive heart failure is frequently seen and may be the presenting feature. Presentation is more common in patients less than 6 years of age, though it is not uncommon in adolescents or preadolescents.[152]

Heart rates in older children vary from 110 to 160 bpm. The rate of the tachycardia varies during the day, accelerating with sympathetic stimuli to as high as 300 bpm.

Although the cause is rarely identifiable, this arrhythmia may be seen in association with myocarditis.

Treatment. Because of the association of congestive heart failure, digoxin is usually the first drug given. It will usually improve symptoms and slow the tachycardia slightly but is rarely effective alone. Class IA agents have been effective in slowing the tachycardia to rates sufficiently low to allow marked improvement in cardiac function. Procainamide may be given intravenously initially and switched to the oral form if it proves effective.[37, 153] Studies have suggested that flecainide or propafenone may be effective. Because these drugs depress cardiac function, they may be contraindicated in patients with congestive heart failure. β-Blockers may also depress cardiac function and should be used cautiously in patients with congestive heart failure. In patients refractory to other forms of treatment, amiodarone has been effective in suppressing the ectopic focus and allowing return of normal sinus rhythm. Cardioversion or atrial pacing is not effective, as the ectopic rhythm resumes immediately. Surgical or catheter ablative therapy may be necessary in patients refractory to medical management.[154, 155]

Junctional Ectopic Tachycardia

Junctional ectopic tachycardia occurs in two distinctly separate settings.[156] First, it occurs in infants in a familial form and is associated with congenital heart defects in 50% of affected individuals. Second, it is seen in the immediate postoperative period after cardiac surgery.

The ECG (Fig. 36–7) shows a narrow QRS complex with a slower atrial than ventricular rate with AV

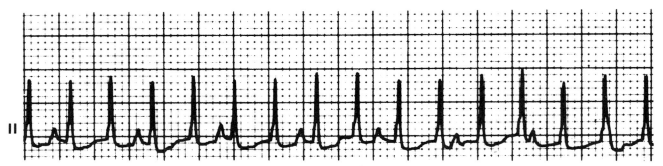

Figure 36–7. Lead II electrocardiogram illustrating junctional ectopic tachycardia with a junctional rate of 240 bpm with AV dissociation and a slower atrial rate of 136 bpm.

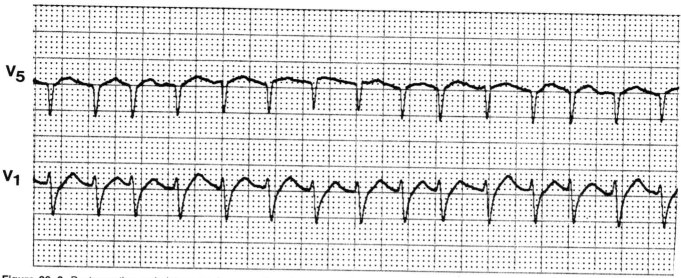

V_5

V_1

Figure 36–8. Postoperative ambulatory monitor recording of electrocardiographic leads V_5 and V_1 immediately after Fontan repair. Note the slightly variable rapid ventricular rate without clearly discernable P waves typical of postoperative accelerated junctional rhythm.

dissociation. As with automatic atrial tachycardia, pacing or cardioversion is ineffective in treating the tachycardia.

Treatment. In the infant form of junctional ectopic tachycardia, digoxin should be used initially. If the rate does not slow sufficiently, the class IA agents may be effective. Amiodarone has been the most successful drug in treating this group of patients.[157] Because the sinus node is suppressed by these drugs and sudden death associated with asystole has occurred, a pacemaker may be needed if amiodarone is used.

The postoperative occurrence of junctional ectopic tachycardia or accelerated junctional rhythm may be fatal. An example is shown in Figure 36–8. In the acute postoperative setting, a number of modalities have been used, including digoxin, class IA agents, surface cooling, and paired pacing. Waldo has described a technique of paired ventricular pacing to decrease the effective ventricular rate and increase the cardiac output.[158] Propafenone has had some limited success. If the rate can be slowed slightly and the patient supported for 24 to 48 hours, the junctional ectopic tachycardia will generally resolve and normal sinus rhythm will resume.

Ventricular Tachycardia

Ventricular arrhythmias are less common than supraventricular arrhythmias in children but appear to be occurring more frequently as the survival of patients with congenital heart defects increases. Other associated conditions are shown in Table 36–7. Postoperatively, the most common associated congenital lesion is tetralogy of Fallot.[160] No known cause may be identified in 30 to 45% of patients, and these cases are classified as idiopathic.

A typical example of ventricular tachycardia is shown in Figure 36–9. Ventricular tachycardia is defined as three or more consecutive wide premature QRS complexes. Although other mechanisms of wide QRS tachy-

cardia have been described, until proved otherwise, a wide QRS tachycardia must be considered to be ventricular tachycardia. The heart rate in ventricular tachycardia in pediatrics varies from 120 to 300 bpm. The T wave vector is divergent from the QRS vector, but

Table 36–7. VENTRICULAR TACHYCARDIA: ASSOCIATED CONDITIONS

CHD*	Tetralogy of Fallot
	Ventricular septal defect, common AV† canal defect
	Complex CHD (single-ventricle, end-stage CHD)
	Aortic stenosis and insufficiency
	Ebstein anomaly
	Mitral valve prolapse
	Eisenmenger syndrome
Acquired heart disease	Myocarditis
	Rheumatic heart disease
	Collagen vascular diseases
	Kawasaki disease
Cardiomyopathies	Hypertrophic
	Dilated, idiopathic
	Dilated, metabolic
	Right ventricular dysplasia
	Marfan syndrome
	Neuromuscular disorders
	Duchenne muscular dystrophy
	Friedreich ataxia
Tumors and infiltrate	Rhabdomyomas
	Oncocytic transformation
	Purkinje cell tumors
	Hemosiderosis
	Thalassemia
	Sickle cell anemia
	Leukemia
Other	Electrolyte imbalance
	Drugs and toxins
	Anesthesia
	Central nervous system lesions
	Long QT syndrome

*CHD = Congenital heart disease.
†AV = atrioventricular.

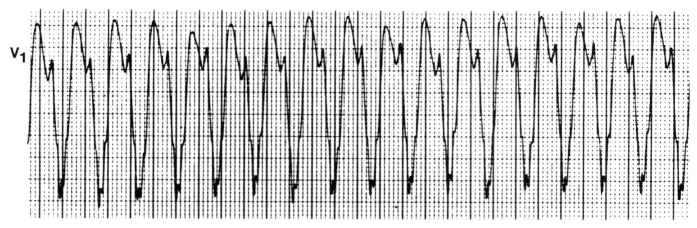

Figure 36–9. Electrocardiographic lead V₁ from a patient with ventricular tachycardia at a rate of 175 bpm.

opposite polarity will not occur in every lead. Left bundle branch block is the most common morphologic feature, but right bundle branch block or alternating right and left bundle branch block may occur. Premature ventricular contractions during sinus rhythm with the same configuration as ventricular tachycardia is a suggestive sign. AV dissociation is suggestive of ventricular tachycardia, but 1:1 ventriculoatrial conduction is common, especially in young children. Fusion beats are commonly noted at the onset or termination of the ventricular tachycardia.

Symptoms include dyspnea, chest or abdominal pain, palpitations, dizziness, syncope, and cardiac arrest. Patients with ventricular tachycardia and heart disease usually have symptoms, whereas only one third with normal hearts and ventricular tachycardia have symptoms. The type of symptoms relates to both the rate of the tachycardia (rare at <150 bpm) and the underlying state of the myocardium. Sudden death occurs most commonly in the presence of an abnormal heart,[161] but it has been reported in patients with normal hearts.[162, 163] The mechanisms of ventricular tachycardia in children include re-entry in 60% of cases and abnormal automaticity in 40% of cases.[164]

Treatment. Ventricular tachycardia should be treated emergently unless the rate is slow and the patient is clinically stable. If an extracardiac cause has been identified, such as an electrolyte abnormality or acidosis, the underlying abnormality should be corrected, usually resulting in conversion of the ventricular arrhythmia to sinus rhythm. In patients with cardiac compromise, intravenous lidocaine at 1 mg/kg should be given immediately. If the lidocaine is effective, a continuous infusion of lidocaine at 10 to 50 μg/kg should be started to maintain an adequate level. Lidocaine levels should be carefully monitored to prevent toxicity. Synchronized cardioversion at 2 to 5 watt-sec/kg should be performed if the lidocaine does not result in immediate conversion or if an intravenous site is not available. Other forms of acute therapy are presented in Table 36–8. Rapid ventricular pacing may be used to convert the rhythm to sinus if pharmacologic therapy fails or is contraindicated. Once the arrhythmia has been converted, choice of an appropriate chronic regimen is essential to maintaining

Table 36–8. ACUTE TREATMENT OF VENTRICULAR TACHYCARDIA

Initial Treatment	IV Dosage	Level
Lidocaine	1–2 mg/kg bolus every 5–15 min	1.5–6.0 mg/l
	Infusion: 10–15 μg/kg/min	
Cardioversion	1–5 watt-sec/kg	—
	Double if ineffective	

Secondary Treatment	IV Dosage	Level
Procainamide	5 mg/kg over 5–10 min	NAPA* 4–10 mg/l
	15 mg/kg over 30–45 min	†PA 4–8 mg/l
	Infusion: 20–100 μg/kg/min	
Propranolol	0.05–0.1 mg/kg over 5 min every 6 hr	
Phenytoin	3–5 mg/kg over 5 min, not to exceed 1 mg/kg/min	10–20 μg/ml
Bretylium	5 mg/kg bolus every 15 min	
	Infusion: 5–10 mg/kg over 10 min every 6 hr	
Amiodarone	1 mg/kg every 10 min every 12 hr × 10 doses	
Propafenone	0.2 mg/kg every 10 min to 2 mg	
	At ventricular rate of 150 bpm start infusion 4–7 μg/kg/min	
Magnesium²⁺	0.25 mEq/kg over 1 min, followed by 1 mEq/kg over 5 hours to achieve Mg²⁺ level of 3–4 mg/dl	

*NAPA = n-acetylprocainamide.
†PA = procainamide.

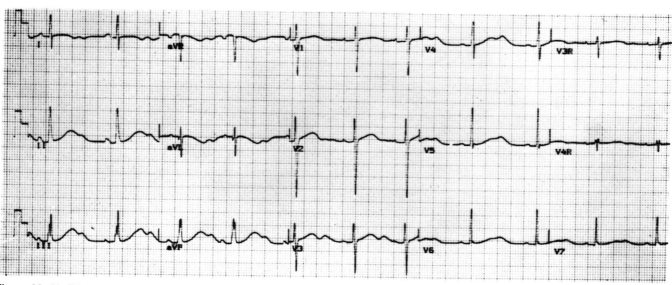

Figure 36–10. Fifteen-lead electrocardiogram in a patient with congenital long QT syndrome. The QTc measures 0.62. Note the bizarre notched T waves.

patient stability. If lidocaine has been successful, it may be maintained until adequate levels of a chronic regimen agent have been obtained or the acute causative agent is no longer present. When switching to mexiletine, the lidocaine should be gradually weaned as the mexiletine is loaded to prevent combined toxicity of these two drugs, as the side effects are similar. Propranolol is especially effective in patients whose arrhythmia is sensitive to sympathetic stimuli.[165] The class I agents and amiodarone are effective in more refractory cases.[43, 166]

Because sudden death occurs in up to 30% of patients with ventricular tachycardia and congenital heart defects, these patients should be placed on a chronic regimen. These life-threatening arrhythmias are most commonly seen in association with tetralogy of Fallot, in defects with long-standing ventricular pressure overload such as single ventricles or D-transposition of the great arteries after intra-atrial repair, and in conditions with abnormal myocardium such as in the Ebstein anomaly or hypertrophic subaortic stenosis. In the immediate postoperative period, this type of arrhythmia is poorly tolerated but generally responds to lidocaine and correction of other underlying hemodynamic and metabolic abnormalities. Studies have shown that patients with early postoperative ventricular tachycardia are likely to acquire this arrhythmia in the late postoperative period, so chronic therapy is generally recommended. The postoperative patient who presents months to years after surgery also requires chronic therapy. A thorough investigation is needed to rule out underlying hemodynamic abnormalities, as ventricular tachycardia is tolerated less well in this group of patients. Electrophysiologic study may be a helpful guide to medical therapy,[167, 168] or in patients refractory to drug therapy it may determine the site of origin of the tachycardia and can direct treatment by surgical ablation. Mexiletine has been shown to be an effective chronic drug after tetralogy of Fallot repair, as have the β-blocker drugs.[169]

The congenital long QT syndrome is a special case. An example of the ECG in long QT syndrome is shown in Figure 36–10. In addition to the prolongation of the QTc, these patients often have bizarre or notched T wave morphologic characteristics, with prominent U waves. This syndrome includes the Jervel and Lange-Nielsen syndrome associated with congenital deafness and the Romano-Ward syndrome without hearing deficit.[170] Sudden death occurs in 73% of patients without treatment.[171] The sudden death is secondary to ventricular arrhythmias (torsades de pointes) of the type shown in Figure 36–11, which frequently degenerate to ventricular fibrillation. A high level of suspicion is needed to diagnose these patients. Any patient who presents with ventricular tachycardia, especially of the polymorphic or torsades de pointes type, should have corrected QT intervals determined.[172] A complete history may reveal a family history of sudden death in young relatives or a history of syncope associated with exercise or emotional stress. Emergent treatment of these patients includes lidocaine and cardioversion. In addition, temporary atrial or ventricular pacing at a rate 10 to 20% faster than the underlying sinus rate may be needed to control the arrhythmia, especially in patients with underlying bradycardia, a common association.[173] Intravenous propranolol and phenytoin have also been successfully used in these patients. The class I agents that prolong the QT interval in normal patients should be avoided in patients with the long QT syndrome. A number of drugs that may produce this form of ventricular tachycardia are shown in Table 36–9. This is felt to be related to QTc prolongation with associated ventricular arrhythmias and has an associated bradycardia. Temporary pacing and removal of the offending agent are effective therapies.

Patients with myocarditis present another special problem. Often these patients have diminished myocardial function and require inotropic support to maintain cardiac output. Although each patient has his or her

Table 36–9. PHARMACOLOGIC AGENTS WITH QTc PROLONGATION

Antiarrhythmic agents
  Quinidine
  Procainamide
  Flecainide
  Encainide
  Amiodarone
  Sotolol
Phenothiazines
Tricyclic antidepressants
Lithium carbonate
Organophosphates
Anthracyclines

own sensitivities, an agent with the least arrhythmogenic characteristics should be chosen if possible. For example, dobutamine is usually less arrhythmogenic than dopamine, which is less arrhythmogenic than epinephrine or isoproterenol. Ventricular arrhythmias may occur in patients with myocarditis and associated complete heart block and slow escape rhythms. In these instances, an increase in the heart rate with a temporary transvenous pacemaker may be all that is needed to control the ventricular arrhythmia. In general, pressor agents should not be used just to increase the heart rate because of the arrhythmogenic potential in this subset of patients.

Bradycardia

Patients with bradycardia present with slow heart rates because of abnormalities of impulse formation in the sinus node or a block of conduction through the atrium or AV node. This is either a primary abnormality or secondary to autonomic nervous system influences. Bradycardia also occurs when subsidiary pacemakers fail to take over when the sinus node fails or when the impulse is not conducted through the AV node because of AV block. A relatively common cause of bradycardia in the neonate is the presence of blocked premature atrial contractions. With blocked premature atrial contractions that produce clinically significant bradycardia, the medical treatment of choice is digoxin, which will suppress the premature atrial contractions and therefore increase the rate.

Sinus Bradycardia

Symptomatic sinus bradycardia may occur with a wide range of clinical settings and systemic diseases as listed in Table 36–3. Treatment of the underlying disorder is indicated. The QTc interval should be determined in all infants with marked sinus bradycardia, as sinus slowing often accompanies the congenital long QT syndrome. Cardiac surgical procedures that may damage the sinus node, such as intra-atrial repair for D-transposition of the great arteries or the Fontan repair, result in sinus node dysfunction and marked sinus bradycardia.[109, 110]

Sinus Node Dysfunction

Sinus node dysfunction may be manifested by bradycardia or tachycardia. The most common arrhythmias include sinus bradycardia (Fig. 36–12), sinus arrest or pause with junctional escape rhythms, wandering atrial pacemakers, severe sinus arrhythmia, sinoatrial block, SVT, and atrial flutter or fibrillation. Syncopal episodes may occur. Although sinus node dysfunction may occur in children with no associated illness, it is most commonly seen in inflammatory illnesses, such as viral myocarditis, or after atrial surgery.[174, 175] The most commonly associated operation is the intra-atrial repair of D-transposition of the great arteries, though it may be seen after other types of atrial surgery, including the Fontan repair; ASD repairs, especially sinus venosus ASD; or repair of total anomalous pulmonary venous return. Congenital causes include the long QT syndrome, asplenia syndrome, and rare familial cases.

Treatment. If the patient is symptomatic, temporary pacing may be used, or pharmacologic agents may be used to increase the rate, as shown in Table 36–10. Acute medical therapy consists of atropine (0.02 to 0.04 mg/kg intravenously) or isoproterenol (0.01 to 2.0 μg/kg/min). Temporary atrial pacing may be performed by the transcutaneous, esophageal, or intracardiac routes. Support of the heart rate and blood pressure with pharmacologic or inotropic agents or temporary pacing may be necessary in extreme cases of sinus bradycardia. Temporary pacing can generally be achieved by the transesophageal route because of the proximity of the esophagus to the atrium. Long-term medical therapy is rarely indicated, and persistent symptomatic bradycardia should be treated with permanent pacing.

Second-degree Atrioventricular Block

Second-degree AV block results from the failure of some impulses to traverse the AV node. This can occur

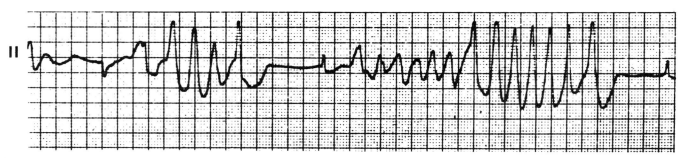

Figure 36–11. Lead II rhythm strip from a patient with long QT syndrome and torsades de pointes. The ventricular tachycardia is polymorphic, rapid, and irregular.

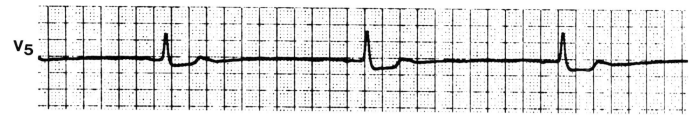

Figure 36–12. Electrocardiographic lead V_5 from a 10-year-old girl 9 years after intra-atrial repair of D-transposition of the great arteries illustrating marked sinus bradycardia at a rate of 27 bpm.

with a progressive increase in the PR interval and an eventual dropped QRS complex as in Wenckebach AV block, or it can occur as a sudden failure of AV conduction without preceding slowing of AV conduction. AV block may occur with digitalis intoxication; inflammatory cardiac diseases such as viral myocarditis, rheumatic fever, or collagen vascular diseases; Kawasaki disease; neuromuscular, metabolic, or hematologic disorders; cardiac tumors or cardiac sclerosis; or with certain types of congenital heart defects either before surgery (as in L-transposition of the great arteries, ASDs, the Ebstein anomaly) or after surgery (as in ventricular septal defect repairs or L-transposition of the great arteries).[176, 177]

The area of delay may be either in the AV node or in the His-Purkinje system, which may be more significant and more likely to progress to complete heart block.

Treatment. Second-degree AV block is generally asymptomatic, but if the ventricular rate is low, especially in a patient with compromised myocardial function, the cardiac output may be insufficient to meet the patient's needs. If a higher rate is needed, pharmacologic agents such as atropine may be helpful, especially if the block is in the AV node and partially mediated by vagal influences. Isoproterenol may increase the rate by increasing the rate of the escape pacemaker. Acutely, temporary transcutaneous or transvenous pacing may be necessary.

Complete Heart Block

Complete heart block is the complete failure of the AV junctional area to conduct the electrical impulse from the atria to the ventricles. An example is shown in Figure 36–13. It is the most common cause of significant bradycardia in children. The atrial rate is faster than the ventricular rate, which is usually 40 to 80 bpm.

Table 36–10. PHARMACOLOGIC TREATMENT OF BRADYCARDIA AND ATRIOVENTRICULAR BLOCK

Drug	Route	Dose
Atropine	IV*	0.02–0.04 mg/kg (max 1–2 mg)
Epinephrine	IV bolus	0.01–0.5 mg/kg
		(0.1 ml/kg of 1:10,000 dilution)
		(0.01 ml/kg of 1:1,000 dilution)
	Infusion	0.1–2.0 µg/kg/min
Isoproterenol	Infusion	0.1–2.0 µg/kg/min

*IV = intravenous.

The QRS morphologic characteristics and heart rate are related to the location of the escape pacemaker. The higher the origin of the pacemaker, the faster the rate and the more narrow the QRS complex. Wider QRS escape complexes usually originate from the His bundle or below.

Complete heart block may be either congenital or acquired. The associated congenital heart defects most commonly include L-transposition of the great arteries or the heterotaxy syndromes.[178] The same causes of acquired heart block discussed previously can cause complete heart block. Postoperative congenital heart lesions include those with ventricular septal defect repairs or complex lesions associated with L-transposition of the great arteries.[179]

Congenital heart block occurs in 1/20,000 live births. A strong association has been noted with connective tissue disease in the mother.[58] Although many infants with congenital complete heart block will be asymptomatic at birth, a subset will experience severe congestive heart failure and cardiovascular collapse. These symptoms are most commonly seen in patients with associated congenital heart defects, ventricular rates less than 50 bpm, or atrial rates greater than 150 bpm.

Treatment. Patients with congenital heart block may require intubation and ventilation, treatment of acidosis, and catecholamine support of heart rate and blood pressure. In emergent situations, immediate transthoracic pacing can be accomplished. The transcutaneous pacemaker may be effective for short-term emergent situations but should be replaced with another pacing method as soon as possible. Placement of a temporary transvenous pacemaker, through either the umbilical vein or the femoral vein under direct fluoroscopic observation is preferred. Although infants with rates lower than 50 bpm or slightly higher rates and associated congenital heart defects or cardiomyopathies may require pacing, this decision should not be made on the basis of rate alone. Only a small percentage of patients with congenital complete heart block need pacemakers, and many of these are not needed until a later age. Pacemakers may be placed because of associated ventricular arrhythmias either during sleep or exercise, easy fatigability or exercise intolerance, or syncope or presyncope.[180–182]

The heart block associated with inflammatory disease may be transient and require only temporary pacing. With postsurgical heart block, temporary pacing is usually performed for 10 to 14 days. Permanent pacing should be performed if a sinus rhythm does not return because of the high incidence of sudden death in this

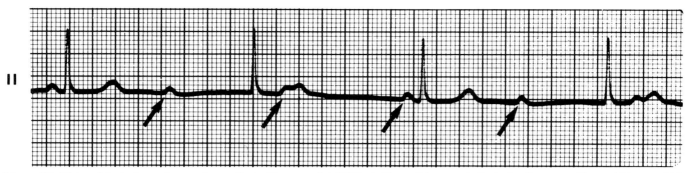

Figure 36–13. Lead II electrocardiogram in a patient with congenital AV block. The solid arrows indicate the P waves with an atrial rate of 93 bpm and a ventricular rate of 38 bpm.

group of postoperative patients if they are not paced.[183] Even the return of sinus rhythm does not ensure that heart block will not return at a later time, and close follow-up is indicated.

DIAGNOSTIC TECHNIQUES AND PROCEDURES

Electrocardiography

The use of the standard 12- or 15-lead ECG may leave questions as to the mechanism of the arrhythmia because P waves may be difficult to visualize. The most prominent P waves in children are usually seen in the right precordial leads and lead II. Amplification of the P wave may be obtained by using the right and left arm leads across the heart. An esophageal lead, an epicardial lead placed at cardiac surgery, or an intracardiac lead can be used to locate atrial activity and distinguish it from the QRS complex or T wave.

Many of the current telemetry and arrhythmia analysis units are helpful in caring for the patient with arrhythmias in the critical care unit. These systems recognize and store electrocardiographic strips for analysis and may quantitate types and numbers of specific arrhythmias.

Transesophageal Pacing

Transesophageal pacing may be accomplished with a lead or capsule placed through the mouth or nose.[141, 184] Older children will swallow a capsule, whereas the lead may be passed in a manner similar to nasogastric tube placement in younger children and infants. Esophageal pacing requires a pulse duration of 10 to 20 msec and a relatively high current amplitude of 10 to 20 mA. This technique is effective in terminating SVT and, to a lesser extent, atrial flutter. To terminate SVT or atrial flutter, a rate approximately 10 bpm faster than the SVT or atrial flutter rate should be chosen, with progressive increases in the rate if the tachycardia is not interrupted at the slower rates. Esophageal pacing may also provide emergency pacing for bradycardia when AV conduction is present. Electrophysiologic studies can be performed

in this manner to evaluate accessory pathway properties in the WPW syndrome and to determine mechanisms of SVT.

Many patients will require sedation for transesophageal studies to be performed. The catheter is positioned behind the heart to record the largest atrial signal possible. Predicted insertion depths can be calculated from charts that relate patient height to the length of catheter insertion depth needed.[184] Descriptions of techniques and information gained from esophageal pacing are available in several excellent texts to which the reader is referred for additional information.

Temporary Pacemakers

Transvenous Pacemakers

In pediatrics, emergent pacing is most commonly needed to treat bradycardia. Transvenous sites are usually the jugular, subclavian, or femoral routes. An appropriate-sized pacing catheter (No. 4 French to No. 7 French) should be chosen and placed by an experienced operator. Fluoroscopic guidance is ideal, but in emergent situations the balloon-tipped pacing catheters may be floated into the ventricle. An external pacemaker is attached to the intracardiac lead, which is secured.[185] The settings vary according to the patient's needs, but they should ensure sensing of the patient's intrinsic rhythm with enough current to allow for changes in threshold (twice diastolic threshold). The rate settings should provide the best cardiac output possible. Rapid atrial pacemakers can pace at extremely fast rates, up to 1,400 bpm, and should be used with extreme care.

Transthoracic Pacemakers

The transthoracic route used in children is the subxyphoid route. The procedure is similar to that used to perform a pericardiocentesis. A pacing wire is inserted through a needle, which is subsequently removed once the wire is inside the heart. This type of pacing should be replaced by a transvenous pacemaker, if possible, once the patient is stable.

External Pacemakers

Although external pacing was first introduced by Zoll in 1952, it has been reintroduced more recently.[186, 187] This technique may be used successfully in critical situations to increase the heart rate, but it should be replaced as soon as possible with another type of pacemaker. In infants, it has been reported to cause third-degree burns.[188]

References

1. James TN: Anatomy of the conduction system of the heart. *In*: Hurst JW (ed): The Heart, 6th ed. New York, McGraw-Hill, 1982, pp. 22–74.
2. Anderson RH and Becker AE: Gross anatomy and microscopy of the conducting system. *In*: Mandel WJ (ed): Cardiac Arrhythmias, Their Mechanisms, Diagnosis, and Management. Philadelphia, JB Lippincott, 1987, pp. 13–52.
3. Zipes DP: Genesis of cardiac arrhythmias: Electrophysiologic considerations. *In*: Braunwald E (ed): Heart Disease: A Textbook of Cardiovascular Medicine, 3rd ed. Philadelphia, WB Saunders, 1988, pp. 581–620.
4. Lev M: The pre-excitation syndrome: Anatomic considerations of anomalous A-V pathways. *In*: Dreifus LS and Koff WS (eds): Mechanisms and Therapy of Cardiac Arrhythmias. New York, Grune & Stratton, 1966, p. 665.
5. Hoffman BF and Cranefield PF: Electrophysiology of the Heart. New York, McGraw-Hill, 1960.
6. Hoffman BF and Rosen MR: Cellular mechanisms of cardiac arrhythmias. Circ Res 49:1, 1981.
7. Reuter H: The dependence of slow inward current of Purkinje fibers on the extracellular calcium concentration. J Physiol (Lond) 192:479, 1967.
8. Cranefield PF: The Conduction of the Cardiac Impulse. Mt. Kisco, NY, Futura, 1975.
9. Zipes DP: Management of cardiac arrhythmias: Pharmacological, electrical, and surgical techniques. *In*: Braunwald E (ed): Heart Disease: A Textbook of Cardiovascular Medicine, 3rd ed. Philadelphia, WB Saunders, 1988, pp. 621–657.
10. Wit AL: Cellular electrophysiologic mechanisms of cardiac arrhythmias. Ann N Y Acad Sci 432:1, 1984.
11. Zipes DP and Jolife J: Cardiac electrophysiology and arrhythmias. New York, Grune & Stratton, 1985.
12. Ferrier GR: Digitalis arrhythmias: Role of oscillatory afterpotentials. Progr Cardiovasc Dis 19:459, 1977.
13. Weidmann S: Passive properties of cardiac fibers. *In*: Rosen MR, Janse MJ, and Wit AL (eds): A Cardiac Electrophysiology: A Textbook. Mt. Kisco, NY, Futura, 1990, pp. 29–35.
14. Mines GR: On dynamic equilibrium in the heart. J Physiol 46:349, 1913.
15. Moe GK, Preston JB, and Burlington H: Physiologic evidence for a dual AV transmission system. Circ Res 4:357, 1956.
16. Singer DH, Lazzara R, and Hoffman BF: Interrelationships between automaticity and conduction in Purkinje fibers. Circ Res 21:537, 1967.
17. Vaughan-Williams EM: Classification of antiarrhythmic drugs. J Pharmacol Ther 1:115, 1975.
18. Vaughan-Williams EM: A classification of antiarrhythmic actions reassessed after a decade of new drugs. J Clin Pharmacol 24:129, 1984.
19. Grant AO, Starmer CF, and Strauss HC: Antiarrhythmic drug action: Blockade of the inward sodium current. Circ Res 55:427, 1984.
20. Koch-Weser J and Frishman WH: Beta-adrenoreceptor antagonists: New drugs and new indications. N Engl J Med 305:500, 1981.
21. Singh BN and Vaughan-Williams EM: The effect of amiodarone: A new antianginal drug on cardiac muscle. Br J Pharmacol 39:657, 1970.
22. Cranefield PF, Aronson RS, and Wit AL: Effect of verapamil on the normal action potential and on a calcium-dependent slow response of canine cardiac Purkinje fibers. Circ Res 34:204, 1974.
23. Bean BP, Cohen CJ, and Tsien RW: Lidocaine block of cardiac sodium channels. J Gen Physiol 81:613, 1983.
24. Hoffman BF, Rosen MR, and Wit AL: Electrophysiology and pharmacology of cardiac arrhythmias. VII: Cardiac effect of quinidine and procainamide. Am Heart J 90:117, 1975.
25. Giardina EG: Procainamide: Clinical pharmacology and efficacy against ventricular arrhythmias. Ann N Y Acad Sci 432:117, 1984.
26. Strasberg B, Schlarovsky S, Erdberg A, et al: Procainamide-induced polymorphous ventricular tachycardia. Am J Cardiol 47:1309, 1981.
27. Garson A Jr, Bink-Boelkens M, Hesslein PS, et al: Atrial flutter in the young: A collaborative study of 380 cases. J Am Coll Cardiol 6:871, 1985.
28. Smith WM and Gallagher JJ: "Les torsades de pointes": An unusual ventricular arrhythmia. Ann Intern Med 93:578, 1980.
29. Eldar M, Griffin JC, Abbott JA, et al: Permanent cardiac pacing in patients with the long QT syndrome. J Am Coll Cardiol 10:600, 1987.
30. Sclarovsky S, Strasberg B, Lewin RF, et al: Polymorphous ventricular tachycardia: Clinical features and treatment. Am J Cardiol 44:339, 1979.
31. Tzivoni D, Keren A, Cohen AM, et al: Magnesium therapy for torsades de pointes. Am J Cardiol 53:528, 1984.
32. Binah O and Rosen MR: The cellular mechanisms of cardiac antiarrhythmic drug action. Ann N Y Acad Sci 432:31, 1984.
33. Singh BN and Vaughan-Williams EM: Investigations of the mode of actions of a new antidysrhythmic drug Ko 1173. Br J Pharmacol 44:1, 1972.
34. Monk JP and Brogden RN: Mexiletine: A review of its pharmacodynamic and pharmacokinetic properties, and therapeutic use in the treatment of arrhythmias. Drugs 40:374, 1990.
35. Bigger JT and Strauss HC: Digitalis toxicity: Drug interactions promoting toxicity and the management of toxicity. Semin Drug Treat 2:147, 1972.
36. Garson A Jr, Kugler JD, Gillette PC, et al: Control of late postoperative arrhythmias with phenytoin in young patients. Am J Cardiol 46:290, 1980.
37. Perry JC, McQuinn R, Smith RT, et al: Flecainide acetate for resistant arrhythmias in the young: Efficacy and pharmacokinetics. J Am Coll Cardiol 14:185, 1989.
38. Chang AC, Zappalla FR, Kürer CC, et al: Clinical outcome in children with the permanent form of junctional reciprocating tachycardia. J Am Coll Cardiol 15:176A, 1990.
39. Fish FA, Gillette PC, and Benson DW: Incidence of death, cardiac arrest and proarrhythmia in young patients receiving flecainide or encainide (Abstract). Circulation 80(Suppl II):II-87, 1989.
40. Gillette PC, Garson A Jr, Eterovic E, et al: Oral propranolol treatment in infants and children. J Pediatr 92:141, 1978.
41. Naccarelli GV, Rinkenberger RL, Dougherty AH, et al: Amiodarone: Pharmacology and antiarrhythmic and adverse effects. Pharmacotherapy 5:298, 1985.
42. Yabek SM, Kato R, and Singh BN: Acute effects of amiodarone on the electrophysiologic properties of isolated neonatal and adult cardiac fibers. J Am Coll Cardiol 5:1109, 1985.
43. Garson A Jr, Gillette PC, McVoy P, et al: Amiodarone treatment of critical arrhythmias in children and young adults. J Am Coll Cardiol 4:749, 1984.
44. Leveque PE: Antiarrhythmic action of bretylium. Nature 207:203, 1965.
45. Heissenbuttel RH and Bigger JT: Bretylium tosylate: A newly available antiarrhythmic drug for ventricular arrhythmias. Ann Intern Med 91:229, 1979.
46. Rosen MR, Wit AL, and Hoffman BF: Electrophysiology and pharmacology of cardiac arrhythmias. VI: Cardiac effects of verapamil. Am Heart J 89:665, 1975.
47. Woelfel A, Foster JR, McAllister RG, et al: Efficacy of verapamil in exercise-induced ventricular tachycardia. Am J Cardiol 56:292, 1985.
48. Epstein MC, Kiel EA, and Victoria BE: Cardiac decompensation following verapamil therapy in infants with supraventricular tachycardia. Pediatrics 75:737, 1985.
49. Gulamhusein S, Ko P, and Klein GJ: Ventricular fibrillation

following verapamil in the Wolff-Parkinson-White syndrome. Am Heart J 106:145, 1983.

50. Pelleg A: Cardiac cellular electrophysiologic actions of adenosine and adenosine triphosphate. Am Heart J 110:688, 1985.
51. DiMarco JP, Sellers TD, Berne RM, et al: Adenosine: Electrophysiologic effects and therapeutic use for terminating paroxysmal supraventricular tachycardia. Circulation 68:1254, 1983.
52. Fozzard HA and Sheets MF: Cellular mechanisms of action of cardiac glycosides. J Am Coll Cardiol 5:10A, 1985.
53. Watanabe AM: Digitalis and the autonomic nervous system. J Am Coll Cardiol 5:35A, 1985.
54. Rosen MR, Wit AL, and Hoffman BF: Electrophysiology and pharmacology of cardiac arrhythmias. IV: Cardiac arrhythmias and toxic effects of digitalis. Am Heart J 89:391, 1975.
55. Byrum C, Wahl RA, Behrendt DM, et al: Ventricular fibrillation associated with the use of digitalis in a newborn infant with Wolff-Parkinson-White syndrome. J Pediatr 101:400, 1982.
56. Sellers TD, Bashore TM, and Gallagher JJ: Digitalis in the preexcitation syndrome: Analysis during atrial fibrillation. Circulation 56:260, 1977.
57. Kornreich HK and Hanson V: The rheumatoid diseases of childhood. Curr Probl Pediatr 4:3, 1974.
58. Chameides L, Truex RC, Vetter VL, et al: Association of maternal systemic lupus erythematosus with congenital complete heart block. N Engl J Med 297:1204, 1977.
59. Wray R and Iveson M: Complete heart block and systemic lupus erythematosus. Br Heart J 37:982, 1975.
60. Ferri C, Bemini L, Bongiorno MG, et al: Noninvasive evaluation of cardiac dysrhythmias and their relationship with multisystemic symptoms in progressive systemic sclerosis patients. Arthritis Rheum 28:1259, 1985.
61. Fernhoff PM and Plotkin SA: Extraintestinal shigellosis: Bacteremia and paroxysmal atrial tachycardia; shigella sonnei in a three year old boy. Clin Pediatr 12:302, 1973.
62. Surawicz B: Electrolytes and the electrocardiogram. Postgrad Med 55:123, 1974.
63. Murphy MC, Sweeney MS, Putnam JB Jr, et al: Surgical treatment of cardiac tumors: A 25 year experience. Ann Thorac Surg 49:612, 1990.
64. Casta A: Tuberous sclerosis and Wolff-Parkinson-White syndrome. J Pediatr 109:399, 1986.
65. Garson A Jr, Gillette PC, Titus JL, et al: Surgical treatment of ventricular tachycardia in infants. N Engl J Med 310:1442, 1984.
66. Roberts WG, Bodey GP, and Wertake PT: The heart in acute leukemia: A study of 420 autopsy cases. Am J Cardiol 21:388, 1968.
67. Gilladoga AC, Manuel C, Tan CTC, et al: The cardiotoxicity of adriamycin and daunomycin in children. Cancer 37(Suppl):1070, 1976.
68. Perloff JK, deLeon AC, and O'Doherty D: The cardiomyopathy of progressive muscular dystrophy. Circulation 33:625, 1966.
69. Perloff JK, Roberts WC, deLeon AC, et al: The distinctive electrocardiogram of Duchenne's progressive muscular dystrophy. Am J Med 42:179, 1967.
70. Perloff JK: Cardiac rhythm and conduction in Duchenne's muscular dystrophy. J Am Coll Cardiol 3:1263, 1984.
71. Woolliscroft J and Tuna N: Permanent atrial standstill: The clinical spectrum. Am J Med 49:2037, 1982.
72. Grigg LE, Chan W, Mond HG, et al: Ventricular tachycardia and sudden death in myotonic dystrophy: Clinical electrophysiologic and pathologic features. Am J Cardiol 6:254, 1985.
73. Zimmermann M, Gabathuler J, Adamee R, et al: Unusual manifestations of heart involvement in Friedreich's ataxia. Am Heart J 111:184, 1986.
74. Child JS, Perloff JK, Bach PM, et al: Cardiac involvement in Friedreich's ataxia. J Am Coll Cardiol 7:1370, 1986.
75. Roberts NK, Perloff JK, and Kark P: Cardiac conduction in Kearns-Sayre syndrome. Am J Cardiol 44:1396, 1979.
76. Buruma OJ, Schipperheyn JJ, and Bots GT: Heart muscle disease in familial hypokalemic periodic paralysis. Circulation 64:12, 1981.
77. Perloff JK: Neurologic disorders and heart disease. In: Braunwald E (ed): Heart Disease: A Textbook of Cardiovascular Medicine, 3rd ed. Philadelphia, WB Saunders, 1988, pp. 1782–1799.
78. Blieden LC and Moller JH: Cardiac involvement in inherited disorders of metabolism. Prog Cardiovasc Dis XVI (No 6):615, 1974.
79. Stanbury JB, Wyngaarden JB, Fredrickson DS, et al (eds): The Metabolic Basis of Inherited Disease, 5th ed. New York, McGraw Hill, 1983.
80. Schieken RM, Kerber RE, Ionasecu VV, et al: Cardiac manifestations of mucopolysaccharidoses. Circulation 52:700, 1975.
81. Mehta J, Tuna N, Moller JA, et al: Electrocardiographic and vectorcardiographic observations in Fabry's disease. Adv Cardiol 21:220, 1978.
82. Fung KP, Lo RNS, and Ho HC: Pompe's disease presenting as supraventricular tachycardia. Aust Paediatr J 25:101, 1989.
83. Hohn AR, Lowe CV, Sokal JE, et al: Cardiac problems in the glycogenoses with specific reference to Pompe's disease. Pediatrics 35:313, 1965.
84. Buchwald H, Lee GB, Amplatz K, et al: Severe atherosclerotic cardiovascular disease in a 14 year old homozygous familial hypercholesterolemic. Minn Med 51:477, 1968.
85. Hudson LD, Kurt TL, Petty TL, et al: Arrhythmias associated with acute respiratory failure in patients with chronic airway obstruction. Chest 63:661, 1973.
86. Engle MA, Eilandson M, and Smith CH: Late cardiac complications of chronic, severe, refractory anemia with hemochromatosis. Circulation 30:698, 1964.
87. Propper RD, Shurin SB, and Nathan DG: Reassessment of the use of desferoxamine B in iron overload. N Engl J Med 294:1421, 1976.
88. Uzsoy NK: Cardiovascular findings in patients with sickle cell anemia. Am J Cardiol 13:320, 1964.
89. Talwar KK, Gupta V, Kaul U, et al: Electrophysiologic studies in thyrotoxicosis with and without associated sick sinus syndrome. Clin Cardiol 10:249, 1987.
90. Kumar A, Bhandari AK, and Rahimtoola SH: Torsades de pointes and marked QT prolongation in association with hypothyroidism. Ann Intern Med 106:712, 1987.
91. Sode J, Getzen LC, and Osborne DP: Cardiac arrhythmias and cardiomyopathy associated with pheochromocytomas. Am J Surg 114:927, 1967.
92. Hayward RP, Emanuel RW, and Nabarro JDN: Acromegalic heart disease: Influence of treatment of the acromegaly on the heart. Q J Med 62:41, 1987.
93. Slovis TL, Oh JE, Teitelbaum DT, et al: Physostigmine therapy in acute tricyclic antidepressant poisoning. Clin Toxicol 4:451, 1971.
94. Scheffer GJ, Jonges R, Holley HS, et al: Effects of halothane on the conduction system of the heart in humans. Anesth Analg 69:721, 1989.
95. Tellez DW, Hardin WD Jr, Takahashi M, et al: Blunt cardiac injury in children. J Pediatr Surg 22:1123, 1987.
96. Langan MNS and Horowitz LN: Cardiac surgery and cardiac trauma. In: Horowitz LN (ed): Current Management of Arrhythmias. Philadelphia, BC Decker, 1991, pp. 272–278.
97. Clarkson PM, Frye RL, DuShane JW, et al: Prognosis for patients with ventricular septal defect and severe pulmonary vascular obstructive disease. Circulation 38:129, 1968.
98. Watson H: Natural history of Ebstein's anomaly of tricuspid valve in childhood and adolescence: An international cooperative study of 505 cases. Br Heart J 36:417, 1974.
99. Martin RP, Radley-Smith R, and Yacoub MH: Arrhythmias before and after correction of transposition of the great arteries. J Am Coll Cardiol 10:200, 1987.
100. Dalienta L, Corrado D, Buja G, et al: Rhythm and conduction disturbances in isolated, congenitally corrected transposition of the great arteries. Am J Cardiol 58:314, 1986.
101. Warnes CA and Somerville J: Tricuspid atresia in adolescents and adults: Current state and late complications. Br Heart J 57:543, 1987.
102. Schwartz LS, Goldfischer J, Sprague GJ, et al: Syncope and sudden death in aortic stenosis. Am J Cardiol 23:647, 1969.
103. James TN and Jackson DA: De subitaneis mortibus. XXVII: Histological abnormalities in the sinus node, AV node and His bundle associated with coarctation of the aorta. Circulation 56:1094, 1977.
104. Deanfield JE, McKenna WJ, Presbitero P, et al: Ventricular arrhythmia in unrepaired tetralogy of Fallot: Relation to age, timing of repair and hemodynamic status. Br Heart J 52:77, 1984.

105. Forfang K, Simonsen S, Andersen A, et al: Atrial septal defect of secundum type in the middle-aged. Am Heart J 94:44, 1977.
106. Clark EB, Roland JMA, Varghese PJ, et al: Should the sinus venosus type ASD be closed? A review of the atrial conduction defects and surgical results in 28 children. Am J Cardiol 35:127, 1975.
107. Vetter VL: What every pediatrician needs to know about arrhythmias in children who havehad cardiac surgery. Pediatr Ann 20:378, 1991.
108. Vetter VL: Postoperative pediatric electrocardiographic and electrophysiologic sequelae. In: Liebman J, Plonsey R, and Rudy Y (eds): Pediatric and Fundamental Electrocardiography. Boston, Martinus Nijhoff Publishing, 1987, pp. 187–206.
109. Vetter VL, Tanner CS, and Horowitz LN: Electrophysiologic consequences of the Mustard repair of d-transposition of the great arteries. J Am Coll Cardiol 10:265, 1987.
110. Kürer CC, Tanner CS, and Vetter VL: Electrophysiologic findings after Fontan repair of functional single ventricle. J Am Coll Cardiol 17:174, 1991.
111. Vetter VL, Tanner CS, and Horowitz LN: Inducible atrial flutter after the Mustard repair of complete transposition of the great arteries. Am J Cardiol 61:428, 1988.
112. Scagliotti D, Strasberg B, Duffy CE, et al: Inducible polymorphous ventricular tachycardia following Mustard operation for transposition of the great arteries. Pediatr Cardiol 5:39, 1984.
113. Vetter VL: Ventricular arrhythmias in patients with congenital heart disease. In: Greenspon AJ and Waxman HL (eds): Contemporary Management of Ventricular Arrhythmias. (Cardiovascular Clinics) Philadelphia, FA Davis, 1991.
114. Gillette PC, Yeoman MA, Mullins CE, et al: Sudden death after repair of tetralogy of Fallot. Circulation 56:566, 1977.
115. Garson A Jr and Gillette PC: Junctional ectopic tachycardia in children: Electrocardiography, electrophysiology and pharmacologic response. Am J Cardiol 44:298, 1979.
116. Kürer CC, Tanner CS, Norwood WI, et al: Perioperative arrhythmias after Fontan repair. Circulation 82(Suppl IV) IV-190-4, 1990.
117. Karjalainen J, Viitasals M, Kala R, et al: 24 hour electrocardiogram recordings in mild acute infectious myocarditis. Ann Clin Res 16:34, 1984.
118. Vikerfors T, Stjerna A, Icén P, et al: Acute myocarditis: Serologic diagnosis, clinical findings and follow-up. Acta Med Scand 223:45, 1988.
119. Clarke M and Keith JD: Atrioventricular conduction in acute rheumatic fever. Br Heart J 34:472, 1972.
120. Belani K and Regelmann WE: Lyme disease in children. Rheum Dis Clin North Am 15:679, 1989.
121. Dale JB and Beachey EH: Multiple, heart cross-reactive epitopes of streptococcal M proteins. J Exp Med 161:113, 1985.
122. Kannel WB, Abbott HRD, Savage DD, et al: Epidemiologic features of chronic atrial fibrillation: The Framingham study. N Engl J Med 306:1018, 1982.
123. Kegel SM, Dorsey TJ, Rowen M, et al: Cardiac death in mucocutaneous lymph node syndrome. Am J Cardiol 40:282, 1977.
124. Surawicz B: Electrolyte solutions. In: Horowitz LN (ed): Current Management of Arrhythmias. Philadelphia, BC Decker, 1991, pp. 322–325.
125. Surawicz B: Role of electrolytes in the etiology and management of cardiac arrhythmias. Prog Cardiovasc Dis 8:364, 1966.
126. Surawicz B: Relation between electrocardiogram: A review. Am Heart J 88:360, 1974.
127. Williams JF, Klocke FJ, and Braunwald E: Studies on digitalis. XIII: A comparison of the effects of potassium on the inotropic and arrhythmia producing actions of ouabain. J Clin Invest 45:346, 1966.
128. Ludomirsky Achi and Garson A Jr: Supraventricular tachycardia. In: Garson A Jr and Gillette PC (eds): Pediatric Arrhythmias: Electrophysiology and Pacing. Philadelphia, WB Saunders, 1990, pp. 380–426.
129. Deal BJ, Keane JF, Gillette PC, et al: WPW syndrome with supraventricular tachycardia during infancy: Management and follow-up. J Am Coll Cardiol 5:130, 1985.
130. Spurell RAJ, Kirkler DM, and Sowton E: Concealed bypasses of the atrioventricular mode in patients with paroxysmal supraventricular tachycardia revealed by intracardiac electrical stimulation and verapamil. Am J Cardiol 33:590, 1974.
131. Critelli G, Gallagher JJ, Monda V, et al: Anatomic and electrophysiologic substrate of the permanent form of junctional reciprocating tachycardia. J Am Coll Cardiol 4(3):601, 1984.
132. Gillette PC: Concealed anomalous cardiac conduction pathways: A frequent cause of supraventricular tachycardia. Am J Cardiol 40:848, 1977.
133. Garson A Jr and Gillette PC: Electrophysiologic studies of supraventricular tachycardia in children. I: Clinical electrophysiologic correlations. Am Heart J 102:233, 1981.
134. Vetter VL: The pediatric electrophysiologic study. In: Liebman J, Plonsey R, and Rudy Y (eds): Pediatric and Fundamental Electrocardiography. Boston, Martinus Nijhoff Publishing, 1987.
135. Vetter VL: Management of arrhythmias in children—Unusual features. In: Dreifus LS (ed): Cardiac Arrhythmias. (Cardiovascular Clinics) Philadelphia, FA Davis, 1985, pp. 329–357.
136. Bisset GS III, Gaum W, and Kaplan S: The ice bag: A new technique for interruption of supraventricular tachycardia. J Pediatr 97:593, 1980.
137. Overholt ED, Rheuban KS, Gutgesell HP, et al: Usefulness of adenosine for arrhythmias in infants and children. Am J Cardiol 61:925, 1988.
138. Rosen KM, Barwolf C, Ehsani A, et al: Effects of lidocaine and propranolol on the normal and anomalous pathways in patients with pre-excitation. Am J Cardiol 30:801, 1972.
139. Klein HO and Hoffman BF: Cessation of paroxysmal supraventricular tachycardia by parasympathomimetic interventions. Ann Intern Med 81:48, 1974.
140. Lister JW, Cohen LS, Bernstein WH, et al: Treatment of supraventricular tachycardia by rapid atrial stimulation. Circulation 38:1044, 1968.
141. Benson DW Jr, Dunnigan A, Sterba A, et al: Atrial pacing from the esophagus in the diagnosis and management of tachycardia and palpitations. J Pediatr 102:40, 1983.
142. Abinader E, Borochowitz Z, and Berger A: A hemodynamic complication of verapamil therapy in a neonate. Hebw Paediatr Acta 36(5):451, 1981.
143. Wellens HJJ, Durer DR, Liem KL, et al: Effects of digitalis in patients with paroxysmal atrioventricular nodal tachycardia. Circulation 52:779, 1975.
144. Wellens HJJ and Durer D: Effect of procainamide, quinidine and admaline in the Wolff-Parkinson-White syndrome. Circulation 30:114, 1974.
145. Dunnigan A, Benson DW Jr, and Benditt DG: Atrial flutter in infancy: Diagnosis, clinical features, and treatment. Pediatrics 75:725, 1985.
146. Garson A Jr, Bink-Boelkens M, Hesslein PS, et al: Atrial flutter in the young: A collaborative study of 380 cases. J Am Coll Cardiol 6:871, 1985.
147. Dreifus LS, Fisch C, and Griffin JC: Guidelines for implantation of cardiac pacemakers and antiarrhythmic devices: A report of the American College of Cardiology/American Heart Association Task Force on Assessment of Diagnostic and Therapeutic Cardiovascular Procedures (Committee on Pacemaker Implantation). J Am Coll Cardiol 18:1, 1991.
148. Fisher JD, Johnston DR, Kim SG, et al: Implantable pacers for tachycardia termination: Stimulation techniques and long-term efficacy. PACE 9:1325, 1986.
149. Radford DJ and Izukawa T: Atrial fibrillation in children. Pediatrics 59:250, 1977.
150. Stafford WJ, Trohman RG, Bilsker M, et al: Cardiac arrest in an adolescent with atrial fibrillation and hypertrophic cardiomyopathy. J Am Coll Cardiol 7:701, 1986.
151. Dreifus LS, Wellens HJ, Wanatabe Y, et al: Sinus bradycardia and atrial fibrillation associated with the Wolff-Parkinson-White syndrome. Am J Cardiol 38:149, 1976.
152. Gillette PC and Garson A Jr: Electrophysiologic and pharmacologic characteristics of automatic ectopic atrial tachycardia. Circulation 56:571, 1977.
153. Zeigler VL, Gillette PC, Ross B, et al: Flecainide for supraventricular and ventricular arrhythmias in children and young adults. Clin Prog Electrophysiol Pacing 4:328:1986.
154. Gillette PC, Garson A Jr, Hesslein PS, et al: Successful surgical treatment of atrial, junctional and ventricular tachycardia unassociated with accessory connections in infants and children. Am Heart J 102:984, 1981.
155. Margolis PO, Roman CA, Moulton KP, et al: Radiofrequency

catheter ablation of left and right ectopic atrial tachycardia (Abstract). Circulation 82:718, 1991.

156. Garson A Jr and Gillette PC: Junctional ectopic tachycardia in children: Electrocardiography, electrophysiology, and pharmacologic response. Am J Cardiol 44:298, 1979.

157. Villain E, Vetter VL, Garcia JM, et al: Evolving concepts in the management of junctional ectopic tachycardia: A multicenter study. Circulation 81:1544, 1990.

158. Waldo AF, MacLean WAH, Karp RB, et al: Entrainment and interruption of atrial flutter with atrial pacing: Studies in man following open heart surgery. Circulation 56:737, 1977.

159. Vetter VL: Ventricular arrhythmias in pediatric patients with and without congenital heart disease. In: Horowitz LN (ed): Current Management of Arrhythmias. Philadelphia, BC Decker, 1990, pp. 208–220.

160. Garson A, Nihill MR, McNamara DG, et al: Status of the adult and adolescent after repair of tetralogy of Fallot. Circulation 59:1232, 1979.

161. Garson A Jr, Smith RT, Moak JP, et al: Ventricular arrhythmias and sudden death in children. J Am Coll Cardiol 5:130B, 1985.

162. Fulton DR, Kyung JC, and Burton ST: Ventricular tachycardia in children without heart disease. Am J Cardiol 55:1328, 1985.

163. Deal BJ, Scott MM, Scagliotti D, et al: Ventricular tachycardia in a young population without overt heart disease. Circulation 73:1111, 1986.

164. Vetter VL, Josephson ME, and Horowitz LN: Idiopathic recurrent sustained ventricular tachycardia in children and adolescents. Am J Cardiol 47:315, 1981.

165. Kornbluth A, Frishman WH, and Ackerman M: β-Adrenergic blockade in children. Cardiol Clin 5:629, 1987.

166. Moak JR, Smith RT, and Garson A Jr: Newer antiarrhythmic drugs in children. Am Heart J 113:179, 1986.

167. Garson A Jr, Porter CJ, Gillette PC, et al: Induction of ventricular tachycardia during electrophysiologic study after repair of tetralogy of Fallot. J Am Coll Cardiol 1:1493, 1983.

168. Horowitz LN, Vetter VL, Harken AH, et al: Electrophysiologic characteristics of sustained ventricular tachycardia occurring after repair of tetralogy of Fallot. Am J Cardiol 46:446, 1980.

169. Malcolm ID, Stubington D, and Gibbons JE: Mexiletine for ventricular arrhythmia after repair of tetralogy of fallot. CMA J 123:530, 1980.

170. Schwartz PJ: Idiopathic long QT syndrome: Progress and questions. Am Heart J 109:399, 1985.

171. Moss AJ, Schwartz PJ, Crompton RS, et al: The long QT syndrome: A prospective international study. Circulation 71:17, 1985.

172. Kay GN, Plumb VJ, Araniegas JG, et al: Torsade de pointes: The long-short initiating sequence and other clinical features: Observations in 32 patients. J Am Coll Cardiol 2:806, 1983.

173. Crawford MH, Karliner JS, O'Rouke RA, et al: Prolonged QT interval syndrome: Successful treatment with combined ventricular pacing and propranolol. Chest 68:369, 1975.

174. Yabek SM and Jamakami JM: Sinus node dysfunction in children, adolescents and young adults. Pediatrics 61:593, 1978.

175. Greenwood RD, Rosenthal A, Sloss LJ, et al: Sick sinus syndrome after surgery for congenital heart disease. Circulation 52:208, 1975.

176. Young D, Eisenberg R, Fish B, et al: Wenckebach atrioventricular block (Mobitz Type I) in children and adolescents. Am J Cardiol 40:393, 1977.

177. Kelly DT, Brodsky SJ, and Krovetz LJ: Mobitz Type II atrioventricular block in children. J Pediatr 79:972, 1971.

178. Michaelsson M and Engle MA: Congenital complete heart block: An international study of the natural history. In: Engle MA (ed): Pediatric Cardiology. Philadelphia, FA Davis, 1972, pp. 85–101.

179. Fryda RJ, Kaplan S, and Helmsworth JA: Postoperative complete heart block in children. Br Heart J 22:456, 1971.

180. Levy AM, Camon AJ, and Keane JF: Multiple arrhythmias detected during nocturnal monitoring in patients with congenital complete heart block. Circulation 55:247, 1977.

181. Winkler RB, Freed MD, and Nadas AS: Exercise induced ventricular ectopy in children and young adults with complete heart block. Am Heart J 9:87, 1980.

182. Dewey RC, Capeles MA, and Levy AM: Use of ambulatory electrocardiographic monitoring to identify high-risk patients with congenital complete heart block. N Engl J Med 316:835, 1987.

183. Lillehei CW, Sellers RD, Bonnaheau, et al: Chronic postsurgical complete heart block. J Thorac Cardiovasc Surg 46:436, 1963.

184. Benson DW Jr, Sanford M, Dunnigan A, et al: Transesophageal atrial pacing threshold: Role of interelectrode spacing, pulse width and catheter insertion depth. Am J Cardiol 40:282, 1977.

185. Hynes JK, Holmes DR, and Harrison CE: Five-year experience with temporary pacemaker therapy in the coronary care unit. Mayo Clin Proc 58:122, 1983.

186. Zoll PM: Resuscitation of the heart in ventricular standstill by external electrical stimulation. N Engl J Med 247:768, 1952.

187. Madsen JK, Meibom J, Videlak R, et al: Transcutaneous pacing: Experience with the Zoll noninvasive temporary pacemaker. Am Heart J 116:7, 1988.

188. Pride HB and McKinley DF: Third degree burns from the use of an external cardiac pacing device. Crit Care Med 18:768, 1952.

37

Maturation of the Respiratory System

James L. Robotham, M.D., Lynn D. Martin, M.D.,
Randall C. Wetzel, M.B., B.S., and
David G. Nichols, M.D.

The prompt recognition and treatment of respiratory failure is essential in the management of any acutely ill infant or child, particularly since developmental physiologic factors predispose these patients to greater risks from respiratory insults than adults who have a comparable injury.[1] This chapter presents an overview of the developmental principles applicable to understanding the pathophysiology of acute respiratory failure in childhood.

GROWTH AND DEVELOPMENT OF AIRWAY ALVEOLI

The conducting airways develop embryologically by the 16th week of gestation.[2,3] Thus, any congenital insult that limits lung development early in gestation may influence not only the normal development of the conducting airways and their subtended gas exchange volumes but also the development of the accompanying pulmonary vascular structures.[2,4]

During the past few years there has been an increasing recognition that lung growth and development may be affected by multiple chemical and mechanical factors independently controlling lung cell number, differentiation, and function in addition to the morphologic complexity of the airspace.[5–7] Thus a small lung may be functionally mature, or a large lung may be immature. This increases the difficulty in understanding the effects of disease processes. Simplifying greatly, it appears that airspace growth and development can often be related to primary mechanical factors, whereas the degree of functional maturity of the individual cell types relates to neurohumoral or hormonal factors acting individually and together. Cooney and Thurlbeck[8] noted that in infants born with anencephaly or hydranencephaly without associated defects known to independently reduce lung growth, normal in utero lung growth without a

pituitary gland is possible. Conversely, the most studied hormonal factors influencing lung growth, corticosteroids, clearly can accelerate surfactant production but may adversely affect short-term and possibly long-term lung growth.[9–11] Whether a prenatal increase in corticosteroids has an immediate positive clinical result in premature newborns because of an increase in surfactant or because of an independent marked structural increase in lung compliance remains to be evaluated.[12]

The primary mechanical variables have been grouped by Kitterman[13] as four physical parameters that may limit the lung's ability to express its full potential for growth with a normal hormonal milieu: (a) an adequate intrathoracic space; (b) fetal diaphragmatic excursions; (c) an adequate volume of amniotic fluid within the uterine cavity; and (d) an adequate volume of liquid within the potential airspaces of the lung.

The intrathoracic space available for lung growth may be limited in utero by a diaphragmatic hernia allowing abdominal contents to fill the thorax, pleural effusions, adenomatoid malformations, or tumors. The marked reduction in the number of airway generations and alveoli in both the ipsilateral and contralateral lungs associated with a diaphragmatic hernia confirms an early insult to both lungs.[3] The pendulum continues to swing between the concept that irreversible respiratory failure observed with a large congenital diaphragmatic hernia (CDH) is associated with a dominant pulmonary vascular lesion producing severe pulmonary hypertension, and the perception that inadequate alveolar development limiting gas exchange is the dominant issue.[14] The use of extracorporeal membrane oxygenation (ECMO) to improve survival in these patients will allow animal and human studies to help understand the dynamic interrelationships between lung airway/airspace growth and growth of the pulmonary vascular bed.[15,16] It is clear that a primary mechanical reduction in space for lung growth proportionately reduces airway and vascular growth, while it is also evident that a substantial primary reduction in fetal pulmonary blood flow leads to diminished overall lung growth.[17-19]

Absence of fetal breathing movements may reflect primary spinal cord lesions, phrenic nerve injury, diaphragm malformations or maternal-fetal environmental factors (e.g., smoking, maternal hypoxia, ethanol) that reduce fetal breathing activity.[13, 20-22] A lack of diaphragmatic tone and activity will allow the abdominal contents to impinge on the thoracic space and limit development of a positive transpulmonary (distending) pressure. Intermittent fetal breathing appears to be an important factor, triggering lung growth that produces a separate message from factors producing static lung distention.[21]

The fetal respiratory tract actively secretes fluid into potential airspaces sufficient to account for the normal postnatal residual capacity. This process appears to be influenced strongly by β-adrenergic stimuli[13] and can be influenced by agents that interfere with ionic pumps.[23]

Given normal control of these secretory processes, mechanical factors regulating the egress of the actively secreted fluid from the lungs will also influence lung growth. At one extreme, laryngeal atresia, which prohibits egress of pulmonary fluid, leads to an abnormal increase in alveolar development, whereas the experimental production of a tracheoesophageal fistula leads to decreased cell numbers, lung distensibility, and alveolar development.[7, 24, 25] These two extremes suggest that an expiratory resistance produced by the normal fetal upper airway may be an important factor in lung growth by producing a positive transpulmonary pressure.[26, 27] This factor appears in studies of fetal lambs to be present mainly during fetal apnea. Paradoxically, during fetal breathing, inspiratory resistance increases greatly such that the predominant effect of fetal respiration is to prevent amniotic fluid from entering the lung during inspiration and then to empty pulmonary liquid into the amniotic fluid during expiration. Thus, the expectation that fetal inspiration would contribute to stretching the lung is not observed. This suggests that the importance of fetal respiration, in addition to exercising the respiratory muscles, is related to pulmonary liquid turnover.

The fourth mechanical factor influencing lung growth is the volume of amniotic fluid that normally surrounds the chest wall. Oligohydramnios, even with persistent fetal breathing activity, may substantially inhibit lung growth.[28, 29] This suggests that one purpose of amniotic fluid is to prevent a potentially greater local contact pressure from the uterine wall over the thoracoabdominal cavity from limiting thoracic expansion. The liquid interface between the fetus and the uterine wall would maintain a constant and even surface pressure over the fetal thorax and abdomen regardless of any acute volume exchanges between the fetal pulmonary, gastrointestinal, or genitourinary systems and the surrounding amniotic fluid.

The role of pulmonary blood flow in determining lung growth has been confirmed both in experimental animal studies and in studies of humans with congenital heart disease (CHD) that profoundly reduce pulmonary blood flow. Experimentally, ligation of one pulmonary artery in utero results in a substantial reduction in lung growth

in the ipsilateral lung.[18] Histologic studies of lungs of patients with tetralogy of Fallot have found reduced lung volume and alveolar number.[30-32] Gaultier and associates performed pulmonary function testing in children with tetralogy of Fallot and found that if complete repair was performed within the first 2 years of life, normal lung volumes, compliance, resistance, carbon monoxide diffusing capacity, and arterial blood gases could be obtained.[17] In contrast, children with initial palliative shunts, followed by intracardiac repair later in life, had reduced lung volumes and carbon monoxide diffusing capacities suggestive of reduced alveolar growth and abnormal vascular development.

Until recently, it was believed that the classic morphologic alveolus, with an extremely thin epithelial and endothelial cell layer, did not appear until birth.[33] Alveolar development was believed to rapidly increase and level out at approximately 8 years of age.[3] Langston and associates challenged this belief, based on a larger number of morphometric studies; they found that substantial numbers of alveoli are indeed present at term.[34] They found a very wide variation, with the term infant having an average of 50 million alveoli compared with 400 million alveoli in the average adult. Further studies by Thurlbeck[35] suggest that the total number of alveoli may be present as early as 2 years of age. This result is consistent with the findings of Gaultier and associates that repair of a tetralogy of Fallot after 2 years of age results in long-term deficits.[17] Thus, there is evidence that early injury to the lung, either in utero or in the early postnatal period, may have a profound effect on alveolar development. The existence of a relatively substantial period of time postnatally in which alveolar development may still be induced from normal lung is strongly supported by many, but not all, animal and human studies in which pneumonectomy or lobar resection early in life allows substantial, if not complete, compensatory alveolar growth from the remaining normal lung.[3, 5, 6, 36-38] Since alveoli grow, whereas conducting airways do not, these children may show evidence of a relative increase in airway resistance for a given alveolar volume.[36, 39] The reason for the hyperplastic growth of the remaining lung is not well understood. One hypothesis suggests that distortion of the remaining lung tissue leads to an elaboration of local growth factors that have been found in the blood of animals postpneumonectomy, whereas an alternative hypothesis suggests that the primary factor is the relative increase in blood flow to the remaining tissue.[6]

Compared with discrete regional disease (e.g., pneumonectomy), a diffuse early lung injury may cause a long-term disruption of normal lung growth and development. Normal airway budding, leading to alveolar sac development, septation, and thus discrete alveoli, requires the physical apposition of endothelium and mesothelium.[40] Presumably, this allows the secretion and reception of small protein growth factors.[3, 6] Thus, any diffuse pathologic process that disrupts this cell-to-cell interaction (e.g., inflammation, interstitial edema, or fibrosis) can produce lung dysplasia. Hakulinen and associates reported on a 6- to 9-year follow-up of 42 prematurely born children and 30 full-term controls.[41]

The most important finding was that ventilator treatment associated with lung disease was more important than prematurity alone in producing long-term abnormalities. During the past few years there has been an increasing appreciation that standard mechanical ventilation, independent of oxygen toxicity, may well be the primary factor producing lung damage in hyaline membrane disease.[42–45] These results suggest that any approach that prevents disruption of the small airways may greatly reduce the pathologic and physiologic consequences of hyaline membrane disease. Thus either surfactant administration that increases lung compliance[46] or appropriate methods of high-frequency ventilation after airway recruitment that minimize overdistention of the airway may reduce both the short- and long-term effects of the disease process.[42, 43]

Severe cases of bronchopulmonary dysplasia are usually associated with hyaline membrane disease; however, meconium aspiration, tracheoesophageal fistula, and other diffuse pulmonary insults in the neonatal period may predispose the child to long-term respiratory problems. Even a minor viral respiratory infection can cause a rapid deterioration in the respiratory status of a child with moderately severe bronchopulmonary dysplasia. These high-risk children require long-term follow-up and care for respiratory difficulties.

Independent of immaturity, viral infections of the respiratory system in the newborn may predispose to long-term deficits in normal lung growth and development. Using a newborn rat model, Castleman and colleagues have studied the long-term influence of neonatal bronchiolitis and pneumonia.[47, 48] They found evidence of viral replication in epithelial cells at all levels of the respiratory tree and in macrophages. Persistence of the virus was observed in neonatal rats compared with 1-month-old rats consistent with a relative immunodeficiency. Follow-up morphologic studies found abnormal alveolar development and bronchiolar hypoplasia associated with reduced compliance and decreased dynamic compliance.

In summary, airway and alveolar development are susceptible to in utero and early postnatal injuries that may produce long-term adverse effects. A careful history of this time period is essential when evaluating the respiratory status of any patient who presents with respiratory disease.

GROWTH AND DEVELOPMENT OF THE PULMONARY CIRCULATION

Over the last decade the structural and functional maturation of the pulmonary vascular bed has taken on a new significance. It has become increasingly well recognized that the interactions between multiple endogenous and exogenous mediators of smooth muscle tone, the vasoregulatory aspects of the endothelium, and intrinsic smooth muscle activity determine the structural and functional features of the pulmonary circulation. This interplay acutely determines both the resistance and reactivity of the pulmonary circulation. These same factors over time result in hyperplasia, hypertro-phy, smooth muscle differentiation, and the pathologic migration into the subendothelium, which cause altered pulmonary vascular structure, resistance, and reactivity. It is important to differentiate "resistance" from "reactivity." Although they are frequently related—that is, high resistance is often associated with high reactivity—this is not necessarily so. A change in smooth muscle tone to a given stimulus (reactivity) depends on the intrinsic muscle response potentially modified by other mediators. These factors may or may not be the determinants of baseline vascular resistance at any given time. As an example, at birth, baseline pulmonary vascular resistance decreases dramatically, but reactivity to bradykinin and many other stimuli may not change. The net effect of the various modulators of pulmonary vascular smooth muscle tone on resistance and reactivity at any given developmental stage may be quite complex. This complex interplay between structure and function has been studied postnatally in newborn sheep.[49] Even though the pulmonary arterioles are highly muscularized at birth, with the onset of ventilation, baseline resistance falls and rapid changes in the biochemical milieu produce a marked attenuation of hypoxic vasoreactivity. At 2 weeks of age, the baseline resistance has decreased further as muscularization involutes. Even so, despite this fall in baseline resistance and decreased muscularization, pulmonary vasoresponsiveness to hypoxia is more pronounced than at birth. Thus, in the perinatal period, biochemical factors appear to blunt reactivity and reduce resistance whereas attenuated muscularization is not necessarily associated with decreased reactivity at 2 weeks of age.[49, 50] In this setting, pulmonary hypertension may result from abnormally increased muscularization, decreased vasodilator activity, increased vasoconstrictor activity, or any combination of these factors.

Recent investigations have clarified many of the factors involved in the decrease in pulmonary vascular resistance that accompanies expansion of the lungs and oxygenation at birth, as the interactions are more fully appreciated. Pulmonary vascular development mirrors the development of the airways with all preacinar arteries present by the 16th week of gestation.[51] Muscular arteries end at the level of the terminal bronchiole in the fetus and newborn (Fig. 37–1). During childhood, the muscular arteries gradually extend to the alveolar level as in adults. Preacinar muscular arteries grow in size throughout gestation; however, there is little change in medial wall thickness.[52] Within minutes of birth, many aspects of the pulmonary circulation change dramatically. Peripheral arteries that were previously closed in utero are recruited.[53] Morphologically, the endothelial cells become less cuboidal and more elongated with fewer surface projections and less overlap.[54] The smooth muscle cells become more fusiform and less globular with decreased density of endoplasmic reticulum and increased density of myofilaments.[54] These structural adaptations result in functionally less compliant arteries and are associated with a dramatic decrease in pulmonary vascular resistance.[53, 55]

In addition to the structural development of the pulmonary circulation, the ability to release specific

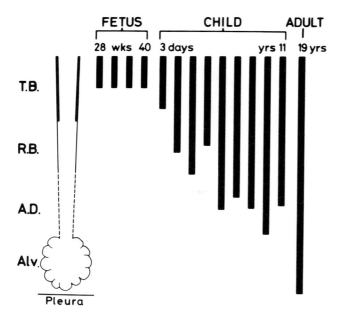

Figure 37–1. The age-related distribution of muscular pulmonary arteries. With increasing age, muscular arteries extend further toward the alveolus. TB = terminal bronchiole; RB = respiratory bronchiole; AD = alveolar duct; Alv = alveolus. (Reprinted with permission from Am Rev Respir Dis 119:531, 1979.)

mediators as well as maturation of specific receptor systems determines the changing response to multiple stimuli. Multiple mediators and various mechanisms have been implicated in modulating the pulmonary circulation during the transition from the fetal environment to the neonatal environment.[56] Eicosanoids form one of the major groups of mediators intimately involved in the regulation of the fetal and transitional pulmonary circulation. Leukotrienes have been implicated in maintaining pulmonary vascular tone in the fetal pulmonary circulation and may play a role in modulating hypoxic pulmonary vasoconstriction.[57–59] Prostacyclin is involved in the normal relaxation of the pulmonary vasculature at birth.[57, 60] Prostaglandin D_2 is a dilator in the fetal lamb and a constrictor in the newborn,[61] and the degree of constriction increases with maturation.[62] The role of endothelial cell mediators such as platelet-activating factor (PAF), endothelium-derived relaxing factor (EDRF), and endothelin in the regulation of the transitional circulation remains to be explored.

Failure of the pulmonary vascular bed to dilate at birth results in the syndrome of persistent pulmonary hypertension in the newborn with hypoxemia and right-to-left shunting through the patent foramen ovale ductus arteriosus. The failure of pulmonary vascular resistance to decrease at birth may result from hypoplasia, which is seen with CDH or oligohydramnios (underdevelopment),[63, 64] abnormal extension of muscle into peripheral arteries caused by an intrauterine insult (maldevelopment),[65, 66] or a perinatal insult such as hypoxia that leads to failure of normal vasodilator mediator systems (maladaptation). Conventional medical management of this syndrome consists of mechanical hyperventilation, muscle relaxation, sedation, and the debatable use of

vasodilators.[67, 68] ECMO is being used more commonly for these critically ill infants with improved survival in patients without CDH.[69] Because the degree of pulmonary hypoplasia determines survival in patients with CDH,[63] attempts at substantially improving survival with supportive care such as ECMO may be limited,[15] and interventions designed to affect the degree of hypoplasia such as fetal surgery or transplantation may be required.[70, 71]

Acute or chronic hypoxia in utero or in the early postnatal period may prevent the fall in pulmonary vascular resistance and produce structural changes in the pulmonary vascular bed at birth.[72, 73] The mediator(s) responsible for this change in pulmonary vascular resistance in response to a change in oxygen tension have not been identified. A complex interaction of vasoconstrictors (thromboxane, leukotrienes, PAF, endothelin),[59, 74–77] vasodilators (prostacyclin, ERDF) or possibly direct effects on the vasculature may contribute to this pathologic response.[78–81] It is clear that the physiologic response to alveolar hypoxia varies with age and is modulated in part by dilator prostaglandins.[49, 50]

Physicians involved in the care of critically ill infants and children frequently encounter patients with CHD such as ventricular and atrioventricular septal defects that cause large left-to-right shunts and result in elevated pulmonary blood flow and pressure. This abnormal hemodynamic state leads to progressive structural changes in the pulmonary circulation and contributes to the increasing functional impairment of the pulmonary circulation.[82] By correlating the vascular structure of lung biopsy tissue and pulmonary hemodynamic data, investigators have been able to identify patients at risk for early postoperative pulmonary hypertension and determine whether pulmonary arterial pressure and resistance eventually would remain elevated or return to normal following repair of the cardiac lesion.[83] The pulmonary hypertension is frequently labile and is usually controlled by mechanical hyperventilation and continued narcotic anesthesia.[84] Evidence suggests that endothelial cell injury leads to altered endothelial-platelet, leukocyte, and endothelial-smooth muscle interactions resulting in increased pulmonary vascular reactivity, abnormal pulmonary vascular smooth muscle growth and differentiation, and increased connective tissue protein synthesis that may be important in the pathogenesis of the progressive pulmonary vascular disease associated with CHD.[85–87]

GROWTH AND FUNCTIONAL DEVELOPMENT OF THE CHEST WALL

The chest wall consists of the rib cage, the intercostal muscle, and the diaphragm. Its purpose is to ventilate the lungs. The functional concept of a respiratory pump for the lungs may be expanded to include abdominal wall musculature that contributes to chest wall motion. The respiratory center in the brain stem integrates the action of these muscles, and impulses to chest wall musculature are conveyed via the spinal cord and phrenic and intercostal nerves (see also Chapter 48).

The shape of the thorax changes with age. During fetal life, the chest is compressed in the transverse axis but becomes approximately circular immediately after birth. With the circular configuration of the chest wall, the ribs are attached perpendicularly to the vertebral column, which significantly limits the elevation of the ribs during inspiration. Thus expansion of the thoracic cavity during inspiration in the newborn depends primarily on diaphragmatic action. As the child develops assuming an upright posture, the shape of the chest becomes elliptical in horizontal cross-section, and the ribs are attached to the vertebral column at an acute angle so that elevation of the rib cage occurs with a "bucket handle" motion at the costal vertebral junction. The left and right hemidiaphragms form the inferior border of the chest cavity and can be divided into costal and crural segments on functional and embryologic grounds.[88] Since the crural segments of the diaphragm are anchored to lumbar vertebrae, crural contraction leads exclusively to a diaphragmatic descent. In contrast, the costal segments of the diaphragm are attached to the seventh to twelfth ribs and the posterior surfaces of the xiphoid process and sternum. Because the ribs are themselves mobile, contraction of the costal segments of the diaphragm may lead either to expansion or contraction of the rib cage, depending on several factors. Coordinated expansion of the rib cage during contraction of the diaphragm in inspiration depends on the patient's position. In the upright position, tonic contraction of the abdominal musculature produces a decrease in abdominal compliance. When the costal segments of diaphragm contract against the stiff abdomen, a lever action exerts an upper pull on the lower ribs, thus enlarging the chest cavity at that level.[89] Infants are at a disadvantage because they spend most of their time in the supine position, which is associated with relaxation of abdominal wall musculature. Thus, the supine infant who also has a soft, cartilaginous rib cage may experience lower rib contraction during retraction of the diaphragm.

Since the diaphragm is the major muscle of respiration, most investigation has concentrated on factors that impair diaphragmatic contractility. Contractile force of the diaphragm depends on fiber length, load, and the intrinsic contractile properties of the diaphragmatic fibers. A reduction in muscle fiber length leads to a fall in diaphragmatic force output for the same degree of neural excitation of the diaphragm. Many common forms of lung disease in infants and young children are associated with increased expiratory resistance, such as asthma, bronchiolitis, and bronchopulmonary dysplasia. During acute increases in expiratory resistance, the resultant hyperinflation reduces diaphragm fiber length and thus force output may fall, contributing to the development of respiratory failure.[90] A variety of compensatory responses may improve diaphragm force output by adjusting the diaphragm fiber length. Tonic recruitment of the expiratory abdominal and intercostal muscles leads to a reduction in functional residual capacity and therefore an increase in diaphragmatic fiber length.[91] Compensation for chronic hyperinflation may include actual sarcomere loss leading to a more favorable relationship between diaphragmatic length and force output.[92] Increased inspiratory resistance or very large reductions in abdominal compliance may produce an enormous load to breathing in infants and result in a fall in tidal volume and minute ventilation.[93] In contrast, the adult who is awake is able to defend tidal volume to a greater extent during loaded breathing, although this is accomplished at the expense of increased diaphragmatic work and energy expenditure.[94]

Intrinsic histochemical and mechanical properties of the various muscle fiber types that make up the diaphragm determine its strength and endurance properties. The type I muscle fiber exhibits a slow contraction velocity and highly oxidative metabolic properties. Therefore, it is a capable of continuous moderate force output and is extremely resistant to fatigue. The diaphragm of the premature is deficient in these efficient type I muscle fibers. In addition the newborn lacks type IIb muscle fibers, which are rapidly contracting and depend on glycolytic metabolism.[95] The rapid contraction velocity of type IIb fibers allows for a large force output but only for a limited time. Instead of type I and IIb muscle fibers present in the adult diaphragm, the premature infant diaphragm consists of fetal IIc (highly oxidative, slow twitch) and IIa (oxidative, fast twitch) fibers that depend on oxidative metabolism. Thus, it is not a lack of oxidative fatigue-resistant fibers that is responsible for the high incidence of respiratory muscle fatigue and respiratory failure in the neonate. It is possible that the overriding determinant of the function of the diaphragm is the diaphragm muscle mass, since it has been shown that force output of the diaphragm rises with increasing mass. Infants who have required mechanical ventilation have evidence of small muscle fiber size or disuse atrophy in the diaphragm.[96–98]

Birth injury or thoracic surgery may produce phrenic nerve injury that leads to paralysis of the ipsilateral hemidiaphragm. Although such an injury is generally asymptomatic in the adult and older child, it may be life-threatening in the infant. Cyanosis and tachypnea develop in the infant, with hemidiaphragm paralysis because, in addition to the flaccid hemidiaphragm, the infant also possesses a highly compliant rib cage such that the fall in pleural pressure during inspiration will not ventilate the ipsilateral lung as the hemidiaphragm and the rib cage move paradoxically inward.[99] Developmental changes in rib cage stability and intercostal muscle activity have profound effects on ventilation. The soft cartilaginous structure of the infant's rib cage necessitates intercostal muscle activity in order to provide stability to the rib cage during even normal respiration. Intercostal muscle activity is inhibited during active rapid eye movement [REM] sleep.[100] When inhibition of the intercostal muscles prevents stabilization of the rib cage, retraction of the rib cage during breathing is noted during the physical examination. Without the synergistic activity of the intercostal muscles to stabilize the rib cage, diaphragmatic contraction becomes highly inefficient, because each contraction distorts the rib cage and reduces its contribution to tidal respiration.[101] Prolonged inhibition of intercostal muscle activity may result in diaphragmatic fatigue and apnea.[102]

Abdominal wall compliance has a critical influence on ventilation. Increased abdominal compliance secondary to abdominal wall relaxation occurs in the supine position. This aggravates the tendency for distortion of the rib cage during REM sleep. When abdominal binding is applied to raise intra-abdominal pressure modestly up to 20 cm of water, chest wall retractions can be abolished with preservation of lung volume and diminished work of breathing.[103, 104] The most extreme example of increased intra-abdominal compliance is provided by prune belly syndrome in which there is an absence of abdominal wall musculature in association with cryptorchidism, urinary tract malformation, and pulmonary hypoplasia. Because of the lack of any abdominal tone, the diaphragm is flat and short, thus impairing force output on inspiration. Because lower rib cage elevation is dependent on a rise in abdominal pressure during diaphragmatic contraction, these patients simply have lower rib cage retraction on inspiration. Finally, since an effective cough to clear lung secretions depends on the expiratory muscle function of the abdominal wall, patients with prune belly syndrome frequently develop atelectasis. The opposite problems are exhibited by patients following gastroschisis and omphalocele repair in which the abdominal wall may become extremely noncompliant. The greatly reduced abdominal compliance forces the diaphragm to contract against an increased load. This rise in energy demands on the diaphragm is compounded by the potential for decreased diaphragmatic perfusion because of raised intra-abdominal pressure.[105] These patients are dependent on mechanical ventilation until abdominal compliance increases sufficiently to allow spontaneous breathing.

GROWTH AND DEVELOPMENT OF THE UPPER AIRWAY

The age at which an infant is no longer an obligate nose breather is uncertain and probably varies.[106] Children with choanal atresia may have life-threatening difficulties despite the patent oropharynx, whereas an upper respiratory infection that provokes copious nasal secretions may lead to mild or moderate respiratory distress in anatomically normal children.

Anatomic factors including mandibular development (micrognathia), neck flexion, a tracheal web, or subglottic stenosis may contribute to upper airway obstruction. The presence of a residual subglottic stenosis or tracheomalacia is particularly common in children who were intubated during the neonatal period. Neural factors are also important in maintaining the structural patency of the upper airway during inspiration.[107] The striated muscles that control the nares, tongue, pharynx, and larynx can be viewed as physiologically linked with the diaphragm and intercostals in providing an integrated system to draw air into the lungs through an upper airway with the minimal resistance compatible with its other roles as humidifier and filter.[108] Thus, with airway obstruction during inspiration, the alar nasae should dilate the nares while the hypoglossal nerve activates the muscles that will pull the tongue forward

and open the pharynx maximally. It is, therefore, not surprising that in human neonates with airway obstruction the submental electromyogram demonstrates activation of the genioglossus prior to any evidence of diaphragmatic activity.[109] A marked increase in the submental electromyogram is noted with obstruction consistent with a role in preventing or ending obstructive apnea. This finely tuned, integrated response appears to be mediated via the superior laryngeal nerve's afferent fibers, which sense pressure, air flow, or local distortion and trigger upper airway dilation.[108] However, in the immediate postnatal period, negative upper airway pressure can lead to apnea,[110] suggesting that the appropriate neural connections for postnatal survival are not established. Thus, it is not surprising that infants with anatomic abnormalities of the upper airway (e.g., micrognathia,[111] cerebral palsy, or increased intracranial pressure affecting brain stem function) appear to be more vulnerable to upper airway obstruction.

Although a history of inspiratory stridor/snoring during sleep or with postural changes may indicate the presence of a upper airway obstruction, the absence of structural anatomic abnormalities does not rule out a dynamic upper airway obstruction severe enough to cause cor pulmonale (i.e., collapse of the pharyngeal soft tissues against the tongue). A carefully done cinefluoroscopy study of a barium swallow in the lateral projection may document an abnormal swallowing pattern, with or without aspiration, that is part of an overall, occasionally subtle neurologic deficit. A positive result on a barium study should be followed by an evaluation of the patient's history and a physical examination for evidence of dynamic airway obstruction during rest or, perhaps more noticeably, during a sleep study. It seems more than coincidental that recurrent or chronic pulmonary disease is found in children with evidence of an abnormal swallowing mechanism. It is important that the barium swallow be recorded at high speed in the lateral view so that the process of deglutition can be evaluated and reviewed at slow speed.

The muscles of the larynx are similarly linked with the diaphragm during respiration, both prenatally and postnatally. At birth, the high positive expiratory pressure with the first breath require laryngeal adduction.[112]

The developmental sensory activity of the upper airway and its interactions with anesthesia require further definition. In the unanesthetized, premature human (less than 35 weeks' gestational age), carinal stimulation can provoke ventilatory depression or apnea; after 35 weeks' gestation, the typical cough is elicited.[113] The interaction of newborns and infants with anesthetics is well known to clinicians; in such infants, life-threatening largyngospasm may occur with minimal airway irritation. This can be demonstrated experimentally in animal models.[114, 115]

VENTILATORY CONTROL

Although there is no question that profound hypoxia depresses the central nervous system respiratory output at all ages, studies of mild-to-moderate hypoxia in humans and animals are frequently unable to separate peripheral affector, central integrator, and peripheral effector dysfunction. Thus, any study that claims hypoxic depression of ventilation must define its end-point and measure the output of peripheral neural activity, peripheral and central chemoreceptor activity, central neural output, electromyograms, and mechanical force. Whether hypoxia in the premature infant fails to stimulate the carotid bodies[116] or depresses the mechanical activity of respiratory muscle,[117] or both, it influences our concepts of monitoring, diagnosis, and therapy. Indeed, even the type of stimulus can be used experimentally to define the component that is affected—for example, a single breath step change in oxygen will essentially influence only the peripheral chemoreceptors, whereas a steady-state challenge may influence all aspects of the loop.

The infant, the growing child, and particularly the premature infant deal less well with hypoxic, hypercarbic, and obstructive stresses than the adult, regardless of the precise cause.[118, 119] Mild hypoxia, which produces hyperventilation in the full-term infant or adult, may produce respiratory depression or even apnea in the otherwise normal premature infant. Alternatively, vagally mediated pulmonary stretch reflexes, which are minimal in the adult, may produce prolonged apnea in the infant.[119] It is likely that these and other improperly modulated airway or chemoreceptor reflexes all lead to a final common pathway of neurally mediated apnea and secondary bradycardia or, less often, a primary cardiac bradyarrhythmia followed by respiratory arrest (i.e., sudden infant death syndrome [SIDS]).

CONGENITAL HEART DISEASE AND AIRWAY OBSTRUCTION

In addition to its well-known etiologic role in the development of pulmonary edema leading to respiratory failure, CHD is less commonly associated with cardiovascular anomalies causing severe large airway obstruction (see also Chapter 33). One such anomaly is vascular rings. Vascular rings often produce some degree of inspiratory stridor in the neonatal period; however, severe symptomatology may not develop until later.[120] Inspiratory stridor or dysphagia is the most common presenting sign of a vascular ring; severe expiratory obstruction with wheezing throughout both lung fields and hyperexpanded lungs suggest a compression of the distal trachea by a vascular ring. There may be clinical, radiologic, or electrocardiographic evidence of intracardiac abnormalities. A plain chest x-ray film may reveal some compression of the distal trachea, which is seen more easily on a lateral film; a barium swallow can show external compression of the esophagus.

Children with tetralogy of Fallot and absent or rudimentary pulmonary valves are born with massively dilated pulmonary arteries, one of which is often much larger than the other. One or both of these enlarged pulmonary arteries can compress the left or right mainstem bronchus, leading to severe airway obstruction and lung overexpansion. Many other forms of congenital

heart disease leading to cardiomegaly and dilated pulmonary arteries may secondarily obstruct one or both bronchi.[121] Thus, an underlying congenital heart lesion may produce unilateral or bilateral lung hyperlucency.

Finally, hypocalcemia resulting from cardiovascular malformations of the aortic arch associated with hypoparathyroidism (DiGeorge syndrome) may also lead to upper airway obstruction due to largyngospasm.

DEVELOPMENT OF COLLATERAL VENTILATION

Adult patients with extensive disease of the small airways or mucus plugging are protected to some degree from diffuse atelectasis by extensive intralobar collateral ventilatory channels between and among the alveoli and bronchi. Thus, within the lobe of an adult's lung there are multiple channels to ventilate the alveoli of an obstructed small airway. However, because collateral ventilation is also a developmental phenomenon that increases with age,[122] the same degree of small airways disease may lead to considerably more atelectasis in the infant.

The high resistance to collateral ventilation that is present in the newborn has a number of physiologic implications. The dynamic functional residual capacity of the newborn is determined by starting inspiration before the end of a passively determined expiration. This is necessary to maintain the end-expiration lung volume close to the closing capacity, thus minimizing the ventilation perfusion mismatch since the flaccid rib cage of the newborn has essentially no elastic recoil. With no rib cage recoil, the newborn maintains a rapid respiratory rate which, when combined with the increased resistance for collateral ventilation that limits expiratory gas flow, will maintain an adequate end-expiratory lung volume. Paradoxically, if atelectasis occurs, the relative absence of collateral ventilations will inhibit re-expansion of the collapsed alveoli. Over time, as the rib cage stability increases, neither a rapid respiratory rate nor increased resistance to collateral ventilation are necessary to maintain end-expiratory lung volume, while the development of collateral ventilation prevents the development of atelectasis.

References

1. Hogg JC: Age as a factor in respiratory disease. *In*: Kendig EL and Chernick V (eds): Disorders of the Respiratory Tract. Philadelphia, WB Saunders, 1977, pp. 177–187.
2. Burri PH: Fetal and postnatal development of the lung. Ann Rev Physiol 46:617, 1984.
3. Reid LM: Structure and function in pulmonary hypertension: New perceptions. Chest 84:279, 1986.
4. Reid LM: Lung growth in health and disease. Br J Dis Chest 78:113, 1984.
5. Thurlbeck WM and Galaugher WJM: Adaptive response to pneumonectomy in puppies. Thorax 36:424, 1981.
6. Rannels DE and Rannels SR: Compensatory growth of the lung following partial pneumonectomy. Exp Lung Res 14:157, 1988.
7. Wigglesworth JS, Desai R, and Aber V: Quantitative aspects of perinatal lung growth. Early Hum Dev 15:203, 1987.

8. Cooney TP and Thurlbeck WM: Lung growth and development in anencephaly and hydranencephaly. Am Rev Respir Dis 132:596, 1985.

9. Adamson IYR and King GM: Postnatal development of rat lung following retarded fetal lung growth. Pediatr Pulmonol 4:230, 1988.

10. Ellington B, McBride JT, and Stokes DC: Effects of corticosteroids on post-natal lung and airway growth in the ferret. J Appl Physiol 68:2029–2033, 1990.

11. Warburton D, Parton L, Buckley S, et al: Combined effects of corticosteroid, thyroid hormones, and β-agonist on surfactant, pulmonary mechanics, and β-receptor binding in fetal lamb lung. Pediatr Res 24:166, 1988.

12. Mitzner W, Johnson JWC, Scott R, et al: Effect of bethamethasone on pressure-volume relationship of fetal rhesus monkey lung. J Appl Physiol 47:377–382, 1979.

13. Kitterman JA: Physiological factors in fetal lung growth. Can J Physiol Pharmacol 66:1122, 1988.

14. Bohn DI, Tamura M, Hosokawa Y, et al: Deterioration of oxygenation and lung compliance associated with repair of congenital diaphragmatic hernia. Am Rev Respir Dis 133:A151, 1986.

15. Langham, Jr. MR, Krummel TM, Bartlett RH, et al: Mortality with extracorporeal membrane oxygenation following repair of congenital diaphragmatic hernia in 93 infants. J Pediatr Surg 22:1150, 1987.

16. Stolar C, Dillon P, and Reyes C: Selective use of extracorporeal membrane oxygenation in the management of congenital diaphragmatic hernia. J Pediatr Surg 23:207, 1988.

17. Gaultier C, Boule M, Thibert M, et al: Resting lung function in children after repair of tetralogy of Fallot. Chest 89:561, 1986.

18. Wallen LD, Perry SF, Alston JT, et al: Morphometric study of the role of pulmonary arterial flow in fetal lung growth in sheep. Pediatr Res 27:122–127, 1990.

19. Wallen LD, Kondo CS, Takahashi Y, et al: Left pulmonary artery ligation impairs fetal lung growth. Pediatr Res 12:239, 1987.

20. Inselman LS, Fisher SE, Spencer H, and Atkinson M: Effect of intrauterine ethanol exposure on fetal lung growth. Pediatr Res 19:12, 1985.

21. Nagai A, Thurlbeck WM, Jansen AH, et al: The effect of chronic biphrenectomy on lung growth and maturation in fetal lambs. Am Rev Respir Dis 137:167, 1988.

22. Larson JE and Thurlbeck WM: The effect of experimental maternal hypoxia on fetal lung growth. Pediatr Res 24:156, 1988.

23. Olver RE and Strang LB: Ion fluxes across the pulmonary epithelium and the secretion of lung liquid in the fetal lamb. J Physiol Lond 241:327, 1974.

24. Silver MM, Thurston WA, and Patrick JE: Perinatal pulmonary hyperplasia due to laryngeal atresia. Human Pathol 19:110, 1988.

25. Fewell JE, Hislop AA, Kitterman JA, et al: Effect of tracheostomy on lung development in fetal lambs. J Appl Physiol 55:1103, 1983.

26. Harding R, Bocking AD, and Sigger JN: Upper airway resistances in fetal sheep: The influence of breathing activity. J Appl Physiol 60:160, 1986.

27. Harding R, Bocking AD, and Sigger JN: Influence of upper respiratory tract on liquid flow to and from fetal lungs. J Appl Physiol 61:68, 1986.

28. Moessinger AC, Singh M, Donnely DF, et al: The effect of prolonged oligohydramnios on fetal lung development, maturation and ventilatory patterns in the newborn guinea pig. J Dev Physiol 9:419, 1987.

29. Blott M and Greenough A: Oligohydramnios in the second trimester of pregnancy, fetal breathing and normal lung growth. Early Hum Dev 17:37, 1988.

30. Hislop A, and Reid L: Structural changes in the pulmonary arteries and veins in tetralogy of Fallot. Br Heart J 35:1178, 1973.

31. Rabinovitch M, Herrera-Deleon V, Castaneda AR, et al: Growth and development of the pulmonary vascular bed in patients with tetralogy of Fallot with or without pulmonary atresia. Circulation 64:1234, 1981.

32. Johnson RJ, and Haworth SG: Pulmonary vascular and alveolar development in tetralogy of Fallot: A recommendation for early correction. Thorax 37:893, 1982.

33. Boyden EA: Development and growth of the airways. In: Hodson WA (ed): Development of the Lung. New York, Marcel Dekker, 1977, pp. 3–36.

34. Langston C, Kida K, Reed M, et al: Human lung growth in late gestation and in the neonate. Am Rev Respir Dis 129:607, 1984.

35. Thurlbeck WM: Postnatal human lung growth. Thorax 37:564–571, 1982.

36. McBride JT, Wohl MEB, Strieder DJ, et al: Lung growth and airway function after lobectomy in infancy for congenital lobar emphysema. J Clin Invest 66:962, 1980.

37. Holmes C, and Thurlbeck WM: Normal lung growth and response after pneumonectomy in rates at various ages. Am Rev Respir Dis 120:1125, 1979.

38. Thurlbeck WM, Galaugher W, and Mathers J: Adaptive response to pneumonectomy in puppies. Thorax 36:424, 1981.

39. Kirchner KK and McBride JT: Changes in airway length after unilateral pneumonectomy in weanling ferrets. J Appl Physiol 68:187, 1990.

40. Spooner BS, and Wessells NK: Mammalian lung development: Interactions in primordium formation and bronchial morphogenesis. J Exp Zool 175:445, 1970.

41. Hakulinen AL, Heinonen K, Lansimies E, et al: Pulmonary function and respiratory morbidity in school-age children born prematurely and ventilated for neonatal respiratory insufficiency. Pediatr Pulmonol 8:226, 1990.

42. Meredith KS, deLemos RA, Coalson JJ, et al: Role of lung injury in the pathogenesis of hyaline membrane disease in premature baboons. J Appl Physiol 66:2150, 1989.

43. Froese A and Bryan AC: High frequency ventilation. Am Rev Respir Dis 135:1363, 1987.

44. Hislop AA, Wigglesworth JS, Desai R, et al: The effects of preterm delivery and mechanical ventilation on human lung growth. Early Hum Dev 15:147, 1987.

45. Hislop AA and Haworth SG: Airway size and structure in the normal fetal and infant lung and the effect of premature delivery and artificial ventilation. Am Rev Respir Dis 140:1717, 1989.

46. Enhorning G, Shennan A, Possmayer F, et al: Prevention of neonatal respiratory distress syndrome by tracheal instillation of surfactant: A randomized clinical trial. Pediatrics 76:145, 1985.

47. Castleman WL, Sorkness RL, Lemanske RF, et al: Neonatal viral bronchiolitis and pneumonia induces bronchiolar hypoplasia and alveolar dysplasia in rats. Lab Invest 59:387, 1988.

48. Castleman WL, Brundage-Anguish LJ, Kreitzer L, et al: Pathogenesis of bronchiolitis and pneumonia induced in neonatal and weanling rats by parainfluenza (Sendai) virus. Am J Pathol 129:277, 1987.

49. Gordon JB, Tod ML, Wetzel RC, et al: Age-dependent effects of indomethacin on hypoxic vasoconstriction in neonatal lamb lungs. Pediatr Res 23:580, 1988.

50. Fike CD, and Hansen TN: Hypoxic vasoconstriction increases with postnatal age in lungs from newborn rabbits. Circ Res 60:297, 1987.

51. Hislop A and Reid L: Intrapulmonary arterial development during fetal life: Branching pattern and structure. J Anat 113:35, 1975.

52. Levin DL, Rudolph AM, Heymann MA, et al: Morphological development of the pulmonary vascular bed in fetal lambs. Circulation 53:144, 1976.

53. Haworth SG, and Hislop AA: Adaptation of the pulmonary circulation to extrauterine life in the pig and its relevance to the human infant. Cardiovasc Res 15:108, 1981.

54. Haworth SG, Hall SM, Chew M, et al: Thinning of fetal pulmonary arterial wall and postnatal remodelling: Ultrastructural studies on the respiratory unit arteries of the pig. Virchows Arch 411:161, 1987.

55. Hall SM, and Haworth SG: Conducting pulmonary arteries: Structural adaptation to extrauterine life in the pig. Cardiovasc Res 21:208, 1987.

56. Lyrene RK. and Philips JB: Control of pulmonary vascular resistance in the fetus and newborn. Clin Perinatol 11:551, 1984.

57. Piper PJ, and Levene S: Generation of leukotrienes from fetal and neonatal porcine blood vessels. Biol Neonate 49:109, 1986.

58. Soifer SJ, Loitz RD, Roman C, et al: Leukotriene end organ antagonists increase pulmonary blood flow in fetal lambs. Am J Physiol 249:H570, 1985.

59. Morganroth ML, Reeves JT, Murphy RC, et al: Leukotriene

synthesis and receptor blockers block hypoxic pulmonary vaso-constriction. J Appl Physiol 56:1340, 1984.

60. Leffler CW, Hessler JR, and Green RS: The onset of breathing at birth stimulates pulmonary vascular prostacyclin synthesis. Pediatr Res 18:938, 1984.

61. Cassin S, Tod M, Philips J, et al: Effects of prostaglandin D_2 on perinatal circulation. Am J Physiol 240:H755, 1981.

62. Perreault T, Coe JT, Olley PM, et al: Pulmonary vascular effects of prostaglandin D_2 in the newborn pig. Am J Physiol 258:H1292, 1990.

63. Bohn D, Tamura M, Perrin D, et al: Ventilatory predictors of pulmonary hypoplasia in congenital diaphragmatic hernia, confirmed by morphologic assessment. J Pediatr 111:423, 1987.

64. Perlman M, William J, and Hirsch M: Neonatal pulmonary hypoplasia after prolonged leakage of amniotic fluid. Arch Dis Child 51:349, 1976.

65. Murphy JD, Rabinovitch M, Goldstein JD, et al: The structural basis of persistent pulmonary hypertension of the newborn infant. J Pediatr 98:962, 1981.

66. Murphy JD, Vawter GF, and Reid LM: Pulmonary vascular disease in fetal meconium aspiration. J Pediatr 104:758, 1984.

67. Fox WW, and Duara S: Persistent pulmonary hypertension in the neonate: Diagnosis and management. J Pediatr 103:505, 1983.

68. Wung JT, James LS, Kilchevsky E, et al: Management of infants with severe respiratory failure and persistence of the fetal circulation, without hyperventilation. Pediatrics 76:488, 1985.

69. O'Rourke PP, Crone RK, Vacanti JP, et al: Extracorporeal membrane oxygenation and conventional medical therapy in neonates with persistent pulmonary hypertension of the newborn: A prospective randomized study. Pediatrics 84:957, 1989.

70. Harrison MR, Adzick NS, Longaker MT, et al: Successful repair in utero of a fetal diaphragmatic hernia after removal of herniated viscera from the left thorax. N Engl J Med 322:1582, 1990.

71. Crombleholme TM, Adzick NS, Hardy K, et al: Pulmonary lobar transplantation in neonatal swine: A model for treatment of congenital diaphragmatic hernia. J Pediatr Surg 25:11, 1990.

72. Abman SH, Accurso FJ, Wilkening RB, et al: Persistent fetal pulmonary hypoperfusion after acute hypoxia. Am J Physiol 253:H941, 1987.

73. Abman SH, and Accurso FJ: Acute and chronic fetal pulmonary hypertension alter pulmonary vasoreactivity. Chest 93:117S, 1988.

74. Stenmark KR, James SL, Voelkel NF, et al: Leukotriene C_4 and D_4 in neonates with hypoxemia and pulmonary hypertension. N Engl J Med 309:77, 1983.

75. Zimmerman GA, McIntyre TM, and Prescott SM: Production of platelet-activating factor by human vascular endothelial cells: Evidence for a requirement for specific agonists and modulation by prostacyclin. Circulation 72:718, 1985.

76. O'Brien RF, Robbins RJ, and McMurtry IF: Endothelial cells in culture produce a vasoconstrictor substance. J Cellular Physiol 132:263, 1987.

77. Yanagisawa M, Kurihara H, Kimura S, et al: A novel potent vasoconstrictor peptide produced by vascular endothelial cells. Nature 332:411, 1988.

78. Green RS, and Leffler CW: Hypoxia stimulates prostacyclin synthesis by neonatal lungs. Pediatr Res 18:832, 1984.

79. Rodman DM, Yamaguchi T, O'Brien RF, et al: Methylene blue enhances hypoxic contraction in isolated rat pulmonary arteries. Chest 93:93S, 1988.

80. Johns RA, Linden JM, and Peach MJ: Endothelium-dependent relaxation and cyclic GMP accumulation in rabbit pulmonary artery are selectively impaired by moderate hypoxia. Circ Res 65:1508, 1989.

81. Sylvester JT, Rock P, Gottlieb JE, et al: Acute hypoxic responses. In: Bergofsky EH (ed): Abnormal Pulmonary Circulation. New York, Churchill Livingstone, 1986, pp. 127–165.

82. Hislop A, Haworth SG, and Reid L: Quantitative structural analysis of the pulmonary vessels in isolated ventricular septal defect in infancy. Br Heart J 37:1014, 1975.

83. Rabinovitch M, Keane JF, Norwood WI, et al: Vascular structure in lung tissue obtained at biopsy correlated with pulmonary hemodynamic findings after repair of congenital heart defects. Circulation 69:655, 1984.

84. Hickey PR, Hansen DD, Wessel DL, et al: Blunting of stress responses in the pulmonary circulation of infants by fentanyl. Anesth Analg 64:1137, 1985.

85. Rabinovitch M, Andrew M, Thom H, et al: Abnormal endothelial factor VIII associated with pulmonary hypertension and congenital heart defects. Circulation 76:1043, 1987.

86. Ilkiw R, Todorovich-Hunter L, Maruyama K, et al: SC-39026, a serine elastase inhibitor, prevents muscularization of peripheral arteries, suggesting a mechanism of monocrotaline-induced pulmonary hypertension in rats. Circ Res 64:814, 1989.

87. Todorovich-Hunter L, and Rabinovitch M: Non-serine elastase-like activity in the pulmonary artery of rats with monocrotaline-induced pulmonary hypertension. Am Rev Respir Dis 137:209, 1988.

88. DeTroyer A, Sampson M, Sigrist S, et al: Diaphragm: Two muscles. Science 213:237, 1981.

89. Hillman DR, and Finucane KE: A model of respiratory pump. J Appl Physiol 63:951, 1987.

90. Sharp JT: The chest wall and respiratory muscles in air flow limitation. In: Roussos C and Macklem PT (eds.): Thorax, Part 2. New York, Marcel Dekker, 1985, pp. 1155–1201.

91. Bazzy AR, and Haddad GG: Diaphragmatic fatigue in unanesthetized adult sheep. J Appl Physiol 57:182, 1984.

92. Farkas GA, and Roussos C: Adaptability of the hamster diaphragm to exercise and/or emphysema. J Appl Physiol 53:1263, 1982.

93. Abbasi S, Duara S, Shaffer T, et al: Effect of external inspiratory loading on ventilation of premature infants. Pediatr Res 18:150, 1984.

94. LaFramboise WA, Standaert TA, Guthrie RD, et al: Developmental changes in the ventilatory response of the newborn to added airway resistance. Am Rev Respir Dis 136:1075, 1987.

95. Maxwell LC, Kuehl TJ, Robotham JL, et al: Temporal changes after death in primate diaphragm muscle oxidative enzyme activity. Am Rev Respir Dis 130:1147, 1984.

96. Scott CB, Nickerson BG, Sargent CW, et al: Developmental pattern of maximum transdiaphragmatic pressure in infants during crying. Pediatr Res 17:707, 1983.

97. Knisely AS, Leal SM, and Singer DB: Abnormalities of diaphragmatic muscle in neonates with ventilated lungs. J Pediatr 113:1074, 1988.

98. Maxwell LC, Kuehl TJ, McCarter RJM, et al: Regional distribution of fiber types in developing baboon diaphram muscles. Anat Rec 224:66, 1989.

99. Robotham JL: A physiologic approach to hemidiaphragm paralysis. Crit Care Med 7:563, 1979.

100. Henderson-Smart DJ, and Read DJC: Depression of respiratory muscles and defective responses to nasal obstruction during active sleep in the newborn. Aust Paediatr J 12:261, 1976.

101. Guslits BG, Gaston SE, Bryan MH, et al: Diaphragmatic work of breathing in premature human infants. J Appl Physiol 62:1410, 1987.

102. Lopes JM, Muller NL, Bryan MH, et al: Synergistic behavior of inspiratory muscles after diaphragmatic fatigue in the newborn. J Appl Physiol 51:547, 1981.

103. Fleming PJ, Muller NL, Bryan MH, et al: The effects of abdominal loading on rib cage distortion in premature infants. Pediatrics 64:425, 1979.

104. Guslits BG, Gaston SE, Bryan MH, et al: Diaphragmatic work of breathing in premature human infants. J Appl Physiol 62:1410, 1987.

105. Masey SA, Koehler RC, Buck JR, et al: Effect of abdominal distension on central and regional hemodynamics in neonatal lambs. Pediatr Res 19:1244, 1985.

106. Swift PGF, and Emery JL: Clinical observations on response to nasal occlusion in infancy. Arch Dis Child 48:947, 1973.

107. Phillipson EA: Control of breathing during sleep. Am Rev Respir Dis 118:909, 1978.

108. Fisher JT, and Sant'Ambrogio G: Airway and lung receptors and their reflex effects in the newborn. Pediatr Pulmonol 1:112, 1985.

109. Carlo WA, Miller MI, and Martin RJ: Differential response of respiratory muscles to airway occlusion in infants. J Appl Physiol 59:847, 1985.

110. Fisher JT, Mathew OP, Sant'ambrogio FB, et al: Reflex effects and receptor responses to upper airway pressure and flow stimuli in developing puppies. J Appl Physiol 58:258, 1985.

111. Roberts JL, Reed WR, Mathew OP, et al: Assessment of pharyngeal airway stability in normal and micrognathic infants. J Appl Physiol 58:290, 1985.
112. Harding R: Function of the larynx in the fetus and newborn. Ann Revu Physiol 46:645, 1984.
113. Fleming P, Bryan AC, and Bryan MH: Functional immaturity of pulmonary irritant receptors and apnea in newborn premature infants. Pediatrics 61:515, 1978.
114. Marchal F, Corke BC, and Sundell H: Reflex apnea from laryngeal chemostimulation in the sleeping premature lamb. Pediatr Res 16:621, 1982.
115. Lawson EE: Prolonged central respiratory inhibition following reflex induced apnea. J Appl Physiol 50:874, 1981.
116. Maloney JE, Alcorn D, Bowes G, et al: Development of the future respiratory system before birth. Sem Perinatol 4:251, 1977.
117. LaFramboise WA, and Woodrum DE: Elevated diaphragm electromyogram during neonatal hypoxic ventilatory depression. J Appl Physiol 59:1040, 1985.
118. Rigatto H: Respiratory control and apnea in the newborn infant. Crit Care Med 5:2, 1977.
119. Kirkpatrick SML, Olinsky A, Bryan MH, et al: Effect of premature delivery on the maturation of the Hering-Breuer inspiratory inhibitory reflex in human infants. J Pediatr 88:1010, 1976.
120. Moss CAF: Vascular rings and anomalies of the aortic arch. In: Keith JD, Rowe RD, and Vlad P (eds): Heart Disease in Infancy and Childhood. New York, Macmillan, 1978, pp. 856–881.
121. Moss AJ, and McDonald LV: Cardiac disease in the wheezing child. Chest 71:187, 1977.
122. Terry PB, Menkes H, and Traystman RJ: Effects of maturation and aging on collateral ventilation. J Appl Physiol 62:1028–1032, 1987.

38

Respiratory Monitoring

David F. Westenkirchner, M.D., and
Howard Eigen, M.D.

Many of the recent improvements in monitoring of critically ill pediatric patients in intensive care units (ICUs) have been in the area of hemodynamic monitoring. However, the ability to monitor variables related to respiratory function may be even more important because patients with respiratory disorders constitute such a large proportion of critically ill pediatric patients. Respiratory monitoring is not limited to patients receiving mechanical ventilation but can include all patients with potentially serious respiratory dysfunction. Respiratory monitoring should serve as an indication of illness severity at one point in time as well as provide serial measure of changes. The goals of any monitoring system are to aid in diagnosis and prognosis, guide and assess therapy, alert caregivers to changes in status, and detect complications. In these ways respiratory monitoring may indicate: (1) an acute need for therapy to treat or prevent respiratory failure, (2) the progression of illness despite therapy, (3) an improvement related to therapeutic intervention, (4) the ability to maintain spontaneous ventilation, or (5) the unfortunate irreversible loss of respiratory function. The ability to achieve these goals is related to the frequency of measurements. Intermittent measures can only provide information about one point in time and may not reflect the true status of a constantly changing system. The fluctuating status of critically ill patients makes real-time measurements more desirable. In this way they may allow earlier intervention and may perhaps improve patient care.

The major function of the respiratory system is that of gas exchange (i.e., provision of oxygen to hemoglobin for delivery to the periphery for cellular metabolism and removal of the carbon dioxide byproduct of that metabolism). Two obvious categories of respiratory variables to be monitored then are oxygenation and carbon dioxide removal via ventilation. In addition, less distinct but perhaps more important variables are those that relate to non-blood gas measures of respiratory system performance. These include respiratory center function, respiratory muscle function, and respiratory mechanics. A last ill-defined category that includes monitors from all of the aforementioned categories is that of estimation of work of breathing. These categories are outlined in Table 38–1. Each category includes variables that easily may be monitored clinically, whereas others are only research tools at this time. Technologic advances in the future may make bedside monitoring of more complex variables feasible. However, it is important to remember that a monitored variable cannot replace and should be used in conjunction with careful and repeated physical examination and bedside evaluation of the patient.

OXYGEN LEVEL

The ability of the respiratory system to contribute oxygen to the blood is important in the maintenance of normal cellular respiration and organ function. Peripheral oxygen delivery is defined as the product of cardiac output and arterial oxygen content ($\dot{V}O_2 = Q_t \times CaO_2$). Arterial oxygen content is determined by the saturation of hemoglobin and oxygen dissolved in plasma ($CaO_2 = [Hgb \times SaO_2 \times 1.34] + [PaO_2 \times 0.003]$). Obviously the ability to monitor PaO_2 and SaO_2 is a key reflection of cellular respiratory function.

Table 38–1. CATEGORIES OF RESPIRATORY MONITORING

Physical examination
Oxygen level
  ABG—PaO_2, SaO_2
  Transcutaneous O_2
  Noninvasive oximetry
  Mixed venous oxygen saturation
Carbon dioxide level
  ABG—$PaCO_2$
  Transcutaneous CO_2
  Capnography
Respiratory drive
  $P_{0.1}$
  V_t/T_I
Respiratory muscle strength
  P_{Imax}, P_{Emax}
  NIF
Respiratory muscle endurance
Respiratory mechanics
  VC, FRC
  Compliance

ABG = arterial blood gas; FRC = functional residual capacity; VC = vital capacity.

Arterial Oxygen Tension

Since the development of the polarographic electrode by Clark, the clinician has been able to measure Pao_2, and arterial blood gases are universally utilized in the evaluation of pulmonary function. Arterial blood can be obtained by intermittent percutaneous collection or by intermittent withdrawal from an indwelling arterial catheter (see also Chapter 27). Intravascular electrodes have been developed to allow continuous display of Pao_2 in an effort to avoid the problems of intermittent collection. However, such devices have not gained wide acceptance because of technical problems that have included slow response time, erroneous values, and calibration difficulties.[1] Pao_2 may not be a specific or sensitive indicator of efficiency of gas exchange because it is influenced by changes in ventilation, changes in the Fio_2, and other nonpulmonary factors. The Pao_2 must always be evaluated with respect to Fio_2, and various oxygenation indices have been used to better assess gas exchange. One such index is the alveolar-arterial oxygen tension difference ($Pao_2 - Pao_2$), which is calculated as Pao_2 minus Pao_2 when $Pao_2 = [(PB - Ph_2O) \times Fio_2] - [Paco_2/R]$ (PB = barometric pressure, $Ph_2O = 47$ mm Hg, R = respiratory exchange ratio). The normal $Pao_2 - Pao_2$ is 5 to 10 mm Hg in room air. Changes in minute ventilation and $Paco_2$ do not affect the $Pao_2 - Pao_2$. However, elevations of the $Pao_2 - Pao_2$ occur on the basis of pulmonary dysfunction. This index changes unpredictably with Fio_2 changes.[2] This variability with changes in Fio_2 limits its value to assess pulmonary function if Fio_2 is changed and does not allow prediction of a change in Pao_2 for a therapeutic change in Fio_2. Therefore, it has limited value in critically ill patients. A better index of oxygenation for use in ICU patients is the Pao_2/Pao_2 ratio. This ratio does remain stable with changes in Fio_2.[3] The lower limit of normal for the Pao_2/Pao_2 of any Fio_2 is reported to be 0.75.[4] A Pao_2/Pao_2 which is less than 0.75 signifies pulmonary dysfunction. The Pao_2/Pao_2 ratio is more helpful for following a patient's status with serial changes in Fio_2 and can be used to predict the Fio_2 required for a desired Pao_2.[5]

Transcutaneous Oxygen Tension

Transcutaneous oxygen electrodes were developed in the early 1970s to measure oxygen values at the skin's surface. The device utilizes a small probe attached to the skin that incorporates a membrane-covered polarographic electrode, a heater, and a temperature-sensing thermistor. Local skin heating causes an increase in the Po_2 from the capillaries to the skin surface, which is measured and displayed. They have been used extensively in newborn intensive care units (NICUs) with good correlation between $Ptco_2$ value and Pao_2 value.[6, 7] However, as skin thickness increases with age, the $Ptco_2$ is proportionally lower than the Pao_2.[8] One disadvantage of transcutaneous oxygen electrodes that has reduced their initial widespread use is a poor approximation of the transcutaneous value to the arterial value when there is poor perfusion and local skin hypoxia.[9] In addition, they require frequent calibration and a change of site to prevent local skin damage. Because of these difficulties, transcutaneous oxygen monitoring has fallen out of favor in most pediatric intensive care units (PICUs) and is used less often even in NICUs.

Arterial Oxygen Saturation

In an effort to have both an accurate and continuous monitor of oxygen, noninvasive pulse oximetry was developed in the middle to late 1970s.[10] Pulse oximetry utilizes the principle of differential light absorption spectra for saturated oxyhemoglobin compared with reduced hemoglobin.[11] The device consists of a probe, usually disposable, and a microprocessor/display unit. The probe is placed around a finger or toe tip and contains a light source on one side that beams red and infrared light through the pulsating arteriovascular bed to a detector placed on the opposite side. Skin, soft tissues, and venous blood absorb a constant amount of light, and that amount represents a reference signal. A varying amount of light is absorbed by arterial blood because the sample thickness changes between systole and diastole, with more absorbed during systole (increased blood volume). The changing ratio of absorbed to transmitted light is measured, and a microprocessor calculates Sao_2, which is continuously displayed. In some of the currently available pulse oximeters, the arterial pulse tracing is also continuously displayed. Under steady state conditions, pulse oximeters measure Sao_2 within 95% confidence limits of $\pm 4\%$ when the Sao_2 is greater than 70%.

The reliability of the pulse oximeter in pediatric patients over a wide age range and a variety of cardiorespiratory disorders has been demonstrated. The devices are able quickly to detect change in Sao_2 that would have otherwise gone unrecognized. One technical point of importance is that the similarity of the pulse oximeter heart rate to an electrocardiogram (ECG) heart rate must be monitored closely. A discrepancy between these two heart rates is an indication of a probable false Sao_2 value. Under dynamic conditions, many variables may interfere with the accuracy of measurements, including blood transit time and the electronics of the system.[12] In some patients with very low cardiac output or peripheral perfusion, the oximeter may not function correctly. Nontechnical factors may also contribute to inaccuracy. Elevated carboxyhemoglobin levels, for example, in a patient with smoke inhalation, can cause the pulse oximeter reading to overestimate the true Sao_2 because the oximeter cannot distinguish between oxyhemoglobin and carboxyhemoglobin.[13] The same is true for the elevated methemoglobin levels.[14] Skin pigmentation is well known to affect the accuracy of pulse oximeters.[15] Fluorescent and Xenon arc surgical lights may cause false-low values, although ambient light can easily be excluded by covering the probed hand or foot with a sheet or a diaper.[16] A large source of error in the pediatric population is that of motion artifact causing poor pulse tracking and false-low values. Conversely, especially in NICUs, elevations of PaO_2 into dangerous ranges for development of retinopathy of prematurity may occur with "acceptable" oximeter SaO_2 values.[17] This is because of the shape of the upper portion of the oxygen dissociation curve in which small SaO_2 changes can correspond to large increases in PaO_2 levels to greater than 100 mm Hg. The utility of pulse oximetry in PICUs has not been investigated extensively. Although they are utilized quite frequently, their dynamic response characteristics and benefits in ICUs have not been well documented.

Mixed Venous Oxygen Saturation

Mixed venous oxygen saturation ($S\bar{v}O_2$) is a frequently monitored cardiopulmonary variable in ICUs. Rather than a specific monitor of pulmonary function, it serves to assess oxygen transport on a global basis. True mixed venous blood is a mixture of blood that is circulated through all systemic vascular beds. Therefore, the $S\bar{v}O_2$ reflects the balance between oxygen delivery and oxygen consumption of perfused tissues. Mixed venous oxygen content is determined by the variables of the Fick equation:

$$\dot{V}O_2 = \dot{Q}T \, (CaO_2 - C\bar{v}O_2)$$

($\dot{V}O_2$ = oxygen consumption, $\dot{Q}T$ = cardiac output, CaO_2 = arterial oxygen content, $C\bar{v}O_2$ = mixed venous oxygen content). By rearranging this equation, $C\bar{v}O_2 = CaO_2 - (\dot{V}O_2/\dot{Q}T)$. Thus, the determinants of mixed venous oxygen content include the principal elements of oxygen supply and demand: arterial oxygen content (which is largely dependent on hemoglobin concentration and arterial oxygen saturation), oxygen consumption, and cardiac output. Measurements of $S\bar{v}O_2$ in the clinical setting can be made by intermittent sampling from the distal port of a typical pulmonary artery catheter. More useful are pulmonary artery catheters designed specifically for continuous measurement and display of $S\bar{v}O_2$. These continuous venous oximeters are based on the principle of reflection spectrophotometry. Three wavelengths of light are passed through fiberoptic bundles in the catheter. The light is reflected from the flowing red blood cells to another fiberoptic bundle that returns the light to a photodetector. The reflection ratio of oxyhemoglobin to total hemoglobin is calculated to yield the fraction of hemoglobin saturated with oxygen. The normal value for $S\bar{v}O_2$ ranges from 70 to 80%.[18] Values above normal indicate an augmented oxygen delivery relative to consumption, which may occur in peripheral left-to-right shunting, marked hyperoxia, or cyanide toxicity. Reduced oxygen extraction (as occurs in sepsis) also results in an elevated $S\bar{v}O_2$. Reduced $S\bar{v}O_2$ values may have many mechanisms including anemia, arterial hypoxemia, increased oxygen consumption, or decreased cardiac output. $S\bar{v}O_2$ of less than 50% is commonly associated with impaired tissue oxygenation,[19] but threshold values have not been determined that result in organ dysfunction or death. The exact cause of the reduction in $S\bar{v}O_2$ requires further detailed analysis of the aforementioned components. The measurement of a normal $S\bar{v}O_2$ can serve as an assurance of stability of the cardiopulmonary system providing adequate oxygen supply-demand balance. Although its clinical utility is unclear and unproven, it does provide a monitor of global oxygen supply-demand balance.[20]

CARBON DIOXIDE LEVEL

Arterial Carbon Dioxide Tension

The measurement of arterial carbon dioxide tension ($PaCO_2$) serves as a measure of the ventilation function of the respiratory system. Elevation of $PaCO_2$ is the hallmark of disorders of the respiratory drive and is one of the criteria for the diagnosis of acute respiratory failure. The need for mechanical ventilation is indicated by an arterial carbon dioxide tension value greater than 65 mm Hg with an associated pH value less than 7.20. As with measurement of arterial oxygen tension level drawn by arterial blood gases, as noted earlier, this monitor suffers from the need for an invasive procedure with a peripheral collection or an indwelling arterial line, requires intermittent sampling, and thus may miss sudden changes. In addition, the deterioration in the arterial carbon dioxide tension occurs late in the evolution of acute respiratory failure. Intravascular arterial carbon dioxide tension electrodes for continuous display have been developed but are even more problematic than oxygen tension electrodes, as noted earlier.[1] A newer fluorescence-based electrode has been shown to measure arterial carbon dioxide tension accurately in critically ill patients,[21] but its inaccurate arterial oxygen tension measure limits its usefulness.

Transcutaneous carbon dioxide tensions can be measured by using a modified Severinghaus electrode.[22] The underlying skin must be heated to 44° C to enhance carbon dioxide diffusion, but this can also cause local carbon dioxide production and resultant falsely elevated transcutaneous carbon dioxide values. Other disadvantages include technical problems, fragility of electrodes, and difficult calibration procedures.[23]

Capnography

In healthy subjects, the end-tidal carbon dioxide ($PetCO_2$) value is normally 1 mm Hg less than $PaCO_2$. Thus, measurement of $PetCO_2$ provides a noninvasive means of monitoring arterial carbon dioxide tension.[24] A device that measures and displays the breath-to-breath numeric values of carbon dioxide is referred to as a capnometer, whereas a device that also displays the wave form of carbon dioxide during the respiratory cycle is called a capnograph. This device operates on the principle that carbon dioxide absorbs infrared light within a narrow wavelength range. The absorption of the light is proportional to the carbon dioxide present. Monitors are of two types, sidestream or mainstream. Sidestream monitors aspirate a small sample of expired gas and transport it by way of a capillary tube to an infrared absorption chamber for measurement of carbon dioxide. A disadvantage of sidestream monitors is the time delay as gas is transported to the analysis chamber. Inaccurate values can be obtained if the capillary tubing is occluded with water or secretions. Mainstream monitors are used more commonly in ICUs because they can be incorporated into the ventilator circuit at the proximal end of the endotracheal tube and allow light to pass through the expired gas before pickup by the detector. In such a device the sensor window is heated to 40° C to prevent condensation, which can lead to falsely elevated values. As noted earlier, in normal, healthy patients, the $PetCO_2$ should be similar to the $PaCO_2$. This requires normal, unchanging metabolism, V/Q matching, and cardiac output. In patients with respiratory dysfunction, who have an uneven distribution of ventilation, the $PetCO_2$ may not reflect $PaCO_2$.[12] With reduced V/Q ratios, the $PetCO_2$ will underestimate the $PaCO_2$, and the worse the lung disease the greater will be the discrepancy. Critically ill patients on ventilators may have continuously changing levels of metabolism, cardiac output, or ventilation.[25] In such cases, the end-tidal carbon dioxide tension may no longer be an accurate measure of the arterial carbon dioxide tension. However, in patients with stable cardiorespiratory status and a regular breathing pattern, the end-tidal carbon dioxide tension may be helpful in monitoring changes in the patient's ventilatory status or in guiding and assessing alterations in ventilator settings.

MONITORING OF RESPIRATORY DRIVE

Normal respiratory center function based on chemoreception allows for the maintenance of normal arterial blood gases. Abnormalities in respiratory center output, therefore, can lead to reduced ventilatory performance with subsequent alveolar hypoventilation and elevation of carbon dioxide. One measure of respiratory drive is airway pressure 0.1 second after the initiation of inspiration against an airway occlusion ($P_{0.1}$).[26] This pressure can be thought of as the intention to initiate inspiration. Although rarely monitored in the ICU, it is possible to measure the $P_{0.1}$ by using a pressure transducer connected to the endotracheal tube and by measuring the inspiratory pressure while the inspiratory circuit is occluded by a one-way valve during the preceding expiration. Another measure of respiratory drive is the mean inspiratory airflow, which can be estimated by dividing the tidal volume by the inspiratory time (V_T/T_I).[27] There has been no systematic attempt to measure respiratory drive by either determination of the $P_{0.1}$ or V_T/T_I measurements in acutely ill patients in ICUs. In fact, with respiratory dysfunction and altered pulmonary mechanics, both values may underestimate respiratory drive. The measurement of $P_{0.1}$ has been used in studies to attempt to predict weaning success, but there has been no clear-cut utility nor a threshold value separating success from failure demonstrated. Although promising, the clinical utility of monitoring respiratory drive for the evaluation and treatment of critically ill patients is unclear at this time.

RESPIRATORY MUSCLE FUNCTION

Abnormalities of respiratory muscle function are often cited in ICUs as justification for mechanical ventilation as well as for problems with inability to wean from mechanical ventilation. This is true particularly for children with chronic respiratory disorders such as bronchopulmonary dysplasia and those who have acute and chronic respiratory insufficiency. The evaluation of respiratory muscle function can be divided into the categories of respiratory muscle strength and respiratory muscle endurance (see also Chapter 48).

Respiratory muscle strength can be evaluated by monitoring maximum respiratory pressures. This is used more commonly in adults and in older pediatric patients. The assessment of respiratory muscle strength is determined by the measure of maximum inspiratory pressure ($PImax$) as well as maximum expiratory pressure ($PEmax$). Such values are dependent on the lung volume at which the measurement is made, with $PImax$ greatest following complete expiration to residual volume, and $PEmax$ greatest following an inspiration to total lung capacity. Obviously, proper performance of these tests requires cooperation and patient effort. A standardized approach to the measurement of respiratory pressures with uncooperative critically ill patients has been described.[28] Such a technique has not been used in the assessment of respiratory muscle strength in critically ill pediatric patients. In an appropriate aged child, the $PImax$ or negative inspiratory force (NIF) is often employed as a criterion of ability to be weaned from mechanical ventilation. Values of NIF that are more negative than -30 cm H_2O are usually accepted as predicting successful weaning. Recent studies, however, have suggested that such criteria are inaccurate and can lead to a high rate of both false-negative and false-positive results.[29] The determination of maximum respiratory pressures is not routinely used in the PICU as a measure of respiratory muscle strength.

In addition to the measures of respiratory muscle strength, there are various techniques to measure respiratory muscle endurance. Reduced endurance is translated into a measure of the fatigability of the respiratory muscles. Respiratory muscle fatigue is often suspected as the cause of inability to wean patients from the mechanical ventilation, especially those with prolonged need for ventilator support or those who are malnourished. Numerous techniques have been utilized for the determination of respiratory muscle fatigue. These include measures of transdiaphragmatic pressure response to phrenic nerve stimulation, electromyographic power spectral analysis of the diaphragm, relaxation rate of respiratory pressures, and maximum sustained ventilation.[30, 31] Even in adult patients, however, these techniques have not proved useful for the clinical diagnosis of respiratory muscle fatigue. This is because these measures are dependent on patient cooperation and motivation. They are also highly invasive techniques. Paradoxic movement of the rib cage and abdomen has been considered to be a clinical marker for respiratory muscle fatigue. This refers to the abnormal inward motion of the abdomen during outward motion of the rib cage during inspiration. However, a study suggested that rib cage abdominal paradoxic motion was related to increased respiratory load rather than to respiratory muscle fatigue.[32] As such, paradoxic motion can be considered a predecessor of respiratory muscle fatigue since it is a direct reflection of respiratory load.

Although clinically attractive, the exact measure of respiratory muscle strength and respiratory muscle fatigue remains elusive, especially for critically ill pediatric patients.

RESPIRATORY MECHANICS

Patients with acute respiratory dysfunction and acute respiratory failure often have abnormalities of respiratory mechanics. In addition to being important in the development of respiratory disease, such abnormalities are also important in the ability to wean patients from mechanical ventilation. In this way their assessment can be helpful for the diagnosis of respiratory dysfunction, the effect of therapeutic intervention, and the need for mechanical ventilation or the ability to discontinue mechanical ventilation. Lung volumes and flow rates are easily measured in the ambulatory patient; however, they are less easily obtained for the critically ill or intubated patient in the ICU.

The determination of vital capacity and functional residual capacity can be obtained at the patient's bedside in the ICU. Vital capacity is the volume from maximum inspiration to maximum expiration. Unfortunately, this value is an effort dependent measurement and is therefore less useful for younger pediatric patients or for those who are sedated, paralyzed, or otherwise unable to cooperate with the test. Vital capacity is reduced in many forms of respiratory dysfunction, including obstructive impairment, restrictive lung disease, and neuromuscular disorders. Measurement of the vital capacity has often been used as a criterion to predict the ability to wean a patient from mechanical ventilation. Vital capacity greater than 10 to 15 ml/kg is said to predict successful weaning. However, because this measurement is dependent on good patient cooperation, its ability to predict successful weaning has been poor.[33] The ability to measure vital capacity should be useful in the ICU because the vital capacity reflects the maximum volume available for inspiratory effort; however, its use is limited to older cooperative patients.

The measurement of functional residual capacity, although theoretically useful in critically ill patients, is difficult to measure during mechanical ventilation. The commonly used helium dilution technique for measurement of functional residual capacity is not easily adapted to a routine bedside monitoring in the ICU. Two methods that have been utilized at the bedside to provide information about functional residual capacity are those of respiratory inductance plethysmography and auto–positive end–expiratory pressure (auto-PEEP) measurement. Respiratory inductance plethysmography uses two bands placed on the abdomen and the rib cage to monitor excursions during inspiration and expiration. Thus estimates can be made of tidal volume and func-

tional residual capacity as changes in ventilatory settings are made.[34] Although not a direct measure of functional residual capacity, the presence of auto-PEEP is an indicator of hyperinflation, air trapping, and an unintentional increase in functional residual capacity. It should be measured routinely in patients with obstructive impairment or high mechanical ventilation requirements. This measurement is made by occluding the expiratory port of the ventilator at the end of the period allowed for exhalation between ventilator breaths. Under these conditions, the ventilator manometer pressure will be equivalent to the alveolar end-expiratory pressure and indicates the level of auto-PEEP.[35] The Siemens Servo 900C ventilator allows prolongation of the expiratory phase with closure of the exhalation valve at the end of the set expiratory time, thus simplifying this measurement. In the ICU auto-PEEP should be measured, and its presence has the same implications for cardiac dysfunction and pulmonary barotrauma as does deliberately applied PEEP.

In many ICUs total thoracic compliance is measured routinely in patients with acute respiratory failure who are receiving mechanical ventilation. Compliance information is used to assess and define the different stages of acute respiratory dysfunction, as well as to optimize mechanical ventilation by allowing the correct application of PEEP and determination of appropriate tidal volume. Compliance is a measure of the distensibility of the lungs and is expressed as volume change per unit pressure change. In the pulmonary function laboratory, static compliance can be measured by using the esophageal pressure to estimate pleural pressure and can yield separate values for lung, chest wall, and total thoracic compliance. During mechanical ventilation of critically ill patients, the respiratory system compliance can be estimated by dividing the tidal volume by the distending transthoracic pressure.[36] Pressure and volume measurements must be made at points of no airflow following delivery of tidal volume at end inspiration. The so-called static or effective compliance refers to the pressure differences between airway plateau pressure during inspiratory hold minus the PEEP divided by the tidal volume. The normal range is stated to be 60 to 100 ml/cm H_2O. This measure of effective compliance reflects the average distensibility of all participating alveoli as well as the chest wall. A decrease in effective thoracic compliance is observed with disorders of the thoracic cage or a reduction in the number of functioning lung units. Various techniques to measure compliance at the bedside have been used, and these are reviewed elsewhere.[34] As noted earlier, compliance data may be used to establish trends in pulmonary status, to adjust the application of PEEP, and to guide the optimal tidal volume delivery. Decreases of the measurement of effective compliance from baseline may indicate the development of pulmonary edema, pneumonia, or atelectasis. Right or left mainstem intubation or a tension pneumothorax will cause an immediate fall in the effective compliance. In addition, the interpretation of compliance data must be made in view of changes in ventilator settings. Any change in the tidal volume or PEEP setting will alter the degree of lung distention and thus alter the measurement of effective compliance. Thus serial measurements of effective compliance can be used to indicate acute changes in respiratory status on an hourly basis. Serial measurement of effective compliance over periods of days can reveal the progression or resolution of respiratory dysfunction. Effective compliance may correlate with peripheral oxygen delivery at varying levels of PEEP and has been used as an index of "best" PEEP,[37] although some investigators question such a correlation.[38] In addition, during application of PEEP, the measure of effective compliance can be a useful indicator of overdistention of alveoli. As PEEP is increased there should typically be some improvement in compliance, but as high levels are applied, there may be overdistention of alveoli that causes the compliance to decrease. Therefore, a decrease in compliance at higher levels of PEEP suggests that the PEEP should be reduced to avoid pulmonary barotrauma. Likewise, the measure of effective compliance may be utilized for the adjustment of the delivered ventilator tidal volume. This may be thought of as a determination of "best" tidal volume. By serially monitoring effective compliance as tidal volume changes are made, it may be useful to determine an effective tidal volume that results in the best compliance as well as to determine tidal volumes that are too great because of a reduction in compliance. Effective compliance measurements may also be useful to predict patients who can be weaned successfully from mechanical ventilation. Patients with compliance values less than 25 to 30 ml/cm H_2O have been shown not to be able to wean from mechanical ventilation in previous studies.[34] The so-called dynamic compliance is determined by using the peak inspiratory pressure rather than the plateau pressure at the end of inspiration for the measurement of compliance. Because this dynamic compliance value includes the resistive pressure component of the applied pressure, it will usually be lower than the effective compliance noted earlier and is normally about 50 to 80 ml/cm H_2O. The dynamic compliance value may be decreased by disorders of the airways, lung parenchyma, or chest wall. If the dynamic compliance is reduced to a greater extent than the effective compliance, it suggests an increase in airway resistance as may occur with secretions plugging the airway, increased bronchospasm, or kinking of the endotracheal tube.[8]

Measurement of thoracic compliance of mechanically ventilated patients can be done at the bedside. As noted earlier, serial measurements of such values can be important as warning signs of alterations in respiratory function, complications of assisted ventilation, and as a criterion for successful weaning from mechanical ventilation. Their application has not been used systematically for patients in the PICU but should provide valuable information for their care.

PHYSICAL EXAMINATION

Despite the availability of various technologic respiratory monitors, their use is presently not widespread in PICUs. Much of this relates to the lack of patient cooperation and patient motivation. Also, the predictive power of many of the monitors is somewhat low when considered individually. It is therefore important to remember that monitoring is only an adjunct to careful clinical evaluation at the patient's bedside. The presence of cyanosis can be a simple measure of arterial oxygenation. When present, cyanosis usually represents an arterial oxygen saturation of less than 80%. The utility of cyanosis is small, however, because it can be a late finding in the assessment of respiratory failure, and there are differences between observers in their ability to detect cyanosis and in the reproducibility of their assessment.[12]

Usually, an examination of the chest is focused on auscultatory findings, but considerable information concerning the work of breathing and adequacy of respiratory muscle function can be obtained by careful observation and inspection of the breathing pattern. Simple measurement of the respiratory rate can be particularly helpful because tachypnea is an early sign of respiratory dysfunction and respiratory compromise. Another very simple marker for the work of breathing is the degree of suprasternal and intercostal retractions. These retractions can provide indirect evidence of increased pleural pressure swings.[39] In addition, patient effort can be estimated by determining the use of accessory muscles of respiration, particularly the sternocleidomastoid muscles. Scalene and parasternal muscle recruitment during inspiration are increased as work of breathing is increased. Likewise, palpable tensing of the abdominal musculature during expiration is a marker for increased work of breathing.[40] Paradoxic abdominal-rib cage movement with inward motion of the abdomen with outward motion of the rib cage during inspiration can be a sign of increased work of breathing.[32] Not only can the physical signs of increased respiratory work be determined in the spontaneously breathing patient, but it is also possible to observe such signs of distress in an intubated patient on mechanical ventilation. Inappropriate ventilator settings can be sources of respiratory embarrassment, and the aforementioned signs of increased work of breathing can be noted in poorly or inappropriately ventilated patients. The physical examination signs of increased respiratory distress should be considered highly valuable in the clinical assessment of patients with respiratory dysfunction. When used in conjunction with appropriate respiratory monitoring, they can provide valuable information regarding respiratory dysfunction.

References

1. Ledingham FA, Macdonald AM, and Douglas HS: Monitoring of ventilation. *In*: Shoemaker WC, Thompson WL, and Holbrook PR (eds): Textbook of Critical Care. Philadelphia, WB Saunders, 1984, pp. 121–136.
2. Kanber GJ, King FW, Eshchar YR, et al: The alveolar-arterial oxygen gradient in young and elderly men during air and oxygen breathing. Am Rev Respir Dis 97:376, 1968.
3. Gilbert R, Auchincloss JH Jr, Kuppinger M, et al: Stability of the arterial/alveolar oxygen partial pressure ratio: The effects of low ventilation/perfusion regions. Crit Care Med 7:267, 1979.
4. Gilbert R and Keighley JF: The arterial/alveolar oxygen tension

ratio: An index of gas exchange applicable to varying inspired oxygen concentrations. Am Rev Respir Dis 109:142, 1974.

5. Hess D and Maxwell C: Which is the best index of oxygenation—$P(A-a)O_2$, PaO_2/PAO_2, or PaO_2/FIO_2? Respir Care 30:961, 1985.

6. Shoemaker WC and Vidyasagar D: Physiological and clinical significance of $PtcO_2$ and $PtcCO_2$ measurements. Crit Care Med 9:689, 1981.

7. Epstein MF, Cohen AR, Feldman HA, et al: Estimation of $PaCO_2$ by two noninvasive methods in the critically ill newborn infant. J Pediatr 106:282, 1985.

8. Tobin MJ: Respiratory monitoring. JAMA 264:244, 1990.

9. Tremper KK and Waxman KS: Transcutaneous monitoring of respiratory gases. In: Nochomovitz ML and Cherniack NS (eds): Non-invasive Respiratory Monitoring. New York, Churchill-Livingstone, 1986, pp. 29–57.

10. Maunder RJ and Hudson LD: Respiratory monitoring in the intensive care unit. In: Shoemaker WC and Abraham E (eds): Diagnostic Methods in Critical Care. New York, Marcel Dekker, 1987, pp. 33–45.

11. Wukitsch MW, Petterson MT, Tobler DR, et al: Pulse oximetry: Analysis of theory, technology, and practice. J Clin Monit 4:290, 1988.

12. Tobin MJ: Respiratory monitoring in the intensive care unit. Am Rev Respir Dis 138:1625, 1988.

13. Barker SJ and Tremper KK: The effect of carbon monoxide inhalation on pulse oximetry and transcutaneous PO_2. Anesthesiology 66:667, 1987.

14. Eisenkraft JB: Pulse oximeter desaturation due to methemoglobinemia. Anesthesiology 68:279, 1988.

15. Ries AL, Farrow JT, and Clausen JL: Accuracy of two ear oximeters at rest and during exercise in pulmonary patients. Am Rev Respir Dis 132:685, 1985.

16. Hanowell L, Eisele JH, and Donns D: Ambient light affects pulse oximeters. Anesthesiology 67:864, 1987.

17. Ries AL: Oximetry: Know thy limits. Chest 91:316, 1987.

18. Barratt-Boyes BG and Wood EH: The oxygen saturation of blood in the venae cavae, right heart chambers, and pulmonary vessels of healthy subjects. J Lab Clin Med 50:93, 1957.

19. Simmons DH, Alpas AP, Tashkin DP, et al: Hyperlactatemia due to arterial hypoxemia or reduced cardiac output, or both. J Appl Physiol 45:195, 1978.

20. Gettinger A: Mixed venous saturation: The puzzle is still incomplete. Chest 98:786, 1990.

21. Shapiro BA, Cane RO, Chomka CM, et al: Preliminary evaluation of an intra-arterial blood gas system in dogs and humans. Crit Care Med 17:455, 1989.

22. McLellan PA, Goldstein RS, Ramcharan V, et al: Transcutaneous carbon dioxide monitoring. Am Rev Respir Dis 124:199, 1981.

23. Leasa WJ and Sibbald WJ: Respiratory monitoring in a critical care unit. In: Simmons DH (ed): Current Pulmonology. Chicago, Year Book Medical Publishers, 1988, pp. 209–266.

24. Rebuck AS and Chapman KR: Measurement and monitoring of exhaled carbon dioxide. In: Nochomovitz ML and Cherniack NS (eds): Noninvasive Respiratory Monitoring. New York, Churchill-Livingstone, 1986, pp. 189–201.

25. Harris K: Noninvasive monitoring of gas exchange. Respir Care 32:544, 1987.

26. Whitelaw WA, DeVenne JP, and Milic-Emili J: Occlusion pressure as a measure of respiratory center output in conscious man. Respir Physiol 23:181, 1975.

27. Milic-Emili J: Recent advances in clinical assessment of control of breathing. Lung 160:1, 1982.

28. Marini JJ, Smith TC, and Lamb V: Estimation of inspiratory muscle strength in mechanically ventilated patients: the measurement of maximal inspiratory pressure. J Crit Care 1:32, 1986.

29. Fiastro JF, Habib MP, Shou BY, et al: Comparison of standard weaning parameters and mechanical work of breathing in mechanically ventilated patients. Chest 94:232, 1988.

30. Rochester DF: Tests of respiratory muscle function. Clin Chest Med 9:249, 1988.

31. Celli BR: Clinical and physiological evaluation of respiratory muscle function. Clin Chest Med 10:199, 1989.

32. Tobin MJ, Perez W, Guenther SM, et al: Does rib cage abdominal paradox signify respiratory muscle fatigue? J Appl Physiol 63:851, 1987.

33. Tahvanainen J, Salenpera M, and Nikki P: Extubation criteria after weaning from intermittent mandatory ventilation and continuous positive airway pressure. Crit Care Med 11:702, 1983.

34. Capps JS and Hicks GH: Monitoring non-gas respiratory variables during mechanical ventilation. Respir Care 32:558, 1987.

35. Pepe PE and Marini JJ: Occult end-expiratory pressure in mechanically ventilated patients with air flow obstruction: The auto-PEEP effect. Am Rev Respir Dis 126:166, 1982.

36. Bone RC: Monitoring ventilatory mechanics in acute respiratory failure. Respir Care 28:597, 1983.

37. Suter PM, Fairley HB, and Isenberg MD: Optimum end-expiratory airway pressure in patients with acute pulmonary failure. N Engl J Med 292:284, 1975.

38. Falke KJ: Do changes in lung compliance allow the determination of "optimal PEEP?" Anaesthetist 29:165, 1980.

39. Heldt GP, Clements JA, McIlroy MB, et al: An intercostal retractometer for estimation of intrapleural pressure changes in infants. J Appl Physiol 52:1667, 1982.

40. Pardee NE, Winterbauer RH, and Allen JD: Bedside evaluation of respiratory disease. Chest 85:203, 1984.

39

Access to the Airway

Constance S. Houck, M.D.

Pediatric intensive care practitioners are frequently called upon to evaluate and establish a secure airway. Occasionally, this requires only proper positioning, clearing of secretions, and bag-mask ventilation. More often, however, endotracheal intubation and mechanical ventilation are needed. Safe, atraumatic endotracheal intubation is a skill that requires practice and a thorough understanding of the principles of pharmacologic therapy with sedatives, anesthetic induction agents, and muscle relaxants. There are many inherent risks with this procedure and, though in most instances endotracheal intubation can be lifesaving, improper techniques can lead to further injury or death. A period should be set aside early in critical care training to practice the techniques of endotracheal intubation. This is often best achieved by perfecting this skill in the operating suite under the supervision of an experienced pediatric anesthesiologist.

ANATOMY

The structures of the larynx are illustrated in Figure 39–1. Several structures deserve particular mention, as they are often unfamiliar to the inexperienced laryngoscopist. The *vallecula* is the space between the base of the tongue and the epiglottis; it serves as the landmark for placement of the curved laryngoscope blade. When pressure is exerted on this space by the tip of the blade, the hyoepiglottic ligament stretches, lifting the epiglottis out of view. The *arytenoids* are the posterior cartilaginous attachments of the true vocal cords. During laryngoscopy, especially when the larynx is anteriorly placed, the arytenoids may be the only structures of the larynx visualized. In this instance, the endotracheal tube can be guided into the larynx by directing it anterior to the arytenoids.

There are several major anatomic differences between the infant airway and that of older children and adults. These differences may increase the risk of airway compromise and make bag-mask ventilation and endotracheal intubation in emergency situations more difficult. First, the oral cavity is small in the infant and young child, whereas the tongue is relatively large. This in itself can cause significant obstruction, which is only worsened in conditions with relative macroglossia, such

as Down and Beckwith-Wiedemann syndromes. Adenoid and tonsillar hypertrophy are also common, adding to the soft tissue obstruction and often making visualization of the larynx more difficult. During bag-mask ventilation, even small amounts of additional pressure placed over the submental area in an attempt to maintain a tight mask seal may worsen pre-existing airway compromise caused by these enlarged soft tissues.

The larynx in the young child is higher in the neck than it is in adults; it is located between the third and fourth cervical vertebrae.[1] As the child grows toward adulthood, the larynx moves caudally in relation to the other structures of the neck to lie between the fourth and fifth cervical vertebrae. On laryngoscopy, therefore, the vocal cords of the infant occupy a more anterior, superficial position in relation to other structures. A stylet may be required to direct the tip of the endotracheal tube anteriorly.

The infant epiglottis is hard and narrow and is angled away from the axis of the trachea, making it difficult to control with a laryngoscope blade.[2] This may further complicate efforts to visualize the glottis. In addition, the vocal cords are more cartilaginous and quite distensible and are easily damaged.

In the young child, the narrowest portion of the airway is at the cricoid ring rather than at the vocal cords.[3] Therefore, an endotracheal tube that slips easily past the vocal cords may not pass any further because of more distal obstruction at the level of the cricoid ring. Significant subglottic swelling may develop if the endotracheal tube passed into the trachea is too large, often resulting in serious postextubation croup.[4]

The trachea of the young child is short, only 4 to 5 cm in the newborn, growing to approximately 7 cm by 18 months of age.[5] The adult trachea is 12 cm long. A rough approximation of the appropriate distance from the tip of the endotracheal tube to the lip should be determined in order to avoid endobronchial intubation (Table 39–1).

INITIAL AIRWAY MANAGEMENT

The pediatric intensive care practitioner should be proficient in bag-mask ventilation of the infant and young child. Initial emergency airway management is

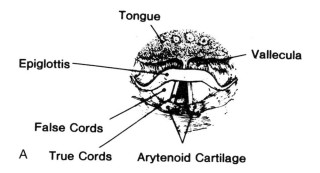

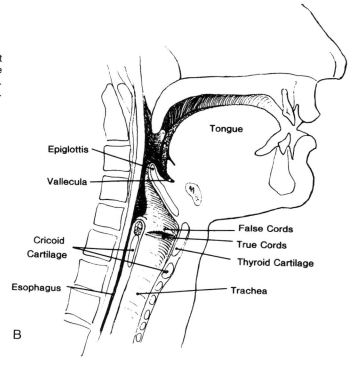

Figure 39–1. *A*, Cross-sectional view of the trachea with pertinent anatomic structures labeled. *B*, Sagittal view of the head showing the position of the epiglottis and vallecula. Please see text for details. (From Natanson C, Shelhamer J, and Parillo J: Endotracheal Intubation. JAMA 253:1160–1165, 1985.)

Table 39–1. ENDOTRACHEAL TUBE SIZE AND APPROXIMATE LENGTH FROM MOUTH OR NOSE TO MIDTRACHEA*

Age	Endotracheal Tube Internal Diameter	Length (OT)† (cm)	Length (NT)‡ (cm)
Premature (<1 kg)	2.5	7–8	9
Premature (>1 kg)	3.0	8–9	9–10
Newborn	3.0	9–10	11–12
3 mo	3.5	10–11	12
3–9 mo	3.5–4.0	11–12	13–14
9–18 mo	4.0–4.5	12–13	14–15
1½–3 yr	4.5–5.0	12–14	16–17
4–5 yr	5.0–5.5	14–16	18–19
6–7 yr	5.5–6.0	16–18	19–20
8–10 yr	6.0–6.5	17–19	21–23
10–11 yr	6.0–6.5 (cuffed)	18–20	22–24
12–13 yr	6.5–7.0 (cuffed)	19–21	23–25
14–16 yr	7.0–7.5 (cuffed)	20–22	24–25

*Modified from Smith RM: Anesthesia for Infants and Children. St. Louis, CV Mosby, 1991.
†OT = orotracheal.
‡NT = nasotracheal.

facilitated by mask ventilation with 100% oxygen to provide adequate oxygenation prior to attempting endotracheal intubation. A tight seal must be achieved to assure adequacy of ventilation. This is accomplished by using the thumb and index fingers to press the mask firmly against the face while the middle and ring fingers are placed at the mandibular ramus to pull the jaw forward and the base of the tongue away from the posterior portion of the pharynx. It is important to avoid external compression of the airway by pressure on the soft tissues of the anterior portion of the neck. When a tight mask fit cannot be achieved with this method, the mask may be held with both hands, applying pressure to the mask with the thumbs while pulling the mandible forward with the other fingers. This method, though quite effective when significant upper airway obstruction is encountered, requires an additional person to squeeze the bag. If no other person is available, one's chin can be used to apply firm downward pressure over the top of the mask, freeing one hand to squeeze the bag. A tight mask fit over the nose, maxilla, and mandible with a seal around the cheeks is necessary in order to ventilate with positive pressure. It may be difficult to adequately ventilate a patient with a large or flat nose, small mandible, facial injuries, burns, or a nasogastric tube in place because of the inability to maintain this tight seal. Padding of the mask or the use of a rubber head strap may make mask ventilation easier in these circumstances.

ENDOTRACHEAL INTUBATION

The important differences in anatomy between the adult larynx and infant larynx require variations in technique when endotracheal intubation is attempted in children of different ages. Because of the infant's relatively large head in proportion to body size, intubation is more easily accomplished with the head in the neutral position. With hyperextension, the larynx rotates anteriorly, and visualization can be more difficult. Con-

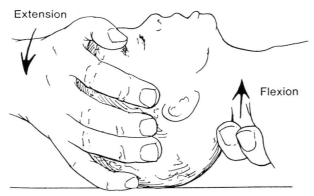

Extension

Flexion

Figure 39–2. "Sniffing position." Extension of the head at the atlanto-occipital joint and elevation of the occiput align the airway structures. A small pillow may be placed under the occiput in order to facilitate this positioning. (From American Academy of Pediatrics/American College of Emergency Medicine: Advanced Pediatric Life Support, Elk Grove Village, IL, American Academy of Pediatrics Press, 1989, p. 4. Copyright 1989. Reproduced by permission.)

Table 39–2. EQUIPMENT NECESSARY FOR ENDOTRACHEAL INTUBATION

Suction with Yankauer or large-suction catheter
Oxygen source with ventilating bag
Mask—appropriate size
Laryngoscope
Endotracheal tubes—0.5 cm larger and 0.5 cm smaller than projected endotracheal tube size
Oropharyngeal airway
Tongue blade
Tape
Stylets in small, medium, or large sizes

versely, in the older child, as in the adult, the "sniffing" position better aligns the oropharyngeal and tracheal planes to provide easier visualization of the larynx. This can be achieved by extension of the head at the atlanto-occipital joint and elevation of the occiput (Fig. 39–2).

Equipment

The equipment needed for endotracheal intubation is listed in Table 39–2. There are many types and sizes of laryngoscope blades suitable for pediatric use. A tray or cart containing laryngoscope handles and blades, endotracheal tubes, stylets, and oral airways should always be readily available in the intensive care unit. Table 39–3 describes the items that are available on the intubation tray at Children's National Medical Center.

Suction must be available at all times when an attempt is made to gain airway access with an endotracheal tube. This is critical for clearing secretions, vomitus, blood, or debris that may obstruct the view of the laryngeal orifice. Oxygenation by either bag-mask ventilation or spontaneous ventilation with 100% oxygen prior to laryngoscopy should provide adequate oxygen reserves for the period of apnea anticipated during placement of the endotracheal tube.

After the proper head position is established, the mouth is opened by exerting firm pressure on the mandible. The laryngoscope is held in the left hand, inserted into the right side of the mouth, and moved toward the midline, pushing the tongue out of the area

Table 39–3. CONTENTS OF INTUBATION TRAY OR CART

Laryngoscope handles, large and small
Extra batteries, AA and C
Laryngoscope blades
    Miller, sizes 0, 1, 2, 3
    Macintosh, sizes 2, 3
    Wis-Hippel, size 1.5
Additional light bulbs, small and large
Endotracheal tubes,
    Uncuffed, 2.5, 3.0, 3.5, 4.0, 4.5, 5.0, 5.5
    Cuffed, 5.0, 6.0, 7.0, 8.0
Stylets, infant, child, and adult sizes
Lubricating jelly
Magill forceps, small and large
Oral airways, sizes 40, 60, 80, 100
Nasal airways, infant to adult sizes
4 × 4 gauze sponges

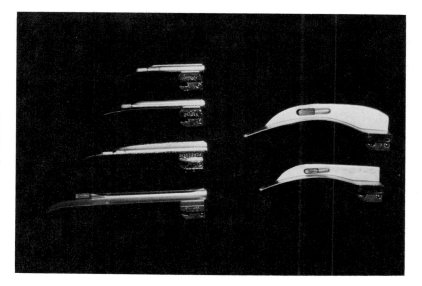

Figure 39–3. Straight (Miller or Wis-Hippel) blades (*left*) and curved (Macintosh) blades (*right*) are available in various sizes to accommodate children of all ages. The straight blades are sized from 0 (neonatal) to 3 (adult) with a 1.5 size between 1 and 2. The curved blades are available only in sizes 2, 3, and 4.

of visualization. The blade is then advanced slowly over the tongue.

Both straight (Miller and Wis-Hippel) and curved (Macintosh) blades are available in various sizes suitable for infants and children (Fig. 39–3). When using a straight blade, the tip is advanced at about a 45-degree angle toward the epiglottis, and the laryngoscope handle is gently lifted forward and upward along its axis. This exposes the larynx, making the vocal cords visible below or behind the epiglottis. If the larynx is not easily visualized, external pressure on the cartilages of the neck may help bring the glottis into view. When a curved blade is used, the tip is placed at the base of the tongue to rest in the vallecula behind the epiglottis. With an upward pull along the axis of the laryngoscope handle, the hyoepiglottic ligament is stretched and the glottis comes into view. The curved blade is wider and better able to keep the tongue out of the line of vision. In addition, there is less trauma to the epiglottis if it is not manipulated during intubation. The straight blade is flatter and fits much more easily into the small child's mouth. It can be used in the same manner as a curved blade by placing the tip into the vallecula when one wishes to avoid trauma to the epiglottis.

Table 39–1 gives a general guide to appropriate endotracheal tube sizes for infants and children based on age. ID refers to the inner diameter of the tube as measured in millimeters. For children more than 2 years of age, the size tends to correlate better with age than with weight and the simplest formula

$$\frac{16 + \text{age (in years)}}{4}$$

is most commonly used.[6] The tube size can also be compared with the width of the patient's little finger. It is important to determine the appropriate size of the endotracheal tube because a tube that is too small can lead to a marked increase in airway resistance. A tube that is too large can cause airway edema and has been closely correlated with problems with postextubation laryngotracheitis.

Most endotracheal tubes are marked at the distal end with either one or several black lines indicating the distance from the tip of the tube. The Mallinckrodt tube illustrated in Figure 39–4 has single, double, and triple markers about a centimeter apart starting 2.5 to 3 cm from the tip. When the middle (double) line is situated at the vocal cords, the tip is usually at the proper depth from the glottis. If a cuffed endotracheal tube is used, the tube is advanced to the point at which the cuff has just passed beyond the vocal cords. Auscultation over both lung fields must be performed to assure proper placement. The depth marker at the lip should also be noted prior to securing the tube with tape. Guidelines for the approximate distance from the lip or nares to the midtrachea in various age groups can be found in Table 39–1. For children older than 3 years of age, the length of the oral endotracheal tube from incisors to midtrachea can also be estimated by the formula[5]

$$\text{Airway length (cm)} = \text{age}/2 + 12$$

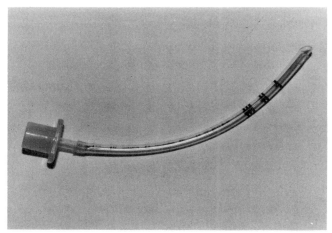

Figure 39–4. Pediatric endotracheal tube illustrating the bold black lines at the distal end of the tube, which should be situated at the vocal cords to ensure proper placement within the trachea. See text for details.

For nasotracheal tubes, the length from the nares to midtrachea can be estimated by

$$\text{Airway length (cm)} = \text{age}/2 + 15$$

Cuffed endotracheal tubes are generally avoided in patients less than 8 years of age unless the airway pressures required to ventilate the patient are so high that a cuffed tube is needed in order to achieve adequate ventilation. The risk of airway edema and laryngeal damage is significantly increased when a cuffed endotracheal tube is used in a small child. The more compliant chest wall of the infant and the resultant lower inflation pressures required for ventilation make the use of a cuffed tube rarely necessary except with severe respiratory failure.

DRUGS USED TO FACILITATE ENDOTRACHEAL TUBE PLACEMENT

Many indications for endotracheal intubation exist beyond that of acute respiratory failure. Intensive care practitioners are often called upon to "electively" intubate and initiate controlled ventilation when patients have suffered acute neurologic or cardiovascular injuries. In these situations, the use of appropriate sedation and muscle relaxation not only can aid in the establishment of an artificial airway but also can prevent the intracranial hypertension and trauma that occurs when this procedure is performed on a struggling patient. Sedatives, anesthetic induction agents, and muscle relaxants can prevent injury during endotracheal intubation, but they are also associated with life-threatening complications if not used with caution. Before instituting their use, one must understand when and how these agents should be used.

Before giving anesthetic induction agents or muscle relaxants, it is important to anticipate those patients in whom there may be potential difficulty with laryngoscopy and endotracheal intubation. Loss of the spontaneous respiratory drive as a result of these agents can be life-threatening if positive-pressure ventilation cannot be achieved with a bag and mask. Table 39–4 gives a list of conditions and syndromes that have been associated with difficult oral or nasotracheal intubation. In general, the abnormalities that make endotracheal intubation difficult in these patients include a small mouth or trismus, a large amount of pharyngeal soft tissue, inability to extend the neck and align the laryngeal structures, obstructions within the trachea, or infectious distortions of the airway. If any of these conditions are present, anesthetic agents and muscle relaxants should be avoided until it is certain that bag-mask ventilation can be easily accomplished. If positive-pressure ventilation with a mask cannot be assured, it is prudent to consider an awake, sedated intubation with or without topical anesthesia (see section on awake intubation in section on methods of intubation).

Neuromuscular Blocking Agents (See also Chapter 78)

There are two types of neuromuscular blocking agents used to facilitate endotracheal intubation. The choice of

Table 39–4. ABNORMALITIES ASSOCIATED WITH DIFFICULT AIRWAY MANAGEMENT

Nasopharynx	Choanal atresia-stenosis
	Foreign bodies
	Trauma
	Adenoidal hypertrophy
Tongue	Hemangioma
	Down syndrome
	Beckwith-Weidemann syndrome
	Mucopolysaccharidosis (Hunter, Hurler, and so on)
	Cystic hygroma
Mandible-Maxilla	Treacher Collins syndrome
	Pierre-Robin syndrome
	Goldenhar syndrome
	Apert syndrome
	Fracture
Neck	Juvenile rheumatoid arthritis
	Turner syndrome
	Klippel-Feil syndrome
	Neck burn with contractures
Pharynx-Larynx	Laryngeal web
	Subglottic stenosis
	Laryngomalacia
	Foreign body
	Laryngotracheitis
	Epiglottitis
	Peritonsillar abscess
	Retropharyngeal abscess
	Laryngeal papillomas

agent is usually dependent on the circumstances surrounding the intubation and any underlying disease processes. Depolarizing muscle relaxants (succinylcholine is the only one commonly used) have a rapid onset and short duration of action, which makes them the most popular agents to use in emergency situations. Nondepolarizing muscle relaxants, with their paucity of side effects, are used in situations in which easy airway access is anticipated and succinylcholine is contraindicated. They have a slower onset and significantly longer duration of action.

Succinylcholine

Succinylcholine consists of two molecules of acetylcholine linked by acetate methyl groups.[7] When given as a single dose, this agent binds to the nicotinic cholinergic receptors and mimics the action of acetylcholine. The hydrolysis of succinylcholine is slow compared with that of acetylcholine, so the postjunctional membrane is maintained in a depolarized, unresponsive state until the molecule diffuses away from the receptor.

Succinylcholine's similarity to the acetylcholine molecule explains its very rapid onset of action and usefulness for emergency intubation. Complete relaxation can usually be achieved in 30 to 60 seconds. It gradually diffuses away from the postjunctional membrane into the extracellular fluid and is rapidly hydrolyzed by plasma cholinesterases. The effects of this drug usually dissipate in less than 10 minutes. Smaller children have a larger extracellular fluid space, so a larger dose is required.[8] Table 39–5 shows the appropriate doses for use in pediatric patients.

Succinylcholine has a number of side effects and

Table 39–5. MUSCLE RELAXANTS USED TO FACILITATE INTUBATION*

	Dose	Onset	Duration	Advantages-Disadvantages
Succinylcholine	2.0 mg/kg (infants) 1.0–2.0 mg/kg (children) 1.0–1.5 mg/kg (adults)	30–60 sec	3–12 min	Rapid onset Short duration Hyperkalemia (see text) Increases intraocular pressure Increases intragastric pressure Increases intracranial pressure Associated with bradycardia and arrhythmias
Pancuronium	30 µg/kg (0–1 wk) 60 µg/kg (1–2 wk) 90 µg/kg (2–4 wk) 0.1–0.15 mg/kg (children, adults)	1–5 min	30–80 min	Less CV† effects Reversible Longer duration of action Tachycardia, secondary to vagolytic effects
Vecuronium	0.1 mg/kg 0.3 mg/kg (for RSI)‡	1.5–4.0 min 60–90 sec	25–60 min 60–180 min	No histamine release No effects on HR§ Reversible
Atracurium	0.4–0.5 mg/kg	2.5–4.0 min	20–45 min	Duration not prolonged in patients with renal or hepatic disease Significant histamine release Hypotension if injected too rapidly

*Modified from Yamamoto LG, Yim GK, Britten AG, et al: Rapid sequence induction for emergency intubation. Pediatr Emerg Care 6:200, 1990. © by Williams & Wilkins, 1990.
†CV = cardiovascular.
‡RSI = rapid sequence induction.
§HR = heart rate.

contraindications that limit its use. Its effects on the cardiovascular system are accentuated in infants and small children and can lead to profound sustained bradycardia, nodal rhythms, and ventricular ectopic beats.[9] Prior or simultaneous administration of atropine can protect against these cardiac dysrhythmias in all age groups. A higher dose is needed in infants (0.02 to 0.03 mg/kg) than in older children who may receive adequate protection from 0.005 mg/kg.[10] It is recommended that atropine either be given prior to or mixed in the syringe with succinylcholine whenever this drug is given to children less than 10 years of age.

Another important consideration when using succinylcholine in the critical care setting is its potential to cause significant hyperkalemia. Use of succinylcholine in normal patients produces an average increase in the serum potassium concentration of 0.5 mEq/l.[7] Whenever motor nerves are less active, either from denervation or traumatized skeletal muscle, extrajunctional cholinergic receptors rapidly form. These extrajunctional receptors are very responsive to depolarizing neuromuscular blockers, and a rapid increase in extracellular potassium concentration can develop after the administration of succinylcholine.[7] This has led to profound hyperkalemia and death.[11] Succinylcholine, therefore, should be avoided in patients with unhealed third-degree burns, denervation injury leading to skeletal muscle atrophy, and upper motor neuron lesions. The potential for hyperkalemia develops within 2 days of an acute injury and may persist for up to several years.[7]

Succinylcholine increases intracranial pressure when administered to anesthetized patients and has been reported to increase intracranial pressure by as much as 9 mm Hg in patients with brain tumors.[12] Caution in its use in patients with head trauma or other causes of intracranial hypertension is advised. Judicious use of an anesthetic induction agent (e.g., thiopental) with ameliorating effects on intracranial pressure is recommended when succinylcholine is used in this circumstance.

Other potential side effects from succinylcholine use are listed in Table 39–5.

Nondepolarizing Neuromuscular Blockers

Pancuronium, vecuronium, and atracurium are the most commonly used nondepolarizing muscle relaxants in the critical care setting. All of these agents initiate a competitive blockade at the neuromuscular junction by binding to the receptors but not activating them. They have a small volume of distribution and few side effects.[7] These agents are primarily used in situations in which the use of succinylcholine is contraindicated. Significantly more time is required to achieve adequate relaxation with these agents, and the duration of paralysis is prolonged compared with succinylcholine. When difficulty in airway access is anticipated, this longer duration of action may be life-threatening. Once the patient's ability to spontaneously ventilate is removed with these agents, difficulty with bag-mask ventilation and endotracheal intubation can lead to hypoxia and death. The appropriate doses of these agents and their side effects are listed in Table 39–5.

Anesthetic Induction Agents

Several anesthetic induction agents can be used to facilitate atraumatic endotracheal intubation. Thiopental or thiamylal are most commonly used and lead to rapid development of unconsciousness and lowering of intracranial pressure.[13] They may have significant effects on the cardiovascular system, however, so the choice of anesthetic agent must be decided only after an assessment of the patient's ability to tolerate these effects is made. Dosing guidelines for these agents can be found in Table 39–6.

Thiopental produces a dose-dependent decrease in blood pressure because of its effects on the medullary

Table 39–6. ANESTHETIC INDUCTION AGENTS*

	Dose	Onset	Duration	Advantages-Disadvantages
Thiopental or thiamylal	5–7 mg/kg (1–6 mo) 4–5 mg/kg (6 mo–16 yr) 2–4 mg/kg (adults)	30 sec	10–30 min	Short-acting Rapid onset Decreases ICP† May cause hypotension May increase bronchospasm in asthmatic patients Contraindicated in patients with porphyria
Ketamine	1–2 mg/kg	30–60 sec	10–20 min	Short-acting Rapid onset of anesthesia Produces significant analgesia and amnesia Maintains BP‡ and HR§ in hypovolemic patients May alleviate bronchospasm Increases ICP Increases airway secretions Associated with hallucinations Increases intraocular pressure
Propofol	2–3 mg/kg	60 sec	4–8 min	Short-acting Rapid onset Less sedation on awakening Dose-dependent CV‖ depression Pain on injection Involuntary skeletal muscle movements Hiccoughs Less propensity for nausea and vomiting

*Modified from Yamamoto LG, Yim GK, Britten AG, et al: Rapid sequence induction for emergency intubation. Pediatr Emerg Care 6:200, 1990. © by Williams & Wilkins, 1990.
†ICP = intracranial pressure.
‡BP = blood pressure.
§HR = heart rate.
‖CV = cardiovascular.

vasomotor center, resulting in a decrease in sympathetic outflow. This leads to peripheral vasodilatation and lowering of the blood pressure.[13] In normal patients, this is well compensated for by an increase in heart rate, maintaining the cardiac output.[13] Critically ill patients, however, often have little cardiovascular reserve because of hypovolemia or sepsis and can manifest profound decreases in blood pressure and cardiac output. An agent that maintains systemic vascular resistance is usually better tolerated by these patients.

Ketamine is a dissociative anesthetic that has the unique ability to increase catecholamine levels. This makes it the drug of choice for patients with hypovolemia or severe reactive airway disease.[14] Administration of this agent to patients with hypovolemia causes either no change in blood pressure and cardiac output or a slight increase.[15] In addition, patients with severe asthma who require endotracheal intubation for uncontrollable hypercarbia or respiratory muscle fatigue often benefit from the bronchodilating effects of ketamine.[16, 17] Appropriate intubating doses of this agent for pediatric patients are found in Table 39–6.

Propofol is an alkyl phenol compound with anesthetic properties in humans. It is used primarily for short anesthetic procedures but is also an excellent anesthetic induction agent for endotracheal intubation. Its main advantage is that it is rapidly eliminated and causes little residual sedative effect.[18] Propofol, like thiopental, causes a dose-related decrease in blood pressure and is limited to use in patients with no cardiovascular compromise.[18] The appropriate dosage requirements for this agent are found in Table 39–6.

Sedative Agents

Benzodiazepines are used primarily as adjunctive agents to provide both sedation and amnesia for endotracheal intubation. Midazolam is a particularly beneficial agent because of its superior amnestic qualities. To achieve adequate sedation,[19] infants and children often require higher doses of these agents than do older patients. Dosing guidelines can be found in Table 39–7.

Fentanyl may also be used as an adjunctive agent to facilitate endotracheal intubation. In appropriate doses, it provides profound sedation and analgesia without significant myocardial depression or peripheral vasodilatation. It does inhibit sympathetic response, however, so mild decreases in heart rate and blood pressure are often seen.[20] The cardiovascular stability noted with this agent makes it the preferred drug to facilitate the endotracheal intubation of patients with congenital heart disease. The sedative effects are variable, so careful titration of this agent is required. Table 39–7 provides further information on the use of this drug.

Additional Agents

Lidocaine administered intravenously decreases the tachycardia and hypertension exhibited during laryngoscopy and intubation.[21] In addition, at 1.5 mg/kg it can ameliorate the increases in intracranial pressure that may occur during endotracheal intubation in patients with intracranial mass lesions.[22] This makes it an excellent additional agent to consider when endotracheal

Table 39–7. SEDATIVE AGENTS*

	Dose	Onset	Duration	Advantages-Disadvantages
Benzodiazepines				
Diazepam	0.1–0.2 mg/kg	1–3 min	10–20 min	Low risk of CV† side effects
Midazolam	0.05–0.1 mg/kg	2–3 min	Approximately 10 min	Excellent amnestic properties (especially midazolam)
				Has anticonvulsant properties
				Dose and effects can be variable (requires titration)
				May cause hypotension (especially when combined with narcotics)
Fentanyl	1–10 μg/kg	30–60 sec	Approximately 30 min (variable)	Minimal CV side effects
				Does not cause myocardial depression
				Preferred to the anesthetic induction agents for patients with cardiac disease
				Reversible with naloxone
				Dose must be titrated, as effects may be variable
				May cause chest wall rigidity
Lidocaine	1.0–1.5 mg/kg	60 sec		Lowers intracranial pressure
				Controls ventricular dysrhythmias
				May precipitate seizures if administered too rapidly

*Modified from Yamamoto LG, Yim GK, Britten AG, et al: Rapid sequence induction for emergency intubation. Pediatr Emerg Care 6:200, 1990. © by Williams & Wilkins, 1990.
†CV = cardiovascular.

intubation is required in a patient with intracranial hypertension. Advantages and disadvantages, along with dosing guidelines for this agent, can be found in Table 39–7.

METHODS OF INTUBATION

Rapid Sequence Induction

When a patient has a full stomach and endotracheal intubation is planned, steps must be taken to reduce the risk of pulmonary aspiration. The use of anesthetic induction agents with muscle relaxants abolishes the protective pharyngolaryngeal reflexes and places the patient at significant risk of aspirating regurgitated stomach contents. Patients considered to have a full stomach include any patient with recent oral intake, bowel obstruction, swallowed blood, increased intra-abdominal pressure, or delayed gastric emptying from recent trauma, pain, peritonitis, or shock.

Sufficient pressure placed over the cricoid cartilage to occlude the esophageal lumen (Sellick maneuver) prior to the institution of anesthetic induction agents can significantly reduce the risk of passive regurgitation of stomach contents.[23] The sequence of steps needed to perform this "rapid sequence" or "crash" induction are outlined in Table 39–8. All preparations must be completed prior to the administration of any drugs. Suction must be available and set to the maximum setting. Preoxygenation should be accomplished either by having the patient take deep inhalations of 100% oxygen or by placing 100% oxygen close to the airway. Positive-pressure ventilation is avoided to prevent gastric distention. The sedatives and muscle relaxants are given in rapid succession while cricoid pressure is applied to compress the esophagus. A defasciculating dose of a nondepolarizing muscle relaxant (one tenth of the intubating dose) is often given prior to the administration of succinylcholine to prevent fasciculations and the ele-

vation in intragastric pressure that can accompany these fasciculations.[24]

Cricoid pressure is maintained until the endotracheal tube is placed and the position is confirmed by auscultation. If a cuffed endotracheal tube is used, the cuff should be inflated until no leak is detected before the cricoid pressure is released. It is important that the person designated to apply and maintain cricoid pressure has experience with this type of intubation and has no other duties during the process of intubation that will distract or prevent him or her from applying cricoid pressure throughout the procedure.

Table 39–8. RAPID SEQUENCE INDUCTION*

Preoxygenation with 100% oxygen
Atropine 20 μg/kg (0.1 mg minimum and 1 mg maximum) for children <10 yr
Obtain mask seal—gentle mask ventilation may be indicated if severe respiratory insufficiency (modified rapid sequence induction)
Slight elevation of the head
Cricoid pressure—dedicated person
Anesthetic-sedative agent (See Table 39–5)
  No hypotension or hypovolemia—thiopental 4–5 mg/kg
  Mild hypotension or hypovolemia with suspected head injury— thiopental 2–4 mg/kg
  Mild hypotension or hypovolemia without head injury—ketamine 1–2 mg/kg
  Severe hypotension or hypovolemia—no sedation or ketamine 0.5 mg/kg
  Status asthmaticus—ketamine 1–2 mg/kg
Muscle relaxant (See Table 39–4)
  Succinylcholine 1.0–2.0 mg/kg (consider many contraindications)
  Vecuronium 0.1–0.3 mg/kg (avoid if difficult intubation is suspected or other airway compromise is present)
Intubate when full relaxation is achieved
Release cricoid pressure only after endotracheal tube position is confirmed
Place oral or nasogastric tube to decompress stomach after endotracheal tube is secured

*Modified from Yamamoto LG, Yim GK, Britten AG, et al: Rapid sequence induction for emergency intubation. Pediatr Emerg Care 6:200, 1990.

Awake Intubation

If there are anatomic abnormalities that may make endotracheal intubation difficult or any evidence of airway compromise, a rapid sequence induction should not be attempted. Rather, an awake, sedated intubation is advised. In smaller children, this can often be accomplished with a sedative dose of a benzodiazepine, such as midazolam, followed by intravenous lidocaine. Older children may benefit from the use of topical anesthetic agents, such as viscous lidocaine applied to the tongue. It should be applied thickly and as far back on the tongue as possible so that the anesthetic can be spread over the tongue and posterior portion of the pharynx by the patient's licking and swallowing movements. Several minutes should be allowed to provide adequate spread of the anesthetic. Immobilization of the head by a trained assistant will make awake intubation far easier and less traumatic.

Nasotracheal Intubation

Nasotracheal intubation can provide a more stable airway for the critically ill patient who requires prolonged intubation. The tube is more easily secured to the nose, is less likely to be dislodged by movements of the tongue, and is protected from becoming obstructed from the patient's biting actions.

Nasotracheal intubation requires more skill than does intubation by the oral route and is more difficult to accomplish in smaller children. The laryngeal opening in the small child is placed more anteriorly, and the pathway of the tube is not as straight. In addition, the oral cavity is smaller, making it harder to maneuver both a laryngoscope and curved forceps. Often, when emergent intubation is required, an oral endotracheal tube is placed first and the patient is hyperventilated with 100% oxygen. This tube is then pulled to the corner of the mouth and another endotracheal tube is lubricated and placed through the naris into the posterior pharynx. Care must be taken to avoid excessive force when placing the endotracheal tube through the naris, as significant bleeding can result. The vocal cords and tip of the endotracheal tube are then visualized with a laryngoscope. If difficulty is noted in visualizing the endotracheal tube as it protrudes from the nasopharynx, the tube should be pushed backward or forward or rotated until the tip is easily seen. The end of the lubricated endotracheal tube is then picked up with a pair of curved Magill forceps and placed directly in front of the vocal cords. The oral endotracheal tube is then removed, and the nasal tube is directed through the vocal cords by having an assistant push the tube forward while the tension is released on the forceps. If difficulty is encountered with sliding the tube into the trachea, directing the tip downward with the forceps may ease this maneuver.

Complications with nasotracheal intubation include epistaxis, trauma to the adenoids, pressure necrosis of the nares, obstruction of the eustachian tubes, and an increased incidence of sinusitis from obstruction of the ostia. Nasotracheal tubes should not be used if there is evidence of a basilar skull fracture or a coagulopathy that may lead to uncontrollable nasal bleeding.

ADVANCED AIRWAY TECHNIQUES

Occasionally, anatomic abnormalities may exist that make placement of an endotracheal tube by the preceding techniques virtually impossible. Patients with Pierre-Robin syndrome and other such abnormalities in which micrognathia is a feature may have enough anterior displacement of the glottis that visualization of the glottic opening cannot be achieved with the typical Macintosh or Miller laryngoscope blades. Several modifications have been made to the Macintosh blade to increase vision anteriorly by lifting the tip of the blade superiorly. An example of this is the Bizzari-Guiffridi blade that is shown in Figure 39–5. In addition, there are several other devices such as the Howland lock and the Bullard laryngoscope that make visualization of the anteriorly placed larynx easier.

When extension of the head may cause spinal cord injury, or visualization cannot be achieved with any of the preceding methods, other techniques may be used in order to place an endotracheal tube without aligning the airway structures. These methods include fiberoptic, lighted stylet, and retrograde catheter techniques.

Fiberoptic Laryngoscopy

Skill and practice are required for fiberoptic laryngoscopy, and it should not be attempted in an emergent situation except by those trained in the technique. It is also not easily performed on an uncooperative, strug-

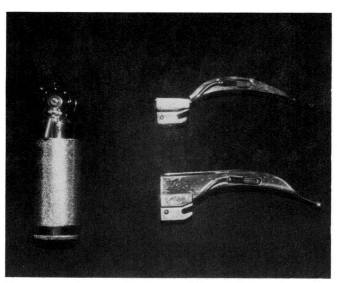

Figure 39–5. Bizzari-Guiffridi blade with the tip lifted superiorly to improve visualization of the anteriorly-placed glottis (*top right*). Standard Macintosh blade is shown for comparison (*bottom right*). Adjustable "polio scope," which permits easier visualization of the anterior portion of the larynx by changing the angle of the blade in relation to the handle, is shown (*left*).

gling patient, so its usefulness in small children is limited. The size of the scope makes it impossible to use in infants, whose endotracheal tube inner diameter is usually smaller than the scope. In older children, this technique can be performed with sedation and topical anesthesia as already described.

Briefly, the fiberoptic scope is lubricated, and the endotracheal tube is placed over it. The end of the scope is then placed in the posterior pharynx and is advanced toward the vocal cords by manipulating the tip with the controls. Once the scope has passed through the vocal cords and tracheal rings are seen, the tube is advanced over the scope into the trachea. Fiberoptic laryngoscopy can be particularly difficult if there are secretions in the airway that cannot be cleared effectively through the suction port of the fiberoptic scope. Hypoxemia commonly occurs if this procedure is prolonged, so it is important to provide oxygen by mask prior to the procedure and by blow-by during the procedure.

Lighted Stylet Intubation

A lighted stylet can be used to provide a blind, guided orotracheal intubation in patients with cervical spine injuries or limited mouth opening.[25] This technique is limited to use in older children (must be able to accommodate a 5-mm endotracheal tube), as the stylet is currently available in only one size. Intubation by this method is accomplished by transillumination of the soft tissues of the neck with a flexible surgical light. The lighted stylet is placed inside the endotracheal tube to within 0.5 cm of the tip. The tube and stylet are then bent to an angle slightly greater than 90 degrees. The tongue is grasped with gauze and gently pulled forward and the tube is advanced along the back of the tongue to the glottic opening. Proper placement can be determined by a bright glow in the midline at the level of the laryngeal prominence. The tube is then advanced off the stylet distally into the trachea. If properly lubricated, the tube should easily pass into the glottic opening. Few complications have been reported with this procedure, but soft tissue bleeding has occurred. Difficulty has been observed when this technique has been used in patients with thick necks and when increased ambient light has been present. Further investigation of the use of this technique with a smaller stylet in younger children appears warranted.

Retrograde Catheter Technique

Although rarely necessary, the retrograde catheter technique has been used in children as young as 30 months old when other efforts to place an endotracheal tube have failed.[26] A 20-gauge needle attached to a saline-filled syringe is placed through the cricothyroid membrane until air is aspirated into the syringe. Lidocaine is often injected through the membrane to lessen the risk of coughing and laryngospasm during this procedure. A long wire such as that used in the cardiac catheterization suite is then placed through the needle and retrieved in the mouth using Magill forceps. The endotracheal tube is then placed over the wire and guided into the trachea while tension is maintained on both ends of the wire. Once placement is confirmed, the wire is cut at the neck and pulled out through the mouth. Special precautions must be exercised to prevent trauma to the soft tissues and laryngeal cartilages when performing this maneuver. Unfortunately, there has been little success with this technique in infants because of difficulty in locating the cricothyroid membrane.

Cricothyrotomy

In an emergent situation, when rapid establishment of airway access is essential, placement of a catheter through the cricothyroid membrane can be lifesaving. This can be accomplished by tilting the head back and palpating the cricothyroid membrane. A large-bore intravenous catheter (12-gauge in adults and 14-gauge in smaller children) can be placed through the cricothyroid membrane and advanced at a caudad angle to avoid injury to the vocal cords. Placement is confirmed by aspiration of air. The catheter is then advanced over the needle into the trachea. A 3-mm endotracheal tube adaptor can then be used to connect the catheter to an oxygen source. Due to the small caliber of the catheter, resistance to flow can be extremely high. Hypoxia can usually be reversed, but CO_2 retention remains a problem. Transtracheal jet ventilation can be instituted to limit CO_2 accumulation until more stable airway access is established.[27] Landmarks useful in the location of the cricothyroid membrane are illustrated in Figure 39–6.

SPECIAL CIRCUMSTANCES

Certain clinical situations call for a specific understanding of the risks and hazards of endotracheal intu-

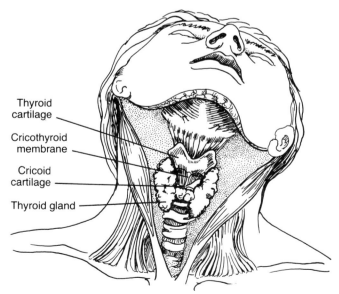

Figure 39–6. The cricothyroid membrane can be located by palpating the membrane between the thyroid and cricoid cartilages in the midline of the neck.

bation to avoid worsening of the underlying pathologic condition. The risk of aspiration when the patient has a full stomach has already been discussed, but certain other disease processes can put the patient at risk of greater injury if proper precautions are not taken. Airway manipulations must be carefully planned in patients with intracranial hypertension, mediastinal masses, and epiglottitis.

Increased Intracranial Pressure

Children with head injuries often require endotracheal intubation to establish mechanical ventilation for the control of pH and P_{CO_2}. In addition, patients with decreased levels of consciousness have an increased risk of pulmonary aspiration and may be unable to protect the airway from their own oral secretions. Pain associated with laryngoscopy and endotracheal intubation, along with the coughing that can occur during the performance of this procedure, can significantly increase intracranial pressure. Therefore, unless difficulty with airway access is suspected because of anatomic abnormalities or facial injuries, intravenous anesthesia should be administered prior to intubation.

If the patient is hemodynamically stable, thiopental or thiamylal will lower intracranial pressure and prevent further increases during laryngoscopy.[28] A muscle relaxant should also be administered to avoid any risk of a cough-induced rise in intracranial pressure. Although succinylcholine may cause a mild increase in intracranial pressure, this increase is offset by the marked lowering in cerebral metabolic rate afforded by thiopental. Because of its rapid onset and short duration of action, it is often the drug of choice for emergent airway access. The intermediate-acting muscle relaxants vecuronium and atracurium may also be used, but their time of onset and duration of action is much longer. A larger dose of vecuronium (up to 0.3 mg/kg) has been used to speed onset time to less than 90 seconds, but the paralysis from this dose may last for several hours.[29, 30] Many authors recommend administering a precurarizing dose (one tenth of the intubating dose) of one of the nondepolarizing muscle relaxants to children older than 4 years of age to prevent the muscle fasciculations that may occur with the use of succinylcholine. Fasciculations may also cause a mild increase in intracranial pressure. Intravenous lidocaine in a dose of 1.5 mg/kg should also be added to this regimen to blunt the hypertensive effects of laryngoscopy.[21]

If the patient is unstable, fentanyl may be used in place of thiopental, but its effects on intracranial pressure are limited, and often a smaller dose of thiopental is preferred. Ketamine should never be used when increased intracranial pressure is suspected. Use of this drug has been associated with an increase in intracranial pressure of as much as 60%.[31]

If difficult airway access is anticipated, sedative agents and local anesthesia should be used. It is more important in this instance to safely secure the airway than to try to lower intracranial pressure.

Mediastinal Masses

Children with Hodgkin disease or other types of lymphomas can present with large mediastinal masses that cause varying degrees of airway obstruction. Endotracheal intubation may be required in these patients to decrease the work of breathing and improve ventilation. In this situation, muscle relaxants must be avoided until the adequacy of ventilation can be assured. There have been a number of case reports describing severe airway obstruction after the administration of muscle relaxants, despite appropriately placed endotracheal tubes.[32–34] These patients are able to maintain airway patency by stenting the airways open with respiratory muscle movements. If muscle tone is impaired, the large mediastinal mass can collapse the proximal airways and lead to nearly complete airway obstruction despite positive-pressure ventilation. Extreme care must be used not to impair respiratory muscle ability with either muscle relaxants or anesthetic agents when endotracheal intubation becomes necessary in these patients.

Epiglottitis

Epiglottitis is an extreme respiratory emergency and care must be taken not to worsen the obstruction prior to securing the upper airway. The patient should be approached quietly, and painful procedures should not be performed unless absolutely necessary. Muscle relaxants should not be used in these patients until the airway is assured. The anesthesiologist and the otolaryngologist should be contacted immediately and preparations made to transport the patient to the operating room for an emergent anesthetized intubation. The anesthesiologist slowly administers halothane by inhalation to the point that respiratory reflexes are obtunded but spontaneous ventilation is maintained. The larynx is then intubated with a frozen, styletted endotracheal tube. If the anesthesiologist feels comfortable with the ease of placement, a muscle relaxant is administered, and the oral endotracheal tube is changed to a more stable nasotracheal tube prior to transport to the intensive care unit.

References

1. Sasaki CT, Levine PA, Laitman JT, et al: Postnatal descent of the epiglottis in man. Arch Otolaryngol 103:169, 1977.
2. Cote CJ and Todres ID: The pediatric airway. *In:* Cote CJ and Todres ID: A Practice of Anesthesia for Infants and Children. New York, Grune & Stratton, 1986, pp 35–37.
3. Eckenhoff J: Some anatomic considerations of the infant larynx, influencing endotracheal anesthesia. Anesthesiology 12:401, 1951.
4. Koka BV, Jeon S, Andre JM, et al: Postintubation croup in children. Anesth Analg 56:501, 1977.
5. Morgan GAR and Steward DJ: Linear airway dimensions in children: Including those with cleft palate. Can Anaesth Soc J 29:1, 1982.
6. Cole F: Pediatric formulas for the anesthesiologist. Am J Dis Child 94:472, 1957.
7. Stoelting RK: Neuromuscular blocking drugs. *In:* Stoelting RK: Pharmacology and Physiology in Anesthetic Practice. Philadelphia, JB Lippincott, 1987.
8. Cook DR and Fischer CG: Neuromuscular blocking effects of

succinylcholine in infants and children. Anesthesiology 42:662, 1975.

9. Craythorne NWB, Turndorf H, and Dripps RD: Changes in pulse rate and rhythm associated with the use of succinylcholine in anesthetized children. Anesthesiology 21:465, 1960.

10. Cook DR and Davis PJ: Pharmacology of pediatric anesthesia. *In*: Smith's Anesthesia for Infants and Children. St. Louis, CV Mosby, 1990.

11. Cooperman LH, Strobel GE, and Kennell EM: Massive hyperkalemia after administration of succinylcholine. Anesthesiology 32:161, 1970.

12. Minton MD, Grosslight K, Stirt JA, et al: Increases in intracranial pressure from succinylcholine: Prevention by prior nondepolarizing blockade. Anesthesiology 65:165, 1986.

13. Stoelting RK: Barbiturates. *In:* Stoelting RK: Pharmacology and Physiology in Anesthetic Practice. Philadelphia, JB Lippincott, 1987.

14. White PR, Way WL, and Trevor AJ: Ketamine—its pharmacology and therapeutic uses. Anesthesiology 56:119, 1982.

15. Reich DL and Silvay G: Ketamine: An update on the first twenty-five years of clinical experience. Can J Anaesth 36:186, 1989.

16. Rock MJ, Reyes de la Rocha S, L'Hommedieu CS, et al: Use of ketamine in asthmatic children to treat respiratory failure refractory to conventional therapy. Crit Care Med 14:514, 1986.

17. Corssen G, Gutierrez J, Reves JC, et al: Ketamine in the anesthetic management of asthmatic patients. Anesth Analg 51:588, 1972.

18. Sebel PS and Lowdon JD: Propofol: A new intravenous anesthetic. Anesthesiology 71:260, 1989.

19. Stoelting RK: Benzodiazepines. *In:* Stoelting RK: Pharmacology and Physiology in Anesthetic Practice. Philadelphia, JB Lippincott, 1987.

20. Stoelting RK: Opioid agonists and antagonists. *In:* Stoelting RK: Pharmacology and Physiology in Anesthetic Practice. Philadelphia, JB Lippincott, 1987.

21. Donegan M, Bedford RF, and Dacey R: IV lidocaine for prevention of intracranial hypertension. Anesthesiology 51:S201, 1979.

22. Sakabe T, Maekawa T, Ishikawa T, et al: The effects of lidocaine on canine cerebral metabolism and circulation related to the electroencephalogram. Anesthesiology 40:433, 1974.

23. Sellick BA: Cricoid pressure to control regurgitation of stomach contents during induction of anesthesia. Lancet 2:404, 1961.

24. Salem MR, Wong AY, and Lin YH: The effect of suxamethonium on the intragastric pressure in infants and children. Br J Anaesth 44:166, 1972.

25. Vollmer TP, Stewart RD, and Paris PM: Use of a lighted stylet for guided orotracheal intubation in the prehospital setting. Ann Emerg Med 14:324, 1985.

26. Borland LM, Swan DM, and Leff S: Difficult pediatric endotracheal intubation: A new approach to the retrograde catheter technique. Anesthesiology 55:577, 1981.

27. Attia RR, Battit GE, and Murphy JD: Transtracheal jet ventilation. JAMA 234:1152, 1975.

28. Shapiro HR, Galindo A, Whyte SR, et al: Rapid intraoperative reduction of intracranial pressure with thiopentone. Br J Anaesth 45:1057, 1973.

29. Lennon RL, Olson RA, and Gronert GA: Atracurium or vecuronium for rapid sequence endotracheal intubation. Anesthesiology 64:510, 1986.

30. Casson WR and Jones RM: Vecuronium induced neuromuscular blockade. The effect of increasing dose on speed of onset. Anesthesia 41:354, 1986.

31. Takeshita H, Okuda Y, and Sari A: The effects of ketamine on cerebral circulation and metabolism in man. Anesthesiology 36:69, 1972.

32. Piro A, Weiss D, and Hellman S: Mediastinal Hodgkin's disease: A possible danger for intubation anesthesia. Int J Radiat Oncol Biol Phys 1:415, 1976.

33. Bittar D: Respiratory obstruction associated with induction of general anesthesia in a patient with mediastinal Hodgkin's disease. Anesth Analg 54:399, 1975.

34. Northrip D, Bohman B, and Tuesada K: Total airway occlusion and superior vena cava syndrome in a child with anterior mediastinal tumor. Anesth Analg 65:1079, 1986.

Mechanical Ventilation

Katsuyuki Miyasaka, M.D.

Respiratory support constitutes a major portion of pediatric critical care. A variety of methods have been developed, including such innovative modes of respiratory support as high-frequency ventilation (HFV),[1] extracorporeal membrane oxygenation (ECMO),[2] and negative-pressure ventilation[3]; however, conventional mechanical ventilation (CMV) has been, and still is, the principal mode of respiratory support in all age groups.

The principal purpose of mechanical ventilation has changed over the past few decades from the respiratory support of totally apneic patients to the pertinent support of spontaneous respiration. Many adult ventilators have been developed to accommodate various kinds of sophisticated synchronized ventilation, but the majority of neonatal ventilators currently available still utilize the simple principle of providing abundant continuous flow.

Ventilators for pediatric critical care have not yet been clearly or definitively designed, and the pediatric critical care specialist is forced to adapt treatment to what is available in either neonatal or adult ventilators. This painful situation is slowly being relieved by better understanding of the pathophysiology of pediatric respiratory care and by advancements in medical engineering.

This chapter will, therefore, deal with the physical characteristics and functional aspects of mechanical ventilation in pediatric critical care.

CHARACTERISTICS OF MECHANICAL VENTILATION IN CHILDREN

Pediatric critical care is unique in the sense that patients range in size from neonates (with the possible exclusion of extremely premature babies) to adults. Patients who are large enough and well enough to have cuffed endotracheal tubes are managed with adult ventilators, and patients who are small enough are managed with neonatal ventilators—both choices involving various degrees of modification. Since there is a wide variety of factors to be considered, it is helpful to have sound understanding of pediatric respiratory mechanics and pediatric ventilators.

Airways

The airways of a child are smaller than those of the adult, and airway conductance may be less than one fifteenth that of the adult. The anteroposterior diameter of the glottis of an infant is less than one third of an adult airway.[4] Thus an endotracheal tube of the same thickness reduces the cross-sectional area of the airway to a greater degree in a child, reducing airway conductance significantly. The narrowest part of the airway in children is not in the glottic region but in the subglottic region.[5] The subglottic region is susceptible to edema and can barely expand due to being surrounded completely by cricoid cartilage. The use of cuffed endotracheal tubes is not common in small children under 8 years of age for this reason.[6] Snugly fitting endotracheal tubes with a small leakage of gas around the outside upon the application of 20 to 30 cm H_2O airway pressure are commonly used to prevent untoward complications.[7]

The glottis opens during inspiration and narrows during expiration in normal breathing. Since the absolute diameter of the airway is small, this small narrowing causes a significant brake on normal expiration, the equivalent of approximately 3 cm H_2O of positive end-expiratory pressure (PEEP).[8] This physiologic PEEP mechanism to keep functional residual capacity (FRC) at the appropriate level may be offset by the use of an artificial airway. It is thus mandatory to modify the endotracheal tube or tracheostomy system when attempting to provide the requisite range of physiologic PEEP in pediatric critical care. Lower airway conductance and varying degrees of air leakage are common due to the anatomy of the pediatric airway.

Respiratory Rate

The respiratory rate of the child is faster than that of the adult. Whereas adults or midadolescents have a normal respiratory rate of 12 to 16 breaths/min, the respiratory rate of small children is 30 to 40 breaths/min.[9] The inspiratory time in an adult may be 1.25 seconds, but smaller children have a substantially shorter inspiratory time of 0.4 to 0.5 seconds.[10] Furthermore, small children tend to increase respiratory rate rather than tidal volume to cope with increased respiratory demand.

Respiratory rates of over 80 breaths/min or inspiratory times of 0.2 to 0.3 seconds are frequently experienced in pediatric critical care. The rapid respiratory rate causes respiratory phase differences between the patient and the ventilator when synchronization to spontaneous respiration is tried.

Mechanical ventilators in pediatric critical care have little time to waste functionally and should be capable of providing fine inspiratory time adjustments.

Inspiratory Time and Expiratory Time

Time constants of the respiratory system are important in determining inspiratory time. The time constant of the respiratory system is the product of compliance and resistance and is measured in seconds. More than 95% of the pressure in the proximal airway (ventilator circuit pressure) is delivered to the alveoli after a period of three time constants. Thus, the shorter the time constant, the quicker the proximal airway and alveolar pressures will become equal. The magnitude of the time constant varies widely in different forms of respiratory illness. There may be a wide spread of inhomogeneity of time constants, particularly those causing uneven obstruction of airways. This fact must be taken into account when deciding how best to determine inspiratory and expiratory time.[10]

The time constant in diseases associated with diffusely decreased compliance and relatively normal resistance, such as acquired respiratory distress syndrome (ARDS) and pulmonary edema, is generally shorter. Inspiratory time can be prolonged since less time is required for expiration. Theoretically, longer inspiratory time, either in the form of inspiratory plateau or inspiratory pause, allows for better distribution of inspired volume into the compartments of the lungs with relatively prolonged time constants. Although better recruitment of collapsed alveoli is helpful in obtaining better oxygenation, there is the associated risk of pulmonary barotrauma.

Prolongation of the time constant in diseases associated with diffusely increased airway resistance, such as asthma or bronchiolitis, particularly during expiration, makes it necessary to prolong expiratory time to minimize gas trapping and alveolar distension. Gas trapping is a kind of "inadvertent PEEP" and is a major cause of alveolar overdistention creating alveolar rupture, an increase in wasted ventilation, and depression of cardiac output due to decreased venous return.[11]

Tidal Volume

Whereas tidal volume relative to body weight changes little, absolute tidal volume is significantly smaller in smaller children. A small infant may have a tidal volume of less than 20 ml compared with over 500 ml in an adult.[12] The relatively large volume of ventilator circuit (breathing tubes, humidifier) relative to tidal volume creates a large and variable compressible volume making precise tidal volume control difficult.[13]

The volume delivered by the ventilator is distributed to the patient and the respiratory circuit according to individual compliance, and it is not uncommon to see more gas being delivered to the respiratory circuit than to the patient! Gross errors may occur when actual tidal volume is estimated by the delivered tidal volume of the ventilator. Thus, volume-controlled ventilation is not common in small children. A pediatric ventilator should have an adjustment mechanism capable of delivering smaller and finer tidal volumes. Use of pressure-limited ventilation can avoid this problem.

Inspiratory Flow

Complete control of the delivery of tidal volume by the ventilator (mandatory breaths) is usually carried out using a specific inspiratory flow pattern, such as a constant (square) or variable flow sinusoidal wave pattern or a decelerating or accelerating flow pattern (ramp). Most ventilators currently available adopt constant inspiratory flow as the principal flow pattern for mandatory breaths, and average inspiratory flow becomes the determining parameter. Average inspiratory flow in this situation can be calculated from the tidal volume and inspiratory time. Smaller infants have approximately 2.0 l/min, and larger children have 25 to 30 l/min of average inspiratory flow.[10]

Peak inspiratory flow becomes the most important parameter to achieve optimal respiratory support when the patient's spontaneous respiratory efforts are preserved. It is natural for most patients in respiratory distress to try to breathe rapidly. Peak inspiratory flow may be only two times higher than that of average inspiratory flow under normal conditions but may become 10 to 20 times higher in a distressed situation. Smaller infants may show a peak inspiratory flow of 20 l/min.[11] Larger children may briefly exceed 300 l/min of peak flow.

Inspiratory flow differs significantly between mandatory breaths and spontaneous breaths. Even a small infant may show a peak inspiratory flow equal to the average inspiratory flow of an adult.

Inspiratory Pressure

Respiratory compliance is the major determinant of the inflating pressure required. However, respiratory resistance to gas flow is a major determinant of inspiratory pressure for the ventilator. Thus both compliance and conductance define the mechanical forces needed to inflate the lungs during mandatory breaths.

The compliance of the total respiratory system is determined by the individual compliance of the lungs and chest wall. The chest wall of small children is very pliable and has a very high compliance compared with that of larger children and adults. However, the compliance of their lungs is substantially lower.

Increased resistance causes a larger pressure gradient between the airway opening and the alveoli. A higher inspiratory pressure is thus required to maintain the same inspiratory flow and to deliver the same tidal volume in a short given time. Even though absolute values of respiratory compliance and conductance are lower in children, they are similar to values found in adults when normalized for body size (e.g., body weight or height). This means that comparable levels of positive inspiratory pressure are required in small children and adults.[10] Inspiratory time and artificial airway size will significantly influence inspiratory pressure in pediatric patients.

The only way to achieve adequate tidal volume when the time constant of the respiratory system is prolonged and a short inspiratory time is used to reduce the amount of air trapping is to deliver high proximal airway pressure. Only a small fraction of the pressure will be transmitted distally to the gas-exchange area. Areas with a shorter time constant will be more evenly aerated, thus decreasing the risk of a partially obstructed area being hyperinflated.

Peak pressure in volume-controlled ventilation is the end-result of factors such as delivered tidal volume and flow rate. However, in pediatric respiratory care in which volume-controlled ventilation is difficult to achieve, peak pressure is not an end-result but is the factor to be controlled. Inspiratory pressure becomes the major determinant of alveolar inflation or tidal volume when inspiratory time and flow are controlled on a patient with a certain compliance. An increase in peak pressure not only increases tidal volume but also may recruit areas of the lung that are collapsed or poorly ventilated.

The safe inspiratory pressure range cannot be defined clearly, but there is classic evidence to suggest that inspiratory pressures above 60 cm H_2O increase the incidence of barotrauma.[14] High inspiratory pressure increases the risk of pulmonary barotrauma and may also impair pulmonary and systemic circulation. These risks are less in patients with severe lung disease; however, as lung compliance improves during the recovery phase of the disease, inspiratory pressure must be reduced appropriately to avoid complications related to high inspiratory pressure. Although attempts to limit the peak inspiratory pressure are common practice, it has never been clearly demonstrated that such maneuvers decrease the incidence of barotrauma. Barotrauma may correlate with the severity of the lung disease rather than with the peak inspiratory pressure.[15]

Mean Airway Pressure

Mean airway pressure (the area under the pressure curve of each respiratory cycle) is frequently used as a standard ruler to compare the effectiveness and complications of a variety of ventilatory modes. In general, the same change of mean airway pressure results in a similar change of PaO_2 regardless of ventilatory mode. However, patients respond quite differently to the same mean pressure with a different ventilatory pattern. Mean inspiratory pressure is the end-result of many variables including inspiratory pressure, expiratory pressure, PEEP, and wave form, all of which produce different effects on ventilation, FRC, and circulation. The effects of individual variables have yet to be elucidated. Mean airway pressure is known to be useful in comparing the effects of positive pressure on pulmonary and systemic circulation.

Positive End-Expiratory Pressure
(Fig. 40–1)

It is possible to increase lung volume (FRC) and avoid alveolar collapse during expiration by applying positive

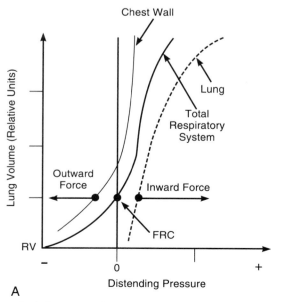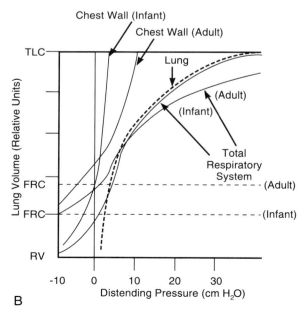

Figure 40–1. Pressure-volume relationship. The total respiratory system pressure-volume relationship has a characteristic sigmoid curve, and compliance decreases at either extreme of lung volume. FRC depends on the balance between the elastic recoil properties of the lungs (inward force) and the chest wall (outward force), as shown in A. The chest wall is significantly pliable and compliant in children. FRC is set relatively low owing to decreased outward force, as shown in B.

pressure throughout the expiratory phase. PEEP has been shown to be effective in treating hypoxemia associated with reduced FRC caused by various conditions.

The increase in FRC by PEEP offers much more than just an increase in lung volume in pediatric patients. Airway closure in young children is said to occur above the FRC level, even under normal conditions, and a slight fall in FRC can cause a significant fall in PaO$_2$.[16, 17] Measures such as PEEP or continuous positive airway pressure (CPAP) (the application of PEEP with spontaneous respiration) that elevate FRC above closing capacity have become extremely useful tools.

FRC is dependent on the balance between the elastic recoil properties of the lungs (inward force) and chest wall (outward force). Outward force is affected significantly in children by the administration of anesthesia or muscle relaxant, resulting in a decrease in FRC. The total respiratory system pressure-volume relationship has a characteristic sigmoid curve with compliance decreasing at either extreme of lung volume. A decrease in FRC will put the respiratory system into the less compliant part of the curve. The application of PEEP makes ventilation occur at the steeper and more compliant portions of the pressure-volume curve. It has been used for internal splinting of the chest wall in cases of chest trauma with flail chest for this reason. PEEP also helps to stabilize and expand fluid filled alveoli, such as occurs in pulmonary edema.

The use of PEEP for unilateral or nondiffuse lung diseases should be evaluated carefully, because it may cause overdistention of unaffected portions of the lungs. The degree of PEEP applied should be carefully determined in patients with normal or already elevated FRC, high intracranial pressure, or decreased pulmonary blood flow.

It is extremely difficult to determine the adverse hemodynamic effects or the exact contribution of PEEP to barotrauma. The effects of PEEP on hemodynamic status are the end-result of many interacting variables, such as mean airway pressure, the existence of spontaneous breaths, intravascular volume status, and underlying cardiac condition. The application of PEEP in excess of 15 cm H$_2$O is not necessarily associated with significant depression of cardiac output in certain conditions of acute respiratory failure in children.[18] Depression of cardiac output can easily be managed by volume expansion or dopamine infusion even if it occurs.[19, 20] The application of PEEP does increase the risk of barotrauma. However, patients who require PEEP may already have lungs with a high risk of barotrauma. The exact contribution of PEEP itself to the risk of barotrauma is again not clearly determined.

The application of PEEP increases FRC and improves compliance of the respiratory system, resulting in less work of breathing. PEEP is applied in the case of most patients in pediatric critical care because of the unique characteristics of respiratory mechanics in children.

Humidification

The absolute amount of heat and moisture loss via the respiratory tract of children is small but can poten-

tially cause significant clinical problems, such as inadvertent hypothermia, impaired mucociliary function, and drying of respiratory secretions leading to airway obstruction.[21] The airways of children have a much smaller diameter than those of adults and are more easily obstructed by dehydrated thick and tenacious secretions.

Inspired gases normally are heated to body temperature and humidified to 100% relative humidity (RH) as they pass through upper respiratory tract. Insertion of artificial airways, either in the form of endotracheal tubes or tracheostomy tubes, bypasses approximately 25% of the humidifying area. Since medical gases used in the hospital are virtually dehumidified, active humidification of respiratory gases is mandatory.

A relative humidity of 100% at 20° C represents less than 40% relative humidity at a body temperature of 37° C, thus a simple humidifier without heating capability is useful in patients without artificial airways. Heated humidifiers are used exclusively in patients with artificial airways.

Controversies still exist over the optimal range for humidity and temperature. Although there is no need to deliver body humidity (37° C 100% RH), 80 to 100% RH at temperatures of 32 to 37° C can be recommended.[10]

Inspired gas temperature should be monitored continuously to prevent thermal injury in the absence of clinically usable hygrometers.[22] However, the extrapolation of inspiratory temperature to humidity when a heating mechanism is incorporated should be done with caution. Condensation or rain out that lowers the temperature and water content can be minimized when a heating wire is used in the breathing tubes.

Condensation causes another problem in that it may become a source of infection. This is a problem especially with the use of a nebulizer in which aerosols consisting of suspended water droplets, rather than water in the gaseous state, are delivered. Nebulizers are used commonly in patients without artificial airways to deliver inhalation medications such as bronchodilators. However, the use of nebulizers in patients with artificial airways carries the potential risk of carrying bacteria into the lower airways and producing bronchospasm in susceptible individuals.[23, 24] The routine use of nebulizers in patients with artificial airways is best avoided without specific indications.[10]

Another factor to be considered in the use of humidifiers is the addition of compressible volume.

Compressible Volume

The relatively large volume of the ventilator circuit compared with tidal volume makes the role of compressible volume in the pediatric ventilatory system rather large.[25] A standard ventilator circuit with a humidifier may have a total gas volume of 1,000 ml, which is relatively small compared with the total lung capacity (TLC) of an adult (5,000 to 6,000 ml). The use of smaller diameter and shorter circuit tubing has made it possible for some infant ventilator circuits to have total gas volumes as small as 200 ml of total gas volume. This is still equal to the TLC of a 3-kg infant.

The volume delivered by the ventilator is distributed to the patient and the respiratory circuit according to their respective compliances. It is not uncommon to see more gas being delivered to the respiratory circuit than to the patient in pediatric critical care. Circuit gas volume is the major determinant of compliance, although the characteristics of circuit tubing also have some effect.[13] The use of shorter and narrower tubing with rigid walls and decreasing humidifier volume (using smaller size reservoir or increasing water level) will contribute to decreasing compressible volume but may be inconvenient.

The characteristics of large circuit compliance mean that more gas must be pulled in to cause a certain negative pressure. This results in a decreased sensitivity to spontaneous breaths in ventilator synchronizing mechanisms and delays in delivery of mandatory respiratory support.

Synchronization (Fig. 40–2)

There are significant psychologic and physiologic differences between mandatory breaths and spontaneous breaths, and they are selected in various ways. Certain mechanisms for synchronizing to spontaneous respiratory breaths must be incorporated when spontaneous respiration is preserved in respiratory support. Ideal synchronization is extremely difficult to achieve in pediatric patients, primarily because the sensing mechanisms of most ventilators are not responsive to small changes in airway pressure and volume.[26] Even though some ventilators are sensitive enough, pressure changes caused by multiple extraneous factors such as cardiogenic oscillation, condensated water in the tubing, or movement of the tubing may result in autocycling. Preservation of spontaneous breaths with inappropriately achieved synchronization will create more hazards than benefits in pediatric critical care.

The most common mechanism of synchronization is pressure sensing with a device that detects changes in pressure caused by spontaneous breaths within the ventilator circuit. Other methods of sensing spontaneous breaths that have been used clinically or experimentally include flow-sensing devices that detect flow changes in the ventilator circuit and devices to detect chest wall movement or phrenic nerve activity.

The pressure-sensing principle has the advantage of being simple. The respiratory efforts of patients of any size can be extrapolated into simple pressure terms; however, the principle may contradict itself during use. The patient has to do active respiratory work against some degree of resistance to create a certain level of negative pressure from the baseline pressure to make the system clearly functional. The work of breathing can be a formidable task to a pediatric patient in respiratory failure. Designing the ventilator to accommodate easier spontaneous breaths means that the negative pressure created will be less, thus making it difficult for the ventilator to recognize the effort of spontaneous

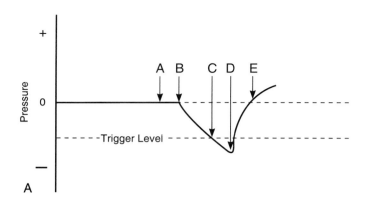

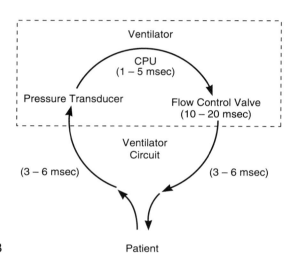

Figure 40–2. Time required for synchronization. *A,* Analysis of delay over the airway pressure curve. The most common mechanism of synchronization is pressure sensing with a device that detects changes in pressure caused by spontaneous breaths. However, there is an inevitable measurable time delay between the patient's initiation of a breath (a), when the airway pressure begins falling (b), when the airway pressure reaches the ventilator's sensory threshold (c), when gas flow starts flowing into the lungs (d), and when the airway pressure reaches the projected pressure (e). *B,* Time required for synchronization. The negative pressure created by the patient trying to breathe is transmitted to the pressure transducer by way of a pressure line (moving at the speed of sound [1 m/3 msec]). Signal processing can be done extremely fast (depending on the speed of the CPU and computer program). But even the fastest electronically controlled flow regulating valves in clinical use have a resolution of 10 to 20 msec (actual resolution may vary significantly owing to mechanical friction). Gases dispatched from the flow control valve reach the patient (after passing through a length of tubing). Thus even the fastest electronically controlled synchronization mechanisms would theoretically have a delay of at least 30 to 40 msec in responding to the patient's immediate respiratory demands (middle).

respiration. The delay in sensing and responding is another problem to be dealt with, and some recently developed ventilators have successfully dealt with this problem (Newport E200, Newport Medical Instruments).

The flow-sensing principle has advantages over pressure sensing in not increasing respiratory work; however, long-term continuous and stable flow sensing in pediatric use is technically difficult at the present time. The flow-sensing principle is also susceptible to the presence of variable leakages and requires great attention. It is quite possible that once these problems are solved, flow-sensing devices may become the principal mode of detecting spontaneous respiration in pediatric critical care. The flow-sensing principle is incorporated into some adult ventilators (7200a, Puritan-Bennett; Elvira, Engstrom).

Use of chest wall movement to detect spontaneous respiration is an attractive alternative and is incorporated into some infant ventilators (InfantStar, Infrasonic). Although use of chest wall movement has theoretical advantages in avoiding many airway gas related problems, it has its own problems such as body movement interferences and delay due to the sensing method used or chest wall distortion.

BASIC PRINCIPLES OF MECHANICAL VENTILATORS

Classification (Fig. 40–3)

Mechanical ventilators may be defined in a variety of ways. Classical and widely used terms of defining the ventilator are based on the way the device terminates mandatory breaths, such as volume-cycled, pressure-cycled, time-cycled, and flow-cycled ventilators. This classification is very comprehensive, but it does not explain the performance of modern ventilators fully. Mainly, it lacks description of the power generators of the mandatory breaths and the gas supply for spontaneous breaths. Pressure wave forms of both mandatory and spontaneous breaths including initiation mode of breaths should also be described.

Power Generators for Mandatory Breaths (Fig. 40–4)

Gas flow may be delivered to the patient with a variety of devices; piston-type, flow-regulating valves, or simple exit portion interruption of high-pressure gas sources. Whatever mechanisms are used, understanding of the basic performance is important.[27]

The actual flow of gas to the alveoli gradually decreases when the lungs are inflated at relatively low pressure (a pressure close to the peak inspiratory pressure) because of a gradual decrease in driving pressure (ventilator pressure minus alveolar pressure). Actual flow also decreases considerably with high respiratory resistance. Gas delivery of the low-pressure type is called "pressure generator." Its use in pediatric critical care is not common because of its weak power.

In contrast, inspiratory flow remains virtually constant throughout the inspiratory phase, regardless of the pressure build up due to high resistance or low compliance of the respiratory system, when gas is delivered at a relatively high pressure (a pressure well over 10 times peak inspiratory pressure). This type of high-pressure

gas delivery is called "flow generator," and because of its strong power, it is the principal power generator in pediatric critical care. Since the flow generator guarantees a set flow to the patient, its use with a time cycle is equivalent to volume-cycled ventilation (VCV). A typical example of this combination is seen in most infant ventilators using continuous flow. However, because of the pressure-limiting features usually incorporated, they give the false impression of being a pressure-cycled ventilator.

Gas Delivery for Mandatory Breaths

Volume-Cycled Ventilation (Fig. 40–5)

In VCV, mandatory breaths end when a preset volume has been delivered from the ventilator. Applied pressure becomes the variable, depending on the patient's characteristics. Inspiratory time and flow may or may not vary with different patient characteristics or with the type of power generator used by the particular ventilator.

Volume-cycled ventilators do not always deliver precise volume to patients with different conditions. The actual volume delivered to patients may differ significantly, mostly due to the compressible volume of the circuit including the internal compressible volume of the ventilator and airway pressure applied. The driving pressure needed to deliver the volume increases as compliance or resistance worsens. In this case, the ventilator terminates inspiration or vents excess gases through a relief valve at a predetermined limit pressure for safety. Most critical care ventilators including infant ventilators are able to deliver in excess of 100 cm H_2O driving pressure without these safety features.

End-inspiratory pause is a variation of VCV in which the exhalation valve is closed for a given period of time (a predetermined number of seconds or percentage of inspiratory time) after the delivery of the set tidal volume before starting exhalation.[28] Proximal airway pressure falls at the onset of inspiratory pause due to the cessation of the bulk of airflow and redistribution of the gases delivered. This typical fall in proximal airway pressure can be used to monitor the quasistatic compliance of the respiratory system. Pressure in the circuit tends to equilibrate with pressure in the patient's alveoli during this period, allowing inspired volume to be discharged into the compartments of the lungs with relatively prolonged time constants, possibly resulting in better oxygenation. Maintenance of end-inspiratory pause causes increased mean airway pressure, and it is quite possible that the effectiveness of end-inspiratory pause may be a nonspecific consequence of this associated elevation of mean airway pressure.[10] Incorporation of end-inspiratory pause into the already short inspiratory time of pediatric patients, in addition to the small amount of leakage due to the use of uncuffed endotracheal tubes, may make this method impractical.

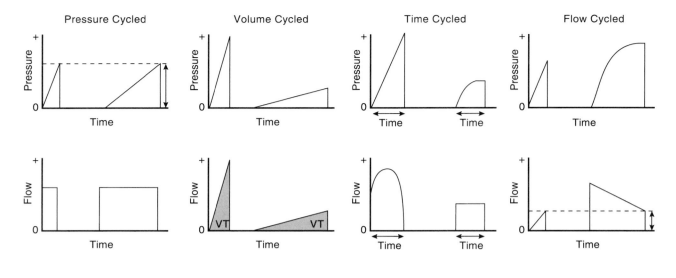

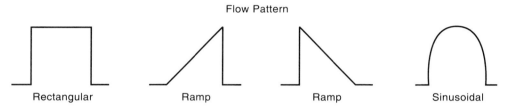

Figure 40–3. Traditional classification of mechanical ventilators. Mechanical ventilators can be classified by the way the devices terminate mandatory breaths. Simplified illustrations are shown here. This classification does not include flow patterns of mandatory breaths. Any kind of flow wave (rectangular, ramp, or sinusoidal) can be incorporated, except rectangular flow wave in flow-cycled ventilation.

In pressure-cycled ventilators, mandatory inspirations are terminated when a preset airway pressure *(arrow)* is reached, regardless of volume or time elapsed.

In volume-cycled ventilators, mandatory breaths end when preset volumes *(hatched area)* have been delivered from the ventilator regardless of airway pressure or time.

Time-cycled ventilators deliver mandatory inspirations for a predetermined time *(arrow)*. Delivering predetermined flow securely in a time-cycled fashion (as is the case in most modern ventilators) is the same as using a volume-cycled ventilator.

Flow-cycled ventilators terminate inspiration when preset flow (either in absolute value or percentage of peak flow value) is reached. This mode is used most frequently in pressure support ventilation.

Pressure-Cycled Ventilation (PCV)

Pressure-cycled ventilators terminate mandatory inspiration when a preset pressure is reached, regardless of the volume delivered or the time elapsed.[29] When lung compliance decreases or flow resistance increases (i.e., accumulation of secretions), the set airway pressure is reached rapidly and inspiration terminates, thus decreasing delivered volume. On the other hand, when compliance is at a maximum (i.e., circuit disconnection), the set airway pressure is never reached and inspiration continues until the time-limiting mechanism functions. Delivered tidal volume can be increased when ventilation is not adequate by increasing the set inspiratory pressure; however, this pressure setting may lead to hyperventilation once the patient improves.

The pressure-cycled mode requires meticulous attention to function properly and is not frequently used in modern critical care, but it can provide better compensation for leakage when the leakage is not great enough to prevent cycling. A larger peak flow can be set safely with pressure-cycled ventilators, unlike VCVs in which flow is predetermined. The advantages of PCV are preserved while some of its disadvantages can be avoided by the use of pressure-limited ventilation (PLV) in the time-cycled ventilation mode (Fig. 40–6).

Time-Cycled Ventilation

Pure time-cycled ventilation implies that mandatory inspiration ends once a preset time has passed, regardless of airway pressure or delivered tidal volume. All of the modern microprocessor controlled critical care ventilators are time cycled. In practice, time-cycled ventilation is used in conjunction with volume-limited or pressure-limited modes. Since time-cycled, volume-limited ventilation acts in a similar fashion to VCV, only time-cycled PLV is discussed here.

Time-Cycled, Pressure-Limited Ventilation

This is the most widely used method of delivering mandatory breaths in pediatric critical care. PLV differs

Pressure Generator

Flow Generator

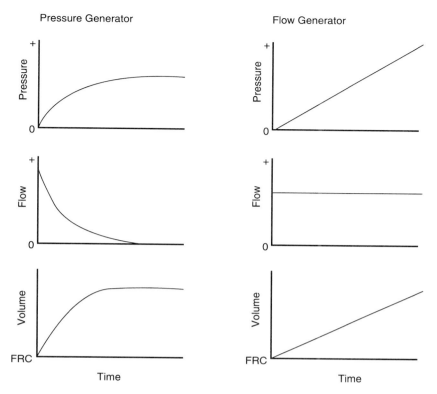

Figure 40–4. Power generators for mandatory breaths. The actual flow of gas to the alveoli in "pressure generator" ventilators gradually decreases when the lungs are inflated, because the driving pressure (ventilator pressure minus alveolar pressure) becomes extremely low. Volume delivered to the lungs decreases as time goes by.

In "flow-generator" ventilators, inspiratory flow remains virtually constant throughout the inspiratory phase regardless of the build-up of pressure, because the driving pressure is relatively high. Volume in the lung increases almost linearly as time goes by.

from PCV in that mandatory breaths are not terminated even when a preset airway pressure is reached. The preset airway pressure is sustained during inspiratory time and produces an inspiratory pressure plateau. This differs from end-inspiratory pause, in which the characteristic drop in airway pressure occurs owing to the cessation of bulk flow from the ventilator. The compliance of the respiratory system in VCV determines the end-inspiratory pause pressure, but the compliance determines the tidal volume in PLV. Given enough time, the applied pressure will equilibrate throughout the lungs and their inflation becomes solely dependent on the compliance of the system. Improved distribution of inspired gases is achieved due to recruitment with relatively prolonged time constants. This helps to eliminate poor oxygenation due to maldistribution of inspired gases caused by disparities in regional time constants. PLV can deliver the same tidal volume with significantly lower inspiratory pressure, because tidal volume is delivered relatively independently of the resistance.

PLV has many advantages in providing mandatory breaths in children. Volume ventilation in small pediatric patients is unreliable because of the variable amounts of leakage caused by the use of uncuffed tubes to minimize tracheal compression injuries and because of unavoidably relatively large compressible volume. Precise control of inspiratory time and a rapid respiratory rate are possible with time-cycled mechanisms incorporated into the PLV ventilators. Rapid flow rate can be safely accommodated because plateaued airway pressures are the major determinant of the ventilation. This is particularly useful in managing larger children who continue to inspire during mandatory breaths. VCV in this situation may cause inadequate flow supply and

inadequate ventilatory support, since inspiratory flow is prefixed based on the delivering tidal volume.

The delivered tidal volume in PLV is influenced by the changes in the patient's respiratory compliance. Precise and meticulous monitoring and control of inspiratory pressures and monitoring of chest excursions are mandatory. Continuous monitoring of tidal volume is also preferable.

PLV can be applied with two different methods: pressure-relief ventilation or pressure-controlled ventilation (Fig. 40–7).

Pressure Relief. This is the simplest and the most common method of delivering PLV in pediatric patients.[30] It has been adopted for use in most infant ventilators (Bear Cub, Bear Medical; InfantStar, Infrasonic; IV100B, Sechrist). Either an exhalation valve or a separate pressure relief valve is used to control inspiratory pressure. Gas actively continues to flow from the ventilator during inspiration. Gas flows into the lung below the set pressure, but as the lung pressure becomes equal to set pressure, gas vents out of the relief valve making pressures in the lung and circuit equal throughout the inspiratory period. Pressure-relief mechanisms should be incorporated into inspiratory tubings because of the possible danger of extremely high pressure caused by the kinking of breathing tubes.[31] In theory, PLV can be applied on most pediatric patients, including small infants using adult ventilators with a pressure-relief modification. However, the safety features based on VCV of some ventilators prevent them from being used in this way.

Most PLV ventilators rely on airway pressure alarms for safety. Thus the major problem associated with the use of PLV is the inability to detect airway obstruction

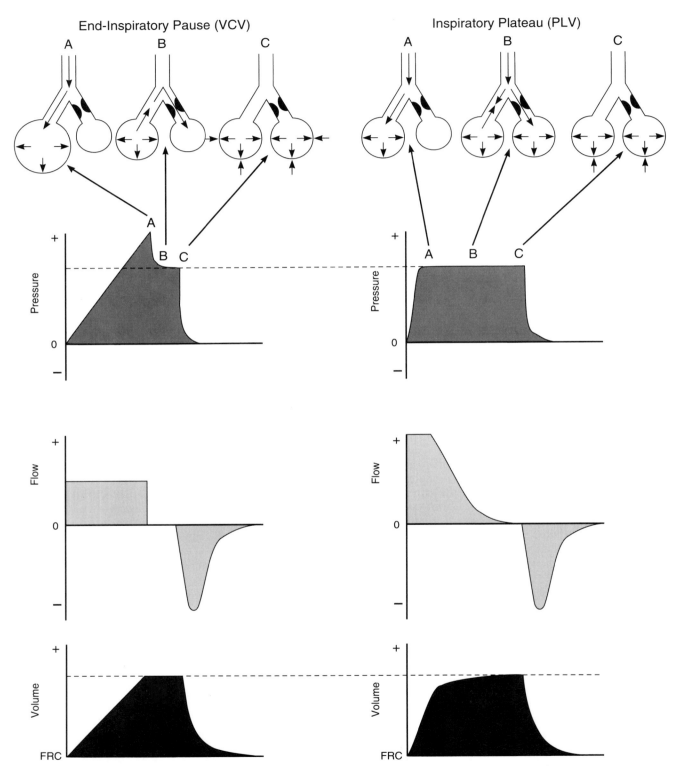

Figure 40–5. End-inspiratory pause in volume-cycled ventilation (VCV) and inspiratory plateau in pressure-limited ventilation (PLV). In VCV, the peak inspiration pressure (a) may be substantially higher than PLV. When the flow from the ventilator ceases briefly before expiration in VCV (end-inspiratory pause), a characteristic drop in airway pressure occurs. The tidal volume delivered may be identical when the end-inspiratory pause pressure (b–c in VCV) and inspiratory plateau pressure (a–c in PLV) are identical.

Thus PLV can deliver the same tidal volume with significantly lower peak inspiratory pressure than VCV.

Volume-Cycled Ventilation

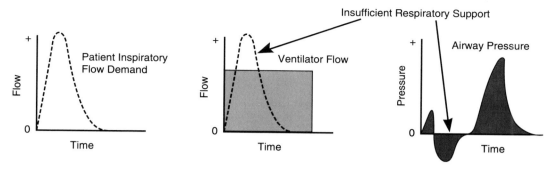

Pressure-Limited Ventilation (Time-Cycled)

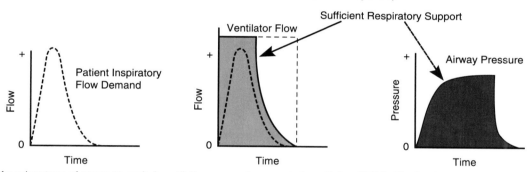

Figure 40–6. An advantage of pressure-cycled ventilation over volume-cycled ventilation (VCV). The inspiratory flow in VCV is predetermined based on the tidal volume being delivered. Insufficient respiratory support can occur if the patient's spontaneous inspiratory flow demand exceeds preselected ventilator flow. This situation occurs less frequently in pressure-limited ventilation (PLV), in which inspiratory flow can be set higher safely.

or kinking. Unlike VCV, complete airway obstruction may not cause a rise in peak inspiratory pressure, and the high pressure alarm may not go off. Similarly, the low-pressure alarm may not go off when small diameter endotracheal tubes are dislodged from the patient while still being connected to the breathing circuit.

Detection of airway obstruction, kinking, or disconnection is a major concern of pediatric respiratory care. Greater attention should be paid to avoid these complications. Tidal volume monitors are useful but are not always practical in small children. The use of capnometers should be encouraged.

Pressure-Controlled Ventilation. This is a relatively new and sophisticated method of applying PLV. Flow rate, peak inspiratory pressure, and inspiratory time are also set in this mode, but it differs from the pressure-relief method in that flow varies during inspiration. Gas flow from the ventilator is decreased once a large initial flow brings airway pressure to the preset level in pressure-controlled ventilation. But the gas flow is used to actively maintain the set airway pressure (Newport E200, Newport Medical Instruments). An extremely large initial flow can be provided without any fear of increased expiratory resistance or gas wasting, because delivered flow can be decreased as much as necessary

toward the end of inspiration and since inspiratory pressure is controlled precisely. The amount of tidal volume delivered can also be monitored.

Pressure-controlled ventilation is very similar to PSV. The biggest technical difference is that inspiratory time and maximum inspiratory flow are preset in pressure-controlled ventilation but are controlled by the patient in PSV. Pressure-controlled ventilation can be considered to be full mechanical support of PSV. On the other hand, PSV can be considered to be partial respiratory support of pressure-controlled ventilation with maximum flow settings.

Flow-Cycled Ventilation (FCV)

In FCV, mandatory breaths end when a preset flow has been achieved. This is typically used in pressure support ventilation (PSV), in which pressure-controlled breaths end when the inspiratory flow decays to one fourth to one half of its peak flow value.

Gas Delivery for Spontaneous Breaths
(Fig. 40–8)

The introduction of intermittent mandatory ventilation (IMV) made ways of supplying gas flow during

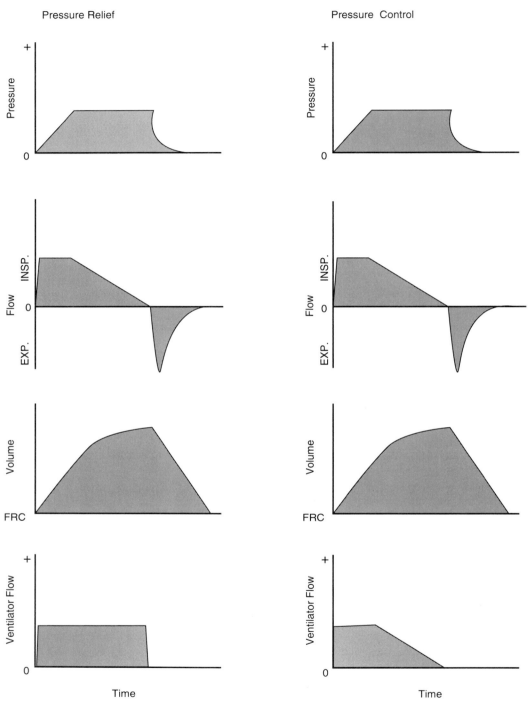

Figure 40–7. Two methods of pressure-limited ventilation. In the pressure relief method, gas actively continues to flow from the ventilator during inspiration. Gas flows into the lung below the set pressure, but as the lung pressure becomes equal to set pressure, gas vents out of the relief valve and makes pressures in the lung and circuit equal throughout the inspiratory period.

In volume-controlled ventilation, gas flow from the ventilator is decreased once a large initial flow brings airway pressure to the preset level. A small amount of gas flow is used to actively maintain set airway pressure.

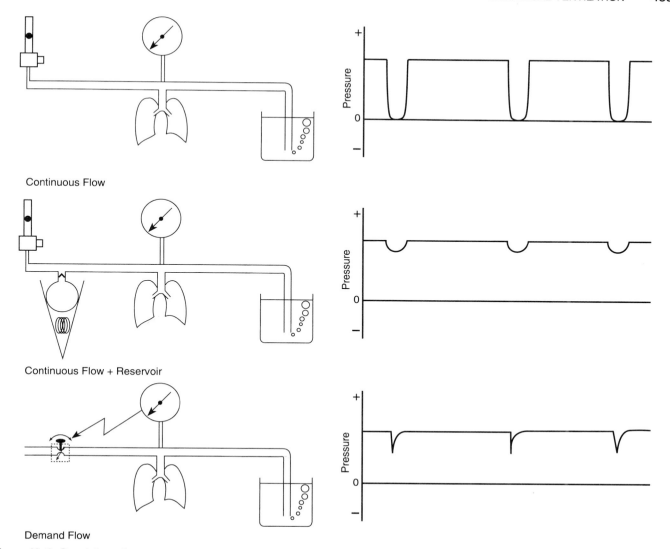

Continuous Flow

Continuous Flow + Reservoir

Demand Flow

Figure 40–8. Gas delivery for spontaneous breaths. Three basic methods of supplying gas flow for spontaneous breaths are illustrated. These methods are used separately or can be combined.

Continuous flow is the simplest method; however, unless a flow rate above the patient's peak flow is delivered, airway pressure swings (respiratory work of breathing) cannot be minimized.

Incorporation of a reservoir bag (or pressurized volume reservoir) via a low-resistance one-way valve eliminates the necessity for supplying peak flow rate gases and decreases pressure swings considerably, but lacks the ability to actively support spontaneous respiratory efforts.

Gases in a demand flow system are delivered only when the patient shows spontaneous respiratory effort. The mechanisms of detecting spontaneous respiration and delivering gases appropriately without delay are not easily achieved.

spontaneous breaths an integral function of mechanical ventilators. Continuous flow, continuous flow with a reservoir bag, demand flow, and a combination of any of these are used.

Continuous Flow

Continuous flow is the simplest method of all and has been used as a principal mode in infant ventilators for the last 2 decades.[31] The patient can inspire gases without mechanical intervention. This system thus offers minimum inspiratory work, especially at the beginning of respiration. Small air leaks will not cause pressure instability because of the presence of a relatively large flow. The flow delivered should be, in theory, at least three times the patient's expected minute ventilation or

above peak flow. The relatively high flow rate required may exceed the ability of the humidifier or increase expiratory resistance. Wasted gas flow and extra rain out in the circuit may add other problems. This method is extremely simple, but its use in larger children is limited.

Continuous Flow with a Reservoir Bag

Many of the shortcomings of the continuous flow method can be eliminated by incorporating a reservoir bag (or pressurized volume reservoir) via a one-way valve into a continuous flow system.[32] The advantages of continuous flow are retained without losing its simplicity. The whole system can be used even in larger children and adults since the brief excess flow rate can be supplemented from gas in the reservoir bag. This system is usually used by modifying ventilators on hand. Only a few ventilators incorporating the reservoir bag are commercially available (Newport E100, Newport Medical Instruments; Mera Humming 2, Senko Medical). Continuous flow with a reservoir system works extremely well in almost all pediatric critical care patients. It does lack, however, the ability to actively support a patient's spontaneous respiratory effort, as PSV does. A demand-flow system is required for this purpose.

Demand Flow

Gases in a demand flow system are delivered only when the patient shows spontaneous respiratory effort. This is ideal since gases are not wasted and monitoring of respiratory volume is easy to perform. The mechanisms of detecting spontaneous respiration and delivering gases appropriately without delay are complex and not easily achieved.[33-35]

Significant delays would still occur even if spontaneous respiratory effort were detected with good sensitivity and processed rapidly electronically. Delays in both pressure tubing (sensing) and breathing tube (delivery of gases) are caused by such physical limitations as the speed of sound (1 m/3 msec). In addition, even the fastest electronically controlled flow regulating valves in clinical use have a resolution of 10 to 20 msec. It is not surprising that a delay in gas delivery of even 40 to 60 msec can cause a significant phase delay in pediatric patients who have relatively large compressible volumes and fast respiratory rates. A system of demand flow is thus very difficult to operate in actual pediatric critical care.

Combination Demand and Continuous Flow

Incorporation of continuous flow or bias flow (continuous flow during the expiratory phase) into a demand flow system is effective in compensating for pressure drift due to variable air leakage and in decreasing the patient's initial respiratory work of breathing. It may, however, decrease the sensitivity of the demand flow sensing mechanisms or cause delays in sensing respiratory movement.[36] Improvement of the demand flow system for pediatric use is being pursued in some ventilators (VIP Bird, Bird Products; Newport E200, Newport Medical Instruments) because of the possible capability of providing PSV to pediatric patients.[37] A combination of demand flow and continuous or bias flow to decrease the patient's work of breathing is used. This approach is suited for pediatric patients, because the patient can institute the early part of inspiration without any mechanical resistance. However, sophisticated complex gas-flow pattern manipulation, such as learning and prediction control is required to prevent increased work of breathing due to phase delay (Newport E200, Newport Medical Instruments) (Fig. 40–9).

PRESSURE WAVE FORMS OF VARIOUS TYPES OF MECHANICAL VENTILATION

Continuous-Flow Ventilation (CFV)
(Fig. 40–10)

CFV provides simple insufflation of continuous oxygen flow into the endobronchial region.[38-40] A relatively large flow of 1 l/kg/min through two endobronchial catheters can maintain $PaCO_2$ at normal levels or keep PaO_2 constant in paralyzed dogs or cats with normal CO_2 production, without any respiratory movement.[38]

The clinical implications of CFV in diseased patients are not clear at the present time since CFV failed to maintain carbon dioxide homeostasis in animals with high CO_2 production. Gas flows greater than 1 l/kg/min caused thoracic distention and a decrease in arterial pressure.

Continuous Positive Airway Pressure
(Fig. 40–11)

CPAP simply indicates that airway pressure stays above ambient pressure throughout the respiratory cycle. It is possible, however, that airway pressure may fall to subatmospheric pressure during a part of the inspiratory phase. This term traditionally refers to the application of PEEP with spontaneous respiration in pediatric critical care. PEEP refers to the level of positive pressure in expiration regardless of ventilatory mode.

CPAP was introduced into pediatric respiratory care in the early 1970s and has been playing a major role ever since.[41] CPAP is of primary importance in dealing with diffuse lung diseases characterized by decreased resting lung volume (FRC) and compliance. It improves oxygenation by increasing FRC and decreases the work of breathing by increasing lung compliance. CPAP is also used in maintaining intrathoracic airway patency in cases such as tracheomalacia. Appropriate CPAP levels may have a beneficial effect on left ventricular overload in infants with increased pulmonary blood flow by increasing pulmonary vascular resistance and decreasing pulmonary blood flow.

The main effects of CPAP involve changes in the mechanics of breathing and cardiovascular function. CPAP stabilizes alveoli that tend to collapse but may simultaneously overexpand those with better compliance, shifting these units to the flatter portion of their pressure-volume curve and reducing distensibility.[10] This may increase the risk of barotrauma and cause increased work of breathing. Subsequent respiratory fatigue leads to hypoventilation and CO_2 retention.

Pressure applied to the airway is partially transmitted to the pleural space and cardiovascular structures within the chest. The amount thus transmitted is directly proportional to the compliance of the lungs and is inversely related to the compliance of the chest wall, suggesting that sicker patients with lower compliances undergo less transmission. Transmitted pressure may impede venous return to the right side of the heart, increase pulmonary resistance, and decrease pulmonary blood flow. Subse-

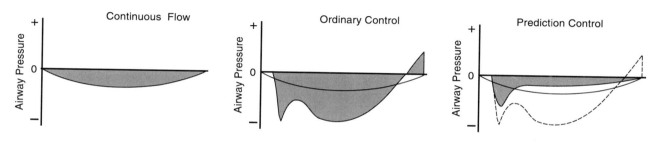

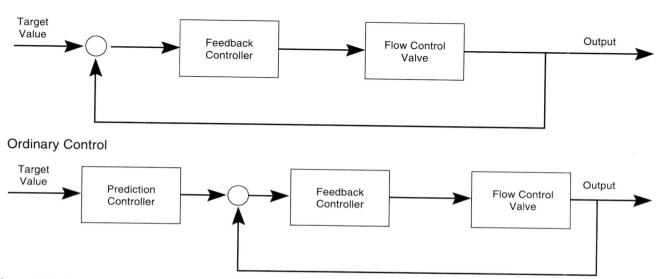

Figure 40–9. Prediction control. A typical airway pressure curve (with a theoretically ideal continuous flow system) during spontaneous inspiration is shown for reference. Ordinary feedback control of the airway pressure may cause excess respiratory work, making the use of prediction control necessary. In ordinary feedback control, the patient's flow demand based on the fall in airway pressure is just delivered, but with a delay causing excess negative pressure. In prediction control, although the initial delay in flow delivery cannot be eliminated, predicted flow based on a learning process is delivered and compensates for the delay.

The outline of control logic is shown for both ordinary and prediction control.

quently cardiac output may decrease. Increased pulmonary artery pressure may worsen an already existing right-to-left shunt. Impeded venous return also contributes to an increase in intracranial pressure.[42]

Airway Pressure Release Ventilation

Airway pressure release ventilation (APRV) can be considered a modification of CPAP and is a relatively new addition to clinical practice.[43–46] APRV involves intermittent release of CPAP in the expiratory limb of the breathing circuit with a release valve. In APRV, CPAP level is adjusted to optimize expiratory lung volume, and the duration and frequency of pressure release are adjusted to optimize CO_2 elimination. The pressure pattern of prolonged sustained pressure with brief pressure release closely resembles an inverse I:E ratio ventilation (IRV); however, it differs from IRV because the patient can breathe in and out freely during

any phase of APRV. The patient breathes spontaneously on CPAP, but the CPAP level is periodically decreased for a brief time to deflate the lungs and eliminate CO_2. Thus APRV delivers CPAP and supports ventilation simultaneously.

APRV differs from CMV in that peak inflation pressure never exceeds the level of CPAP and airway pressure decreases, rather than increases, when tidal volume is delivered. The risk of pulmonary barotrauma and adverse hemodynamic effects associated with conventional mechanical ventilation (CMV) may thus be decreased because of lower peak inflation and mean airway pressures. APRV can provide ventilation and oxygenation similar to CMV, but at a lower peak airway pressure. A laboratory model of acute lung injury comparing APRV and CPAP showed that APRV maintained comparable oxygenation but showed augmented alveolar ventilation suggesting decreased physiologic dead space ventilation in APRV.[46] The occasional deflation that occurs during APRV provides for passive

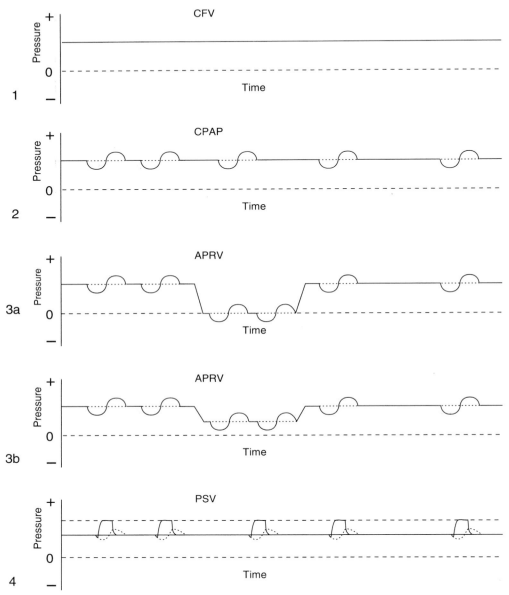

Figure 40–10. Pressure wave forms of various types of mechanical ventilation.

1. Continuous flow ventilation (CFV)

This is a simple insufflation of gases into the endobronchial region. No mechanical support is involved.

2. Continuous positive airway pressure (CPAP)

CPAP refers to the application of PEEP with spontaneous respiration.

3. Airway pressure release ventilation (APRV)

APRV can be considered a modification of CPAP. APRV involves intermittent release of CPAP to ambient pressure (APRV [A]) or a lower PEEP level (APRV [B]).

4. Pressure support ventilation (PSV)

PSV is a pressure assist during spontaneous inspiration. The work of each spontaneous inspiration receives a certain level of relief from partial ventilatory support to full respiratory support, depending on the pressure level. End of pressure support is terminated by the patient's own respiratory cycle rather than a preset inspiratory time.

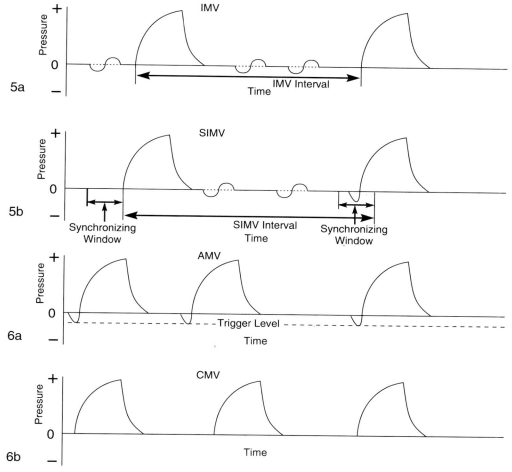

Figure 40–10 *Continued* 5. Intermittent mandatory ventilation/synchronized IMV (IMV/SIMV)
   a. IMV delivers mandatory breaths at a fixed mechanical rate (IMV interval) while allowing simultaneous free spontaneous breaths.
   b. In SIMV, mandatory breaths occur during synchronizing windows (usually set at the last 25% of the IMV interval) that can be synchronized with spontaneous breaths.
   6. Assist/control mechanical ventilation
   a. Assisted mechanical ventilation (AMV)
   In AMV, preset mandatory breaths are delivered on all spontaneous efforts. The initiation of inspiration is usually sensed as a pressure fall below trigger level and is determined by the patient, but the pattern of mandatory breaths is predetermined by the ventilator.
   b. Controlled mechanical ventilation (CMV)
   CMV also provides predetermined mandatory breaths but with predetermined timing. The patient's spontaneous respiratory effort is either absent or abolished intentionally.

ventilation with a released volume determined by the releasing pressure and time, compliance, and resistance. APRV should thus be useful in patients on CPAP who need supplemented ventilatory assistance and for whom intermittent positive inflation is either detrimental or not effective.

APRV is an attractive new concept, but its clinical role in pediatric critical care has not yet been established.

Pressure Support Ventilation

PSV is a form of spontaneous inspiration with assistance in the application of pressure, which is very similar to the well-trained manual assist type of ventilation during spontaneous respiration. Spontaneous inspiration is sensed in PSV, and a variable flow of gas is delivered until airway pressure reaches a preset pressure that is then actively sustained throughout the patient's inspiration.[47] Thus, the work of each spontaneous inspiration receives a certain level of relief from partial ventilatory support to full respiratory support depending on the pressure level. Most of the respiratory work is done by the ventilator when pressure support level is increased adequately. This situation is quite similar to PLV in the assisted mechanical ventilation (AMV) mode; however, PSV differs by terminating pressure support by the patient's own respiratory cycle rather than preset inspiratory time. Weaning from ventilatory support to spontaneous respiration may be facilitated since PSV provides self-adjusting respiratory support from breath to breath and since the level of inspiratory support can be adjusted from full to partial to none (the equivalent of

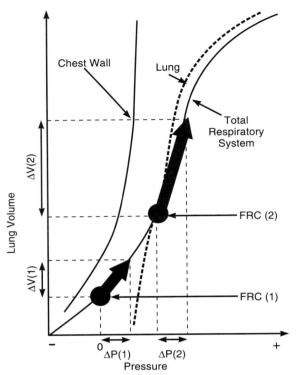

Figure 40–11. Effect of positive end-expiratory pressure (PEEP) on the pressure-volume curve. The application of PEEP not only produces an increase in functional residual capacity (FRC) from FRC (1) to FRC (2) but may also allow ventilation to take place in a more compliant part of the respiratory system owing to the characteristic sigmoid relationship of the pressure-volume curve. Larger volumes (ΔV2>ΔV1) are moved with identical ΔP (ΔP1 = ΔP2).

CPAP) in a gradual fashion.[48] It is reported that PSV up to 30 cm H_2O can be safely applied without hemodynamic embarrassment in patients with good left ventricular ejection fraction.[49] Iatrogenically induced respiratory alkalosis and fighting against the ventilator should also be less likely since the patient establishes the duration of inspiration and respiratory frequency.

Partial inspiratory assist with PSV is an attractive concept in letting pediatric patients breathe spontaneously as the effects of unavoidable resistive work caused by artificial airways can effectively be eliminated.[50] But little is known about the usefulness of PSV in pediatric patients.[51] The major reason for this is technical. Only a few commercially available ventilators provide PSV function for pediatric use (Newport E200, Newport Medical Instruments; Servo 900C, Siemens; VIP Bird, Bird Products). PSV should have extremely sensitive spontaneous respiration detection, but it should also be able to adequately sense the termination of inspiration; otherwise, spontaneous expiration could be impeded significantly.[52] PSV for pediatric use demands not only sensitive respiration detection but also sophisticated gas delivery mechanisms (flow control system) that work extremely fast and over a broad range of flow.

Problems associated with the termination criteria of pressure support are unique to PSV. Inspiratory pressure support should ideally be sustained throughout the inspiratory cycle but should be terminated completely when the patient is ready to exhale. The termination criterion of patient demand for inspiratory flow is usually determined by the percentage of peak flow attained, such as a decrease to the 25 or 50% level of initial peak flow.[52] Flow rate is a good measure of lung filling during pressure-generated inflation; however, pediatric patients in distress characteristically have shorter inspiratory times (faster respiratory frequency with active respiratory drive) and lower compliance making it more complicated to determine adequate termination criteria.

Patients in distress with lower compliance may require a rapid initial peak flow to reach PSV pressure. This sets a higher termination flow rate. A higher flow rate in low compliance lungs also causes a rapid fall in flow rate because of faster filling. As a result, pressure support may be terminated prematurely in the middle of inspiration causing insufficient pressure support or autocycling due to reactivation of PSV.

Preset pressure can be achieved with relatively low-peak pressure when airway resistance is high and compliance is normal or high. This causes a relatively low flow terminating threshold pressure. Inspiratory pressure support may be sustained for an extremely long period since high compliance causes a slow decrease in flow rate. The same situation may occur with air leakage (Fig. 40–12).

Adjustable or very sophisticated termination criteria combined with specific inspiratory flow characteristics are needed for pediatric use (Newport E200, Newport Medical Instruments).

Intermittent Mandatory Ventilation

IMV is the most widely used ventilatory technique in pediatric critical care at the present time. IMV delivers mandatory breaths at a fixed mechanical rate while allowing simultaneous free spontaneous breaths.[53, 54] Mandatory breaths can be synchronized with spontaneous breaths (synchronized IMV: SIMV), but not all spontaneous breaths are assisted. This is the major difference between IMV and assist/control mechanical ventilation. IMV can be combined with CPAP or PSV. The level of mechanical support that can be supplied during IMV ranges from minimum to full depending on the patient's spontaneous respiratory effort. IMV can thus be used on almost all patients.

The presence of spontaneous breaths has great clinical significance. Inspired gas is predominantly distributed to the dependent (posterior) lungs during spontaneous breathing, but mechanically ventilated gas tends to be distributed to the nondependent (anterior) lungs, causing a mismatch of ventilation and perfusion in the supine position.[55] Mechanical ventilation may be necessary to ensure CO_2 elimination, but spontaneous breathing ensures a better matching of ventilation and perfusion. The presence of spontaneous ventilation also contributes to reducing mean airway pressure, minimizing the adverse effects on hemodynamic status. Preserving spontaneous respiratory movement avoids iatrogenic hyperventilation, and this may help to maintain normocarbia. Respiratory muscle strength and coordination are better

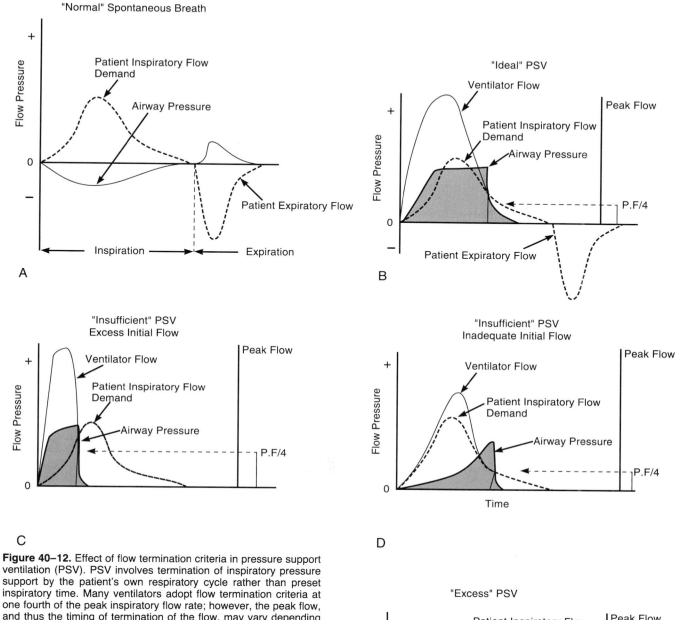

"Normal" Spontaneous Breath

A

"Ideal" PSV

B

"Insufficient" PSV
Excess Initial Flow

C

"Insufficient" PSV
Inadequate Initial Flow

D

"Excess" PSV

E

Figure 40–12. Effect of flow termination criteria in pressure support ventilation (PSV). PSV involves termination of inspiratory pressure support by the patient's own respiratory cycle rather than preset inspiratory time. Many ventilators adopt flow termination criteria at one fourth of the peak inspiratory flow rate; however, the peak flow, and thus the timing of termination of the flow, may vary depending on the patient's condition and flow-control logic. *A*, "Normal" spontaneous breath. Normal inspiration produces slight negative pressure during inspiration and slight positive pressure during expiration *(solid line)*. The *dotted curve* represents the patient's flow demand. *B*, "Ideal" PSV. Ventilator flow exceeds the patient's spontaneous flow demand, and airway pressure is well sustained throughout the inspiratory phase. Ventilator flow is terminated when ventilator flow decreases to one fourth of peak flow value. The airway pressure falls to the baseline before the patient starts exhaling. *C*, "Insufficient" PSV. Two examples are shown here. Excess initial flow: Peak flow becomes relatively high when the ventilator is designed to deliver extremely high initial flow. This sets the terminating flow threshold high and causes pressure support that is too short, or recycling of PSV during one inspiration. *D*, Inadequate initial flow. The patient's inspiratory flow demand exceeds ventilator flow, and airway pressure will not be raised until the end of the inspiration phase when the ventilator is designed to deliver lower initial flow. *E*, "Excess" PSV. Preset pressure can be achieved with relatively low peak pressure when airway resistance is high and compliance is normal or high. This causes a relatively low-flow terminating threshold pressure. Inspiratory pressure support may be sustained for an extremely long period, since high compliance causes a slow decrease in flow rate. The same situation may occur with air leakage.

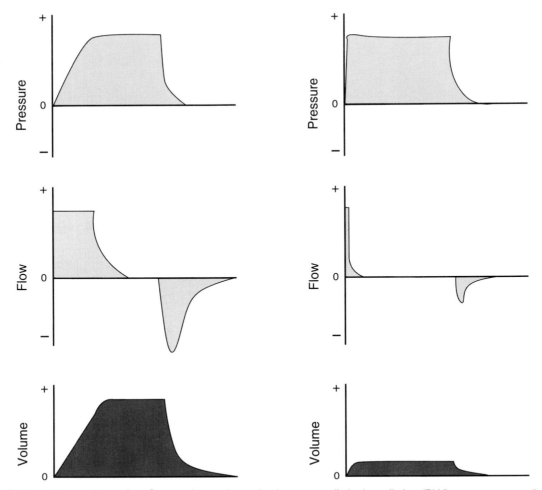

Figure 40–13. PLV and airway obstruction. Severe airway obstruction in pressure-limited ventilation (PLV) may cause a rather rapid rise in airway pressure but may not cause a rise in peak inspiratory pressure. Pressure monitoring alone cannot detect severe obstruction or kinking of endotracheal tubes in PLV.

maintained, although this has not been clearly proven in children. IMV also demands less sedatives and muscle relaxants, which facilitates the safety of respiratory care.

An important consideration in applying IMV to pediatric patients is to ensure that extra work of breathing is not added during spontaneous breaths. The patient's respiratory condition does not always allow for the spontaneous work of breathing, and full mechanical support may be indicated. Characteristics of ventilator performance play an important role. Ventilators with high-flow resistance, low-flow capacity, and a poorly functioning demand flow system are best avoided. Most of the demand flow systems designed for adults do not function properly in children.

SIMV is a variation of IMV, in which mandatory breaths are synchronized with the child's own breathing. The ventilator sets a period of time for sensing the patient's spontaneous breath before delivering a mandatory breath. If the child does not initiate a breath, the ventilator will then deliver a breath (IMV). SIMV is superior to IMV in theory, but it may reintroduce the problem of asynchrony, avoidance of which was the reason why IMV became common in pediatric critical care.

Mandatory minute ventilation (MMV) is another variation of IMV. The machine measures the volume of gas breathed by the patient over a certain time and determines the volume of gas that should be mandatorily delivered.[56] A predetermined minute volume will be delivered to the patient in a variable ratio of spontaneous breaths or mandatory breaths. This mode is primarily designed for automatic weaning. The major drawback of MMV is the fact that the amount of mandatory breaths delivered is determined solely by the amount of spontaneous breaths. The patient can have normal or increased minute ventilation in a distress phase, but the ventilator will stop ventilatory support automatically. Impracticality of measuring minute volume in children also makes MMV not that useful a tool in pediatric patients.

IMV Ventilators for Pediatric Use (Fig. 40–13)

Since IMV involves both spontaneous breaths and mandatory breaths, the ventilator should provide a separate gas supply for both demands. Differences in the requirements for these two types of breaths may be quite significant. A combination of intermittent gas supply for mandatory breaths and a separate gas supply for spontaneous breaths either in the form of a demand or continuous flow system is used for this purpose. A continuous flow system (with or without a reservoir bag) works very well in pediatric patients. However, the function and control mechanisms of the demand valve play essential roles in a demand flow system to achieve successful operation.

Most infant ventilators currently available use just one set of continuous flow for both requirements (Bear Cub, Bear Medical; Sechrist 100B, Sechrist).[30, 57] Although this is quite simple in design, problems may arise when the discrepancy in the two types of breaths becomes larger, which is the case in larger children.

Assist/Control Mechanical Ventilation

Assisted Mechanical Ventilation

AMV is a ventilatory mode in which preset mandatory breaths are delivered on all spontaneous efforts to breathe by the patient. The initiation of inspiration is determined by the patient, but the pattern of mandatory breaths is predetermined by the ventilator.[58] Patients on AMV tend to continue their spontaneous inspiratory efforts beyond the triggering of mandatory breaths, resulting in inadequate ventilatory support when preselected gas flow is less than the patient's spontaneous respiratory demands. This situation tends to occur more frequently when mandatory breaths are delivered in VCV than in PCV, in which inspiratory flow can be increased generously.

The use of AMV in pediatric critical care is not advantageous, because only a preset pattern of mandatory breaths is delivered and because triggering by all spontaneous breaths, which is not always easily obtainable in pediatric patients, is involved. Triggering or synchronization mechanisms, when they do not function properly, will increase the work of breathing considerably. Thus, at the present time, IMV is used as the principal means of respiratory support preserving spontaneous respiration. Advances in medical microprocessor technology may result in more widespread use of an improved version of AMV, namely PSV, in pediatric critical care.

Controlled Mechanical Ventilation

CMV also provides predetermined mandatory breaths but with predetermined timing. The patient's spontaneous respiratory effort is either absent or abolished intentionally.[59] Respiration is fully supported by CMV. This may be the only clinical option in patients with limited cardiorespiratory function. Patients with severe asynchrony in other types of ventilation may benefit from CMV. However, the administration of sedatives or relaxants and the use of hyperventilation to control spontaneous ventilation may in themselves produce adverse effects.

Mandatory breaths can be delivered in a variety of forms, such as VCV and PCV. Inversed ratio ventilation (IRV) is one option of CMV, in which the inspiratory to expiratory time ratio (I/E ratio) exceeds one. Extension of inspiratory time takes various forms, such as end-inspiratory pressure pause and inspiratory pressure plateau. The improvement in oxygenation obtained is due mostly to increased mean airway pressure. Complications due to air trapping and intrinsic PEEP are the major drawbacks of IRV since the time available for expiration is extremely short. Routine use of IRV is best avoided.

High-Frequency Ventilation

HFV refers to a mode of ventilation involving ventilatory frequencies substantially higher than physiologic respiration. Respiratory phasic swings in the airways and alveoli during HFV are much less than those with conventional mechanical ventilation because a relatively small volume is delivered during each cycle. A variety of methods are grouped under the name of HFV, but it is important to recognize that HFV refers a heterogenous group of techniques in which different physiology is involved. High-frequency jet ventilation (HFJV) and high-frequency oscillation are the two major techniques of HFV used in pediatric critical care. The precise role of these two types of HFV in the management of respiratory failure in pediatric critical care is not clearly established, but their definite role in selected cases is appreciated (Fig. 40–14).

High-Frequency Jet Ventilation

HFJV uses intermittent bursts (2 to 5 Hz) of high-pressure gas into the airway through a small diameter needle or catheter.[60] A specially designed endotracheal tube with an intramural lumen for the delivery of jet gases down into the trachea distally may be used for this purpose. Negative pressure caused by the Bernoulli effect results in entrainment of gases, and various degrees of gases can be delivered to the patient as tidal volume. The possibility of maintaining ventilation with an open airway is the major advantage of HFJV. Peak inflation pressure is also lowered.[61]

Expiration occurs passively, and owing to the extremely short expiratory time, intrinsic air trapping is a major concern. Limited access to ventilation monitoring and lack of efficient humidification make the use of HFJV in critical care of value in limited cases only, such as bronchopleural fistulas with massive air leak.[10, 62] HFJV has been used successfully for the anesthetic management of patients with complicated airway surgery in the operating room.

High-Frequency Oscillatory Ventilation (HFOV)

HFOV differs clearly from HFJV because HFOV produces active expiration with a piston-pump mechanism and has a relatively higher frequency (10 to 20 Hz).[63] A high-frequency sinusoidal piston pump is incorporated into a continuous flow CPAP system with a

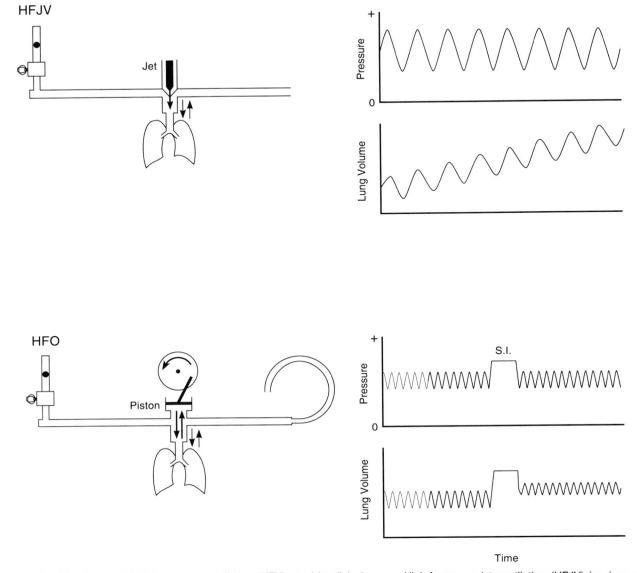

Figure 40–14. Two types of high-frequency ventilation (HFV) used in clinical cases. High-frequency jet ventilation (HFJV) involves active inspiration but passive expiration. Lung volume may increase gradually (air trapping). High-frequency oscillatory ventilation (HFOV) involves both active inspiration and active expiration. S.I. indicates sustained inflation for lung volume recruitment. Lung volume is maintained after S.I. with HFOV.

low-pass filter (Hummingbird BMO2ON, Senko Medical).[64] This system allows a patient to breathe spontaneously (low frequency), yet the high-frequency oscillatory component is retained. Adequate humidification is readily obtained, and air trapping is minimized due to active expiration.

HFOV can be considered a combination of CPAP to obtain oxygenation and oscillation to obtain CO_2 removal. The two parameters can be adjusted independently: PaO_2 by mean airway pressure and $PaCO_2$ by oscillation. A frequency of 15 Hz is commonly used; however, oscillation amplitudes are adjusted subjectively based on the degree of chest vibration and objectively by the $PaCO_2$ of the patient.[64] Lung volume remains stationary in HFOV so adequate lung volume recruitment at the beginning of application is essential.

Brief sustained inflation (S.I.) followed by HFOV keeps lung volume on the deflated limb (lower pressure) of the pressure-volume curve.[65–68] Maintenance of relatively higher mean airway pressure is also useful in using HFOV; however, this is compensated for by a great reduction in peak inflation pressure.[69] Previous methods of treating respiratory failure concentrated on enhancing convection, but the principle of augmented diffusion as demonstrated by HFOV offers hope in cases in which the strategy of enhancing convection failed. HFOV is considered a less invasive way of ventilating fragile lungs since it does not involve intermittent stretching of alveolar walls. Clinical and basic physiologic evidence to support these points has been presented in neonatal critical care, but its clinical role in pediatric critical care has not yet been studied.

References

1. Marchak BE, Thompson WK, Duffy P, et al: Treatment of RDS by high frequency oscillation. J Pediatr 99:287, 1981.
2. Bartlett RH, Andrews AF, and Toomasian JM: Extracorporeal membrane oxygenation for newborn respiratory failure: Forty-five cases. Surgery 92:425, 1982.
3. Sills JH, Cvetnic WG, and Pietz J: Continuous negative pressure in the treatment of infants with pulmonary hypertension and respiratory failure. J Perinatol 9:43, 1989.
4. Fearon B and Whalen JS: Tracheal dimensions in the living infant. Ann Otol 76:964, 1967.
5. Fearon B and Cotton R: Subglottic stenosis in infants and children: The clinical problem and experimental surgical correction. Can J Otolaryngol 1:281, 1972.
6. Downes JJ and Heiser MS: Status asthmatics in children. In: Gregory GA (ed): Respiratory Failure in the Child. New York, Churchill Livingstone, 1981, pp 107–133.
7. Ellington MI: Respiratory care of the pediatric patient. In: Nussbaum E (ed): Pediatric Intensive Care, 1st ed. New York Futura Publishing Company, 1984, pp 339–368.
8. Berman LS, Fox WW, Raphaely RCR, et al: Optimum levels of CPAP for tracheal extubation of newborn infants. J Pediatr 89:109, 1976.
9. Motoyama EK: Respiratory physiology in infants and children. In: Motoyama EK and Davis PJ (eds): Smiths's Anesthesia for Infants and Children. St. Louis, CV Mosby, 1990, pp 11–76.
10. Gioia FR, Stephenson RL, and Alterwitz SA: Principles of respiratory support and mechanical ventilation. In: Rogers M (ed): Textbook of Pediatric Intensive Care. Baltimore, Williams & Wilkins, 1987, pp 113–169.
11. Auld PAM: Pulmonary physiology of the neonate. In: Scarpelli EM (ed): Pulmonary Physiology of the Fetus, Newborn and Child. Philadelphia, Lea & Febiger, 1975, pp 140–145.
12. Doershuk CF, Fisher BJ, and Matthews LW: Pulmonary physiology of the young child. In: Scarpelli EM (ed): Pulmonary Physiology of the Fetus, Newborn and Child. Philadelphia, Lea & Febiger, 1975, pp 133–139.
13. Robbins L, Crocker D, and Smith RM: Tidal volume losses of volume-limited ventilators. Anesth Analg 46:294, 1967.
14. Bone RC, Francis PB, and Pierce AK: Pulmonary barotrauma complicating positive end-expiratory pressure. Am Rev Respir Dis 11:921, 1975.
15. Cohen DJ, Baumgart S, and Stephenson LW: Pneumopericardium in neonates. Is it PEEP or PIP? Ann Thorac Surg 35:179, 1983.
16. Mansell A, Bryan C, and Levison H: Airway closure in children. J Appl Physiol 33:711, 1972.
17. Zapatel A, Paul T, and Samanek M: Pulmonary elasticity in children and adolescents. J Appl Physiol 33:11, 1976.
18. Pollack MM, Fields AI, and Holbrook PR: Cardiopulmonary parameters during high PEEP in children. Crit Care Med 8:372, 1980.
19. Zvist J, Pnotopiddan H, Wilson RS, et al: Hemodynamic responses to mechanical ventilation with PEEP. Anesthesiology 42:45, 1975.
20. Hemmer M and Suter PM: Treatment of cardiac and renal effects of PEEP with dopamine in patient with acute respiratory failure. Anesthesiology 50:399, 1979.
21. Egan DF: Aerosol and humidity therapy. In: Fundamentals of Respiratory Therapy, 3rd ed. St. Louis, CV Mosby, 1977, pp 213–221.
22. Klein EFJ and Graves SA: "Hot pot" tracheitis. Chest 65:225, 1974.
23. Lilker ES and Janregui R: Airway response to water inhalation: A new test for "bronchial reactivity." N Engl J Med 305:702, 1981.
24. Sheppard D, Rizk NW, Boushey HA, et al: Mechanism of cough and bronchoconstriction induced by distilled water aerosol. Am Rev Respir Dis 127:691, 1983.
25. Haddad D and Richards CC: Mechanical ventilation of infants: Significance of compression volume. Anesthesiology 29:365, 1968.
26. Martin LD, Rafferty JF, Wetzel RC, et al: Inspiratory work and response times of a modified pediatric volume ventilator during synchronized intermittent mandatory ventilation and pressure support ventilation. Anesthesiology 71:977, 1989.
27. Mushin WW, Rendell-Baker L, Thompson PW, and Mapleson WW (eds): Automatic ventilation of infants. In: Automatic Ventilation of the Lungs. Oxford, Blackwell Scientific, 1980, pp 167–177.
28. Lindahl S: Influence of an end-inspiratory pause on pulmonary ventilation, gas distribution, and lung perfusion during artificial ventilation. Crit Care Med 7:540, 1979.
29. Spearman CB and Sanders HG: Physical principles and functional designs of ventilators. In: Kirby RR, Smith RA, and Desauteles SA (eds): Mechanical Ventilation, 1st ed. New York, Churchill Livingstone, 1985, pp 59–113.
30. Kirby RR, Robison EJ, Schulz J, et al: Continuous-flow ventilation as an alternative to assisted or controlled ventilation in infants. Anesth Analg 51:871, 1971.
31. Hall MW and Peevy KJ: Infant ventilator design: Performance during expiratory limb occlusion. Crit Care Med 11:26, 1983.
32. Cane RD and Shapiro BA: Mechanical ventilatory support. JAMA 254:87, 1985.
33. Katz JA, Kraemer RW, and Gjerde GE: Inspiratory work and airway pressure with continuous positive airway pressure delivery systems. Chest 88:519–526, 1985.
34. Gibney RTN, Wilson RS, and Pontoppidan H: Comparison of work of breathing on high gas flow and demand valve continuous airway pressure system. Chest 82:692, 1982.
35. Cox D and Niblett, DJ: Studies on continuous positive airway pressure breathing systems. Br J Anaesth 56:905, 1984.
36. Beaty CD, Ritz RH, and Benson MS: Continuous in-line nebulizers complicate pressure support ventilation. Chest 96:1360, 1989.
37. Nakagawa S, Miyasaka K, Sakai H, et al: A new demand flow type ventilator with learning and prediction control logic. Jap J Respir Care 7:202, 1990.
38. Perl A, Whitwam JG, Chakrabarti MK, et al: Continuous flow ventilation without respiratory movement in cat, dog and human. Br J Anaesth 58:544, 1986.
39. Vettermann J, Brusasco V, and Rehder K: Gas exchange and intrapulmonary distribution of ventilation during continuous-flow ventilation. J Appl Physiol 64:1864, 1988.
40. Obermiller T, Lakshminarayan S, Willoughby S, et al: Influence of lung volume and left atrial pressure on reverse pulmonary venous blood flow. J Appl Physiol 70:447, 1991.
41. Gregory GA, Kitterman JA, Phibbs RH, et al: Treatment of the idiopathic respiratory distress syndrome with continuous positive pressure ventilation. N Engl J Med 284:1333, 1971.
42. Duncan AW, Oh TE, and Hillman DR: PEEP and CPAP. Anaesth Intensive Care 14:23, 1986.
43. Stock MC, Downs JB, and Frolicher DA: Airway pressure release ventilation. Chest 93:911, 1987.
44. Garner W, Downs JB, Stock MC, et al: Airway pressure release ventilation (APRV): A human trial. Chest 94:779, 1988.
45. Florete OG, Banner MJ, Banner TE, et al: Airway pressure release ventilation in a patient with acute pulmonary injury. Chest 96:679, 1989.
46. Martin LD, Wetzel RC, and Bilenki AL: Airway pressure release ventilation in a neonatal lamb model of acute lung injury. Crit Care Med 19:373, 1991.
47. MacIntyre NR: Respiratory function during pressure support ventilation. Chest 89:677, 1986.
48. Brochard L, Harf A, Lorino H, et al: Inspiratory pressure support prevents diaphragmatic fatigue during weaning from mechanical ventilation. Am Rev Respir Dis 139:513, 1989.
49. Dries DJ, Kumar P, and Mathru M: Hemodynamic effects of pressure support ventilation in cardiac surgery patients. Am Surg 57:122, 1991.
50. LeSouef PN, England SJ, and Bryan AC: Total resistance of respiratory system in preterm infants with and without an endotracheal tube. J Pediatr 104:108, 1984.
51. Stewart KG: Clinical evaluation of pressure support ventilation. Br J Anaesth 63:362, 1989.
52. MacIntyre NR and Ho LI: Effects of initial flow rate and breath termination criteria on pressure support ventilation. Chest 99:134, 1991.
53. Downs JB, Klein EFJ, Desautels D, et al: Intermittent mandatory ventilation: A new approach to weaning from patients from mechanical ventilation. Chest 64:331, 1973.
54. Downs JB, Perkins HM, and Modell JH: Intermittent mandatory ventilation. Arch Surg 109:519, 1974.

55. Froese AB and Bryan AC: Effects of anesthesia and paralysis on diaphragmatic mechanics in man. Anesthesiology 41:242, 1974.

56. Hewlett AM, Plott AS, and Terry VG: Mandatory minute volume ventilation: A new concept in weaning from mechanical ventilation. Anaesthesia 32:163, 1977.

57. Bancalali E and Eisler E: Neonatal respiratory support. *In*: Kirby RR, Smith RA, and Desauteles SA (eds): Mechanical Ventilation, 1st ed. New York, Churchill Livingstone, 1985, pp. 243–291.

58. Heenan TJ, Downs JB, Douglas ME, et al: Intermittent mandatory ventilation—Is synchronization important? Chest 77:598, 1980.

59. Shapiro B: General principles of airway pressure therapy. *In*: Shoemaker WC, Ayers S, Grenvik A, et al (eds): Textbook of Critical Care. Philadelphia, WB Saunders, 1989, pp. 505–515.

60. Klein M and Smith RB: High frequency percutaneous transtracheal jet ventilation. Crit Care Med 5:280, 1977.

61. Carlo WA, Chatburn RL, and Martin RJ: Randomized trials of high-frequency jet ventilation versus conventional ventilation in respiratory distress syndrome. J Pediatr 110:275, 1987.

62. Mammel MC, Ophoven JP, Lawallen PK, et al: High-frequency ventilation and tracheal injuries. Pediatrics 77:608, 1986.

63. Bohn DJ, Miyasaka K, Marehak BE, et al: Ventilation by high frequency oscillation. J Appl Physiol 48:710, 1980.

64. Tamura M, Tsuchida Y, Kawano T, et al: Piston-pump-type high frequency oscillatory ventilation for neonates with congenital diaphragmatic hernia: A new protocol. J Pediatr Surg 23:478, 1988.

65. Kolton M, Cattran CB, Kent G, et al: Oxygenation during high frequency oscillatory ventilation with conventional mechanical ventilation in two models of lung injury. Anesth Analg 61:323, 1982.

66. Walsh MC and Carlo WA: Sustained inflation during HFOV improves pulmonary mechanics and oxygenation. J Appl Physiol 65:368, 1988.

67. Byford LJ, Finker JH, and Froese AB: Lung volume recruitment during high-frequency oscillation in atelectasis-prone rabbits. J Appl Physiol 64:1607, 1988.

68. McCulloch PR, Forkert PG, and Froese AB: Lung volume maintenance prevents lung injury during high frequency oscillatory ventilation in surfactant-deficient rabbits. Am Rev Respir Dis 137:1185, 1988.

69. Bryan AC and Froese AB: Reflections on the HIFI trial. Pediatrics 87:565, 1991.

Cardiopulmonary Interactions

Desmond Bohn, M.B., B.Ch., F.R.C.P.(C.)

To suggest that the heart and lungs are closely connected in more than the merely anatomic sense may seem like stating the obvious. Yet the great physiologists of the late 19th and early 20th centuries who defined for us the laws that govern our understanding of cardiovascular physiology were largely unaware of the major hemodynamic changes that we now know occur during the passage of venous blood to the arterial side of the circulation. The classic observations of Starling on the effect of the changes in filling pressure on cardiac output presumed that the right heart pumped blood to the left side without taking into account the hemodynamic changes associated with respiration. For many years, the pulmonary circulation was referred to as the minor circulation, and it was thought that pulmonary disease was important only in the respect that it limited the full oxygenation of the blood. We know now that the heart and lungs function as more than two independent but connected circulations. Pulmonary parenchymal disease can result in major circulatory changes because of alterations in mechanical forces within the thorax, and heart disease with ventricular dysfunction can result in both changes in pulmonary blood flow and the way that changes in intrathoracic pressure (ITP) directly modulate cardiac performance. In addition, with the development of our ability to measure hemodynamic changes in critically ill patients has come the realization that the passage of venous return through the thoracic cavity is associated with major hemodynamic changes during the respiratory cycle, whether during spontaneous or positive pressure ventilation. These interactions between the heart and the lungs may be influenced by either the primary disease process or the therapies used in intensive care treatment, and it is thus important that we have a fundamental understanding of the normal physiology of cardiopulmonary interactions as a prelude to an explanation of how they may change because of disease or therapeutic interventions in the critically ill patient.

CARDIOPULMONARY CIRCULATION

Perhaps the easiest way of understanding the fundamentals of the complex interaction between the systemic and pulmonary circulations is to use a model of two pumps connected in series enclosed within a chamber in which the pressure is constantly changing. The reservoir for the right side of the heart (venous return) lies entirely outside the thorax and is consequently subject to atmospheric pressure, though the venous connections are intrathoracic and subject to changes in pleural pressure. In contrast, the reservoir (the pulmonary circulation) and the pumping chamber for the left heart lie entirely within the thorax, though the pump ejects against a high-impedance circulation that is largely extrathoracic (Fig. 41–1). Since intrapleural pressure is constantly changing during the respiratory cycle, it follows that intrathoracic pressures will affect the output from the pump by fluctuations in the amount of filling or preload. In addition, alterations in pressure across the wall of the pumping chamber (transmural pressure), which is the difference between intracavity and intrapleural pressure, have significant effects on pump function. Two further factors govern the performance of the two pumping chambers: (1) We now know that they do not function as merely two separate pumping chambers connected in series; because there are muscle fibers that interconnect both ventricles and because they share a common septum, changes in the contractile state of one ventricle will be reflected in the other, a phenomenon known as ventricular interdependence.[1] (2) Both pumping chambers are also constrained within viscoelastic membrane (the pericardium), which, although it does not normally have a significant influence on function, may inhibit contraction in situations in which intrapericardial pressure increases.

The interaction between respiratory and cardiac function will be discussed in relation to the sequence of events in the cardiac cycle and the effect of ventilation on each phase of blood flow from the venous to the

465

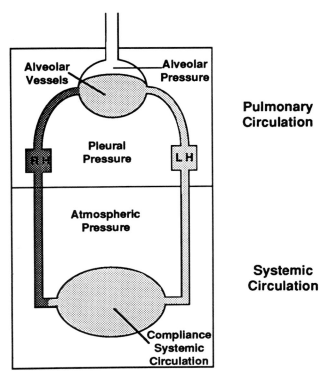

Alveolar
Vessels

Alveolar
Pressure

**Pulmonary
Circulation**

Pleural
Pressure

RH   LH

Atmospheric
Pressure

**Systemic
Circulation**

Compliance
Systemic
Circulation

Figure 41–1. The two compartment model of the circulation. Both the right heart (RH) and left heart (LH) are subjected to pleural (intrathoracic) pressure, while the systemic vasculature is subjected to atmospheric pressure. The filling pressure for both LV and RV serve as back pressure to drainage and as preload. (Reprinted from Permutt S, Wise RA, and Brower RG: How changes in pleural pressure cause changes in afterload and preload. In: Scharf SM and Cassidy SS [eds]: Lung Biology in Health and Disease: Heart-Lung Interactions in Health and Disease. Courtesy of Marcel Dekker Inc., New York, 1989.)

arterial side of the circulation, namely, (1) venous return and right atrial (RA) filling (right ventricular [RV] preload), (2) RV ejection, (3) the pulmonary vascular bed, and (4) left ventricular (LV) output.

RIGHT HEART

Systemic Venous Return

A fundamental principle of normal cardiovascular physiology is the ability to balance the output of the left and right heart and that in the event of a sudden change in either venous return or cardiac output, the balance is restored within a few heartbeats. Although the normal heart will pump all the blood returned to it from the venous side of the circulation, differing changes in venous return to the right atrium occur during the inspiratory and expiratory phases of respiration. The forces that govern venous return and how they are influenced by respiration have been defined in the classic experiments of Guyton and associates.[2] The pressure generated for return of blood flow to the heart is the driving pressure (mean systemic pressure) minus the back pressure to venous return, which in this instance is the RA pressure. The pressure within the venous

system is determined by the compliance and the volume of the vascular bed. With the total circulation arrested, this mean systemic pressure has been measured at 7 mm Hg.[2] Acute elevations in RA pressure will result in a fall in cardiac output until compensated for by a change in compliance in the venous capacitance system.

The negative pleural pressure that occurs during a normal spontaneous inspiration produces a fall in RA pressure, and hence the back pressure that the venous capacitance sees, resulting in increased RA filling (Fig. 41–2). The filling pressure gradient for venous return to the right atrium is usually around 5 mm Hg and is determined by the difference between the extrathoracic and intrathoracic venous pressures. Negative intrapleural pressure increases the transmural pressure of the intrathoracic veins and increases their caliber. One might suppose that a dramatic increase in venous return might occur if there was a reduction in RA pressure produced by a deep inspiration. In the normal human, when flow limitation conditions exist, this augmentation of venous return by negative intrathoracic pressures is limited by the fact that venae cavae collapse at the thoracic inlet. In these conditions, maximum venous return occurs at RA pressures of zero, and decreasing the RA pressure to less than zero relative to the periphery will not result in any further increase in venous return. Although negative pressures in relation to atmosphere can be measured in the right atrium, the transmural RA pressure, which is the difference between the intracavity RA pressure and pleural pressure, is always positive. Collapse of the intrathoracic superior and inferior venae cavae is prevented by a system of valves. Similarly, the rise in intra-abdominal pressure that occurs during inspiration will result in collapse of the abdominal portion of the inferior vena cava. When conditions of flow limitation do not exist, a rise in intra-abdominal pressure will cause an increase in venous return to the right atrium, but this rise in pressure on the inferior vena cava will result in an increase in impedance for venous return from the peripheral veins.[3]

Although these concepts are straightforward, the total effect of respiration on the right side of the heart is somewhat more complicated. The increase in venous return to the right atrium that occurs during inspiration increases preload to the right ventricle, but at the same time that the RA pressure rises, the gradient for venous return decreases, so that there are differing and opposite effects. One can draw function curves for both venous return and cardiac output based on RV preload (Fig. 41–3). It is evident that an increase in RA pressure tends to reduce venous return but increase cardiac output, and vice versa. There is an "ideal" point at which these two curves intersect when the demands for venous return and cardiac output are satisfied.[3] Either an underlying pathologic condition or therapeutic manipulations may alter the shape and position of these curves. In addition, there may be important neurohumoral reflexes that affect venous capacitance vessels in response to a change in venous return. α-Adrenergic stimulation results in constriction of peripheral veins and a fall in venous compliance, increasing the upstream pressure for blood flow toward the right atrium.

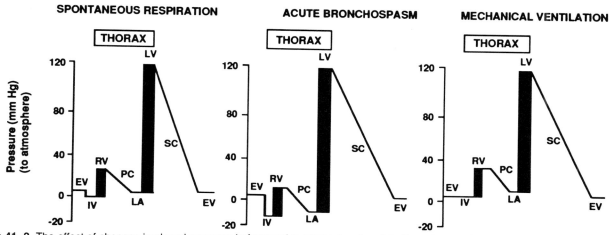

Figure 41–2. The effect of changes in pleural pressure (referenced to atmosphere) on intrathoracic vascular structures associated with normal respiration and with increased negative and positive ITP. EV = extrathoracic veins; IV = intrathoracic veins (including RA); RV = right ventricle; PC = pulmonary circulation; LA = left atrium; LV = left ventricle; SC = systemic circulation. (From Weber KT, Janicki JS, Hunter WC, et al: The contractile behaviour of the heart and its functional coupling to the circulation. Prog Cardiovasc Dis 24:375, 1982.)

Right Ventricular Ejection

The right ventricle must pump desaturated venous blood with a high CO_2 content through what is normally a low-resistance pulmonary vascular bed. To accomplish this requires only 20 to 30 mm Hg at rest, though this may rise to 50 mm Hg with severe exercise at which time venous return may increase to three to four times normal.[4] The morphometry of the right ventricle shows that its structure reflects this function well in that it is a

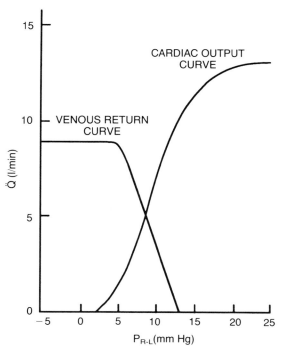

Figure 41–3. Cardiac output and venous return curves plotted on the same abscissa. An increase in right atrial pressure tends to reduce venous return but increase cardiac output. There is a single point where the curves intersect that satisfies the conditions for both. (From Sylvester JT, Goldberg HS, and Permutt S: The role of the vasculature in the regulation of cardiac output. Clin Chest Med 4:111, 1983.)

relatively flat, crescent-shaped, heavily trabeculated, thin-walled chamber that serves as a low-pressure, high-volume displacement pump. It can be considered to be made up of four anatomically distinct components: (1) the RV free wall, (2) the septal wall, anchored to the left ventricle, (3) the inflow portion of the RV cavity, and (4) the outflow portion. The geometry of the right ventricle is entirely different from that of the left ventricle as can be seen by comparing the two chambers in cross section (Fig. 41–4). It is closely integrated with the left ventricle by being directly attached to the septal wall and by an anatomic attachment of muscle fibers that cross between the free walls of the left and right ventricles. The left ventricle, in comparison, has an entirely different configuration. The chamber is thick-walled and ellipsoid, which allows for an efficient and homogeneous contraction capable of generating high pressures. Contraction of the right ventricle is anything but homogeneous by comparison, as it functions like two different chambers connected in series. The heavily trabeculated inflow portion at the apex is electrically activated and contracts before the outflow tract, giving rise to an almost peristaltic action when visualized angiographically. The close anatomic arrangement of the right ventricle with the left ventricle in fact enhances the efficiency of its contraction. The continuity of muscle fibers between the two free walls means that they are pulling together toward a common center of gravity, thereby enhancing contraction.[5] As stated previously, this symbiotic relationship has been termed *ventricular interdependence.*[1] In addition, the presence of a common septum may further influence the function of one ventricle in conjunction with the other. The septum acts as a fixation point for the RV free wall as it contracts, and it also shifts in relation to the different diastolic pressures in either chamber, and by encroaching upon the lumen of the left ventricle it may alter its diastolic compliance (see Fig. 41–4). The septum also contracts during systole and, depending on its radius of curvature, could help or hinder ventricular ejection. There is good evidence that RV ejection is enhanced by left ventricular (LV) con-

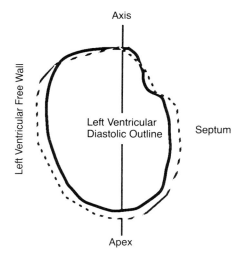

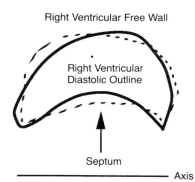

Figure 41–4. Left *(top panel)* and right ventricular profiles before (-----) and after (———) increasing the volumes of the opposite ventricle. (From Santamore WP, Lynch PR, Meier GM, et al: Myocardial interaction between the ventricles. J Appl Physiol 41:362, 1976.)

traction. Isolated heart studies have shown that increasing LV volume increases the pressure generated by the right ventricle.[6–8] In addition, there are angiographic studies that show rightward displacement of either a normal muscular or artificial septum associated with LV contraction.[9–13]

The fact that the right ventricle and pulmonary circulation is essentially a low-pressure system with the generation of modest systolic pressures has led some investigators to question the importance of the right ventricle in the maintenance of normal circulatory homeostasis. Several studies have shown that experimental destruction of myocardium in the RV free wall, its replacement with artificial material,[14–18] or removal of intraventricular septum[12] do not result in alteration in cardiac output or a rise in RA pressure. The introduction of the Fontan procedure for the surgical correction of obstructive lesions of the right heart, whereby the right atrium is connected to the pulmonary artery, has also shown that effective pulmonary blood flow can be sustained when no right ventricle is present. However, in diseases associated with sustained elevations in pulmonary vascular resistance (PVR), which demand an increase in driving pressure to sustain pulmonary blood

flow, the right ventricle hypertrophies and performs as a thick-walled pressure chamber capable of generating pressures up to and greater than systemic levels. Blood flow through the lung to the left atrium is sustained by the pressure differentials among the pulmonary artery, the downstream pressure in the pulmonary circulation, and the intracavity pressure in the left atrium.

The muscle fiber alignment of the intraventricular septum closely resembles that of the LV free wall.[11] The septum can therefore be considered functionally to be an extension of the LV free wall, and its important contribution to LV systolic ejection can be seen angiographically when both the free wall and ventricular septum move inward toward the center of the chamber as the ventricle contracts.

The conformation of the septum also aids systolic ejection of the right ventricle by anchoring the RV free wall and thereby creating a radial force that draws the free wall toward the septum (see Fig. 41–4). The position and curvature of the septum also depend upon the balance of forces between the two chambers, which create an axial force. Normally, high pressures within the LV chamber result in an axial force that bows the septum toward the right ventricle during systole, whereas the radial forces produced by the alignment of muscle fibers within the septum predominate in the direction of the LV free wall. Any acute change in either the volume or pressure of the right ventricle can result in a shift in septal position. This may be particularly pronounced in advanced pulmonary vascular disease in which it is not uncommon for pressures in the right ventricle to approach or even exceed systemic pressures. In this situation, the septal muscle hypertrophies and its motion is altered.[19] Left-sided deviation of the septum, especially at the base of the right ventricle, can result in encroachment on the LV outflow tract and compromise of LV function. This may explain the acute falls in cardiac output and pulmonary edema occasionally seen with the use of vasodilator therapy in pulmonary hypertension. Similar distortions in ventricular geometry are seen in patients with cor pulmonale and RV enlargement. Septal shift alters the distensibility of the left ventricle, thereby reducing its compliance. This will have an adverse effect on LV function, leading to the erroneous assumption that the left heart is also abnormal. Abnormal septal shift can also be produced physiologically by a forced inspiration with the glottis closed (Mueller maneuver), which generates a large negative ITP without a change in lung volume. Pleural pressure becomes markedly negative without a change in alveolar pressure, whereas the increase in diastolic filling shifts the septum leftward.[20]

PULMONARY VASCULAR BED

The pulmonary vasculature bridges the right and left heart, and changes in its caliber influence the performance of both ventricles. The afterload against which the right ventricle contracts is influenced by alterations in PVR produced by changes in either pulmonary blood flow or ventilation. The pulmonary vasculature has a great capacity to dilate in response to increased pulmonary blood flow. The fact that the pulmonary artery pressure does not rise significantly in situations of increased cardiac output is attributable to recruitment of previously nonperfused vessels. In conditions with excessively high pulmonary blood flow associated with left-to-right intracardiac shunting, the pulmonary vasculature will become abnormally muscularized which will result in a rise in PVR and increased RV afterload. PVR and RV afterload will also be increased in situations in which there is a fixed arteriolar obstruction, as in primary pulmonary hypertension, or in response to acute and chronic hypoxemia, though whether this vasoconstriction occurs at the level of the capillary, venule, or arteriole remains a matter of some dispute. However, as well as responding to variations in systemic output, PVR is also governed by changes in alveolar pressure during respiration.

It has been convenient to think of the pulmonary vasculature as being divided into two functional groups: (1) vessels that behave as if they were exposed to an extravascular pressure, which reflects pleural pressure (extra-alveolar vessels) and (2) vessels that are exposed to an extravascular pressure, which reflects alveolar pressure (intra-alveolar vessels). An increase in lung volume during inspiration increases radial traction on extra-alveolar vessels, increasing their caliber and causing a fall in PVR and a decrease in RV afterload. The change in blood flow in the intra-alveolar vessels depends on their position within the different zones of the lung as defined by West and Dollery[21] and the relationship between pressures in alveolus (PA) and pulmonary artery (Pa) and left atrium (Pla). When zone I conditions apply (PA > Pa > Pla), the pressure within the arterial end of the vessel is less than the alveolar pressure and is therefore insufficient to open the vessels, which remain collapsed. The behavior of these vessels can be described in terms of a Starling resistor in which there is no flow regardless of LA pressure.[22] These conditions exist in the uppermost parts of the lung in the upright human. When zone II conditions apply (Pa > PA > Pla), arterial pressure is higher than alveolar pressure, and the intra-alveolar vessels behave like Starling resistors surrounded by alveolar pressure, in which flow depends on the difference between arterial and alveolar pressures and is independent of changes in LA pressure. These conditions predominate in the midzone of the lung in the upright human. In zone II conditions, the back pressure to RV ejection is alveolar rather than LA pressure, and the relevant resistance is only that between the pulmonary artery and the downstream end of the alveolar vessels. An increase in lung volume produces an increase in back pressure to RV ejection compared with the pressure around the heart and increased afterload. This requires that an approximately equal increase in pressure be produced in the pulmonary artery and alveolus to maintain pulmonary blood flow, which translates into increased RV wall stress. Thus, an increase in alveolar pressure relative to pleural pressure increases RV afterload, and this change in alveolar pressure relative to arterial pressure can produce a marked degree of RV afterload seen in acute asthma.[23] In the zone

II state, lung inflation also produces a transient fall in LV preload because of the increase in volume of the extra-alveolar vessels.[24]

When zone III conditions exist (Pa > Pla > PA), the pressure in the venous side of the capillary is higher than the alveolar pressure, and pulmonary blood flow behaves like a Starling resistor in which flow is independent of alveolar pressure and is governed by the difference between arterial and venous pressures. In these situations, there is a transient increase in RV afterload and LV preload but no steady state changes.[25]

The net effect of these various changes is that PVR is lowest at functional residual capacity (FRC) and rises in situations in which vessels are compressed during lung collapse or when there is overdistention of the lung[26] (Fig. 41–5). Loss of FRC (e.g., as seen with the development of pulmonary edema or atelectasis) will result in a rise in PVR, as will overdistention of the lung due to airway obstruction or high peak airway pressure ventilation, which puts the lung on the flat portion of the pressure volume curve. In this situation, zone I conditions would predominate throughout the lung (PA > Pa > Pla), and PVR would be increased. Changes in transpulmonary pressure will have the same effect on PVR whether they are produced by positive or negative changes in pleural pressure.

LEFT VENTRICLE

The left ventricle differs from the right ventricle not only in its anatomic configuration, being a thick-walled, spherical chamber capable of supporting high systemic

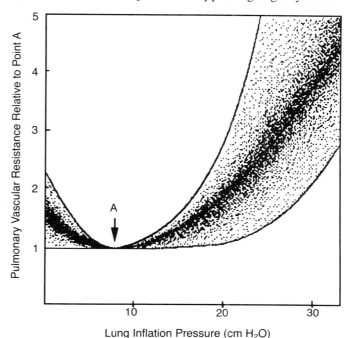

Figure 41–5. The mean and range of response of PVR in relation to changes in lung inflation pressure relative to point A, which represents FRC. Pulmonary vascular resistance rises with increasing distention of the lung and with loss of FRC. (From Nunn JF: Applied Respiratory Physiology. London, Butterworths, 1977, p 269.)

pressures, but also in the important respect that because its filling reservoir (the left atrium) and the chamber lie within the thorax, its preload and afterload are both subject to changes in ITP (see Fig. 41–1). The preload for input into the left ventricle comes from pulmonary venous return and LA filling, and it ejects against an afterload consisting of aortic pressure and the forces acting across the chamber wall. The predominant afterload forces against which the left ventricle ejects are outside the thorax.

LV preload will be affected to some extent by changes in the diastolic pressure volume relationship of the LV secondary to RV function, enhanced by the constraint produced by an intact pericardium (ventricular interdependence).[1] In addition, direct mechanical compression of the chamber from inflation of the lung (mechanical heart-lung interactions) will also affect LV preload.[27] Systolic function of the left ventricle is governed by contractility, heart rate, and the afterload against which the ventricle contracts. In the normal situation in which there is no gradient between the left ventricle and aorta, this pressure is the major component of LV afterload and correlates well with LV end-systolic volume.[28, 29]

VENTRICULAR INTERDEPENDENCE

Although the two ventricles are different in terms of their morphometry and the preload and afterload forces to which they are subjected, the function of one ventricle is related to the other by muscle fibers that encircle both chambers, a common deformable septum, and the pericardium that surrounds both chambers. The right and left heart are so intimately connected that it is not surprising that changes in systolic and diastolic performance of one side will be reflected in the other, though to what extent is a matter of some controversy. Since the end-diastolic pressure and volume in one ventricle is a function of the end-diastolic pressure and volume in the other, the degree to which direct interdependence is a significant factor in changing LV function is difficult to separate from those in series effects, particularly in the intact circulation. Santamore and colleagues[30] have shown a decrease in LV diastolic volume and an increase in RV volume with inspiration. In the isolated heart, Janicki and coworkers[31] have demonstrated that if LV end-diastolic volume is held constant while RV end-diastolic volume is increased, LV end-diastolic pressure will rise. Therefore, if LV filling pressure remains constant during acute distention of the right ventricle, the stroke volume of the left ventricle will decrease. This diastolic interdependence is thought to be responsible for some of the decrease in LV stroke volume seen during inspiration. In contrast, studies in intact humans and experimental animals have shown that though diastolic compliance of the left ventricle is altered by septal wall shift during RV filling, this does not inhibit systolic function when there is no cardiopulmonary disease.[32, 33] Robotham[34] has suggested that both acute changes in LV afterload and RV volume, which are seen to occur as a consequence of diastolic interdependence during negative ITP, contribute to the decrease in LV stroke

volume and the increase in end-diastolic pressure seen with inspiration.

The corollary of this is the finding of systolic interdependence. As the RV volume rises, the end-systolic volume of the left ventricle decreases,[35] indicating that the LV stroke volume is maintained by decreased afterload. Thus, systolic interdependence is a compensatory mechanism to any reduction in LV output due to diastolic interdependence.[36]

PERICARDIUM

Because it surrounds the heart and limits acute changes in chamber size, the pericardium will influence cardiac function directly and will also affect output through the mechanism of ventricular interdependence. In the normal situation, the pericardium has some minor influence on both diastolic and systolic function of the ventricles in that ventricular interaction is enhanced during diastole by transmission of pressures throughout the myocardium. In situations in which there is an increase in intrapericardial pressure, as in the dilated, failing heart or with the development of pericardial fluid accumulation, there can be major alterations in systolic and diastolic performance of both ventricles. However, changes in intrapericardial pressure cannot be examined in isolation without making reference to pressure changes in the thorax produced by ventilation. Any influence that the pericardium may have on the function of either ventricle is related to a change in transmural pressure across the wall of the myocardium, which in this instance is the difference between intracavity and intrapleural-intrapericardial pressure. Constraint on ventricular function because of changes in intrapericardial pressure will always be more pronounced in diastole than in systole. The change in transmural pressure that occurs with the development of a pericardial effusion will interfere with diastolic filling, and the larger the effusion and the more rapidly it develops, the greater will be the compromise to ventricular function.[37] The intrapericardial pressure also contributes to ventricular interdependence, being increased in situations of cardiac tamponade[38] and reduced following pericardectomy.[39] As the majority of coronary blood flow occurs during diastole, the pericardial constraint on the RV free wall may limit coronary perfusion in situations in which the ventricle has hypertrophied.[40, 41] The dilated and failing heart will also become constrained within the pericardial cavity, resulting in a rise in intrapericardial pressure and interference with diastolic filling.

LEFT VENTRICULAR FUNCTION AND SPONTANEOUS RESPIRATION

The most commonly observed change in left heart function that occurs with spontaneous respiration is a fall in arterial pressure during inspiration because of a decrease in LV stroke volume.[34] The reasons for this have been attributed mainly to events occurring on the right side of the circulation but also include effects of negative ITP on the function of the left ventricle. The explanations advanced for this fall in output include (1) the pooling of blood in the pulmonary circulation because of lung expansion, (2) a phase lag between RV and LV output, (3) the stimulation of systemic baroreceptors or pulmonary stretch receptors, (4) right heart filling causing a change in LV diastolic compliance or ejection mediated through ventricular interdependence, and (5) an increase in LV afterload caused by a change in ITP.

In order to determine the significance of these various forces and the effect of positive or negative ITP on LV preload and afterload, it is important to understand the changes in transmural pressure produced by alterations in ITP. If LA and ventricular diastolic pressures were measured relative to atmosphere (see Fig. 41–2), one could demonstrate a fall in these pressures relative to atmosphere during inspiration, which would support the concept that the principal cause of the decrease in left-sided output during inspiration was pooling of blood in the lungs. However, it has been shown in both the intact animal and the isolated lung preparation that during inspiration, pulmonary venous return actually increases at the same time that LV stroke volume is falling.[42, 43] This apparent contradiction is explained when these pressures are related to intrapleural pressure; transmural filling pressures on the left side are shown to actually increase during inspiration.[44, 45] Thus, it is more accurate to define the pressure load as being equal to the pressure gradient across the wall of the ventricle (transmural pressure), which in this instance is the intracavity pressure minus the intrapleural pressure.

Studies of pulmonary transit time have shown that it takes one to two cardiac cycles for a change in right-sided output to be reflected in the left side.[46, 47] However, the phase lag theory is also unlikely to explain the decrease in LV ejection associated with a fall in ITP. In experiments in which preload through the pulmonary circulation was maintained constant by replacing the right ventricle with a roller pump in closed chested, spontaneously breathing dogs, stroke volume still declined during inspiration.[48] This finding does not mean that changes in right heart output must not at some stage affect the left side, as the two circulations are connected in series, which accounts for the observation that blood pressure and LV stroke volume rise after an initial fall.[49] In this situation, the increase in venous return eventually overides the other factors that tend to impede LV output.

Neural receptors that have been suggested to influence LV function include stretch receptors in the lung supplied by the vagus nerve and intra- and extrathoracic baroreceptors that are mediated by the autonomic system. There is reliable experimental data to suggest that neither of these is likely to be a major mechanism in the fall of left-sided output. Robotham and colleagues[48] found that there were still significant falls in LV stroke volume in vagotomized animals during Meuller maneuver, in which intrapleural pressure falls but lung volume remains unchanged. A decrease in LV stroke volume during inspiration is still seen even with autonomic blockade of vagal and sympathetic efferent nerves. Di-

astolic ventricular interdependence does influence LV preload, but any reduction is offset by the increased LV output due to systolic interdependence.[50]

There is abundant experimental evidence that negative ITP has a significant inhibitory effect on LV ejection by increasing afterload and that this is particularly pronounced in lung disease in which there are increasingly negative swings in ITP. In addition, increases in pulmonary lymph flow have been shown to occur with increased respiratory loads in experimental animals.[51] The observation that afterload increases with negative ITP has been confirmed by studies of LV function during spontaneous breathing with increased inspiratory loads in which both LV end-diastolic and end-systolic volumes are increased.[49, 52] However, though LV end-systolic volumes increase when ITP falls during normal inspiration, they also increase when a negative ITP is not associated with a change in lung volume during a Mueller maneuver.[45, 53] This would suggest that ventricular interdependence plays a minor role in the increase in LV afterload. Alternatively, echocardiographic studies would suggest that interdependence does influence LV function. Both Brinker and Guzman and their associates[54, 55] have shown septal wall displacement during the Mueller maneuver that is associated with decreased diastolic compliance and volume of the LV.

Sustained decreases in ITP have also been shown clinically to produce mild degrees of LV dysfunction in the setting of ischemic heart disease.[56] Since the generation of large negative ITP can impede both diastolic and systolic performance of the left ventricle, it is not surprising that this may result in acute LV failure and the development of pulmonary edema. This has been well documented to occur following acute upper airway obstruction with laryngospasm during anesthesia[57-60] and with croup and epiglottitis.[61-63] It may also occur following the relief of upper airway obstruction[64] and during status asthmaticus, when at the peak of inspiration, a negative ITP of up to -40 cm H_2O can be produced.[65]

Various mechanisms have been invoked to explain the marked fall in LV stroke volume arterial blood pressure that occurs with large, negative ITP generated by spontaneous respiration (pulsus paradoxus) during severe airway obstruction. It has been difficult to determine whether it is due to decreased LV filling or increased afterload because repeated LV filling and emptying may occur contemporaneously with a single inspiration that extends over several cardiac cycles. In a series of experiments, Peters and colleagues[66, 67] attempted to clarify this issue by synchronizing negative ITP with systole and diastole independently in experimental animals. Their findings would suggest that negative ITP with the airway obstructed during systole reduces LV stroke volume predominantly by increasing afterload and impedance to blood flow out of the thorax. Similar changes were noted with the airway unobstructed. When negative ITP was synchronized with diastole, LV output fell because of ventricular interdependence.

Changes in lung volume also affect LV function independent of the change in ITP. Lung expansion changes the capacitance of the pulmonary venous sys-

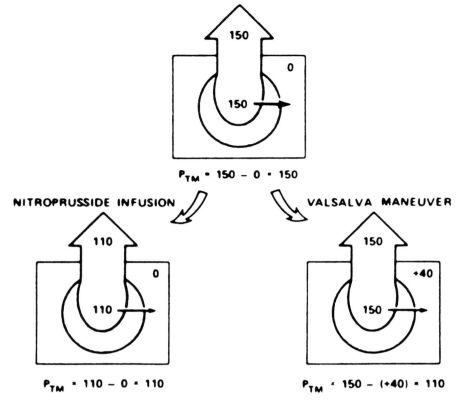

Figure 41–6. A schematic diagram of the left ventricle *(crescent)*, thoracic cavity *(box)*, and aorta *(arrow)*. Similar changes in left ventricular transmural pressure (PTM) can be produced by decreasing aortic pressure (nitroprusside) or by raising ITP (Valsalva maneuver). (From Snyder JV and Pinsky MR [eds]: Oxygen Transport in the Critically Ill. Chicago, Year Book Medical Publishers, 1987.)

tem, thereby altering pulmonary blood flow depending on the underlying pulmonary blood volume and vascular tone.[24, 68] Increasing lung volume also restricts cardiac filling in a fashion similar to cardiac tamponade by encroachment of the lung on the cardiac fossa.[27] The overall effect of a negative ITP on LV function is therefore a balance between its effect on the preload and LV systolic ejection.

SPONTANEOUS RESPIRATION AND ABNORMAL HEART FUNCTION

Left Ventricular Failure

Since decreases in ITP tend to both augment cardiac output by increased systemic venous return and diminish it by increasing LV afterload, the net result will be a balance between these opposite effects. Negative ITP may adversely affect LV performance, but whether the increase in afterload becomes hemodynamically significant depends on the underlying pump function. We have seen that in the normovolemic state in which flow limitation conditions exist, any increase in venous return is limited by collapse of the large veins as they enter the thorax. Similarly, if LV function is normal, even sustained negative ITP will result in little or no readily identifiable adverse hemodynamic change.[69, 70] Some of the studies that have examined the magnitude of the afterload effect produced by increased negative or positive ITP have tended to underestimate its significance because of different methods of measuring afterload.

Considering the left ventricle in isolation, in situations in which there is a major change in ITP associated with increasing negative intrapleural pressures secondary to lung disease or positive intrapleural pressures secondary to mechanical ventilation, aortic pressure does not reflect LV afterload. This was confirmed in a study by Buda and associates of eight patients[71] in whom ventricular volumes were measured and plotted against aortic pressure and transmural aortic pressure (aortic pressure minus intrapleural pressure). Physiologically, more consistent function curves for the left ventricle were obtained when transmural pressure was used for the pressure load for LV ejection. If the LV filling pressure is unchanged, similar changes in LV afterload can result from either reducing aortic pressure by vasodilator therapy or increasing ITP if the net result is no change in transmural pressure (Fig. 41–6).

Although some diminution of LV ejection can be demonstrated when ventricular function is normal,[49, 52, 71] it is only comparatively recently that worsening LV function in the presence of LV failure has been shown to be associated with negative ITP in the clinical situation. Rasanen and associates[72] first showed that changing from spontaneous to positive-pressure breathing in patients with myocardial infarction resulted in a decrease in the pattern of injury seen on the electrocardiogram and subsequently confirmed that the myocardial sparing occurred only when the negative swings in ITP were abolished.[73, 74] Similarly Beach and colleagues[75] described a series of patients with LV failure supported with positive pressure ventilation who could not tolerate being weaned to spontaneous ventilation until LV function was improved with inotropic support. Based on these findings, we can conclude that in patients with overt cardiac failure or borderline LV function, the increased afterload associated with the negative ITP generated during spontaneous respiration will result in worsening heart failure. Furthermore, in situations in which pulmonary edema develops following myocardial infarction, the pulmonary venous congestion and alveolar flooding that occur lead to a fall in lung compliance, which translates into increased respiratory work and greater negative ITP. Under these conditions, a positive ITP with the use of positive pressure ventilation or continuous positive airway pressure (CPAP) may result in rapid improvement in the situation with interruption of the cycle of increasingly negative ITP producing an ever-decreasing lung compliance. Therefore, changing ITP has differing effects on LV ejection, depending on whether function is normal or compromised. Increasing ITP with positive pressure in the setting of LV failure, far from adversely affecting cardiac output, as has been widely assumed, may in fact enhance cardiac performance in certain circumstances.

Congenital Heart Disease

The presence of congenital cardiac disease in children will frequently produce changes within the lung that result in respiratory symptoms that sometimes make it difficult to distinguish whether the primary disease process is within the lung or the heart. In the case of congenital heart disease, lesions that produce abnormal patterns of pulmonary blood flow through the lungs can produce changes in mechanics that can both mimic lung disease and, by increasing respiratory work and oxygen consumption, aggravate heart failure. The extent of these changes depends on whether pulmonary blood flow is increased, as in the situation of a left-to-right intracardiac shunt, or decreased, as in right-to-left shunts.

Cardiac lesions with left-to-right intracardiac shunting produce pulmonary changes that result from a combination of increased pulmonary blood flow and increased pulmonary artery pressure. These lesions include the most common cardiac defects such as atrial septal defects and patent ductus arteriosus, and though these conditions permit increased blood flow through the lungs, they are unlikely to produce pulmonary hypertension or respiratory symptoms unless they remain undiagnosed for a prolonged period. When the communication for the left-to-right shunt is large and occurs at the level of the ventricles or great vessels (ventricular septal defect, aortopulmonary window, or single ventricle), high flows and pressures may be transmitted to the pulmonary circulation, and changes to the pulmonary vascular bed will occur that result in alterations in lung mechanics. The amount of shunting that will occur depends on the relative resistances of the pulmonary and systemic circulations, which change with age. In the normal newborn, PVR is high at birth but then declines significantly with age. The factors associated with this fall in PVR in the newborn period are an increase in the alveolar P_{O_2}

and expansion of the lung. Beyond the neonatal period, a more gradual reduction in PVR occurs secondary to growth and remodeling of the pulmonary vascular bed, with regression of smooth muscle in the media of the arterial wall.[76] In addition, the intra-acinar pulmonary arteries develop in conjunction with alveoli, increasing the overall area of the pulmonary vascular bed. Factors such as a decrease in lung water after birth[77] and a reduction in blood viscosity with the fall in hemoglobin[78] may contribute to this reduction in PVR. The importance of this last effect on the degree of left-to-right shunting has been shown in the study by Lister and associates.[78] These investigators were able to demonstrate a significant reduction in systemic-to-pulmonary shunting in infants with congestive heart failure and ventricular septal defects by increasing the hemoglobin concentration from 10 to 15 g/dl with blood transfusion, while the blood volume was kept constant. These observations would suggest that in the newborn period, even in the presence of large systemic to pulmonary communications, only a small amount of shunting will occur because the resistances in the two circulations are balanced. Shunting will increase and signs of congestive heart failure occur as PVR falls beyond the newborn period.

Increases in pulmonary blood flow due to left-to-right shunting will result in an elevated pulmonary venous return and enlargement of the left atrium. These, in turn, will aggravate the increase in PVR produced by the increased flow through the lungs and further elevate pulmonary artery pressure (Fig. 41–7). The combination of increased pulmonary blood flow and pulmonary hypertension is well recognized as producing severe respiratory symptoms.[79] Respiratory distress and atelectasis in the spontaneously breathing child can result from compression of the large bronchi by an enlarged left atrium or pulmonary artery dilatation and can be responsible for the sudden increase in airway resistance seen in ventilated children who have a reactive pulmonary vascular bed. The left atrium lies immediately inferior to both main stem bronchi and the left main stem bronchus. The left upper lobe bronchus and the right middle lobe bronchus are the most common sites of obstruction.[80] Infantile lobar emphysema has also been described in association with pulmonary stenosis.[79] Rabinovitch and colleagues[81] have described compression of large bronchi by dilated main pulmonary arteries and compression of intrapulmonary bronchi by tufts of abnormal pulmonary vessels in the absent pulmonary valve syndrome. Any of these abnormalities can result in lobar atelectasis, emphysema, intermittent attacks of wheezing, and blood gas abnormalities. These respiratory symptoms are more likely to occur after the first 2 months of life, when the PVR drops and left-to-right shunting increases, and before the end of the first year, when the airways become more cartilaginous and less susceptible to compression.[80]

In addition to compression of large airways, children with left-to-right shunts may be susceptible to bronchiolar narrowing owing to the high flows and pulmonary venous pressure producing interstitial and alveolar edema. Hordof and associates[82] have described clinical

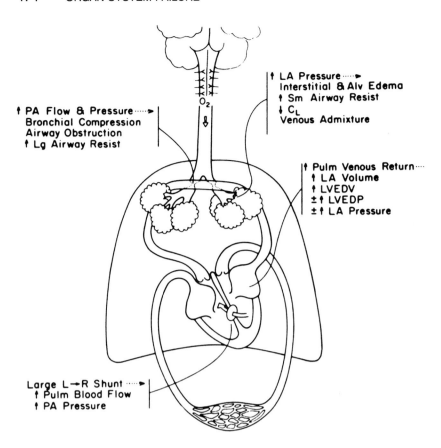

↑ PA Flow & Pressure ┈┈➤
Bronchial Compression
Airway Obstruction
↑ Lg Airway Resist

O₂

↑ LA Pressure ┈┈➤
Interstitial & Alv Edema
↑ Sm Airway Resist
↓ C_L
Venous Admixture

↑ Pulm Venous Return ┈┈
↑ LA Volume
↑ LVEDV
±↑ LVEDP
±↑ LA Pressure

Large L→R Shunt ┈┈➤
↑ Pulm Blood Flow
↑ PA Pressure

Figure 41–7. Potential sites where left to right shunting in congenital heart disease may adversely affect respiratory system mechanics. The increased pulmonary blood flow and pulmonary artery pressure may lead to increased airways resistance owing to compression of large or small bronchi while alveolar and interstitial edema may result in decreased lung compliance. (From Lister G and Talner N: Management of respiratory failure of cardiac origin. *In*: Gregory GA [ed]: Respiratory Failure in the Child. New York, Churchill Livingstone, 1981.)

and radiologic manifestations of peripheral airway obstruction in infants with ventricular septal defect associated with increased pulmonary: systemic flow ratios, which regressed with closure of the defect. Motoyama and colleagues[83] have demonstrated increased airway resistance measured by expiratory flow volumes in patients with large left-to-right shunts prior to corrective cardiac surgery. These changes were reversed following closure of the defect. In a more recent study, the same authors[84] have measured expiratory flows ($FEF_{75\%}$) in children under general anesthesia at the time of corrective cardiac surgery. They found that increased pulmonary blood flow, secondary to left-to-right shunts, was associated with a decrease in $FEF_{75\%}$. Furthermore, when they performed a morphometric analysis on lung biopsy material taken at the time of surgery, they observed that patients with medial hypertrophy of the small pulmonary arteries showed prominent smooth muscle hypertrophy and narrowing of the lumen of alveolar ducts and respiratory bronchioles. Those observations may explain the finding of a sudden increase in airway resistance commonly seen in patients who experience a rapid rise in pulmonary artery pressure following corrective cardiac surgery for lesions such as ventricular and atrioventricular septal defects. It is possible that some of the bronchoconstrictor response seen in pulmonary hypertension may be mediated, at least in part, by the leukotriene products of arachidonic metabolism. Leukotrienes C4 and D4, previously known as the slow-reacting substance of anaphylaxis, which is known to be a mediator of bronchoconstriction in

asthma, have been shown to be present in large quantities in the lung lavage fluid of infants with persistent pulmonary hypertension.[85]

There are also changes in lung compliance seen in congenital cardiac disease.[86-88] Bancalari and coworkers[86] have found that both total and specific lung compliance was significantly lower in children with congenital heart disease in whom there was increased pulmonary blood flow, compared with lesions with a normal or decreased pulmonary blood flow. When pulmonary blood flow was increased but pulmonary artery pressure was normal, compliance was unchanged, suggesting that it was the pressure level rather than the increased flow within the lung that actually caused the alteration in compliance. Decreased pulmonary compliance has also been described in newborn infants with persistent pulmonary hypertension.[89] These changes in compliance are responsible for the increased respiratory rate and decreased tidal volume seen during spontaneous respiration in children with left-to-right intracardiac shunts.[90] In the infant or small child with a highly compliant chest wall, this is frequently associated with chest wall retraction and intercostal recession. With increasing age, these conditions become less prominent as PVR rises, secondary to increased flow, and left-to-right shunting diminishes.

In congenital heart lesions associated with right-to-left intracardiac shunts, desaturated blood passes from the venous to the arterial side of the circulation, bypassing the lungs. These lesions fall into three different categories: (1) isolated right-to-left shunts such as those that occur in tetralogy or critical pulmonary stenosis in which the shunt is proximal to the obstruction; (2) bidirectional shunts seen in transposition of the great arteries and double-outlet right ventricle, in which systemic venous blood returns to the aorta and pulmonary venous blood returns to the pulmonary artery; and (3) common mixing lesions such as truncus arteriosus and pulmonary atresia with intact intraventricular septum, in which systemic and pulmonary venous blood mix in a common chamber before ejection from a functionally common ventricle. In this last group of lesions, the pulmonary and systemic circulations behave as two parallel circulations with shunt-dependent pulmonary blood flow, rather than two systems in series, and the ratio of blood flow in the parallel circuits depends on the relative balance between the pulmonary and the systemic vascular resistance. Another example of this type of lesion with parallel circulations is the infant with hypoplastic left heart syndrome who frequently presents with cyanosis and heart failure beyond the immediate newborn period when the PVR falls and the ductus closes. In truncus arteriosus, the fall in PVR results in increased runoff into the pulmonary circulation and myocardial ischemia from poor coronary perfusion. Changes within the lung can alter the delicate balance between these two circulations. An increase in inspired oxygen and arterial pH can lead to a decrease in PVR in hypoplastic left heart syndrome, with increased shunting across the ductus arteriosus and a fall in systemic output with a rise in PaO_2. A similar sequence of events can occur if PVR is abruptly changed in truncus arteriosus.[91] In pulmonary atresia with intact interventricular septum, normal pulmonary blood flow is obstructed at the pulmonary valve. Infants with this condition require left-to-right ductal flow to perfuse the lungs. When this is replaced by a systemic-to-pulmonary surgical shunt, a similar physiology of a shunt-dependent pulmonary blood flow with parallel circulations exists, and the balance may be altered significantly by changing ventilation.

SUMMARY OF CARDIOPULMONARY INTERACTIONS DURING SPONTANEOUS RESPIRATION

In the normal heart, a decrease in pleural pressure during inspiration results in increased venous return and RV preload. At the same time, RV afterload (increased wall stress during systole) increases during inspiration because of increased pulmonary arterial transmural pressure and an increase in RV volume without a change in shape, producing increased wall tension. In conditions in which lung volume at FRC is greatly increased, a rise in PVR will further increase RV afterload. LV stroke volume and aortic pressure fall during inspiration partly because of decreased LV preload, which is mediated partly by the effects of RV distention working through the ventricular interdependence mechanism and partly through lateral compressive forces from the lung, both decreasing LV volume. LV afterload also increases during inspiration and is particularly exaggerated during the generation of large negative inspiratory forces. The increased afterload produced by negative ITP may precipitate cardiac failure in the setting of underlying LV ischemia or dysfunction, and this cardiac failure can be reversed by the use of positive ITP. In the setting of congenital heart disease, increased pulmonary blood flow resulting from left-to-right intracardiac shunting can produce significant changes in compliance and resistance within the lung that may mimic pulmonary disease.

POSITIVE INTRATHORACIC PRESSURE AND THE NORMAL HEART

It has been recognized from the very outset of the widespread use of positive pressure ventilation that there are major effects on hemodynamics associated with its use. Courand and associates[92] were the first to show the association between the decreased cardiac output and increased airway pressure in normal humans more than 40 years ago. The widely accepted explanation for this finding was that increased ITP is transmitted to the systemic venous system and reduces the gradient for RA filling; this has been confirmed in numerous studies since then.[93–99] However, the mechanisms involved are much more complex than a simple reduction in venous return. With the more widespread use of positive pressure ventilation and positive end-expiratory pressure (PEEP) it has become increasingly obvious that there may be other mechanisms involved that produce different responses depending on the underlying pathophysiology. Although positive ITP reduces cardiac output in the normovolemic or hypovolemic state, significantly different effects are produced when positive-pressure ventilation and PEEP are applied in the setting of cardiac or pulmonary disease, when changes in lung mechanics, PVR, or ventricular function will modify the hemodynamic responses. In order to understand these differences, it is important to examine the complex cardiopulmonary interactions that occur in the normal state with an increase in ITP.

In positive-pressure ventilation, increased airway pressure is transmitted to the pleural space (see Fig. 41–2). The increase in ITP reduces the pressure gradient for venous return to the right atrium. As has been clearly shown in the studies of Morgan and co-workers[100, 101] caval blood flow was shown to decrease during inflation of the lungs. At the same time that systemic venous return decreases, the increase in pleural pressure causes the right heart volume to decrease because of the decreased transmural RA pressure, which, in turn, leads to a fall in RV stroke volume. In the normovolemic and, to a greater extent, the hypovolemic state, the pulmonary venous blood flow to the left atrium would be significantly reduced with positive ITP, whereas in the hypervolemic state, pulmonary venous return would be increased because of augmented antegrade flow. These same principles also apply during spontaneous respiration if the increase in pleural pressure occurs without a change in lung volume as in the Valsalva maneuver.[102–104] What has been less widely appreciated is that in the normal situation there is an initial increase in both aortic pressure and LV output early in the inspiratory phase of positive pressure ventilation before they fall toward the end of inspiration.[96, 98, 101] Scharf and associates[98] have shown that this increase in aortic pressure is more pronounced at faster respiratory rates (see Fig. 41–8). In contrast, changes in respiratory rate have little effect on pulmonary artery flow, which declines during inspiration and rises during expiration. It appears, therefore, that increased pleural pressure will have different effects on the right and left heart output at different phases of the respiratory cycle, in which a fall in pulmonary artery flow and a rise in pulmonary arterial pressure are seen at the same time, as there is a rise in both pressure and flow in the aorta early in the inspiratory phase of intermittent positive-pressure ventilation (IPPV).

These differing effects require more detailed analysis. Among the theories that have been advanced to account for them are (1) a phase lag resulting from pulmonary transit time, (2) a reduction in LV afterload associated with positive pleural pressure, (3) increased LV preload resulting from forward flow of pulmonary venous blood due to lung expansion, and (4) increased LV compliance through ventricular interdependence. The fact that pulmonary transit time has little or no bearing on the asynchrony between right and left heart has been demonstrated in the intact animal by Robotham and associates.[105] In these experiments, right heart output was replaced by a roller pump to maintain a constant left-sided preload. Aortic flow still increased during the early phase of inspiration despite the elimination of the variation in RV output. In a further series of experiments in open chest animals in which pleural pressure was no longer a factor, and with the right heart decompressed, which eliminated the ventricular interdependence factor, Robotham and Mitzner[106] were also able to show that the application of positive pressure to the lung still results in increased LV output. They were also able to demonstrate that following a sustained inspiration with a constant flow into the pulmonary artery, aortic flow abruptly drops with the following inspiration and rises again with the first lung inflation following an expiratory apneic pause. The conclusion that could be drawn from these studies is that changes in lung volume and PVR are the major influences on the variation in LV output.

Although the alterations in preload produced by raised ITP are the predominant mechanism for the reduction in cardiac output with IPPV, it has been suggested that the addition of PEEP may adversely affect ventricular contractility[107–110] and cause ventricular compression by lung distention.[27, 111] Several studies[48, 112, 113] have shown that LV dimensions are altered by both intermittent positive-pressure ventilation and PEEP in that the septal to free wall and anterior to posterior minor axis dimensions diminish, which is consistent with an overall decrease in LV end-diastolic volume. These changes tend to be more pronounced with IPPV than with PEEP,[112] and the effect is greater in the septal to free wall dimension, which suggests that ventricular interdependence is an important mechanism contributing to the decreased LV preload seen in posi-

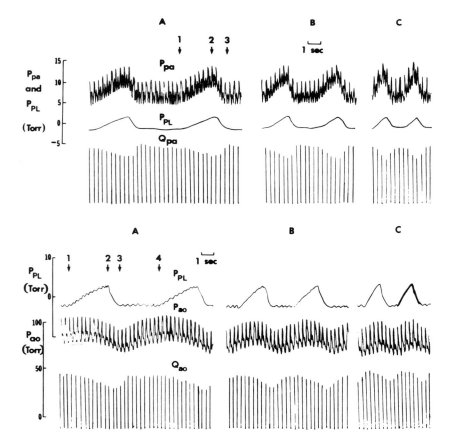

Figure 41–8. Pulmonary *(top panel)* and systemic *(lower panel)* hemodynamic changes associated with positive pressure ventilation in the anesthetized dog at (A) slow, (B) medium, and (C) fast respiratory rates. Pa = pulmonary artery pressure; PPL = pleural pressure; QPA = pulmonary arterial flow; QAO, aortic flow. Pulmonary artery pressure and flow increase with the rise in pleural pressure associated with inspiration. At the same time aortic pressure and flow fall, reaching a minimum early in expiration (A). With increasing respiratory rates aortic pressure and flow increase during inspiration, reaching a minimum late in expiration. (From Scharf SM, Brown R, Saunders N, et al: Hemodynamic effects of positive pressure inflation. J Appl Physiol 49:124, 1980.)

tive-pressure ventilation. The septal to free wall changes are perhaps more likely to represent laterally acting forces produced by mechanical heart-lung interactions[27, 114] than actual septal wall shift per se. There is evidence that the pressure within and the size of the ventricular chambers may be directly affected by lung inflation. This observation has been confirmed in a study in which intraventricular pressures were directly measured during IPPV with PEEP. It was shown that the intracavity pressures rose slightly at the end-expiratory point and were even more exaggerated at end-inspiration.[115] PEEP, in addition to increasing pleural pressure, will increase lung volume and FRC, depending on lung and chest wall compliance. If this overdistends the lung and increases PVR, an increase in RV volume will occur, which will adversely affect LV compliance through interventricular dependence. However, in the common situation in which PEEP is being used, the RV volume will diminish, and therefore any decrease in LV size cannot be attributed to ventricular interdependence.

It has also been suggested that PEEP may reduce cardiac output and LV stroke volume by a depression of the contractile state of the left ventricle,[107–110] perhaps through the release of a circulating myocardial depressant factor. With the introduction of more sophisticated measurement techniques of LV function, there is no evidence to support the notion that the contractile state of the left ventricle is decreased with increased ITP, either in the setting of a normal lung or in acute pulmonary edema.[116, 117] However, raised ITP has the potential to adversely affect contractility in the setting of marginal coronary blood flow. PEEP has been reported to cause a decrease in myocardial blood flow in experimental animals.[118, 119] Tittley and colleagues[120] have shown that the application of 15 cm H_2O after coronary artery bypass surgery resulted in small but measurable amounts of markers of marginal coronary perfusion in half the patients without a change in ventricular function.

POSITIVE INTRATHORACIC PRESSURE IN CARDIAC DISEASE

Right Heart

Independent of changes in RV preload, increased ITP associated with positive pressure ventilation will have differing effects on RV function, depending on the presence or lack of underlying cardiac or pulmonary disease and the level of inspiratory and end-expiratory pressure used. For example Rankin and associates[32] found that the application of PEEP in the normal human and animal heart resulted in a fall in cardiac output resulting from decreased preload (venous return) and increased afterload (PVR). The net result was a decrease in LV end-diastolic volume resulting from decreased preload but no change in systolic RV function. Further evidence that suggests that PEEP has no effect on RV contractility comes from a study of the application of increasing increments of PEEP up to 25 cm H_2O in the setting of adult respiratory distress syndrome

(ARDS).[121, 122] There was no change in RV ejection even at the highest PEEP levels, though stroke volume did decrease because of reduced preload. However, in the situation of severely depressed baseline RV ejection in humans, the application of PEEP can be shown to depress contractile function.[123] The reason for this difference may lie in the presence or lack of underlying RV ischemia.[124] Schulman and colleagues[125] have shown differing effects of PEEP before and after coronary ligation in the intact animal. In the normal heart, there was no change in RV volume or systolic performance, but following right coronary artery ligation, the RV ejection fraction declined in association with an increase in end-systolic volume. PEEP can further compromise flow in a marginal right coronary circulation because of decrease in flow associated with the rise in RV systolic pressure[126, 127] and intrapericardial pressure.[128] Similar observations on the differing effects of PEEP on RV ejection fraction have been made on adults with ischemic heart disease after cardiopulmonary bypass.[129] Patients with pronounced right coronary artery stenosis had diminished RV ejection fraction and RV end-diastolic volume, whereas there was no effect in patients with minor coronary artery stenosis. Paradoxically, in situations in which severe RV failure results in profoundly low cardiac output, ventilation with high peak inflation pressures at rapid rates may result in a rapid improvement in hemodynamics. Serra and colleagues[130] have reported a dramatic improvement in four children with severe RV failure after corrective cardiac surgery when they were switched from conventional ventilator settings to higher frequency (50/min), high-volume-tidal volume, (30 ml/kg) ventilation. The increase in ITP in this situation probably works as an RV assist, acting as an auxiliary pump to increase forward flow from a dilated and noncontractile right ventricle. We have observed a similar response in three children with severe right-sided failure, two cases of which occurred after the Fontan procedure in which pulmonary blood flow is entirely supported by the right atrium.[131]

Left Heart

Although there is substantial experimental and human data to suggest that in the setting of normal cardiac function, preload factors are the predominant forces responsible for the respiratory variation in LV function during IPPV, with or without PEEP, and that they may be compensated for by volume infusion[92, 132–134] the situation is clearly very different in the presence of the failing left ventricle in which increased pleural pressure may, in fact, reduce LV afterload.[73, 74] The extreme example of this is the discovery that during ventricular fibrillation in which there is no LV output, raising intrathoracic pressure by coughing results in forward blood flow out of the thorax, the phenomenon commonly referred to as "cough cardiopulmonary resuscitation (CPR)."[135] Although this may be the ultimate example of the reduction of LV afterload with increased ITP, there is now abundant clinical data to show that although increased pleural pressure will result in decreased cardiac output in hypo- or normovolemic individuals, cardiac output may be significantly improved in individuals with evidence of LV failure.[136, 137]

Some of the most interesting insights into the effects of elevations in ITP in the setting of LV failure come from the work of Pinsky and colleagues.[138] In their animal model, LV failure was induced with large doses of β-blockade, while adequate venous return was maintained by volume infusion. In order to study the effects of large increases in ITP cardiac function without overdistending the lung and causing increased PVR and pulmonary barotrauma, they reduced thoracic cage compliance by applying a thoracoabdominal binder. Tidal volumes of 35 ml/kg were used to produce a "phasic high intrathoracic pressure support" ventilation (PHIPS) (Fig. 41–9). The study showed that there was an improvement in both LV and RV function curves with increased ITP, a finding that they attributed to a decrease in LV wall stress analogous to the use of vasodilator therapy in congestive heart failure (see Fig. 41–6). The same technique was applied to a group of patients with cardiogenic shock, and when conventional ventilator settings were changed to PHIPS, there was an improvement in cardiac output and mean arterial pressure[139] (Fig. 41–10).

Although it is clear that these large changes in ITP augment cardiac output in the failing heart, the mechanism reponsible for this action is a balance between the effect on LV preload and afterload. Large changes in lung volume will affect intra- and extra-alveolar blood volume[24] and result in increased forward flow in a

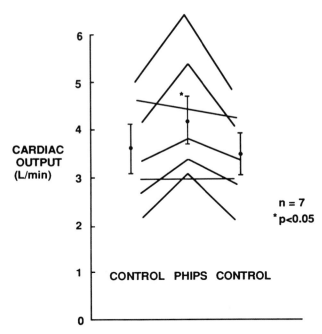

Figure 41–10. Effect of phasic high intrathoracic pressure support (PHIPS) plus thoracoabdominal binding on cardiac output in human subjects with cardiogenic shock. *Circles* represent mean values for the group. Cardiac output increases significantly with PHIPS. (From Pinsky MR and Summer WR: Cardiac augmentation by phasic high intrathoracic pressure support in man. Chest 84:370, 1983.)

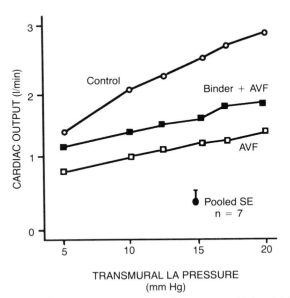

Figure 41–9. Relationship between cardiac output and left atrial (LA) pressure in the setting of acute LV failure (AVF) induced by β-blockade in animals ventilated with high tidal volume, rapid rate ventilation. Both mean values and slopes of AVF are significantly less than control. When thoracoabdominal binding was used to decrease thoracic cage compliance, thus allowing for an increase in ITP without overdistending the lung, the mean values for for binder-AVF are significantly greater than AVF (p<0.05). (From Pinsky MR, Summer WR, Wise RA, et al: Augmentation of cardiac function by elevation of intrathoracic pressure. J Appl Physiol 54:950, 1983.)

manner analogous to cough CPR. At the same time, increased ITP will reduce LV afterload. These differing mechanisms were studied in a further series of experiments by Pinsky and associates[93] in which they varied respiratory frequency, percent inspiratory time, mean ITP, and swings in ITP using a jet ventilator under normal conditions and during acute LV failure. They found that despite a decrease in transmural LA pressure, a rise in ITP resulted in an increase in LV stroke volume (Fig. 41–11). Furthermore, this increase in stroke volume continued until a lower limit of LA pressure was reached, after which there was no further augmentation of LV stroke volume. This demonstrates that when cardiac function is reduced and filling pressures are elevated, an increase in ITP can result in an improvement in cardiac output despite a fall in filling pressures. However, this augmentation becomes limited once filling pressures fall to less than a critical value when cardiac output again becomes dependent upon filling pressures. A similar effect has been described when ITP is increased by the addition of PEEP in the setting of LV dysfunction in humans.[136] The application of PEEP in this situation did not result in a decrease in cardiac output until the filling pressure fell to less than 15 mm Hg. These data, as well as data from human studies that show enhanced cardiac performance with increased pressure ITP in the setting of cardiogenic shock,[72, 73] would suggest that this aspect of the beneficial effect of increased ITP on LV performance was preload-dependent, being least beneficial when LV filling was reduced and most marked when LV filling pressures were elevated. The predominant hemodynamic effect of in-

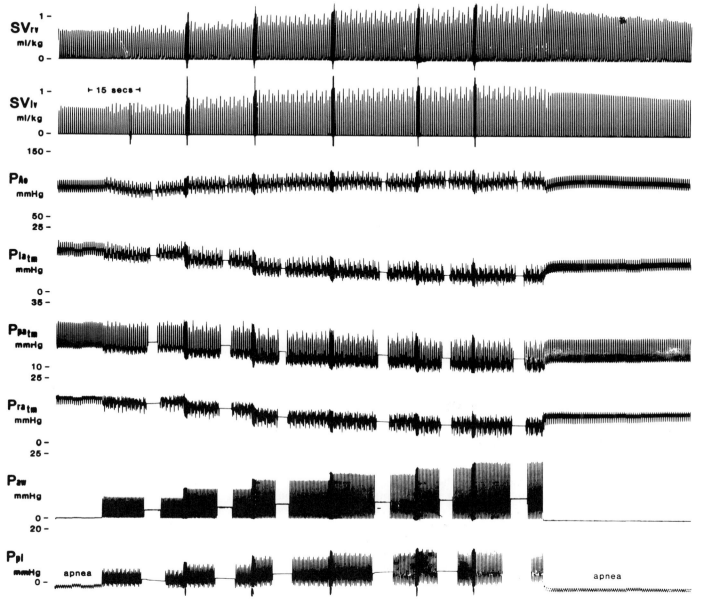

Figure 41–11. Effect of increased ITP produced by high frequency jet ventilation in an animal model of acute ventricular failure (AVF) induced by β-blockade. The trend recordings are for right ventricular stroke volume (SV$_{RV}$), left ventricular stroke volume (SV$_{LV}$), aortic pressure (P$_A$), transmural left atrial pressure (Platm), right atrial pressure (Pratm), airway pressure (Paw), and pleural pressure (Ppl). ITP is increased in a stepwise fashion from apnea while the LV filling pressure falls but the SV$_{LV}$ increases until the filling pressure falls below 14 mm Hg. (From Pinsky MR, Matuschak GM, and Klain M: Determinants of cardiac augmentation by elevations in intrathoracic pressure. J Appl Physiol 58:1189, 1985.)

creased ITP will result from changes in preload if contractility and circulating volume are normal, whereas in situations of reduced LV function, in which filling pressures are frequently elevated, the principal hemodynamic change will be changes in LV wall stress (afterload).

It has recently become evident that hemodynamic changes that occur with increased ITP also vary according to different phases in the cardiac cycle. This has been demonstrated in the recent studies by Pinsky and associates[140] in which positive pressure ventilation was linked to the cardiac cycle by the use of a jet ventilator in animals with LV failure. When positive pressure was timed to occur early in diastole in normal animals, LV stroke volume was decreased, whereas when it was timed to coincide with early systole, there was no effect. They also found that when positive pressure was phased with early diastole, the reduction in stroke volume of the right ventricle preceded that of the left ventricle by one to two heartbeats, suggesting that the cause of the reduction was due to reduced venous return. In the animals with LV failure, increased ITP in phase with systole increased LV stroke volume compared with diastole, though the increased ITP in either phase was associated with increased stroke volume when compared with apnea (Fig. 41–12). These investigators then compared the hemodynamic effects of increases in ITP synchronized with early and late systole. They found that although increased ITP in both phases of the systolic cycle was associated with an increase in stroke volume when compared with apnea, early systolic phase ventilation resulted in an increase in stroke volume without a change in aortic pressure, whereas late systolic ventilation increased both stroke volume and pressure (Fig 41–13). These findings would suggest that positive-pressure ventilation synchronized with early cardiac systole allows for LV ejection into a volume-depleted thoracic aorta. They have applied these principles in the clinic arena for the ventilatory management of patients with severe congestive cardiomyopathy who are undergoing heart transplantation.[141] They compared the effects of high-frequency jet ventilation synchronized with cardiac systole, high-frequency jet ventilation asynchronous with the cardiac cycle, and conventional ventilation at similar levels of ITP. They found that changing to synchronous high-frequency jet ventilation was associated with an increase in cardiac output compared with the other modes of ventilation. Similar improvements in cardiac output with synchronized high-frequency jet ventilation have been reported by McIntyre in patients with heart failure who required ventilation.[142]

Positive Intrathoracic Pressure and Congenital Heart Disease

Changing the PVR by positive pressure ventilation can profoundly affect the amount of either right-to-left or left-to-right shunting. In the setting of the shunt-dependent parallel circulations, positive pressure ventilation by changing PVR can radically alter the balance between the systemic and pulmonary circulations. The abnormal pulmonary vascular bed is also highly susceptible to changes in both blood gases and lung mechanics. The former has been used to advantage in infants with persistent pulmonary hypertension. Drummond and associates[143] have shown that hyperventilation down to a $PaCO_2$ less than 25 mm Hg and a pH greater than 7.6 resulted in marked increases in PaO_2 secondary to a reduction in pulmonary arterial pressure: systemic arterial pressure ratio. Similarly Peckham and Fox[144] have been able to demonstrate a reduction in pulmonary arterial pressure with hyperventilation to a $PaCO_2$ of less than 30 mm Hg in a group of newborn infants with primary pulmonary hypertension. Whether the pulmonary vasodilator effect of hyperventilation is due to a change in $PaCO_2$ or pH, or both, has been a subject of some dispute since the original observations of Rudolph and Yuan[145] that showed increases in PVR with hypoxia and acidosis. Schreiber and associates have shown that metabolic and respiratory alkalosis were equally effective at attenuating hypoxic vasoconstriction, but that hypocapnia alone (normal pH with hypocapnia) had no effect.[146] Although hyperventilation is widely accepted as a method of treating increases in pulmonary arterial pressure in infants, until recently little information was

available on the response of the pulmonary vascular bed beyond the newborn period. Salmenpera and Heinonen[147] have shown that the pulmonary vascular bed in the adult may respond in a similar fashion. They examined the effect of hypocarbia and hypercarbia on PVR in a group of patients undergoing coronary artery bypass surgery and showed that pulmonary arterial pressure increased significantly with a rise in $PaCO_2$ and decreased during hypocarbia. This effect of CO_2 occurred independent of any change in tidal volume or FRC. In a subsequent study, they evaluated RV performance in response to various $PaCO_2$ levels following bypass surgery.[148] They found that a $PaCO_2$ of 50 mm Hg was associated with a 54% increase in PVR and a 34% increase in pulmonary arterial pressure. In addition there were significant increases in RV end-diastolic volume and a decrease in RV ejection. Morray and associates[149] have also shown a similar beneficial effect on RV function in acutely reducing $PaCO_2$ in children with congenital heart disease and pulmonary hypertension.

As well as the actual changes in blood gases, there is additional evidence that there is a beneficial effect of positive pressure on lung mechanics that helps in controlling pulmonary arterial pressure. Mechanical ventilation by stretching the lung releases prostaglandins,[150, 151] which cause pulmonary vasodilatation and help explain the rapid reductions in pulmonary arterial pressure that are seen immediately after the onset of hyperventilation before there has been any time for a change in $PaCO_2$. Changes in lung volume may also account for the abrupt rises in pulmonary arterial pressure when weaning the patient from mechanical ventilation to CPAP. Jenkins and colleagues[152] have shown in a group of children following cardiac surgery that when weaning from a low ventilatory rate to CPAP there is a fall in FRC and a rise in pulmonary arterial pressure and PVR, especially in children with underlying pulmonary hypertension. Studies in newborn infants following corrective surgery for congenital heart disease show that compliance is low in the postoperative period and the application of CPAP frequently results in improvements in FRC and PaO_2.[153, 154]

POSITIVE INTRATHORACIC PRESSURE AND PULMONARY FAILURE

Postive Pressure Ventilation (PPV)

Positive-pressure ventilation and PEEP are frequently used in pulmonary failure associated with pulmonary edema and low lung compliance as a method of increasing FRC and improving oxygenation. If this were the only consideration, it would simply be a case of increasing PEEP until the best PaO_2 was achieved. However, the adverse effects of PEEP on cardiac output mean that the most important therapeutic goal is the level of PEEP that gives the best combination of oxygenation and cardiac output, thereby achieving maximum oxygen delivery (oxygen content × cardiac output). This concept has been termed *best* or *optimal PEEP* by Suter

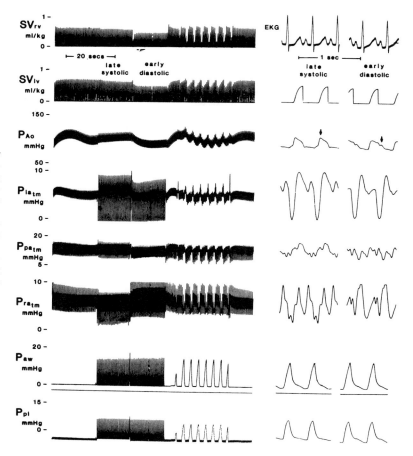

Figure 41–12. The effect of increased ITP, produced by high-frequency jet ventilation, synchronised with late systolic and early diastolic phases of the cardiac cycle in control-binder conditions compared with apnea. Early diastolic synchronous HFJV resulted in a decrease in LV stroke volume, whereas there was no change with early systole. SVrv = right ventricular stroke volume; SVlv = left ventricular stroke volume; PAO, Pla$_{tm}$ = transmural left atrial pressure; Pra$_{tm}$ = transmural right atrial pressure; Ppa$_{tm}$ = transmural pulmonary artery pressure; Paw = airway pressure; Ppl = pleural pressure. (From Pinsky MR, Matuschak GM, Bernardi L, et al: Hemodynamic effects of cardiac cycle specific increases in intrathoracic pressure. J Appl Physiol 60:604, 1986.)

and associates.[155] In their study on patients with ARDS, they found that the optimal PEEP level in each individual was that which produced the highest static lung compliance; this level varied between 0 and 15 cm H_2O. It is a simple exercise to apply increasing amounts of PEEP in the setting of ARDS, but to define the changes in hemodynamics that are produced by this therapy has proved more difficult. The magnitude of these changes will depend partly on factors that influence the underlying cardiovascular status (circulating volume, ventricular dysfunction, increased PVR) and on factors within the lung that may modulate the transmission of airway pressure to the pleural space, such as decreased lung compliance, which will reduce it,[156] or increased thoracic compliance, which will enhance it.[157] Taking all these factors into consideration, it is still common to see a fall in cardiac output and stroke volume with high levels of positive-pressure ventilation with PEEP in ARDS, primarily because of a decrease in LV preload, which can be compensated for by volume expansion.[117, 122, 133, 158, 159] The mechanisms that have been invoked as a cause for this decrease include decreased venous return, increased RV afterload, decreased LV compliance, and decreased ventricular contractility. There are conflicting data on what the most important factors are depending on how the various measurements were made. As is seen with positive-pressure ventilation in the normal lung, the increase in pleural pressure with PEEP reduces venous return to the right heart in ARDS,[121, 122, 133] and there is

little dispute that this is a major factor in the reduction of RV preload. Levels of PEEP greater than 10 cm H_2O are also associated with a slight increase in RV afterload in human studies of ARDS,[117, 122, 133, 158] but there is little effect on RV contractility.[160, 161]

Severe ARDS is frequently associated with acute pulmonary artery hypertension caused by acute vasoconstriction and intravascular thrombosis. The increased RV afterload may alter RV performance. Sibbald and colleagues have shown that RV end-diastolic volume increases with increasing pulmonary arterial pressure.[162] Patients with ARDS have a higher RV end-diastolic volume and a decrease in RV ejection fractions when compared with controls.[163] Further observations on the effect of increased ITP on RV function in the setting of acute respiratory failure have been made that show an adverse effect on RV systolic function by the mechanism of increased RV impedance. This has been confirmed in a recent study by Jardin and associates[164] in which they examined the effect on RV function of changes in ITP at different phases of the respiratory cycle produced by positive pressure ventilation. Lung inflation during inspiration was associated with reduced RV ejection fraction and end-systolic volume, thus increasing RV wall stress or afterload. Decreased output from the right heart, in turn, reduces LV preload and LV end-diastolic volume.[33, 71] These changes are frequently compensated for by expansion of circulating volume, which, by increasing RV preload, can compensate for RV overload-

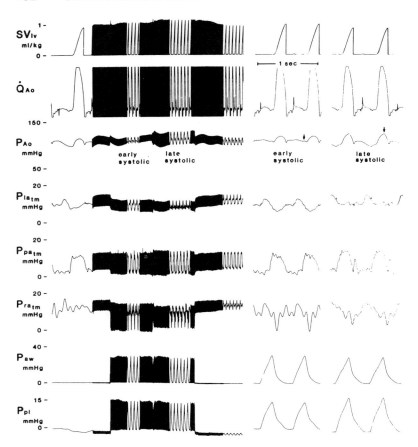

Figure 41-13. The effect of increased ITP produced by HFJV synchronised with early and late systole in an animal with AVF. Although both were associated with an increase in SVlv, early systolic synchrony did not increase aortic pulse pressure over apnea whereas late systolic did, suggesting that the increased stroke volume was being ejected into a volume depleted aorta. SVlv = left ventricular stroke volume; Pao, Pla$_{tm}$ = transmural left atrial pressure; Pra$_{tm}$ = transmural right atrial pressure; Ppa$_{tm}$ = transmural pulmonary artery pressure; Paw = airway pressure; Ppl = pleural pressure; Q̇ao. (From Pinsky MR, Matuschak GM, Bernardi L, et al: Hemodynamic effects of cardiac cycle specific increases in intrathoracic pressure. J Appl Physiol 60:604, 1986.)

ing by increasing myocardial segment length.[134] Positive pressure applied to the lung is also known to alter PVR by compression of the intra-alveolar vessels and at the same time increasing the cross-sectional diameter of extra-alveolar vessels by radial traction. The former effect will increase PVR, whereas the latter effect will cause a decrease. Which effect predominates depends on the underlying condition of the lung. Jardin and colleagues[165] have shown that PVR increases with positive intrathoracic pressure in humans with normal lungs, thus increasing RV afterload. However, in the setting of acute respiratory failure, the underlying PVR is increased,[166] and compliance is reduced. These changes will modify the effect of positive-pressure ventilation, as only part of the increased airway pressure will be transmitted to the pleural space.[157]

Decreased ventricular compliance due to direct mechanical heart-lung interaction from lung inflation has been advanced as an explanation for the decrease in LV preload in ARDS.[118, 167] This would reduce diastolic compliance and impede filling. However, more sophisticated measurements using direct measurements of pressure at the surface of the heart showed little change in compliance.[168] Another of the suggested mechanisms for the reduction in cardiac output with PEEP in ARDS comes from the observations of Jardin and colleagues that there is a left-sided shift of the ventricular septum with the application of PEEP in ARDS and that this is responsible for the reduction in LV preload. Filling pressures were restored with volume infusion in this

study, but LV size failed to return to normal, suggesting a reduction in compliance of the left ventricle. Indeed, flattening of the intraventricular septum was noted at high PEEP levels, suggesting that ventricular interdependence plays a part in the hemodynamic effects of PEEP. However, this effect was seen only at PEEP levels of more than 25 cm H$_2$O at which the degree of lung inflation will result in a marked increased RV afterload and flattening of the intraventricular septum.

LV contractility seems to be unaffected by acute lung injury. Studies of experimental lung injury in animals have shown that there are changes in end-diastolic volume and compliance rather than systolic performance.[169, 170] Although there are data in experimental animals to suggest that PEEP reduces myocardial contractility,[110, 119] human studies of patients with ARDS do not support this finding.[133, 171] On the contrary, Jardin and colleagues[158] have shown an increase in contractility with PEEP in ARDS. The situation may be different when there is underlying coronary ischemia in which contractility may be adversely affected by the addition of PEEP.

Continuous Positive Airway Pressure (CPAP)

Patients who are capable of maintaining adequate spontaneous ventilation in ARDS with use of CPAP will achieve better oxygenation for the same level of

PEEP with less adverse hemodynamic effect and therefore better oxygen delivery[172–174] because of lower mean airway pressures. Dhainaut and colleagues[175] have observed that patients with ARDS show a decrease in RV end-systolic and end-diastolic volumes, suggesting a fall in RV afterload, when patients were changed from spontaneous respiration to CPAP. Jardin and colleagues[165] have observed the opposite effects in normal subjects without lung disease. This discrepancy is explained by the fact that when FRC is normal, PVR is at its lowest and RV afterload is minimal. The application of CPAP increases lung volume to greater than FRC and compresses the extra-alveolar vessels, thus increasing RV afterload. In contrast, FRC is considerably reduced in ARDS and PVR is increased at these low lung volumes, a situation that can be reversed by the application of CPAP. Dhainaut and coworkers have also been able to demonstrate both a cardiac output and oxygen consumption decrease during CPAP, but with volume expansion cardiac output increases, whereas oxygen consumption remains low, suggesting decreased oxygen demand. They have suggested that the explanation for the reduced demand is the reduced oxygen consumed by the work of breathing following the application of CPAP.

SUMMARY OF CARDIOPULMONARY INTERACTIONS DURING POSITIVE-PRESSURE VENTILATION

The inspiratory increase in pleural pressure that occurs during positive-pressure ventilation results in decreased venous return and reduced RV preload. Changes in RV volume and RV ejection that alter pulmonary venous return will do so in a manner determined by the underlying characteristics of the lung. Aortic pressure and blood flow increase during the initial phase of increased intrathoracic pressure, whereas LV afterload tends to decrease. In the setting of LV failure, significant reductions in LV afterload can be achieved with positive pressure ventilation, especially if it is linked to the systolic phase of cardiac contraction. Positive-pressure ventilation can be used to rapidly alter PVR resistance in the setting of congenital heart disease in which pulmonary blood flow is very sensitive to changes in pH mediated through $Paco_2$ levels. The use of PEEP in acute respiratory failure leads to increased FRC, a rise in pulmonary compliance, and improved oxygenation. Although there may be adverse effects on venous return and LV preload, these effects may be minimized by applying ventilatory support in the CPAP mode rather than by intermittent positive-pressure ventilation with PEEP.

References

1. Bove AA and Santamore WP: Ventricular interdependence. Prog Cardiovasc Dis 23:365, 1981.
2. Guyton AC, Lindsey AW, Abernathy B, et al: Venous return at various right atrial pressures and the normal venous return curve. Am J Physiol 189:609, 1957.
3. Sylvester JT, Goldberg HS, and Permutt S: The role of the vasculature in the regulation of cardiac output. Clin Chest Med 4:111, 1983.
4. Ekelund LG and Holmgren A: Central hemodynamics during exercise. Circ Res 20 and 21:33, 1967.
5. Robotham JL and Scharf S: Effects of positive and negative pressure ventilation on cardiac performance. Clin Chest Med 4:161, 1983.
6. Oboler AA, Keefe JF, Gaasch WH, et al: Influence of left ventricular isovolumic pressure upon right ventricular pressure transients. Cardiology 58:32, 1973.
7. Santamore WP, Lynch PR, Meier GD, et al: Myocardial interaction between the ventricles. J Appl Physiol 41:362, 1976.
8. Santamore WP, Lynch PR, Heckman JL, et al: Left ventricular effects of right ventricular developed pressures. J Appl Physiol 41:925, 1976.
9. Badke FR, Boinay P, and Covell JW: Effects of ventricular pacing on regional left ventricular performance in the dog. Am J Physiol 238:H858, 1980.
10. Little WC, Barr WK, and Crawford MH: Altered effect of the Valsalva maneuver on left ventricular volume in patients with cardiomyopathy. Circulation 71:227, 1985.
11. Pearlman AS, Clark CE, Henry WL, et al: Determinants of ventricular septal motion: Influence of relative right and left ventricular size. Circulation 54:83, 1976.
12. Shimazaki Y, Kawashima Y, Mori T, et al: Ventricular function of single ventricle after ventricular septation. Circulation 61:653, 1980.
13. Weymann AE, Wann S, Feigenbaum H, et al: Mechanism of abnormal septal motion in patients with right ventricular volume overload: A cross-sectional echocardiographic study. Circulation 54:179, 1976.
14. Bakos ACP: The question of the function of the right ventricular myocardium: An experimental study. Circulation 1:724, 1950.
15. Donald DE and Essex HE: Pressure studies after inactivation of the major portion of the canine right ventricle. Am J Physiol 176:155, 1954.
16. Kagan A: Dynamic responses of the right ventricle following extensive damage by cauterization. Circulation 5:816, 1952.
17. Starr I, Jeffers WA, and Meade RH Jr: The absence of conspicuous increments of venous pressure after severe damage to the right ventricle of the dog, with a discussion of the relation between clinical congestive failure and heart disease. Am Heart J 26:291, 1943.
18. Sawatani S, Mandell G, Kusaba E, et al: Ventricular performance following ablation and prosthetic replacement of right ventricular myocardium. Trans Am Soc Artif Intern Organs 20:629, 1974.
19. Likoff MJ, Sutton MG St J, Weber KT, et al: The effect of chronic pulmonary hypertension on left ventricular size and dynamics. Circulation 66:327, 1982.
20. Weiss JL, Eaton LW, Maughan WL, et al: Ventricular size and shape by two-dimension echocardiography. Fed Proc 40:2031, 1981.
21. West JB and Dollery CT: Distribution of blood flow and the pressure-flow relations of the whole lung. J Appl Physiol 20:175, 1965.
22. Hughes JMB, Glazier JB, Maloney JE, et al: Effect of lung volume on the distribution of pulmonary blood flow in man. Respir Physiol 4:58, 1968.
23. Permutt S: Relation between pulmonary artery pressure and pleural pressure during the acute asthmatic attack. Chest 63(Suppl.):25, 1973.
24. Brower R, Wise RA, Hassapoyannes C, et al: Effect of lung inflation on lung blood volume and pulmonary venous flow. J Appl Physiol 58:954, 1985.
25. Permutt S, Wise RA, and Brower RG: How changes in pleural and alveolar pressure cause changes in afterload and preload. In: Scharf SM and Cassidy SS (eds): Heart Lung Interactions in Health and Disease. New York, Marcel Dekker, 1989, p. 243.
26. Nunn JF: Applied Respiratory Physiology, 2nd ed. London, Butterworths, 1977, p. 213.
27. Lloyd TC Jr: Mechanical cardiopulmonary interdependence. J Appl Physiol 52:333, 1982.
28. Suga H and Sagawa K: Instantaneous pressure-volume relationships and their ratio in the excised, supported canine left ventricle. Circ Res 35:117, 1974.

29. Grossman W, Braunwald E, Mann T, et al: Contractile state of the left ventricle in man as evaluated from end-systolic pressure-volume relations. Circulation 56:845, 1977.

30. Santamore WP, Bove AA, and Heckman JL: Right and left ventricular pressure-volume response to positive end-expiratory pressure. Am J Physiol 246:H114, 1984.

31. Janicki JS, Reeves RC, Weber KT, et al: Application of a pressure servo system developed to study ventricular dynamics. J Appl Physiol 37:376, 1974.

32. Rankin JS, Olsen CO, Arentzen CE, et al: The effects of airway pressure on cardiac function in intact dogs and man. Circulation 66:108, 1982.

33. Olsen CO, Tyson GS, Maier GW, et al: Dynamic ventricular interaction in the conscious dog. Circ Res 52:85, 1983.

34. Robotham JL: Cardiovascular disturbances in chronic respiratory insufficiency. Am J Cardiol 47:941, 1981.

35. Weber KT, Janicki JS, Shroff S, et al. Contractile mechanisms and interaction of the right and left ventricles. Am J Cardiol 47:686, 1981.

36. Slinker BK and Glantz SA: End-systolic and end-diastolic ventricular interdependence. Am J Physiol 251:H1062, 1986.

37. Janicki JS and Weber KT: The pericardium and ventricular interaction, distensibility and function. Am J Physiol 238:H494, 1980.

38. Reddy PS, Curtis EL, O'Toole JD, et al: Cardiac tamponade: Hemodynamic observations in man. Circulation 58:265, 1971.

39. Taylor RR, Covell JW, Sonnenblick EH, et al: Dependence of ventricular distensibility on filling of the opposite ventricle. Am J Physiol 213:711, 1967.

40. Jarmakani JMM, McHole PA, and Greenfield JC Jr: The effect of the cardiac tamponade on coronary hemodynamics in the awake dog. Cardiol Res 9:112, 1973.

41. O'Rourke RA, Fischer DP, Escobar EE, et al: Effect of acute pericardial tamponade on coronary blood flow. Am J Physiol 212:549, 1967.

42. Guntheroth WG, Morgan BC, and Mullins GL: Effect of respiration on venous return and stroke volume in cardiac tamponade. Circ Res 20:381, 1967.

43. Howell JBL, Permutt S, Proctor DF, et al: Effect of inflation of the lung on different parts of pulmonary vascular bed. J Appl Physiol 16:71, 1961.

44. Robotham JL, Lixfield W, Holland L, et al: The effects of respiration on cardiac performance. J Appl Physiol 44:703, 1978.

45. Summer WR, Permutt S, Sagawa K, et al: Effects of spontaneous respiration on canine left ventricular function. Circ Res 45:719, 1979.

46. Franklin DL, Van Citters RL, and Rushmer RF: Balances between right and left ventricular output. Circ Res 10:17, 1962.

47. Maloney JE, Bergel DH, Glazier JB, et al: Transmission of pulsatile blood pressure and flow through the isolated lung. Circ Res 23:11, 1968.

48. Robotham JL, Rabson J, Permutt S, et al: Left ventricular hemodynamics during respiration. J Appl Physiol 47:1295, 1979.

49. Scharf SM, Brown R, Tow DE, et al: Cardiac effects of increased lung volume and decreased pleural pressure in man. J Appl Physiol 47:257, 1979.

50. Janicki JS, Shroff SG, and Weber KT: Ventricular interdependence. In: Scharf SM and Cassidy SS (eds): Heart-Lung Interactions in Health and Disease. New York, Marcel Dekker, 1989, p 285.

51. Loyd JE, Nolop KB, Parker RE, et al: Effects of inspiratory resistance loading on lung fluid balance in awake sheep. J Appl Physiol 60:198, 1986.

52. Scharf SM, Brown R, Saunders N, et al: Effects of normal and loaded spontaneous inspiration on cardiovascular function. J Appl Physiol 47:582, 1979.

53. Robotham JL, Badke FR, Kindred MK, et al: Regional left ventricular performance during normal and obstructed spontaneous respiration. J Appl Physiol 55:569, 1983.

54. Brinker JA, Weiss JL, Lappe DL, et al: Leftward septal displacement during right ventricular loading in man. Circulation 61:623, 1980.

55. Guzman PA, Maughan WL, Lin FCP, et al: Transseptal pressure gradient with leftward septal displacement during the Mueller maneuver in man. Br Heart J 46:657, 1981.

56. Scharf SM, Bianco JA, Tow DE, et al: The effects of large negative intrathoracic pressure on left ventricular function in patients with coronary artery disease. Circulation 63:871, 1981.

57. Conzanitis DA, Leijala M, Pesoner E, et al: Acute pulmonary edema due to laryngeal spasm. Anesthesia 37:1198, 1982.

58. Lee KWT and Downes JJ: Pulmonary edema secondary to laryngospasm in children. Anesthesiology 59:347, 1983.

59. Jackson FN, Rowland V, and Corssen G: Laryngospasm-induced pulmonary edema. Chest 78:819, 1980.

60. Poulton TJ: Laryngospasm-induced pulmonary edema. Chest 80:762, 1981.

61. Travis KW, Todrea ID, and Shannon DC: Pulmonary edema associated with croup and epiglottitis. Pediatrics 59:695, 1977.

62. Stradling JR and Bolton P: Upper airways obstruction as cause of pulmonary edema. Lancet 1:1353, 1982.

63. Oswalt CE, Gates GA, and Holstrom FMG: Pulmonary edema as a complication of acute upper airway obstruction. JAMA 238:1833, 1977.

64. Sofer S, Bar-Ziv J, and Scharf SM: Pulmonary edema following relief of upper airway obstruction. Chest 86:401, 1984.

65. Stalcup SA and Mellins RB: Mechanical forces producing pulmonary edema in acute asthma. N Engl J Med 297:592, 1977.

66. Peters J, Kindred MK, and Robotham JL: Transient analysis of cardiopulmonary interactions. I: Diastolic events. J Appl Physiol 64:1506, 1988.

67. Peters J, Kindred MK, and Robotham JL: Transient analysis of cardiopulmonary interactions. II: Systolic events. J Appl Physiol 64:1518, 1988.

68. Sylvester JT, Mitzner W, Ngeow Y, et al: Hypoxic constriction of alveolar and extra-alveolar vessels in isolated pig lungs. J Appl Physiol 54:1660, 1983.

69. Polianski JM, Huchon GJ, Gaudebout CC, et al: Pulmonary and systemic effects of increased negative inspiratory intrathoracic pressure in dogs. Am Rev Respir Dis 133:49, 1986.

70. Rebuck AS and Read J: Assessment and management of severe asthma. Am J Med 51:788, 1971.

71. Buda AJ, Pinsky MR, Ingels NB, et al: Effect of intrathoracic pressure on left ventricular performance. N Engl J Med 301:453, 1979.

72. Rasanen J, Nikki P, and Heikkila J: Acute myocardial infarction complicated by respiratory failure. The effects of mechanical ventilation. Chest 85:21, 1984.

73. Rasanen J, Heikkila J, Downs J, et al: Continuous positive airway pressure by face mask in acute cardiogenic pulmonary edema. Am J Cardiol 55:296, 1985.

74. Rasanen J, Vaisanen IT, Heikkila J, et al: Acute myocardial infarction complicated by left ventricular dysfunction and respiratory failure. Chest 87:158, 1985.

75. Beach T, Millen E, and Grenvik A: Hemodynamic response to discontinuance of mechanical ventilation. Crit Care Med 1:85, 1973.

76. Rabinovitch M and Reid LM: Quantitative structural analysis of the pulmonary vascular bed in congenital heart defects. In: Engle MA (ed): Pediatric Cardiovascular Disease. Philadelphia, FA Davis, 1981.

77. Bland RD, Hansen TN, Haberkern CM, et al: Lung fluid balance in lambs before and after birth. J Appl Physiol 53:992, 1982.

78. Lister G, Hellenbrand WE, Kleinman CS, et al: Physiologic effects of increasing hemoglobin concentration in left-to-right shunting in infants with ventricular septal defects. N Engl J Med 306:502, 1982.

79. Stanger P, Lucas RV Jr, and Edwards JE: Anatomic factors causing respiratory distress in acyanotic congenital cardiac disease: Special reference to bronchial obstruction. Pediatrics 43:760, 1969.

80. Lister G and Pitt BR: Cardiopulmonary interactions in the infant with congenital heart disease. Clin Chest Med 4:219, 1983.

81. Rabinovitch M, Grady S, David I, et al: Compression intrapulmonary bronchi by abnormally branching pulmonary arteries associated with absent pulmonary valves. Am J Cardiol 50:804, 1982.

82. Hordof AJ, Mellins RB, Gersony WM, et al: Reversibility of chronic obstructive lung disease in infants following repair of ventricular septal defect. J Pediatr 90:187, 1977.

83. Motoyama EK, Laks H, Oh T, et al: Deflation flow-volume (DFV) curves in infants with congenital heart disease (CHD): Evidence for lower airway obstruction. Circulation 58:107, 1978.

84. Motoyama EK, Tanaka T, Fricker FJ, et al: Peripheral airway obstruction in children with congenital heart disease and pulmonary hypertension (PAH). Am Rev Respir Dis 133:A10, 1986.
85. Stenmark KR, James SL, Voelkel NF, et al: Leukotriene C4 and D4 in neonates with hypoxemia and pulmonary hypertension. N Engl J Med 309:77, 1983.
86. Bancalari E, Jesse MJ, Gelband H, et al: Lung mechanics in congenital heart disease with increased and decreased pulmonary blood flow. J Pediatr 90:192, 1977.
87. Wallgren G, Geubelle F, and Koch G: Studies of the mechanics of breathing in children with congenital heart lesions. Acta Paediatr 49:415, 1960.
88. Howlett G: Lung mechanics in normal infants and infants with congenital heart disease. Arch Dis Child 47:707, 1972.
89. Yeh TF and Lilien LD: Altered lung mechanics in neonates with persistent fetal circulation syndrome. Crit Care Med 9:83, 1981.
90. Lees MH, Burnell RH, Morgan CL, et al: Ventilation-perfusion relationships in children with heart disease and diminished pulmonary blood flow. Pediatrics 42:778, 1968.
91. Wong RS, Baum VC, and Sangwan S: Truncus arteriosus: Recognition and therapy of intraoperative cardiac ischemia. Anesthesiology 74:378, 1991.
92. Courand A, Motley HL, Werko L, et al: Physiological studies of the effects of intermittent positive-pressure breathing on cardiac output in man. Am J Physiol 152:162, 1948.
93. Pinsky MR, Matuschak GM, and Klain M: Determinants of cardiac augmentation by elevations in intrathoracic pressure. J Appl Physiol 58:1189, 1985.
94. Brecker GA and Hubay CA: Pulmonary blood flow and venous return during spontaneous respiration. Circ Res 3:210, 1955.
95. Guyton AC: Effect on cardiac output by respiration, opening the chest, and cardiac tamponade. In: Guyton AC, Jones CE, and Coleman CE (eds): Circulatory Physiology: Cardiac Output and its Regulation. Philadelphia, WB Saunders, 1973, pp. 378–386.
96. Morgan BC, Crawford EW, and Guntheroth WG: The hemodynamic effects of changes in blood volume during intermittent positive-pressure ventilation. Anesthesiology 30:297, 1969.
97. Scharf SM, Caldini P, and Ingram RH Jr: Cardiovascular effects of increasing airway pressure in the dog. Am J Physiol 232:H35, 1977.
98. Scharf SM, Brown R, Saunders N, et al: Hemodynamic effects of positive pressure inflation. J Appl Physiol 49:124, 1980.
99. Charlier AA, Jaumin PM, and Pouleur H: Circulatory effects of deep inspirations, blocked expirations and positive pressure inflations at equal transpulmonary pressures in conscious dogs. J Physiol 241:589, 1974.
100. Morgan BC, Abel FL, Mullins GL, et al: Flow patterns in cavae, pulmonary artery, pulmonary vein, and aorta in intact dogs. Am J Physiol 20:865, 1966.
101. Morgan BC, Martin WE, and Hornberger JF: Intermittent positive pressure respiration. Anesthesiology 27:584, 1966.
102. Parisi AF, Harrington JJ, Askenazi J, et al: Echocardiographic evaluation of the Valsalva maneuver in healthy subjects and patients with and without heart failure. Circulation 54:921, 1976.
103. Brooker JZ, Alderman EL, and Harrison DC: Alterations in left ventricular volumes induced by Valsalva maneuver. Br Heart J 36:713, 1974.
104. Korner PI, Tonkin AM, and Uther JB: Reflex and mechanical circulatory effects of graded Valsalva maneuvers in normal man. J Appl Physiol 40:434, 1976.
105. Robotham JL, Cherry D, Mitzner W, et al: A re-evaluation of the hemodynamic consequences of positive pressure ventilation. Crit Care Med 11:783; 1983.
106. Robotham JL and Mitzner W: A model of the effects of respiration on left ventricular performance. J Appl Physiol 46:41, 1979.
107. Ashton JH and Cassidy SS: Reflex depression of cardiovascular function during lung inflation. J Appl Physiol 58:137, 1985.
108. Grindlinger GA, Manny J, Justice R, et al: Presence of negative inotropic agents in canine plasma during positive end-expiratory pressure. Circ Res 45:460, 1979.
109. Manny J, Grindlinger G, Mathe AA, et al: Positive end-expiratory pressure, lung stretch, and decreased myocardial contractility. Surgery 84:127, 1978.
110. Liebman PR, Patten MT, Manny J, et al: The mechanism of depressed cardiac output on positive end-expiratory pressure (PEEP). Surgery 83:594, 1978.
111. Scharf SM and Brown R: Influence of the right ventricle on left ventricular function with PEEP. J Appl Physiol 52:254, 1982.
112. Robotham JL, Bell RC, Badke FR, et al: Left ventricular geometry during positive end-expiratory pressure in dogs. Crit Care Med 13:617, 1985.
113. Visner MS, Arentzen CE, O'Conner MJ, et al: Alterations in left ventricular three-dimensional dynamic geometry and systolic function during acute right ventricular hypertension in conscious dog. Circulation 67:353, 1983.
1 4. Wallis TW, Robotham JL, Compean R, et al: Mechanical heart-lung interactions with positive end-expiratory pressure. J Appl Physiol 54:1039, 1983.
115. Robotham JL, Lixfield W, Holland L, et al: The effects of positive end expiratory pressure on right and left ventricular performance. Am Rev Respir Dis 121:667, 1980.
116. Johnston WE, Vinten-Johansen J, Santamore WP, et al: Mechanism of reduced cardiac output during positive end-expiratory pressure in the dog. Am Rev Respir Dis 140:1257, 1989.
117. Calvin JE, Driedger AA, and Sibbald WJ: Positive end-expiratory pressure (PEEP) does not depress left ventricular function in patients with pulmonary edema. Am Rev Respir Dis 124:121, 1981.
118. Cassidy SS, Mitchell JH, and Johnson RL Jr: Dimensional analysis of right and left ventricles during positive-pressure ventilation in dogs. Am J Physiol 242:H549, 1982.
119. Manny J, Patten MT, Liebman PR, et al: The association of lung distention, PEEP and biventricular failure. Ann Surg 187:151, 1978.
120. Tittley JG, Fremes SE, Weisel RD, et al: Hemodynamic and myocardial metabolic consequences of PEEP. Chest 88:496, 1985.
121. Potkin R, Hudson L, Weaver J, et al: Effect of positive end-expiratory pressure on right and left ventricular function in patients with the adult respiratory distress syndrome. Am Rev Respir Dis 135:307, 1987.
122. Viquerat C, Righetti A, and Suter P: Biventricular volumes and function in patients with ARDS ventilated with PEEP. Chest 83:509, 1983.
123. Schulman DS, Biondi JW, Matthay RA, et al: Effect of positive end-expiratory pressure on right ventricular performance: Importance of baseline right ventricular function. Am J Med 84:57, 1988.
124. Vlahakes GJ, Turley K, and Hoffman JI: The pathophysiology of failure in acute right ventricular hypertension: Hemodynamic and biochemical correlations. Circulation 63:87, 1981.
125. Schulman DS, Biondi JW, Zohgbi S, et al: Coronary flow limits right ventricular performance during positive end-expiratory pressure. Am Rev Respir Dis 141:1531, 1990.
126. Brooks H, Kirk E, Vokonas P, et al: Performance of the right ventricle under stress: Relation to right coronary flow. J Clin Invest 50:2176, 1971.
127. Bishop S, White F, and Bloor C: Regional myocardial blood flow during acute myocardial infarction in the conscious dog. Circ Res 38:429, 1976.
128. Fessler J, Braver R, Wise R, et al: Effect of positive pleural pressure on myocardial perfusion (Abstract). Am Rev Respir Dis 37:293, 1988.
129. Boldt J, Kling D, Bormann B, et al: Influence of PEEP ventilation immediately after cardiopulmonary bypass on right ventricular function. Chest 94:566, 1988.
130. Serra J, McNicholas KW, Moore R, et al: High frequency, high volume ventilation for right ventricular assist. Chest 93:1035, 1988.
131. Paret G, Taylor RH, Williams W, et al: Augmentation of right ventricular function by elevation of intrathoracic pressure. Am Rev Respir Dis 141:A68, 1990.
132. Braunwald E, Binion JT, Morgan WL, et al: Alterations in central blood volume and cardiac output induced by positive-pressure breathing and counteracted by metaraminol (Aramine). Circ Res 5:670, 1957.
133. Dhainaut JF, Devaux JY, Monsallier JF, et al: Mechanisms of decreased left ventricular preload during continuous positive-pressure ventilation in ARDS. Chest 90:74, 1986.
134. Qvist J, Pontoppidan H, Wilson RS, et al: Hemodynamic re-

sponses to mechanical ventilation with PEEP. Anesthesiology 42:45, 1975.

135. Criley JM, Balfuss AH, and Vissel GL: Cough-induced cardiac compression: Self-administered form of cardiopulmonary resuscitation. JAMA 236:1246, 1976.

136. Grace MP and Greenbaum DM: Cardiac performance in response to PEEP in patients with cardiac dysfunction. Crit Care Med 10:358, 1982.

137. Mathru M, Rao TLK, El-etr AA, et al: Hemodynamic response to changes in ventilatory pattern in patients with normal and poor left ventricular reserve. Crit Care Med 10:423, 1982.

138. Pinsky MR, Summer WR, Wise RA, et al: Augmentation of cardiac function by elevation of intrathoracic pressure. J Appl Physiol 54:950, 1983.

139. Pinsky MR and Summer WR: Cardiac augmentation by phasic high intrathoracic pressure support in man. Chest 84:370, 1983.

140. Pinsky MR, Matuschak GM, Bernardi L, et al: Hemodynamic effects of cardiac cycle-specific increases in intrathoracic pressure. J Appl Physiol 60:604, 1986.

141. Pinsky MR, Marquez J, Martin D, et al: Ventricular assist by cardiac cycle-specific increases in intrathoracic pressure. Chest 91:709, 1987.

142. MacIntyre NR: The effects of jet ventilation synchronized to cardiac systole in MICU patients. Chest 92:665, 1987.

143. Drummond WH, Gregory GA, Heymann MA, et al: The independent effects of hyperventilation, tolazoline, and dopamine on infants with persistent pulmonary hypertension. J Pediatr 98:603, 1981.

144. Peckam GJ, and Fox WW: Physiologic factors affecting pulmonary artery pressure in infants with persistent pulmonary hypertension. J Pediatr 93:1005, 1978.

145. Rudolph AM and Yuan S: Response of the pulmonary vasculature to hypoxia and H^+ ion concentration changes. J Clin Invest 45:399, 1966.

146. Schreiber MD, Heymann MA, and Soifer SJ: Increased arterial pH, not decreased $PaCO_2$, attenuates hypoxia-induced pulmonary vasoconstriction in newborn lambs. Pediatr Res 20:113, 1986.

147. Salmenpera M and Heinonen J: Pulmonary vascular responses to moderate changes in $PaCO_2$ after cardiopulmonary bypass. Anesthesiology 64:311, 1986.

148. Viitanen A, Salmenpera M, and Heinonen J: Right ventricular response to hypercarbia after cardiac surgery. Anesthesiology 73:393, 1990.

149. Morray JP, Lynn AM, and Mansfield PB: Effect of pH and PCO_2 on pulmonary and systemic hemodynamics after surgery in children with congenital heart disease and pulmonary hypertension. J Pediatr 113:474, 1988.

150. Berend N, Christopher KL, and Voelkel NF: The effect of positive end-expiratory pressure on functional residual capacity: role of prostaglandin production. Am Rev Respir Dis 126:646, 1982.

151. Berry EM, Edmonds JF, and Wyllie JH: Release of prostaglandin E2 and unidentified factors from ventilated lungs. Br J Surg 58:189, 1971.

152. Jenkins J, Lynn A, Edmonds J, et al: Effects of mechanical ventilation on cardiopulmonary function in children after open-heart surgery. Crit Care Med 13:77, 1985.

153. Hatch DJ, Taylor BW, Glover WJ, et al: Continuous positive airway pressure after open-heart operations in infancy. Lancet 9:469, 1973.

154. Gregory GA, Edmunds LH Jr, Kitterman JA, et al: Continuous positive airway pressure and pulmonary and circulatory function after cardiac surgery in infants less than three months of age. Anesthesiology 43:426, 1975.

155. Suter PM, Fairley HB, and Isenberg MD: Optimum end-expiratory airway pressure in patients with acute pulmonary failure. N Engl J Med 292:284, 1975.

156. Pontoppidan H, Wilson RS, Rie MA, et al: Respiratory intensive care. Anesthesiology 47:96, 1977.

157. Jardin F, Genevray B, Brun-Ney D, et al: Influence of lung and chest wall compliances on transmission of airway pressure to the pleural space in critically ill patients. Chest 88:653, 1985.

158. Jardin F, Farcot JC, Boisante L, et al: Influence of positive end-expiratory pressure on left ventricular performance. N Engl J Med 304:387, 1981.

159. Prewitt RM, Oppenheimer L, Sutherland JB, et al: Effect of positive end-expiratory pressure on left ventricular mechanics in patients with hypoxic respiratory failure. Anesthesiology 55:409, 1981.

160. Neidhart PP and Suter PM: Changes of right ventricular function with positive end-expiratory pressure (PEEP) in man. Intensive Care Med 14:471, 1988.

161. Zwissler B, Forst H, and Messmer K: Local and global function of the right ventricle in a canine model of pulmonary microembolism and oleic acid edema: Influence of ventilation with PEEP. Anesthesiology 73:964; 1990.

162. Sibbald WJ, Driedger AA, Cunningham DG, et al: Right and left ventricular performance in acute hypoxemic respiratory failure. Crit Care Med 14:852; 1986.

163. Brunet F, Dhainaut JF, Devaux MF, et al: Right ventricular performance in patients with acute respiratory failure. Intensive Care Med 14:474, 1988.

164. Jardin F, Delorme G, Hardy A, et al: Reevaluation of hemodynamic consequences of positive pressure ventilation: emphasis on cyclic right ventricular afterloading by mechanical lung inflation. Anesthesiology 72:966, 1990.

165. Jardin F, Farcot JC, Gueret P, et al: Echocardiographic evaluation of ventricles during continuous positive airway pressure breathing. J Appl Physiol 56:619, 1984.

166. Zapol WM and Snider MT: Pulmonary hypertension in severe acute respiratory failure. N Engl J Med 296:476, 1977.

167. Scharf SM, Brown R, Saunders N, et al: Changes in canine left ventricular size and configuration with positive end-expiratory pressure. Circ Res 44:672, 1979.

168. Fewell JE, Abendschein DR, Carlson J, et al: Continuous positive-pressure ventilation does not alter ventricular pressure volume relationship. Am J Physiol 240:H821, 1981.

169. Calvin JE, Baer RW, and Glantz SA: Pulmonary injury depresses cardiac systolic function through the Starling mechanism. Am J Physiol 251:H722; 1986.

170. Qvist J, Mygind T, Crottogini A, et al: Cardiovascular adjustments to pulmonary vascular injury in dogs. Anesthesiology 68:341, 1988.

171. Van Trigh P, Spray TL, Pasque MK, et al: The effect of PEEP on left ventricular diastolic dimensions and systolic performance following myocardial revascularization. Ann Thorac Surg 33:585, 1982.

172. Shah DM, Newell JC, Dutton RE, et al: Continuous positive airway pressure versus positive end-expiratory pressure in respiratory distress syndrome. J Thorac Cardiovasc Surg 14:557, 1977.

173. Simmoneau G, Lemaire F, Harf A, et al: A comparative study of the cardiorespiratory effects of continuous positive airway pressure breathing and continuous positive pressure ventilation in acute respiratory failure. Intensive Care Med 8:61, 1982.

174. Schlobohm, RM, Falltrick RT, Quan SF, et al: Lung volumes, mechanisms and oxygenation during spontaneous positive pressure ventilation: The advantage of CPAP over EPAP. Anesthesiology 55:416, 1981.

175. Dhainaut JF, Aoute P, Monsallier JF, et al: Improvement of RV performance by continuous positive airway pressure in ARDS. J Crit Care 2:15, 1987.

Extracorporeal Techniques

P. Pearl O'Rourke, M.D.

Clinical support of gas exchange has recently undergone a number of advances. Basic management remains increased ambient oxygen and various modes of pressure ventilation, ranging from continuous positive airway pressure (CPAP) to delivery of mechanical breaths by either positive or negative pressure ventilation. Although routine support is effective in the majority of clinical situations, there are limitations and risks. Conventional methods of support can be inadequate in patients with extremely severe lung disease: These patients can die of hypoxemia or hypercarbia, or both, in spite of maximal conventional support. In addition, conventional mechanical ventilation (CMV) has the associated morbidity of barotrauma and oxygen toxicity.[1, 2]

In recognition of these clinical limitations, investigators have developed methods of gas exchange that obviate the lungs. At present, these methods include extracorporeal membrane oxygenation (ECMO), extracorporeal CO_2 removal (ECCO$_2$R), and intravascular oxygenation (IVOX). Each of these technologies will be discussed.

EXTRACORPOREAL MEMBRANE OXYGENATION

The development of ECMO followed the development of cardiopulmonary bypass technology used in the operating room for cardiothoracic surgery. The first oxygenators were bubble oxygenators that were characterized by a direct blood-gas interface, causing hemolysis that limited the duration of safe exposure.[3] The development of membrane oxygenators with a physical separation between the blood and gas phase minimized hemolysis and introduced the potential for long-term support.[4] As soon as these oxygenators became available, they were used to support adult patients with acute respiratory failure (ARF). By the mid-1970s, 150 patients treated with ECMO had a reported 10% survival rate.[5] In response to these early reports, the National Institutes of Health sponsored a multicentered study to compare the effects of ECMO and CMV in an adult population with terminal ARF. Ninety-six patients with an 80% predicted mortality rate were selected and

randomized into CMV or ECMO. Unexpectedly, the results showed no difference—an 8.7% survival rate with CMV versus a 9.3% survival rate with ECMO.[6] These disappointing results halted the use of ECMO in patients with ARF.

Critics of the study felt that ECMO was effective support but that the entry criteria selected a group of patients who already had fibrosis and irreversible lung disease. Furthermore, they thought that ECMO would still prove beneficial if applied to a group of patients with reversible lung disease. Neonates with persistent pulmonary hypertension of the newborn were identified as a potential group. The first experience with neonatal ECMO was reported by Dorson and colleagues in 1969: He described partial venoarterial ECMO using umbilical vessels in five neonates; all died.[7] In 1973, White and coworkers reported the use of ECMO in three premature infants; all experienced fatal intracranial hemorrhages.[8] Bartlett and associates reported the first successful ECMO support of a full-term neonate in 1975.[9] At present, there are more than 70 centers in the United States that have offered neonatal ECMO to more than 5,000 full-term neonates whose predicted mortality rate was in excess of 80%.[10]

The neonatal experience has been systematically collected since 1981 in a national registry. This registry is sponsored by the Extracorporeal Life Support Organization (ELSO). Although patient reporting is voluntary, it is estimated that the registry captures at least 95% of the ECMO cases in the United States. The data from October 1991 given in Table 42–1 describe the national experience and show an overall survival rate of 83% with ECMO.

At present, the children selected for ECMO are infants who have completed at least 35 weeks' gestation and who have no more than a grade I or II intraventricular hemorrhage, no evidence of severe congenital heart disease, and a predicted fatality rate of at least 80%. Venoarterial ECMO is standard in these children. This procedure has been described elsewhere[11] and is illustrated in Figure 42–1. In venoarterial ECMO, the blood is drained from the child via a large catheter placed in the right internal jugular vein. Blood then flows through the circuit (pump, oxygenator, heat exchanger) and back into the baby through a catheter that is placed in the right common carotid artery and advanced into the

Table 42–1. NEONATAL ELSO* REGISTRY
OCTOBER 1991

Diagnosis	Survived		Died		Total
	Count	%	Count	%	
Meconium aspiration syndrome	1,919	93	148	7	2,067
Congenital diaphragmatic hernia	608	61	388	39	996
Respiratory distress syndrome	666	85	122	15	788
Primary persistent pulmonary hypertension of the newborn	606	88	86	12	692
Sepsis pneumonia	578	77	174	23	752
Other	145	79	39	21	184
Total	4,522	83	957	17	5,479

*ELSO = Extracorporeal Life Support Organization.

ascending aorta. While ECMO is in progress, the child and the ECMO circuit are heparinized to an activated clotting time approximately twice that of normal (200 to 220 seconds). ECMO flow in the range of 100 ml/kg/min is adequate to support oxygenation and ventilation. The native lungs are not expected to participate in gas exchange and are rested with a rate of 4 breaths/minute, FIO_2 of 0.21, and low ventilator pressures. The usual time course for an ECMO run is 5 to 8 days and is dependent on the cause of the lung disease. Infants with meconium aspiration have the shortest runs, and patients with congenital diaphragmatic hernia have the longest. It is important to remember that ECMO does

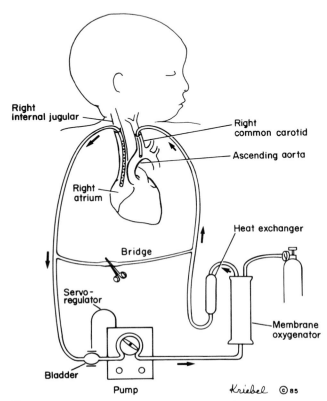

Figure 42–1. Venoarterial extracorporeal membrane oxygenation.

not cure lung disease, it merely supports gas exchange until the disease resolves. Another approach is to use venovenous ECMO, which can be performed with either a single- or double-catheter system. In two-catheter venovenous ECMO, outflow is through a catheter placed in the right atrium via the right internal jugular vein. Blood is then returned through a catheter placed in the femoral vein.[34] Single-catheter ECMO is usually carried out with a double-lumen catheter placed in the right atrium; the proximal lumen provides the outflow and the distal lumen provides the return.[35] There has been some experimentation of single-lumen venovenous ECMO. It requires a system of valves or pumps that allow time- or tidal flow–gated inflow-outflow cycles.[36]

Regardless of which system is used, venovenous ECMO has some basic differences when compared with venoarterial ECMO. Perhaps most important is the fact that venovenous ECMO does not support cardiovascular function. Second, the patient's PaO_2 is less in venovenous ECMO than in venoarterial ECMO. This reflects the fact that there is some degree of recirculation of oxygenated blood back into the ECMO circuit. Because the efficiency of gas exchange in venovenous ECMO is less than in venoarterial ECMO, often the patient's lungs have to be used to augment oxygenation. This obviates the ability to totally rest the lungs, which potentially has an impact on the ability of the patient's lungs to heal.

The infants selected for ECMO meet institutional criteria for an 80% predicted mortality rate. Most institutions have created their criteria via retrospective chart review of historical control populations.[12, 13] Common criteria are PAO_2-PaO_2 or an oxygenation index, which is calculated as the product of the FIO_2 and the mean airway pressure divided by the PaO_2. Oxygenation indices of 0.40 to 0.55 are generally used as predictors of high mortality. The use of historical controls has been criticized for potentially overestimating mortality. Cole and associates reported that when ECMO criteria were prospectively applied to a neonatal population, a predicted 80% mortality rate was only a 23% true mortality rate.[14] Dworetz and associates reported a similar study and found only a 17% true mortality rate.[15]

Historical control data are always problematic. Retrospective studies evaluate the therapy used during a prescribed period, and relevance to the present standard of care is questionable. A concurrent control population would be the obvious way to compare ECMO and conventional management.

There have been two prospective randomized studies comparing ECMO and CMV. One was reported by Bartlett and colleagues in 1985.[16] This study supported ECMO but was criticized[17] for the study design: "Play the winner" randomization was used and resulted in 11 patients in the ECMO arm and only 1 patient in the CMV arm. All ECMO patients survived, and the CMV patient died. A second study was reported by O'Rourke and colleagues.[18] This study also supported ECMO but was again criticized[19, 20] for the adaptive study design. A first stage of 50:50 randomization was followed by a second nonrandomized stage in which all patients received the "better" therapy. Ten patients were sup-

Table 42–2. RISKS OF EXTRACORPOREAL MEMBRANE OXYGENATION

Cannulation and ligation of the right common carotid artery
Cannulation and ligation of the right internal jugular vein
Systemic heparinization
Return of unfiltered blood to the ascending aorta
Exposure to blood products
Technical misadventures
Being sick enough to meet ECMO* entry criteria

ECMO = extracorporeal membrane oxygenation.

ported with CMV; six of them survived. Twenty-nine patients received ECMO; 28 of them survived.

Despite the limitations of patient selection and paucity of controlled studies, ECMO is now considered the standard of care for a number of diseases in full-term neonates. There are complications of ECMO, however. The basic risk categories are listed in Table 42–2. Perhaps of greatest interest and concern is the long-term neurologic outcome of these infants. It is estimated that 15 to 30% of the children treated with ECMO will suffer some degree of neurologic injury.[21-24] At present, however, ECMO graduates are a young group and it will be valuable to methodically evaluate them as they reach school age.

Pediatric ECMO: Pulmonary Support

The history and success of neonatal ECMO introduces the topic of pediatric ECMO. As the technology for neonatal ECMO became routine in many pediatric services, ECMO was soon applied to older children who were seemingly dying of pulmonary disease. In most situations it was offered as rescue therapy on a case-by-case basis.[25-30] Before discussing this in any greater detail, it must be again stated that ECMO does not cure lung disease; therefore, it should be offered only to patients who not only have a high likelihood of dying but also most likely have reversible disease. Although selection criteria have been difficult in the neonatal group, it is significantly more difficult in the pediatric population. This older group presents the clinician with an extreme heterogeneity of diseases and ages. Although much lung disease shares a final common pathophysiology, the inciting events can be remarkably different. In addition, the following questions arise: Is acute respiratory failure (ARF) from hydrocarbon ingestion the same as ARF from aspiration with near drowning or

ARF from viral pneumonia? Are these patients comparable? Can predictors of mortality be elucidated from this heterogeneous group of patients? In addition, these patients represent a spectrum of ages. It is well known that lungs undergo growth and maturation in the first years of life. Does this mean that the child is more likely to recover in the first years of life? Do equivalent injuries have the same morbidity and mortality in a 10-month-old infant as in a 10-year-old child?

Another problem is the lack of understanding of the natural history of ARF in the older pediatric patient. Why do these children die? Studies of adult patients with adult respiratory distress syndrome show that fewer than 20% die of inadequate gas exchange from respiratory failure.[31] The cause of death is more often multiple organ system failure (MOSF), with particularly high mortality in the presence of sepsis or malignancy.[32] The data in pediatric patients, though limited, point to the same observation.[33] Therefore if, in fact, death is not commonly a direct cause of hypoxia or hypercarbia, would support of gas exchange with ECMO have any impact on the survival of pediatric patients with ARF? Perhaps ECMO should be offered earlier before MOSF occurs. Perhaps MOSF should be a contraindication for the institution of ECMO support.

To date, most pediatric ECMO has used the same technologic approach as routine neonatal venoarterial ECMO, with cannulation of the right internal jugular vein and the right common carotid artery. Because there is a greater concern about ligation and cannulation of the common carotid in the older child and adult, alternative arterial cannulation sites have been tried, namely, the axillary artery and the subclavian artery. Both have potential problems. There may be inadequate collateral flow to the arm after cannulation of the axillary artery, and isolation of the subclavian artery can require a difficult dissection, and control of bleeding can be problematic.

The existing experience of pediatric ECMO for ARF is documented in a series of small case reports,[25-30] as well as in the ELSO registry. The entry criteria for these patients are institution-specific and not standardized. The ELSO registry reports that 285 children (non-neonates) received ECMO for pulmonary support; 47% of these children survived.[10] This is a very heterogeneous group representing a variety of patient ages and primary diseases. There are also a number of case reports and small patient series in the literature; the more recent ones are summarized in Table 42–3. This limited patient experience suggests that a longer ECMO course may be

Table 42–3. PEDIATRIC EXTRACORPOREAL MEMBRANE OXYGENATION FOR PULMONARY SUPPORT

Reference	No.	Patient Age	Diagnosis	Duration of ECMO* (Hr)	% Survival
Redmond et al,[25]	3	2 mo–6 yr	Mixed	20–116	33
Steinhorn and Green[26]	12		Respiratory syncytial virus disease	98–428	58
Scalzo et al,[27]	2	15–16 mo	Hydrocarbon ingestion	168–288	100
Anderson et al,[28]	5	1–17 yr	Trauma	140–527	60

*ECMO = extracorporeal membrane oxygenation.

required in the older child, and this prolonged exposure to ECMO may introduce a higher rate of ECMO complications.

The status of ECMO for support of ARF in older children and adults is still evolving. A better understanding of the pathophysiology and prognosis of these diseases is needed in order to better identify inclusion as well as exclusion criteria for this group of patients.

Pediatric ECMO: Cardiovascular Support

ECMO has also been used to primarily support cardiac function in pediatric patients with cardiovascular dysfunction. Obviously only venoarterial ECMO can provide this support. The majority of these patients are children who have low cardiac output syndrome or severe pulmonary artery reactivity after surgical repair of congenital heart defects, or both. There are also a few children who have been put on ECMO support preoperatively either by design or mistake. The children placed on ECMO by mistake are neonates who were misdiagnosed as having persistent pulmonary hypertension of the newborn rather than a structural heart defect to explain their hypoxemia—that is, total anomalous pulmonary venous return. There are also a few children with myocarditis or myocardiopathy for whom ECMO support was provided until their disease resolved or as a bridge to transplantation.

The ELSO registry reports 494 children (non-neonates) who were treated with ECMO for cardiac failure. Forty-six per cent survived.[10] There are also case reports in the literature, which are summarized in Table 42–4.[25, 37–42] For the purposes of discussion, general comments will be made about the postoperative patients only.

Although the numbers are small, there are a few general trends that have been observed. Those patients requiring ECMO support either in the operating room or within 4 hours of surgery had an increased mortality rate; death was often secondary to uncontrollable hemorrhage. In contrast, those children who could be medically supported for 4 to 6 hours after surgery before being placed on ECMO had a higher survival rate. The higher mortality in the group placed on ECMO in the operating room suggests that the myocardia in this group were more diseased or these patients were less stable, their blood not having had time to adequately coagulate before systemic heparinization was restarted. Again,

because the numbers are small, these are only observed trends. More patients must be studied before any generalizations can be made.

The duration of ECMO support is shorter for children with cardiac failure than for children with respiratory failure. Venoarterial ECMO is the only mode used, and there is controversy in cardiac support regarding the indications for intrathoracic cannulation and the need for a left ventricular vent in the case of left ventricular failure.

The future of pediatric ECMO for both pulmonary and cardiac support requires a better understanding of the target populations. Unfortunately, these populations are "moving targets." As conventional therapy changes, associated morbidity and mortality change, and as ECMO technology improves, ECMO will become a safer method of support and its earlier use will be justified.

EXTRACORPOREAL CARBON DIOXIDE REMOVAL

Another approach to extracorporeal gas exchange is extracorporeal CO_2 removal or $ECCO_2R$. This mode of support disassociates oxygenation and carbon dioxide elimination into essentially two separate functions. The lungs are used for oxygenation, whereas the ECMO circuit maintains ventilation or removal of carbon dioxide. Because the circuit only supports ventilation, a relatively small portion of the cardiac output is obligated to go through the ECMO circuit. This can be accomplished by using venovenous ECMO either with a single catheter placed in the internal jugular system or via a two-catheter system using a combination of the jugular-to-femoral or femoral-to-femoral systems. Oxygenation is then supported with the lungs. Low-frequency positive pressure ventilation is used and is incorrectly called "apneic oxygenation." In the described series, a catheter delivers low-flow 100% oxygen directly at the level of the carina, whereas the ventilator delivers 4 to 12 bpm with peak inspiratory pressures of 45 to 50 cm H_2O and positive end-expiratory pressure of 8 to 15 cm H_2O. Heparinization is required while a patient is on this support.[43]

The advantage of this system over routine venoarterial ECMO is the fact that the arterial system does not need to be entered. This is particularly important when con-

Table 42–4. POSTOPERATIVE PEDIATRIC EXTRACORPOREAL MEMBRANE OXYGENATION SUPPORT FOR CARDIAC FAILURE

| Reference | Year | No. | Duration of ECMO (Hr) | Survival | ECMO Within 4 Hr Postoperatively | |
					No. of Patients	Survival
Bartlett et al,[37]	1977	3	7–36	1 (33%)	2 (67%)	0
Cullen et al,[38]	1986	1	94	1 (100%)		
Redmond et al,[25]	1987	4	6–96	1 (25%)	2 (50%)	0
Kanter et al,[39]	1987	13	12–214	6 (46%)	1 (8%)	0
Trento et al,[40]	1988	7	70–190	4 (57%)	1 (14%)	0
Weinhaus et al,[41]	1989	14	6–269	6 (36%)	4 (29%)	0
Klein et al,[42]	1990	36	61–162	22 (61%)	9 (25%)	2/9 (22%)

sidering the fact that the standard arterial approach has involved the common carotid artery or, in older patients, another vessel through which a catheter can be advanced into the ascending aorta. One of the benefits of this support over CMV is the fact that there is less barotrauma.

$ECCO_2R$ depends on the ability to use the patient's lungs for oxygenation. This implies that $ECCO_2R$ should be instituted before the lung damage is too severe. If the lungs cannot support any oxygenation, $ECCO_2R$ is not possible.

There has been reported clinical experience with $ECCO_2R$. In 1986, Gattinoni and colleagues presented the results of $ECCO_2R$ in 43 patients who had an expected mortality rate greater than 90% with conventional therapy.[43] These patients were placed on $ECCO_2R$ as rescue therapy. Thirty-one patients (72.8%) showed improved lung function, and 21 patients (48.8%) survived. Although this was an uncontrolled study, it was stated that $ECCO_2R$ was a safe and effective method to support gas exchange, and it should be considered as an alternative to standard methods of mechanical ventilation.[43]

INTRAVASCULAR OXYGENATION

A new investigational method of gas exchange is the intracorporeal intravenous mechanical gas exchange system which has been dubbed IVOX (intravenous oxygenation). Developed by Cardiopulmonics of Salt Lake City, this system has already undergone laboratory evaluation and is now in a phase I multi-institutional evaluation in human subjects.

The concept is simple: A small-diameter holofiber membrane oxygenator is placed in the inferior vena cava, thereby obviating the need for an extracorporeal circuit. The oxygenator itself is inserted through a sheath placed via a common femoral venotomy. It is advanced in a cephalad direction with the distal tip lying in the superior vena cava or the right atrial appendage. Once inserted, the oxygenator unfurls, exposing the expanded surface area necessary for gas exchange. The oxygenator has a double-lumen gas transport tube that allows for an inflow and an outflow limb. Oxygen passes through the inflow limb driven by suction and provides oxygenation while it washes out carbon dioxide. The oxygenators are made in three different sizes, with surface areas that range from 225 to more than 9,000 cm^2 and external diameters of 1.8 to 10.8 mm. Gas exchange is a function of the oxygenator surface area, the sweep gases through the oxygenator, the mixed venous PO_2 and PCO_2, and the patient's cardiac output. The oxygenator surface area is perhaps the most important factor: Oxygen transfer capability is 3.4 ml/min/100 cm^2, and carbon dioxide transfer capability is 4.2 ml/min/100 cm^2.[44, 45]

IVOX has been used successfully for gas exchange in 20- to 40-kg dogs and 60-kg sheep. There have been no reportable complications. There was little or no hemodynamic effect in central venous pressure or cardiac output after insertion. There was no evidence of gas emboli or bubbling. Finally, neither clotting nor thrombi deposition was observed in any of these animals. It is of note that all animals were fully heparinized.

At present, clinical trials are in process under surveillance of the Food and Drug Administration. In the phase I trial, IVOX support is being offered to patients with at least a 90% predicted mortality rate with continued conventional methods of support. If there is benefit with no significant IVOX-related complications, further studies will be performed in less ill patients with ARF. The phase I trials are nearly completed.[46]

Intracorporeal membrane oxygenation is an obvious extension of ECMO. This method of gas exchange may avoid some of the complications of ECMO but may also invoke new risks. The continued problem will be the identification of appropriate patients for this support.

The common goal for each of these technologies is twofold: more effective and safer support of gas exchange. Interest in these therapies has been driven by the recognition and appreciation of the morbidity associated with aggressive positive-pressure ventilation. A word of caution is necessary, however. Although ECMO, $ECCO_2R$, and IVOX are attractive alternatives, each has associated morbidity and mortality. These forms of support must be critically assessed and compared with routine methods of ventilation. Prospective randomized studies, although optimal, would be difficult in view of the multifactorial heterogeneity of the populations. At the least, we must carefully collect and review the evolving clinical experience.

References

1. Haake R, Schlichtig R, Ulstad DR, et al: Barotrauma: Pathophysiology, risk factors and prevention. Chest 91:608, 1987.
2. Jackson RM: Pulmonary oxygen toxicity. Chest 88:900, 1988.
3. Kenedi RM, Courey JM, Gaylor JDS, et al: Artificial Organs. Baltimore, University Park Press, 1976 pp. 11–19.
4. Clowes GHA, Hopkins AL, and Neville WE: An artificial lung dependent upon diffusion of oxygen and carbon dioxide through plastic membranes. J Thorac Surg 32:630, 1956.
5. Short BL and Pearson GD: Neonatal membrane oxygenation: A review. J Intensive Care Med 1:47, 1986.
6. Zapol WM, Snider MT, Hill DJ, et al: Extracorporeal membrane oxygenation in severe acute respiratory failure: A randomized prospective study. JAMA 242:2193, 1979.
7. Dorson W Jr, Meyer B, Baker E, et al: Response of distressed infants to partial bypass lung assist. Trans Am Soc Artif Int Organ 16:345, 1970.
8. White JJ, Andrews HG, Risenberg H, et al: Prolonged respiratory support in newborn infants with a membrane oxygenator. Surgery 70:288, 1971.
9. Bartlett RH, Gazzaniga AB, Jefferies MR, et al: Extracorporeal membrane oxygenation (ECMO) cardiopulmonary support in infancy. Trans Am Soc Artif Int Organ 22:80, 1976.
10. Extracorporeal Life Support Organization (ELSO): National Registry, Ann Arbor, MI, October, 1990.
11. Bartlett RH, Andrews RF, Toomasian JM, et al: Extracorporeal membrane oxygenation for newborn respiratory failure: Forty-five cases. Surgery 92:425, 1982.
12. Beck R, Anderson KD, Pearson GD, et al: Criteria for extracorporeal membrane oxygenation in a population of infants with persistent pulmonary hypertension of the newborn. J Pediatr Surg 21:297, 1986.
13. Marsh TD, Wilkerson SA, and Cook LN: Extracorporeal membrane oxygenation selection criteria: Partial pressure of arterial oxygen versus alveolar arterial oxygen gradient. Pediatrics 82:162, 1988.

14. Cole CH, Jillson E, and Kessler D. ECMO: Regional evaluation of need and applicability of selection criteria. Am J Dis Child 142:1320, 1988.
15. Dworitz AR, Moya FR, Sabo B, et al: Survival of infants with persistent pulmonary hypertension of the newborn without extracorporeal membrane oxygenation. Pediatrics 84:1, 1989.
16. Bartlett RH, Roloff DW, Cornell RG, et al: Extracorporeal circulation in neonatal respiratory failure: A prospective randomized study. Pediatrics 76:479, 1985.
17. Ware JH and Epstein MF. Extracorporeal circulation in neonatal respiratory failure: A prospective randomized study (Editorial). Pediatrics 76:849, 1985.
18. O'Rourke PP, Crone RK, Vacanti JP, et al: A prospective randomized study of extracorporeal membrane oxygenation (ECMO) and conventional medical therapy in neonates with persistent pulmonary hypertension of the newborn. Pediatrics 84:957, 1989.
19. Chalmers TC: A belated randomized control trial. Pediatrics 86:366, 1990.
20. Meinert CL: Extracorporeal membrane oxygenation trials (Editorial). Pediatrics 85:365, 1990.
21. Andrews AF, Nixon CA, and Cilley RE: One-to-three-year outcome for 14 neonatal survivors of extracorporeal membrane oxygenation. Pediatrics 78:692, 1986.
22. Krummel TM, Greenfield LJ, Kirkpatrick BV, et al: The early evaluation of survivors after extracorporeal membrane oxygenation for neonatal pulmonary failure. J Pediatr Surg 19:585, 1984.
23. Glass P, Miller M, and Short B: Morbidity for survivors of extracorporeal membrane oxygenation: Neurodevelopment outcome at 1 year of age. Pediatrics 83:72, 1989.
24. Towne BH, Lott IT, Hicks DA, et al: Long-term follow-up of infants and children treated with extracorporeal membrane oxygenation (ECMO): A preliminary report. J Pediatr Surg 20:410, 1985.
25. Redmond CR, Graves ED, Falterman KW, et al: Extracorporeal membrane oxygenation for respiratory and cardiac failure in infants and children. J Thorac Cardiovasc Surg 93:199, 1987.
26. Steinhorn RH and Green TP: Use of extracorporeal membrane oxygenation in the treatment of respiratory syncytial virus bronchiolitis: The national experience 1983–1988. J Pediatr 116:338, 1990.
27. Scalzo AJ, Weber TR, Jaeger RW, et al: Extracorporeal membrane oxygenation for hydrocarbon aspiration. Am J Dis Child 144:867, 1990.
28. Anderson HL III, Coran AG, Schmeling DJ, et al: Extracorporeal life support (ECLS) for pediatric trauma: Experience with five cases. Pediatr Surg Int 5:302, 1990.
29. Goulon M, Raphael JC, Gajdos PH, et al: Membrane oxygenators for acute respiratory insufficiency. Intensive Care Med 4:173, 1978.
30. Hill JD, O'Brien TG, Murray JJ, et al: Prolonged extracorporeal oxygenation for acute post-traumatic respiratory failure (shock-lung syndrome). N Engl J Med 286:629, 1972.
31. Fowler AA, Hamman RF, Zerbe GO, et al: Adult respiratory distress syndrome: Prognosis after onset. Am Rev Respir Dis 132:472, 1985.
32. Bell RC, Coalson JJ, Smith JD, et al: Multiple organ system failure and infection in adult respiratory distress syndrome. Ann Intern Med 99:293, 1983.
33. DeBruin W, Notterman D, and Greenwald B: Mortality of ARDS in infants and children. Crit Care Med 17:S111, 1988.
34. Andrews AF, Klein MD, Toomasian JM, et al: Venovenous extracorporeal membrane oxygenation in neonates with respiratory failure. J Pediatr Surg 18:339, 1983.
35. Andrews AF, Zwishenberger JB, Cilley RE, et al: Venovenous extracorporeal membrane oxygenation (ECMO) using double-lumen cannula. Artif Organs 11:265, 1987.
36. Durandy Y, Chevalier JYU, and Lecompte Y: Single-cannula venovenous bypass for respiratory membrane lung support. J Thorac Cardiovasc Surg 99:404, 1990.
37. Bartlett RH, Gazzaniga AB, Fong SW, et al: Extracorporeal membrane oxygenation support for cardiopulmonary failure. J Thorac Cardiovasc Surg 73:375, 1977.
38. Cullen M, Splittgerber F, Sweezer W, et al: Pulmonary hypertension postventricular septal defect repair treated by extracorporeal membrane oxygenation. J Pediatr Surg 21:675, 1986.
39. Kanter KR, Pennington DG, Weber TR, et al: Extracorporeal membrane oxygenation for post operative cardiac support in children. J Thorac Cardiovasc Surg 93:27, 1987.
40. Trento A, Thompson A, Siewers R, et al: Extracorporeal membrane oxygenation in children: New trends. J Thorac Cardiovasc Surg 96:542, 1988.
41. Weinhaus L, Canter C, Noetzel M, et al: Extracorporeal membrane oxygenation for circulatory support after repair of congenital heart defects. Ann Thorac Surg 48:206, 1989.
42. Klein MD, Shaheen KW, Whittlesey GC, et al: Extracorporeal membrane oxygenation for the circulatory support of children after repair of congenital heart disease. J Thorac Cardiovasc Surg 100:498, 1990.
43. Gattinoni L, Pesenti A, Mascheroni D, et al: Low frequency positive pressure ventilation with extracorporeal CO_2 removal in severe acute respiratory failure. JAMA 256:881, 1986.
44. Mortensen JD: An intravenacaval blood gas exchange (IVCBGE) device: A preliminary report. Trans Am Soc Artif Organ 33:570, 1987.
45. Mortensen JD and Berry G: Conceptual and design features of a practical, clinically effective intravenous mechanical blood oxygen/carbon dioxide exchange device (IVOX). Int J Artif Organ 12:384, 1989.
46. Cardiopulmonics News Brief, 5th ed. Salt Lake City, UT.

43

Hyperbaric Oxygen Therapy*

James W. Thorp, Capt., M.C., U.S.N.

For hyperbaric oxygen therapy (HBO), the patient is enclosed in a hyperbaric chamber and breathes 100% oxygen while the pressure in the chamber is greater than the atmospheric pressure. During the hyperbaric exposure, 100% oxygen may be breathed continuously; for prolonged exposures, however, the patient must breathe air for brief periods in order to minimize the risk of oxygen toxicity. A common use for this therapy is to treat decompression sickness or gas embolism in divers and fliers (persons subjected to sudden changes in environmental pressure). Several other medical conditions also are treated with HBO.

Many of the basic concepts for HBO have evolved from experience and research in underwater diving. Some terminology reflects this evolution. The units of pressure most commonly used are atmospheres absolute (ATA) and equivalent feet of sea water (fsw). To calculate ATA under water, the pressure of the atmosphere and the depth of the water above the diver are combined. Each 33 fsw is equivalent to 1 ATA. The pressure at 33 feet under water then is 33 fsw or (33 + 33)/33 = 2 ATA. Similarly, the pressure at 60 feet under water would be 60 fsw or (60 + 33)/33 = 2.8 ATA. One hundred sixty-five fsw would be 6 ATA.

The partial pressure of oxygen to which a tissue is exposed determines what effect oxygen will have on that tissue. At sea level, at which air is 21% oxygen, the partial pressure of oxygen is (0.21 × 1) ATA or 0.21 ATA. At a pressure of 60 fsw the partial pressure of oxygen in air would be (0.21 × 2.8) = 0.58 ATA, while the partial pressure of 100% oxygen would be (1.0 × 2.8) = 2.8 ATA.

For prolonged exposure to hyperbaric conditions, the goal is to limit oxygen exposure to 0.4 ATA or less. During a saturation dive at 800 fsw with a gas mixture of helium and oxygen, then, the gas mixture would be 1.58% oxygen with the rest helium in order to keep oxygen exposure at less than 0.40 ATA. For HBO or very short duration exposures, the goal is to not exceed 2.8 ATA of oxygen.

BASIC MECHANISMS
Increased Pressure

For diseases caused by the presence of gas bubbles in tissue (gas embolism and decompression sickness), the increased pressure (P) of HBO forces the bubble volume (V) to shrink as expected by Boyle's law ($P_1V_1 = P_2V_2$). In addition, the increased environmental pressure enhances oxygenation as expected by Henry's law (the volume of a gas absorbed into a liquid is proportional to the partial pressure of the gas surrounding the liquid).

Increased Oxygenation

The combination of increased pressure and 100% oxygen in the breathing gas increases the oxygen content of the blood. With air (21% oxygen) at normal atmospheric pressure (1 ATA), the hemoglobin is nearly saturated and the oxygen dissolved in plasma is about 0.32 vol%. Increased partial pressure has little effect on the hemoglobin, but the plasma content of oxygen increases to 2.09 vol% with 100% oxygen at 1 ATA and 6.6 vol% with 100% oxygen at 3 ATA. With the latter, it is possible to sustain life without red blood cells.

Besides increasing the oxygen content of the blood, increased pressure further enhances the tissue supply of oxygen by increasing oxygen diffusion into tissue. Air at 1 ATA gives oxygen diffusion of 64 μm compared with 250 μm at 3 ATA with 100% oxygen.

Increased oxygenation causes vasoconstriction in the central nervous system. However, the net supply of oxygen is increased because the increased oxygen in the blood and the increased diffusion more than compensate for decreased blood flow caused by vasoconstriction. The vasoconstriction may be beneficial by decreasing the potential for cerebral edema. Vasoconstriction probably does not occur in other tissues.

EFFECTS OF HYPERBARIC OXYGENATION
Bubble Elimination

For diseases caused by gas bubbles in tissue, the pressure of HBO helps to shrink the bubbles and relieve

---

*The opinions and assertions contained herein are the private ones of the author and are not to be construed as official or reflecting the views of the Navy Department or the naval service at large.

493

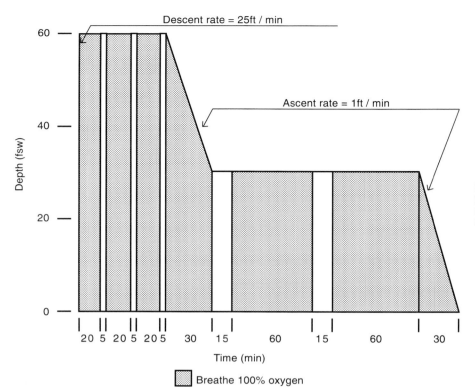

Figure 43–1. The patient breathes 100% oxygen during the period marked O₂ and air during other periods. (From U.S. Navy Treatment Table 6 depth/time profile.)

their immediate effects. The elimination of bubbles is further enhanced by eliminating inert gas from the breathing mix. Bubbles consist primarily of inert gas (nitrogen if the patient was breathing air, helium, or other gas in some diving operations). By providing 100% oxygen during therapy, the diffusion gradient for inert gas out of the bubble increases so that the gas is eliminated and the bubble shrinks more rapidly.

Hyperoxygenation

Hyperoxygenation provides increased oxygen to tissues that are damaged or compromised by poor blood supply. The improved oxygenation enhances (1) the normal function and metabolism of the tissue, (2) the antimicrobial effects of the immune system, (3) growth of new tissue (osteogenesis), and (4) development of new blood vessels (neovascularization).

CLINICAL USES

Decompression Sickness

Decompression sickness (the bends, caisson disease) occurs when the subject moves too rapidly to an environment with a lower surrounding pressure (i.e., ascent from diving, ascent to altitude, or exiting a hyperbaric chamber). Astronauts who work in space are exposed to the risk of decompression sickness and must undergo staged decompression to leave their space vehicle.

Ambient pressure determines the amount of gas dissolved in tissues. If someone moves to a lower ambient pressure more rapidly than the gas can be eliminated by the normal processes of diffusion, circulation, and respiration, then the accumulated gas may form bubbles. The bubbles accumulate in vessels and other tissues to cause ischemia and other effects. The results of the ischemia include local pain, usually in an extremity, but more serious effects of neurologic dysfunction or cardiovascular collapse are possible from the presence of bubbles in the cerebral or cardiovascular circulation.

Based on severity, decompression sickness is usually categorized as type I or type II. Type I includes the relatively minor forms with limb pain, lymphatic obstruction, and skin rashes. There are no neurologic signs or symptoms. Type II includes the more serious forms characterized by respiratory distress, numbness and paraplegia, inner ear dysfunction, shock, extreme fatigue or pain of the abdomen, chest, or back. Symptoms usually develop within the first 2 or 3 hours after a dive or other depressurization, but symptoms can be delayed up to 24 hours.

Immediate treatment with recompression to 60 fsw and periodically breathing 100% oxygen are mandatory. If adequate treatment is initiated early, complete recovery usually occurs. Appropriate treatment tables are available from various sources; Table 6 of the *U.S. Navy Diving Manual* is used with good success by many treatment facilities (Fig. 43–1).

Supportive care includes 100% oxygen for breathing and intravenous hydration. If transport is necessary, these must be provided during transport. If air transport is required, cabin pressures should be maintained at sea level, if possible, or the craft should fly at the lowest possible altitude.

Difficult cases of decompression sickness may require modification of the treatment regimen. This might occur if there was a delay in treatment and the patient manifests neurologic abnormalities that do not resolve completely with a normal length of treatment. If Table 6 of the *U.S. Navy Diving Manual* is used, it is possible to provide additional oxygen breathing periods at the 60 and 30 fsw depths. To avoid oxygen toxicity, there should be no more than two extra periods at each depth. In cases in which there is no improvement at 60 fsw or if conditions worsen during treatment, it may be necessary to increase the pressure at which treatment is provided (i.e., 100 or 165 fsw). Another alternative is to provide repeated treatments according to Table 6 of the *U.S. Navy Diving Manual* with 6 to 24 hours between treatments to minimize the possibility for oxygen toxicity symptoms.

Symptoms of decompression sickness may recur several hours or days after apparently successful HBO has been completed. Retreatment according to Table 6 may be indicated.

Assistance for locating the best treatment facility or guidance in patient management may be available through the Diving Accident Network (DAN) at Duke University—(919) 684-8111. This type of consultation should also be obtained when faced with the complicated types of cases described earlier.

Gas Embolism

In contrast to decompression sickness in which bubble formation develops from dissolved gas, gas embolism develops from either the iatrogenic introduction of air during medical procedures such as catheterizations or from the pulmonary overinflation syndrome (POIS) in divers. POIS may develop at depths as shallow as 4 to 5 feet below the surface; in fact, student divers in pools no more than 10 feet deep have developed gas embolism when they panicked during training and ascended rapidly to the surface without properly exhaling during ascent. The sequence of events leading to gas embolism from POIS is: the diver breathes at depth and holds his or her breath during ascent; the lungs become overinflated; alveolar pressure increases; and gas escapes to the pulmonary veins, travels to the heart, and then to the cerebral circulation to cause sudden loss of consciousness or other neurologic symptoms. Other complications of POIS are pneumothorax, subcutaneous emphysema, or mediastinal emphysema. HBO is not necessarily required for the latter complications, but the patient with any sign or symptom of chest discomfort from POIS should be evaluated carefully for the presence of neurologic abnormalities that indicate the need for HBO.

In contrast to decompression sickness with involvement of the central nervous system, arterial gas embolism in divers is characterized by more sudden onset during ascent or within less than 10 minutes after surfacing. The patient usually experiences seizures or sudden loss of consciousness.

As with decompression sickness, immediate recompression and oxygen therapy are mandatory. Cardiopulmonary resuscitation and life support may be required. The current recommendation for gas embolism is to recompress to 165 fsw on air for 30 minutes and then decompress to 60 fsw for subsequent oxygen therapy. Table 6A of the *U.S. Navy Diving Manual* (Fig. 43–2) is frequently used. Because the symptoms of gas embolism are serious and are caused by a bubble, it is standard practice to begin treatment at the relatively greater pressure of 165 fsw compared with 60 fsw or less used for other diseases. The purpose is to maximize the mechanical effect to cause the bubble to shrink as rapidly as possible. Occasionally, in serious cases of type II decompression sickness, HBO also is started at 165 fsw for the same reasons. Pure oxygen cannot be used at 165 fsw, but some facilities do provide a combination of 50% oxygen with 50% nitrogen. Although not yet accepted as standard, there is evidence that it may be possible to treat embolism at 60 fsw as effectively as at 165 fsw; further evaluation of this possibility is needed.[1]

For patients with serious symptoms or recurrences of symptoms, repetitive treatments or modifications may be required as discussed for the treatment of decompression sickness.

Diving Casualties

Diving is a popular sport, and the critical care unit may be challenged with the patient who has trauma or other illness complicated by the need to treat or consider the possibility of concurrent decompression sickness or gas embolism. As indicated earlier, gas embolism may occur in the diver who has gone no deeper than 4 or 5 feet below the surface.

Any diver who spends significant time under water may need to stop at various levels in water to allow off-gassing of nitrogen and avoid decompression sickness; the number and duration of these stops are determined by the depth and time spent under water before ascent. A diver who has escaped trauma, animal attack, or equipment malfunction from underwater diving may have ascended too fast to avoid decompression sickness. The most common cause of decompression sickness, though, is that divers do not follow recommended guidelines—they dive repeatedly without considering residual nitrogen that is present from diving earlier the same day, their watch or depth gauge is inaccurate, or they do not complete in-water decompression as recommended.

For decompression sickness and gas embolism, there is a high risk that the patient may have significant neurologic impairment that may not be readily apparent. Frequently these impairments develop and progress before treatment can be started. It is crucial, therefore, to have a complete neurologic evaluation before, during, and after therapy, while being careful to minimize any delay in starting therapy. Even with a detailed, accurate history, it may be impossible to determine whether

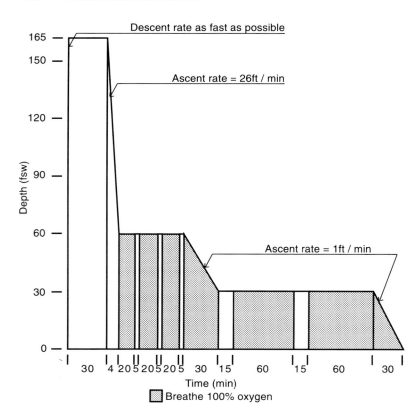

Figure 43–2. The patient breathes 100% oxygen during the period marked O$_2$ and air during other periods. (From U.S. Navy Treatment Table 6A depth/time profile.)

neurologic impairment is caused by decompression sickness, gas embolism, trauma, or some combination of these.

Carbon Monoxide Poisoning

HBO counters the toxicity of carbon monoxide (CO) poisoning through two mechanisms. HBO enhances the elimination of CO from hemoglobin to allow better oxygenation of tissue; the half-life of carboxyhemoglobin decreases from 5 hours 20 minutes in room air to 23 minutes with 100% oxygen at 3 ATA. In addition, hyperoxia counters CO's direct toxic effect on cytochrome A$_3$.

The manifestations of CO poisoning usually appear as flu-like symptoms. Early symptoms are headache, nausea, vomiting, and weakness that may progress to collapse, coma, and death. Indications for HBO include any electrocardiogram (ECG) change, any focal neurologic abnormality, shock, severe acidosis, or carboxyhemoglobin level more than 40%. Patients with significant symptoms may need HBO with carboxyhemoglobin levels as low as 25%. The patient's clinical status reflects toxicity at the tissue level and may be worse than reflected by carboxyhemoglobin levels. It is crucial to follow the patient's clinical status in addition to carboxyhemoglobin levels.

The victim of CO poisoning requires protection of the airway and adequate ventilation, treatment of acidosis as necessary, and HBO when indicated. HBO is provided with compression to 2.4 to 3 ATA and adequate

oxygen breathing to relieve symptoms. U.S. Navy Treatment Table 5 (Fig. 43–3) is similar to the protocols used at most centers. For severe illness, a more extended treatment (e.g., U.S. Navy Table 6) may be needed, and repeat treatments may be required if neurologic symptoms persist.

Smoke Inhalation

Smoke inhalation usually causes CO and, frequently, cyanide poisoning. Pneumonitis complicates the poisoning. HBO helps to overcome the hypoxia and to counter the tissue toxic effects of CO and cyanide. Indications for HBO are similar to those used for CO poisoning.

Necrotizing Infections and Gas Gangrene

HBO is used as an adjunct to surgical and antibiotic treatment of clostridial infections and other mixed soft-tissue infections. HBO halts the production of the α-toxin of *Clostridia* and enhances the effectiveness of leukocytes. With peripheral ischemia, leukocyte function is not possible if the tissue Po$_2$ is less than 30 mm Hg; HBO provides the oxygen free radicals needed for phagocytosis.

HBO should always be considered an adjunct to appropriate surgical therapy, not a replacement for it. For gas gangrene, early use of HBO is considered

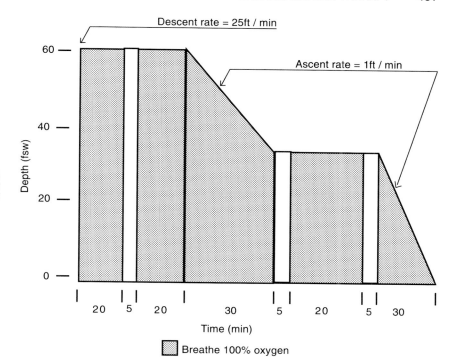

Figure 43–3. The patient breathes 100% oxygen during the period marked O₂ and air during other periods. (From U.S. Navy Treatment Table 5 depth/ time profile.)

necessary to counter the effect of toxins and to improve the patient's ability to tolerate surgery.

Crush Injuries

Acute crush injuries (as seen in wringer or roller injuries) disrupt large vessels and capillaries. The result is compromised blood flow, tissue hypoxia, and edema. HBO is used as an adjunct to the surgical repair of large vessels to improve healing by hyperoxygenation of damaged tissue, especially during the period of revascularization.

Refractory Osteomyelitis

With osteomyelitis, there may be complete anoxia in the center of the affected tissue such that leukocytes are ineffective and osteogenic cells are unable to generate new tissue. As an adjunct to adequate treatment with antibiotics and surgery, HBO enhances the function of the body's immune system and healing processes.

Osteoradionecrosis

After radiation therapy for head and neck tumors there may be aseptic degeneration of soft tissues and bone in the area, primarily from destruction of fibroblasts and osteoblasts. Patients are likely to develop destructive loss of tissue, especially if tooth extraction is required. HBO appears to facilitate healing by stimulating development of new tissue and vessels. The condition may be preventable by appropriate use of HBO before tooth extraction.

Problem Wounds

When surgery alone is ineffective, the adjunctive use of HBO may help to induce healing of compromised skin grafts and flaps. Intermittent periods of hyperoxia may stimulate the function of leukocytes and the proliferation of fibroblasts. The alternate periods of relative hypoxia also may stimulate neovascularization.

It appears that patients are most likely to benefit if it can be demonstrated by transcutaneous monitoring or by other means that HBO does indeed give increased oxygenation of the damaged tissue. Without this effect, there is low probability that HBO will be useful.

Blood Loss Anemia

When blood transfusion cannot be used to correct significant blood loss, adequate oxygen can be dissolved in plasma to support life by using HBO. Treatment must be applied intermittently to avoid the complications of oxygen toxicity.

Burns

The efficacy and appropriate application of HBO to treat burn patients have not yet been defined. HBO should be used for burn patients only by following strict protocols in appropriate medical centers.

SYSTEMS FOR APPLICATION

Multiplace Chamber

The multiplace chamber is a large vessel (somewhat like a small room) that can be pressurized with air. There is room for several people in the chamber, and there are personnel locks to move people into and out of the chamber without losing pressurization. There is room, therefore, for more than one patient and for medical attendants and equipment in the chamber. The atmosphere in the chamber is compressed air, so the patient breathes 100% oxygen by use of face mask or hood.

Monoplace Chamber

The monoplace chamber is much smaller than the multiplace chamber. It is a clear cylinder about 2 to 3 feet in diameter and about 6 to 8 feet long, large enough for a patient to lie on a stretcher slid into the cylinder. In this chamber the entire atmosphere is 100% oxygen, thus the patient does not use a face mask or hood. The walls are transparent so the patient can see his or her surroundings and can be seen by medical attendants.

Compared with the monoplace chamber, the multiplace chamber has the following advantages: greater pressures (6 ATA or more versus less than 3 ATA) can be used; thus this is the preferred equipment to treat decompression sickness or gas embolism; attendants and equipment can be in the chamber to support the more critically ill patients; and, because the atmosphere is air instead of oxygen, there is less risk of fire in the chamber. The relative disadvantages of multiplace chambers are: several personnel must be present to operate the chamber and its support equipment; they require more space and support facilities; they are significantly more expensive to install and maintain; and medical personnel are subjected to the risks of pressurization.

CONTRAINDICATIONS TO HBO

Untreated Pneumothorax

Untreated pneumothorax is an absolute contraindication to HBO. Air accumulated in the pneumothorax during pressurization will expand during decompression. If pneumothorax develops during treatment, it must be relieved before decompression.

Prematurity

Premature infants should not receive HBO because of the risk of retinopathy of the premature. HBO may be used safely with full-term infants if the retinal vessels are fully developed to a mature pattern.

Pregnancy

There are theoretical risks that HBO might induce closure of the ductus arteriosus in the fetus of the pregnant woman. In clinical practice, however, when the risk of not treating was considered greater than the risk of ductus closure (i.e., severe CO poisoning), HBO was used without injury to the fetus.

RELATIVE CONTRAINDICATIONS

Pulmonary Disease

When administering HBO to a patient with pulmonary disease characterized by air trapping, the medical attendants must be prepared to treat pneumothorax and related complications (including gas embolism) that may develop during decompression.

Upper Airway Obstruction

The patient with upper respiratory infections, a history of middle ear surgery, or other hindrances to equalization of pressure with the middle ear or sinuses may suffer barotrauma during compression or decompression. The medical attendant should be prepared to deal with these complications. It may be necessary to compress and decompress at slower than normal rates, and decongestants or tympanostomy tubes may be needed.

Seizure Disorders

One manifestation of oxygen toxicity is seizures. Patients with seizure disorders may be more susceptible to this complication. Additional premedication may be needed.

COMPLICATIONS

The major complications of HBO develop from barotrauma and oxygen toxicity.

Barotrauma

Barotrauma occurs when an air-filled space cannot equalize with changes in ambient pressure. The most common sites are the middle ear and sinuses when they are blocked by congestion. Pneumothorax may develop in patients with disease conditions that cause air trapping.

Oxygen Toxicity

Central Nervous System Oxygen Toxicity

Whenever oxygen is breathed at increased pressure, central nervous system toxicity can occur. Symptoms are especially likely when breathing 100% oxygen at depths greater than 60 fsw. The most dramatic manifestation is a grand mal type of seizure that can occur without prodromal signs. If they do occur, prodromal signs may include visual disturbances, tinnitus, nausea, muscle twitching, irritability, or dizziness. There are no known sequelae in patients who have had seizures during HBO. HBO regimens require periodic interruption of the oxygen breathing to avoid this complication, and treatment regimens limit the amount of oxygen to 2.8 ATA or less.

The basis for treating oxygen-induced seizures is to reduce the partial pressure of oxygen (i.e., switch to breathing air). If the patient truly needs oxygen therapy (e.g., treatment of decompression sickness or gas embolism), then it is possible to resume treatment with oxygen 15 minutes after all symptoms have resolved. Anticonvulsant drugs generally should not be used, because symptoms resolve without them and they may cause respiratory depression that is difficult to manage in a hyperbaric chamber.

Pulmonary Oxygen Toxicity

Prolonged exposure to high partial pressures of oxygen is toxic to the lungs. In general, oxygen partial pressures less than 0.5 to 0.7 ATA cause damage slowly if at all. Partial pressures greater than 3.0 ATA frequently cause central nervous system symptoms before pulmonary toxicity develops. For most treatment regimens, including the U.S. Navy treatment tables used for decompression sickness and gas embolism, there generally will be no evidence of pulmonary damage. If, however, therapy is extended beyond the amount defined as standard, (as might be done in treatment of severe decompression sickness that is improving slowly during treatment), there might be some evidence of pulmonary damage. Symptoms are similar to progressive bronchitis and include substernal chest pain that begins as mild irritation and progresses to burning pain; this may be followed by progressive development of cough and dyspnea. The more severe symptoms are unlikely, and the changes are reversible when managed by reducing the partial pressure of oxygen.

Other Complications

Serous Otitis Media

Serous otitis media is a relatively minor problem that may develop when HBO is used daily. It can be treated by use of decongestants.

Increased Myopia

Myopia may increase by up to 3 diopters after repeated treatments with HBO. Visual acuity returns to its pretreatment status about 6 weeks after treatments end. In patients with pre-existing lens opacities, however, there may be increased rate of maturation of the cataract. This would be a more significant problem in older adults than in pediatric patients.

Chamber Complications

Fire can be catastrophic in the enclosed chamber with its high oxygen atmosphere. All equipment, clothing, and supplies must be selected carefully and used properly to minimize this risk. All gas-filled cavities such as tube cuffs tend to expand during decompression, and appropriate management is required to avoid injury to the patient. Attendants in the chamber under pressure may experience nitrogen narcosis that impairs their ability to think and execute fine motor tasks.

SPECIAL CONSIDERATIONS

Pediatric patients may require HBO for any of the conditions described. For younger children, gas embolism from medical procedures, CO poisoning, crush injury, and osteomyelitis are the most likely. In older adolescents, diving injuries also are possible.

The only age group that generally should not be exposed to HBO is the premature infant or the rare term infant who has an immature pattern of development of the retinal vessels. However, there might be no alternative therapy for a premature infant with gas embolism as a complication of a medical procedure. The potential risks of retinopathy must be balanced against the potential benefit of some type of modified HBO to treat the embolism. It is impossible to give set guidelines for making that decision. If HBO is recommended, the parent or guardian must be fully informed of the potential risk of retinopathy.

The younger child and infant require special attention and, possibly, sedation and restraint to help deal with the frightening experience of being confined in a chamber. This is true for both the multiplace and monoplace chamber, but especially for the latter. Young children will not tolerate face masks, and special hoods are needed to provide 100% oxygen to these patients in the multiplace chamber.

Pulmonary maturation continues for 8 to 10 years, and pulmonary oxygen toxicity is a frequent complication in neonates who have required ventilator support. There is no information about the relative susceptibility to pulmonary oxygen toxicity in this age group, but the clinician should be especially alert to detect signs of pulmonary symptoms in young children and infants who require HBO.

The pediatric patient is more susceptible to the complications of barotrauma, especially to the ears. The younger child and infant have relatively smaller eustachian tubes, and upper respiratory infections are common. Furthermore, it is difficult to teach them how to perform the Valsalva maneuver to equalize middle ear pressure with ambient pressure changes in the chamber. Compression and decompression of the chamber must be accomplished at relatively slow rates for these patients.

Reference

1. Leitch D, Greenbaum L, and Hallenbeck J: Cerebral arterial air embolism. I: Is there a benefit to beginning HBO treatment at 6 bar? Undersea Biomed Res 11:221, 1984.

General References

Clark JM: Oxygen toxicity. *In:* Bennett PB and Elliott DH (eds): Physiology and Medicine of Diving, 3rd ed. London, Bailliere Tindall, 1982, p. 200.

Francis TJ, Dutka AJ, and Hallenbeck JM: Pathophysiology of decompression sickness. *In:* Bove AA and Davis JC (eds): Diving Medicine. Philadelphia, WB Saunders, 1990, p. 170.

Grim PS, Gottlieb LJ, Boddie A, and Batson E: Hyperbaric oxygen therapy. JAMA 263:2216, 1990.

Hyperbaric Oxygen Therapy: A Committee Report. Bethesda, MD, Undersea and Hyperbaric Medical Society, 1986.

Kindwall EP and Goldman RW (eds): Hyperbaric Medical Procedures. Milwaukee, WI, St. Lukes Medical Center, 1988.

U.S. Navy Diving Manual. Superintendent of Documents, U.S. Government Printing Office, Washington, DC, 1988.

Pharmacologic Adjuncts to Mechanical Ventilation in the Adult Respiratory Distress Syndrome in Children

Aaron R. Zucker, M.D.

In 1967, the appellation adult respiratory distress syndrome (ARDS) was given to the lung disease causing hypoxemia after various nonpulmonary insults in a group of adult patients.[1] Approximately 150,000 cases occur each year.[2] In the 1980s, a similar entity in pediatric patients was increasingly recognized, and mortality rates consistent with the adult experience (30 to 90%) were reported.[3–6] In both populations, the most common inciting events have been sepsis, shock, pneumonia, trauma, liquid aspirations, and near-drownings, although many other catalysts have been described. The hallmarks of the syndrome include:

1. Protein-rich alveolar edema causing intrapulmonary shunt that is refractory to oxygen therapy. Most often, the lungs are previously normal, and an inciting clinical event can be identified.
2. Diffuse pulmonary infiltrates on a chest x-ray film and poor lung compliance.
3. Normal cardiac function, as demonstrated by normal heart-filling pressures (pulmonary capillary wedge pressure of 18 mm Hg or less).

In the early exudative phase, histologic alterations called "diffuse alveolar damage" occur, characterized by destruction of type I and type II pneumocytes and also by abnormalities of the microvascular endothelium and basement membranes.[7, 8] This causes a capillary leak state with flooding of the pulmonary interstitium and alveoli with protein-rich edema derived from plasma. This exudative phase lasts for several days[9]; thereafter, a reparative proliferative phase ensues with hyperplasia of type II pneumocytes. These cells are deficient in their ability to secrete pulmonary surfactant. Fibroblasts invade the alveolar walls, and hyaline membranes form from cellular debris. This phase lasts for several weeks, and lung disease may resolve or progress to fibrosis with pulmonary dysfunction or death.

As the capillaries initially leak, other intravascular substances enter the lung interstitium and alveoli. Activated white blood cells become trapped in the lungs and release granular contents or generate oxygen-derived free radical species, all of which may augment lung injury.[7, 10, 11] Components of damaged cellular membranes serve as substrates for formation of arachidonic acid metabolites, which may cause acute pulmonary hypertension and also promote capillary injury.[12, 13] These mediators and alveolar flooding itself lead to the derangements of gas exchange and lung mechanics characteristic of ARDS.

Even if a child survives ARDS, he or she is likely to have clinical or laboratory evidence of chronic pulmonary dysfunction, including cough and exertional dyspnea, reduced lung volumes, ventilation/perfusion mismatching, and obstructive airways disease.[4, 14] The overall dismal results have prompted clinicians to search for a cure for ARDS, but, not surprisingly, its multiple causes and many involved mediator systems have thwarted the efforts. In the meantime, treatment with supplemental oxygen and positive end-expiratory pressure (PEEP) have been therapeutic mainstays. Although these modalities provide support during the acute stage of disease, their benefits are balanced by potential complications. Prolonged use of high concentrations of oxygen causes absorption atelectasis and amplifies structural damage by oxygen-derived free radical species.[15, 16] These highly reactive compounds may also inhibit the formation of pulmonary surfactant.[7] As alveolar flooding increases, the resultant intrapulmonary shunt causes hypoxemia resistant to supplemental oxygen therapy. PEEP must then be used to recruit alveoli by redistributing edema to the interstitial space, where it interferes little with gas exchange.[17, 18] This has the benefit of allowing a reduction in the inspired oxygen concentraton, theoretically reducing the amount of oxygen toxicity that otherwise might occur. However, PEEP can also have significant adverse effects. Barotrauma results from overdistention of alveoli and subsequent dissection of gas along tissue planes to form pneumomediastinum, pneumothorax, or pneumopericardium. The reported incidence of such air leak is 40 to 60% in children with severe ARDS.[19] In addition, high levels of PEEP (>10 cm H_2O) may decrease cardiac output due either to compression of right heart structures by increased intrathoracic pressures or to a left-sided shift of the cardiac septum that compromises left ventricular filling.[20] It seems prudent, therefore, to use the least possible PEEP and oxygen to reach a desired endpoint. We have accepted that endpoint to be associated with more than 90% arterial saturation of an adequate circulating hemoglobin concentration at an FIO_2 of less than or equal to 0.5.

The unavailability of a cure for ARDS, the potential adverse effects of supportive measures, and the consistently high mortality rates have prompted investigations of surfactants and fluorocarbons as pharmacologic adjuncts to mechanical ventilation. In a textbook, one usually attempts to explain the known clinical utility of therapies for given conditions. In this case, laboratory investigations in these areas have had encouraging results, but the paucity of anecdotal patient data, much less controlled clinical trials, does not allow recommendation for their use at this time. Still, it is valid to discuss their theoretical benefits while awaiting the results of studies on humans.

EXOGENOUS SURFACTANT REPLACEMENT THERAPY FOR ARDS

Normal Surfactant Composition and Physiology

Pulmonary surfactant is a combination of lipids and proteins that adsorbs at the alveolar air-liquid interface and reduces surface tension. The composition of surfactant is shown in Table 44–1. Phospholipids comprise approximately 90% by weight, the majority of which

Table 44–1. COMPOSITION OF NORMAL SURFACTANT

Component	% Composition by Weight
Surfactant	
Phospholipids	90
Neutral lipids	6
Proteins	4
Surfactant phospholipids	
Phosphatidylcholine	80
Phosphatidylglycerol	7
Phosphatidylethanolamine	5
Phosphatidylinositol	3
Sphingomyelin	2
Others	3

consists of the primary active compound, dipalmatoylphosphatidylcholine (DPPC). Other lipids (phosphatidylethanolamine, phosphatidylserine, and sphingomyelin) are present in small amounts, much less than the fractions they represent in cell membranes. Two groups of surfactant-related proteins have been described, both of which are present in small amounts (2% by weight). Surfactant apoprotein A (SP-A) can be subdivided into two subunits with molecular weights approximately 26 to 36 kDa and appears to have a role in surfactant recycling or secretion.[21, 22] Perhaps more important is its promotion of tubular myelin formation in the presence of proteins SP-B and SP-C, which aids in spreading along the air-liquid interface. These smaller hydrophobic proteins appear to be essential for optimum surfactant function, even in the absence of SP-A.

Surfactant is synthesized in the type II alveolar cell.[23] The phospholipids are made in the endoplasmic reticulum and stored in the type II cell's lamellar inclusion bodies, where they are joined by the apoproteins. After stimuli such as adrenergic agents and prostaglandins, lamellar bodies undergo exocytosis into the alveolar space.[24, 25] After secretion, the structure of surfactant changes so that tubular myelin and the characteristic monolayer form and confer alveolar stability. Surfactant is cleared from normal alveoli primarily by type II pneumocytes and by macrophages with a half-life of 6 to 24 hours.[26–28] After lung injury from chronic hyperoxic exposure, this clearance is considerably prolonged.[29]

Normal surfactant lining the airspaces causes surface tension to vary with lung volume, so that minimum surface tension occurs at functional residual capacity. This prevents alveolar collapse at low lung volumes and minimizes work of breathing.[30] Additionally, surfactant's presence protects against edema formation in normal lungs. The mechanism underlying its role in edema formation is embodied in the Starling equation governing liquid flux across the capillary membrane:

$$\text{Edema flux} = K_f [(Pmv - Pis) - \sigma (\pi mv - \pi is)],$$

in which K_f is the filtration coefficient for water, Pmv and Pis are the hydrostatic pressures of the microvascular lumen and interstitium, respectively, σ is the protein reflection coefficient, and πmv and πis are the respective oncotic pressures. These factors are shown in Figure 44–1. When surface tension increases due to surfactant inactivation (upper alveolus), increased static recoil of the lung parenchyma results in decreased (more negative) Pis. If other factors are unchanged, the hydrostatic contribution to edema formation (Pmv − Pis) increases. In normal lungs, surfactant inactivation by detergent aerosol,[31] ventilation with high tidal volumes from low functional residual capacity,[32] or norepinephrine administration[33] causes pulmonary edema, although capillary permeability is unchanged. Surfactant may also have a role in mitigating increases in alveolar permeability after lung injury. In a rabbit model of chronic hyperoxic lung injury in rabbits (described in detail later), disappearance of a radiolabelled tracer from the alveoli was reduced after surfactant instillation.[34] The authors speculated that this could be caused by decreased lung inflammation or by scavenging of toxic oxygen species.

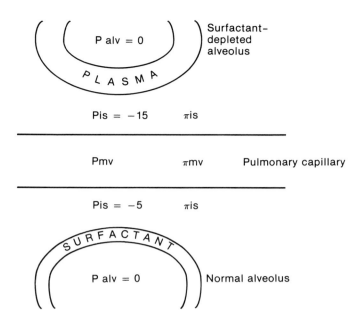

Figure 44–1. Schematic diagram of the Starling forces governing edema flux across the pulmonary capillary membrane. In the normal alveolus (bottom), surfactant lines the airspace and maintains low surface tension. The local interstitial hydrostatic pressure, Pis, is normal (-5 cm H_2O). In the upper injured alveolus, edema derived from plasma replaces surfactant and the increased surface tension generates lower interstitial pressure (-15 cm H_2O). This increases the hydrostatic gradient (Pmv $-$ Pis) for edema formation.

These latter considerations have great significance in the following sections concerning surfactant's potential utility as a treatment of ARDS. The intuition that minimizing edema formation in the early phase of pulmonary capillary leak would reduce the need for potentially dangerous supportive therapies has been corroborated by recent studies. In animal models of ARDS, reduction of pulmonary vascular pressures by plasmapheresis or by partial lung bypass reduced edema formation by minimizing the contribution of Pmv in the Starling equation (see earlier).[35–37] Extrapolations of this concept to the intensive care unit showed increased survival in patients with ARDS.[38, 39] To the extent that surfactant replacement also reduces edema formation by increasing Pis, it might have a place in the clinical arena.

Surfactant System in Pediatric Disease

The association between surfactant deficiency and neonatal hyaline membrane disease (HMD) was first described in 1959.[40] In that syndrome, premature newborns developed refractory hypoxemia from atelectasis and intrapulmonary shunting due to developmental lack of surfactant. It seemed reasonable that exogenous surfactant administration would be beneficial for this primary deficiency, and studies have verified this.[41, 42] Surfactant replacement has been performed with several different mixtures. Natural surfactants, such as calf lung surfactant extract (CLSE), are collected from alveolar lavages of animal lungs or amniotic fluid. These solutions contain all the apoproteins. Modified natural surfactants are organically extracted from alveolar lavage or tissue minces and reconstituted in normal saline. These preparations contain only the hydrophobic apoproteins, and selective removal of cell membrane lipid contaminants may be necessary to retain surface activity. Artificial surfactants are mixtures of protein-poor active phospholipids and chemical additives that improve surface activity. In HMD, various doses (typically 50 to 100 mg/kg of phospholipid) and treatment schemes (prophylactic prior to first breath, "rescue" after illness onset) have been used successfully and become standard practice in some nurseries.

The many histologic and pathophysiologic similarities between HMD and ARDS prompted investigation of the surfactant system in the latter syndrome. In patients who died of ARDS, lung minces had abnormally high minimum surface tensions.[1] Other investigators showed low lung volumes and compliance in a patient with ARDS. Bronchoalveolar lavage fluid (BALF) from this patient had normal lipid levels but increased protein concentration and abnormal surface tension characteristics.[43] In another study, BALF from patients who died of ARDS had total phospholipid concentrations comparable with those of normal persons, but the fractional composition was different.[44] Furthermore, BALF from injured patients had high minimum surface tensions, precluding significant surface activity. These findings have been corroborated by Holm and associates in a model of pulmonary capillary permeability from chronic hyperoxic exposure in rats.[45] These animals developed hypoxemia, protein-rich pulmonary edema, and abnormal surface activity in BALF. These findings and others led, in turn, to investigations of the mechanisms responsible for the surface tension abnormalities in various scenarios. Type II cells may themselves be destroyed in models such as viral pneumonia,[46] causing a reduced surfactant pool. In addition, after chronic hyperoxic exposure or during sepsis induced with *Escherichia coli* in rats,[47, 48] phospholipid turnover by type II pneumocytes is depressed. Finally, regardless of the cause, surfactant may be inactivated after synthesis by the type II cell, either directly by agents such as kerosene,[49] which may be aspirated into the lungs, or by alveolar proteins and blood components derived from the pulmonary circulation during a capillary leak.[50–52] The inhibition of surfactant function by proteins in vivo is greatest when surfactant concentration is low; when it is sequentially increased, inhibition is abolished. It is important to note that some artificial surfactant preparations have an in vitro sensitivity to protein inhibition that is an order of magnitude greater than that of natural surfactants.[53]

In addition to previous knowledge, these findings led to the proposed pathogenetic sequence for ARDS seen in Figure 44–2. The concepts that surfactant dysfunction occupies a crucial place in this scheme and its inhibition can be overcome by a threshold concentration of administered surfactant led to further speculation that surfactant therapy would ameliorate the pulmonary dysfunction in ARDS.

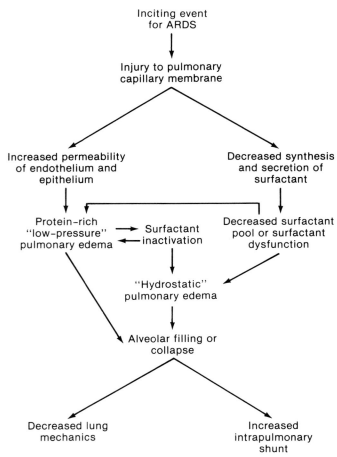

Figure 44–2. Proposed pathogenic sequence for ARDS. Surfactant destruction or inactivation exacerbates the forces promoting edema formation, leading to hypoxemia and abnormal lung mechanics.

Exogenous Surfactant Replacement Therapy for ARDS

Almost all the experience with surfactant replacement during pulmonary capillary leak states has been gained in the laboratory. In a guinea pig model, Berggren and associates induced surfactant deficiency with repeated lung lavage and found large decrements in lung compliance and gas exchange that did not respond to mechanical ventilation with 100% oxygen for 8 hours.[54] After intratracheal administration of 100 mg of natural surfactant, these abnormalities were significantly improved for 5 hours. This model was initially criticized for resembling HMD more than ARDS; in retrospect, this may not be so. It was shown subsequently both that the lavage process itself can increase pulmonary capillary permeability,[55] and HMD is associated with alveolar edema, not just atelectasis.[56] In any event, this was one of the earliest studies showing efficacy of surfactant in treating such a pulmonary problem.

In a model of surfactant dysfunction after bilateral cervical vagotomy in rabbits, Berry and associates noted severe hypoxemia and respiratory distress within hours.[57] Histologic examination of lung parenchyma showed areas of hemorrhage, hyaline membrane formation, and alveolar edema that were not seen in control animals.

Increased microvascular permeability was confirmed by increased recovery of both a radiolabelled intravenous tracer and plasma proteins from BALF. Although surface tension characteristics of these fluids were abnormal, total phospholipid content was not, making surfactant inactivation by alveolar proteins a likely mechanism. These physiologic abnormalities were significantly improved by intratracheal administration of natural surfactant, although the changes were smaller than those in studies of HMD. The authors speculated this may have been due to inhomogeneous surfactant distribution of the administered surfactant in these atelectatic lungs. We will review this distribution question later.

Lachmann and associates caused increased alveolar-capillary permeability with antilung serum in a guinea pig model of ARDS.[58] Gross alveolar edema and decrements in lung mechanics occurred within minutes of injury. Airway fluid contained increased amounts of protein, decreased phospholipid concentration, and increased surface tension. Intratracheal natural bovine surfactant significantly improved all tested parameters of gas exchange and lung mechanics, and survival. However, an extremely large dose of surfactant (approximately 300 mg/kg of phospholipid) was used. This corresponds to 9 ml/kg of a typical surfactant suspension, which is quite an airway volume load in a subject already suffering from increased alveolar fluid! In addition, this experimental lesion developed more rapidly than clinical ARDS (minutes versus hours to days); thus again this model's clinical relevance has been questioned. Nevertheless, this study showed that exogenous surfactant therapy could have beneficial effects in the setting of severe pulmonary capillary leak.

In the model of hyperoxic lung injury,[45] pulmonary derangements develop temporally and physiologically like ARDS. Rabbits exposed to 100% oxygen had increased alveolar permeability and hypoxemia that reached a peak at 64 hours. If hyperoxic breathing continued, a 90% mortality rate occurred. If oxygen exposure was stopped, respiratory distress, pulmonary edema formation, and decreased lung compliance and volumes developed insidiously. Total lavageable alveolar protein increased dramatically, whereas total phospholipid decreased by 50%. In a subsequent study in this model, rabbits were given intratracheal CLSE after permeability increased, but before significant edema formed.[59] Unlike control rabbits, surfactant-treated animals had significant increments in PaO_2 values while breathing 100% oxygen, demonstrating that they suffered primarily from ventilation-perfusion mismatching rather than from an intrapulmonary shunt. Pulmonary edema formation was reduced after surfactant, and BALF exhibited normal surface tension characteristics, both unlike the findings in control animals. A similar pattern of pulmonary abnormalities and responses to exogenous surfactant was found in rats treated 4 days after lung injury with N-nitroso-N-methylurethane.[60]

Not all studies have shown benefits from surfactant, however. Sheep pretreated with artificial surfactant (Exosurf) underwent lung injury with intravenous oleic acid. No acute beneficial effects on gas exchange or lung mechanics were noted.[61] It is possible the negative results of that study were due to the increased sensitivity of synthetic surfactant preparations to inactivation by edema proteins.[53] Alternatively, the authors speculated that penetration of aerosolized surfactant into edematous alveoli might have been prevented. We shared this concern when we devised experiments to evaluate the effects of CLSE in a canine oleic acid model of ARDS. We reasoned that surfactant given intratracheally might not get to the terminal airways if alveoli were already flooded and speculated that the addition of adequate PEEP to the ventilator circuit prior to surfactant administration would potentiate its beneficial effects. This could be due to improved surfactant dispersion or to minimized inactivation by redistribution of proteinaceous edema to the pulmonary interstitium.[17, 18] In addition, PEEP would temporarily decrease shunt and protect against transient additional hypoxemia at the time when surfactant emulsion was placed in the airways. Twelve normovolemic dogs underwent acute lung injury with oleic acid.[62] PEEP of 8 cm H_2O was begun 1.5 hours later, intentionally at a time when peak edema had already formed in this model. This was followed by administration of 1.5 ml/kg (50 mg/kg) of CLSE into each mainstem bronchus in six dogs. In the other six dogs, an equal volume of saline placebo was given in a similar manner. Measurements of hemodynamic variables in both groups were similar at all times for 5 hours after injury. Although surface tension was reduced dramatically to a normal value in the treated group, no significant differences in shunt, edema in excised lungs, or lung mechanics were found. The lack of surfactant effects in this study has several possible explanations. Although unlikely, surfactant dysfunction may be unimportant in this model.[61] Alternatively, inadequate amounts of surfactant or PEEP may have been used in a model in which so much lung water (three to four times normal) forms so quickly; recall that we gave surfactant after maximum edema had formed in order to mimic a frequent clinical scenario.

We concluded that surfactant might be ineffective after large amounts of alveolar fluid were present. In light of surfactant's protective effects against edema formation in normal lungs, we next evaluated its efficacy in a canine model of tracheal hydrochloric acid (HCl) aspiration, in which edema forms progressively over many hours.[35] We speculated that intervention early after injury in this model would facilitate normalization of alveolar surface tension. This, in turn, would minimize edema formation by the mechanisms previously discussed. Twelve normovolemic dogs ventilated with 60% oxygen received 0.5 ml/kg of 0.1N HCl into each mainstem bronchus.[63] At 1 hour after injury, dogs were randomized into two equal groups. The first group received PEEP of 8 cm H_2O at 1 hour, followed by 100 mg/kg of CLSE. The second group received PEEP, followed by an equal volume of saline placebo. The group receiving both PEEP and surfactant had a decrease of 6% in Qva/Qt at 5 hours after intervention, which was significantly different from the 8% increase seen in the saline group. The final edema in excised lungs and surface tension of BALF in this group were

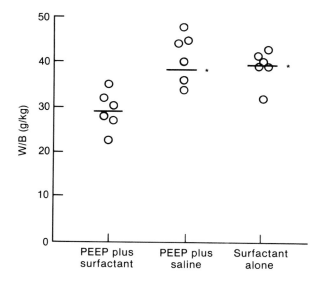

*p < 0.05 compared with PEEP plus surfactant group

Figure 44–3. Edema from 18 dogs' lungs (wet lung weight to body weight ratios [g/kg]) excised 5 hours after injury with hydrochloric acid. Dogs receiving intratracheal CLSE after 8 cm H_2O PEEP had significantly less edema than dogs receiving either PEEP plus saline placebo or surfactant without PEEP.

also significantly lower. We conclude that surfactant reduces edema by restoring normal surface forces and by increasing lung interstitial hydrostatic pressure when delivered early after injury in canine HCl aspiration. In subsequent work, we have learned that PEEP is necessary in this model if surfactant is to be beneficial, since dogs receiving CLSE without PEEP had no improvements in lung water or gas exchange (Figs. 44–3 to 44–5).

Clinical Studies of Surfactant Replacement Therapy for ARDS

Surfactant has also been administered to a very small number of patients with ARDS. Transient improve-

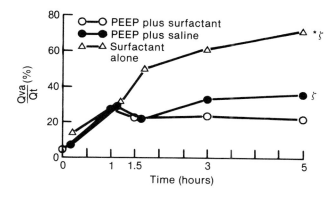

* p < 0.05 from 1 hr value in same group
ʃ p < 0.05, change between 1 and 5 hr different from PEEP plus surfactant group

Figure 44–4. Pulmonary venous admixture (Qva/Qt; %) versus time in the three groups. Dogs receiving PEEP plus surfactant had a mean decrease of 6% between 1 and 5 hours, significantly different from the increases seen in the other two groups.

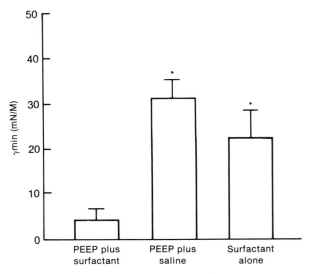

Figure 44–5. Minimum surface tension (γ min; mN/M) of BALF obtained at 5 hours as determined with a pulsating bubble surfactometer. In dogs receiving PEEP plus surfactant, normal values were found, indicating airway fluid could act as a normal surfactant. This was significantly different from the other two groups, in which surface tension was too high for function as an active surfactant.

ments in gas exchange, but not lung mechanics, were found in three patients who received 50 mg/kg of porcine surfactant into each bronchus with a bronchoscope.[64] A 4-year-old patient with sepsis and ARDS received 300 mg/kg of exogenous surfactant and had a rapid, significant improvement in gas exchange.[65] The scarcity of human experience is at least partially due to uncertainty about which surfactant preparation, dose, and route of administration is necessary or optimum in a particular situation. Concerns exist about potential antigenicity of foreign proteins if natural surfactants are used. Although artificial surfactants do not have this problem, they do not resist protein inactivation as well; therefore larger doses may be necessary in ARDS. However, it is disturbing to contemplate administration of large amounts of surfactant into the trachea of a patient who already has alveolar edema. These concerns and others make it clear that many questions must be answered before surfactant replacement can be considered safe and effective adjunctive therapy for ARDS.

ROLE OF FLUOROCARBON EMULSIONS IN ACUTE RESPIRATORY FAILURE

The synthetic fluorocarbon emulsions were originally developed to restore systemic oxygen-carrying capacity in Jehova's Witnesses, who refuse blood product administration on religious grounds. These oil mixtures have a solubility for oxygen that is approximately 20 times greater than that of water, so that 65 ml/dl of oxygen can be dissolved. In addition, they also have low surface tensions (15 mNewt/M) and were shown to eliminate interfacial surface forces, increase pulmonary blood

flow, and support gas exchange in premature animals with respiratory failure.[66] In this way, they might be useful in situations when ARDS or HMD are complicated by barotrauma or by hemodynamic compromise from ventilation with high airway pressures, as proposed for surfactants. In contrast with administering one or two boluses of surfactant, fluorocarbon ventilation is a continuous process. Results of the first clinical trial of such liquid ventilation in premature infants not responding to aggressive therapies with high-frequency ventilation or surfactant instillation have been reported.[67] Three patients received two brief (3 to 5 minutes) periods of liquid ventilation with oxygenated fluorocarbon. In all three, significant improvements in lung compliance were found without cardiovascular compromise. In two, PaO₂ also increased significantly. Although all three infants eventually died, this landmark clinical study showed that brief ventilation with fluorocarbons is feasible, and the authors speculated that earlier intervention would improve outcome. Concerns about development of high alveolar pressures during fluorocarbon ventilation were addressed by Curtis and associates, who showed these pressures to be unimportant. They demonstrated large resistive pressure drops between central airways and alveoli, supporting a strategy of long inspiratory and expiratory times, low flow rates, and minimal fluid viscosity during fluorocarbon ventilation.[68] This modality requires further study and may prove useful when patients do not respond to aggressive conventional mechanical ventilation.

The most completely studied available fluorocarbon is Fluosol-DA, an emulsion containing the maximum attainable concentration of 20% wt/vol of fluorocarbon. Rather than using it for liquid ventilation, Fluosol-DA has been evaluated as a vascular volume expander during ARDS in dogs.[69] The emulsion had not been previously used in this scenario for two reasons; first, it can carry significant volumes of oxygen only at high PaO₂, which is difficult to accomplish during ARDS. In addition, many physicians avoid administration of large volumes of intravenous fluids to patients with ARDS since this increases edema formation, as discussed earlier. Dogs with oleic acid lung injury received 400 ml of whole blood or Fluosol, which achieved a "fluorocrit" of 5%. Similar increases in cardiac output, pulmonary and systemic pressures, and shunt occurred in the two groups. Although arterial PaO₂ increased significantly in treated dogs, CaO₂ decreased due to hemodilution. This decrement was outweighed, however, by a four-fold increase in efficiency of oxygen delivery by the fluorocarbon. This study demonstrated that Fluosol-DA can be useful as a volume expander and oxygen carrier in ARDS, and its effects on oxygen transport and utilization are complex. Again, further study is required before clinical application can be recommended.

References

1. Ashbaugh DG, Bigelow DB, Petty TL, et al: Acute respiratory distress in adults. Lancet 2:319, 1967.
2. Shale D: The adult respiratory distress syndrome 20 years on. Thorax 42:642, 1987.

3. Holbrook PR, Taylor G, Pollack MM, et al: Adult respiratory distress syndrome in children. Pediatr Clin North Am 27:677, 1980.
4. Lyrene R and Truog WE: Adult respiratory distress syndrome in a pediatric intensive care unit: Predisposing conditions, clinical course, and outcome. Pediatrics 67:790, 1981.
5. Nussbaum E: Adult-type respiratory distress syndrome in children: Experience with seven cases. Clin Pediatr 22:401, 1983.
6. Pfenninger J and Rogers R: Adult respiratory distress syndrome in children. J Pediatr 101:352, 1982.
7. Rinaldo JE and Rogers RM: Adult respiratory distress syndrome: Changing concepts of lung injury and repair. N Engl J Med 306:900, 1982.
8. Coalson JJ: Pathophysiologic features of respiratory distress in the infant and adult. In: Shoemaker WC and Thompson WL (eds): Critical Care: State of the Art. Fullerton, CA, Society for Critical Care Medicine, 1982, pp. A1–28.
9. Pratt PC, Vollmer RT, Shelburne JD, et al: Pulmonary morphology in a multihospital collaborative extracorporeal membrane oxygenation project. I: Light microscopy. Am J Pathol 95:191, 1979.
10. Tate R and Repine J: Neutrophils and the adult respiratory distress syndrome. Am Rev Respir Dis 128:552, 1983.
11. Taylor A, Martin D, and Parker J: The effect of oxygen radicals on pulmonary edema formation. Surgery 94:433, 1983.
12. Seeger W, Menger M, Walmrath D, et al: Arachidonic acid lipoxygenase pathways and increased vascular permeability in isolated rabbit lungs. Am Rev Respir Dis 136:964, 1987.
13. Williams T and Piper P: The action of chemically pure SRS-A on the microcirculation in vivo. Prostaglandins 19:779, 1980.
14. Fanconi S, Kraemer R, Weber J, et al: Long term sequellae in children surviving adult respiratory distress syndrome. J Pediatr 106:218, 1985.
15. Shapiro BA, Cane RD, Harrison RA, et al: Changes in intrapulmonary shunting with administration of 100% oxygen. Chest 77:138, 1980.
16. Deneke S and Fanburg B: Normobaric oxygen toxicity of the lung. N Engl J Med 303:76, 1980
17. Malo J, Ali J, and Wood LDH: How does positive end-expiratory pressure reduce intrapulmonary shunt in canine pulmonary edema? J Appl Physiol 57:1002, 1984.
18. Pare PD, Warriner B, Baile EM, et al: Redistribution of pulmonary extravascular water with positive end-expiratory pressure in canine pulmonary edema. Am Rev Respir Dis 127:590, 1983.
19. Royall J and Levin DL: Adult respiratory distress syndrome in pediatric patients. II: Management. J Pediatr 112:335, 1988.
20. Prewitt RM, Oppenheimer L, Sutherland JB, et al: Effects of positive end-expiratory pressure on left ventricular mechanics in patients with acute hypoxemic respiratory failure. Anesthesiology 55:409, 1981.
21. Weaver TE, Whitsett JA, Hull WM, et al: Identification of canine pulmonary surfactant associated glycoprotein A precursors. J Appl Physiol 58:2091, 1985.
22. Wright JR, Wager RE, Hagwood S, et al: Surfactant apoprotein M = 26,000–36,000 enhances uptake of liposomes by type II cells. J Biol Chem 262:2888, 1987.
23. Wright JR and Clements JA: Metabolism and turnover of lung surfactant. Am Rev Respir Dis 135:426, 1987.
24. Ryan US, Ryan JW, and Smith DS: Alveolar type II cells: Studies on the mode of release of lamellar bodies. Tissue Cell 7:597, 1975.
25. Oyarzun MJ and Clements JA: Control of lung surfactant by ventilation, adrenergic mediators, and prostaglandins in the rabbit. Am Rev Respir Dis 117:879, 1978.
26. Jobe A, Kirkpatrick E, and Gluck L: Labelling of phospholipids the surfactant and subcellular fractions of rabbit lung. J Biol Chem 253:3810, 1978.
27. Miles PR, Bowman L, and Castranova V: Incorporation of [H^3] palmitate and [C^{14}] choline into disaturated phosphatidylcholines in rat alveolar macrophages. Biochem Biophys Acta 833:342, 1985.
28. Jacobs H, Jobe A, Ikegami M, et al: Surfactant phosphatidylcholine source, fluxes, turnover times in 3-day old, 10-day old, and adult rabbits. J Biol Chem 257:1805, 1982.
29. Holm BA, Tonucci D, and Matalon S: Clearance of exogenous surfactant in hyperoxic lung injury. FASEB J 3:546A, 1989.
30. Notter RH and Finkelstein JN: Pulmonary surfactant: An interdisciplinary approach. J Appl Physiol 57:1613, 1984.
31. Nieman G and Bredenberg C: High surface tension pulmonary edema induced by detergent aerosol. J Appl Physiol 58:129 1985.
32. Albert R, Lakshminarayan S, Hildebrandt J, et al: Increased surface tension favors pulmonary edema formation in anesthetized dogs' lungs. J Clin Invest 63:1015, 1979.
33. Rao GJ, Ramnarayan K, Rao AK, et al: Experimental production of high surface tension pulmonary edema. Indian J Pathol Microbiol 31:1, 1988.
34. Engstrom PC, Holm BA, and Matalon S: Surfactant replacement attenuates the increase in alveolar permeability in hyperoxia. J Appl Physiol 67:688, 1989.
35. Sznajder JI, Zucker AR, Wood LDH, et al: The effects of plasmapheresis and hemofiltration on canine acid aspiration pneumonitis. Am Rev Respir Dis 134:222, 1986.
36. Zucker AR, Sznajder JI, Becker CJ, et al: The pathophysiology and treatment of canine kerosene pulmonary injury: Effects of plasmapheresis and positive end-expiratory pressure. J Crit Care 4:184, 1989.
37. Zucker AR, Wood LDH, Curet-Scott M, et al: Partial lung bypass reduces pulmonary edema induced by kerosene aspiration in dogs. J Crit Care 6:29, 1991.
38. Eisenberg PR, Hansbrough JR, Anderson D, et al: A prospective study of lung water measurements during patient management in an intensive care unit. Am Rev Respir Dis 136:662, 1987.
39. Humphrey H, Hall J, Sznajder JI, et al: Improved survival in ARDS patients associated with a reduction in pulmonary capillary wedge pressure. Chest 97:1176, 1990.
40. Avery ME and Mead J: Surface properties in relation to atelectasis and hyaline membrane disease. Am J Dis Child 97:517, 1959.
41. Kendig JW, Notter RH, Cox C, et al: Surfactant replacement therapy at birth: Final analysis of a clinical trial and comparison with other trials. Pediatrics 82:756, 1988.
42. Soll RF, Hoekstra RE, Fangman JJ, et al: Multicenter trial of single-dose modified bovine surfactant extract (Survanta) for prevention of respiratory distress syndrome. Pediatrics 85:1092, 1990.
43. Petty TL, Silvers GW, Paul GW, et al: Abnormalities in lung elastic properties and surfactant function in adult respiratory distress syndrome. Chest 75:571, 1979.
44. Hallman M, Spragg R, and Harrell JH: Evidence of lung surfactant abnormality in respiratory failure: Study of bronchoalveolar lavage phospholipids, surface activity, phospholipase activity, and plasma myoinositol. J Clin Invest 70:673, 1982.
45. Holm BA, Notter RH, Seigle J, et al: Pulmonary physiological and surfactant changes during injury and recovery from hyperoxia. J Appl Physiol 59:1402, 1985.
46. Stinson SF, Ryan DP, Hertweck MS, et al: Epithelial and surfactant changes in influenza pulmonary lesions. Arch Pathol Lab Med 100:147, 1976.
47. Holm BA, Matalon S, Finkelstein JN, et al: Type II pneumocyte changes during hyperoxic lung injury and recovery. J Appl Physiol 65:2672, 1988.
48. Oldham KT, Guice KS, Stetson PS, et al: Bacteremia-induced suppression of alveolar surfactant production. J Surg Res 47:397, 1989.
49. Giammona GT: Effects of furniture polish on pulmonary surfactant. Am J Dis Child 113:658, 1967.
50. Seeger W, Stohr G, and Wolf HRD: Alteration of surfactant function due to protein leakage: Special interaction with fibrin monomer. J Appl Physiol 58:326, 1985.
51. Holm BA, Enhorning GE, and Notter RH: A biophysical mechanism by which plasma proteins inhibit surfactant activity. Chem Phys Lipids 49:49, 1988.
52. Li JJ, Sanders RL, McAdam KP, et al: Impact of C-reactive protein (CRP) on surfactant function. J Trauma 29:1690, 1989.
53. Holm BA, Venkitaraman AR, Enhorning GE, et al: Biophysical inhibition of synthetic lung surfactants. Chem Phys Lipids 52:243, 1990.
54. Berggren P, Lachmann B, Curstedt T, et al: Gas exchange and lung morphology after surfactant replacement in experimental adult respiratory distress syndrome induced by repeated lung lavage. Acta Anaesthesiol Scand 30:321, 1986.
55. Kobayashi T, Kataoka H, Ueda T, et al: Effect of surfactant supplement and end-expiratory pressure in lung-lavaged rabbits. J Appl Physiol 57:995, 1984.

56. Jobe A, Ikegami M, Jacobs H, et al: Permeability of premature lamb lungs to protein and the effect of surfactant on that permeability. J Appl Physiol 55:169, 1983.
57. Berry D, Ikegami M, and Jobe A: Respiratory distress and surfactant inhibition following vagotomy in rabbits. J Appl Physiol 61:1741, 1986.
58. Lachmann B, Hallman M, and Bergmann KC: Respiratory failure following anti-lung serum: Study on mechanisms associated with surfactant system damage. Exp Lung Res 12:163, 1987.
59. Matalon S, Holm BA, and Notter RH: Mitigation of pulmonary hyperoxic injury by administration of exogenous surfactant. J Appl Physiol 62:756, 1987.
60. Harris JD, Jackson F Jr, Moxley MA, et al: Effect of exogenous surfactant instillation on experimental acute lung injury. J Appl Physiol 66:1846, 1989.
61. Zelter M, Escudier BJ, Hoeffel JM, et al: Effects of aerosolized artificial surfactant on repeated oleic acid injury in sheep. Am Rev Respir Dis 141:1014, 1990.
62. Zucker AR, Holm BA, Nahum A, et al: Exogenous surfactant reduces pulmonary edema and shunt in canine oleic acid lung injury. Am Rev Respir Dis 137:A226, 1988.
63. Zucker AR, Wood LDH, Crawford G, et al: Early surfactant replacement reduces aspiration pneumonitis in dogs ventilated with PEEP. J Appl Physiol (in press).
64. Richman PS, Spragg RG, Robertson B, et al: The adult respiratory distress syndrome: First trials with surfactant replacement. Eur Resp J 2(Suppl):109, 1989.
65. Lachmann B: Animal models and clinical pilot studies of surfactant replacement in adult respiratory distress syndrome. Eur Respir J 2(Suppl):98, 1989.
66. Wolfson MR and Shaffer TH: Liquid ventilation during early development: Theory, physiologic process and application. J Dev Physiol 13:1, 1990.
67. Greenspan JS, Wolfson MR, Rubenstein SD, et al: Liquid ventilation of human preterm neonates. J Pediatr 117:106, 1990.
68. Curtis SE, Fuhrman BP, and Howland DF: Airway and alveolar pressures during perfluorocarbon breathing in infant lambs. J Appl Physiol 68:2322, 1990.
69. Light RB, Perez-Padilla R, and Kryger MH: Perfluorocarbon artificial blood as a volume expander in hypoxemic respiratory failure in dogs. Chest 91:444, 1987.

45

Disorders of the Proximal Airway

Richard E. Weibley, M.D., M.P.H.

Pathologic conditions of the airway requiring admission to a pediatric intensive care unit are a common problem. This chapter will discuss disorders of the proximal airway, defined here as that portion from the nares to the carina. The sections that follow relate relevant concerns regarding anatomy, physiology, pathology, and treatment of proximal airway disorders in the pediatric patient.

ANATOMY

The structural anatomy of the airway begins very early in fetal development.[1, 2] At approximately 24 days of gestation, the tracheobronchial groove is complete and two primitive lung buds exist. Continued development of the airway occurs throughout pregnancy and early childhood, finally ceasing sometime around adolescence. The process of development, as well as absolute size differences, is important to understand the causes of proximal airway failure and their appropriate treatment in infants, children, and adolescents.

Because the newborn infant has a relatively small mandible and a large tongue that crowds and fills the oropharynx, they are primarily obligate nose breathers during quiet respiration.[3] With crying, when the mouth is wide open and the tongue is thrust forward and down, infants can easily exchange air via the oropharynx. As the midface and mandible grow, the relative difficulties of oropharyngeal breathing in infancy disappear.

The epiglottis in infancy is relatively long and stiff, U- or V-shaped, and angulated approximately 45 degrees from the anterior pharyngeal wall because of the close proximity of the hyoid bone and thyroid cartilage.[4] As growth occurs, separation of the hyoid bone and the thyroid cartilage results in the epiglottis assuming a more erect position. By adolescence, the epiglottis assumes the flattened and flexible shape of adult anatomy, positioned parallel to the base of the tongue.

The laryngeal structures also change with growth, moving lower in the neck with age.[3] In the term infant, the laryngeal inlet is at the level of the intervertebral space between C3 and C4, whereas in adults it rests at the space between C4 and C5 (Fig. 45–1).[4] As the infant grows, the vocal cords change direction and shape, increasing length primarily from growth of the anterior ligamentous portion. Because the infant vocal cord is approximately half cartilaginous and the vocal process of the arytenoid cartilage is angled inward and downward, the infant vocal cord is concave when viewed from above. With growth, as the thyroid cartilage inclines anteriorly, the vocal cord attachments also move forward, which tends to straighten them.

In the adult, the laryngeal inlet is generally the most narrow portion of the respiratory tract. In infants and young children, the narrowest point in the proximal respiratory tract is usually the laryngeal outlet, the inferior ring portion (arch) of the cricoid cartilage. With growth, the ring enlarges, the cricoid plate assumes a more vertical position, and this anatomic point of narrowing disappears (Fig. 45–2).

The histologic characteristics of the larynx remain constant from infancy to adulthood.[3] Squamous epithelium covers the upper portion of the epiglottis, the lateral walls of the vestibule, and the vocal cords.

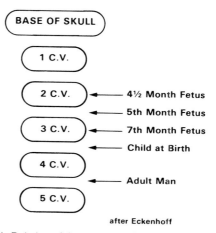

Figure 45–1. Relation of the aperture of the larynx to the base of the skull and vertebral column. (From Shoemaker WC, Ayres S, Grenvik A, et al: Textbook of Critical Care, 2nd ed. Philadelphia, WB Saunders, 1989.)

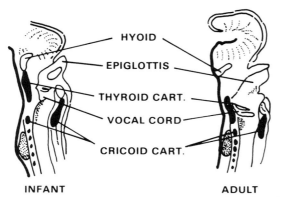

Figure 45–2. The infant and adult larynx in sagittal section. (From Shoemaker WC, Ayres S, Grenvik A, et al: Textbook of Critical Care, 2nd ed. Philadelphia, WB Saunders, 1989.)

Ciliated columnar epithelium lines the ventricle, inferior portion of the vestibules, and the entire laryngeal cavity below the laryngeal inlet. Attached by loose connective tissue, the columnar epithelium easily becomes edematous when irritated, an important process in the pathophysiology of several obstructive disorders.

At birth, the formation of the cartilaginous airways is complete.[1, 2, 5] In the postnatal period, alveolar growth converts nonrespiratory bronchioles to respiratory bronchioles and decreases the number of conducting airways so that by approximately 3 to 4 years of age, the system of branching remains constant. Infants have fewer, smaller, and thicker alveoli than do older children and adults, increasing from approximately 25 million at term gestation to 300 million at full maturation, sometime between the fourth and eighth years of life.[2, 6]

Airway diameter decreases progressively with branching of the conducting airways, but total airways area steadily increases at each successive level of the tracheobronchial tree.[1, 2, 5] Little decrease in individual airways diameter occurs with branching distal to the bronchiole. As the air stream moves peripherally, increases in cross-sectional area sharply reduce air flow velocity, with important physiologic implications for the distribution of airway resistance in normal and disease states.

PHYSIOLOGY

The proximal airway performs many functions, including filtering, warming, and humidifying air in its passage from the atmosphere to the alveoli. Perhaps the most critical physiologic characteristic of the proximal airway is its substantial contribution to total functional resistance secondary to tissue and gas movements.[5, 7] This has implications for both acute and chronic disease states.

Airway resistance is affected by changes in airway dimension, number, pressure, and flow. A simple formula for resistance is:

$$resistance = \frac{change\ in\ pressure}{flow}$$

Thus, resistance is directly proportional to pressure changes and is inversely proportional to flow changes. The Poiseuille law describes the pressure produced by laminar gas flow through a tube.[1, 5] The equation,

$$P = \frac{V\ (8\ l)\ n}{r^4}$$

demonstrates that the radius, raised to the fourth power in the denominator, is the most important determinant of pressure and, thus, resistance.

Airways resistances normally change at differing lung volumes.[1, 5, 7] At large volumes, the airways are distended and resistance is low. After forced expiration and near residual volume, resistance becomes infinitely high as pleural pressures close airways and flow ceases. Estimates of total lung resistance (airway and tissue) have been obtained using dynamic pressure-volume curves and plethysmography.[5, 7] Measurements in children younger than 2 years of age range from 18 to 29 cm H_2O/l/sec, in contrast to adults with larger airways and resistances of 1 to 3 cm H_2O/l/sec at resting lung volumes. Average infant nasal resistance by indirect measurements is 13 cm H_2O/l/sec, nearly half of total respiratory resistance.

Because of the rapid increase in total cross-sectional area with successive branching of conducting airways, nearly all airway resistance occurs proximal to small bronchioles. Hence, even modest reductions in the size of the most proximal airways significantly increase airway resistance, producing signs and symptoms of obstruction. This is particularly important in the smallest and youngest patients.

PATHOPHYSIOLOGY

Abnormalities associated with proximal airway obstruction may be either acute or chronic. They include changes in respiratory rate, depth, inspiratory:expiratory ratio, nasal flaring, retractions, wheezing or stridor, or both, right or left heart failure, or both, and pulmonary edema. In severe obstruction, patients may exhibit agitation, irritability, confusion, or somnolence. Cyanosis, hypercarbia, and uncompensated respiratory or metabolic acidosis indicate imminent collapse.

Stridor and wheezing are the hallmarks of respiratory obstruction.[8–10] Understanding the pathophysiology of the symptoms helps the clinician localize the obstructive lesion and direct therapy most effectively.

Stridor, derived from the Latin "stridulus," means creaking, whistling, or grating.[11] It may be loud or soft, high-pitched or low, musical or harsh. Stridor occurs overwhelmingly in the proximal airway between the laryngeal inlet and the thoracic inlet of the trachea. In this portion of the airway, the individual forces of a relatively positive atmospheric pressure and a negative intraluminal airway pressure combine to cause the airway to collapse and obstruct air flow at the site of the pathologic condition during inspiration. The resulting air flow turbulence creates the characteristic noise termed *stridor*.

Wheezing,[10, 11] derived from the Old Norse, means

"to hiss" and is most often associated (by clinicians) with asthma and reactive airway disease. Wheezing is predominantly an expiratory sound involving obstruction of the intrathoracic conducting airways. In contrast to the dynamics of the extrathoracic airway during inspiration, during expiration the intrathoracic airways are collapsed and obstructed by positive thoracic pressures and tissue elastic forces. Wheezing is usually associated with obvious expiratory effort and is not synonymous with bronchospasm, as it also arises from other obstructive airway pathologic conditions.

Under rare circumstances, an inspiratory wheeze or expiratory stridor may be described. Generally, a careful physical examination coupled with a thorough history will allow localization of the obstructive site.[5, 9] Normal breathing is not audible because even during maximal inspiration and expiration, linear air flow velocity is too low to produce sound. Breathing becomes audible when narrowed air passages change the linear velocity and air flow characteristics, creating turbulence and noise. Supracarinal lesions should commonly reveal symmetric changes throughout the respiratory cycle, whereas an obstructive pathologic condition beyond the carina creates evidence of unilateral signs and symptoms. Similarly, lesions of the extrathoracic airway are evident during the inspiratory phase of respiration and those of an intrathoracic conducting airway are evident during expiration. A good general rule is that lesions causing stridor will be found above the clavicle (thoracic inlet), whereas those associated with wheezing will be located below the clavicle (intrathoracic).

Chronic obstruction of proximal airways was linked to cardiac disease in 1965. Several authors[12, 13] reported the finding of cor pulmonale in patients with various types of chronic airway obstruction, such as hypertrophied lymphoid tissue or laryngotracheomalacia, (LTM). Other authors even reported finding left heart failure caused by airway obstruction.[14, 15] In all cases, the patient had experienced airway obstruction for many months prior to evaluation. Relief of the obstruction improved the heart failure in all cases. Recurrent hypoxia and hypercarbia were felt to be the cause of the heart failure through increases in pulmonary artery smooth muscle tone.[14] Wide fluctuations in intrathoracic pressure and hypoxia were also thought to play a role, particularly in left heart failure.[15]

Pulmonary edema has also been described in association with acute airway obstruction.[16] In the 1970s and 1980s, pulmonary edema was reported in association with croup or epiglottis,[17–19] strangulation,[20] laryngospasm or laryngeal edema,[21–23] and foreign bodies.[16, 24] The presence of the pulmonary edema was noted both before and after relief of the obstructive lesion. The question of whether it is often present (but not recognized) before the airway obstruction is relieved is of some controversy.[25] It is clear that acute pulmonary edema may be a complicating factor of both acute and chronic airway obstruction. Long-term obstruction leads to cor pulmonale and, less frequently, to biventricular disease.

Pulmonary edema exists when pulmonary interstitial fluid accumulates and overflows into the alveoli. The flow of fluid in the pulmonary interstitium is described by the Starling equation.[26] Every variable in the equation can be affected by airway obstruction, resulting in excessive build-up of pulmonary interstitial fluid and pulmonary edema.

Chronic airway obstruction can also lead to pulmonary hypertension. As the right ventricle hypertrophies, encroachment of the left ventricle occurs via ballooning of the interventricular septum. Left ventricular end-diastolic pressures increase, followed by elevated left atrial pressures, resulting in biventricular failure and pulmonary edema.[27–29]

Acute pulmonary edema from proximal airway obstruction is more difficult to conceptualize pathophysiologically. Two mechanisms may be related to its development. The Mueller maneuver (inspiration against a closed glottis) has been shown to increase left ventricular afterload.[30] The Valsalva maneuver (expiration against a closed glottis) raises intrathoracic pressures and diminishes left ventricular end-diastolic volume, left ventricular systolic volume, and ejection fraction via similar but opposite transmural forces.[30, 31]

DIFFERENTIAL DIAGNOSIS AND TREATMENT

Congenital Problems

Airway obstruction in pediatric patients can be easily divided into acquired and congenital causes, which are summarized in Table 45–1.[11] Among the congenital lesions, three craniofacial anomalies occur most frequently: choanal atresia, Pierre-Robin anomalad, and Treacher Collins syndrome.

Bilateral choanal atresia, evident in the newborn in whom respiratory distress develops when the mouth is closed, is easily diagnosed by failure of a suction catheter to pass from the nare through the nasopharynx and into the posterior pharynx. Treatment involves the placement of an oral airway followed by surgical removal of the obstructing tissue or bony plate. The Pierre-Robin and Treacher Collins syndromes both cause airway obstruction resulting from mandibular hypoplasia and relative macroglossia with posterior positioning of the tongue into the nasopharynx and oropharynx. Management goals are to maintain an adequate airway until mandibular growth occurs.[32] In the most severely affected infants, tracheostomy may be necessary to prevent the development of cor pulmonale.

Laryngotracheomalacia (LTM), also called congenital laryngeal stridor, is a common, transient, and generally self-limited cause of stridor resulting from cartilaginous immaturity and laxness in the laryngeal framework and epiglottis. The stridor gradually resolves with growth. Endotracheal intubation or tracheostomy is rarely necessary, though symptoms may worsen dramatically with the occurrence of otherwise trivial viral upper respiratory tract infections. LTM reportedly accounts for as much as 75% of congenital laryngeal pathologic conditions; however, it is probably overdiagnosed because of a lack of precise diagnostic criteria.[11] The patient with

LTM with persistent symptoms that do not resolve with growth and maturation or the patient in whom symptoms are severe, should be carefully evaluated for an alternative pathologic condition.

Congenital subglottic stenosis usually has its most significant point of narrowing in the area of the cricoid cartilage, 2 to 3 mm below the infant glottis. Inflammation and swelling from secondary causes superimposed on the fixed lesion will further decrease airway diameter.[33] In airways of this size, as little as 1 mm of uniform edema can reduce the airway cross-sectional area by 70%, seriously limiting the child's ability to breathe.[4]

Table 45–1. CAUSES OF OBSTRUCTION IN THE PEDIATRIC PATIENT

Congenital
Craniofacial dysmorphologic features (with micrognathia and glossoptosis)
  Pierre-Robin syndrome
  Treacher Collins syndrome (mandibulofacial dysostosis)
  Hallermann-Streiff syndrome (oculomandibular)
  Möbius syndrome
  De Lange syndrome
  Freeman-Sheldon syndrome (whistling face)
Choanal atresia
Macroglossia
  Beckwith syndrome
  Congenital hypothyroidism
  Glycogen storage diseases
  Down syndrome
  Diffuse muscular hypertrophy of the tongue
  Localized lingual tumors
Laryngotracheomalacia
Congenital subglottic stenosis
Congenital vocal cord paralysis
Laryngotracheoesophageal webs
Vascular rings and slings
Congenital tracheal anomalies
Congenital calcification of tracheal cartilages
Congenital tumors and cysts
  Subglottic hemangioma
  Laryngeal lymphangioma and cystic hygroma
  Cysts and laryngoceles
  Miscellaneous congenital tumors
Birth trauma-edema
Metabolic: laryngismus stridulus–hypocalcemia
Immunologic-hereditary angioneurotic edema
Neurogenic-reflex laryngospasm

Acquired Obstruction
Infectious
  Supraglottitis
  Laryngotracheobronchitis
  Acute spasmodic laryngitis
  Diphtheria
  Retropharyngeal abscess
  Bacterial tracheitis–necrotizing tracheobronchitis
Immunologic-juvenile rheumatoid arthritis
Trauma
  Foreign bodies
  Iatrogenic
    Postextubation
    Postinstrumentation
    Postoperative
  External trauma
  Thermal and chemical burns
Neoplasia
  Laryngeal papillomatosis
  Miscellaneous tumors and nodes

Table 45–2. EMBRYOLOGIC ANOMALIES ASSOCIATED WITH ABNORMAL DEVELOPMENT OF THE AORTIC ARCH

Anomalous innominate artery: most common and generally associated with mild tracheal compression
Double aortic arch: associated with severe tracheal compression requiring surgical correction of the arch
Right aortic arch with left ductus or ligamentum arteriosus
Anomalous right subclavian artery
Anomalous left common carotid artery
Anomalous left pulmonary artery

Congenital vocal cord paralysis may account for up to 10% of congenital laryngeal disorders.[11] Bilateral or unilateral paralysis generally corresponds to central or peripheral nerve pathologic conditions. The left recurrent laryngeal nerve is more susceptible to damage associated with surgery or other congenital lesions, often cardiovascular lesions. Bilateral vocal cord paralysis is associated with increased intracranial pressure caused by caudal brain stem displacement and nerve root traction.[3, 11] Birth trauma may also be responsible, though in most cases the cause remains unknown. Congenital vocal cord paralysis has a good prognosis for spontaneous recovery.

Aberrant aortic arch remnant vessels create vascular rings and slings with subsequent compression of the esophagus or trachea (Table 45–2).[11, 34–36] They may be present as either intermittent or persistent wheezing or stridor, often in association with eating. Surgical correction is necessary for lesions causing moderate to severe obstruction associated with recurrent pneumonia, atelectasis, or failure to thrive.[5] Preoperatively, an endotracheal tube will provide a secure airway. Operative mortality is highest in infants less than 6 months of age. Pulmonary artery slings are the most problematic because of associated tracheobronchial tract anomalies, particularly areas of tracheomalacia caused by poor cartilaginous support. This may take weeks to heal after removing the vascular sling, requiring the use of positive end-expiratory pressure or constant positive airway pressure and stints for the softened airway segment while healing and growth occurs.[37]

Acquired Pathologic Conditions

Beyond the newborn period, infectious causes of upper airway obstruction are most common. Adenoidal and tonsillar hypertrophy may cause acute or chronic obstruction.[38–42] Potential spaces defined by fascial planes serve as sites for abscess formation and airway obstruction. These occur most commonly in the child older than 1 to 2 years of age and are generally bacterial, although a notable exception is the lymphoid hypertrophy associated with Epstein-Barr virus infection.[40, 41] Acute epiglottitis (AE), laryngotracheobronchitis (LTB), and bacterial tracheitis (BT) are the most common presenting infectious causes of upper airway obstruction (Table 45–3).[43]

Acute epiglottitis, also called supraglottitis, is most

Table 45–3. COMPARISON OF LARYNGOTRACHEOBRONCHITIS, ACUTE EPIGLOTTITIS, AND BACTERIAL TRACHEITIS*

	LTB†	AE‡	BT§
History			
Age	2mo–3yr	3–7 (usually)	All ages
Onset	Gradual	Rapid	Gradual
Respiratory disease	None to moderate	Marked	Moderate to marked
Symptoms			
Dysphagia	0	2+	±
Dyspnea	±	2–3+	2+
Sore throat	±	4+	±
Signs			
Sound	Bark, stridor	Muffed, guttural	Bark, stridor
Secretions	Normal for age	Drooling	Normal for age
Position	Lying, sitting, standing	Sitting, leaning	Sitting
Fever	37–38° C	38°+ C	38°+ C
Facies	Normal	Anxious, distressed, toxic reaction	Anxious

*Modified from Holbrook PR: Issues in airway management, 1988. Crit Care Clin 4:789, 1988.
†LTB = laryngotracheobronchitis.
‡AE = acute epiglottitis.
§BT = bacterial tracheitis.

often caused by *Haemophilus influenzae*, type B. The spectrum of supraglottitis also includes viral agents[44] and group A β-hemolytic streptococci.[45]

The clinical picture of AE is classically one of extreme respiratory distress, high fever, drooling, and dysphagia, all of abrupt onset. Unfortunately, supraglottic infections may not present with the classic picture, symptomatology often mimicking LTB or BT.[46–48]

The unacceptably high mortality and morbidity associated with failure to diagnose AE has led to a systemized approach to diagnosis and treatment in suspected cases.[49–50] Patients should always be attended by someone skilled in airway management. Radiologic procedures such as lateral neck films should be used only for the exceptional case. At present, the accepted plan is to take the child to the operating room for visual inspection of the airway and nasotracheal intubation. Specimens of the epiglottis and blood should be obtained for culture after the airway is secured, and antibiotic therapy should be instituted to ensure coverage against β-lactamase–positive *H. influenzae*. Other sites of infection due to *H. influenzae* should also be screened, such as lungs, joints and, rarely, the central nervous system.[51] Hopefully, the vaccination of infants against *H. influenzae* disease beginning at 2 months of age will significantly decrease the incidence of epiglottitis.

After intubation, the patient should remain in an intensive care unit so that proper maintenance of the airway can be accomplished. An issue of some controversy is when to extubate the patient and whether to visualize the epiglottis to aid in the decision. Although numerous studies have been performed to address this issue, none has really provided justification for the need or predictive value of visualization.[52–55] Resolution of airway obstruction does not appear to correlate with resolution of fever[52] or the size of the epiglottis.[52–54] A definitive answer about when to safely extubate patients with AE remains elusive, though all studies indicate a time frame of greater than 12 hours. Until a more

scientific method is defined, this author's general rule is, "The tube should be removed by the time of the second sunrise."

LTB is usually a mild illness not resulting in critical care services. The clinical features are well recognized (see Table 45–3).[43] For those with symptoms severe enough to warrant admission to the pediatric intensive care unit, the use of a scoring system provides an objective measure of the degree of respiratory difficulty. Several different scoring systems have been developed.[56–57] A relatively simple one is found in Table 45–4.

A host of viral agents cause LTB.[58] Parainfluenza viruses account for most cases. Adenoviruses, respiratory syncytial virus, influenza, and measles viruses are other identifiable agents. Viral LTB usually has a less rapid onset, lower fever, and a less toxic appearance than does AE. It also tends to occur in younger infants and children, primarily those 3 months to 5 years of age.

Treatment of viral LTB is symptomatic. Mist therapy, though historically used, has never been shown to be beneficial.[59–61] Oxygen is indicated because hypoxemia is often present.[57, 62, 63] The use of α-adrenergic agents, primarily racemic epinephrine, is common and beneficial, though it is associated with a rebound of symptoms.[64] Corticosteroid therapy has been debated for the past 25 years and remains controversial.[65, 66] Helium and oxygen mixtures have been used for LTB and other obstructive lesions.[67, 68] Helium and oxygen mixtures are of lower viscosity than nitrogen and oxygen mixtures and reduce airway resistance and the work of breathing. At least one study has suggested a risk of hypoxemia in small infants.[68] Antibiotics are of no benefit in uncomplicated viral LTB. BT, with features that overlap both LTB and AE (See Table 45–3),[43] probably represents a bacterial superinfection complicating viral LTB.[69–73] Clinical symptoms begin with a gradual onset of upper respiratory tract complaints progressing to fever, toxic-

Table 45–4. CROUP SEVERITY SCORING SYSTEM

Rating	0	1	2	Individual Rating
Sign				
Inspiratory breath sounds	Normal	Harsh rhonchi	Delayed	
Stridor	None	Inspiratory	Inspiratory and expiratory	
Cough	None	Hoarse cry	Seal-like bark	
Retractions–nasal flaring	None	Nasal flaring, suprasternal retractions	Flaring, suprasternal and intercostal retractions	
Cyanosis	None	In room air	40% O_2	
			Total score	

ity, and marked distress. Laryngoscopy reveals a normal epiglottis with mucopurulent edema and copious thick secretions requiring tracheal intubation for airway toilet and relief of obstructive symptomatology. The usual pathogens are *Staphylococcus aureus, H. influenzae,* or α-hemolytic streptococci. A few patients have been reported to experience toxic shock syndrome,[74] and BT may occur more frequently in children with trisomy 21, a population with underlying airway anatomic differences.[75] Despite the concern about BT, antibiotics should not be used routinely in patients with LTB as prophylaxis.

Occasionally, patients who have required tracheal intubation and mechanical ventilation experience a necrotic, inflammatory process of the distal trachea known as necrotizing TB.[76–78] Although its exact cause is unclear, it appears that barotrauma, low humidification, and infection may all play a role. The clinical diagnosis should be suspected when patients with previous stability and normocarbia experience hypercarbia that is otherwise unexplainable. Bronchoscopy reveals occlusive debris histologically composed of sloughed mucosal epithelium, inspissated secretions, and few polymorphonuclear cells.[78] Morbidity and mortality are unacceptably high.

Trauma follows infection as the second most common cause of upper respiratory tract obstruction in the pediatric population.[79, 80] Included are injuries such as those caused by foreign bodies, iatrogenic instrumentation injury to the laryngeal airway or recurrent laryngeal nerve, facial and laryngeal impact injuries, and chemical or thermal burns. Foreign bodies and iatrogenic postextubation obstructive symptoms are most common.

Foreign bodies in children lodge most commonly in the major bronchi.[81–84] Nuts, especially peanuts, and miscellaneous food particles are frequent offenders. Toddlers are most often affected, though foreign bodies may be found in individuals from 6 months of age into adulthood. Obstruction distal to the larynx usually causes not stridor but wheezing. Esophageal foreign bodies produce stridor or wheezing by secondary airway compressions.[82–85] When no history of aspiration is obtained, tracheal foreign bodies are often initially misdiagnosed as viral LTB.

Foreign body removal requires close teamwork among the intensive care practitioner, pulmonologist or surgeon, and anesthesiologist. The use of inhaled broncho-

dilators, postural drainage, and percussion are not recommended for foreign body removal because dislodgement of a distal foreign body into the subglottic space may cause severe or total airway occlusion, a life-threatening complication.[81, 83, 84]

The mechanical trauma associated with intubation, instrumentation, and surgery usually causes stridor because of localized mucosal edema. Less commonly, ulceration, granuloma formation, webs, membranes, stenosis, necrosis, infection, or vocal cord paralysis occur.[79, 86] Severe acquired subglottic stenosis most commonly occurs after prolonged endotracheal intubation and mechanical ventilation.[86–88] Traditional therapy has included tracheostomy for long-term airway support, repeated dilatation, and reconstructive laryngotracheoplasty, all of which can cause significant morbidity and morality.[89–91] The anterior cricoid split operation offers an alternative to the preceding treatment in selected patients and does not preclude subsequent tracheostomy if unsuccessful.[92, 93]

Facial blows and neck injuries can precipitate acute respiratory difficulty through dislocation of the cricoarytenoid cartilage, hematoma, soft tissue swelling and airway compression, and laryngeal or trachea edema or disruption.[3, 5, 94–97]

Acute upper airway obstruction resulting from laryngeal and tracheal edema follows the ingestion of acids, alkalis, and corrosive chemical substances, as well as the inhalation of hot air, steam, smoke, or chemicals.[98, 99] Patients should be admitted to the hospital for observation in a setting in which they can be closely monitored for signs or symptoms of airway compromise. Endoscopic examination of the airway and esophagus may be indicated in some patients.[99–100] Intravenous fluids, oxygen, and racemic epinephrine may relieve obstructive symptoms and alleviate the need for mechanical airway support. Corticosteroids, although used by some clinicians, are probably of no benefit.

Finally, children with mediastinal tumors may present with symptoms of airway obstruction caused by extrinsic compression from the mass lesion.[38, 39, 101, 103] Airway support is often necessary until irradiation or chemotherapy can be instituted to shrink the tumor.

In childhood, early intubation is recommended before edema or obstruction from any proximal airway lesion becomes life-threatening. It is important to realize that laryngoscopy in the infant will demonstrate a larynx located superiorly, a large tongue, and a hyoid bone positioned to depress the epiglottis.[3, 4, 104] The epiglottis is relatively large, stiff, and U-shaped and the airway's narrowest portion is not the glottic inlet but the subglottic space in the region of the cricoid cartilage. An endotracheal tube that passes easily between the vocal cords but not through the cricoid ring should be replaced with a smaller tube to avoid irritating the mucous membranes, a precipitating factor for the development of postextubation stridor and obstruction. In selected circumstances, flexible fiberoptic bronchoscopy may be the method of choice for intubation and evaluation of the airway.[105, 106]

References

1. Murray JF: The normal lung. In: Prenatal Growth and Development of the Lung, 2nd ed. Philadelphia, WB Saunders, 1986, pp. 1–16.
2. Brody JS and Thurlbeck WM: Development, growth and aging of lung. In: Fishman AP (ed): Handbook of Physiology. Section 3: The Respiratory System (American Physiologic Society). Baltimore, Williams & Wilkins, 1986.
3. Adams GL, Boies LR, and Paparella MM (eds): Fundamentals of Otolaryngology. Philadelphia, WB Saunders, 1978.
4. Eckenhoff JE: Some anatomic considerations of the infant larynx influencing endotracheal anesthesia. Anesthesiology 12:401, 1951.
5. Wohl MEB and Mead J: Age as a factor in respiratory disease. In: Chernick V (ed): Kendig's Disorders of the Respiratory Tract, 5th ed. Philadelphia, WB Saunders, 1990, pp. 175–181.
6. Dunhill MS: Postnatal growth of the lung. Thorax 17:329, 1962.
7. Bryan AC and Wohl MD: Respiratory mechanics in children. In: Fishman AP (ed): The Respiratory System: Handbook of Physiology. Section 3, Vol 3 (American Physiologic Society). Baltimore, Williams & Wilkins, 1986.
8. Tunnessen W: Signs and Symptoms in Pediatrics, 2nd ed. Philadelphia, JB Lippincott, 1968.
9. Respiratory noises. In: Phelan PD, Landau LI, and Olinsky A (eds): Respiratory Illness in Children, 2nd ed. Boston, Blackwell Scientific Publications, 1982, pp. 104–131.
10. Schley WS and Krauss AN: Diseases of the upper airways. In: Scarpelli EM, Auld PAM, and Goldman HS (eds): Pulmonary Disease of the Fetus, Newborn and Child. London, Henry Kimpton Publishers, 1978, pp. 254–273.
11. Maze A and Bloch E: Stridor in pediatric patients. Anesthesiology 50:132, 1979.
12. Cox MA, Schiebler GL, Taylor WJ, et al: Reversible pulmonary hypertension in a child with respiratory obstruction and cor pulmonale. J Pediatr 67:192, 1965.
13. Menashe VD, Farrchi C, and Miller M: Hypoventilation and cor pulmonale due to chronic upper airway obstruction. J Pediatr 67:198, 1965.
14. Luke MJ, Mehrizi A, Golger EH, et al: Chronic nasopharyngeal obstruction as a cause of cardiomegaly, cor pulmonale and pulmonary edema. Pediatrics 37:762, 1966.
15. Levin DL, Muster AJ, Pachman LM, et al: Cor pulmonale secondary to upper airway obstruction—cardiac catheterization, immunologic and psychometric evaluation in nine patients. Chest 68:166, 1975.
16. Capitanio MA and Kirkpatric JA: Obstruction of the upper airway in children as reflected on the chest radiograph. Pediatr Radiol 107:159, 1972.
17. Galvis AG, Stool SE, and Bluestone DC: Pulmonary edema following relief of acute upper airway obstruction. Ann Otolaryngol 89:124, 1980.
18. Hurley RM and Kearns JR: Pulmonary edema and croup. Pediatrics 59:695, 1977.
19. Travis KW, Todres ID, and Shannon DC: Pulmonary edema associated with croup and epiglottitis. Pediatrics 59:695, 1977.
20. Oswalt CE, Gates GA, and Holmstrom FMG: Pulmonary edema as a complication of acute airway obstruction. JAMA 238:1833, 1977.
21. Jackson FN, Rowland V, and Corssen G: Laryngospasm-induced pulmonary edema. Chest 78:819, 1980.
22. Lee KW and Downes JJ: Pulmonary edema secondary to laryngospasm in children. Anesthesiology 59:347, 1983.
23. Weissman C, Damask MC, and Yang J: Noncardiogenic pulmonary edema following laryngeal obstruction. Anesthesiology 60:163, 1984.
24. Izsak E: Pulmonary edema due to acute upper airway obstruction from aspirated foreign body. Pediatr Emerg Care 2:235, 1986.
25. Kanter RK and Wacehko JF: Pulmonary edema associated with upper airway obstruction. Am J Dis Child 138:356, 1984.
26. Allen SJ, Drake RE, Williams JP, et al: Recent advances in pulmonary edema. Crit Care Med 15:963, 1987.
27. Kelly DT, Spotnitz HM, and Beiser D: Effects of chronic right ventricular volume and pressure loading on left ventricular performance. Circulation 44:403, 1971.
28. Ladbrook PA, Byrne JD, and McKnight RC: Influence of right ventricular hemodynamics on left ventricular diastolic pressure-volume relations in man. Circulation 59:21, 1979.
29. Ross J: Editorial. Acute displacement of the diastolic pressure-volume of the left ventricle: Role of the pericardium and the right ventricle. Circulation 59:32, 1979.
30. Buda AJ, Pinsley MR, Ingels NB, et al: Effect of intrathoracic pressure on left ventricular performance. N Engl J Med 301:453, 1979.
31. Pinsky MR, Summer WR, Wise RA, et al: Augmentation of cardiac function by elevation of intrathoracic pressure. J Appl Physiol 54:950, 1983.
32. Bull MJ, Given DC, Sandove AM, et al: Improved outcome in Pierre Robin sequence: Effect of multidisciplinary evaluation and management. Pediatrics 86:294, 1990.
33. Phillips JJ and Sansone AJ: Acute infective airway obstruction associated with subglottic stenosis. Anesthesia 45:34, 1990.
34. Colquhoun IW and Pollock JC: Distal tracheal stenosis in two children with double aortic arch and associated tracheomalacia. Eur J Cardiothorac Surg 4:287, 1990.
35. Fletcher BD and Cohn RC: Tracheal compression and the innominate artery. MR evaluation in infants. Radiology 170:103, 1989.
36. Dupuis C, Vaksman G, Pernot C, et al: Asymptomatic form of left pulmonary artery sling. Am J Cardiol 61:177, 1988.
37. Mair EA, Parsons DS, and Lally KP: Treatment of severe bronchomalacia with expanding endobronchial stents. Arch Otolaryngol Head Neck Surg 116:1087, 1990.
38. Guarisco JL, Littlewood SC, and Butcher RB: Severe upper airway obstruction in children secondary to lingual tonsil hypertrophy. Ann Otol Rhinol Laryngol 99:621, 1990.
39. Kraus DH, Rehm SJ, Orlowski JP, et al: Upper airway obstruction due to tonsillar lymphadenopathy in human immunodeficiency virus infection. Arch Otolaryngol Head Neck Surg 116:738, 1990.
40. Woolf DC and Diedericks RJ: Airway obstruction in infectious mononucleosis: A case report. S Afr Med J 75:584, 1989.
41. Kielmovitch IH, Keleti G, Bluestone CD, et al: Microbiology of obstructive tonsillar hypertrophy and recurrent tonsillitis. Arch Otolaryngol Head Neck Surg 115:721, 1989.
42. Sofer S, Weinhouse E, Tal A, et al: Cor pulmonale due to adenoidal or tonsillar hypertrophy or both. Chest 93:119, 1988.
43. Holbrook PR: Issues in airway management, 1988. Crit Care Clinics 4:789, 1988.
44. Grattan-Smith T, Forer M, Kilham H, et al: Viral supraglottitis. J Pediatr 110:434, 1987.
45. Lacroix J, Ahronheim G, Arcand P, et al: Group A streptoccal supraglottitis. J Pediatr 109:20, 1986.
46. Shackleford GD, Siegel MJ, McAllister WH, et al: Subglottic edema in acute epiglottitis in children. Am J Roentgenol 131:603, 1978.
47. Brilli RJ, Benzing G, and Cotcamp DH: Epiglottitis in infants less than two years of age. Pediatr Emerg Care 5:16, 1989.
48. Gershan WM, Gillman K, Baxter M, et al: Acute airway obstruction in a seven month old infant with epiglottitis. Pediatr Emerg Care 4:197, 1988.
49. Bass JW, Fajardo JE, Brien JH, et al: Sudden death due to acute epiglottitis. Pediatr Infant Dis 4:447: 1987.

50. Kantrell RW, Bell RA, Morioka WT, et al: Acute epiglottitis: Intubation versus tracheostomy. Laryngoscope 88:994, 1978.
51. Friedman EM, Healy GB, Damioh J, et al: Supraglottitis and concurrent *Haemophilus* meningitis. Ann Otol Rhinol Laryngol 94:470, 1985.
52. Rothstein P and Lister G: Epiglottitis—duration of intubation and fever. Anesth Analg 62:785, 1983.
53. Oh TH and Motoyama EK: Comparison of nasotracheal intubation and tracheostomy management of acute epiglottitis. Anesthesiology 46:214, 1977.
54. Rowe LD: Advances and controversies in the management of supraglottitis and laryngotracheobronchitis. Am J Otholaryngol 1:235, 1980.
55. Wolf M, Strauss B, Kronenberg J, et al: Conservative management of adult epiglottitis. Laryngoscope 100:183, 1990.
56. Leipzig B, Oski FA, Cummings CW, et al: A prospective randomized study to determine the efficacy of steroids in croup. J Pediatr 94:194, 1979.
57. Taussig LM, Castro O, and Beaudry AC: The respiratory status of children with croup. J Pediatr 81:1068, 1975.
58. Tooley WH: The respiratory system. *In* Rudolf AM and Hoffman JIE (eds): Pediatrics, 18th ed. Norwalk, CN, Appleton & Lange, 1987, pp. 1359–1444.
59. Bourchier D, Dawson KP, and Fergusson DM: Humidification in viral croup: A controlled trial. Aust Pediatr J 20:289, 1984.
60. Henry R: Moist air in the treatment of laryngotracheitis. Otolaryngol Head Neck Surg 88:207, 1980.
61. Corkey CWB, Barker GA, Edmonds DF, et al: Radiographic tracheal diameter measurements in acute infections croup: An objective scoring system. Crit Care Med 9:587, 1981.
62. Taussig L, Castro O, Beaudry PH, et al: Treatment of laryngotracheobronchitis (croup). Am J Dis Child 29:790, 1975.
63. Newth CJL, Levision H, and Bryan AC: The respiratory status of children with croup. J Pediatr 81:1068, 1972.
64. Fogel, JM, Berg IJ, Gerber MA, et al: Racemic epinephrine in treatment of croup: Nebulization alone versus nebulization with intermittent positive pressure breathing. J Pediatr 101:1028, 1982.
65. Tunnessen WW Jr and Feinstein AR: The steroid-croup controversy: An analytic review of methodologic problems. J Pediatr 96:751, 1980.
66. Freezer N, Butt W, and Phelan P: Steroids in croup: Do they increase the incidence of successful extubation? Anaesth Intensive Care 18:224, 1990.
67. Skrinkas GJ, Hyland RH, and Hutcheon MA: Using helium-oxygen mixtures in the management of acute airway obstruction. Can Med Assoc J 128:555, 1983.
68. Butt WW, Koren G, England S, et al: Hypoxia associated with helium-oxygen therapy in neonates. J Pediatr 106:474, 1985.
69. Sofer S, Duncan P, and Chernick V: Bacterial tracheitis—an old disease rediscovered. Clin Pediatr 22:407, 1983.
70. Edwards KM, Dundon MC, and Altemeier WA: Bacterial tracheitis as a complication of viral croup. Pediatr Infect Dis 2:390, 1983.
71. Navi SH and Dunkle LM: Bacterial tracheitis and viral croup. Pediatr Infect Dis 3:282, 1984.
72. Dubin AA, Tholji A, and Rambaud-Cousson A: Bacterial tracheitis among children hospitalized for severe obstructive dyspnea. Pediatr Infect Dis J 9:293, 1990.
73. Kasian GF, Bingham WT, Steinberg J, et al: Bacterial tracheitis in children. Can Med Assoc J 140:46, 1989.
74. Chenaud M, Leclere F, and Martinot A: Bacterial croup and toxic shock syndrome. Pediatrics 145:306, 1986.
75. Caut AJ, Gibson PJ, and West RJ: Bacterial tracheitis in Down's syndrome. Arch Dis Child 62:962, 1987.
76. Metlay LA, MacPherson TA, Doshi N, et al: A new iatrogenous lesion in newborns requiring assisted ventilation (Letter). N Engl J Med 309:111, 1983.
77. Kirpalani H, Higa T, Perlman M, et al: Diagnosis and therapy of necrotizing tracheobronchitis in ventilated neonates. Crit Care Med 13:792, 1985.
78. Pietsch JB, Hirikati SN, Groff DB, et al: Necrotizing tracheobronchitis: A new indication for emergency bronchoscopy in the neonate. J Pediatr Surg 20:391, 1985.
79. Touloukian RJ (ed): Pediatric Trauma. New York, John Wiley & Sons, 1978.
80. Kissoon N, Dreyer J, and Walia M: Pediatric trauma: Differences in pathophysiology, injury patterns and treatment compared with adult trauma. Can Med Assoc J 142:27, 1990.
81. Lima JA: Laryngeal foreign bodies in children: A persistent, life-threatening problem. Laryngoscope 99:415, 1989.
82. Freidman EM: Foreign bodies in the pediatric aerodigestive tract. Pediatr Ann 17:640, 1988.
83. Humphries CT, Wagener JS, and Morgan WJ: Fatal prolonged foreign body aspiration following an asymptomatic interval. Am J Emerg Med 7:669, 1988.
84. Laks Y and Barzilay Z: Foreign body aspiration in childhood. Pediatr Emerg Care 4:102, 1988.
85. Adachi K, Hayashida M, and Toyoshima K: Airway obstruction in a child with esophageal achalasia. Acta Paediatr Jpn 31:600, 1989.
86. Koka BV, Jeon IS, Andre JM, et al: Postintubation croup in children. Anaesth Analg 56:501, 1977.
87. Sherman JM, Lowitt S, Stephenson C, et al: Factors influencing acquired subglottic stenosis in infants. J Pediatr 109:322, 1986.
88. Hawkins DB: Pathogenesis of subglottic stenosis from endotracheal intubation. Ann Otol Rhinol Laryngol 96:116, 1987.
89. Catlin FL and Spanksy EM: Management of subglottic stenosis in children. Otolaryngol Head Neck Surg 93:585, 1985.
90. Burnstein FD, Canalis R, and Ward H: Composite hyoidsternohyoid interposition graft revisited: UCLA experience 1974–1984. Laryngoscope 96:516, 1986.
91. Crysdale WS, Feldman RI, and Naito K: Tracheostomies: A 10 year experience in 319 children. Ann Otol Rhinol Laryngol 97:439, 1988.
92. Cotton RT, Myer CM, Bratcher GO, et al: Anterior cricoid split, 1977–1987. Evolution of a technique. Arch Otolaryngol Head Neck Surg 114:1300, 1988.
93. Anderson GL, Tom LW, Wetmore RF, et al: The anterior cricoid split: The Children's Hospital of Philadelphia experience. Int J Pediatr Otorhinolaryngol 16:31, 1988.
94. Shepherd RT: Accidental self-strangulation in a young child—a case report and review. Med Sci Law 30:119, 1990.
95. Nakayama DK, Gardner MJ, and Rowe MI: Emergency endobronchial intubation in pediatric trauma. Ann Surg 211:218, 1990.
96. Myer CM and Fitton CM: Vocal cord paralysis following child abuse. Int J Pediatr Otorhinolaryngol 15:217, 1988.
97. Fitz-Hugh GS and Powell JB: Acute traumatic injuries of the oropharynx, laryngopharynx, and cervical trachea in children. Otolaryngol Clin North Am 3:375, 1970.
98. Fein A, Lefe A, and Hopewell PC: Pathophysiology and management of complications resulting from fire and the inhaled products of combustion: Review of the literature. Crit Care Med 8:94, 1980.
99. Charnock EL and Meehan J: Postburn respiratory injuries in children. Pediatr Clin North Am 27:661, 1980.
100. Bingham HG, Gallagher TJ, and Powell MD: Early bronchoscopy as a predictor of ventilatory support of burned patients. J Trauma 27:1286, 1987.
101. Abdulla F and Dietrich KA: Endobronchial tuberculosis manifested as obstructive airway disease in a 4 month old infant. South Med J 83:715, 1990.
102. Zarella JT and Finberg FJ: Obstruction of the neonatal airway from teratomas. Surg Gynecol Obstet 170:126, 1990.
103. Pelton JJ and Ratner IA: A technique of airway management in children with an obstructed airway due to tumor. Ann Thorac Surg 48:301, 1989.
104. Salem MR, Mathrubhutham M, and Bennett EJ: Difficult intubation. N Engl J Med 295:789, 1976.
105. Fan LL, Sparks LM, and Fix FJ: Flexible fiberoptic endoscopy for airway problems in a pediatric intensive care unit. Chest 93:556, 1988.

Lower Airway Disease

Howard Eigen, M.D., and Karla M. Gerberding, M.D.

Lower airway disease occurs in pediatric patients of all ages and is particularly characterized by airway obstruction. This is usually caused by bronchoconstriction, airway wall edema, and obstruction of the airway by secretions. Diseases that are characterized by these elements and that are often the cause for admission to the pulmonary intensive care unit (PICU) include asthma and bronchiolitis. Similar processes may occur as well in patients with pneumonia, foreign body aspiration, and inhalation injuries.

Asthma is the leading cause of school absenteeism due to chronic disease.[1] Bronchiolitis affects 2.2/100 children under 2 years of age and results in hospitalization in 1/100 children in the first year of life.[2] Care of patients with these conditions in the pediatric intensive care unit (ICU) warrants a thorough understanding of the pathophysiology and therapy of lower airway disease.

PATHOPHYSIOLOGY

In lower airway disease any of the elements of bronchoconstriction, airway wall edema, and obstruction of the airway lumen by secretions can predominate. The presence of secretions and wall edema may, for example, be more prominent than bronchospasm in infants with bronchiolitis. The musculature of distal airways is relatively poorly developed until 2 to 3 years of age.[3] However, airway obstruction is definitely reversible in young infants.[4]

The combination of these elements results in narrowing of the lumen in both central and peripheral airways. In more distal airways, the lumen may become completely obstructed. At first, obstruction occurs during expiration due to increased pressure compressing the airway and resulting in air trapping. As the degree of obstruction progresses the lumen becomes occluded during inspiration as well, resulting in areas of poorly ventilated alveoli that are distributed throughout the lung. The resultant ventilation perfusion inequality first manifests itself as arterial hypoxemia. Ventilation perfusion inequality has been demonstrated in 83% of a group of asymptomatic patients with asthma by Wagner and associates.[5] In a similar study, Rodriguez-Rosin and associates demonstrated an abnormal ventilation perfusion distribution in 6 of 8 patients with status asthmaticus.[6] Blood flow distribution in this study was bimodal in all patients, suggesting an uneven distribution of pathology within the lung. The degree of airway obstruction leading to ventilation perfusion inequality is assessed clinically by monitoring arterial oxygenation and by pulmonary function testing. The impact of the changes in the airways is magnified by characteristics of the respiratory system unique to infants and young children. The diameter of the tracheal lumen in the newborn infant is one-third that of the adult, whereas that of the bronchiole in the infant is one-half the adult size.[7] Airway edema, airway secretions, or bronchoconstriction in the smaller airway of the infant obstruct a greater percentage of the lumen. Because resistance to airflow is related to the fourth power of the radius of the airway, a small decrease in effective airway diameter can cause a significant increase in resistance and decrease in flow. In infants and young children, this increases significantly the work of breathing.[8] The lower airways contribute a greater portion of total airway resistance in the infant and child than in the adult. Thus an increase in peripheral airway resistance has a greater influence on total airway resistance and causes greater symptomatology.[9]

The pliable sternum and soft ribs of infants and young children cause the chest wall to have a higher compliance than those of older children, and the horizontal relationship of the ribs to the sternum and diaphragm places them at a mechanical disadvantage in infants.[10, 11] These factors add to the work of breathing in the patient with airway obstruction. The diaphragm of infants has been shown to contain more fast-twitch muscle fibers that fatigue easily.[12] When combined, these factors make the infant and young child highly susceptible to respiratory failure.

Impairment of other organ systems may significantly affect the infant with airway disease. Factors that impair tissue oxygenation or increase metabolic demands or impair nutrition such as congenital heart disease or bronchopulmonary dysplasia may cause the patient with airway obstruction to progress to respiratory failure more rapidly.

517

EVALUATION

Evaluation of the child with airway obstruction should begin with a brief physical examination to assess the adequacy of air exchange and oxygenation. After air exchange is deemed adequate and supplemental oxygen is administered, details of the history should be elicited from the caregivers. Important historical data include onset, duration, progression, and relative severity of the current episode, presence of fever, and signs of concurrent illness. In addition, the medications received chronically and on an acute basis during the current episode should be determined. It is important as well to obtain a history of past admissions, noting particularly the need for intensive care therapy, mechanical ventilation, and any history of adverse drug reactions.

The physical examination should begin with a general assessment of the degree of respiratory distress. This includes noting the use of accessory muscles, anxious appearance, and combativeness or agitation. Galant and associates found that increasing pulsus paradoxus correlated with worsening airway obstruction, as does increased use of the accessory muscles of inspiration.[13] In patients with PCO_2 above 40, the pulsus paradoxus was significantly greater than in patients with PCO_2 below 40; however, measurement of pulsus in a distressed child may be difficult.

Auscultation of the chest of the wheezing patient allows further assessment of the degree of air entry and of wheezes or crackles. This information is important not only during initial assessment but also as a serial evaluation during therapy. Auscultatory findings may be difficult to interpret in the child with severe airway obstruction and quiet breath sounds. Patients who have signs of respiratory distress but minimal wheezing on physical examination likely have airway obstruction so severe that flow is not sufficient to generate a wheeze. In a patient with respiratory distress, the absence of wheezing should be interpreted as a sign of severe airway obstruction warranting immediate intervention.

The predictive value of parameters obtained during the initial evaluation for determining the likelihood of admission was studied by Commey and Levison.[14] They found that auscultatory findings, dyspnea, and subjective wheezing were not of value. However, supraclavicular retractions, sternocleidomastoid contraction, and increased pulsus paradoxus were associated with forced expiratory volume in 1 second (FEV_1), forced vital capacity (FVC), and maximal expiratory flow rate (MEFR) below 50% of predicted.

The evaluation of the patient with lower airway disease and respiratory distress must include an assessment of oxygenation and of alveolar ventilation. Pulse oximetry can be used as a rapid initial assessment of oxygenation and as a part of continuous monitoring during inpatient therapy. Oximetry does not replace the arterial blood gas as part of the evaluation of the wheezing child. Its measurement allows an accurate assessment of the adequacy of alveolar ventilation as well as of the level of oxygenation. Serial measurement of arterial blood gases in the patient with severe airway obstruction may require placement of an intra-arterial catheter.

The patient who presents with symptoms of wheezing and respiratory distress should receive humidified supplemental oxygen at a known inspired concentration without delaying therapy until blood gases or oximetry can be obtained. Patients in the pediatric population with respiratory disease do not rely on hypoxic drive to breathe. The danger that supplemental oxygen will cause PCO_2 retention should not preclude institution of therapy in this population.

A chest radiograph should be obtained in all patients who present with severe respiratory distress, especially if the child does not carry a diagnosis of asthma, and should be repeated in any patient who develops a change in the level of oxygenation or degree of respiratory distress. Typical findings on the chest x-ray in patients with asthma or bronchiolitis include air trapping and atelectasis. A review of radiographs in children with asthma has demonstrated abnormalities in 43 to 75% of cases.[15-17] Brooks and associates reviewed the x-ray findings and care of 128 patients hospitalized with asthma and found that no change in the plan of treatment was required as a result of the x-rays in the seven patients with abnormal radiographs or in the 14 patients with normal x-rays in whom abnormalities were suspected clinically.[18]

The removal of free air noted on x-ray is recommended by some people, but a more conservative course may be adopted in the absence of cardiac compromise or as evidence of tension pneumothorax.[19]

THERAPY

The goals of therapy of the child with disease of the lower respiratory tract are maintenance of adequate oxygenation and ventilation, and reversal of airway obstruction. Initial therapy of the patient with respiratory distress from lower airway obstruction involves oxygen, β-adrenergic agonists, and intravenous hydration.

In some patients who experience impaired gas exchange secondary to lower airway disease, therapy and observation in the ICU are required. Patients who demonstrate significant ventilation perfusion inequality manifested by a requirement for more than 50% supplemental oxygen should be monitored in an ICU. Patients who have severe bronchospasm requiring administration of β_2-agonists on a frequent basis (more than every 2 to 3 hours) by inhalation or require intravenous β-agonists due to signs of impending respiratory failure should be hospitalized in an ICU as well.

The best agents for reversal of bronchospasm are β-adrenergic agonists. Agents with the greatest specificity for the β_2-receptor are advantageous and may be delivered by the oral, inhaled, and intravenous routes. These agents are divided into three classes by structure: catecholamines, resorcinols, and saligenins. Catecholamines, including epinephrine, isoproterenol, and isoetharine, are taken up into cells and inactivated rapidly by catechol-O-methyl transferase (COMT). As a result they have a short duration of action and are not as effective by the oral route. Resorcinols (metaproterenol, terbutaline, and fenoterol) and saligenins (albuterol) are not degraded by COMT, are effective when given orally, and have a longer duration of action.[20, 21]

Epinephrine was the first sympathomimetic used in the treatment of asthma. Agents with greater specificity for the β_2-receptor of bronchial smooth muscle are available and have replaced epinephrine. Among the agents those with the most selective β_2 action are terbutaline and albuterol. Because these agents are less active at the β_1- and α-receptors, the incidence of side effects is reduced considerably. Metaproterenol, terbutaline, and albuterol are available for delivery by inhalation and form the basis for therapy in the PICU.[21]

These agents are as effective as subcutaneous epinephrine when given orally or by inhalation and can be given in high doses.[22-24] In the patient with severe airway obstruction the inhaled route is preferred because higher doses can be delivered and the problem of inconsistent absorption is avoided.[25, 26] The degree of β_2-receptor specificity, relative potency and duration of action vary among the β-agonist agents. Available routes of delivery and appropriate doses for these agents are summarized in Table 46–1. The frequency of administration of inhaled bronchodilators is determined by the patient's physical examination including an assessment of air exchange and the degree of respiratory distress and by serial measurements of P_{CO_2} and pH. In the patient with severe airway obstruction manifested by marked respiratory distress and an elevation of the P_{CO_2}, administration of aerosolized β-agonists on a frequent (every 1 to 2 hours) or continuous basis is required. Clinical studies have demonstrated efficacy of inhaled β-agonists in reversing airway obstruction when used in this manner,[27, 28] but patients in the PICU should be monitored for side effects by continuous cardiac and blood pressure monitoring, continuous oximetry, and serial measurement of blood gases and serum electrolytes. Side effects associated with these agents include tachy-cardia, tachydysrhythmias, hypokalemia, and hypertension.[29, 30] These agents act at β_2-receptors in the pulmonary vasculature as well as in the airways, and their frequent use may increase blood flow to areas of poorly ventilated lung resulting in an increase in ventilation perfusion inequality and a decrease in arterial oxygenation. This effect may appear before an improvement in airway obstruction, leading to a transient but significant increase in requirement for supplemental oxygen. This effect is observed whether the drug is given intravenously or by inhalation. Acute mobilization of secretions has also been reported as a side effect of frequent β-agonist administration.[31]

Theophylline is the second bronchodilator commonly used in the treatment of asthma. Theophylline blocks adenosine receptors. This activity may cause cardiac and central nervous system (CNS) side effects. Intravenous aminophylline causes bronchodilation.[32] The degree to which airway obstruction is relieved is related to the logarithm of the plasma concentration between serum concentrations of 5 and 20 μg/dl.[33] The occurrence of side effects in association with theophylline coupled with its low therapeutic index make this necessary as well. The incidence of side effects increased when theophylline was given in combination with β-agonists in studies of children with asthma by Siegel and associates[34] and Galant and associates.[35]

Use of theophylline in pediatric patients is complicated by the many factors that influence its absorption and metabolism. In the intensive care setting, theophylline is generally administered by continuous intravenous infusion, which is thought to provide continuous therapeutic serum drug concentrations. Intermittent boluses of theophylline have been shown to be effective when given every 4 to 6 hours. Administration by bolus infusion may be associated with a greater risk of side effects due to transiently high serum drug levels. In a study of 11 asthmatic children requiring bronchodilators,

Table 46–1. TREATMENT REGIMENS FOR ASTHMA

	Systemic Administration			Inhaled Administration	
	Oral	Subcutaneous	IV	Metered Dose	Nebulizer*
Catecholamine Base					
Epinephrine	—	0.01 ml/kg (1:1,000)	—	—	
Epinephrine suspension	—	0.005 ml/kg	—	—	
Isoproterenol	—	—	—	2 puffs 4 times daily	0.1 ml (1% solution)
Isoetharine	—	—	—	2 puffs 4 times daily	0.24 ml (1% solution)
Resorcinol Base					
Metaproterenol	0.5 mg/kg/dose 3–4 times/daily	—	—	2 puffs 4 times daily	0.01–0.02 ml/kg
Terbutaline	0.035 mg/kg/dose 3–4 times/daily	0.005 mg/kg (0.1% solution)	—	2 puffs 4 times daily	0.1–0.3 ml/kg (0.1% solution or 1 mg/ml)
Fenoterol	0.1 mg/kg/dose 3–4 times daily	—	—	2 puffs 4 times daily	0.03 ml/kg (0.5% solution)
Salinigen Base					
Albuterol	0.15 mg/kg/dose 3–4 times daily	—	0.2–2.0 μg/kg/min	2 puffs 4 times daily	0.1 ml (5% solution)

*Doses are diluted with saline to 2 to 3 ml total volume. Nebulized doses are given every 4 to 6 hours, but the dosage frequency may be increased in the case of a very severe attack.

Goldberg and associates demonstrated better pulmonary function in patients receiving continuous infusion of aminophylline than in those receiving intermittent boluses.[36]

Administration of theophylline is complicated additionally by interindividual variability in metabolism. The clearance of theophylline decreases with increasing age in the pediatric population. The average half-life of theophylline in children from 1 to 16 years of age has been shown to have an average between 3.0 and 3.69 hours.[37, 38] The hepatic metabolism and clearance of theophylline may be influenced further by the presence of viral infection or by the concurrent use of other medications. In the presence of viral infection, the half-life of theophylline may be decreased. In the presence of erythromycin the half-life of theophylline is increased whereas in the presence of isoproterenol and aminophylline its half-life is shortened.[39]

In the patient with severe airway obstruction, aminophylline is administered by bolus followed by continuous infusion. A bolus is administered to achieve a serum theophylline level of 15 to 20 μg/dl. A bolus of 1 mg/kg is assumed, in a patient with an average volume of distribution, to raise the serum concentration by 2 μg/dl. Ideally, the bolus is given after the theophylline serum concentration is known, but this is rarely the case in practice. The maintenance infusion rate is calculated by conversion of the total daily dose of theophylline to an equivalent amount of aminophylline in patients who have documented therapeutic theophylline levels and are known to be compliant. In patients for whom these data are not available, the continuous infusion rate should be based on the patient's age and weight (Table 46–2).[40]

Serum theophylline levels must be monitored closely in any patient receiving the drug by continuous infusion. A level is generally obtained 1 hour following the initial bolus. The level is then repeated after four to five half-lives. These levels are then used to determine the patient's clearance rate. The continuous infusion rate may be adjusted based on this information. Additional levels should be obtained in the presence of any signs of toxicity including tachycardia, irritability, vomiting, nausea, or seizure activity.

Resolution of airway obstruction in the lower respiratory tract involves a reversal of bronchospasm as well as a decrease in the secretions and wall edema resulting from local inflammation. The use of steroids in the treatment of bronchiolitis has not been shown to improve patient outcome.[41] In the patient with bronchiolitis and impending respiratory failure, steroids may be used with the goal of reversing airway inflammation and avoiding the need for mechanical ventilation.

The use of steroids to treat acute exacerbations of asthma is more widely accepted. Controlled studies have not shown persistent benefit from their use. In controlled trials of intravenous steroid use in children with status asthmaticus, Pierson and associates found no significant improvement in pulmonary function parameters or clinical score in patients treated with steroids.[42] Kattan and associates found no significant improvement in pulmonary function parameters or clinical score in steroid-treated patients compared with controls, though, unlike Pierson, he excluded patients already receiving steroids from his study.[43] In contrast, Shapiro and associates[44] found that nonhospitalized children with wheezing who received methylprednisolone in addition to standard therapy had more rapid return of FEV_1 to normal. Younger and associates found that in 49 nonsteroid-dependent children with status asthmaticus, the addition of methylprednisolone to regimens of aminophylline and β-agonists resulted in significantly greater improvement in FEF 25 to 75% and clinical score after 36 hours of therapy as well as fewer episodes of relapse within 4 weeks of hospitalization when compared with control patients.[45] In none of these studies were side effects related to steroid use noted.

Patients who have persistent airway obstruction and PCO_2 elevation (more than 45 to 50) despite the use of continuous aerosolized β-agonists, intravenous aminophylline and corticosteroids are in danger of respiratory failure. The use of intravenous β-agonists should be considered in this group of patients. Downes and associates reported the use of intravenous isoproterenol in a group of patients with PCO_2 of greater than 55 despite conventional therapy.[46] In these patients a rapid, persistent decrease in PCO_2 was observed. Other studies comparing inhaled and intravenous administration of terbutaline[47] and albuterol[48, 49] did not show greater improvement in FEV_1 with intravenous administration.

In patients with persistent PCO_2 elevation who do not respond to conventional therapy and aerosolized β-agonists given every 30 to 60 minutes or continuously, intravenous β-agonists may be used in an effort to prevent respiratory failure and the need for mechanical ventilation.[26, 27] Isoproterenol is given in a dosage of 0.05 to 0.1 μg/kg/min. The infusion is increased if a decrease in PCO_2 does not occur and side effects are not present. Side effects commonly associated with intravenous isoproterenol include tachycardia, tachydysrhythmias, increased ventilation perfusion inequality, and increased theophylline clearance. Other side effects reported in association with its use include elevation of myocardial creatine kinase and myocardial ischemia.[50–52] Thus it is not recommended.

Terbutaline is given by continuous intravenous infusion at a dosage of 25 to 50 ng/kg/min. In the absence of side effects, including tachycardia and tachydysrhythmias, this dose may be increased gradually until a persistent decrease in PCO_2 occurs. Although tachycardia and tachydysrhythmias may occur with the use of intravenous terbutaline, we believe that side effects are less common with this medication than with intravenous isoproterenol.

Table 46–2. AMINOPHYLLINE INFUSION

Age	Dosage
0–1 month	0.15 mg/kg/hr
1–6 months	0.5 mg/kg/hr
6–12 months	1.0 mg/kg/hr
1–9 years	1.2 mg/kg/hr
10–16 years	1.0 mg/kg/hr
>16 years	0.7 mg/kg/hr

MECHANICAL VENTILATION

Respiratory failure from acute asthma has been reported in 5 to 6% of patients. In a study of 19 episodes of respiratory failure in 13 patients with status asthmaticus, Simons and associates found that delayed or inappropriate therapy was a contributing factor in most cases.[53]

Patients with severe airway obstruction who, despite maximal medical therapy, develop progressive Pco_2 retention and or metabolic acidosis, suggesting impending respiratory failure may require intubation and mechanical ventilation. Intubation of an asthmatic child should be approached with care and should be performed by a physician skilled and experienced in intubation. Intubation of these patients poses risks, including worsening of the hypoxemia and acidosis already present and worsening of bronchospasm due to vagal stimulation.

A number of different intubation regimens are acceptable. Suggested regimens include premedication with valium or a related benzodiazepine such as midazolam (0.1 mg/kg to a maximum of 3 mg) and atropine (0.01 to 0.02 mg/kg). This avoids the danger involved in paralyzing patients with respiratory compromise. However, the addition of a neuromuscular paralyzing agent may be considered based on the experience of the institution and physicians involved. With either regimen, the intubation must be completed quickly and in a controlled, calm manner.

Mechanical ventilation of the patient with lower airway obstruction due to asthma or bronchiolitis may be challenging. Reported mortality for asthmatics requiring mechanical ventilation is low.[54] A volume-limited ventilator should be used to ensure adequate alveolar ventilation during periods of changing airway resistance. Inspiratory flow, respiratory rate, and inspiratory time should be adjusted to allow sufficient time for exhalation. Auscultation of the chest allows the physician to determine the adequacy of breath sounds at a given tidal volume. Listening for the end of exhalation prior to the delivery of the next breath from the ventilator provides evidence that expiratory time is adequate, preventing iatrogenic elevation of FRC and impairment of alveolar emptying.

Several studies have investigated the use of controlled hypoventilation in adult patients with severe asthma. This approach treats hypoxemia but does not correct hypercarbia. Acidosis is corrected by bicarbonate infusion.[55, 56] Sedation and muscle relaxants were used for ventilator synchronization. No deaths or pneumothoraces were reported. No controlled studies of this technique have been completed in pediatric patients. It may be considered in the most severely ill mechanically ventilated asthmatic patients whose disease does not improve with conventional mechanical ventilation and who require high airway pressures for ventilation and are at risk for air leak.

The use of positive end-expiratory pressure (PEEP) has traditionally been contraindicated in mechanical ventilation of patients with expiratory airflow obstruction because of its effect of elevating further the FRC in patients with air trapping. PEEP has been used in select patients with the goal of decreasing airway closure and improving emptying of gas from the lungs. Several reports exist of the use of PEEP in severely ill patients who could not be ventilated or oxygenated with minimal PEEP.[57] The use of PEEP in the patient with severe expiratory airflow obstruction should be considered when conventional therapy is not sufficient to meet needs of ventilation or oxygenation, but PEEP should not be considered a part of routine therapy.

Comfort of the child requiring mechanical ventilation is an important part of patient management. Sedation and paralysis are important in this group of patients. Agents commonly used for sedation include midazolam, valium, and seconal. Midazolam has the advantage when given by continuous infusion of providing a constant level of sedation. Neuromuscular paralysis is an important part of management during mechanical ventilation of the patient with lower airway obstruction. Agents commonly used for paralysis include pancuronium and vecuronium (0.1 mg/kg intravenously as needed).

As the patient's condition improves mechanical ventilation should be weaned as the first step in reducing support. Pharmacologic therapy instituted prior to mechanical ventilation should be continued at the same level when ventilation is instituted. Pharmacologic support can be gradually reduced after the patient has progressed to extubation.

References

1. Stempel DA and Mellon MM: Management of acute severe asthma. Pediatr Clin North Am 31:879–890, 1984.
2. Wright PF: Bronchiolitis. Pediatr Rev 7:219–222, 1986.
3. Matsuba K and Thurlbeck WM: A morphometric study of bronchial and bronchiolar walls in children. Am Rev Respir Dis 105:908, 1972.
4. Hughes DM, Lesouef PN, and Landau LI: Effect of salbutamolon respiratory mechanics in bronchiolitis. Pediatr Res 22:83, 1987.
5. Wagner PD, Dantzker DR, Iacovoni VE, et al: Ventilation-perfusion inequality in asymptomatic asthma. Am Rev Respir Dis 118:511–524, 1978.
6. Rodriguez-Rosin R, Ballister E, Roca J, et al: Mechanisms of hypoxemia in patients with status asthmaticus requiring mechanical ventilation. Am Rev Respir Dis 138:732–739, 1985.
7. Engel S: The Child's Lung: Developmental Anatomy, Physiology, and Pathology. London, Edward Arnold, 1947.
8. Eckenhoff JE: Some anatomical considerations of the infant larynx influencing endotracheal anesthesia. Anesthesiol 12:401, 1951.
9. Hogg JC, Williams J, Richardson JB, et al: Age as a factor in the distribution of lower airway conductance and in the pathologic anatomy of obstructive lung disease. N Engl J Med 282:1283–1287, 1970.
10. Agostoni E: Volume pressure relationships of the thorax and lungs in the newborn. J Appl Physiol 14:909, 1959.
11. Richards CL and Bachman L: Lung and chest wall compliance of apneic paralyzed infants. J Clin Invest 40:273, 1961.
12. Keens TG, Bryan AL, Levison H, et al: Development of fatigue-resistant muscle fibers in the human diaphragm and intercostal muscles. Physiologist 20:50, 1977.
13. Galant ST, Groncy CE, and Shaw KC: The value of pulsus paradoxus in assessing the child with status asthmaticus. Pediatrics 61:46–51, 1978.
14. Commey JOO and Levison H: Physical signs in childhood asthma. Pediatrics 58:537–541, 1976.
15. Cooper DM, Cutz E, and Levison H: Occult pulmonary abnormalities in asymptomatic asthmatic children. Chest 71:361–365, 1977.

16. Gilles JD, Reed MH, and Simons FER: Radiographic findings in acute childhood asthma. J Can Assoc Radiologists 29:28, 1978.
17. Eggleston PA, Ward BH, Pierson WE, and Bierman CW: Radiographic abnormalities in acute asthma in children. Pediatrics 54:442–490, 1974.
18. Brooks LJ, Cloutier MM, and Afshani E: Significance of Roentgenographic abnormalities in children hospitalized for asthma. Chest 82:315–318, 1982.
19. Nelson HS: Beta adrenergic agonists. Chest 82:33S–38S, 1982.
20. McFadden ER Jr: Beta-2 receptor agonist: Metabolism and pharmacology. J Allergy Clin Immunol 68:91–97, 1981.
21. Becker AB, Nelson NA, and Simons FER: Inhaled salbutamol vs injected epinephrine in the treatment of acute asthma in children. J Pediatr 102:465, 1983.
22. Uden DL, Goetz DR, Kohen DP, and Fifield GL: Comparison of nebulized terbutaline and subcutaneous epinephrine in the treatment of acute asthma. Ann Emerg Med 14:229–232, 1985.
23. Ben-Zvi Z, Lam C, Hoffman J, et al: An evaluation of the initial treatment of acute asthma. Pediatrics 70:348–353, 1982.
24. Shim C and Williams H Jr: Bronchial response to oral versus aerosol metaproterenol in asthma. Ann Intern Med 93:428–431, 1980.
25. Lee HS: Comparison of oral and aerosol adrenergic bronchodilators in asthma. J Pediatr 99:805–807, 1981.
26. Roth MJU, Wilson AF, and Novey HS: A comparative study of the aerosolized bronchodilators isoproterenol, metaproterenol, and terbutaline in asthma. Ann Allergy 38:16–21, 1977.
27. Colacone A, Wolkove N, Stern E, et al: Continuous nebulization of albuterol in acute asthma. Chest 97:693–697, 1990.
28. Laaban JP, Iuny B, Chauvet JP, et al: Cardiac arrhythmias during the combined use of intravenous aminophylline and terbutaline in status asthmaticus. Chest 94:496–502, 1988.
29. Kolshki GB, Cunningham AS, Niemec PW, et al: Hypokalemia and respiratory arrest in an infant with status asthmaticus. J Pediatr 116:304–307, 1988.
30. Parry WH, Martorano F, and Cotton EK: Management of life threatening asthma with intravenous isoproterenol infusions. Am J Dis Child 130:39–42, 1976.
31. Rossing TH, Fanta CH, McFadden ER Jr, et al: A controlled trial of the use of single versus combined drug therapy in the treatment of acute episodes of asthma. Am Rev Respir Dis 123:190–194, 1981.
32. Levy G and Koysooko R: Pharmacokinetic analysis of the effect of theophylline on pulmonary function in asthmatic children. J Pediatr 86:789–793, 1975.
33. Mitenko PA and Ogilvie RI: Rapidly achieved plasma concentration plateaus with observations on theophylline kinetics. Clin Pharm Ther 13:329–335, 1972.
34. Siegel D, Sheppard D, Gelb A, and Weinberg PF: Aminophylline increases the toxicity but not the efficacy of an inhaled beta-adrenergic agonist in the treatment of acute exacerbations of asthma. Am Rev Respir Dis 132:283–286, 1985.
35. Galant SP, Groncy CE, Duriseti S, and Strick L: The effect of metaproterenol in chronic asthmatic children receiving therapeutic doses of theophylline. J Allergy Clin Immunol 61:73–79, 1978.
36. Goldberg P, Leffert F, Gonzalez M, et al: Intravenous aminophylline therapy for asthma. Am J Dis Child 134:596–599, 1980.
37. Loughman PM, Sitar DS, Ogilvie RI, et al: Pharmacokinetic analysis of the disposition of intravenous theophylline in young children. J Pediatr 88:874–879, 1976.
38. Ellis EF, Koysooko R, and Levy G: Pharmacokinetics of theophylline in children with asthma. Pediatrics 58:542–547, 1976.
39. Hemstreet MP, Miles MV, and Rutland RO: Effect of intravenous isoproterenol on theophylline kinetics. J Allergy Clin Immunol 69:360–364, 1982.
40. Eigen H and McWilliams B: Treatment of the life threatening asthma attack in children. In: Murphy S and Jeene JW (eds): Bronchodilators. New York, Marcel Dekker, 1987.
41. Springer C, Bar-Yishayy E, Uwayyed K, et al: Corticosteroids do not affect the clinical or physiological status of infants with bronchiolitis. Pediatr Pulmonol 9:181–185, 1990.
42. Pierson WE, Bierman CW, and Kelley VC: A double blind trial of corticosteroid therapy in status asthmaticus. Pediatrics 54:282–288, 1974.
43. Kattan M, Gurwitz D, and Levison H: Corticosteroids in status asthmaticus. J Pediatr 96:596–599, 1980.
44. Shapiro GG, Furukawa CT, Pierson WE, et al: Double blind evaluation of methylprednisolone versus placebo for acute asthma episodes. Pediatrics 71:510–514, 1983.
45. Younger RE, Gerber PS, Herrod HG, et al: Intravenous methyl prednisolone efficacy in status asthmaticus of childhood. Pediatrics 80:225–230, 1987.
46. Downes JJ, Wood DW, Harwood I, et al: Intravenous isoproterenol infusion in children with severe hypercapnia due to status asthmaticus. Crit Care Med 1:63–68, 1973.
47. Pierce RJ, Payne CR, Williams SJ, et al: Comparison of intravenous and inhaled terbutaline in the treatment of asthma. Chest 79:506–511, 1981.
48. Hetzel MR and Clark THJ: Comparison of intravenous and aerosol salbutamol. Br Med J 2:16:919, 1976.
49. Lawford P, Jones BJM, and Milledge JS: Comparison of intravenous and nebulized salbutamol in initial treatment of severe asthma. Br Med J 1:84, 1978.
50. Maguire JF, Geha RS, and Umetsu DT: Myocardial specific creatine phosphokinase isoenzyme elevation in children with asthma treated with intravenous isoproterenol. J Allergy Clin Immunol 78:631–636, 1986.
51. Matson JR, Loughlin GM, and Strunk RC: Myocardial ischemia complicating the use of isoproterenol in asthmatic children. J Pediatr 92:776–778, 1978.
52. Kurland G, Williams J and Lewiston NJ: Fatal myocardial toxicity during continuous infusion intravenous isoproterenol therapy of asthma. J Allergy Clin Immunol 63:407–411, 1979.
53. Simons FER, Pierson WE, and Bierman W: Respiratory failure in childhood status asthmaticus. Am J Dis Child 131:1097–1101, 1977.
54. Richards W, Lew C, Carney J, et al: Review of intensive care unit admission for asthma. Clin Pediatr 18:345–352, 1979.
55. Davioli R and Perrett C: Mechanical controlled hypoventilation in status asthmaticus. Am Rev Respir Dis 129:385–387, 1984.
56. Menitove SMK and Goldring RM: Combined ventilator and bicarbonate strategy in the management of status asthmaticus. Am J Med 74:898–901, 1983.
57. Martin JG, Shore S, and Engel LA: Effect of continuous positive airway pressure on respiratory mechanics and pattern of breathing in induced asthma. Am Rev Respir Dis 126:812–817, 1982.

Lung Parenchyma

Samuel J. Tilden, M.S., M.D., and James J. Logan, M.D.

ATELECTASIS

Atelectasis (collapsed normal lung parenchyma) is probably the most frequently encountered pulmonary parenchymal abnormality found in the intensive care unit (ICU). The incidence may be as high as 30% following thoracic surgery. Its importance is generally overlooked because segmental, or subsegmented, collapse does not produce significant physiologic derangements. Failure to consider atelectasis, however, may lead to an erroneous diagnosis of pneumonia and inappropriate treatment. The causes of atelectasis generally fall into two broad categories: bronchial obstruction and direct parenchymal compression. In certain conditions, both factors may be important. The causes of atelectasis are listed in Table 47–1. Bronchial obstruction may be associated with entities that directly block the bronchial lumen (e.g., foreign body, right main stem intubation), injury and diseases of the bronchi, or extrabronchial compression.

The classic findings of lobar or pulmonary atelectasis include retractions, decreased or lacking breath sounds and dullness to percussion over the involved lung, and shift of the heart toward the affected side. The trachea will be shifted toward the side of the collapsed lung (Fig. 47–1). These findings are generally dependent on complete large airway obstruction, including sites at the carina, main stem bronchi, and larger segmental bronchi. Causes of this type of atelectasis most commonly include endotracheal tube malposition, intrabronchial foreign bodies, mucous plug, granuloma or stricture, or extrinsic compression at the carina or main stem bronchus from a vascular ring, bronchogenic cyst, enlarged lymph nodes, or esophageal foreign body.

Atelectasis in small infants and toddlers (4 weeks to 2 years of age) presents more frequently with acute respiratory illnesses. In this population, roentgenologic examination reveals multiple focal areas of opacity (mainly subsegmental), implying scattered areas of complete small airway obstruction. These opacities are discrete in nature, such as strings, bands, and patches; are well defined; and frequently can be traced to the periphery of the lung.

Multiple projections (e.g., lateral view), which are often underutilized in the ICU setting, are more likely to unmask the discreteness and typical appearance of focal atelectasis. An interesting observation is that often areas of focal atelectasis are seen anteriorly involving the right middle lobe, lingula, and right and left anterior segments of both upper lobes. This may be helpful in differentiation between atelectasis and pulmonary edema, which is usually generalized but may concentrate posteriorly in patients kept in the supine position. The number and size of focal atelectatic regions do not necessarily correlate well with the severity of clinical disease. The radiographic findings frequently lag behind clinical improvement in the disease process.

Several factors associated with anesthesia and surgery promote atelectasis with resulting hypoxemia (Table 47–2).[1] They include progressive ascent of the diaphragm associated with supine positioning, induction of anesthesia, muscle paralysis, and direct surgical displacement of thoracic viscera. Loss of inspiratory muscle tone following induction of anesthesia also occurs. Following the decrease in functional residual capacity (FRC) from the preceding, a pathophysiologic sequence of events ensues. Tidal ventilation occurs near or less than volumes associated with small airway closure (i.e., closing capacity), and regions of low ventilation-perfusion mismatch occur with resulting hypoxemia. Decreased lung compliance (resulting from decreased FRC) increases work of breathing and may also contribute to hypoxemia.

Lobar atelectasis results in a compensatory response of the pulmonary vascular bed, which shunts blood away from hypoxic lung regions, thus preventing systemic

Table 47–1. CAUSES OF ATELECTASIS

Foreign Body	Extrabronchial	Parenchymal Compression
Mucous plugs	Enlarged heart	Cardiothoracic surgery
Cystic fibrosis	Tumors	Upper abdominal surgery
Asthma	Vascular rings	Anesthesia, muscle paralysis
Airway inflammation	Enlarged great vessels	
Bronchial stenosis	Enlarged lymph nodes	Pleural effusion pneumothorax
Granuloma, papilloma		Tumors

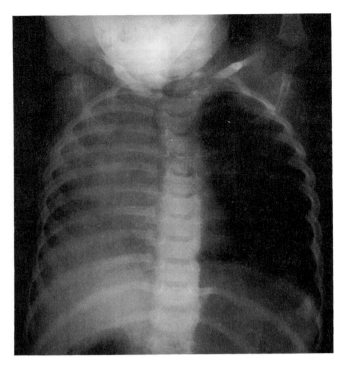

Figure 47-1. A 17-month-old infant with a peanut in the right mainstem bronchus. Note: atelectasis of the right lung, with volume loss, elevation of the right hemidiaphragm, shift of the trachea and mediastinum toward the side of the lesion, and compensatory hyperexpansion of the left lung.

hypoxemia caused by intrapulmonary shunting. Reductions in lobar blood flow of as much as 60% may occur following lobar atelectasis. This reduction is due to an increase in pulmonary vascular resistance of the hypoxic lobe. This response is fairly modest, however, and is altered by many factors, including systemic hypoxemia, vasodilators such as sodium nitroprusside, alkalosis, excessive fluid resuscitation, and pulmonary hypertension (mean pulmonary artery pressures greater than 25 mm Hg).

The mainstay of treatment for lobar atelectasis is aimed at reversing its major underlying causes—intrabronchial obstruction and lung compression—using respiratory therapy maneuvers.[2] Mobilization of secretions is promoted by administration of bronchodilators, chest percussion, postural drainage, and frequent repositioning of the patient. Maneuvers to expand compressed lung include deep cough and incentive spirometry. In addition, for ventilated patients, relatively large insufflations with an anesthesia bag before tracheal suctioning to promote cough are helpful. Care must be taken to avoid mucosal injury during suctioning. Use of positive

Table 47-2. PATHOPHYSIOLOGIC FACTORS IN ATELECTASIS

Decreased functional residual capacity
Increased closing volume
Increased airway resistance
Increased expiratory muscle tone
Altered diaphragmatic position

end-expiratory pressure (PEEP) and continuous positive airway pressure may be of benefit as both a therapeutic and prophylactic therapy, though this is controversial. Intermittent positive-pressure breathing may be useful in patients with neuromuscular weakness. The optimal timing for such treatment is not known; however, 4-hour intervals seem to be common. Frequently, improvement can be seen following the first respiratory treatment. The presence or lack of an x-ray air bronchogram feeding the atelectatic lobe is an important distinction. Atelectasis occurring without an air bronchogram is more likely to signify intrabronchial obstruction and tends to resolve more quickly with therapy than if an air bronchogram is present.

Although use of flexible fiberoptic bronchoscopy (FFB) has been known to resolve atelectasis in selected cases, there is no evidence to support its general use as an initial or preventive mode of treatment.[3] FFB seems most appropriate in the setting in which atelectasis is refractory to 3 or 4 days of intensive respiratory therapy and no air bronchogram is present. In critically ill patients with lobar or total lung collapse, FFB can be useful for definitively identifying patients who require rigid bronchoscopy, and thereby a potentially unnecessary transport to the operating room can be avoided.

Absorption atelectasis and re-expansion pulmonary edema are related to lung collapse and have relevance to the practice of intensive care. Use of 100% oxygen over a period of 10 to 30 minutes promotes atelectasis and intrapulmonary shunting in lung regions with low ventilation:perfusion ratios.[4] Replacing nitrogen with oxygen increases the gas absorption rate across the alveolar membrane and may exceed the net ventilation of poorly ventilated lung, causing collapse. In addition, elevated alveolar oxygen concentrations inhibit hypoxic pulmonary vasoconstriction, increasing blood flow to these regions and gas absorption. These mechanisms provide the basis for the practice of minimizing unnecessary exposure to high levels of oxygen in critically ill patients with significant pulmonary dysfunction.

Pulmonary edema following re-expansion of collapsed lung is a well-known event and occurs after resolution of pneumothorax, pleural effusion, or bronchial obstruction.[5] The onset of symptoms is rapid, occurring immediately or over a few hours and includes tachypnea, intercostal retractions, tachycardia, and cyanosis. Radiographic examination reveals unilateral pulmonary edema in the re-expanded lung. Endotracheal intubation and PEEP may be necessary to control the production of pulmonary edematous fluid and arterial hypoxemia. The mechanism by which re-expansion pulmonary edema occurs is not well understood. Proposed mechanisms include increased negative interstitial and alveolar pressure associated with re-expansion, increased pulmonary vascular endothelial permeability, loss of surfactant, and increased pulmonary artery pressure. Rapid re-expansion of the lung with mechanical strain of lung parenchyma seems to be important. Recent evidence in a rabbit model suggests that other factors, such as release of oxygen free radicals following reperfusion of the re-expanded lung, are also present.[6] Pretreatment with the antioxidants dimethylthiourea and catalase significantly

$$O_2 \xrightarrow{\ e^-\ } O_2^- \xrightarrow{\ e^- + 2H^+\ } H_2O_2 \xrightarrow{\ e^- + H^+\ } OH\cdot \xrightarrow{\ e^- + H^+\ }$$

$$H_2O \qquad\qquad H_2O$$

$$O_2^- + O_2^- + 2H^+ \longrightarrow H_2O_2 + O_2 \quad \} \quad \text{Superoxide dismutases}$$

$$H_2O_2 + H_2O_2 \longrightarrow 2H_2O + O_2 \quad \} \quad \text{Catalases}$$

$$H_2O_2 + RH_2 \longrightarrow 2H_2O + R \quad \} \quad \text{Peroxidases}$$

Figure 47–2. The univalent pathway of oxygen reduction and the enzymatic defenses against the intermediates encountered. (From Fridovich I: The biology of oxygen radicals. Science 201:875, 1978. Copyright 1978 by the AAAS.)

reduced pulmonary edema and inflammation on reexpansion.

OXYGEN TOXICITY

Supplemental oxygen represents one of the most frequently used therapies in the intensive care unit and is an essential component of treatment for most critically ill patients. Its use is tempered by the fact that high levels of oxygen produce lung injury. Use of high oxygen concentrations occurs most often in patients with underlying acute or chronic lung injury; in this instance, the unenviable circumstance of causing ongoing injury to an already damaged lung is present. Currently, there is no effective means of assessing the degree of ongoing injury or of treating oxygen toxicity in the clinical arena; thus, strict attention must be paid to providing a minimum effective dose. Because supplemental oxygen use is so prevalent, oxygen toxicity is an area of intense investigation. This area has been reviewed recently.[7] In this section we will discuss the physiology, simple concepts of its biochemical mechanism, and prospects for the future therapy of oxygen toxicity.

Exposure to greater than 90 to 95% oxygen in humans results in a progressive decline in pulmonary function. Changes during the first 24 hours include mild chest pain, decreased tracheal mucus velocity, development of tracheobronchitis, and evidence of increased alveolar permeability to albumin and transferrin. Alveolar macrophage function may also be altered. After 24 to 48 hours, detectable changes in vital capacity, lung compliance, and diffusing capacity are present but are usually clinically insignificant. During this period, increased dead space and intrapulmonary shunting may be evident. These pathophysiologic changes have been found for the most part in subjects without underlying lung disease. Underlying disease or injury may render the lungs more or less tolerant to oxygen exposure. Usually, oxygen levels less than 50% are considered safe, but the effects of long-term exposure at these concentrations are not known.

Primates who breathe pure oxygen experience severe respiratory distress and signs of pulmonary edema after approximately 7 days. This is associated with significant decreases in total lung capacity and an increase in pulmonary vascular resistance.

Pathologic changes of oxygen toxicity involve all elements of the alveolar-capillary unit. Type I alveolar cells gradually diminish, and type II cells proliferate. The interstitium swells and becomes infiltrated with mono-

nuclear and neutrophilic infiltrates. The capillary endothelial cells become markedly reduced. This process undergoes gradual resolution with fibroblastic proliferation and fibrosis. These pathologic findings are nonspecific, and similar findings are seen in adult respiratory distress syndrome (ARDS).

Biophysical and biochemical studies in animals reveal decreased surfactant activity after exposure to 95% oxygen.[8] The factors responsible include diminished synthesis of phospholipids by type II pneumocytes, as well as increased levels of extruded plasma proteins. Serum proteins such as albumin inactivate surfactant and adversely affect surface tension. On discontinuation of the oxygen exposure, surfactant activity gradually returns to normal.

For clinicians, an elementary understanding of the theory of oxygen radicals is useful to gain insight into potential therapeutic advances to alleviate oxygen toxicity. Although most oxygen is converted directly to water by the mitochondrial cytochrome oxidase system, a small portion of oxygen undergoes reduction through a series of biochemical pathways that have oxygen radicals as intermediates (Fig. 47–2). Some intermediates, in order of their reactivity, include the hydroxyl radical (OH), superoxide (O_2^-), and hydrogen peroxide (H_2O_2). Other highly reactive species have been identified, including singlet oxygen and peroxynitrite. These reactive oxygen species can attack cellular constituents, such as lipids, proteins, and nucleic acids, rendering them functionally ineffective. Hyperoxia is generally assumed to produce injury by increased oxygen radical production via the law of mass action. Its effects on the lung include decreased synthesis of surfactant proteins and deoxyribonucleic acid (DNA), and decreased cellular respiration, resulting in cell death. Several pharmacologic agents such as epinephrine, norepinephrine, and thyroid hormone may increase the lung's sensitivity to oxygen toxicity.

Various intracellular mechanisms are available to combat and neutralize the effect of oxygen radicals. They have been termed the *antioxidant defense.* Included in this classification are the enzymes superoxide dismutase, catalase, glutathione peroxidase, and glutathione reductase, as well as many nonenzymatic compounds, including hemoglobins, glutamine, β-carotene, α-tocopherol, and ascorbate. The neutralization of free radicals by antioxidants is seen in Table 47–3. Antioxidant enzymes have specificity for certain oxygen radicals: Superoxide dismutase converts superoxide to H_2O_2, and catalase and glutathione peroxidase convert H_2O_2 to H_2O and oxygen. Glutathione peroxidase also reduces lipid hydroperoxides.

Table 47–3. MECHANISMS OF REDUCTION OF REACTIVE OXYGEN SPECIES*

Enzymatic	Nonenzymatic
Superoxide dismutase $2O_2^- + 2H^+ \rightarrow H_2O_2 + O_2$	α-Tocopherol Vitamin E + ROO• $\rightarrow$ Vitamin E• + ROOH
Catalase $2H_2O_2 \rightarrow 2H_2O + O_2$	Ascorbate $O_2^- + H^+ + $ Ascorbate $\rightarrow$ Semidehydroascorbate• + H_2O
Glutathione peroxidase ROOH + 2GSH† $\rightarrow H_2O$ + GSSG + ROH	β-Carotene $O_2 + $ β-carotene $\rightarrow$ O + β-carotene•
Glutathione reductase GSSG‡ + NADPH + H$^+$ $\rightarrow$ 2GSH + NADP$^+$	Glutathione GSH + O$^-$ + H$^+$ $\rightarrow$ GS•§ + H_2O

*From Jackson RM: Molecular, pharmacologic and clinical aspects of oxygen induced lung injury. Clin Chest Med 11:73, 1990.
†GSH = reduced glutathione.
‡GSSG = oxidized glutathione.
§GS• = glutathione free radical.

As one might expect, susceptibility or resistance to cellular injury by hyperoxia can be related to intracellular levels of antioxidant enzymes. Following pretreatment with sublethal concentrations of oxygen, increased levels of manganese-containing superoxide dismutase are generated and result in increased resistance to subsequent exposure to 100% oxygen. Pretreatment with low-dose endotoxin, interleukin-1 (IL-1) or tumor necrosis factor (TNF) confers increased resistance to hyperoxic exposure by a similar mechanism. In contrast, methylprednisolone, by inhibiting synthesis of antioxidant enzymes, can increase susceptibility to hyperoxic exposure.[9]

The understanding of cellular biochemical events has led to novel therapeutic approaches for hyperoxic lung injury. In animal experiments, exogenous administration of superoxide dismutase and catalase, encapsulated in lipid vesicles (liposomes) or covalently bound to polyethylene glycol (PEG), enhanced survival in 100% oxygen and diminished pathologic lung changes.[10] The in vivo delivery system—that is, liposomes or PEG—increases intracellular levels of antioxidant enzymes by retarding their extracellular degradation and increasing cell membrane permeability. It will be interesting to see the results of clinical trials of PEG–superoxide dismutase in ameliorating proposed oxygen free radical injury in various types of disease states.

Since surfactant deficiency is a component of hyperoxic lung injury, intratracheal instillation of surfactant could potentially improve oxygenation by stabilizing alveoli and allowing a decrease in inspired oxygen levels. Experimental evidence in animals indicates that repeated surfactant administration significantly increases survival in 100% oxygen, improves lung mechanics, and lessens lung edema.[11] With the present capability to produce surfactant in large amounts, there is significant interest in its clinical application to disease states other than hyaline membrane disease. It is likely that clinical trials with artificial surfactant will soon begin in children with acute lung injury who are exposed to high levels of oxygen for prolonged periods.

PULMONARY EDEMA

Pulmonary edema is a frequent problem in pediatric critical care because of the varied causes that have as one of their end points the production of excessive amounts of water in the lung. Most systemic disease processes have some adverse effect on the lung. A listing of all of the causes of pulmonary edema is nearly equal to the index of *Nelson's Textbook of Pediatrics*. A shortened version is provided in Table 47–4. The lung is affected so often because of its basic anatomic design. It is the only organ to filter the entire cardiac output. This makes it more vulnerable to circulating toxins and inflammatory mediators that initiate inflammatory cascades, magnifying their effect. The lung also has extensive exposure to the outside environment. Each day an adult inhales an average of 9,000 l of air, exposing the large, fragile surface area of the alveoli to toxic substances.

Table 47–4. CLASSIFICATION OF PULMONARY EDEMA*

Edema Produced by Increased Pressure Across the Microvasculature
Hydrostatic microvascular pressure becomes more positive
  Left heart failure
  Mitral stenosis
  Expansion of the microvascular space by overtransfusion
  Obliteration of pulmonary veins
Hydrostatic interstitial pressure becomes more negative
  Acute atelectasis (drowned lung)
  Rapid re-expansion of hydro- or pneumothorax
Microvascular colloid osmotic pressure decreased
  Overtransfusion with crystalloid
  Hypoalbuminemia due to liver or renal disease
  Starvation
Interstitial colloid osmotic pressure increased
  Obstructed lymphatics
Edema Due to a Damaged Microvascular Membrane (Endothelium or Epithelium)
Infectious agents
  Viruses, mycoplasma, other (especially in immunocompromised patients)
Inhaled substances
  Gases: Oxygen, nitrogen dioxide, sulfur dioxide, smoke, other noxious gases and fumes
  Liquid aspiration: gastric contents, salt and fresh water drowning
Ingestants
  Chemotherapeutic agents: azathioprine, BCNU, bleomycin, bisulfan, chlorambucil, cytosine arabinoside, cytoxan, melphalan, methotrexate, mitomycin
  Other medications: amphotericin B, colchicine, gold, hexamethonium, hydrochlorothiazide, nitrofurantoin, placidyl, practolol, salicylate, penicillamine, phenylbutazone
  Other: heroin, kerosene, paraquat
Shock, trauma, and sepsis
Radiation
Miscellaneous
  Acute pancreatitis, cardiopulmonary bypass, fat or air embolism, uremia, heat, molar pregnancy, systemic lupus erythematosus, postlymphangiography
Edema due to Undetermined Origin
High altitude
Neurogenic

*Reprinted with permission from Hogg JC and Kazanstein AA: Pulmonary edema and diffuse alveolar injury. *In:* Thurlbeck WM (ed): Pathology of the Lung. Copyright 1988, Thieme Medical Publishers, Inc., New York.
BCNU = 1,3-Bis [chlorethyl]-1 nitrosurea.

The Starling equation, describing the forces governing fluid movement across a semipermeable membrane, provides a framework for classifying the causes of pulmonary edema, since an aberration in any one of the variables can be responsible for edema. It is convenient to think in terms of diseases that affect one variable—for example, pulmonary vascular hydrostatic pressure, even though this rarely happens. For the purpose of discussion, however, we will treat a process as though it affects mainly one variable, realizing that at the same time an opposing affect on a second variable may occur.

The Starling equation states that the flow of fluid across a semipermeable membrane is governed by the pressure and osmolarity on either side of the membrane, as well as the relative permeability of the membrane to the solute and to the solvent.

Q_f = K_f (Pmv − Ppmv) − σ (π mv − π pmv) where

Q_f = net transvascular flow
K_f = filtration coefficient
Pmv = microvascular hydrostatic pressure
Ppmv = perimicrovascular hydrostatic pressure (interstitial)
πmv = microvascular colloid osmotic pressure
πpmv = perimicrovascular colloid osmotic pressure
σ = reflection coefficient (relative resistance to the flow of colloid)

Increased Microvascular Pressure

The first term of the equation deals with the difference between the microvascular pressure and the interstitial pressure. Pulmonary edema may be produced by either increasing the microvascular pressure or decreasing the interstitial pressure. Causes of increased pulmonary microvascular pressure are relatively common. Volume overload secondary to excessive intravenous fluid administration (though this also affects osmotic pressure) is a common example. Cardiac defects that usually present with signs of pulmonary edema include large left-to-right shunts, pulmonary venous and left atrial obstruction, and left ventricular dysfunction (Table 47–5).

Decreased Interstitial Pressure

Pulmonary edema may also result from increasing the negative interstitial pressure. Values for interstitial pressures have been estimated as between −5 to −10 mm Hg, but during certain circumstances they may be increased markedly, such as during the increased respiratory effort associated with an obstructed upper airway. The negative pleural pressure generated is transmitted to the interstitial space in a fairly uniform fashion, widening the pressure gradient across the vascular membrane and encouraging interstitial fluid formation. Upper airway obstruction in conditions such as tonsillar and adenoidal hypertrophy has been known to produce pulmonary edema. An acute form of this is seen when laryngospasm occurs following extubation. Clinically significant pulmonary edema may arise even if a patent

Table 47–5. CARDIOVASCULAR LESIONS ASSOCIATED WITH PULMONARY EDEMA

Increased Pulmonary Arterial Pressure
PDA*
VSD†
AV‡ canal
ASD§ (late)
Truncus arteriosus

Increased Pulmonary Venous Pressure
Left atrial myxoma
Restrictive pericarditis
Mitral stenosis
Mitral regurgitation
Cor triatriatum
Myocarditis
Coarctation of the aorta
Aortic stenosis

*PDA = patent ductus arteriosus.
†VSD = ventricular septal defect.
‡AV = arteriovenous.
§ASD = atrial septal defect.

airway is quickly established, as the edema may take hours to resolve.

The pathophysiology of pulmonary edema secondary to upper airway obstruction is probably a more complicated process than simply an increase in the negative pleural pressure pulling fluid into the interstitial space. High protein content has been found in the edematous fluid obtained by bronchoalveolar lavage, suggesting a vascular permeability defect.[12] The exact cause of the vascular injury is unknown, but mechanical stress imposed by the approximately −80 mm Hg of pleural pressure that can be generated by forceful breathing against an obstructed airway, along with inflammatory responses to hypoxia and acidosis, are likely mechanisms. Other potential contributory mechanisms include increased venous return and left ventricular afterload. The relative contributions of the mechanisms are unknown. Occasionally, relief of upper airway obstruction results in pulmonary edema. It is hypothesized that this occurs by relieving auto-PEEP, which had previously counterbalanced the forces of pulmonary edema.[18]

Decreased Colloid Osmotic Pressure

A decrease in the plasma colloid osmotic pressure will also result in a tendency toward edema formation. This is seen in volume overload with crystalloid solutions, as previously mentioned, and in hypoproteinemic conditions, such as nephrotic syndrome, protein-losing enteropathy, and malnutrition. Increased interstitial protein content, and thus increased interstitial osmotic pressure, results from permeability defects.

Increased Vascular Permeability

Injury to the pulmonary vasculature is the presenting feature in a variety of insults. In terms of the Starling equation, this amounts to an increase in the filtration coefficient (K_f) and a decrease in the reflection coefficient. This results in a relatively protein-rich edematous fluid.

Pulmonary edema resulting from increased permeability is discussed further on.

Lymphatic Drainage

Pulmonary edema resulting from lymphatic insufficiency is the only cause of pulmonary edema so far not described by the Starling equation. Pulmonary lymph flow has been estimated at between 10 and 20 ml/hr in adults with the ability to handle an increase of a factor of 10 without significant change in the accumulation of interstitial fluid. The relative contribution of factors within the lymphatics, such as lymphatic valves and smooth muscles, acting as a pump to overcome increased systemic venous pressure is of some debate. It has been noted experimentally that lymph flow stops when the central venous pressure (CVP) approaches 20 mm Hg,[14] though when the CVP is elevated to this extent, pulmonary capillary pressures are usually also elevated. An elevated CVP is probably the most common cause of lymphatic obstruction; other rarer causes include silicosis, lymphangitis carcinomatosa, congenital pulmonary lymphangiectasis, and pulmonary lymphangioleiomyomatosis.

Unknown Causes

As in any listing of causes for diseases, a category in which the exact mechanism is not well understood remains. This is the case for high-altitude and neurogenic pulmonary edema. Respiratory distress due to pulmonary edema occurring in conjunction with cerebral injury is a well-recognized but poorly understood phenomenon. The edematous fluid has a high protein content as shown by BAL and thus presumably is secondary to a vascular permeability defect.[15] However, hemodynamic monitoring has shown transient increases in systemic and pulmonary blood pressures, considered to be secondary to the increased adrenergic output during central nervous system dysfunction, which is suggestive of a hemodynamic cause for edema formation. Neurogenic pulmonary edema can be produced experimentally in animals by inducing nonspecific cerebral injury, and the effect can be blocked by pulmonary denervation, cervical cord transection, or adrenergic blocking agents. Neurogenic pulmonary edema is presumably the cause of pulmonary edema seen in the postictal period in some patients after a generalized tonic-clonic seizure, though upper airway obstruction may also be evident.

Clinical Findings

The specific findings of pulmonary edema on physical examination vary according to the severity of respiratory distress and the underlying cause of the edema. In general, some degree of respiratory distress is manifested by an increased respiratory rate, labored breathing, intercostal retractions, and use of accessory muscles of respiration. Cyanosis may be noted, and there may be crackles on auscultation, especially in dependent lung fields. An increased P_2 or even an S_3 and a "flow" murmur may be noted, along with jugular venous distention and hepatomegaly. Excessive frothy, pink-tinged sputum is noted in fairly severe pulmonary edema with alveolar flooding. Wheezing has been noted early in the course of pulmonary edema in children, along with pulmonary hyperexpansion.

Other findings pertinent to the underlying cause are anasarca (especially with hypoproteinemia), specific cardiac murmurs suggestive of congenital heart disease, and stridor associated with upper airway obstruction.

Radiographic Appearance

Hyperexpansion secondary to air trapping is an early nonspecific finding of pulmonary edema seen on chest radiographs in children. This may precede other more specific findings of interstitial edema and is hard to distinguish from other causes of air trapping such as reactive airway disease and bronchiolitis.

Perivascular cuffing occurs with excess fluid accumulation in the interstitium surrounding vascular and lymphatic structures. Bronchial wall edema probably also contributes to the thickening of pulmonary markings.

Septal thickening (edema of the interlobular septa) is seen as thin, straight lines, 2 to 6 cm in length. In the perihilar region they are referred to as Kerley "A" lines. Similar lines no longer than 2 cm found in the peripheral lung fields perpendicular to the pleural lining are referred as Kerley "B" lines. Kerley "C" lines are shorter and form a reticular pattern in the central basilar portion of the lungs and are usually best appreciated on a lateral chest film.

Fluid may be found in the pleural space, but the amount is usually minimal and is confined to the fluid seen in the major fissures and, with some blunting of the costophrenic angles, on an upright chest x-ray film. Occasionally, however, moderate or even large pleural fluid collections occur with pulmonary edema.

These signs are usually present with mild to moderate pulmonary edema prior to the onset of alveolar filling. When alveolar filling occurs, it appears as patchy densities in both lung fields, usually in the perihilar region, giving the typical "butterfly" appearance with relatively clear peripheral lung fields.

Cardiomegaly and prominent pulmonary vascularity are also frequent radiographic findings when pulmonary edema is associated with left ventricular dysfunction or volume overload (Fig. 47–3). In upright individuals, an inversion of the usual relationship of the caliber of pulmonary vessels between upper and lower lung fields is found. Normally, the more dependent lung has relatively larger vessels because of gravitational effects. The vascular congestion associated with hydrostatic causes of pulmonary edema causes an increase in the size of all pulmonary vessels, with the relative size of the upper lobe vessels increased to a greater extent. This is a more consistent finding in older children and adults with pulmonary edema than in infants, who usually remain supine and whose chest x-ray films are taken in the supine position. Portable chest x-ray films taken in a pediatric ICU are also usually taken in a supine position.

The previously described findings on chest x-ray film apply to pulmonary edema from hydrostatic causes. However, when the edema results from increased vascular permeability such as in adult respiratory distress syndrome (ARDS), the appearance on x-ray film is slightly different. In this case, the vascular injury is diffuse and is likely to be peripherally distributed. Alveolar filling appears earlier in the course of the disease, producing a diffuse haze. The interstitial and alveolar fluid has a high protein content and clears slowly.

Kerley's lines, peribronchial cuffing, inversion of pulmonary vessels, and cardiomegaly are generally not found in this form of pulmonary edema and thus can aid in differentiating the two categories.

Management

The treatment of hydrostatic pulmonary edema is directed toward first reversing hypoxia and then addressing the cause of edema formation. Supplemental oxygen, alone or with mechanical ventilation, and PEEP may be necessary. Diuretics, inotropes, and afterload reducing agents, as well as narcotics, may be beneficial, depending on the cause of the pulmonary edema. In the case of pulmonary edema caused by congenital heart disease, successful preoperative management may improve survival following palliative or definitive surgical correction.

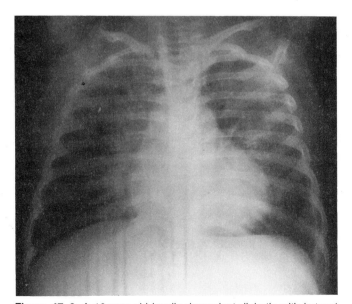

Figure 47–3. A 10-year-old insulin-dependent diabetic with ketoacidosis and an oxygen requirement after fluid resuscitation. Note: cardiomegaly, increased vascular markings, perihilar infiltrates, and Kerly "B" lines of pulmonary edema.

Table 47–6. CRITERIA FOR DIAGNOSING ADULT RESPIRATORY DISTRESS SYNDROME*

Clinical Setting
Catastrophic event
  Pulmonary
  Nonpulmonary (e.g., shock)
Exclusions
  Chronic pulmonary disease
  Left heart abnormalities
Respiratory distress (judged clinically)
  Tachypnea usually >40
  Labored breathing
X-ray: Diffuse Pulmonary Infiltrates
Interstitial (initially)
Alveolar (later)
Physiologic
PaO_2 <50 with FIO_2 >0.6
Overall compliance <50% normal, usually 20 to 30% normal
Increased shunt fraction Q_S/Q_T and dead space ventilation V_D/V_T
Pathologic
Heavy lungs, usually >1000 g
Congestive atelectasis
Hyaline membranes
Fibrosis

*Adapted from Petty TL: Adult respiratory distress syndrome: Definition and historical perspective. Clin Chest Med 3:3, 1982.

ADULT-TYPE RESPIRATORY DISTRESS SYNDROME

Clinical Manifestations

ARDS is a clinical syndrome based on the pathophysiologic consequences of diffuse alveolar disease of the lung. Clinically, patients present with tachypnea, retractions, tachycardia, sometimes cyanosis, and relative hypoxemia despite a high minute ventilation. Frequently auscultation of the chest reveals quiet breath sounds with or without crackles. Hypoxemia that is refractory to supplemental oxygen therapy is a characteristic finding in the full-blown condition. The onset of ARDS may be insidious (e.g., shock), abrupt (e.g., aspiration symptoms), or variable (e.g., sepsis), and recurrence has been known to occur.

The epidemiology of ARDS in children is not well defined. In one study from Switzerland, its incidence accounted for approximately 1% of admissions to the pediatric ICU.[16] Similar data for the United States are not available. Several retrospective studies of ARDS in children suggest an overall mortality rate of approximately 60%, a figure strikingly similar to that in adults.[17] This figure is highly variable, however, and depends on how ARDS is defined and the presence or lack of other organ system failure. It is unknown whether certain specific causes carry a better or worse prognosis independent of multiple organ system involvement.

The diagnosis of ARDS rests on the demonstration of a constellation of clinical, chest radiographic, physiologic and, when available, pathologic findings (Table 47–6). A variety of clinical conditions involving direct lung injury, pulmonary infection, extrapulmonary infection, or severe systemic insult, or a combination, are associated with ARDS. Table 47–7 lists associated conditions linked to the development of ARDS. In children,

Table 47–7. CONDITIONS ASSOCIATED WITH ADULT RESPIRATORY DISTRESS SYNDROME*

Direct Injury to the Lung	Secondary Injury to the Lung
Pulmonary infections	Shock—any cause
Inhalation	Sepsis
NO_2	Trauma
Cl_2	Multiple trauma
SO_2	Fractures
NH_3	Burns
Phosgene	Head trauma
Smoke	Blood disorders
Oxygen toxicity	Diffuse intravascular
Aspiration	coagulation
Gastric fluid	Massive blood transfusion
(especially if pH <2.5)	Drug overdose
Near drowning	Heroin
(fresh or salt water)	Methadone
Hydrocarbons	Barbiturates
Emboli	Ethychlorvynol
Air	Salicylates
Fat	Propoxyphene
Amniotic fluid	Metabolic disorders
Pulmonary contusion	Diabetic ketoacidosis
Radiation pneumonitis	Uremia
	Pancreatitis
	Increased intracranial
	pressure
	Postcardiopulmonary bypass
	Posthemodialysis
	Postcardioversion
	Paraquat ingestion

*Reprinted with permission from Royall JA and Levin DL: Adult respiratory distress syndrome. I. Clinical aspects, pathology, and mechanism of lung injury. J Pediatr 112:169, 1988.

the most common conditions precipitating ARDS include sepsis with bacteremia, pneumonia, near drowning, pulmonary aspiration, cardiopulmonary arrest, and trauma. Patients with underlying malignancy or acquired immunodeficiency disease (AIDS) appear to have a higher predisposition to ARDS.

Because of the large numbers of clinical conditions associated with ARDS, several authorities have questioned the use of this terminology altogether. Lumping together diverse disease entities may obscure important clinical, pathophysiologic, and pathogenic variables involved in specific types of lung injury. Conversely, use of the single category ARDS serves to emphasize the similarities in pathophysiology and mechanisms of injury in the later stages of acute respiratory failure independent of the inciting event. In spite of its limitations, the term ARDS is well entrenched and will continue to be used widely.

Radiographic findings in ARDS evolve from increased interstitial markings early in the disease process to a diffuse alveolar filling pattern over several hours to days. It is not uncommon (e.g., aspiration syndromes) for diffuse alveolar filling to be present on the initial chest radiograph. Occasionally ARDS may present as isolated unilateral pulmonary edema with or without extension bilaterally.

Extravascular accumulation of water in the lung is responsible for the altered physiology seen in ARDS. Isolated respiratory failure is associated with decreased lung compliance, decreased FRC, increased dead space, and increased intrapulmonary shunting. Furthermore, pulmonary hypertension is usually present and, along with PEEP, predisposes the child to circulatory dysfunction. The combination of hypoxemia and inadequate circulatory function leads to decreased tissue oxygenation and metabolic derangements associated with hypoxic hypoxia or stagnant hypoxia, or both.

Pathologic features of the lung in ARDS reveal diffuse alveolar damage. During the first few days of injury, the lung parenchyma exhibits pulmonary edema, hyaline membranes, microatelectasis, capillary plugging with thrombi and platelets, and an acute inflammatory infiltrate. This process has been labeled the exudative phase. Three to 10 days following injury, the histologic examination reveals type II epithelial cell hyperplasia, mononuclear infiltrates in the interstitium, and fibroblastic proliferation in and around alveoli. Following this reparative phase, the pulmonary parenchyma returns toward normal, but evidence of fibrosis around the alveolar ducts may remain. In some instances, fibroblastic proliferation proceeds onward to pulmonary fibrosis and permanent lung dysfunction.

Pathophysiology

In their review in 1982, Renaldo and Rogers[18] suggested that improved survival in ARDS would have to await increased understanding of the mechanisms occurring in acute lung injury and repair rather than advances in clinical intensive care. A decade later, with overall survival in ARDS substantially unchanged, that statement remains true. The exact mechanisms of acute alveolar injury are unknown, though significant advances have been made in understanding the cellular pathobiology potentially related to ARDS. Some of the proposed pathogenic mechanisms associated with ARDS are listed in Table 47–8. There is considerable evidence that endogenously released products from macrophages and neutrophils and their intercellular communication are important elements of tissue injury. Initial inciting events, such as endotoxemia, activate macrophages that release cytokines such as TNF and IL-1. Once elaborated, TNF preferentially binds to kidney, liver, and lung. Acting singly or together, these bioactive compounds can cause direct vascular injury and induce adherence and activation of neutrophils, complement, and coagulation proteins by vascular endothelial cells (Fig. 47–4). Activated neutrophils may initiate or amplify injury through the release of oxygen radicals, proteolytic enzymes, and products of arachidonic acid metabolism (leukotrienes and thromboxanes). Many of these reactions may participate in positive feedback loops, which enhance tissue injury.

The body also produces endogenous substances to counteract or oppose the actions of the preceding mediators. Thus, superoxide dismutase, catalase, and glutathione peroxidase scavenge oxygen radicals, and α_1-antitrypsin binds to the proteolytic enzyme elastase. Prostaglandin E_2 (PGE_2), a vasodilator, antagonizes the vasoconstrictor effects of thromboxane A_2. Currently no

Table 47–8. POSSIBLE PATHOGENIC MECHANISMS IN ADULT RESPIRATORY DISTRESS SYNDROME*

May cause or amplify the initial lung injury: cellular mediators
  Polymorphonuclear leukocytes
  Mononuclear-phagocytes (monocytes and macrophages)
  Platelets
  Lymphocytes
  Fibroblasts
May cause or amplify the initial lung injury: circulating mediators
  Bacterial toxins (endotoxin)
  Oxygen radicals
  Cytokines (tumor necrosis factor, interleukin-1)
  Eicosanoids (prostaglandins, thromboxane, leukotrienes)
  Free fatty acids
  Fat emboli
  Serotonin
  Histamine
  Activated complement
  Proteases
  Platelet activating factor
  Fibrin-platelet microthrombi
  Fibrin degradation products
  Tissue thromboplastin
  Hageman factor (Factor XII)
  Bradykinin
Secondary results of lung injury
  Surfactant deficiency
  Pulmonary fibrosis
  α_1-antitrypsin deficiency
Iatrogenic factors
  Oxygen toxicity
  Barotrauma
  Malnutrition

*Reprinted with permission from Royall JA: Adult respiratory distress syndrome in children. Semin Respir Med 11:223, 1990.

cytokine that directly opposes the effects of TNF has been identified, though prostaglandin E_2 inhibits production and release of TNF and IL-1.

Therapy aimed at the endogenous mediators of tissue injury offers the hope for more successful treatment and improved outcome in ARDS. Potential novel approaches to therapy include treatment with α_1-antitrypsin, oxygen free radical scavengers (superoxide dismutase, catalase, n-acetyl cysteine), and cyclooxygenase inhibitors. Pentoxifylline, a compound that decreases TNF production and inhibits neutrophil adhesion, may have potential benefit. Passive immunization with TNF antibodies significantly improves survival in mice given lethal doses of endotoxin and offers exciting future possibilities.[19] In addition, artificial surfactant has been shown to increase oxygenation in animals with diffuse lung injury and could potentially reduce secondary pulmonary injury from oxygen toxicity [20](see Chapter 44).

In certain instances, unproven forms of supportive therapy have been reported to be beneficial in selected patients with ARDS. High-frequency ventilation and extracorporeal membrane oxygenation are currently available clinical examples of this (see Chapters 40 and 42). Exact criteria for when these interventions may be suitable are lacking. Clearly, however, one would expect better outcome when there is no evidence of multiple organ failure (e.g., pulmonary aspiration).

Secondary pulmonary infection is difficult to accurately diagnose in patients with acute lung injury and requires a high index of suspicion by the clinician. The typical findings of pneumonia, such as fever, tachypnea, crackles, infiltrates on chest radiograph, and evidence of inflammation in tracheal secretions, are all found in acute lung injury. In addition, increased bacterial adherence to epithelial cells results in colonization of the respiratory tract by gram-negative bacteria; therefore, the presence of organisms in the respiratory tract does not imply an active infectious process. Bronchial washings, protected brush catheter specimens, BAL fluid, and open lung biopsy have increased sensitivity and specificity for diagnosis of pneumonia over culture of tracheobronchial secretions.[21] Transthoracic lung aspiration and transbronchial biopsy are commonly avoided because of the associated high incidence of pneumothorax. Because BAL has good sensitivity (approximately 80%) and specificity (approximately 100%) for viral, fungal, and mycobacterial diseases, it is the most clinically useful procedure, along with open lung biopsy, for diagnosis of pneumonia. From a clinical standpoint it seems reasonable to initiate antimicrobial therapy in patients suspected of having secondary lung infection based on Gram stain results, culture results of tracheobronchial secretions, and blood culture results. If the patient continues to exhibit signs of infection or deteriorates on antimicrobial therapy, flexible bronchoscopy for BAL should be performed to exclude unusual pathogens. If the patient is rapidly deteriorating, proceeding directly to open biopsy is indicated.

Management

The cornerstone of intensive care management in ARDS is primarily supportive. The discovery that PEEP improves oxygenation has been the most important contribution to improving survival. Since PEEP does not restore normal oxygenation in some severely affected patients with ARDS and may adversely affect cardiac function (see Chapter 41), provision of adequate

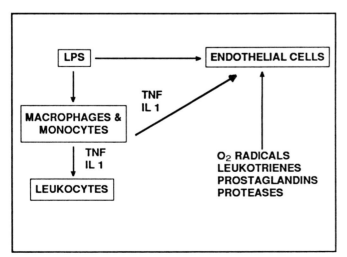

Figure 47–4. Biochemical derangements in sepsis and ARDS. (From Wheeler AP and Bernard GR: Preventive strategies and innovative therapy for sepsis syndrome and adult respiratory distress syndrome. Pulm Crit Care Update 6:1, 1991.)

tissue oxygenation has recently evolved as the primary goal of therapy. Other important aspects of care include specific therapy for underlying associated conditions, appropriate fluid and nutritional support, and early identification of nosocomial infections.

PEEP is the only known intervention that clearly counteracts the hypoxemia in ARDS, though the main determinant may be elevation in mean airway pressure. Some patients with ARDS are refractory to PEEP (>20 cm H_2O), however, and show no clear benefit. PEEP acts by decreasing intrapulmonary shunting, which results in improved oxygenation; simultaneously, increased dead space ventilation occurs, which can result in CO_2 retention at excessive levels (Fig. 47–5). These effects are purported to occur by stinting open fluid-filled alveoli throughout the respiratory cycle and recruiting microatelectic lung units. Use of PEEP may result in increased extravascular lung water. Cardiac effects attributable to PEEP include increased right ventricular afterload and decreased venous return and decreased left ventricular afterload and contractility. Decreases in cardiac output may independently lead to decreased intrapulmonary shunting at the expense of tissue oxygen delivery. Thus, knowledge of the cardiac output is important in determining the direct effects of PEEP in pulmonary function.

From a clinical perspective, PEEP is titrated in increments of 3 to 5 cm H_2O until FIO_2 is less than or equal to 60%. Deleterious effects on cardiac output are not usually seen at levels of PEEP less than 15 cm H_2O unless the patient is hypovolemic or pulmonary compliance is only mildly decreased. Other principles of mechanical ventilation include the use of large tidal volumes (10 to 15 ml/kg) over long inspiratory times (0.8 to 1.2 sec) and slow ventilatory rates to improve distribution of ventilation and minimize peak airway pressures. Intermittent mandatory ventilation is a commonly used mode of ventilation, though its potential advantage of increasing venous return compared with controlled ventilation is probably overestimated because at the height of their illness many patients with ARDS are given muscle relaxants, which prevents spontaneous respiration.

More recently, the focus of treatment in ARDS has centered on the provision of adequate tissue oxygenation. This is a rational approach and highlights the relationship of ARDS to multiple organ system failure (see Chapter 15). It also provides a framework that gives equal consideration to cardiopulmonary physiology and end organ dysfunction in ARDS. Determining adequate tissue oxygenation, however, is difficult because there is no universally acceptable test to measure adequate tissue oxygen metabolism. Thus, we are left with indirect estimates of adequate tissue function. In precise physiologic experiments using healthy animals, oxygen consumption in regional tissue beds is independent of oxygen delivery.[22] As oxygen supply is reduced, a certain critical level is attained. At levels less than this, oxygen consumption begins to decrease in a linear fashion. This is the critical inflection point. At levels greater than this, oxygen supply is adequate and tissue oxygenation is optimal (Fig. 47–6). In patients with ARDS, controversy exists as to the presence of a critical inflection point in the oxygen supply-consumption relationship. If such a

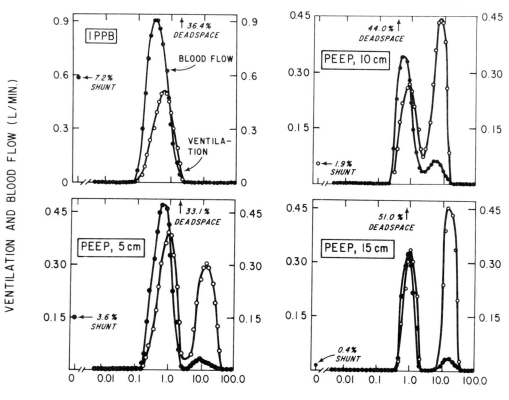

Figure 47–5. The effect of PEEP on the ventilation-perfusion distribution in a normal dog. The very high $\dot{V}_A/\dot{Q}$ units are likely to represent continued perfusion through corner vessels in lung units whose alveolar capillaries have been shut by the high pressure. (From Dueck R, et al: Effects of positive end-expiratory pressure on gas exchange in dogs with normal and edematous lungs. Anesthesiology 47:359, 1977.)

VENTILATION-PERFUSION RATIO

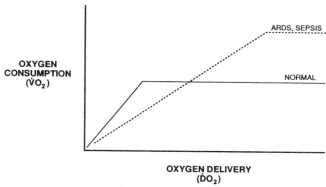

Figure 47–6. Classical $\dot{D}O_2/\dot{V}O_2$ relationship as described in animal models and in ARDS and sepsis. (From Clarke C, Edwards JD, Nightingale P, et al: Persistence of supply dependency of oxygen uptake at high levels of delivery in adult respiratory distress syndrome. Crit Care Med 19:497, 1991. © by Williams & Wilkins, 1991.)

point occurs, does it happen at such a high value of oxygen delivery that the cardiopulmonary system would not be able to reach or sustain it?[23] Future studies will have to clarify these questions. At the present time, achieving a cardiac index of 4.5 l/min/m² and an oxygen delivery of 600 ml/min/m² or greater has been recommended.[17]

Fluid therapy in ARDS usually requires acute resuscitation to maintain blood pressure and circulation in the face of capillary leak and any adverse effects of PEEP. The type of fluid recommended, crystalloid versus colloid, is controversial and neither fluid has a distinct advantage over the other. Frequently, both are used to obtain different effects—for example, packed red blood cells to increase arterial oxygen capacity, 25% salt-poor albumin to maintain colloid oncotic pressure, and isotonic saline for hypotension.

Malnourished children are at higher risk of morbidity and mortality from acute illness. Since children with ARDS can stay in the ICU for weeks or months, proper nutritional support is essential to prevent malnutrition. Because excessive caloric supplementation can increase

carbon dioxide production and mechanical ventilatory requirements, measurement of energy requirements is desirable. Accurate data for caloric requirements can be obtained by inspired and expired gas analysis in patients requiring an FIO_2 of less than 0.6. Nutritional support is provided via enteral feeding, if possible. When parenteral nutrition is necessary, a mixed fuel source of intravenous glucose and lipid is used.

The major complications associated with ARDS include barotrauma and secondary infection. Barotrauma, precipitated by decreased lung compliance, can result in pneumothorax, pneumomediastinum and, in severe cases, pneumoperitoneum and subcutaneous emphysema. Pneumothorax and pneumoperitoneum may worsen hypoxemia and hypercarbia even after appropriate placement of a thoracostomy tube or peritoneal catheter because of shunting of ventilation through the site of the air leak. In such an instance, unconventional ventilatory approaches (e.g., high-frequency ventilation) may be beneficial.

PARENCHYMAL INFECTIONS (PNEUMONIAS)

Lower respiratory tract infections are common in the pediatric age group, with the frequency reaching as high as 240 episodes/1,000 infants less than 1 year of age. A significant percentage of infantile pneumonias result in hospitalization, and as many as 25% of hospitalized children require intensive care.[24] The vast majority of admissions to the pediatric ICU for primary pneumonia have a nonbacterial cause, reflecting the prevalence of pneumonias in the population at large.

The cause of nonbacterial pneumonia varies with age and the time of year. Table 47–9 lists the major causative agents for different age groups. Respiratory syncytial virus (RSV) pneumonia is a frequent cause of admission to the pediatric ICU for respiratory failure requiring

Table 47–9. RELATION OF AGE TO MOST LIKELY PATHOGEN FOR LOWER RESPIRATORY TRACT INFECTIONS*

	Bacteria	Virus	Other
Neonate:	Group B *Streptococci* + + + +	RSV +	
	E. coli + + + +	HSV +	
	Other enterics + +	CMV +	
	S. aureus + +	Enteroviruses +	
1–3 mo	*S. pneumoniae* + +	RSV + + + +	*Chlamydia* + +
	H. influenzae B + +		
4 mo–5 yr	*S. pneumoniae* + +	RSV + + + +	
	H. influenzae B + +	Parainfluenza + + +	
		Influenza + +	
		Adenoviruses + +	
>5 yr	*M. pneumoniae* + + + +		
	S. pneumoniae + +		
At any age	Less likely pathogens—but reflecting environment and patient status		
	M. tuberculosis	HIV	*C. immitis*
	Legionella		*H. capsulatum*
	B. pertussis		*Pneumocystis*

*From Florman AL, Cushing AH, and Umland ET: Rapid noninvasive techniques for determining etiology of bronchitis and pneumonia in infants and children. Clin Chest Med 8:670, 1987.
+ + + + = most common, + + + = very common, + + = common, + rare.

mechanical ventilation. RSV infections typically occur during midwinter epidemics; however, sporadic cases can occur all year. Parainfluenza viruses, though mainly causing croup, may also cause pneumonia in infants and toddlers. Parainfluenza virus infections are most prevalent during the fall and spring. Influenza virus infections tend to cause pneumonia in older children and adults during the winter months. Adenovirus infections have no seasonal predilection and appear to cause a lower incidence of pneumonia than do other respiratory viruses. Pneumonia caused by adenovirus, particularly types 3, 7, 11, and 21, can be especially severe and may result in bronchiolitis obliterans. In contrast to the respiratory viruses, which are spread via direct contact or airborne transmission, chlamydial pneumonia occurs by contamination from the mother's genital tract at birth; thus, infection occurs during the first 3 months of life.

Except for signs and symptoms referable to the respiratory tract, the clinical features of nonbacterial pneumonitis are quite variable. Fever may or may not be present; other nonspecific findings include lethargy, irritability, and vomiting. Significant respiratory findings include tachypnea and intercostal retractions. Crackles and wheezes may be present, and occasionally apnea is the presenting sign. Radiographic findings include hyperinflation, bronchial wall thickening, irregular pulmonary markings, and patchy atelectasis. Rarely, a diffuse alveolar filling pattern suggestive of ARDS occurs.

The development of rapid diagnostic tests in clinical virology has markedly enhanced the clinical management of patients with nonbacterial pneumonia. Decisions such as appropriate isolation precautions, introduction of specific antiviral therapy, and reduction or discontinuance of empirical antibacterial therapy are all possible within the first few hours of hospital admission. Accurate diagnosis is dependent on adequate collection and transport of the specimen to the laboratory. Specimens should be collected as soon as possible in the course of the patient's illness. Nasopharyngeal specimens (nasopharyngeal swabs or washings) are best for RSV and parainfluenza viruses, whereas throat swabs are adequate for adenovirus. Combined throat and nasopharyngeal specimens are best for influenza viruses. Since many laboratories may grow cultures for viruses, as well as perform rapid diagnostic tests, specimens should be inoculated in a viral transport medium and transported in crushed ice or refrigerated at 4° C before processing to maintain the viability of organisms.

Rapid diagnostic studies using immunofluorescent staining of infected epithelial cells, and direct fluorescent antibody or enzyme-linked immunosorbent assays (ELISA) for viral antigens are the most commonly used techniques in clinical application. The use of monoclonal antibodies to specific viral antigens has led to the development of sensitive (>85%) and specific (>99%) assays for RSV, parainfluenza, influenza, and adenovirus. The time-resolved fluoroimmunossay and ELISA technique for direct antigen detection are illustrated in Figure 47–7. Commercial kits are available for RSV and *Chlamydia*. When compared with culture techniques, they

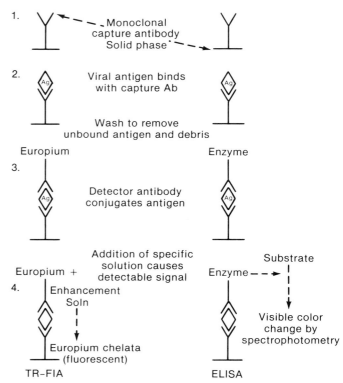

Figure 47–7. Direct fluorescent antibody technique with time-resolved fluorescent immunoassay (TR-FIA) and enzyme-linked immunosolvent assay (ELISA). (Adapted from Walls HH, et al: Time-resolved fluoroimmunoassay with monoclonal antibodies for rapid detection of influenza infections. J Clin Microbiol 24:907, 1986.)

have sensitivities and specificities of greater than 80 and 90%, respectively.

Specific therapy for nonbacterial pneumonitis depends on the causative agent. Ribavirin via aerosol appears effective for RSV pneumonia and results in increased survival in certain high-risk populations (e.g., those with pulmonary hypertension) when compared with patients treated with placebo. Some concern was initially voiced about the safety of ribavirin administration in mechanically ventilated children because of the fouling of components in the ventilator circuit. Most pediatric ICUs, however, have been able to devise mechanical ventilator circuits that allow ribavirin use without precipitating ventilator malfunction. The exact duration of ribavirin treatment is uncertain and should be correlated with clinical response over 3 to 7 days. Relapse of RSV pneumonitis may occur, necessitating additional ribavirin therapy. Erythromycin effectively eradicates *Chlamydia trachomatis* and *Mycoplasma pneumoniae* from the respiratory tract and prevents disease transmission; its effect on the clinical course of disease resulting from these pathogens is less certain, however. Intravenous trimethoprim-sulfamethoxazole or pentamidine provides effective treatment in *Pneumocystis carinii* pneumonia.

Primary bacterial pneumonias are an infrequent cause of admission to the pediatric ICU except under circumstances in which patients have significant underlying disease. Patients with diabetic ketoacidosis who do not respond to insulin treatment may have an associated

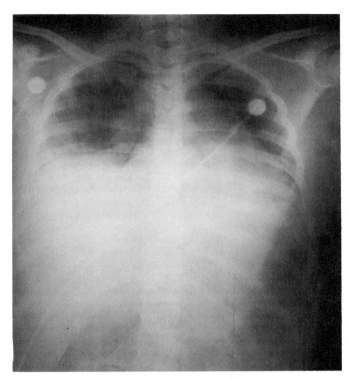

Figure 47-8. A 12-year-old patient with pneumonia and previously undiagnosed hemoglobin SC disease unresponsive to 1 week of antibiotic therapy. The patient responded to an exchange transfusion and appropriate intravenous antibiotics.

bacterial pneumonia, or patients with sickle cell disease may experience fulminant pneumonia associated with community-acquired organisms (Fig. 47-8). Occasionally, extrapulmonary manifestations of bacterial pneumonia, such as the triad of fever, vomiting, and obtundation with normal results on cerebrospinal fluid examination, result in patient admission to the pediatric ICU, and subsequent examination and chest radiographs demonstrate the diagnosis. Primary pneumonias are commonly caused by *Streptococcus pneumoniae*, *Haemophilus influenzae*, and *Staphylococcus aureus*. Less frequent causes include *Neisseria meningitidis* and *Streptococcus pyogenes*.

Chills and fever associated with tachypnea, intercostal retractions, lacking or tubular breath sounds over the affected area, and purulent sputum compose the classic presentation. Frequently, especially in younger infants and children, nonspecific complaints predominate. Pleural effusions are not uncommon and occasionally are the major feature of the disease. Typical chest radiographic findings include lobar consolidation or multiple, patchy, round infiltrates. A white blood cell count greater than 15,000 mm^3 (higher in pneumococcal disease) is usual. Blood culture results are diagnostic but are positive in only 10 to 25% of cases. Bacterial antigen studies in blood or urine, or both, may increase the diagnostic yield. Empirical management of severe bacterial pneumonia should include therapy for penicillinase-producing organisms such as *S. aureus* and β-lactamase–producing *H. influenzae*. Usually a semisynthetic penicillin in combination with a third-generation ceph-

alosporin is effective. In some areas, methicillin-resistant *S. aureus* is increasingly prevalent and, in such instances, vancomycin is recommended instead of a semisynthetic penicillin.

References

1. Foltz BD and Benumof JL: Mechanisms of hypoxemia and hypercapnia in the perioperative period. Crit Care Med 3:269, 1987.
2. Marini JJ: Postoperative atelectasis: Pathophysiology, clinical importance and principles of management. Respir Care 29:516, 1984.
3. Jaworski A, Goldberg SK, Walkenstein MD, et al: Utility of immediate postlobectomy fiberoptic bronchoscopy in preventing atelectasis. Chest 94:38, 1988.
4. Wagner PD, Laravuso RB, Uhl RR, et al: Continuous distribution of ventilation-perfusion ratios in normal subjects breathing air and 100% O$_2$. J Clin Invest 54:54, 1974.
5. Sprung CL, Loewenherz JW, Baier H, et al: Evidence for increased permeability in reexpansion pulmonary edema. Am J Med, 71:497, 1981.
6. Jackson RM, Veal CF, Alexander CB, et al: Re-expansion pulmonary edema: A potential role for free radicals in its pathogenesis. Am Rev Respir Dis 137:1165, 1988.
7. Jackson RM: Molecular, pharmacologic and clinical aspects of oxygen-induced lung injury. Clin Chest Med 11:73, 1990.
8. Matalon S and Nickerson PA: Alterations in mammalian blood-gas barrier exposed to hyperoxia. *In*: Taylor AF, Matalon S, and Ward P (eds): Physiology of Oxygen Radicals. Bethesda, MD, American Physiological Society, 1986, p. 55.
9. Gross N and Smith D: Methylprednisolone increases the toxicity of oxygen in adult mice. Mechanical and biochemical effects on the surfactant system. Am Rev Respir Dis 129:805, 1984.
10. Freeman B, Young S, and Crappo J: Liposome-mediated augmentation of superoxide dismutase in endothelial cells prevents oxygen injury. J Biol Chem 258:12534, 1983.
11. Matalon S, Holm BA, and Notter RH: Mitigation of pulmonary hyperoxic injury by administration of exogenous surfactant. J Appl Physiol 62:756, 1987.
12. Kollef MH, and Pluss J: Noncardiogenic pulmonary edema following upper airway obstruction: 7 cases and a review of the literature. Medicine 70:91, 1991.
13. Lang SA, Duncan PG, Shephard DAE, et al: Pulmonary edema associated with airway obstruction. Can J Anesth, 37:210, 1990.
14. Allen SJ, Drake RE, Williams JP, et al: Recent advances in pulmonary edema. Crit Care Med 15:963, 1987.
15. Colice GL: Neurogenic pulmonary edema. Clin Chest Med 6:473, 1985.
16. Pfenniger J, Gerber A, Tschäppeler H, et al: Adult respiratory distress syndrome in children. J Pediatr 101:352, 1982.
17. Royall JA and Levin DL: Adult respiratory distress syndrome in pediatric patients. I: Clinical aspects, pathophysiology, pathology, and mechanism of lung injury; II: Management. J Pediatr 112:169, 1988.
18. Rinaldo JE and Rogers RM: Adult respiratory-distress syndrome: Changing concepts of lung injury and repair. N Engl J Med 306:900, 1982.
19. Butler B, Milsark IW, and Cerami A: Passive immunization against cachectin/tumor necrosis factor protects mice from the lethal effects of endotoxin. Science 229:869, 1985.
20. Holm BA, Notter RH, Siegle J, et al: Pulmonary physiological and surfactant changes during injury and recovery from hypoxia. J Appl Physiol 59:1402, 1985.
21. Tobin MJ: Diagnosis of pneumonia: Techniques and problems. Clin Chest Med 8:513, 1987.
22. Cain SM: Oxygen delivery and uptake in dogs during anemic and hypoxic hypoxia. J Appl Physiol, Respir Environ Exercise Physiol 42:228, 1977.
23. Clarke C, Edwards JD, Nightingale P, et al: Persistence of supply dependency of oxygen uptake at high levels of delivery in adult respiratory distress syndrome. Crit Care Med 19:497, 1991.
24. Stagno S, Brasfield DM, Brown MB, et al: Infant pneumonitis associated with cytomegalovirus, Chlamydia, Pneumocystis, and ureaplasma: A prospective study. Pediatrics 68:322, 1981.

48

Diseases of the Chest Wall

Marc B. Hershenson, M.D.

The unique shape and deformability of the immature chest wall hinder the normal function of the immature respiratory system. Only by understanding such mechanical disadvantages may the clinician appreciate the normal function of the immature respiratory system and understand the propensity of the infant to develop ventilatory failure and apnea.

The chest wall consists of the thorax and those muscles capable of influencing intrathoracic pressure. This includes the rib cage and rib cage muscles, diaphragm, abdomen and abdominal muscles, and the accessory muscles of respiration, such as the sternocleidomastoid and scalene muscles.

DEVELOPMENTAL PHYSIOLOGY

Diaphragm

The diaphragm is composed of two principal parts: the crural diaphragm and the costal diaphragm (Fig. 48–1). Contraction of the crural part of the diaphragm causes piston-like, axial movement of the diaphragmatic dome, increasing the vertical dimension of the thoracic cavity and lowering intrathoracic pressure. (Shortening of the crural diaphragm also increases abdominal pressure.) Contraction of the axially placed fibers of the costal diaphragm raises and expands the lower rib cage. This has been called the insertional component of the diaphragm's action on the rib cage.

A large portion of the costal diaphragm lies in direct apposition to the inner surface of the rib cage. This area, the zone of apposition, holds major significance for diaphragmatic function (Fig. 48–2).[1] Because the abdominal contents lie adjacent to the lower rib cage, increases in abdominal pressure generated by contraction of the crural diaphragm may expand the lower rib cage. This is the appositional component of the diaphragm's action on the rib cage.

The capability of the diaphragm to expand the upper rib cage as well as the lower rib cage depends on mechanical coupling between the upper and lower rib cages. The diaphragm will have an expanding influence on the upper rib cage as well as lower rib cage only if

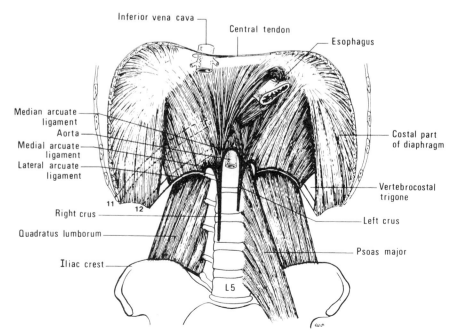

Figure 48–1. Schematic drawing of the coronal section of the diaphragm. The costal diaphragm arises from the lower rib cage and likewise inserts onto the central tendon. The crural diaphragm originates from the lumbar vertebrae and inserts onto the central tendon. The positions of eleventh and twelfth ribs are indicated. (From Osmond DG: Functional anatomy of the chest wall. *In*: Roussos C and Maclem PT [eds]: The Thorax. New York, Marcel Dekker, 1985, p. 221.)

Inferior vena cava

Central tendon

Esophagus

Median arcuate ligament

Aorta

Medial arcuate ligament

Lateral arcuate ligament

Costal part of diaphragm

Vertebrocostal trigone

11 12

Right crus

Left crus

Quadratus lumborum

Psoas major

Iliac crest

L5

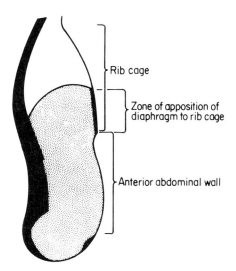

Figure 48–2. Schematic drawing of the zone of apposition (sagittal view). Through the zone of apposition, the diaphragm may expand the lower rib cage through the agency of abdominal pressure. (From Mead J, Smith JC, and Loring SH: Volume displacements of the chest wall and their mechanical significance. *In*: Roussos C and Maclem PT [eds]: The Thorax. New York, Marcel Dekker, 1985, p. 373.)

the rib cage is relatively stiff, due either to contraction of the intercostal muscles or mechanical properties of the rib cage itself. The inspiratory effect of the diaphragm on the upper rib cage is limited in the newborn infant. First, the zone of apposition is smaller in newborns than in adults,[2] limiting the capability of the diaphragm to expand the lower rib cage by increasing abdominal pressure. Second, because the rib cage of the newborn infant is highly compliant, the diaphragm's

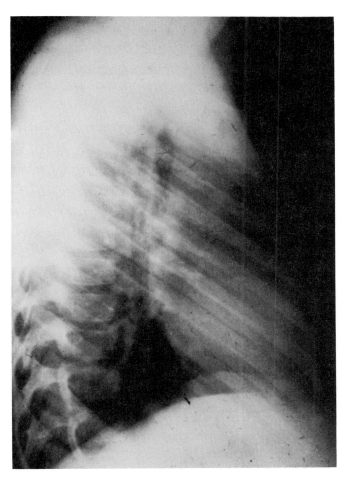

Figure 48–4. Lateral chest radiograph of a 4-year-old child. Because of the usual caudal inclination of the ribs, raising the ribs increases thoracic volume and is inspiratory.

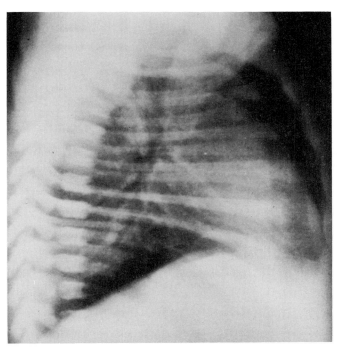

Figure 48–3. Lateral chest radiograph of a newborn infant. In the newborn, the ribs are horizontal, limiting the mechanical advantage of the intercostal muscles.

expanding influence on the lower rib cage is unlikely to be conveyed to the upper rib cage without recruitment of the intercostal muscles.

Rib Cage

The inspiratory action of the rib cage muscles is based on elevation of the ribs to a more horizontal position. Because of the usual inclination of the ribs, raising the ribs increases thoracic volume. Three groups of muscles occupy the intercostal space. The external intercostal muscles and the interchondral internal intercostal muscles (parasternal muscles) raise the ribs and are inspiratory. The interosseous internal intercostal muscles lower the ribs and are expiratory.

The ribs are relatively horizontal in the newborn infant, limiting the potential increase in thoracic cross-sectional area (Fig. 48–3). This mechanical disadvantage limits the contribution of the rib cage to tidal volume,[3] leading to the common observation that newborns are "abdominal (diaphragmatic) breathers." With development, gravity and the change to the upright posture tend to pull the ribs downward, orienting them more diagonally (Fig. 48–4).

The outward recoil of the chest wall is reduced in infants; in the newborn, it is close to zero.[4] The diminished outward recoil of the newborn chest wall is related primarily to a lack of mineralization of the ribs. Reduced outward recoil of the chest wall is opposed by an inward recoil of the lung that is similar to that of the adult. Accordingly, functional residual capacity (FRC), the volume of the respiratory system under equilibrium conditions, decreases to approximately 10% of total lung capacity (Fig. 48–5). As this volume is below closing capacity, breathing at or around passively determined FRC would predispose to significant atelectasis. Measurements in newborn infants have demonstrated an end-expiratory volume substantially greater than passively determined FRC, however. There are several mechanisms by which newborn infants maintain end-expiratory volume above passively determined FRC. Kosch and Stark showed that expiratory flow rates at end-expiration are substantial, suggesting an active interruption of expiration (Fig. 48–6).[5] Expiratory "braking" may be accomplished by contraction of laryngeal adductors. End-expiratory volume is also increased by respiratory timing changes that decrease expiratory time below the expiratory time constant of the respiratory system. Finally, inspiratory influences are maintained during expiration via increasing tonic activity of the diaphragm.

In addition to compelling the infant to develop strategies to maintain end-expiratory volume above passively determined FRC, the highly pliant chest wall predisposes the newborn infant to paradoxic inward movement of the rib cage during inspiration. Diaphragmatic contraction, by generating a negative intrathoracic pressure, may have an expiratory effect on the upper rib cage. Contraction of the inspiratory rib cage muscles reduces rib cage deformation, as evidenced by the exaggerated paradoxic rib cage motion during active rapid eye movement (REM) sleep, a state in which intercostal muscle activity is diminished or absent (Fig. 48–7).[6]

The repercussions of paradoxic rib cage movement are substantial in the newborn. During active sleep (in part defined by paradoxic inward movement of the rib cage), end-expiratory volume decreases by more than

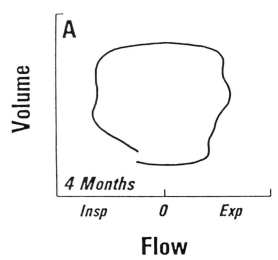

Figure 48–6. Flow-volume representation of a newborn tidal breath. The latter portion of expiration is interrupted by inspiration. Inspiratory interruption occurs at a substantial expiratory flow rate. Thus, end-expiratory volume is not determined by the passive characteristics of the lungs and chest wall in infants. (From Colin AA, Wohl MEB, Mead J, et al: Transition from dynamically-maintained to relaxed end-expiratory volume in human infants. J Appl Physiol 67:2108, 1989.)

30% and transcutaneous P_{O_2} decreases. Because diaphragmatic contraction draws in the rib cage instead of air, the diaphragm must increase its activity to maintain tidal volume. During paradoxic rib cage movement, abdominal motion, the diaphragmatic electromyogram, and diaphragmatic work all increase considerably (see Fig. 48–7).[6, 7] Therefore, increased chest wall compliance and deformability, by allowing paradoxic rib cage motion, predispose the infant to diaphragmatic fatigue.

Increased chest wall compliance and deformability also influence regional ventilation in infants. Normally, a gravitational pleural pressure gradient exists outside

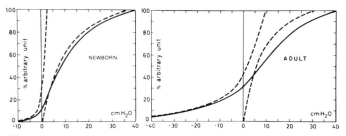

Figure 48–5. Volume-pressure (V-P) characteristics of the newborn and adult respiratory system *(solid lines)*. The dashed lines represent the V-P characteristics of the chest wall and lung. In the newborn, the reduced outward recoil of the chest wall reduces passively determined functional residual capacity (the volume at which the pressure of the respiratory system is equal to zero). (From Agostoni E and Mead J: Statics of the respiratory system. *In*: Fenn WO and Rahn H [eds]: Handbook of Physiology, Respiration. Washington DC, American Physiological Society, 1964, Sec. 3, Vol. 1, p. 401.)

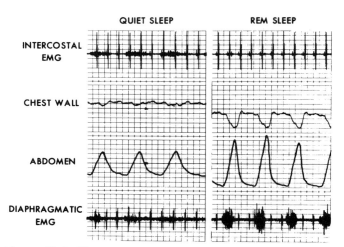

Figure 48–7. Effect of sleep state on intercostal muscle activity. During REM sleep, intercostal muscle activity decreases. Reduced intercostal muscle activity results in paradoxic rib cage motion, increased diaphragmatic displacement, and increased electromyographic activity of the diaphragm. (From Muller N, Gulston G, Cade D, et al: Diaphragmatic muscle fatigue of the newborn. J Appl Physiol 46:692, 1979.)

the lung, with the alveolar distending pressure being highest (least negative) at the bottom. Accordingly, basal alveoli are less inflated than apical alveoli at end-expiration and reside at a lower portion of their volume-pressure characteristic. With an increase in distending pressure, the alveolar volume change is greater for basal alveoli. Thus, ventilation is greatest to lower regions of the lung. When adults are placed in the decubitus position, ventilation is redistributed to the dependent lung. In the infant, however, ventilation is redistributed away from the dependent lung,[8] likely because the deformable chest wall cannot fully support the weight of the thorax.

Chest Wall and Airway Obstruction

Pathophysiology. Chronic obstructive pulmonary disease (COPD) occurs in infants and children with bronchopulmonary dysplasia, cystic fibrosis, recurrent aspiration or infection, and congenital anomalies involving the respiratory tract (tracheoesophageal fistula, diaphragmatic hernia, prune belly syndrome). A larger number of children have reversible airways obstruction (asthma). Air flow limitation has several implications for the chest wall. The first involves the length-tension characteristics of skeletal muscle. Active tension increases as muscle length approximates L_o (resting length). Thus, longer muscles usually have increased force-generating capacity. Conversely, reductions in the length of the diaphragm and intercostal muscle accompanying hyperinflation would decrease pressure-generating capacity, demanding increased neural activation to maintain inspiratory pressure generation.

Second, air flow limitation-induced hyperinflation alters the mechanical advantage of the respiratory muscles. As described earlier, shortening of the axially placed fibers of the costal diaphragm raises and expands the lower rib cage (insertional effect of the diaphragm on the rib cage). Hyperinflation, by orienting the costal diaphragmatic fibers horizontally, may actually cause the diaphragm to pull the lower rib cage inward. Hyperinflation also decreases the size of the zone of apposition, decreasing the appositional effect of the diaphragm on the rib cage. Finally, hyperinflation decreases the mechanical advantage of the inspiratory intercostal muscles by elevating the ribs (a situation similar to that of the newborn infant). Like muscle shortening, reductions in mechanical advantage increase the neural activation of the inspiratory muscles required for a given change in intrathoracic pressure.

In children with COPD, inspiratory muscle work must be increased to overcome changes in both airways resistance and lung elasticity. In addition, increments in negative inspiratory pressure required to overcome airways resistance may paradoxically pull in the upper rib cage, further increasing diaphragmatic work. Muscle shortening, loss of mechanical advantage, and paradoxic rib cage motion all predispose to fatigue of the diaphragm.

Diagnosis. The distinguishing characteristic of altered chest wall function in patients with obstructed airways is subcostal retraction. Retraction of the lower costal margins results from contraction of a flattened diaphragm. Patients with airways disease commonly have a "barrel chest," a consequence of both hyperinflation and increased inspiratory muscle tone. The explanation for tonic inspiratory muscle activity in asthma, which paradoxically fosters further hyperinflation, is unclear. Increased paradoxic movement of the rib cage has been observed in children with COPD and in adolescents with asthma. Continual inward movement of the anterior rib cage due to chronic airway obstruction may cause a lasting depression deformity of the lower part of the sternum. This "acquired" pectus excavatum has been noted in infants with long-standing upper airway obstruction and in infants with severe COPD. Finally, the chest radiograph of patients with airways obstruction shows a flattened diaphragm, hyperinflation, horizontal orientation of the ribs, and an increased anteroposterior diameter of the chest.

Treatment. There are no specific approaches to the chest wall dysfunction in patients with obstructive airways disease. Treatment should be directed toward the underlying airways obstruction.

Diaphragmatic Fatigue and Apnea

Pathophysiology. The frequent occurrence of respiratory failure and apnea in premature infants has led to deliberation regarding the capacity of immature skeletal muscle to resist fatigue. An initial report demonstrating a deficiency of oxidative fibers in the diaphragm of premature and newborn infants suggested that the ventilatory muscles of these infants were more susceptible to fatigue than those of older subjects. These studies were flawed, however, by a delay in the collection of autopsy samples. Maxwell and coworkers examined the respiratory muscles of freshly killed baboons.[9] Although the diaphragm and intercostal muscles of premature and term baboons possessed a lower percentage of type I fibers, they were replaced by highly oxidative type IIc fibers that would not be expected to fatigue easily. These data were verified by physiologic studies demonstrating that fetal muscle strips maintained 83% of their peak tension after a series of tetanic stimuli, significantly greater than the 50% in adult strips.

Nevertheless, most investigators believe that diaphragmatic fatigue is common in infants, especially in those born prematurely. As described earlier, diaphragmatic work increases dramatically during rib cage deformation, predisposing the newborn infant to fatigue of the diaphragm. Muller and colleagues demonstrated a shift in the electromyogram (EMG) power spectrum (see Diagnosis, later) during breaths with rib cage distortion in infants of 26 to 40 weeks' gestational age. This shift was followed either by intercostal muscle recruitment or by apnea, evidence that changes in the power spectrum were indicative of fatigue of the diaphragm.

Although most apnea in infants is thought to be central in origin, the aforementioned data suggest that apneic episodes may sometimes represent a response to rib cage deformation or fatigue of the diaphragm. It has been shown that rib cage distortion in cats elicits a reflex that terminates inspiration. Similarly, rib cage deformation induced by airway occlusion or by manual compression decreases inspiratory time and tidal volume in newborn infants. Apnea in infants with extreme rib cage deformation might represent an exaggerated form of this reflex. This reflex may also play a role in the apnea observed in infants with viral bronchiolitis.

Diagnosis. Muscle fatigue may be diagnosed when, at a constant level of neural activation, the tension generated by that muscle decreases. Thus, the determination of fatigue of the diaphragm requires some knowledge of muscular electrical activity (electromyography). Diaphragmatic electromyographic activity is not easy to assess, however. EMGs obtained using skin electrodes placed on the lower ventrolateral surface of the rib cage may be contaminated by rib cage muscle activity, and esophageal electrodes are preferred. In addition, it has been shown that the EMG signal from the diaphragm may be reduced by increases in the length of the diaphragm, suggesting that the EMG may not be an accurate reflection of the diaphragm's activity.

Fatigue of the diaphragm has been identified by a shift in the power spectrum of the EMG from high to low frequencies. Low-frequency muscle fatigue (i.e., fatigue produced by successive submaximal contractions) may not be associated with a shift in the power spectrum, however. Also, the effects of changes in muscle load, length, and activation on the power spectrum of an EMG of the diaphragm are unclear.

If an EMG of the diaphragm cannot be obtained, maximal respiratory efforts, in which neural activation (phrenic nerve output) is assumed to be constant, are substituted. Measurements of maximal inspiratory pressure are employed to diagnose respiratory muscle fatigue in older children and adults and to assess patients' capacity to wean from mechanical ventilation. A maximal inspiratory pressure of -20 cm H_2O has been said to be a predictor of successful weaning; however, the utility of maximal inspiratory pressure measurements is limited. First, inadequate effort on the part of the subject may lead to misleading results. Second, patients with "acceptable" maximal inspiratory pressures often fail to wean from ventilatory support. Finally, the diaphragm may not be maximally active during such efforts, suggesting that maximal inspiratory pressure measures the strength of the inspiratory muscles of the rib cage, not the strength of the diaphragm.[10]

The diaphragm is fully active during maximal open-glottis expulsive efforts or combined maximal inspiratory and expulsive efforts performed with the glottis closed.[10] A reduction in the transdiaphragmatic pressure (P_{di}) generated during such efforts (P_{di}max) is evidence of diaphragmatic fatigue. Drawbacks to this routine include the requirement of esophageal and gastric catheters for the measurement of P_{di} and the complexity of the respiratory maneuvers involved, which are often difficult for the untrained subject.

P_{di}max, like maximal inspiratory pressure, is often an unreliable predictor of ventilator weaning. Both measurements fail to take into account the duration and magnitude of pressure generation required for tidal breathing (i.e., respiratory work). Successful weaning can occur only if the P_{di} generated during tidal breathing is a nominal fraction of P_{di}max. (The P_{di} required during tidal breathing, in turn, is inversely related to lung compliance.) The time · tension index (fraction of each breath spent in inspiration · P_{di}/P_{di}max) takes such factors into account, has been employed to assess respiratory muscle fatigue, and may be used to predict ability to wean. A time · tension index greater than ≈ 0.15 has been associated with respiratory failure. If transdiaphragmatic pressure measurement cannot easily be accomplished, P_{di}/P_{di}max may be estimated by the fraction tidal inspiratory pressure/maximal inspiratory pressure.

Attempts to diagnose respiratory muscle fatigue in children have been hindered by the incapacity of infants and small children to generate reproducible respiratory efforts and by the appropriate reluctance of parents and investigators to perform invasive studies on children. As noted earlier, noninvasive measures (i.e., the EMG power spectrum using skin electrodes) may be unreliable.

Finally, extreme diaphragmatic fatigue may be diagnosed by observing inward motion of the abdomen and negative gastric pressure fluctuation and reduced P_{di} swings during inspiration.

Treatment. Methylxanthines (theophylline, caffeine) induce a shift to the left in the force-frequency relationship of skeletal muscle (Fig. 48–8), thus increasing developed force at submaximal ($\sim < 120$ Hz) stimulation frequencies.[11] Such increments in force presumably result from an increase in intracellular calcium flux.

On the other hand, methylxanthines have no effect on tension development at high stimulation frequencies. During maximal tetanic stimulation, cytoplasmic calcium levels are sufficiently high that actin-myosin cross-bridge interaction is completely uninhibited, precluding methylxanthine-induced increases in force. Thus, one should not expect methylxanthines to increase the strength of

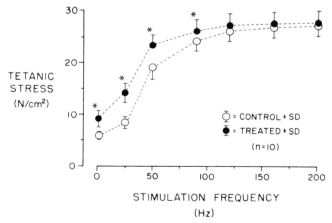

Figure 48–8. Treatment with methylxanthines induces a left-sided shift in the force-frequency relationship of skeletal muscle, thus increasing developed force at submaximal stimulation frequencies. Methylxanthines have no effect on tension development at high stimulation frequencies. (From Reid MB and Miller MJ: Theophylline does not increase maximal tetanic force or diaphragm endurance in vitro. J Appl Physiol 67:1658, 1989.)

the diaphragm during a truly maximal respiratory effort.[11]

Normal diaphragm function includes a wide range of firing frequencies, from less than 30 Hz during quiet breathing to 400 Hz during vigorous respiratory efforts. The effect of methylxanthines on the contractility of the diaphragm depends therefore on the firing frequency (central respiratory drive) of the patient in question; if drive is increased (such as in most patients with reduced lung compliance), methylxanthines may have little effect on the strength of the diaphragm. On the other hand, methylxanthines are likely to increase developed force when neural drive is abnormally depressed.

Deformities of the Chest Wall in Children

A complete review of thoracic deformities may be found elsewhere.[12] We focus on idiopathic (nonparalytic) scoliosis, pectus excavatum, congenital narrow thorax, congenital diaphragmatic hernia, and abdominal wall defects.

Scoliosis. Idiopathic scoliosis (i.e., that not associated with muscle weakness or paralysis) rarely causes significant respiratory compromise. Only when the spinal angle exceeds 50 degrees does lung volume decrease significantly. In the developed countries, children with idiopathic scoliosis are braced or repaired during adolescence, before respiratory symptoms occur. Adult patients with untreated kyphoscoliosis may experience severe restrictive lung disease, respiratory failure, and cor pulmonale. Reductions in both maximal inspiratory pressure and P_{di}max have been found in adults with severe scoliosis, evidence of reduced muscle strength. The mechanism of reduced muscle strength (mechanical disadvantage, limitation of physical activity, malnutrition) is unclear.

The diagnosis of scoliosis and other chest wall deformities relies chiefly on the physical examination and chest radiograph. The severity of restrictive lung disease in scoliosis may be determined by pulmonary function testing. Reductions in vital capacity and residual volume are directly proportional to the angle of scoliosis.[13] Harrington rod instrumentation and spinal fusion appear to modestly increase lung volume in patients with either idiopathic or paralytic scoliosis; the more severe the original deformity, the greater will be the increase in lung volume with treatment.

Pectus Excavatum. Persons with pectus excavatum may infrequently experience symptoms of exercise intolerance during adolescence. Such individuals may have minimally reduced lung volumes and greater than predicted oxygen uptake at high work loads, suggesting a mild restrictive defect. Although most individuals with pectus excavatum are asymptomatic, significant deformities are often repaired for cosmetic reasons.

Narrow Thorax. Respiratory insufficiency associated with a narrow chest has been described in conditions such as asphyxiating thoracic dystrophy, short-limbed dwarfism (e.g., achondroplasia), and giant (liver-containing) omphalocele. Respiratory failure in infants with a narrow chest may result from the severe restrictive

defect or from associated pulmonary hypoplasia. There is no specific therapy for congenital narrow thorax. Some infants experience significant chest growth in infancy, allowing prolonged survival. In such cases, continuous positive airway pressure or mechanical ventilation may be required.

Congenital Diaphragmatic Hernia. Bilateral pulmonary hypoplasia is the chief cause of respiratory failure in infants born with a diaphragmatic hernia. Little is known, however, about the function and development of the diaphragm in these infants. Studies have demonstrated decreased excursion and electromyographic activity of the hemidiaphragm on the side of the hernia.

Survival in infants with diaphragmatic hernia depends on the degree of pulmonary hypoplasia. Fatal pulmonary hypoplasia may be predicted by a preoperative Pa_{CO_2} greater than 40 mm Hg despite mechanical ventilation or the absence of a single preductal Pa_{O_2} greater than 100 mm Hg (despite breathing 100% oxygen). In the perioperative period, reversible pulmonary hypertension is a frequent complication. Pulmonary hypertension has been associated with excessive muscularization of the peripheral pulmonary arteries. The presence of reversible pulmonary hypertension has led to the use of extracorporeal membrane oxygenation (ECMO) in patients with congenital diaphragmatic hernia. The number of survivors of ECMO who would not have done so with only conventional management is probably small, however.

Abdominal Wall Defects. Typically, newborns with gastroschisis or small omphalocele have little respiratory difficulty. Generally, a few days of postoperative mechanical ventilatory support is all that is required. As mentioned earlier, newborns with a giant (liver-containing) omphalocele fare poorly due to an associated narrow chest deformity. These infants often die of respiratory failure or require long-term respiratory care. Prune belly syndrome (abdominal muscle deficiency, cryptorchidism, and urinary tract malformations) is thought to result from early congenital obstruction of the fetal bladder. Infants with prune belly syndrome may have chronic respiratory problems due to pulmonary hypoplasia, diaphragmatic weakness, and inability to cough. Diaphragmatic weakness results from the lack of abdominal tone, which allows the diaphragm to flatten and shorten, thus impairing its function. Inability to cough leads to recurrent respiratory tract infections and reactive airways disease. Bronchodilators, chest physiotherapy, and antibiotics are the mainstays of treatment. In some cases, reconstruction of the abdominal wall has improved respiratory function, owing to enhancement of the diaphragm's mechanical advantage and improved cough.

Chest Wall and Neuromuscular Disease

Generalized Neuromuscular Disease. A variety of congenital and acquired neuromuscular diseases cause respiratory insufficiency in infants and children. A partial list includes Werdnig-Hoffman disease, Guillain-Barré syndrome, myasthenia gravis, Duchenne muscular dystrophy, and myotonic dystrophy. In each case, respiratory insufficiency is distinguished by reduced lung volumes. The restrictive defect in patients with muscle weakness is magnified by the scoliosis that usually accompanies it. Although the relative contributions of the diaphragm and intercostal muscles to tidal breathing have not been measured in children with neuromuscular disease, diaphragm function is typically spared until late in the illness. Paradoxic inward motion of the rib cage during inspiration is commonly seen in infants with neuromuscular disease, owing to the loss of intercostal muscle activity and the high compliance and deformability of the immature chest wall. This further compromises the remaining diaphragm function. Reduced expiratory muscle strength decreases the ability to cough and clear secretions from the respiratory tract.

Patients with significant neuromuscular disease are tachypneic and have small tidal volumes. Intercostal retractions are absent, even in the face of CO_2 retention. Paradoxic inward motion of the rib cage during inspiration is commonly seen.

Spirometry in patients with neuromuscular disease is characterized by reductions in vital capacity, inspiratory reserve volume, expiratory reserve volume, and tidal volume. Reductions in vital capacity are a result of decreased lung and chest wall compliance as well as muscle weakness.[14] Maximal inspiratory and expiratory pressures are also decreased. There is often a blunted ventilatory response to CO_2. A reduced ventilatory response cannot be taken as evidence of respiratory center dysfunction in the presence of neuromuscular disease, however.

Unfortunately, there is no specific treatment for most children with respiratory insufficiency due to neuromuscular disease. Care is supportive and consists primarily of spinal instrumentation, mechanical hyperventilation of the lung, and assisted ventilation.

Although Harrington rod instrumentation and spinal fusion increase lung volume in patients with paralytic scoliosis, surgery should be performed before severe weakness supervenes. Repair in patients with a preoperative vital capacity less than 35% predicted has been associated with prolonged postoperative respiratory failure.

As noted earlier, reductions in vital capacity in patients with neuromuscular disease are due in part to reductions in lung and chest wall compliance. Mechanical hyperventilation of the lung (intermittent positive pressure breathing [IPPB]) might be useful in preventing such changes. Although studies of IPPB in patients with long-standing muscle weakness have failed to show an effect, a prophylactic regimen of IPPB starting early in the course of the illness has yet to be evaluated.

In patients with CO_2 retention, nocturnal ventilation with a cuirass shell, and negative-pressure ventilator has successfully reduced both nocturnal and daytime $Paco_2$.[15] The mechanism by which patients improve is unclear. Nighttime ventilation might rest fatigued muscles or improve lung and chest wall compliance. Alternatively, improved nocturnal blood gases might reset central chemoreceptors and reduce serum bicarbonate, leading to more appropriate ventilatory responses to

CO_2 during the day. The usefulness of negative-pressure ventilation may be limited by airway obstruction during negative-pressure development and kyphoscoliosis (which hinders the fit of the cuirass shell). The former patients may require a tracheostomy, which also serves to improve tracheobronchial toilet.

More and more frequently, children with severe muscle weakness are being treated with full-time positive-pressure mechanical ventilation. The appropriateness of such treatment depends on the ability of the patient to enjoy an acceptable quality of life despite mechanical ventilation.

Cervical Spinal Cord Injuries. Spinal cord lesions involving the phrenic nerve roots (C3–C5) result in respiratory failure requiring mechanical ventilation. Cervical spinal cord injury below C5 causes intercostal muscle paralysis and quadriparesis. Physiologic alterations in intercostal muscle paralysis resemble those in generalized neuromuscular disease.

Pacing of the diaphragm has been used to treat respiratory failure in patients with lesions of the cervical spinal cord or above. Pacing has no value if respiratory failure is due to damaged lower motor neurons of the phrenic nerve, muscular dystrophy, or lung disease.

Unilateral Diaphragmatic Paralysis. Paralysis of one hemidiaphragm may result from brachial plexus injury at birth or arise as a complication of cardiac surgery.[16] Paradoxic movement of the involved hemidiaphragm often accompanies paralysis, a consequence of negative pleural pressure generated by the inspiratory muscles of the rib cage and uninvolved hemidiaphragm and positive abdominal pressure generated by the functioning hemidiaphragm. In adults, unilateral diaphragmatic paralysis has little significance, although vital capacity and maximal inspiratory pressure are reduced. In infants, however, unilateral diaphragmatic paralysis may cause prolonged ventilator dependence. The increased clinical severity relates to several factors. First, the ability of the rib cage to contribute to tidal volume is limited in infants. As discussed earlier, the ribs are relatively horizontal at rest, limiting the potential increase in thoracic cross-sectional area. This mechanical disadvantage restricts the ability of the inspiratory rib cage muscles to compensate for the loss of hemidiaphragmatic function. Second, the infant's mediastinum is very mobile, so that paradoxic elevation of the paralyzed hemidiaphragm during inspiration causes a shift in the mediastinum to the contralateral side, limiting pulmonary expansion on the side opposite the paralysis. Third, the supine posture allows the abdominal viscera to promote upward displacement of the paralyzed hemidiaphragm.

Unilateral diaphragmatic paralysis is typically diagnosed by chest radiograph; an elevated hemidiaphragm, often accompanied by lower lobe atelectasis, is found. Further evidence of paralysis may be found at the bedside. First, paradoxic inward motion of the abdomen may be seen on the affected side. This tendency toward paradoxic motion may be accentuated by placing the infant with the side of the paralyzed hemidiaphragm up (this prevents stabilization of the affected hemidiaphragm by gravity). Second, one can examine the patient's nasogastric tube (if present) for respiratory fluctuations in the air-fluid level. During normal inspiration, descent of the crural diaphragm increases gastric pressure, and the air-fluid interface rises. In some infants with unilateral diaphragmatic paralysis, gastric pressure decreases during inspiration, indicating a net expiratory movement of the diaphragm during inspiration. (For abdominal pressure fluctuations to become negative, the expanding influence of the rib cage muscles on the abdominal compartment must predominate over the compressive effect of the unaffected hemidiaphragm.) Finally, paradoxic motion may be confirmed by fluoroscopy or ultrasonography.

The time course for recovery after phrenic nerve injury is variable, making treatment decisions difficult. Spontaneous recovery has been observed more than 6 months after injury, convincing some workers to delay surgical plication therapy until that time. It seems unreasonable, however, to delay plication therapy for that period of time in infants requiring ventilatory support. Plication of the involved hemidiaphragm to prevent paradoxic motion has consistently been shown to allow extubation of previously ventilator-dependent infants with unilateral diaphragmatic paralysis. Plication does not appear to interfere with the return of normal diaphragmatic function. On the other hand, immediate plication may fail to permanently prevent paradoxic motion. After phrenic nerve injury, progressive loss of diaphragmatic muscle tone may loosen what was previously a tight plication.[17] I recommend early, but not immediate plication of the diaphragm after phrenic nerve injury.

Diseases of the Pleura

Pneumothorax

Pathophysiology. A pneumothorax is defined as gas in the pleural space (the pleural space is normally gas-free). Pneumothorax or pneumomediastinum occur when overexpansion of alveoli causes gas to leak into the pulmonary interstitium and along interlobular septa. The gas may then migrate centrally to produce a pneumomediastinum or peripherally to create a subpleural bleb and pneumothorax. Alveolar overexpansion is particularly hazardous in newborn infants, in whom the pores of Kohn, which usually allow interalveolar gas dispersion, are underdeveloped. The term pulmonary interstitial emphysema refers to air leak that is confined to the interstitium of the lung.

Because alveolar pressure is always greater than pleural pressure (due to the recoil pressure of the lung), any opening between the lung and pleural space will cause gas to move into the pleural space. As gas enters, the lung collapses. Most commonly, the leak seals as lung volume decreases, resulting in only partial collapse. With highly emphysematous or fibrotic lungs, however, the leak often fails to seal, leading to a tension pneumothorax. In this event, gas enters the pleural space during inspiration but fails to exit during expiration, and pleural pressure increases over atmospheric. This leads to shifting of the mediastinum, compression of the

contralateral lung, reduced venous return, and the associated respiratory and hemodynamic compromise.

The magnitude of hypoxia accompanying a pneumothorax depends on whether appropriate hypoxic pulmonary vasoconstriction follows lung collapse. Alterations in gas exchange also depend on the severity of underlying lung disease.

Typically, the pressure of gas in a pneumothorax is atmospheric (760 mm Hg); the usual pressure of gas in the tissues is less (P_{CO_2}, 45 mm Hg; P_{O_2}, 40 mm Hg; P_{H_2O}, 47 mm Hg; P_{N_2}, 570 mm Hg; total, 702 mm Hg). Thus, there is a driving pressure favoring gas absorption. The rate of gas absorption may be hastened by breathing 100% oxygen, which washes out tissue nitrogen without substantially increasing tissue oxygen tension (P_{CO_2}, 45 mm Hg; P_{O_2}, 50 mm Hg; P_{H_2O}, 47 mm Hg; P_{N_2}, 0 mm Hg; total, 142 mm Hg).

Diagnosis. Pneumothorax may occur in four settings. Primary spontaneous pneumothorax occurs in patients without apparent underlying lung disease. Pneumothorax results from the rupture of a bleb located near the apex of the lung. The cause of primary spontaneous pneumothorax is obscure. Secondary spontaneous pneumothorax occurs in patients with underlying lung disease, such as bronchopulmonary dysplasia, asthma, or cystic fibrosis. Alveolar collapse and small airways obstruction each increase the risk of pneumothorax because they predispose to overinflation of normal alveoli. The most common variety of pneumothorax encountered by the critical care specialist is iatrogenic; that is, consequent to procedures such as thoracentesis, bronchoscopy, central venous catheter insertion, and mechanical ventilation. Although air leak during mechanical ventilation is widely perceived to result from excessive pressure, inadvertent intubation of the right mainstem bronchus and excessive ventilatory rates (with mechanical exhalation times shorter than the patient's own) are responsible for a substantial number of pneumothoraces. Finally, pneumothorax may occur in association with chest trauma.

Children with pneumothorax may experience sudden chest or shoulder pain and dyspnea. On physical examination, there is decreased chest wall motion, chest bulging, and reduced breath sounds on the affected side. Pneumothorax may also cause reductions in blood pressure, pulse pressure, and heart rate. It should be emphasized, however, that these signs and symptoms are often unreliable or absent. First, signs of pneumothorax may be obscured in patients with underlying lung disease, which may cause signs and symptoms similar to those found with pneumothorax. Second, in the infant, breath sounds from ventilated areas may be transmitted throughout the chest. If a pneumothorax is suspected, a chest radiograph should be obtained. If, in a critically ill patient, the suspicion of pneumothorax is high, a diagnostic thoracentesis should be performed.

The diagnosis of pneumothorax is best made by chest radiograph. The classic finding is lucency between the lung and chest wall. At times a bright light is needed to confirm the absence of lung markings. Differentiation of a pneumothorax from a skinfold, pulmonary cyst, or lobar emphysema may be difficult. Lung markings should be present lateral to a skinfold line; in cystic disease, the inner margins of the radiolucency are concave to the chest wall. In supine patients, air frequently accumulates anteriorly, around the heart. These collections of air are particularly hard to identify. In such instances, a cross-table lateral view of the chest may be helpful.

Treatment. In patients with primary spontaneous pneumothorax, lasting re-expansion of the lung is often accomplished by thoracentesis alone, although some workers prefer introduction of a standard chest tube. In patients with underlying lung disease, however, the frequent occurrence of respiratory embarrassment and ongoing air leak makes placement of an anteriorly positioned chest tube and suction mandatory. Obviously, emergency thoracentesis, with the needle directed into the second or third intercostal space at the midclavicular line, may be performed prior to chest tube insertion.

Pulmonary interstitial emphysema has been treated by lowering the level of ventilatory support, shortening inspiratory time, and high-frequency ventilation. For unilateral interstitial emphysema, selective bronchial intubation of the unaffected lung and positioning of the infant with the affected side down have been tried. Finally, muscle paralysis may be helpful in preventing air leak in patients undergoing mechanical ventilation.

Complications. A bronchopleural fistula may be defined as persistent air leak lasting longer than 5 to 7 days. Such fistulas are not uncommon, especially in patients with severe lung disease (e.g., adult respiratory distress syndrome) undergoing high-pressure mechanical ventilation. Resolution of bronchopleural fistulas in patients undergoing mechanical ventilation may take weeks; the leak often persists until just prior to extubation. If the air leak should continue in an extubated patient, surgical closure of the fistula and pleurodesis should be contemplated. Opinions vary as to the appropriate time for thoracotomy. (Thoracotomy with obliteration of the pleural space should also be performed in patients with bilateral or recurrent spontaneous pneumothorax.)

Pneumomediastinum rarely causes respiratory or hemodynamic embarrassment. Infrequently, a pneumomediastinum will fail to decompress into the pleural space, requiring placement of a mediastinal tube.

Pneumopericardium occurs when air dissects from the mediastinum to the pericardial space. Most workers assert that pericardiocentesis is not indicated unless hemodynamic compromise occurs.

Air may also dissect out of the thorax along tissue planes to cause pneumoperitoneum or subcutaneous emphysema. Although massive pneumoperitoneum requires paracentesis to prevent respiratory difficulty, treatment is usually unnecessary. Pneumoperitoneum must be differentiated from a perforated viscus, however. Paracentesis of gas from a perforated viscus yields the oxygen tension of room air, whereas paracentesis of a true pneumoperitoneum yields an oxygen tension proportional to the inspired oxygen concentration. Subcutaneous emphysema, although transiently disfiguring, does not require specific treatment.

Pleural Effusions

Pathophysiology. The pleural membranes cover the outer surface of the lung (visceral pleura) and the inner surfaces of the rib cage, diaphragm, and mediastinum (parietal pleura). A layer of blood vessels and lymphatics is located below the pleural mesothelium. The blood supply to the parietal pleura is systemic; the blood supply to the visceral pleura is from the pulmonary circulation. Although subatmospheric pressure in the pleural space (due to the recoil pressure of the chest wall) favors fluid accumulation, the volume of fluid in the pleural space is small (1 to 5 ml). This situation is primarily the result of differences in capillary hydrostatic pressure between the parietal pleura and the visceral pleura. Because the visceral pleura is supplied by pulmonary capillaries, hydrostatic pressure is decreased, favoring movement of fluid from the parietal pleura to the pleural space to the visceral pleura. Excess water and protein in the pleural space resulting from alterations in capillary hydrostatic pressure, plasma oncotic pressure, or capillary permeability are drained by the pulmonary lymphatics.

Normally, the composition of fluid between the parietal and viscera pleura is that of an ultrafiltrate of plasma. The concentration of albumin and other macromolecules is lower in pleural fluid than in plasma.

Transudative effusions (see Diagnosis, later) occur when capillary hydrostatic pressure is increased (e.g., congestive heart failure), plasma oncotic pressure decreased (hypoalbuminemia) or lymphatic inflow increased (abdominal surgery, ascites of hepatic cirrhosis, pancreatitis).

Pleural effusions due to increased capillary permeability may be induced by pulmonary infection, infarction, or neoplasm. Pulmonary infection adjacent to the visceral pleura may precipitate either a parapneumonic effusion or empyema. The term parapneumonic effusion refers to fluid that is culture-negative with characteristics of a transudate. If the infection in the pulmonary parenchyma continues, the infectious agent invades the pleural space to create an empyema. Empyema is defined as bacteria in the pleural space or culture-negative fluid with characteristics of an effusion.

When lymphatic outflow is obstructed (mediastinal lymphadenopathy, disruption of the thoracic duct, lymphangiectasia), the resultant pleural effusion is often chylous, although transudates and exudates may also ensue.

Prospective studies of adult patients with pneumonia report a 30 to 50% incidence of pleural effusion.[18] In children hospitalized with pneumonia, however, the incidence of effusion is said to be less than 1%.[19] The reasons for this disparity may relate to differences in study design (prospective versus retrospective) and difficulties encountered in diagnosing small pleural effusions in children.

Diagnosis. The historical features of pleural disease are fever, pain, and breathlessness. The physical findings of a pleural effusion include ipsilateral restriction of chest wall motion, dull or flat percussion, and decreased breath sounds. A pleural friction rub occurs in 10% of children with empyema. On upright chest radiograph, the costophrenic angle is lost and a stripe of pleural fluid is frequently seen along the inner aspect of the chest wall. In critically ill patients, diagnosis is made difficult by the fact that most radiographs are taken in the supine position. A stripe of pleural fluid is infrequently seen. Instead, the hemithorax appears diffusely hazy. In the intensive care unit, the diagnosis of pleural effusion often requires decubitus films or ultrasonography.

Thoracentesis is performed to define the cause of an effusion. Transudates are generally clear with a slight yellow tint. The fluid usually contains less than 10,000 white blood cells/mm³ and small amounts of protein (total protein less than 3 g/dl, pleural fluid to serum ratio of less than 0.5). The lactate dehydrogenase is usually less than 200 IU (pleura fluid to serum ratio of less than 0.6), the pH greater than 7.20, and the glucose greater than 60 mg/dl. Exudates are characterized by a high white blood cell count, high protein concentration, low pH, and low glucose concentration. The results of the Gram stain and culture are often positive and are more reliable than endotracheal tube aspirates for the diagnosis of underlying pneumonia. Chylothorax due to injury to lymphatic channels is distinguished by its milky appearance (seen in infants only during milk feedings) and high triglyceride concentration (> 110 mg/dl). Hemorrhagic pleural fluid results from trauma or malignancy.

For patients in whom tuberculosis or malignancy are suspected, improved diagnostic accuracy may be obtained when a needle biopsy of the pleura is performed.

Treatment. When pleural effusion is accompanied by significant respiratory distress, a thoracentesis is indicated. For drainage of empyema, a tube thoracostomy is required to prevent fibrothorax, a thick layer of fibrous tissue on the visceral pleura that restricts lung expansion. Tubes should be placed posteriorly and inferiorly in order to drain as much of the fluid as possible. If purulent drainage persists, placement of more than one tube, and rarely, open drainage, may be necessary. Treatment of chylothorax requires not only chest tube placement or repeated thoracentesis but must also include reduction of oral fat intake and replacement with medium-chain triglycerides.

The bacteriology of empyema has changed during the years of antibiotic therapy; the incidence of staphylococcal empyema has decreased and infections due to anaerobic bacteria and aerobic gram-negative rods have increased considerably, with multiple infecting organisms now common.[20] Antibiotic coverage should be altered appropriately. The possibility of tuberculous effusion should not be overlooked. Finally, effusions due to adenovirus, cytomegalovirus, Epstein-Barr virus, herpes simplex virus, and *Mycoplasma* are occasionally seen, particularly in immunocompromised hosts.

Hemothorax

Hemothorax is a frequent consequence of chest trauma. The diagnosis of hemothorax should be considered in any patient with chest trauma and a pleural effusion. Most hemothoraces are caused by bleeding from low-pressure, pulmonary parenchymal vessels. Accordingly, adequate chest tube drainage and re-expansion of the lung stops the bleeding in approximately 90% of the cases. Like empyema, the mainstay of treatment is the introduction of a large, posteriorly placed chest tube. Adequate drainage is required to prevent fibrothorax. Finally, hemothorax is often associated with pneumothorax.

References

1. Mead J: Functional significance of the area of apposition of diaphragm to rib cage. Am Rev Respir Dis 119:31, 1979.
2. Devlieger H: The Chest Wall in the Preterm Infant. Belgium, K.U. Leuven, 1987, pp. 136–140.
3. Hershenson MB, Colin AA, Wohl MEB, et al: Changes in the contribution of the rib cage to tidal breathing during infancy. Am Rev Respir Dis 141:922, 1990.
4. Agostoni E and Mead J: Statics of the respiratory system. In: Fenn WO and Rahn H (eds): Handbook of Physiology, Respiration. Washington, DC, American Physiological Society, 1964, Sec. 3, Vol. 1, pp. 387–409.
5. Kosch PC and Stark AR: Dynamic maintenance of end-expiratory volume in full-term infants. J Appl Physiol 57:1126, 1984.
6. Muller N, Gulston G, Cade D, et al: Diaphragmatic muscle fatigue of the newborn. J Appl Physiol 46:688, 1979.
7. Heldt GP and McIlroy MB: Distortion of the chest wall and work of the diaphragm in preterm infants. J Appl Physiol 62:164, 1987.
8. Heaf DP, Helms P, Gordon I, et al: Postural effects of gas exchange in infants. N Engl J Med 308:1505, 1983.
9. Maxwell LC, McCarter RJ, Kuehl TJ, et al: Development of histochemical and functional properties of baboon respiratory muscles. J Appl Physiol 54:551, 1983.
10. Hershenson MB, Kikuchi Y, and Loring SH: Relative strengths of the chest wall muscles. J Appl Physiol 65:852, 1988.
11. Reid MB, and Miller MJ: Theophylline does not increase maximal tetanic force or diaphragm endurance in vitro. J Appl Physiol 67:1655, 1987.
12. Wohl MEB, Stark AR, and Stokes DC: Thoracic disorders of childhood. In: Roussos C and Macklem PT (eds): The Thorax. New York, Marcel Dekker, 1985, pp. 1203–1251.
13. Kafer E: Idiopathic scoliosis: Gas exchange and age dependence of arterial blood gases. J Clin Invest 58:825, 1976.
14. DeTroyer A, Borenstein S, and Cordier R: Analysis of lung volume restriction in patients with respiratory muscle weakness. Thorax 35:603, 1980.
15. Goldstein RS, Molotiu N, Skrastins R, et al: Reversal of sleep-induced hypoventilation and chronic respiratory failure by nocturnal negative pressure ventilation in patients with restrictive ventilatory impairment. Am Rev Respir Dis 135:1049, 1987.
16. Lynn AM, Jenkins JG, Edmonds JF, et al: Diaphragmatic paralysis after pediatric cardiac surgery: A retrospective analysis of 34 cases. Crit Care Med 11:280, 1982.
17. Hershenson MB: Unpublished observations.
18. Taryle DA, Potts DE, and Sahn SA: The incidence and clinical correlates of parapneumonic effusions in pneumococcal pneumonia. Chest 74:170, 1978.
19. Chonmaitree T and Powell KR: Parapneumonic pleural effusion and empyema in children. Clin Pediatr 22:414, 1983.
20. Varkey B, Rose HD, Cutty CPK, et al: Empyema thoracic during a 10 year period: Analysis of 72 cases in comparison to a previous study (1952–1967). Arch Intern Med 141:1771, 1981.

49

Respiratory Disease in the Newborn

Dharmapuri Vidyasagar, M.D., and
Michael R. Uhing, M.D.

The transition from intrauterine to extrauterine life involves marked changes in the respiratory system. Within minutes after birth, the fluid filling the lungs in utero is reabsorbed and an adequate functional residual capacity (FRC) is established. Pulmonary blood flow increases to 8 to 10 times the intrauterine level as a result of a decrease in pulmonary vascular resistance. With these complex changes occurring, it is not surprising that respiratory diseases are a leading cause of morbidity and mortality in the newborn period.

The signs of respiratory disease in newborns are different from those in older pediatric patients because of differences in physiology. Cyanosis does not occur in newborns until the oxygen tension falls to 30 to 40 mm Hg, because of the presence of a high percentage of fetal hemoglobin with a high oxygen affinity. Retractions are more pronounced in newborns, especially premature infants, because the chest wall is extremely compliant. Since nasal resistance in newborns contributes up to 50% of the total pulmonary resistance, nasal flaring, which leads to a significant reduction in nasal resistance, becomes an important compensatory mechanism. Expiratory grunting, caused by breathing against partially closed vocal cords, results in improved FRC and oxygenation. This improvement in FRC is significant in the neonatal period because the highly compliant chest wall of the newborn is unable to keep the lungs expanded in diseases causing alveolar collapse and atelectasis. Finally, respiratory rates are higher, and thus tachypnea is defined as a respiratory rate greater than 60 bpm.

Laboratory evaluation is essential in the management of newborns with respiratory disease. At a minimum, a complete blood count, serum glucose determinations, blood culture, and arterial blood gas analysis are required. Chest radiographs are especially important in the diagnosis of respiratory disease. The need for further investigation is determined by the history and findings on physical examination.

The differential diagnosis of respiratory distress in the newborn is long and includes disorders of many different organ systems (Table 49–1). In this chapter, only diseases of pulmonary origin will be discussed. Diseases of nonpulmonary origin are discussed in other chapters, as are bronchopulmonary dysplasia and diaphragmatic abnormalities.

In this chapter, respiratory diseases have been separated into two groups. The first group is composed of diseases that are acquired at or after birth. The second group consists of diseases resulting from disorders of lung development.

ACQUIRED DISORDERS

Respiratory Distress Syndrome

Neonatal respiratory distress syndrome (RDS) is the most common cause of respiratory distress in premature infants. RDS occurs in 10 to 16% of infants weighing less than 2,500 g at birth. The incidence varies inversely with gestational age, occurring in up to 80% of newborns between 28 and 30 weeks' gestation and occurring rarely after 37 weeks' gestation.[1] In addition, RDS is responsible for 11% of perinatal deaths.[2]

The primary risk factor for the development of RDS is prematurity. Other significant risk factors include maternal diabetes, perinatal asphyxia, male gender, white race, second-born twin, and history of previous siblings with RDS. Factors that are protective against the development of RDS are maternal narcotic addiction, chronic placental insufficiency, and chronic maternal hypertension.

The disease is caused by a deficiency of pulmonary surfactant, a surface-active substance that prevents alveolar collapse by reducing the surface tension of the alveoli. Surfactant is 90% lipid; 80% of the total surfactant is phospholipid, with phosphatidylcholine and phosphatidylglycerol accounting for 80% and 10%, respectively.[3]

Surfactant deficiency leads to alveolar collapse, resulting in hypoxemia, acidosis, and pulmonary hypoperfusion. These factors lead to further decrease in surfactant production, epithelial cell damage, and increased capillary permeability, with consequent development of pulmonary edema.

At autopsy, the lungs are heavy and have a liver-like consistency. Microscopic inspection reveals atelectasis, congested capillaries, distended lymphatics, and air spaces lined with eosinophilic material containing fibrin and cellular debris ("hyaline membranes").

It is possible to predict infants at risk of developing RDS prenatally by using the lecithin:sphingomyelin (L:S) ratio of the amniotic fluid. A ratio of greater than 2 indicates pulmonary maturity. As the ratio decreases, the incidence of RDS increases. The ratio is less reliable in diabetic mothers, with ratios of 2 to 3 occasionally associated with RDS in the infant.[4] The presence of phosphatidylglycerol and phosphatidylinositol in amniotic fluid may give a better assessment of pulmonary maturity.

Clinically, infants with RDS have varying degrees of tachypnea, nasal flaring, retractions, grunting, and cyanosis. Apnea may occur secondary to hypoxemia and respiratory failure. In moderate to severe disease, breath sounds will be diminished because of atelectasis. Onset

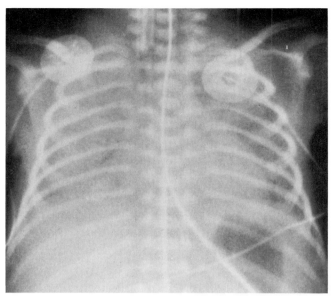

Figure 49–1. Anteroposterior chest x-ray demonstrating severe respiratory distress syndrome with complete opacity and an obscure cardiac border on the right and diffuse haziness on the left.

Table 49–1. DIFFERENTIAL DIAGNOSIS OF RESPIRATORY DISTRESS IN THE NEWBORN

Pulmonary Disorders
  Acquired disorders
    Respiratory distress syndrome
    Meconium aspiration syndrome
    Pneumonia
    Transient tachypnea of the newborn
    Pulmonary hemorrhage
    Air leaks
    Bronchopulmonary dysplasia
  Developmental anomalies
    Pulmonary hypoplasia
    Congenital lobar emphysema
    Chylothorax
    Cystic adenomatoid malformation
    Congenital lung cysts
    Pulmonary lymphangiectasis
Upper Airway
  Choanal atresia
  Micrognathia, Pierre-Robin syndrome
  Laryngeal obstruction (vocal cord paralysis,
    stenosis, malacia, web)
  Tracheal obstruction
Diaphragmatic Abnormalities
  Diaphragmatic hernia
  Eventration
  Phrenic nerve injury
Cardiovascular
  Arrhythmias
  Structural heart disease
  Cardiomyopathies
Hematologic
  Polycythemia
  Anemia
Neuromuscular Disease
Infection-Sepsis
Chest Wall Deformities
Metabolic Diseases
  Hypoglycemia
  Inborn errors of metabolism
Miscellaneous
  Asphyxia
  Hypothermia
  Hyperthermia

of RDS usually occurs in the first 6 hours after birth. If untreated, the disease gradually worsens over the next 2 to 3 days, and if there are no complications, recovery usually begins at 72 hours and is invariably associated with diuresis.

Chest x-ray studies typically show a diffuse reticulogranular pattern ("ground glass" appearance), with superimposed air bronchograms and decreased lung volume. In severe disease, the lung fields may be totally opaque (Fig. 49–1). The radiographic findings may not be present initially but may appear in follow-up films.

Pulmonary function studies are also abnormal. FRC and lung compliance are decreased. Resistance is usually normal. Alveolar minute ventilation is decreased secondary to large areas of atelectasis. Large areas of uneven ventilation and perfusion are also present.

Antenatal glucocorticoid administration has been shown to be effective in reducing the incidence of RDS, especially when used between 28 and 34 weeks' gestation.[5] The steroids are given 24 to 48 hours prior to, but not earlier than 7 days before, delivery. Recent studies suggest that extremely premature infants also benefit from prenatal steroid therapy.[6]

Treatment of infants with RDS begins with prevention of asphyxia and hypothermia, which have been shown to increase the severity of the disease. Frequent blood gas monitoring or continuous transcutaneous oxygen saturation monitoring is important to prevent both hypoxia and hyperoxia. Because these infants are usually premature and thus susceptible to retinopathy of prematurity, it is important to keep the arterial oxygen tension between 50 and 80 mm Hg. If inspired oxygen concentrations of greater than 0.40 are needed, infants should be treated with continuous positive airway pressure administered by nasal prongs or face mask. Early introduction of continuous positive airway pressure may eliminate the need for intubation and assisted ventilation.

Mechanical ventilation is indicated if the P_{CO_2} is greater than 50 to 60 mm Hg, the pH is less than 7.25, or severe apnea or gasping are present. Most centers use intermittent positive pressure ventilation with time-cycled, pressure-limited ventilators. Peak inspiratory pressures between 20 and 40 cm H_2O are usually required initially. Maintenance of positive end-expiratory pressure between 3 and 5 cm H_2O is required to prevent alveolar collapse and maintain an adequate FRC. This type of conventional mechanical ventilation usually uses frequencies of 60 to 70 bpm or less.

New modes of ventilation, including high-frequency oscillation and high-frequency jet ventilation, have been developed in an attempt to reduce the airway pressure required for ventilation. Preliminary studies of high-frequency ventilation have shown no benefit over conventional ventilation in infants with uncomplicated RDS.[7, 8] Further data are needed to determine whether these modes of ventilation may be beneficial, however, if the disease is complicated by pulmonary interstitial emphysema (PIE) or intractable air leaks or if the infant does not respond to conventional ventilation.

Many studies now have shown that intratracheal administration of surfactant is efficacious in reducing the severity of the disease. An artificial surfactant preparation (Exosurf) and a bovine surfactant (Survanta) currently have Federal Drug Administration approval for use in newborns with RDS. Other preparations are being studied, including porcine surfactant and human amniotic fluid surfactant. Surfactant solutions in doses of 100 mg/kg of phospholipid have been instilled into infants' lungs in the delivery room as prophylactic treatment, with good results. Similarly, administration of surfactant as rescue therapy after the onset of the disease has been shown to improve lung compliance and arterial oxygen tension. Because of the improved clinical status, earlier extubation has been possible. Thus, surfactant treatment has reduced hospitalization costs, as well as morbidity and mortality.[9]

Complications of RDS are numerous and often are compounded by the associated prematurity. A patent ductus arteriosus with significant left-to-right shunting occurs in 40 to 60% of infants with RDS. These infants have higher mortality and a higher incidence of bronchopulmonary dysplasia.[10] The incidence of bronchopulmonary dysplasia ranges between 20 and 40%.[11] Other pulmonary complications include pulmonary hemorrhage and air leakage syndromes. Prematurity predisposes the infant to intracranial hemorrhage and retinopathy of prematurity.

Meconium Aspiration Syndrome

The incidence of meconium staining of the amniotic fluid is between 8 and 20% of all deliveries.[12, 13] The incidence is as high as 44% in deliveries of infants greater than 42 weeks' gestation and is uncommon prior to 37 weeks' gestation.[14] Meconium aspiration syndrome occurs in approximately 2% of infants with meconium-stained amniotic fluid.[12]

The passage of meconium in utero has been associated with fetal distress, but there may be other causes.[15] The intestinal response to an episode of hypoxia is hyperperistalsis and relaxation of the anal sphincter, resulting in the passage of meconium into the amniotic fluid. No evidence of fetal distress can be identified in 12 to 25% of deliveries complicated by meconium-stained amniotic fluid, leading some investigators to postulate that the passage of meconium in utero may only be a sign of gastrointestinal maturity or an indication of compensated fetal distress. Additionally, meconium passage may be secondary to a vagal response caused by umbilical cord compression.

Once present in the amniotic fluid, meconium may be aspirated either in utero or at the time of delivery. Hypoxemia and acidemia can cause increased fetal breathing movements, with deep gasping and movement of meconium into the trachea or lungs. Conversely, meconium-stained fluid in the nasopharynx and oropharynx may be aspirated with the newborn's initial breaths after delivery.

The aspiration of particulate meconium leads to mechanical obstruction of both the upper and lower airways. Obstruction of the upper airway leads to acute hypoventilation, and the resultant hypoxemia, hypercapnea, and acidosis may cause pulmonary hypertension. Obstruction of the lower airway leads to atelectasis if the obstruction is complete. Partial obstruction may produce a ball-valve effect, with air trapping and overdistention and possible rupture of air sacs, leading to air leakage. In addition, a chemical pneumonitis, sometimes with bacterial superinfection, develops, leading to worsening oxygen diffusion over the next 24 to 48 hours.[16]

Pulmonary mechanics may become abnormal. The FRC is increased secondary to the air trapping. Airway resistance is increased secondary to the inflamed bronchial mucosa or obstruction from the meconium itself, or both. There is also a decrease in lung compliance, which may be secondary to the displacement of surfactant by the free fatty acid portion of the meconium.[17]

Clinical manifestations of meconium aspiration syndrome can vary from mild tachypnea to severe respiratory distress and cyanosis. The anteroposterior diameter of the chest often is increased because of the hyperinflation. Because infants with meconium aspiration syndrome may have experienced asphyxia, signs of central nervous system damage may be prominent.

The chest x-ray film shows patchy, often fluffy areas of increased density with areas of hyperinflation (Fig. 49-2). Even asymptomatic infants may have radiographic changes consistent with aspiration.

Management of meconium-stained amniotic fluid consists of a combined obstetric and pediatric approach at the time of delivery. The obstetrician should use a No. 8 French or larger catheter to suction the infant's nasopharynx, hypopharynx, and mouth when the head is at the perineum but prior to the delivery of the shoulders. Immediately after delivery, the pediatrician should suction the trachea under direct laryngoscopic visualization. Finally, the stomach should be emptied to prevent the possible regurgitation and aspiration of meconium that has been swallowed.

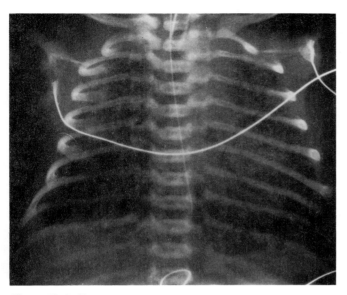

Figure 49–2. Chest x-ray showing severe meconium aspiration pneumonitis. Patchy areas of atelectasis with hyperinflation and depression of the diaphragm can be seen.

Some investigators believe that tracheal suctioning may not be indicated in cases in which the meconium is thin or in infants who have had no evidence of fetal distress and are vigorous at the time of delivery.[18]

Saline amnioinfusion has been used by some investigators, essentially to thin or even wash out the meconium from the uterus before it can be aspirated by the infant.[19] At present, however, no large prospective studies have been conducted to evaluate the effectiveness of amnioinfusion in reducing the incidence of meconium aspiration.

Management centers on respiratory care and support for infants with the meconium aspiration syndrome. If only mild respiratory distress is present, oxygen may be given by hood or nasal cannula. Blood gases and arterial oxygen saturation should be monitored closely for purposes of immediate detection of episodes of hypoxemia, hypercapnea, and acidosis, which may lead to worsening respiratory distress or the development of persistent pulmonary hypertension (PPH) (see also Chapter 34), or both. Antibiotics should be initiated along with chest physiotherapy.

If severe respiratory distress or respiratory acidosis is present, the infant will require mechanical ventilation. Arterial oxygen tension should be maintained at levels greater than 100 mm Hg, if possible, because these infants are at low risk for the development of retinopathy of prematurity but are at high risk for the development of PPH. Frequently, high peak inspiratory pressures are required to achieve adequate oxygenation because of the high airway resistance and decreased lung compliance. Fluids should be restricted to prevent pulmonary and cerebral edema.

PPH is a frequent complication of meconium aspiration syndrome. Acidosis, hypercapnea, and hypoxemia lead to pulmonary vasoconstriction and hypertension. This produces right-to-left shunting through the ductus arteriosus or foramen ovale, or both. Diagnosis of PPH can be made by (1) an improvement in arterial P_{O_2} as a result of hyperventilation, (2) a preductal and postductal P_{O_2} differential greater than 20 mm Hg, or (3) echocardiography showing right-to-left shunting.

Infants who experience PPH should be hyperventilated to keep the P_{CO_2} between 25 and 30 mm Hg. Arterial P_{O_2} should be maintained at levels greater than 100 mm Hg. Sodium bicarbonate should be given to maintain a pH of greater than 7.5 if this cannot be accomplished by hyperventilation. Inotropic agents, such as dopamine, may be needed to support the systemic blood pressure and minimize the pressure gradient between the pulmonary and systemic arterial systems. Sedation or paralysis, or both, often are required to minimize the infant's response to stimuli and decrease his or her agitation.

Tolazoline, an α-adrenergic blocker with pulmonary vasodilatory effects, can be used in infants who are unresponsive to the preceding therapy. An initial dose of 1 to 2 mg/kg by intravenous bolus is followed by a continuous infusion of 1 to 2 mg/kg/hr. Many infants with PPH have an unfavorable response to tolazoline because of the severe systemic hypotension it can cause. Consequently, a dopamine infusion should be started, and 10 ml/kg of 5% albumin should be drawn up before giving the tolazoline bolus, regardless of the infant's initial systemic blood pressure.

Extracorporeal membrane oxygenation is reserved for those infants who fail medical management (see Chapter 42). To qualify, an infant with PPH must have a predicted mortality rate of 80% or greater based on the alveolar-arterial oxygen differential and mean airway pressure. Contraindications for extracorporeal membrane oxygenation include birth weight less than 2 kg, gestational age less than 34 weeks, postnatal age greater than 7 days, the presence of an intracranial hemorrhage, or the presence of congenital heart disease.

The ultimate prognosis of infants with meconium aspiration syndrome depends largely on the degree of the oxygen desaturation and parenchymal disease. Approximately 40% of these infants will experience air leakage. Prolonged hyperventilation in infants with PPH can lead to deafness.[20] The mortality rate is approximately 30% in those infants requiring mechanical ventilation.[21]

Neonatal Pneumonia

The incidence of neonatal pneumonia is less than 1% in full-term infants. In premature infants, however, the incidence may be as high as 10%. The mortality rate from neonatal pneumonia is between 20 and 50%; it is one of the leading causes of mortality in neonates.[22]

The infant can become infected by a variety of mechanisms in utero, during delivery, or after delivery. Infection acquired in utero is primarily caused by organisms ascending the birth canal, leading to chorioamnionitis. The infected fluid is then swallowed or aspirated. This most commonly occurs when there is prolonged rupture of membranes, usually longer than 24 hours, but organisms can invade through intact membranes. Organisms causing disease consist primarily of maternal vaginal flora. Group B streptococcus and *Escherichia coli* are the most common organisms, but bacterial pneumonia caused by other streptococci (especially groups A, D, and G), *Klebsiella pneumoniae,* and *Proteus* are also important.

Transplacental infections are uncommon. The bacterial pathogens acquired by this mode are *Listeria monocytogenes* and those causing syphilis and tuberculosis. Usually, infections acquired in this fashion are not primarily pulmonary in nature. The infants are often stillborn or have other congenital anomalies. Viral infections, including cytomegalovirus, rubella, influenza A, adenovirus, echovirus, coxsackievirus, and herpes simplex, are acquired in this fashion.

During delivery, the infant may become infected either by aspiration of infected secretions in the birth canal or by becoming colonized with virulent organisms that invade later. The organisms responsible for this type of infection also consist primarily of vaginal flora.

The neonate's susceptibility to infection is higher when compared with other pediatric and adult patients because of an immature host defense system (see Chapter 11). Other predisposing factors to infection are prematurity, prolonged rupture of membranes, prolonged labor, incompetent cervix, asphyxia, and maternal infection such as urinary tract infection and amnionitis.

Clinically, neonates with pneumonia have more generalized symptoms of infection, such as temperature instability, jaundice, poor feeding, vomiting, and lethargy, in addition to respiratory distress. Neonates with viral intrauterine pneumonia usually have other associated abnormalities, such as petechiae, microcephaly, or hepatosplenomegaly. Bacterial pneumonia (group B streptococcus is the most common) may present with either early-onset disease, occurring at less than 1 week of age, or late-onset disease, occurring after 1 week of age. Early-onset disease is usually fulminant, with respiratory distress as its usual manifestation. Late-onset disease is more insidious, has a lower mortality rate, and is more often associated with meningitis and bone and skin manifestations.

The radiographic appearance is variable but most often shows a diffuse or patchy consolidation. In premature infants, the appearance may be very similar to hyaline membrane disease, especially with group B streptococcal pneumonia. The presence of effusions is suggestive of pneumonia and may be associated with *E. coli* and staphylococcal and streptococcal disease.

In neonates suspected of having pneumonia, culture specimens should be obtained from blood, urine, and cerebrospinal fluid. The blood culture may be negative if there has not been systemic invasion. Tracheal aspirate cultures may be helpful, especially if obtained within 8 hours of intubation. Urine latex agglutination tests may provide quicker results for certain organisms. If an effusion is present and a bacterial pathogen has not been identified, a thoracentesis may be considered. If a viral pathogen is suspected, viral specimens should be sent for culture, including specimens from the naso-pharynx and stool, and blood should be sent for serologic titers, particularly for specific IgM titers if available.

The complete blood count is also useful for identifying infected neonates. Neutropenia ($<1,500$ cells/mm^3), neutrophilia ($>15,000$ cells/mm^3), an immature to total neutrophil ratio greater than or equal to 0.2, and thrombocytopenia are all suggestive of infection.[23]

Initial therapy usually includes ampicillin with either an aminoglycoside, usually gentamicin, or a third-generation cephalosporin such as cefotaxime. Upon identification of an organism, the initial therapy should be reevaluated and tailored to the specific organism. Duration of therapy depends on the causative agent but usually lasts 7 to 10 days.

Transient Tachypnea of the Newborn

A frequent cause of respiratory distress is transient tachypnea of the newborn, also called respiratory distress syndrome, type II or wet lung syndrome. It occurs in 1.1% of neonates,[24] most commonly in infants born by cesarean section or precipitous vaginal delivery. Other predisposing factors are prematurity, asphyxia, and male gender.

Delayed resorption of lung fluid is the supposed cause. Infants delivered by cesarean section do not experience the thoracic compression with the subsequent expulsion of lung fluid that occurs in vaginally delivered infants. In addition, the high fetal catecholamine levels that inhibit fluid secretion by the lungs is not as great in infants delivered by cesarean section. Both of these factors may be associated with the high lung fluid volume in infants delivered by cesarean section.

Both Milner and Boon and their associates have shown that the thoracic gas volume is decreased in infants delivered by cesarean section.[25, 26] This difference lasts up to 48 hours and is postulated to be a result of increased interstitial and alveolar fluid.

Other possible causes for delayed lung fluid resorption include a transient period of left ventricular failure associated with asphyxia or an excessive placental transfusion.[27] Both of these factors lead to increased vascular hydrostatic pressure and thus less resorption of extravascular fluid.

Transient tachypnea of the newborn is usually a benign, self-limited disease. Infants present in the first few hours of life with tachypnea. Other symptoms of respiratory distress, such as grunting and retractions, are usually mild. Oxygen concentrations greater than 40 to 50% are rarely required to correct the hypoxemia. The symptoms usually resolve within 24 hours but may last up to 72 hours. Rarely, an infant may require mechanical ventilation or PPH may develop.

Laboratory evaluation usually reveals a normal pH and P_{CO_2}. Lung compliance is decreased, but the FRC is usually normal.

Radiographically, perihilar streaking is present along with fluid in the interlobar fissures. The lung fields usually appear hyperinflated. Occasionally, small pleural effusions or mild cardiomegaly may be present.

Treatment is supportive only. Treatment with furosemide does not alter the course of the disease. It is important that the possibility of sepsis, especially group B streptococcal sepsis, be considered in the evaluation, since the presenting symptoms may be very similar to transient tachypnea of the newborn.

Air Leakage Syndromes

One to 2% of all newborns experience a spontaneous pneumothorax or pneumomediastinum. These air leaks occur more frequently in males, postmature infants, and infants with meconium-stained amniotic fluid, even without evidence of aspiration. Spontaneous air leaks are rare prior to 34 weeks' gestation. Only 0.05% of newborns have symptomatic pneumothoraces or pneumomediastinums.[28]

The incidence of air leaks in the presence of underlying lung disease is greatly increased. Pneumothoraces occur in up to 40% of infants with RDS and meconium aspiration syndrome. They occur in up to 10% of infants with transient tachypnea of the newborn.[29] Pneumopericardium is rare and almost always occurs in infants receiving positive-pressure ventilation. Pulmonary interstitial emphysema (PIE) occurs in 20% of premature infants with RDS and occasionally occurs in full-term infants requiring mechanical ventilation.[31]

Spontaneous pneumothorax or pneumomediastinum at birth results from the high transpulmonary pressures generated during the initial breaths along with uneven inflation of alveoli. This uneven alveolar inflation is exaggerated in the newborn period by the decreased size and number of intra-alveolar pores, which help to equilibrate ventilation. Overinflation results in alveolar rupture with air dissecting down the perivascular sheaths to the hilum at which point it can rupture into the pleural or mediastinal space. Alternatively, air can rupture directly into the pleural space at the periphery of the lung.

PIE develops when air dissects along the perivascular sheaths and becomes trapped. Preterm infants are more susceptible to PIE because they have increased interstitial connective tissue with a looser texture when compared with full-term infants. Thus, air is more likely to become trapped in this tissue. Pathologically, PIE is characterized by irregularly shaped, gas-filled spaces with bronchovascular elements projecting into their lumina. These spaces are surrounded by variable amounts of fibrous tissue and multinucleated giant cells.

Most infants with spontaneous pneumothorax or pneumomediastinum are asymptomatic. In addition to the typical symptoms of respiratory distress, the symptoms of pneumothorax include an increased anteroposterior chest diameter, displacement of the apical pulse, and hypotension with narrowing of the pulse pressure.

A small pneumopericardium may be asymptomatic. If cardiac tamponade occurs, hypotension, bradycardia, and muffled heart sounds are present, and immediate drainage is required.

PIE leads to increased hypoxia secondary to increased ventilation and perfusion abnormalities. The interstitial air compresses alveoli and separates them from their blood vessels. PIE is frequently a precursor for the occurrence of other air leaks. Seventy-five per cent of preterm infants with RDS and PIE acquire other types of air leaks.[30]

Radiographically, a pneumothorax appears as a hyperlucent area without lung markings. The shadow of the collapsed lung can usually be seen. A pneumomediastinum appears as a "sail" sign secondary to elevation of the thymus (Fig. 49–3). On lateral views, the pneumomediastinum appears as a lucent area between the sternum and the heart. A pneumopericardium is characterized by gas surrounding the heart, especially the inferior surface (Fig. 49–4).

PIE may be either localized or diffuse. Diffuse disease is characterized by hyperinflation and multiple gas-filled cysts, usually less than 0.3 cm in diameter, in all lobes of the lung but more pronounced in the hilar regions. Localized disease may occur in one or more lobes, with cysts up to 3 cm in diameter leading to mediastinal shift and atelectasis of normal lung tissues (Fig. 49–5).

Mildly symptomatic pneumothoraces can be treated by administering 100% oxygen. This results in increased absorption of the trapped gas by nitrogen washout. Needle aspiration of the pneumothorax may also be performed to drain it. A chest tube should be inserted if the infant is on assisted ventilation, has severe respiratory distress, or has a tension pneumothorax.

Pneumomediastinum rarely requires drainage. If cardiac tamponade occurs as a result of a pneumopericardium, immediate pericardiocentesis is required.

PIE is usually treated by reducing ventilatory pressures as much as tolerated. High-frequency ventilation has been advocated because of the ability to ventilate infants at lower airway pressures. If PIE is unilateral, selective intubation of the less affected side may be considered. If localized PIE is leading to multiple recurrent pneumothoraces, atelectasis, or dependency on assisted ventilation, resection of the affected lobe may

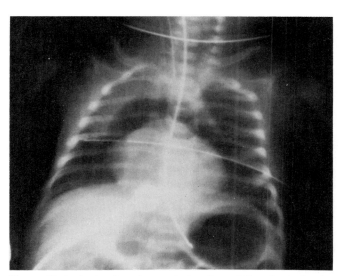

Figure 49–3. A classic anteroposterior view of the chest showing pneumomediastinum. The lifted thymic shadow above the heart is a typical presentation of pneumomediastinum.

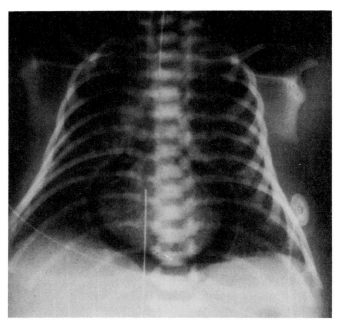

Figure 49–4. A typical chest x-ray showing pneumopericardium. The air is trapped in the pericardium as demonstrated by the radiolucent area surrounding the heart.

improve lung function. Less than 2% of infants with PIE require surgical resection.[31]

Pulmonary Hemorrhage

Fedrick and Butler estimated that the incidence of massive pulmonary hemorrhage is 1 in 1,000 live births and is present in 9% of neonatal autopsies.[32] Almost all cases occur in infants suffering from other major illnesses. Massive pulmonary hemorrhage is associated with RDS, asphyxia, congenital heart disease, infection, hypothermia, and coagulation disorders.

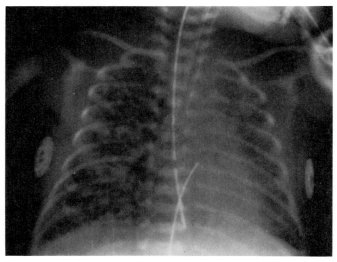

Figure 49–5. Anteroposterior chest x-ray showing unilateral right-sided pulmonary interstitial emphysema. Radiolucent areas of various sizes can be seen.

Clinically, patients present with sudden deterioration, shock, and cyanosis. Pink or red frothy liquid can be suctioned from the mouth or endotracheal tube. The peak age of incidence is between 2 and 4 days of age. Chest radiographs may show diffuse infiltrates or complete opacification of the lung fields.

Cole and associates proposed that massive pulmonary hemorrhage occurred secondary to increased pulmonary capillary pressure and left ventricular failure, resulting in hemorrhagic edema.[33] Left ventricular failure is caused by hypoxia or acidosis. Predisposing factors in the pathogenesis of pulmonary hemorrhage are decreased plasma oncotic pressure and lung tissue damage from the underlying disease process.

DEVELOPMENTAL ANOMALIES

Pulmonary Hypoplasia

Pulmonary hypoplasia can be found in 7.8 to 10.9% of neonatal autopsies.[34] Primary pulmonary hypoplasia without other abnormalities is rare. Secondary pulmonary hypoplasia may occur as a result of (1) oligohydramnios from premature rupture of membranes or renal abnormalities, (2) diaphragmatic hernia, (3) neuromuscular disorders such as anencephaly, and (4) thoracic skeletal abnormalities.

The degree of pulmonary hypoplasia associated with premature rupture of membranes depends on the gestational age of the fetus. Rotschild and colleagues found pulmonary hypoplasia in 16% of newborns with premature rupture of membranes longer than 7 days prior to delivery at less than 29 weeks' gestation.[35] Moessinger and colleagues showed that the effect of oligohydramnios on pulmonary development is most pronounced in the canalicular stage of development in guinea pigs. This corresponds to 16 to 26 weeks' gestation in human pregnancies.[36]

Pulmonary hypoplasia is quantitatively defined at autopsy as a lung weight:body weight ratio of less than 0.012 or by decreased alveolar number as determined by radial alveolar counting.[34]

The pathologic features of pulmonary hypoplasia vary depending on the amount of amniotic fluid. Hypoplasia associated with oligohydramnios is associated with immature structure with poor saccular branching, delayed vascularization, narrow airways, and decreased development of epithelial and interstitial tissue. In addition, phospholipid levels are low. Hypoplastic lungs associated with normal or increased amniotic fluid tend to have decreased lung growth but are structurally mature and contain normal phospholipid levels.[37]

Clinically, infants with pulmonary hypoplasia show varying degrees of respiratory distress. These infants are very prone to the development of air leaks and persistent fetal circulation.

Radiographic studies show small, clear lung fields. If the hypoplasia is unilateral, the mediastinum may be shifted to the affected side.

Chylothorax

Chylothorax is rare but is a common cause of pleural effusion in the first days of life. Boys are affected twice as often as are girls. The right side is affected more often than is the left.

The cause of chylothorax is not known. Suggested causes include (1) rupture of the thoracic duct secondary to birth trauma, (2) maldevelopment of the lymphatic ducts, and (3) presence of a fistula between the pleural cavity and the thoracic duct.

Respiratory distress develops in 50% of infants with chylothorax within 24 hours of birth and in 75% by the end of the first week of life.[28] Breath sounds are usually diminished on the affected side, and the mediastinum may be shifted to the contralateral side. In unilateral disease, chest x-rays films show a large pleural effusion with depression of the diaphragm and a shift of the mediastinum contralaterally. In bilateral disease, bilateral pleural effusions without mediastinal shift may be seen (Fig. 49–6).

Final diagnosis is made by thoracentesis. The fluid may be serous if the infant has not been fed but will turn milky once feedings have been initiated. The fluid has elevated protein and lipid levels and contains a high number of leukocytes. More than 80% of the leukocytes will be lymphocytes. Cultures of the fluid are negative.

Treatment begins with thoracentesis to drain the fluid. If repeated thoracentesis is required, placement of a chest tube should be considered. Affected newborns may be fed formula containing medium chain triglycerides, which are absorbed directly into the portal venous system. If the infant does not tolerate feedings or if the effusion reaccumulates, total parenteral nutrition should be started and the infant fed nothing by mouth for 2 weeks. Some infants may not tolerate feeding for a longer period.

The mortality rate is approximately 25%. In 15% of infants, a single thoracentesis leads to resolution.[28] If

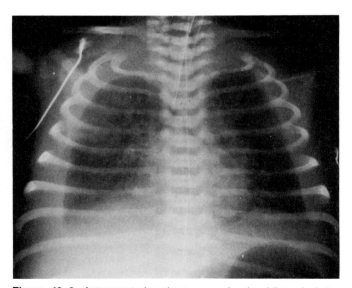

Figure 49–6. Anteroposterior chest x-ray showing bilateral chylothorax. Note the bilateral filling of the costophrenic angles with fluid.

the chylothorax is diagnosed prenatally by ultrasound, the mortality rate is greater than 50% because of pulmonary hypoplasia.[38]

Infantile Lobar Emphysema

Overdistention of a pulmonary lobe secondary to a ball-valve obstruction at the level of the bronchus results in infantile lobar emphysema. This overinflation results in atelectasis of the surrounding lung tissue, with shifting of the mediastinum to the contralateral side. Usually only one lobe is affected: Involvement in the left upper lobe occurs in 40% of patients, the right upper lobe is involved in 20% of patients, and the right middle lobe is affected in 30% of patients.[39]

The most common cause is bronchial obstruction, either intrinsically or extrinsically. The most common intrinsic obstruction is congenital deficiency or dysplasia of the bronchial cartilages, which occurs during the fourth to sixth weeks of embryonic development. Other intrinsic causes include redundant mucosal tissue, mucous plugs, or bronchial atresia. Extrinsic bronchial obstruction can be caused by mediastinal masses, esophageal duplication cysts, bronchogenic cysts, or vascular compression. In approximately 50% of cases, however, no cause can be identified.[40]

Microscopically, the affected lobe has distended alveoli with ruptured walls. The vasculature is usually normal.

Usually full-term infants are affected and may either be asymptomatic or have severe respiratory distress. One half of these infants are symptomatic in the first month of life, and almost all have symptoms by 6 months of age. The patients have typical symptoms of respiratory distress with decreased chest excursion and breath sounds on the affected side. The apical pulse is usually shifted contralaterally. Approximately 10 to 20% of these infants have associated congenital heart disease.[39]

The diagnosis can usually be made radiographically. Computed tomography scanning may detect the specific cause of obstruction. In addition, an esophagram may show anomalous vessels and bronchogenic cysts. Bronchoscopy can be both diagnostic and therapeutic if obstruction is secondary to a mucous plug or other intrabronchial process.

Treatment in the majority of cases consists of removal of the affected lobe. If bronchoscopy can relieve an intrinsic obstruction, or an isolated extrinsic obstruction can be removed (e.g., a bronchogenic cyst or anomalous vessel), lobectomy may not be required.

Cystic Adenomatoid Malformation

Cystic adenomatoid malformation (CAM) of the lung is a rare condition in which there is abnormal proliferation of terminal bronchiolar tissue beginning in the fourth and fifth weeks of gestation. Usually only one lobe is affected. Each lobe is affected with equal frequency.

The affected lobe contains multiple, smooth-walled

cysts lined with cuboidal or columnar epithelium resembling terminal bronchioles. There is a lack of cartilage and alveolar development. Stocker and coworkers described three types of CAM. Type I is the most common and has large, widely spaced cysts. Type II has smaller cysts usually measuring less than 1.2 cm. Type III is the least common, with the affected lobe appearing large and solid macroscopically and small cysts apparent microscopically.[41]

In a review by Wolf and associates, one third of cases presented in the neonatal period and two thirds were seen within the first year of life.[42] Infants may have varying degrees of respiratory distress. Older children may present with chronic pulmonary infections. CAM has been associated with polyhydramnios and fetal hydrops.

The radiographic findings show multiple radiolucent areas of varying sizes in the affected lobe, with shifting of the mediastinum contralaterally and depression of the ipsilateral hemidiaphragm. The presence of a normally placed stomach and intestinal gas pattern can help differentiate CAM from diaphragmatic hernia.

Excision of the affected lobe is the only treatment.

Congenital Lung Cysts

Congenital lungs cysts may be central or may occur at the lung periphery. Central bronchogenic cysts are usually solitary and are lined with pseudostratified columnar epithelium. They are the result of abnormal budding of the tracheal diverticulum between the third and sixth weeks of gestation.

Peripheral lung cysts result from separation of distal bronchiolar tissue from the bronchial tree between the 6th and 16th weeks of gestation. These cysts are usually multiple and may involve the entire lobe.

The symptoms of congenital lung cysts depend on the extent of lung involvement, the presence and level of obstruction, and the presence of tension. If a cyst has a bronchial communication, it may expand secondary to a ball-valve mechanism, resulting in atelectasis of normal lung tissue and a mediastinal shift. A central bronchogenic cyst may cause tracheal obstruction, leading to stridor, or bronchial obstruction, leading to wheezing. Severe respiratory distress can result from tension or obstruction. Cysts that are asymptomatic in the neonatal period may later become infected.

Treatment consists of surgical removal.

Congenital Pulmonary Lymphangiectasia

Congenital pulmonary lymphangiectasia is a rare disease that may occur (1) as part of a generalized lymphangiectasia with anasarca; (2) secondary to obstruction of pulmonary venous drainage resulting from congenital heart disease, especially total anomalous pulmonary venous return; or (3) as a primary obstruction of the pulmonary lymphatic drainage caused by maldevelopment of the main lymphatic ducts.[40]

Microscopically, there is diffuse dilatation of the lymphatic vessels and thickening of the interlobular septa. Macroscopically, the lungs are heavy and firm.

Radiographically, this disease is difficult to differentiate from other causes of respiratory distress. A diffuse granular pattern may be seen with prominent interstitial markings. Variable degrees of hyperinflation may also be present.

Prognosis is poor with a mortality rate of greater than 90%.[43]

References

1. Farrel PM and Avery ME: Hyaline membrane disease. Am Rev Respir Dis 111:657, 1975.
2. Ohlsson A, Shennan AT, and Rose TH: Review of causes of perinatal mortality in a regional perinatal center, 1980 to 1984. Am J Obstet Gynecol 157:443, 1987.
3. Wright JR and Clements JA: Metabolism and turnover of lung surfactant. Am Rev Respir Dis 135:426, 1987.
4. Gluck L, Kulovich MV, Borer RC, et al: The interpretation and significance of the lecithin/sphingomyelin ratio in amniotic fluid. Am J Obstet Gynecol 120:142, 1974.
5. Collaborative Group on Antenatal Steroid Therapy: Effect of antenatal dexamethasone administration on the prevention of respiratory distress syndrome. Am J Obstet Gynecol 141:276, 1981.
6. Doyle LW, Kitchen WH, Ford GW, et al: Effects of antenatal steroid therapy on mortality and morbidity in very low birth weight infants. J Pediatr 108:287, 1986.
7. HIFI Study Group: High-frequency oscillatory ventilation compared with conventional mechanical ventilation in the treatment of respiratory failure in preterm infants. N Engl J Med 320:88, 1989.
8. Bancalari E and Goldberg RN: High-frequency ventilation in the neonate. Clin Perinatol 14:581, 1987.
9. Vidyasagar D, Raju TNK, Shimada S, et al: Surfactant replacement therapy: Clinical and experimental studies. Clin Perinatol 14:713, 1987.
10. Dudell GG and Gersony WM: Patent ductus arteriosus in neonates with severe respiratory distress. J Pediatr 104:915, 1984.
11. O'Brodovich HM and Mellins RB: Bronchopulmonary dysplasia. Am Rev Respir Dis 132:694, 1985.
12. Davis RO, Phillips JB, Harris BA, et al: Fatal meconium aspiration syndrome occurring despite airway management considered appropriate. Am J Obstet Gynecol 151:731, 1985.
13. Gregory GA, Gooding CA, Phibbs RH, et al: Meconium aspiration in infants—a prospective study. J Pediatr 85:848, 1974.
14. Knox GE, Huddleston JF, and Flowers CE: Management of prolonged pregnancy: Results of a prospective randomized trial. Am J Obstet Gynecol 134:376, 1979.
15. Mitchell J, Schulman H, Fleischer A, et al: Meconium aspiration and fetal acidosis. Obstet Gynecol 65:352, 1985.
16. Tyler DC, Murphy J, and Cheney F: Mechanical and chemical damage to lung tissue caused by meconium aspiration. Pediatrics 62:454, 1978.
17. Clark DA, Nieman GF, Thompson JE, et al: Surfactant displacement by meconium free fatty acids: An alternative explanation for atelectasis in meconium aspiration syndrome. J Pediatr 110:765, 1987.
18. Linder N, Aranda JV, Tsar M, et al: Need for endotracheal intubation and suction in meconium-stained neonates. J Pediatr 112:613, 1988.
19. Wenstrom KD and Parsons MT: The prevention of meconium aspiration in labor using amnioinfusion. Obstet Gynecol 73:647, 1989.
20. Hendricks-Munoz KD and Walton JP: Hearing loss in infants with persistent fetal circulation. Pediatrics 81:650, 1988.
21. Vidyasagar D, Yeh TF, Harris V, et al: Assisted ventilation in infants with meconium aspiration syndrome. Pediatrics 56:208, 1975.

22. Dennehy PH: Respiratory infections in the newborn. Clin Perinatol 14:667, 1987.
23. Monroe BL, Weinberg AG, and Rosenfeld CR: The neonatal blood count in health and disease. I: Reference values for neutrophils cells. J Pediatr 95:89, 1976.
24. Rawlings JS and Smith FR: Transient tachypnea of the newborn. Am J Dis Child 138:869, 1984.
25. Milner AD, Saunders RA, and Hopkin IE: Effects of delivery by caesarean section on lung mechanics and lung volume in the human neonate. Arch Dis Child 53:545, 1978.
26. Boon AW, Milner AD, and Hopkin IE: Lung volumes and lung mechanics in babies born vaginally and by elective and emergency lower segmental cesarean section. J Pediatr 98:812, 1981.
27. Halliday HL, McClure G, and McCreid M: Transient tachypnea of the newborn: Two distinct clinical entities. Arch Dis Child 56:322, 1981.
28. Chernick V and Reed M: Pneumothorax and chylothorax in the neonatal period. J Pediatr 76:624, 1970.
29. Madansky DL, Lawson EE, Chernick V, et al: Pneumothorax and other forms of pulmonary air leak in newborns. Am Rev Respir Dis 120:729, 1979.
30. Greenough A, Dixon AK, and Robertson NRC: Pulmonary interstitial emphysema. Arch Dis Child 59:1046, 1984.
31. Schneider JR, St Cyr JA, Thompson TR, et al: The changing spectrum of cystic pulmonary lesions requiring surgical resection in infants. J Thorac Cardiovasc Surg 89:332, 1985.
32. Fedrick J and Butler NR: Certain causes of neonatal death: IV, massive pulmonary hemorrhage. Biol Neonate 18:243, 1971.
33. Cole VA, Normand ICS, Reynolds EOR, et al: Pathogenesis of hemorrhagic pulmonary edema and massive pulmonary hemorrhage in the newborn. Pediatrics 51:175, 1973.
34. Askenazi SS and Perlman M: Pulmonary hypoplasia: Lung weight and radial alveolar count as criteria of diagnosis. Arch Dis Child 54:614, 1979.
35. Rotschild A, Ling EW, Puterman ML, et al: Neonatal outcome after prolonged preterm rupture of the membranes. Am J Obstet Gynecol 162:46, 1990.
36. Moessinger AC, Collins MH, Blan WA, et al: Oligohydramnios-induced lung hypoplasia: The influence of timing and duration in gestation. Pediatr Res 20:951, 1986.
37. Wigglesworth JS, Desai R, and Guerrini P: Fetal lung hypoplasia: Biochemical and structural variations and their possible significance. Arch Dis Child 56:606, 1981.
38. Longaker JT, Laberge JM, Danereau J, et al: Primary fetal hydrothorax: Natural history and management. J Pediatr Surg 24:573, 1989.
39. Hendren WH and McKee DM: Lobar emphysema of infancy. J Pediatr Surg 1:24, 1966.
40. Berlinger NT, Porto DP, and Thompson TR: Infantile lobar emphysema. Ann Otol Rhinol Laryngol 96:106, 1987.
41. Stocker JT, Madewell JE, and Drake RM: Congenital cystic adenomatoid malformation of the lung. Hum Pathol 8:155, 1977.
42. Wolf SA, Hertzler JH, and Philippart AI: Cystic adenomatoid dysplasia of the lung. J Pediatr Surg 15:925, 1980.
43. Noonan JA, Walters LR, and Reeves JT: Congenital pulmonary lymphangiectasis. Am J Dis Child 120:314, 1970.

Bronchopulmonary Dysplasia in the Pediatric Intensive Care Unit

Bennie McWilliams, M.D., and Robert Katz, M.D.

Bronchopulmonary dysplasia (BPD) is an important cause of chronic respiratory disease in infants and children. The wide clinical spectrum of BPD ranges from minimal or no respiratory symptoms to crippling pulmonary function abnormalities and significant respiratory morbidity. Based on the current literature, the diagnosis of BPD implies significant respiratory and medical problems, frequent hospitalizations, and ongoing financial and psychosocial strain in the family. Although innovations in neonatal care such as artificial surfactant and extracorporeal membrane oxygenation have improved neonatal care, the number of patients with BPD does not seem to be decreasing and may actually be increasing. Infants and children with BPD are admitted to the pediatric intensive care unit (PICU) for various reasons, including acute deterioration of their chronic lung disease, direct transfer from a newborn intensive care unit (NICU) for long-term ventilatory management, or postoperative care after a surgical procedure. Pediatric intensivists, therefore, should have an understanding of the pathophysiology, treatment, and outcome of patients with BPD.

EPIDEMIOLOGY

BPD is a chronic lung disease of infancy characterized by respiratory distress and oxygen dependency persisting beyond 1 month of age in children requiring oxygen and ventilator therapy in the newborn period.[1] First described by Northway and colleagues in 1967,[2] it is most commonly seen after treatment of respiratory distress syndrome, but also occurs following meconium aspiration syndrome, persistent fetal circulation, and conditions requiring surgery, such as tracheoesophageal fistula or diaphragmatic hernia.

In addition to mechanical ventilation, birth weight under 1,500 g is a risk factor for the development of BPD. The incidence of BPD in infants with birth weight of under 1,500 g who require mechanical ventilation is between 15 and 38%.[3] In addition to weight, male sex and white race appear to be independent risk factors. It has been assumed that the incidence of BPD is similar in most level III nurseries. However, a study comparing the incidence of chronic lung disease at 28 days of age in eight NICUs showed a very low rate in one institution,[4] and this difference persisted even after adjusting for weight distribution, race, and sex, raising the possibility that the management of low birth weight infants may vary significantly among institutions.

Since 1974, numerous studies have documented considerable medical problems in infants with BPD following discharge from the hospital. In a prospective study of survivors of hyaline membrane disease (HMD), Myers and coworkers found that those infants who developed residual lung disease had a greater risk of both more frequent and more severe subsequent lower respiratory illnesses compared to infants with normal chest films.[5] Rehospitalization rates for lower respiratory tract disease have approached 50% during the first 2 years of life in several studies. In a recently completed survey of infants with BPD, 49% of the children required hospitalization at least once, and 18% were hospitalized at least three times in the first 2 years of life for a severe chest illness.[6] Thus, available studies suggest that premature infants who develop BPD during their initial hospitalization have significant respiratory morbidity after discharge.

PATHOPHYSIOLOGY

Since Northway's first description of BPD showing extensive lung parenchymal and airway damage,[2] numerous reviews have further characterized the pathologic damage.[7-9] Although most commonly seen following HMD in children requiring mechanical ventilation and high inspired oxygen concentrations (FiO_2), BPD can occur in infants receiving high FiO_2 without mechanical ventilation as well as mechanically ventilated infants receiving low FiO$_2$ values. In addition, BPD may be seen in infants without HMD, full-term infants, and adults.[10, 11] There is a typical pathologic progression of HMD to BPD,[12] from the initial surfactant deficiency to the reparative stage. As a result of surfactant deficiency, there is widespread atelectasis, hyaline membrane formation, pulmonary edema, and lymphatic dilatation.

In addition to surfactant deficiency other factors involved in the development of BPD are barotrauma, oxygen toxicity, and inflammation. Barotrauma is caused by alveolar rupture with resultant extra-alveolar air; this can lead to pulmonary interstitial emphysema (PIE), pneumothorax, pneumopericardium, pneumoperitoneum, and intravascular air. The marginal alveoli (alveoli adjacent to nondistendable structures, such as pulmonary arterioles) are usually the first to rupture. This forces air into the connective tissue sheaths surrounding the airways (PIE) and pulmonary vessels, resulting in compression of the airways and increased airway resistance, clinically manifested by hyperinflation. In addition, impaired lymphatic drainage from the compression contributes to pulmonary edema. Once extra-alveolar air develops, it may extend in a number of directions, causing pneumomediastinum, pneumothorax, pneumoperitoneum and other extra-alveolar collections of air, and resultant recovery is slow with a very high incidence of BPD.

Oxygen toxicity plays a role in the development of BPD. Oxygen increases capillary permeability, releases fibroblast stimulatory factors, impairs ciliary motility, and decreases the metabolic function of endothelial cells.[13] Anti-inflammatory agents, including corticosteroids, cromolyn sodium, and vitamin E, have been used with equivocal results to reduce the inflammatory response.[14, 15]

Abnormal inflammatory response to injury may also be an important contributory factor. In HMD there is increased permeability of the lung to solutes.[16] Additional disruption of the integrity of the alveoli and terminal airways leads to the development of hyaline membranes. Protein leak into the alveoli from abnormal permeability of the lungs also contributes to pulmonary edema in HMD. This abnormal permeability returns to normal in patients recovering from HMD but remains abnormal in patients developing BPD. Bronchoalveolar lavage in patients at risk of developing BPD has demonstrated impaired neutrophil-derived elastase in patients who subsequently develop BPD.[17, 18] In addition, there is a predominance of polymorphonuclear cells in bronchoalveolar lavage in patients with BPD, which may increase pulmonary permeability, proteases, and oxygen radicals, all of which contribute to lung injury.[19]

Numerous other factors are felt to be related to the development of BPD. Since infants lack pores of Kohn and Lambert channels, they have poor collateral ventilation and a greater tendency to develop atelectasis.[17] Additionally, infants have very compliant chest walls, which increases the risk of atelectasis. Also, infants with lung disease have a tendency to maintain a state of persistent fetal circulation. When this happens, instead of the usual decrease in pulmonary vascular resistance, the resistance remains high. Thus, right-to-left shunting

may continue through the foramen ovale and patent ductus arteriosus, resulting in increased hypoxemia. Lastly, infants receiving positive pressure ventilation develop barotrauma, as described previously, to a greater degree than older patients.

The pulmonary damage results in both increased airway resistance and decreased lung compliance. Airway resistance in patients with BPD is higher than in those with uncomplicated HMD. The widespread fibrosis and decreased number of alveolar units result in decreased lung compliance in BPD, while infants with uncomplicated HMD have normal lung compliance. Since the respiratory bronchioles and alveoli continue to grow in number until approximately 6 years of age and in size until adolescence, children with BPD tend to improve with age. Thus, even in the most severe cases, if the patient is aggressively supported the prognosis for significant improvement is good.

The pulmonary pathology of BPD causes increased pulmonary vascular resistance and pulmonary hypertension, and this may lead to right ventricular hypertrophy and cor pulmonale. Systemic hypertension is occasionally seen in patients with BPD, although the etiology is unclear.

PULMONARY ASPECTS

Pulmonary Function Abnormalities

The amount of pulmonary function data on patients with BPD has been scant because measurement of pulmonary function is difficult in this population and few patients with severe BPD are old enough for standard pulmonary function tests. There are, however, a growing number of studies addressing pulmonary function tests in these infants.

Partial expiratory flow volume maneuvers in infants with BPD have demonstrated marked concavity in the loops with tidal breathing, approaching expiratory flow limitation.[20] Infants with BPD have significantly lower absolute and size-corrected flows than control infants of the same age and size. The persistently low forced expiratory rates demonstrate that the smaller airways are probably not growing normally and that the significantly decreased expiratory reserve places these infants at high risk for recurrent episodes of respiratory deterioration when stressed by otherwise minor illnesses.

Other studies of infants with BPD requiring mechanical ventilation have demonstrated decreased functional residual capacity (FRC) and pulmonary conductance soon after birth but near-normal values at 36 months of age.[21] Minute ventilation and respiratory effort, however, remained elevated throughout the follow-up period, presumably as a result of persistently elevated pulmonary resistance with resultant increased work of breathing. This partially accounts for the higher oxygen consumption observed in infants with BPD.[22, 23]

The forced deflation technique has been used to examine the response of premature infants with chronic lung disease to bronchodilators. Premature infants as young as 12 days old and 26 weeks postconception had improved flows following the administration of a nebulized β-agonist. Studies in older infants with BPD have documented similar results.[24]

Follow-up studies of older children with BPD have demonstrated a wide spectrum of pulmonary function abnormalities, ranging from normal to reversible and nonreversible airway obstruction and bronchial hyperreactivity.[24] Earlier studies on small groups of infants with BPD have shown that many infants with BPD have high airway resistance, low dynamic compliance, and increased work of breathing.[25] Persistent ventilation/perfusion mismatching, as demonstrated by the need for long-term oxygen therapy has also been documented.

Medical Therapy

A better understanding of the pathophysiology of BPD enables the physician to approach therapy more rationally. The major pathophysiologic abnormalities involved in BPD are ventilation-perfusion mismatching, hypertrophy of peribronchial smooth muscles with increased bronchial hyperactivity and increased air resistance, inflammation, interstitial edema and fibrosis, and increased pulmonary vascular resistance. Management of patients with BPD, therefore, needs to be directed toward treating these abnormalities. Thus, pulmonary therapy can be divided into the following categories: O_2 therapy, bronchodilator therapy, anti-inflammatory therapy, diuretic therapy, and vasodilator therapy. Additionally, these patients may require chronic mechanical ventilation because of chronic pulmonary insufficiency, which is addressed later in the chapter.

Oxygen

Oxygen is one of the most important medications in patients with BPD. Since $\dot{V}/\dot{Q}$ mismatching is a major cause of hypoxemia in these infants, the hypoxemia is at least partially responsive to O_2 therapy. In addition, O_2 therapy decreases the required minute ventilation and thus the oxygen cost of breathing. Also, O_2 functions as a pulmonary vasodilator, minimizing the oxygen-sensitive increased pulmonary vascular resistance in these patients. Oxygen is usually administered via nasal cannula or tracheostomy in sufficient amounts to maintain Sa_{O_2} at greater than 90.

Bronchodilators

Bronchodilators are frequently used to decrease airway obstruction and decrease the work of breathing. Bonikos and colleagues demonstrated that infants who died of BPD had hypertrophied peribronchial smooth muscle even at a young age.[26] In the last several years, physiologic data have been gathered that support this empiric approach. Bronchodilator therapy similar to that used in patients with asthma may be instituted; thus, bronchodilator medications are divided into β-adrenergic agents, anticholinergic agents, and methylxanthines.

β-Adrenergic Agents. Selective β-adrenergic agonists

are playing an increasingly greater role in the management of bronchospasm in children with BPD. Kao and associates studied the effect of inhaled isoproterenol, a nonselective β-agonist, on lung mechanics in 10 infants with BPD and a mean age of 41 weeks.[27] Thirty minutes after inhalation of the drug, airway resistance dropped by 28% and specific conductance increased by an average of 53%. Logvinoff studied eight infants 5 to 43 months of age who had moderate to severe BPD and found that inhaled isoproterenol decreased work of breathing as well as pulmonary resistance.[28] Similar improvements in pulmonary function have been seen with subcutaneous terbutaline, oral metaproterenol, and inhaled salbutamol (albuterol). Of these, the route of choice for the delivery of β-adrenergic agents is the inhaled route, since it is rapid and provides greater bronchoselectivity compared with systemic administration.[29] The medication of choice for aerosol administration in the United States is currently albuterol since it has the greatest β_2 selectivity and is available in a nebulizer form. Preparations and starting doses for nebulized β-agonists are listed in Table 50–1. It is important to remember that in many instances higher doses may need to be given due either to the severity of the patient's condition or to decreased delivery to the lungs, as in the case of the infant on mechanical ventilation.[30]

For young infants and children, β-agonists are most commonly delivered with a jet nebulizer driven by air or oxygen. Although the aerosol route of delivery has the greatest β_2-adrenergic selectivity and minimal systemic side effects when compared with other delivery methods, it is a relatively inefficient method of delivery in terms of the lost medication. There are relatively few data on the delivery of aerosolized drugs to the lungs in patients receiving mechanical ventilation.[30] However, it has been shown that much of the drug is retained in the endotracheal tube, with only a small fraction reaching the lungs. Endotracheal tube size, inspiratory flow rate, and aerosol size all have an effect on the percentage of drug actually delivered to the lungs.[31]

Side effects from β-agonists are largely due to adrenoreceptor stimulation and depend on dose, selectivity, and route of administration. The most common adverse effects include tachycardia, tremor, central nervous system stimulation, and occasional gastrointestinal upset.

Table 50–1. β-ADRENERGIC AEROSOLS

Drug	Preparation	Dosage
Metaproterenol	5% (50 mg/ml) solution for nebulization	0.25–0.5 mg/kg every 2–4 hr
Terbutaline	0.1% (1 mg/ml) solution in 0.9% NaCl for injection (not approved for this use)	0.1–0.3 mg/kg every 2–6 hr
Albuterol	0.5% (5 mg/ml) solution for nebulization	0.05–0.15 mg/kg every 2–4 hr (may increase to 0.6 mg/kg/hr by continuous nebulizer as clinically indicated)

Increases in serum glucose and decreases in serum potassium may also be seen. Overall, side effects are minimal and rarely require discontinuation of therapy.

Anticholinergic Agents. Evidence points to the importance of the parasympathetic system in the control of airway caliber and the possible ability of inhibiting these cholinergic mechanisms pharmacologically.[32] Numerous double-blind controlled studies have been reported in the last 10 years documenting the beneficial effect of inhaled atropine or ipratropium bromide (a synthetic congener of atropine) in asthma and chronic obstructive pulmonary disease.

In addition, nebulized glycopyrrolate, a quaternary ammonium derivative of atropine (similar to ipratropium bromide), is also used to treat bronchospasm. Since ipratropium bromide is available in the United States only as a metered-dose inhaler, nebulization of atropine or glycopyrrolate is a practical way to administer anticholinergic therapy to small infants and children (Table 50–2).

Logvinoff and colleagues demonstrated increased dynamic compliance and a trend toward decreased work of breathing following nebulized atropine (0.05 mg/kg) in six children with BPD.[28] Likewise, nebulized ipratropium bromide may produce improved resistance and compliance in infants with BPD. Thus, it appears that at least some of the increased airway tone in infants with BPD is secondary to increased vagal activity.

Atropine is well absorbed from the gastrointestinal tract and mucosa. It is distributed throughout the body and crosses the blood-brain barrier. It is largely excreted in the urine and its serum half-life is 3 hours in young adults and is two to three times as long in children.[33] Side effects, which are dose related,[34] include dryness of the mouth, difficulty with voiding, flushing of the skin, and less commonly, tachycardia, blurred vision, gastrointestinal disturbances, and mental changes. Inhaled nebulized atropine produces optimal bronchodilatation at a dose of 0.05 mg/kg in children and 0.025 mg/kg in adults with airway obstruction.[34] After inhalation, atropine absorption from the respiratory and gastrointestinal tracts is erratic and blood levels are highly variable. However, in adult dose-response studies, the smallest dose of inhaled atropine that produces significant bronchodilatation is about 0.4 mg, which is the level at which side effects may occur. After an optimal dose of atropine most subjects will experience side effects. Side effects of ipratropium bromide have been less troublesome, presumably due to less systemic absorption.[35]

Methylxanthines. Although their use is decreasing, methylxanthines, in the form of theophylline or aminophylline, are also used in the treatment of BPD. Theophylline has several potential effects in BPD. Since it is a mild bronchodilator, it may decrease airway resistance. Additionally, it may improve diaphragmatic contractility, stimulate the central nervous system, and serve as a mild diuretic agent. Caffeine is also used in infants with BPD, but mostly for its stimulation of the central nervous system in children with apnea.

There have been few objective measurements of the effect of theophylline in infants with BPD. Rooklin and coworkers performed serial pulmonary function measurements in 11 neonates with BPD after intravenous aminophylline therapy.[36] In those infants less than 30 days of age, there was a trend (although not statistically significant) toward increased compliance and decreased inspiratory and expiratory resistance. Infants older than 30 days had no change in their pulmonary functions. Kao and associates studied 18 infants with BPD treated with theophylline and/or a diuretic.[37] At the end of the 4-day study period, oral theophylline produced significant improvements in airway resistance, specific conductance, compliance, and maximal expiratory flow. When a diuretic was administered with the theophylline, an additive effect was noted in most pulmonary functions.

Theophylline may have other beneficial effects in patients with chronic lung disease. In adults with chronic obstructive pulmonary disease, theophylline improves diaphragmatic function and decreases pulmonary artery pressure. Infants have been shown to have fewer fatigue-resistant (type 1) fibers in their diaphragm (see also Chapter 48), and respiratory muscle fatigue (see also Chapter 51) may play a role in the respiratory manifestations of BPD. The reduction of pulmonary artery pressure may decrease transvascular filtration and has the potential to minimize pulmonary edema in BPD patients.

The elimination half-life of theophylline is considerably longer in infants under 6 months of age than in older children. Elimination increases in a linear fashion during the first year of life. However, there have been no specific studies on the pharmacokinetics of theophylline in infants with BPD. This lack of knowledge, combined with the potential for hepatic or cardiac failure, calls for careful monitoring of plasma theophylline levels.

In an acute attack of wheezing, a loading dose of theophylline is used to obtain a desired plasma concentration quickly. General loading dose recommendations when the current theophylline concentration is unknown are given in Table 50–3. The loading doses are based on a mean volume of distribution for theophylline of 0.5 l/kg (range 0.3 to 0.7 l/kg).[38] This relationship would give a 2 mg/l increase in serum theophylline concentration for every 1 mg/kg increment in dose. After the loading dose is given, maintenance theophylline dosages can be given orally or as aminophylline infusions. Recommended infusion rates are listed in Table 50–3 based on the amount of intravenous aminophylline (80% theophylline) required to achieve a steady-state theophylline concentration of 15 μg/ml.

Regardless of the route of administration, the wide interpatient variability in theophylline clearance mandates that plasma concentrations be routinely monitored and dosages adjusted accordingly. This is particularly

Table 50–2. AEROSOLIZED ANTICHOLINERGIC AGENTS IN BRONCHOPULMONARY DYSPLASIA

Atropine	0.05–0.1 mg/kg every 4–6 hr
Glycopyrrolate	0.025–0.05 mg/kg every 4–6 hr
Ipratropium bromide	40–250 μg by metered dose inhaler; nebulizer solution not available in the United States

Table 50–3. THEOPHYLLINE AND AMINOPHYLLINE DOSING*

Age	Oral Dosage (Theophylline) (mg/kg/day)	Infusion Rate (Aminophylline) (mg/kg/hr)
Neonates	3–9	
1 mo–6 mo†	10	0.5
6 mo–1 yr	15	1.0
1 yr–9 yr	24	1.5

*These are approximate doses and the final dose should be determined by serum theophylline concentrations and clinical symptoms.
†This age range has the widest interpatient variability and is based on the fewest number of patients.

true in light of the paucity of pharmacokinetic data in infants with BPD. There are numerous approaches to monitoring plasma theophylline concentrations. Most children will be within 95% of their steady-state concentration within 12 to 16 hours on continuous dosing. In patients receiving continuous intravenous infusions, dosages can be adjusted on one steady state level. Alternatively, one can obtain a level 30 minutes after the loading dose and then a second level at 4 to 8 hours. This will indicate to the clinician the loading dose achieved, and a rise or fall in the second level will suggest whether the infusion rate should be increased or decreased (see also Chapter 28).

Multiple factors may affect the metabolism and elimination of theophylline. The changes in theophylline clearance occurring with age have been mentioned. Of particular relevance to infants with BPD is the fact that theophylline clearance may be reduced in the presence of cor pulmonale and during febrile viral respiratory tract infections. Therapeutic drugs also affect theophylline clearance, but the clinical relevance of these interactions is variable. For example, the concurrent administration of erythromycin decreases theophylline clearance. In contrast, chronic administration of phenobarbital or phenytoin increases theophylline clearance, and dosages may have to be readjusted accordingly.

Theophylline has the potential for a wide range of adverse effects. Caffeine-like side effects, including minor degrees of central nervous system stimulation and gastrointestinal upset occur frequently after a loading dose and appear to have little direct relationship to serum concentrations. More severe and persistent adverse effects generally are associated with serum concentrations above 20 µg/ml and include nausea, vomiting, headache, diarrhea, irritability, and at higher levels hyperglycemia, hypokalemia, hypotension, cardiac arrhythmias, seizures, and death.[64] Among infants and children, severe toxicity most commonly has resulted from administration of inappropriate dosages.

Anti-Inflammatory Therapy

Anti-inflammatory therapy is an important aspect of BPD treatment. As previously mentioned, studies have examined the potential role of inflammation in the development of BPD, and as a result, steroid and cromolyn sodium therapy have been suggested as a means of reducing the inflammatory process and thus improving the clinical course of infants with BPD. Steroids also may be helpful in treating the bronchospasm that occurs in these infants.

Since 1983, multiple studies (mostly retrospective and uncontrolled) have looked at the effect of steroids on the ventilator-dependent infant with BPD. Two randomized prospective studies have documented improvement in clinical symptoms following the administration of steroids. Mammel and colleagues administered dexamethasone (0.5 mg/kg) to six infants with long-established BPD and noted a marked improvement in clinical status and pulmonary function.[39] Ventilator-determined respiratory rate, peak inspiratory pressure, and alveolar-arterial gradient improved significantly in all infants receiving steroids. Although the study was double-blind and randomized, the use of sequential analysis and marked short-term improvement resulted in a very small study group. In addition, three of the six infants died of "septic" complications after the acute part of the study was completed while they were on "weaning" doses of dexamethasone.

Avery and coworkers used a shorter course of steroids in a group of premature infants who remained ventilator dependent at 2 weeks of age.[14] The patient population consisted of seven pairs of matched infants of less than 1,500 g and less than 6 weeks postnatal age who were refractory to weaning from ventilatory support despite diuretic therapy and fluid restriction. All seven pairs favored dexamethasone therapy in weaning from ventilatory support within 72 hours. Dynamic pulmonary compliance improved significantly compared with that in the control group. There were few complications in this short-term study, which demonstrated that dexamethasone was relatively safe and resulted in extubation within 3 days. However, the number of infants studied was small, the steroid group tended to require less ventilatory support, criteria for extubation were not defined, and the study was not blind.

It appears from these two controlled studies and other uncontrolled trials that steroid therapy leads to acute significant improvements in pulmonary mechanics and gas exchange in infants with BPD and facilitates weaning from ventilatory support and supplemental oxygen. However, significant morbidity may occur, including infectious complications, systemic hypertension, and possible adrenal suppression. Furthermore, the application of the results of these studies to older infants with BPD in a pediatric intensive care unit is problematic in that most of the steroid studies involved young premature infants whose chronic lung disease was evolving. Whether older infants with BPD would demonstrate such dramatic improvements in pulmonary function is unknown.

Many studies on asthma and chronic obstructive pulmonary suggest that steroids may also be helpful in treating the bronchospasm that occurs in infants with BPD. Steroids have been shown to be beneficial in treating an acute episode of asthma, avoiding admission to the hospital, and preventing relapses of an acute episode. The authors are unaware of any specific studies in infants with BPD, but based on clinical experience, steroids may be useful in selected infants with persistent or recurrent bronchospasm that has not responded to other bronchodilators.

Cromolyn sodium is another anti-inflammatory agent used in infants with BPD. It has been available for the treatment of asthma in the United Kingdom since 1968 and in the United States since 1973; the nebulizer solution of cromolyn has been available since 1982. The primary mode of action is stabilization of mast cells, which prevents the subsequent release of mediators. Early laboratory studies of antigen challenge of tissues presensitized with IgE antibodies demonstrated that cromolyn sodium inhibited the release of biologically active chemical mediators.

In a small uncontrolled study, cromolyn sodium (20 mg nebulized every 6 hours) was administered to 10 ventilator-dependent infants with BPD.[40] Eight of the 10 demonstrated clinical improvement with decreased oxygen requirement, decreased wheezing, and improvement in pulmonary mechanics. Bronchial lavage in four of four infants after treatment showed a decrease in total white blood cell counts, neutrophil counts, and alveolar macrophage counts.

The anti-inflammatory activity of cromolyn and the rarity of adverse reactions make it an attractive drug to use in infants with BPD. Elucidation of the exact role of cromolyn in the acute and chronic management of BPD awaits further controlled clinical trials.

Diuretic Therapy

Pathologic studies in infants with BPD have demonstrated dilated lymphatics, interstitial pulmonary edema, and increased water content in addition to pulmonary fibrosis and other alterations in the architecture of the lung. This accumulation of fluid may contribute to the narrowed terminal airways, altered pulmonary mechanics, and impaired gas exchange. Diuretics are used frequently in infants with BPD in hopes of decreasing this accumulation of fluid and improving pulmonary functions.

Several studies have examined both the acute and the chronic effects of diuretics in infants with BPD. In an acute study Kao and coworkers administered furosemide 1 mg/kg to 10 infants with BPD and measured pulmonary functions 1, 4, 6, and 24 hours later.[41] Airway resistance, conductance, and compliance all improved significantly compared to the placebo group, while thoracic gas volume was unchanged. By 4 hours all measurements had returned to baseline. In a subsequent double-blind crossover study, the same authors demonstrated that chronic (1 week) administration of an oral diuretic resulted in significant improvement in pulmonary mechanics.[42] The changes in pulmonary function were associated with a significant diuretic-induced increase in urine output and a decrease in retention of fluid. This temporal relationship probably indicates that the improvement in pulmonary mechanics in infants with BPD is partly explained by diuresis and removal of edema fluid from the pulmonary interstitium. In a similarly designed study, McCann and colleagues docu-

mented improvements in venous admixture and ventilatory requirements as well as pulmonary mechanics in 17 infants with chronic lung disease.[43] However, Englehardt and coworkers in a study of 16 infants with BPD were unable to demonstrate a consistent improvement in gas exchange, although pulmonary mechanics did improve after a 6- to 10- day course of furosemide.[44] In addition, there was no correlation between improvements in pulmonary mechanics and changes in blood gases.

It appears that diuretic therapy consistently improves lung mechanics and should decrease the work of breathing in infants with BPD; this effect is seen acutely and is maintained during chronic therapy. The effects on gas exchange are not as consistent, and therefore, clinicians should not always expect improvement in blood gases in all patients receiving long-term diuretic therapy.

Furosemide and chlorothiazide are the most commonly used diuretics in infants with BPD. The dose of furosemide in the studies of infants with BPD was 1 mg/kg intravenously or 2 mg/kg orally twice a day. In their study of chronic diuretic effects, Kao and colleagues used 20 mg/kg of chlorothiazide plus spironolactone 1.5 mg/kg twice a day. Side effects of diuretics are largely related to loss of electrolytes in the urine. Furosemide in particular has been associated with hypercalciuria, renal calcifications, and rickets.[45] Thiazide diuretics, although less potent than furosemide, do not have the same effect on calcium excretion and may be the diuretic of choice for long-term use in infants with BPD.

CARDIOVASCULAR ASPECTS

The cardiovascular effects of BPD can be divided into changes in pulmonary vascular resistance, right heart function, and the systemic circulation. Pulmonary vascular disease has been well documented in BPD.[26] In earlier studies, medial hypertrophy of the pulmonary arteries was found, although these studies were mainly looking at the airway and alveolar pathology. The pulmonary vascular muscular hypertrophy and muscle extension are considered to be secondary to hypoxia and to hypoplasia and delayed maturity of the fetal circulation. Tomashefski and coworkers studied the pulmonary vascular changes using morphometric methods. In addition to the changes caused by chronic lung disease, there were systemic-to-pulmonary anastomoses representing an adaptation to the injury.[46]

The increase in pulmonary vascular resistance leads to pulmonary hypertension, right ventricular hypertrophy, and in severe cases, right ventricular failure.[47] The incidence of this complication seems to be declining, probably secondary to more aggressive oxygen therapy. The importance of maintaining adequate PaO_2 values in minimizing right ventricular failure has been well documented. If oxygen therapy fails to improve pulmonary artery hypertension, chronic mechanical ventilation often will lessen the right ventricular strain and improve pulmonary hypertension.

Pharmacologic intervention to reduce pulmonary vascular resistance has also been studied. Vasodilators, such as nifedipine and hydralazine, have been used with variable success.[48, 49] More studies will be necessary to determine the role of vasodilators in the management of infants with BPD.

There is relatively little published information on the long-term follow-up of pulmonary hypertension in patients with BPD. The most commonly used methods of assessing cardiac function are electrocardiography (ECG), echocardiography (ECHO), and cardiac catheterization. Currently, ECHOs are the most commonly used means of following the course of BPD.[50] ECHO evaluation of pulmonary hypertension is sensitive but may overestimate the degree of pulmonary hypertension. The most sensitive and specific method of assessing cardiac function is cardiac catheterization.[47] In general, cardiac catheterization should be considered in a child with BPD who is not thriving, is developing worsening pulmonary hypertension by ECHO, or is being considered for vasodilator therapy. Because pulmonary artery pressures may vary with different interventions and may not immediately respond, a pulmonary artery catheter is usually placed and pulmonary artery pressures monitored over a 24-hour period in the PICU while various therapeutic interventions are used (oxygen, ventilation, vasodilators).

In addition to pulmonary hypertension and right ventricular dysfunction, systemic hypertension has been seen in patients with BPD. The etiology is unclear, and the elevation in blood pressure is usually transient. It is very important to follow this complication because systemic hypertension may result in left ventricular hypertrophy and cerebrovascular accidents in patients with BPD.

NUTRITION

The importance of nutrition in patients with a variety of chronic lung diseases has been the subject of recent investigations, and both animal and human studies have demonstrated that malnutrition can have a profound impact on a number of pulmonary functions, including surfactant production, immune defense mechanisms, respiratory muscle function, and respiratory control.

Numerous studies have documented a high incidence of acute and chronic malnutrition in BPD. In a study of infants with BPD followed as outpatients, 13% were found to be suffering from acute protein-calorie malnutrition and 30% demonstrated growth retardation or chronic protein-calorie malnutrition.[51] Studies have also shown that many infants with BPD are below the third percentile for height and weight during the first 2 years of life.

Children with BPD have higher basal caloric requirements than children of the same age without chronic lung disease.[22] In addition, their chronic respiratory symptoms and associated neurodevelopmental delays may interfere with caloric intake.[52] Repeated hospitalizations for acute exacerbations of their chronic lung disease may also contribute to their failure to thrive.

Therefore, it is not surprising that a number of these infants are suffering from malnutrition.

Given the deleterious effects malnutrition has on critically ill patients in general and the potential effects on the patient with chronic lung disease, aggressive nutritional therapy is indicated for the infant with BPD admitted to a PICU. Although there are specific problems of nutritional support of infants with BPD, there are general principles that apply to any critically ill child.

Nutritional therapy should begin as soon as practical after admission to the PICU, and whenever possible the gastrointestinal tract is the preferred route. It is more physiologic, efficient, and cost effective than the parenteral route and safer since it avoids the necessity of indwelling catheters. In general, infants less than 12 months old should receive infant formulas, whereas those over 12 months may be given adult preparations. All the formulas may be modified with the use of additives such as carbohydrate polymers, medium-chain triglycerides, or corn oil. This is frequently necessary in infants with BPD.

Although caloric needs may be estimated from a number of equations, numerous studies in critically ill adults have demonstrated that these estimations are frequently incorrect. If possible, oxygen consumption should be measured and caloric requirements calculated taking into account the caloric need for growth. Commercially available metabolic carts are capable of measuring oxygen consumption and carbon dioxide production in ventilated infants and children. Meticulous technique is mandatory when measuring oxygen uptake and carbon dioxide in the critically ill patient.[53]

If the enteral route cannot be utilized, the intravenous route is indicated. When some of the calories can be given by the enteral route, peripheral vein supplementation with intralipids and 10 to 12% glucose/amino acid solution can be given. If the combination of peripheral plus enteral nutrition is not sufficient or if the enteral route cannot be utilized, central vein parenteral nutrition is indicated early in the child's stay in the intensive care unit.

Planning nutritional therapy for infants with BPD presents unique challenges. These include:

1. *Fluid restriction.* Because of lung disease or other medical problems, fluid intake often has to be restricted in these infants. By using additives such as polycose and medium-chain triglycerides, the caloric density of formulas may be increased up to, and occasionally exceeding, 30 calories/oz.

2. *Carbohydrate intake.* Excessive carbohydrate calories in critically ill patients can cause excessive CO_2 production, which is particularly deleterious to the patient with chronic lung disease, who has limited pulmonary reserve. In adults with chronic lung disease, a diet with a low percentage of calories derived from carbohydrates results in decreased CO_2 production and arterial P_{CO_2}.[54] Although there are no specific studies in infants with BPD, it may be beneficial for them to receive up to 60% of the calories from fat. By modifying infant formulas with additives or by using high-fat, low-carbohydrate formulas designed for patients with chronic lung disease in older children, this caloric goal can be achieved under most circumstances.

3. *Increased caloric need.* Numerous studies have documented that infants with BPD have increased oxygen consumption due to the work of breathing.[22, 23] Although the etiology of the increased metabolic rate is unclear, these infants require high caloric intakes to achieve adequate growth. This, combined with the fact that many of these infants may be malnourished upon admission to the PICU, accounts for their large caloric requirements. In our experience, many infants with moderate to severe BPD may require 140 to 160 calories/kg to grow.

4. *Gastroesophageal reflux (GER).* GER occurs frequently in infants with BPD and may cause a significant deterioration in pulmonary function.[55] If an infant has persistent vomiting or worsening respiratory status or fails to gain weight while receiving adequate calories, GER must be suspected, and a diagnostic work-up including barium swallow and pH monitoring should be considered.

5. *Effects of diuretics.* Diuretics can cause significant loss of electrolytes in the urine. Furosemide in particular has been associated with hypercalciuria and rickets.[56] These losses need to be taken into consideration when planning nutritional therapy.

DEVELOPMENTAL AND NEUROLOGIC ISSUES

Although a considerable amount is known about the cardiopulmonary and nutritional aspects of BPD, little is known of the neurologic and developmental outcomes in patients with severe BPD. There is, however, reason for considerable concern. Northway and colleagues found 34% of patients with BPD had significant handicaps including cerebral palsy, mental retardation, deafness, or blindness.[2] Although the developmental delays improve, one follow-up study found that 52% had abnormal neurodevelopment, 24% had suspected abnormal neurodevelopment, and 24% had normal neurodevelopment.[52] The neurodevelopmental abnormalities included quadriplegia, dysplasia, blindness, seizures, hydrocephalus, ataxia, aphasia, and developmental delay. In longer term studies, children with BPD had learning difficulties and required special education. In a 2-year follow-up study, Goldson also found significant developmental delay in children with BPD.[57] Abnormal shoulder girdle muscle tone, decreased arm midline activity, poor head control, and retention of infant reflexes have also been seen in patients with BPD. When shoulder girdle retraction, elevation, and axial extension are present, feeding may be difficult.

Thus, it is important to begin early assessments of movement disorders and sensorimotor and development disturbances. Aggressive therapy should be instituted, but with the understanding that children with BPD often have increased oxygen requirements during therapy and are susceptible to fractures secondary to osteoporosis. Guidelines for assessment and therapy have been developed.[58] An organized and systematic approach to therapy is important because, with aggressive intervention, developmental delays in these children usually improve.

Occupational therapy, physical therapy, and speech therapy are instituted as soon as the child's medical condition allows. These services also play an integral role in the general care of the patient. If treatment causes undue stress, the overall therapeutic plan should be re-evaluated and medical management possibly escalated.

TRANSITION FROM NICU TO PICU

With improved understanding of the pathophysiology and treatment modalities in HMD, there is an increasing number of patients with very severe BPD requiring long-term mechanical ventilation. Since most NICUs are not equipped to manage patients on a chronic basis, there is an increasing number of patients transferred from NICUs to PICUs and chronic respiratory units for chronic care. In a review by Kettrick and Donar, 37% of chronically ventilated pediatric patients required ventilation because of BPD.[59] These patients required mechanical ventilation an average of 12 months (range 1 to 47 months) with a 73% survival rate. Thus, a significant number of chronically ventilated pediatric patients have BPD as their primary pathologic process. In addition, the prognosis for successful weaning from mechanical ventilation is good, although it may take a long time.

When patients are transferred to a PICU or chronic respiratory unit, a systematic team approach to chronic care must be taken. The first step is to make a smooth transition from the neonatal service to the pediatric service. Often there are differences in philosophies and approaches to therapy between the services in addition to the differences in caretakers. In our institution, prior to transferring a patient from the NICU for chronic care, the primary neonatologist, NICU nurse, pulmonary/ICU physician, and pulmonary/ICU nurse all meet with the patient's family to discuss issues regarding the change in caretakers and location of care. With families often ambivalent about changing the child's caretakers and unit, an explanation of the reasons for transfer and reassurance by the NICU staff facilitate a smooth transition. It is important to assign a primary attending physician, nurse, and possibly respiratory therapist to orchestrate the overall care of these children. This creates a consistent team with whom the family can discuss management issues; this is especially important in large institutions with rapid house staff turnover. Regular meetings among the primary attending physician, staff (nurses, respiratory therapists, occupational therapists, developmental team, and social worker), and the family should be instituted. How often these meetings should take place and which members of the health team should be present depend on individual patient and family needs. Since these patients are usually hospitalized for months, it is important that major changes in management do not occur when new house staff and attending physicians rotate on the service.

One of the first issues to be addressed is the maintenance of a stable airway in the chronically ventilated patient. In our institution we require a child to have a tracheostomy placed prior to transfer from the NICU for chronic ventilator care. Tracheostomies in these children have several advantages. First, compared with endotracheal tubes, tracheostomies are more stable and safer for long-term management in terms of accidental extubation and minimizing the incidence of subglottic stenosis. This allows the patient to be admitted to a subacute care unit rather than an intensive care unit. Second, since a tracheostomy bypasses the upper airway, there is a significant reduction in the work of breathing, which may facilitate weaning from mechanical ventilation. A tracheostomy allows the child to nipple feed, thus providing pleasant oral stimulation and avoiding the noxious stimulation of intubation. Lastly, because the patient has a stable airway, he or she is more mobile and can receive more aggressive occupational and physical therapy.

MANAGEMENT OF CHRONIC RESPIRATORY FAILURE

Mechanical ventilation in chronic respiratory failure can be divided into acute, subacute, and weaning phases. The first goal in ventilatory support is to establish stable oxygen delivery by adequate cardiac output and ventilation (acute phase of ventilation). This includes the use of appropriate levels of FiO_2, positive pressure ventilation, tidal volume, and positive end-expiratory pressure (PEEP), preferably with a volume ventilator.[60]

Next, the subacute phase of mechanical ventilation is entered. Since the lung pathology will only improve slowly, this phase may last much longer in patients with BPD than in other ventilated pediatric patients. At this time, other respiratory and nonrespiratory issues must be addressed, namely nutrition, development, and infection problems.

The increased caloric needs and methods of supplementation have been reviewed. Usually, children at this stage are receiving their nutrition by the enteral route. Children with BPD have several specific practical problems with enteral feedings. First, most of these children have been maintained on nasogastric feedings for an extended period and nipple feed poorly even after a tracheostomy is in place. The administration of adequate calories is essential, so if the child is not able to nipple feed adequate calories, chronic nasogastric, gastrostomy, or jejunostomy feedings should be instituted. Very frequently, these children will improve greatly with gastrostomy feedings because a gastrostomy eliminates the irritation of chronic nasogastric tubes, a major source of noxious oral stimulation. Prior to the placement of a feeding gastrostomy, the child should be evaluated for GER by a barium swallow, 24-hour esophageal pH monitoring, or both. Children with BPD have an increased incidence of GER and may require a Nissen fundoplication at the time of gastrostomy placement.[55] Alternatively, jejunostomies have been used in these patients. However, even when a gastrostomy or jejunostomy is in place, the child should be encouraged to nipple feed as much as possible, and the gastrostomy feedings should be decreased accordingly. This arrangement will allow aggressive therapy directed at instituting normal feedings while maintaining adequate caloric supplementation. The combination of mechanical ventilation and aggressive caloric supplementation should enable these children to achieve normal weight gain.

Children with BPD are at a high risk for deterioration with intercurrent infections, both respiratory and nonrespiratory. Because pulmonary reserves are marginal or absent in patients with BPD, any infection, such as otitis media or viral gastroenteritis, can precipitate respiratory failure. Thus, aggressive diagnosis and therapy should be instituted at the first sign of an infectious process. This is especially important with viral respiratory tract infections, which frequently result in considerable worsening in the patient's pulmonary status.

Once adequate respiratory stability and weight gain are achieved, a plan for weaning from mechanical ventilation may be instituted. Whatever weaning approach is taken in these children, the process will be slow and lung mechanics will improve with time and good nutrition. Thus, if adequate weight gain ceases at any time during weaning, even if blood gases are normal, the child is possibly being weaned too quickly and the weaning plan should be reevaluated.

The ability to be successfully liberated from mechanical ventilation is dependent on the balance between the energy demands of ventilation and the energy supplied to the respiratory muscles, most importantly the inspiratory respiratory muscles. There must be adequate oxygen and substrate delivered to the respiratory muscles. Thus, adequate cardiac output, adequate PaO_2, and hemoglobin in conjunction with ample caloric supplementation are essential prior to considering weaning from mechanical ventilation, and these parameters need to be reassessed throughout the weaning process.

Energy demand, or oxygen cost of breathing, comprises two aspects: the work of breathing and the efficiency of breathing. The major determinants of the work of breathing are lung mechanics, and the most important factors in improving lung mechanics are time and good nutrition. Therapy to optimize lung mechanics, such as bronchodilators, anti-inflammatory agents, and diuretics, should be used, as discussed previously. There are other factors that can be modified to minimize the work of breathing. As mentioned, a tracheostomy will bypass the upper airways and thus decrease the work of breathing. In addition, different ventilator circuits have different impedance characteristics, and manipulation of ventilator circuits can minimize the work of breathing for the patient.

The efficiency of breathing may play a major role in ventilator weaning. The chest wall of infants is very compliant and predisposes infants with lung disease to paradoxic respirations, which are inefficient and greatly increase oxygen demand. Time and growth will improve the chest wall mechanics in these infants. In addition, infants with BPD may have areas of high ventilation-perfusion ratios and increased dead space ventilation. There are several controllable factors that may be modified to minimize the dead space ventilation and thus maximize the efficiency of breathing. A tracheostomy decreases both dead space ventilation and the work of breathing. Creating a slower, deeper ventilatory pattern will also decrease the dead space ventilation. This may be accomplished by ventilatory maneuvers that decrease circuit impedance (e.g., continual flow circuits) and pressure support ventilation.

In addition to oxygen and substrate delivery and the oxygen cost of breathing, diaphragmatic function should be addressed. Methods of preparing, or training, the diaphragmatic muscles for independent functioning should be considered.

The ventilatory methods most commonly used in the weaning process in children with BPD include intermittent mandatory ventilation (IMV), T tube or continuous positive airway pressure (CPAP) trials, pressure support, or a combination of the above methods.

The most commonly used ventilator weaning method in children with BPD is slow weaning of IMV. In this method, the IMV is decreased very slowly (often by one breath per minute every 7 to 14 days). If weaning occurs too rapidly, the patient will not necessarily develop worsening in blood gases initially, but may simply be more irritable and have a poorer weight gain. Such patients may have chronic respiratory muscle fatigue and eventually develop obvious respiratory failure over the course of days to weeks. If these signs develop, the weaning process should be slowed because if the patient develops respiratory failure, ventilatory support usually has to be increased and there is a considerable strain on the patient.

Another method of weaning is the progressive use of periods completely off mechanical ventilation with either a T tube (T tube trials) or, more commonly in infants, CPAP (CPAP trials). Once the IMV rate is in the 10 to 15 breath/min range the patient is taken off IMV for progressively increasing amounts of time and then placed back on the previous IMV. This method allows "training" periods for the diaphragm with resting periods in between. This method has gained popularity in recent years, especially in light of the knowledge of diaphragmatic fatigability. These training periods initially occur four times a day for 15 minutes and are progressively increased in length of time. In order to allow adequate rest, these trials are not conducted at night and the trials are progressively increased to a point where the child is being ventilated at night and on a tracheostomy collar during the day. Then the child may be weaned from nighttime ventilation. If blood gas levels worsen during these trials, they are too stressful and they should be shortened or discontinued altogether. At this institution, we measure the heart rate, respiratory rate, tidal volume, oxygen saturation, and end-tidal CO_2 at the beginning and end of these trials so that early signs of stress are noticed. The theoretical advantage of this method is that between trials the diaphragms are allowed to rest and the levels of high-energy compounds may be restored rather than creating a situation of chronic low-grade diaphragmatic fatigue.

A newer method that is becoming popular in patients with BPD is pressure support ventilation. Pressure support delivers a predetermined positive pressure each time a spontaneous breath is initiated by the patient, thus supplementing spontaneous breathing. Usually spontaneous breathing in these patients is relatively fast and shallow (tachypneic breathing), which increases dead space ventilation and is inefficient. By the use of pressure support, deeper, more efficient breaths are generated. In addition to helping to overcome abnormal lung mechanics, pressure support ventilators help to overcome ventilator tubing resistance to air flow. There are studies of the use of pressure support in adults but not in small children.[61, 62] The addition of pressure support is generally recommended to supplement synchronized intermittent mandatory ventilation (SIMV) breaths when a patient is spontaneously breathing. This minimizes the work of breathing and promotes spontaneous breathing.

Another parameter to consider is the ventilator's delivery circuit. The two main ventilator circuits in use clinically are demand valve and continuous flow. The characteristics of each have been reviewed.[60] Continual flow circuits offer the least circuit impedance and minimize the work of breathing, although many of the newer demand-valve circuits have very efficient demand valves and only slightly higher impedance than continuous-flow circuits.[63] Demand-valve circuits have the advantage of enabling pressure support ventilation to be used.

The most important principle is to use a slow, consistent wean and to stop weaning at the first sign of intolerance. If at any point in the weaning process the child has inadequate weight gain, worsened cardiac function, increased irritability, or decreased tolerance to therapy, the weaning process may be going too fast or the child may be developing an intercurrent infection. At this time the entire weaning process must be re-evaluated and work-up for infection considered. Early intervention is important because if weaning is occurring too fast, when the child develops respiratory failure, he or she often has a considerable setback not only in pulmonary aspects but in all aspects of care. Also, any time an intercurrent infection develops, weaning usually is discontinued and respiratory support is often escalated. Thus, a mild gastroenteritis in a child with severe BPD may set back the weaning schedule by weeks to months. These issues make it essential that a primary attending physician supervise the overall care of the individual patient and that a consistent, although constantly re-evaluated, plan be followed.

MANAGEMENT OF ACUTE RESPIRATORY FAILURE

Infants with BPD are frequently readmitted to the hospital during the first 2 years of life. The most common cause for rehospitalization is an acute viral lower respiratory tract illness superimposed on the chronic lung disease.

Respiratory syncytial virus (RSV) is the most important cause of lower respiratory tract illness in children; however influenza virus, adenovirus, parainfluenza virus and other agents may be responsible (see Chapter 72). Data on the impact of RSV on children with BPD and therapy for this virus have been collected in the last few years. It appears that, like children with congenital heart disease, infants with BPD are at special risk for serious disease with RSV. In a prospective study, Groothius and coworkers found a 90% incidence of upper respiratory tract infection per winter in BPD patients with 59% being caused by RSV.[64] Eleven of the children required hospitalization with four admitted to the intensive care unit and two requiring mechanical ventilation.

In 1985 ribavirin aerosol was approved for use in moderate to severely ill infants with RSV infections. In controlled clinical trials, ribavirin aerosol has been shown to speed recovery from RSV infections both in normal infants and in those with BPD.[65, 66] The benefit however, was not dramatic, possibly because treatment was initiated relatively late (3 to 5 days into the illness). The early use of ribavirin in BPD infants infected with RSV was examined by Groothius and colleagues in a multicenter study.[67] The drug appeared to have only a moderate effect on the course of the disease in this high-risk group of infants. Ribavirin is administered in aerosol for 12 to 18 hours/day for 3 to 5 days. It can also be administered to mechanically ventilated patients.[68] The use of ribavirin in children with RSV bronchiolitis is still controversial. The diagnosis of RSV can be made on clinical grounds plus the presence of the virus in the community. Fluorescent antibody slide tests are available in most viral laboratories for rapid diagnosis.

Typically, lower respiratory infections in infants with BPD are accompanied by wheezing, tachypnea, retractions, and feeding intolerance. Hypoxemia is inevitable and in more severe cases acute hypercarbia may be present. Since many of these infants have chronic respiratory distress, it is important to compare the respiratory rate, degree of retractions, presence of wheezing, and other respiratory findings to those prior to the current illness. Similarly, arterial blood gas values must be interpreted with the knowledge that some of these infants may have chronic carbon dioxide retention, hypoxemia, or both when they are in their usual state of health. Interpretation of chest roentgenograms may be difficult in that many of these patients have chronic atelectasis and fibrotic changes. An increase in the amount of hyperinflation is frequently the only significant finding.

The management of acute lower respiratory tract illness in infants with BPD should follow the same guidelines as for any child in respiratory distress. Admission to the PICU should be considered for younger infants and those patients showing signs of impending respiratory failure. Serial arterial blood gas analyses should be performed and compared to baseline levels. Pulse oximetry has been shown to be accurate in infants with chronic lung disease and can be used to continuously monitor oxygenation.

There are no absolute criteria for endotracheal intubation and mechanical ventilation for acutely ill infants with BPD. As in normal children, acute elevations of P_{CO_2} with respiratory acidosis, P_{O_2} of less than 60 mm Hg (with $F_{IO_2} > 60\%$), and clinical findings such as lethargy, apnea, and increasing respiratory distress all point to the need for mechanical ventilation.

Management of Bronchospasm

Many of these infants exhibit prolonged expiration and wheezing that contribute to their respiratory distress. Aggressive bronchodilator therapy is indicated in the infant with BPD and a lower respiratory tract illness who is wheezing.

Presence of Pulmonary Hypertension

Right ventricular enlargement and cor pulmonale occur in some infants with BPD. An episode of acute respiratory failure may cause further increases in pulmonary hypertension and complicate fluid and ventilatory management. Echocardiographic assessment of ventricular function and estimation of pulmonary artery pressure using acceleration times provide useful hemodynamic information in this clinical setting. In stable infants with BPD, studies have shown decreases in pulmonary vascular resistance when the concentration of inhaled oxygen was increased. Presumably, during an acute illness further increases in pulmonary vascular resistance will also respond to oxygen therapy. However, there are no studies on the pulmonary vascular response in infants with BPD during an acute respiratory illness.

Potential Upper Airway Damage

Abnormal upper airway anatomy has been documented in infants with BPD who required mechanical ventilation in the newborn period.[69] Subglottic stenosis is a well-known complication of prolonged endotracheal intubation. These potential problems should be taken into account when securing the airway and at the time of extubation in the PICU.

Psychosocial Concerns

For the parents of an infant with BPD, readmission may be a particularly trying time. Feelings of guilt are often present because parents may feel they "failed" because their child became ill. In addition, they may be unfamiliar with the staff, procedures, and the environment of the PICU. There may be difficulties with interactions between the physicians, nurses, respiratory therapists, and other staff and the parents who are frequently strong advocates of their child's specific needs. Anticipation of these potential problems and an honest and supportive approach are the best way to help the family and avoid problems in communication.

OUTCOME

Because bronchopulmonary dysplasia is a relatively new disease, the overall outcome is to a large extent unknown. As mentioned, numerous studies have documented progressive improvement in pulmonary function as these children grow. Since lung growth continues through adolescence, the prognosis for improvement of symptoms is very good in small children even with very severe BPD. Many patients with severe BPD, however, have a fixed obstructive pulmonary impairment that remains unresponsive to either bronchodilators or anti-inflammatory agents. There is concern that these patients may be more prone to chronic obstructive pulmonary disease in adulthood, but there have been no studies documenting this since the oldest of these patients are only in very early adulthood. With the advent of improved overall care of BPD, children with more severe pulmonary disease are surviving and they very likely will enter adulthood with significant pulmonary impairment.

Although patients with bronchopulmonary dysplasia have a higher incidence of reactive airway disease, it differs from that in asthma in that patients with BPD, even when they are at their best clinically, do not have normal pulmonary function or normal gas exchange.

References

1. O'Brodovich HM and Mellins RB: Bronchopulmonary dysplasia: Unresolved neonatal lung injury. Am Rev Respir Dis 132:694, 1985.
2. Northway WH, Rosan RC, and Porter DY: Pulmonary disease following respirator therapy of hyaline-membrane disease. N Engl J Med 276:357, 1967.
3. Tooley WH: Epidemiology of bronchopulmonary dysplasia. J Pediatr 95:851, 1979.
4. Avery ME, Tooley WH, Keller JB, et al: Is chronic lung disease in low birth weight infants preventable? A survey of eight centers. Pediatrics 79:27, 1987.
5. Myers MG, McGuiness GA, and Lachenbruch PA: Respiratory illness in survivors of infant respiratory distress syndrome. Am Rev Respir Dis 133:1011, 1986.
6. Katz RW and Samet J: Longitudinal study of respiratory morbidity of infants with bronchopulmonary dysplasia (Abstract).
7. Anderson WR and Engel RR: Cardiopulmonary sequelae of reparative stages of bronchopulmonary dysplasia. Arch Pathol Lab Med 107:603, 1983.
8. Barnes ND, Glover WJ, Hull D, et al: Effects of prolonged positive pressure ventilation in infants. Lancet 2:1096, 1969.
9. Fitzhardinge PM, Pape K, Arstikatis M, et al: Mechanical ventilation of infants of less than 1,501 gm birth weight: Health, growth and neurologic sequelae. J Pediatr 88:531, 1976.
10. Churg A, Golden J, Fligiel S, et al: Bronchopulmonary dysplasia in the adult. Am Rev Respir Dis 127:117, 1983.
11. Edwards DK, Dyer WM, and Northway WH Jr: Twelve years' experience with bronchopulmonary dysplasia. Pediatrics 59:839, 1977.
12. Taghizadeh A and Reynolds EOR: Pathogenesis of bronchopulmonary dysplasia following hyaline membrane disease. Am J Pathol 82:241, 1976.
13. Clark JM and Lambertsen CJ: Pulmonary oxygen toxicity: A review. Pharmacol Rev 28:37, 1971.
14. Avery GB, Fletcher AB, and Brudno DS: Controlled trial of dexamethasone in respirator-dependent infants with bronchopulmonary dysplasia. Pediatrics 75:106, 1985.
15. Ehrenkranz RA, Ablou RC, and Warshaw JB: Prevention of bronchopulmonary dysplasia with vitamin E administration during the acute stages of respiratory distress syndrome. J Pediatr 95:873, 1979.
16. Jefferies AL, Coates G, and O'Brodovich H: Pulmonary epithelial permeability in hyaline-membrane disease. N Engl J Med 311:1075, 1984.
17. Merrit TA, Cochrane CG, Holcomb K, et al: Elastase and A1

proteinase inhibitor activity in tracheal aspirates during respiratory distress syndrome. J Clin Invest 72:656, 1983.
18. Ogden BE, Murphy SA, Saunders GC, et al: Neonatal lung neutrophils and elastase/proteinase inhibitor imbalance. Am Rev Respir Dis 130:817, 1984.
19. Repine JE, Bowman CM, and Tate RM: Neutrophils and lung edema. Chest 81:47S, 1982.
20. Tepper RS, Morgan WJ, Cota K, et al: Expiratory flow limitation in infants with bronchopulmonary dysplasia. J Pediatr 109:1040, 1986.
21. Gerhardt T, Hehre D, Feller R, et al: Serial determination of pulmonary function in infants with chronic lung disease. J Pediatr 110:448, 1987.
22. Weinstein MR and Oh W: Oxygen consumption in infants with bronchopulmonary dysplasia. J Pediatr 99:958, 1981.
23. Kurzner S, Gars M, Bautiota D, et al: Growth failure in bronchopulmonary dysplasia: Elevated metabolic rates and pulmonary mechanics. J Pediatr 112:73, 1988.
24. Smyth JA, Tabachnik E, Duncan WJ, et al: Pulmonary function and bronchial hyperactivity in long-term survivors of bronchopulmonary dysplasia. Pediatrics 68:336, 1981.
25. Bryan MH, Hardie MJ, Reilly BJ, et al: Pulmonary function studies during the first year of life in infants recovering from respiratory distress syndrome. Pediatrics 52:169, 1973.
26. Bonikos DS, Bensch KG, and Northway WH: Bronchopulmonary dysplasia: The pulmonary pathologic sequel of necrotizing bronchiolitis and pulmonary fibrosis. Hum Pathol 7:643, 1976.
27. Kao LC, Warburton D, Platzker ACG, et al: Effect of isoproterenol inhalation on airway resistance in chronic bronchopulmonary dysplasia. Pediatrics 73:509, 1984.
28. Logvinoff MM, Lemen RJ, Taussig LM, et al: Bronchodilators and diuretics in children with bronchopulmonary dysplasia. Pediatr Pulmonol 1:198, 1985.
29. Shim C, Williams MH: Bronchial response to oral versus aerosol metaproterenol in asthma. Ann Intern Med 93:428, 1980.
30. Watterberg KL, Clark AR, Kelly HW, et al: Delivery of aerosolized medication to intubated babies. Pediatr Pulmonol 10:136, 1991.
31. Ahrens RC, Ries RA, Popendorf W, et al: The delivery of therapeutic aerosols through endotracheal tubes. Pediatr Pulmonol 2:19, 1986.
32. Gross NJ and Skorodin MS: Anticholinergic, antimuscarinic bronchodilators. Am Rev Respir Dis 129:865, 1984.
33. Virtanen R, Kanto J, Tisaol F, et al: Pharmacokinetic studies on atropine with special reference to age. Acta Anaesthesiol Scand 26:297, 1982.
34. Cavanaugh MJ and Cooper DM: Inhaled atropine sulfate: Dose response characteristics. Am Rev Respir Dis 114:517, 1976.
35. Pabes GF, Brogdin RN, Heel RC, et al: Ipratropium bromide: A review of its pharmacological properties and therapeutic efficacy in asthma and chronic bronchitis. Drugs 20:237, 1980.
36. Rooklin AR, Momjiian AS, and Fox WW: Theophylline therapy in bronchopulmonary dysplasia. J Pediatr 95:882, 1979.
37. Kao LC, Durand DJ, Phillips BL, et al: Oral theophylline and diuretics improve pulmonary mechanics in infants with bronchopulmonary dysplasia. J Pediatr 111:439, 1987.
38. Hendeles L and Weinberger M: Disposition of theophylline after a single intravenous infusion of aminophylline. Am Rev Respir Dis 118:97, 1978.
39. Mammel MC, Green TP, and Johnson DE: Controlled trial of dexamethasone therapy in infants with bronchopulmonary dysplasia. Lancet 1:1356, 1983.
40. Stenmark KE, Eyzaguirre M, Remigio L, et al: Recovery of platelet activating factor and leukotrienes from infants with severe bronchopulmonary dysplasia: Clinical improvement with cromolyn treatment. Am Rev Respir Dis 131(Pt4):236, 1985.
41. Kao LC, Warburton D, Sargent CW, et al: Furosemide acutely decreases airways resistance in chronic bronchopulmonary dysplasia. J Pediatr 103:624, 1983.
42. Kao LC, Warburton D, Cheng MH, et al: Effect of oral diuretics on pulmonary mechanics in infants with chronic bronchopulmonary dysplasia: Results of a double-blind crossover sequential trial. Pediatrics 74:37, 1984.
43. McCann EM, Lewis K, Deming DD, et al: Controlled trial of furosemide therapy in infants with chronic lung disease. J Pediatr 106:957, 1985.

44. Engelhardt B, Elliott S, and Hazinski TA: Short- and long-term effects of furosemide on lung function in infants with bronchopulmonary dysplasia. J Pediatr 109:1034, 1986.

45. Patel H, Yeh T, Jain R, et al: Pulmonary and renal responses to furosemide in infants with stage III-IV bronchopulmonary dysplasia. Am J Dis Child 139:917, 1985.

46. Tomashefski JR Jr, Oppermann HC, Vawter GF, et al: Bronchopulmonary dysplasia: A morphometric study with emphasis on the pulmonary vasculature. Pediatr Pathol 2:469, 1984.

47. Berman W Jr, Yabek SM, Dillon T, et al: Evaluation of infants with bronchopulmonary dysplasia using cardiac catheterization. Pediatrics 70:708, 1982.

48. Kochanek P and Zartisky A: Nifedipine in the treatment of a child with pulmonary hypertension associated with severe bronchopulmonary dysplasia. Clin Pediatr 25:214, 1986.

49. Goodman G, Perkin R, Anas N, et al: Pulmonary hypertension in infants with bronchopulmonary dysplasia. J Pediatr 112:67, 1988.

50. Newth CJ, Gow RM, and Rowe RD: The assessment of pulmonary arterial pressures in bronchopulmonary dysplasia by cardiac catheterization and M-mode echocardiography. Pediatr Pulmonol 1:58, 1985.

51. Katz RW and Smith JC: Acute and chronic protein energy malnutrition in O_2 dependent infants with bronchopulmonary dysplasia (Abstract). Am Rev Respir Dis 133(Suppl.):A207, 1986.

52. Vohr BR, Bell EF, and Oh W: Infants with bronchopulmonary dysplasia: Growth pattern and neurologic and developmental outcome. Am J Dis Child 136:443, 1982.

53. Weissman C: Measuring oxygen uptake in the clinical setting. In: Christopher W, Bryan-Brown CW, and Ayres, VS: Oxygen Transport and Utilization. Fullerton, CA, Society of Critical Care Medicine, 1980.

54. Angelillo VA, Sukhdarshan B, Durfee D, et al: Effect of low and high carbohydrate feedings in ambulatory patients with chronic obstructive pulmonary disease and chronic hypercapnia. Ann Intern Med 103:883, 1985.

55. Giuffre RM, Rubin S, and Mitchell I: Antireflux surgery in infants with bronchopulmonary dysplasia. Am J Dis Child 141:648, 1987.

56. Hurnagle KG, Shadid NK, Penn D, et al: Renal calcifications: A complication of long-term furosemide therapy in preterm infants. Pediatrics 70:360, 1982.

57. Goldson E: Severe bronchopulmonary dysplasia in the very low birth weight infant: Its relationship to developmental outcome. J Dev Behav Pediatr 5:165, 1984.

58. Chandler L, Andrews MS, and Swanson M: The movement assessment of infants. P.O. Box 4631. Rolling Bay, WA, 1980.

59. Kettrick RG and Donar ME: The ventilator-dependent child: Medical and social care. Critical Care Medicine. State of the Art 6:F1-F38. Fullerton, CA, Society of Critical Care Medicine, 1985.

60. McWilliams B: Mechanical ventilation in pediatric patients. Clin Chest Med 8:1, 1987.

61. Brochard L, Harf A, Lorino H, et al: Pressure support decreases work of breathing and oxygen consumption during weaning from mechanical ventilation. Am Rev Respir Dis 135:A51, 1987.

62. Brochard L, Harf A, Lorino H, et al: Optimal level of pressure support in patients with unsuccessful weaning from mechanical ventilation. Am Rev Respir Dis 115:A51, 1987.

63. Gibney RT, Wilson R, and Pontoppidan H: Comparison of work of breathing in high gas flow and demand valve continuous positive airway pressure systems. Chest 82:692, 1982.

64. Groothuis JR, Gutierrez KM, and Lauer BA: Respiratory syncytial virus infection in children with bronchopulmonary dysplasia. Pediatrics 82:199, 1988.

65. Hall CB, McBride JT, Gala CL, et al: Ribavirin treatment of respiratory syncytial viral infection in infants with underlying cardiopulmonary disease. JAMA 254:3047, 1985.

66. Hall CM, McBride JT, Walsh EE, et al: Aerosolized ribavirin treatment of infants with respiratory syncytial viral infection. N Engl J Med 308:114, 1983.

67. Groothuis JR, Woodin KA, Katz R, et al: Early ribavirin treatment of respiratory syncytial viral infection in high-risk children. J Pediatr 117:792, 1990.

68. Foy T, Marion J, and Harris TR: Isoproterenol and aminophylline reduced lung capillary filtration during high permeability. J Appl Physiol 46:146, 1979.

69. Tover B, Ball F, and Hack: Changes in tracheobronchial width in bronchopulmonary dysplasia: A result of altered transmural pressures? Ann Radiol 29:691, 1986.

70. Bose C, Corbet A, Bose G, et al: Improved outcome at 28 days of age for very low birth weight infants treated with a single dose of a synthetic surfactant. J Pediatr 117:947, 1990.

71. Corbet A, Bucciarelli R, Goldman S, et al: Decreased mortality rate among small premature infants treated at birth with a single dose of synthetic surfactant: A multicenter controlled trial. J Pediatr 118:277, 1991.

Neuromuscular Disorders

Robert K. Kanter, M.D.

Respiratory failure is a common complication of neuromuscular disorders. Impairment of breathing may occur as the result of ineffective motor nerve stimulation or intrinsic muscle disease. In addition, weakness often occurs in critically ill patients without primary neuromuscular problems. Respiratory fatigue develops as a terminal process when the work of breathing exceeds muscle capabilities, whether due to abnormally high respiratory workload or to neuromuscular disease. In Chapter 24, recognition and specific therapy of primary neuromuscular disorders are reviewed. In this chapter, the factors limiting respiratory muscle strength and endurance in critically ill patients are considered, general principles in the evaluation of muscle strength and reserve are outlined, and the chapter concludes with suggestions for the care of patients with respiratory insufficiency due to weakness.

PRIMARY NEUROMUSCULAR DISORDERS LEADING TO RESPIRATORY FAILURE

Ineffective motor nerve input to muscles may originate in disorders of the brain, spinal cord, anterior horn cell, peripheral nerve, or neuromuscular junction. Ineffective contraction of muscle may result from primary myopathy. Chapter 24 provides an overview of the diagnostic approach and specific therapy for neuromuscular disorders. In Chapter 51 specific comments are made relating to resultant respiratory failure. Severe encephalopathies, which can impair upper motor neuron signals to respiratory muscles as well as cause loss of consciousness, are considered in Chapters 20 and 80. Traumatic spinal cord and phrenic nerve injuries are discussed in Chapters 22 and 48. Table 51–1 summarizes the diagnostic features of neuromuscular disorders according to anatomic site. Table 51–2 lists the neuromuscular disorders likely to cause respiratory failure according to the patient's age.

Selected Conditions

In addition to the diseases discussed in Chapter 24, other conditions can affect respiratory function. The acute onset of weakness, paresthesias, and loss of sensation along with bowel or bladder dysfunction suggests *transverse myelitis*.[1] A thoracic level is usually definable, but higher involvement can compromise respiration. An autoimmune process, vascular occlusion, or viral infection may be responsible for this rare disorder. The diagnosis is established after ruling out compressive lesions of the spinal cord such as epidural abscess (often staphylococcal), tumors, and vertebral or intervertebral disk disorders. These mass lesions require urgent treatment to salvage spinal cord function. Radiologic studies may be helpful in clarifying the diagnosis. As in Guillain-Barré syndrome, muscle tone is reduced in the early stages of transverse myelitis. Spasticity develops later. Transverse myelitis has a clearer level of sensory deficit and earlier loss of bowel and bladder function than Guillain-Barré syndrome. A cerebrospinal fluid (CSF) pleocytosis is present in some but not all cases of transverse myelitis. Partial or complete recovery is the norm, but specific therapy is not available.

Tetanus presents with a distinct pattern of muscle rigidity and spasms after a brief interval of irritability, painful stiffness of the jaw and back, and difficulty in swallowing. The toxin from *Clostridium tetani* reduces inhibitory input to motor neurons, resulting in painful and dangerous reflex contractions in response to even minor stimuli. The toxin may also stimulate, as well as block, neuromuscular transmission directly. Trismus, laryngeal spasm, and rigidity of respiratory muscles can all lead to respiratory insufficiency. Swallowing dysfunction causes aspiration. Abnormal function of the autonomic nervous system frequently results in lability of the cardiovascular system. Unimmunized individuals are at risk from accidental puncture wounds, lacerations, and burns, as well as surgical wounds. The umbilical stump is the usual source of infection in newborns whose mothers have not been immunized. There is usually little diagnostic uncertainty as the clinical presentation of tetanus is unique. Treatment includes local wound care. Although the neuropathic effect of toxin cannot be acutely reversed, administration of tetanus immune globulin and treatment with penicillin G may limit progression. Since muscle spasms can cause an abrupt and life-threatening respiratory crisis, a period of mechanical ventilation, sedation, analgesia, and sometimes

Table 51–1. CLINICAL SIGNS ASSOCIATED WITH SITE OF NEUROMUSCULAR DISORDER

Clinical Observations	Spinal Cord	Anterior Horn Cell	Peripheral Nerves	Neuromuscular Junction	Muscle
Pattern of weakness	Below lesion	Proximal extremity	Initially distal, then ascending	Cranial nerve distribution, then descending	Axial, proximal extremity
Tone	Increased (flaccid in early spinal shock)	Decreased	Decreased	Decreased	Decreased
Tendon reflexes	Present (decreased in early spinal shock)	Decreased	Decreased	Present	Present
Sensation	Deficit below lesion	Normal	Variable	Normal	Normal
Fasciculation	No	Yes	Occasionally	No	No

neuromuscular blockade is usually warranted. Early respiratory support is important in reducing mortality.[2]

Organophosphates inhibit the activity of acetylcholinesterase at synapses and the neuromuscular junction, resulting in sustained stimulation of acetylcholine receptors (see also Chapter 80). Nicotinic effects include weakness and decreased muscle tone. Muscarinic effects include myosis, salivation, nausea, vomiting, bradycardia, wheezing, diaphoresis, lacrimation, abdominal pain, and bowel and bladder incontinence. Central nervous system dysfunction results from central nervous system penetration of toxin. Diagnosis may be difficult in children, since ingestion or transcutaneous absorption of an improperly used or stored insecticide may not have been observed by parents. Salivation, lacrimation, and bowel and bladder incontinence are nonspecific findings in crying, sick infants and young children. The signs of organophosphate poisoning in children differ in important ways from those in adults, leading to delays in the diagnosis. In one report, tachycardia was present in 49% of pediatric patients compared with only 19% having bradycardia from muscarinic effects.[3] Seizures occurred in 22%, possibly as a result of hypoxia, a rate far greater than that reported in adults. Fifty-nine per cent had respiratory distress, occasionally leading to the erroneous diagnosis of lower respiratory tract infection. Weakness was common, occurring in 68%. Impaired level of consciousness and pulmonary dysfunction, often in combination with weakness, led to respiratory insufficiency in 38%. The diagnosis is supported by a limited response to usual doses of atropine and can be confirmed by measuring a low level of cholinesterase activity in serum or red blood cells. In addition to the acute manifestations, delayed toxicity at 24 to 96 hours may manifest with muscle weakness in proximal extremities, neck, and cranial nerve distributions as the predominant effect.[4] Respiratory failure is a common occurrence in this delayed presentation, which may be specific to certain organophosphate agents.

Treatment of organophosphate poisoning includes general supportive care and specific therapy with atropine to antagonize cholinergic effects (0.02–0.05 mg/kg). Pralidoxime (Protopam), a cholinesterase reactivator, is indicated for organophosphate poisoning. Phenothiazines and succinylcholine potentiate cholinergic toxicity and should be avoided.

Disorders of Autonomic Function

Autonomic nervous system dysfunction frequently accompanies neuromuscular disorders. Extremely labile heart rate and blood pressure and dysrhythmias are common with Guillain-Barré syndrome,[5] tetanus,[2] polio,[6] and spinal cord injury.[7] Unopposed vagal reflexes can cause bradycardia and asystole, which can alternate in the same patient with exaggerated sympathetic responses causing hypertension and tachydysrhythmias. Dysautonomia has become the leading cause of death in Guillain-Barré syndrome and tetanus, as aggressive respiratory intensive care prevents respiratory insufficiency.

WEAKNESS AND MUSCLE FATIGUE IN CRITICAL ILLNESS

The systemic factors discussed in the following section may exacerbate weakness of a patient with primary

Table 51–2. NEUROMUSCULAR CAUSES OF RESPIRATORY WEAKNESS AND INSUFFICIENCY: TIME OF ONSET

Neonatal Period and Early Infancy	Children	
	Gradual Onset	Acute Onset
Acute brain injury	Spinal muscular atrophy	Brain injury
Hypotonic cerebral palsy	Myasthenia gravis	Transverse myelitis
Spinal cord injury	Muscular dystrophy	Spinal cord injury
Spinal muscular atrophy	Other myopathies	Tetanus
Tetanus		Guillain-Barré syndrome
Myasthenia gravis		Tick paralysis
Botulism		Myasthenia gravis
Myopathy		Botulism
		Organophosphate poisoning
		Some metabolic myopathies

neuromuscular disease or any critical illness. Recognition of these factors allows their correction or timely initiation of mechanical ventilation in a high-risk patient to avert a respiratory crisis. In the ventilator-dependent patient, correcting reversible systemic factors may aid in ventilator weaning.

Muscle strength refers to the tension that a muscle can generate during a contraction. Determinants of greater contracting muscle tension include longer resting fiber length, slower velocity of fiber shortening, and greater intensity of stimulation by the motor nerve. Factors intrinsic to the muscle, such as metabolism and fatigue, also affect strength.

Endurance is the ability of a muscle to continue generating a given tension during sustained or repeated contractions. Thus, fatigue is a cause of weakness as the muscle fails to sustain tension during periods of work. Fatigue develops more rapidly when contracting muscle tension is near its maximum. The longer the duty cycle (the per cent of time spent actively contracting), the more rapidly repetitive contractions cause fatigue.

The tendency of respiratory muscles to fatigue can be quantitatively described. Pressure generated by the contracting diaphragm is expressed as the transdiaphragmatic pressure (Pdi), the difference between gastric and esophageal pressures. The pressure-time index is an empirical quantity defined as

$$Pdi/Pdi\ max \times TI/TT$$

Higher values for the pressure-time index occur when respiratory muscles are working near their maximum (Pdi max), and when inspiratory time (TI) is long relative to total respiratory cycle time (TT). For adults, respiratory muscle fatigue tends to develop when the pressure-time index exceeds 0.2, while levels below 0.15 can be sustained indefinitely.[8] Transdiaphragmatic pressure less than 40% of the Pdi max can be sustained indefinitely with typical breathing patterns. While fatigue should be thought of as one cause of weakness, underlying weakness also increases the likelihood that a given respiratory workload will result in fatigue, since the weak muscle must work near its maximum capability.

The cellular basis of muscle fatigue remains the subject of investigation. The inability of oxygen delivery to meet aerobic metabolic demands of working muscle appears to be an important factor in fatigue. In an experimental model involving diaphragm pacing, increasing frequency of diaphragm contraction resulted in increased diaphragmatic blood flow, oxygen transport, and oxygen consumption.[9] At 100 stimulations per minute, simulating rapid breathing, lactate efflux from the diaphragm rose out of proportion to the increase in oxygen consumption. These metabolic changes accompanied a diminution in contractile force. These observations support the hypothesis that failure to sustain aerobic metabolism accounts for fatigue.

Strategies to Delay the Onset of Fatigue

When the organism is presented with a large respiratory workload, the breathing pattern tends to minimize muscle tension,[10] which usually results in rapid shallow breathing. Before the muscle actually fatigues, it appears that neural stimulus to breathe becomes attenuated. In experimental models of loaded respiration, reductions in effort[11] or respiratory frequency[12, 13] preceded muscle fatigue. Alternating use of diaphragmatic and thoracic muscles may also give the diaphragm an opportunity to rest during its fatiguing load.[14] Such strategies may have survival value, delaying the onset of fatigue even though ventilation may be sacrificed to some extent.

Inefficient Function of Muscle

Hyperexpansion of the lung and diaphragmatic flattening shorten resting diaphragm fiber length and limit the tension that can be generated even if the muscle is healthy. Thus patients with air trapping have a smaller respiratory reserve than healthy individuals.[15, 16] The floppy chest wall of infants poses another mechanical disadvantage. Large inspiratory efforts are partially wasted as sternal retractions reduce the amount of gas inhaled. Forced expiration in the dyspneic patient uses more energy than passive expiration, especially when the forced expiration results in dynamic collapse of intrathoracic airways. Sleep poses a particular problem for infants with incipient respiratory failure. The highly compliant thorax of infants is responsible for a lung volume that is partly dependent on inspiratory muscle tone and rapid breathing. Sleep reduces thoracic muscle tone and increases periodic breathing with a resultant drop in expiratory lung volume.[17, 18] Lung volume may fall enough to allow collapse of basal alveoli and hypoxia in some cases. Therefore, sleep is a time when respiratory crises are more likely to occur in sick infants. Likewise, deterioration of respiratory function may be present during sleep in adults with chronic weakness long before respiratory insufficiency is noted in the waking state.[19, 20] While sleep is a hazardous period, sleep deprivation is counterproductive, resulting in impaired respiratory muscle endurance[21] and increased obstructive sleep apnea.[22]

Factors Impairing Contractility of Muscle

The susceptibility of infants to respiratory failure has long been noted by pediatricians, but it remains unclear whether intrinsic deficiencies of immature muscle are responsible. Maximum pressure generated by the human diaphragm appears to be lower at a younger age.[23] Data are conflicting on developmental differences in muscle endurance in experimental models.[24, 25] Mild experimental respiratory loads revealed slightly better defense of ventilation by older animals than newborns, but no difference in blood gases was noted.[26] It may be that inefficient respiration due to the infant's compliant chest wall is a more important developmental determinant of respiratory failure than is muscle immaturity.

In severe circulatory collapse, oxygen supply to the respiratory muscles becomes a limiting factor in their function.[27] Patients in congestive heart failure have respiratory muscle weakness out of proportion to weakness in other muscle groups.[28] In bacterial septic shock[29, 30] and viral illnesses,[31] other factors may directly impair muscle strength and endurance even before oxygen transport has been affected. Circulating peptides in sepsis and trauma appear to induce muscle proteolysis, potentially accounting for impaired muscle function.[32]

Malnutrition reduces the maximal pressures that can be generated by inspiratory and expiratory respiratory muscles,[33] in addition to its adverse effect on wound healing and immune competence.

In severe pulmonary disease, abnormality of gas exchange contributes to the patient's rapidly deteriorating condition as hypoxia and hypercapnia interfere with respiratory muscle contractility.[34, 35] Hypocalcemia may reduce respiratory muscle strength directly, in addition to its tendency to cause seizures.[36] Severe hypokalemia is known to cause muscle weakness and may rarely contribute to respiratory muscle failure.[37] Likewise, hypophosphatemia is a reversible cause of diaphragm weakness.[38] Hypomagnesemia is seen in some patients with respiratory muscle weakness; however clinical hypomagnesemia often accompanies hypokalemia and hypocalcemia, making it difficult to attribute weakness to a single factor in such cases.[39, 40] Finally, the myopathy of hyperthyroidism contributes to muscle weakness and is reversible with medical therapy.[41]

A variety of therapeutic agents and modalities used in critically ill patients can also interfere with respiratory function. Aminoglycosides and magnesium decrease the release of acetylcholine at the neuromuscular junction.[42] Succinylcholine action, normally diminishing over minutes, can be somewhat prolonged by alkalosis, hyperkalemia, hypermagnesemia, aminoglycosides, liver disease, and malnutrition and greatly prolonged in the rare patient with deficiency of cholinesterase activity. Nondepolarizing neuromuscular blockers can have their action prolonged by acidosis, hypokalemia, hypermagnesemia, aminoglycosides, myasthenia gravis, and renal or hepatic dysfunction.[43] Occasional protracted weakness lasting for days after administration of nondepolarizing muscle relaxants[44, 45] may be due to accumulation of the blocker or a metabolite. In addition, patients on prolonged mechanical ventilation with or without neuromuscular blockers may have muscle atrophy associated with disuse.[46, 47] Steroids cause myopathy, which can contribute to muscle weakness.[48] Nutritional therapy is vital in the recovery of critically ill patients, but hypophosphatemia with muscle weakness can occur during the course of nutritional therapy.[49] Finally, muscle rigidity can impair respiration. In addition to the occasional incidence of succinylcholine-induced generalized rigidity with malignant hyperthermia, some patients have isolated trismus.[50] Opiates occasionally cause increased muscle tone, especially when used in anesthetic doses.[51] The muscle rigidity, which may be severe enough to impair respiration, appears to result from a supraspinal mechanism. Other drugs used in the critical care setting, such as phenothiazines and metoclopramide, occasionally cause milder dystonic movement disorders. Distinguishing these from seizures is important in order to avoid unnecessary use of anticonvulsants.

EVALUATION OF THE PATIENT

Some generalizations can be made about the systematic evaluation of respiration in patients with weakness, whether due to primary neuromuscular disease or other factors.

Acute Illness

During an acute illness, progression of all the usual signs of respiratory distress provides warning of an impending crisis. A subjective evaluation of the patient's ability to cough and breathe deeply can be made quickly at the bedside. Neuromuscular weakness commonly leads to atelectasis,[52] with further impairment of gas exchange and pulmonary mechanics. When weakness involves the pharyngeal muscles, airway obstruction and aspiration are common. Noisy snoring inspiratory sounds, difficulty in swallowing, and an impaired gag reflex indicate an urgent need to improve airway patency. Blood gas analysis typically shows impaired oxygenation with ventilation-perfusion mismatching early in the course of respiratory muscle weakness. Shallow rapid respiration allows the patient to maintain a normal or low $PaCO_2$ until weakness becomes severe. When $PaCO_2$ begins rising during an acute illness, it suggests that all compensatory mechanisms have been exhausted and a crisis is evolving rapidly. More direct pulmonary function tests should be undertaken in the older child if time allows. The nose must be occluded to prevent erroneous underestimates of function when respiratory measurements are carried out through a mouthpiece. Vital capacity can be compared to predicted values relative to the patient's height (height is estimated by the armspan if the patient has scoliosis). Inspiratory muscle strength can also be measured as the negative inspiratory pressure generated when the patient inhales forcefully against an obstructed airway. Values under 30 cm H_2O suggest severe weakness. So many factors can affect gas exchange that only a fair correlation exists between measured respiratory muscle strength and blood gas values.

Mechanical ventilation should be considered if the patient is distressed or has impaired pharyngeal muscle function, acutely rising $PaCO_2$, persistent hypoxia (PaO_2 ≤ 60 mm Hg on FIO_2 ≥ 0.6), atelectasis on chest radiography, or a rapidly worsening vital capacity and negative peak inspiratory pressure. In shock, respiratory muscle oxygen consumption diverts oxygen transport from other ischemic organs.[53] Mechanical ventilation of the patient with circulatory impairment may improve the relationship between limited oxygen supply and excessive demands. A decision to defer intubation and continue other medical support with close monitoring may be justified if the patient is comfortable, has good cough and swallowing reflexes, maintains $PaCO_2$ under 45 mm Hg and PaO_2 over 80 mm Hg, has a stable vital capacity at least twice the resting tidal volume, and has a negative inspiratory pressure of at least 30 cm H_2O. The spontaneously breathing patient with respiratory weakness should be allowed to sleep, but monitoring must be especially close during that time. Sleep hypoxia may be an indication for intubation even if respiration is adequate in the waking state. Pulse oximetry is useful in the detection of sporadic hypoxia.

Chronic Respiratory Insufficiency

In the patient with chronic weakness and respiratory insufficiency, therapeutic goals should be formulated well in advance of a crisis. In some cases respiratory intensive care may improve the patient's comfort and survival; in other cases, mechanical ventilation will only prolong the process of dying. In the terminally ill patient, a decision to provide comfort care without mechanical ventilation may be warranted.

When the decision is made to carry out respiratory intensive care for the patient with chronic weakness, indications for mechanical ventilation include worsening of airway protective reflexes, impaired level of consciousness, progression of hypercapnia, life-threatening hypoxia, and intractable dyspnea. It is especially useful to know the patient's baseline status, as dyspnea, poor cough, hypercapnia, mild hypoxia, and low vital capacity may be chronic conditions that have been well tolerated. When no previous blood gas values are available for comparison, a compensatory metabolic alkalosis suggests that hypercapnia has been present for more than a day.

Evaluation for Ventilator Weaning and Extubation during Recovery

Coordination and function of the upper airway are crudely assessed by testing the gag reflex. If the gag is vigorous in the alert patient, upper airway control will seldom be the limiting factor in the patient's recovery. More objective methods to evaluate pharyngeal and laryngeal function prior to extubation would be desirable. Occult aspiration due to swallowing dysfunction is common after endotracheal intubation even in patients without primary neuromuscular disease.[54]

When a decision must be made about whether to discontinue mechanical ventilation and remove the endotracheal tube in a patient with weakness of respiratory muscles, a 30- to 60-minute trial of spontaneous breathing with the endotracheal tube still in place provides important insights. Respirations should be regular and comfortable without apnea. $PaCO_2$ under 45 mm Hg with pH over 7.35 and safe oxygenation confirm that drive to breathe and muscle strength are adequate to allow withdrawal of mechanical ventilation. If the patient becomes tachypneic, uses accessory respiratory muscles, or complains of dyspnea, it is likely that respiratory muscle strength is not adequate. Failure to cough, to at least double resting tidal volume, and to generate peak inspiratory negative pressures of at least 30 cm H_2O all suggest that muscle strength is inadequate to accomplish the necessary work of spontaneous breathing. Used alone, tests of vital capacity and peak inspiratory negative pressure are not reliable predictors of the patient's ability to breathe without ventilator support.[55–59] These tests may be useful if unexpectedly normal values are encountered or a consistently rising trend reveals a patient to have better strength than was presumed. Likewise, unexpectedly poor performance on these tests suggests the need for caution to avoid premature and unsuccessful extubation.

Newer methods to evaluate strength and to identify the patient likely to fatigue after extubation have been explored recently in adult patients. A value of Pdi measured during resting spontaneous breathing that is high relative to Pdi max indicates that the patient is working near the limits of muscle capacity. This identifies patients who are likely to fail ventilator weaning better than conventional criteria.[60] In another approach, an estimate of neural drive to breathe is assessed. Pressure measured at the airway after 0.1 second of inhalation against an airway obstruction (before conscious or reflex response to obstruction occurs) reflects the baseline respiratory neural output; this measurement is referred to as the P0.1. The P0.1 was high at the onset of respiratory failure in all patients, associated with stress and increased neural stimulus to breathe in these patients. Those whose P0.1 fell tended to be successfully weaned from mechanical ventilation, while those whose P0.1 remained high tended to need more extended periods of respiratory support because their respiratory drive was still highly stimulated as the result of an imbalance between respiratory work and muscle capabilities.[61] Diaphragm electromyographic (EMG) findings suggestive of fatigue have been described in infants and adults; however, their sensitivity is inadequate in detecting fatigue after submaximal contractions.[62] When present, the EMG pattern changes only during the development of fatigue, providing little advance warning of an impending problem in the clinical setting. Direct formal testing of diaphragm strength requires the removal of voluntary effort as a variable. This may be accomplished by measuring Pdi in response to supramaximal phrenic nerve electrical stimulation. In another approach, Pdi is measured relative to the amplitude of diaphragm EMG, an index of neural excitation of the diaphragm.[63] These methods have been explored mainly in the laboratory, and experience in the pediatric critical care setting is unavailable. Even direct testing of the diaphragm will provide incomplete information to the clinician since different respiratory muscle groups may be recruited independently[14] and their fatigue may not occur simultaneously.[64]

TREATMENT

For the patient with incipient respiratory failure due to weakness, recognition of specific risk factors allows their timely correction. Monitoring should include frequent assessment of vital signs, direct observation of the patient, and continuous electrocardiographic, apnea, and pulse oximetry monitoring. In addition to the methods of evaluation outlined in the previous section, these observations may reveal subtle signs of respiratory failure before a sudden respiratory crisis develops. Monitoring should be especially close during sleep, but undisturbed sleep should be allowed as much as possible. In the patient with weakness, the reserve to compensate for respiratory mechanical disorders is small. Abdominal distention, bronchospasm, pulmonary edema, and infection should all be treated promptly. In addition, the various factors discussed earlier contributing to weakness should be corrected when possible. When hemodynamic disorders limit blood flow to respiratory muscles, circulatory support (e.g., with dopamine) may improve muscle strength.[65] Sedating drugs should be used cautiously, as reduction of the drive to breathe is likely to compromise the patient with severe weakness. When progression of respiratory failure is anticipated, enteral feedings should be interrupted to avoid aspiration.

When indicated, mechanical ventilation in the acute crisis should be handled in conventional fashion, as discussed elsewhere in this text. An interval of mechanical ventilation rests the respiratory muscles, potentially relieving fatigue and improving muscle performance.[66] In planning the approach to endotracheal intubation, note that patients with myopathies have an increased incidence of malignant hyperthermia when exposed to succinylcholine and inhalation anesthetics.[67] Lesions of upper or lower motor neurons as well as muscle injury predispose to dangerous release of potassium from muscle in response to succinylcholine. Hyperkalemia may reach levels high enough to cause cardiac arrest.[43]

As already noted, many patients with neuromuscular disorders have abnormal autonomic nerve function. Management of the patient with potential autonomic instability involves continuous cardiovascular monitoring. Antihypertensive treatment and adrenergic blockade are ideally carried out with short-acting drugs such as nitroprusside or esmolol. Since tachydysrhythmias and hypertensive crises typically do not last long and may give way to bradycardia or hypotensive spells, short-acting drugs facilitate adjustment of therapy. Hypotension associated with vasodilatation responds well to intravenous fluid loading.

Efforts to stimulate muscle contractility directly with agents such as theophylline and digoxin have been investigated with conflicting results.[68] The lack of convincing evidence does not allow strong recommendations in this area.

Chronic Illness

In the patient with chronic weakness and borderline respiratory insufficiency, attention to all the details of general medical care discussed previously is vital. Efforts should be made to avoid contractures, scoliosis, and pressure sores.

Enteral or parenteral nutrition may improve respiratory muscle strength and exercise tolerance and reduce dyspnea in poorly nourished patients with respiratory disorders.[69, 70] The patient should be monitored for complications of nutritional therapy including increased CO_2 production and hypercapnia with carbohydrate loads,[71] hypophosphatemia,[49] and aspiration.

Dyspnea, the sensation of labored and uncomfortable breathing, may be troubling to the patient with chronic respiratory insufficiency and can cause exercise intolerance and sleep problems. Sensory mechanisms contributing to dyspnea are not well understood. The sensation of dyspnea does not depend on chemoreceptors, as it may occur with normal blood gases; neither is perception of forceful muscle contraction necessary, since patients with profound muscle weakness experience dyspnea. Afferent signals do not depend on spinal pathways since patients with cervical cord transection can have the sensation of dyspnea. It may be that perception of dyspnea arises from ascending neural impulses generated by respiratory centers in the brain stem.[72] Unfortunately, no available pharmacologic therapy can alleviate dyspnea without depressing respiratory drive. As weakness progresses, dyspnea and exercise intolerance may become incapacitating.

Occasional patients with central nervous system causes of respiratory insufficiency may benefit from diaphragm pacing[73] if the phrenic nerve and diaphragm function are intact. Although pacing is often successful, failure of some internal component (e.g., wire or insulation breakage) tends to occur after a mean of 56 months. Pacer-associated phrenic nerve injury is an occasional complication.

As deterioration progresses, tracheostomy without mechanical ventilation may improve the clearance of secretions.[20] Part-time positive-pressure breathing by noninvasive methods may improve the patient's functional state. Nasal or oral interface for assisted ventilation during sleep has been used successfully in older children and adults.[20, 74] Positive-pressure breathing may actually improve pulmonary mechanics in some cases, increasing vital capacity as atelectatic lung areas reexpand[75]; however, scarring in areas of previous pneumonia make such improvement inconsistent.[76] Full-time mechanical ventilation via tracheostomy may allow an individual to attend school, remain employed, and contribute to society.[75] When the patient has some respiratory muscle activity, ventilator frequency should be set low enough to allow some spontaneous breathing activity in hopes of avoiding disuse atrophy of respiratory muscles.

The alert ventilator-dependent patient with profound weakness or paralysis experiences an extraordinary level of stress. Discomfort, confusion, anxiety, and anger are constant problems, and systematic efforts must be made to deal with these in an age-appropriate fashion. Repeatedly orienting the patient to time and place and providing a schedule of activities are helpful. If possible, the patient should be allowed intervals of time during which no uncomfortable procedures will be carried out and should be given means to signal for help, communicate, and vent emotions. Involvement of family and friends and resumption of school activities and play are important in the chronic care of a pediatric ventilator-dependent patient.[77, 78]

In some cases, mechanical ventilation may have been initiated in a crisis only to result in permanent ventilator dependency. Progressive discomfort and disability may severely compromise the patient's quality of life, and the patient, family, and health care staff may agree that discontinuing mechanical ventilation is appropriate even though death may ensue.[79, 80] When this is the case, opiates or barbiturates should be administered in sufficient doses to provide comfort as mechanical ventilation is withdrawn. Intensive care unit staff have a vital role in emotionally supporting the patient and family during this difficult time and in adjusting therapy to optimize comfort.

References

1. Novak RW, Jones G, and Ch'ien LT: Acute transverse myelopathy in childhood. Clin Pediatr 17:894, 1978.
2. Trujillo MH, Castillo A, Espana J, et al: Impact of intensive care management on the prognosis of tetanus. Chest 92:63, 1987.
3. Zwiener RJ and Ginsburg CM: Organophosphate and carbamate poisoning in infants and children. Pediatrics 81:121, 1988.
4. Senanayake N and Karalliedde L: Neurotoxic effects of organophosphorus insecticides: An intermediate syndrome. N Engl J Med 316:761, 1987.
5. Lichtenfeld P: Autonomic dysfunction in the Guillain-Barré syndrome. Am J Med 50:772, 1971.
6. Auld PAM, Kevy SV, and Eley RC: Poliomyelitis in children. N Engl J Med 263:1094, 1960.
7. Mansel JK and Norman JR: Respiratory complications and management of spinal cord injuries. Chest 97:1447, 1990.
8. Bellemare F and Grassino A: Effect of pressure and timing of contraction on human diaphragm fatigue. J Appl Physiol 53:1190, 1982.
9. Nichols DG, Howell S, Massik J, et al: Relationship of diaphragmatic contractility to diaphragmatic blood flow in newborn lambs. J Appl Physiol 66:120, 1989.
10. Mead J: Control of respiratory frequency. J Appl Physiol 15:325, 1960.
11. Scardella AT, Santiago TV, and Edelman NH: Naloxone alters the early response to an inspiratory flow-resistive load. J Appl Physiol 67:1747, 1989.
12. Watchko JF, Standaert TA, Mayock DE, et al: Ventilatory failure during loaded breathing: The role of central neural drive. J Appl Physiol 65:249, 1988.
13. Kanter RK and Fordyce WE: Slowing of respiratory frequency accompanies respiratory failure with resistive loads. Pediatr Res 25:39A, 1989.
14. Lopes JM, Muller NL, Bryan MH, et al: Synergistic behavior of inspiratory muscles after diaphragmatic fatigue in the newborn. J Appl Physiol 51:547, 1981.
15. Tzelepis G, McCool FD, Leith DE, et al: Increased lung volume limits endurance of inspiratory muscles. J Appl Physiol 64:1796, 1988.
16. Gaultier C, Boule M, Tournier G, et al: Inspiratory force reserve of the respiratory muscles in children with chronic obstructive pulmonary disease. Am Rev Respir Dis 131:811, 1985.
17. Kosch PC and Stark AR: Dynamic maintenance of end expiratory lung volume in full-term infants. J Appl Physiol 57:1126, 1984.
18. Bryan AC and England SJ: Maintenance of an elevated FRC in the newborn: Paradox of REM sleep. Am Rev Respir Dis 129:209, 1984.
19. Smith PEM, Edwards RHT, and Calverley PMA: Ventilation and breathing pattern during sleep in Duchenne muscular dystrophy. Chest 96:1346, 1989.
20. Baydur A, Gilgoff I, Prentice W, et al: Decline in respiratory function and experience with long-term assisted ventilation in advanced Duchenne's muscular dystrophy. Chest 97:884, 1990.
21. Chen H and Tang Y: Sleep loss impairs inspiratory muscle endurance. Am Rev Respir Dis 140:907, 1989.
22. Canet E, Gaultier C, D'Allest AM, et al: Effects of sleep deprivation on respiratory events during sleep in healthy infants. J Appl Physiol 66:1158, 1989.
23. Scott CB, Nickerson BG, Sargent CW, et al: Developmental pattern of maximal transdiaphragmatic pressure in infants during crying. Pediatr Res 17:707, 1983.
24. Maxwell LC, McCarter R, Kuehl T, et al: Development of histochemical and functional properties of baboon respiratory muscles. J Appl Physiol 54:551, 1983.
25. Le Souef PN, England SJ, Stogryn HAF, et al: Comparison of diaphragmatic fatigue in newborn and older rabbits. J Appl Physiol 65:1040, 1988.
26. Laframboise WA, Standaert TA, Guthrie RD, et al: Developmental changes in the ventilatory response of the newborn to added airway resistance. Am Rev Respir Dis 136:1075, 1987.
27. Aubier M, Trippenbach T, and Roussos C: Respiratory muscle fatigue during cardiogenic shock. J Appl Physiol 51:499, 1981.
28. Hammond MD, Bauer KA, Sharp JT, et al: Respiratory muscle strength in congestive heart failure. Chest 98:1091, 1990.
29. Hussain SNA, Simkus G, and Roussos C: Respiratory muscle fatigue: A cause of ventilatory failure in septic shock. J Appl Physiol 58:2033, 1985.
30. Boczkowski J, Dureuil B, Branger C, et al: Effects of sepsis on diaphragmatic function in rats. Am Rev Respir Dis 138:260, 1988.
31. Mier-Jedrzejowicz A, Brophy C, and Green M: Respiratory muscle weakness during upper respiratory tract infections. Am Rev Respir Dis 138:5, 1988.
32. Clowes GHA, George BC, Villee CA, et al: Muscle proteolysis induced by a circulating peptide in patients with sepsis or trauma. N Engl J Med 308:545, 1983.
33. Arora NS and Rochester DF: Respiratory muscle strength and maximal voluntary ventilation in undernourished patients. Am Rev Respir Dis 126:5, 1982.
34. Jardim J, Farkas G, Prefaut C, et al: The failing inspiratory muscles under normoxic and hypoxic conditions. Am Rev Respir Dis 124:274, 1981.
35. Juan G, Calverley P, Talamo C, et al: Effect of carbon dioxide on diaphragmatic function in humans. N Engl J Med 310:874, 1984.
36. Aubier M, Viires N, Piquet J, et al: Effects of hypocalcemia on diaphragmatic strength generation. J Appl Physiol 58:2054, 1985.
37. Kolski GB, Cunningham AS, Niemec PW, et al: Hypokalemia and respiratory arrest in an infant with status asthmaticus. J Pediatr 112:304, 1988.
38. Aubier M, Murciano D, Lecocguic Y, et al: Effect of hypophosphatemia on diaphragmatic contractility in patients with acute respiratory failure. N Engl J Med 313:420, 1985.
39. Molloy DW, Dhingra S, Sloven F, et al: Hypomagnesemia and respiratory muscle power. Am Rev Respir Dis 129:497, 1984.
40. Zaloga GT: Interpretation of the serum magnesium level. Chest 95:257, 1989.
41. Mier A, Brophy C, Wass JAH, et al: Reversible muscle weakness in hyperthyroidism. Am Rev Respir Dis 139:529, 1989.
42. L'Hommedieu CS, Nicholas D, Armes DA, et al: Potentiation of magnesium sulfate–induced neuromuscular weakness by gentamicin, tobramycin, and amikacin. J Pediatr 102:629, 1983.
43. Nugent SK, Laravuso R, and Rogers MC: Pharmacology and use of muscle relaxants in infants and children. J Pediatr 94:481, 1979.
44. Partridge BL, Abrams JH, Bazemore C, et al: Prolonged neuromuscular blockade after long-term infusion of vecuronium bromide in the intensive care unit. Crit Care Med 18:1177, 1990.
45. Pascucci RC: Prolonged weakness after extended mechanical ventilation in a child. Crit Care Med 18:1181, 1990.
46. Rutledge ML, Hawkins EP, and Langston C: Skeletal muscle growth failure induced in premature newborn infants by prolonged pancuronium treatment. J Pediatr 109:883, 1986.
47. Knisely AS, Leal SM, and Singer DB: Abnormalities of diaphragmatic muscle in neonates with ventilated lungs. J Pediatr 113:1074, 1988.
48. Janssens S and Decramer M: Corticosteroid-induced myopathy and the respiratory muscles. Chest 95:1160, 1989.
49. Mezoff AG, Gremse DA, and Farrell MK: Hypophosphatemia in the nutritional recovery syndrome. Am J Dis Child 143:1111, 1989.
50. Van Der Spek AFL, Fang WB, Ashton-Miller JA, et al: The effects of succinylcholine on mouth opening. Anesthesiology 67:459, 1987.
51. Benthuysen JL, Smith NT, and Sanford TJ: Physiology of alfentanil-induced rigidity. Anesthesiology 64:440, 1986.
52. Schmidt-Nowara WW and Altman AR: Atelectasis and neuromuscular respiratory failure. Chest 85:792, 1984.
53. Magder S, Lockhat D, Luo BJ, et al: Respiratory muscle and

organ blood flow with inspiratory elastic loading and shock. J Appl Physiol 58:1148, 1985.

54. DeVita MA and Spierer-Rundback L: Swallowing disorders in patients with prolonged orotracheal intubation or tracheotomy tubes. Crit Care Med 18:1328, 1990.

55. Malsch E: Maximal inspiratory force in infants and children. Southern Med J 71:428, 1978.

56. Shoults D, Clarke TA, Benumof JL, et al: Maximum inspiratory force in predicting successful neonatal tracheal extubation. Crit Care Med 7:485, 1979.

57. Andreou A, Keh E, Bhat R, et al: Critical care problems in the newborn: CVC in infants on assisted ventilation. Crit Care Med 8:291, 1980.

58. Shimada Y, Yoshiya I, Tanaka K, et al: Crying, vital capacity, and maximal inspiratory pressure as clinical indicators of readiness for weaning of infants less than a year of age. Anesthesiology 51:456, 1979.

59. Belani KG, Gilmour IJ, McComb RC, et al: Pre-extubation ventilatory measurements in newborns and infants. Anesth Analg 59:467, 1980.

60. Pourriat JL, Lamberto C, Hoang PH, et al: Diagraphmatic fatigue and breathing pattern during weaning from mechanical ventilation in COPD patients. Chest 90:703, 1986.

61. Murciano D, Boczkowski J, Lecocguic Y, et al: Tracheal occlusion pressure: A simple index to monitor respiratory muscle fatigue during acute respiratory failure in patients with chronic obstructive pulmonary disease. Ann Intern Med 108:800, 1988.

62. Moxham J, Edwards RHT, Aubier M, et al: Changes in EMG power spectrum (high to low ratio) with force fatigue in humans. J Appl Physiol 53:1094, 1982.

63. Roussos C and Macklem PT: The respiratory muscles. N Engl J Med 307:786, 1982.

64. Hershenson MB, Kikuchi Y, Tzelepis GE, et al: Preferential fatigue of the rib cage muscles during inspiratory resistive loaded ventilation. J Appl Physiol 66:750, 1989.

65. Aubier M, Murciano D, Menu Y, et al: Dopamine effects on diaphragmatic strength during acute respiratory failure in chronic obstructive pulmonary disease. Ann Intern Med 110:17, 1989.

66. Rochester DF: Does respiratory muscle rest relieve fatigue or incipient fatigue? Am Rev Respir Dis 138:516, 1988.

67. Sessler DI: Malignant hyperthermia. J Pediatr 109:9, 1986.

68. Aubier M: Pharmacologic strategies for treating respiratory failure. Chest 97:98S, 1990.

69. Kelly SM, Rosa A, Field S, et al: Inspiratory muscle strength and body composition in patients receiving total parenteral nutrition therapy. Am Rev Respir Dis 130:33, 1984.

70. Efthimiou J, Fleming J, Gomes C, et al: The effect of supplementary oral nutrition in poorly nourished patients with chronic obstructive pulmonary disease. Am Rev Respir Dis 137:1075, 1988.

71. Covelli HD, Black JW, Olsen MS, et al: Respiratory failure precipitated by high carbohydrate loads. Ann Intern Med 95:579, 1981.

72. Chen Z, Wagner PG, and Eldridge FL: Respiratory related rhythmic firing of midbrain neurons: Relation to level of respiratory drive. FASEB J 4:405A, 1990.

73. Weese-Mayer DE, Morrow AS, Brouillette RT, et al: Diaphragm pacing in infants and children. Am Rev Respir Dis 139:974, 1989.

74. Bach JR, Alba AS, and Shin D: Management alternatives for post polio respiratory insufficiency: Assisted ventilation by nasal or oral nasal interface. Am J Phys Med Rehab 68:264, 1989.

75. Gilgoff IS, Kahlstrom E, MacLaughlin E, et al: Long term ventilatory support in spinal muscular atrophy. J Pediatr 115:904, 1989.

76. DeTroyer A and Desser P: The effects of intermittent positive pressure breathing on patients with respiratory muscle weakness. Am Rev Respir Dis 124:132, 1981.

77. McBride MM and Sach WH: Emotional management of children with acute respiratory failure in the intensive care unit. Heart Lung 9:98, 1980.

78. Parker MM, Schubert W, Shelhamer JH, et al: Perceptions of a critically ill patient experiencing therapeutic paralysis in an ICU. Crit Care Med 12:69, 1984.

79. Schneiderman LJ and Spragg RG: Ethical decisions in discontinuing mechanical ventilation. N Engl J Med 318:984, 1988.

80. Leikin S: A proposal concerning decisions to forego life sustaining treatment for young people. J Pediatr 115:17, 1989.

52

Oxygen Transport

James D. Wilkinson, M.D.

One of the fundamental goals of critical care medicine is to ensure the delivery of sufficient oxygen to metabolically active tissues to subserve cellular energy production and, thus, maintain vital organ integrity and function in the seriously ill patient.

The role of the lung and the cardiovascular system in the delivery of inspired oxygen to various organs is described elsewhere in this text. This chapter reviews the physiologic and biochemical aspects of the movement of oxygen from the alveolus to the pulmonary capillary erythrocyte, its binding and subsequent release by hemoglobin, and its uptake and utilization by the cells of peripheral tissues. Clinical methods of monitoring tissue oxygenation are also reviewed.

ALVEOLAR-PULMONARY CAPILLARY OXYGEN TRANSPORT

Oxygen moves from the alveolus to the pulmonary capillary by a process of diffusion. The diffusion of a gas through a tissue phase is described by Fick's law:

$$V \text{ gas} = \frac{A}{T} \cdot D \cdot (C_1 - C_2)$$

in which A is the alveolar-capillary membrane area; T is the thickness of the alveolar-capillary membrane; D is constant $\alpha \sqrt{\dfrac{\text{solubility}}{\text{molecular weight of gas}}}$ and $(C_1 - C_2)$ is the concentration gradient of the gas across the tissue. Diffusion is directly proportional to the partial pressure gradient, the alveolar-capillary membrane area, and the gas solubility; it is inversely proportional to the thickness of the membrane and the molecular weight of the gas. In the lung, A is extremely large and T is less than 0.5 μm, which efficiently maximizes diffusion capacity. Using Henry's law, $C \text{ gas} = K \cdot P \text{ gas}$, partial pressures may be substituted in the aforementioned equation for clinical convenience. The resultant equation becomes:

$$V \text{ gas} = \frac{A}{T} \cdot D \cdot (P_1 - P_2)$$

Specifically, for the diffusion of oxygen we can write:

$$V_{O_2} = \frac{A}{T} \cdot D_{O_2} \cdot (P_{A O_2} - P_{C O_2})$$

in which $P_{A O_2}$ and $P_{C O_2}$ are the alveolar and capillary partial pressures of oxygen, respectively.

Since normally A, T, and oxygen solubility are relatively constant, the most important variable influencing alveolar-capillary oxygen exchange is the partial pressure gradient, $(P_{A O_2} - P_{C O_2})$. Alveolar partial pressure of oxygen, $P_{A O_2}$, can be determined using the simplified *alveolar gas equation*[1]:

$$P_{A O_2} = P_{I O_2} - \frac{P_{a C O_2}}{RQ}$$

The inspired partial pressure of oxygen, $P_{I O_2}$, can be calculated using a derivation of Dalton's law for gas mixtures, corrected for water vapor pressure (47 mm Hg):

$$P_{I O_2} = (P_{bar} - 47) \cdot F_{I O_2}$$

For room air ($F_{I O_2} = 0.21$), at normal barometric pressure, 760 mm Hg,

$$\begin{aligned} P_{I O_2} &= (760 - 47) \cdot 0.21 \\ &= 149.7 \text{ mm Hg} \end{aligned}$$

Substituting this value into the alveolar gas equation along with a normal $P_{a C O_2}$ of 40 mm Hg and a respiratory quotient of 0.8:

$$\begin{aligned} P_{A O_2} &= 149.7 \text{ mm Hg} - 50.0 \text{ mm Hg} \\ &= 99.7 \text{ mm Hg} \end{aligned}$$

For clinical purposes, the mixed venous partial pressure of oxygen, normally about 40 mm Hg, may be used for the $P_{C O_2}$. Therefore, the usual diffusion gradient for oxygen, $P_{A O_2}$-$P_{C O_2}$, is about 60 mm Hg. By comparison, this is about 12 times the pulmonary capillary-alveolar partial pressure gradient for carbon dioxide. However, carbon dioxide is more than 20 times as soluble as oxygen, so that it diffuses across the capillary-alveolar interface slightly less than twice as fast as oxygen.

Physiologically, diffusion of alveolar oxygen into the pulmonary capillaries is actually a two-step process: (1) the nearly instantaneous physical diffusion of gaseous oxygen across the alveolar-capillary membrane into the erythrocyte (a distance of 1 to 2 μm), and (2) the relatively slow chemical reaction of oxygen and deoxyhemoglobin, which takes about 0.2 second.[2] In the person at rest, red blood cell transit time through a pulmonary capillary is quite brief, about 0.75 second. Given a normal P_{AO_2} of 100 mm Hg, oxygen uptake is essentially complete about one third of the way through the erythrocyte's capillary transit. With increases in blood flow (as with exercise or other hyperdynamic cardiac states), the capillary transit time may be reduced by up to two thirds to about 0.25 second.[2] This means that oxygen-hemoglobin binding, taking 0.2 second, still should not be a rate-limiting step in pulmonary capillary oxygen uptake. In other words, since the normal diffusion time is less than the pulmonary capillary transit time, even at high cardiac outputs, pulmonary oxygen uptake is mostly limited by perfusion rather than by diffusion.

From the discussion earlier, it is apparent that disease states that create diffusion defects can limit pulmonary capillary oxygen uptake. Again by Fick's law, the volume of oxygen transported from the alveolus to the capillary may be limited by decreases in alveolar-capillary membrane area (atelectasis), increases in alveolar-capillary membrane distance (fibrosis, interstitial edema), or decreased partial pressure gradients, usually by decreased P_{AO_2} (hypoxia). The latter is most easily corrected simply by increasing inspired oxygen, F_{IO_2}.

As already noted, in the absence of diffusion defects, pulmonary capillary O_2 uptake is mostly perfusion, or cardiac output, dependent. Increases in pulmonary blood flow facilitate gas exchange by providing more deoxygenated blood to the proximal pulmonary capillary per unit time, thus maximally maintaining the alveolar-proximal pulmonary capillary oxygen diffusion gradient. Significant decreases in pulmonary perfusion alone (shock, pulmonary artery occlusion) may result in decreased pulmonary oxygen uptake or may worsen the effects of a diffusion defect.

Clinically, decreases in pulmonary oxygen uptake may result from either diffusion or perfusion defects. The magnitude of these deficits can be described by the alveolar-arterial ($P_{AO_2} - P_{aO_2}$) oxygen gradient, in the absence of intracardiac or aortopulmonary artery shunts. Large $P_{AO_2} - P_{aO_2}$ values are most likely the result of low alveolar O_2 partial pressures, ventilation-perfusion mismatching, or low cardiac output states.

OXYGEN TRANSPORT BY BLOOD

The *arterial oxygen content*, CaO_2, is calculated using the following equation:

$$CaO_2 \text{ (ml/dl)} = (1.34 \times Hgb \times SO_2) + (0.003 \times PO_2)$$

(SO_2 = oxygen saturation). For a normal hemoglobin concentration of 15 g/100 ml of blood, an arterial SO_2 of 1.00 (100%), and a PO_2 of 80 mm Hg:

$$
\begin{aligned}
CaO_2 \text{ (ml/dl)} &= (1.34 \cdot 15 \cdot 1.00) + (0.003 \cdot 80) \\
&= 20.1 + 0.24 \\
&= 20.34 \text{ ml/dl}
\end{aligned}
$$

By combining CaO_2 with a measure of flow, cardiac output (C.O.), we obtain the amount of oxygen delivered to the tissues per unit time, or *oxygen delivery*, $\dot{D}O_2$:

$$\dot{D}O_2 = CaO_2 \cdot C.O.$$

Oxygen delivery, $\dot{D}O_2$, may also be called oxygen availability or oxygen transport.

The arterial oxygen content equation demonstrates that only a minimal amount (<1%) of oxygen is transported dissolved in blood. It is only oxygen's singular affinity for hemoglobin that allows oxygen delivery to meet even normal resting tissue oxygen demands (or O_2 consumption, $\dot{V}O_2$), about 120 to 160 ml/min/m².[3]

OXYGEN-HEMOGLOBIN AFFINITY

The concentration of hemoglobin in the erythrocyte is extremely high, about 32 g/dl.[4] Its intracellular location allows maximizing hemoglobin's oxygen-carrying capacity while minimizing its plasma osmotic effects. Each hemoglobin A molecule (molecular weight = 64,400 daltons) consists of four monomers (2 α and 2 β), each composed of a peptide chain and an iron-containing heme moiety. The iron atoms, in the ferrous [Fe^{2+}] state, are capable of a reversible binding reaction with a molecule of oxygen, without any resultant change of valence.

In the deoxygenated, or tense conformational, state, the hemoglobin molecule is resistant to oxygen binding. However, the binding of a single oxygen molecule to an α subunit results in conformation changes in the other monomers toward the more relaxed oxyhemoglobin state. This results in increasing affinity for binding of each subsequent oxygen molecule up to a total of four, representing complete oxygen saturation of that individual hemoglobin molecule. The facilitation of subsequent oxygen binding by the already bound oxygen is called heme-heme interaction.[4]

Human fetal hemoglobin, hemoglobin F, is made up of 2 α and 2 γ subunits. The switch from production of fetal to adult hemoglobin occurs just before birth in the full-term infant and is usually complete by about 6 months of age. Hemoglobin F has a lower organic phosphate affinity relative to hemoglobin A, resulting in an increased oxygen affinity (see later).

Oxyhemoglobin Dissociation Curve

As noted earlier, nearly all oxygen is carried in the blood bound to hemoglobin. In other words, the oxygen-carrying capacity of blood is directly related to the hemoglobin concentration and to oxygen's affinity for that hemoglobin. The affinity of hemoglobin for oxygen is related to the blood PO_2 and is described by the oxygen dissociation curve (ODC) (Fig. 52–1).[5] Oxygen-hemoglobin affinities are most commonly described or compared by the P_{50}, the PO_2 at which hemoglobin is 50% saturated. The normal in vivo P_{50} for hemoglobin A is 27 mm Hg (at pH 7.4, 37° C).[6] By contrast, hemoglobin F, with its increased oxygen affinity mentioned earlier, has a P_{50} of 19 mm Hg.

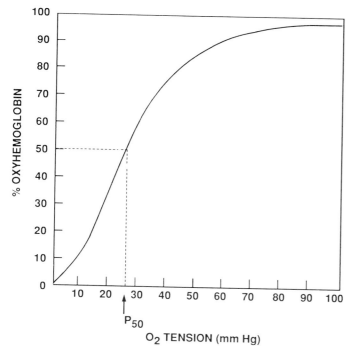

Figure 52–1. The standard oxyhemoglobin dissociation curve.

The sigmoidal shape of the curve is advantageous for both pulmonary capillary uptake and tissue release of oxygen. At the upper, flattened part of the curve, hemoglobin is nearly 100% saturated over the range of P_{O_2} (70 − >100 mm Hg) commonly found in the pulmonary capillary. The steeper portion of the curve corresponds to increasingly enhanced dissociation of oxygen from hemoglobin at the lower P_{O_2} values of tissue capillary blood. Evidence indicates that oxygen may not be available to tissues at a mixed venous (end capillary) value of less than 20 mm Hg.[7] Oxygen delivery may be adjusted to account for this finding:

$$\dot{D}_{O_2} = (Ca_{O_2} - [(S20\bar{v}O_2 \cdot 1.34 \cdot Hgb) + 0.063]) \times C.O.$$

in which $S20\bar{v}O_2$ is the oxygen saturation of blood at a P_{O_2} of 20 mm Hg. This concept is called "consumable oxygen."[8]

In terms of the ODC, conditions that *increase* the affinity of oxygen for hemoglobin cause *"shifts to the left"* in the curve's position. Conversely, conditions that *decrease* oxygen affinity result in *"shifts to the right"* (Fig. 52–2).[9, 10] The principal modulators of oxygen-hemoglobin affinity are temperature, pH (Bohr effect), and the 2,3-diphosphoglycerate (DPG) concentration in the erythrocyte.

Temperature. Increasing temperature results in a decreased oxygen affinity for hemoglobin, a "shift to the right" of the ODC. Conversely, with decreasing temperature, oxygen affinity increases.[11, 12] In vitro, a 10° C increase in temperature almost doubles the P_{50}. Clinically, this effect favors off-loading of oxygen to tissues in hypermetabolic states, such as fever.

Bohr Effect. The effect on O_2 binding of CO_2 in the blood is known as the Bohr effect, a combination of

fixed acid [H^+] and direct CO_2 effects.[13, 14] The Bohr effect describes the "shift to the right" of the ODC, which is predominantly the result of increased H^+ ion concentration (decreased pH) produced from hydration of CO_2 to carbonic acid catalyzed by erythrocyte carbonic anhydrase. The binding of carbon dioxide to deoxyhemoglobin, creating carbamino-hemoglobin, also decreases oxygen affinity, but the effect is minor compared with the effect of increases in H^+ concentration.[15] Both of the aforementioned effects of CO_2 on oxygen affinity favor the release of oxygen for aerobic metabolism in the more acidic, CO_2-rich blood of the tissue capillaries. Moreover, the Bohr effect is not constant along the ODC but increases at lower oxygen saturations, further favoring the off-loading of oxygen in the tissue capillaries.[16]

Red Blood Cell Organic Phosphates. In the red blood cell, glycolysis is anaerobic and results in the production of 2,3-DPG via the Rapoport-Luebering shunt, without net production of adenosine triphosphate (ATP).[4] The concentration of 2,3-DPG in the erythrocyte is essentially equimolar with hemoglobin (about 5 mM). It decreases hemoglobin's affinity for oxygen in two ways: (1) through direct binding to deoxyhemoglobin, forming salt bridges between peptide chains, and (2) through its multiple acid groups, which lower intraerythrocyte pH relative to that of plasma.[17, 18] The effects of 2,3-DPG on oxygen affinity are not immediate, as are those of temperature and pH. The effects of 2,3-DPG are dependent on both saturation and temperature. Increased concentrations of 2,3-DPG in the erythrocyte may be found with respiratory alkalosis, anemia, cyanotic car-

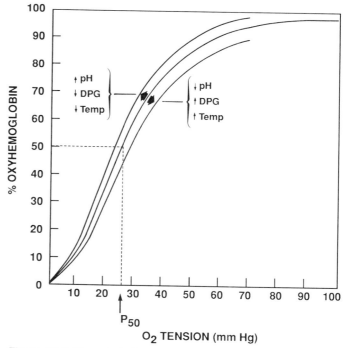

Figure 52–2. The principal modulators of oxygen-hemoglobin affinity and their effect on the position of the oxyhemoglobin dissociation curve.

diac disease, and chronic lung disease. 2,3-DPG concentrations decrease with advanced red blood cell age, particularly in banked blood products. The abnormally high oxygen affinity of 2,3-DPG–depleted banked blood may persist for up to 24 hours after transfusion. Inorganic phosphate deficiency may also result in lowered 2,3-DPG concentrations.

METHEMOGLOBIN, CARBOXYHEMOGLOBIN, AND MYOGLOBIN

Oxidation of the 4 heme iron atoms to the ferric state, Fe^{3+}, creates methemoglobin, which binds oxygen ***irreversibly***, making it unavailable at the tissue cellular level for aerobic metabolism. Exposure to various oxidants (aniline dyes, nitrites) may result in clinically significant methemoglobinemia. The normally limited endogenous red blood cell (nicotinamide-adenine dinucleotide [NADH]-dependent) capacity for the reduction of methemoglobin may be augmented by the administration of methylene blue, which serves as an electron acceptor for another, usually nonfunctioning, nicotinamide-adenine dinucleotide phosphate (NADPH)-dependent pathway.[4]

Carboxyhemoglobin binds reversibly to hemoglobin with an affinity more than 200 times that of oxygen.[19] Carbon monoxide's increased affinity is not a result of faster binding to hemoglobin, but rather of a much slower dissociation rate when compared with that of oxygen. Therefore, the presence of carbon monoxide decreases available binding sites for oxygen. Carbon monoxide also decreases available oxygen by increasing the affinity of any remaining hemoglobin monomers, functionally shifting the ODC to the left.[20, 21]

Myoglobin has a high affinity for oxygen and may represent a skeletal muscle reserve store of oxygen that is available for release at the very low tissue PO_2 (<15 mm Hg) resulting from exercise.

STROMA-FREE HEMOGLOBIN

Development of a stroma-free hemoglobin (SFH), an acellular solution of hemoglobin from which all other erythrocyte components have been removed, has many potential advantages: ease of storage, long shelf-life, decreased cost, avoidance of immune or infectious patient complications, relatively unlimited availability, and perhaps, low cost. Purified SFH solutions have several disadvantages that have limited their clinical usefulness: high oncotic load, brief plasma half-life (<4 hours), and very high oxygen affinity (P_{50} < 20 mm Hg) due to low 2,3-DPG levels.[22]

Recently, polymerized, pyridoxilated SFH solutions have been produced resulting in plasma concentrations around 14 g/dl, almost normal oncotic pressure, and plasma half-lives of 40 to 46 hours.[23] The P_{50} remains low for these compounds (about 20 mm Hg) but in animal experiments, off-loading of oxygen has occurred even in the presence of erythrocytes with a more normal

P_{50} of 27 mm Hg. Moreover, polymerized, pyridoxilated SFH solutions have been shown to have significantly fewer deleterious effects on cardiovascular function and global oxygen consumption than purified SFH.[24] These improvements, plus increasing concerns with transfusion-associated infections with hepatitis B virus, cytomegalovirus, and human immunodeficiency virus, hold promise for future clinical applicability in critically ill patients.

TISSUE OXYGEN TRANSPORT: CAPILLARY TO CELL

Several characteristics of the microcirculation are important to oxygen transport, although their clinical significance in various disease states is not well defined. Arteriolar and precapillary sphincter tone, under both neural and humoral control, as well as cardiac output affect both capillary recruitment and transit time. These may be important, particularly in conditions such as septic shock, or central nervous system injuries. Capillary hematocrit also has important implications for capillary oxygen availability.

In tissue capillaries, oxygen moves from the red blood cell through the plasma into tissues by diffusion governed by Fick's law as described earlier for the pulmonary capillary. Specifically,

$$\dot{V}O_2 = Dt \times (PcO_2 - PmitO_2)$$

in which Dt is the Krogh diffusion coefficient and PcO_2 and $PmitO_2$ represent the partial pressures of oxygen in the capillary and mitochondrion, respectively.[25] The classic geometric model to describe tissue oxygenation was developed by Krogh early in the present century. In this model, each capillary is at the center of a cylinder of tissue whose long axis is parallel to the capillary (Fig. 52–3). Several assumptions are implicit in this model: (1) adjacent cylinders are independently perfused, with an intercapillary distance of twice the cylinder radius; (2) oxygen diffusion is dependent only on radial oxygen gradients; and (3) all capillaries are simultaneously patent.

The radial oxygen diffusion gradient, the partial pressure of oxygen at any point in the tissue, is described by the Krogh-Erlang equation:

$$PO_2 x = PO_2 - \frac{\dot{V}O_2}{2K^2} \left(R2 \ln \frac{x}{r} - \frac{x^2 - r^2}{2} \right)$$

in which x is the distance from the capillary, R is the radius of tissue cylinder, r is the capillary's radius, $\dot{V}O_2$ is the tissue oxygen consumption, and K is a diffusion constant.[26, 27] If tissue oxygen consumption is uniform, the O_2 saturation drops linearly along the capillary. The PO_2 drops off more sharply, as predicted from the ODC (Fig. 52–4). As PO_2 drops along the capillary, the radial diffusion gradient ***decreases***, exposing "lethal corners" that are outside the effective radius for oxygen diffusion at the venous end of the cylinder (see Fig. 52–3). This model, which may have some anatomic validity in tissues such as skeletal muscle, is mostly of conceptual value in describing the movement of oxygen from the microcir-

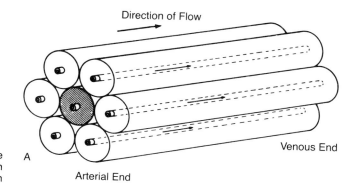

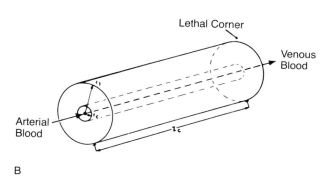

Figure 52–3. *A,* The geometric model used by Krogh to describe tissue oxygen transport. *B,* A single capillary-tissue cylinder from the Krogh model. The "lethal corner" lies outside the effective radius for oxygen diffusion. (Reprinted with permission from Fletcher JE: Mathematical modeling of the microcirculation. Math Biosci 38:159–202, 1978. Copyright 1978 by Elsevier Science Publishing Co., Inc.)

culation to the individual organ cells. The Krogh model does not account for redundant or corollary capillary supply to tissue cylinders, nonlinear capillary arrangement, or microcirculatory conformational changes in contractile tissues. Also, decreased intercapillary distances at the venous end of the capillary beds could potentially protect tissue oxygenation in the "lethal corners."

CELLULAR OXYGEN METABOLISM

Cellular survival, as well as specific metabolic function, depends on the continuous synthesis of high-energy compounds, particularly ATP. About 80 to 90% of cellular oxygen consumption occurs in the mitochondria, with molecular oxygen serving as the final electron acceptor in the electron transport chain that provides the energy to drive oxidative phosphorylation.

Glucose is metabolized in the cytosol to 2 molecules of pyruvate and is then converted into acetyl-CoA and 2 electron pairs. Metabolism of amino acids or fatty acids also results in the production of acetyl-CoA. The acetyl-CoA enters into the tricarboxylic, or citric, acid cycle in the mitochondria with the production of carbon dioxide and 4 more electron pairs (Fig. 52–5). Each electron pair moves along the electron transport chain in which its final acceptor is oxygen. In the presence of inorganic phosphate and adenosine diphosphate (ADP),

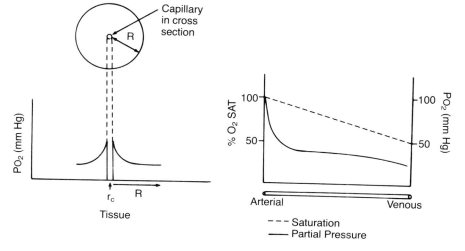

Figure 52–4. Radial oxygen diffusion gradients around a single capillary. (Reprinted with permission from Siesjo BK: Brain Energy Metabolism. New York, John Wiley, 1978. Copyright 1978. Reprinted by permission of John Wiley & Sons, Inc.)

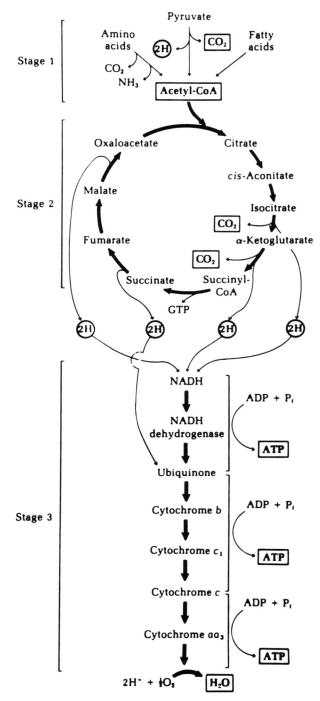

Figure 52–5. Cell respiration with the production of ATP. Stage 1: Production of acetyl-CoA. Stage 2: The tricarboxylic acid cycle. Stage 3: Electron transport coupled with oxidative phosphorylation. (Reprinted with permission from Lehninger A: Biochemistry: The Molecular Basis of Cell Structure and Function. New York, Worth Publishers, 1975.)

the transport of each pair of electrons produces 3 molecules of ATP.[28]

The phosphorylation of ADP to ATP at normal body temperature and pH creates a high-energy bond that stores about 12,000 calories. The oxidation of each molecule of glucose, requiring 6 molecules of oxygen,

results in the production of 36 molecules of ATP, representing stores of 432,000 kcal of bioavailable energy.

In the absence of sufficient mitochondrial oxygen, or in the presence of electron transport poisons such as cyanide ion, there is a marked decrease in electron transport activity, and the cell produces ATP anaerobically from the conversion of pyruvate to lactate. This process is less than 20% as efficient as aerobic glycolysis.[28] In addition to the marked decrease in ATP production, the accumulated lactic acid lowers tissue pH and depletes cellular NAD^+ necessary for aerobic glycolysis. Another anaerobic energy (ATP)–producing pathway found in brain and cardiac muscle involves the degradation of creatine phosphate by creatine kinase.

Oxygen is necessary for several nonenergy-producing chemical reactions of importance to mammalian cells involving enzymes such as mixed function oxidases, cytochrome P_{450}, and ceruloplasmin. Specifically important in critically ill patients is the requirement for oxygen by the phagocyte respiratory burst[29]:

$$A + NADPH + O_2 \; NADPH \; oxidase \rightarrow AH + NADP+ + O_2^- \; (\text{where A is one of several substrates}).$$

The superoxide produced is converted to other active oxygen radicals (singlet $^1O_2$ and OH·) and hydrogen peroxide formed subsequently, all of which are actively involved in the killing of phagocytosed bacteria.[28] Cytosolic superoxide dismutase and catalase are present to detoxify the reactive oxygen species, thus protecting phagocytic cell integrity. Patients with chronic granulomatous disease, who have a congenital deficiency of NADPH oxidase, often have serious, life-threatening bacterial infections.[30]

OXYGEN TRANSPORT MONITORING

Oxygen delivery, $\dot{D}o_2$, is a function of both arterial oxygen content and flow:

$$\dot{D}o_2, \; ml/min = Cao_2 \cdot C.O.$$

This measurement gives no information, however, regarding tissue oxygen demand or distribution. In specific conditions, such as septic shock, "optimal values" for $\dot{D}o_2$ and other transport measurements (e.g., $\dot{V}o_2$, O_2ER) have been derived and validated clinically and associated positively with increased survival.[31] Their applicability outside of the specific study conditions is less well confirmed.

Mixed venous oxygen partial pressure, $P\bar{v}o_2$, and saturation, $S\bar{v}o_2$, have been advanced as accurate representations of tissue oxygenation.[32] This relationship is based on the Krogh model and assumes normal blood flow distribution, steady-state oxygen consumption, and a physiologic P_{50}. Redistribution of normal blood flow patterns or shunting, derangements in global and regional oxygen consumption patterns, and alterations in modulators of oxygen affinity in various pathologic states may account for the failure of mixed venous oxygen measurements to consistently correlate with clinical organ function. Continuous monitoring of mixed venous oxygen saturations, while technically convenient, has the same intrinsic limitations as indicators of tissue oxygenation as the $P\bar{v}_{O_2}$. Regional venous oxygen measurements might be more accurate indicators of local oxygen conditions but are technically difficult.

Oxygen consumption, $\dot{V}_{O_2}$, is independent of oxygen delivery at normal or high levels but becomes dependent on oxygen delivery at low values of $\dot{D}_{O_2}$.[33, 34] This biphasic relationship has been questioned in some pathologic states, such as adult respiratory distress syndrome, which appear to exhibit a "pathologic oxygen supply dependency" even under physiologic oxygen delivery conditions.[35]

The oxygen extraction ratio, O_2ER, compares the supply-demand relationship between oxygen delivery and consumption:

$$O_2 \text{ extraction ratio} = \frac{\dot{V}_{O_2}}{\dot{D}_{O_2}} = \frac{(Ca_{O_2} - Cv_{O_2}) \cdot C.O.}{Ca_{O_2} \cdot C.O.}$$

and therefore represents a measure of global oxygen transport efficiency. The usual value is around 20 to 25%. Extraction ratios rise under conditions of inadequate oxygen delivery; sustained extraction ratios of 70 to 80% may be inconsistent with survival in humans. O_2ER may be low in conditions of significant shunting or, theoretically, cellular respiratory poisoning.

Several biochemical markers of tissue oxygen transport have been suggested, with $[H^+]$ concentration and serum lactate being the most common.[36–38] Once again, based on the Krogh model, some investigators have suggested venous, rather than arterial, $[H^+]$ concentrations as more representative of tissue anaerobic states.[36] Serum lactate's usefulness as an accurate measure of tissue anaerobic states may be limited by variations in clearance of lactate due to hepatic dysfunction, as well as altered lactate utilization as substrate in pathologic states such as multiple organ failure.[39] With normal hepatic function, prolonged serum lactate half-lives (normally about 40 minutes) probably represent significant anaerobic metabolism.[40]

References

1. Dantzker DR: Pulmonary gas exchange. *In*: Dantzker DR (ed): Cardiopulmonary Critical Care. Philadelphia, WB Saunders, 1986, p. 27.
2. West JB: Respiratory Physiology, 4th ed. Baltimore, Williams & Wilkins, 1990, pp. 21–30.
3. Shoemaker WC: Physiologic monitoring of the critically ill patient. *In*: Shoemaker WC, Ayres S, Holbrook PR, et al (eds): Textbook of Critical Care, 2nd ed. Philadelphia, WB Saunders, 1989, pp. 145–159.
4. Ranney HM and Rapaport SI: The red blood cell. *In*: West JB (ed): Physiological Basis of Medical Practice, 11th ed. Baltimore, Williams & Wilkins, 1985, pp. 398–408.
5. Nunn JF: Applied Respiratory Physiology, 2nd ed. London, Butterworths, 1977, p. 441.
6. Severinghaus JW: Simple accurate equations for human blood O_2 dissociation computations. J Appl Physiol 46:599, 1979.
7. Lennox W, Gibbs F, and Gibbs E: Relationship of unconsciousness to cerebral blood flow and to anoxemia. Arch Neurol Psychol 34:1001, 1935.
8. Bryan-Brown CW, Baek SM, Makabali G, et al: Consumable oxygen: Oxygen availability in relation to oxyhemoglobin dissociation. Crit Care Med 1:17, 1973.
9. Shappell SD and Lenfant C: Adaptive, genetic and iatrogenic alterations of the oxyhemoglobin dissociation curve. Anesthesiology 37:127, 1972.
10. Malmberg PO, Hlastala MP, and Woodson RD: Effect of increased blood-oxygen affinity on oxygen transport in hemorrhagic shock. J Appl Physiol 47:891, 1979.
11. Reeves RB: The effect of temperature on the oxygen equilibrium curve of human blood. Respir Physiol 42:317, 1980.
12. Zwart A, Kwant G, Oeseburg B, et al: Human whole-blood affinity: Effect of temperature. J Appl Physiol 57:429, 1984.
13. Bohr C, Hasselbalch K, and Krogh A: Uber einen biologische Beziehung wichtigen Einfluss den die Kohlensaurespannung des Blutes auf dessen Sauerstoffbindung abt. Skand Arch Physiol 16:402, 1904.
14. Margaria R and Green AA: The first dissociation constant, pK1, of carbonic acid in hemoglobin solutions and its relation to the existence of a combination of hemoglobin with carbon dioxide. J Biol Chem 103:611, 1933.
15. Hlastala MP: Physiological significance of the interaction of oxygen and carbon dioxide in blood. Crit Care Med 7:374, 1979.
16. Hlastala MP and Woodson RD: Saturation dependency of the Bohr effect: Interactions among H^+, CO_2, and DPG. J Appl Physiol 38:1126, 1975.
17. Benesch R and Benesch RE: The effect of organic phosphates from the human erythrocyte on the allosteric properties of hemoglobin. Biochem Biophys Res Commun 26:162, 1967.
18. Bauer C, Klocke A, Kamp D, et al: Effect of 2,3-diphosphoglycerate and H^+ on the reaction of O_2 and hemoglobin. Am J Physiol 224:838, 1973.
19. Collier CR: Oxygen affinity of human blood in the presence of carbon monoxide. J Appl Physiol 40:487, 1976.
20. Hlastala MP, McKenna HP, Franada RL, et al: Influence of carbon monoxide on hemoglobin-oxygen binding. J Appl Physiol 41:893, 1976.
21. Coburn RF: Mechanisms of carbon monoxide toxicity. Prev Med 8:310, 1979.
22. Rabiner SF, Helbert JR, Lapos H, et al: Evaluation of a stroma free hemoglobin solution as a plasma expander. J Exp Med 126:1127, 1967.
23. Sehgal LR, Gould SA, Rosen AL, et al: Polymerized pyridoxilated hemoglobin: A red cell substitute with normal oxygen capacity. Surgery 95:433, 1984.
24. Gould SA, Sehgal LR, Rosen AL, et al: The efficacy of polymerized pyridoxilated hemoglobin solution as an oxygen carrier. Ann Surg 211:397, 1990.
25. Krogh A: The number and distribution of capillaries in muscle with calculations of the oxygen pressure head necessary for supplying the tissue. J Appl Physiol 52:409, 1919.
26. Krogh A: Anatomy and Physiology of Capillaries. New Haven, Yale University Press, 1922.
27. Cone JB: Oxygen transport from capillary to cell. *In*: Snyder JV and Pinsky MR (eds): Oxygen Transport in the Critically Ill. Chicago, Year Book Medical Publishers, 1987, p. 153.
28. Cone JB: Cellular oxygen utilization. *In*: Snyder JV and Pinsky MR (eds): Oxygen Transport in the Critically Ill. Chicago, Year Book Medical Publishers, 1987, pp. 157–163.
29. Babior BM: Oxygen dependent microbial killing by phagocytes. N Engl J Med 298:659, 1978.
30. Hohn DC and Rehrer RI: NADPH oxidase deficiency in x-linked chronic granulomatous disease. J Clin Invest 55:707, 1975.
31. Shoemaker WC, Appel P, and Bland R: Use of physiologic monitoring to predict outcome and to assist in clinical decision making in critically ill postoperative patients. Am J Surg 146:43, 1983.
32. Tenney SM: A theoretical analysis of the relationship between venous blood and mean tissue oxygen pressures. Respir Physiol 20:283, 1974.

33. Cain SM: Peripheral oxygen uptake and delivery in health and disease. Clin Chest Med 4:139, 1983.

34. Shibutani K, Komatsa T, Kubal K, et al: Critical level of oxygen delivery in anesthetized man. Crit Care Med 11:640, 1983.

35. Danek SJ, Lynch JP, Weg JG, et al: The dependence of oxygen uptake on oxygen delivery in the adult respiratory distress syndrome. Am Rev Respir Dis 122:387, 1980.

36. Weil MH, Rackow EC, Trevino R, et al: Difference in acid-base state between venous and arterial blood during cardiopulmonary resuscitation. N Engl J Med 315:153, 1986.

37. Cain SM: Oxygen deficit incurred during hypoxia and its relation to lactate and excess lactate. Am J Physiol 213:57, 1967.

38. Connett RJ, Gayeski TE, and Honig CR: Lactate accumulation in full aerobic working dog gracilis muscle. Am J Physiol 246:H120, 1984.

39. Cerra FB: Hypermetabolism-organ failure syndrome: A metabolic response to injury. Crit Care Clin 5:289, 1989.

40. Cady LD Jr, Weil MH, Afifi AA, et al: Quantification of severity of critical illness with special references to lactate. Crit Care Med 1:75, 1973.

53

Diagnosis and Management of Acute Renal Failure in the Critical Care Unit

Jose Ramon C. Ongkingco, M.D., and
Glenn H. Bock, M.D.

Acute renal failure (ARF) is a sudden impairment of renal function that results in the retention of nitrogenous wastes regardless of the specific etiology. The kidney's excretory and autoregulatory functions are governed by distinct anatomic structures and physiologic processes. Therefore, the clinical and biochemical manifestations of ARF vary, often depending on the site and nature of the primary renal injury. Since the severity of the renal injury is determined, to a great extent, by the type and duration as well as magnitude of the insult, a thorough understanding of pathophysiology as well as etiology will ensure the optimal diagnostic and therapeutic management of the patient with ARF.

Standards of living and quality of health care exert an influence on the epidemiology of ARF. Its incidence in industrialized countries is lower than that of Third-World nations. While surgical and traumatic events, the hemolytic-uremic syndrome, and nephrotoxicity from drugs constitute the major pediatric etiologies in industrialized nations, infectious illness is the predominant underlying cause in underdeveloped regions.

The occurrence of ARF is commonly associated with oliguria. Since the classic descriptions of ARF occurring in combat casualties during World War II, oliguria (<500 ml/m²/day; in infants < 0.5 ml/kg/hr) has often been considered a component of ARF. During the past several decades, however, cases of nonoliguric ARF have been reported with increasing frequency. Currently, the incidence ranges from 25 to 80% of the reported cases of ARF. The rise in the incidence of nonoliguric ARF is likely the result of several factors, including the more frequent recognition of ARF by routine biochemical monitoring of hospitalized patients, its occurrence as a result of nephrotoxicity from aminoglycoside and heavy-metal–containing drug treatments, early aggressive resuscitation of traumatized patients and, possibly, the increasing use of potent diuretics, vasodilators, and volume expanders in patients at high risk for ARF.[1]

Approximately 65 to 85% of ARF cases in the adult population are due to acute tubular necrosis (ATN) of various etiologies.[1] In contrast, more than 50% of cases in children are secondary to acute glomerulonephritis and the hemolytic-uremic syndrome (HUS).[2] In neonates, most episodes of ARF are secondary to major perinatal insults, which include perinatal asphyxia, hypoxia, and sepsis.[3–6]

The mortality rates of children suffering from ARF vary widely, relating to a great extent to underlying causative factors. Overall, mortality may exceed 50%, a rate similar to that reported in the adult population.[7, 8] Poorer outcome is associated with young age; postcardiac surgery; presence of a serious, underlying medical illness; and poor nutritional state.[9–11] Similarly, mortality rates in neonates with ARF range from 14 to 73%, those with congenital heart disease and congenital renal anomalies being at greatest risk.[2] In general, the occurrence of nonoliguric renal failure is considered to have a better prognosis.[1, 3, 5]

RENAL PHYSIOLOGY

Some knowledge of the mechanisms by which renal autoregulation occurs is necessary to understand the pathophysiologic disturbances that occur in ARF. The major physiologic considerations in the understanding of renal function are blood flow to the nephron, filtration, and tubular secretion and reabsorption.

The kidneys receive approximately 20% of the cardiac output. After flowing through the renal artery and its intrarenal branches, blood enters the glomerulus via the afferent arteriole. Blood cells and unfiltered plasma leave the glomerulus via the efferent arteriole, entering the postglomerular capillaries that run in proximity to the renal tubules of the glomerulus of origin. Blood flow to the kidney is a function of the mean arterial pressure (MAP) and renal vascular resistance. Changes in systemic MAP are followed by concomitant changes in renal vascular resistance which attempt to preserve a constant renal blood flow. The major sites of renovascular resistance in the kidney are the afferent (preglomerular) and efferent (postglomerular) arterioles. As a result of this autoregulation, the glomerular filtration rate (GFR) is also held constant since glomerular capillary hydraulic pressure is dependent on perfusion pressure (see later).

The intrarenal autoregulatory mechanisms include myogenic responses via stretch receptors in vessel walls, tubuloglomerular feedback (TGF), and neurohormonal factors. Myogenic responses refer to the dilatation or constriction of the afferent arteriole as a result of decreased or increased systemic blood pressure, respectively. TGF refers to modulation of GFR as a result of the rate of tubular flow. This process results from changes of delivered chloride ion concentration to the macula densa (Fig. 53–1). These changes cause alterations of preglomerular vascular resistance, which are postulated to be mediated by a direct effect of high interstitial chloride concentration on the vessel wall[12] and to some extent by angiotensin II. Thus, increased chloride delivery and reabsorption would lead to afferent arteriolar vasoconstriction. A decrease in chloride

delivery produces the opposite effect. Neurohormonal factors that have active roles in renal autoregulation include the renin-angiotensin system (RAS) and prostaglandins. Renin release by the juxtaglomerular cells of the afferent arteriole is stimulated by renal hypoperfusion resulting from hypotension or volume contraction with increased sympathetic activity. Renin initiates a cascade of events that leads to the increased production of angiotensin II, an octapeptide that induces both systemic and intrarenal vasoconstriction, as well as the secretion of aldosterone. Intrarenally, angiotensin II has a disproportionately greater effect on the efferent arteriole, resulting in increased glomerular capillary hydraulic pressure. This serves to maintain GFR. At the same time, the RAS-stimulated vasodilator prostaglandin synthesis may play a role in modulating the renal vasoconstrictive effects of angiotensin II.

Glomerular filtration is the initial renal event that permits excretion of nitrogenous wastes and regulation of the constituents of the internal environment. Since the glomerular hydraulic pressure is greater than the sum of the hydraulic pressure in Bowman's space and colloid osmotic pressure, blood flowing through the glomerular capillary loses fluid through the permeable endothelial fenestrae, basement membrane, and slits of the podocytes that comprise the glomerular capillary wall. These filtration barriers are normally only permeable to water molecules, hydrated ions, and low molecular weight solutes. Thus, the glomerular filtrate that is formed is essentially protein-free and contains crystalloids in concentrations similar to that of plasma.

The integrity and efficiency of glomerular filtration in a given individual is frequently expressed as the GFR. This is a measure of the average volume of fluid filtered from the plasma into the Bowman's capsule per unit time (ml/min) and is governed by the Starling forces operating across the glomerular capillary. Mathematically, GFR is the product of the filtration coefficient (K_f) and the net filtration pressure (NFP). K_f is the product of the hydraulic permeability of the capillaries and the total surface area available for filtration. NFP is the algebraic sum of the hydraulic and colloid oncotic pressures inducing and opposing filtration across the glomerular capillary. Perturbations directly or indirectly affecting any of these components affect GFR.

$$GFR = K_f \times NFP$$
$$K_f = \text{hydraulic permeability} \times \text{surface area}$$
$$NFP = (P_{GC} + \pi_{BC}) - (P_{BC} + \pi_{GC}),$$

in which P_{GC} = glomerular capillary hydraulic pressure

π_{BC} = oncotic pressure in Bowman's capsule (is equal to zero in the absence of proteinuria)

P_{BC} = hydraulic pressure in Bowman's capsule

π_{GC} = oncotic pressure in glomerular capillary plasma.

There are certain points to keep in mind regarding GFR. First, in the clinical setting, the rate of endoge-

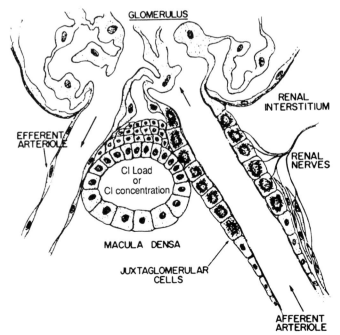

Figure 53–1. Diagram of the glomerulus showing the juxtaglomerular apparatus. (From Davis JO: Relation of renal blood supply to diuresis. Am J Med 55:333, 1973.)

nously produced creatinine has been generally used to estimate GFR. Although, overall, the creatinine clearance (Cl_{Cr}) is a satisfactory measure of GFR, caution must be exercised in certain clinical settings, such as nephrotic syndrome and chronic renal failure when Cl_{Cr} may overestimate true GFR. In ARF, a changing serum creatinine may also prevent an accurate estimate of GFR. Second, whole kidney GFR is the product of single nephron GFR and the number of filtering nephrons. Therefore, improvement in the GFR after an acute insult does not necessarily mean recovery of *all* previously functioning nephrons. Hyperfiltration, occurring in the surviving nephrons, may mask an underlying loss of functioning renal mass.[13]

Because of tubular reabsorption of varying degrees along the entire length of the tubule, the volume and composition of the urine are normally less than the ultrafiltrate volume and contains little or none of the originally filtered plasma components needed by the body. In contrast, urea and other waste products that are excreted represent relatively sizable fractions of the filtered amounts. The bulk of water and electrolyte reabsorption occurs in the proximal tubule via passive and active transport mechanisms. Subsequent movement of these molecules from the interstitium into the peritubular capillaries is favored by the low hydrostatic pressure within the capillaries and high oncotic pressure of the plasma emerging from the glomerulus relative to that of the interstitium. The ability of the tubular epithelium to reabsorb water and electrolytes plays an important role in the TGF mechanism of autoregulation and in the differential diagnosis of ARF (see later).

Tubular secretion is the process by which substances may be added to the glomerular filtrate. The tubular secretion of creatinine accounts for the overestimation of the true GFR. Among the most important secretory processes are those for hydrogen ions and potassium.

PATHOGENESIS AND ETIOLOGY

ARF has been traditionally classified as prerenal, intrinsic renal, and postrenal. These categories imply different pathologic processes of renal hypoperfusion, parenchymal damage, and obstruction, respectively. However, the boundaries between these categories are not well defined. One can view ARF as a continuum in that prolonged prerenal or postrenal states can lead eventually to intrinsic renal damage. In addition, more than one distinct pathologic process can occur *simultaneously* at the onset to cause ARF secondary to several etiologies. For example, significant volume contraction can result in prerenal azotemia but at the same time predispose to renal dysfunction in a patient with chronic intake of nonsteroidal anti-inflammatory drugs. Amphotericin toxicity not only causes tubular damage but also ischemia from renal vasoconstriction. Nevertheless, this simplified classification is useful in understanding the pathologic processes, and in the rapid diagnosis and initial approach to the management of ARF.

Prerenal Acute Renal Failure

This condition, also referred to as functional renal failure, occurs when the autoregulatory capacity of a functionally intact kidney is unable to compensate for decreases of systemic blood pressure that result in severe renal hypoperfusion. Under normal circumstances, autoregulation is operative within the MAP range of 80 to 180 mm Hg (Fig. 53–2). Afferent arteriolar dilatation is maximal at a MAP of 80 mm Hg and GFR ceases at 40 to 50 mm Hg.

Severe renal hypoperfusion results in exaggeration of the previously discussed mechanisms which maintain GFR, although the precise physiologic responses vary in different clinical settings. True intravascular depletion due to external losses or internal fluid translocation ("third spacing") predominantly results in efferent arteriolar vasoconstriction mediated by angiotensin II, catecholamines, and vasopressin.[13–15] The acute reduction in renal blood flow (RBF) and GFR results in avid tubular water and sodium reabsorption that is further facilitated by the increased secretion of aldosterone and vasopressin. This conservation of water and sodium is an attempt to restore the circulatory volume or cardiac output. By contrast, a diminished effective circulating volume, such as that which occurs in congestive heart failure and advanced liver disease, results in a significantly increased afferent arteriolar vasoconstriction which is mediated by a still-unknown substance.[16] The acute reduction in RBF and GFR in this circumstance is also associated with an enhanced reabsorption of water and sodium in an attempt to re-expand the intravascular space. This retention of water and sodium may be inappropriate to the patient's volume status and could, therefore, be detrimental in this setting. The avidity for water and sodium is possible only with an intact tubular epithelium and, therefore, differentiates prerenal azotemia from other causes of ARF. An essential feature of prerenal ARF is that GFR recovers once RBF to the intact kidneys is restored to normal.

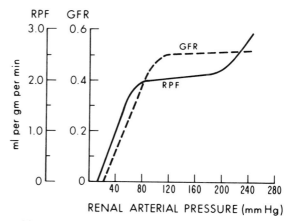

Figure 53–2. Autoregulation of renal blood flow and glomerular filtration rate. (Data from Ochwadt B: Prog Cardiovasc Dis 3:501, 1961. Reproduced from Spitzer A: Renal physiology and functional derangement. *In:* Edelmann CM, Jr [ed]: Pediatric Kidney Disease. Reproduced with permission from 1st edition, Little, Brown, and Company, copyright 1978.)

Table 53–1. CAUSES OF PRERENAL FAILURE IN INFANTS AND CHILDREN

Total Body Volume Depletion
   Gastrointestinal losses (vomiting or diarrhea)
   Increased insensible losses (fever)
   Osmotic diuresis (e.g., diabetes mellitus, mannitol infusion)
   Diabetes insipidus
   Burns

Intravascular Volume Depletion
   Hemorrhage
   "Third spacing" (e.g., sepsis, nephrotic syndrome, after
     surgery, or trauma)

Diminished Effective Circulating Volume
   Cardiogenic shock
   Cardiomyopathies
   Decreased cardiac output
   Pharmacologic vasodilatation

Renal Vasoconstriction
   Prostaglandin synthetase inhibitors
   Cyclosporine
   Hepatorenal syndrome

Other conditions that may impair the efficiency of renal autoregulation are listed in Table 53–1.

Parenchymal Acute Renal Failure

Many of the conditions that can result in renal parenchymal injury can be grouped into several broad categories (Table 53–2).

Large Vessel Occlusion

Thromboembolic events can lead to occlusion of the main or segmental renal arteries. This occurs infrequently in the pediatric age group but can develop as a complication of umbilical artery catheterization, bacterial endocarditis, atrial fibrillation in the presence of cardiac disease, and renal artery angiography. Renal artery stenosis, when bilateral, can result in ARF with the use of angiotensin-converting enzyme inhibitor therapy or from hypotension induced by aggressive treatment during periods of accelerated hypertension. Arterio-occlusive disease should be considered if a patient suddenly becomes anuric.

Thrombosis of the renal veins can occur in the presence of a hypercoagulable state, such as in nephrotic syndrome and sickle cell disease, as well as in infants with dehydration and hemoconcentration, birth asphyxia, sepsis, maternal diabetes mellitus, and cyanotic heart disease following angiography. It can also arise from an impairment of RBF caused by trauma to the renal veins or from external compression by tumors.

The pathogenesis of impaired GFR in arterial occlusive diseases is the direct consequence of diminished RBF and renal infarction. Although little is known about the rate of development of collateral circulation following arterial occlusion, successful revascularization after prolonged intervals has been reported.[17] Renal failure from renal vein thrombosis is due to vascular congestion and hemorrhagic necrosis. The development of venous collaterals and the recanalization of the thrombi may be associated with the subsequent improvement of GFR.[18]

Microvascular Disease

This category refers to injury of the arterioles and glomerular capillaries from intravascular thrombi, inflammation, or barotrauma. HUS is the most common cause of oliguric ARF in children younger than 4 years of age. This syndrome is characterized by the onset of an acute hemolytic anemia, thrombocytopenia, and ARF. As a syndrome, HUS encompasses a group of disorders with similar but varying degrees of illness, resulting from different causes and multiple pathogenic mechanisms. Recurrent and familial forms have been described. HUS is typically preceded by a respiratory or gastrointestinal illness. The precise cause is unknown in many cases, but there is accumulating evidence that has linked verocytotoxin-producing *Escherichia coli* to some cases of HUS.[19] Viral infection has been frequently associated with the occurrence of HUS, but a precise causal relationship has not been established. Microvascular occlusion by intraluminal platelet-fibrin thrombi deposition occurs following endothelial cell damage by the cytotoxic agent. Presumably, the passage of red blood cells through the intraluminal fibrin strands results in the hemolytic anemia. Decreased prostacyclin production by the damaged endothelial cells and increased thromboxane A_2 are also suggested to play a role in the

Table 53–2. CAUSES OF PARENCHYMAL ACUTE RENAL FAILURE IN INFANTS AND CHILDREN

Large Vessel Occlusion
   Renal vein thrombosis
   Renal artery occlusion (thrombus, embolus)
   Renal artery stenosis

Microvascular Disease
   Hemolytic-uremic syndrome
   Thrombotic thrombocytopenic purpura
   Acute nephritis (post-infectious, idiopathic)
   Vasculitis (e.g., Henoch-Schonlein purpura, Wegener
     granulomatosis, periarteritis nodosa)
   Malignant hypertension

Tubulointerstitial Disease
Ischemic
   Shock syndromes
   Respiratory distress syndromes
   Severe cardiac failure

Nephrotoxic
   Antibiotics (e.g., aminoglycosides, amphotericin)
   Heavy metals
   Organic solvents (e.g., glycols, carbon tetrachloride,
     methanol, toluene)
   Salicylates
   Fluorinated hydrocarbon anesthetics
   Prostaglandin synthetase inhibitors
   Cisplatin
   X-ray contrast media
   Rhabdomyolysis
   Massive hemolysis
   Uricosuric/hyperuricemic agents (e.g., pancreatic enzymes,
     antineoplastics, x-ray contrast media, loop diuretics)

Acute interstitial nephritis
Fulminant pyelonephritis

decrease of GFR.[20] The diminished GFR, therefore, is secondary to both the reduction of capillary blood flow and the loss of effective filtration surface area. Habib has proposed that the primary site of vascular injury as determined by renal biopsy can influence the clinical manifestations and prognosis of this disease.[21] This study suggested that patients with predominantly preglomerular arteriolar involvement presented with more severe disease compared with those with predominantly glomerular capillary involvement. A more recent report supports this observation.[22]

As a result of improved supportive management in terms of early dialysis and control of hypertension, the mortality rate has decreased substantially during the past several decades and currently ranges from 5 to 10% in most series.[20, 23] In patients who recover, the duration of oliguria is usually less than 2 weeks although renal function may take months to completely return to normal.[24] Other investigators have reported that 12 to 15% of cases may develop chronic renal failure, end-stage renal disease, hypertension, or proteinuria.[23]

Thrombotic thrombocytopenic purpura, although more common in adults, has also been reported in older children. Like HUS, it is characterized by hemolytic anemia, thrombocytopenia, and renal failure in 50% of the cases. In addition, neurologic involvement is a major feature. Also like HUS, renal dysfunction is a result of intravascular platelet aggregation with microvascular thrombosis.

Microvascular inflammation as a cause of ARF can be secondary to glomerulonephritis or vasculitic syndromes. The specific etiologic entities are numerous and cannot be covered in this discussion. Although the pathogenesis may vary, the renal injury usually includes extensive glomerular capillary wall injury, which is often associated with fibroepithelial crescent formation within Bowman's space. The reduction in GFR is the result of diminished RBF due to increased resistance of the injured microvasculature as well as to loss of filtration surface area.

Barotrauma to the renal vasculature occurs in malignant hypertension. Histologic examination of the kidneys shows concentric thickening of the intima of the interlobular arteries and arterioles referred to as nephrosclerosis. Necrotizing arteriolitis and glomerulitis are also seen.

Tubular Ischemic and Nephrotoxic

ARF has long been equated with ATN. In actuality, ATN is only one of the causes of ARF, although it accounts for the majority of adult cases. As the term implies, ATN is histomorphologically characterized, in most cases, by areas of tubular cell necrosis caused by ischemia or nephrotoxic agents.

The development of ARF in this setting has three phases: the initiation phase in which the primary insult from ischemia or a toxin occurs; the maintenance phase in which GFR remains low for a variable period of time depending on the severity and type of insult; and the recovery phase in which GFR may or may not return to baseline. Pathophysiologic mechanisms implicated in the

impairment of GFR include hemodynamic disturbances, tubular cell disruption, and metabolic/cellular factors. There is experimental evidence to support roles of each of these mechanisms and undoubtedly, they are of variable importance in different settings.

Hemodynamic factors refer to alterations in RBF as well as K_f. The kidney's paradoxical susceptibility to an ischemic injury despite a relatively enormous blood supply and thus, oxygen delivery, stems from a poorly understood nonhomogeneous intrarenal oxygen distribution.[25] In perfused kidney models, the proximal tubule and thick ascending limb of the loop of Henle are the principal foci of hypoxic injury.[25] This vulnerability has been attributed to the high energy demands of their transport work. However, since it is likely that tubular work is reduced following the drop in tubular load that results from diminished perfusion pressure in vivo, the occurrence of an inappropriate and intense vasoconstriction as the initiating event in some settings has been proposed.

Diminished blood flow appears to be the initiating event in ischemic and myoglobinuric injuries.[26] While a preferential decrease in blood flow to the outer cortical nephrons has been demonstrated by radioactive microsphere studies,[27] the identity of the vasoactive hormone responsible for the afferent arteriolar vasoconstriction remains controversial. Recognition of the importance of sodium and of chloride ions in modulating TGF has been previously discussed. The role of the RAS has been considered in the pathogenesis since both plasma and intrarenal renin levels rise following renal artery clamping. This is further supported by the finding that volume depletion predisposes to ARF and may be prevented by sodium chloride loading.[28] However, the inability of angiotensin-converting enzyme inhibition and angiotensin antagonist administration to prevent ARF in experimental models suggests the importance of other humoral substances, including intrarenal prostaglandins, catecholamines, adenosine, and vasopressin.[15, 16, 29] There is increasing interest also in the role of endothelin, a potent vasoconstrictor peptide probably released by endothelial cells, in potentially contributing to the maintenance of the hemodynamic alterations of ARF.[30] The vasodilatory effects of furosemide and mannitol treatments in preventing ARF (see Management), when given prior to the insult, lends further credence to the vascular theory of ARF.[31, 32]

While hemodynamic factors undoubtedly contribute to the manifestations of ARF, alterations in K_f appear to be a major pathophysiologic component in some experimental settings, including models of uranyl and aminoglycoside nephrotoxicity.[26] Morphologic changes in the glomeruli that occur in these settings include endothelial cell swelling and reduction in the density and size of endothelial fenestrae. Furthermore, RAS-mediated mesangial cell contraction with resultant decreased filtration surface has also been demonstrated.[33]

Injury to the proximal tubules results in cellular necrosis and loss of structural tubular integrity.[34] Sloughed epithelial cells can obstruct distal tubular lumina with a concomitant rise in intratubular pressure. In addition, the loss of tubular basement membrane integrity can permit the "backleak" of substances (e.g., creatinine) that are not normally reabsorbed as well as water into the peritubular fluid and plasma.[34] Morphologic evidence of tubular obstruction and clearance studies in support of the "backleak theory" have demonstrated the importance of these factors as major determinants of the diminished GFR in certain experimental models including those resulting from mercuric chloride, uranyl nitrate, and ischemia.[26] The inconsistent observation of increased intratubular pressure observed by micropuncture techniques suggests that reduced filtration pressure results in diminished ultrafiltrate formation.[35] From a somewhat different viewpoint, this interaction between decreased tubular reabsorptive ability and hemodynamically mediated reduction in GFR can be regarded as an important adaptive response to prevent massive water and electrolyte losses that would occur in the setting of unrestricted ultrafiltrate formation and poor tubular function. This concept has been referred to as "acute renal success."[36]

Various cellular and metabolic factors have also been proposed in an attempt to explain the cause of the persisting diminished GFR during the maintenance phase of ARF. The production of oxygen-free radicals has been demonstrated to further aggravate the ischemic injury and can conceivably perpetuate tissue injury following reflow.[2, 37] The injurious effects of cellular calcium influx has been attributed to the uncoupling of oxidative phosphorylation, activation of membrane-bound phospholipases, activation of intracellular proteases, inhibition of Na/ATPase, and direct effects on intracellular pH.[2, 37, 38] This role of calcium is interesting in that endothelin appears to exert its effects by activating transmembrane calcium flux into vascular tissue.[30] An exception to this is the protective role of calcium in experimental aminoglycoside nephrotoxicity.[39] Finally, the adenine nucleotide system is currently under investigation. Decreased mitochondrial production of ATP following a hypoxic insult impairs homeostatic regulation of the intracellular environment.[2] The possible role of increased adenosine levels in renal vasoconstriction has been mentioned.

From the currently available data presented here, the critical pathophysiologic determinants of ARF in ATN are still unsettled. It is likely that both vascular and tubular mechanisms contribute, in varying degrees, to the overall impairment in renal function at different stages of renal failure.

Postrenal Acute Renal Failure

Urinary obstruction causing ARF is uncommon in children. When present, it is usually congenital and may be associated with other physical abnormalities such as that of an infant with features of Potter's syndrome and a history of oligohydramnios. More frequently, patients with milder degrees of obstruction and azotemia, which might occur with posterior urethral valves, may remain undiagnosed until ARF is precipitated by a complicating event like urinary infection.

Urinary obstruction may occur at any point in the

urinary collecting system from the renal pelvis to the urethra. It may be intraluminal or extrinsic to the urinary tract. It may be anatomic or functional (e.g., as a result of bladder dyssynergy) in nature. Obstruction may be unilateral or bilateral. The major causes of urinary tract obstruction are listed in Table 53–3.

When obstruction is unilateral, the normally functioning contralateral kidney is usually capable of preventing significant accumulation of nitrogenous wastes. Thus, the syndrome of ARF, except in cases of solitary kidneys, is usually the result of obstruction bilaterally or distal to the urinary bladder. Regardless of the site of obstruction, urinary volumes often vary. In the early phase of acute obstruction when ultrafiltrate flow is low, solute load not excessive, and tubular epithelium still undamaged, obstruction may actually be associated with enhanced water and salt reabsorption. This is of clinical significance, because early obstruction may mimic a prerenal disorder. By contrast, impaired renal-concentrating ability has also been observed in experimental acute obstruction.[40] Partial obstruction or recently relieved partial or complete obstruction is associated with defects in tubular handling of water, electrolytes, and acid. Urine is isotonic or hypotonic because of an impaired urinary concentrating ability secondary to a number of causes that include (1) decreased water reabsorption by the juxtaglomerular nephrons, (2) decreased medullary tonicity from "washout" of solutes due to increased medullary blood flow and impaired NaCl reabsorption by the thick ascending limb of Henle, and (3) decreased collecting duct sensitivity to vasopressin.[41, 42] Aside from the inability to reabsorb sodium and chloride, hydrogen ion and potassium secretion are impaired due to damaged distal tubular intercalated cells and decreased sensitivity to aldosterone in the collecting tubules.[41]

Our current understanding of the pathophysiology of the diminished GFR during urinary obstruction is derived mostly from animal studies. This reduction of

Table 53–3. CAUSES OF POSTRENAL ACUTE RENAL FAILURE IN INFANTS AND CHILDREN

Intraluminal
    Intrarenal: Calculi
    Extrarenal: Structural
            Urethral strictures
            Posterior urethral valves
            Ureteroceles
            Duplicated collecting system
            Ureteropelvic junction strictures

        Functional
            Neuropathic bladder
            Bladder dyssynergy

        Nonstructural
            Nephrolithiasis
            Foreign body in urethra
            Intraureteral blood clots
            Edema following urinary tract infection
            Pelvic inflammatory disease

    Extrinsic
        Retroperitoneal/intra-abdominal tumors
        Aortic/iliac aneurysms
        Retroperitoneal fibrosis

GFR is the result of both hydrodynamic and, more significantly, hemodynamic alterations.[41, 42] The initial fall in GFR during acute unilateral and bilateral obstruction is primarily due to the increased hydrostatic pressure that is transmitted to the proximal tubules, thus decreasing the net pressure gradient favoring filtration across the glomerular capillary wall. This fall in GFR is blunted by the simultaneous increase in RBF that occurs during the first few hours following obstruction. This has been attributed to afferent arteriolar dilatation presumably mediated by vasodilator prostaglandins (prostacyclin), which in turn activate the RAS.[41–44] Thus, progressive renal vasoconstriction eventually sets in if the obstruction is not relieved. Besides angiotensin II, thromboxane may play a role in these hemodynamic changes.[41, 42] A decrease in K_f secondary to angiotensin II- and thromboxane-induced mesangial contraction further contributes to the decline in GFR.

In experimental unilateral obstruction of the affected kidney, dominant preglomerular vasoconstriction accounts for the persistently abnormal GFR despite the return of intraluminal hydrostatic pressure to near-normal levels; the latter occurs partly as a result of a slowly evolving TGF.[40] With bilateral obstruction, the site of altered vascular resistance is thought to be postglomerular since glomerular capillary pressures remain normal even with the reduction of total RBF. The abnormal GFR in this setting is secondary to persistently elevated hydrostatic pressures and, possibly, to the decline in RBF. The hemodynamic differences between unilateral and bilateral obstruction remain incompletely understood.

During partial obstruction, GFR may remain unaffected or may decrease depending on the duration and severity of obstruction. The increase in glomerular capillary hydraulic pressure that results from a predominantly efferent arteriolar vasoconstriction tends to maintain GFR in this setting. The accompanying decrease in K_f, however, and progressive nephron injury contribute to an eventual decline in GFR with prolonged obstruction.

Early recognition and correction of obstruction is important since functional recovery is related to the duration of obstruction. In children with severe congenital lesions, however, it appears that progression to end-stage renal disease frequently occurs despite prompt surgical treatment.[40]

Kidney Transplant and Acute Renal Failure

The reported incidence of ARF in kidney transplants ranges from 25 to 75% in cadaver allografts and is approximately 10% in living related grafts.[45] This difference in frequencies is influenced by the donor's clinical state, the period of ischemia from the time of organ removal to revascularization, the mode of preservation, the degree of immunologic compatibility, and surgical complications that may occur. The first four of these would, generally, be greater risk factors in cadaveric transplants.

Although the causes of ARF in this setting can also be considered as prerenal, intrinsic renal, and postrenal (Table 53–4), the boundaries between these are often extremely difficult to define in a denervated, invariably ischemic kidney often subjected to complex polypharmacologic regimens. Therefore, a high index of suspicion for many potential causes must be maintained. In the presence of the profuse diuresis that may occur immediately post-transplant, there is risk of hypovolemia. The inability of the recently transplanted kidney to volume autoregulate increases the risk for ischemic injury.

In addition, the post-transplant diuresis may be aggravated by the high glucose solute load that arises from rapid urine volume replacement with 5% dextrose solutions.

Surgical complications causing perfusion or drainage problems are less common and can be detected by appropriate radiographic studies. A major problem is the importance of and difficulty in differentiating renal failure from transplant rejection and other related causes. Systemic manifestations of rejection (e.g., fever, allograft tenderness) are not always present. For the reasons outlined earlier, conventional laboratory tests, including urinary indices, may not be particularly helpful in the post-transplant period. Imaging modalities become valuable diagnostic aids in this situation, and angiography or renal biopsy may sometimes be required. If the patient is receiving cyclosporine, possible nephrotoxicity from this drug should be considered. The risk of acquiring viral infections, primarily from cytomegalovirus, during the second and third months post-transplant is another cause of renal dysfunction that may, at the onset, mimic rejection. The availability of T cell marker surveillance may become a useful diagnostic tool in differentiating infection from rejection and in monitoring recovery or treatment response.[46]

DIAGNOSTIC EVALUATION

The outcome of acute renal failure is greatly influenced by the institution of early renal resuscitation and subsequent medical management. Therefore, an aggressive approach to the early diagnosis and appropriate management of the ARF should be undertaken (Fig. 53–3).

Clinical Considerations

A thorough history and clinical examination of the patient with ARF are essential and useful in determining

Table 53–4. CAUSES OF KIDNEY TRANSPLANT ACUTE RENAL FAILURE

Early Causes	Late Causes
Hypovolemia	Rejection
Thrombosis	Cyclosporine toxicity
Ureteral obstruction	Ureteral obstruction
Urinary leak	Artery stenosis
Acute tubular necrosis	Viral infection
Rejection	

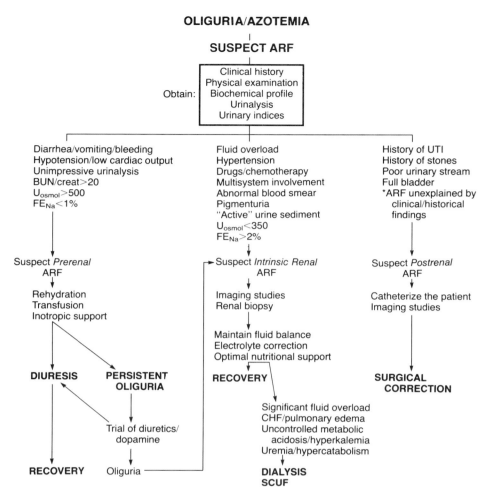

Figure 53–3. Suggested approach to the basic diagnostic and therapeutic management of acute renal failure in infants and children.

the etiology of ARF. The possibility of previously underlying renal disease might be suggested by the presence of signs and symptoms that include pre-existing anorexia, poor growth, pallor, rachitic bone changes, and nocturia. A history of urinary tract infection or an abnormal voiding pattern in a male child suggests a urologic disorder. In a female, the possibility of underlying chronic reflux nephropathy must be considered. Access to potentially nephrotoxic drugs or poisons in a child and drug abuse in a teenager must be investigated. The occurrence of a recent respiratory infection or diarrheal illness suggests an acute glomerulonephritis or the HUS. Diarrhea and vomiting, in themselves, with accompanying volume depletion can be a prelude to the development of ATN or renal vein thrombosis. In hospitalized patients who develop unexplained ARF, a review of previous hospitalizations can provide vital information of antecedent risk factors, such as exposure to nephrotoxic agents, surgery, and trauma. Inspection of fluid balance and the drug regimen records of the current hospitalization is equally vital.

The physical examination also provides important information, pertaining not only to the possible cause of the ARF but also to the severity of the condition. The state of hydration should be assessed in any oliguric patient. The findings of tachycardia, dry mucous mem-

branes, poor skin turgor, and orthostatic hypotension favor a prerenal type of azotemia. It must be kept in mind, however, that a prerenal condition may also be associated with an ongoing renal parenchymal disease. Persistence of oliguria even after normalization of intravascular volume is more consistent with the latter. Bilateral obstruction or cortical necrosis should be considered in anuric cases. Signs of fluid overload such as peripheral or pulmonary edema and jugular venous distention with or without hypertension suggest an acute nephritic process. In addition to historical evidence, the presence of the extrarenal findings of lymphadenopathy, arthritis, rash, vasculitic skin changes, and organomegaly suggest a multisystem disorder. Abdominal examination should always include a careful bimanual palpation of the kidneys. Enlarged kidneys may suggest hydronephrosis, cystic disease, or venous infarction. The finding of a full bladder by palpation and percussion suggest infravesical obstruction.

Kussmaul respiration, ecchymoses, hand tremors, or Chovstek sign indicate severe metabolic abnormalities that require immediate attention.

Laboratory Investigation

Determination of hemoglobin and white blood cell and platelet counts has potential value. Anemia may be indicative of a chronic illness. When associated with thrombocytopenia or fragmented erythrocytes, HUS, renal vein thrombosis, and septicemia must be considered. The latter may exhibit leukocytosis or leukopenia. Serum determinations of electrolytes, urea, creatinine, calcium, magnesium, and phosphorus reveal the severity of the biochemical disturbances and in turn help to guide appropriate therapy. For example, a serum urea measurement disproportionately elevated when compared with the serum creatinine is compatible with prerenal azotemia during which increased passive reabsorption of urea accompanies the avid water reabsorption. This commonly results in a urea-creatinine ratio of more than 20. On the other hand, a creatinine rising disproportionately to urea may direct attention to the possibility of rhabdomyolysis. A rapidly rising creatinine on serial determinations that is unexplained may also indicate the need for an early diagnostic renal biopsy. Elevated serum SGOT and LDH are associated with renal infarction. Uric acid level determinations may be useful in patients with tumor lysis syndromes or other causes of severe hyperuricemia. When there is suspicion of drug-induced nephrotoxicity, serum specimens should be saved for subsequent drug screens, particularly if dialysis is to be performed.

A urine specimen should be obtained as soon as possible and prior to any diuretic administration, even if catheterization is required. In anuric patients, catheterization may yield some residual urine. The urinalysis can provide immediate diagnostic information. In prerenal azotemia, the urine specific gravity is usually high, typically approaching the maximal value of 1.035. However, maximal concentration in this setting may not be achieved as a result of diminished distal tubular solute delivery and a consequently diminished medullary tonicity. In fact, polyuria has also been described in this setting, likely a result of a similar process.[47] Detection of urinary glucose in the presence of normal serum levels suggests proximal tubular damage. Detection of blood by urine dipstick can indicate hemoglobinuria, myoglobinuria, or hematuria. The latter is verified by the presence of more than 10 erythrocytes per high power field on microanalysis. This, however, does not necessarily rule out the possibility of myoglobinuria. The relative absence of erythrocytes by microscopic inspection in the face of a strongly positive blood dipstick result suggests a hemolytic or myolytic process and should be pursued with more specific biochemical studies if the cause is not immediately evident. Hematuria associated with proteinuria ($\geq 2+$ by dipstick) suggests underlying glomerulonephritis. In addition, pyuria may be indicative of infection, interstitial nephritis, and some forms of glomerulonephritis. Although a value of more than 5 WBC per high power field in a midstream urine sample is regarded as abnormal, the quantitative count of more than 2,000 WBC/ml offers more accuracy. Urine culture is required for a definitive diagnosis of urinary infection. Coarse granular or red blood cell casts are more suggestive of nephritis, while casts of tubular origin are more consistent with nephrotoxic or ischemic parenchymal damage. WBC casts are frequently associated with pyelonephritis and severe interstitial nephritis.

Several tests for the integrity of renal tubular function have evolved in an attempt to differentiate parenchymal from functional ARF. In this regard, their *diagnostic* value is applicable almost exclusively to oliguric and oligoanuric situations. Since the accurate interpretation of these tests is often limited by indeterminate values between these two categories of ARF[48] and potentially confounding variables often coexist, a general understanding of the specificity of several tests is necessary.

One of the primary functions of the tubular epithelium is the reabsorption of sodium against a concentration gradient. In the absence of urinary obstruction, the urinary sodium (U_{Na}) concentration is commonly less than 20 mEq/l in cases of functional ARF. In the presence of significant tubular injury of any cause, the U_{Na} is generally more than 40 mEq/l. Due to the considerable number of intermediate nondiagnostic values obtained with this test, the fractional excretion of sodium (FE_{Na}) is recommended because of its greater discriminatory ability.[48-50] The FE_{Na} is an index of total sodium reabsorption as reflected by the amount of sodium that is excreted. Since the total amount of Na^+ excreted is equal to the urine [Na] $\times$ urine volume and the total amount of filtered Na^+ is equal to the serum [Na] $\times$ $U_{Cr}V/P_{Cr}$ (or GFR), then the FE_{Na} is calculated as:

$$\frac{([U_{Na}])(U_{vol})}{([P_{Na}])\,(U_{vol})([U_{Cr}])/[P_{Cr}]} \times 100$$

which, after rearrangement of the equation, is

$$([U/P]_{Na})/([U/P]_{Cr}) \times 100.$$

Using a cut-off value of <1% ($\geq 99\%$ reabsorption) to indicate a prerenal state and more than 2% ($\leq 98\%$ reabsorption) to indicate ATN will correctly distinguish prerenal ARF from oliguric ATN in more than 90% of cases. Some authors use more than 1% as the critical value for ATN. Although prior diuretic therapy has an effect on sodium excretion, a value of less than 1% still strongly suggests a prerenal etiology. Because of the lower tubular reabsorptive capacity for sodium among premature infants, a higher cut-off value of more than 2.5% has been suggested for ATN in this setting.[51, 52]

Prerenal azotemia is physiologically associated with stimulated antidiuretic hormone secretion and, thus, normal tubules tend to reabsorb a greater amount of water than solute. As a result, both urine specific gravity and osmolality (relative to that of the plasma) are high. Since the urine specific gravity is affected by solute diuresis, diuretic therapy, heavy proteinuria, and preexistent chronic renal failure, urine osmolality is a more reliable measure of tubular water reabsorption. Generally, a value of more than 500 mOsm/l suggests prerenal azotemia whereas less than 350 mOsm/l suggests parenchymal disease. Equivocal values may be further analyzed by determining the ratio of urine to plasma osmolality.[53] A ratio of more than 1.35 suggests a prerenal (functional) disturbance whereas less than 1.1 is compatible with ATN.

The ratio of urine$_{[Cr]}$/serum$_{[Cr]}$ is another quantitative index of total water reabsorption by the kidney.[16] Since creatinine in the tubular fluid is not reabsorbed, its concentration is related primarily to the amount of water that is removed from the glomerular ultrafiltrate. A ratio of more than 40 represents more than 97.5% water reabsorption, suggestive of prerenal azotemia, whereas a ratio of less than 20 (<95% water reabsorption) suggests ATN.

The clearance of solute-free water has also been shown to be useful in differentiating prerenal from parenchymal renal failure.[54] It denotes the volume of pure water that has to be either removed from or added to the urine to make it iso-osmotic to plasma. Free-water clearance (C_{H_2O}) is "positive" when urine is hypo-osmotic and is "negative" when urine is hyperosmotic. The former indicates free-water excretion, and the latter indicates free water reabsorption. Therefore, a negative C_{H_2O} is seen in prerenal ARF while the value approaches or exceeds zero in ATN. The actual value can be calculated as follows:

$$C_{H_2O} = V - \left(\frac{U_{osm} V}{P_{osm}}\right)$$

where V is the urine volume per unit time, U_{osm} is the urine osmolality, and P_{osm} is the plasma osmolality. The second term of the right side of the equation is also referred to as the osmolar clearance and represents the volume of isotonic urine needed to excrete a given solute load.

When renal failure is unexplained or its course is unrelenting, radiographic imaging studies of the kidneys often become necessary. Because of the risk of furthering renal parenchymal damage with the use of radiocontrast material[55] and the availability of alternative noninvasive techniques, excretory urography has been largely replaced by sonography and renal nuclear imaging as initial diagnostic modalities in many pediatric centers. Information regarding kidney size and number, the state of the renal parenchyma (echogenicity), presence of vascular thrombi, congenital abnormalities, or obstructive lesions can be obtained reliably by ultrasonography in experienced hands. With the addition of the Doppler-flow component to the sonographic capabilities, alterations in RBF can now be assessed as well. In situations when additional information regarding renal perfusion and the integrity of urinary drainage are needed, a ^{99m}Tc-diethylenetriamine penta-acetic acid (DTPA) renal scan can be obtained. Computed tomography and magnetic resonance imaging are diagnostic modalities, although available, that are usually not necessary in the initial diagnostic evaluation of ARF. In the immediate post-transplant period, early imaging of the transplanted kidney is necessary to assess the integrity of renal perfusion and also serves as a baseline study for future diagnostic purposes.

Percutaneous renal biopsy is not required frequently for diagnostic evaluation of ARF. Nevertheless, there are specific circumstances when it should be strongly considered. These include a clinical picture of rapidly progressive glomerulonephritis of unknown etiology, a nonstreptococcal acute nephritis associated with systemic signs and symptoms, suspected nephrotoxic ATN that is not improving, and primary nonfunction of a transplanted kidney in which differentiation from rejection is crucial.

SPECIFIC APPROACHES TO MANAGEMENT

The fundamental goals of ARF management are (1) early recognition and treatment of the underlying disorder, (2) maintenance of the body's fluid and biochemical composition close to normal, and (3) anticipatory management to obviate the onset of other potential complications.

Fluid and Electrolyte Balance

Correction of any fluid and electrolyte imbalance in a patient with ARF demands close monitoring of certain parameters that include the patient's weight (daily or more frequently as needed), hourly fluid volume delivery from all sources, hourly urine volume measurements, accurate measurements of fluid losses from other sources, and serial determinations of the electrolyte concentration of serum and, if needed, of other body fluids (e.g., gastrointestinal losses, urine). The goal is to attain a stable clinical state by providing appropriate replacements despite constantly changing patient requirements.

An individual's daily fluid requirement can be calculated with some degree of accuracy by making relative estimates of ongoing measurable and insensible fluid losses. Several methods for determining the fluid requirements of hospitalized patients have been reviewed by Holliday and Segar.[56] In their analysis, during the resting state in a comfortable environment, the average net water requirement as a function of energy expenditure after correcting for endogenous water production (~ 16.7 ml/100 kcal) is approximately 100 ml/100 kcal/day. This daily water requirement is the sum of insensible water losses (estimated to be 50 ml/100 kcal expended) and the obligate urinary losses for the excretion of solute load (~ 66.7 ml/100 kcal expended) minus the water of oxidation. Inherent in this approach is the need to determine the individual's basal caloric expenditure according to weight. Estimation of water requirement is then based on the *corresponding* daily caloric needs for the hospitalized infant and child as reported by previous studies (Fig. 53–4).[56]

Although this estimate is useful for the average patient, the clinician must make appropriate adjustments for conditions that may alter insensible water losses such as fever and respiration of humidified air. *In addition, fluid replacement must be adjusted for the altered urinary volumes of the patient with ARF, particularly in the presence of an oliguric state.* In our experience, failure to adjust so-called "maintenance" fluid requirements for altered urine production rates is a common management error in patients with ARF.

Provided the measurable fluid losses are monitored accurately, total fluid requirement can be modified by readjusting the initial estimate of insensible water loss. In effect, the approach should be individualized and guided by frequent clinical evaluation of the patient's weight and functional intravascular volume status. However, this clinical assessment may be limited by the

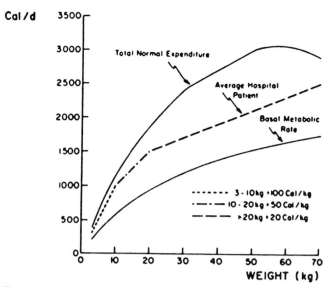

Figure 53–4. Estimated caloric expenditures under basal conditions *(bottom curve)* under conditions of bed rest *(middle curve)*, and under conditions of full activity *(top curve)*. The middle curve can be divided into three segments according to slope: from 3 to 10 kg = 100 Cal/kg; from 10 to 20 kg = 50 Cal/kg; and over 20 kg = 20 Cal/kg. These slopes can be used to formulate reasonable estimates of caloric expenditure for maintenance fluid therapy without use of the graph. (Data from Holliday MA and Segar WE: Pediatrics 19:823, 1957. Reproduced from Winters RW: Maintenance fluid therapy. *In:* Winters RW [ed]: The Body Fluids in Pediatrics, 1st ed, p. 117. Reprinted with permission from Little, Brown, and Company, copyright 1973.)

development of edema or by abnormal vascular tone and capacitance such that invasive intravascular monitoring may become necessary. Since an intensive care patient with ARF is usually in a hypercatabolic state and frequently has inadequate caloric intake, a weight loss of about 0.25 to 0.5% of lean body mass per day is common. Therefore, a patient whose weight remains stable could actually be retaining significant amounts of fluid.

Maintenance requirements for sodium, chloride, and potassium in the normal individual are approximately 3.0, 2.0, and 2.0 mEq/100 kcal/day, respectively. In a patient with ARF, electrolyte replacement should be based on measurable losses that are primarily urinary in the absence of abnormal gastrointestinal or other cavity drainage. Since insensible fluids contain relatively small amounts of these electrolytes, this can be replaced by electrolyte-free solutions. Hyponatremia, when present, is usually from fluid overload rather than from total body sodium depletion and can be corrected by appropriate fluid restriction.

Hyperkalemia, as a life-threatening complication of ARF, more commonly occurs in oliguric states and may be aggravated by ongoing infection, ischemic tissue damage, acidemia, gastrointestinal damage, and so forth. Early dietary and parenteral potassium restriction should be instituted and, when hyperkalemia is mild (<6.5 mEq/l), sodium polystyrene sulfonate may be given orally as a 70% sorbitol solution or as a retention enema as a 30% sorbitol solution (Table 53–5). Higher elevations of the serum potassium concentration may be

accompanied by potentially fatal electrocardiographic abnormalities. In this setting, urgent dialysis should be considered. It is important that dialysis be considered early on in the course of an uncontrolled rising potassium concentration since there may be insufficient time for its implementation once life-threatening electrocardiogram (ECG) abnormalities occur. Hemodialysis is the modality of choice since it can significantly improve hyperkalemia within hours.[57] If hemodialysis is not feasible because of the patient's size, hemodynamic instability, or other relative contraindications, continuous arteriovenous hemofiltration, preferably with dialysate flow, can be as effective.[58–60] While awaiting potassium *removal* by dialysis, recommended treatments for acute hyperkalemia should be carried out (see Table 53–5).

The usual endogenous generation of hydrogen ions (primarily from dietary proteins) is 1 mEq/kg/day but can be significantly greater in catabolic patients. Metabolic acidosis in patients with ARF can be treated with sodium bicarbonate administered with caution since it can exacerbate hypocalcemia and fluid overload.

Hyperphosphatemia (5 to 8 mg/dl) and symptomatic hypermagnesemia (>5 mg/dl) may present early in ARF and are usually associated with hypocalcemia (5 to 8 mg/dl). Oral phosphate binders will slowly lower serum phosphorus followed by an elevation of calcium levels. In symptomatic hypocalcemia, intravenous calcium gluconate is administered. Magnesium-containing antacids should be avoided.

Other Complications

In a previously normotensive patient, significant hypertension is more characteristic of ARF due to acute glomerulonephritis. However, volume-dependent elevations of blood pressure are common in non-nephritic, oliguric ARF. Vasodilator antihypertensive agents may produce short-term control of moderate-to-severe hypertension associated with volume overload when response to diuretic treatment is poor. Definitive management of poorly controlled hypertension may require fluid removal by dialysis.

Bleeding diatheses occurring during ARF may be accentuated by the platelet and factor VIII dysfunctions associated with uremia. In addition to the use of plasma, platelet, or clotting factor transfusions, better control of uremia by dialysis can ameliorate these bleeding distur-

Table 53–5. TREATMENT REGIMEN FOR HYPERKALEMIA*

Agent	Dose
Calcium gluconate (10%)	50–100 mg/kg IV (0.5–1 ml/kg)
Glucose (50%)/insulin	Glucose, 1 ml/kg IV; reg. insulin, 0.1 unit/kg
Sodium bicarbonate (7.5%)	1–2 mEq/kg IV
Sodium polystyrene sulfonate	0.5–1 g/kg PO or PR

*Modified from Ruley EJ and Bock GH: Acute renal failure in infants and children. *In:* Shoemaker WC, Ayres S, Grenvik A, et al (eds): Textbook of Critical Care, 2nd ed. Philadelphia, WB Saunders, 1989, p. 728 (with permission).

bances. The infusion of desmopressin acetate (DDAVP) at a dose of 0.3 μg/kg has also been shown to temporarily correct the bleeding time in uremic adult patients.[61]

Infections significantly increase the morbidity and mortality rates of patients with ARF. More than 70% of adults with ARF, mostly from traumatic or postoperative causes, are complicated by bacterial infections.[27, 62] Of these, more than half result in deaths. Although the incidence of infection in the pediatric population with ARF is not available, a similar situation most likely exists. Urinary tract infections account for approximately 31 to 89% of all cases, followed by pulmonary infections, septicemia, and infections related to indwelling lines.[27] This emphasizes the importance of (1) scrupulous avoidance of indwelling urinary catheters for prolonged periods in favor of intermittent catheterization, (2) pulmonary physiotherapy in the critically ill, and (3) aseptic handling of wounds and indwelling devices. The use of routine antibiotic prophylaxis is not recommended since it may actually be associated with an overall frequency of infection in patients with ARF.[63]

Dialysis

Dialytic therapies of various forms are important adjuncts in the management of ARF. The goals of dialysis should be defined clearly at the onset in order to institute the most appropriate dialytic modality and avoid indiscriminate use. Absolute indications for the initiation of dialysis are:

1. Symptomatic fluid overload unresponsive to conservative management
2. Life-threatening or medically uncontrolled metabolic disturbances, such as hyperkalemia, hyperuricemia, hyperphosphatemia, hypocalcemia, acidemia
3. Uremic pericarditis
4. Dangerous poisoning with dialyzable or hemofilterable compounds

Edema, in itself, is not an indication for dialysis. In specific situations, one can justify institution of "anticipatory" dialysis treatment in order to avoid or prevent complications in an unstable patient whose renal function is not expected to improve soon. Some data suggest that "prophylactic dialysis" with the goal of keeping the blood urea nitrogen concentration below 70 to 100 mg/dl in acute situations reduces morbidity and mortality.[27] In other conditions, in which optimal nutritional care is hindered by the fluid restriction imposed on an oliguric patient who does not require dialysis, elective slow continuous ultrafiltration facilitates administration of the volume of fluid necessary to infuse hyperalimentation or other necessary solutions. Since it takes time to set up and plan for any dialysis procedure, these acute situations require the early involvement of the nephrology team in order to ensure synchronized medical care.

From a nephrology standpoint, the choice of dialysis treatment should take into consideration the patient's age and size, cardiopulmonary status, adequacy of vascular access, history of a recent or previous intra-abdominal surgical procedure, and the specific goals for dialysis as well as the technical support available. Life-threatening metabolic disturbances, pulmonary edema, and the removal of dialyzable poisons are best managed by efficient hemodialysis (HD). However, HD may pose considerable risks for the hemodynamically unstable patient. In this setting, vasopressors and volume replacement are often needed. Other risks include the occurrence of the disequilibrium syndrome if dialysis is done briskly and the need for systemic heparinization in the patient who is already at risk for bleeding. The risk of bleeding can be minimized by careful monitoring of the activated clotting time.

Peritoneal dialysis (PD), although less hemodynamically destabilizing, is not as efficient as HD in the management of acute situations. Nevertheless, it is generally preferred in the pediatric age group and is as effective in most situations when implemented in the early stages of ARF. There are several strategies for the use of PD, but continuous 24-hour dialysis is preferred in acute treatments. Compared with HD, its other advantages are (1) lesser need for highly trained dialysis personnel, (2) continuous dialysis and fluid removal, and (3) greater safety in patients with coagulation disorders. On the other hand, PD may be complicated by seepage around the PD catheter, blockage of the catheter, exit site infection, hollow viscus perforation, and peritonitis. The development of fluid leaks around the PD catheter, particularly in infants, is not an unusual event in acute settings when insufficient time is allowed for the exit site to heal completely. In our experience, this risk can be minimized by initially using small PD fluid volume infusions with rapid cycles. Fluid leaks not only predispose to exit site infection but may require a decrease of the PD fluid volumes per cycle, thus reducing dialysis efficiency and even temporarily stopping dialysis. The catheter can be aseptically flushed in the case of fibrin clots that can lead to drainage problems. At times, surgical revision of catheter placement may be required because of omental wraps. Early diagnosis of hollow viscus perforation and peritonitis, particularly in the early stages prior to the appearance of clinical signs, requires regular PD fluid cell counts (increased index of suspicion when >100 WBC/mm³ with predominance of polymorphonuclears) and cultures. The latter should include fungal cultures, particularly in immunocompromised patients. The microorganisms usually isolated are listed in Table 53–6. When suspected, broad antibiotic coverage should be commenced intraperitoneally (dosing found in Table 53–7) and subsequently modified according to the sensitivity profile. Intraperitoneal installation of antibiotics, as listed, generate therapeutic serum levels without the need for intravenous administration.

Hypotension and reduced splanchnic blood flow may limit the efficiency of PD. The increased intra-abdominal pressure created by significant PD fluid volumes can potentially accentuate pre-existing hemodynamic instability due to preload reduction in patients with marginal cardiac function.[64] In this condition, the use of rapid-cycle (1- to 2-hourly), small-volume PD exchanges may be better tolerated. In addition, increased intra-abdom-

Table 53–6. ORGANISMS CAUSING
PERITONITIS IN CAPD*

Organism	%
Staphylococcus epidermidis	45
Staphylococcus aureus	14
Streptococci	9
Streptococcus faecalis	4
Diphtheroids	1.5
Escherichia coli	8
Enterobacter sp.	1.5
Klebsiella sp.	2.5
Acinetobacter sp.	2
Pseudomonas aeruginosa	4.5
Fungi	2
Miscellaneous	6

*From Gokal R: Continuous ambulatory peritoneal dialysis. *In:* Maher JF (ed): Replacement of Renal Function by Dialysis, 3rd ed. Dordrecht, Holland, Kluwer Academic Publishers, 1989, p. 602.

inal pressure can further compromise respiratory function in infants and small children who are already on ventilatory assistance. Finally, PD may be associated with either hypernatremia or hyponatremia. The occurrence of these disturbances depend, to a large extent, on the rapidity of the PD cycle and on the amount of ultrafiltration.*

Despite the major technical improvements that have been achieved over the years with HD and PD, these modalities may not always be feasible in very small infants. Likewise, seriously ill patients with cardiovascular instability and multiple organ failure may not always tolerate critically needed HD sessions. These situations have led to the recent re-evaluation of hemofiltration as an alternative extracorporeal therapy in ARF. When first described by Kramer, continuous arteriovenous hemofiltration (CAVH) was intended for fluid overloaded patients who did not respond to diuretics.[65] Currently, this modality has been performed successfully in infants and children for the management not only of fluid overload but also the metabolic abnormalities of ARF.[58, 66–68] In addition to its use for ATN, this technique has been used successfully for rhabdomyolysis,[69] the tumor lysis syndrome,[70] and the treatment of ARF in neonates during extracorporeal membrane oxygenation.[71]

Classic CAVH requires the passive flow of blood through a hemofilter driven by the arterial-venous pressure gradient. Generally, a MAP greater than 50 mm Hg to achieve a blood flow rate of 50 to 100 ml/min/m² is the minimum needed for CAVH.[72] This requirement, however, has been overcome by the use of pump-

*The passive transport mechanisms operating in PD are diffusion and convection. Diffusion accounts primarily for solute movement and is, therefore, dependent on a chemical gradient. Convection involves both solvent movement (ultrafiltration) and solvent drag of solutes. Convection is dependent on an osmolar gradient. It results in ultrafiltrate losses in which solute concentrations may be below that of plasma because of sieving effects along the peritoneal membrane capillaries. This occurs when exchange times are relatively brief. Large ultrafiltration volumes can, therefore, lead to hypernatremia. Hyponatremia can occur during longer cycles, when sodium equilibration is nearly complete. As a result, net sodium loss can be significant by virtue of the large total ultrafiltrate volumes, particularly if sodium replacement is inadequate.

assisted extracorporeal circulation.[73, 74] This modification, in turn, has made continuous venovenous hemofiltration (CVVH) possible, equally effective, and often preferred because of the risks involved with arterial cannulation. Longer hemofilter use and more precise regulation of the ultrafiltration rate are added advantages in a pump-assisted set-up. Despite these advances that make hemofiltration technically and clinically convenient, it must be kept in mind that the convective clearance of low molecular weight solutes achieved in hemofiltration (urea clearance of approximately 12 ml/min using a 0.6 m² polyamide hemofilter)[75] is not as high as the diffusive low molecular weight solute clearance attained in HD (urea clearance range of 90 to 130 ml/min using a 0.5 m² cellulose hollow fiber dialyzer at a blood flow of 100 to 200 ml/min). Patients whose primary clinical indication for hemofiltration is fluid overload can undergo slow continuous ultrafiltration (SCUF),[76] which generates a low rate of continuous fluid removal, but little molecular clearance. This technique causes little disruption of electrolyte balance since the electrolyte composition of the ultrafiltrate closely approximates that of the serum and requires no ultrafiltrate replacement. On the other hand, conventional hemofiltration requires large ultrafiltration volumes, as much as 6 to 10 l/day, in order to generate adequate molecular clearance. These volumes must be replaced with a balanced crystalloid solution in an amount equal to the ultrafiltrate volume (minus the desired fluid deficit). Improper electrolyte or fluid replacement may quickly lead to severe disturbances. The composition of a standard bicarbonate-based replacement solution is shown in Table 53–8. Lactate-based and acetate-based replacement solutions can also be used, although hepatic or cardiovascular instability, respectively, may make the bicarbonate-based solution preferable.

In order to further improve solute (e.g., urea, creatinine) clearances, dialysis can be added to continuous hemofiltration.[59, 60] In continuous hemofiltration/dialysis (CAVHD; CVVHD), dialysate is administered by an infusion pump at the rate of 15 ml/min in a countercur-

Table 53–7. ANTIBIOTIC DOSAGE FOR USE IN CAPD (PER LITER OF DIALYSATE UNLESS SPECIFIED OTHERWISE)*

Antibiotic	Loading Dose	Maintenance Dose
Tobramycin	1.7 mg/kg/bag	8 mg
Cephazolin	500 mg	250 mg
Ampicillin	500 mg	50 mg
Cloxacillin	1,000 mg	100 mg
Penicillin	1,000,000 units	50,000 units
Ticarcillin	1,000 mg	100 mg
Cotrimoxazole		
Sulfamethoxazole	400 mg	25 mg
Trimethoprim	80 mg	5 mg
Clindamycin	300 mg	50 mg
Amikacin	125 mg	25 mg
Vancomycin	500 mg	30 mg
5-Fluorocytosin		100 mg

*Modified from Balfe JW: Peritoneal dialysis. *In:* Holliday MA, Barratt TM, and Vernier RL (eds): Pediatric Nephrology, 2nd ed, p. 823. © 1987, the Williams & Wilkins Co., Baltimore.

Table 53–8. COMPOSITION OF BICARBONATE-BASED REPLACEMENT SOLUTION FOR CAVH

Solute	Concentration
Sodium	147 mEq/l
Chloride	112 mEq/l
Bicarbonate	35 mEq/l
Potassium	0–4 mEq/l
Calcium	2.4 mEq/l
Magnesium	1.4 mEq/l
Glucose	1.2 g/l

rent fashion in the hemofilter. Standard peritoneal dialysis solution containing 1.5 g/dl dextrose can be used.

Reported patient complications during hemofiltration are uncommon and mostly involve hemorrhage or infection at the blood access site. Heparinization of the extracorporeal circuit may be minimized or may not even be necessary in patients with coagulopathies. However, most patients require an infusion of 5 to 15 units/kg/hr of heparin in order to avoid the need for frequent hemofilter changes. As previously mentioned, accurate fluid replacement is necessary in order to avoid untoward hypotensive episodes during hemofiltration and also during rapid cycling PD, since underperfusion may have an adverse effect on the recovering kidney. Although the experimentally observed "tolerance" to second injury of already damaged kidney tissue remains controversial and may be true for some nephrotoxic ARF models, resistance does not seem to develop in ischemic models particularly in the presence of predisposing nephrotoxic insult.[77]

Nutritional Considerations

The provision of adequate nutrition is essential in the recovery of patients with ARF who are, in general, hypercatabolic. Aside from azotemia and metabolic acidosis, other factors that underlie the catabolic state of patients with ARF have been described and include infection, dialysis treatments and surgical interventions.[78] However, fluid limitations in an oliguric patient and the risk of excessive nitrogen retention can make the maintenance of a positive caloric and nitrogen balance difficult to achieve.

An estimate of the protein nitrogen balance provides information regarding the nutritional requirements of a patient. A catabolic state exists when the rate of endogenous protein catabolism estimated by the urea nitrogen appearance (UNA) exceeds nitrogen intake (NI). UNA is the sum of the urinary nitrogen and nitrogen from other fluids plus the change in body urea nitrogen during a 24-hour period without dialysis. Assuming that the volume of distribution of urea is equal to total body water (TBW = body weight in kg × 0.60 for children and adults, × 0.70 to 0.75 for infants), the change in body urea nitrogen is calculated as:

$$[\text{TBW (l)}_{final} \times \text{BUN (mg/l)}_{final}] - [\text{TBW (l)}_{initial} \times \text{BUN (mg/l)}_{initial}].$$

Since protein nitrogen balance is equal to NI (g) −

UNA (g), a negative nitrogen balance results when UNA is greater than NI. A UNA that exceeds NI by more than 5 g/day of nitrogen represents significant protein degradation.[79]

The role of early nutritional support in reducing postoperative morbidity and mortality in patients *without* renal failure is well recognized.[80, 81] However, the outcome of nutritional manipulations in patients *with* ARF including the effect of supplemental protein and the value of essential amino acids (AA), branched-chain essential AA, nonessential AA, and ketoanalogues of AA have been generally equivocal.[78, 79, 82–84] While aggressive protein-calorie supplementation seems sensible, experimental data suggest that amino acid infusions may predispose the kidney to ischemic or nephrotoxic injury.[85] While some protein is probably indicated, the general approach has been to restrict total protein intake. However, modifications should be made during hypercatabolic states within the limits of the patient's fluid tolerance while recognizing the risk of worsening the degree of azotemia.

For children, it has been suggested that protein catabolism can be minimized by providing 50 to 60 kcal/kg/day from nonprotein sources (glucose) and by restricting protein to approximately 0.5 g/kg/day in the form of high-quality protein or as a mixture of essential and nonessential amino acids (3 to 4:1, 40% of the essential AA as branched-chain) for those unable to tolerate oral feeding.[83, 84] Patients receiving HD or PD have particularly large protein deficits and should be provided a more liberal protein intake of 1.0 to 1.5 g/kg/day.[79] Calories (averaging 8.4 ± 2.7 kcal/kg/day) derived from intraperitoneally absorbed glucose during PD must also be taken into account in determining caloric replacement.[86] Hyperglycemia, if it occurs, can be managed with regular insulin (0.5 to 1.0 IU/kg). Fat emulsions should be given with caution since patients with ARF can be hyperlipidemic.

Drug Dosing in Acute Renal Failure

Drugs that are primarily excreted by the kidneys should be avoided, if possible, in ARF. If no alternative drug is available, the dose or time interval of administration must be adjusted according to the patient's renal function. Several drug dose-modification formats for this purpose are available.[87] However, these are generally constructed for the adult patient, and some extrapolation is often necessary. These dosing guidelines use Cl_{Cr} as an estimate of renal function. For practical purposes, the patient's Cl_{Cr} can be estimated using Schwartz formulas based on the patient's height[88, 89]:

$$Cl_{Cr}\ (\text{ml/min/1.73 m}^2) = \frac{\text{height or length (cm)} \times 0.55}{P_{Cr}\ (\text{mg/dl})}\ (\text{or } 0.45 \text{ if} <1 \text{ yr})$$

The accuracy of these formulas can be limited by a serum creatinine that is changing. In these situations, the nomogram developed by Hallnyck and associates can be useful for estimating the Cl_{Cr}.[90]

Patients receiving dialysis or hemofiltration may also require supplemental drug dosing if an appreciable amount of the drug is removed by the procedure. Information on the dialyzability of some drugs are available.[87, 91] In general, a drug that is highly protein bound is poorly dialyzed. Whenever possible, actual drug levels should be monitored.

PREVENTIVE MANAGEMENT

Prevention is a key element in the management of ARF. Prevention takes the form of (1) the identification of patients at risk in order to eliminate potential insults; (2) the institution of pharmacologic measures in an attempt to reverse imminent ARF; and (3) attenuation of the severity of the ARF by conversion of an oliguric form to one that is nonoliguric. In the pediatric setting, some of the commoner clinical conditions that *predispose* to the development of ARF include prematurity, asphyxia, septic conditions, shock, trauma, burns, postsurgical states, severe heart failure, liver failure, and the presence of pre-existing renal disease including renovascular disorders and nephrotic syndrome. In the majority of these conditions, maintenance of an effective intravascular volume with the preservation of a high urinary flow rate can prevent or correct renal hypoperfusion and, thus, the progression of prerenal azotemia to established ARF. In addition, the use of potentially nephrotoxic agents (e.g., antibiotics, chemotherapeutic drugs, x-ray contrast media), particularly in the presence of prerenal azotemia or pre-existing renal disease, should be avoided or at the very least minimized.

The three pharmacologic agents that have most frequently been advocated for the prevention or amelioration of ARF are mannitol, furosemide, and low-dose intravenous dopamine. Conflicting data exist regarding the efficacy of these agents, from both experimental models and clinical studies. Nevertheless, their use can generally be considered as one of potential benefit rather than risk.

The proposed mechanisms by which mannitol can lessen ischemic renal injury include a vasodilatory effect on the postischemic kidney possibly via intrarenal vasodilator prostaglandin synthesis; diuretic action with resultant decrease in both intratubular obstruction and tubular reabsorptive work; diminished tubular cell swelling (as a nonpermeant solute); improved mitochondrial energetics during the reflow period; and diminished cellular damage due to the scavenging of oxygen-free radicals.[32, 92] The efficacy of mannitol in improving GFR when administered prior to the ischemic or nephrotoxic event has been demonstrated in several experimental models. There is limited evidence that supports its usefulness when given once ARF is established. A number of clinical studies have demonstrated a preventive role in the settings of *cis*-platinum, amphotericin, and radiocontrast nephrotoxicity, biliary tract surgery, and transplant ARF.[27] Beneficial effects of mannitol in other conditions are equivocal since it appears to increase urine flow rather than improve GFR. Most likely, the potential clinical benefit of mannitol occurs when it is administered prophylactically or in the very early phase of ARF.

The preventive role of loop diuretics when administered prior to the injurious agent in experimental ARF has been attributed to a combination of its natriuretic properties as well as the suppression of TGF, dislodgement of intratubular obstruction, and renal vasodilatation most likely mediated by prostaglandins.[90, 91] Several studies, however, have failed to support this benefit, and furosemide has been shown to increase renal insufficiency in rats when administered with cephaloridine and glycerol.[92, 93–95] Nonetheless, furosemide has been found to be beneficial in transforming oliguric ARF into a nonoliguric state and possibly reducing the number of dialytic treatments in some cases.[92, 96] Response in these cases appeared to be influenced by the magnitude of the dose and the schedule of administration. Return of renal function and overall mortality, however, when compared with controls, were unchanged by furosemide treatment. As with mannitol, the benefit that may be derived from loop diuretics may depend on its prophylactic or early administration.

There is evidence that "low-dose" dopamine infusion (1 to 3 μg/kg/min) can reverse oliguric ARF because of its renal vasodilatory action.[97–99] In addition, a synergistic effect of dopamine with diuretics has been proposed since oliguric patients unresponsive to diuretics alone have been shown to respond to the concomitant infusion of dopamine.[100–102] This synergistic effect, if real and greater than dopamine alone, is most likely multifactorial, initially mediated by renal vascular dilatation allowing more diuretic to reach the loop of Henle and the macula densa followed by an increase in solute excretion, urine flow rate, and inhibition of TGF.[103]

Although it is evident that the success of pharmacologic prevention or attenuation of ARF depends on early intervention, it is unfortunate that most patients are referred to the nephrologist or intensivist having already reached the established phase of renal failure. This is further complicated by the difficulty in distinguishing early from established ARF, especially if nephrotoxin-induced. Because toxicity from diuretics is low, it seems appropriate to give oliguric ARF patients who have been adequately hydrated a trial of intravenous mannitol (0.5 g/kg) or furosemide (1 to 2 mg/kg).[90] Patients who do not respond may benefit from a concomitant infusion of low-dose dopamine. Unfortunately, *there is limited experience with children in the current literature that can provide us with dosing guidelines.* Diuresis may be sustained by larger furosemide doses (3 to 5 mg/kg/day) given slowly over 30 minutes as a single daily infusion in order to minimize the risk of ototoxicity. An equivalent oral dose can also be used. With a response of urine output, this regimen may be discontinued in 48 to 72 hours with a continued diuresis in the majority of cases. The earlier discontinuation of these agents must be based upon the physician's clinical judgement and the awareness of the risks of fluid overload, electrolyte imbalance, transient or permanent ototoxicity, and even aggravation of ARF from failure to replace fluid losses.

The ability to respond to diuretics is regarded by some authors as merely identifying cases that are intrinsically less severe; that transformation to a nonoliguric state carries the same prognosis as a *primary* nonoliguric ARF is only speculation. Furthermore, a lag period of as long as 48 hours, the same time interval given for a diuretic response, has been observed between fluid replacement and the onset of diuresis.[94] Although it is true that an improved urine volume facilitates fluid and nutritional management of ARF, it must be reiterated that aggressive diuretic administration does not lower the mortality rate in these patients nor does it appear to significantly alter the course of the disease.

Other pharmacologic approaches of potential use in the future for the prevention or reversal of ARF include combined norepinephrine–low dose dopamine therapy, calcium channel blockers, antagonists of platelet activating factor, analogues of prostanoids, xanthine compounds, and *p*-chlorophenylalanine.

References

1. Dixon BS and Anderson RJ: Nonoliguric acute renal failure. Am J Kidney Dis 6:71, 1985.
2. Gaudio KM and Siegel NJ: Pathogenesis and treatment of acute renal failure. Pediatr Nephrol 34:771, 1987.
3. Stapleton FB, Jones DP, and Green RS: Acute renal failure in neonates: Incidence, etiology and outcome. Pediatr Nephrol 1:314, 1987.
4. Jones AS, James E, Bland H, and Groshong T: Renal failure in the newborn. Clin Pediatr 18:286, 1979.
5. Chevalier RL, Campbell F, and Brenbridge AN: Prognostic factors in neonatal acute renal failure. Pediatrics 74:265, 1984.
6. Norman ME and Asadi FK: A prospective study of ARF in the newborn infant. Pediatrics 63:475, 1979.
7. Van der Merwe WM and Collins JF: Acute renal failure in a critical care unit. NZ Med J 102:96, 1989.
8. Hodson EM, Kjellstrand CM, and Mauer SM: Acute renal failure in infants and children: Outcome of 53 patients requiring hemodialysis treatment. J Pediatr 93:756, 1978.
9. Chaundry VP, Srivastava RN, Vellodi A, et al: A study of acute renal failure. Indian J Pediatr 17:405, 1980.
10. Niaudet P, Haj-Ibrahim M, and Gignadous MF: Outcome of children with acute renal failure. Kidney Int 28(Suppl.):S-148, 1985.
11. Anand SK: Acute renal failure in the neonate. Pediatr Clin North Am 29:791, 1982.
12. Rose BD: Clinical Physiology of Acid-Base and Electrolyte Disorders, 3rd ed. New York, McGraw-Hill, 1989, pp. 40–75.
13. Kon V and Ichikawa I: Research seminar: Physiology of acute renal failure. Pediatrics 105:351, 1984.
14. Kon V, Yared A, and Ichikawa I: Role of renal sympathetic nerves in mediating hypoperfusion of renal cortical microcirculation in experimental heart failure and acute extracellular fluid volume depletion. J Clin Invest 76:1913, 1985.
15. Goldsmith SR: Vasopressin as a vasopressor. Am J Med 82:1213, 1987.
16. Bidani A and Churchill PC: Acute renal failure. Dis Mon 35:63, 1989.
17. Patterson LT, Bock GH, Guzzetta PC, and Ruley EJ: Restoration of kidney function after prolonged renal artery occlusion. Pediatr Nephrol 4:163, 1990.
18. Humphreys MH and Alfrey AC: Vascular diseases of the kidney. In: Brenner BM and Rector FC Jr (eds): The Kidney, 3rd ed. Philadelphia, WB Saunders, 1986, pp. 1175–1220.
19. Smith HR and Scotland SM: Vero cytotoxin-producing strains of Escherichia coli. J Med Microbiol 26:77, 1988.
20. Kaplan BS and Proesmans W: The hemolytic uremic syndrome of childhood and its variants. Semin Hematol 24:148, 1987.
21. Habib R, Levy M, Gagnadoux MF, and Broyer M: Prognosis of the hemolytic uremic syndrome in children. Adv Nephrol 11:99, 1982.
22. Argyle JC, Hogg RJ, Pysher TJ, et al: A clinicopathological study of 24 children with hemolytic uremic syndrome. Pediatr Nephrol 4:52, 1990.
23. Van Dyck M, Proesmans W, and Depraetere M: Hemolytic uremic syndrome in childhood: Renal function ten years later. Clin Nephrol 29:109, 1988.
24. Gusmano R, Perfumo F, Ciardi MR, and Sarperi M: Long-term prognosis of haemolytic-uraemic syndrome in children. Adv Exp Med Biol 212:199, 1987.
25. Ratcliffe RJ, Tange EJ, and Ledingham JG: Ischemic acute renal failure: Why does it occur. Nephron 52:1, 1989.
26. Hostteter TH and Brenner BM: Renal circulatory and nephron function experimental acute renal failure. In: Brenner BM and Lazarus JM (eds): Acute Renal Failure, 2nd ed. New York, Churchill Livingstone, 1988, pp. 67–89.
27. Brezis M, Rosen S, and Epstein FH: Acute Renal Failure. In: Brenner BM and Rector FC Jr (eds): The Kidney, 3rd ed. Philadelphia, WB Saunders, 1986, pp. 735–799.
28. Schrier RW and Conger JD: Acute renal failure: Pathogenesis, diagnosis and management. In: Schrier RW (ed): Renal and Electrolyte Disorders, 3rd ed. Boston, Little, Brown, 1986, pp. 423–460.
29. Gouyon JB and Guingard JP: Functional renal insufficiency: Role of adenosine. Biol Neonate 53:237, 1988.
30. Firth JD, Ratcliffe PJ, Raine AE, and Ledingham JG: Endothelin: An important factor in acute renal failure? Lancet ii:1179, 1988.
31. Brown CB, Ogg CS, and Cameron JS: High dose furosemide in acute renal failure: A controlled trial. Clin Nephrol 15:90, 1981.
32. Zager RA, Mahan J, and Merola AJ: Effects of mannitol on the postischemic kidney. Lab Invest 53:433, 1985.
33. Ausiello DA, Kreisberg JF, Roy C, and Karnovsky MJ: Contraction of cultured rat glomerular cells of apparent mesangial origin after stimulation with angiotensin II and arginine vasopressin. J Clin Invest 65:754, 1980.
34. Donohoe JF, Venkatachalam MA, Bernard DB, and Levinsky NG: Tubular leakage and obstruction after renal ischemia: Structural-functional correlations. Kidney Int 13:208, 1978.
35. Oken DE: Hemodynamic basis for human acute renal failure (vasomotor nephropathy). Am J Med 76:702, 1984.
36. Thurau K and Boylan JW: Acute renal success. Am J Med 61:308, 1976.
37. Canavese C, Stratta P, and Vercellone A: The case for oxygen radicals in the pathogenesis of ischemic acute renal failure. Nephron 49:9, 1988.
38. Schrier RW and Hensen J: Cellular mechanism of ischemic acute renal failure: Role of Ca^{2+} and calcium entry blockers. Klin Wochenchr 66:800, 1988.
39. Ernest S: Model of gentamicin-induced nephrotoxicity and its amelioration by calcium and thyroxine. Medical Hypotheses 30:195, 1989.
40. Wilson DR and Schrier RW: Obstructive uropathy: Pathophysiology and management. In: Schrier RW (ed): Renal and Electrolyte Disorders, 3rd ed. Boston, Little, Brown, 1986, pp. 495–526.
41. Klahr S, Harris K, and Purkerson ML: Effects of obstruction on renal function. Pediatr Nephrol 2:34, 1988.
42. Wilson DR: Pathophysiology of obstructive uropathy. Kidney Int 18:281, 1980.
43. Olsen UB, Magnussen MP, and Eilersten E: Prostaglandins: A link between renal hydro- and hemodynamics in dogs. Acta Physiol Scand 97:369, 1976.
44. Nishikawa K, Morrison A, and Needleman P: Exaggerated prostaglandin biosynthesis and its influence on renal resistance in the isolated hydronephrotic rabbit kidney. J Clin Invest 59:1143, 1977.
45. Leichtman AB, Goldzer RC, Strom TB, and Tilney NL: Acute renal failure associated with renal transplantation. In: Brenner BM and Lazarus JM (eds): Acute Renal Failure, 2nd ed. New York, Churchill Livingstone, 1988, pp. 659–673.
46. Siegel DL, Fox I, Dafoe DC, and Power M: Discriminating rejection from CMV infection in renal allograft recipients using flow cytometry. Clin Immunol Immunopathol 51:157, 1989.
47. Miller PD, Krebs RA, Neal BJ, and McIntyre DO: Polyuric prerenal failure. Arch Intern Med 140:907, 1980.
48. Miller TR, Anderson RJ, Linas SL, et al: Urinary diagnostic indices in acute renal failure: A prospective study. Ann Intern Med 89:47, 1978.

49. Espinal CH: The FE Na test: Use in the differential diagnosis of acute renal failure. JAMA 236:579, 1976.
50. Espinal CH and Gregory AW: Differential diagnosis of acute renal failure. Clin Nephrol 13:73, 1980.
51. Shaffer SE and Norman ME: Renal function and renal failure in the newborn. Clinics Perinatol 16:199, 1989.
52. Ellis EN and Arnold WC: Use of urinary indices in renal failure in the newborn. Am J Dis Child 136:615, 1982.
53. Eliahou HE and Bata A: The diagnosis of acute renal failure. Nephrology 2:287, 1967.
54. Rudnick MR, Bastl CP, Elfinbein IB, and Narins RG: The differential diagnosis of acute renal failure. *In*: Brenner BM and Lazarus JM (eds): Acute Renal Failure, 2nd ed. Philadelphia, WB Saunders, 1988, pp. 177–232.
55. Fontanarosa PB: Radiologic contrast-induced renal failure. Emerg Clin North Am 6:601, 1988.
56. Holliday MA and Segar WE: Maintenance need for water in parenteral fluid therapy. Pediatrics 19:823, 1957.
57. Chan JCM: Peritoneal dialysis of renal failure in childhood: Clinical aspects and electrolyte changes as observed in 20 cases. Clin Pediatr 17:349, 1978.
58. Lopez-Herce J, Dorao P, Delgado MA, et al: Continuous arteriovenous hemofiltration in children. Intensive Care Med 15:224, 1989.
59. Schneider NS and Geronemus RP: Continuous arteriovenous hemodialysis. Kidney Int 33(Suppl.):S-159, 1988.
60. Siglar MH and Teehan BP: Solute transport in continuous hemodialysis: A new treatment for acute renal failure. Kidney Int 32:562, 1987.
61. Mannucci PM, Remuzzi G, Pusineri F, et al: Deamino-8-D-arginine vasopressin shortens the bleeding time in uremia. N Engl J Med 308:8, 1983.
62. McMurray SD, Luft FC, Maxwell DR, et al: Prevailing patterns and predictor variables in patients with acute tubular necrosis. Arch Intern Med 138:950, 1978.
63. Zech P, Bouletreau R, Moskovchenko JF, et al: Infection in acute renal failure. *In*: Hamburger J, Crosnier J, and Maxwell MH (eds): Advances in Nephrology from the Necker Hospital, Vol 1. Chicago, Year Book Medical Publishers, 1971, p. 231.
64. Franklin JO, Alpert MA, Twardowski ZJ, et al: Effect of increasing intra-abdominal pressure and volume on left ventricular function in continuous ambulatory peritoneal dialysis (CAPD). Am J Kidney Dis 12:291, 1988.
65. Kramer P, Wigger W, Rieger J, et al: Arteriovenous hemofiltration: A new and simple method for treatment of over-hydrated patients resistant to diuretics. Klin Wschr 55:1121, 1977.
66. Weiss L, Danielson BG, Wikstrom B, et al: Continuous arteriovenous hemofiltration in the treatment of 100 critically ill patients with acute renal failure: Report on clinical outcome and nutritional aspects. Clin Nephrol 31:184, 1989.
67. Lieberman KV, Nardi L, and Bosch JP: Treatment of acute renal failure in an infant using continuous arteriovenous hemofiltration. J Pediatr 106:646, 1985.
68. Zobel G, Ring E, and Muller W: Continuous arteriovenous hemofiltration in premature infants. Crit Care Med 17:534, 1989.
69. Winterberg B, Tenschert W, Rolf N, et al: CAVH in myorenal syndrome. Adv Exp Med Biol 252:385, 1989.
70. Heney D, Essex-Cater A, and Brocklebank JT: Continuous arteriovenous hemofiltration in the treatment of tumor lysis syndrome. Pediatr Nephrol 4:245, 1990.
71. Sell LL, Cullen ML, Whittlesey GC, et al: Experience in renal failure during extracorporeal membrane oxygenation: Treatment with continuous hemofiltration. J Pediatr Surg 22:600, 1987.
72. Golper TA: Continuous arteriovenous hemofiltration in acute renal failure. Am J Kidney Dis 6:373, 1985.
73. Canaud B, Garrel LJ, and Christol JP: Pump assisted continuous venovenous hemofiltration for treating acute uremia. Kidney Int 33(Suppl.):S-154, 1988.
74. Chanard J, Milcent T, Toupance O, et al: Ultrafiltration-pump assisted continuous arteriovenous hemofiltration (CAVH). Kidney Int 33(Suppl.):S-157, 1988.
75. Zobel G, Ring E, Trop M, and Stein JI: Arteriovenous hemofiltration in children. Int J Pediatr Nephrol 7:203, 1986.
76. Paganini EP and Nakamoto S: Continuous slow ultrafiltration in oliguric acute renal failure. Trans Am Soc Artif Intern Organ 26:201, 1980.
77. Honda N, Hishida A, Ikuma K, et al: Acquired resistance to acute renal failure. Kidney Int 31:1233, 1987.
78. Teschner M and Heidland A: Hypercatabolism in acute renal failure—mechanism and therapeutic approaches. Blood Purif 7:16, 1989.
79. Mitch WE and Wilmore DW: Nutritional considerations in the treatment of acute renal failure. *In*: Brenner BM and Lazarus JM (eds): Acute Renal Failure. New York, Churchill Livingstone, 1988, p. 743.
80. Mullen JL: Consequences of malnutrition in the surgical patient. Surg Clin North Am 61:465, 1981.
81. Starker PM, LaSala PA, Askanazi J, et al: The influence of preoperative total parenteral nutrition upon morbidity and mortality. Surg Gynecol Obstet 162:569, 1986.
82. Andrews PM and Bates SB: Dietary protein prior to renal ischemia dramatically affects postischemic kidney function. Kidney Int 30:299, 1986.
83. Feinstein EI, Kopple JD, Silberman H, and Massry SG: Total parenteral nutrition with high or low nitrogen intakes in patients with acute renal failure. Kidney Int 26(Suppl.):S-319, 1983.
84. Abitbol CL and Holliday MA: Total parenteral nutrition in anuric children. Clin Nephrol 5:153, 1976.
85. Zager RA and Venkatachalam MA: Potentiation of ischemic renal injury by amino acid infusion. Kidney Int 24:620, 1983.
86. Steinman TI and Mitch WE: Nutrition in dialysis patients. *In*: Maher JF (ed): Replacement of Renal Function by Dialysis, 3rd ed. Leiden, Netherlands, Kluwer Academic Publishers, 1989, pp. 1088–1106.
87. Bennett WM, Aronoff GR, Golper TA, et al: Drug Prescribing in Renal Failure. Philadelphia, American College of Physicians, 1987.
88. Schwartz GJ, Feld LG, and Langford DJ: A simple estimate of GFR in full-grown infants during the first year of life. J Pediatr 104:849, 1984.
89. Schwartz GJ, Haycock GB, Edelman CM Jr, and Spitzer A: A simple estimate of GFR in children derived from body length and plasma creatinine. Pediatrics 58:259, 1976.
90. Hallnyck T, Soep HH, Thomis J, et al: Prediction of creatinine clearance from serum creatinine concentration based on lean body mass. Clin Pharmacol Ther 30:414, 1981.
91. Choi L and Johnson CA: Removal of drugs by hemodialysis and peritoneal dialysis. Dial Transplant 16:538, 1987.
92. Levinsky NG and Bernard DB: Mannitol and loop diuretics. *In*: Brenner BM and Lazarus JM (eds): Acute Renal Failure, 2nd ed. New York, Churchill Livingstone, 1988, pp. 875–918.
93. Kleinknecht D, Ganeval D, Gonzalez-Duque LA, and Fermanian J: Furosemide in acute oliguric renal failure: A controlled trial. Nephron 17:51, 1976.
94. Lucas CE, Zito JG, Carter KM, et al: Questionable value of furosemide in preventing renal failure. Surgery 82:314, 1977.
95. Fink M: Are diuretics useful in the treatment or prevention of acute renal failure? South Med J 75:329, 1982.
96. Cantarovich F, Galli C, Benedetti L, et al: High dose furosemide in established acute renal failure. Br Med J 4:449, 1973.
97. Polson RJ, Park GR, Lindop MJ, et al: The prevention of renal impairment in patients undergoing orthotopic liver grafting by infusion of low dose dopamine. Anaesthesia 42:15, 1987.
98. Henderson IS, Beattie TJ, and Kennedy AC: Dopamine hydrochloride in oliguric states. Lancet ii:827, 1980.
99. Davis RF, Lappas DG, Kirklin JK, et al: Acute oliguria after cardiopulmonary bypass: Renal functional improvement with low dose dopamine infusion. Crit Care Med 12:852, 1982.
100. Lindner A: Synergism of dopamine and furosemide in diuretic-resistant oliguric acute renal failure. Nephron 33:121, 1983.
101. Baquero A, Morris M, Om A, et al: Dopamine and furosemide infusion for prevention of post-transplant oliguric renal failure. Transplantation 16:327, 1987.
102. Graziani G, Cantaluppi A, Casati S, et al: Dopamine and furosemide in oliguric acute renal failure. Nephron 37:39, 1984.
103. Lindner A, Cutler RE, and Goodman WG: Synergism of dopamine plus furosemide infusion in preventing acute renal failure in the dog. Kidney Int 16:158, 1979.

54

Hypertension

Edward J. Ruley, M.D.

Elevated blood pressure (BP) is not an uncommon problem in pediatric patients in the intensive care unit (ICU). BP elevation may be (1) the primary problem necessitating intensive care, (2) a secondary complication of a different primary pathologic process, or (3) the consequence of a therapeutic program. Regardless, elevated BP is an important clinical problem because it may directly contribute to morbidity and mortality or may be responsible for sequelae that persist beyond recovery from the acute process. Furthermore, significantly elevated BP may indirectly complicate the patient's course by necessitating modifications in the treatment plan or by producing side effects from the antihypertensive medications.

NORMAL VALUES FOR BLOOD PRESSURE AND DEFINITION OF TERMS

Normative values for BP have been determined for newborns, infants, children, and adolescents and are presented in Figure 54–1. Application of these norms presumes that the same conditions and parameters used in the development of the normal ranges are applied to the patient in question. In the intensive care setting, such a situation is unlikely because the normative studies were derived from a clinically well outpatient population. Regardless, these population studies provide useful ranges to be considered in the individual patient.

The normal BP ranges for newborns were derived from the first BP measurement in quiet, awake infants using a Doppler instrument. Since BP is lower in the sleeping infant, it is recommended that 7 mm Hg be added to the systolic blood pressure (SBP) and 5 mm Hg to the diastolic blood pressure (DBP) before comparison with the standard curves.[1]

The normal BP ranges for infants, children, and adolescents were based on the first auscultatory BP determination in supine infants or seated children and adolescents, with the measurement taken in the forearm using a cuff that completely encircled the circumference of the arm and covered greater than 75% of the length of the upper arm. The first Korotkoff sound was taken as the SBP. The fourth Korotkoff sound (muffling) was taken as the DBP for infants and children aged 3 to 12

years. The fifth Korotkoff sound (absence) was considered the DBP for adolescents between 13 and 18 years of age. The current standard curves not only portray the variations of BP with age and gender but also provide body mass (height and weight) information at each age so that patients whose growth is markedly less than or greater than that of their peers can be compared with the norms of children of comparable size.

By definition, *normal BP* is an SBP and DBP less than the 90th percentile for age and gender. *High normal BP* is the term used for average SBP and DBP between the 90th and 95th percentiles, whereas *high BP* is a value greater than the 95th percentile measured on at least three occasions. The terms *accelerated* or *malignant hypertension* are applied when there is a rapid increase in BP associated with microvascular damage that is evident on ocular fundoscopic examination.[2] Accelerated hypertension is associated with grade III Keith-Wagener retinopathy, which is characterized by the presence of retinal exudates and hemorrhages. Malignant hypertension occurs when there is grade IV Keith-Wagener retinopathy (papilledema).

MEASUREMENT OF BLOOD PRESSURE

In the ICU, BP is often measured by a direct intra-arterial (IA) catheter. The accuracy of direct measurements varies with catheter location. Brachial artery BP tends to be 10 mm Hg higher than the central aortic pressure.[3] Although direct measurements of BP in the brachial, femoral, and radial arteries are comparable,[3, 4] direct measurements of SBP in pedal arteries in children tend to be significantly higher.[5] This is the result of the summation of the incident and reflected pressure waves in small vessels, a phenomenon that occurs with increasing distance from the heart.

Indirect BP measurements can be made by auscultatory, Doppler, and oscillometric techniques. Although the upper arm is the customary site for auscultatory measurements, the forearm and leg can also be used. BP cuff size needs to be adapted to these sites.[1, 4] Comparisons of upper arm auscultatory BP measurements with direct IA measurements have shown a correlation coefficient of 0.87 for both SBP and DBP.[6] It

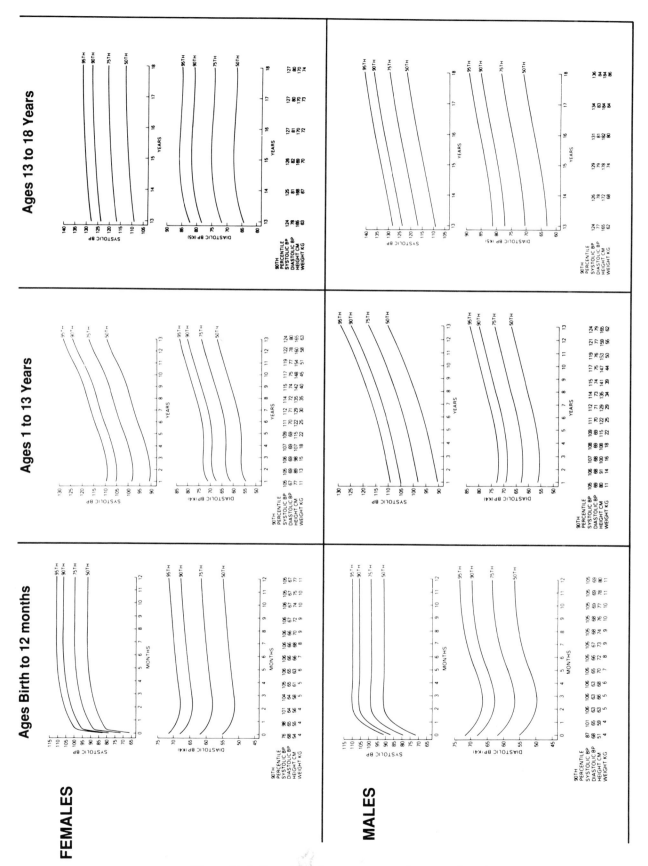

Figure 54–1. Normal blood pressure ranges by age and gender.

should be noted, however, that muscle movement and observer variation may result in significant inaccuracy.

The accuracy of Doppler devices varies with the manufacturer.[6] Although the correlation coefficient for SBP with direct IA measurements is high in optimal circumstances, the Doppler cannot measure DBP. The best correlation is achieved with a device that has the detector separated from the BP cuff. This is more awkward to use and is not automated.

Oscillometric devices depend on the detection of pressure oscillation rather than sound. They have the advantage of being able to measure BP in patients with faint Korotkoff sounds or in noisy ambient environments. Their correlation coefficient compared with direct IA measurements is 0.97 for SBP and 0.90 for DBP.[7] Oscillometric measurement has also proved to be accurate in neonates.[8] At the present time, oscillometry is the optimal automated indirect method for BP measurement.

There is no place for palpated or "flush" BP determination in the intensive care setting.

PATHOPHYSIOLOGIC CONSIDERATIONS

Although there are a variety of physiologic and pathologic interactions that determine the level and course of BP elevation, a highly simplified concept of etiology has been proposed and is of clinical usefulness.[9] This concept classifies all hypertensive states as being mediated by expansion of *intravascular volume* (preload) or an increase in *systemic vascular resistance* (afterload). Preload is determined by sodium balance, water excretion, and plasma oncotic pressure. It represents the load on myocardial fibers at the end of diastole and can be inferred from measurements of pulmonary wedge pressure or left ventricular end-diastolic volume or pressure. Afterload is the impedance the left ventricle must overcome during ejection. Afterload is determined by a variety of vasoconstrictive mediators such as catecholamines, angiotensin, and sympathetic vascular tone. Normotension is maintained by the homeostatic interplay of these two factors. Although such a classification ignores many of the nuances of BP homeostasis and pathophysiology, most clinical hypertension is dominated by either one or the other of these mechanisms. This concept is useful in the consideration of pathogenesis and in choosing antihypertensive therapy.

Regardless of the cause, elevated BP can result in a variety of symptoms that most often involve the brain or cardiovascular system. The severity and type of symptoms depend on the degree of BP elevation, the rate at which the pressure increases, and the pre-existing normal BP for the individual. For example, a sudden moderate rise in BP in a previously normotensive child can result in hypertensive encephalopathy or congestive heart failure (CHF). In contrast, a more gradual rise of BP to very high levels, particularly in a patient who has a history of chronic hypertension, may fail to produce symptoms. The pre-existing BP in a patient is of impor-

tance in setting therapeutic goals, as well as in the production of symptoms.

A related pathophysiologic consideration is the effect of hypertension on certain end organs, specifically the brain, heart, kidney, and eye. Under normal circumstances, the brain maintains cerebral blood flow (CBF) over a wide range of systemic BP through autoregulatory mechanisms (Fig. 54–2).[10, 11] If the BP decreases, arterioles in the brain respond by dilating so that the CBF is maintained in the normal range. In addition, as the lower limit of CBF is reached, cerebral oxygen extraction increases to preserve the metabolic viability of the central nervous system cells. Conversely, when the BP increases, there is progressive cerebral vasoconstriction so that normal CBF is again maintained. In a healthy adult, this autoregulation serves to keep the intracranial pressure (ICP) normal over a range of mean BP of about 60 to 150 mm Hg. When the upper limit of vasoconstrictive control is exceeded, there is forced dilatation of arteriolar segments so that leakage of plasma protein occurs and focal and then generalized cerebral edema develops.[12, 13] This brain edema causes the symptoms of hypertensive encephalopathy. These events increase the ICP, which further reduces CBF. Extreme BP elevations can cause intracerebral bleeding, producing the symptoms of a stroke.

In a patient with chronic systemic hypertension, the autoregulatory system in the brain adapts in such a way that the autoregulation curve shifts to the right to diminish the adverse effects of higher systemic BPs.[10, 11, 14] In this circumstance, however, the breadth of the plateau narrows so that the range over which autoregulation is physiologically effective is reduced (see Fig. 54–2). This shift to the right to modulate CBF at higher systemic pressures accounts for the tolerance of patients with chronic hypertension to sustained BP elevation with a minimum of symptoms.

Hypertension affects the cardiovascular system by increasing cardiac work. In its most simplistic form, cardiac work is the product of heart rate and systemic BP. Studies of children with early essential hypertension[15] have shown an increase in cardiac output (CO),

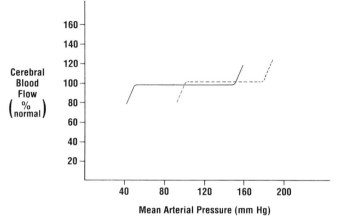

Figure 54–2. Autoregulation of cerebral blood flow at different systemic arterial mean blood pressures. (*Solid line* = normal; *dashed line* = right shift with chronic hypertension.)

heart rate, and oxygen consumption associated with a normal total peripheral resistance (TPR). With sustained BP elevation, the CO tends to normalize, whereas the hypertension is maintained by an increase in TPR. Gradually, left ventricular mass increases and is manifested by cardiac hypertrophy, a phenomenon most readily demonstrated by echocardiography.[16] In rapidly progressive hypertension in which there may be insufficient time for the functional adaptation of cardiac muscle, the CO may fall, and the patient experiences CHF. This may also occur in a child with chronic hypertension if the functional capacity of the hypertrophied myocardium is exceeded.

Hypertension and the kidney have a somewhat confusing interrelationship in pediatric patients. Renal disease is frequently the cause of hypertension through its production of renin and its pivotal role in the maintenance of vascular volume. Conversely, the kidney can undergo adverse secondary effects from hypertension due to any other cause by means of a vasoconstrictive response that decreases renal blood flow, resulting in azotemia and fluid retention. These latter acute changes are usually reversible. However, uncontrolled chronic hypertension can produce morphologic changes in the structure of the kidney that are irreversible. Such changes are unlikely to be permanently established during a limited stay in the ICU.

Uncontrolled hypertension can also cause cortical blindness or ocular muscle dysfunction, leading to diplopia and amblyopia. Although the acute effects are usually reversible, chronic uncontrolled hypertension can produce severe, irreversible visual impairment resulting from damage to the retina.

ETIOLOGY

Severe hypertension in the pediatric age group is usually due to secondary (i.e., specific) causes. Secondary hypertension should be suspected in patients with a greater degree and more rapid (hours to days) rate of BP elevation—two factors that also determine the presence of symptoms. It may occur at any age. In contrast, primary (i.e., essential) hypertension usually begins in adolescence, often being discovered as part of well child care. The BP elevation is usually mild to moderate, becomes worse very slowly (months to years), and is rarely associated with symptoms. It almost never is the reason for an ICU admission, though its pre-existence may complicate the management of an acutely ill patient.

Although there are a large number of possible causes for acute hypertension in pediatric patients, disorders of a few specific systems account for the vast majority. The frequency of causes varies by age. Rather than provide an encyclopedic list, it is more practical to approach elevated BP by considering causes in two categories: (1) those conditions in which the hypertension is the reason for ICU admission and (2) those situations in which hypertension may occur concomitantly with a separate acute life-threatening condition.

Conditions that may cause hypertensive emergencies

necessitating ICU admission are listed in Table 54–1. In all pediatric age groups, renal parenchymal and renovascular abnormalities are the most common cause of hypertension. Hypertension in the neonate can be caused by a variety of cystic[17] and cystic-dysplastic renal anomalies[18, 19] or by urinary obstruction.[20, 21] In some patients, these malformations may not be discovered until childhood. Although congenital renal artery stenosis in infants is very uncommon, renal artery stenosis caused by idiopathic fibromuscular dysplasia or as a complication of renal artery trauma is more common in older children and adolescents.[22] There is a high association of neurofibromatosis with intimal hyperplasia.[23] In older children and adolescents, acquired renal parenchymal diseases such as poststreptococcal glomerulonephritis, hemolytic-uremic syndrome, or unspecified chronic glomerulonephritis are not uncommonly associated with elevated BP. Although acute pyelonephritis may be associated with hypertension, elevated BP is more often a complication of renal scarring from previous infections. Acquired tubulointerstitial diseases are much less likely to produce hypertension than are acquired glomerular diseases. When oliguric renal failure is not present, the hypertension seen in these renal and renovascular diseases is usually mediated by increased renin secretion.

The principal cardiovascular cause of hypertension is coarctation of the aorta. It is often discovered during the neonatal period or infancy, though an occasional patient will have a delayed diagnosis. The age of discovery depends in large part on the degree of aortic narrowing. Neonates and infants with more severe coarctation usually have severe hypertension and are

Table 54–1. CONDITIONS THAT MAY PRESENT WITH HYPERTENSION AS THE PRIMARY PROBLEM

Renal
  Congenital renal structural anomalies
    Cystic kidney disease
    Cystic-dysplastic developmental disorders
    Obstructive uropathies
  Renal artery stenosis
    Congenital
    Post-traumatic
  Acquired renal parenchymal diseases
    Poststreptococcal glomerulonephritis
    Hemolytic-uremic syndrome
    Henoch-Schönlein purpura–IgG-IgA glomerulonephritis
    Rapidly progressive glomerulonephritis
    Chronic glomerulonephritis of unknown cause
    Renal scarring from pyelonephritis

Cardiovascular
  Coarctation of the aorta
  Arteritis
    Takayasu arteritis
    Polyarteritis nodosa

Tumors
  Neuroblastoma
  Pheochromocytoma
  Nephroblastoma (Wilms' tumor)

Endocrine (rare)
  Thyrotoxicosis
  Cushing syndrome
  Adrenal enzymatic deficiencies

symptomatic. Less severe degrees of narrowing are usually unassociated with symptoms, so the abnormality is discovered as part of the evaluation for hypertension in the older child or adolescent. The mechanism of hypertension is complex, particularly in the adolescent who has had long-standing BP elevations. It has been proposed that the primary mechanism corresponds to the one-kidney Goldblatt model in which an excessive production of aldosterone causes an increased plasma volume associated with normal plasma renin levels.[24, 25] Hypertension usually resolves with coarctation repair. Resolution is said to be inversely related to the age of the patient at repair. Hypertension may occur paradoxically after the repair, particularly in older patients whose disease has a more complicated pathophysiology.[26] Acquired forms of arteritis, particularly Takayasu's arteritis, may also cause severe hypertension. These are relatively uncommon.[27, 28]

Tumors, particularly neural crest tumors such as neuroblastomas, ganglioneuroblastomas, or ganglioneuromas, may cause hypertension in infants.[29] High BP may be mediated through (1) stimulation of the renin-angiotensin system, resulting from compression of the aorta or renal vasculature by a mass effect of the tumor or (2) catecholamines secreted by the tumor itself. In older children and adolescents, the most common neural crest tumor is pheochromocytoma.[29, 30] Hypertension is sometimes seen in Wilm's tumor in which it is most often mediated by renin-angiotensin hypersecretion.[31]

Endocrine causes are very uncommon at all ages but should always be considered in the differential diagnosis. They include thyrotoxicosis, Cushing syndrome, hyperaldosteronism, and adrenal deficiencies of enzymes such as 11-β-hydroxylase or 17-α-hydroxylase. With the exception of hyperaldosteronism and the adrenal enzyme deficiencies, endocrinopathies almost never present with hypertension as the *only* manifestation. The more generalized effects of excesses of thyroid and adrenocortical hormone production are usually quite obvious. Although a secondary cause for severe hypertension can usually be discerned in the child and adolescent, approximately half of neonates with significant hypertension will not have a discernible cause.[32, 33]

Another way of viewing hypertension is to consider those situations in which children admitted to the ICU for a life-threatening problem may experience hypertension during the course of their care. Many of these cases will be iatrogenic. Some of the more common situations encountered in the ICU setting are listed in Table 54–2.

The most common cause of secondary hypertension in neonates and infants is thromboembolism occurring as a complication of vascular catheterization. Obviously, this may occur in patients of any age. However, the incidence of clinically significant thromboembolism in neonates in particular has risen over recent years to 2 to 10% because of the increased use of umbilical artery catheters (UACs).[34–36] Using a UAC "pull-out" arteriogram, Neal and colleagues[37] found a 95% incidence of arterial thromboses, most of which were asymptomatic. The incidence of UAC thromboembolism increases with shock, infection, or the injection of hyperosmotic solu-

Table 54–2. INTENSIVE CARE SITUATIONS IN WHICH HYPERTENSION MAY OCCUR AS A COMPLICATING FACTOR

Renal
  Renal artery thromboembolism
    Catheter-associated
    Thrombosed PDA*
  Oliguric acute renal failure
  Acute urinary obstruction
  Renal trauma

Increased intracranial pressure
  Head injury
  Intracranial bleeding
  Meningitis-encephalitis
  Tumor

Iatrogenic-pharmacologic
  Vascular volume overload
  Postresuscitation
  Upper airway obstruction
  Bronchopulmonary dysplasia
  Abdominal surgery-distention
  Transfusion in a patient with chronic renal failure
  Extracorporeal membrane oxygenation
  Corticosteroid administration
  Bronchodilator administration
  Cyclosporine administration
  Illicit drug use

Immobilization
  Hypercalcemia
  Idiopathic

Burns

*PDA = patent ductus arteriosus.

tions, particularly antibiotics.[38] There is no consensus about the relative risks of high (T7 to T8) versus low (aortic bifurcation) catheter tip positioning.[39] Although most thromboembolic renal infarcts are too small to be identified with imaging techniques, occasionally renal segmental thrombosis[40] or complete or partial aortic thrombosis[41] will occur. Thromboembolism with hypertension can also occur secondary to thrombosis of a patent ductus arteriosus.[40]

Oliguric acute renal failure can be associated with fluid retention that can produce hypertension on a volume expansion basis. In contrast, when acute urinary obstruction is associated with hypertension, it is usually mediated by the renin-angiotensin system. Acute renal trauma, more common in older infants, children, and adolescents, may produce transient BP elevation, usually on a renin-mediated basis.[42] Furthermore, sustained hypertension can be a post-traumatic complication developing weeks to months after the injury.[43]

Increased ICP from any cause may produce hypertension by means of the Cushing reflex.[44, 45] In infants, this is most often the result of an intracranial bleeding episode or meningitis. In the child or adolescent, the most common cause is head injury.[46] Meningitis and meningoencephalitis, as well as brain tumors, may also cause hypertension.

Iatrogenic causes of high BP occur frequently in the acutely ill or injured child. Excessive fluid or colloid administration can lead to intravascular volume expansion and hypertension. This may be a particular problem in oliguric acute renal failure or in unrecognized chronic renal failure in which excessive fluid administration in a misguided attempt to increase urine flow may worsen edema and increase BP (see Chapter 53). Hypertension may also occur in the recovery phase of an acute cardiac arrest after successful resuscitation. This is thought to result from reabsorption of sequestered fluid with the consequent sudden expansion of intravascular volume.[47] Upper airway obstruction in children can be associated with severe hypertension.[48] The association of hypertension with bronchopulmonary dysplasia[49] and pneumothorax in the neonate[50] is also well known. Increased abdominal pressure has been associated with elevated BP,[51, 52] presumably by increasing venous return and intrathoracic pressure. Finally, hypertension is a frequent complication in infants treated with extracorporeal membrane oxygenation for respiratory failure. The elevated BP in this condition is multifactorial and is highly associated with increased ICP from intracranial bleeding, as well as stimulation of the renin-angiotensin system.[53] Blood transfusions in pediatric patients with chronic renal failure are a special circumstance. This phenomenon seems to result from an aberration in fluid distribution in chronic renal failure wherein infused fluid preferentially remains in the intravascular compartment.[54] A variety of pharmacologic agents, both legal and illegal, may elevate BP.

Another cause of hypertension is immobilization, and it may result from the development of hypercalcemia[55] or be of unknown cause.[56] Significantly elevated BP has been observed in 54% of immobilized children compared with only 12% of nonimmobilized hospitalized children.[56] It may be severe enough to precipitate seizures.

Finally, there is the hypertension frequently seen in patients with thermal burns. This hypertension has been proposed to be a result of the neuroendocrine response to trauma.[57, 58]

CLINICAL SYMPTOMATOLOGY

As previously mentioned, the severity and type of symptoms a patient experiences depend on the severity

Table 54–3. CAVEATS FOR THE TREATMENT OF HYPERTENSIVE EMERGENCIES

Parenteral or sublingual hypertensive medications are preferred for the initial treatment of hypertensive emergencies in order to achieve a prompt, controlled response and to avoid the unknowns of intestinal absorption

Sudden normalization of blood pressure may be hazardous; a reduction of 25–30% is a better goal

Plasma renin and aldosterone specimens should be obtained *before* instituting antihypertensive therapy

Blood pressure should be controlled *before* more complicated tests are performed or the patient is transported for diagnostic procedures (e.g., radiographs)

Oral medications should replace parenteral antihypertensive medications as soon as the patient's condition permits

of BP elevation, its rate of rise, the presence of pre-existing hypertension, and the age of the patient.

Acute hypertension in the neonate or infant usually causes irritability, feeding problems, and vomiting. Uncontrolled elevations may produce CHF with respiratory distress and cyanosis. Seizures can occur.[59]

In the child and adolescent, elevated BP produces headache, irritability, lethargy, nausea, vomiting, and visual disturbances (blurred vision and diplopia). Severe elevations most often produce encephalopathy with seizures and cranial nerve palsies, particularly of the fifth cranial nerve. Heart failure can occur. The most serious consequence of severe hypertension is stroke.

TREATMENT

Some general caveats for the treatment of hypertensive emergencies are given in Table 54–3. The clinician should make a working diagnosis as to the cause of hypertension so that the most likely pathogenesis can be considered. Presuming the pathogenesis, one can then select the antihypertensive agent most likely to be effective, taking into account the mechanism of action, as well as the contraindications, side effects, and inter-

Table 54–4. CLASSIFICATION OF SELECTED ANTIHYPERTENSIVE MEDICATIONS BY PRINCIPAL MODE OF ACTION

Principal Mechanism of Action	Parenteral Preparations	Oral Preparations
β-Adrenergic blockade	Propranolol	Propranolol Atenolol Metoprolol Nadolol
Vasodilatation	Nitroprusside Diazoxide Hydralazine	Minoxidil Hydralazine Prazosin
Converting enzyme inhibition	Enalaprilat	Captopril Enalapril Lisinopril
Calcium channel blockade	Nifedipine	Nifedipine Verapamil
Central α-stimulation		Clonidine
α-Adrenergic blockade	Phentolamine	Phenoxybenzamine Prazosin
Combined α-β-adrenergic blockade	Labetalol	Labetalol

Table 54–5. ANTIHYPERTENSIVE DRUGS FOR PARENTERAL AND SUBLINGUAL ADMINISTRATION

	Administration			Effect		
Drug	*Route*	*Preparation*	*Dosage*	*Onset*	*Peak*	*Duration*
Diazoxide	IV* rapid push (minibolus)	20 ml ampule (15 mg/ml)	1–3 mg/kg; may repeat after 15 min	1–5 min	1–5 min	Variable usually <12 hr
Enalaprilat‡‡	IV >5 min	2 ml vials (1.25 mg/ml)	0.04–0.8 mg/kg/dose Neonate: 0.01 mg/kg/dose	15 min	1–4 hr	Variable
Hydralazine	IV over 30 min or IM††	1 ml ampule (20 mg/ml)	0.15–0.2 mg/kg/dose, q 6 hr	10–20 min	10–90 min	3–6 hr
Labetalol‡‡	IV, slow bolus or infusion	20- and 40-ml vials (5 mg/ml)	0.25 mg/kg over 2 min; may double dose and repeat q 10 min to maximum cumulative dose = 5 mg/kg. Infusion dose = 1–3 mg/kg/hr	2–5 min	5–15 min	Variable usually 2–4 hr
Nifedipine	Sublingual	10- and 20-mg capsules	0.25 mg/kg/dose q 4–6 hr	10–15 min	60–90 min	Variable usually 2–4 hr
Nitroprusside	IV infusion	Lyophilized powder, 50 mg Dilute with D5W	0.5 µg/kg/min, titrate; max dose = 10/µg/kg/min	Within 30 sec	Within 30 sec	Duration of infusion
Phentolamine	IV rapid bolus	Lyophilized powder, 5 mg Reconstitute with diluent	0.05–0.1 mg/kg	Within 30 sec	2 min	15–30 min

*IV = intravenous.
† = supplemental dose after dialysis is not necessary.
‡Sx = symptoms.
§Vasodilatation Sx—sweating, flushing, feelings of warmth, tachycardia, palpitations.
‖Neurologic Sx—headache, blurred vision, dizziness, lightheadedness.
**ECFV = extracellular fluid volume.
††IM = intramuscular.
‡‡Manufacturer's warning—safety in children not established.
§§HPLC = high-pressure liquid chromatography.
Note: "Removal by dialysis" relates to the need for a supplemental dose after dialysis treatment, not to the use of dialysis to treat drug overdosage.

Removal by Dialysis				
(Hemodialysis)	(Peritoneal Dialysis)	Adverse Effects	Relative Contraindications	Comments
−†	−	Hyperglycemia Na$^+$ and H$_2$O retention Vasodilatation Sx‡§ Neurologic Sx‖	Thiazide sensitivity Tachycardia Diabetes Coarctation of aorta	Hypoproteinemia potentiates effect Use diuretics for Na$^+$ retention Ineffective for pheochromocytoma
+	−	Hypotension when ECFV** is contracted Hyperkalemia Oliguria	Renal failure Dehydration	Rx hypotension with volume expansion
−	−	Headache Vasodilation Sx§	Tachycardia Sensitivity to hydralazine	Color change in IV fluids does not indicate loss of potency

−	−	Neurologic Sx‖
		Scalp tingling
		  (bronchospasm)
			Asthma
			Pheochromocytoma
			Diabetes
			Hepatic insufficiency
				False + urine catecholamine by
				  fluorometric assay, not HPLC§§
				Synergistic with halothane anesthesia
				  (hypotension)

−	−	Headache
		Vasodilatation Sx§
			Concomitant use of β-
			  blocking drugs and
			  cimetidine
				Dose can be withdrawn from capsule
				  with 1-ml syringe and squirted
				  sublingually

−	−	Nausea-vomiting
		Vasodilatation Sx§
			Hepatic insufficiency
			Coarctation of aorta
				Photosensitive, solution good for 24 hr;
				  monitor blood thiocyanate after 72
				  hr, discontinue for thiocyanate >10
				  mg/dl; acidosis + tachyphylaxis =
				  cyanide poisoning

?	?	Tachycardia Hypotension Nausea, vomiting Abdominal pain	Peptic ulcer Gastritis	Specific for pheochromocytoma

actions. A listing of selected antihypertensive medications by their principal mode of action is given in Table 54–4. Specifics about preparations, dosages, pharmacokinetics, adverse effects, and relative contraindications for some of the more useful parenteral drugs are given in Table 54–5. Therapy should be adjusted, taking into account the time of onset and peak action of the drug's effect and the patient's response in relation to the therapeutic goals. Pharmacopeias should be consulted for further details about the drugs selected.

The following specific conditions deserve special comment.

Pre-encephalopathic Severe Hypertension

Attempts should be made to reduce the peak of BP by 25 to 30% in the pediatric patient who is symptomatic from severe hypertension but is not yet encephalopathic. Although the patient's underlying problems must be taken into consideration, no particular class of antihypertensive drug need be avoided in trying to achieve this goal.

Hypertensive Encephalopathy

It is generally advised that antihypertensive medications that act primarily by vasodilatation (e.g., nitroprusside and hydralazine) or calcium channel blockade (e.g., nifedipine) are not preferred in encephalopathic patients because of their potential to increase intracranial blood flow and raise ICP.[11, 60] Diazoxide does not cross the blood-brain barrier and therefore can be used in patients with encephalopathy as long as the "minibolus" regimen is carefully followed to prevent excessive BP reduction. Medications that act by inhibition of angiotensin II converting enzyme (enalaprilat), combined α-β-blockade (labetalol), or β-blockade (propranolol) can also be used.

Poststreptococcal Glomerulonephritis

The mechanism of hypertension in poststreptococcal glomerulonephritis is intravascular volume expansion; renin is usually suppressed.[60, 61] Although diuretics theoretically should be the drugs of choice, the diuretic response of the patient is usually markedly impaired by the decreased glomerular filtration that is part of this disease. Calcium channel blockers and vasodilators usually are effective.

Renal Artery Stenosis

The mechanism of high BP in unilateral renal artery stenosis is usually associated with elevated renin values.[25] Although converting enzyme inhibitors are usually very effective for controlling BP in this abnormality, the

kidney can suffer damage from the diminished blood flow when there is medically induced normotension over a long period. Definitive therapy includes relief of the vascular obstruction by transluminal angioplasty or arterial reconstruction.[63] In bilateral renal artery stenosis, there is volume expansion with normal peripheral renin activity. However, in the presence of hypertension, a normal value for renin is not "normal." In the chronic steady state, these patients have a volume-maintained hypertension from the effects of increased aldosterone production, which is driven by ongoing renin production.[25] Diuretics will lower the BP somewhat, and the institution of a converting enzyme inhibitor regimen will usually normalize it further. The same caveat concerning renal damage from chronic medical therapy in unilateral renal artery stenosis also applies to bilateral stenosis.

Urinary Tract Obstruction

Since high BP in urinary obstruction is most often mediated by the renin-angiotensin system, converting enzyme inhibitors are usually the drugs of choice. Surgical correction of the obstruction usually produces resolution of the hypertension. Diuretics should be avoided because an increase in urine volume may worsen the obstruction by causing increased kinking of the redundant ureters.

Oliguric Acute Renal Failure

Hypertension in oliguric acute renal failure can be treated with nearly any class of antihypertensive medication. Careful management so as not to aggravate fluid overload is important in minimizing the severity of the BP elevation. This is sometimes difficult because of the obligatory fluid required to deliver medications and hyperalimentation. In these circumstances, fluid control can be achieved with peritoneal dialysis, continuous arteriovenous hemofiltration, continuous venovenous hemofiltration, or conventional hemodialysis. The former three methods are preferred because they provide "around-the-clock" volume control.

Closed Head Injury

In closed head injury, there is usually an increased TPR resulting from catecholamine secretion and increased sympathetic tone. Therefore, combined α-β-adrenergic blocking drugs (labetalol, phentolamine, prazosin) or centrally acting drugs that reduce sympathetic tone (clonidine) are most likely to be effective.

Pheochromocytoma

The use of α-adrenergic blocking agents is preferred in pheochromocytoma, a disorder of excessive catecholamine secretion. With control, the intravenous preparation can be changed to orally administered phenoxybenzamine.

SEQUELAE OF ACUTE HYPERTENSION

The most severe sequelae of a hypertensive crisis are residual brain damage from a stroke and cerebral edema. Prompt treatment should minimize these complications. Some children will continue to be hypertensive after the acute phase of their illness and will require chronic antihypertensive medications. Although uncontrolled hypertension is a major cause of chronic renal failure in adults, it is much less so in children.

References

1. Report of the Second Task Force on Blood Pressure Control in Children–1987. Pediatrics 79:1, 1987.
2. Grossman SH and Gunnells JC: Recognition and treatment of hypertensive emergencies. Cardiovasc Clin 3:97, 1981.
3. Kroeker EJ and Wood EH: Comparison of simultaneously recorded central and peripheral arterial pressure pulse during rest, exercise and tilted position in man. Circ Res 3:623, 1955.
4. Park MK and Guntheroth WG: Direct blood pressure measurements in brachial and femoral arteries in children. Circulation 41:231, 1970.
5. Park MK, Robotham JL, and German VF: Systolic pressure amplification in pedal arteries in children. Crit Care Med 11:286, 1983.
6. Reder RF, Dimich I, Cohen ML, et al: Evaluating indirect blood pressure measurement techniques: A comparison of three systems in infants and children. Pediatrics 62:326, 1978.
7. Park MK and Menard SM: Accuracy of blood pressure measurement by the dinamap monitor in infants and children. Pediatrics 79:907, 1987.
8. Friesen RH and Lichtor JL: Indirect measurement of blood pressure in neonates and infants utilizing an automatic noninvasive oscillometric monitor. Anesth Analg 60:742, 1981.
9. Izzo JL: Labile hypertension, vasomotor instability, and postural syndromes. In: Laragh JH and Brenner BM (eds): Hypertension: Pathophysiology, Diagnosis, and Management. New York, Raven Press, 1990, p 1418.
10. Paulson OB, Waldemar G, Schmidt JF, et al: Cerebral circulation under normal and pathologic conditions. Am J Cardiol 63:2C, 1989.
11. Strandgaard A and Paulson OB: Hypertensive disease and the cerebral circulation. In: Laragh JH and Brenner BM (eds): Hypertension: Pathophysiology, Diagnosis, and Management. New York, Raven Press, 1990, pp 399–416.
12. MacKenzie ET, Strandgaard S, Graham DI, et al: Effects of acutely induced hypertension in cats on pial arteriolar caliber, local cerebral blood flow, and the blood-brain barrier. Circ Res 39:33, 1976.
13. Tamaki K, Sadoshima S, Baumbach GL, et al: Evidence that disruption of the blood-brain barrier precedes reduction in cerebral blood flow in hypertensive encephalopathy. Hypertension 6 (Suppl I):I-75, 1984.
14. Heistad DD: Protection of the blood-brain barrier during acute and chronic hypertension. FASEB J 43:205, 1984.
15. Zahka KG, Neill CA, Langford H, et al: Cardiac involvement in adolescent hypertension. Hypertension 3:664, 1981.
16. Reichek N and Devereux RB: Left ventricular hypertrophy: Relationship of anatomic, echocardiographic and electrocardiographic findings. Circulation 63:1391, 1981.
17. Cole BR, Conley SB, and Stapleton FB: Polycystic kidney disease in the first year of life. J Pediatr 111:693, 1987.
18. Gilboa N, Bartoletti A, and Urizar RE: Severe hypertension in a newborn associated with increased renin production by a hypoplastic kidney. J Urol 128:570, 1982.
19. Chen Y-H, Stapleton FB, Roy S, et al: Neonatal hypertension from a unilateral multicystic dysplastic kidney. J Urol 133:664, 1985.
20. Weidmann P, Beretta-Piccoli D, Hirsch D, et al: Curable hypertension with unilateral hydronephrosis: Studies on the role of circulating renin. Ann Intern Med 87:437, 1977.
21. Abramson M and Jackson B: Hypertension and unilateral hydronephrosis. J Urol 132:746, 1984.
22. Guzzetta PC, Potter BM, Ruley EJ, et al: Renovascular hypertension in children: Current concepts in evaluation and treatment. J Pediatr Surg 24:1236, 1989.
23. Tilford DL and Kelsch RC: Renal artery stenosis in childhood neurofibromatosis. Am J Dis Child 126:665, 1973.
24. Alpert BS, Bain HH, Balfe JW, et al: Role of the renin-angiotensin-aldosterone system in hypertensive children with coarctation of the aorta. Am J Cardiol 43:828, 1979.
25. Nabel EG, Gibbons GH, and Dzau VJ: Pathophysiology of experimental renovascular hypertension. Am J Kidney Dis 5:A111, 1985.
26. Sealy WC: Paradoxical hypertension after repair of coarctation of the aorta: A review of its causes. Ann Thorac Surg 50:323, 1990.
27. Dillon MJ: Classification and pathogenesis of arteritis in children. Toxicol Pathol 17:214, 1989.
28. Lagneau P and Michel JB: Renovascular hypertension and Takayasu's disease. J Urol 134:876, 1985.
29. Weinblatt ME, Heisel MA, and Siegel SE: Hypertension in children with neurogenic tumors. Pediatrics 71:947, 1983.
30. Hull CJ: Phaeochromocytoma: Diagnosis, preoperative preparation and anaesthetic management. Br J Anaesth 58:1453, 1986.
31. Yokomori K, Hori T, Takemura T, et al: Demonstration of both primary and secondary reninism in renal tumors in children. J Pediatr Surg 23:403, 1988.
32. Buchi KF and Siegler RL: Hypertension in the first month of life. J Hypertens 4:525, 1986.
33. Friedman AL and Hustead VA: Hypertension in babies following discharge from a neonatal intensive care unit. Pediatr Nephrol 1:30, 1987.
34. Wigger HJ, Bransilver B, and Blanc WA: Thromboses due to catheterization in infants and children. J Pediatr 76:1, 1970.
35. Plumer LB, Kaplan GW, and Mendoza SA: Hypertension in infants—a complication of umbilical arterial catheterization. J Pediatr 89:802, 1976.
36. Bauer SB, Feldman SM, Gellis SS, et al: Neonatal hypertension: A complication of umbilical-artery catheterization. N Engl J Med 293:1032, 1975.
37. Neal WA, Reynolds JW, Jarvis CW, et al: Umbilical artery catheterization: Demonstration of arterial thromboses by aortography. Pediatrics 50:6, 1972.
38. Brooks WG and Weibley RE: Emergency department presentation of severe hypertension secondary to complications of umbilical artery catheterization. Pediatr Emerg Care 3:104, 1987.
39. Mokrohisky ST, Levine RL, Blumhagen JD, et al: Low positioning of umbilical-artery catheters increases associated complications in newborn infants. N Engl J Med 299:561, 1978.
40. Durante D, Jones D, and Spitzer R: Neonatal renal arterial embolism syndrome. J Pediatr 89:978, 1976.
41. Malin SW, Baumgart S, Rosenberg HK, et al: Nonsurgical management of obstructive aortic thrombosis complicated by renovascular hypertension in the neonate. J Pediatr 106:630, 1985.
42. Elias AN, Anderson GH, Dalakos TG, et al: Renin angiotensin involvement in transient hypertension after renal injury. J Urol 119:561, 1978.
43. Monstrey SJM, Beerthuizen GIJM, vander Werken C, et al: Renal trauma and hypertension. J Trauma 29:65 1989.
44. Jones JV: Differentiation and investigation of primary versus secondary hypertension (Cushing reflex). Am J Cardiol 63:10C, 1989.
45. Kaiser AM and Whitelaw AGL: Hypertensive response to raised intracranial pressure in infancy. Arch Dis Child 63:1461, 1988.
46. Simard JM and Bellefleur M: Systemic arterial hypertension in head trauma. Am J Cardiol 63:32C, 1989.
47. Dawson CW, Lucas CE, and Ledgerwood AM: Altered interstitial fluid space dynamics and postresuscitation hypertension. Arch Surg 116:657, 1981.
48. Serratto M, Harris V, and Carr I: Upper airways obstruction: Presentation with systemic hypertension. Arch Dis Child 56:153, 1981.

49. Abman SH, Warady BA, Lum GM, et al: Systemic hypertension in infants with bronchopulmonary dysplasia. J Pediatr 104:929, 1984.

50. Goldberg RN: Sustained arterial blood pressure elevation associated with pneumothoraces: Early detection via continuous monitoring. Pediatrics 68:775, 1981.

51. Adelman RD and Sherman MP: Hypertension in the neonate following closure of abdominal wall defects. J Pediatr 97:642, 1980.

52. Sinkin RA, Phillips BL, and Adelman RD: Elevation in systemic blood pressure in the neonate during abdominal examination. Pediatrics 76:970, 1985.

53. Sell LL, Cullen ML, Lerner GR, et al: Hypertension during extracorporeal membrane oxygenation: Cause, effect, and management. Surgery 102:724, 1987.

54. Koomans HA, Geers AB, Boer P, et al: A study on the distribution of body fluids after rapid saline expansion in normal subjects and in patients with renal insufficiency: Preferential intravascular disposition in renal failure. Clin Sci 64:153, 1983.

55. Rosen JF, Wolin DA, and Finberg L: Immobilization hypercalcemia after single limb fractures in children and adolescents. Am J Dis Child 132:560, 1978.

56. Turner MC, Ruley EJ, Buckley KM, et al: Blood pressure elevation in children with orthopedic immobilization. J Pediatr 95:989, 1979.

57. Falkner B, Roven S, DeClement FA, et al: Hypertension in children with burns. J Trauma 8:213, 1978.

58. Popp MB, Silberstein EB, Srivastava LS, et al: A pathophysiologic study of the hypertension associated with burn injury in children. Ann Surg 193:817, 1981.

59. Mace S and Hirschfeld S: Hypertensive encephalopathy: A cause of neonatal seizures. Am J Dis Child 137:32, 1983.

60. Barry DI: Cerebrovascular aspects of antihypertensive treatment. Am J Cardiol 63:14C, 1989.

61. Fleisher DS, Voci G, Garfunkel J, et al: Hydrodynamic findings in acute glomerulonephritis. J Pediatr 69:1054, 1966.

62. Rodriguez-Itrube B, Baggio B, Colina-Chourio J, et al: Studies on the renin-aldosterone system in acute nephritis syndrome. Kidney Int 19:47, 1981.

63. Guzzetta PC, Potter BM, Kapur S, et al: Reconstruction of the renal artery after unsuccessful percutaneous transluminal angioplasty in children. Am J Surg 145:647, 1983.

55

Renal Transplantation

Philip C. Guzzetta, M.D.

BACKGROUND

Although solid organ transplantation has been contemplated since antiquity, serious scientific studies have only been performed during the 20th century. The development of vascular suturing techniques by Carrel (for which he was granted the Nobel Prize in 1912) established the methods by which solid organs could be transplanted. Attempts at renal xenografts from animals to the arms of uremic humans early in the 20th century were met with rapid graft failure despite technical success of the vascular anastomoses, suggesting an unknown barrier to transplantation among species.[1]

These early failures convinced many physicians that solid organ transplantation was not possible, and little clinical experimentation was done until after 1950. In 1953, Michon and associates reported a renal transplant from a mother to her son who had suffered the loss of his solitary kidney in an accident.[2] The kidney allograft functioned for 22 days, then acutely failed and the recipient died. The first successful renal transplant between identical twins was performed in 1954 by Murray and associates in Boston.[3] For this transplant and other pioneering work in transplantation, Murray received the Nobel Prize in Medicine in 1990.

Extension of this lifesaving modality to all uremic patients required the development of potent immunosuppressive therapies. Attempts at total body irradiation as a method of immunosuppression led to lethal consequences of radiation illness and infection.[4] Development of immunosuppressive medication protocols using 6-mercaptopurine, its derivative azathioprine, and prednisone in the early 1960s made genetically disparate living-related donor (LRD) and cadaver renal transplants a viable alternative to dialysis.[5, 6] Interestingly, it was not until 1964 that tissue typing of the human leukocyte antigens (HLA) was utilized to select recipients for kidney allografts.[7]

The next major advance in immunosuppression occurred with the use of polyclonal antibodies to human lymphocytes.[8] The release of cyclosporine in 1984 dramatically improved the kidney allograft success rates, most notably in those receiving cadaver kidneys.[9] The development of OKT3, a murine monoclonal antibody to a surface antigen on all human T cells, has significantly improved the treatment results with steroid-resis-

tant acute rejection.[10] More potent and specific immunosuppressive agents are being developed, and attempts to induce a form of tolerance by infusion of bone marrow from the kidney donor are undergoing clinical trials.[11]

PREOPERATIVE MANAGEMENT

Almost all renal transplant patients are on dialysis at the time of their transplant. Patients on daily peritoneal dialysis, the preferred method of dialysis in children, are usually in good fluid and electrolyte status when they arrive at the hospital for the transplant. This may not be the case with hemodialysis patients, who may have significant fluid shifts and electrolyte imbalances between dialysis sessions. The most critical issues for the operative procedure are the patient's acid-base status, serum potassium, and degree of anemia.

Most renal failure children have a chronic acidosis that increases their risk with anesthesia by shifting the oxygen dissociation curve to the right, thus aggravating poor tissue oxygenation to which they are already predisposed because of chronic anemia (see later). If the acidosis is severe (pH < 7.2 or serum HCO_3 < 14), this should be corrected with base infusion or dialysis before surgery.

Hyperkalemia may develop between hemodialysis sessions, thus increasing anesthetic risks because of the potential for cardiac dysrhythmias. It is unwise to force the serum potassium intracellularly with an infusion of insulin and glucose immediately preoperatively, because the hyperkalemia is likely to recur and possibly worsen during surgery. It is much safer to delay the procedure for a few hours and dialyze the patient to a potassium level of less than 5 mEq/l.

The anemia associated with renal failure is a chronic, hemodynamically stable one, although it does have negative effects on the oxygen-carrying capacity of the blood. We do not preoperatively transfuse the renal transplant patients if their hematocrits are above 20%, although we always type and cross-match three units of blood for the procedure. Whenever a blood product is given to a transplant patient, it must be washed. If the recipient is cytomegalovirus (CMV) negative, the blood should also be CMV negative. Fortunately, the use of

Table 55–1. LIVING-RELATED DONOR RENAL TRANSPLANT IMMUNOSUPPRESSION PROTOCOL

Day −1	Cyclosporine 10 mg/kg po at midnight
Day 0	Azathioprine 2 mg/kg/ IV in the OR*
	Methylprednisolone 5 mg/kg IV in the OR
	Cyclosporine 1 mg/kg IV q 8 hr

Good renal function?

Yes	No
(With oral intake established)	Begin Minnesota ALG† as in cadaver donor protocol

Day 1	Azathioprine, 2 mg/kg po qd
	Prednisone, 2 mg/kg po bid
	Cyclosporine, 5 mg/kg po bid
	(check cyclosporine level qd)
Day 2	Azathioprine, 2 mg/kg po qd
	Prednisone, 1.5 mg/kg po bid
	Cyclosporine, 5 mg/kg po bid
Day 3	Azathioprine, 2 mg/kg po qd
	Prednisone, 1 mg/kg po bid
	Cyclosporine, 5 mg/kg po bid
	If the cyclosporine level is in the therapeutic range for days +2 and +3 continue prednisone taper
Days 4, 5, and 6	Azathioprine, 2 mg/kg po qd
	Prednisone, 0.75 mg/kg po bid
	Cyclosporine dose given po bid dependent on keeping the level in the therapeutic range
Days 7, 8, and 9	Azathioprine, 2 mg/kg po qd
	Prednisone, 0.5 mg/kg po bid
	Cyclosporine dose given po bid dependent on keeping the level in the therapeutic range
Days 10, 11, and 12	Azathioprine 2 mg/kg po qd
	Prednisone 0.5 mg/kg po qd
	Cyclosporine dose given po bid dependent on keeping the level in the therapeutic range
Days >12	Same medications as for day 12

*OR = operating room.
†ALG = antilymphoblastglobulin.

human recombinant erythropoietin has made chronic anemia less of a problem in patients with renal failure.

INTRAOPERATIVE MANAGEMENT

Intraoperative Monitoring. A urinary catheter is placed, the bladder is distended with an antibacterial irrigant, and the drainage tubing is clamped until the neoureterocystostomy is completed. A single large-bore peripheral intravenous (IV) catheter is placed for administration of medications, fluids, and blood. A percutaneous central venous catheter is placed for intraoperative monitoring of the central venous pressure (CVP) and postoperative administration of Minnesota antilymphoblast globulin (ALG) in patients receiving a kidney from a cadaver. We prefer a subclavian approach for placement of a double-lumen CVP line, because the patients are more comfortable with the line in that position than in the internal jugular vein when it must be maintained for several days.

Transcutaneous pulse oximetry is also routinely obtained. We have not found routine arterial line placement to be necessary, and we have avoided it. Almost all of our patients have near-normal cardiopulmonary function, and therefore Swan-Ganz catheters are rarely used.

Fluid Replacement. IV fluids should be normal saline or D5 normal saline, and depending on the length of the procedure these fluids may be alternated. Lactated Ringer's solution is avoided because of its small amount of potassium. Almost all patients have the kidney placed in a retroperitoneal position, which minimizes intraoperative fluid losses. The operative procedure takes 3 to 4 hours, and fluid replacement should be approximately 15 ml/kg/hr. We routinely use mannitol (1 g/kg up to 50 g) just before reperfusing the kidney. The exact amount of fluid used depends substantially on the CVP and on the turgor of the kidney after the vascular clamps have been released. Ideally the CVP should be 12 to 15 mm Hg, and the kidney should be firm. Fluid boluses to accomplish these goals should be given before starting the ureteral anastomosis. Any blood products must be washed and should also be CMV negative in the CMV-negative recipient.

Medications. The immunosuppressive medications are different for LRD and cadaveric transplants; our protocols are seen in Tables 55–1 and 55–2. All patients receive prophylactic antibiotics once the IV is placed in the operating room (OR). We use cefazolin in a dose of 25 mg/kg, up to 1 gram. All patients receive azathioprine and methylprednisolone intravenously in the OR as seen in Tables 55–1 and 55–2, and as mentioned earlier all patients receive mannitol. No other medications are routinely given in the OR.

Technical Considerations. Almost all patients will have the transplant placed in a retroperitoneal position. Even when a large kidney is placed into a small recipi-

Table 55–2. CADAVERIC RENAL TRANSPLANT IMMUNOSUPPRESSION PROTOCOL

Day 0	Azathioprine, 2 mg/kg IV in the OR
	Methylprednisolone, 5 mg/kg IV in the OR
	Minnesota ALG, 15 mg/kg IV via CVP line over 6 hours (given immediately after surgery)
Day 1	Azathioprine, 2 mg/kg po qd
	Prednisone, 2 mg/kg po bid
	ALG, 15 mg/kg IV via CVP
Day 2	Azathioprine, 2 mg/kg po qd
	Prednisone, 1.5 mg/kg po bid
	ALG, 15 mg/kg IV via CVP
Day 3	Azathioprine, 2 mg/kg po qd
	Prednisone, 1.0 mg/kg po bid
	ALG, 15 mg/kg IV via CVP

When serum creatinine is less than 50% of preoperative value or after 14 days of ALG if the serum creatinine is still high, the patient is changed to cyclosporine therapy in the following manner:

Day 4	Azathioprine, 2 mg/kg po qd
	Prednisone, 1.0 mg/kg po bid
	ALG, 15 mg/kg IV via CVP
	Cyclosporine, 5 mg/kg po bid
Day 5	Azathioprine, 2 mg/kg po qd
	Prednisone, 1.0 mg/kg po bid
	Cyclosporine, 5 mg/kg po bid

Once the cyclosporine level is therapeutic for 3 consecutive days the prednisone is tapered in the following manner, while maintaining the azathioprine and cyclosporine doses the same:

Prednisone, 0.75 mg/kg po bid × 3 days
Prednisone, 0.50 mg/kg po bid × 3 days
Prednisone, 0.50 mg/kg po qd thereafter

ALG = antilymphoblast globulin; CVP = percutaneous central venous catheter; IV = intravenous; OR = operating room.

ent, it can be placed in the right retroperitoneum. Generally we place the right kidney in the left iliac fossa and the left kidney in the right iliac fossa so that the renal artery and vein do not cross after anastomosing them to the recipient vessels. Our preferred method for vascular anastomoses are end-to-side renal vein to external iliac vein and end-to-side renal artery to external iliac artery.

The incidence of renal artery stenosis is generally higher in the pediatric population than in the adult population,[12] and we believe that not using end-to-end renal artery–to–internal iliac artery anastomosis should minimize that problem.

In small children (<20 kg) receiving adult kidneys, the renal artery and vein must be anastomosed to the side of the recipient aorta and inferior vena cava, respectively, with the kidney placed in the retroperitoneum. It is surprisingly easy to place the large kidney into the small child,[13] particularly if the child has been on peritoneal dialysis, and we have had no difficulty with renal transplant perfusion nor hypotension due to diversion of the arterial flow away from the aorta and into the renal transplant.

Our usual method of neoureterocystostomy, the Litch procedure, minimizes bladder dissection and postoperative hematuria. In the very thick bladder, such as the patient with chronic obstructive uropathy due to posterior urethral valves, or the patient who has had several operative procedures on the bladder, a procedure to tunnel the ureter necessitating an opening into the bladder, a Politano-Ledbettor procedure, is performed.

IMMEDIATE POST-TRANSPLANT MANAGEMENT

Monitoring and Care of the Immunosuppressed Child. Stringent isolation procedures for the moderately immunosuppressed patient are unnecessary.[14] In our hospital, good hand washing and restricting contact with people with active infections, including upper respiratory infections (URI), are enforced for all transplanted children. The child is confined to the room for 1 week, when maximally immunosuppressed, but thereafter the child is allowed access to the rest of the hospital. Viral infection is the greatest risk in these patients, particularly if the patient has been treated for rejection with steroid boluses, ALG, or OKT3. A discussion of the management of these problems follows.

Monitoring on the first day after transplantation is focused primarily on urine output, serum creatinine, blood pressure, and CVP. Most patients coming to renal transplantation today have not had bilateral nephrectomies, and thus urine output may not accurately reflect renal allograft function. It is mandatory to know the patient's usual urine output prior to the transplant. In the LRD transplant, a large urine output is anticipated in all patients immediately. As a rule, at least 2 ml/kg/hr is expected if the transplant is functioning properly.

Serum creatinine is measured immediately postoperatively and every 6 hours thereafter for the first day. To prevent the problem of early kidney dysfunction due to cyclosporine toxicity, in the cadaver kidney recipient we utilize the Minnesota ALG until the kidney is functioning well (see Table 55–2). If the creatinine is decreasing steadily, it is measured daily. If the transplant works well immediately, the serum potassium may drop precipitously since IV fluid replacement will be with normal saline without potassium; thus, serum potassium should also be measured every 6 hours. In the patient with a promptly functioning allograft, it is not unusual to see the serum creatinine level fall below 1.0 mg/dl within 24 hours.

The kidney transplant is very sensitive to hypotension, and thus prevention of low blood pressure is necessary to obviate delayed graft function from acute tubular necrosis (ATN). More commonly, patients have problems with hypertension because many of the patients were hypertensive prior to surgery, and they have received a large amount of fluid in the OR.

Postoperative CVP monitoring is important only in the patient with inadequate urine output. If the CVP is low (< 10 mm Hg) and the urine output is low, we give a 10-ml/kg bolus of normal saline unless there is evidence that blood replacement is necessary. If the CVP is high (>12 mm Hg) and the urine output is low, we give a single dose of furosemide (1 mg/kg, with a maximum dose of 50 mg). If the urine output is good, we base the fluid management on the urine output and make no effort to maintain the CVP at any certain level.

Fluid Management. The goals of fluid replacement following renal transplant are to keep the kidney well perfused without causing complications of fluid overload. The CVP port is perfused at 2 ml/hr of one-half normal saline (NS) + 1 unit/ml of heparin. When a double-lumen CVP line is placed, one port is used to measure CVP and the other is used for medications. The peripheral IV is used for fluid replacement by the following method:

The previous hour's urine output is replaced with D5 ½ NS + 5 mEq NaHCO$_3$/500ml. If the urine output is less than 4 ml/kg, it is replaced milliliter for milliliter. If the urine output is greater than 4 ml/kg, 75% of the urine output is replaced that hour. If the urine output is less than the calculated hourly maintenance fluid rate, the latter is given. This formula is used only for the first 24 hours after surgery, because either the transplant is functioning well and maintenance fluids are adequate or the kidney has delayed function and fluids have to be restricted to prevent fluid overload.

Medications. All patients receive cefazolin 25 mg/kg, with a maximum dose of 1 gram, every 8 hours for three doses. Mycostatin, 100,000 units by mouth three times per day, is also given. The majority of our patients over 5 years of age are placed on patient-controlled analgesia (PCA), using morphine for relief of pain. Younger children or those who cannot use PCA are given IV meperidine 1 mg/kg every 2 hours as necessary for pain. All recipients of cadaver kidneys are started on a dopamine drip of 3 µg/kg/min for the first postoperative day.

The immunosuppressive medications are written daily by protocol (see Tables 55–1 and 55–2). Although children with chronic renal failure usually have an impressive list of medications, only those not directly related to their renal disease, such as seizure medications, are continued immediately after surgery. Because

almost all kidneys are placed in a retroperitoneal position, oral medications can be given even on the first day. Hypertension is usually treated with hydralazine or nifedipine.

Radiographic Studies. As soon as the patient has been stabilized in the intensive care unit (ICU), the patient is transferred to the nuclear medicine department for a diethylenetriamine penta-acetic acid (DTPA) renal scan. The obtaining of a baseline renal scan has proved to be very important when making decisions about the management of low urine output, as well as when confirming good perfusion of the kidney (which is particularly important in patients who made a significant amount of urine prior to transplantation). The scan is done within 2 hours of the surgery; thus if there is any question about renal perfusion, the patient can be taken back to surgery immediately.

Within 24 hours of surgery, a renal transplant ultrasound and Doppler flow study are obtained. These studies localize any fluid collection and also give important baseline information on renal artery flow, renal parenchymal flow, and size of the ureter and renal pelvis.

Dialysis. Post-transplant dialysis is necessary in fewer than 20% of our cadaver kidney recipients and has not been necessary in an LRD kidney recipient in the last 10 years in our hospital. In patients requiring dialysis, it is preferable to delay the dialysis until the second postoperative day. Hemodialysis immediately after surgery predisposes the patient to bleeding in the retroperitoneum adjacent to the transplanted kidney, and careful fluid and electrolyte management should prevent the need for dialysis on the first postoperative day, even if there is no renal function. It is best to avoid peritoneal dialysis (PD) immediately after surgery to prevent pain at the surgical site, although PD is less hazardous than hemodialysis.

COMPLICATIONS THAT REQUIRE MANAGEMENT IN THE PEDIATRIC INTENSIVE CARE UNIT

Primary Nonfunction of the Kidney Transplant. Primary nonfunction of the kidney transplant refers to kidneys that never function. According to the 1989 report of the North American Pediatric Renal Transplant Cooperative Study (NAPRTCS), this problem occurs in approximately 4% of children.[15] The etiology of primary nonfunction may be related to kidney procurement problems, such as prolonged warm ischemia, although some investigators have postulated that acute rejection is the cause in many patients.[16]

As mentioned earlier, we routinely evaluate the kidney function and perfusion with a renal scan using DTPA, immediately following the transplant. When perfusion is poor, Doppler ultrasound and in selected cases, renal transplant arteriography, are necessary to rule out a technical cause for the poor perfusion. When perfusion is good but function is poor, it is assumed that the patient has ATN and he or she is treated accordingly. When function remains poor for more than 4 days despite good perfusion, the kidney is biopsied to confirm viability and to rule out rejection superimposed on ATN. Return of function as late as 1 month after the onset of ATN may occur, but usually diuresis begins within 2 weeks of surgery.

The management of the immunosuppressive medications becomes a challenge when there is delayed renal function. As noted in the protocol for cadaveric kidney recipients (see Table 55–2), Minnesota ALG is continued to a maximum of 14 days and then cyclosporine is begun. Our approach with the patient who has a prolonged delay in allograft function has been to begin cyclosporine cautiously after a kidney biopsy and to maintain levels in the low therapeutic range.

The decision to perform a transplant nephrectomy for primary nonfunction is based on a renal biopsy and on the general status of the patient. If the patient is developing infectious complications from the immunosuppressive medications and the biopsy shows questionable viability, the kidney should be removed. If the patient is well on maintenance immunosuppression, it is reasonable to wait 6 to 8 weeks before removing the kidney. If another kidney became available for the patient before a transplant nephrectomy was done, a second transplant would be recommended.

Severe Rejection. Rejection of a renal allograft may be hyperacute, acute, or chronic. Hyperacute rejection occurs within 1 hour of the time when the kidney is perfused with the recipient's blood and is recognized when the kidney becomes hemorrhagic and appears cyanotic. The hyperacute rejection is caused by the recipient's preformed antibodies reacting with the donor kidney's antigens. With the advent of routine crossmatching of the recipient's serum and the donor's cells prior to transplant, hyperacute rejection has become rare.

Acute rejection can occur any time after transplantation but is unusual in the first week post transplant. In the 1989 NAPRTCS report, the median time for a rejection episode in LRD recipients was 196 days, compared with 42 days for cadaveric kidney recipients.[15] Rejection in the first several days after transplant is called accelerated acute rejection and is associated with a poor outcome.[17]

Acute rejection may be evidenced by fever, graft tenderness, malaise, decreased urine output, hypertension, and rising blood urea nitrogen (BUN) and serum creatinine. In children with adult donor kidneys treated with cyclosporine, signs of rejection can be quite subtle because of the large renal parenchyma reserve. We routinely obtain serum creatinine daily and aggressively evaluate any rise greater than 0.2 mg/dl. Fever is the most common sign of rejection in our patients, and careful assessment of the patient is mandatory to rule out another source of fever. The DTPA renal scan is very sensitive in detecting decreased function due to rejection, and a renal scan is done weekly for the first 3 weeks to have a current baseline study.

Doppler ultrasound has also been recommended to diagnose rejection,[18] but we have not found it to be helpful in our limited experience with the technique. Percutaneous needle renal biopsy and fine needle aspiration have proved to be very helpful if we are differentiating rejection from other causes of decreased renal allograft function. The biopsy is done under local anesthesia with sonographic guidance, and the permanent sections are available for reading within 8 hours.

Measurement of T cell subsets has been useful in evaluating the renal transplant child with a rising serum creatinine. When the CD4+/CD8+ (helper/suppressor) ratio is close to the control ratio (2:1), the patient is inadequately immunosuppressed and the risk of rejection is increased. To differentiate rejection from viral infection, one must consider the CD4+/CD8+ ratio (increased in rejection, decreased in viral infection), the IL-2 receptor–positive cells (increased in rejection, normal in viral infection), and the B cell percentage (increased in rejection, normal in viral infections).

Management of rejection is seen in Table 55–3. Acute rejection is reversible in more than half of the patients with steroid boluses. In steroid-resistant rejection, the rejection can be reversed in 85% of patients with OKT3, a mouse monoclonal antibody against the human T cell receptor.[10] As noted in Table 55–3, special attention to the patient's fluid balance is mandatory prior to initiating OKT3 therapy because of the possible complication of pulmonary edema if the patient is overloaded with fluid. The side effects of the first dose of OKT3 can be quite impressive with temperature elevation over 40° C, shaking chills, and a flu-like syndrome. Pretreatment with acetaminophen, steroids, and diphenhydramine may lessen these side effects, but in our experience fever and chills are common despite pretreatment with these medications. Fortunately, these side effects are much milder after the first dose of OKT3.

Chronic rejection is the slow, progressive destruction of the kidney transplant, and its mechanism is poorly understood. Most patients show evidence of vascular changes that may contribute to the fibrosis and loss of functional renal mass over time. Usually patients with several bouts of acute rejection develop chronic rejection, but some patients develop chronic rejection with little history of acute rejection. There is no effective treatment, and some authors have recommended a second kidney transplant in children with chronic rejection before they return to dialysis.[19]

Infection. Infection in the renal transplant patient is the result of the nonspecific immunosuppression that prevents the allograft from being rejected. With the use of prophylactic antibiotics and mycostatin in the perioperative period, the incidence of early bacterial infection or fungal infection is quite low. Unfortunately, as immunosuppressive medications have become more effective in altering T cell function, particularly CD4+ (helper) T cells, viral infections have become quite common.

The viruses that most commonly affect renal transplant patients are CMV and Ebstein-Barr Virus (EBV). CMV generally occurs after a CMV-positive kidney is transplanted into a CMV-negative recipient; however, if the recipient is CMV positive prior to transplantation, the CMV may become reactivated whether the donor is CMV positive or negative. We routinely administer CMV-negative blood to our CMV-negative renal trans-

Table 55–3. PROTOCOL FOR MANAGEMENT OF ACUTE REJECTION

Days 1, 2, and 3—methylprednisolone, 20 mg/kg (up to 1 g) IV* qd
If the patient continues to show evidence of rejection or has a second rejection episode within several days of the first rejection and the cyclosporine level is therapeutic, OKT3 is begun using the following protocol:

Preparation
1. The patient must be euvolemic (< 3% over dry weight) to prevent pulmonary edema. Obtain a chest x-ray.
2. OKT3 may be given through a good peripheral IV.
3. Medications to prevent severe symptoms from OKT3 damage to the T cells with massive lymphokine release:
   a. Acetaminophen, 10 mg/kg po or pr
   b. Diphenhydramine, 1 mg/kg (up to 50 mg) IV or po
   c. Methylprednisolone, 10 mg/kg IV over 20 minutes (first two doses of OKT3 only)
   d. Hydrocortisone, 2 mg/kg IV 30 minutes after OKT3 started (first dose of OKT3 only)

OKT3 Administration
1. 5 mg IV push qd for patients >30 kg
2. 2.5 mg IV push qd for patients <30 kg
3. 0.1 mg/kg IV push qd for small infants
4. Usual length of therapy is 10 days

Monitoring
1. Most severe symptoms occur with the first dose so a physician should be available to treat anaphylaxis or pulmonary edema. Temperature elevation to 41° C may occur, thus appropriate equipment to treat fever must be available. Vital signs, including temperature, should be measured every 15 minutes for 2 hours for the first 2 doses.
2. Blood for T lymphocyte subset panel should be drawn before starting therapy, the next day, and twice weekly thereafter.
3. Draw blood for anti-OKT3 antibodies before starting therapy, at the end of therapy, and 6 weeks later.

Other Therapy
1. Prednisone, 0.50 mg/kg po qd (withheld when IV steroids are given)
2. Azathioprine, 2 mg/kg po qd unless WBC† is low
3. Cyclosporine: Continue at doses necessary to keep at a low therapeutic blood level
4. Acyclovir, 100–200 mg po tid (after OKT3 is discontinued, should be given for 3 months)
5. The next to the last day of OKT3 treatment, the prednisone and cyclosporine doses should return to prerejection doses.

*IV = intravenous.
†WBC = white blood cell count.

plant recipients when a transfusion is necessary. When the patient is at risk of developing CMV, which includes all patients receiving a CMV-positive kidney,[20] the patient receives immunoglobulin IV on the day of transplantation, at 1 week post transplant, and monthly for 3 months thereafter (see also Chapter 63).

If the patient develops symptomatic CMV infection, the immunosuppression is reduced and the patient is begun on ganciclovir. High-titer anti-CMV immunoglobulin is also available for use in the patient with CMV infection. It is critical to monitor the patient's immune status with T cell subset analysis during a viral infection to prevent excessive immunosuppression, because the CMV infection may profoundly immunosuppress the patient. Although death from CMV infection may occur after renal transplantation, it is uncommon in our experience.

Infection with EBV is less common in renal transplant patients than in those receiving liver transplants, probably because the renal transplant recipients are generally less immunosuppressed. EBV infection has been associated with lymphoproliferative disorders following transplantation. EBV infection is treated by reducing the immunosuppressive medications and by administering acyclovir.

It is important to realize that when any infection develops following renal transplant, the first priority is always to clear the infection and rescue the patient, even if that means removing the kidney transplant. This philosophy and improved immunosuppression are responsible for the excellent patient survival following renal transplantation today compared with 20 years ago.

Hypertension. The development of hypertension in the early period following renal transplantation may be due to rejection, a side effect of medications, renal artery stenosis, or disease within the native kidneys. In the cyclosporine era, more than 70% of children receiving a renal transplant are hypertensive on a long-term basis.[21] In the first few days after the transplant, exogenous fluid overload and the retention of fluid by steroids contribute to the hypertension. Thereafter, the development of hypertension must be investigated to determine the etiology.

If a patient has poorly controlled hypertension, bilateral nephrectomy is done before the transplant; however, most patients have their native kidneys retained and this is not the usual cause of severe post-transplant hypertension. The diagnosis of rejection is discussed earlier, but it must always be kept in mind as a potential cause of hypertension.

Renal artery stenosis is more common in the pediatric patient than in adults.[12] In the last 100 renal transplants at our hospital, seven have developed renal artery stenosis, four from technical problems and three from chronic rejection. The diagnosis of renal artery stenosis may be suggested by Doppler ultrasound or by a DTPA renal scan, particularly if the patient is pretreated with captopril.[22] The definitive diagnostic test for renal artery stenosis remains selective angiography.

Treatment of the stenosis may be by percutaneous transluminal angioplasty (PTA), if the patient is at least 1 month post transplant, or by surgical correction. The success rate with PTA appears to be less in children[23] than in adults.[24] Surgical repair of transplant renal artery stenosis in adults has an excellent success rate.[25] In our own patient population at the Children's National Medical Center (CNMC), five of seven children with transplant renal artery stenosis required surgical correction of the stenosis, and four of five had control of their hypertension and preservation of the allograft. One kidney was lost owing to renal artery occlusion following repair. One child had control of the hypertension with PTA alone, and the seventh patient lost the kidney from renal artery occlusion after PTA.

OUTCOME

Several factors have an impact on the patient and kidney transplant survival rates. Results for LRD transplants should be separated from those for cadaver donors. Since the introduction of cyclosporine in 1984, there has been a significant improvement in kidney allograft survival. Thus, for series that include patients transplanted before 1984, the results should be evaluated according to whether the patients received cyclosporine or not. Children younger than 5 years of age have a poorer kidney transplant survival than those older than 5 years of age (particularly for cadaveric kidneys[15]), although some contend that young children do as well as older ones.[13] When the donor of a cadaveric kidney is younger than 5 years of age, the graft survival is less than when the donor is older, regardless of the age of the recipient.[15, 26, 27] Taking all these factors into consideration, the following results were generated from various published studies and were compared with the results from the CNMC.

The most important statistic is patient survival, and in most series the patient survival rate at 1 year is greater than 90% for both LRD and cadaver kidney recipients.[13, 28, 29] In the 1989 report of NAPRTCS, the patient survival at one year was 96% for LRD and 92% for cadaver transplants.[15] At CNMC, all 26 children receiving an LRD transplant in the last 10 years are living, whereas 59 of 65 (91%) receiving a cadaver kidney were alive 1 year after the transplant.

The 1-year kidney allograft function rate for all children receiving LRD kidneys is excellent,[13, 28, 29] and in the 1989 NAPRTCS report the function rate for this group was 88% at 1 year.[15] The 1-year graft function rate for LRD at CNMC has been 100% for the last 5 years. Despite the use of cyclosporine, the overall function rate for cadaveric kidneys remains substantially lower than for LRD and the 1-year function rate for cadaver kidneys in the 1989 NAPRTCS was 71%.[15] The 1-year function rate for cadaver kidneys at CNMC has been 60% for the last 5 years, which is a reflection of the large number of kidneys used from donors younger than 5 years of age as is discussed later.

Although some transplant teams have had excellent results with renal transplants in children younger than 6 years of age,[13] the overall success rate continues to be less than for older children with a 66% 1-year function rate for children 6 years old or younger compared with 73% for older children receiving cadaver kidneys.[15] At CNMC, the 1-year function rate for children receiving

a cadaver kidney is 56% for children younger than 6 years of age and 62% for older children.

It has been recognized that patients receiving cadaver kidneys from young donors have a higher graft failure rate than patients receiving kidneys from older donors.[15, 26, 27] In children, kidneys from cadaver donors younger than 6 years old are functioning at 1 year in only 55% of patients compared with 79% of patients receiving kidneys from cadaver donors older than 10 years.[15] This donor age-related graft failure has been particularly noteworthy in CNMC, in which 60% of the cadaver kidneys transplanted in the last 5 years have been from donors younger than 6 years old, resulting in an allograft function rate of only 60% at 1 year.

The shortage of cadaver kidneys is an ever-increasing problem with more patients being placed on the waiting list than kidneys transplanted each year (see Chapter 94). Currently, there are nearly 18,000 patients awaiting a cadaver kidney. Children often do not effectively compete for the available organ because most children have relatively low panel reactive antibody (PRA) titers, and patients with high PRAs are preferentially given the organ. Although efforts are being made by United Network for Organ Sharing (UNOS) to enhance a child's likelihood of receiving an organ, the organs offered for our patients continue to be from young pediatric donors who unfortunately have a worse 1-year function rate. Because of the 100% function rate of our LRD transplants in the last 5 years and the distressing shortage of cadaver kidneys from donors older than 5 years, we support LRD transplantation whenever possible.

Renal transplantation in children is a most rewarding endeavor because of the possibility of converting a chronically ill child into a robust one, free from the restrictions of dialysis in a matter of weeks. Attention to technical detail and meticulous management of the immunosuppressive medications are demanded because of the small safety margin in these patients. Despite early doubts about the advisability of recommending transplantation to the pediatric patient with renal failure, it is now clear that renal transplantation is the treatment of choice in this patient population.

References

1. Jaboulay M: Greffe de reins au pli du coude par soudures arterielles et veineuses. Lyon Med 107:575, 1906.
2. Michon L, Hamburger J, Oeconomos N, et al: Une tentative de transplantation renale chéz l'homme; aspects médicaux et biologiques. Presse Med 61:1419, 1953.
3. Murray JE, Merrill JP, and Harrison JH: Renal homotransplantation in identical twins. Surg Forum 6:432, 1955.
4. Murray JE, Merrill JP, Dammin GJ, et al: Study on transplantation immunity after total body irradiation: Clinical and experimental investigation. Surgery 48:272, 1960.
5. Calne RY: The rejection of renal homografts; inhibition in dogs by 6-mercaptopurine. Lancet 1:417, 1960.
6. Murray JE, Merrill JP, Dammin GJ, et al: Kidney transplantation in modified recipients. Ann Surg 156:337, 1962.
7. Terasaki PI, Vredevoe DL, Mickey MR, et al: Serotyping for homotransplantation-VI, selection of kidney donors for thirty-two recipients. Ann N Y Acad Sci 129:500, 1966.
8. Starzl TE, Marchioro TL, Porter KA, et al: The use of heterologous antilymphoid agents in canine renal and liver transplantation

and in human renal homotransplantation. Surg Gynecol Obstet 124:301, 1967.

9. Canadian Multicentre Transplant Study Group: A randomized clinical trial of cyclosporine in cadaveric renal transplantation: Analysis at three years. N Engl J Med 314:1219, 1986.

10. Ortho Multicenter Transplant Study Group: A randomized clinical trial of OKT3 monoclonal antibody for acute rejection of cadaveric renal transplants. N Engl J Med 313:337, 1985.

11. Barber WH, Diethelm AG, Laskow DA, et al: Use of cryopreserved donor bone marrow in cadaver kidney allograft recipients. Transplantation 47:66, 1989.

12. Henning PH, Bewick M, Reidy JF, et al: Increased incidence of renal transplant arterial stenosis in children. Nephrol Dial Transplant 4:575, 1989.

13. Najarian JS, Frey DJ, Matas AJ, et al: Renal transplantation in infants. Ann Surg 212:353, 1990.

14. Nausef WM and Maki DG: A study of the value of simple protective isolation in patients with granulocytopenia. N Engl J Med 304:448, 1981.

15. Alexander SR, Arbus GS, Butt KMH, et al: The 1989 report of the North American Pediatric Renal Transplant Cooperative Study. Pediatr Nephrol 4:542, 1990.

16. Halloran P, Aprile M, Farewell V, et al: Factors influencing early renal function in cadaver kidney transplants: A case-control study. Transplantation 45:122, 1988.

17. Williams GM: Clinical course following renal transplantation. *In*: Morris PJ (ed): Kidney Transplantation: Principles and Practice, 2nd ed. London, Grune & Stratton, 1984, pp. 342–343.

18. Drake DG, Day DL, Letourneau JG, et al: Doppler evaluation of renal transplants in children: A prospective analysis with histopathologic correlation. AJR 154:785, 1990.

19. Kaiser BA, Polinsky MS, Palmer J, et al: Successful kidney retransplantation of children with stable but chronically rejecting allografts prior to dialysis. Transplantation 49:1009, 1990.

20. Pollak R, Barber PL, Prusak BF, et al: Cytomegalovirus as a risk factor in living-related renal transplantation: A prospective study. Ann Surg 205:302, 1987.

21. Gordjani N, Offner G, Hoyer PF, et al: Hypertension after renal transplantation in patients treated with cyclosporine and azathioprine. Arch Dis Child 65:275, 1990.

22. Miach PJ, Ernest D, McKay J, et al: Renography with captopril in renal transplant recipients. Transplant Proc 21:1953, 1989.

23. Aliabadi H, McLorie GA, Churchill BM, et al: Percutaneous transluminal angioplasty for transplant renal artery stenosis in children. J Urol 143:569, 1990.

24. Lohr JW, MacDongall ML, Chonko AM, et al: Percutaneous transluminal angioplasty in transplant renal artery stenosis: Experience and review of the literature. Am J Kidney Dis 7:363, 1986.

25. Dickerman RM, Peters PC, Hull AR, et al: Surgical correction of posttransplant renovascular hypertension. Ann Surg 192:639, 1980.

26. Ilstadt ST, Tollerud DJ, Noseworthy J, et al: The influence of donor age on graft survival in renal transplantation. J Pediatr Surg 25:134, 1990.

27. Rao KV, Kasiske BL, Odlund MD, et al: Influence of cadaver donor age on posttransplant renal function and graft outcome. Transplantation 49:91, 1990.

28. Potter D, Feduska N, Melzer J, et al: Twenty years of renal transplantation in children. Pediatrics 77:465, 1986.

29. Najarian JS, So SKS, Simmons RL, et al: The outcome of 304 primary renal transplants in children (1968–1985). Ann Surg 204:246, 1986.

Digestive System

56

Hepatic Failure

Parvathi Mohan, M.B.B.S., M.D., and
Benny Kerzner, M.D.

Fulminant hepatic failure (FHF) is a severe, sudden hepatocellular injury directed at a previously healthy organ. It is a medical emergency that warrants immediate admission to the intensive care unit (ICU), and the condition stands in contrast to the more insidious end-stage hepatic failure (HF), which complicates chronic liver disease. By definition, FHF occurs within 8 weeks after the onset of symptomatic liver disease, and though it is rapidly progressive, it is a potentially reversible condition.[1] Some cases, labeled as subfulminant or late-onset HF, occur beyond the 8-week limit, but ascites and a milder cerebral edema are also generally present.[2] Patients with chronic liver disease tend to have a relatively mild intermittent encephalopathy; they are admitted to the ICU for devastating complications such as gastrointestinal hemorrhage, renal failure, and sepsis. Wilson's disease is an exception, as it is a chronic disorder that is known to present with a sudden progressive illness clinically indistinguishable from FHF.

The epidemiology of liver disease is in flux. Reye syndrome, a dreaded cause of FHF prior to the 1980s, has virtually vanished since the use of aspirin in the course of viral illnesses was implicated in its pathogenesis. Diagnostic tests for the hepatitis C virus (HCV) and the hepatitis D virus (HDV) have narrowed the residual spectrum of "idiopathic liver diseases" that cause FHF. Acquired immunodeficiency syndrome predisposes more children to opportunistic liver infections and is itself associated with a hepatopathy.[3] Moreover, we are witnessing an increase in drug- and toxin-induced liver disease. This increase is in part related to hepatotoxic medications developed in immunology, oncology, and other areas experiencing rapid medical advances. In addition, recreational and suicidal use of drugs contribute to this upswing. Fortunately, a positive outlook is now possible, as liver transplantation can rescue a substantial number of individuals with severe FHF.

Two comprehensive reviews on HF have recently been published.[4, 5] In this chapter, we examine the pathophysiology of FHF and the implications of the physiology for management in an intensive care setting. A section is devoted to pediatric liver transplantation, the most dramatic breakthrough in the management of FHF and end-stage liver disease.

ETIOLOGY

FHF is uncommon. Fewer than 2,000 cases are reported each year in the United States, and the most prominent causes continue to be viruses and drugs as indicated in Table 56–1.[6] Age-related causes are outlined in Table 56–2.

Infections

In the United States and other Western countries, HBV, alone or in combination with HDV, is the most prevalent infectious cause of FHF in adults. The high incidence is primarily the result of intravenous drug abuse. FHF occurs in approximately 1% of patients with symptomatic hepatitis B.[7] However, with the decline in transfusion-related transmission, HBV is becoming a rarer cause of FHF in children. The δ virus, which is the causative agent of HDV, is a hepatotropic ribonucleic acid (RNA) virus that requires the presence of HBV to cause disease. It may occur as a superinfection in an HBV carrier or as a coinfection with HBV.[8] Coinfection with the δ agent increases the incidence of HF to 20% in HBV-infected patients. Thus, δ infection should be sought in high-risk patients, such as those

Table 56–1. RELATIVE FREQUENCY OF CAUSES OF HF*

Cause	% of Cases
Hepatitis A	2–4
Hepatitis B	60–75
Hepatitis non-A, non-B	24–34
Drugs	6–15
Poisoning	1–2
Miscellaneous	0–10

*Adapted from Yanda RJ: Fulminant hepatic failure (Medical staff conference). West J Med 149:586, 1988.

621

Table 56–2. ETIOLOGY OF HEPATIC FAILURE

	Perinatal	Infancy	Childhood
Infection	TORCH,* hepatitis B		
		EBV,† CMV‡ ————————————————→	
		Hepatitis A,B,C,D ————————————————→	
		Bacterial ————————————————→	
Drugs and toxins		Acetaminophen, phenytoin ————————→	
		Ampicillin, sulfa drugs	
		Valproate, antimetabolites	
Metabolic	Galactosemia ————————————————→		
	Neonatal iron ————————————————→		
	Storage disease		
	Tyrosinemia ————————————————→		
	Glycogen storage disease ————————————————————————→		
	Zellweger syndrome ————————→		
		Hereditary fructose intolerance ————————————→	
			Wilson disease
			α₁-antitrypsin deficiency
Anatomic		Biliary atresia ————————————————→	
		Alagille syndrome ————————————————→	
		Byler syndrome	
Miscellaneous	Anoxia ————————————————————————————→		
		Parenteral nutrition ————————————————→	
		Niemann-Pick disease ————————————→	
			Chronic active hepatitis
			Reye syndrome

*TORCH = toxoplasmosis, rubella, cytomegalovirus, and herpes simplex.
†EBV = Epstein-Barr virus.
‡CMV = cytomegalovirus.

with hemophilia or drug addiction.[6, 7] Immunity against HBV assures protection against HDV.

The prevalence of the hepatitis A virus (HAV) is low, and the risk of FHF developing from it is less than 0.1%. Yet, as a cause of FHF, its incidence varies remarkably from 2 to 31% of cases.[6, 9] The recently defined HCV generally causes a mild illness that may gradually progress to cirrhosis.[10] Its incidence as a cause of FHF is yet to be defined but is suspected to be low. This stands in contrast to the relatively high incidence of FHF from non-A non-B hepatitis, possibly because this nondescript category of illness includes other idiopathic causes of hepatitis.[9]

In most cases of hepatitis caused by the Epstein-Barr virus (EBV) liver involvement is mild, but severe cases are well documented. White and Juel-Jensen reported 12 cases of FHF resulting from EBV; only one patient survived.[11] Severe EBV hepatitis should prompt a search for an immunodeficiency state and, conversely, hepatitis in an immune-deficient patient warrants a search for unusual viral causes, notably EBV, adenovirus, and cytomegalovirus.[12] The advent of both organ transplantation and acquired immunodeficiency syndrome is especially relevant in this regard.[3] Herpesvirus plays a small but significant role as a cause of pediatric FHF. Mothers transmit herpes simplex type 2 to the neonate, resulting in disseminated infection and severe hepatitis.[13] In older children, fatal cases of FHF result from herpes simplex type 1 infection, mostly but not exclusively in immunocompromised patients.[14]

Drugs

Mitchell and associates reported that 2% of pediatric hospital admissions are for drug-related illnesses, but drug-induced FHF is relatively rare in children.[15] The explanation is not known but is presumably the result of underdiagnosis, faster or alternate metabolism of drugs by the younger liver, and the relative infrequency of drug use among the pediatric population.[16]

The damage from drugs can result from a direct, dose-related injury to the cell organelles (e.g., carbon tetrachloride), an idiosyncratic type of reaction (e.g., sulfonamides and phenytoin), and occasionally a combination of direct cell damage followed by an induced host immune response (e.g., halothane).[17, 18] A primary cholestatic picture is also seen, either associated with hepatocellular changes (e.g., chlorpromazine) or with minimal enzyme elevations (e.g., contraceptive steroids).[19] Antimetabolites such as methotrexate, cis-platinum, cytosine arabinoside, dactinomycin, and cyclophosphamide are potential hepatotoxins and often produce enzyme elevations without other indications of liver damage.[20] Hepatic fibrosis with steatosis leading to cirrhosis has been reported with chronic low-dose administration of methotrexate, and acute hepatitis may occur with high doses of the drug.[21] Severe but reversible hepatotoxicity with steatosis and necrosis has been reported with L-asparaginase.[22] Veno-occlusive disease with acute enlargement of the liver, ascites, and jaundice is seen with thioguanine, carmustine (BCNU), busulfan, and cytosine arabinoside administration.[23] Table 56–3 provides a classification of some of the commonly used drugs based on the pathologic changes they produce in the liver.[24] Histologic features in the liver suggestive of drug-induced hepatitis include discrete zonal necrosis, bile duct involvement, steatosis, eosinophilia, granuloma, and necrotic changes that are out of proportion to the clinical and laboratory features.[25, 26]

Table 56–3. DRUG-INDUCED LIVER DISEASES*

Type of Involvement	Drug
Hepatitis	Methyldopa, isoniazid, halothane, phenytoin
Hepatitis and cholestasis	Erythromycin, nitrofurantoin chlorpromazine, azathioprine, cimetidine
Cholestasis	Cyclosporine, contraceptive steroids
Zonal cell necrosis	Acetaminophen
Microvesicular steatosis	Valproate, tetracycline
Granuloma	Sulfonamides, carbamazepine
Vascular changes	Estrogens, senecio alkaloids, busulfan
Biliary cirrhosis	Practolol, chlorpromazine

*Adapted from Roberts EA and Spielberg SP: Drug induced hepatotoxicity in children. *In:* Walker WA, Durie PR, Hamilton JR, et al (eds): Pediatric Gastrointestinal Disease, Vol. 2. Philadelphia, BC Decker, 1990, pp. 898–914.

Chronic Liver Diseases

Metabolic Causes

Wilson disease may present as FHF in children who have no antecedent history of liver disease or neurologic signs to distinguish the condition.[27] Timely diagnosis is, however, essential because the patients do not respond to conventional therapy, and liver transplantation must be promptly considered. Clues to the diagnosis are low hemoglobin levels caused by hemolysis, mild transaminasemia and alkaline phosphatasia, and intense jaundice. As a consequence, the ratio of alkaline phosphatase:bilirubin is less than 2 and that of aspartate aminotransferase (AST):alanine aminotransferase (ALT) is greater than 4.[28] Ceruloplasmin, being an acute phase reactant, can be falsely elevated into the normal range and therefore cannot be depended upon for diagnosis. The major distinguishing characteristic of Wilson disease is the extremely high hepatic copper content. α_1-*Antitrypsin* deficiency may progress to cirrhosis and liver failure in childhood or adolescence, especially if the patient has experienced neonatal cholestasis.[29] Other metabolic liver diseases that cause HF are tyrosinemia, galactosemia, glycogen storage diseases, and hereditary fructose intolerance. More recent additions to this list include neonatal hemochromatosis and defects in bile salt metabolism.[30, 31]

Anatomic lesions

Biliary atresia is the most common indication for liver transplantation in children.[32] About 400 to 600 new cases of biliary atresia are diagnosed in the United States each year, and the children survive because Kasai portoenterostomy establishes bile flow in 50 to 90% of patients for a finite period of time. Nonetheless, HF is expected in almost all patients between 2 and 10 years after the original surgery, and a failed Kasai operation constitutes the most common indication for liver transplantation in children less than 2 years of age.[33] *Paucity of the intrahepatic biliary system* is a pathologic finding in some of the important neonatal cholestatic conditions that progress to liver failure: Alagille, Byler, and Zellweger syndromes are examples. The Alagille syndrome is recognized by jaundice and pruritis coupled with characteristic morphologic features, including peripheral pulmonic stenosis and the typical triangular face with a prominent forehead.[34] Most patients follow a benign course but others ultimately develop HF. The Byler syndrome, first described in Amish immigrants to the United States, is characterized by a unique biochemical profile with normal or near-normal γ-glutamyl transpeptidase (GGT) levels and relatively low alkaline phosphatase and cholesterol levels in the face of severe cholestasis.[35] It follows a rapidly deteriorating course ending in early death. The Zellweger syndrome is a diffuse disorder of peroxisomes and, therefore, the hepatic pathology is accompanied by cerebral dysgenesis, pigmentary retinopathy, and cystic changes in the kidneys, which are hallmarks of the disease.[36]

Miscellaneous

Chronic active hepatitis, especially the immune variety, is an important cause of cirrhosis and HF in childhood. This category of immune hepatitis has recently been expanded by the identification of a subgroup of patients with positive anti–liver-kidney microsomal antibodies, as opposed to the classic anti–smooth muscle antibodies that have traditionally been used to identify these patients.[37] The anti–liver-kidney microsomal–positive children are believed to carry a greater predilection for cirrhosis and HF, and both subgroups of immune hepatitis have been shown to respond to steroids or azathioprine.[37] Prolonged use of *total parenteral nutrition* is a common cause of liver disease in children who require intravenous nutrition to survive conditions such as short gut syndrome or intractable diarrhea. HF and sepsis are the major causes of mortality in children who remain dependent on intravenous nutrition.

PATHOPHYSIOLOGY

Hepatic Injury and Failure

The hepatocyte membrane injury that allows transaminases to leak from the cell may also contribute to failed hepatic function: Calcium gains access to the cytoplasm in which it potentiates the injurious action of a variety of toxins, leading to further disruption of the cell membrane and eventual cell death.[38, 39] Hepatic injury may be a direct cytopathic toxic effect, as indicated by the paucity of the inflammatory reactions often evident in viral hepatitis and characteristic of Reye syndrome. Alternatively, the liver pathology may be immune-mediated. An example is the FHF in type A hepatitis, in which T8 lymphocytes predominate in the liver and are thought to target viral antigens expressed on the hepatocyte cell surface.[40] The very complexity of the hepatic parenchymal cell renders it vulnerable to damage by drugs and toxins. Fixed elements can be covalently bound and injured. The Na^+, K^+-ATPase pump on the plasma membranes of hepatocytes may be inhibited by endotoxins, resulting in cholestasis.[41] The deoxyribonucleic acid (DNA)–RNA axis responsible for protein production can be disrupted, as exemplified by the ability of tetracycline to bind transfer RNA and mushroom toxins to inhibit RNA polymerase.[42]

The hepatocyte is poised to deal with toxins, and its integrity depends on a balance between the elaboration of toxic products by cytochrome P-450 and other systems and neutralizing mechanisms such as conjugation with glutathione. Toxicity may, therefore, be accentuated by nonspecific induction of the P-450 system by drugs such as phenobarbital and alcohol, exhaustion of the glutathione supply, and malnutrition, which deprives the liver of essential nutrients, including vitamin E and the constituent amino acids of glutathione.[43, 44]

The following are illustrative examples of the mechanisms of drug-induced hepatic injury: For *acetaminophen*, the basic step initiating the noxious process is its conversion to a toxic metabolite, *N*-acetyl-*p*-benzoquinoneimine.[45] This noxious product causes harm by reacting with cell protein and is prevented from doing so by conjugation with glutathione. Damage follows the exhaustion of the glutathione content and is prevented by early provision of *N*-acetylcysteine, a substrate for glutathione production[46] (see also Chapters 74 and 80). *Phenytoin* toxicity is the consequence of a hypersensitivity type of reaction. An inherent defect in detoxification of an intermediary metabolite is postulated, and immunologic mechanisms involving sensitized lymphocytes are also believed to play a role.[47] Histologic examination of the liver shows cholestasis and granuloma formation in addition to hepatocellular injury.[48] *Valproic acid* injury appears to be another example of a pathologic condition caused by the accumulation of a toxic intermediary metabolite under the influence of the P-450 system.[49] Consequently, those most at risk are young children with neurologic conditions requiring the use of other anticonvulsants that act as nonspecific stimulants of the P-450 system. The target organelle is the mitochondrion, and patients present with perturbations reminiscent of Reye syndrome.[50] Early on, there is hyperammonemia without the presence of liver failure. Later, there may be severe hepatic dysfunction, massive hepatocellular necrosis and, characteristically, microvesicular steatosis.[51] Serum carnitine levels may be low, but carnitine has not been shown to positively influence the outcome of the toxic injury despite its ability to improve mitochondrial fatty acid metabolism.[52] *Halothane* hepatotoxicity may present as a relatively mild hepatitis with elevated transaminase levels in the first 2 weeks after exposure to the drug or as severe liver failure caused by diffuse cell necrosis.[53] The mechanism again hinges on the generation of toxic metabolites by the cytochrome P-450 system. These chemicals engage in lipid peroxidation, disturbances in calcium homeostasis, and acetylation of the cellular membrane, all of which contribute to cell damage.[54, 55] Recently, an immunologic mechanism has also been invoked. Halothane-specific antibodies have now been described, and they may help in the diagnosis of halothane hepatitis[56] (see also Chapter 76).

Complications of Hepatic Failure

Hepatic Encephalopathy and Altered Consciousness

The hallmark of FHF, hepatic encephalopathy (HE) is a frequent complication of portosystemic shunting in cirrhosis and has a characteristic progression. At first, forebrain dysfunction results in behavioral changes and abnormal sleep patterns. Ultimately, brain stem disturbances cause a loss of consciousness. In parallel, neuromuscular abnormalities become evident, ammonia levels increase, and there is a characteristic progressive decrease in frequency and an increase in the amplitude of the electroencephalographic tracings. Triphasic waves are considered specific.[57] Agitation and seizures may be present, but they are variable features of the encephalopathy.

Toxins, hypoxia, and acid-base disturbances that alter hepatic function may also affect neurocytes and contribute to the induction of HE, but more fundamental to the altered sensorium are the metabolites that are normally eliminated by a healthy liver. These "toxins" are thought to originate, at least in part, from bacterial action on protein and amino acids in the lumen of the bowel.[58] This postulate was first proposed to explain why dogs experience an encephalopathy following the construction of a portosystemic shunt (Eck fistula), which can be reversed by administering oral antibiotics.[59] In FHF, the blood bypasses dysfunctional hepatic parenchymal cells through normal sinusoids, whereas in cirrhosis, the channeling of blood is through fibrotic bands. Either way, "toxins" reach the systemic circulation and persist.

The induction of HE is the subject of an ongoing debate that others have detailed and we summarize. There are three competing hypotheses regarding relevant toxins: (1) Some claim that ammonia alone is responsible; (2) some that ammonia acts in synergy with other neurotoxins, notably mercaptan and short chain fatty acids (SCFAs); and (3) others implicate false neurotransmitters, derivatives of aliphatic amino acids such as tryptophan or alternatively γ-aminobutyric acid (GABA).[60] *Ammonia* is suspected not only because removal of protein from the diet and sterilization of the bowel ameliorates HE but also because of additional indirect evidence, notably a similar type of encephalopathy that accompanies the metabolic defects of the urea cycle.[61] In experiments, however, the encephalopathy induced by high levels of exogenous ammonia is unlike that of HF in that it is characterized by hypertonicity and seizures and lacks the distinctive electroencephalographic and visual evoked responses of HE.[62] *Mercaptans*, which are thought to produce the characteristic odor of fetor hepaticus, are generated by the action of bacteria on methionine in the gut.[63] They are normally cleared by the liver, and very low serum concentrations can cause reversible coma.[64] This may be due to inhibition of brain microsomal Na^+, K^+-ATPase activity or an indirect effect as the result of impaired clearance of ammonia by depressing urea cycle enzymes.[60] As with ammonia, mercaptans produce a hyperkinetic state. Furthermore, experimental intoxication requires much higher levels of mercaptans than are actually found in hepatic coma. *SCFAs* have also been implicated in the pathogenesis of HE. Infusion of octanoate in experimental animals leads to reversible coma, central hyperventilation, increased ammonium levels, and inhibition of Na^+, K^+-ATPase activity in brain microsomes.[60] Moreover, SCFAs may have a synergistic role with other coma-producing substances involved in the production of HE. A positive correlation between the tissue or serum levels of SCFAs and the severity of HE has not been established.[62]

The *neurotransmitter theory* envisages a balance between excitatory and inhibitory brain impulses. In the model of Fisher and Baldessarini, excitation is blocked by the presence of false neurotransmitters.[65] The hypothesis starts from the observation that in HF there is an amino acid imbalance in serum; aromatic amino acid (AAA) levels are high and branched chain amino acid (BCAA) levels are low. The AAAs enter the blood from injured hepatocytes and catabolic muscle, whereas the BCAAs are preferentially used by muscle and fat under the influence of insulin.[65] When excess AAAs enter the brain, tryptophan is converted to serotonin, which is inhibitory, and phenylalanine and tyrosine are converted to octopamine, a false neurotransmitter that blocks excitatory impulses.[60] The most compelling evidence for this theory is the coma induced in dogs with a 6-hour intracarotid infusion of a solution of phenylalanine and free tryptophan, which is avoided by simultaneous infusion of BCAAs.[5] Jones postulates that an excess of GABA, the principal inhibitory neurotransmitter in brain in mammals, is mainly responsible for the genesis of HE.[66] GABA is synthesized from glutamate in presynaptic neurons, stored in cytoplasmic vesicles, and released across the synaptic cleft to bind to specific receptors on the postsynaptic neurons. This binding sets up a biochemical sequence that increases chloride entry into the postsynaptic cell and thereby generates an inhibitory postsynaptic potential. Increased levels of GABA-like activity in serum prior to the onset of encephalopathy have been reported in a rabbit model of FHF, thereby corroborating the role of GABA in HE.[66, 67] Drugs that increase GABA-mediated neurotransmission—that is, benzodiazepine and barbiturates, can produce visual evoked potentials similar to those seen in HE, and GABA antagonists induce both clinical and electrophysiologic remission in HE.[68, 69]

The endothelial lining of the cerebral capillaries is an effective blood-brain barrier (BBB) that prevents toxins and marker molecules like D-sucrose, L-glucose, and trypan blue from entering the brain substance.[70] These markers do, however, enter prior to and in the course of the encephalopathy of HF, indicating a loss of the integrity of the BBB. A vicious cycle is possible as accumulation of toxic substances such as mercaptans further damages this barrier. The entry of "false neurotransmitters" helps to explain the encephalopathy, and the entry of an excess of fluids causes cerebral edema.

The evolution and outcome of HE are influenced by concurrent *metabolic disturbances*, which offer an opportunity for positive therapeutic intervention. *Hypoglycemia* is especially relevant given that glucose is a critical fuel for brain function. Hypoglycemia complicates the massive hepatic necrosis of FHF, presumably because of depleted hepatic glycogen stores and raised serum insulin levels that result from impaired hepatic destruction of the hormone. Disordered mitochondrial function, as seen in Reye's syndrome and other defects of

fatty acid oxidation, is also associated with hypoglycemia and in addition results in aberrant fatty acid oxidation and energy production.[71] *Impaired synthesis of protein* by the chronically failing liver limits the availability of albumin to bind toxins and drugs, a process that normally prevents free access of these agents into brain. *Hypoxemia* increases the severity of the encephalopathy and results from intrapulmonary arteriovenous shunting, reduced pulmonary vascular resistance, and peripheral vasodilatation, known effects of HF.[72] HF also results in a centrally driven respiratory alkalosis, which may compromise cerebral blood flow and encourage hypokalemia, which, in turn, results in a metabolic alkalosis. *Alkalosis* promotes the conversion of ammonium to ammonia, which can now enter the blood from the gut and more readily pass the BBB.[73]

Cerebral Edema

The most common cause of death in FHF is cerebral edema; it is reported in 25 to 81% of cases.[74, 75] The onset is not directly correlated with the presence of other complications of HF—that is, hemorrhage, hypotension, and hypoglycemia—nor is its relationship to encephalopathy and the stages of coma entirely consistent. There may be a very early change in the BBB permeability, but the signs and symptoms of edema are evident only when intracranial pressure (ICP) increases beyond 30 mm Hg.[76] The pathogenesis of cerebral edema in HF may be *vasogenic*—that is, the consequence of damage to the endothelial cell junctions of the cerebral capillaries.[70] Alternatively, it may be *cytotoxic* when the edema is the result of cell wall injury and a maldistribution of intracellular fluids and electrolytes. Vasogenic edema is compounded by generalized vasodilatation and fluid overload.[70] In a rabbit model, it is induced by the FHF caused by galactosamine, but hypoxia and hypoglycemia do not occur in this condition.[77] Depressed Na^+, K^+-ATPase activity may be a factor in the genesis of cytotoxic edema.[76] Other factors that contribute to both forms of edema are a reduction in cerebral blood flow and oxygenation secondary to systemic hypotension or a progressive increase in ICP.[78]

Coagulopathy

Fatal bleeding, especially from the gastrointestinal tract, is a prominent cause of death in HF.[79] The coagulopathy responsible for the hemorrhage is not merely due to failed production of clotting factors but is also the consequence of inadequate clearance of coagulation activating factors, thrombocytopenia, and impaired platelet function.[79] Decreased synthesis of *coagulation factors* and fibrinogen is a hallmark of severe liver failure. The earliest change is a decrease in the circulating levels of Factor VII, which has a short half-life.[80] Impaired synthesis of vitamin K–dependent Factors II, VII, IX, and X account for the prolongation of prothrombin time (PT). Factor V levels are independent of vitamin K and account for the persistently abnormal partial thromboplastin time (PTT) in liver disease. In contrast, levels of Factor VIII, an acute phase reactant that is synthesized in the spleen and lymph nodes, as well as in the liver, may actually be increased.[81] The origin of *thrombocytopenia* in HF is also multifactorial, being the result of bone marrow depression, hypersplenism, the presence of platelet-associated antibodies, and disseminated intravascular coagulopathy (DIC).[82] In FHF, plasma and platelet lipids, prostaglandins, thromboxanes, and endoperoxidases may indicate changes in platelet aggregation and adhesion.[83] Low-grade DIC causes increased catabolism of fibrinogen and raised circulating fibrin split products, changes that are partially blocked by infusion of antithrombin III, an inhibitor of the coagulation cascade.[84] Its levels are decreased in FHF because of decreased production by the liver and increased consumption in intravascular coagulation.[82] Finally, in chronic liver disease, fibrin may polymerize to cause dysfibrinogenemia.[85]

Renal Dysfunction in Hepatic Failure

Renal salt retention is a characteristic response to deteriorating hepatic function and is explained by two contrasting theories:[86] The *underfill theory*, which proposes that fluid shifts to form ascites in response to portal hypertension and low oncotic pressure, and the result is a decrease in the effective blood volume of the systemic circulation. The *overflow theory* stresses primary renal sodium and water retention caused by a decrease in hepatic synthesis of natriuretic hormone or decreased hepatic clearance of a salt-retaining hormone. An increase in blood volume in conjunction with portal hypertension and a decrease in oncotic pressure leads to ascites and a reduction in the effective blood volume. In both theories, the volume depletion acts via baroreceptors to stimulate the sympathetic nervous system and renin angiotensin aldosterone system to cause a further secondary salt retention.[4] Both of these theories envisage the formation of ascites prior to the onset of salt retention, but ascites is not usual in FHF. A more convincing cascade of events starts with the recently described decrease in peripheral arterial resistance.[87] The mechanism proposed is failure of clearance of endogenous vasodilators, presumably glucagon, vasoactive intestinal polypeptide, and other chemical mediators. In response to vasodilatation, there is decreased effective arterial blood volume, an increase in cardiac output and sympathetic tone, and stimulation of the renin angiotensin system. Salt is retained, and the plasma volume expands prior to the formation of ascites.

Oliguria, which has ominous implications in hepatic failure, has three important, readily distinguished causes: (1) acute tubular necrosis, prerenal azotemia, and *hepatorenal syndrome* (HRS) (Table 56–4). HRS is caused by a functional impairment of renal function in which there is sodium retention but no associated histologic abnormality.[88] The renal dysfunction is severe, and mortality from this virtually irreversible condition is very high; however, when the kidneys are transplanted into a new host, they function normally.[89] The sodium retention can be explained by either the underfill or overflow theory already discussed, and in addition there is a redistribution of blood in the renal cortex to the

Table 56–4. DIFFERENTIATION OF HEPATORENAL SYNDROME FROM OTHER CAUSES OF OLIGUREA*

	Prerenal Failure	Hepatorenal Syndrome	Acute Tubular Necrosis
Urine sodium (mEq/l)	<10	<10	>30
Urine sediment	Normal	Normal	Casts
Urine-plasma creatinine	>30:1	>30:1	<20:1
Urine-plasma osmolality	>1	>1	1
Volume expansion	Diuresis	None	None

*Modified from Epstein M, Berk DP, Hollenberg NK, et al: Renal failure in the patient with cirrhosis: The role of active vasoconstriction. Am J Med 49:175, 1970.

juxtamedullary glomuleri. Fluid filtered through these glomeruli is subjected to the concentrating action of the loop of Henle but not the dilutional contribution of the convoluted tubules; hence, salt and water are retained.[90] The redistribution of blood in HRS is presumed to be mediated by an imbalance of the vasoconstricting and vasodilating prostaglandins, as suggested by an increase in thromboxane B_2 and a decrease in prostaglandin F_2 in the urine.[91]

Infections

The infections that are prone to occur in HF are responsible for a substantial proportion of the morbidity and mortality of the condition. Among the predisposing causes are the patient's unconscious state, which favors hypostasis and impaired ventilation; the presence of venous and arterial lines and catheters; and the use of steroids. More fundamentally, there are specific defects in the host immune system in advanced liver disease, including impaired serum bactericidal activity, opsonization by phagocytes such as the Kupffer cells in the liver, and low plasma fibronectin levels.[92] The consequence is a tendency to bacteremia caused by bacteria such as *Staphylococcus aureus*, *Streptococcus pneumoniae*, and *Escherichia coli*, and soft tissue infections such as phlebitis and wound sepsis, pneumonia, and urinary tract infections.[93]

CLINICAL FEATURES

Systemic Manifestations

Progressively deepening jaundice is often the initial reason for seeking the counsel of a specialist in the diagnosis and management of FHF. With rare exceptions (e.g., acetaminophen toxicity), massive cell necrosis accompanied by a rapid increase in jaundice occurs well before the signs of HE appear.[94] Persistent anorexia, fevers, and vomiting are frequent but nonspecific symptoms. Physical examination reveals jaundice, hepatomegaly with or without splenomegaly, evidence of coagulopathy such as ecchymosis or purpura, neurologic deficits and fetor hepaticus, which is a peculiar fruity, sweet, and musty breath odor.[63] A generalized rash, joint swelling, and fever should alert one to the possibility of a hypersensitivity reaction to drugs.

Table 56–5. STAGES OF HEPATIC ENCEPHALOPATHY*

Stage	Mental State	Tremor	EEG
Stage I: prodrome	Euphoria, occasional depression, mild confusion, slow mentation and affect, slurred speech, change in sleep rhythm	Slight	None
Stage II: impending coma	Accentuation of stage I, drowsiness, inappropriate behavior, loss of sphincter control	Present	Abnormal (slowing)
Stage III: stupor	Mostly sleeping but rousable, incoherent, marked confusion	Usually present	Abnormal
Stage IV: coma	May (IV A) or may not (IV B) respond to noxious stimuli	Usually lacking	Abnormal

*Adapted from Jones AE: Fulminant hepatic failure. *In:* Zakim D and Boyer TD (eds): Hepatology: A Textbook of Liver Disease, Vol 1, 2nd ed. Philadelphia, WB Saunders, 1990, pp. 460–475.

Hepatic Encephalopathy

HE, the most significant complication of FHF, is divided into the stages detailed in Table 56–5, and the "staging of coma" is a critical element in choosing a management strategy because stages I and II, and even stage III, are potentially reversible, whereas stage IV coma carries high mortality.[95] The encephalopathy can follow a variety of courses: It may improve steadily; it may progress to an unresponsive coma over a period of days, as is typical of hepatitis A; or it may wax and wane, as in Wilson disease. Furthermore, progression through the various stages may be extremely rapid. It can also be so slow and subtle that the early stages are detected by teachers because of a notable deterioration in handwriting and increasing combativeness.[4] A helpful differentiating sign is the development of asterixis, a flapping movement of the fingers and hands upon dorsiflexion at the wrist with the arm fixed in extension. This tremor may be lacking at rest and may disappear in deep coma. The flap may also be seen in other conditions such as congestive heart failure and uremia.[96]

Cerebral Edema

Normal ICP ranges between 0 and 15 mm Hg, and clinical signs of cerebral edema generally appear when pressure rises to levels greater than 30 mm Hg.[97] Early on, there is increased muscle tone, myoclonus, hyperventilation, dilated or unequal pupils that react sluggishly to light, and in some patients, focal seizures. Later features of greater severity include papilledema, decerebrate posturing, loss of the oculocephalic and oculovestibular reflexes, and fixed dilated pupils; these changes herald severe and often fatal consequences of cerebral edema. One must bear in mind that these valuable signs of progressive disease can be masked by the use of sedatives and muscle paralyzing drugs (see also Chapters 16 and 17).

Reye Syndrome

Reye syndrome presents in a unique manner. Following or at the end of a prodromal illness such as chickenpox or influenza, there is an abrupt onset of persistent emesis followed by mental changes and irritability or lethargy, or both, which at a variable rate progress to coma and even death. The serum bilirubin level is less than 1 mg/dl in the majority of cases, with AST and ALT levels 3 to 30 times normal values. Serum ammonia levels are variably elevated, and hypoglycemia can be a significant feature.[98] Urea cycle and fatty acid oxidation defects closely mimic Reye syndrome. These defects assume greater importance now that Reye syndrome is rarely encountered. Characteristic pathologic features in the liver biopsy specimen help to confirm the diagnosis; there is a virtual lack of cell necrosis and inflammatory cells in the presence of diffuse microvesicular steatosis. The organelle believed to be the primary site of injury in Reye syndrome is the mitochondrion, as indicated by its pleomorphism, enlargement with disruption of cristae, and the reduction of dense bodies.[98] The presence of dicarboxylic acids in the serum and urine confirms mitochondrial injury and the consequent disruption of β-oxidation.[99] Because Reye syndrome almost invariably occurs in the recuperative phase of a viral illness, a viral cause seems obvious, but because relatively few children experience the syndrome, a further factor must be involved. Because a decrease in the use of aspirin correlates with a dramatic fall in the incidence of Reye syndrome, this relationship seems relevant, even if not conclusively proved. Salicylates are known to uncouple mitochondrial respiration, impair adenosine triphosphate formation, and induce mitochondrial swelling.[100] Secondary insults such as hyperammonemia, acid-base balance disturbances, hypoglycemia, and free fatty acidemia probably play a synergistic role by promoting cerebral edema.

LABORATORY TESTS

Liver Function Studies

Hepatocellular Damage

Serum elevations of AST and ALT are sensitive indices of hepatocyte cell wall injury but do not necessarily indicate cell death, as noted in Reye syndrome, in which minimal cell necrosis is associated with dramatic elevations of the serum transaminases. Markedly increased transaminase activity to levels beyond 2,000 IU, accompanied by an increasing bilirubin level to greater than 20 mg/dl, are usually encountered in progressive

FHF; however the height of the elevation does not correlate directly with prognosis. Moreover, occasionally the source of the enzyme (especially AST) is muscle, and elevated levels may reflect myocardial damage or a myopathy.[101] ALT is a more specific indicator of liver injury than is AST; however, hemolysis, which is often seen in FHF, may be associated with elevated levels of ALT.[101]

Cholestasis

A rapidly increasing serum *bilirubin* level is indicative of advancing hepatocellular damage and is especially ominous when coupled with falling transaminase levels in patients with worsening encephalopathy. Care must be taken to fractionate the bilirubin, as a high indirect fraction may be due to the hemolysis that can accompany FHF rather than from hepatocyte injury. Injury of the biliary canaliculi and bile ducts can be monitored by following alkaline phosphatase, GGTP, and 5'-nucleotidase levels in addition to serum bilirubin levels. Determination of *alkaline phosphatase* activity is a simple, widely applied test that is valuable if the additive effect of its isoenzymes are taken into account. The fractions originate in liver, intestine, placenta, and bone; the latter accounts for elevations associated with growth in the newborn and at puberty, when levels greater than 300 U/γ are frequently achieved.[102] Therefore, simultaneous determination of additional enzymes such as GGTP and fractionation of alkaline phosphatase are helpful to determine the source of an elevated enzyme level. γ-*Glutamyltranspeptidase* is expressed on the biliary canalicular membrane and bile duct epithelium; in addition, the renal tubular epithelium and pancreatic acini are rich sources of the enzyme. In practice, raised serum levels are quite specific reflections of biliary tract dysfunction. The serum value is particularly sensitive for monitoring the canalicular injury that is seen with hepatic rejection following transplantation and with cholangitis.[103] GGTP is, however, an inducible enzyme, and confusion is possible when serum levels are boosted by drugs such as phenytoin and alcohol.[104] 5'-*Nucleotidase* is also a specific enzyme of hepatobiliary dysfunction but is not widely used because of its poor sensitivity.[103]

Synthetic Functions

When synthetic function is well preserved, the potential for recovery from HF is good, even in the face of extremely high transaminase values. A low *albumin* level indicates excessive protein loss from the gut or urine or decreased production by the liver. Since albumin has a relatively long half-life of 21 days, normal serum values in the presence of severe hepatic injury suggest a recent onset of illness rather than a chronic disease. Assessing the integrity of the *clotting mechanism* is a sensitive means of monitoring the progression and predicting the outcome of hepatic disease. The PT and PTT are both prolonged in liver failure. The PT is a measurement of vitamin K–dependent Factors II, VII, IX, and X. A prolonged PT that is not corrected by the administration of vitamin K has prognostic value. Factor VII has a very

short half-life and therefore serves as a sensitive index of hepatic function. Coagulation-related indices of poor prognosis in HF include a Factor V level persistently less than 20% of the control, a low antithrombin III level, and a prolonged PT that is unresponsive to vitamin K; a value greater than 50 seconds is used to predict the need for liver transplantation.[105]

Miscellaneous

Bromsulphalein uptake was employed in the past as a sensitive test of liver function and integrity but has become obsolete because of hypersensitivity reactions to the drug.[106] *Indocyanine green* excretion has been offered as a substitute but is not widely used because of its complex kinetics. More recently, *xenobiotics* such as lignocaine are being used to test liver function.[107] Lignocaine is transformed to monothylglyanexylidide under the influence of the P-450 system. The level of this substance in the blood 1 hour after intravenous administration of lignocaine appears to be a useful adjunct in the selection of children for liver transplantation. It may also serve as a more accurate monitor of changing hepatocellular function than either endogenous metabolites or hepatic enzyme values.

The magnitude and duration of *hyperammonemia* have little bearing on the prognosis of hepatic disease, but ammonia levels do serve to confirm a hepatic contribution to the origin of encephalopathy. *Hypoglycemia* is anticipated in liver failure, and blood glucose levels must be monitored because, even without massive cell necrosis, patients with liver disease have asymptomatic hypoglycemia. With progressive liver failure, the hypoglycemia becomes more profound and may contribute to the severity of HE.

Specific Diagnostic Tests to Establish a Viral Cause

The presence of HAV is confirmed by finding IgM anti-HAV in serum, though serial measurement of IgG anti-HAV by commercial immunoassays is also advocated.[109] A molecular hybridization assay for HAV RNA in stool samples is a highly specific but clinically impractical test that is currently used exclusively for research purposes.[110] The patient with type B hepatitis who goes into HF could be in the throes of an initial attack of hepatitis B, may be entering the end-stage of chronic active hepatitis and cirrhosis, or could have a coinfection with HDV. Hepatitis B surface antigen (HB_sAG) levels rise before the clinical and chemical evidence of the disease and are well established at the height of an acute attack. By this time, markers of viral replication hepatitis B e antigen (HB_eAG), and the more sensitive HBV DNA are also found in serum and they will remit before the HB_sAG will. HB_sAG subsides with the appearance of hepatitis B_s antibody (HB_sAb). The most consistently positive test for HBV infection is the presence of IgM anti–hepatitis B core antibody (HB_cAb), which peaks within several weeks of the onset of the disease and persists beyond the disappearance of the HB_sAg. This is the only marker of the infection during the "window" period between the loss of HB_sAg and the appearance of HB_sAb.[110, 111] *HDV* infection, without the presence of HB_sAg, is extremely rare and its presence is confirmed with commercially available assays for IgM and IgG antibodies against hepatitis D. Currently, tests to detect the viral antigen and RNA are restricted to research facilities.[112] During acute coinfection, the IgM antibody appears transiently for a few weeks and is followed by the IgG. In HDV superinfection, a brisk and sustained IgM and IgG response is found that correlates with the presence of the viral antigen in the liver.[113] The presence of *HCV* can be determined with the IgM anti–hepatitis C assay now commercially available. There may be a prolonged period before the test results are positive, and false-positive results are noted in patients with hypergammaglobulinemia—for example, in chronic active hepatitis. HCV RNA can be detected in the sera to confirm the diagnosis, but this test is not yet available for routine use. Assays for the enterically transmitted, epidemic form of hepatitis E are now being developed.[114] IgM antibodies to other viruses such as herpes simplex and EBV are routinely performed tests in most clinical laboratories. Detection of viral inclusions in the liver biopsy tissue using immunofluorescent techniques is also valuable, especially when the progression of the disease is rapid and decisions regarding treatment options have to be made quickly.

PROGNOSIS AND OUTCOME

As the name implies, FHF is a dangerous condition. The leading causes of death are herniation of the brain from cerebral edema, cardiorespiratory arrest secondary to arrhythmias and electrolyte abnormalities, uncontrolled sepsis, intractable bleeding, and renal failure.[115] Mortality in adults is approximately 60%, and despite the superior regenerative capacity of the young liver, the mortality in childhood is still daunting at approximately 40%.[116] If the outlook is to be improved, ominous features must be recognized so that patients requiring as heroic a measure as liver transplantation can be more rapidly selected. The features used to prognosticate outcome are imprecise, but taken together they offer fair insight into the potential for recovery. Important factors are clinical attributes suggesting rapid onset and progression, specific causes known to follow a perilous course, and biochemical features of exhausted synthetic hepatic function as opposed to those indicating regeneration of the parenchyma.

In general, increased mortality is associated with a longer duration of HE and electroencephalographic changes.[117] A high mortality rate is associated with stage IV coma. Patients with halothane intoxication have a particularly severe illness.[118] The rapidity of onset of jaundice, male gender, and obesity add greater risk to the severity of halothane hepatitis.[119] Associated complications such as infection and renal failure greatly reduce the chance of survival, regardless of the causative agent.[120] A small liver or rapid reduction in the liver span, associated symptoms such as seizures, or signs

such as arrhythmias and ascites herald a poor outcome.[121, 122] Histologic examination can also be helpful but has limited application because of the danger of bleeding. The hepatocyte volume as a percentage of the total needle biopsy volume is a measure of hepatic regenerative capacity. Normal is $85 \pm 5\%$, and a volume less than 40% indicates a poor prognosis.[123] The extent of hepatocellular necrosis on a biopsy specimen may correlate with mortality but not with the duration or the stage of HE.[120]

Laboratory tests have predictive value when used in conjunction with the developing clinical condition. A rapid reduction in the aminotransferase value in the face of deepening jaundice indicates a preterminal state with massive cell destruction.[124] Similarly, altered coagulation factors as discussed in the section on synthetic functions and low serum complement (C3) levels also point to severe hepatic dysfunction.[125] The finding of increased plasma levels of α-fetoprotein has been used as an indicator of hepatic regeneration, but it does not necessarily predict the ultimate outcome.[126]

MANAGEMENT

The management of HE can be divided into three categories: (1) supportive measures applied piecemeal to address the multiple problems that develop in response to deteriorating hepatic failure, (2) the establishment of a liver support system analogous to dialysis in renal failure, and (3) the replacement of the liver with a new organ.

General Supportive Measures

In most instances, successful outcome of HF relates to the meticulous management of the individual complications as detailed in Table 56–6.

Fluid and Electrolytes

Strict monitoring and judicious use of *fluid and electrolyte* solutions cannot be overemphasized, especially in a state of impending cerebral edema and compromised renal function. Furthermore, as discussed in the section on complications of renal failure, the associated *hyponatremia* of HF is largely caused by fluid retention; sodium balance is actually positive in most instances. Therapy, therefore, depends on fluid restriction. The provision of sodium only aggravates water retention. Fluid volumes should be on the order of two thirds of maintenance or 60 to 80 ml/kg. Intravenous fluids should not contain sodium, and total sodium intake should not exceed total losses; urine losses can be promoted by using spironolactone. Generally, the sodium intake is kept at less than 2 mEq/kg/day, but rarely hyponatremia is due to the excessive use of diuretics or vomiting, so estimating sodium balance by measuring levels in urine and nasogastric aspirates can be extremely helpful. As renal function deteriorates, fluid replacement is restricted to calculated obligatory losses plus the total

Table 56–6. GENERAL SUPPORTIVE MEASURES IN THE MANAGEMENT OF FULMINANT HEPATIC FAILURE*

Complications	Treatment
Fluid and electrolytes	
Hyponatremia	Restrict sodium to 1–2 mEq/kg/day
	Restrict fluids to 60–80 ml/kg or ⅔ of maintenance
	Spironolactone 3–5 mg/kg/day orally or by nasogastric tube
Hypokalemia	IV† K⁺ to 3 mEq/kg as KCl or KPO4
	Minimize diuretics
Acidosis	Maintain intravascular volume intravenous albumin, 25% 1 g/kg
	Dialysis if unresponsive
Hypoglycemia	IV dextrose, 10%
Azotemia	Dialysis
Hyperkalemia	Dialysis
Intravascular volume	Assess and maintain adequate circulating volume
Gastrointestinal bleeding	H₂ blockers—ranitidine 2 mg/kg/day or cimetidine 30 mg/kg/day intravenously
	Keep gastric pH >5
	Nasogastric aspiration or lavage to clear blood
	Transfusion
Sedation	Avoid oversedation
	IV midazolam
Infection	Broad-spectrum antibiotics—cephalosporins, aminoglycosides
Coagulopathy	Fresh frozen plasma only for active bleed—10 ml/kg
	Vitamin K (0.2 mg/kg up to 10 mg/day IM‡ or IV)
Hypoxemia	Oxygen to keep O₂ saturation >90%
	Intubate and protect airway in stages III and IV coma
	Ventilatory support when indicated
Reduce nitrogenous waste production	Withdraw dietary protein
	Nasogastric aspiration of blood or protein
	Cleansing enemas
	Lactulose via nasogastric tube 15–30 ml every 6 hr or neomycin, 50 mg/kg/day orally or by nasogastric tube

*Modified from Treem WR: Hepatic failure. *In:* Walker WA, Durie PR, Hamilton JR, et al (eds): Pediatric Gastrointestinal Disease, Vol 1. Philadelphia, BC Decker, 1990, pp 146–192.
†IV = intravenous.
‡IM = intramuscular.

urine output/day. *Hypokalemia* is prone to occur from diuretic treatment and vomiting. It requires prompt therapy because it causes a metabolic alkalosis that can aggravate encephalopathy by increasing serum ammonia levels.[4, 173] Administration of potassium as the chloride salt will tend to reverse the alkalosis, and given as the phosphate salt, it is useful for the treatment of hypophosphatemia. To avoid *hypoglycemia* and prevent gluconeogenesis, fluids are administered as a 10% dextrose solution.

The intrusion of *oliguria* into the clinical picture may indicate the development of prerenal failure, HRS, or ATN. Distinguishing among the three conditions (see Table 56–4) is essential for correct fluid management. *Prerenal failure* is identified by noting measures of intravascular volume—that is, central venous pressure and pulmonary capillary wedge pressure. When necessary, the volume is repleted with normal saline or

colloid. In contrast, *HRS* requires fluid and sodium restriction. Dialysis may improve the chances of survival by maintaining homeostasis until hepatic dysfunction is reversed.

In the context of more chronic liver disease, the treatment of *ascites* has an impact on fluid and electrolyte therapy. Traditional modalities such as albumin infusions to enhance oncotic pressure and diuretics are giving way to alternatives. Newer diuretics, such as muzolimine provide a longer, more gradual diuresis that tends to avoid development of HRS.[127] Moreover, in adults, large-volume paracentesis (up to 5 I within a 20- to 40-minute period) supported by albumin infusion is once more being advocated.[128]

Reduction in Nitrogenous Waste Production and Drug Treatment of Hepatic Encephalopathy

The realization that nitrogenous waste products emanating from the intestine play an integral role in the production of HE is the basis for much of the standard therapy of HF. Protein is withheld from the diet or eliminated from the gastrointestinal tract with the aid of laxatives, enemas and, in the event of bleeding, nasogastric aspiration. The bacterial contribution to toxin production from protein is blocked with the use of nonabsorbed antibiotics, such as neomycin, or acidification of the colon by nonabsorbed sugars, notably lactulose, a disaccharide 4-β-D-galactosido-D-fructose, or more recently lacitol (β-galactosidosorbitol). These sugars are especially useful, as they are laxatives, and in the colon they are metabolized to acids that suppress the bacterial enzymes producing the toxins believed to cause HE. In addition, the acid environment converts ammonia to nonabsorbed ammonium.[129, 130] The dose of lactulose is 15 to 30 ml every 4 hours by nasogastric tube, orally, or as an enema until the stools are loose, whereupon the dose is adjusted to produce two to four loose stools/day. Because the actions of these sugars depend on their bacterial metabolism, they should not be given in conjunction with oral neomycin or other broad-spectrum antibiotics. Neomycin alone is effective. To ensure rapid evacuation of the colon, saline enemas may be given initially, but they are generally not favored when fluid balance is difficult.

Drugs are becoming available to counter encephalopathy by their direct action on the brain. In anecdotal reports, L-DOPA is said to have had dramatic effects, but these results could not be confirmed in controlled trials.[131] Recently, patients with grade III coma who did not respond to L-DOPA were shown to have an improved level of consciousness following administration of naloxone.[132] Even more encouraging are the preliminary data on flumazenil, the benzodiazepine receptor antagonist that reduces GABAergic transmission in the brain. Improvements in clinical status and the electroencephalograms are described, and a response to flumazenil has good prognostic implications.[133, 134]

Ventilatory Support

The incidence of pulmonary complications in FHF is high and includes pneumonia, atelectasis, and pulmonary edema; all of these problems contribute to the development of hypoxia, which, in turn, can aggravate cerebral dysfunction.[135] Therefore, prevention of hypoxia is mandatory. In an awake patient with minimal respiratory distress, oxygen administration with pulse oximetry to monitor the oxygen saturation will suffice. As soon as the patient moves into stage IV coma, an endotracheal tube is placed to prevent aspiration and clear secretions from the bronchial tree.[136] If hypoxemia worsens or if pulmonary edema is suspected, early institution of positive end-expiratory pressure will reduce the morbidity.[137] Care should be taken to avoid hypocapnia, which will aggravate the lactic acidosis commonly found in FHF.[138]

Sepsis

Infections are frequent complications of FHF; often they are iatrogenic, resulting from the aggressive and invasive measures that are necessary to maintain life, including arterial and central venous lines, urinary catheters, and ICP monitors. Intensive microbiologic monitoring by frequent culturing of blood, urine, tracheal aspirates, and stools is recommended, but prophylactic antibiotic therapy is not necessary.[139] The infections should be aggressively treated with appropriate antibiotics, based on the culture and sensitivity of the isolated organism, or with a combination of broad-spectrum antibiotics, if the sensitivities are not known. Some of these antibiotics are toxic to vulnerable organ systems (e.g., gentamicin and the kidneys), and therefore drug levels must be meticulously adjusted.

Gastrointestinal Bleeding and Coagulopathy

Hemorrhage, particularly from the gastrointestinal tract, is one of the most common causes of mortality in FHF. Therefore, if bleeding occurs, coagulopathy must be aggressively corrected. The use of H_2 blockers sufficient to keep the intragastric pH at greater than 5 reduces the intensity of bleeding and the need for transfusions.[140] Furthermore, continuous infusion of the H_2 blocker should be used to maintain the gastric pH at greater than 5 without fluctuations in acid production. We advocate cimetidine, 30 mg/kg/day, or ranitidine, 2 to 4 mg/kg/day, as a continuous infusion added to the total parenteral nutrition solution, with which the drugs are compatible. Newer H_2 blockers, ranitidine and famotidine, are credited with fewer side effects than cimetidine and may be favored. Since complex coagulation abnormalities are compounded by platelet dysfunction in FHF, maintenance of platelet counts at greater than 50,000 is important, particularly during invasive procedures. Vitamin K given as a slow infusion in the first few days after detecting a coagulopathy is beneficial, but prophylactic administration of fresh frozen plasma does not reduce morbidity in patients who are not bleeding.[141] Desmopressin has been used to shorten bleeding and PTTs and increase the levels of factors VII, VIII, IX, and XII.[142] Similarly, antithrombin III has been used to counter DIC, but only in a few patients, and the efficacy of these drugs has not been validated by controlled studies.[143]

Sedation

Great caution has to be exercised in the use and choice of sedatives and tranquilizers to deal with symptoms like delirium and anxiety. Depression of centers in the brain that control consciousness and vital functions such as respiration and blood pressure are the major concerns. Opiates, benzodiazepines, and barbiturates are contraindicated, but there may be a place for milder agents such as midazolam or promethazine for control of symptoms.[144]

Nutrition

The administration of nutrients in the course of liver failure must take into account the perturbations in hepatic nutrient metabolism that are a consequence of both acute and chronic liver damage. In FHF, the most dramatic effects are in protein and carbohydrate processing, and the most pressing need is the avoidance of hypoglycemia. In chronic liver failure, the most consistent requirement is attention to the nitrogenous wastes leading to encephalopathy and the correction of the effects of cholestasis on fat and fat-soluble vitamin absorption.[145] Furthermore, there is a need to avoid an excessive load of trace metals, especially in patients who are intravenously fed.[146]

The anorexia that accompanies viral and drug-induced hepatitis is usually short-lived, and a high-calorie diet is encouraged as soon as appetite returns. At least 1 g protein/kg is given and fat is not restricted, though it is preferable to give it as eggs and dairy products rather than fried foods. Oral feedings are not tolerated in patients with FHF, and from the time of admission, intravenous glucose is given to avoid hypoglycemia and muscle breakdown for gluconeogenesis.[147] If oral nutrients cannot be provided for 3 days, the danger of aggravating the outcome by compromised nutrition mandates a consideration of intravenous feedings; however, the need for nitrogen and the form in which it should be given remains an area of controversy. One must reconcile the benefits of positive nitrogen balance with the knowledge that high doses of protein administered orally to patients with cirrhosis and portosystemic shunting cause a reversible coma.[148] Failing to establish positive nitrogen balance results in gluconeogenesis and an imbalance of aliphatic amino acids and BCAAs, similar to that caused by HF. A positive effect of nitrogen on survival in FHF is difficult to demonstrate but seems logical, more especially as amino acids provided intravenously rather than orally have little danger of aggravating the coma. The administration of a branched chain–enriched solution that has less phenylalanine and methionine and increased quantities of arginine and BCAAs offers the hope of an improvement in the encephalopathy, better nitrogen balance, and survival.[150] Unfortunately, improvement in encephalopathy is only anecdotally reported and not confirmed by controlled trials, and there is no consistent improvement in survival. Disappointing results with BCAA-enriched solutions for FHF are anticipated because in contrast to cirrhosis, BCAA levels are normal and the distortion in the amino acid profile is caused mainly by hepatocellular necrosis with the release of aliphatic amino acids.[151] In FHF, treatment with BCAAs fails to normalize serum amino acids; hemodialysis is needed and there is virtually no evidence that dialysis makes a substantial difference to the outcome. In chronic HF, there is evidence of improved survival when positive nitrogen balance is accomplished, but the absolute need for BCAAs as opposed to standard amino acid solutions is still an open question.[152, 153] Proponents for BCAAs point to animal experiments that show improved nitrogen balance and brain stem activity.[154] Nonetheless, in controlled human studies, the improvements were not consistently found, possibly because of related factors in the study design, notably the use of intravenous fat, which the two negative studies have in common.[155, 156] In summary, intravenous amino acids are indicated in FHF, but there is little objective data on morbidity and mortality to substantiate the use of a branched chain–enriched solution.

Management of Increased Intracranial Pressure

Successful management of raised ICP is accomplished with meticulous planning aimed at ensuring prompt coordinated responses by those at the bedside. In anticipation of the swings in pressure that are possible, the parameters that will mandate hyperventilation and the initiation of a mannitol bolus must be agreed upon. It is preferable that the neurosurgeon be consulted in advance of the need for an intracranial monitor so that plans can be made for prompt placement when it becomes necessary. Systematic close monitoring at regular intervals by experienced personnel who will recognize and immediately respond to signs such as altered pupil size, a change in sensorium, or the occurrence of extensor tone is mandatory.[157] The need to follow these clinical signs is not diminished by establishing continuous monitoring of ICP because inconsistencies and device failures are possible. Clinical monitoring is especially important if the patient is to be transported for computed tomography scans and so on, and a manual ventilation bag and mannitol should always be on hand.

As soon as deterioration of neurologic status indicates progression beyond stage II coma, a monitoring device should be placed, and continuous recording of ICP is commenced. Subdural hemorrhage or infection may complicate the placement of the device and compromise an already perilous clinical state. Hence, the decision to insert the monitor cannot be taken lightly. The aim of monitoring ICP is to maintain the cerebral perfusion pressure (calculated by subtracting the ICP from the mean arterial pressure) at greater than 40 mm Hg.[97] Reducing the P_{CO_2} to between 25 and 30 mm Hg produces a cerebral vasoconstriction that controls the cerebral edema and delays fatal coning of the brain.[158] Controlled trials with mannitol have shown significant reduction of ICP in 80% of patients, as well as improved

survival.[5] Additional approaches to the control of ICP—employing agents such as barbiturates, anesthetics, and steroids—remain controversial.[159] ICP management is discussed further in Chapter 17.

Temporary Hepatic Support Systems

We use artificial liver support systems in an attempt to supplant the liver's deranged homeostatic mechanisms by removing potential toxins and supplementing the serum with substances normally synthesized by the liver. The aim is to give the injured liver time to regenerate and resume its role. Unfortunately, no consistent improvement in survival has as yet been demonstrated as a result of these methods. Two major problems have offset the potential benefits of hepatic support: (1) failure of the liver to regenerate and resume its functions and (2) technical limitations that result in inefficient clearing of toxins. *Charcoal hemoperfusion* is perhaps the most extensively studied modality. It works on the principle that charcoal adsorbs a wide range of water-soluble molecules and toxins such as mercaptans and GABA. The technique involves passage of blood through a column containing charcoal granules coated with an ultrathin cellulose nitrate membrane.[160] Improved survival with decreased cerebral edema has been reported in series from the United Kingdom and Japan, but these findings have been disputed by others.[161] The technique may offer temporary lifesaving support to patients in end-stage HF while they await liver transplantation. *Plasmapheresis* is a method by which the patient's plasma is exchanged with that of a donor—a process that could be useful for the replacement of coagulation factors. As with hemoperfusion, however, it has not added significantly to the survival rate in FHF, and the exposure to blood adds a significant risk of transmission of non-A, non-B hepatitis.[162] *Hemofiltration* has temporarily improved mental status in HF, particularly in coincident renal failure, but the technique is significantly complicated by the development of coagulopathies.[163] It is thus reasonable to conclude that at the present time, artificial liver support systems do not offer a reliable avenue for improving the outcome of FHF.

Liver Transplantation

The decision to treat hepatic failure with a liver transplant is always onerous given the radical nature of the surgery, the scarcity of donor livers, the exorbitant expense, and the need for lifelong immunosuppression with the related risks of infection and rejection. Nonetheless, the determination to transplant is fairly obvious for patients with end-stage chronic, progressive liver disease, given that the short-term survival for transplantation is 80% and the liver disease is almost invariably fatal.[32, 164] The situation in FHF is more complex: Most of these patients have the potential to recover completely if they can be maintained until their livers spontaneously recuperate; however, the mortality rate for FHF is close to 50% and even greater for those with advanced disease. Furthermore, the deterioration in the patient's condition may be very rapid and the "window of opportunity" for transplantation can be very brief.

The timing of the transplantation has to be tailored to each case. The cause of FHF is an important consideration; metabolic diseases such as α-antitrypsin deficiency, Wilson disease, and tyrosinemia with irreversible damage to the liver merit consideration for transplantation at the onset of HF, whereas in potentially reversible conditions such as hepatitis A, pushing conservative management to the limit may save the patient an unnecessary transplantation procedure. Clinical indications for imminent transplantation include persistent gastrointestinal bleeding, hypoglycemia, and acidosis, as well as progressive renal failure and encephalopathy in the face of maximal supportive measures.[32] It is a paradox that stage IV hepatic coma, which carries a very high mortality rate, is also a contraindication to liver transplantation because of the high incidence of permanent neurologic damage in those who survive this degree of encephalopathy. The key to the management of FHF with liver transplantation, therefore, is the timely identification of those patients likely to need liver transplantation and their referral to an appropriate center before they progress beyond stage III coma. Laboratory tests are often used to assist in these deliberations, and tests of hepatic synthetic functions are particularly helpful: A steadily falling serum albumin level, a factor VII level less than 10% of normal, a factor V level less than 20% of normal, and a PT longer than 50 seconds strongly point to the need for immediate liver transplantation.[80]

In principle, relative contraindications to liver transplantation for HF include the availability of an alternative therapy, an anticipated suboptimal outcome, a poor chance for recovery, functional impairments of other organ systems that may affect the success of the liver transplantation, massive sepsis, and the expectation that the primary disease will recur in the new liver. Some of the severe neurologic dysfunctions may be reversed by the transplant, but complete recovery without neurologic impairment cannot be guaranteed once there is inadequate cerebral perfusion pressure consequent on cerebral edema.[32] Similarly, the presence of intrapulmonary shunts secondary to chronic liver disease can lead to respiratory failure and a poor prognosis for hepatic transplantation.[165] These patients need careful evaluation of pulmonary and cardiac functions prior to the surgery but are still potential candidates for liver transplantation, because recently extracorporeal mechanical oxygenation has been successfully used to manage this complication. Even congenital anomalies of portal veins, which have been an absolute contraindication in the past, do not now preclude patients from being successful recipients of a transplanted liver.[166]

Postoperative Management

The first few days following liver transplantation are fraught with the potential for significant, often life-threatening, complications and therefore require intense monitoring and management in the ICU.

Immediately after the liver transplantation procedure,

the patient is allowed to recover from anesthesia in the ICU because the anesthetic is not reversed in the operating room.[167] Mortality from the liver transplant primarily results from technical complications related to the biliary and vascular anastomosis. Massive hemorrhage, bile leaks, and obstruction of blood vessels and bile duct can occur. To monitor progress, urine output, coagulation status, standard liver function tests, and, more specifically, hepatobiliary scintiscans, abdominal ultrasound, and T-tube cholangiograms are needed.

A vigorous intravenous immunosuppressive regimen is initiated at the onset of the transplant surgery and continued through the first few postoperative days. The mainstay of immunosuppressive therapy is steroids and cyclosporine, a cyclic endecapeptide that inhibits generation of interleukin-2 and proliferation of T cells bearing the interleukin-2 receptors. A more potent immunosuppressive drug, FK506, a macrolide extracted from Streptomyces tsukubaenis, which has similar immune suppressing qualities but avoids hypertension and other side effects of cyclosporine, has been introduced. Episodes of rejection confirmed by biopsies are treated with pulses of steroids and, if necessary, 6-mercaptopurine, monoclonal antibodies such as OKT3, and polyclonal antilymphocyte or antithymocyte antibodies. The indications for their use have been discussed in detail in two reviews.[167, 168]

An immediate and dreaded complication following liver transplantation is primary graft nonfunction of the transplanted liver, the cause of which is unknown. The graft fails to perfuse well despite patency of all of the major vessels. Failure of the transplanted liver to rapidly restore its functions, particularly coagulation, heralds the onset of this event. Prompt retransplantation is required.[167]

The more commonly encountered early postoperative complications include hypertension, oliguria, infections, and rejection. The exact cause of the postoperative hypertension is not clear; it may be multifactorial. Occasionally, hypertension precipitates encephalopathy, and often a continuous nitroprusside drip is needed initially. Oliguria is frequent despite preservation of normal urine output and an adequate intravascular volume during surgery. Intensive monitoring of central venous and pulmonary artery wedge pressures is the key to the successful management of this complication, since excessive fluid administration to counter this oliguria may lead to pulmonary edema and ascites.[168]

During the first few days of ICU care, the patient continues to be susceptible to significant gastrointestinal bleeding from gastritis, peptic ulcers, or the anastomosis. Overwhelming infections can occur as a result of immunosuppression. Seizures are possible because of infections, air embolism, and vascular compromise. Vascular complications such as thrombosis of the portal vein or hepatic artery continue to be a threat.

The demand for livers to be transplanted is growing rapidly as physicians and patients realize that individuals with FHF or chronic nonreversible liver diseases can be saved. The need in small infants has been met by transplanting a segment of a larger organ.[32] The success of segmental transplantation, plus the remarkable regenerative capacity of the liver, has led to the development of living donor transplantation, a controversial procedure that may markedly increase the donor pool. The future holds even greater promise with the development of immunosuppressing agents such as FK506 and the possibility of intraperitoneal transplantation of hepatocytes.

References

1. Trey C and Davidson CS: The management of fulminant hepatic failure. *In*: Popper H and Schaffner F (eds): Progress in Liver Disease. New York, Grune & Stratton, 1970, pp 292–298.
2. Gimson AES, O'Grady J, Ede RJ, et al: Late onset hepatic failure: Clinical, serological and histological feature. Hepatology 6:288, 1986.
3. Wilzleben CL, Marshall GS, Wenner W, et al: HIV as a cause of giant cell hepatitis. Hum Pathol 19:603, 1988.
4. Treem WR: Hepatic failure. *In*: Walker WA, Durie PR, Hamilton JR, et al (eds): Pediatric Gastrointestinal Disease, Vol 1. Philadelphia, BC Decker, 1990, pp. 146–192.
5. Jones AE: Fulminant Hepatic Failure. *In* Zakim D and Boyer TD (eds): Hepatology—A Textbook of Liver Disease, Vol. 1, 2nd ed. Philadelphia, WB Saunders, 1990, pp. 460–475.
6. Yanda RJ: Fulminant hepatic failure (Medical staff conference). West J Med 149:586, 1988.
7. Martin P and Maddrey WC: Fulminant hepatic failure. Pract Gastroenterol 14:50, 1990.
8. Govindarajan S, Chin KP, Redeker AG, et al: Fulminant B viral hepatitis: Role of delta agent. Gastroenterology 86:1417, 1984.
9. Gimson AES, White YS, Eddleston ALWF, et al: Clinical and prognostic differences in fulminant hepatitis type A, B, and non-A, non-B. Gut 24:1194, 1983.
10. Realdi G, Alberti A, Rugge M, et al: A long term follow up of acute and chronic non-A, non-B hepatitis: Evidence of progression to liver cirrhosis. Gut 23:270, 1982.
11. White NJ and Juel-Jensen BE: Infectious mononucleosis hepatitis. Semin Liver Dis 4:301, 1984.
12. Deutsch J, Wolf H, Becker H, et al: Demonstration of Epstein-Barr virus DNA in a previously healthy boy with fulminant hepatic failure. Eur J Pediatr 145:94, 1986.
13. Nahmias AJ, Josey WE, and Naib ZM: Neonatal herpes infection. Role of genital infection in mother as the source of virus in the newborn. JAMA 199:164, 1967.
14. Moedy JCA, Lerman SJ, and White RJ: Fatal disseminated herpes simplex virus infection in a healthy child. Am J Dis Child 135:45, 1981.
15. Mitchell AA, Lacouture PG, Sheehan JE, et al: Adverse drug reactions in children leading to hospital admission. Pediatrics 82:24, 1988.
16. Schmucker DL and Wang RK: Age-related changes in liver drug metabolism: Structure as function. Proc Soc Exp Biol Med 165:178, 1980.
17. Smith MT, Thor H, and Orrenius S: The role of lipid peroxidation in the toxicity of foreign compounds to liver cells. Biochem Pharmacol 32:763, 1983.
18. Ransohoff DF and Jacobs G: Terminal hepatic failure following a small dose of sulfamethoxazole-trimethoprim. Gastroenterology 80:816, 1981.
19. Maddrey WC and Zimmerman HJ: Toxic and drug induced hepatitis. *In*: Schiff L and Schiff ER (eds): Diseases of the Liver, 6th ed. Philadelphia, JB Lippincott, 1987, p. 591.
20. Menard DB, Gisselbrecht C, Marty H, et al: Antineoplastic agents and the liver. Gastroenterology 78:142, 1980.
21. Jolivet J, Cowan KH, Curt GA, et al: The pharmacology and clinical use of methotrexate. N Engl J Med 5:323, 1983.
22. Pratt CB and Johnson WW: Duration and severity of fatty metamorphosis of the liver following L-asparaginase therapy. Cancer 28:361, 1971.
23. Rollins BJ: Hepatic veno-occlusive disease. Am J Med 81:297, 1986.
24. Roberts EA and Spielberg SP: Drug induced hepatotoxicity in

children. *In*: Walker WA, Durie PR, Hamilton JR, et al (eds): Pediatric Gastrointestinal Disease, Vol 1. Philadelphia, BC Decker, 1990, pp. 898–914.
25. Zimmerman HJ and Ishak KG: Hepatic injury due to drugs and toxins. *In*: MacSween RNM, Antony PP, and Scheuer PJ (eds): Pathology of the Liver, 2nd ed. London, Churchill Livingstone, 1987, p. 503.
26. Bianchi L, DeGroute J, Desmet VJ, et al: Guidelines for diagnosis of therapeutic drug-induced liver injury in liver biopsies: Analysis of 77 cases. Hepatology 6:1163, 1985.
27. McCullough AJ, Fleming CR, Thistle JL, et al: Diagnosis of Wilson's disease presenting as fulminant hepatic failure. Gastroenterology 84:161, 1983.
28. Berman DH, Leventhal RI, Gavaler JS, et al: Clinical differentiation of fulminant Wilsonian hepatitis from other causes of hepatic failure. Gastroenterology 100:1129, 1991.
29. Alagille D: Alpha-1-antitrypsin deficiency. Hepatology 4:115, 1984.
30. Setchell KDR and Street JM: Inborn errors of bile acid synthesis. Semin Liver Dis 7:85, 1987.
31. Witzleben CL and Uri A: Perinatal hemochromatosis: Entity or end result? Hum Pathol 20:335, 1989.
32. Whitington PF and Balistreri WF: Liver transplantation in pediatrics. J Pediatr 118:169, 1991.
33. Ohi R, Hanamatsu M, Mochizuki I, et al: Progress in the treatment of biliary atresia. World J Surg 9:285, 1985.
34. Alagille D, Estrada A, Hadchouel M, et al: Syndromatic paucity of interlobular bile ducts (Alagille syndrome or arteriohepatic dysplasia): Review of 80 cases. J Pediatr 110:195, 1987.
35. Maggiore G, Bernard O, Riely CA, et al: Normal serum gammaglutamyltransferase activity identifies groups of infants with idiopathic cholestasis with poor prognosis. J Pediatr 111:251, 1987.
36. Kelley RI: Review: The cerebrohepatorenal syndrome of Zellweger, morphology and metabolic aspects. Am J Med Genet 16:503, 1983.
37. Maggiore G, Bernard O, Homberg JC, et al: Liver disease associated with anti liver-kidney microsome antibody in children. J Pediatr 108:399, 1986.
38. Popper H and Keppler D: Networks of interacting mechanisms of hepatocellular degeneration and death. *In*: Popper H and Schaffner F (eds): Progress in Liver Diseases, Vol 8. New York, Grune & Stratton, 1986, p. 209.
39. Schanne FAX, Kaner AB, Young EE, et al: Calcium dependence of toxic cell death: A final common pathway. Science 206:700, 1979.
40. Mathieson LR, Linglof T, Moller AM, et al: Fulminant hepatitis A. J Infect Dis 11:303, 1979.
41. Nolan JP: The role of endotoxin in liver injury. Gastroenterology 69:1346, 1975.
42. Zimmerman HJ: Hepatotoxicity. The Adverse Effects of Drugs and Other Chemicals on the Liver. New York, Appleton-Century Crofts, 1978.
43. Pascoe GA, Fariss MW, Olafsdottir K, et al: A role of vitamin E in protection against cell injury: Maintenance of intracellular glutathione precursors and biosynthesis. Eur J Biochem 166:241, 1987.
44. Ketterer B: Detoxification reactions of glutathione and glutathione transferases. Xenobiotica 16:957, 1986.
45. Miner DJ and Kissinger PT. Evidence for the involvement of N-acetyl-p-quinoneimine in acetaminophen metabolism. Biochem Pharmacol 28:3285, 1979.
46. Corcoran GB, Racz WJ, Smith CV, et al: Effects of N-acetylcysteine on acetaminophen covalent binding and hepatic necrosis in mice. J Pharmacol Exp Ther 232:864, 1985.
47. Spielberg SP, Gordon GB, Blake DA, et al: Predisposition to phenytoin hepatotoxicity assessed in vitro. N Engl J Med 305:722, 1981.
48. Mullick FG and Ishak KG: Hepatic injury associated with diphenylhydantoin therapy. Am J Clin Pathol 74:442, 1980.
49. Dreifuss FE, Santilli N, Langer DH, et al: Valproic acid hepatic fatalities. Neurology 37:379, 1987.
50. Gerber N, Dickinson RG, Harland RC, et al: Reye-like syndrome associated with valproic acid therapy. J Pediatr 95:142, 1979.
51. Zimmerman HJ and Ishak KG: Valproate-induced hepatic injury: Analysis of 23 fatal cases. Hepatology 2:591, 1982.

52. Böhles H, Richter K, Wagner-Thiessen E, et al: Decreased serum carnitine in valproate induced Reye syndrome. Eur J Pediatr 139:185, 1982.

53. Moult PJ and Sherlock S: Halothane-related hepatitis: A clinical study of twenty-six cases. Q J Med 44:99, 1975.

54. DeGroot H and Noll T: Halothane hepatotoxicity: Relation between metabolic activation pyrexia, covalent binding, lipid peroxidation and liver cell damage. Hepatology 3:601, 1983.

55. Farrell GC, Mahoney J, Bilous M, et al: Altered hepatic calcium homeostasis in guinea pigs with halothane-induced hepatotoxicity. J Pharmacol Exp Ther 247:751, 1988.

56. Hassall E, Israel DM, Gunasekharan T, et al: Halothane hepatitis in children. J Pediatr Gastroenterol Nutr 11:553, 1990.

57. Karnaze DS and Bickford RG: Triphasic waves: A reassessment of their significance. Electroencephalogr Clin Neurophysiol 57:193, 1984.

58. Weber FL and Veach GI: The importance of the small intestine in gut ammonium production in the fasting dog. Gastroenterology 77:235, 1979.

59. Nance FC, Kaufman HJ, Kline DG, et al: Role of urea in the hyperammonemia of germ-free Eck fistula dogs. Gastroenterology 66:108, 1974.

60. Fraser CL and Arieff AI: Hepatic encephalopathy. N Engl J Med 313:865, 1985.

61. Snodgrass PJ and Delong GR: Urea-cycle enzyme deficiencies and an increased nitrogen load producing hyperammonemia in Reye's syndrome. N Engl J Med 294:855, 1976.

62. Zieve L: The mechanism of hepatic coma. Hepatology 1:360, 1981.

63. Challenger F and Walshe JM: Methyl mercaptan in relation to foetor hepaticus. Biochem J 59:372, 1955.

64. Foster D, Ahrnad K, and Zieve L: Action of methanethiol on Na$^+$K$^+$ATPase: Implications for hepatic coma. Ann NY Acad Sci 242:573, 1974.

65. Fischer JE and Baldessarini RJ: Neurotransmitter metabolism in hepatic encephalopathy. N Engl J Med 293:1152, 1975.

66. Jones EA, Schafer DF, Ferenci P, et al: The neurobiology of hepatic encephalopathy. Hepatology 4:1235, 1984.

67. Ferenci P, Colev D, and Schafer DF: Metabolism of the inhibitory neurotransmitter γ-aminobutyric acid in a rabbit model of fulminant hepatic failure. Hepatology 3:507, 1983.

68. Jones DB, Mullen KD, Roessle M, et al: Hepatic encephalopathy: Application of visual evoked responses to test hypotheses of its pathogenesis in rats. J Hepatol 4:118, 1987.

69. Bassett ML, Mullen KD, Skolnick P, et al: Amelioration of hepatic encephalopathy by pharmacological antagonism of the GABA$_A$/benzodiazepine receptor complex in a rat model of fulminant hepatic failure. Gastroenterology 93:1069, 1987.

70. Zaki AEO, Ede RJ, Davis M, et al: Experimental studies on blood brain barrier permeability in acute hepatic failure. Hepatology 4:359, 1984.

71. Treem WR, Witzleben CA, Piccoli DA, et al: Medium-chain and long-chain acyl-CoA dehydrogenase deficiency: Clinical, pathologic, and ultrastructural differentiation from Reye's syndrome. Hepatology 6:1270, 1986.

72. Warren KS and Schenker S: Hypoxia and ammonia toxicity. Am J Physiol 199:1105, 1960.

73. Hoyumpa AM, Desmond PV, Avant GR, et al: Hepatic encephalopathy. Gastroenterology 76:184, 1979.

74. Psacharopoulos HT, Mowat AP, Davies M, et al: Fulminant hepatic failure in childhood: An analysis of 31 cases. Arch Dis Child 55:252, 1980.

75. Ware AJ, D'Agostino A, and Combes B: Cerebral edema: A major complication of massive hepatic necrosis. Gastroenterology 61:877, 1971.

76. Ede RJ and Williams R: Hepatic encephalopathy and cerebral edema. Semin Liver Dis 6:107, 1986.

77. Horowitz ME, Scafer DF, Molnar P, et al: Increased blood-brain transfer in a rabbit model of acute liver failure. Gastroenterology 84:1003, 1983.

78. Trewby PN, Hanid MA, Mackenzie RL, et al: Effects of cerebral oedema and arterial hypotension on cerebral blood flow in an animal model of hepatic failure. Gut 19:1999, 1978.

79. Gazzard BG, Rahe MO, Flute PT, et al: Bleeding in relation to the coagulation defect of fulminant hepatic failure. In: Williams R and Murray-Lyon IM (eds): Artificial Liver Support. London, Pittman Medical Publishing, 1975, p. 143.

80. Dymock IW, Tucker JS, Woolf IL, et al: Coagulation studies as a prognostic index in acute liver failure. Br J Haematol 29:385, 1975.

81. Langley PG, Hughes RD, and Williams R: Increased factor VIII complex in fulminant hepatic failure. Thromb Haemost 54:693, 1985.

82. Weston MJ, Langley PG, Rubin MH, et al: Platelet function in fulminant hepatic failure and effect of charcoal hemoperfusion. Gut 18:897, 1977.

83. Rubin MH, Weston MJ, Bullock G, et al: Abnormal platelet function and ultrastructure in fulminant hepatic failure. Q J Med 46:339, 1977.

84. Fujiwara K, Ogata I, Ohta Y, et al: Intravascular coagulation in acute liver failure in rats and its treatment with antithrombin III. Gut 29:1103, 1988.

85. Green FB, Thomson JM, Dymock JW, et al: Abnormal fibrin polymerization in liver disease. Br J Haematol 34:427, 1976.

86. Epstein M: The hepatorenal syndrome. Hosp Pract 24(4):65, 1989.

87. Arroyo V, Bernardi M, Epstein M, et al: Pathophysiology of ascites and functional renal failure in cirrhosis. J Hepatol 6:239, 1988.

88. Papper S: Renal failure in cirrhosis (the hepatorenal syndrome). In: Epstein M (ed): The Kidney in Liver Disease, 2nd ed. New York, Elsevier Science, 1983, p. 87.

89. Koppel MH, Coburn JW, Mims MM, et al: Transplantation of cadaveric kidneys from patients with hepatorenal syndrome. Evidence for the functional nature of renal failure in advanced liver disease. N Engl J Med 280:1367, 1969.

90. Epstein M, Berk DP, Hollenberg NK, et al: Renal failure in the patient with cirrhosis: The role of active vasoconstriction. Am J Med 49:175, 1970.

91. Zipser RD, Radvan GH, Kronborg IJ, et al: Urinary thromboxane B$_2$ and prostaglandin E$_2$ in the hepatorenal syndrome: Evidence for increased vasoconstrictor and decreased vasodilator factors. Gastroenterology 84:697, 1983.

92. Rimola A, Soto R, Bory F, et al: Reticuloendothelial system phagocytic activity in cirrhosis and its relation to bacterial infections and prognosis. Hepatology 4:53, 1984.

93. Larcher VF, Wyke RJ, Mowat AP, et al: Bacterial and fungal infection in children with fulminant hepatic failure: Possible role of opsonisation and complement deficiency. Gut 23:1037, 1982.

94. Russell GJ, Fitzgerald JF, and Clark JH: Fulminant hepatic failure. J Pediatr 111:313, 1987.

95. Trey C, Lipworth L, and Davidson CS: Parameters influencing survival in the first 318 patients reported to the fulminant hepatic failure surveillance study. Gastroenterology 58:306, 1970.

96. Conn HO: Asterixis in non-hepatic disorders. Am J Med 29:647, 1960.

97. Basha MA and Popovich Jr: Managing intracranial hypertension to avoid neurological sequelae. J Crit Illness 6:68, 1991.

98. Heubi JE, Partin JC, Partin JS, et al: Reye's syndrome: Current concepts. Hepatology 7:155, 1987.

99. Partin JC, Schubert WK, and Partin JS: Mitochondrial ultrastructure in Reye's syndrome (encephalopathy and fatty degeneration of the viscera). N Engl J Med 285:1339, 1971.

100. Martens ME and Lee CP: Reye's syndrome: Salicylates and mitochondrial functions. Biochem Pharmacol 33:2869, 1984.

101. Reichling JJ and Kaplan MM: Clinical use of serum enzymes in liver disease. Dig Dis Sci 33:1601, 1988.

102. Kovar IZ and Mayne PD: Postnatal and gestational age and the interpretation of plasma alkaline phosphatase activity in preterm infants. Ann Clin Biochem 26:193, 1989.

103. Nemesanszky E and Lott JA: Gamma-glutamyltransferase and its iosenzymes: Progress and problems. Clin Chem 31:797, 1985.

104. Keefe EB, Sunderland MC, and Gabourel JD: Serum gamma-glutamyl transpeptidase activity in patients receiving chronic phenytoin therapy. Dig Dis Sci 31:1056, 1986.

105. Ekindjian OG, Devanley M, Duchassaing D, et al: Multivariate analysis of clinical and biological data in cirrhotic patients: Application of prognosis. Eur J Clin Invest 11:213, 1981.

106. Walker CH and Kozalka MF: Fatal bromsulphthalein reaction. Ann Intern Med 47:362, 1957.

107. Oellerich M, Burdelski M, Ringe B, et al: Lignocaine metabolite formation as a measure of pre-transplant liver function. Lancet 1:640, 1989.

108. Decker RH, Kosakowski SM, Vanderbilt AS, et al: Diagnosis of acute hepatitis A by HAVAB-M, a direct radioimmunoassay for IgM anti HAV. Am J Clin Pathol 76:140, 1981.
109. Sjogren M, Tanno H, Fay O, et al: Hepatitis A virus in stool during clinical relapse. Ann Intern Med 106:221, 1987.
110. Hoofnagle JH and Schafer DF:Serological markers of hepatitis B virus infection. Semin Liver Dis 6:1, 1986.
111. Mushawar IK, Dienstag JL, Polesky HF, et al: Interpretation of serological profiles of hepatitis B virus infection. Am J Clin Pathol 76:773, 1981.
112. Rasshofer R, Buti M, Esteban R, et al: Demonstration of hepatitis D virus RNA in patients with chronic hepatitis. J Infect Dis 157:191, 1987.
113. Aragona M, Caredda F, Lavarini C, et al: Serological response to the hepatitis delta virus in hepatitis D. Lancet 1:478, 1987.
114. Dienstag JL: Non-A, non-B hepatitis. I: Recognition, epidemiology, and clinical features. Gastroenterology 85:439, 1983.
115. De Knegt RJ, Schalm SW, Van Der Berg B, et al: Causes of death in fulminant hepatic failure. Neth J Med 29:235, 1986.
116. Rakela J, Lange SM, Ludwig J, et al: Fulminant hepatitis: Mayo Clinic experience with 34 cases. Mayo Clin Proc 60:289, 1985.
117. Van Der Rijt C and Schalm SW: Quantitative EEG analysis and survival in liver disease. Electroencephalogr Clin Neurophysiol 61: 502, 1985.
118. Trey C, Lipworth L, and Davidson CS: Parameters influencing survival in the first 318 patients reported to the Fulminant Hepatic Failure Surveillance Study. Gastroenterology 58:306, 1970.
119. Walton B, Simpson BR, Strunin L, et al: Unexplained hepatitis following halothane. Br Med J 1:1171, 1976.
120. Desmet VJ, de Groote J, and van Damme B: Acute hepatocellular failure. A study of 17 patients treated with exchange transfusion. Hum Pathol 3:167, 1972.
121. Sherlock S: Acute (fulminant) hepatic failure. In: Sherlock S (ed): Diseases of the Liver and the Biliary System, 6th ed. Oxford, Blackwell Scientific Publications, 1981, pp. 107–113.
122. Weston MJ, Talbot IC, Howorth PJN, et al: Frequency of arrhythmias and other cardiac abnormalities in fulminant hepatic failure. Br Heart J 38:1179, 1976.
123. Scotto J, Opolon P, Eteve J, et al: Liver biopsy and prognosis in acute liver failure. Gut 14:927, 1973.
124. Sawhey VK, Knauer CM, and Gregory PB: Rapid reduction of transaminase levels in fulminant hepatitis. N Engl J Med 302:970, 1980.
125. Mackenjee MK, Kiepiela P, Cooper R, et al: Clinically important immunological processes in acute and fulminant hepatitis, mainly due to hepatitis B virus. Arch Dis Child 57:277, 1982.
126. Bloomer JR, Waldmann TA, McIntire KR, et al: Serum alpha-fetoprotein in patients with massive hepatic necrosis. Gastroenterology 72:479, 1977.
127. Bernardi M, DePalma R, Trevisani F, et al: Effects of a new loop diuretic (muzolimine) in cirrhotics with ascites: Comparison with furosemide. Hepatology 6:400, 1986.
128. Pinto PC, Amerian J, and Reynolds TB: Large volume paracentesis in nonedematous patients with tense ascites: Its effect on intravascular volume. Hepatology 8:207, 1988.
129. Conn HO, Leevy CM, and Vlahcevic ZR: Comparison of lactulose and neomycin in the treatment of chronic portal-systemic encephalopathy: A double blind controlled trial. Gastroenterology 72:573, 1977.
130. Uribe M, Toledo H, Perez F, et al: Lactitol, a second generation disaccharide for treatment of chronic portal-systemic encephalopathy. Dig Dis Sci 32:1345, 1987.
131. Ozsoylu S and Kocak N: Levodopa in hepatic coma in children. Turk J Pediatr 17:5, 1975.
132. Ozsoylu S and Kocak N: Naloxone in hepatic encephalopathy. Am J Dis Child 139:749, 1985.
133. Bansky G, Meier PJ, and Riederer E: Effect of a benzodiazepine antagonist in hepatic encephalopathy in man (Abstract). Hepatology 7:1103, 1987.
134. Grimm G, Ferenci P, Katzenschlager R, et al: Improvement of hepatic encephalopathy treated with flumazenil. Lancet 2:1392, 1988.
135. Warren R, Trewby PN, Laws JW, et al: Pulmonary complications in fulminant hepatic failure: Analysis of serial radiographs from 100 consecutive patients. Clin Radiol 29:363, 1978.
136. Berk PD and Popper H: Fulminant hepatic failure. Annotated abstracts of a workshop held at the National Insitutes of Health, 1977. Am J Gastroenterol 69:349, 1978.
137. Ede RJ and Williams R: Hepatic encephalopathy and cerebral edema. In: Williams R (ed): Seminars in Liver Disease, Vol. 6, No. 2. New York, Thieme, 1986, p. 107.
138. Bihari D, Gimson AE, Lindridge J, et al: Lactic acidosis in fulminant hepatic failure. Crit Care Med 13:1034, 1985.
139. Mummary RV, Bradley JM, and Jefferies DJ: Microbiological monitoring of patients in hepatic failure with particular reference to extracorporeal porcine liver perfusion. Lancet 2:60, 1971.
140. Macdougall BRD and Williams R: H₂ receptor antagonist in the prevention of acute upper gastrointestinal hypertension in fulminant hepatic failure. Gastroenterology 74:464, 1978.
141. Gazzard BG, Henderson JM, and Williams R: Early changes in coagulation following a paracetamol overdose and a controlled trial of fresh frozen plasma therapy. Gut 16:617, 1975.
142. Agnelli G, DeCunto M, Berritini M, et al: Desmopressin improvement of abnormal coagulation in chronic liver disease. Lancet 1:645, 1983.
143. Braude P, Arias J, Hughes RD, et al: Antithrombin III infusion during fulminant hepatic failure (Abstract). Thromb Haemost 46:369, 1981.
144. Saunders SJ, Seggie J, Kirsch RE, et al: Acute liver failure. In: Wright R, Alberti KGMM, Karan S, et al (eds): Liver and Biliary Disease. Philadelphia, WB Saunders, 1979, p. 569.
145. Farrell MK, Balistreri WF, and Suchy FJ: Serum sulfated lithocholate as an indicator of cholestasis during parenteral nutrition in infants and children. J Parent Enteral Nutr 6:30, 1982.
146. Sokol RJ: Medical management of the infant or child with chronic liver disease. Semin Liver Dis 7:155, 1987.
147. Munro HN, Fernstrom JD, and Wurtman RJ: Insulin, plasma amino acid imbalance and hepatic coma. Lancet 1:722, 1975.
148. Thompson JS, Schafer DF, Haun J, et al: Adequate diet prevents hepatic coma in dogs with Eck fistulas. Surg Gynecol Obstet 162:126, 1986.
149. Marchesini G, Zoli M, and Dondi C: Anticatabolic effect of branched-chain amino acid-enriched solutions in patients with liver cirrhosis. Hepatology 2:420, 1982.
150. Rossi-Fanneli F, Freund H, Krause R, et al: Induction of coma in normal dogs by the infusion of aromatic amino acids and its prevention by the addition of branched chain amino acids. Gastroenterology 83:664, 1982.
151. Chase RA, Davis M, Trewby PN, et al: Plasma amino acid profiles in patients with fulminant hepatic failure treated by repeated polyacrylonitrate membrane haemodialysis. Gastroenterology 75:1033, 1987.
152. Wahren J, Denis J, Desurmont P, et al: Is intravenous administration of branched-chain amino acids effective in the treatment of hepatic encephalopathy? A multicenter study. Hepatology 3:475, 1983.
153. Horst D, Grace ND, Conn HO, et al: Comparison of dietary protein with an oral, branched chain-enriched amino acid supplement in chronic portal systemic encephalopathy: A randomized controlled trial. Hepatology 4:279, 1984.
154. Beaubernard C, Delorme ML, Opolon P, et al: Effect of oral administration of branched chain amino acids on hepatic encephalopathy in the rat. Hepatology 4:288, 1984.
155. Cerra FB, Cheung NK, Fischer JE, et al: Disease-specific amino acid infusion (F080) in hepatic encephalopathy: A prospective, randomized, double-blind controlled trial. J Parent Enteral Nutr 9:288, 1985.
156. Naylor CD, O'Rourke K, Detsky AS, et al: Parenteral nutrition with branched-chain amino acids in hepatic encephalopathy. Gastroenterology 97:1033, 1989.
157. Hanid MA, Davies M, Mellon PJ, et al: Clinical monitoring of intracranial pressure in fulminant hepatic failure. Gut 21:866, 1980.
158. Ede RJ, Gimson AES, Bihari D, et al: Controlled hyperventilation in the prevention of cerebral edema in fulminant hepatic failure. J Hepatol 2:43, 1986.
159. Ware AJ, Jones RE, Shorey JW, et al: A controlled trial of steroid therapy in massive hepatic necrosis. Am J Gastroenterol 62:130, 1974.
160. O'Grady JG, Gimson AES, O'Brien CJ, et al: Controlled trials of charcoal hemoperfusion and prognostic factors in fulminant hepatic failure. Gastroenterology 94:1186, 1988.

161. Matsubara S, Okabe K, Ouchi K, et al: Temporary metabolic support by extracorporeal blood therapy for liver failure after surgery. Trans Am Soc Artif Intern Organs 34:266, 1988.
162. Winikoff S, Glassman MS, and Spivak G: Plasmapheresis in a patient with hepatic failure awaiting liver transplantation. Lancet 2:681, 1982.
163. Davenport A, Will EJ, Davison AM, et al: Changes in intracranial pressure during hemofiltration in oliguric patients with grade IV hepatic encephalopathy. Nephron 53:142, 1989.
164. Starzl TE, Demetrius AJ, and Van Thiel D: Liver transplantation. N Engl J Med 321:1014, 1092, 1989.
165. Mews CF, Dorney SF, Sheil AG, et al: Failure of liver transplantation in Wilson's disease with pulmonary arteriovenous shunting. J Pediatr Gastroenterol 10:230, 1990.
166. Woodle ES, Thislethwaite JR, Emond JC, et al: Successful orthotopic liver transplantation in congenital absence of the portal vein. Surgery 107:475, 1990.
167. Paradis KJ, Freese DK, and Sharp HL: A pediatric perspective on liver transplantation. Pediatr Gastroenterol 35:409, 1988.
168. Shaw BW Jr, Wood RP, Kaufman SS, et al: Liver transplantation therapy for children. Part 2. J Pediatr Gastroenterol Nutr 7:797, 1988.

Gastrointestinal Dysfunction and Failure

Lynn F. Duffy, M.D., and Benny Kerzner, M.D.

The manifestations of failed gastrointestinal function are remarkably varied because of the diverse functions of the intestine. The integrated function of the intestine involves appropriate propagation of food; addition of secretions providing acid, alkali, and potent digestive enzymes; absorption of nutrients; packaging and timely passage of waste products. Therefore, the scope of intestinal failure includes cessation of intestinal motility causing gastroparesis and paralytic ileus, failure of the normal protective mucosal functions leading to ulceration and inflammation, and malabsorption or uncontrolled secretion resulting in diarrhea. The severely ill patient is at higher risk for the development of these problems.

In this chapter, we focus on intestinal dysfunction and failure in terms of these manifestations, and we have described a differential diagnosis for each symptom. The emphasis is placed on the implications of etiology and pathogenesis for management of a selection of the more common disease entities seen in the intensive care unit (ICU).

ABDOMINAL DISTENTION

It is unlikely that a child with the insidious onset of distention will present to the ICU. Rather, in the critically ill patient acute and rapid progression of distention is more likely. The causes of abdominal distention in childhood are shown in Table 57-1 and may be the result of accumulation of gas, fluid, or solid material. A physical examination will usually distinguish among these three possibilities.

When intestinal obstruction is the cause of gaseous distention, it is imperative to immediately make the diagnosis to ensure rapid treatment. The physical signs of obstruction are readily confirmed by the gas pattern on x-ray. Contrast material should be added when further definition is needed. Nonobstructive gaseous distention in the ICU patient will most likely be secondary to paralytic ileus (see later), although other causes of distention, such as malabsorption syndromes, should be considered. When fluid is causing abdominal disten-

tion in an ICU trauma patient, hemorrhage must be considered. In other patients, ascites is more likely. The presence of abdominal fluid is readily confirmed by ultrasound, but the determination of its character is made by abdominal paracentesis. The fluid must be appropriately examined to determine if it a transudate or exudate, of hepatic, pancreatic, or lymphatic origin, infected, or hemorrhagic. When abdominal distention is due to enlargement of a solid mass, admission to the ICU is prompted by additional factors, such as respiratory distress and organ compromise that mandate immediate attention. The key to management lies in determining the origin and nature of the mass.

Paralytic Ileus

Paralytic ileus, adynamic ileus, and intestinal pseudo-obstruction are terms used to describe a dysmotility resulting in a loss of propulsion leading to the accumulation of gas and fluid in the intestine.[1] The ileus is a nonspecific response to a variety of insults (Table 57-2), and in the ICU patient, drugs, biochemical aberrations, infectious peritonitis, and referred pain are important causes.

Just as the etiologies of a paralytic ileus are diverse, so also are the pathogenetic mechanisms.[1] This is not surprising if the complexity of the intestine's motility and the variety of ways in which it can be influenced are taken into consideration. There are two distinct patterns of contraction—propulsive waves and segmental contractions.[2] Propulsive waves sweep down the intestine linked to the migrating motor complexes (MMC), which are recurrent bursts of electrical activity that occur in the fasted state. Segmental contractions, which allow for the mixing of products of digestion, occur independently of MMCs during the fed state. In paralytic ileus, both contractile patterns are lost. Intestinal motility is under the control of the enteric nervous system (ENS) and the autonomic nervous system (ANS) and is also influenced by hormones and regulatory peptides in the gut.[2] The ENS innervates the intestinal smooth muscle through neurons in the myenteric plexus and receives modulating input from the ANS. In general, the ANS establishes control through parasympathetic fibers from the vagus that stimulate motility, and sympathetic fibers from the celiac, superior, and inferior mesenteric ganglia that inhibit motility.[1] The inhibition of intestinal motility in paralytic ileus is the result of adrenergic nervous impulses that act through the enteric plexuses.[1, 3] The pattern of autonomic innervation, that is, the number of α- and β-receptors, varies in different parts of the intestine. The stomach has a combination of both α- and β-receptors; the small intestine contains primarily α-receptors, and the colon contains β-receptors. Potential treatment of the ileus in different areas of the bowel relates to this nervous innervation. Postoperative ileus mainly affects the colon.[4] When myoelectric activity is recorded postoperatively in animals, small bowel and antral function return within a short period of time, whereas colonic activity remains depressed for up to 72 hours.[4] Theoretically, treatment aimed at blocking β-adrenergic receptors should prevent ileus; however, when agents such as guanethidine have been tried, the results have been disappointing.[5] Isolated colonic ileus can occur without surgery. In 1948, Ogilvie described cases of cecal dilatation without mechanical obstruction that he ascribed to inhibition of parasympathetic stimulation.[6]

The biochemical basis of ileus remains obscure. Intestinal peptides are important modulators of gut motility. Enteroglucagon and motilin are hormones that have stimulatory effects, whereas neurotensin (a neurotransmitter) and peptide YY (a hormone) are inhibitors. Even prostaglandin metabolism may be involved; administered prostaglandin F has counteracted experimental ileus.[7] The diagnosis of an ileus is based on the finding of abdominal distention, decreased or absent bowel sounds, and tympany on examination. In contrast to mechanical obstruction, air fluid levels are seen throughout the small intestine and the colon on abdominal radiographs.[8] Once an ileus has been diagnosed, the evaluation should focus on ascertaining its cause (see Table 57–2). To implicate drugs, a medication history and toxicology screen are useful. Electrolyte and other biochemical aberrations are readily detected by

Table 57–1. CAUSES OF ABDOMINAL DISTENTION IN CHILDHOOD

Intestinal	Extraintestinal
Pseudo-obstruction syndrome	Ascites
Paralytic ileus	Nonchylous
Chronic idiopathic intestinal	Chylous
pseudo-obstruction	Visceromegaly
Obstruction	Hepatomegaly
Partial	Splenomegaly
Complete	Hydronephrosis
Constipation	Tumors
Fecal impaction	Neuroblastoma
Malabsorption syndromes	Wilms tumor
Celiac disease	Cysts
Cystic fibrosis	Mesenteric
Aerophagy	Pancreatic
	Ovarian
	Urinary bladder retention
	Skeletal muscle defect

Table 57–2. ETIOLOGIES OF PARALYTIC ILEUS

Drugs	Peritonitis
Opioids	Perforated viscus
Ganglionic blockers	Primary infection
Antidepressants	Appendicitis
Phenothiazines	**Referred Pain**
Anticholinergics	Biliary and renal colic
Biochemical Aberrations	Spinal and rib fractures
Hyponatremia	Basilar pneumonia
Hypochloremia	Myocardial infarction
Hypokalemia	**Bowel Ischemia**
Hypomagnesemia	
Retroperitoneal Pathology	
Bleeding	
Pancreatitis	
Tumors	

routine laboratory studies. Retroperitoneal masses, biliary stones, and renal stones are best identified with abdominal ultrasonography or by computed tomography (CT).

Despite the onslaught of new investigative modalities that allow us to visualize and study intestinal motility, the management of the patient with a paralytic ileus has not changed and remains conservative.[9] Nasogastric or nasojejunal intubation, which decompresses the bowel and relieves distention, affords symptomatic relief. Medical therapy with agents known to enhance motility has been disappointing to date. In particular, the use of the cholinergic agent bethanechol,[10] adrenergic neuronal blockers,[4] and the prokinetic agents metoclopramide[11] and domperidone[12] have neither prevented nor shortened the course of postoperative ileus. There are encouraging reports of chemical therapy that must still be confirmed. The newer prokinetic agent, cisapride, which is still under investigation, has reduced the length of postoperative ileus in a small number of patients.[13] Intravenous infusion of exogenous motilin was used successfully to stimulate contractile activity in an infant with an intestinal pseudo-obstruction.[14]

GASTROINTESTINAL BLEEDING

Gastrointestinal bleeding is a frightening experience for the pediatric patient and his or her parents. But, because of the child's resilient cardiovascular system, the bleeding usually stops with conservative treatment.[15] This outcome is in sharp contrast to adults, in which the mortality reaches 10%.[16] The differential diagnosis of gastrointestinal (GI) bleeding varies over the pediatric age range as indicated in Table 57–3, and the extent of the hemorrhage is strongly influenced by the cause. Bleeding may therefore be minor or serious, and a stepwise approach to the diagnosis and intervention is needed to avoid unnecessary procedures.[17] The first step is to confirm that the patient has in fact had a bleeding episode; the second step is to determine the severity of the bleeding by evaluating the patient's hemodynamic and mental status; and the third step is to discover the source of the blood.

Many substances that children ingest can mimic blood

Table 57–3. ETIOLOGIES OF UPPER AND LOWER GASTROINTESTINAL BLEEDING

Upper Gastrointestinal			
Neonate	Infant–2 yr old	3–12 yr old	Adolescent
Swallowed maternal blood	Erosive gastritis	Erosive gastritis	PUD*
Stress ulcer	Peptic esophagitis	Stress ulcer	Mallory-Weiss tear
Hemorrhagic gastritis	Stress ulcer	Peptic esophagitis	Stress ulcer
Hemorrhagic disease of the newborn	Gastric volvulus	Foreign body	Esophageal varices
	Foreign body	Mallory-Weiss tear	
	Mallory-Weiss tear	Esophageal varices	
	Esophageal varices		

Lower Gastrointestinal Bleeding			
Neonate	Infant–2 yr old	3–12 yr old	Adolescent
Swallowed maternal blood	Milk protein colitis	Anal fissure	Infectious colitis
NEC†	Anal fissure	Polyp	Hemorrhoids
Milk protein colitis	Infectious colitis	Infectious colitis	Anal fissure
Infectious colitis	Intussusception	HUS‡	IBD§
Anal fissure	Meckel diverticulum	IBD	
Midgut volvulus	Polyp		
Hemorrhagic disease of the newborn	Duplication cysts		
	HUS‡		
	IBD§		

*PUD = peptic ulcer disease.
†NEC = necrotizing enterocolitis.
‡HUS = hemolytic-uremic syndrome.
§IBD = inflammatory bowel disease.

because they are red or cause the stool to turn black. Red-colored foods, iron compounds, and bismuth are common offenders. Stool and emesis must therefore be tested to confirm the presence of blood. It is important to be aware that certain products may interfere with the interpretation of the results with hemoccult testing (SmithKline Diagnostics). Red meat and iron preparations will give false-positive results, whereas excessive amounts of ascorbic acid will give false-negative results.

It is important to consider whether or not the bleeding is dangerous and warrants aggressive investigation. A serious blood loss is generally greater than 10% of blood volume. In these patients, hemodynamic stabilization is a priority. Assessment for shock, and intravascular resuscitation with fluid, colloid, and blood products are necessary, and the details are presented elsewhere. Once the patient is stabilized, an investigation for the etiology of the hemorrhage should take place. In the patient with hematemesis, once epistaxis has been ruled out, the source is usually located in the upper intestine proximal to the ligament of Treitz. Melena (black tarry stool) can originate from either the upper intestine or the right colon. Melenic stools contain at least 200 ml of denatured blood. Maroon and red-colored stools usually denote a lower GI lesion. However, in the patient with massive hemorrhage from the upper tract, the blood acts as a cathartic, decreasing transit time and its conversion to the characteristic black color. When a distinction of an upper GI bleed from a lower GI bleed cannot be made, passage of a nasogastric tube and gastric lavage can be performed. A large bore Salem sump tube should be used if lavage is necessary. The presence of gross blood or Hemoccult positive material is indicative of a bleeding source above the ligament of Treitz. A negative aspirate usually signifies bleeding below the second portion of the duodenum.[18]

Nasogastric (NG) suction and lavage are utilized to control bleeding, prevent aspiration, and make visualization by endoscopy possible. Normal saline is used for lavage to prevent hyponatremia. Room temperature saline lavage is as effective[19] as "iced" saline and should be used in the small child who may otherwise develop hypothermia. After gastric lavage, investigation should proceed as shown in Figure 57–1.

Lower GI bleeding can be more difficult to evaluate. Proctoscopy is very safe, and a limited evaluation to exclude colitis can be completed in very ill patients. It is more sensitive than barium contrast studies and should be done before contrast material is instilled. If a cause cannot be found in the rectosigmoid, then colonoscopy is necessary. However, massive bleeding makes endoscopy difficult, and under these circumstances bleeding scans, contrast studies, and arteriograms may yield better results.[20]

Stress-Related Mucosal Damage

With the current status of life support technology, patients in critical care settings are surviving longer and have a greater opportunity to develop stress-related mucosal damage (SRMD) of the upper GI tract. It occurs in approximately 80% of ICU patients.[21] The causes are multifactorial and include severe head trauma, extensive burns, and multiorgan system failure[22] (Table 57–4).

The inflammation and ulceration of SRMD reflect a breakdown between mucosal protection and gastric acid production, and therefore the old adage of "no acid, no ulcer" still holds true.[23] Understanding and finding the means to interrupt acid production is still the mainstay of therapy. The final step in gastric acid production is

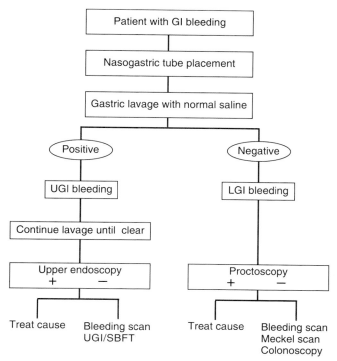

Figure 57–1. Algorithm for evaluation of gastrointestinal bleeding. GI = gastrointestinal; LGI = lower gastrointestinal; UGI = upper gastrointestinal.

the release of hydrogen ions via the H^+/K^+ exchange pump in the parietal cell. Histamine augments this hydrogen release through adenylate cyclase. The parietal cell is governed by neural, endocrine, and paracrine systems, mediated by acetylcholine and gastrin, and for the paracrine system, histamine and somatostatin.[24, 25] Gastric mucosal mast cells release histamine, and enterochromaffin-like cells release both histamine and somatostatin. Gastrin has a dominant effect on acid production by positively influencing the parietal cell directly and by augmenting the release of histamine from the paracrine system.[26] A negative feedback turning off gastrin production is mediated by the release of somatostatin. In contrast, acetylcholine has a lesser but entirely positive effect; it acts directly on the parietal cell, augments histamine release from histamine containing cells, and inhibits the release of somatostatin.[24, 25] The aforementioned physiology explains the three mo-

Table 57–4. ETIOLOGIES OF STRESS-RELATED MUCOSAL DAMAGE

Central nervous system injury
    Cushing ulcer
Extensive burns (>35%)
    Curling ulcer
Multiple organ failure
    Renal failure
    Liver failure
Sepsis
Trauma
Shock
Mechanical ventilation
Coagulopathy

dalities utilized in pharmacology to interrupt acid production: H^+/K^+ pump inhibition (proton pump inhibitors), inhibition of cell activation (prostaglandins), and receptor blockade (H_2 and muscarinic antagonists).

The remarkable ability of the gastroduodenal mucosa to defend itself against not only acid but also other potentially injurious agents such as pepsin, bile, drugs, and ischemia is described as cytoprotection and entails multiple mechanisms.[27–30] Surface epithelial cells secrete an insoluble water-mucous gel layer and bicarbonate, which prevents hydrogen ions from reaching the epithelial cell. As a result there is a pH gradient across the mucous layer between the gastric lumen and the mucosal cell surface. Further aspects of the cytoprotective ability of the mucosa are the rapid replacement of the injured epithelial cell and the enhancement of blood flow to remove toxic products. Prostaglandins are known to enhance all the aspects of this defense mechanism.[31, 32]

The most common presentation of SRMD is bleeding. Abdominal pain or tenderness is found only in 25% of the cases.[33] The bleeding may manifest as coffee ground or bright red emesis, melena, hematochezia, or a falling hematocrit. The rate and extent of bleeding vary but may be severe enough to require transfusion.

In adults with SRMD significantly higher mortality rates have been reported in bleeding as opposed to nonbleeding patients, 50 to 77% versus 9 to 22%,[34] a finding that suggests that early diagnosis and intervention should be beneficial. Conservative monitoring of NG aspirates for the presence of occult bleeding and increased gastric acid output have not been helpful as a means of early diagnosis. Endoscopy is the gold standard and has been effective in both the bleeding and nonbleeding patient. The diagnosis is readily made because (as opposed to chronic peptic ulceration in which the lesions are single and deep), the erosions of SRMD are multiple and superficial and occur in the acid-producing portions of the stomach.[35] Histologically, the lesions are often not true ulcers, because they do not extend beyond the mucosa.

Since gastric acid is the primary factor in the development of SRMD, its suppression is imperative in the treatment. Maintenance of gastric pH at more than 4.5 is associated with decreased morbidity and mortality.[36, 37] Many agents are available that control acid production (Table 57–5). Antacids are very effective when titrated to maintain gastric pH above 4.0.[38] However, the availability of H_2 antagonists for prophylaxis has revolutionized the treatment of SRMD. They are as effective as antacids, avoid troublesome side effects like diarrhea, and are more convenient to use.[39] In addition, these agents can be used parenterally as well as enterally. Continuous infusion of H_2 antagonists has been proposed to constantly suppress acid; however, there are no data supporting the greater efficacy of this route of administration. Proton pump inhibitors are a new class of drugs that cause profound acid suppression by blocking the H^+/K^+ exchange pump. Intermittent parenteral administration of omeprazole was more effective than continuous infusion of the H_2 antagonist ranitidine.[40] Antimuscarinic agents, such as dicyclomine, are weaker acid suppressors and are reserved for use in the outpa-

Table 57–5. MEDICATIONS USED FOR THE TREATMENT OF STRESS-RELATED MUCOSAL DAMAGE

Drug	Dosage	Mechanism of Action
Antacids	30 ml/1.73m^2 every 1 and 3 hr p.c.*	Acid neutralization Mucosal protection
Cimetidine	40 mg/k/day every 6 hr	Acid suppression by antagonism of the H$_2$ receptor
Ranitidine	2 mg/k/day every 8 hr IV 12 mg/k/day every 8 hr po	
Omeprazole	40–80 mg/day	Acid suppression by inhibition of the H$^+$ pump
Sucralfate	1 g q.i.d.$^+$	Adheres to denuded mucosa preventing back-diffusion of H$^+$ and pepsin Stimulates HCO$_3$ and mucus secretion, and prostaglandin synthesis
Misoprostol	Dosage for children not determined	Acid suppression via parietal cell membrane receptors; decrease gastrin production; mucosal protection
Enprostol		

*p.c. = after meals.
†q.i.d. = four times a day.

tient with chronic acid peptic disease (APD). In addition to acid suppression, therapies aimed at controlling the balance of mucosal defenses and acid production have been proposed. Sucralfate and prostaglandins do not suppress acid production, but they do enhance mucosal defenses. Studies regarding their efficacy in the ICU setting are limited. Current data do not indicate their superiority over H$_2$ antagonists in the treatment of SRMD, but they may be beneficial for prophylaxis.[41]

Rupture of Esophageal Varices

Esophageal varices are due to increased pressure in the portal vein and develop in patients with fibrotic liver disease and cirrhosis, or obstruction in the portal venous system. Ruptured varices are the most common cause of massive upper GI hemorrhage in children, although the bleeding can also be subtle.

The mortality in children is substantial, although less than in adults, in whom one third of patients die with the initial bleeding episode and a further third have a recurrence within 6 months.[42, 43] Because of the potential risk of massive bleeding, much interest has been paid to the grading of varices and to the establishment of criteria to predict a bleed. Varices 5 mm or larger denote high portal venous pressure and are more likely to rupture. A red wale sign, seen on endoscopic inspection, is also ominous. In contrast, the presence of esophagitis does not increase the risk of bleeding.[44, 45]

Endoscopy is most accurate for the diagnosis of varices; however, in the patient who is not actively bleeding, less invasive methods are utilized. Large varices can be detected directly by both barium contrast studies and ultrasonography. An increased ratio of omental thickness to aortic diameter on ultrasound is consistent with the presence of varices.[46, 47]

Prophylactic treatment to prevent bleeding from esophageal varices is difficult to assess because there are no criteria that will predict bleeding in 100% of cases. Sclerotherapy should be reserved for the bleeding patient and should not be used as a preventive measure in a patient who has never bled.[48, 49] Propranolol, which decreases portal venous pressure, has been advo-

cated but its efficacy in the prevention of bleeding is unclear.[50–53] When first studied, propranolol was shown to have a beneficial effect.[50] However, follow-up studies failed to corroborate this finding.

There is much more agreement on the treatment of acute variceal bleeding, and the available methods are shown in Table 57–6. As indicated earlier, conservative measures suffice for most pediatric patients.[43] The patient is stabilized with intravascular fluids, NG lavage, and intravenous vasopressin when necessary. Intravenous resuscitation should not be too vigorous because slight hypotension is well tolerated in the pediatric patient and promotes hemostasis. More aggressive therapy, placement of a Sengstaken-Blakemore tube, or sclerotherapy is needed when bleeding persists or when hypertension develops preventing further use of vasopressin.[54] The Sengstaken-Blakemore tube is virtually obsolete because of the high complication rate associated with its use and the availability of effective sclerotherapy.

Sclerotherapy has its own hazards: fever, chest pain secondary to mediastinitis, ulceration at the site of injection, and increased bleeding. Long-term side effects include the development of esophageal stricture.[43] The approach to rebleeding is also evolving. Portasystemic shunts were virtually replaced by sclerotherapy in the last decade, because injection treatment avoids the risk of encephalopathy and is a simpler procedure. However,

Table 57–6. TREATMENT OF RUPTURED ESOPHAGEAL VARICES

1. **Stabilization of the patient**
   a. Establish good intravenous access
   b. Insert arterial and CVP* lines for close monitoring
   c. Infuse crystalloid and blood products to maintain low normal intravascular volumes (do not overtransfuse)

2. **Cessation of bleeding**
   a. Nasogastric lavage with normal saline until clear
   b. Intravenous vasopressin (4 units/kg/min) until bleeding stops or until side effects noted (hypertension, SIADH†)
   c. Emergency sclerotherapy
   d. Insertion of a Sengstaken-Blakemore tube

*CVP = central venous pressure.
†SIADH = syndrome of inappropriate antidiuretic hormone.

shunts may be more effective in the elective treatment of variceal hemorrhage[55] and certainly deserve consideration in conditions like portal vein thrombosis, congenital hepatic fibrosis, and cystic fibrosis in which encephalopathy is unlikely.

ABDOMINAL PAIN

Severe acute abdominal pain must be regarded as a potential surgical emergency, whereas chronic abdominal pain (even if severe) rarely requires an immediate surgical remedy. The patient in the ICU usually presents with acute signs that are very often difficult to assess because of the patient's level of consciousness and the confounding effects of multiple ongoing therapies. It is therefore important to have a systematic approach to these patients that allows one to be comprehensive in determining the etiology. In addition, one must be cautious not to focus on the abdomen alone without considering the extra-abdominal causes of pain (Table 57–7). A physical examination is frequently the best method of identifying the surgical abdomen. The presence of localized tenderness, guarding, and rebound all indicate peritonitis, which should be considered surgical unless an obvious alternative explanation can be found. Such explanations include primary peritonitis associated with nephrotic syndrome, chronic liver disease, and collagen vascular disorders. In the critically ill patient, who is in coma or paralyzed, a physical examination may not be definitive, and the physician must depend on laboratory tests and imaging. Blood studies are valuable in pancreatitis, metabolic processes, and toxic processes. Abdominal paracentesis can define the origin of the fluid and the presence of infection. Ultrasonography is safe and versatile and is especially suited for the assessment of pancreatic, gallbladder, and renal disease.[56] CT scanning is excellent for retroperitoneal masses and spinal cord processes. Ultimately, when a surgical problem cannot be excluded, exploratory laparotomy is indicated. Surgery must be prompt to reduce morbidity and mortality of an abdominal catastrophe.

Once a surgical abdomen has been ruled out, the patients remaining with persistent abdominal pain may be evaluated more slowly. Functional abdominal pain due to irritable bowel syndrome or nonulcer dyspepsia is not frequently seen in the ICU but is nonetheless the most common cause of abdominal pain in the pediatric population. To avoid an elaborate and unnecessary work-up, a positive diagnosis is made based on the following symptom complexes: In irritable bowel syndrome the pain is vague, poorly localized, crampy, and often relieved by defecation.[57] There is alternating constipation and diarrhea and frequently associated headaches, dizziness, and fatigue.[58] The child's growth and development are normal. Nonulcer dyspepsia identifies a group of children with upper intestinal symptoms, no definite pathology, and a demonstrated response to H_2 antagonists.[59] The differential diagnosis of this condition includes three important causes of upper abdominal pain that may prompt admission to the ICU: APD, pancreatitis, and cholecystitis.

Table 57–7. ETIOLOGIES OF ABDOMINAL PAIN

Intra-abdominal	Extra-abdominal
Retroperitoneal	Pulmonary
Pancreatitis	Pneumonia
Spinal cord disease	Pleural effusion
Renal disease	Diabetes
Tumors	Lead poisoning
Mechanical obstruction	Porphyria
Cholelithiasis/cholecystitis	Epilepsy
Peptic ulcer disease	
Inflammatory bowel disease	
Appendicitis	

Acid Peptic Disease

As opposed to SRMD, which presents with bleeding, APD from other causes usually presents with abdominal pain (Table 57–8). In the ICU setting, APD is either the primary reason for the patient's admission to the hospital or secondary to other illnesses. Common etiologies for APD include drug exposure (in particular, corticosteroids, aspirin, nonsteroidal anti-inflammatory agents [NSAIDs], and chemotherapeutic agents) and peptic ulcer disease (PUD).

The pathogenesis of drug-induced APD may be local, owing to topical contact of the drug with the mucosa, or systemic, as a consequence of prostaglandin synthetase inhibition.[60, 61] The topical lesions are acute and include hemorrhages, erosions, and ulcers of the stomach. The systemic lesions are more chronic and comprise solitary ulcers most often located on the incisura of the gastric antrum.

Gastric acidity has an important role in the pathogenesis of APD, as it does in SRMD.[27, 62] Basal, peak, and maximal acid outputs have been shown to be elevated in at least 50% of patients.[27] High maximal acid outputs have been most often associated with recurrent disease in adults.[63] Reasons for elevated acid output include increases in parietal cell mass, basal secretory drive, and food-stimulated acid secretion. In cases in which acid production is not increased, other factors affecting the mucosal barrier have been suggested. These include hyperpepsinogenemia, and infection with the recently identified bacterium *Helicobacter pylori,* a gram-negative, nonsporulated, microaerophilic, motile bacterium.[64] To survive the acid barrier of the stomach, this bacterium produces a large amount of the enzyme urease, which incorporates the acid in ammonium. This organism is found in 20 to 30% of adults and in 5 to 20% of children and is strongly identified with

Table 57–8. INCIDENCE OF SYMPTOMS IN CHILDREN WITH ACID PEPTIC DISEASE

Symptom	Incidence (%)
Abdominal pain	90
Epigastric	50
Periumbilical	30
Vomiting	40
Hematemesis or melena	50
Occult bleeding	10
Perforation	10

APD.[65-68] *Helicobacter* infection is associated with chronic gastritis in 55% of children, gastric ulcer in 54% of adults, and duodenal ulcer in 60% of adults. It is now believed that treatment of *H. pylori* in patients with PUD significantly reduces the high recurrence rate of 75%.[64, 65]

Age influences the presentation of APD in children. In infants hematemesis and perforation are most common; in the older age groups, 90% have abdominal pain.[27] In half of these children, the pain is localized to the epigastrium and is associated with meals. On examination tenderness is common. It ranges from mild to severe and is often located in the epigastrium; however, it can be diffuse. Other symptoms such as vomiting, hematemesis, and melena occur in a significant number of patients as detailed in Table 57–8.

Upper endoscopy is the definitive test for suspected APD.[69] Visualization of the ulcer crater allows for diagnosis and also enables the endoscopist to establish if bleeding is active or impending. The presence of a visible vessel indicates a poor prognosis and suggests the need for surgery. Immediate endoscopic therapy with electrocoagulation can prevent hemorrhage and can be used to stop an active bleed.[70-72] Endoscopic biopsy is an accurate method for detecting *H. pylori*. Radiologic investigation of the stomach and small intestine using barium has been shown to be diagnostic in only 50 to 89% of cases in which an ulcer was seen by an endoscopist.[69]

The aim of APD therapy is threefold: removal of the offending agent when applicable; suppression of acid production; and re-establishment of normal mucosal defenses when it has been compromised. The agents discussed and listed in Table 57–5 accomplish these aims. These agents may be used singly or in combination. Prophylactic therapy with H_2 antagonists may be instituted for patients at high risk for APD, such as the critically ill patient. Although patients with *H. pylori* respond to H_2 antagonist therapy symptomatically, the probability of a recurrence is high unless the infection is eradicated.[73] Treatment with an antimicrobial agent is therefore necessary. Table 57–9 lists two of the currently recommended regimens for this infection.

Pancreatitis

Pancreatitis in the pediatric population is a rare occurrence, probably because alcohol abuse and biliary tract disease are not common.[74, 75] The etiologies in

Table 57–9. TREATMENT REGIMENS FOR *HELICOBACTER PYLORI*

Study	Treatment
Drumm et al[73]	Bismuth subsalicylate 30 ml q.i.d.* × 6 wk
	Ampicillin 250 mg q.i.d. × 6 wk
Marshall[74]	Colloidal bismuth 1 tablet q.i.d. × 14 days
	Tetracycline 500 mg q.i.d. × 14 days†
	Metronidazole 250 mg q.i.d. × 10 days

*q.i.d. = four times a day.
†Contraindicated for use in children less than 7 years of age.

Table 57–10. ETIOLOGIES OF PANCREATITIS

Infection	Pancreaticobiliary Abnormalities
Bacterial	Bile reflux
Mycoplasma	Pancreas divisum
Leptospirosis	Outflow obstruction
Salmonella typhi	Gallstones
Verocytotoxin-producing	Choledochal cyst
Escherichia coli	Biliary stricture
Viral	**Systemic Diseases**
Hepatitis A and B	Shock/hypovolemia
Mumps	Inflammatory disorders
Coxsackie B	Collagen vascular disease
Influenza A and B	Inflammatory bowel disease
ECHO*	
Varicella	**Miscellaneous**
EBV	Trauma
Rubella	Hereditary
Rubeola	Idiopathic
Parasitic	Hyperlipidemia
Malaria	Cystic fibrosis
Ascariasis	Hyperparathyroidism
Clinorchis sinensis	

Drugs
Corticosteroids
Chemotherapeutic agents
  6-Mercaptopurine
  L-Asparaginase
Diuretics
  Chlorothiazides
  Furosemide
Antibiotics
  Tetracycline
  Sulfonamides
  Metronidazole
Anticonvulsants
  Valproic acid
Analgesics
  Acetaminophen
  NSAIDs†

*ECHO = enteric cytopathogenic human orphan virus.
†NSAIDs = nonsteroidal anti-inflammatory drugs.

children are more diverse (Table 57–10) and commonly include infection, trauma, drug reaction, and congenital anomalies of the pancreaticobiliary tree.[75] In a study of 61 patients with pancreatitis,[76] Weizman and associates found that 35% of the patients had multisystem disease. Pancreatitis occurred as part of the disease process or as a result of its therapy.

Pancreatitis is the result of autodigestion of pancreatic tissue by activated proteolytic enzymes in the parenchyma.[75, 77] The trigger for this inappropriate release of enzymes has not been fully elucidated for many of the causes listed. Under normal conditions, pancreatic enzymes, except for amylase and lipase, are stored in their inactive forms in zymogen granules. The pancreas is protected from their premature activation by protease inhibitors in the pancreatic tissue and in the circulation. Protease activation occurs in response to a meal and involves a cascade of events. First, trypsinogen is activated to trypsin by intestinal enterokinase or by trypsin itself. Trypsin then activates the remaining enzymes: chymotrypsinogen, proelastase, procarboxypeptidase, procolipase, and prophospholipase. Under aberrant conditions, the activated enzymes are released into pancreatic tissue, and edema, necrosis, and hemorrhage occur.[74] In response to the localized reaction, systemic

Table 57–11. EXTRAPANCREATIC COMPLICATIONS OF PANCREATITIS

Peripancreatic	Systemic
Splenic vein thrombosis	Shock
Splenic vein infarction	Cardiac failure
Retroperitoneal abscess	Respiratory distress
Peritonitis	Renal failure
Intestinal necrosis	Vascular damage
Ascites	
Fat necrosis	
Bleeding	

Table 57–12. CONSERVATIVE MEASURES FOR THE TREATMENT OF PANCREATITIS

General
1. Maintenance of adequate hydration by fluid replacement
   a. Colloid bolus for hypovolemia and shock
   b. Blood replacement for hemorrhage
2. Electrolyte and mineral replacement
3. Intravenous hyperalimentation

Specific
1. Nothing by mouth
2. Continuous nasogastric suctioning
3. Antacid or H_2 antagonist therapy

complications follow.[75] They include inflammation in surrounding tissues as well as more generalized system failures (Table 57–11).

Abdominal pain is the cardinal symptom of acute pancreatitis. It is most often located in the epigastrium and right upper quadrant with radiation to the back. However, in a small number of patients, diffuse abdominal pain is described, and in others no pain occurs at all.[76] Vomiting, which may be bilious, is a frequent complaint. It occurs in two thirds of patients. On physical examination, epigastric tenderness and decreased or absent bowel sounds are common. Guarding of the upper abdomen, rebound, abdominal distention, and ascites can also be present. In the unconscious patient, abdominal distention, decreased bowel sounds, and laboratory studies indicative of pancreatitis may be all that are available for the physician to make the diagnosis.

Although an elevated serum amylase is considered the hallmark of pancreatitis, the differential diagnosis also includes renal failure, biliary tract disease, intestinal problems, and macroamylasemia. Confirmatory tests are, therefore, important. The urine amylase/creatinine ratio is no longer considered reliable. Serum lipase and serum cationic trypsinogen are more dependable but are usually not immediately available.[76] Imaging techniques, in particular ultrasonography, are most helpful; not only do these techniques confirm the presence of pancreatitis in most cases, but they also identify etiologies of the disease (e.g., gallstones) and complications (e.g., pseudocyst formation).[78, 79] CT scanning is utilized in cases in which ultrasonography is not definitive or when a pancreatic tumor is suspected.

Endoscopic investigation of the patient with pancreatitis may be useful to define peptic ulceration or ampullary abnormalities that may lead to pancreatitis. Endoscopic retrograde cholangiopancreatography (ERCP), performed most frequently in the adult population, is a valuable test to assess patients with recurrent or chronic pancreatitis[80] or to relieve obstruction in the biliary tree caused by gallstones in the acute setting. With the development of smaller instruments, this test becomes a safe and practical consideration in the child with pancreatitis and has added a great deal to assessing the patient with persistent disease. Identification of ductal abnormalities as well as presurgical evaluation of pseudocysts are two of the primary conditions that can be delineated by ERCP.

Although most physicians agree based on experience that treatment of pancreatitis is beneficial, this has not been proved by clinical trials. The proposed objective of therapy is to arrest the autodigestive process. This is accomplished in two ways: first, elimination of the cause of the inflammatory process such as treatment of infection, removal of the insulting drug, or correction of the structural abnormality; and second, implementation of measures that allow the pancreas to be placed at rest. Table 57–12 lists the measures that help to accomplish the second goal. In theory, agents that decrease pancreatic stimulation should be beneficial. However, agents such as anticholinergics, glucagon, somatostatin, vasopressin, and protease inhibitors have performed poorly and have for the most part been discarded.[75]

The outcome of acute pancreatitis depends on the severity of the inflammation and on the presence of an underlying condition. In the adult population, morbidity is high primarily as a result of the significant degree of alcoholism in these patients. In children, data are scant. In Weizman's study of 61 children, 13 had a fatal outcome.[76] In all cases, multisystem disease was present. Poor prognostic indicators have been developed in adults, and these apply to the pediatric population as well (Table 57–13). They include hypocalcemia, hyperglycemia, elevated hemoglobin, hematocrit, and urea nitrogen. In the face of these, admission to the ICU for closer monitoring is recommended. These patients constitute the group that may ultimately require pancreatectomy as a last resort. For patients who recover from an acute episode of pancreatitis, only a small percentage go on to develop recurrent problems.

Cholecystitis

Ninety per cent of adult patients with gallbladder disease have cholelithiasis[81] compared with the pediatric

Table 57–13. POOR PROGNOSTIC INDICATORS FOR PANCREATITIS

Clinical Indicators	Laboratory Indicators
Coma	Hyperglycemia
Hypotension	Hypocalcemia
Renal failure	Anemia
Pulmonary edema	Leukocytosis
Shock	Azotemia
Hemorrhage	Hypoxemia
	Hypoalbuminemia

population in which acalculous cholecystitis is more common.[81, 82] The acalculous cholecystitis can be caused by childhood infections, particularly viral gastroenteritis, but also by salmonella, shigella, *E. coli,* and streptococci. Other causes include opiate administration, total parenteral nutrition, trauma, surgery, burns, and vascular or metabolic diseases.[82] The initial event in the pathogenesis of cholecystitis is believed to be inflammation and obstruction of the cystic duct. This inflammatory response can result from a spasm of the sphincter of Oddi with reflux of infected pancreatic secretions into the bile duct[83]; increased prostaglandin synthesis secondary to lysolecithin production from phospholipase A[84–86]; and release of chemical mediators by distention, ischemia, or infection. An obstructed duct is followed by gallbladder mucosal inflammation with the threat of necrosis and perforation.

The cardinal features of cholecystitis include fever, right upper quadrant tenderness, and jaundice.[81] Leukocytosis and elevated serum transaminases are usually present. Initially, it may be difficult to distinguish this condition from pancreatitis. The diagnosis of acalculous cholecystitis is confirmed with ultrasonography or by cholescintigraphy. Distention of the gallbladder with evidence of intraluminal sludge, mural thickening, and subserosal edema (halo sign) in the absence of gallstones is noted.[81] The gallbladder does not visualize with cholescintigraphy.[87] The treatment of choice for acute cholecystitis is cholecystectomy if surgery is feasible, and the surgical risk may be decreased with laparoscopic cholecystectomy.[88, 89] However, currently the laparoscopic approach is recommended only for patients with symptomatic cholelithiasis without cholecystitis. As experience with this procedure increases and indications are broadened, it may offer an alternative for the patient in the ICU who is a poor surgical risk.

DIARRHEA

Diarrhea is the most frequent manifestation of intestinal failure, and it is an important cause of death in young children. However, as patients who receive simple rehydrating solutions have an excellent prognosis, there is little reason to admit them to an ICU. In this setting, diarrhea is almost invariably a secondary or intercurrent event. The incidence for a pediatric ICU has not been documented, but the adult experience suggests that it is not rare. Kelly found that 41% of adult patients developed diarrhea at approximately 7 days after entry into the ICU.[90]

Pathophysiology

The intestine handles more fluids than the amount taken orally might suggest. In 1 day, an adult drinks 2 liters; 7 more liters are added by salivary, pancreatic, biliary, and intestinal secretions. The small intestine reduces this 9-liter load to 1 liter, which the colon converts to 0.15 liter of stool. The colon has a reserve capacity for a further 3 liters and therefore only when

small intestinal function is reduced beyond 40% is there a marked increase in stool volume. Under normal circumstances on a per-kilogram basis, the child's small bowel absorbs twice that of an adult and presents two to three times more fluid (60 ml/kg versus 25 ml/kg) to the colon. Therefore there is little colonic reserve, and a reduction in small intestinal function by even 10% causes conspicuous diarrhea.[90, 91] The proximal intestine absorbs the bulk of Na^+, K^+, Cl^-, HCO_3^-, carbohydrates (CHO), amino acids, vitamins, and trace elements, and in the distal ileum there are highly efficient Na^+/H^+ and Cl^-/HCO_3^- exchange mechanisms to assimilate residual sodium, chloride, and water. In addition, there is a critical sodium-coupled bile salt absorption mechanism and a receptor-mediated B_{12} uptake process. The colon salvages residual Na^+, Cl^-, H_2O and considerable quantities of unabsorbed carbohydrates. Bacterial fermentation converts the sugars to short-chain fatty acids (SCFA) that stimulate Na^+ and water absorption.[93]

The *Na^+-K^+ ATPase pump* at the basolateral border of the enterocyte facilitates both absorption and secretion by decreasing intracellular sodium concentration[94] (see also Chapter 4). Na^+ is drawn into the enterocyte from the bowel lumen, and Cl^- is driven from the cell by electrochemical forces. The energy for the pump is derived primarily from glutamine (75%), acetoacetate, betahydroxyacetate, SCFA, and to a lesser degree glucose. *Na^+ absorption* is rate limited at the enterocyte brush border, but at least three mechanisms are available to facilitate its uptake: (1) a sodium conductance channel under the influence of steroids that is mainly located in the ileum and colon; (2) a Na^+/Cl^- electroneutral entry point under the influence of the intracellular "second messengers," notably adenylate and guanylate cyclase and Ca^{2+} ions; and (3) nutrient enhanced Na^+ entry stimulated by glucose and various amino acids. *Chloride secretion* occurs because the "second messengers" induce phosphorylation of the membrane proteins that open brush border chloride channels.[92, 95, 96]

Electrolyte transport is regulated by three systems: (1) The enteric nervous system that includes extrinsic nerves of the ANS, Auerbach and Meissner plexus, and mucosal endocrine cells. Many peptides of the system including acetylcholine, serotonin, and vasoactive intestinal polypeptide (VIP) mediate a secretory action, and somatomedin mediates powerful inhibition of the secretory flux. (2) The endocrine system that acts via glucocorticoids and mineralocorticoids. (3) The immune system that releases—from macrophages, neutrophils, eosinophils, and mast cells—prostaglandins, leukotrienes, platelet-activating factor, and reactive oxygen species.[97–99]

Malabsorption of water causes diarrhea and, as the movement of water is passive and osmotically driven, diarrhea implies a breakdown in the absorption or active secretion of solutes.

Diarrhea results from a relative increase in intestinal luminal osmolality, diminished mucosal absorptive capacity, altered motility, active anion secretion, and usually a combination of more than one of these mechanisms. The addition to the diet of nonabsorbed ingredients such as magnesium sulfate or sorbitol, failure of digestion of osmotically active molecules like lactose and sucrose, or poor absorption of the products of digestion, which occurs with mucosal injury, all cause an *osmotic diarrhea*.[100] The tendency toward secretion may also be enhanced by hypoalbuminemia, which frequently complicates the course of the patient under stress.[101]

A prototype of *mucosal injury* resulting in diarrhea is viral enteritis. The virus invades and destroys the mature enterocytes, which are rapidly replaced by crypt-like cells. These cells lack surface area and brush border transport systems and have low levels of Na^+/K^+-ATPase activity. Therefore, in the involved intestinal segment nutrient, sodium and water absorption is suboptimal and there is no enhancement of sodium and water uptake in the presence of glucose and amino acids.[102] An affected infant under 6 months of age who becomes malnourished is likely to develop a persistent monosaccharide malabsorption.[103] Enterotoxigenic diarrhea as exemplified by cholera is the prototype of *secretory diarrhea*. The extrinsic toxin, which acts as the "first messenger," induces the production of the intrinsic "second messenger," which strongly induces the Cl^-

secretory pathway. Mucosal structure and absorption are intact, and this allows for glucose stimulated Na^+ transport, which is a factor that is the basis for oral rehydrating solutions.[104]

Etiology

The mechanisms underlying the production of diarrhea can be used to develop a systematic approach to diarrhea as indicated in Table 57–14. The incidence of these conditions has not been well documented in a pediatric ICU, but the adult experience shows that pharmaceutical agents, enteral feedings, and possibly hypoalbuminemia are important causes. Up to 10% of patients taking *antibiotics* develop severe diarrhea, and the effect is usually not related to the presence of *Clostridium difficile* toxin. Diarrhea may result because antibiotics eliminate the colonic flora that produce the SCFAs needed to enhance colonic sodium assimilation. *Antacids*, especially those containing magnesium hydroxide, are commonly used in the ICU and cause osmotic diarrhea. H_2 *blockers* may cause diarrhea by allowing bacterial overgrowth in the stomach and small

---

Table 57–14. ETIOLOGY OF DIARRHEA—A MECHANISTIC CLASSIFICATION

Absorptive Defect	**Secretory Defects (Classified according to the mediating chemical)**

1. Selective malabsorption: osmotic type diarrhea with mucosal structure preserved (e.g., magnesium hydroxide ingestion)
    Adult onset lactose intolerance
2. Generalized malabsorption: (often associated with villous atrophy and crypt hyperplasia)
    Infectious agents
        Viruses
            Rotavirus
            Adenovirus
            CMV
        Bacteria
            Enteroadhesive *Escherichia coli*
            Salmonella
            Yersinia enterocolitica
            Campylobacter jejuni
        Parasites
            Giardia lamblia
            Strongyloides
        Fungi
            Cryptosporidia
    Food intolerance
        Celiac disease
        Cow's milk, soy, and egg protein allergy
    Immune related
        Crohn disease
        Autoimmune enteropathy
        Eosinophilic enteropathy
    Nutritional defects
        Kwashiorkor
        Congenital folate and B_{12} deficiency
        Acrodermatitis enteropathica (zinc deficiency)
    Drugs
        Chemotherapeutic agents (e.g., cytosine arabinoside, methotrexate)
        Ipecac
        Neomycin
        Para-amino salicylic acid
    Short bowel syndrome
    Irradiation
    Ischemia
	1. VIP
	        Endocrine tumors
	        Ganglioneuroma and neuroblastoma
	        Non-β cell islet neoplasia
	2. Bile salts
	        Ileal resection
	        Congenital malabsorption
	3. Long-chain fatty acids: (The cause of diarrhea in steatorrhea; the diarrhea stops when feeding is withdrawn.)
	        Lack of pancreatic secretions
	            Cystic fibrosis
	            Shwachman syndrome
	        Inadequate bile salt concentrations
	            Cholestasis
	        Mucosal injury
	            Celiac disease
	            Lymphangiectasia
	            Abetalipoproteinemia
	4. Bacterial enterotoxins
	        Via adenylate cyclase (AMP)
	        Cholera toxina
	            Heat-labile *Escherichia coli*
	            Salmonella
	            Campylobacter jejuni
	            Pseudomonas aeruginosa
	            Shigella
	        Via guanylate-cyclase (GMP)
	            Heat-stable *Escherichia coli*
	            Yersinia enterocoliticae
	            Klebsiella pneumoniae
	5. Laxative agents
	        Ricinoleic acid
	        Bisacodyl
	        Dioctyl sodium sulfosuccinate

intestine. A host of other drugs cause diarrhea including *flucytosine*, the antifungal agent that is associated with the development of ulcerative enteritis as well as strictures and perforation of the bowel; *chemotherapeutic agents* that induce necrotizing enteritis when neutropenia develops; and medications important in *cardiopulmonary support* such as digoxin and antihypertensive and antiarrhythmic agents.[90, 105, 107]

The role of *enteral feeding* as a cause of diarrhea is debated. Early claims that lactose-containing formulations frequently cause diarrhea probably exaggerate the present role of these formulas because they have been modified, are infused progressively in terms of concentration and volume, and are delivered in a closed sterile system. They are more likely to cause diarrhea if there is underlying mucosal damage, and mucosal atrophy is likely to evolve if the patient is not given food enterally over a protracted period. Hypertonic solutions in the face of mucosal injury may cause osmotic diarrhea, but this is not a consistent finding. Often no obvious explanation for the diarrhea is evident.[107, 108] One possibility is that hypoalbuminemia, which commonly complicates the course of a severe illness resulting in a catabolic state, in combination with various mediators of inflammation allows for protein-rich fluid to accumulate in the interstitium resulting in an alteration in mucosal permeability and a protein-losing enteropathy.[101]

The growing population of patients who are *immune compromised* by diseases like acquired immunodeficiency syndrome (AIDS) or are receiving immunosuppressing medications has made infection an important cause of diarrhea in the ICU. As a result, other than commonly anticipated infections like *Clostridium difficile*, organisms that generally are not suspected such as *Mycobacterium avium intracellulare* (MAI), *Cytomegalovirus* (CMV), and *Cryptosporidia* must be sought.[109] Furthermore, a large proportion of immunocompromised patients have diarrhea caused by pathogens amenable to treatment, pathogens that can be identified by routine stool evaluation and, when necessary, endoscopy as indicated in Table 57–15.[110]

Diagnostic Evaluation

Most diarrheal illnesses are acute intercurrent events that require a search for a removable or reversible cause. In the ICU, this entails a careful review of orally administered nutrients and medications and a search for potential infections. The passage of liquid stools that are *heme negative* should prompt a consideration of osmotic causes of diarrhea or small bowel injury as seen with *Rotavirus* or *Giardia*. These patients are likely to have carbohydrate malabsorption that can be readily detected by screening the stools for an *acid pH* and the presence of *reducing substances*. A more definitive diagnosis is made with hydrogen breath testing. To find reducing substances, fresh stool must be promptly tested because stool in the diaper ferments rapidly. A Clinitest tablet is added to ten drops of water plus five drops of liquid stool, and anything more than a trace indicates excessive losses. A more definitive diagnosis is made

Table 57–15. PROCEDURES TO IDENTIFY INFECTIOUS ORGANISMS

Stool Examination
1. Culture for routine bacterial pathogens: *Campylobacter*, *Shigella*, *Salmonella*, and *Yersinia*.
2. Assay for *Clostridium difficile* cytotoxin.
3. Examine three fresh stool and concentrated specimen for ova and parasites.
4. Do an acid-fast stain for *Cryptosporidium*, *Mycobacterium avium* (MAI) complex, and *Isospora belli*.
5. Enzyme-linked immunosorbent assay (ELISA) for viral antigens of rotavirus and adenovirus.

Endoscopic Examination
1. Tissue inspection for inflammation, ulcers, nodules, and pseudomembranes
2. Biopsy culture—Colon: cytomegalovirus (CMV), MAI, adenovirus, and herpes simplex
   —Duodenum: CMV, MAC, and bacteria
3. Biopsy histology—Hematoxylin-eosin: CMV, adenovirus, *Cryptosporidia*, and *Isospora*
   —Giemsa: *Giardia*
   —Methenamine silver: Fungi
   —Acid-fast or Fite: *Cryptosporidium*, *Isospora*, MAC
   —Electron microscopy: *Microsporidia*, adenovirus
4. Duodenal fluid—Culture for bacteria
   —Examine for ova and parasites

Hydrogen Breath Testing
1. Carbohydrate malabsorption
2. Bacterial overgrowth

with hydrogen breath testing. The presence of *blood and polymorphonuclear cells* warrants consideration of bacterial pathogens and *Clostridium difficile* toxin—causes of a colitis that may be promptly identified by sigmoidoscopy.

Treatment

The major sequelae of prolonged diarrhea are dehydration, malnutrition, and discomfort. The primary goal of therapy is therefore to restore and limit further fluid losses, encourage nutritional intake, and deal with symptoms like abdominal pain. Supportive measures are particularly relevant in acute self-limiting diarrheal illness but are also important in chronic diarrhea when a specific diagnosis cannot be made or when specific treatment is not available.

Oral fluids should include electrolytes and glucose or glucose polymers but not the sorbitol, fructose, fructose corn solids, and caffeine that are found in many sodas. *Bulk-forming agents* such as kaolin and pectin, attapulgite, methylcellulose, and psyllium are worthy only of a trial in mild diarrhea. *Bismuth subsalicylate* has both antimicrobial and antisecretory effects and is effective in traveler's diarrhea but less so in chronic diarrhea and the immunocompromised patient. The chronic use of salicylate can cause toxicity, and levels should be monitored. *Cholestyramine*, a chelating agent capable of binding various salts and toxins, is most useful for the secretory diarrhea caused by bile salts entering the colon and is also helpful in enterotoxigenic diarrheas. *Antimotility agents* are helpful in chronic diarrhea without a treatable cause. They are not advised for patients with bloody diarrhea for fear that they will diminish the clearance of infectious agents and therefore exacerbate or aggravate the illness. In patients with ulcerative colitis, they can precipitate toxic megacolon. The preferred drug is loperamide hydrochloride (Imodium), which has an antimotility effect and also blocks the calcium channels that mediate secretion. It is preferred to the alternative phenoxylate hydrochloride (Lomotil), which has anticholinergic effects. Patients who use opiate-based agents like paregoric frequently develop tolerance to their effect. *Somatostatin* is finding a role for the reversal of diarrhea caused by vasoactive intestinal peptide (VIP)-secreting tumors, but its antisecretory effect has been used in a wide variety of situations. Unfortunately, its use is limited by the need to give it by injection.

Nutritional measures are consequential because malnutrition frequently complicates chronic diarrhea and is itself an important cause of diarrhea. Because enteral nutrition is safer, cheaper and circumvents villous atrophy, it is preferred. A simple diet containing complex carbohydrates like rice and avoiding lactose and possibly gluten is more readily accepted. NG or G tube feeding that allows continuous administration of a defined diet is likely to be best tolerated. Semi-elemental formulations only have a limited place; they are indicated for the management of pancreatic insufficiency and protein sensitivity. It is suggested that they may have positive effects in patients with hypoalbuminemia and short bowel syndrome but controlled trials are still needed to confirm these findings. Severe diarrhea can preclude reliance on enteral infusions to support nutrition, but even under these circumstances a limited volume of nutrients should be introduced enterally for their trophic effect on the intestine.[111]

Treatment of Specific Pathogens in the Immunocompromised Host

The treatment of specific organisms in healthy individuals has been standardized. For the immunocompromised patient, this therapy is still evolving.[112]

Bacterial Infections. Organisms like *Shigella* and *Campylobacter* that usually cause a benign illness will in immunocompromised individuals result in prolonged and relapsing diarrhea. Shigella, which is normally confined to the mucosa, becomes a cause of bacteremia.[113–115] Antibiotics are therefore commonly used, preferably once sensitivities are determined. For *Salmonella* species amoxicillin is used, and in resistant cases ciprofloxacin or chloramphenicol is administered. Trimethoprim sulfamethoxazole is reserved for *Pneumocystis carinii*. Resistance to erythromycin and tetracyclines is common; in *Campylobacter* infection, good alternatives are ciprofloxacin and norfloxacin. For *Shigella*, ampicillin is preferred but again in resistant cases ciprofloxacin or nor-floxacin are used. *Clostridium difficile* may be more prevalent than appreciated in immunocompromised hosts because it is acquired in hospitals. It affects patients needing antibiotics, and the cytotoxin is detected in only 65 to 70% of the patients

tested. It is therefore important to also culture for the organism; it can be identified in 95% of infected patients who test negative for the toxin. Vancomycin, metronidazole, and bacitracin are all effective, but a 15% relapse rate is anticipated.[116, 117] *MAI* causes weight loss, fever, and often diarrhea. There is a minimum inflammatory reaction, but macrophages contain large numbers of the organisms. Combinations of amikacin, ethambutol, rifampin, ciprofloxacin, rifabutin, clofazamine, and isoniazid have been tried, but the efficacy of the treatment is not well established.[118–120]

Viral Infections. *CMV* can infect any part of the intestinal mucosa to cause esophagitis, gastritis, enteritis, or colitis. In addition, acalculous cholecystitis, sclerosing cholangitis, and pancreatitis are described.[121] *Herpes simplex* causes perianal ulcerations, proctitis, and esophagitis. Gancyclovir is used to treat CMV and acyclovir for herpes, but resistant forms of both viruses are described.[121–124] *Adenovirus*, an important cause of enteritis in children, involves the colon of patients with AIDS, resulting in a chronic, watery, nonbloody, nonmucoid diarrhea. To date no specific treatment is available.

The treatment of *Cryptosporidium* is difficult. Experience with spiromycin is disappointing.[125] The success reported with efluornithine and bovine transfer factor is more promising.[126, 127] Patients with hypogammaglobulinemia are most likely to have protracted symptoms from *Giardia lamblia*, but the parasite is also common in normal children. Asymptomatic patients should not be treated, and metronidazole is very effective for those with diarrhea. *Entamoeba histolytica* is rare in the United States, but it occurs among patients with AIDS in U.S. institutions. Fortunately, most cases are mild and amenable to treatment with metronidazole. *Isospora belli* can also cause symptoms in patients with AIDS, and it responds to treatment with TMP-SMX. An alternative choice is sulfadoxine with pyrimethamine. The role of *Blastocystis hominis* in the pathogenesis of diarrhea is controversial, but at least in the immunocompromised patient it should be treated. The obligate intracellular protozoan *Microsporidium* causes AIDS enteropathy, but unfortunately there is no known treatment available.[128]

Fungal Infections. *Candida albicans*, the cause of thrush is, in the immunocompromised patient, an important cause of esophagitis, dysphagia, and inanition. When the unpleasant taste of nystatin reduces compliance, treatment with clotrimazole troches can be helpful. An alternative is ketoconazole, but it requires an acid pH for absorption (it cannot be used if gastric acid is being neutralized), and its complications include vomiting, hepatotoxicity, and hypersensitivity. Fluconizole is not dependent on an acid pH for absorption, it has a longer half-life than ketoconazole and a higher cure rate. Patients with neutropenia are especially susceptible to fungemia, and they require treatment with amphotericin.[129] *Histoplasma capsulatum* is increasingly recognized as an opportunistic infection that in immunocompromised patients causes GI symptoms including diarrhea. Most of these patients have colitis that is identified on proctoscopy. Treatment with amphotericin is successful.[130]

References

1. Nadrowski L: Paralytic ileus: Recent advances in pathophysiology and treatment. Curr Surg 40:260, 1983.
2. Scott B: Motility disorders. *In:* Walker WA, Durie PR, Hamilton JR, et al (eds): Pediatric Gastrointestinal Disease, 1st ed. Philadelphia, BC Decker, 1991, pp. 784–799.
3. Furness JB and Costa M: Adynamic ileus: Its pathogenesis and treatment. Med Biol 52:82, 1974.
4. Woods JH, Erikson LF, Condon RE, et al: Post-operative ileus: A colonic problem? Surgery 80:527, 1978.
5. Heimbach DM and Crout JR: Treatment of paralytic ileus with adrenergic neuronal blocking drugs. Surgery 69:582, 1971.
6. Ogilvie H: Large intestine colic due to sympathetic deprivation. Br Med J 2:671, 1948.
7. Lee JB: The prostaglandins. *In:* Williams RH (ed): Textbook of Endocrinology, 5th ed. Philadelphia, WB Saunders, 1974, pp. 854–868.
8. Franken EA, Smith WL, and Smith JA: Paralysis of the small bowel resembling mechanical intestinal obstruction. Gastrointest Radiol 5:161, 1980.
9. Canton MO: Ileus. Am J Gastroenterol 47:461, 1967.
10. Schuffler MD: Chronic intestinal pseudo-obstruction syndromes. Med Clin North Am 65:1331, 1981.
11. Davidson ED, Hersh T, Brinner RA, et al: The effects of metoclopramide on postoperative ileus. Ann Surg 190:27, 1979.
12. Spino M: Pharmacologic treatment of gastrointestinal motility. *In:* Walker WA, Durie PR, Hamilton JR, et al (eds): Pediatric Gastrointestinal Disease, 1st ed. Philadelphia, BC Decker, 1991, pp. 1741–1742.
13. Camilleri M, Brown ML, and Malagalada JR: Impaired transit of chyme in chronic intestinal pseudo-obstruction: Correction by cisapride. Gastroenterology 91:619, 1986.
14. Aynsley-Green A: Endocrine function of the gut in early life. *In:* Walker WA, Durie PR, Hamilton JR, et al (eds): Pediatric Gastrointestinal Disease, 1st ed. Philadelphia, BC Decker, 1991, p. 251.
15. Silverman A and Roy CC: Pediatric Clinical Gastroenterology, 3rd ed. St. Louis, CV Mosby, 1983, pp. 181–185.
16. Savino JA, Berman HL, and Del Guercio LRM: A multidisciplinary approach to gastrointestinal bleeding. *In:* Shoemaker WC, Ayres S, Grenvik A, et al (eds): Textbook of Critical Care, 2nd ed. Philadelphia, WB Saunders, 1989, pp. 703–710.
17. Hyams JS, Leichtner AM, and Schwartz AN: Recent advances in diagnosis and treatment of gastrointestinal hemorrhage in infants and children. J Pediatr 106:1, 1985.
18. Luk GD, Bynum TE, and Hendrin TR: Gastric aspiration in localization of gastrointestinal hemorrhage. JAMA 241:576, 1979.
19. Ponsky JL, Hoffman M, and Swayngim DS: Saline irrigation in gastric hemorrhage: The effect of temperature. J Surg Res 28:204, 1980.
20. Markisz JA, Front D, Royal HD, et al: An evaluation of ^{99m}Tc-labeled red blood cell scintigraphy for the detection and localization of gastrointestinal bleeding sites. Gastroenterology 83:394, 1982.
21. Lucas CE, Sugawa C, Riddle J, et al: Natural history and surgical dilemma of "stress" gastric bleeding. Arch Surg 102:266, 1971.
22. Schuster DP, Robley H, Feinstein S, et al: Prospective evaluation of the risk of upper gastrointestinal bleeding admission to a medical intensive care unit. Am J Med 76:623, 1984.
23. Silen W, Merhav A, and Simonson JNL: The pathophysiology of stress ulcer disease. World J Surg 116:597, 1981.
24. Berglindh T and Soll AH: Physiology of isolated gastric glands and parietal cells: Receptors and effectors regulating function. *In:* Johnson LR, Christensen J, Jackson MJ, et al (eds): Physiology of the Gastrointestinal Tract, 2nd ed. New York, Raven Press, 1987, pp. 883–909.
25. Soll AH: Gastric mucosal receptors. *In:* Schultz SG, Makhlouf GM, and Rauner BB (eds): Handbook of Physiology. Section 6: The Gastrointestinal System. Bethesda, American Physiological Society, 1989, pp. 193–214.
26. Soll AH: Treatment strategies for peptic diseases. Presented at the American Gastroenterological Association 1991 Postgraduate Course. Pharmacology and Therapy of Digestive Diseases.
27. Eastham EJ: Peptic ulcer. *In:* Walker WA, Durie PR, Hamilton JR, et al (eds): Pediatric Gastrointestinal Disease, 1st ed. Philadelphia, BC Decker, 1991, pp. 438–451.
28. Silen W: What is cytoprotection of the gastric mucosa? Gastroenterology 94:232, 1988.
29. Oates PJ and Hakkinen JP: Studies on the mechanism of ethanol-induced gastric damage in rats. Gastroenterology 94:10, 1988.
30. Wallace JL: Increased resistance of the rat gastric mucosa to hemorrhagic damage after exposure to an irritant. Gastroenterology 94:22, 1988.
31. Kessler KM: Peptic ulcer disease, cytoprotection, and prostaglandins. Arch Intern Med 148:2112, 1988.
32. Miller T: Protective effects of prostaglandins against gastric mucosal damage: Current knowledge and proposed mechanisms. Am J Physiol 245:601, 1983.
33. Czaja AJ, McAlhany JC, and Pruitt BA: Acute gastroduodenal disease after thermal injury: An endoscopic evaluation of incidence and natural history. N Engl J Med 291:925, 1974.
34. Vorder Bruegge WF and Peura DA: Stress-related mucosal damage: Review of drug therapy. J Clin Gastroenterol 12(Suppl. 2):S35, 1990.
35. Peura DA: Stress and drug-induced ulcer disease. Presented at the American Gastroenterological Association 1991 Postgraduate Course. Pharmacology and Therapy of Digestive Diseases.
36. Silen W: Stress ulcers. Viewpoints Dig Dis 3:5, 1971.
37. Curtis LF, Simonian S, Buerck CA, et al: Evaluation of the effectiveness of controlled pH in management of massive upper gastrointestinal bleeding. Am J Surg 125:474, 1973.
38. Hastings PR, Skillman JJ, Bushnell LS, et al: Antacid titration in the prevention of acute gastrointestinal bleeding. N Engl J Med 298:1041, 1978.
39. Peura DA and Johnson LF: Cimetidine for prevention and treatment of gastroduodenal mucosal lesions in patients in an intensive care unit. Ann Intern Med 103:173, 1985.
40. Brunner G and Chang J: Intravenous therapy with high doses of ranitidine and omeprazole in critically ill patients with bleeding peptic ulcerations of the upper intestinal tract: An open randomized controlled trial. Digestion 45:217, 1990.
41. Peura DA: Prophylactic therapy of stress-related mucosal damage: Why, which, who and so what? Am J Gastroenterol 85:935, 1990.
42. Koransky JR, Galambos JT, Hersh T, et al: The mortality of bleeding esophageal varices in a private university hospital. Am J Surg 136:339, 1978.
43. Graham DY and Smith JL: The course of patients after variceal hemorrhage. Gastroenterology 80:800, 1981.
44. Lebrec D, Defleury P, Rueff B, et al: Portal hypertension, size of esophageal varices, and risk of gastrointestinal bleeding in alcoholic cirrhosis. Gastroenterology 79:1139, 1980.
45. Eckardt VF and Grace ND: Gastroesophageal reflux and bleeding esophageal varices. Gastroenterology 76:39, 1979.
46. De Giacomo C, Tomasi G, Gatti C, et al: Ultrasonographic prediction of the presence and severity of esophageal varices in children. J Pediatr Gastroenterol Nutr 9:431, 1989.
47. Rabinowitz SS, Norton KI, Benkov KJ, et al: Sonographic evaluation of portal hypertension in children. J Pediatr Gastroenterol Nutr 10:395, 1990.
48. Piai G, Cipolletta L, Claar M, et al: Prophylactic sclerotherapy of high-risk esophageal varices: Results of a multicentric prospective controlled trial. Hepatology 8:1495, 1988.
49. Triger DR, Smart HL, Hosking SW, et al: Prophylactic sclerotherapy for esophageal varices: long-term results of a single-center trial. Hepatology 13:117, 1991.
50. Lebrec D, Poynard T, Bernon J, et al: A randomized controlled study of propranolol for prevention of recurrent gastrointestinal bleeding in patients with cirrhosis: A final report. Hepatology 4:355, 1984.
51. Burroughs A, Jenkins W, Sherlock S, et al: Controlled trial propranolol for the prevention of recurrent variceal hemorrhage patients with cirrhosis. N Engl J Med 309:1539, 1983.
52. Villeneuve JP, Pomier-Layrargues G, Infante-Rivard C, et al: Propranolol for the prevention of recurrent variceal hemorrhage controlled trial. Hepatology 6:1239, 1986.
53. Colombo M, De Franchis R, Tommasini M, et al: β-Blockade prevents recurrent gastrointestinal bleeding in well-compensated patients with alcoholic cirrhosis: A multicenter randomized controlled trial. Hepatology 9:433, 1989.

54. Rikkers LF: Bleeding esophageal varices. Surg Clin North Am 67:475, 1987.
55. Planas R, Boix J, et al: Portacaval shunt versus endoscopic sclerotherapy in the elective treatment of variceal hemorrhage. Gastroenterology 100:1078–1086, 1991.
56. Stringer DA: Pediatric Gastrointestinal Tract Imaging. Philadelphia, BC Decker, 1989.
57. Apley J and Nash N: Recurrent abdominal pains: A field survey of 1000 school children. Arch Dis Child 33:165, 1958.
58. Oster J: Recurrent abdominal pain, headache and limb pains in children and adolescents. Pediatrics 50:429, 1972.
59. Silverberg M: Chronic abdominal pain in adolescents. Pediatr Ann 20:179, 1991.
60. McCarthy DM: Nonsteroidal anti-inflammatory drug-induced ulcers: Management by traditional therapies. Gastroenterology 96:662, 1989.
61. Soll AH, Weinstein WM, Kurata J, et al: Non-steroidal anti-inflammatory drugs and peptic ulcer. Ann Intern Med 114(4):307, 1991.
62. Richardson CT: Pathogenetic factors in peptic ulcer disease. Am J Med 79:1, 1985.
63. Battaglia G, Farini R, Di Mario F, et al: Is maximal acid output useful in identifying relapsing duodenal ulcer patients? J Clin Gastroenterol 7:375, 1985.
64. Antonescu CG and Marshall BJ: *Helicobacter pylori:* A potentially curable form of peptic ulcer disease. Gastroenterol J Club Jan 1990, p. 3.
65. Kilbridge PM, Dahms BB, and Czinn SJ: *Campylobacter pylori*—associated gastritis and peptic ulcer disease in children. Am J Dis Child 142:1149, 1988.
66. Czinn SJ, Dahms BB, Jacobs GH, et al: *Campylobacter*-like organisms in association with symptomatic gastritis in children. J Pediatr 109:80, 1986.
67. Drumm B, Sherman P, Cutz E, et al: Association of *Campylobacter pylori* on the gastric mucosa with antral gastritis in children. N Eng J Med 316:1557, 1987.
68. Marshall BJ: Peptic ulcer disease: role of *H. pylori*. Contemp Gastroenterol May/Jun 1990, p 8.
69. Ament ME and Christie DL: Upper gastrointestinal fiberoptic endoscopy in pediatric patients. Gastroenterology 72:1244, 1977.
70. Swain CP, Mills TN, Shemesh E, et al: Which electrode? A comparison of four endoscopic methods of electrocoagulation in experimental bleeding ulcers. Gut 25:1424, 1984.
71. O'Brien JD, Day SJ, and Burnham WR: Controlled trial of small bipolar probe in bleeding peptic ulcers. Lancet i:464, 1986.
72. Laine L: Multipolar electrocoagulation in the treatment of active upper gastrointestinal tract hemorrhage. 316:1613, 1987.
73. Drumm B, Sherman P, Chiasson D, et al: Treatment of *Campylobacter pylori*-associated antral gastritis in children with bismuth subsalicylate and ampicillin. J Pediatr 113:908, 1988.
74. Geokas MC: Acute pancreatitis. Ann Intern Med 103:86, 1985.
75. Durie PR: Pancreatitis. *In:* Walker WA, Durie PR, Hamilton JR, et al (eds): Pediatric Gastrointestinal Disease, 1st ed. Philadelphia, BC Decker, 1991, pp. 1209–1236.
76. Weizman Z and Durie PR: Acute pancreatitis in childhood. J Pediatr 113:24, 1988.
77. Steer ML: Search for the trigger mechanism of pancreatitis. Gastroenterology 86:764, 1984.
78. Fleischer AC, Parker P, and Kirschner SC: Sonographic findings of pancreatitis in children. Radiology 146:151, 1983.
79. Coleman BG, Arger PH, Rosenberg HK, et al: Gray-scale sonographic assessment of pancreatitis in children. Radiology 146:145, 1983.
80. Allendorph M, Werlin SL, Geenen JE, et al: Endoscopic retrograde cholangiopancreatography in children. J Pediatr 110:206, 1987.
81. Shaffer EA: Gallbladder disease. *In:* Walker WA, Durie PR, Hamilton JR, et al (eds): Pediatric Gastrointestinal Disease, 1st ed. Philadelphia, BC Decker, 1991, pp. 1163–1170.
82. Williamson RCN: Acalculous disease of the gallbladder. Gut 29:860, 1988.
83. Thurston WA, Kelly EN, and Silver MM: Acute acalculous cholecystitis in a premature infant treated with parenteral nutrition. Can Med Assoc J 135:332, 1985.
84. Thornell E: Mechanisms in the development of acute cholecystitis and biliary pain: A study on the role of prostaglandins and effects of indomethacin. Scand J Gastroenterol 17(Suppl. 76):1, 1982.
85. Neiderhiser D, Thornell E, Bjorck S, et al: The effect of lysophosphatidylcholine on gallbladder function in the cat. J Lab Clin Med 101:699, 1983.
86. Thornell E, Jivegard L, Bukhave K, et al: Prostaglandin E_2 formation by the gallbladder in experimental cholecystitis. Gut 27:370, 1986.
87. Paré P, Shaffer EA, and Rosenthal L: Nonvisualization of the gallbladder by ^{99m}Tc-HIDA choléscintigraphy as evidence of cholecystitis. Can Med Assoc J 118:384, 1978.
88. Reddick EJ and Olsen DO: Laparoscopic laser cholecystectomy: A comparison with mini-lap cholecystectomy. Surg Endosc 3:131, 1989.
89. Perissat J, Collet D, and Belliard R: Gallstones: Laparoscopic treatment—cholecystectomy, cholecystostomy, and lithotripsy: Our own technique. Surg Endosc 4:1, 1990.
90. Kelly TWJ, Patrick MR, and Hillman KM: Study of diarrhea in critically ill patients. Crit Care Med 11:7, 1983.
91. Phillips SF: Diarrhea: A current view of the pathophysiology. Gastroenterology 63:495, 1972.
92. Rhoads JM and Powell DW: Diarrhea. *In:* Walker WA, Durier PR, Hamilton JR, et al (eds): Pediatric Gastrointestinal Disease, 1st ed. Philadelphia, BC Decker, 1991, pp 62–78.
93. Binder HJ and Mehta P: Short-chained fatty acids stimulate active Na and Cl absorption in vitro in the rat distal colon. Gastroenterology 96:989, 1989.
94. Harms V and Wright EM: Some characteristics of Na/K-ATPase from rat intestinal basal lateral membranes. J Membr Biol 74:85, 1983.
95. Powell DW: Intestinal water and electrolyte transport. *In:* Johnson LR (ed): Physiology of the Gastrointestinal Tract, 2nd ed. New York, Raven Press, 1987, p. 1267.
96. Field M: Intracellular mediators of secretion in the small intestine. *In:* Binder HJ (ed): Mechanisms of Intestinal Secretion. New York, Alan R. Liss, 1979, p. 37.
97. Cooke HJ: Neural and humoral regulation of small intestinal electrolyte transport. *In:* Johnson, LR (ed): Physiology of the Gastrointestinal Tract, 2nd ed. New York, Raven Press, 1987, p. 1307.
98. Castro HJ: Immunological regulation of epithelial function. Am J Physiol (Gastrointest Liver Physiol 6) 243:G321, 1982.
99. Bern MJ, Sturbaum CW, Karayalcin SS, et al: Immune system control of rat and rabbit colonic electrolyte transport: Role of prostaglandins and enteric nervous system. J Clin Invest 83:1810, 1989.
100. Fordtran JS: Speculations on the pathogenesis of diarrhea. Fed Proc 26:1405, 1967.
101. Brinson RB and Kolts BE: Hypoalbuminemia as an indicator of diarrheal incidence in critically ill patients. Crit Care Med 15:506, 1987.
102. Kerzner B, Kelly MH, Gall DG, et al: Transmissible gastroenteritis: Sodium transport and the intestinal epithelium during the course of viral enteritis. Gastroenterology 72:457, 1977.
103. Sack DA, Rhoads M, Molla A, et al: Carbohydrate malabsorption in infants with rotavirus diarrhea. Am J Clin Nutr 36:1112, 1982.
104. Levine MM and Edelman R: Enteropathogenic *Escherichia coli* of classic serotypes associated with infant diarrhea: Epidemiology and pathogenesis. Epidemiol Rev 6:31, 1984.
105. Tabibian N: Diarrhea in critically ill patients. Am Fam Physician 40:135, 1989.
106. Ruddell WSJ and Losowsky MS: Severe diarrhea due to small intestinal colonization during cimetidine treatment. Br Med J 281:273, 1980.
107. Jones ES and Peaston MJT: Metabolic care during acute illnesses. Practitioner 196:271, 1966.
108. Pesola GR, Hogg JE, Eissa N, et al: Hypertonic nasogastric tube feedings: Do they cause diarrhea? Crit Care Med 18:1378, 1990.
109. Hauger SB and Powell KR: Infectious complications in children with HIV infection. Pediatr Ann 19:421, 1990.
110. Guerrant RL, Lohr JA, and William EK: Acute infectious diarrhea: Epidemiology, etiology and pathogenesis. Pediatr Infect Dis J 5:353, 1986.
111. Binder HJ: Treatment strategies for diarrheal disorders. American Gastroenterological Association Course 1990: Principles of Therapy. Presented at the American Gastroenterological Asso-

ciation 1991 Postgraduate Course. Pharmacology and Therapy of Digestive Diseases.

112. Smith P and Janoff E: Management of gastrointestinal lesions in AIDS and immunocompromised hosts. Gastroenterological Association Course 1990 Principles of Therapy. Presented at the American Gastroenterological Association 1991 Postgraduate Course. Pharmacology and Therapy of Digestive Diseases.

113. Celum CL, Chaisson RE, Rutherford GW, et al: Incidence of salmonellosis in patients with AIDS. J Infect Dis 156:998, 1987.

114. Perlman DM, Ampel NM, Schifman RB, et al: Persistent *Campylobacter jejuni* infections in patients with the human immunodeficiency virus (HIV). Ann Intern Med 108:540, 1988.

115. Blaser MJ, Hale TL, and Forman SB: Recurrent shigellosis complicating human immunodeficiency virus infection: Failure of pre-existing antibodies to confer protection. Am J Med 86:105, 1989.

116. Peterson LR, Olson MM, Shanholtzer CJ, et al: Results of a prospective, 18-month clinical evaluation of culture, cytotoxin testing, and culturette brand (CDT) latex testing in the diagnosis of *Clostridium difficile*-associated diarrhea. Diagn Microbiol Infect Dis 10:85, 1988.

117. Teasley DG, Gerding DN, Olson MM, et al: Prospective randomized trial of metronidazole versus vancomycin for *Clostridium difficile*-associated diarrhea and colitis. Lancet 2:1043, 1983.

118. Horsburgh CR Jr and Selik RM: The epidemiology of disseminated nontuberculous mycobacterial infection in the acquired immunodeficiency syndrome (AIDS). Am Rev Respir Dis 139:4, 1989.

119. Hoy J, Mijch A, Sandland M, et al: Quadruple-drug therapy for *Mycobacterium avium-intracellulare* bacteremia in AIDS patients. J Infect Dis 161:801, 1990.

120. Chiu J, Nussbaum J, Bozzette S, et al: Treatment of disseminated *Mycobacterium avium* complex infection in AIDS with amikacin, ethambutol, rifampin and ciprofloxacin. Ann Intern Med 113:358, 1990.

121. Chachoua A, Dieterich D, Krasinski K, et al: 9-(1,2-dihydroxy-2-propoxymethyl) guanine (Ganciclovir) in the treatment of cytomegalovirus gastrointestinal disease with the acquired immunodeficiency syndrome. Ann Intern Med 107:133, 1987.

122. Erice A, Sunwenn C, Biron KK, et al: Progressive disease due to gancyclovir-resistant cytomegalovirus in immunocompromised patients. N Engl J Med 320:289, 1989.

123. Engel JP, Englund JA, Fletcher CV, et al: Treatment of resistant herpes simplex virus with continuous-infusion acyclovir. JAMA 263:1662, 1990.

124. Erlich KS, Mills J, Chotis P, et al: Acyclovir-resistant herpes simplex virus infections in patients with the acquired immunodeficiency syndrome. N Engl J Med 320:293, 1989.

125. Soave R, Moskovitz B, Mulhall A, et al: Intravenous spiramycin therapy of AIDS-related cryptosporidial diarrhea. Abstract presented at the 30th Annual Interscience Conference of Antimicrobial Agents and Chemotherapy, Atlanta, GA, Oct 1990.

126. Rolston KVI, Fainstein V, and Bodey GP: Intestinal crytosporidiosis treated with eflornithine: A prospective study among patients with AIDS. J AIDS 2:426, 1989.

127. Ouie E, Borkowsky W, Klesius PH, et al: Persistent *Campylobacter jejuni* infections in patients with the human immunodeficiency virus (HIV). Ann Intern Med 108:540, 1988.

128. Orenstein JM, Chaing J, Steinberg W, et al: Intestinal microsporidiosis as a cause of diarrhea in human immunodeficiency virus-infected patients: A report of 20 cases. Hum Pathol 21:475, 1990.

129. DeWit S, Weerts D, Doossens H, et al: Comparison of fluconazole and ketoconazole for oropharyngeal candidiasis in AIDS. Lancet 1:746, 1989.

130. McKinsey DS, Gupta MR, Riddler SA, et al: Long-term amphotericin B therapy for disseminated histoplasmosis in patients with acquired immunodeficiency syndrome. Ann Intern Med 111:655, 1989.

58

Fluid and Electrolyte Therapy

J. Alan Paschall, M.D., and Tyrone Melvin, M.D.

"Probably, the proper use of water and electrolyte solutions is responsible for saving more lives of seriously ill patients than is the use of any other group of substances."[1] This statement by two pediatricians from Yale University in 1950 seems very bold when the entire range of patient problems and therapeutic modalities is considered, but the concept is accepted by the authors of this chapter and is the impetus behind its scope and topical organization. The goal has been to create a comprehensive data base with regard to questions of body fluid compartments, their composition, and control over them in health and disease. To do this has meant reorganizing a chronology of understanding and therapeutic modalities. The use of intravenous fluids, for example, preceded reproducible studies of body fluid compartments by several decades.

HISTORY

Cholera was the event that led to the first use of intravenous fluids. Cholera was confirmed in England during the second world pandemic with the death of William Sproat, a 60-year-old keelman living in Fish Quay, Sunderland, on October 26, 1831. (The responsible British medical authorities recognized its appearance November 1, 1831).[2] The epidemic in England led Dr. William Brooke O'Shaughnessy (an Irishman, aged 22 years) to investigate the change in the blood and stool in cholera. Having arrived in Sunderland December 11, 1831 (9 days after the Frenchman Francois Magendie, who was intent upon the same study), O'Shaughnessy was able to determine that the blood had a reduced water and alkali content and that the stool had an increased alkali content. He reasoned that replacement of these fluids intravenously would restore health, though it would not necessarily correct the proximate cause of the disorder.[3] The salts and amounts of injection he proposed have been translated into current units by Carpenter,[4] as seen in Table 58–1. They

are remarkably close to the World Health Organization recommendations made in 1976.

Acknowledging O'Shaughnessy, Dr. Thomas Latta from Leith reported on June 2, 1832 the recovery of a woman from cholera-induced hypovolemic shock, accomplished by use of intravenous fluids, the composition of which was suggested by O'Shaughnessy. However, having witnessed the recovery he stated, "I fancied my patient secure, and from my great need of a little repose, left her in charge of the hospital surgeon; but I had not been gone long, ere the vomiting and purging recurring, soon reduced her to her former state of disability . . . and she sunk in five and a half hours after I had left her . . . ."[5]

Such reports were not greeted with acceptance. More published space was given to disputing the priority of Latta's claim than to attempts to reproduce it. Markus,[6] medical secretary to Russian Prince Dimitri Galitzin's Temporary Medical Council (ad hoc for cholera), suggested that in 1831 in Moscow, a German expatriate physician, Dr. Jaehnichen, injected 6 ounces of water into the vein of a woman symptomatic from cholera, resulting in the appearance of the radial pulse for 15 minutes, though death ensued within 2 hours. Markus indicated his purpose in reporting was specifically to ensure priority for Russian physicians over English and French claims of priority. (Indeed, O'Shaughnessy him-

Table 58–1. INTRAVENOUS FLUIDS FOR CHOLERA*

	(mEq/l)	
	1831 O'Shaughnessy	1976 WHO
Na	178	140
Cl	144	110
HCO$_3$	34	40
K	0	10

*From Carpenter CJC: Treatment of cholera—tradition and authority versus science, reason, and humanity. Johns Hopkins Med 139:153, 1976.

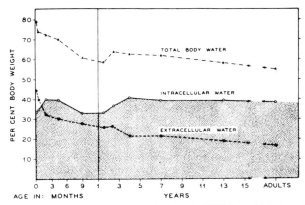

Figure 58–1. Change in TBW, ICW, and ECW from birth to adult, expressed as a percentage of body weight. (From Friis-Hansen BJ: Body water compartment in children changes during growth and related changes in body composition. Reproduced by permission of Pediatrics Vol. 28, p. 170. Copyright 1961.)

self seems to have been "scooped" by a London weekly medical magazine, which had reported the potential intravenous therapy just prior to the *Lancet* article. O'Shaughnessy suggested that his ideas may have been "embezzled" from a notification he had made a week before his Westminster Medical Society lecture from which the *Lancet* article came.)

These prescient observations and intrepid experiments document the 160-year history of intravenous fluid use, though it lay fallow from 1832 to 1900. This was in large part due to criticism from acknowledged medical leaders of the day. A world in which anesthesia for surgery was 15 years off, and in which Princess Victoria, Florence Nightingale, and Joseph Lister were children of 12, 8, and 4 years of age, respectively, could not embrace this

radical therapy.[7] (O'Shaughnessy left medicine in 1833 to join the East India Company, was knighted in 1856 for establishing telegraph service among the main centers of India, and dropped the Irish O'Shaughnessy, using Brooke as his surname. Latta died in 1833.)[7]

BODY FLUID COMPARTMENTS

The modern history of defining body fluid compartments began only 40 years ago with the measurements by Friis-Hansen.[8–11] (Previous measurements completed in the 19th century had been made using desiccated cadavers relative to fresh postmortem weights.)[12, 13] The advent of substances such as deuterium oxide and salts of thiocyanate and thiosulfate allowed for calculation of total body water (TBW), extracellular water (ECW), and derivation of the intracellular water (ICW) compartment. Friis-Hansen's laborious, tedious human experiments form the basis for our knowledge of these compartments. Figure 58–1 reproduces these values given from birth to 15 years, in which deuterium oxide has been used for TBW measurement, thiocyanate has been used for the ECW compartment, and the ICW compartment is derived by subtracting ECW from TBW. These data are extended in Figure 58–2 in which Friis-Hansen has added data from chemical analysis of fetal cadavers.[12, 14–20] These same data are also displayed converted for use in l/m² body surface area in Figure 58–3. When the ECW and ICW compartments are subdivided, the newborn data may be compared with adult human data as in Figure 58–4, in which it is apparent that ECW as a percentage of TBW decreases with age.

Many substances have been used as markers for different body compartments, each adopted to refine

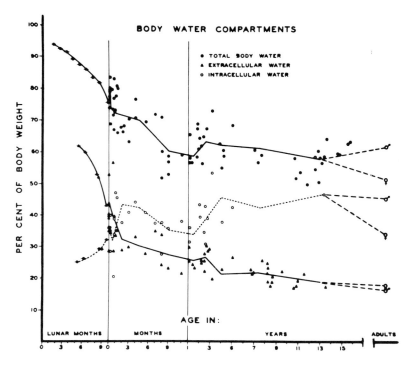

Figure 58–2. Change in TBW, ICW, and ECW as in Figure 58–1, with additional fetal data added, expressed as percentage body weight. (From Friis-Hansen BJ: Body water compartment in children changes during growth and related changes in body composition. Reproduced by permission of Pediatrics Vol. 28, p. 171. Copyright 1961.)

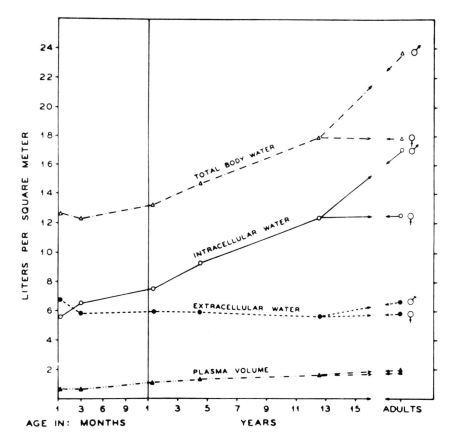

Figure 58–3. Same data as in Figure 58–2 plotted as l/m² body surface area. (From Friis-Hansen BJ: Body water compartment in children changes during growth and related changes in body composition. Reproduced by permission of Pediatrics Vol. 28, p. 174. Copyright 1961.)

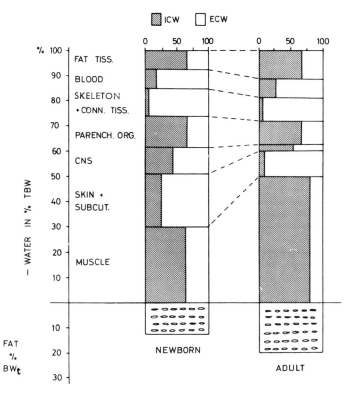

Figure 58–4. Proportion of TBW in organs of the newborn compared with the adult, with relative size of ECW and ICW for each organ. (From Friis-Hansen BJ: Body water compartment in children changes during growth and related changes in body composition. Reproduced by permission of Pediatrics Vol. 47, p. 264, 1961.)

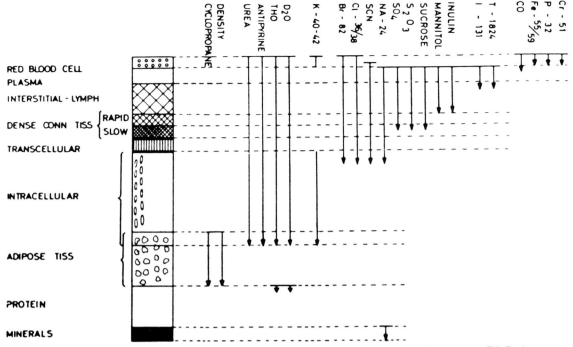

Figure 58–5. Substances used to define the indicated body fluid space and its composition. (From Friis-Hansen BJ: Body water compartment in children changes during growth and related changes in body composition. Reproduced by permission of Pediatrics Vol. 47, p. 266. Copyright 1971.)

the original measurements. No marker is perfect, and different types of error in measurement are introduced with each. Figure 58–5 summarizes the list of substances used and the compartments for which measurement they are relevant. The ECW compartment is particularly difficult to measure, and Figure 58–6 shows the different measurements of ECW obtained with several methods. Problems include a substance failing to penetrate dense

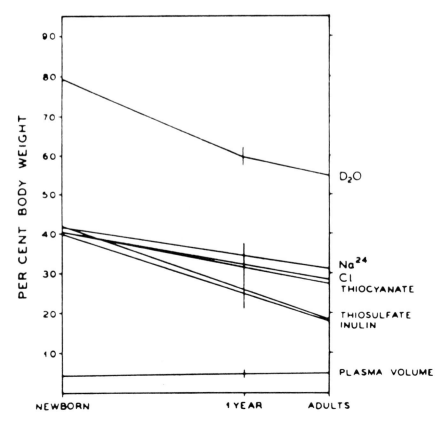

Figure 58–6. Comparison of various means of defining ECW in newborn, at 1 year and in adults. There is increasing variation in ECW measured by these methods, with age. TBW (D_2O) and plasma volume are also shown. (From Friis-Hansen BJ: Body water compartment in children changes during growth and related changes in body composition. Reproduced by permission of Pediatrics Vol. 28, p. 172. Copyright 1961.)

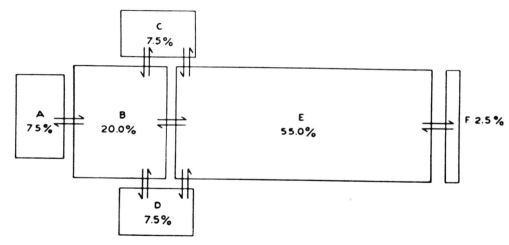

Figure 58–7. Box diagram of body water compartments. (Reproduced with permission from Edelman IS and Leibman J: Anatomy of body water and electrolytes. Am J Med 27:261, 1959.)

A. PLASMA WATER–7.5% OF BODY WATER
B. INTERSTITIAL–LYMPH WATER–20.0%
C. DENSE CONNECTIVE TISSUE AND CARTILAGE WATER–7.5%
D. BONE WATER–7.5%
E. INTRACELLULAR WATER–55.0%
F. TRANSCELLULAR WATER–2.5%

connective tissue, metabolism of the indicator substance, or renal excretion after introduction but prior to final measurement. Much of the quoted data in textbooks are based on thiocyanate distribution.

Despite such methodologic concerns, Edelman and Leibman[21] developed a useful consensus depiction of human body fluid subcompartments (Fig. 58–7). They highlighted the "heterogeneity of the extracellular fluids which are not a direct part of the plasma-interstitial-lymph pool."[21] The arrows in the figure indicate that "in disease states transductions of fluid and electrolytes among these subdivisions may be of vital importance."[21]

In addition, the concept of a transcellular space is introduced, which is defined as the luminal contents of the gastrointestinal and urinary tracts. Although this compartment is relatively small in health, it represents an enormous trafficking of fluid (e.g., saliva secretion is 1.5 l/day and gastric secretion is 2 l/day) in adults.[22] It is easy to see how a small change in reabsorption in this system could lead to it becoming the critical body fluid compartment (e.g., in cholera).

Electrolyte Composition of Body Fluid Compartments

The electrolyte composition of these body spaces has been determined by similar laborious experimentation. Winters[23] published a consensus illustration in "Gamble-gram" form (named for Dr. James Gamble). The electrolyte composition of plasma, interstitial fluid, and intracellular fluid in adults (virtually the same as in children) is depicted. The comparison of electrolyte content of human plasma is often made to sea water and is erroneously considered to be similar. Table 58–2 points out this error and provides a reference for these quantities that is useful in salt water ingestion or near-drowning victims, or both.[24]

To complete the data base with regard to electrolyte content, box diagrams and tables of sodium, potassium, and chloride spaces are shown in Figures 58–8 to 58–10 and Tables 58–3 to 58–5. These figures and tables introduce the concept of exchangeable pools relative to stable pools with respect to individual electrolyte content. Table 58–6 and Figure 58–11 provide representations of the electrolyte content of various transcellular fluids. In addition, it is often useful to be able to compare the composition of body compartments with respect to ionic or osmolar composition. Figures 58–12 and 58–13 provide these data for plasma.

It will be recognized that no mention is made of bicarbonate space. This is avoided because the ECW is only one space in which bicarbonate exists. The intracellular buffering capacity may be small or so large, depending upon disease states, as to make ECW bicarbonate content insignificant.

Table 58–2. COMPOSITIONS OF SEA WATER AND HUMAN EXTRACELLULAR FLUID*

	(mEq/Kg H₂O)		
Chemical	Sea Water Today	Sea Water Proportionately Reduced to 290 mOsm/kg H₂O	Extracellular (Interstitial) Fluid
Sodium	475	138	144
Potassium	10	3	4
Calcium	20	6	3
Magnesium	108	31	1.5
Chloride	554	161	114
Sulfate	56	8	1
Phosphate	Trace	Trace	2
Bicarbonate	2	1	28
Water (mOsm/kg H₂O)	1,000	290	290

*From Maffly R: The body fluids: Volume, composition, and physical chemistry. In: Brenner BM and Rector FC (eds): The Kidney. Philadelphia, WB Saunders, 1976, p. 67.

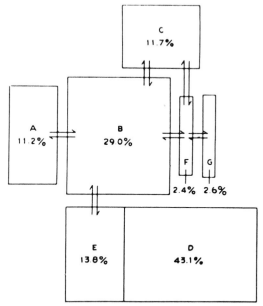

A   PLASMA SODIUM - 11.2% OF TOTAL
     BODY SODIUM.
B   INTERSTITIAL - LYMPH SODIUM - 29.0%
C   DENSE CONNECTIVE TISSUE AND
     CARTILAGE SODIUM - 11.7%
D   TOTAL BONE SODIUM (INCLUDING E) 43.1%
E   EXCHANGEABLE BONE SODIUM - 13.8%
F   INTRACELLULAR SODIUM 2.4%
G   TRANSCELLULAR SODIUM 2.6%

Figure 58–8. Box diagram of body sodium distribution in the adult male. (Reproduced with permission from Edelman IS and Leibman J: Anatomy of body water and electrolytes. Am J Med 27:266, 1959.)

Figure 58–9. Box diagram of body potassium distribution in the adult male. (Reproduced with permission from Edelman IS and Leibman J: Anatomy of body water and electrolytes. Am J Med 27:269, 1959.)

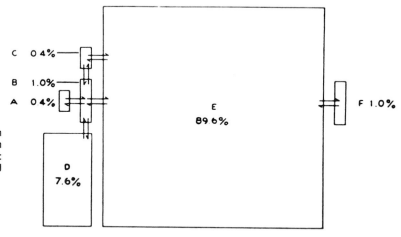

A   PLASMA POTASSIUM - 0.4% OF TOTAL BODY POTASSIUM
B   INTERSTITIAL - LYMPH POTASSIUM - 1.0%
C   DENSE CONNECTIVE TISSUE AND CARTILAGE POTASSIUM - 0.4%
D   BONE POTASSIUM - 7.6%
E   INTRACELLULAR POTASSIUM - 89.6%
F   TRANSCELLULAR POTASSIUM - 1.0%

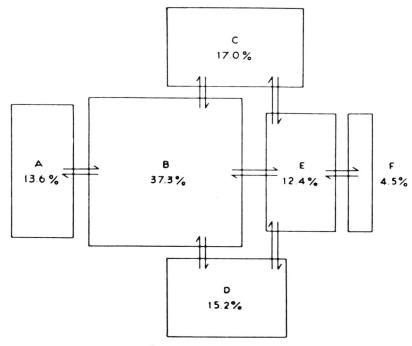

A   PLASMA CHLORIDE - 13.6% OF TOTAL BODY CHLORIDE
B   INTERSTITIAL-LYMPH CHLORIDE - 37.3%
C   DENSE CONNECTIVE TISSUE AND CARTILAGE CHLORIDE - 17.0%
D   BONE CHLORIDE - 15.2%
E   INTRACELLULAR CHLORIDE 12.4%
F   TRANSCELLULAR CHLORIDE   4.5%

Figure 58–10. Box diagram of body chloride distribution. (Reproduced with permission from Edelman IS and Leibman J: Anatomy of body water and electrolytes. Am J Med 27:272, 1959.)

Control of Body Fluid Compartment Size and Content

The forces controlling size and content of body fluid compartments will now be examined. This discussion deals with local forces at the cell membrane: fluid interface. Overall volume and content control of the entire body will be discussed later in the chapter.

The discussion of the control of composition of fluid compartments is complex, and its full treatment is beyond the scope of this chapter; however, examination of some of its elements will develop a working knowledge, that is useful in clinical problem-solving. The phenomenon of Gibbs-Donnan equilibrium may be seen in Figure 58–14.[25] In the figure, two compartments, A and B, have identical ionic compositions. In A, 10 molecules of albumin, necessitating 180 cationic Na^+ to

Table 58–3. BODY SODIUM DISTRIBUTION IN AN "AVERAGE" NORMAL YOUNG ADULT MALE*

	mEq/Kg of Body Weight	% of Total Exchangeable Sodium	% of Total Body Sodium
Plasma	6.5	15.9	11.2
Interstitial-lymph	16.8	41.0	29.0
Dense connective tissue and cartilage	6.8	16.5	11.7
Exchangeable bone	8.0	19.5	13.8
Total bone	25.0	—	43.1
Transcellular	1.5	3.7	2.6
Total exchangeable extracellular	39.6	96.6	68.3
Total extracellular	56.6	—	97.6
Total body sodium	58.0	142.9	100.0
Total intracellular	1.4	3.4	2.4

*From Edelman IS and Leibman J: Anatomy of body water and electrolytes. Am J Med 27:256, 1959.

Table 58–4. BODY POTASSIUM DISTRIBUTION IN AN "AVERAGE" NORMAL YOUNG ADULT MALE*

	mEq/Kg of Body Weight	% of Total Exchangeable Potassium	% of Total Body Potassium
Plasma	0.2	0.4	0.4
Interstitial-lymph	0.5	1.0	1.0
Dense connective tissue and cartilage	0.2	0.4	0.4
Total bone	4.1	—	7.6
Transcellular	0.5	1.0	1.0
Total extracellular	5.5	—	10.4
Total body potassium†	53.8	110.0	100.0
Total intracellular	48.3	98.8	89.6

*From Edelman IS and Leibman J: Anatomy of body water and electrolytes. Am J Med 27:268, 1959.

†Estimate is based on the assumption that the exchangeable potassium content of young males, 48.9 mEq/kg of body weight is 90% of total body potassium.

Table 58–5. DISTRIBUTION OF BODY CHLORIDE IN HUMANS*

	mEq/Kg of Body Weight	% of Total Exchangeable Chloride	% of Total Body Chloride
Plasma	4.5	14.5	13.6
Interstitial-lymph	12.3	39.7	37.3
Dense connective tissue and cartilage	5.6	17.8	17.0
Bone	5.0	15.9	15.2
Transcellular	1.5	4.8	4.5
Total extracellular	28.9	92.7	87.6
Total body chloride	33.0	104.8	100.0
Total intracellular	4.1	13.0	12.4

*From Edelman IS and Leibman J: Anatomy of body water and electrolytes. Am J Med 27:272, 1959.

counterbalance the total albumin negative charge, are present, leading to Na^+ movement down a concentration gradient from A to B, along with Cl^-. This occurs until an equilibrium is reached, with each compartment being balanced for charge but A having a greater number of osmotically active particles. The important point is, therefore, that this compartment will exert an osmotic force increasing its water content. This will always occur in the side containing the impermeant anion.

Also, the ions will be distributed unevenly, with the cationic species higher in the compartment with the impermeant anion and correspondingly fewer Cl^- anions. The actual ratio is given by the following equation:

$$\left(\frac{[A^z]p}{[A^z]int} \right)^z = \left(\frac{[X^s]int}{[X^s]p} \right)^z$$

where A and X are ionic species of valence z or q and p = plasma and int = interstitium. The Donnan ratio for Na^+ is 1.05, with Na^+ levels higher in plasma relative to interstitium.

Another consequence of this distribution is to generate a membrane potential governed by the following:

$$\begin{aligned}
E \text{ (in mV)} &= \frac{RT}{zF} \cdot \ln \frac{Xo}{Xi} \\
&= (61) \log \frac{Xo}{Xi} \\
&= (61) \log 1.05 = 1.3 \text{ mV}
\end{aligned}$$

R	=	8.31 joules/mol	o = outside
T	=	310°K at 37°C	i = inside
	=	1.987 cal/mol K°	
F	=	96,500 coulombs/mol	
	=	23 kcal/V • mol	

The last relevant point given the Donnan distribution is to quantify the pressure difference attributable to the impermeant protein. The van't Hoff equation describes this force:

$$\Delta\pi = \Delta CRT \qquad C = \text{colloid osmotic pressure in mOSm/Kg } H_2O$$

1 mOSm/kg H_2O therefore exerts in millimeters of mercury the following pressure:

$$\Delta\pi = \frac{1}{1,000} \cdot \frac{mole}{liter} \times \left(0.0821 \cdot \frac{liter \cdot atm}{degree \cdot mole} \right) \times 310°K$$

$$= (0.0254 \text{ atm}) \times (760 \text{ mm Hg/atm})$$
$$= 19.3 \text{ mm Hg}$$

This enables one to express the normal osmotic pressure difference between plasma and interstitium.

osmolar difference due to electrolyte =
$[Na^+ + Cl^-]$ plasma − $[Na^+ + Cl^-]$ interstitium = 0.4 mm/l
protein difference (given value) = 0.9 mm/l
total osmolar difference = 0.4 mm/l + 0.9 mm/l = 1.3 mm/l
therefore, the total osmotic pressure gradient =
1.3 mm/l • 19.3 mm Hg/mm/l = 25 mm Hg
= normal colloid osmotic pressure (plasma greater than interstitium)

This force allows for the delicate balance whereby an organism keeps body fluids in the vascular compartment while under the hydrostatic pressure head generated by the heart. It was not always recognized so clearly as it is today. In 1896, Starling[26] published his discussion of colloid osmotic pressure refuting the widely held notion that force generated by plasma protein was negligible. This erroneous assumption was held in large part because of the knowledge that albumin's contribution was very small relative to the contribution of electrolytes. It took Starling to directly measure the oncotic pressure and relate it to the capillary hydrostatic pressure. His recognition that the plasma colloid oncotic pressure virtually matched capillary hydrostatic pressure (while electrolyte forces were essentially equal between plasma

Table 58–6. TRANSCELLULAR FLUID VOLUME IN MAN*

Source	Ml/Kg of Body Weight	% of Body Water	Remarks
Intraluminal, gastrointestinal	7.4	1.4	Obtained at postmortem examination
Intraluminal, gastrointestinal (dog)	19.0	3.0	Normal dogs sacrificed after 24-hr fast
Cerebrospinal fluid	2.8	—	—
Biliary tree	2.1	—	Calculated from the average gallbladder volume (50 ml) and 5% of total liver water
Remainder	3.0	—	Calculated as 15% of organ weights, including the mucosal layer of the gastrointestinal tract plus aqueous and vitreous humor

*From Edelman IS and Leibman J: Anatomy of body water and electrolytes. Am J Med 27:260, 1959.

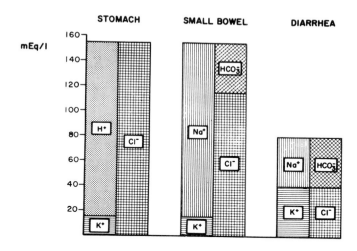

Figure 58–11. Electrolyte composition of stomach, small bowel, and diarrheal fluids. (Reproduced with permission from Winters RW [ed]: Body Fluids in Pediatrics, p. 130. Boston, Little, Brown and Company, copyright 1973.)

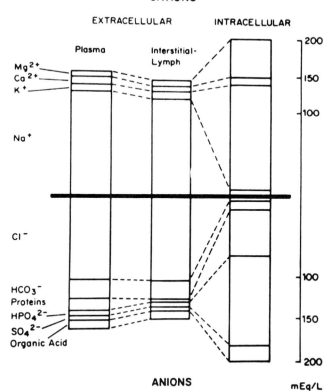

Figure 58–12. Ionic composition of the EC and IC compartments with cations above the dark horizontal line and anions below the line. (Reproduced with permission from Yoshioka T, Iitaka K, and Ichikawa I, In: Ichikawa I [ed]: Pediatric Textbook of Fluids and Electrolytes, p. 16. © 1990, the Williams & Wilkins Co., Baltimore.)

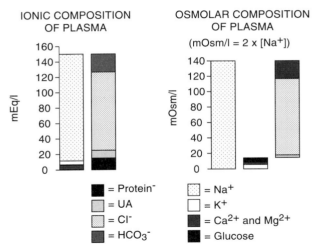

Figure 58–13. Comparison of ionic and osmolar composition of plasma. (Reproduced with permission from Winters RW [ed]: Body Fluids in Pediatrics, p. 104. Boston, Little, Brown and Company, copyright 1973.)

and interstitium) really broke the ground for the explanation of edema and glomerular filtration.

MAINTENANCE REQUIREMENTS FOR ENERGY, WATER, AND ELECTROLYTES

All maintenance requirements for energy, water, and electrolytes may be understood in the context of energy expenditure. Talbot[27] performed a series of measurements to define basal caloric expenditure in children of various ages. Estimates were made of the requirement

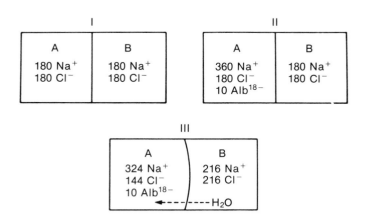

Figure 58–14. Gibbs-Donnan effect. In this example, compartments A and B are separated by a semipermeable membrane (impermeable to albumin). In II, 10 albumin molecules have been added with the required 180 Na^+ molecules to balance the added $10 \times ^-18 = 180$ negative charges from the albumin. The resulting concentration gradient for Na^+ causes it to move from A to B. To maintain charge neutrality Cl^- moves also from A to B, until as in III, an equilibrium is reached such that Na^+ and Cl^- diffusion from A to B is balanced by the concentration gradient driving Cl^- from B to A. As a consequence, greater total solute is present on the side with the impermeant anion (albumin) and water, therefore, flows from B to A. (Reproduced with permission from Fanestil DD. *In:* Maxwell MH, Kleeman CR, and Narins RG [eds]: Clinical Disorders of Fluid and Electrolyte Metabolism. New York, McGraw-Hill, 1987, p. 2.)

in situations of normal activity. Holliday and Segar,[28] lamenting the availability of a reliable, easy to use reference for caloric need based on weight, plotted Talbot's data using weight at the 50th percentile for age and added a line for caloric expenditure of the hospitalized patient. The system is arbitrary and may, depending on the clinical situation, be seriously in error, but is often reproduced as in Figure 58–15 and remains a convenient starting point. It must always be used in tandem with a checklist of conditions that may greatly alter an individual's metabolic rate, as summarized in Table 58–7.

Defining caloric needs of patients is still not by itself useful in defining the quantity of water and electrolytes required for homeostasis. Fortunately, nature sees to it that losses of water are a function of energy expenditure; therefore, water needs may be broken down into constituent parts, the first being the relation of insensible water loss to caloric expenditure. At the time Holliday and Segar put forth their convenient system, it was known from direct measurement[29, 30] that insensible water loss in the resting state is a constant function of basal energy expenditure, averaging 45 ml of water lost for each 100 kcal of energy used. Direct measurements by Heeley and Talbot[31] corroborated these findings. They were able to show that certain clinical conditions could dramatically alter this value, as shown in Figure 58–16 (shown in ml/m^2 surface area [SA]/24 hr). Although these observations were in the controlled clinical research environment, it was Gamble[32] who measured such losses under real life extremes in his bold, colorful experiments on human adult male volunteers living on a raft in Cotuit Bay, MA (Fig. 58–17). Table 58–8 reconciles these insensible losses in relation to both caloric expenditure and body SA.

If insensible losses account for 45 to 50 ml of water loss/100 kcal expended, what makes up the rest? Obviously urine water is the next major component. Although it seems obvious that this urine water is a consequence of glomerular filtration, and the excretion of exogenous wastes is a fortuitous consequence, the conditions of thirsting and fasting allow for a quick examination of the actual sources of urine water.

Again the elegant, unique experiments of Gamble[32] illustrate the point. Figure 58–18 shows three sets of parallel bars: thirsting, fasting, and access to glucose as an energy source only. The left-hand bar of each pair is the source of water, and the right-hand bar indicates the form in which water leaves the body. It can be appreciated that in the thirsting state, water is derived from both intracellular space, extracellular space, and from what is termed *water of oxidation*, or that derived from the end of the electron transport chain. In the fasting states, with free access to water, there is a significant reduction in loss from intracellular and extracellular compartments, but not until energy substrate is provided in the form of glucose do these losses really decrease.

These bars gave Gamble clues as to the nature of what drove urine losses. It became apparent that there was a constant but variable production of osmotically active solute daily, which had to be removed to prevent

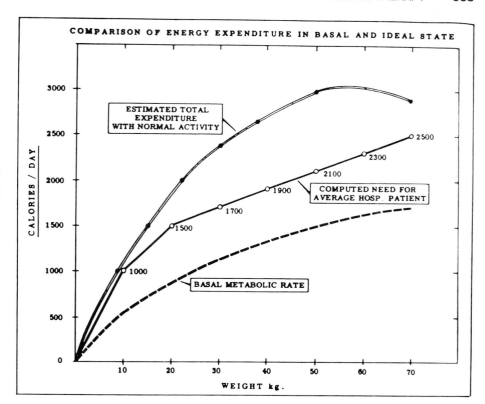

Figure 58–15. Energy expenditure in calories (kcal)/day at various body weights, under basal, hospital, and normal activity states. (Reproduced with permission from Segar W: Parenteral fluid therapy. Curr Probl Pediatr 3(2):4, 1972.)

dangerous changes in extra-and intracellular osmolality. The variability in osmolar production depends upon energy state, with a usual diet producing the greatest number of osmoles, followed by the fasting state, which, in turn, is greater than the consumption of glucose alone. Figure 58–19 illustrates this point in relation to the concentrating and diluting capacity of the kidney. It can be seen from the graph that at a usual food intake in adults, 1,200 mOsm/day are produced that need to be eliminated. At the maximal concentrating ability of the kidney (1400 mOsm/l), this will require a minimum of 750 ml of urine/day to avoid increasing osmolality. At an osmolality of 600 mOsm/l, much less work is

required by the kidney, but now the 1,200 mOsm requires 2 l of urine to be eliminated. Figure 58–20 provides a convenient reference for urine water required given the osmoles created through energy expenditure (the renal solute load) and the osmolality of the urine.

The relationship of renal solute load to energy expenditure and its variation with food intake is seen in Table 58–9. Note the dramatic changes both over time (on constant regimen) and with diet.

Putting this all together provides a convenient method of calculating maintenance water requirements. Paraphrasing Holliday and Segar,[28] assuming a minimal solute load of 10 mOsm/100 kcal excreted at a twofold

Table 58–7. CONDITIONS ALTERING USUAL ESTIMATE OF METABOLIC RATE*

Condition	Type of Adjustment to be Made
Increase in metabolic rate	
Fever	Increase caloric estimate by 12% per °C rise in body temperature
Hypermetabolic states (hyperthyroidism, salicylism, and so on)	Increase caloric estimate by 25–75%
Decrease in metabolic rate	
Hypothermia	Reduce caloric estimate by 12% per °C fall in body temperature
Hypometabolic states	Reduce caloric estimate by 10–25%

*From Winters R (ed): Body Fluids in Pediatrics, p. 118. Boston, Little, Brown and Company, copyright 1973.

Table 58–8. RELATION OF INSENSIBLE LOSS OF WATER TO SURFACE AREA AND TO ESTIMATED CALORIC EXPENDITURE FOR VARIOUS AGE GROUPS*

Age Groups	Ml/m²	Ml/100 cal†	% Deviation of Each Age Group from Mean for All Ages‡ Ml/m²	Ml/100 cal
0–3 yr	1,150	59	124	118
3–8 yr	950	49	102	102
8–16 yr	700	45	75	90
All ages	930	50	—	—

*From Holliday MA and Segar WE: The maintenance need for water in parenteral fluid therapy. Reproduced by permission of Pediatrics Vol. 19, p. 823. Copyright 1957.

†Data of Heeley and Talbot[31] recalculated from weight, estimated caloric expenditure, and observed insensible loss.

‡Mean for all ages taken as 100% and mean for each age group expressed as a percentage of this figure.

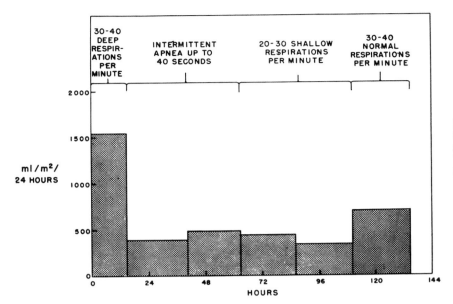

Figure 58–16. Alteration in insensible water loss with different respiratory patterns in a 14-month-old infant. (Reproduced with permission from Heeley AM and Talbot NB: Insensible water losses per day by hospitalized infants and children. Am J Dis Child 90:254, 1955. Copyright 1955, American Medical Association.)

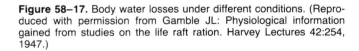

Figure 58–17. Body water losses under different conditions. (Reproduced with permission from Gamble JL: Physiological information gained from studies on the life raft ration. Harvey Lectures 42:254, 1947.)

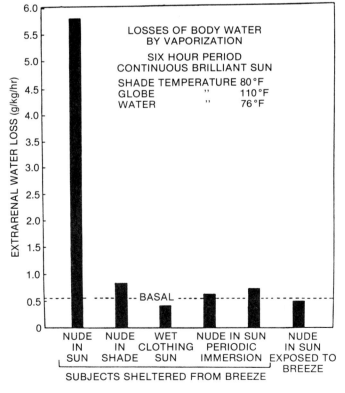

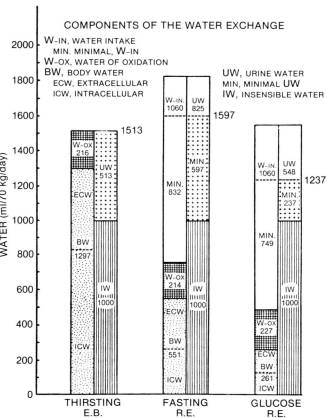

Figure 58–18. Components of water exchange under conditions of thirsting, fasting, and access to water and glucose. Source of water is in the left hand bars, and the form in which it leaves the body is in the right hand bars of each set. (Reproduced with permission from Gamble JL: Physiological information gained from studies on the life raft ration. Harvey Lectures 42:249, 1947.)

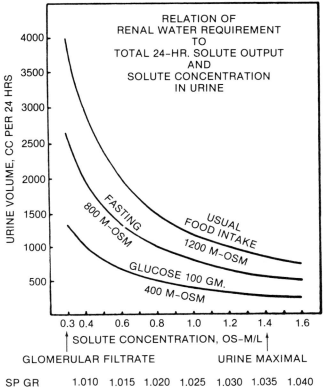

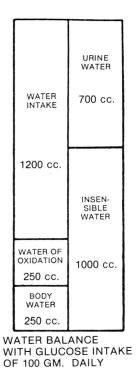

WATER BALANCE
WITH GLUCOSE INTAKE
OF 100 GM. DAILY

Figure 58–19. Renal water requirement in relation to solute generated and concentration of urine. Arrows along the x-axis indicate the osmolality of the initial glomerular filtrate and the maximum osmolality of urine. The bar graph shows this renal water requirement in the context of daily water balance. (Reproduced with permission from Gamble JL: Physiological information gained from studies on the life raft ration. Harvey Lectures 42:272, 1947.)

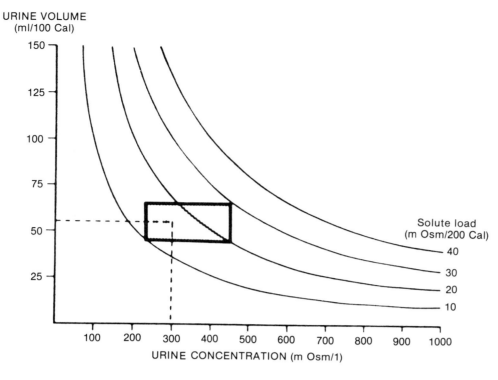

URINE VOLUME
(ml/100 Cal)

Solute load
(m Osm/200 Cal)

URINE CONCENTRATION (m Osm/1)

Figure 58–20. Urine volume and osmolality required to excrete solute load for normal daily activity. (Data from Figure 58–19 as modified by Winters RW [ed]: Body Fluids in Pediatrics, p. 125. Boston, Little, Brown and Company, copyright 1973.)

concentration (75 mOsm/l being minimum = 150 mOsm/l), requires 10 mOsm/150 mOsm/l × 1,000 ml/l = 66.7 ml. At a maximum solute load of 40 mOsm/100 kcal and excreting it at 600 mOsm/l (safe maximum expected in hospitalized patients), requires 40 mOsm/600 mOsm/l × 1,000 ml/l = 66.7 ml. An average renal solute load of 25 mOsm/100 kcal in 66.7 ml of urine would easily achieve an osmolarity of 25 mOsm/66.7 ml × 1,000 ml/l = 375 mOsm/l. So providing 66.7 ml H_2O/100 kcal covers the expected range of solute load that the average kidney can achieve. In addition, 50 ml/100 kcal will be required to cover insensible losses, leading to a total need of 66.7 + 50 = 116.7 ml/100 kcal; however, the water provided by oxidation probably approaches 16.7 ml/100 kcal. Hence, the familiar 100 ml H_2O/100 kcal required for maintenance is derived.

Maintenance needs for electrolytes are more difficult

Table 58–9. AVERAGE DAILY EXCRETION OF SOLUTES ON VARIOUS REGIMENS*

Subjects	Regimen	Day of Study	mOsm/100 Cal/ Day
Infants	Glucose	1	24.2
Infants	Glucose	2–5	14.5
Infants	Glucose	6–10	10.3
Adults	Glucose	Adjusted†	12.5
Infant	Human milk	Adjusted	11.0
Infant	Cow's milk	Adjusted	41.0
Adult	Average diet (1,200 mOsm/ day)	Adjusted	48.0

*From Holliday MA and Segar WE: The maintenance need for water in parenteral fluid therapy. Reproduced by permission of Pediatrics Vol. 19, p. 827. Copyright 1957.

†Observation made when diet had been constant so that excretion of solutes was relatively constant.

to glean from the literature. The composition of the various body compartments are not useful, as they vary enormously. Rather, direct observation of balance in human subjects in various metabolic states is the preferred guide, and the literature does fill in some of these gaps. These measurements are subject to several sources of error.

Gamble and colleagues[33] articulated the obstacles to attaining reproducible maintenance quantities for sodium, chloride, and potassium. Of particular concern was the inability to accurately measure loss of electrolytes from the skin and the large oscillations in daily balance that necessitate a long period of observation. This is illustrated in Figure 58–21 for a 1-month-old infant on breast milk fed on demand. It is readily apparent that balance really has no meaning on a given day. In addition, the attempt to use interval body weight gain with respect to different sodium loads to measure sodium retention is flawed because of variation in water balance. Therefore, rough estimates have been retained in the literature as rules of thumb. These were made up as a concoction from balance studies and theoretical retentions based on the obscure values for body content in infants published in 1900 and 1902 by Camerer and Soldner.[34] Gamble and associates[33] used these data to construct the graph showing theoretical retentions (Fig. 58–22). The maintenance values from these types of studies are 3 mEq Na^+/100 kcal/day, 2 mEq K^+/100 kcal/day, and 2 mEq Cl/100 kcal/day. It should be noted that normal breast milk consumption probably provides somewhat less than this, necessitating virtually complete Na^+ reabsorption by the kidney. Although these values allow for body maintenance, frequently the bodies of normal and ill individuals are subjected to great swings of surfeit and deficit. It is useful to have some reference data on the maximum tolerance for electrolyte loading

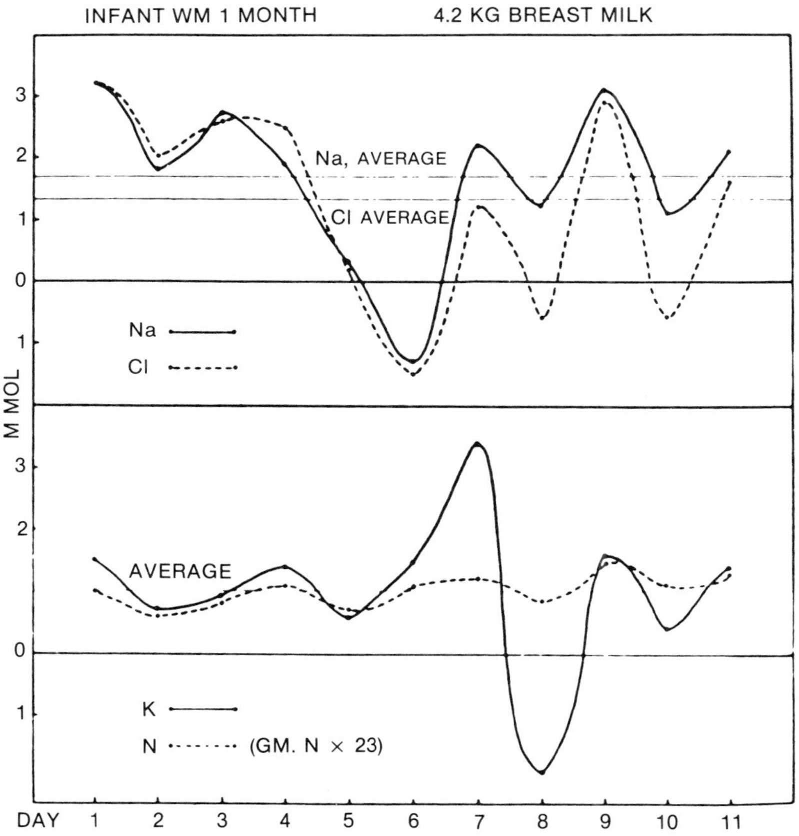

INFANT WM 1 MONTH
4.2 KG BREAST MILK
Na, AVERAGE
Cl AVERAGE
Na
Cl
AVERAGE
K
N (GM. N × 23)
M MOL
DAY

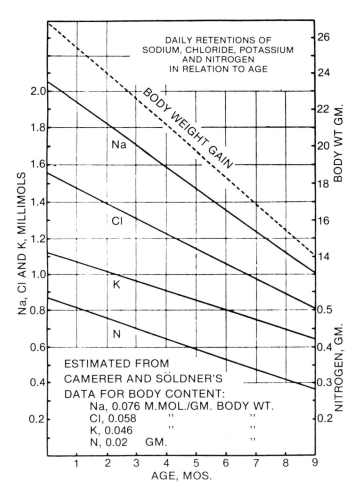

Figure 58–21. Daily balances for sodium chloride, potassium, and nitrogen (corrected for insensible losses). Wallace WM, Eliel L, et al: Effects of large loads of electrolytes. (Reproduced with permission from Gamble JL, Wallace WM, Eliel L, et al: Effects of large loads of electrolytes. Reproduced by permission of Pediatrics Vol. 7, p. 306. Copyright 1951.)

DAILY RETENTIONS OF SODIUM, CHLORIDE, POTASSIUM AND NITROGEN IN RELATION TO AGE
BODY WEIGHT GAIN
Na
Cl
K
N
Na, Cl AND K, MILLIMOLS
BODY WT GM.
NITROGEN, GM.
AGE, MOS.
ESTIMATED FROM CAMERER AND SÖLDNER'S DATA FOR BODY CONTENT:
Na, 0.076 M.MOL./GM. BODY WT.
Cl, 0.058 " "
K, 0.046 " "
N, 0.02 GM. "

Figure 58–22. Daily retentions of sodium, chloride, and potassium in relation to age. (Reproduced with permission from Gamble JL, Wallace WM, Eliel L, et al: Effects of large loads of electrolytes. Reproduced by permission of Pediatrics Vol. 7, p. 310. Copyright 1951.)

and deprivation as a companion to the preceding data on diluting and concentrating capacity.

Figure 58–23 illustrates cumulative balances under conditions of NaCl loading in a 7-month-old infant. The sodium load was 10 mEq/kg/day. Balance was not achieved even at 8 days with persistent sodium retention. ICW decreased in sodium chloride loading and increased dramatically in sodium bicarbonate loading because of increased sodium entry into cells. Potassium similarly accumulated through 6 days of loading, accompanied by a loss of sodium as seen in Figure 58–24.

Such studies led several investigators to define the absolute limit for sodium, potassium, and water for humans. Talbot and associates summarize these limits as follows[35]: Maximum tolerance of sodium is 250 mEq/m²SA/day, potassium is 250 mEq/m²SA/day, and water is 15.7 l/m² SA/day (15 l of urine and 1 l insensible loss − 0.3 l water of oxidation and water of catabolism). Potassium excretion rates can increase to 200 mEq/m² SA/day in about 3 hours, and sodium may be excreted at a rate of 10 to 12 mEq/kg/day.

At the other extreme of total deprivation, sodium excretion is generally reduced to a minimum of 10 mEq/m² SA/day. The process of sodium conservation takes 3 to 5 days to become maximal. Similarly, the urine may be made relatively free of potassium over the same period.[35] The limits of dehydration have been cited by Gamble[32] as 30 to 40% dehydration being incompatible with life.

These data are all based on adult volunteers and patients with a variety of illnesses and should not be routinely applied as reasonable tolerance limits within

which to prescribe parenteral fluids—that is, the tolerance for error in infants and children is not as great as it is in adults.

Barnett and colleagues[36] have shown that even premature infants have no limitations in their ability to dilute urine but rather are limited in water tolerance by the glomerular filtration rate (GFR; discussed later). However, sodium tolerance in the premature infant and newborn is reduced. In a series of studies, Aperia and associates[37–39] showed that the full-term infant was less tolerant to salt administration than was the adult, having about 25% the capacity/kilogram body weight to excrete sodium, with a theoretical maximum of 12 mEq/kg/day. The natriuretic response is somewhat higher in preterm infants but further limited because of an even lower GFR.

It should be mentioned in this discussion of homeostatic limits of water and electrolytes how parenteral glucose came into use. It is not by chance or manufacturing necessity that intravenous solutions frequently contain 5 g of dextrose/100 ml. Gamble,[32] in investigating the renal solute loads of a variety of states was also able to determine that glucose ingestion spared protein catabolism and, surprisingly, reduced sodium losses. He defined the maximum benefit at about 100 g/day in a 70-kg adult, as illustrated in Figure 58–25, which shows cumulative catabolism of protein and intracellular fluid losses (*top*) under conditions of fasting and different glucose intakes and the conservation of sodium and ECW loss (*bottom*). If we use the value of 2,500 ml of water as maintenance, 100 g/2,500 ml = 4 g/100 ml, which is close to the most frequently used intravenous

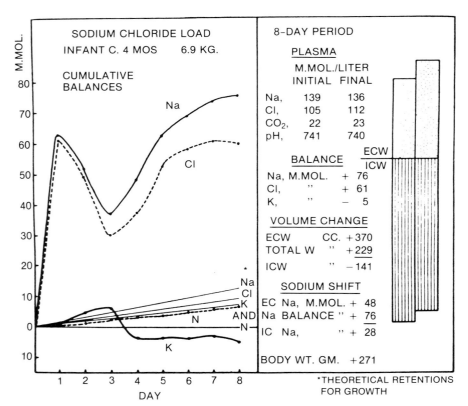

Figure 58–23. Balance of Na⁺, Cl⁻, and K⁺ during NaCl loading (10 mEq/kg/day) of a 4-month-old infant. Note persistent Na⁺ retention at 8 days and loss of K⁺. The fluid balance for ECW and ICW is shown at the beginning and end of experimental period (*left and right bars* respectively). (Reproduced with permission from Gamble JL, Wallace WM, Eliel L, et al: Effects of large loads of electrolytes. Reproduced by permission of Pediatrics Vol. 7, p. 311. Copyright 1951.)

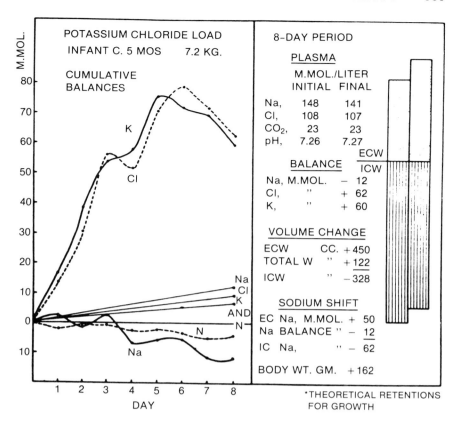

Figure 58–24. Balance of Na⁺, K⁺, and Cl⁻ in KCl loading (10 mEq/kg/day) in a 5-month-old infant, showing potassium retention up through 5 days. *Bars at right* depict ECW and ICW changes (pre-experiment and post experiment conditions on *right and left,* respectively). (Reproduced with permission from Gamble JL, Wallace WM, Eliel L, et al: Effects of large loads of electrolytes. Reproduced by permission of Pediatrics Vol. 7, p. 312. Copyright 1951.)

solution of D_5 today, the manufacturers adding a small buffer of 1 g/100 ml. It should be noted, as stated by Gamble,[32] that this level of intake provides maximum benefit but is capable of reducing protein catabolism by only 50%.

A number of clinical situations occur that may change water, electrolyte, and energy needs. They are summarized in Tables 58–10 and 58–11. A special situation that is often ignored is the renal solute load imposed by physicians using parenteral medications. Table 58–12 lists several medications and the predominant renal solute involved.

Although the concept of GFR has yet to be integrated into systemic mechanisms controlling volume, it is essential to using the preceding graphs and tables as clinical guides, and therefore Table 58–13 is provided as a companion to the other maintenance and homeostatic limit data. It provides a quick reference for creatinine value, GFR, osmolar limits, and fractional excretion of sodium. In addition, a formula developed by Schwartz and associates,[40] based on direct observation, for creatinine clearance is reproduced here:

$$\frac{\text{Creatinine clearance (Ccr)}}{\text{(corrected to 1.73m}^2 \text{ SA)}} = \frac{\text{(height or length in cm) (K)}}{\text{serum creatinine in mg/dl}}$$

$$K = 0.45 \text{ in infants} <1 \text{ year}$$
$$= 0.55 >1 \text{ year}$$

CONTROL OF NORMAL FLUID AND ELECTROLYTE HOMEOSTASIS

Body fluid volume regulation is required for maintainance of life. Although its narrow limits are not intui-

tive, practically they are respected because of the disastrous consequences apparent to clinicians when they are exceeded. Since the 19th century, a unifying hypothesis has been sought that might be verified experimentally and allow for a rational approach to all clinical derangements. It is only in the late 20th century that the number of physical and neurohumoral mediators of volume control has risen to the point at which investigators in the field believe that such hypotheses may be constructed. To pick any comprehensive scheme is risky, however, since many more mediators may yet be discovered, any one of which may be pivotal in the entire scheme. Even for those mediators and mechanisms known, there are few human experimental data in health, let alone disease. However, there must be a starting point to allow for practice in relating clinical situations to the known forces governing body volume and composition.

The starting point will be that proposed by Schrier[41] in which the central hypothesis states that the

arterial circulation is the primary body fluid compartment modulating renal sodium and water excretion. In a 70-kg man, total body water approximates 42 l, of which only 0.7 l or 1.7% resides in the arterial circulation. From a teleologic viewpoint, it is attractive to propose that the primacy for regulation of renal sodium and water excretion (and thus body fluid homeostasis) is modulated by a very small body fluid compartment, such as the arterial circulation. This endows the volume regulatory system with exquisite sensitivity to relatively small changes in body fluid volume, and locates it in the fluid compartment that is responsible for arterial perfusion of the body's vital organs and tissues.

The hypothesis stipulates further that there are two controls on under- or overfilling the arterial circulation:

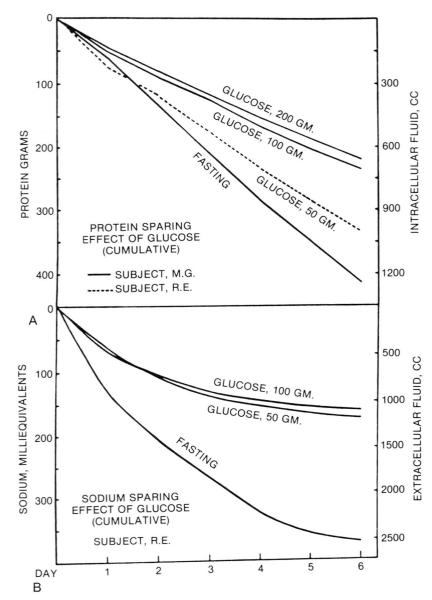

Figure 58–25. *A,* The effect of glucose on sparing catabolism of body protein and reduction in intracellular water loss. *B,* Sodium losses are concomitantly reduced by the addition of glucose to break the fasting state. (Reproduced with permission from Gamble JL: Physiological information gained from studies on the life raft ration. Harvey Lectures 42:264, 1947.)

Table 58–10. CONDITIONS AFFECTING ABNORMAL MAINTENANCE REQUIREMENTS*

Factor Affected	Type of Adjustment to be Made
Insensible water loss requirements	
High environmental humidity	Reduce IWL† to 0–15 ml/100 cal
Hyperventilation	Increase IWL to 50–60 ml/100 cal
Sweat requirements	
Mild to moderate thermal sweating in cystic fibrosis	Increase water allowance by 10–25 ml/100 cal; increase Na⁺ and Cl⁻ allowance by 1–2 mEq/100 cal
Mild to moderate thermal sweating in otherwise normal subject	Increase water allowance by 10–25 ml/100 cal; increase Na⁺ and Cl⁻ allowance by 0.5–1.0 mEq/100 cal
Gastrointestinal losses	
Gastric loss	Replace volume for volume with appropriate solution
Small intestinal loss	Replace volume for volume with appropriate solution
Diarrheal loss	Replace with equal volume of appropriate solution
Mild (10–25 ml/kg/day)	
Moderate (25–50 ml/kg/day)	
Severe (50–75 ml/kg/day)	

*From Winters RW: Regulation of normal water and electrolyte metabolism. *In:* Winters RW (ed): Body Fluids in Pediatrics, p. 131. Boston, Little, Brown and Company, copyright 1973.
†IWL = insensible water loss.

Table 58–11. CONDITIONS RESULTING IN THE ABNORMAL LOSS OF WATER AND ELECTROLYTES*

	Approximate Composition of Fluid Lost in these Circumstances		
	Na (mEq/l)	Cl (mEq/l)	K (mEq/l)
Sweating—heat exhaustion, fever	70	60	15
Gastric fluid—vomiting, fistula, gastric suction	80	150	20
Intestinal fluid—fistula, intestinal, suction diarrhea	130	50	15
Obligatory renal loss of sodium chloride—Addison's disease, salt losing nephritis, (diuresis of ECF†)	140	100	10–30
Acute renal failure	50–150	40–100	20–100
Obligatory renal loss of potassium—diabetes mellitus, chloride deficiency, high sodium–low potassium intake, adrenal overactivity	Low	Low	High
Obligatory renal loss of base-sodium and potassium—specific renal tubular disease, advanced nephritis, acute acidosis Na + K = 110–140	High	Low	High

*From Segar W: Parenteral fluid therapy. Curr Probl Pediatr 3(2):34, 1972.
†ECF = extracellular fluid.

Table 58–12. DRUGS WITH SIGNIFICANT METABOLIC LOADS*

Acid
  Acetazolamide, NH_4Cl, aspirin, methenamine mandelate, ethanol, paraldehyde
Alkali
  Antacids, carbenicillin, plasma protein concentrates, licorice, oral hyperalimentation, tobacco
Creatinine
  Anabolic and androgenic steroids
Magnesium
  Laxatives, antacids
Potassium
  Potassium penicillin (3 mEq/million units), salt substitutes, K-sparing diuretics, neuromuscular blocking agents, blood transfusions, oral hyperalimentation fluid
Sodium
  Ampicillin (3.0 mEq/g), azlocillin (2.7 mEq/g) Carbenicillin (4.7 mEq/g), cephalothin (2.4 mEq/g) Kayexalate (1.5 mEq/g), mezlocillin (1.9 mEq/g) Moxalactam (3.8 mEq/g), piperacillin (1.9 mEq/g) Ticarcillin (5.2 mEq/g), antacids, oral hyperalimentation fluids
Urea
  Glucocorticosteroids, tetracyclines, hyperalimentation, protein
Water
  Nonsteroidal anti-inflammatory drugs, oral hypoglycemics, clofibrate, cyclophosphamide, carbamazepine, vincristine, narcotics

*From Golper T and Bennett W. Drug usage in dialysis patients. *In:* Nissenson AR, Fine RN, and Gentile DE: Clinical Dialysis. Norwalk CT, Appleton & Lange, 1990, p. 613.

cardiac output and perpherial arterial resistance. (It should be noted that it is assumed in the hypothesis that no intrinsic renal disease exists.)

It follows then that all sodium and water retaining states will result from decreased cardiac output or reduced peripheral arterial resistance. These situations and their consequences are schematized, respectively, in Figures 58–26 and 58–27. Many clinical conditions seen in patients in ward and intensive care units may be reviewed in the context of these figures. It is clear that arterial underfilling in either scenario will be followed by rapid activation of the renin-angiotensin-aldosterone system, increased sympathetic nervous system activity, and nonosmotically stimulated release of vasopressin. The sympathetic nervous system is likely the major integrator because it is involved in stimulating the supraoptic and paraventricular nuclei of the hypothala-

mus,[42] as well as the renin-angiotensin-aldosterone system via β-adrenergic activity.[43] Differentiating between which sequence of events is occurring in a given patient is critical to appropriate intervention, but this may be very difficult to do based on conventional clinical approaches such as measurement of mean arterial pressure, cardiac output, and peripheral vascular resistance. This is because they are measured after compensatory responses have occurred.

Schrier[41] outlines the clinical dilemma as follows: "volume expansion with arterial overfilling is associated with an increase in cardiac output and a secondary decrease in peripheral vascular resistance so that the steady state mean arterial pressure may be within the normal range. On the other hand, primary peripheral arterial vasodilation may cause arterial underfilling with a secondary increase in cardiac output and a steady state

Table 58–13. NORMAL VALUES OF RENAL FUNCTION*

Age	GFR (Ml/min/1.73 m²)	Renal Blood Flow (Ml/min/1.73 m²)	Maximal Urine Osmolality (mOsm/kg)	Serum Creatinine (Mg/dl)	Fractional Excretion† of Sodium (%)
Newborn					
Premature‡	14 ± 3	40 ± 6	480	1.3	2–5
Full term	21 ± 4	88 ± 4	800	1.1	<1
1–2 wk	50 ± 10	220 ± 40	900	0.4	<1
6 mo–1 yr	77 ± 14	352 ± 73	1,200	0.2	<1
1–3 yr	96 ± 22	540 ± 118	1,400	0.4	<1
Adult	118 ± 18	620 ± 92	1,400	0.8–1.5	<1

*From Avner ED, Ellis D, Ichikawa I, et al: Normal neonates and the maturational development of homeostatic mechanisms. *In:* Ichikawa I (ed): Pediatric Textbook of Fluids and Electrolytes, p. 109. © 1990, the Williams & Wilkins Co., Baltimore.
†Fractional excretion of sodium (Fe Na$^+$ %) = $\frac{Una/Pna}{Uu/Pcr} \times 100\%$
‡Of 32 to 34 weeks' gestation.

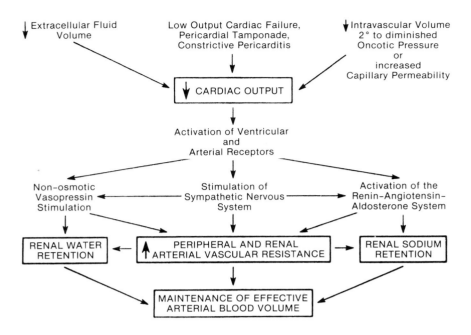

Figure 58–26. The sequence of physiologic changes in which reduced cardiac output is the initiating event. (Reproduced with permission from Schrier RW: Body fluid volume regulation in health and disease: A unifying hypothesis. Ann Intern Med 113:156, 1990.)

blood pressure within the normal range," that is, they are clinically indistinguishable. However, in arterial overfilling, the neurohumoral profile will be suppressed, whereas in the circumstance of arterial underfilling, the neurohumoral profile will be stimulated (Fig. 58–28). (Note this does not deal with differentiating arterial underfilling as a result of decreased cardiac output or increased arterial vasodilatation.) The neurohumoral

mechanisms outlined are rapid in onset. The renal sodium and water retention is slower to make a contribution to restoration of the arterial volume. It is logical to assume that the neurohumoral stimulation leads to this salt and water retention as a consequence of renal vasoconstriction. This leads to decreased sodium and water delivery to the distal nephron, allowing more complete sodium and water retention via aldosterone

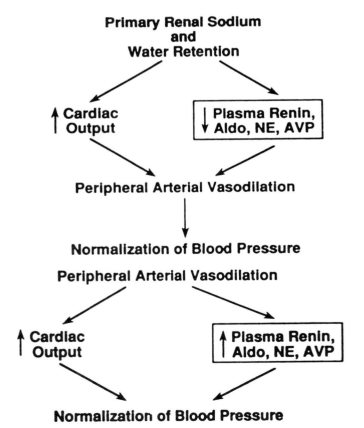

Figure 58–27. Sequence of physiologic changes in which peripheral arterial vasodilatation is the initiating event. (Reproduced with permission from Schrier RW: Body fluid volume regulation in health and disease: A unifying hypothesis. Ann Intern Med 113:156, 1990.)

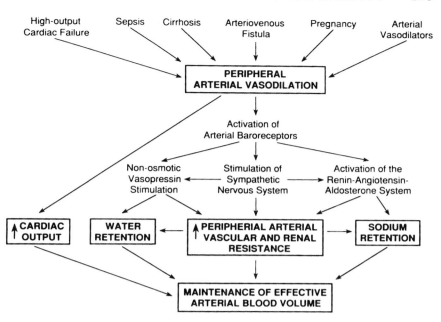

Figure 58–28. Neurohumoral and hemodynamic profiles. *Top sequence* for increased arterial blood volume. *Bottom sequence* for reduced arterial blood volume. While the blood pressure, cardiac output, and vascular resistance may be the same in the two states, the neurohumoral profile and urinary sodium and water excretion distinguish the two conditions. (Aldo = aldosterone; NE = norepinephrine; AVP = arginine vasopressin.) (Reproduced with permission from Schrier RW: Body fluid volume regulation in health and disease: A unifying hypothesis. Ann Intern Med 113:157, 1990.)

and vasopressin effects. It also causes the action of atrial natriuretic peptide, which exerts its natriuretic activity at the level of the collecting duct, to be less evident.

To carry this further, normal individuals encounter states leading to arterial underfilling—for example; dehydration—which activates the neurohumoral mechanisms that lead to salt and water retention. However, escape from aldosterone activity takes place as the increased circulatory volume leads to increased cardiac output. This leads to increased filtered sodium and subsequent increased distal sodium delivery overcoming and reducing aldosterone, whereas the filling of the arterial circuit decreases stimulation of the neurohumoral mechanisms. In edema-forming states, the cardiac output never increases, so the neurohumoral profile remains that of intense sodium and water retention and increasing edema. Figure 58–29 illustrates these two

sequences. The nature of the mediators that cause persistence of vasodilatation in a broad range of clinical states remains to be identified. Many have been proposed, including prostaglandin, endotoxin, and endorphin.

Guyton[22] has provided a relevant figure (Fig. 58–30) that serves as a reminder of the rapidity of onset of the different mechanisms the body has to combat arterial underfilling. Some of the individual clinical parameters and neurohumoral effectors will now be examined in more detail.

Blood Pressure

Without detailing the determinants of arterial and venous pressure, some sense of the normal pressures is

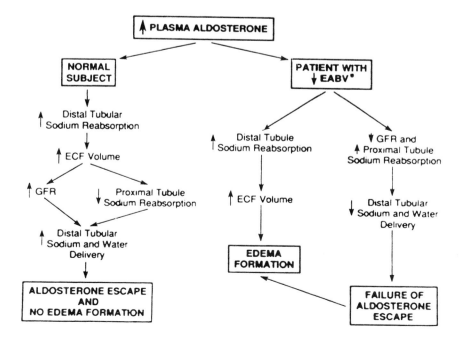

Figure 58–29. Summary of physiologic changes involved in "escape" from aldosterone effect in normal subjects *(left)* and inability to "escape" in patients with arterial underfilling *(right)*. (Reproduced with permission from Schrier RW: Body fluid volume regulation in health and disease: A unifying hypothesis. Ann Intern Med 113:158, 1990.)

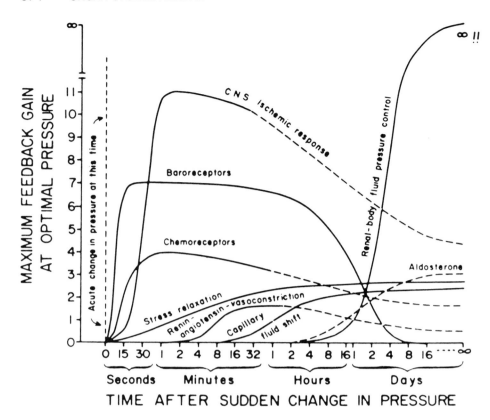

Figure 58–30. Time of onset and relative strength of various control mechanisms for arterial pressure. (Reproduced from Guyton AC: Textbook of Medical Physiology, 5th ed., Philadelphia, WB Saunders, 1976, p. 279.)

useful, as is the effect of posture on them. Figure 58–31 provides a convenient schematic of changes in pressure based solely on body position, and the progressive decline in pressure through the entire circulatory system is illustrated in Figure 58–32.

Arginine Vasopressin

Increased plasma osmolality with or without hypotension leads to arginine vasopressin (AVP) release. Figure 58–33 shows the relationship of AVP release to increasing plasma osmolality in healthy adults, with the line defining both a threshold and measure of sensitivity (slope) of this mechanism. Figure 58–34 illustrates the change in both threshold and sensitivity of osmolality that volume changes exert. It can be appreciated that volume depletion lowers the threshold and increases the sensitivity and that the converse is true of volume expansion. High osmolality and volume depletion are the most potent stimuli to AVP release.

Thirst is an ironic clinical phenomenon in the context of the volume and osmolal stimuli to AVP release. Thirst is apparent when osmolality has already risen to

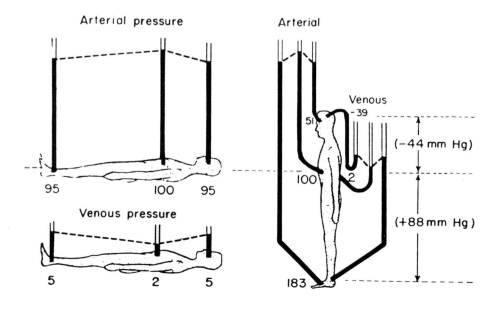

Figure 58–31. Effect of posture on arterial and venous pressures (in mm Hg). (Reproduced with permission from Burton AC: Physiology and Biophysics of the Circulation, 2nd ed, Chicago, Year Book Medical Publishers, 1972.)

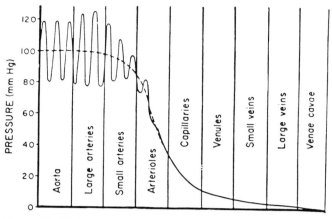

Figure 58-32. Blood pressure across the entire circulatory circuit. (Reproduced with permission from Guyton AC: Textbook of Medical Physiology, 5th ed. Philadelphia, WB Saunders, 1976, p. 238.)

a point at which AVP is released and causes maximum urine osmolality. It is possible that the thirst receptor is distinct from hypothalamic osmoreceptors. This is supported by experiments in which volume is reduced, with osmolality remaining unchanged.[44] The common mediator may be angiotensin.[45] Several stimuli are also known to release AVP without osmolality changes. Table 58-14 provides a reference checklist covering a large range of medications and clinical states that may cause or suppress release of AVP.

A nonhomeostatic increase in AVP is termed *the syndrome of inappropriate antidiuretic hormone (SIADH)*, whereas the lack of AVP is known as *diabetes insipidus (DI)*. These conditions will now be examined.

Syndrome of Inappropriate Diuretic Hormone

SIADH is usually identified as a diagnosis of exclusion. It is self-evident that it represents a nonphysiolog-

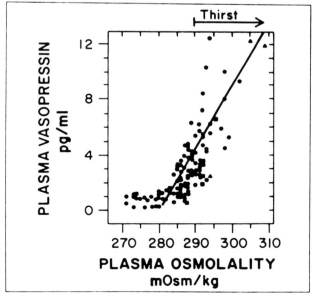

Figure 58-33. Plasma vasopressin plotted against plasma osmolality. Note that vasopressin levels are already significantly elevated prior to awareness of thirst. (Reproduced with permission from Robertson GL, et al: Am J Med 72:334, 1982.)

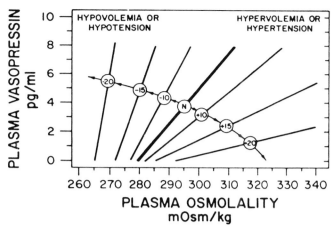

Figure 58-34. Influence of volume on osmoregulation of vasopressin release. The thick line is the relationship with normal blood volume. Note the threshold and sensitivity *(slope)*. Hypovolemia decreases the threshold and increases the sensitivity, whereas volume overload has the opposite effect. (Reproduced with permission from Robertson GL et al: Neurogenic disorders of osmoregulation. Am J Med 72:339, 1982.)

ically increased release of adrenocorticotropic hormone (ADH). Hyponatremia is a constant feature. Persistent elevation of AVP renders the urine inappropriately concentrated and causes retention of ingested water; clinically, however, this is not reflected in edema because most of the water increase occurs in the intracellular space. Urine sodium losses reflect intake and generally exceed 20 mEq/l, but if sodium is restricted in these individuals, urinary sodium levels may be less than 10 mEq/l. It is impossible to isolate a discussion of SIADH from the overall approach to hyponatremic states. There are many satisfactory algorithms and one of them is reproduced in Figure 58-35. This figure takes the clinician stepwise through the possibilities. Tables 58-15 and 58-16 overlap and expand upon Table 58-14, classifying antidiuretic drugs according to clinical action and a rather exhaustive list of clinical conditions in which SIADH should be considered.

Therapy for this disorder consists of eliminating known nonphysiologic stimuli that are augmenting secretion of AVP. To deal with the hyponatremia itself is

Table 58-14. NONOSMOLAL FACTORS AFFECTING THE RELEASE OF ARGININE VASOPRESSIN*

Stimulatory	Inhibitory
Hypovolemia	Hypervolemia
Pain	α-Adrenergic agonists
Emotional stress	Atrial tachycardia
Nausea	Left atrial distention
Hypoxia	Ethanol
β-Adrenergic agonists	Phenytoin
Renin-angiotensin system	Chlorpromazine
Portal hypertension	Reserpine
Cholinergic agonists	
Vincristine	
Clofibrate	
Chlorpropamide	
Tricyclic antidepressants	
Nicotine	

*From Yared A: Regulation of plasma osmolality. *In:* Ichikawa I: Pediatric Textbook of Fluids and Electrolytes, p. 68. © 1990, the Williams & Wilkins Co., Baltimore.

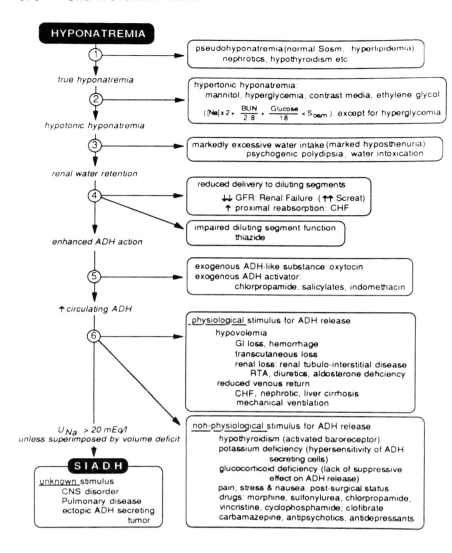

Figure 58–35. Diagnostic evaluation of hyponatremia, showing a stepwise approach to the diagnosis of syndrome of inappropriate ADH (SIADH). (Reproduced with permission from Yared A, et al: *In*: Ichikawa I [ed]: Pediatric Textbook of Fluids and Electrolytes, p. 176. © 1990, the Williams & Wilkins Co., Baltimore.)

a more tedious process. First fluid is restricted; the total fluid allowed does not exceed urine output plus a reasonable estimate of insensible loss. If the urine sodium level is less than 20 mEq/l, the patient may have been on reduced sodium intake, and extra care must be used to ensure adequate and usually supranormal sodium amounts. In practice, fluid restriction using isotonic saline with dextrose as a fluid source allows for a slow rise in the sodium level. Hypertonic NaCl solutions are reserved for the symptomatic patient. They may be used in conjunction with loop diuretics that increase free water excretion as a function of larger urine volumes (furosemide actually impairs the maximal free water clearance, but when the total urine output is very high, the absolute amount of free water excreted increases). These hypertonic saline and loop diuretic combinations are extremely dangerous. Regardless of which therapy is chosen, it will be the responsibility of the physician to control the rate of sodium rise to no more than 1 to 2 mEq/hr. Rates in excess of this have led to severe neurologic deterioration and death.[45] Modest goals should be to increase sodium levels in symptomatic patients quickly to greater than 120 mEq/l. In those patients in whom the sodium level is greater than 120

mEq/l, the rate of rise should not exceed the guidelines given previously.

Volume expansion has been suggested to cause aldosterone suppression in SIADH, and deoxycorticosterone acetate has been advocated as an additional therapy[46] but is not routinely recommended. Most of the volume expansion is not extracellular.

Usually the process is transient, and these therapeutic maneuvers suffice. Occasionally there is a patient in whom the problem is persistent. Fluid restriction in infants and children under these conditions is intolerable in the long term because of caloric deprivation. This has led to sodium supplementation of formula as a more reasonable long-term regimen. This has been augmented with loop diuretics as well. Lithium and demeclocycline, which have effectively suppressed AVP in adults with SIADH, are not routinely prescribed in childhood.

Diabetes Insipidus

The opposite problem is created with a lack of AVP or lack of responsiveness to it. The acute onset of DI is at times seen in the ICU, generally as a result of recent brain injury. This can occur as a result of accidental

Table 58-15. ANTIDIURETIC DRUGS*

Antidiuretic Hormones and Analogues
  Vasopressin
  Oxytocin
  1-Desamino-8-D-arginine vasopressin (dDAVP)

Diuretics
  Thiazide
  Furosemide
  Ethacrynic acid
  Bumetanide

Central Nervous System Active Drugs
  Vincristine
  Carbamazepine
  Psychotropic drugs
  Opiates
  Isoproterenol
  Nicotine

Inhibitors of Prostaglandin Synthesis
  Chlorpropamide and other sulfonylureas
  Salicylates
  Nonsteroidal anti-inflammatory drugs

Others
  Clofibrate
  Cyclophosphamide
  Colchicine

*From Morrison G and Singer I: Hyperosmolal states. In: Maxwell MH, Kleeman CR, and Narins RG (eds): Clinical Disorders of Fluid and Electrolyte Metabolism. New York, McGraw-Hill, 1987, p. 467. © 1987, reproduced with permission of McGraw-Hill, Inc.

injury, surgical trauma, or brain ischemia and is frequently associated with increased intracranial pressure. A striking increase in output of an extremely dilute-appearing urine is often the presenting manifestation. This is associated with a rapid rise in serum sodium levels, at times to extreme levels.

Early diagnosis and aggressive treatment is required to prevent the large swings in sodium and fluid balance frequently seen. Hourly urine replacement with an equal volume of dilute IV fluid (e.g., 0.20% NS) in addition to maintenance fluids may be undertaken, but often becomes problematic as tremendous volumes of fluid replacement may be required. Dextrose-containing solutions should not be used as hyperglycemia will ensue leading to further diuresis.

Cautious therapy with hormonal replacement (see Table 58–20) has become increasingly accepted and is less cumbersome than fluid replacement. The dose of hormone given should be titrated upward to decrease urine output to that normally expected. As urine output falls, IV fluids should be decreased to provide renal and insensible losses with a small additional amount as necessary to correct hypernatremia and the previously accumulated fluid deficit. Frequent accounting of fluid balance and serum electrolyte values is mandatory as therapy proceeds. As usual the underlying process responsible for DI should be treated if possible.

Chronic DI is relatively more easy to diagnose because the hallmarks are hypernatremia, thirst, polydipsia, polyuria, and failure to thrive. Frequently in childhood, DI is hereditary. There are many hereditary forms of nephrogenic DI, x-linked recessive being the most frequent. The obligate heterozygote mothers may be partially affected. It is important to make the diagnosis early because prevention of dehydration is critical to preventing neurologic damage. If the history and initial clinical laboratory presentation are not striking, a water deprivation test should be performed. This test is dangerous; it must be done in the hospital and if all water sources are not controlled (for the ambulatory child), it is often inconclusive because of surreptitious water ingestion. The patient is placed on a nothing by mouth regimen; and after initial weight determination, plasma and urine osmolality and plasma and urine sodium measurements are done hourly, along with weight and urine volume determinations. The test is terminated if more than or equal to 3% of body weight is lost, the sodium level is greater than or equal to 150 mEq/l, serum osmolality is greater than 300 mOsm/kg, or urine osmolality does not increase by 30 mOsm/kg in two successive collections. At this time, the serum ADH level is checked and 5 units aqueous pitressin is given subcutaneously, or with careful administration, 10 µg of 1-desamino-8-D-arginine vasopressin (DDAVP) is given intranasally. This is followed by two consecutive 30-minute urine collections for specific gravity and osmo-

Table 58-16. DISORDERS ASSOCIATED WITH THE SYNDROME OF INAPPROPRIATE ANTIDIURETIC HORMONE SECRETION*

Neoplasms
  Bronchogenic carcinoma
  Carcinoma of the duodenum
  Carcinoma of pancreas
  Thymona
  Carcinoma of the ureter
  Lymphoma
  Ewing sarcoma
  Mesothelioma
  Carcinoma of the bladder
  Prostatic carcinoma

Pulmonary Disorders
  Pneumonia (viral or bacterial)
  Pulmonary abscess
  Tuberculosis
  Aspergillosis
  Positive pressure breathing
  Asthma
  Pneumothorax
  Cystic fibrosis

Central Nervous System Disorders
  Encephalitis (viral or bacterial)
  Meningitis (viral, bacterial, tuberculous, fungal)
  Head trauma
  Brain abscess
  Brain tumors
  Guillain-Barré syndrome
  Acute intermittent porphyria
  Subarachnoid hemorrhage or subdural hematoma
  Cerebellar and cerebral atrophy
  Cavernous sinus thrombosis
  Neonatal hypoxia
  Hydrocephalus
  Shy-Drager syndrome
  Rocky Mountain spotted fever
  Delirium tremens
  Cerebrovascular accident (cerebral thrombosis or hemorrhage)
  Acute psychosis
  Peripheral neuropathy
  Multiple sclerosis

*From Morrison G and Singer I: Hyperosmolal states. In: Maxwell MH, Kleeman CR, and Narins RG (eds): Clinical Disorders of Fluid and Electrolyte Metabolism. New York, McGraw-Hill, 1987, p. 468. © 1987, reproduced with permission of McGraw-Hill, Inc.

lality with accompanying serum osmolality determinations.

The response determines the diagnosis, as shown in Figure 58–36. If central DI is suspected, studies looking for a central nervous system (CNS) lesion should then be performed. Many cases of central DI are idiopathic; however, some have a defined inheritance pattern, usually autosomal dominant or x-linked recessive. A more exhaustive list of central DI disease associations is seen in Table 58–17.

Of the patients with nephrogenic DI, the history may again point toward an x-linked recessive pattern. Table 58–18 expands the list to include many clinically important conditions.

In the older child, particularly if CNS injury is present, compulsive water drinking may be difficult to discern from nephrogenic DI. Table 58–19 provides several criteria to help discriminate compulsive water drinking from central and nephrogenic DI.

Treatment in all cases of DI may be helped by restricting sodium but not water intake. The less sodium filtered, the less obligatory urinary water loss. In central DI, hormonal replacement is the key, as shown in Table 58–20. Specific treatment of nephrogenic DI does not exist; however, diuretics have made an improvement (used at customary doses for diuretic effect, usually thiazides) because volume depletion may lead to more avid proximal tubular resorption of sodium. Prostaglandin synthetase inhibitors are also useful, but the precise mechanism of action remains unknown.

Renin-Angiotensin-Aldosterone System

The active substrates and products of the renin-angiotensin-aldosterone system are shown in Figure 58–37. The action of the enzyme renin on angiotensinogen

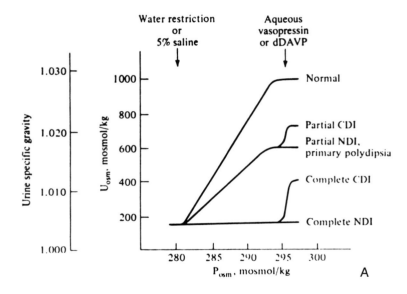

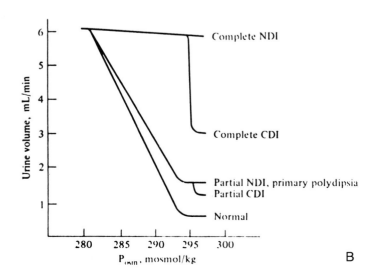

Figure 58–36. Evaluation of water deprivation test in suspected cases of diabetes insipidus. A, The changes in urine osmolality with aqueous pitressin administration are shown. B, The change in urine volume with the pitressin administration is shown. (Reproduced with permission from Rose BD: Clinical Physiology of Acid-Base and Electrolyte Disorders. New York, McGraw-Hill, 1989, p. 532.)

Table 58–17. ETIOLOGY OF CENTRAL DIABETES INSIPIDUS (CDI)*

Acquired	Granulomas
Posthypophysectomy	Histiocytosis X
Post-trauma	Eosinophilic granuloma
Tumors (intracranial):	Schüller-Christian disease
Primary	Sarcoidosis
Craniopharyngioma	Drugs
Pinealoma	Clonidine
Pituitary adenoma	Phencyclidine
Secondary (metastatic)	Idiopathic syndromes
Breast	Autoimmune diseases
Leukemia	Hereditary
Infections	X-linked
Encephalitis	Congenital anomalies
Meningitis	
Guillain-Barré syndrome	
Vascular disorders	
Hypoxia	
Aneurysms	
Sheehan syndrome	

*From Morrison G and Singer I: *In:* Maxwell MH, Kleeman CR, and Narins RG (eds): Clinical Disorders of Fluid and Electrolyte Metabolism. New York, McGraw-Hill, 1987, p. 492. © 1987, reproduced with permission of McGraw-Hill, Inc.

causes angiotensin I to be formed and subsequently angiotensin II via the action of converting enzyme.

Many stimuli influence renin release, as seen in Table 58–21. The action of angiotensin II is that of a potent vasoconstrictor, which increases renal efferent arteriolar resistance, restoring glomerular capillary hydraulic pressure and GFR.

Aldosterone secretion is dependent upon angiotensin II, adrenocorticotropin, sodium depletion, and hemorrhagic or other acute volume losses.

The GFR is a prime determinant of volume control. The forces acting on the individual glomerular capillaries are illustrated in Figure 58–38. Both schematic and diagrammatic forms are seen, showing the relative contribution of hydrostatic pressure and colloid osmotic

Table 58–18. CAUSES OF NEPHROGENIC DIABETES INSIPIDUS*

Congenital
Acquired
  Chronic renal disease
    Polycystic kidney disease
    Medullary cystic disease
    Pyelonephritis
    Obstruction
    Chronic renal failure
    Uric acid or calcium nephropathy
  Electrolyte disorders
    Hypokalemia
    Hypercalcemia
  Sickle cell trait
  Adrenal insufficiency
  Drugs (lithium, colchicine, vinblastine, radiocontrast agents, diuretics)
  Dietary abnormalities
    Protein starvation
    Chronic salt depletion
    Chronic high water intake

*From Yared A, Foose J, and Ichikawa I: Disorders of osmoregulation. *In:* Ichikawa I (ed): Pediatric Textbook of Fluids and Electrolytes, p. 172. © 1990, the Williams & Wilkins Co., Baltimore.

Table 58–19. CLINICAL FEATURES IN THE DIFFERENTIAL DIAGNOSIS OF DIABETES INSIPIDUS VERSUS PSYCHOGENIC POLYDIPSIA*

Feature	CDI†	NDI‡	PWD§
Onset of polyuria	Sudden	Variable	Variable
Urine volume	Large	Variable	Variable
Nocturine	+ + + +	+ + +	+
Preference for iced water	+ + + +	±	±
Serum osmolality	N/high	N/high	N/low

*From Yared A, Foose J, and Ichikawa I: Disorders of osmoregulation. *In:* Ichikawa I (ed): Pediatric Textbook of Fluids and Electrolytes, p. 169. © 1990, the Williams & Wilkins Co., Baltimore.
  †CDI = central diabetes insipidus.
  ‡NDI = nephrogenic diabetes insipidus.
  §PWD = psychogenic water drinking.

pressure. One essential feature is the balance of forces such that there is no net ultrafiltration at the efferent arteriolar end. A dramatic consequence of this balance is the clinical situation in which the plasma colloid osmotic pressure is artificially increased because of infusion of dextran[47] or hyperoncotic albumin solution.[48] This leads to total anuria when the colloid osmotic pressure exceeds 35 mm Hg. Urine formation resumes within minutes of the colloid osmotic pressure decreasing to less than 30 mm Hg.

Atrial Natriuretic Peptide

Atrial natriuretic peptide (ANP) is a recently discovered peptide with profound influence on volume control. It results in natriuresis, decrease in arterial pressure, and inhibition of the renin-angiotensin-aldosterone system.[49] The control of its secretion from cardiac atria seems to be governed in part by cardiac filling pressure.[50] In the spectrum from normal through cardiovascular disease without increased filling pressure to cardiovascular disease with increased filling pressure to increased filling pressure and congestive heart failure, there is a steady increase in ANP (Fig. 58–39). The failure of this increase in ANP to cause natriuresis has remained unexplained. It is clear that ANP inhibits angiotensin II–stimulated proximal sodium and water reabsorp-

Table 58–20. DRUGS USED IN THE TREATMENT OF CENTRAL DIABETES INSIPIDUS*

Drug	Dose	Duration of Action
Hormone replacement		
Aqueous vasopressin	5–10 units SC†	3–6 hr
Lysine vasopressin	2–4 units IV‡	4–6 hr
Vasopressin tannate in oil	1–5 units IM§	24–72 hr
DDAVP	5–20 μg IN‖	12–24 hr
Nonhormonal agents		
Chlorpropamide	1 g/m²/day	Divided tid

*From Yared A, Foose J, and Ichikawa I: Disorders of osmoregulation. *In:* Ichikawa I (ed): Pediatric Textbook of Fluids and Electrolytes, p. 173. © 1990, the Williams & Wilkins Co., Baltimore.
  †SC = subcutaneous.
  ‡IV = intravenous.
  §IM = intramuscular.
  ‖IN = intranasal.

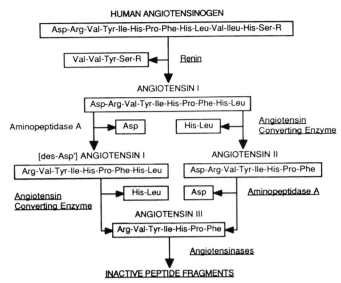

Figure 58–37. Renin-angiotensin metabolic pathway in man. (Reproduced with permission from Ingelfinger J. *In:* Ichikawa I [ed]: Pediatric Textbook of Fluids and Electrolytes, p. 59. © 1990, the Williams & Wilkins Co., Baltimore.)

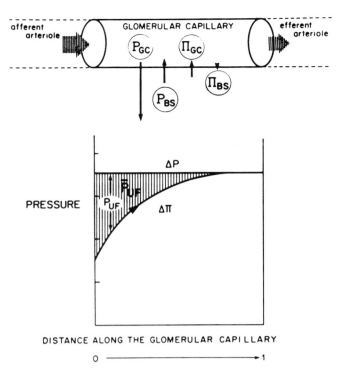

Figure 58–38. Schematic of glomerular capillary filtration. In the top figure, filtration is seen to be a result of the sum of forces including glomerular capillary hydraulic pressure (P_{GC}), hydraulic pressure in Bowman's space (P_{BS}), glomerular capillary oncotic pressure (πGC), and Bowman's space oncotic pressure (πBS). The arrow length reflects the relative potency of each force. In the bottom graph, the net ultrafiltration pressure (*shaded area*) is greatest at the beginning of the glomerular capillary and decreases along it due to loss of colloid-free solution from plasma as filtrate. This leads to increasing πGC, balancing P_{GC} and therefore no net ultrafiltration pressure near the efferent arteriole. (Reproduced with permission from Ichikawa I and Yared A. *In:* Holliday MA, Barratt TM, and Vernier RL [eds]: Pediatric Nephrology, 2nd ed, p. 47. © 1987, the Williams & Wilkins Co., Baltimore.)

tion;[51] however, therapeutic trials of exogenous ANP[52, 53] have shown decreased vascular resistance and increased GFR but no substantial diuretic-natriuretic response. Berg and colleagues[54] have provided an elegant explanation for this, showing that ANP is rapidly metabolized by a nonsaturable degradative neutral endopeptidase (NEP) present in brush border vesicles of the proximal tubule. Inhibition of this degradative enzyme is now

Table 58–21. FACTORS INFLUENCING RENIN RELEASE*

Increase in Renin Release
Drugs
  Vasodilators
  Diuretics
  β-Adrenergic stimulators
  EDTA (via calcium efflux)
Hormones
  Glucagon
  Prostaglandins
  Norepinephrine and other catecholamines
Diet
  Na deprivation or loss

Decrease in Renin Release
Drugs
  β-Adrenergic blockers
  Mineralocorticoids
  α-Adrenergic stimulators
  Lanthanum
Hormones
  Mineralocorticoids
  Vasopressin
  Angiotensin
  Atrial natriuretic factor (ANF)
Diet
  Salt load

*From Ingelfinger JR. Hypertension and hypotension. *In:* Ichikawa I (ed): Pediatric Textbook of Fluids and Electrolytes, p. 60. © 1990, the Williams & Wilkins Co., Baltimore.

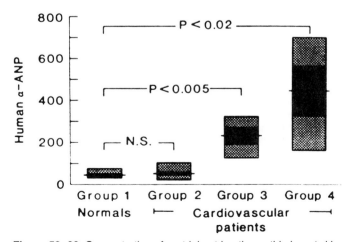

Figure 58–39. Concentration of α-atrial natriuretic peptide in pg/ml in normal adults and in patients with heart disease. Group 1 = heart disease without increased atrial filling pressure; group 2 = heart disease with increased atrial filling pressure; group 3 = heart disease with increased filling pressure and congestive heart failure. (Reproduced with permission from Burnett JC, et al: Atrial natriuretic peptide elevation in congestive heart failure in the human. Science 231:1146, 1986. Copyright 1986 by the AAAS.)

possible, and designer enzyme inhibitors have been synthesized (e.g., NEP-I [SQ28,603], Squibb Institute for Medical Research, Princeton, NJ). In an animal model of congestive heart failure, NEP-I produced a significant diuresis-natriuresis that was not dependent on increased GFR or renal blood flow and did not parallel increases in serum ANP and did not lead to any significant change in renal hemodynamics (Fig. 58–40).

Endothelin

A peptide that has recently been discovered and characterized is endothelin,[55] which is secreted from vascular endothelium. It is perhaps the most potent vasoconstrictor yet known. Its interaction and relative importance compared with angiotensin II and other mediators remains to be sorted out. It may also play an important role in perpetuating ischemia in acute renal failure.[56]

ROUTINE INTENSIVE CARE UNIT REQUIREMENTS

Although some may consider fluid and electrolyte homeostasis a mundane aspect of pediatric critical care,

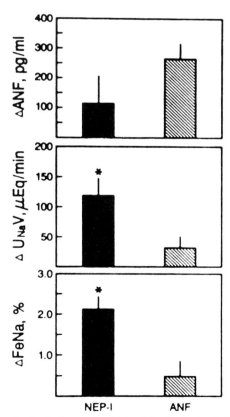

Figure 58–40. Peak change in atrial natriuretic factor (ANF), urinary Na⁺ excretion (U$_{Na}$V), and fractional excretion of Na⁺ (FE$_{Na}$) in patients with congestive heart failure when given neutral endopeptidase inhibitor (NEP-I). (Reproduced with permission from Cavero PG, Margulies KB, Winaver J, et al: Cardiorenal actions of ventral endopeptidase inhibition in experimental congestive heart failure. Circulation 82:199, 1990. By permission of the American Heart Association, Inc.)

Table 58–22. PEDIATRIC FLUID AND ELECTROLYTE REQUIREMENTS

Fluid
(1) 100 ml/kg for first 10 kg +
    50 ml/kg for next 10 kg +
    20 ml/kg greater than 20 kg = daily requirement
                        OR
(2) 4 ml/kg for first 10 kg +
    2 ml/kg for next 10 kg
    1 ml/kg greater than 20 kg = hourly fluid requirement
                        OR
(3) 1500 ml/m²/day

Electrolytes
Sodium, 3–4 mEq/kg/day
Potassium, 2–3 mEq/kg/day
Chloride, 2–3 mEq/kg/day
Calcium, 150–500 mg/kg/day
Phosphorus, 0.5–2 mmol/kg/day
Magnesium, 0.25–0.5 mEq/kg/day

it represents the mileau in which all physiologic activities are carried out. Minor aberrations of fluid and electrolyte balance, though apparently tolerated by the routine patient, may have serious impact on the outcome of the severely ill child. The morbidity associated with prolonged admission to the intensive care unit (ICU) and maintenance of invasive support measures may not be apparent to the casual observer; however, they are at times striking to the bedside intensive care specialist. The child who becomes markedly hypokalemic as a result of excessive diuresis has suffered an iatrogenic event. Likewise, the child who did not undergo a proper diuresis, leading to an extra day of mechanical ventilation and acquisition of a nosocomial pneumonia, has also suffered an iatrogenic event, with increased use of limited resources, along with morbidity and potential mortality. Meticulous attention to fluid and electrolyte homeostasis may lessen physiologic fluctuations and result in a more stable and shortened course in the ICU.

Table 58–22 outlines the commonly used methods of calculating routine fluid and electrolyte requirements for the pediatric patient. They are derived from estimation of caloric requirements, as described earlier in this chapter. The observations in Table 58–22 were made on healthy children with normal activity levels, and as can be seen from Figure 58–15, they differ from those of the hospitalized pediatric patient. These variations are even further magnified in the critically ill pediatric patient by a number of physiologic and pathologic considerations.

Fluid balance must be evaluated for each patient on a daily basis because alterations from predicted requirements occur commonly in the ICU. The acutely ill patient may require even more frequent assessment. Hourly running totals of measured intake and output with a consideration of insensible fluid losses are essential for precise fluid management. Although daily patient weight determinations are perhaps helpful in determining TBW changes, they may be unrelated to the most important variable—adequacy of intravascular volume. Moving patients from the bed to a scale not only risks loss of indwelling devices and monitors but also may result in unwanted physiologic changes in the critically ill child. Repeated careful physical examination of the severely ill patient should allow diagnosis of increased or decreased TBW without measuring weight. Adequacy of intravascular volume must be assessed independantly by clinical examination and laboratory and invasive measurements.

An appreciation of the significance and variability of insensible water loss is required to fully assess fluid homeostasis in the ICU setting. Insensible losses, normally accounting for approximately one third of calculated maintenance fluid requirements, may vary substantially in pathologic conditions. Respiratory losses, which routinely account for one third of insensible losses, increase with tachypnea and in dry environmental settings and may double in these situations (see Fig. 58–16). Provision of humidified gas by tent or face mask markedly decreases respiratory losses. Fully humidified gases, generally provided with mechanical ventilation, should ablate respiratory losses and may result in net positive fluid balance. Therefore, after fluid homeostasis has been obtained, the ventilated child should require 10 to 15% less than calculated maintenance requirements. A SIADH-like syndrome has been noted in some mechanically ventilated patients and may require even further reductions in fluid administration.

Transdermal water loss accounts for two thirds of normal insensible losses. Fever increases losses by 10% per degree Centigrade. Radiant warmers and exposure of the skin to air movement increase both evaporative and conductive losses. Loss of skin integrity as a result of abrasions, toxic epidermal necrolysis, Stevens-Johnson syndrome, and particularly burns can lead to massive losses, which diminish with artificial coverings and grafts. Respiratory and skin losses consist largely of free water, though perspiration contains approximately 45 mEq Na^+ and 4.5 mEq K^+/l. When skin integrity is lost, an electrolyte solution similar to plasma H_2O, often with large quantities of albumin, may be lost. These insensible losses must be considered when evaluating measured input and output in the assessment of daily fluid balance, as they may represent up to 50% or more of daily losses.

Often unappreciated are the large quantities of fluids and electrolytes lost through cerebrospinal fluid, chest tube and wound drainage, as well as upper and lower gastrointestinal secretions. In order to maintain fluid balance, these secretions will require partial to complete replacement in addition to maintenance requirements. Electrolyte content may be estimated from Table 58–23. With large volume output and electrolyte abnormal-

ities, actual measurement of electrolyte content of these fluids allows more precise replacement therapy.

Excessive renal losses frequently occur with hormonal (in DI), metabolic (in glucosuria), and intrinsic renal dysfunction (in the high-output phase of acute renal failure). Dehydration may ensue quickly unless these losses are accounted for and replaced. Diagnosis and treatment of the underlying condition should be undertaken initially. Isovolumetric fluid therapy with an electrolyte solution mimicking losses is often required in addition to maintenance fluid balance during this period. Following correction of the underlying disease state, the cycle of high urine output and vigorous replacement therapy is occasionally hard to escape. Cautious attempts to decrease replacement with frequent assessment of volume status should be carried out. Assessment of central venous pressure may be extremely beneficial in the management of this and similar fluid management challenges.

Although fluid input appears appropriate or even excessive based on measured intake or patient weight, many disorders seen in pediatric critical care lead to severe third spacing of intravascular volume into the interstitial space. Intravascular volume may be decreased in this case despite the appearance of edema and an obviously increased TBW. Frequently in sepsis and other such disease states, an increased intravascular volume is required to maintain optimal cardiovascular function. Thus one cannot assess fluid requirements simply based on the balance of measured inputs or patient weight. Fluid therapy will be necessary to a degree to adequately maintain intravascular volume until capillary integrity is restored. This may require several days and is at times associated with marked edema. As the underlying disease process resolves, resorption of the interstitial fluid into the vascular space can exacerbate congestive heart failure and pulmonary edema. Although a spontaneous diuresis should ensue, this often seems to be delayed by several days, especially in the more seriously ill patient. Cautious administration of diuretics, initially in low doses (e.g., 0.25 to 0.5 mg/kg of furosemide), may hasten the loss of interstitial, intravascular, and pulmonary water, thereby more quickly returning the patient to euvolemia and shortening the duration of ICU care. One must be careful, however, to ensure adequacy of intravascular volume to maintain perfusion. In addition, electrolytes should be determined frequently, especially for the development of hypokalemia. This more interventional approach to the patient with a resolving capillary leak, varies greatly from the traditional "wait and see" philosophy. With shortened requirements for intubation and invasive monitoring, nosocomial infection rates decline, potentially decreasing the duration and need for intensive care.

The frequency of serum electrolyte determination should be individualized to each patient and the clinical condition. The patient's diagnosis, along with changes in physiology and treatment, should be considered when ordering laboratory tests. Timely care of the child with life-threatening illness is frequently dependent on the rapid availability of physiologic and laboratory evaluations. Continuous electrocardiographic and pressure

Table 58–23. APPROXIMATE VOLUMES AND ELECTROLYTE COMPOSITION OF GASTROINTESTINAL FLUIDS IN A 7-kg INFANT*

	Volume (Ml)	Na (mEq/l)	K (mEq/l)	Cl (mEq/l)	HCO$_3$ (mEq/l)
Salivary glands	200	50	20	30	40
Stomach	1,440	35	10	180	—
Gallbladder	400	150	10	90	40
Pancreas	450	150	10	50	110
Small intestine	800	140	5	70	75
Colon (stool)	(100)	40	90	15	30

*From Awazu M, Kon V, and Barakat AY: Volume disorders. *In:* Ichikawa I (ed): Pediatric Textbook of Fluids and Electrolytes. © 1990, the Williams & Wilkins Co., Baltimore.

monitoring, in addition to pulse oximetry and capnography, have revolutionized anesthesia and critical care. Real-time displays of pH, PO_2, PCO_2, and serum electrolytes by indwelling intravascular probes, though under development, are not widely available at this time. The hospital laboratory must therefore strive to provide clinically important data to the bedside practitioner in a time frame necessary to optimally care for the critically ill patient. Clinically significant turnaround time begins when a sample is obtained from the patient and ends when test results are seen by the practitioner and acted upon. Although large, centralized hospital laboratories may report apparently reasonable turnaround times, these are often significantly extended by transportation of samples to the laboratory, triage, processing, and actual reporting of data to the physician who may have left the bedside in the interim. This time can equal or exceed 150 minutes for immediate electrolyte determinations of patients in the ICU of a large teaching hospital. These delays may alter the quality of patient care, as well as frustrate caregivers. As economically feasible alternatives to centralized laboratory services become increasingly available, the clinical laboratory will be judged increasingly on timeliness, as well as accuracy.

Unit-based or even bedside analytic systems that make common laboratory data accessible nearly instantaneously have become available in recent years, allowing therapeutic interventions to be carried out in a nearly continuous manner.[57] These devices, using automated microanalytic techniques, have decreased turnaround times to less than 3 minutes in many systems.[58] Decreased specimen sizes (0.5 to 1 ml of whole blood) may also decrease the incidence of anemia related to phlebotomy, an increasingly common problem in the ICU. The cost of these systems, though prohibitive years ago, now approaches that of specimen analysis in a central laboratory with adequate volume and consistent usage.[59, 60] The accuracy of these units has steadily improved, and advancements in automation allow nontechnologists (ICU nurses, physicians, respiratory therapists) to analyze samples with reasonable reproducibility.[60]

Caregivers must understand the operation and limitations of bedside systems to avoid errors that are possible in any laboratory evaluation.[61] In addition, federal and state regulation of laboratory services, as well as medicolegal concerns, require documented accuracy and quality control measures designed to prevent errors in patient care. A partnership with laboratory personnel to provide daily quality assurance checks of equipment, as well as routine monitoring of results for quality control, is essential.[62] Assistance in developing a program to evaluate quality control of equipment and personnel under the auspices of a consultant from the hospital laboratory is advocated, with provision of accurate and timely results motivating cooperation among health care professionals.[63]

CONDITIONS SEEN IN THE INTENSIVE CARE UNIT

Dehydration

Dehydration is the leading cause of death in children worldwide. Severe dehydration occurs most often as a result of increased gastrointestinal losses through vomiting or diarrhea. Excessive losses may also occur via the kidneys as a result of inadequate renal conservation. Increased insensible losses via the skin with fever or increased ambient temperature and respiratory losses may exacerbate dehydration in the pediatric patient. The intensive care practitioner must master the assessment of fluid deficit in the patient with routine illness, as well as the wide array of abnormalities in fluid and electrolyte balance occurring in the critically ill child.

The clinical assessment of dehydration is a familiar subject to pediatricians. Although weight loss may be the most objective measure of acute fluid deficit, one must remember to account for loss of lean body mass secondary to inadequate nutrition during periods of prolonged illness. Table 58–24 lists the clinical findings

Table 58–24. CLINICAL ASSESSMENT OF SEVERITY OF DEHYDRATION*

Signs and Symptoms	Mild Dehydration	Moderate Dehydration	Severe Dehydration
General appearance and condition:			
Infants and young children	Thirsty; alert; restless	Thirsty; restless or lethargic but irritable to touch or drowsy	Drowsy; limp, cold, sweaty, cyanotic extremities; may be comatose
Older children and adults	Thirsty; alert; restless	Thirsty; alert; postural hypotension	Usually conscious; apprehensive; cold, sweaty, cyanotic extremities; wrinkled skin of fingers and toes; muscle cramps
Radial pulse	Normal rate and volume	Rapid and weak	Rapid, feeble, sometimes impalpable
Respiration	Normal	Deep, maybe rapid	Deep and rapid
Anterior fontanel	Normal	Sunken	Very sunken
Systolic blood pressure	Normal	Normal or low	Less than 90 mm; may be unrecordable
Skin elasticity	Pinch retracts immediately	Pinch retracts slowly	Pinch retracts very slowly (>2 sec)
Eyes	Normal	Sunken (detectable)	Grossly sunken
Tears	Present	Absent	Absent
Mucous membranes	Moist	Dry	Very dry
Urine flow	Normal	Reduced amount and dark	None passed for several hours; empty bladder
% body weight loss	4–5%	6–9%	10% or more
Estimated fluid deficit	40–50 ml/kg	60–90 ml/kg	100–110 ml/kg

*From Nelson W (ed): Textbook of Pediatrics. Philadelphia, WB Saunders, 1983, p. 234.

associated with varying degrees of dehydration in the pediatric patient. Corresponding estimates of TBW deficit are given for infants and children. Note that infants tolerate larger fluid losses because of their larger proportion of body H_2O as compared with that of the older child. The practitioner must remember that these findings are somewhat subjective and will vary from patient to patient.

The appropriate therapy for dehydration requires replacement of fluid and electrolyte deficits in addition to replacement of ongoing excessive losses and provision of maintenance requirements. Because electrolyte abnormalities are most closely related to derangements in sodium balance, dehydration is generally characterized as hyponatremic (Na^+ <130 mEq/l), isonatremic ($130 < Na^+ < 150$ mEq/l), or hypernatremic (Na^+ >150 mEq/l). Initial therapy in all patients with dehydration is designed to rapidly correct deficits in intravascular volume to restore adequate perfusion to tissue beds. The assessment and acute management of shock is discussed in greater detail in Chapter 12. A 20 ml/kg bolus of isotonic solution such as 0.9% NaCl or lactated Ringer's solution should be administered rapidly (5 to 10 minutes) and repeated as necessary until the patient is resuscitated from the shock state. These isotonic, high sodium content solutions should be used to initially treat shock in all forms of dehydration because administration of hypotonic, hyponatremic solutions may lead to inadequate intravascular volume expansion and symptomatic hyponatremia.

Hypernatremic dehydration represents a particularly serious abnormality in fluid and electrolyte balance between the intracellular and extracellular spaces and has been associated with significant CNS morbidity and mortality.[64-67] Seizures may occur before or during therapy and are believed to result from intracellular dehydration, changes in membrane electrical potentials, and intracranial bleeding. Long-term neurologic disability and death may occur as sequelae of neuronal damage. Rapid changes in the tenuous balances mentioned have been implicated in further exacerbating CNS injury; thus, correction of serum Na^+ at a rate of 0.5 to 1.0 mEq/l/hr has been recommended, with restoration of the fluid deficit over 48 hours. As there is usually only a small total body fluid deficit of Na^+, an intravenous (IV) solution of D_5 in 0.20% normal saline (NS) is recommended. The hourly rate is calculated as maintenance rate plus the estimated fluid deficit evenly replaced over 48 hours. It is imperative that serum sodium values be monitored frequently (every 2 to 4 hours) until it is clear that they are normalizing appropriately. Too rapid a fall in serum Na^+ requires a decrease in the rate of rehydration or an increase in the Na^+ content of the IV solution. Too slow a decline indicates the need for an increase in the rate of hydration. Frequent evaluation and adjustment of therapy are mandatory. Any decline in neurologic status requires prompt investigation into the possibility of cerebral edema with elevated intracranial pressure or seizure activity, or both (Table 58–25). Treatment of the child with severe hypernatremia should be undertaken in a facility with staff having pediatric critical care expertise.

Table 58–25. TREATMENT OF HYPERNATREMIC DEHYDRATION

Resuscitate from shock with isotonic solution (NS* or LR†)
Estimate fluid deficit (see Table 58–24)
Calculate hourly IV‡ rate = maintenance + deficit/48 hr
Infuse D_5 0.20% NS at preceding rate
Add 10–20 mEq KCl/l based on renal function and serum K^+ level
Follow serum Na every 2–4 hr initially, less frequently as normonatremia is steadily approached
If Na^+ falls >0.5 mEq/hr, slow IV rate
If Na^+ falls <0.5 mEq/hr, increase IV rate
Follow neurologic examination closely

*NS = normal saline.
†LR = lactated Ringer's.
‡IV = intravenous.

Rehydration of the pediatric patient with a normal or decreased serum Na^+ level is less complex in general than that of the hypernatremic patient, yet there are several potential difficulties that may be encountered. Frequently, there is an ongoing loss of fluids and electrolytes caused by the primary illness, such as is seen in diabetic ketoacidosis, burns, persistent vomiting, or diarrhea. These fluid losses, along with their associated electrolyte constituents, must be replaced in addition to calculated deficit and maintenance requirements. The electrolyte composition of these ongoing losses may be estimated from Table 58–23, or a specimen may be sent to the laboratory for exact determination. Frequent re-examination of the patient and a running hourly total of all intake and output will alert the physician to inadequate or overzealous rehydration. Serum electrolytes, urine output, and renal function, as well as neurologic status and overall perfusion, should be frequently re-evaluated until the patient is adequately rehydrated. Adjustments in IV infusion rate and electrolyte composition will be required, as therapy must be individualized to the specific patient.

Hyponatremic dehydration (serum Na^+ <130 mEq/l) most commonly occurs when the fluid replacement children receive is inadequate because the Na^+ content is less than that of ongoing losses. This may occur in the home setting when gastrointestinal losses are replaced with hypotonic fluids such as water, fruit juice, soda, or jello water. It may also occur iatrogenically with the administration of dilute Na^+ solutions, especially D_5W, by the inexperienced physician. Rapid or severe decreases in serum Na^+ may be associated with generalized seizure activity, and prompt correction is required to achieve a serum Na^+ level of 120 to 125 mEq/l (see Table 58–30). Rehydration should be continued with a solution of D_5 NS + 10 to 20 mEq KCl/l at a rate designed to replace one half of the calculated fluid deficit over the first 8 hours and the remainder over the next 16 hours. The clinical assessment of fluid deficit is frequently less than the actual deficit in hyponatremic dehydration. Abnormal ongoing losses must also be taken into account and replaced appropriately (Table 58–26).

Normonatremic dehydration is also corrected by replacement of calculated deficits and maintenance requirement, with one-half given in the first 8 hours and

Table 58–26. TREATMENT OF HYPONATREMIC DEHYDRATION

Resuscitate from shock with isotonic solution (NS* or LR†)
If seizures suspected secondary to hyponatremia, calculate acute Na⁺ deficit:
  (125 − observed Na⁺) × weight (kg) × 0.6 = mEq Na⁺
  Give 2 ml of 3% saline/mEq Na⁺
    deficit as calculated intravenously over 5 min
    to 1 hr based on acuteness of situation
Estimate fluid deficit (see Table 58–24)
Calculate hourly IV‡ rate = maintenance
  + deficit/24 hr (consider replacing deficit over 48 hr if chronic hyponatremia)
Infuse D₅ 0.45% to D₅ NS (or D₅ LR) at calculated rate
Add 10–20 mEq KCl/l based on renal function and serum K⁺ level
Follow serum Na⁺ every 4–8 hr initially, less often as normalizes

*NS = normal saline.
†LR = lactated Ringer's.
‡IV = intravenous.

the remainder over the subsequent 16-hour period. A solution of D₅ in 0.45% NS + 10 mEq KCl/l will usually suffice as the initial rehydration solution. Abnormal ongoing losses will need replacement as well.

The meticulous physician may wish to calculate not only fluid deficit but also Na⁺ deficit in order to tailor IV solutions to the individual patient. It is essential that the intensive care practitioner understand this approach and apply it to situations deviating from routine care or when laboratory values reveal an unexpected abnormality. Without undue losses, the child requires 3 to 4 mEq of Na⁺/kg/day as a maintenance requirement. Loss of fluid from the extracellular space represents the greatest portion of the calculated fluid deficit in dehydration and is essentially isonatremic with a sodium content of 140 mEq/l. The total body Na⁺ deficit in hyponatremia may be calculated by the formula (140 − Na⁺ observed) × weight (kg) × per cent TBW. Thus, a 10-kg child with a 10% fluid deficit (1 l fluid, 140 mEq Na⁺), a serum Na⁺ of 125 mEq/l (Na⁺ deficit = (140−125) × 10 × 0.6 = 90 mEq) and a maintenance requirement of 1,000 ml and 30 mEq Na⁺/day will require 2 l of IV fluid over the first 24 hours with a Na⁺ content of approximately 120 mEq/l, in addition to excessive ongoing abnormal losses.

Hemorrhage

Acute severe hemorrhage is an uncommon problem in the pediatric patient, most often seen in traumatic injuries, especially of the solid intra-abdominal organs. Cardiovascular surgery, liver transplantation, and chronic medical conditions with coagulopathy and gastrointestinal bleeding, as encountered in the critically ill pediatric patient, may also be associated with acute, large-volume blood loss. The homeostatic mechanisms that attempt to compensate for bleeding have been studied almost exclusively in animal models and adult patients, therefore, the physiology of acute blood loss in small children is poorly understood.

Rapid loss of volume from the intravascular space due to hemorrhage in the adult patient quickly incites compensatory mechanisms in order to restore tissue perfusion. A small amount of intracellular fluid (60 to 150 ml) and potassium is exchanged from the intracellular space to the vascular space, especially with cell injury and breakdown. A far more significant fluid and electrolyte shift occurs among the extracellular, interstitial, and vascular spaces. A brisk influx of interstitial water and sodium into the vascular space occurs initially at rates of 90 to 120 ml/hr in adults with moderate blood loss[68–70] and up to 160 ml/hr in dogs with severe hemorrhage. Over the next 6 to 8 hours, plasma volume refill continues at 40 to 60 ml/hr at the expense of interstitial water. This transcapillary fluid shift then continues at a slower rate over the next 1 to 2 days until intravascular volume is restored.

Numerous hormonal changes occur with acute hemorrhage to restore intravascular content. Although cortisol levels change minimally,[68, 71] aldosterone levels are dramatically increased to promote intense renal sodium conservation.[72, 73] ADH levels also rise quickly, increasing free water retention by the kidney.[74] Atrial natriuretic factor levels fall with intravascular volume depletion, leading to further retention of sodium and water. The release of renin and endogenous catecholamines with this degree of stress serves to improve perfusion pressure, though it may result in an actual loss of vascular water secondary to increased intravascular pressure.[75, 76]

Isotonic solutions such as NS or Ringer's lactate are the appropriate crystalloid forms of resuscitation in the treatment of hemorrhagic shock. Interest in hypertonic saline as a resuscitation fluid is re-emerging and continues under study. The usual electrolyte content of colloid solutions are listed in Table 58–27. As a general rule, 3 ml of isotonic crystalloid solution is required to replace each milliliter of whole blood lost.

Despite concerns of hyperkalemia and hypocalcemia associated with large-volume blood transfusions, these electrolyte abnormalities are in general seen only with massive replacement. It is imperative, however, to closely monitor the ongoing changes of fluid balance and distribution, as well as electrolyte abnormalities that may arise with aggressive volume replacement therapy.

Burns

Severe burn injuries represent one of the most acute challenges to fluid and electrolyte balance in the young patient (see also Chapter 91). Early resuscitation of fluid deficits has perhaps been the largest factor in increasing survival of burned children to nearly 95%.[77] Burns of less than 30% of the body surface generally result in localized tissue edema with loss of intravascular volume into the surrounding interstitial tissues. More extensive burns are associated with a systemic loss of capillary integrity, with histamine, bradykinin, leukotrienes, free radicals, and tumor necrosis factor being implicated as causative mediators. This loss of capillary integrity is greatest in the first 1 to 2 days after injury, resolving over several days.[78–80] Initial fluid losses result in marked hypovolemia acutely and require vigorous fluid replacement with isotonic solution to maintain intravascular

Table 58–27. ELECTROLYTE CONCENTRATION OF COMMON INTRAVENOUS AND ENTERAL FLUIDS

Fluid	Na+ (mEq/l)	K+ (mEq/l)	Cl (mEq/l)	HCO3- (mEq/l)	Ca2+ (mg/dl)	P (mg/dl)	CHO (gm/dl)	Protein (gm/dl)	Osmolality (mOsm/l)
D5W	0	0	0	0	—	—	5	—	266
D5 25% NS*	38	—	38	—	—	—	5	—	340
D5 50% NS	77	—	77	—	—	—	5	—	405
D5 NS	154	—	154	—	—	—	5	—	558
NS	154	—	154	—	—	—	5	—	292
3% Saline	513	—	513	—	—	—	—	—	969
5% Saline	855	—	855	—	—	—	—	—	1,616
LR†	130	4	109	28	3	—	—	—	261
D5 LR	130	4	109	28	3	—	5	—	531
FFP‡	145	4	100	—	—	—	—	—	—
5% Albumin	145	1	100	50	—	—	—	5	300
Plasmanate	145	0.25	100	50	—	—	—	5	300
Human/whole milk	7/21	13/39	—	—	30/79	14/40	6.9/4.7	1.0/3.3	273/260
Pedialyte	45	20	35	—	0	0	2.5	0	250
ENF/Sim/SMA 20	8/8/7	19/19/14	12/12/11	—	46/51/42	32/39/28	7.2	1.5	30
Nutramagin/portagen	14/16	19/22	14/16	—	64	43	7.8–9.1	1.9/2.3	320/230
Vivonex TEN	20	20	—	—	500	500	20	3.8	630
Pregestimil	12	19	16	—	64	43	6.9	1.9	340
Enrich	36	43	—	—	708	708	16	3.9	480
Ensure	36	43	—	—	521	521	14	3.7	470
Isocal	23	34	—	—	630	530	13	3.4	300
Jevity	40	39	35	—	896	746	15	4.4	310
Osmolite	27	26	21	—	521	521	14	3.7	300
Pediasure	16	33	—	—	970	800	11	3.0	325
Pulmocare	57	49	45	—	1,057	1,057	11	6.3	520
Sustacal	41	54	—	—	1,010	930	14	6	620
Vital Hn	20	34	—	—	120	667	18.5	4.2	500

*NS = normal saline.
†LR = lactated Ringer's.
‡FFP = fresh frozen plasma.

volume and support vital organ perfusion. As acute losses are replaced and resolve over the first 48 hours, a chronic phase of hypermetabolism and evaporative losses (1 to 2 ml/kg/day/per cent burn) ensues, peaking several days after injury and with surgical débridement.[81, 82] Thus, fluid and electrolyte maintenance remains an integral and ongoing component of therapy.

The goals of fluid resuscitation in burn injuries are (1) to correct hypovolemia and maintain intravascular volume; (2) to prevent abnormalities in plasma electrolytes, protein, and pH; and (3) to minimize tissue and pulmonary edema.[83] Numerous schedules for fluid replacement have been advocated for adult patients. These have been adapted to pediatric patients with moderate success (Table 58–28). When to replace colloid losses and the use of hypertonic resuscitation fluids remain controversial topics.[84, 85]

Regardless of the replacement schedule used, continuous adjustments of fluid rate and electrolyte content are necessary to individualize therapy, especially in the small child in whom pulmonary injury or respiratory insufficiency exists or when large SAs are involved. Maintenance of tissue perfusion is the objective in the acute phase and is best assessed by urine output of approximately 1 ml/kg/hr, adequacy of skin perfusion, neurologic function, and resolution of metabolic acidosis. At times more invasive monitoring may be helpful. Continuing fluid therapy is guided by daily weight, renal function, serum Na+ levels, and assessment of tissue perfusion.

Electrolyte abnormalities are generally well controlled by the early administration of appropriate quantities of isotonic fluids. Serum sodium levels tend to be slightly less than normal initially, becoming elevated in the days after resuscitation and necessitating decreased sodium administration. Sodium loss may occur through burned skin at daily rates up to 0.5 mEq/kg/per cent burn.[86] Potassium is rarely required in the first day; however, requirements may increase significantly over the next several days as diuresis ensues. Calcium and phosphorus levels may fall, and with marked abnormalities in serum albumin content, measurement of ionized calcium levels may be required. Silver nitrate therapy may also leach out calcium,[87] as well as chloride.[88] Hyperglycemia is common secondary to elevated stress hormones and can exacerbate fluid losses resulting from glucosuria. Hypoglycemia may occur in the infant. Sodium bicarbonate or other buffers may be required to correct severe metabolic acidosis, in addition to appropriate fluid replacement.

Surgery

Neuroendocrine effects on fluid and electrolyte homeostasis associated with the preoperative through the postoperative periods have been studied extensively in the adult surgical patient.[89] Surgical trauma presents even greater challenges to maintenance of physiologic balance in the young child and in the child undergoing major surgical procedures, especially when associated disease processes complicate management. Cameron[90] noted in 1986 that "all too many cases of acute renal failure arise through positive action (nephrotoxic drugs, volume depletion, etc.) or delay and neglect on the part of doctors." A lack of understanding and application of these principles to the critically ill child may contribute to increased postoperative morbidity.

The rise in levels of ADH, renin, angiotensin, and aldosterone often begins in the preoperative period as a consequence of fluid restriction prior to a surgical procedure. Induction of general anesthesia results in a number of complex cardiovascular and neuroendocrine responses in order to maintain adequacy of intravascular volume and tissue perfusion.[91, 92] Intraoperative and early postoperative fluid losses provide continued stimulation to fluid and sodium retention. Elevated levels of ADH and aldosterone and decreased levels of atrial natriuretic factor may be present for several days after major surgical procedures. Restriction of water and salt replacement has been advocated by some clinicians in response to the preceding physiologic events. This may be well tolerated after routine, uncomplicated procedures, as interstitial water is quickly drawn into the vascular space over the first postoperative day to maintain plasma volume.[93, 94] Extravascular water deficit is then gradually replenished over the next week. With more severe surgical trauma, blood loss, tissue injury, cardiopulmonary bypass procedures, or prolonged anesthesia (especially when exacerbated by infection and sepsis), translocation of fluids is reversed because of increased capillary permeability and loss of oncotic pressure. Loss of capillary integrity has been associated with tissue ischemia, activation of complement and white

blood cells, free radicals, and a number of mediators of capillary permeability, including kinins, interleukins, and tumor necrosis factor. This third spacing of water and electrolytes from the vascular space to the interstitial space may result in severe intravascular volume depletion. In addition, external fluid losses from drains and wounds may become highly significant challenges to fluid and electrolyte homeostasis in the patient postoperatively. The normal daily volume and electrolyte content of various body fluids is listed in Table 58–23. These losses, along with plasma and blood losses from wounds and drains, must be accurately quantified and considered in fluid replacement therapy.

Failure to replace third space and external fluid losses with the provision of only normal maintenance fluid requirements may lead to marked intravascular volume depletion with inadequate tissue perfusion. The assessment of intravascular volume status is carried out as for other pediatric patients. In addition, central venous pressure, pulmonary capillary wedge pressure, and cardiac output measurements may be of benefit in major surgical procedures, especially when sepsis or cardiopulmonary abnormalities complicate postoperative care. Replacement of volume deficits with hypotonic solutions such as D_5W is commonly associated with dilutional hyponatremia and hypo-osmotic states and may result in seizure activity, especially in the small pediatric patient. Fluid replacement therapy, therefore, requires the use of electrolyte solutions that mimic losses: NS or lactated Ringer's for third space losses and as shown in Table 58–23 for external losses. Immediate postoperative electrolyte values should be checked in all but the most stable patient. With routine intraoperative fluid and electrolyte losses and replacement therapy, major

Table 58–28. FLUID THERAPY STRATEGIES IN PEDIATRIC BURN THERAPY*

	Brooke (Modified)†	Parkland	Evans	Hypertonic Saline (Monafo)
Day 1				
Colloid (ml/kg/% burn)	None	None	1 ml	None
Crystalloid, lactated Ringer's (ml/kg/% burn)	Adult: 2 ml Child: 3 ml	4 ml	1 ml	Sodium (220–250 mEq/l) Lactate (150 mEq/l) Chloride (100 mEq/l)
5% dextrose in water	None	None	1,600–2,000 ml/m² total body surface area	Change to lactated Ringer's orally in 5% dextrose water if $S_{Na} < 160$ mEq/l
Volume	Total of the above	Total of the above	Total of the above calculation up to 50% burn‡	Constant infusion
Rate	Volume 1st 8 hr, volume next 16 hr	Volume 1st 8 hr, volume next 16 hr	Volume 1st 8 hr, volume next 16 hr	To maintain urine volume 50 ml/hr for adult, 1 ml/kg/hr for child
Day 2				
Colloid (ml/kg/% burn)	0.3–0.5 ml	10–20 ml/kg/day to maintain urine output	0.5 ml	None
Crystalloid (ml/kg/% burn)	None	None	0.5 ml	None
5% dextrose in water	Sufficient to maintain urine flow 50 ml/hr for adult, 1 ml/kg/hr for child	1,600–2,000 ml/m² total body surface area volume distributed evenly over 24 hr	1,600–2,000 ml/m² total body surface area volume distributed evenly over 24 hr	Continue as day 1

*From Ichikawa I (ed): Pediatric Textbook of Fluids and Electrolytes, p. 398. © 1990, the Williams & Wilkins Co., Baltimore.
†Original Brooke formula provided colloid at 0.5 ml/kg/% burn surface area and crystalloid at 1.5 ml/kg/% burn surface area. Crystalloid is usually provided as lactated Ringer's solution or isotonic saline. Colloid is usually provided as 5% albumin or fresh frozen plasma.
‡Thus, a 28-kg patient (1 m² total body surface area) with 75% burn surface area requires in 24 hr a total fluid volume of $1 \times 28 \times 50 + 1 \times 28 \times 50 + 1,800 = 4600$ ml.

shifts in electrolyte values are uncommon. With unusual fluid losses or vigorous replacement therapy, electrolyte levels should be monitored frequently to prevent wide variations from baseline values. Laboratory assessment may be required as often as every 2 to 4 hours, less often in the stable patient. Serum potassium levels may rise slightly because of tissue trauma or large-volume blood replacement, but with establishment of good renal function postoperatively, these levels tend to fall, at times significantly when postoperative diuresis is brisk. Hyperglycemia is often encountered after the stress of major surgical procedures and may result in excessive urine output secondary to glucosuria. Postoperative hyperglycemia normally resolves within several hours. Treatment with insulin is rarely required and may result in severe hypoglycemia as gluconeogenesis subsides. Very young infants, especially those with severe malnutrition or cardiovascular disease, may become hypoglycemic postoperatively and require close monitoring until stable.

Exacting fluid management is required following neurosurgical procedures and in CNS injury where the potential for brain swelling exists. Excessive fluid administration may exacerbate intracranial hypertension. Severe fluid restriction may lead to inadequate perfusion of vital organ systems, including traumatized brain tissue. In general, fluids and electrolytes should be provided at or slightly less than maintenance requirements and adjusted frequently to maintain a urine output of 0.5 to 1 ml/kg/hr. Adequacy of intravascular volume to maintain systemic perfusion must be evaluated and supplemented as necessary. Invasive monitoring to more carefully assess the sufficiency of intravascular volume may be helpful in the patient with underlying disease or in the face of multiple injuries. Hypo-osmolar states should be avoided, and vigilance for the development of SIADH or DI must be maintained by following urine output and serum sodium levels.

Cardiovascular procedures using cardiopulmonary bypass may be associated with large absolute fluid increases and extreme shifts in the normal distribution of TBW.[95, 96] Hypothermia, hemodilution, pump oxygenators, ischemia, and activation of the inflammatory response interact to disrupt normal homeostatic mechanisms.[97] Clinical studies of adult patients reveal an increase in TBW of up to 2,500 ml/m² with cardiopulmonary bypass, averaging 800 ml/m²/hr while the procedure is in progress.[98] Because of the severe capillary leak syndrome that ensues, the extracellular fluid compartment may be enlarged by 20 to 33% at the expense of intravascular volume.[98–101] These changes at times appear to be even more significant in the pediatric patient with poor cardiac function and complex congenital heart disease, leading to marked interstitial edema. In adult studies, failure to replace these intravascular losses during surgery have been associated with high mortality due to cardiovascular insufficiency.[102–105] The loss of intravascular fluid may continue for several hours to days following complex repairs and may not fully resolve until 1 to 2 weeks postoperatively.[97] Maintenance of adequate (often increased) intravascular volume is therefore essential to maintain the function of the heart postoperatively as well as sufficient perfusion of vital organ systems. Hypokalemia is common during cardiopulmonary bypass, with potassium levels increasing in the immediate postoperative period and falling again with diuresis. Calcium and magnesium stores may become depleted and, together with potassium abnormalities, may exacerbate arrhythmias. In addition to routine electrolyte studies, magnesium and ionized calcium levels should be assessed frequently in the postoperative period until they are stable.

The writing of postoperative fluid orders requires an estimation of preoperative as well as intraoperative balance, maintenance requirements, and an appreciation of expected third space and external losses. Constant reassessment and adjustments are mandatory to attain appropriate fluid and electrolyte balance in the critically ill child. Interaction with organ system function of the entire patient must be considered in order to provide optimal ongoing therapy. Eventually, as third space fluid is resorbed from the interstitial space postoperatively, fluids may need to be decreased to less than maintenance requirements or the use of diuretics may be considered, or both, especially with associated cardiopulmonary or CNS disease. Expectant management individualized to each patient will prevent extremes of fluid and electrolyte imbalance and associated morbidity and mortality.

Sodium

Hyponatremia

Hyponatremia is a common finding in patients in the ICU, occurring in up to 27% of patients in an adult ICU. This is usually a reflection of increased TBW with dilution of normal total body sodium content and results from elevated ADH levels as a response to perceived intravascular volume deficiency. This may represent an appropriate physiologic response in many forms of critical illness and should signal the physician that perhaps even more fluid and sodium should be provided in order to maintain cardiovascular sufficiency. Other forms of hyponatremia occur as pathologic responses to systemic illness, iatrogenically caused by inappropriate fluid administration, or simply as a reflection of measurement difficulties as seen in pseudohyponatremia. The most common causes of hyponatremia in the critical care unit are listed in Table 58–29. SIADH is discussed in detail in a previous section.

Normal serum Na⁺ levels are defined as 137 to 145 mEq/l in the pediatric patient. Even minor deviations from this range will affect total body H_2O and, more importantly, the distribution of water between the intracellular and extracellular spaces. Hyponatremia of acute onset or in the presence of CNS disease is associated with cerebral edema, progressive neurologic dysfunction, seizure activity, and the potential for herniation syndromes. Although mortality is reportedly low even with acute hyponatremia, morbidity from seizure activity and exacerbation of cerebral edema in the critically ill patient probably occur more frequently than realized. Symptomatic hyponatremia is most commonly associ-

Table 58–29. CAUSES OF HYPONATREMIA*

Depletion of extracellular fluid volume
  Congenital adrenal hypoplasia
  Renal fluid loss with replacement by hypotonic fluid
  Extrarenal fluid loss with replacement by hypotonic fluid

Extracellular fluid volume near normal
  Hormone deficiency
    Addison disease
    Hypothyroidism
  Hormone excess (inappropriate secretion of antidiuretic hormone)
  Drugs that limit the ability of the kidney to excrete water
  Postsurgical nonosmotic stimuli to retain water

Extracellular fluid volume expanded
  Effective arterial volume decreased
    Hepatic cirrhosis
    Nephrotic syndrome
    Congestive heart failure
  Renal failure
  Acute water intoxication

Extracellular fluid volume status uncertain
  Chronic renal failure with renal salt wasting
    Obstructive uropathy
    Interstitial nephropathy
    "Cerebral" salt-wasting syndrome
  Idiosyncratic reaction to thiazide or thiazide-like diuretics

*Adapted from Arieff AI and DeFronzo RA (eds): Fluid Electrolyte and Acid Base Disorders. London, Churchill Livingstone, 1985, p. 992.

ated with a rapid decrease in serum Na$^+$ levels. Overt symptoms are rarely seen until serum Na$^+$ falls to less than 120 to 125 mEq/l, though more subtle manifestations of neurologic dysfunction may become apparent as sodium levels fall. Generalized tonic-clonic seizure activity represents the classic and most striking manifestation of severe acute hyponatremia. Although difficult to control with anticonvulsants, seizures and lesser alterations in neurologic function should respond quickly to elevation of serum Na$^+$ levels. When seizure activity secondary to symptomatic hyponatremia occurs, serum Na$^+$ should quickly be elevated to 120 to 125 mEq/l, most often by infusion of hypertonic 3% saline solution intravenously.[106, 107] The amount of 3% saline necessary to correct serum levels of Na$^+$ to 125 mEq/l is approximated as (125 mEq/l − observed Na$^+$ mEq/l) × body weight (kg) × 0.6 l/kg. Three per cent saline contains 512 mEq NaCl/l, or approximately 0.5 mEq Na$^+$/ml, and should be administered via a reliable IV line over 30 minutes to 1 hour, more quickly with ongoing symptoms. Serum sodium levels should be measured following therapy, as additional supplements may be required if symptoms persist (Table 58–30). The cause of the hyponatremia should be determined and treated. A more gradual yet progressive correction to normal levels should be ensured. Congestive heart failure or intravas-

Table 58–30. TREATMENT OF SYMPTOMATIC HYPONATREMIA

Calculate Na$^+$ deficit required to bring serum Na$^+$ to 125 mEq/l (125 − observed Na$^+$) × weight (kg) × 0.6 = mEq
Administer 2 ml of 3% NaCl/mEq required as calculated above over 5 to 30 minutes, based on acuteness of situation
Follow serum Na$^+$ level and potential for fluid overload closely

cular volume overload syndromes may be exacerbated by the rapid infusion of a hyperosmolar solution such as 3% saline. In these instances, a loop diuretic such as furosemide may be used to increase water removal. Continuous monitoring of filling pressures and fluid balance should be considered in this situation. When renal function is inadequate, dialysis or partial exchange transfusion may be required to control intravascular volume overload with rapid correction of hyponatremia.

Chronic hyponatremia, occurring over several days to weeks, may become well compensated, with minimal brain edema resulting from loss of cellular and extracellular solute. Neurologic sequelae may in fact occur most commonly with rapid correction of the chronic compensated state. Central pontine myelinosis, or the *osmotic demyelination syndrome*, has been well described in the adult literature.[108, 109] An altered level of consciousness, behavioral abnormalities, and seizure activity may evolve to quadriparesis and pseudobulbar palsy. These changes may be permanent and have been associated pathologically with demyelination in the pons and other deep CNS structures.[110] Although these changes are poorly documented in the pediatric age range, correction of nonsymptomatic hyponatremia, especially when chronic, is recommended at less than or equal to 0.5 mEq/l/hr. Diagnosis and treatment of the underlying condition is of initial importance. Restriction of free water intake has been described as the cornerstone of fluid therapy but must take into account adequacy of intravascular volume. Repletion of total body Na$^+$ stores may require sodium administration, and in the nonedematous patient the deficit may be approximated by the formula (140 mEq/l − observed Na$^+$ mEq/l) × body weight (kg) × 0.6 l/kg = mEq deficit Na$^+$. Measurement and replacement of excessive external losses (urine, cerebrospinal fluid, gastric, and so on) may be required in addition to the replacement of maintenance and deficit needs. Laboratory analysis of the Na$^+$ content in excessive external losses may allow the use of more appropriate replacement solutions with similar electrolyte content.

Hypernatremia

Hypernatremia in the pediatric age range is usually associated with an inadequate intake of free water and progressive dessication. This occurs most often in the very young or debilitated patient who cannot satisfy thirst, a powerful stimulus to the maintenance of normal osmolarity and sodium concentration. The variable intake of free water, as dictated by thirst and the maintenance of serum osmolarity, is also denied in most critically ill patients. Increased loss of free water from insensible losses (fever, radiant heater, tachypnea, and so on) or external losses of hyponatremic fluids will lead to increased serum Na$^+$ levels. Vigorous diuresis with loop diuretics may also lead to contraction of intravascular volume and hypernatremia. Excessive Na$^+$ levels may be seen following the administration of NaHCO$_3$ or hypertonic saline solutions during resuscitative efforts. Ingestion of large quantities of sea water (Na$^+$ content 450 to 500 mEq/l), inappropriately prepared infant formulas, and intentional or accidental salt poisoning have also been described. DI of renal and CNS origin is described earlier. Several CNS lesions have been reported to cause hypernatremia.[11, 112] Rarely, a resetting of the osmostat at the CNS level may occur with maintenance of chronically elevated Na$^+$ levels (Table 58-31).

Symptoms of hypernatremia and associated hyperosmolarity occur as serum Na$^+$ levels rise to greater than 160 mEq/l. The rapidity of rise appears to affect mortality as well as symptomatology. The largely neurologic changes that occur are believed to be secondary to intracellular dehydration and subsequent dysfunction, increased blood viscosity as osmolarity rises to more than 320 to 330 mOsm/l with decreased microvascular perfusion, and intracranial bleeding as the brain substance is drawn away from the skull and bridging veins are disrupted. These changes lead to alterations in neurologic function characterized by varying degrees of depression of consciousness with intermittent irritability, high-pitched cry, normal to increased muscle tone, and seizure activity that may be difficult to control.[113, 114] Pathologic changes occurring in the CNS have been associated with the high mortality of acute (>40%) and chronic (>10%) hypernatremia in older studies.[115, 116] Long-term CNS morbidity is prominent in both groups. Hypoglycemia, hypocalcemia, hyperkalemia, and metabolic acidosis often accompany severe hypernatremia and may contribute to the increased morbidity and mortality.[114, 117, 118]

As in hypernatremic dehydration, our current understanding of the therapy of hypernatremia calls for administration of hypotonic fluid, typically D$_5$ in 0.20% NS at a rate sufficient to decrease serum Na$^+$ by 0.5 mEq/l/hr. More rapid reduction of serum Na$^+$ has been associated with increased neurologic symptomatology and mortality, especially in chronic forms of hypernatremia. Replacement of free water deficit, estimated roughly as: Weight (kg) × per cent TBW × (1 − [140 mEq/l ÷ observed Na$^+$ mEq/l]) in addition to routine requirements, should be carried out over 48 hours.

Table 58-31. CAUSES OF HYPERNATREMIA*

Too much salt
  Oral intake of NaCl
  Administration of NaCl or NaHCO$_3$
Too little water
  Excessive losses
    Insensible
      Increased sweating (fever, exposure to high temperature)
    Burns
    Respiratory infections
  Renal
    Central diabetes insipidus
    Nephrogenic diabetes insipidus
  Gastrointestinal
Inadequate intake
  No access to water
  Restrained expression of thirst
  Abnormalities of thirst
  Essential hypernatremia

*From Ichikawa I: Pediatric Textbook of Fluids and Electrolytes, p. 167. © 1990, the Williams & Wilkins Co., Baltimore.

Serum Na$^+$ levels should be followed every 2 to 4 hours initially. The physician must be alert to the potential for cerebral edema with fluid repletion, as well as the onset of seizure activity. These occurrences may require a reduction in the rate of correction of hypernatremia and in some instances administration of small amounts of isotonic or hypertonic saline in order to mitigate symptoms and slow the decline in serum Na$^+$ levels and osmolarity for a brief period. Seizure activity may also necessitate standard anticonvulsant therapy.

Potassium

While sodium serves as the major ion in the extracellular space, potassium exists as the major cation in the intracellular compartment, with concentrations of approximately 150 mEq/l. Physiologic alterations frequently seen in critical illness often alter the normal distribution between intracellular and extracellular potassium; thus, serum potassium values may not reflect total body stores. Rapid changes in acid-base status may lead to marked alterations in serum potassium levels. With each fall in pH of 0.1 units, serum K$^+$ increases by up to 0.6 mEq/l as H$^+$ ions are driven intracellularly in exchange for K$^+$.[119-121] Alkalosis leads to a decrease in serum K$^+$ by 0.3 mEq/0.1 pH unit increase. B-adrenergic stimulation with agents such as isoproterenol, dobutamine, and many of the β-adrenergic agents used as bronchodilators cause activation of the Na$^+$/K$^+$ pump with a fall in serum K$^+$ levels.[122] Alpha agents tend to increase serum K$^+$ levels.[123] Epinephrine initially increases serum K$^+$ followed by an overall decline. Increasing serum osmolarity results in elevation of serum K$^+$ by 0.6 mEq/l/10 mOsm/kg H$_2$O change. Exercise and insulin deficiency cause a rise in serum K$^+$ levels, whereas insulin excess results in diminished levels.

Daily potassium requirements range from 1 to 2 mEq/kg/day, with growth largely accounting for the increased needs as compared with adult requirements. Nearly 90% of excreted potassium is removed by the kidneys; the remainder is excreted in stool losses, and a small proportion (approximately 9 mEq/l) is lost in sweat. Potassium losses may increase substantially with increased oral, gastric, and intestinal losses, brisk diuresis, and in response to diuretic therapy. Gastrointestinal excretion of potassium seems to increase substantially when renal failure exists, though it is frequently inadequate. Normal adult K$^+$ levels are quoted as 3.5 to 5 mEq/l, increasing to 5.5 mEq/l in the child and 6 mEq/l in the newborn.

Hypokalemia

Hypokalemia may occur by three basic mechanisms. Inadequate intake alone is unusual as a cause except during periods of rapid cell growth, as the kidney efficiently conserves potassium. Extrarenal losses, in particular from the gastrointestinal tract with external drainage of gastrointestinal juices or diarrhea, are associated with substantial potassium wasting. Renal excretion of potassium may be markedly increased in the critically ill patient experiencing brisk diuresis or with a variety of medications, in particular potassium-wasting diuretics. Although in the healthy child, a serum K^+ of 3 to 3.5 mEq/l is rarely problematic, the critically ill patient (especially in the presence of digoxin) may experience symptomatology in this range. Systemic effects of hypokalemia described in the adult patient are listed in Table 58–32. Lower absolute K^+ levels may be necessary in the pediatric age range. Electrocardiographic findings include progressive flattening of the T wave, ST segment depression, and the appearance of prominent U waves, though these findings may not be universally present.

Treatment of hypokalemia is indicated whenever serum K^+ falls to less than 3 mEq/l or when physiologic alterations are suspected secondary to hypokalemia. The rapidity of correction should reflect the severity of the situation and associated symptoms. Excessive correction may result in problematic hyperkalemia or bradycardia

Table 58–32. CLINICAL SEQUELAE OF HYPOKALEMIA*

Cardiac

Predisposition to digitalis intoxication
Abnormal electrocardiogram
Ventricular ectopic rhythms
Cardiac necrosis

Neuromuscular

Gastrointestinal:	Constipation
	Ileus
Skeletal muscle:	Weakness, cramps
	Tetany
	Paralysis (including respiratory)
	Rhabdomyolysis

Renal

Decreased renal blood flow
Decreased GFR†
Renal hypertrophy
Pathologic alterations (interstitial nephritis)
Predisposition to urinary tract infection

Fluid and Electrolyte

Polyuria and polydipsia
  Renal concentrating defect
  Stimulation of thirst center
  ADH‡ release (?)
Increased renal ammonia production
  Predisposition to hepatic coma
  Altered urinary acidification
Renal chloride wasting
Metabolic alkalosis
Sodium retention
Hyponatremia (with concomitant diuretic therapy)

Endocrine

Decrease in aldosterone
Increase in renin
Altered prostaglandin metabolism
Decrease in insulin secretion
  Carbohydrate intolerance

Systemic Hemodynamics

Decreased peripheral vascular resistance
Decreased blood pressure

*From Kokko JP and Tannen RL (eds): Fluids and Electrolytes. Philadelphia, WB Saunders, 1990, p. 214.
†GFR = glomerular filtration rate.
‡ADH = antidiuretic hormone.

with intravenous administration of concentrated potassium salts. Whenever possible oral potassium replacement is preferred, and despite concerns of gastric ulceration, is quite safe in the pediatric population. A 0.5 to 1 mEq/kg dose (maximum 20 mEq) will frequently correct hypokalemia if ongoing losses are controlled. This dose may be repeated every 4 to 8 hours as needed. Smaller amounts may be added to enteral feeds (1 to 6 mEq/100 ml) to maintain normokalemia when continued losses are expected. Excessive enteral replacement may result in diarrhea. Intravenous replacement of potassium salts at concentrations of up to 40 mEq/l are generally considered safe and are well tolerated. Many advocate electrocardiographic monitoring and central venous administration with replacement concentrations of 40 to 80 mEq/l, though there is little documented danger in this range. At times, more rapid correction of hypokalemia may be required, yet fluid restriction will require administration of even more concentrated solutions. Concentrations of up to 2 mEq/10 ml have been used, with administration of 0.5 to 1 mEq K^+/kg body weight (maximum 20 mEq) over a 1 to 2 hour period. Continuous electrocardiographic monitoring and observation, central venous administration (preferably distant from the right atrium), as well as frequent potassium level determinations are mandatory to avoid the significant potential complications associated with this therapy. A 1 mEq/kg dose of KCl will raise the serum K^+ in a moderately hypokalemic pediatric patient with normal renal function by approximately 1 mEq/l. Exact calculation of potassium deficit is not possible, as serum potassium may not reflect the intracellular pool.

Hyperkalemia

Hyperkalemia, with its potential for lethal cardiovascular dysfunction, is observed by many pediatric critical care practitioners to be less problematic than in adult critical care, especially when serum K^+ is in the 5 to 7 mEq/l range. A serum K^+ level greater than 5 mEq/l is consistent with hyperkalemia in the adult; however, a level greater than 5.5 mEq/l in the child and 6 in the newborn defines hyperkalemia in the pediatric age group. Observed causes of hyperkalemia are listed in Table 58–33. The most common causes in the critical care setting include improper collection of blood with hemolysis of red blood cells and liberation of intracellular K^+, acute acidosis, and tissue injury with cellular breakdown. Frequently, renal insufficiency or failure is a primary or accompanying abnormality exacerbating hyperkalemia. Iatrogenic hyperkalemia may occur with excessive potassium administration in intravenous fluids or potassium-containing antibiotics and with inadequate mixing of IV fluids. Although blood transfusion has been stated as a common cause of hyperkalemia, properly handled blood products contain less than 30 mEq potassium/l. Acute acidosis results in a transcellular shift of potassium in exchange for hydrogen ion, except in the case of organic acidemias (lactate and so on), which equilibrate freely across the cell wall.

The clinical manifestations of hyperkalemia result from a decreased intracellular to extracellular potassium

Table 58–33. ETIOLOGY OF HYPERKALEMIA*

Pseudohyperkalemia

Hemolysis of drawn blood
Increased WBC† or platelet count

Hyperkalemia with Potassium Excess

Abnormal distal nephron
    Inhibitors of aldosterone (K⁺-sparing diuretics such as
      spironolactone)
    Certain renal diseases, such as sickle cell disease, interstitial
      nephritis, and so on
Decreased mineralocorticoid secretion
    Addison disease
    Hypoaldosteronism
    Some adrenogenital syndromes
    Hyporeninemic hypoaldosteronism
Decreased delivery distally
    Vascular collapse
    Severe salt depletion
    Oliguric renal failure
Increased intake (oral and intravenous)
    Salt substitutes
    Stored blood

Hyperkalemia Without Potassium Excess

Metabolic acidosis
Increased plasma tonicity
Insulin deficiency
Tissue necrosis (including hemolysis)
Drugs (e.g., digitalis, succinylcholine)
Periodic paralysis—hyperkalemic form
Prolonged exercise

*From Kokko JP and Tannen RL (eds): Fluids and Electrolytes. Philadelphia,
WB Saunders, 1990, p. 25.
†WBC = white blood cell.

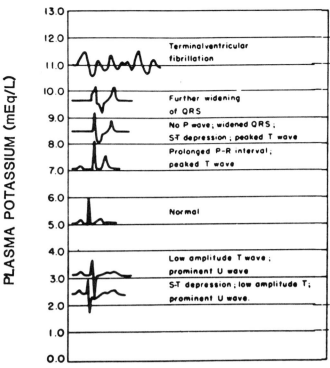

Figure 58–41. ECG changes with increasing serum potassium level. (Reprinted with permission from Winters RW: The Body Fluid in Pediatrics, p. 548. Boston, Little, Brown and Company, copyright 1973.)

gradient, with a subsequent reduction in tissue excitability. Primarily cardiac in nature, clinical findings develop as potassium levels exceeds 7 mEq/l. Peaked or tented T waves are a well-known sequela of hyperkalemia. Although suggestive when present, this finding may be nonspecific on the bedside electrocardiogram monitor without standard lead placement and is best observed in the precordial leads of a 12-channel electrocardiogram. As potassium levels increase, the PR interval lengthens followed by lengthening of the QRS interval and a decrease in P wave amplitude. With progressive hyperkalemia, a sine wave pattern may occur as the QRS complex merges with the peaked T wave. Potassium levels greater than 10 mEq/l are eventually associated with ventricular fibrillation or asystole (Fig. 58–41). Dysfunction of implanted pacemakers has also been observed with inability of the myocardium to generate muscle contraction. Neuromuscular changes, including skeletal muscle weakness, as well as decreased gastrointestinal motility, may occur secondary to hyperkalemia. Endocrine changes include an increase in aldosterone, insulin, and glucagon levels, and some have observed a fall in blood pressure as a result of decreased vascular tone.

Treatment of symptomatic hyperkalemia is accomplished by restoration of the cell's electrical membrane potential, driving potassium into the intracellular space and removing potassium from total body stores (Table 58–34). The intensity of therapy should mirror the

assessed clinical severity of the observed hyperkalemia. Continuous electrocardiographic monitoring is requisite. Removal of K⁺ supplements from enteral and parenteral solutions with immediate repetition of potassium level determinations may be appropriate if no clinical abnormalities are detected. Any electrocardiographic changes or a nonhemolyzed K⁺ level greater than 7 mEq/l should provoke prompt therapy aimed at driving serum potassium levels downward. Calcium gluconate (10% solution) administered intravenously in a dose of 0.5 to 1 ml/kg over 5 to 15 minutes will quickly improve cardiac membrane potential. If no effect is seen in 5 to 10 minutes, a second dose may be given, though it is less

**Table 58–34. TREATMENT OF SYMPTOMATIC
HYPERKALEMIA**

Discontinue potassium administration
Give 50 mg/kg calcium gluconate (0.5 ml/kg of 10% solution) IV* over 5–15 min with electrocardiographic monitoring, slow infusion rate if bradycardia develops
Give 1–2 mEq/kg NaHCO₃ IV over several minutes
Administer 4 ml/kg, glucose-insulin as bolus, then at 4–8 ml/kg/hr (4 units regular insulin/100 ml D₂₅); insulin may require increase to 6 units/100 ml D₂₅ if hyperglycemia develops; for prolonged therapy consider addition of sodium + potassium, i.e., D₂₅ 0.20% NS + 4–6 units regular insulin/100 ml
Sodium polystyrene sulfonate 1 g/kg via rectum in sorbitol, or by mouth with water or sorbitol
Dialysis (hemodialysis most effective acutely)
Loop diuretics may be effective with adequate renal function
Monitor K⁺ frequently to avoid overcorrection and rebound when treatment discontinued

*IV = intravenous

likely to be beneficial. As calcium is quickly absorbed by bone, its effect will decrease over 30 to 60 minutes.[124] It should be remembered that elevated calcium levels may exacerbate digitalis toxicity.

Administration of 1 to 2 mEq/kg $NaHCO_3$ (in an IV line well cleared of calcium) will lead to alkalinization of the extracellular fluid and a shift of K^+ into the intracellular space. A period of hyperventilation, if easily accomplished, will serve the same purpose in the mechanically ventilated patient. Administration of glucose with (or without) insulin will also lead to intracellular transfer of potassium. Four to six units of regular insulin combined with 100 ml of D_{25}, infused at 4 ml/kg over 5 to 10 minutes and then 4 to 8 ml/kg/hr, is effective within 30 minutes and may last for several hours. Serum glucose levels must be determined frequently. Na^+ may be added when this fluid is used for maintenance fluid therapy. One must be cautious to avoid fluid overload when renal failure exists. In patients with adequate renal function, removal of total body potassium may be augmented with loop diuretics such as furosemide. β-Adrenergic agents administered intravenously or by nebulization have been reported to decrease serum K^+ but are not currently considered standard therapy.[125]

Sodium polystyrene sulfonate (Kayexalate), a K^+/Na^+ exchange resin, will bind approximately 1 mEq/l of K^+ when given at a dose of 1 g/kg. Rectal administration with sorbitol as a vehicle is the preferred route, though oral administration with sorbitol or water is also effective. Rectal sodium polystyrene sulfonate should be retained for 15 to 30 minutes and may be administered with a Foley catheter via the rectum with careful inflation of the balloon to aid retention. Resin therapy is usually effective within 4 to 6 hours and may be repeated four to six times/day.[124, 126] Magnesium and calcium may also be inadvertently removed, and frequent monitoring is required. A necrotizing enterocolitis-like syndrome has been described with rectal administration in small infants.

Hemodialysis remains the most effective method of potassium removal. Up to 1 mEq/kg of K may be removed hourly with dialysis across a low K^+ bath; however, caution must be used to prevent overly rapid changes in serum levels.[127] An upward rebound in serum levels may occur following hemodialysis and should be monitored for. Peritoneal dialysis is less effective at potassium removal. Rapid passes with a 30 minute to 1 hour dwell will optimize K^+ removal. Continuous arteriovenous hemofiltration is also less efficient, but K^+ removal may be improved by predilution or countercurrent dialysis.[128]

Prevention of hyperkalemia in the ICU may be aided by maintenance of renal function and urine output. As renal function declines, supplemental potassium should be removed from enteral and parenteral fluids. A progressive increase in serum K^+ levels should prompt a decrease in administered K^+ well before hyperkalemia occurs. Extreme caution must be used in treating hypokalemia, especially when the potential for renal dysfunction exists. Physicians, pharmacists, and nursing staff must be ever-vigilant for tenfold errors in ordering, mixing, or administration of parenteral potassium-containing solutions. Potassium levels should be monitored in accordance with the patient's clinical condition.

Calcium

Serum calcium exists in three forms. Ionized or free calcium composes approximately 47% of the total and serves as the metabolically available form. Forty per cent of serum calcium is protein-bound, primarily by albumin. The remaining 13% forms complexes with phosphate, sulfate, and citrate. Free or ionized calcium, therefore, composes approximately 50% of the total serum calcium. Correction of measured total serum calcium for hypoalbuminemia (increase Ca^+ 0.8 mg/dl for each 1 g/dl decrease in albumin) and acidosis (increase Ca^{2+} 0.2 mg/dl for each 0.1 unit decrease in pH) allows improved estimation of the adequacy of serum calcium, though it may not always accurately reflect physiologically active calcium content. Ionized calcium levels should be measured when any significant clinical question exists.

The homeostasis of total body calcium is dependent on the effects of regulatory hormones on intestine, kidney, and bone. Parathyroid hormone promotes bone resorption, stimulates production of 1, 25-dihydroxyvitamin D by the kidneys, and enhances renal tubular reabsorption of calcium. 1, 25-Dihydroxyvitamin D stimulates bone resorption, increases intestinal absorption of calcium, and improves renal tubular absorption. These actions all serve to increase serum calcium levels. Calcitonin, secreted by the thyroid gland, inhibits bone resorption and facilitates renal calcium excretion. 24, 25-Dihydroxyvitamin D stimulates calcium absorption by bone. These actions serve to decrease serum calcium levels. Hypocalcemia or hypercalcemia may occur when these regulatory control mechanisms are overwhelmed or pathologically affected.

Hypocalcemia

Hypocalcemia is frequently encountered in the critical care setting and appears to be associated with increased mortality.[129–132] Hypocalcemia (<8.5 mg/dl) should be confirmed by measuring ionized calcium, with a level < 4 mg/dl consistent with the diagnosis. Clinical manifestations of hypocalcemia result from increased neuromuscular excitability and initially include perioral tingling, which also may be noted in the fingertips and hands. The Chvostek sign (tapping on the facial nerve anterior to the ear resulting in facial twitching) or the Trousseau sign (carpal spasm induced by inflation of a blood pressure cuff just above systolic blood pressure for 2 to 3 minutes) may be present. Tetany is most notable as carpal spasm, with fingers extended, thumb abducted, and wrist flexed. Tremors, twitches, and seizures may occur, most notably in infants, and laryngospasm has been reported. Cardiovascular changes may include decreased vascular tone and contractility, as well as prolongation of the QT interval.

The causes of hypocalcemia are listed in Table 58–35. Treatment of hypocalcemia in the acute care setting is accomplished by careful administration of calcium salts. Although calcium gluconate traditionally has been the preferred IV solution, some report a more rapid, reliable response with calcium chloride. Elemental calcium, 3 to 6 mg/kg, given intravenously over several minutes with electrocardiographic monitoring for bradycardia or ventricular irritability may be necessary to correct symptomatic hypocalcemia. This represents approximately 0.1 to 0.2 ml/kg of 10% CaCl solution (36 mg of elemental calcium/ml) or 0.4 to 0.8 ml/kg of 10% calcium gluconate (9.3 mg of elemental calcium/ml). Calcium gluconate tends to cause less thrombophlebitis and tissue necrosis with tissue extravasation. Repeated administration of calcium chloride may exacerbate metabolic acidosis. Care must be taken not to administer calcium with bicarbonate- or phosphate-containing solutions, as precipitation may occur. Severe hypocalcemia may require repeated dosing guided by ionized calcium levels (Table 58–36). Hypomagnesemia can impede correction of hypocalcemia and should be considered if hypocalcemia is severe or persistent. With severe hyperphosphatemia, calcium administration may result in soft tissue calcification, and hemodialysis to remove phosphorous may be warranted to prevent this potentially serious complication. A calcium phosphorous product greater than 80 mg/dl should be avoided (total serum calcium × phosphorous). Supplemental calcium in IV or enteral form may be given continuously thereafter to prevent hypocalcemia. Enteral calcium supplementation may be helpful in treating less severe hypocalcemia or in maintaining normocalcemia. The liquid preparation, neocalglucon (23 mg of elemental Ca^{2+}/ml) may be given at 0.25 to 1 ml/kg up to four times/day. Calcium citrate or calcium carbonate are the preferred tablet forms, given as 40 mg/kg/day up to 1 to 2 g of elemental Ca^{2+}/day in divided doses. 1, 25-Dihydroxyvitamin D (Rocaltrol, 0.25 to 1 μ/day) may also be helpful in maintaining

Table 58–35. CAUSES OF HYPOCALCEMIA*

Hypoalbuminemia
Disturbance in parathyroid hormone metabolism
Decreased production: hypoparathyroidism (surgical, infiltrative, and idiopathic)
Ineffective hormone: pseudoidiopathic hypoparathyroidism
Receptor dysfunction: pseudohypoparathyroidism
Hypomagnesemia
Disturbance in vitamin D metabolism
Decreased intake: nutritional malabsorption
Decreased 25-OH D production: parenchymal liver disease
Accelerated 25-OH D catabolism: anticonvulsant therapy, nephrotic syndrome
Decreased 1,25(OH)²D production: renal failure, vitamin D–dependent rickets
End-organ resistance to 1,25(OH)²D
Hyperphosphatemia
Acute pancreatitis
Hungry bone syndrome
Neonatal hypocalcemia
Miscellaneous

*From Arieff AI and DeFronzo RA (eds): Fluid Electrolyte and Acid Base Disorders. London, Churchill Livingstone, 1985, p. 539.

Table 58–36. TREATMENT OF SYMPTOMATIC HYPOCALCEMIA

10–20 mg elemental calcium/kg infused over 5–30 min IV* (secure IV access with continuous electrocardiographic monitoring)
  = 0.1–0.2 ml/kg 10% calcium chloride
        OR
  = 0.3–0.6 ml/kg 10% calcium gluconate
Slow infusion rate if bradycardia develops
Recheck ionized calcium level after 30 min and repeat as necessary; monitor phosphorus levels

*IV = intravenous.

normocalcemia, especially with decreased intestinal resorption and parathyroid hormone deficiency. Serum calcium levels must be followed closely, as potential for hypercalcemia exists with overtreatment.

Recently, concern has been raised that calcium replacement therapy may exacerbate cellular injury following tissue damage or ischemia.[133, 134] Intracellular influx of calcium ions is associated with proteolysis and lipolysis, leading to further loss of cell membrane integrity and cellular injury. It is unclear at this time whether the hypocalcemia frequently seen and associated with increased mortality in critically ill patients is a protective mechanism or a pathologic condition that should be corrected. Mild to moderate asymptomatic hypocalcemia should probably not be rapidly corrected or rapidly treated until this issue is resolved. However severe, symptomatic hypocalcemia may require acute therapy in order to maintain cardiovascular function.[135]

Hypercalcemia

Hypercalcemia, occurring frequently in the adult population as a result of malignancy and hyperparathyroidism, is an uncommon occurrence in the pediatric age range. A serum level greater than 10.5 mg/dl remains the traditional definition of hypercalcemia, though symptoms are rarely noted until the serum calcium level exceeds 12 mg/dl. Measurement of ionized calcium levels should be used increasingly to diagnose abnormalities in serum Ca^{2+} concentration, as free Ca^{2+} may not be directly related to total levels, especially with abnormalities in serum albumin levels or alterations in acid-base status. Hypercalcemia is usually the result of an underlying disease process, or excess administration of Ca^{2+} salts. The causes of hypercalcemia are listed in Table 58–37.

Symptoms attributable to hypercalcemia occur as Ca^{2+} increases exceeding 12 mg/dl. At levels greater than 15 mg/dl, severe toxicity may be encountered. CNS changes are most prominent and include lethargy, delusions, stupor, and eventually coma, which may be associated with seizure activity. Anorexia, nausea, vomiting, and pancreatitis may develop. Electrocardiographic changes with shortening of the QT interval, "coving" of the ST-T wave,[136] and ventricular tachyarrhythmias have been observed. Soft tissue calcifications of the cornea, blood vessels, and kidney (nephrolithiasis, nephrocalcinosis) are reported with severe hypercalcemia. Chronic hypercalcemia is associated with an increased incidence of

Table 58–37. CAUSES OF HYPERCALCEMIA*

Malignancy
  Metastatic bone resorption
  Ectopic PTH† production (pseudohyperparathyroidism)
  Osteolytic factor production
    Osteoclast activating factor
    Osteolytic sterols
    Prostaglandins
Primary hyperparathyroidism
  Adenoma
  Hyperplasia
    Familial
    Multiple endocrine neoplasia syndromes
Familial hypocalciuric hypercalcemia
Hyperthyroidism
Acromegaly
Pheochromocytoma
Adrenal insufficiency
Granulomatous disorders
  Sarcoidosis
  Berylliosis
  Tuberculosis
  Histoplasmosis
  Coccidioidomycosis
Immobilization
Paget disease
Milk-alkali syndrome
Hypervitaminosis D
Hypervitaminosis A
Thiazide administration
Post-transplant hypercalcemia
Recovery phase of acute renal failure (predominantly
  rhabdomyolysis)
Tertiary hyperparathyroidism
Lithium administration
Idiopathic hypercalcemia of infancy

*From Arieff AI and DeFronzo RA (eds): Fluid, Electrolyte and Acid Base Disorders. London, Churchill Livingstone, 1985, p. 516.
†PTH = parathyroid hormone.

hypertension. The neonate may exhibit hypotonia, lethargy, respiratory distress, and failure to thrive with hypercalcemia.[137]

Therapy begins with identification and treatment of the underlying disease. Acute serum calcium reduction may be necessary in the interim, with acute therapy appropriate to the degree of toxicity, as overzealous correction may lead to hypocalcemia. Because many patients with hypercalcemia are volume-depleted, rehydration will improve calcium excretion and lessen the potential for renal dysfunction associated with severe hypercalcemia. Large quantities of calcium may be excreted with brisk urine output and natriuresis. Thus, a normal saline solution with supplemental potassium at 4 to 10 ml/kg/hr should be instituted. Furosemide, 1 to 2 mg/kg every 4 hours, enhances calcium excretion by decreasing calcium reabsorption in the thick ascending limb of the renal tubule, as well as increasing sodium and fluid excretion. Serum Ca^{2+} levels begin to decline within 4 hours and may be significantly decreased with continuing therapy. Fluid overload, hypokalemia, and hypomagnesemia may result with aggressive therapy and should be monitored closely (Table 58–38).

Additional therapy may be necessary with severe or persistent hypercalcemia. Calcitonin inhibits bone resorption and may effectively decrease serum calcium within 2 hours of administration. The standard dose is 4 medical research units/kg subcutaneously every 12 hours. The decrease in serum calcium is generally slight, 1 to 2 mg/dl, and the effect may not be sustained. The antineoplastic agent mithramycin has also been used to inhibit bone resorption. The intravenous administration of 15 to 25 μg over 3 to 8 hours leads to a significant decrease (average 3 mg/dl) in serum calcium within 24 hours, peaking at 3 to 4 days. Its effects are most significant when hypercalcemia results from bone resorption caused by hyperparathyroidism or malignancy. In the dose range given, few complications have been reported with mithramycin, though hemorrhagic disorders, hepatic toxicity, and renal impairment may be observed with higher doses. Steroids tend to decrease serum calcium levels most notably in malignancy, granulomatous disease, and vitamin D toxicity by decreasing vitamin D synthesis and activity, thereby decreasing intestinal calcium absorption. The usual dose is 10 mg/kg/day of hydrocortisone equivalent.

Hemodialysis remains an effective method of calcium removal and may be used to rapidly reduce serum calcium levels.[138] Peritoneal dialysis is significantly less effective. Hemofiltration with predilution or dialysis may be effective, but little clinical literature exists. Rebound hypercalcemia may occur several hours following termination of dialysis.

Binding of serum calcium with chelators and phosphate may be effective but has been associated with soft tissue deposition of calcium complexes and should be used as a last resort (30 to 50 mg/kg/day of elemental phosphorus may be given). Prostaglandin synthesis inhibitors such as indomethacin have been advocated; however, they are not currently accepted as standard therapy.

Magnesium

Abnormalities in magnesium homeostasis, once thought to be rare, have been noted in up to 20 to 65% of critically ill adult patients.[139–141] Magnesium is the second most common intracellular cation and is stored mainly in cells (31%) and bone (67%). Approximately 60% of serum magnesium exists in the ionized form, with 25% being protein-bound and 15% in complexes with serum buffers. Because only 1% of total body magnesium is distributed in the extracellular space, serum levels may poorly reflect tissue stores.[142] Normal serum values range from 1.6 to 2.8 mg/dl. Assessment of ionized or free serum magnesium has also been undertaken.[143]

Table 58–38. TREATMENT OF SYMPTOMATIC HYPERCALCEMIA

Hydrate as possible with normal saline
Furosemide, 1 mg/kg IV* every 4 hr (monitor fluid balance and serum potassium level)
Calcitonin, 4 medical research units, subcutaneously every 12 hr
Hemodialysis
Mithramycin and steroids have been used (see text)

*IV = intravenous.

Table 58–39. CAUSES OF HYPOMAGNESEMIA*

Gastrointestinal Disorders	Renal Disorders
Malabsorption syndromes	Hereditary renal magnesium wasting
Short-bowel syndrome	Acquired causes
Bowel and biliary fistulas	Insulin-dependent diabetes mellitus
Prolonged nasogastric suction	Alcohol
Parenteral hyperalimentation	Antibiotics
Prolonged diarrhea	Aminoglycosides
Laxative abuse	Viomycin
Alcoholism	Capreomycin
Protein-calorie malnutrition	*Cis*-platinum
Pancreatitis	Diuretics
	Cyclosporine
Endocrine Disorders	
Hyperparathyroidism	
Hyperthyroidism	
Primary hyperaldosteronism	
Diabetes mellitus	

*From Kokko JP and Tannen RL (eds): Fluids and Electrolytes. Philadelphia, WB Saunders, 1990, p. 214.

Hypomagnesemia

Hypomagnesemia generally occurs secondary to increased gastrointestinal losses or with renal wasting from diuretics, aminoglycosides, *cis*-platinum, or cyclosporine administration. Other causes of hypomagnesemia are listed in Table 58–39.

The signs and symptoms of hypomagnesemia are often complicated by the coexistence of hypocalcemia or hypokalemia, or both. Tetany, muscle weakness, and tachycardia with shortening of the QT interval are most suggestive of severe hypomagnesemia (Table 58–40). Persistent, difficult to correct hypocalcemia or hypokalemia may be a clue to hypomagnesemia and should prompt assessment of the serum magnesium level.

Severe or symptomatic hypomagnesemia is treated with an initial dose of 40 mg/kg $MgSO_4 \cdot 7H_2O$ given intravenously over several minutes (Table 58–41). Blood pressure and electrocardiographic monitoring are required, as flushing, sweating, warmth, and electrocardiographic changes may be seen and should prompt slowing of the infusion rate. If hypomagnesemia persists, the dose may be repeated. Supplemental magnesium,

Table 58–41. TREATMENT OF SYMPTOMATIC HYPOMAGNESEMIA

Twenty-five–50 mg/kg $MgSO_4$ intravenously over 5–15 min with continuous electrocardiographic monitoring = 0.05–0.1 ml/kg of 50% solution
Recheck serum magnesium level after 30 min and repeat as necessary

40 mg/kg/day in divided doses, will likely be required for several days to replete total body stores. Magnesium should be administered with extreme caution when renal insufficiency is present, as hypermagnesemia may develop. Magnesium, calcium, and potassium levels should be monitored frequently with magnesium replacement therapy.

Hypermagnesemia

Hypermagnesemia is suggestive of excessive magnesium administration, otherwise occuring only in the occasional patient with renal failure. Causes of hypermagnesemia may be found in Table 58–42. Clinical signs and symptoms develop as magnesium concentration exceeds 5 mg/dl and are characterized by muscle weakness progressing to paralysis (Table 58–43).[144–147]

Treatment consists of discontinuation of magnesium administration with augmentation of diuresis, especially with loop diuretics. Intravenous calcium chloride, 10 to 20 mg/kg, or calcium gluconate 40 to 80 mg/kg given slowly with electrocardiographic monitoring, will frequently reverse the acute cardiac manifestations of hypermagnesemia. Hemodialysis or peritoneal dialysis may be required to acutely reduce life-threatening hypermagnesemia and significantly reduce total body stores.

Phosphorus

As a critical molecule for energy maintenance and cellular function, phosphorus exists largely in the phosphate form. Serum levels may inadequately reflect total body stores because 85% of phosphate is contained in

Table 58–40. CLINICAL PICTURE OF MAGNESIUM DEFICIENCY AND ASSOCIATED ABNORMALITIES OF CALCIUM AND POTASSIUM

Hypomagnesemia			
		Hypocalcemia and Hypokalemia	
Cerebellar	*Mental*	*Neuromuscular*	*Cardiac*
Vertigo	Delirium	Muscle tremor	↑ QT interval
Ataxia	Apathy	Twitching	↓ ST segment
Nystagmus	Depression	Weakness	Broad, flat T waves
Athetoid and choreiform movements	Personality changes	Hyperreflexia	Digitalis toxicity
	Coma	Chvostek sign	Arrhythmias
	Irritability	Carpopedal spasm	
		Tetany and seizures	

*From Arieff AI and DeFronzo RA (eds): Fluid, Electrolyte and Acid Base Disorders. London, Churchill Livingstone, 1985, p. 610.

Table 58–42. CAUSES OF HYPERMAGNESEMIA*

Renal failure with impaired glomerular filtration rate
  Acute
  Chronic

Reduced renal excretion without impaired glomerular filtration rate
  Salt depletion
  Deficiency of mineralocorticoid
  Deficiency of thyroid hormone
  ? Chronic hypercapnia

Administration of pharmacologic doses of Mg
  Antacid or laxative abuse
  Purgatives or enemas
  Overzealous treatment of eclamptic mothers
  Inadvertent administration of high Mg dialysate

Increased tissue breakdown
  Rhabdomyolysis
  Burn and tissue trauma
  Severe diabetic ketoacidosis

*From Arieff AI and DeFronzo RA (eds): Fluid, Electrolyte and Acid Base Disorders. London, Churchill Livingstone, 1985, p. 596.

bone, 14% is found in soft tissues, and only 1% is distributed in the extracellular space. Eighty-five per cent of blood phosphate exists in the free form, the remainder being bound to serum proteins. Regulation of total body phosphate content is dependent on the degree of gastrointestinal absorption and the rate of renal excretion. Maintenance of normal serum levels (infants 3.7 to 8.5 mg/dl, children 3.7 to 5.9 mg/dl, and adults 2.7 to 4.7 mg/dl) takes place through complex interplay of several hormonal and nonhormonal mechanisms.[148–152]

Hypophosphatemia

The existence of underlying phosphate depletion may be manifested by acute hypophosphatemia in the critical care unit. Initiation of high-density caloric support in the malnourished patient, parenteral hyperalimentation in particular, is often the precipitating factor in acute hypophosphatemia. Other causes of hypophosphatemia

Table 58–43. CLINICAL FINDINGS IN HYPERMAGNESEMIA*

Depressed neuromuscular function
  Reduction or loss of deep tendon reflexes (serum Mg >7.5 mg/dl)
  Paralysis of voluntary muscle (flaccid quadriplegia, respiratory failure, or apnea) (serum Mg >12 mg/dl)
  Narcosis, stupor, and coma (serum Mg >15 mg/dl)

Cardiovascular dysfunction
  Hypotension, caused by dilation of resistance vessels (serum mg >5 mg/dl)
  Increased PR interval and intraventricular conduction defects (serum Mg >8 mg/dl), increased QRS and QT interval
  Complete heart block or cardiac arrest in asystole (serum Mg >18 mg/dl)

*From Arieff AI and DeFronzo RA (eds): Fluid, Electrolyte and Acid Base Disorders. London, Churchill Livingstone, 1985, p. 599.

Table 58–44. CAUSES OF HYPOPHOSPHATEMIA*

Those with excessive renal losses as primary cause
  Primary hypophosphatemic rickets
  Hereditary hypophosphatemic rickets with hypercalciuria
  Renal tubular acidosis
  Fanconi syndrome
  Potassium deficiency
  Oncogenic osteomalacia or rickets
  Vitamin D deficiency and dependency (also related to decreased intestinal absorption)
  Primary hyperparathyroidism

Those with negative intestinal balance as primary cause
  Breast-fed premature infants
  Term infants fed with low phosphate source
  Use of phosphate-binding antacids
  Decreased dietary intake (rare)
  Vomiting

Acute flux of plasma phosphate to intracellular and skeletal pools†
  Nutritional recovery, usually TPN‡-associated
  Therapy of diabetic ketoacidosis
  Alkalosis
  Androgen therapy
  Burn therapy
  "Hungry bone" phenomenon
  Increased tumor burden

*From Ichikawa I (ed): Pediatric Textbook of Fluids and Electrolytes, p. 256. © 1990, the Williams & Wilkins Co., Baltimore.
†The serum phosphate is maintained but total body pools are depressed (in many of these conditions recovery results in restoration of intracellular phosphate, precipitating acute hypophosphatemia).
‡TPN = total parenteral nutrition.

Table 58–45. PHOSPHATE DEPLETION SYNDROME*

Insidious and Gradual Onset of Signs and Symptoms
Neuropsychiatric
  Decreased mentation, memory loss, neuropathy, ataxia
Constitution
  Lethargy, malaise, debility
Musculoskeletal
  Weakness, myalgia, and subclinical myopathy
  Arthalgia, joint stiffness
  Bone disease and subclinical osteomalacia
Hematologic
  Dysfunctions of platelets, red and white blood cells
Endocrine-Metabolic
  Diminished tissue sensitivity to insulin
  Increased production of 1,25 di(OH)D$_3$
Renal
  Glycosuria, hypercalciuria, hypermagnesuria, RTA†
Gastrointestinal
  Anorexia, dysphagia
Cardiopulmonary
  Tachypnea, shallow respiration, decreased vital capacity
  Decreased cardiac contractility, reduced sensitivity by peripheral vessels to vasoactive hormones

Acute and Sudden Onset of Signs and Symptoms
Confusion, seizure, delirium, and coma
Acute cardiac decompensation, hypotension
Rhabdomyolysis
Pulmonary insufficiency
Generalized systemic decompensation due to tissue hypoxia and ATP‡ deficiency

*From Kokko JP and Tannen RL (eds): Fluids and Electrolytes. Philadelphia, WB Saunders, 1990, p. 539.
†RTA = renal tubular acidosis.
‡ATP = adenosine triphosphate.

Table 58–46. TREATMENT OF SYMPTOMATIC HYPOPHOSPHATEMIA

0.16 mmol phosphorus/kg = 5 mg of elemental phosphorus/kg
Infused over approximately 1 hr IV*
  (secure IV access with continuous electrocardiographic monitoring)
  = 0.05 ml/kg NaPHOS [94 mg PHOS/ml, 4 mEq Na/ml]
      OR
  = 0.05 ml/kg KPHOS [94 mg PHOS/ml, 4.4 mEq K/ml]
Recheck phosphorus level after 30 min and repeat as necessary;
  follow calcium, Na+ and K+ levels closely; hypocalcemia may ensue

*IV = intravenous.

Table 58–47. CLINICAL CAUSES OF HYPERPHOSPHATEMIA*

Redistribution
Severe hemolytic anemia
Rhabdomyolysis
Cancer cell lysis
Diphosphonate therapy
Hyperthyroidism

Positive Phosphate Balance
Acute PO_4 poisoning
  Phosphate-containing enemas
  Phosphate-containing laxatives
  Intravenous administration
Renal retention
  Renal failure
  Hypoparathyroidism
  Tumoral calcinosis
  Acromegaly

*From Kokko JP and Tannen RL (eds): Fluids and Electrolytes. Philadelphia, WB Saunders, 1990, p. 571.

may be found in Table 58–44 and are discussed in detail elsewhere.[153] Chronic phosphate deficiency may be manifested by a wide array of alterations in numerous body systems. The symptoms of acute, severe hypophosphatemia (serum P < 1 mg/dl) are attributable to a deficiency of intracellular adenosine triphosphate, erythrocyte 2, 3-diphosphoglycerate, or both, and may be life-threatening (Table 58–45).

Treatment should be undertaken based on the severity of hypophosphatemia and related symptoms (Table 58–46). Unless acute symptoms are present, PO_4 depletion is generally treated by enteral administration of phosphorus 10 to 20 mg/kg/day divided into several doses to minimize diarrhea. Several days of therapy may be required to replete body stores. Potassium phosphate

Table 58–48. CLINICAL MANIFESTATIONS OF ELECTROLYTE ABNORMALITIES*

Electrolyte Abnormality	Central Nervous System	Musculoskeletal	Electrocardiogram	Arrhythmias	Other	Vascular Tone
↑ Na	Lethargy, stupor, coma	Muscle weakness, myoclonus, cramps			Nausea	↓
↓ Na	Lethargy, stupor, coma, seizures, headache	Myoclonus, fasciculations, cramps			Anorexia, nausea, vomiting	
↑ K		Muscle weakness, fasciculations	Flattened P, lengthened PR, widened QRS, depressed ST, shortened QTc	Bradycardia, asystole, PAC, PVC, junctional	Increased insulin, growth hormone, glucagon, aldosterone, and catechols	↓
↓ K	Lethargy	Muscle weakness, fasciculations, cramps	Shortened PR, depressed ST	PAC, PVC, atrial and ventricular tachycardia, junctional	Constipation; decreased gastrointestinal motility and abdominal pain; decreased aldosterone, insulin, growth hormone	↑
↑ Ca	Lethargy, stupor, coma, seizures	Muscle weakness	Lengthened PR, shortened QTc	Bradycardia, PVC, ventricular tachycardia	Anorexia, nausea, vomiting, constipation, abdominal pain pancreatitis	↑
↓ Ca	Lethargy, seizures	Muscle weakness	Lengthened QTc		Diarrhea	↓
↑ Mg	Lethargy	Muscle weakness	Lengthened PR, increased QRS width	Bradycardia Asystole PVC	Nausea, vomiting	↓
↓ Mg	Seizures, nystagmus	Muscle weakness, myoclonus, cramps, fasciculations	Shortened PR	PVC, ventricular tachycardia	Anorexia, nausea, vomiting, decreased release of parathyroid hormone, elevated cholesterol	↑
↑ PHOS	PO_4					↓
↓ PHOS	Seizures, lethargy, stupor, coma	Muscle weakness			Anorexia, hemolytic anemia, platelet and WBC† dysfunction, decreased 2,3-DPG‡	

*Data from Arieff AI and DeFronzo RA (eds): Fluid, Electrolyte and Acid Base Disorders. London, Churchill Livingstone, 1985, pp. 1087–1144.
†WBC = white blood cell.
‡2,3-DPG = 2,3-diphosphoglycerate.

may be used to partially or completely replace KCl in IV solutions to treat mild to moderate hypophosphatemia. Acute symptomatic hypophosphatemia should be treated with 5 mg/kg elemental phosphorous given slowly via the intravenous route with electrocardiographic and blood pressure monitoring.[155] Repetition of this dose may be required several times until the serum phosphorus level exceeds 2 mg/dl and acute symptomatology is resolved. Electrolyte balance, including calcium, magnesium, and potassium, as well as fluid balance, must be carefully monitored. Enteral replenishment should be undertaken following acute therapy.

Hyperphosphatemia

Hyperphosphatemia may occur when the kidneys' ability to excrete a normal or increased phosphate load is exceeded. Common causes of hyperphosphatemia are listed in Table 58–47 and are fully described elsewhere.[156]

Clinical manifestations of hyperphosphatemia may be both acute and chronic. Acutely, symptoms of hypocalcemia (tetany, seizures, shock, and cardiac arrhythmias) may be precipitated as serum calcium levels fall in response to hyperphosphatemia. Formation of $Ca\text{-}PO_4$ precipitants may occur as the $Ca\text{-}PO_4$ product (Ca^{2+} mg/dl $\times$ P mg/dl) exceeds 65 to 70, leading to acute and chronic deposition of hydroxyapatite crystals in the cornea, lungs, kidneys, heart, and gastrointestinal tract. Hyperphosphatemia, most commonly encountered in the setting of renal insufficiency, may further exacerbate renal failure by these mechanisms, with further elevation in serum phosphorous levels.

The therapy of hyperphosphatemia relies on removal of PO_4 via the gastrointestinal tract or renal system, or both. Phosphate binders such as Ca^{2+} and Mg^{2+} salts (cathartic) and aluminum salts (constipating) have been given enterally with good success. The choice of agents and dose vary widely in relation to the cause of hyperphosphatemia. Magnesium and aluminum may accumulate with prolonged use in patients with renal failure. Maintenance of renal function allows greatly improved clearance of phosphate. Restoration of extracellular fluid volume, bicarbonate diuresis, and administration of acetazolamide and xanthine oxidase inhibitors all may serve to preserve renal function and improve phosphate excretion. If renal function is severely compromised, or in cases of severe hyperphosphatemia, dialysis may be indicated (Tables 58–48 and 58–49).

References

1. Darrow DC and Pratt EL: Fluid therapy. JAMA 143:365, 1950.
2. Van Heyningen WE and Seal JR: Cholera—The American Scientific Experience 1947–1980. Boulder, CO, Westview Press, 1983, pp. 1–25.
3. O'Shaughnessy WB: Proposal of a new method of treating the blue epidemic cholera by the injection of highly oxygenated salts into the venous system. Lancet, 1: 366, 1831–1832.
4. Carpenter CJC: Treatment of cholera—tradition and authority versus science, reason, and humanity. Johns Hopkins Med J 139:153, 1976.
5. Latta T: Malignant Cholera: Documents communicated to the Central Board of Health, London, relative to the treatment of cholera by the copious injection of aqueous and saline solutions. Lancet 2: 274, 1831–1832.
6. Markus FCM: In Rapport sur le cholera—Morbus de Moscow. Semen, Moscow, 1832.
7. Cosnett JE: The origins of intravenous fluid therapy. Lancet 1: 768, 1989.
8. Friis-Hansen BJ, Holliday M, Stapleton T, et al: Total body water in children. Pediatrics 7:321, 1951.
9. Friis-Hansen BJ: The extracellular fluid volume in infants and children. Acta Paediatrica Scand 43:444, 1954.
10. Friis-Hansen BJ: Changes in body water compartments during growth. Acta Paediatr Scand 43 (Suppl 110): 1, 1957.
11. Friis-Hansen BJ: Body water compartment in children changes during growth and related changes in body composition. Pediatrics 28:169, 1961.
12. Von Bezold A: Untersuchungen uber die verteilung von wasser, organische materie und anorganische verbindungen in Tierreiche. Ztsch wissen sch zool 8:487, 1857.
13. Bischoff E: Einige Gervichts—und Trocken-Bestimmungen der Organe des menschlichen Korpers. Ztsch f rationelle Med Reihe III 20:75, 1863.
14. Fehling H: Beitrage zur physiologic des placenten stoffwerkehrs. Arch Gynak 11:523, 1877.
15. Givens MH and Macy JG: The chemical composition of the human fetus. J Biol Chem 102:7, 1933.
16. Harrison HE, Darrow DC, and Yannet H: The total electrolyte content of animals and its probable relation to the distribution of body water. J Biol Chem 113:515, 1936.
17. Iob V and Swanson WW: Mineral growth of the human fetus. Am J Dis Child 47:302, 1934.
18. Michel MC: Sur la composition chimique de l'embryon et du fretus humains aux différentes périodes de la grossesse. Comptes Rendus Soc Biol 51:422, 1899.
19. Stearns G: The mineral metabolism of normal infants. Physiol Rev 19:415, 1939.
20. Shol AT: Mineral Metabolism. New York, Reinhold Publishing, 1939.
21. Edelman IS and Leibman J: Anatomy of body water and electrolytes. Am J Med 27:256, 1959.
22. Guyton AC: Textbook of Medical Physiology, 5th ed. Philadelphia, WB Saunders, 1976, pp. 238, 279.
23. Winters RW: Regulation of normal water and electrolyte metabolism. In: Winters RW (ed): Body Fluids in Pediatrics. Boston, Little, Brown, 1973, p. 101.
24. Maffly R: The body fluids: Volume, composition, and physical chemistry. In: Brenner BM and Rector FC (eds): The Kidney. Philadelphia, WB Saunders, 1976, p. 67.

Table 58–49. FACTORS FOR CONVERSION OF CONCENTRATION EXPRESSED IN MILLIEQUIVALENTS/ LITER TO MILLIGRAMS/DECILITER (100 ml), AND VICE VERSA, FOR COMMON IONS THAT OCCUR IN PHYSIOLOGIC SOLUTIONS*

Element or Radical	mEq/l to mg/dl		mg/dl to mEq/l	
Sodium	1	2.30	1	0.4348
Potassium	1	3.91	1	0.2558
Calcium	1	2.005	1	0.4988
Magnesium	1	1.215	1	0.8230
Chloride	1	3.55	1	0.2817
Bicarbonate (HCO_3)	1	6.1	1	0.1639
Phosphorus valence 1	1	3.10	1	0.3226
Phosphorus valence 1.8	1	1.72	1	0.5814
Sulfur valence 2	1	1.60	1	0.625

Example: To convert milliequivalents of magnesium/l to mg/dl (100 ml), multiply by the factor 1.215.

To convert milligrams of potassium/dl (100 ml) to mEq/l, multiply by the factor 0.2558.

*From Behrman RE, Vaughan VC, and Nelson WE (eds): Textbook of Pediatrics. Philadelphia, WB Saunders, 1983, p. 1853.

25. Fanestil DD: Compartmentation of body water. *In*: Maxwell MH, Kleeman CR, and Narins RG (eds): Clinical Disorders of Fluid and Electrolyte Metabolism. New York, McGraw-Hill, 1987, p. 2.

26. Starling EH: On the absorption of fluids from the connective tissue spaces. J Physio 19:312, 1896.

27. Talbot FB: Basal metabolism in children. *In*: Brenneman's Practice of Pediatrics, Chapter 22. Hagerstown, 1949.

28. Holliday MA and Segar WE: The maintenance need for water in parenteral fluid therapy. Pediatrics 19:823, 1957.

29. Newbaugh LH and Johnston NW: The insensible loss of water. Physiol Rev 22:1, 1942.

30. Levine SZ, Wilson JR, and Kelly M: The insensible perspiration in infancy and in childhood. Am J Dis Child 37:791, 1929.

31. Heeley AM and Talbot NB: Insensible water losses per day by hospitalized infants and children. Am J Dis Child 90:251, 1955.

32. Gamble JL: Physiological information gained from studies on the life raft ration. The Harvey Lecture Series, No. 42, Lancaster, PA, Science Press Printing, 1947, pp. 242–273.

33. Gamble JL, Wallace WM, Eliel L, et al: Effects of large loads of electrolytes. Pediatrics 7:305, 1951.

34. Camerer W Jr. and Soldner: Die chemische zusamnrensetzung des neugeboreneu. Zeitsch f Biologie 39:173, 1900; 40:529, 1900; 43:1, 1902.

35. Talbot NB, Crawford JD, and Butler AM: Homeostatic limits to safe parenteral fluid therapy. N Engl J Med 248:1100, 1953.

36. Barnett HL, Vesterdal J, McNamara H, et al: Renal water excretion in premature infants. J Clin Invest 31:1069, 1952.

37. Aperia A, Broberger O, Thodenius K, et al: Renal response to an oral sodium load in newborn full term infants. Acta Paediatr Scand 61:670, 1972.

38. Aperia A, Berg U, Broberger O, et al: The renal response to an oral salt and fluid load in children with coarctation of the aorta. Acta Paediatr Scand 62:241, 1973.

39. Aperia A, Broberger O, Thodenius K, et al: Developmental study of the renal response to an oral salt load in pre-term infants. Acta Paediatr Scand 63:517, 1974.

40. Schwartz GJ, Haycork GB, Edelmann CM, et al: A simple estimate of glomerular filtration rate in children derived from body length and plasma creatinine. Pediatrics 58:259, 1976.

41. Schrier RW: Body fluid volume regulation in health and disease: A unifying hypothesis. Ann Intern Med 113:155, 1990.

42. Sklar AH and Schrier RW: Central nervous system mediators of vasopressin release. Physiol Rev 63:1243, 1983.

43. Berl T, Henrich WL, Erickson AL, et al: Prostaglandins in the beta-adrenergic and baroreceptor mediated secretion on renin. Am J Physiol 235:F472, 1979.

44. Yared A: Regulation of plasma osmolality. *In:* Chikawa I (ed): Pediatric Textbook of Fluids and Electrolytes. Baltimore, Williams & Wilkins, 1990, p. 176.

45. Sterns RH, Riggs JE, and Schochet SS: Osmotic demyelination syndrome following correction of hyponatremia. N Engl J Med 314:1535, 1986.

46. Weizman Z, Goitein K, Amit Y, et al: Combined treatment of severe hyponatremia due to inappropriate antidiuretic hormone secretion. Pediatrics 69:610, 1982.

47. Morau M and Kapsner C: Acute renal failure associated with elevated plasma oncotic pressure. N Engl J Med 317:150, 1987.

48. Melvin T: Unpublished observation, 1989.

49. Burnett JC, Kao PC, Hu DC, et al: Atrial natriuretic peptide elevation in congestive heart failure in the human. Science 231:1145, 1986.

50. Thrasher TN, Lee ME, Metzler CH, et al: Elevated left atrial pressure (LAP) in conscious dogs increases plasma levels of atrial natriuretic factor like immunoreactivity. Fed Proc Fed Am Soc Exp Biol 44:7711, 1985.

51. Harris PJ, Thomas D, and Morgan TO: Atrial natriuretic peptide inhibits angiotensin-stimulated proximal tubular sodium and water reabsorption (letter). Nature 326:697, 1987.

52. Saito Y, Nakao K, Nishimura K, et al: Clinical application of atrial natriuretic polypeptide in patients with congestive heart failure: Beneficial effects on left ventricular function. Circulation 76:115, 1987.

53. Molina CR, Fowler MB, McCrory S, et al: Hemodynamic, renal and endocrine effects of atrial natriuretic peptide infusion in severe heart failure. J Am Coll Cardiol 12:175, 1988.

54. Berg JA, Hyashi M, Fugu Y, et al: Renal metabolism of atrial natriuretic peptide. Am J Physiol 255:F466, 1988.

55. Yanigasawa M, Kurihara H, Kimura S, et al: A novel potent vasoconstrictor peptide produced by vascular endothelial cells. Nature 332:411, 1988.

56. Firth JD, Raine AEG, Ratcliffe PJ, et al: Endothelin: An important factor in acute renal failure? Lancet 2:1179, 1988.

57. Zaloga GP: Evaluation of bedside testing options for the critical care unit. Chest 97:S185, 1990.

58. Misiano DR, Meyerhoff ME, and Collison ME: Current and future directions in the technology relating to bedside testing of critically ill patients. Chest 97:S204, 1990.

59. Statland BE and Brzys K: Evaluating stat testing alternatives by calculating annual laboratory costs. Chest 97:S198, 1990.

60. Zaloga GP, Hill TR, Strickland RA, et al: Bedside blood gas and electrolyte monitoring in critically ill patients. Crit Care Med 17:920, 1989.

61. Baer DM and Belsey RE: The evolving regulatory environment and bedside metabolic monitoring of the acute care patient. Chest 97:S191, 1990.

62. Belsey RE, Baer DM, and Sewell D: Laboratory test analysis near the patient. JAMA 255:775, 1986.

63. Baer DM and Belsey RE: Managing quality and risk of bedside testing. Perspect Healthcare Risk Management 1990, pp. 3–7.

64. Morris-Jones PH, Houston IB, Evans RC, et al: Prognosis of the neurological complications of acute hypernatremia. Lancet 2:1385, 1967.

65. Simmons MA, Adcock EW, Bard H, et al: Hypernatremia and intracranial hemorrhage in neonates. N Engl J Med 291:6, 1974.

66. Finberg L: Pathogenesis of lesions in the nervous system in hypernatremic states. I: Clinical observation of infants. Pediatrics 23:40, 1959.

67. Macaulay D and Watson M: Hypernatremia as a cause of brain damage. Arch Dis Child 42:284, 1967.

68. Moore FD: Metabolic Care of the Surgical Patient. Philadelphia, WB Saunders, 1959.

69. Skillman JJ, Awwad HK, Moore FD, et al: Plasma protein kinetics of the early transcapillary refill after hemorrhage in man. Surg Gynecol Obstet 125:983, 1967.

70. Moore FD: The effects of hemorrhage on body composition. N Engl J Med 273:567, 1965.

71. Moore FD: Hormones and stress: Endocrine changes after anesthesia, surgery and unanesthetized trauma in man. Recent Progr Hormone Res 13:511, 1957.

72. Bartter FC: Symposium: Water and electrolytes: Role of aldosterone in normal homeostasis and in certain disease states. Metabolism 5:369, 1956.

73. Bartter FC, Mills IH, Biglieri EG, et al: Studies on control and physiologic action of aldosterone. Rec Progr Hormone Res 15:311, 1959.

74. Share L: Vascular volume and blood level of antidiuretic hormone. Am J Physiol 202:791, 1962.

75. Finnerty FA Jr, Buchholz JH, Guillaudeu RL, et al: Blood volumes and plasma protein during levarterenol-induced hypertension. J Clin Invest 37:425, 1958.

76. Schmutzer KJ, Rashke E, Maloney JV Jr, et al: Intravenous 1-norepinephrine as cause of reduced plasma volume. Surgery 50:452, 1961.

77. Harms BA, Bodai BI, Kramer GC, et al: Microvascular fluid and protein flux in pulmonary and systemic circulations after thermal injury. Microvasc Res 23:77, 1982.

78. Iskrant AP: Statistics and epidemiology of burns. Bull NY Acad Med 43:636, 1967.

79. Cotran RS: The delayed and prolonged vascular leakage in inflammation. Am J Pathol 46:589, 1965.

80. Cotran RS and Remensnyder JP: The structural basis of increased vascular permeability after graded thermal injury-light and electron microscopic studies. Ann NY Acad Sci 150:495, 1968.

81. Moyer CA: *In*: Artz CP (ed): Research in Burns. Washington, DC, American Institute of Biological Science, 1962, pp. 113–120.

82. Barr PO, Birke G, Liljedahl SO, et al: Studies on burns. Scand J Plast Reconstr Surg 3:30, 1969.

83. Carvajal HF and Goldman AS: *In*: Nelson WE (ed): Textbook of Pediatrics. Philadelphia, WB Saunders, 1983.

84. Monafo WM, Chuntrasakul C, Ayvazian VH, et al: Hypertonic sodium solutions in the treatment of burn shock. Am J Surg 126:778, 1973.

85. Caldwell FT and Bowser BH: Clinical evaluation of hypertonic and hypotonic solutions to resuscitate severely burned children. Ann Surg 189:546, 1979.

86. Baxter CR: Fluid volume and electrolyte changes in the early postburn period. Clin Plast Surg 1:693, 1974.

87. Szyfelbein SK, Drop LJ, Martyn JA, et al: Persistent ionized hypocalcemia in patients during resuscitation and recovery phase of body burns. Crit Care Med 9:454, 1981.

88. Burke JF, Bondoc CC, Morris PJ, et al: Metabolic effects of topical silver nitrate therapy in burns covering more than fifteen percent of the body surface. Ann NY Acad Sci 150:674, 1968.

89. Greco BA and Jacobsen HR: Fluid and electrolyte problems in surgery, trauma, and burns. In: Kokko JP and Tannen RL (eds): Fluids and Electrolytes. Philadelphia, WB Saunders, 1990, p. 993.

90. Cameron JS: Acute renal failure in the intensive care unit today. Intensive Care Med 12:64, 1986.

91. Hug CC Jr.: Pharmacology-anesthetic drugs. In: Kaplan JA (ed): Cardiac Anesthesia: Cardiovascular Pharmacology. New York, Grune & Stratton, 1983, pp. 3–37.

92. Chambers D: Anesthesia. Methods, effects, and risks in the medical patient. In: Tubin MF, Walker HK, and Smith RB III (eds): Medical Management of the Surgical Patient. Boston, Buttersworths, 1982, pp. 81–137.

93. Zollinger RM Jr, Skillman JJ, Moore FD, et al: Alterations in water, colloid and electrolyte distribution after hemorrhage. In: Fox CL Jr and Nahas GG (eds): Body Fluid Replacement in the Surgical Patient. New York, Grune & Stratton, 1969, pp. 2–9.

94. Lister J, McNeill IF, Marshall VC, et al: Transcapillary refilling after hemorrhage in normal man: Basal rates and volume; effect of norepinephrine. Ann Surg 158:698, 1963.

95. Pacifico A, Digerness S, and Kirklin J: Acute alterations of body composition after open intracardiac operations. Circulation 41:331, 1970.

96. Beattie H, Evans G, Garnett ES, et al: Sustained hypovolemia and extracellular fluid volume expansion following cardiopulmonary bypass. Surgery 71:891, 1972.

97. Utley JR and Stephens DB: Fluid balance during cardiopulmonary bypass. In: Utley JR (ed): Pathophysiology and Techniques of Cardiopulmonary Bypass, Vol II. Baltimore, Williams & Wilkins, 1983, pp. 23–35.

98. Breckenridge IM, Digerness SB, and Kirklin JW: Increased extracellular fluid after open intracardiac operation. Surg Gynecol Obstet 131:53, 1970.

99. Cleland J, Pluth JR, Tauxe WN, et al: Blood volume and body fluid compartment changes soon after closed and open intracardiac surgery. J Thorac Cardiovasc Surg 52:698, 1966.

100. Berger RL, Boyd TF, and Marcus PS: A pattern of blood-volume response to open-heart surgery. N Engl J Med 271:59, 1964.

101. Beattie HW, Evans G, Garnett ES, et al: Albumin and water fluxes during cardiopulmonary bypass. J Thorac Cardiovasc Surg 67:926, 1974.

102. Litwak RS, Slonim R, Keim I, et al: Alterations in blood volume during "normovolemic" total body perfusion. J Thorac Cardiovasc Surg 42:477, 1961.

103. Kaplan S, Edwards FK, Helmsworth JA, et al: Blood volume during and after extracorporeal circulation. Arch Surg 80:31, 1960.

104. McClenahan JB, Yamauchi H, and Roe BB: Blood volume studies in cardiac surgery patients. JAMA 195:356, 1966.

105. Neville WE, Thomason RD, and Hirsch DM: Postoperative hypervolemia after hemodilution cardiopulmonary bypass. Arch Surg 93:715, 1966.

106. Arieff AI: Osmotic failure: Physiology and strategies for treatment. Hosp Pract 23:173, 1988.

107. Covey CM and Arieff AI: Disorders of sodium and water metabolism and their effects on the central nervous system. In: Brenner BM and Stein JH (eds): Sodium and Water Homeostasis. New York, Churchill Livingstone, 1978, pp. 212–241.

108. Sterns RH, Riggs JE, and Schochet SS Jr.: Osmotic demyelination syndrome following correction of hyponatremia. N Engl J Med 314:1535, 1986.

109. Sterns RH: Severe symptomatic hyponatremia: Treatment and outcome. A study of 64 cases. Ann Intern Med 107:656, 1987.

110. Wright DG, Laureno R, and Victor M: Pontine and extrapontine myelinolysis. Brain 102:361, 1979.

111. Ross EJ and Christie SBM: Hypernatremia. Medicine 48:441, 1969.

112. Zierler KL: Hyperosmolarity in adults: A critical review. J Chronic Dis 7:1, 1958.

113. Finberg L: Hypernatremic (hypertonic) dehydration in infants. N Engl J Med 289:196, 1973.

114. Bruck E, Abal G, and Aceto T: Pathogenesis and pathophysiology of hypertonic dehydration with diarrhea. Am J Dis Child 115:122, 1968.

115. Finberg L: Pathogenesis of lesions in the nervous system in hypernatremic states. I: Clinical observations of infants. Pediatrics 23:40, 1959.

116. Macauley D and Watsom M: Hypernatremia as a cause of brain damage. Arch Dis Child 42:485, 1967.

117. Katzman R and Pappius HM: Hypernatremia and hyperosmolarity. In: Katzman R and Pappius HM (eds): Brain Electrolytes and Fluid Metabolism. Baltimore, Williams & Wilkins, 1973, p. 278.

118. Stevenson RE and Bowyer FP: Hyperglycemia with hyperosmolar dehydration in non diabetic infants. J Pediatr 77:818, 1970.

119. Burnell JM, Villamil MF, Uyeno BT, et al: The effect in humans of extracellular pH change on the relationship between serum potassium concentration and intracellular potassium. J Clin Invest 35:935, 1965.

120. Adrogue HJ and Madias NE: Changes in plasma potassium concentration during acute acid-base disturbances. Am J Med 71:456, 1981.

121. Perez GO, Oster JR, and Vaamonde CA: Serum potassium concentration in acidemic states. Nephron 27:233, 1981.

122. Silva P and Spokes K: Sympathetic system in potassium homeostatis. Am J Physiol 241:F151, 1981.

123. Williams ME, Rosa RM, Silva P, et al: Impairment of extrarenal potassium disposal by α-adrenergic stimulation. N Engl J Med 311:145, 1984.

124. Smith JD, Bia MJ, DeFronzo RA, et al: In: Arieff Al, DeFronzo RA (eds): Fluid, Electrolyte, and Acid-Base Disorders. New York, Churchill Livingstone, 1985, p. 413.

125. Montoliu J, Lens XM, and Revert L: Potassium-lowering effect of albuterol for hyperkalemia in renal failure. Arch Intern Med 147:713, 1987.

126. Physician's Desk Reference, 39th ed. Oradell, NJ, Medical Economics Company, 1985.

127. Lazarus JM: Complications in hemodialysis: An overview. Kidney Int 18:783, 1980.

128. Melvin T, Powell B, Pillere D, et al: Continuous arteriovenous hemofiltration—pre-dilution technique used in ornithine transcarbamylase deficiency. Pediatr Res 27:4: 334A, 1990.

129. Caroenas-Rivero N, Chernow B, Stoiko MA, et al: Hypocalcemia in critically ill children. J Pediatr 114:946, 1989.

130. Sanchez GJ, Venkataraman PS, Pryor RW, et al: Hypercalcitoninemia and hypocalcemia in acutely ill children: Studies in serum calcium, blood ionized calcium and calcium-regulating hormones. J Pediatr 114:952, 1989.

131. Chernow B, Zaloga G, McFadden E, et al: Hypocalcemia in critically ill patients. Crit Care Med 10:848, 1982.

132. Zaloga GP and Chernow B: Hypocalcemia in critical illness. JAMA 256: 1924, 1986.

133. White BC, Aust SC, Arfors KE, et al: Brain injury by ischemic anoxia: Hypothesis extension—a tale of two ions? Ann Emerg Med 251:1586, 1984.

134. Siesjo BK: Mechanisms of ischemic brain injury. Crit Care Med 16:954, 1988.

135. Chernow B: Calcium: Does it have a therapeutic role in sepsis? Crit Care Med 18:895, 1990.

136. Bronsky D, Dubin A, Waldstein SS, et al: Calcium and the electrocardiogram. II: The electrocardiographic manifestations

of hyperparathyroidism and marked hypercalcemia from various etiologies. Am J Cardiol 7:833, 1961.

137. Anast CS: Disorders of mineral and bone metabolism. *In*: Avery ME and Tausch HW (eds): Schaffer's Diseases of the Newborn, 5th ed. Philadelphia, WB Saunders, 1984, pp. 464–479.

138. Strauch BS and Ball MF: Hemodialysis in the treatment of severe hypercalcemia. JAMA 235:1347, 1976.

139. Ryzen E, Wagers PW, and Singer FR: Magnesium deficiency in a medical ICU population. Crit Care Med 13:19, 1985.

140. Reinhart RA and Desbiens NA: Hypomagnesemia in patients entering the ICU. Crit Care Med 13:506, 1985.

141. Chernow B, Bamberger BS, Stoiko M, et al: Hypomagnesemia in patients in postoperative intensive care. Chest 95:391, 1989.

142. Fiaccadori E, DelCanale S, and Coffrini E: Muscle and serum magnesium in pulmonary intensive care unit patients. Crit Care Med 16:751, 1988.

143. Munoz R, Khilnani P, and Salem M: Ionized hypomagnesemia: A frequent problem in critically ill neonates. Crit Care Med 19:548, 1991.

144. Mordes JP and Wacker WE: Excess magnesium. Pharmacol Rev 29:273, 1978.

145. Brady JP and Williams HC: Magnesium intoxication in a premature infant. Pediatrics 40:100, 1967.

146. Ebel H and Gunther T: Magnesium metabolism: A review. J Clin Chem Clin Biochem 18:257, 1980.

147. Lipsitz PJ: The clinical and biochemical effects of excess magnesium in the newborn. Pediatrics 47:501, 1971.

148. Lee DBN, Brautbar N, and Kleeman CR: Disorders of phosphorus metabolism. *In*: Bronner F and Coburn JW (eds): Disorders of Mineral Metabolism, Vol 3. New York, Academic Press, 1981, p. 283.

149. Ritz E: Acute Hypophosphatemia. Nephrology forum. Kidney Int 22:84, 1982.

150. Knochel JP: The pathophysiology and clinical characteristics of severe hypophosphatemia. Arch Intern Med 127:203, 1977.

151. Parfitt AM and Kleerekoper M: The divalent ion homeostatic system—physiology and metabolism of calcium, phosphorus, magnesium, and bone. *In*: Maxwell MH and Kleeman CR (eds): Clinical Disorders of Fluid and Electrolyte Metabolism. New York, McGraw-Hill, 1979, p. 269.

152. Parfitt AM and Kleerekoper M: Clinical disorders of calcium, phosphorus and magnesium metabolism. *In*: Maxwell MH and Kleeman CR (eds): Clinical Disorders of Fluid and Electrolyte Metabolism. New York, McGraw-Hill, 1979, p. 947.

153. Lau K: Phosphate disorders. *In*: Kokko JP and Tannen RL (eds): Fluids and Electrolytes. Philadelphia, WB Saunders, 1990, p. 505.

154. Lichtman MA, Miller DR, and Cohen J: Reduced red cell glycolysis, 1,2-diphosphoglycerate and adenosine triphosphate concentration and increased hemoglobin-oxygen affinity caused by hypophosphatemia. Ann Intern Med 74:562, 1971.

155. Lentz DR, Brown DM, and Kjellstrand CM: Treatment of severe hypophosphatemia. Ann Intern Med 89:941, 1978.

156. Lau K: Phosphate disorders. *In*: Kokko JP and Tannen RL (eds): Fluids and Electrolytes. Philadelphia, WB Saunders, 1990, p. 571.

157. Golper W and Bennett W: Drug usage in dialysis patients. *In*: Nissensen AR, Fine RN, and Gentile DE (eds): Clinical Dialysis. Norwalk CT, Appleton & Lange, 1990.

158. Avner ED, Ellis D, Ichikawa I, et al: Normal neonates and the maturational development of homeostatic mechanisms. *In*: Ichikawa I (ed): Pediatric Textbook of Fluids and Electrolytes. Baltimore, Williams & Wilkins, 1990, pp. 107–120.

159. Morrison G and Singer I: Hyperosmolal states. *In*: Maxwell MH, Kleeman CR, and Narins RG (eds): Clinical Disorders of Fluid and Electrolytes, 4th ed. New York, McGraw-Hill, 1987.

160. Yared A, Foose J, and Ichicawa I: Disorders of osmoregulation. *In*: Ichikawa I (ed): Pediatric Textbook of Fluids and Electrolytes. Baltimore, Williams & Wilkins, 1990, pp. 165–186.

161. Ingelfinger JR: Hypertension and hypotension. *In*: Ichikawa I (ed): Pediatric Textbook of Fluids and Electrolytes. Baltimore, Williams & Wilkins, 1990, pp. 130–164.

162. Yoshioka T, Sitaka K, and Ichikawa I: Body fluid compartments. *In*: Ichikawa I (ed): Pediatric Textbook of Fluids and Electrolytes. Baltimore, Williams & Wilkins, 1990, pp. 14–20.

163. Segar W: Parenteral fluid therapy. Curr Prob Pediatr 3(2):34, 1972.

164. Burton AC: Physiology and Biophysics of the Circulation, 2nd ed. Chicago, Year Book Medical Publishers, 1972, p. 54.

165. Robertson GL, Aycinena P, and Zerbe RL: Neurogenic disorders of osmoregulation. Am J Med 72:339, 1982.

166. Rose BD: Clinical Physiology of Acid Base and Electrolyte Disorders. New York, McGraw-Hill, 1984.

167. Ichikawa I and Yared A: Renal blood flow and glomerular filtration rate. *In*: Holliday MA, Barrett TM, and Vernier RL (eds): Pediatric Nephrology, 2nd ed. Baltimore, Williams & Wilkins, 1987.

168. Cavero PG, Margulies KB, Winaver J, et al: Cardiorenal actions of neutral endopeptidase inhibition in experimental congestive heart failure. Circulation 82:190, 1990.

59

Endocrine Disorders

Leticia Castillo, M.D., and Bart Chernow, M.D.

The field of endocrine disorders leading to critical illness has grown considerably during the past decade. With the identification and isolation of growth factors, cytokines, nitric oxide, and other elements that participate in cell-to-cell communication, a "microendocrine" system was discovered. This aspect of the endocrine system is widely discussed in another section of this book (see Chapter 3). This chapter focuses on the pathologic features of the "macroendocrine" system that lead to critical illness.

DIABETIC KETOACIDOSIS

Diabetic ketoacidosis (DKA) is a catabolic process that affects glucose, lipid, and protein metabolism, resulting in life-threatening disease. DKA is responsible for 16% of the total mortality rate in diabetes and is the most frequent cause of death in diabetic children.[1-4] Approximately 20% of patients with type I diabetes mellitus present with DKA as the initial manifestation of disease.[5] Insulin exerts its metabolic effects throughout the body (with the exception of the nervous system, blood cells, and renal medulla); however, the adipose tissue, muscle, and liver become the "target" organs during DKA.

Etiology

Type I diabetes mellitus (insulin-deficient or insulin-dependent diabetes mellitus) is the most frequent form of diabetes mellitus in children. Type II diabetes mellitus (non–insulin dependent) is unusual in children. Although diabetes mellitus has been thought to have a multifactorial cause (genetic predisposition, viral infections, autoimmune processes, and so on), it is now evident through the widespread use of molecular biology techniques that different kinds of molecular defects (such as abnormal membrane receptors for insulin; intracellular uncoupling of the insulin-receptor complex, resulting in defective signal transduction; defective conversion of proinsulin to insulin; or abnormal structure of the insulin molecule[6-8] may result in diabetes mellitus.

Pathophysiology

Insulin is a polypeptide hormone that plays an important role in the regulation of fuel metabolism. Insulin has an overall anabolic effect, promoting the cellular uptake of glucose, amino acids, potassium, and magnesium. It induces glycogen and protein synthesis and lipogenesis. Conversely, it inhibits glycogenolysis, protein breakdown, and lipolysis (Table 59–1). The actions of insulin are mediated via increasing levels of cyclic adenosine monophosphate.[9, 28] Although insulin deficiency is the initial and key event in DKA, many of the pathophysiologic events observed in this state are mediated by increased levels of counterregulatory hormones, which include glucagon, epinephrine, norepinephrine, growth hormone, and cortisol.[10-14] Plasma concentrations of arginine vasopressin, renin, angiotensin, and aldosterone are increased,[15, 16, 27, 59, 60] whereas circulating atrial natriuretic peptide levels are decreased.[17-19] Plasma and urinary prostaglandin E_2 and prostaglandin F_1 values are increased during DKA. This finding probably represents an activation of systemic prostaglandin E metabolism during DKA, though the physiologic importance of this observation remains to be established.[20, 21] Thyroid hormone levels are also increased (Table 59–2).[22, 46, 47]

Hyperglycemia

As mentioned previously, the liver, muscle, and adipose tissues become the primary target organs during DKA. In the liver, a decrease or lack of insulin and an increased glucagon:insulin ratio activate protein kinase through a cyclic adenosine monophosphate mechanism.

Table 59–1. PHYSIOLOGIC EFFECTS OF INSULIN IN "TARGET" ORGANS

Liver	Muscle	Fat
Uptake of glucose, amino acids	Uptake of glucose, amino acids	↑ Lipogenesis
K, Mg	K, Mg	↑ Gylcerol products
↑ Glycogenesis	↑ Glycogenesis	
Protein synthesis	↑ Protein synthesis	

703

Table 59–2. PLASMA CONCENTRATIONS OF DIFFERENT HORMONAL SYSTEMS DURING DIABETIC KETOACIDOSIS

Glucagon ↑	Vasopressin ↑	Atrial natriuretic peptide ↓
Epinephrine ↑	Renin ↑	Thyroid hormone ↓
Growth hormone ↑	Angiotensin ↑	Prostaglandin E₂ ↑
Cortisol ↑	Aldosterone ↑	Prostaglandin F₂ ↑

Increased activity of protein kinase, in turn, decreases fructose 2,6-diphosphate, which is a key metabolite that regulates fructose phosphorylation. When fructose 2,6-diphosphate levels are low, fructose 1,6-diphosphatase is stimulated and phosphofructokinase is inhibited. The net result is a metabolic shift toward increased gluconeogenesis and decreased glycolysis (Fig. 59–1).[23, 26, 28–30, 31–54] Gluconeogenesis is the process by which amino acids, lactate, and glycerol precursors are converted to glucose. Glycolysis is the process by which glucose is converted to pyruvate with the concomitant production of adenosine triphosphate (ATP). Pyruvate undergoes oxidation to form acetylcoenzyme A (acetyl CoA), which enters the citric acid cycle and the electron transport chain. This metabolic sequence represents the final common pathway for fuel metabolism, as well as a source of precursors for biosynthetic reactions. During DKA, therefore, fuel-energy metabolism is impaired.[18, 23, 26] Glycogenolysis is increased during DKA, though this mechanism of hyperglycemia is limited, given the relatively small glycogen reserves.

There is increased protein breakdown in DKA, with massive output of alanine and glutamine from the muscle. Plasma concentrations of branched-chain amino acids increase, whereas plasma alanine concentrations decrease because of accelerated gluconeogenesis.[31] Protein synthesis and glucose uptake are inhibited. Although muscle is the major source of glycogen storage, it lacks glucose-6-phosphatase (a key enzyme in glucose metabolism) and therefore is unable to export glucose to the circulation.[8] In muscle, glycogen is converted to lactate, which then leaves the muscle cell and is taken up by the liver to be used as a precursor for gluconeogenesis.[29, 30] Hyperglycemia during DKA is the result of uncontrolled gluconeogenesis and glycogenolysis.

Ketogenesis

In adipose tissue, the lack of insulin and the increased levels of counterregulatory hormones promote lipolysis—a massive breakdown of triglycerides into free fatty acids and glycerol, which are then released into the circulation and taken up by the liver.[29, 30, 33] Glycerol enters the gluconeogenic pathway and is converted to glucose. The free fatty acids are activated to acyl CoA molecules in the cytosol of hepatocytes and are then oxidized in the mitochondria. Because long-chain acyl CoA fatty acids do not readily tranverse the mitochondrial membrane, a transport mechanism is required. Carnitine carries these molecules into the mitochondria in the form of fatty acyl carnitine derivatives.[32, 34] Glucagon enhances the production of carnitine and inhibits malonyl CoA, which prevents the linkage of fatty acids with carnitine.[25, 32, 34] The massive release of fatty acids leads to an excessive production of acetyl CoA precursors for the tricarboxylic acid cycle. Ketone bodies are

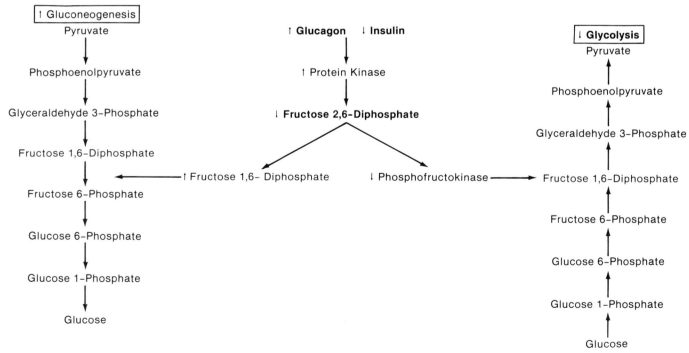

Figure 59–1. Control of gluconeogenesis and glycolysis. Increased glucagon/insulin ratio will decrease activity of fructose 2,6-diphosphate through cAMP and protein kinase mechanism, resulting in stimulation of fructose 1,6-diphosphate, which mediates a key step in gluconeogenesis, and inhibition of phosphofructokinase, which mediates a key step in glycolysis.

formed when the excess acetyl CoA can no longer enter the overwhelmed tricarboxylic acid cycle (Fig. 59–2).[9, 30]

The ketone bodies β-hydroxybutyrate and acetoacetate are strong acids that induce acidosis by releasing hydrogen ions into the circulation; they are eventually oxidized or excreted in the urine. However, their presence in the circulation contributes to the metabolic acidosis seen in DKA. Acetone is a derivative of acetoacetate and is excreted by the lungs and to a lesser extent by the urine.

Despite the fact that β-hydroxybutyrate is the main contributor to ketoacidosis, it is not detected by the nitroprusside reaction frequently used to identify serum ketones. This problem may result in underestimation of the degree of ketosis.[35–37] Likewise, salicylates, valproic acid, phenothiazine, and L-DOPA will react with the nitroprusside reagent and yield false-positive results.[30] The possibility of drug ingestion should always be considered in the ketotic patient.

Hypovolemia and alterations in the erythrocyte morphologic appearance induced by hyperosmolarity will result in impaired or decreased blood flow, which further increases acidosis.

Hyperosmolality

Hyperosmolality in DKA is the result of hyperglycemia, dehydration, and an increased blood urinary nitrogen level. Plasma osmolality is increased by 1 mOsm/kg/H_2O for each 18 mg of glucose/dl and for each 2.8 mg of urea nitrogen/dl.[38, 40] Sodium also contributes to serum osmolality, though true determination of serum sodium in DKA is difficult because hyperlipidemia displaces plasma water, inducing a falsely low value of sodium. In addition, hyperglycemia induces dilution of serum sodium levels by promoting entry of water from the intracellular space into the extracellular space. It has been calculated that every 100 mg/dl increase in glucose will reduce 1.6 mEq/l of plasma sodium.[40–42] Hyperosmolality has consequences in the central nervous system. The blood-brain barrier is "opened" by a hyperosmolar infusion, enabling molecules to penetrate the brain cells. Also, during hyperosmolar states there is an increased solute concentration in the brain cell, which attempts to "osmoprotect" cell integrity and function. These osmoprotective molecules in the cytosol of brain cells favor movement of water into the cell.[15, 62–64] Factors as yet undetermined may exacerbate this process and result in cerebral edema.

Dehydration

Hyperglycemia results in glucosuria. When the amount of glucose in the urine exceeds the reabsorptive capacity of the proximal tubules, an osmotic diuresis ensues with the loss of free water and various electrolytes. This process is the major source of fluid deficit in DKA. Other causes of fluid loss include increased insensible losses from hyperventilation and fever, and loss from ongoing vomiting, a common symptom of ketosis.

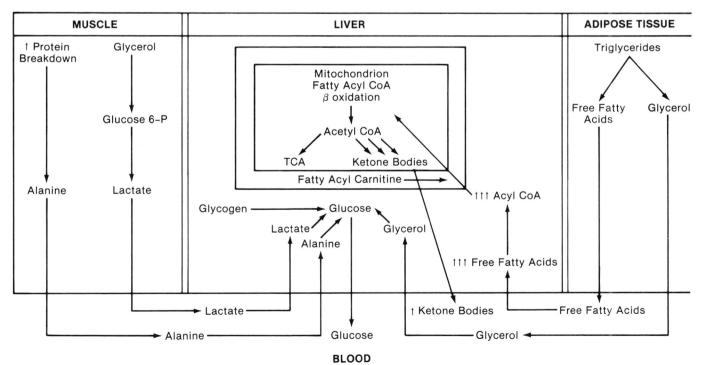

Figure 59–2. Schematic representations of metabolic events during DKA. In muscle, protein breakdown and glycogenolysis provide precursors for gluconeogenesis. In the adipose tissue, lipolysis results in release of glycerol for gluconeogenesis and free fatty acids. These are transported into the mitochondrion through the carnitine transport system and a decrease in malonyl CoA. Fatty acyl CoA is oxidized to acetyl CoA that enters the TCA cycle. The excessive supply of acetyl CoA is converted to ketone bodies, which are released to the circulation.

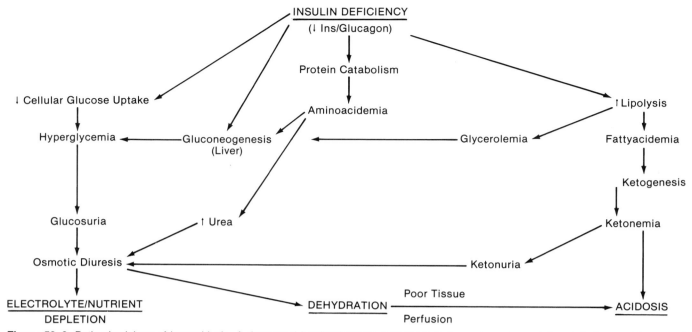

Figure 59–3. Pathophysiology of ketoacidosis. A decreased insulin/glucagon ratio leads to hyperglycemia, protein catabolism and increased lipolysis. Hyperglycemia occurs via a decreased cellular glucose uptake and increased gluconeogenesis, and to a lesser extent via glycogenolysis. Hyperglycemia results in glucosuria, osmotic diuresis, dehydration, and acidosis. Protein catabolism, with the resultant release of amino acids and urea, will provide substrate for gluconeogenesis, and the increase in urea production will contribute to osmotic diureses. Increased lipolysis results in excessive production of glycerol, which is a substrate for gluconeogenesis and a large load of fatty acids, resulting in production of ketone bodies and acidosis. Excretion of ketones in urine contributes to osmotic diureses.

Electrolytes

If severe dehydration is induced by osmotic diuresis, hemoconcentration and hypernatremia may be found. However, it is not unusual to find a normal, low, or high serum sodium concentration in patients with DKA.

Increased osmotic pressure in the extracellular fluid and volume depletion are the two major stimuli for the release of arginine vasopressin into the circulation. During DKA, however, osmoregulation of vasopressin is altered, resulting in persistently high levels of this hormone.[15, 16, 27, 43] Other systems—for example, the renin-angiotensin-aldosterone system—are stimulated in an attempt to retain sodium and water.[30, 34]

Hyperkalemia or hypokalemia is frequently found during the acute stage of DKA; however, total body potassium levels are usually depleted. Insulin promotes the uptake of potassium by the cell, and during DKA the lack of insulin and increased levels of counterregulatory hormones (mainly glucagon) lead to intracellular potassium depletion. In addition, ions are shifted from the intracellular to the extracellular space as a result of the intracellular buffering of hydrogen ions. Osmotic diuresis causes increased loss of water and potassium. Once dehydration results, aldosterone release increases as a compensatory mechanism, increasing renal tubular sodium resorption and increased urinary excretion of potassium.[23, 30, 40, 46] Hypokalemic respiratory arrest has been reported during the course of DKA, and caution should be exercised when hypokalemia is found during the initial evaluation of a patient with DKA. Administration of insulin favors the entry of potassium into the intracellular space and decreases the serum potassium concentration. These insulin-induced actions may increase the risk of arrhythmia or respiratory arrest.[49–51] Phosphate levels may also be decreased because of insulin administration, osmotic diuresis, acidosis, and tubular dysfunction. Decreased levels of diphosphoglycerate may occur during DKA and may impair oxygen transport.[30, 48, 52, 53] Hypocalcemia and hypomagnesemia may also occur in children with DKA, particularly as a complication of aggressive phosphate repletion.[30, 47]

Blood urea nitrogen values may be increased as a result of a decreased glomerular filtration rate. Serum creatinine concentrations may be normal or increased. An increased plasma creatinine determination should be judiciously interpreted because increased serum concentrations of acetoacetate interfere with creatinine analysis.[55, 56]

The pathophysiologic characteristics and clinical events of DKA are illustrated in Figure 59–3.

Clinical Characteristics

DKA is frequently the initial manifestation of diabetes mellitus in pediatric patients. Precipitating factors such as infection or poor compliance with insulin therapy may be found in patients with a long-standing history of diabetes.[40] Salicylate intoxication may resemble DKA; hyperventilation, acidosis, vomiting, dehydration, a positive nitroprusside test result for ketoacids in urine and serum, and the presence of a wide anion gap may therefore be misleading. These patients, however, should have a history of exposure to aspirin or related compounds such as salicylic acid or methylsalicylate, and plasma glucose concentrations should be normal. Alcoholic ketoacidosis and pancreatitis in adolescents may also present with similar chemical characteristics.[30]

In general, the patient with DKA who requires admission to the pediatric intensive care unit is usually in a state of moderate to severe illness. Careful attention must be paid to an integral assessment. Often there is some degree of drowsiness or obtundation and a high risk of aspiration. Progressive obtundation or coma in a patient with DKA may be a manifestation of cerebral edema, a dreaded complication that carries a high rate of morbidity. Tachypnea or frank respiratory distress as a compensatory response to metabolic acidosis is found. Dehydration and even varied degrees of overt shock may be present. The laboratory findings of DKA are summarized in Table 59–3. Once the diagnosis of DKA has been established, treatment should be instituted without delay.

Treatment

The initial therapeutic approach in DKA, as in any other critical illness, is to pay close attention to the patient's airway, breathing, and circulation. A comatose or poorly responsive patient will require endotracheal intubation for airway protection. Most patients, however, become alert and responsive quickly once fluid repletion and insulin therapy is initiated. If progressive lethargy or obtundation occurs, further assessment of neurologic status with a computed tomography scan of the head is warranted. Necessary therapeutic decisions should not be delayed by invasive procedures or specialized testing. If the patient requires endotracheal intubation, sedation should be accomplished with drugs that do not induce hypotension in an already compromised patient; morphine and barbiturates should be avoided for this reason. Likewise, cerebral edema has been described even before therapy has been initiated;[60] therefore, ketamine, a drug that increases both cerebral blood flow and oxygen utilization, should be avoided. A benzodiazepine (diazepam 0.1 mg/kg) and lidocaine (1 mg/kg) or fentanyl (3 to 5 μg/kg) and lidocaine are more appropriate choices. If muscle relaxation is required, it should be considered that hypovolemia and cerebral edema may be present in DKA. The use of a depolarizing muscle relaxant such as succinylcholine (1 mg/kg) should be preceded by a defasciculating dose of pancuronium bromide (0.01 mg/kg).[61, 62] The major toxic effects of succinylcholine result from the initial depolar-

ization and subsequent muscle contraction. A small increase in the plasma potassium concentration occurs when succinylcholine is used, as potassium is released from muscle into the circulation. Severe hyperkalemia and cardiac arrest have rarely occurred in succinylcholine-treated patients with conditions predisposing to increased potassium levels. In these, a nondepolarizing muscle relaxant (vecuronium, 0.1 mg/kg intravenously or atracurium 0.4 mg/kg intravenously) should be used. The generalized muscle contraction elicited by succinylcholine may also induce an increase in intracranial pressure. Atropine (0.02 mg/kg intravenously) should be given before succinylcholine, given that bradycardia may occur as a result of muscarinic receptor stimulation, unless the patient already has tachycardia (>200 bpm).

Fluid and Electrolyte Therapy

At the same time that airway management is handled, appropriate venous access should be secured. A fluid bolus of 10 to 20 ml/kg of an isotonic solution should be given by rapid intravenous infusion and repeated as necessary until hemodynamic stabilization is demonstrated by a decrease in the heart rate, normal blood pressure, and improved tissue perfusion. If the patient with DKA is dehydrated but not in shock, the extent of dehydration should be carefully assessed. The hyperosmolar state in these patients at presentation may result in an underestimation of the severity of dehydration. Usually the patient who is dehydrated but not in shock will require one or two fluid "loads" to achieve stability. Good clinical judgment must prevail in fluid replacement in these patients. Although there is controversy about the reliability of predictive factors in the development of cerebral edema, the administration of large amounts of hypotonic fluids over a short time has been considered a predisposing factor for this complication. Based on these circumstances, some authors have recommended the intravenous solution not exceed 4.2 l/m²/day in the first 24 hours;[47, 65–68] however, inadequate correction of hypovolemic shock may set the stage for complications such as bacterial translocation from an ischemic gut, with activation of endogenous mediators and a systemic inflammatory response that may lead to adult respiratory distress syndrome or multiple organ failure.[69–71] The recommendation of 4.2 l/m²/day without considering the degree of dehydration or body size is limiting and may bring inadequate results under some circumstances.

The objective in fluid therapy is to provide maintenance fluids and correct the fluid deficit slowly over a period of 48 hours.

After initial fluid resuscitation with an isotonic solution, and once the degree of dehydration has been established, maintenance fluids and half of the deficit should be administered in the next 24 hours. The remaining deficit should be administered during the second 24 hours after admission. One must remember to subtract the amount of fluid required for initial resuscitation from the total deficit. Ongoing excessive losses will decrease once insulin therapy is initiated. Monitoring central venous pressure, particularly if the patient presents with shock, provides useful information to guide

Table 59–3. LABORATORY ABNORMALITIES IN DIABETIC KETOACIDOSIS

Blood sugar ↑	Ca ↓ or normal	Plasma triglyceride ↑
Plasma ketones ↑	Mg ↓ or normal	pH ↓ bicarbonate ↓
Na ↑ Normal or ↓	BUN* ↑ or normal	Urine + glucose
K ↑ Normal or ↓	Creatinine ↑ or normal	+ ketones
Phosphate ↓	White blood cell count ↑	± protein

*BUN = blood urea nitrogen.

fluid therapy but, rather than a specific value, the trend should be closely followed. Maintenance fluids with a glucose-free, isotonic solution providing 150 mEq Na/l (0.9% NaCl solution with 30 to 40 mEq/l of potassium; 15 to 20 mEq/l of potassium phosphate; and 15 to 20 mEq/l of potassium chloride) should be adequate. Patients with DKA present with hypertonic dehydration, and administration of a hypotonic solution may be a contributing factor in the development of cerebral edema.[65, 67, 68, 72, 73]

As already stated, the serum sodium concentration may be low, normal, or high; however, false lower values of plasma sodium will often be obtained because of hyperglycemia and hyperlipidemia. To correct for this artifact, plasma sodium levels should be calculated by adding 1.6 mEq Na for every 100 mg/dl of glucose greater than 100 mg/dl (Table 59–4). Plasma sodium concentration should increase as therapy progresses. Failure of the sodium value to increase may alert the clinician to excessive fluid administration. A component of excessive secretion of vasopressin is usually present.[27, 57, 58]

Potassium replacement should be initiated with fluid resuscitation. Caution should be exercised if the patient has plasma values of potassium at both extremes. Hypokalemia will worsen with the administration of insulin because of facilitation of potassium uptake by the cell. If hypokalemia is present, replacement with 10 to 20 mEq/hr of potassium via a central venous catheter may be required. Hyperkalemia may result in life-threatening cardiac arrhythmias. Continuous cardiorespiratory monitoring is required in patients with DKA.

Although initial studies based on sound physiologic principles emphasize the need for phosphate replacement, controlled trials have shown no difference in outcome between patients treated with and those treated without phosphate supplementation.[34, 74, 76, 77] We advocate the judicious use of phosphate until more conclusive clinical trials are conducted.

Hypocalcemia (and hypomagnesemia) may occur if aggressive phosphate replacement therapy is given. In this case, calcium and magnesium supplementation is indicated. Once the blood glucose concentration has decreased to 250 to 300 mg/dl, a 5% glucose-containing solution should be initiated.

Table 59–4. Formulas for Common Calculations in Diabetic Ketoacidosis

Correction of Serum Sodium During Hyperglycemia

$$NA^+ = NA^+ \text{ measured} + 1.6\frac{\text{glucose} - 100}{100}$$

Calculation of Serum Osmolality

$$\text{Serum osmolality (mOsm/l)} = 2(Na^+) + \frac{\text{glucose}}{18} + \frac{BUN\dagger}{2.8}$$

Calculation of Anion Gap

$$\text{Anion gap (mEq/l)} = Na^+ - (Cl^- + HCO_3^-)$$

*Modified from Krane E: Diabetic ketoacidosis: Biochemistry, physiology, treatment, and prevention. Pediatr Clin North Am 34:935, 1987.
†BUN = blood urea nitrogen.

Insulin Therapy

Administration of insulin is *not* urgent in DKA and should be initiated once fluid resuscitation has begun and when potassium homeostasis is assessed and therapy is under way. Although an initial intravenous bolus of insulin, 0.1 units/kg, has been long advocated based on the fact that adequate concentrations can be achieved immediately,[66, 78–82] no difference in the decline of glucose levels, change in osmolality, or time required to achieve a glucose level less than 250 mg/dl has been found[83, 84] in patients who did not receive an initial intravenous bolus of insulin when compared with those patients who did receive an intravenous bolus of insulin. Despite this fact, we recommend giving a bolus dose between 0.05 and 0.1 units/kg. Higher doses of insulin are no longer used except in selected cases of insulin resistance. A continuous intravenous insulin infusion of 0.1 units/kg/hr is recommended. This low-dose insulin has proved to be adequate to control hyperglycemia, with fewer complications of hypoglycemia when compared with higher insulin doses.[79–84] If there is no change in plasma blood glucose levels in 2 hours, the continuous infusion rate should be increased. If, in contrast, the blood glucose level rapidly decreases, the insulin infusion rate should be cut in half. A target for decreasing glucose levels should be no more than 100 mg/dl/hr. The insulin infusion may need to be titrated up or down to achieve this goal. Initially, *no* glucose should be infused—even in intravenous additives. Once the blood glucose level is less than or equal to 250 ml/dl, a fixed substrate (glucose) solution is administered. A concentration of 1 to 10 units of insulin/ml normal saline should be prepared as needed. It should be infused through a separate intravenous catheter to avoid an inadvertent insulin bolus. The plastic catheter tubing should be flushed with 25 ml of the insulin solution to prevent possible insulin absorption by the tubing. Once a glucose-containing solution is started, the insulin infusion rate may need to be adjusted to maintain a stable blood glucose value. Adjustment of the insulin infusion rate should be based on serial bedside blood glucose determinations.

Subcutaneous administration of insulin is not recommended in the critical care setting because of less precise control.

The intravenous insulin infusion may be discontinued 1 or 2 hours after the first dose of long-acting subcutaneous insulin when the plasma glucose value is less than 180 mg/dl, when ketonemia and acidosis have resolved, and when the patient is tolerating enteral feedings. In general, ketonuria continues for 24 to 36 hours after plasma glucose levels and acidosis are under control. The need for increasing requirements of insulin may be associated with the presence of complications such as infection. Decreased sensitivity to insulin has been reported in association with hypophosphatemia.[86] Hemodialysis has proved to be useful in a case of severe resistance to insulin.[87] When serum glucose values have decreased to 250 to 300 mg/dl, 5% dextrose should be added (at a fixed infusion rate) to the running intravenous fluids. Many clinicians find it useful to "match" insulin dosing to glucose values and to create what is known as an "insulin-glucose clamp."

Bicarbonate

Correction of acidosis is accomplished by insulin and fluid replacement. In the past, there has been controversy regarding the use of sodium bicarbonate.[23, 35, 93-95] Animal studies had suggested impairment in myocardial function during acidosis; however, conclusions have been conflicting, depending on the mechanism of induction of acidosis and the animal model used.[87-90] A randomized, prospective, controlled study demonstrated that the administration of bicarbonate to patients with severe DKA (with arterial pH values in the range of 6.9 to 7.14) did not provide beneficial effects in terms of clinical or biochemical recovery.[99]

Bicarbonate therapy may cause some hazards:

1. A rapid correction of acidosis with bicarbonate may cause displacement of potassium into the intracellular space, resulting in hypokalemia and leading to tissue refractoriness to insulin and other hormones.[35, 93, 95]

2. Rapid correction of acidosis may result in deranged tissue oxygen delivery through a diminished oxygen dissociation form of hemoglobin, leading to tissue hypoxia.[30, 66, 97]

3. A paradoxic cerebrospinal fluid acidosis[30, 66, 98] may follow bicarbonate therapy, as has been demonstrated in animal models and humans. This problem probably results in decreased function of intracellular enzymatic systems and possibly enhances further tissue hypoxia.[91, 99, 100]

4. Sodium bicarbonate may also contribute to hypernatremia, resulting in a greater increase of osmolality.

We do not recommend the routine use of sodium bicarbonate for a pH greater than 7. However, in the setting of extreme acidosis (pH of 7 or less, we recommend the use of an intravenous infusion of sodium bicarbonate at a dose of 0.5 to 1 mEq/kg over 10 minutes.

Supportive Care

A central venous catheter may more reliably guide fluid management and may provide a secure venous access for these critically ill patients. An indwelling arterial catheter should be placed for monitoring blood pressure and for serial drawing of blood samples. An indwelling bladder catheter should be placed if the patient is obtunded and an accurate urinary volume is not obtainable by other means (condom catheter, urine bag, and so on). A nasogastric tube may need to be placed depending on the individual patient's circumstances. Functional ileus and gastric atony is common, with risk of vomiting and aspiration. Stress ulcer prophylaxis may be needed if the gastric pH is lower than 4. Blood glucose, electrolyte, amylase, blood gas, serum osmolarity, and urine ketone determinations should be performed hourly during the initial stage of DKA. Once hyperglycemia and metabolic acidosis begin to improve, monitoring laboratory tests may be decreased to every 2 to 4 hours. The use of bedside microchemistry techniques provides close monitoring in critically ill patients without the disadvantage of excessive phlebotomy.[264]

Infection should be ruled out through a careful medical history and physical examination. Blood, urine, and throat cultures and chest x-ray studies should be obtained when indicated.

Judicious fluid administration, close monitoring of "corrected" serum sodium concentration, avoiding indiscriminate use of bicarbonate, as outlined previously, and a smooth decrease in serum glucose levels should be the objectives of therapy.

Involvement of a multidisciplinary team (pediatric intensive care practitioner, pediatric endocrinologist, and social worker) will ensure adequate follow-up. The family and patient need to be thoroughly informed, and referral to diabetic support groups should be offered.

Complications

The most feared complication of DKA is cerebral edema. Headache or lethargy in a patient with DKA should be a warning sign. Hyponatremia and failure of the plasma sodium concentration to increase during the treatment of DKA have been considered risk factors for the development of cerebral edema.[15, 30, 65-67, 72] However, this complication has been reported during hypernatremia and hyponatremia[110] and in patients who were treated with high or low doses of insulin therapy with or without bicarbonate replacement.[15, 67, 72, 110] There may be radiologic evidence of subclinical cerebral edema in patients with DKA before and after treatment with fluids and insulin.[60, 111] It appears that DKA per se is a predisposing risk factor for cerebral edema, and precautions should be taken to avoid progression of subclinical cerebral edema from a subclinical to a clinical state. Intracerebral formation of "idiogenic osmols" such as taurine and glutamate have been implicated in the pathophysiology of cerebral edema.[63, 64] They function as osmoprotective molecules that attract water into the cell but may lead to cerebral edema if the cell becomes relatively hyperosmolar compared with plasma as a result of hypotonic or excessive fluid administration. Abnormal endothelial capillary permeability is also considered a possible contributing factor.[62] Excessive secretion of vasopressin during DKA may also contribute to the development of cerebral edema.[57, 58] A rapid decrease in osmolality, whether induced by excessive free water and hypotonic solutions or a rapid decrease in blood glucose levels, should be avoided. If cerebral edema is suspected, endotracheal intubation, hyperventilation, and monitoring of intracranial pressure (with ventriculostomy catheter or subdural bolt if needed) are indicated. Higher doses of mannitol (1 g/kg) have been successfully used to reverse this state.[103]

Brain stem herniation is an important problem responsible for the mortality associated with DKA. Neurologic sequelae may vary from a vegetative state to subtle learning disabilities. Although they often consist of cerebral atrophy, brain infarcts of the thalamus and hypothalamus, panhypopituitarism, optical atrophy, and blindness have been reported.[103-107] Lateral sinus and arterial thromboses have been described in DKA, and clotting abnormalities have been reported in diabetic

Table 59–5. COMPLICATIONS OF DIABETIC KETOACIDOSIS

Cerebral edema
Intracerebral arterial or venous thrombosis
Adult respiratory distress syndrome
Hyperchloremic metabolic acidosis
Clotting abnormalities
Rhabdomyolysis

patients.[30, 106] These possibilities should be excluded in the patient with DKA who presents with neurologic deterioration. Adult respiratory distress syndrome and rhabdomyolysis have also been reported in these patients (Table 59–5).

HYPERGLYCEMIC NONKETOTIC COMA

Hyperglycemic nonketotic coma, which is seen in adults with type II diabetes,[113] is rarely seen in children.[114] This entity is similar to DKA; however, ketogenesis is minimal. The cause of decreased ketogenesis is unclear, but it is likely that there is decreased availability of sufficient substrate for ketogenesis. Circulating free fatty acid concentrations in these patients are only moderately increased. It is likely that diminished, but not lacking, insulin secretion is enough to prevent lipolysis but is insufficient to inhibit glycogenolysis and gluconeogenesis.[115, 116] These patients also have decreased levels of counterregulatory hormones when compared with patients DKA. In the pediatric group, hyperglycemic nonketotic coma is seen without the presence of diabetes mellitus and is associated with the intake of drugs that induce hyperglycemia—that is, corticosteroids, epinephrine, or thiazides—and has also been reported after the use of high glucose concentrations in total parenteral nutrition.

HYPOGLYCEMIA

Hypoglycemia is a critical state that requires immediate correction. It is frequently seen in the pediatric intensive care unit either as a primary event or as a concomitant manifestation of a serious condition. Regardless of its cause, it carries a high risk of neurologic sequelae if not treated promptly.[117–120]

Hypoglycemia has been traditionally defined as a blood glucose level 40 mg/dl or less in infants, children, and adults, regardless of the presence of symptoms. In neonates and premature infants, 30 mg/dl or less and 20 mg/dl or less, respectively, are considered to be hypoglycemia.[121, 122] This definition, however, is derived from observations made from neonates and premature infants who underwent prolonged periods of fasting (24 and 72 hours, respectively). Although these data are statistically accurate, concerns have been raised about the physiologic impact of these low values.[119–124]

Pathophysiology

In either the feeding or fasting state, the plasma glucose value is the result of a balance between the entry of glucose into the blood and the rate of its removal.[130] During the fasting state, glycogenolysis is often the main mechanism maintaining plasma glucose levels; however, if the fasting state continues, the major source of glucose becomes gluconeogenesis. Glucose homeostasis depends upon a functional endocrine system that regulates substrate utilization, fully active enzymatic systems that allow interconversion of substrates, and an appropriate supply of precursors (Table 59–6).[124–130]

Insulin decreases the plasma glucose concentration by inducing uptake of glucose by the peripheral tissues, mainly liver and muscle. When hypoglycemia occurs, the counterregulatory hormones glucagon, catecholamines, cortisol, and growth hormones are released. Glucagon plays a major role in glycogenolysis, gluconeogenesis, and ketogenesis.

The mechanisms that maintain glucose homeostasis are similar in adults and children. However, newborns and young infants exhibit unique characteristics in glucose regulation that make them more susceptible to hypoglycemia. During the newborn period and early infancy, the large proportion of brain to body weight imposes a large fuel metabolic demand given the fact that the brain, which constitutes only 2% of body weight, is responsible for 20% of the total consumption of oxygen. In addition, in young infants the rate of glucose consumption/100 g of brain is higher than in the adult.[131] The brain utilizes glucose at a rate of 5.5 mg/100 g of tissue/min.[132] Although glucose is an obligatory substrate for the brain, ketones can be utilized if necessary. In this population, the glycogenolytic response to exogenous glucagon is decreased, as shown by the failure of the plasma glucose concentration to increase after glucagon is given to neonates.[121] This fact has led to the assumption that the response to endogenous glucagon may also be diminished in this population.[124] The hepatic glycogen reserve in newborns and young infants is limited to 12 to 18 hours, and though the human neonate is capable of activating the glyconeogenic pathway, the activity of key step-limiting enzymes has not been fully determined.[124, 126] Studies on the fetuses of experimental animals have shown decreased or lacking enzymatic activity for gluconeogenesis and, depending on the species studied, adult enzymatic activity is manifested after a variable period of extrauterine

Table 59–6. FACTORS REQUIRED FOR GLUCOSE HOMEOSTASIS*

Functional endocrine system
 Insulin, glucagon, growth hormone, catecholamine, cortisol, and thyroid hormone
Fully active enzymatic systems
Appropriate supply of precursors
 Amino acids, lactate, and glycerol

*Modified from Tazer H, Given B, and Baldwin I: A structurally abnormal insulin causing human diabetes. Reprinted by permission of *Nature* vol. 281, p 122; copyright © 1979 Macmillan Magazines Limited.

Table 59–7. ETIOLOGY OF HYPOGLYCEMIA IN THE PEDIATRIC INTENSIVE CARE UNIT

Deficient Supply of Substrate
Abrupt discontinuation of intravenous glucose infusion
Decreased concentrations of infused glucose
Prolonged fasting before surgery in invasive procedures
Ketotic hypoglycemia

Defects in Substrate Utilization
Late stages of sepsis
Hepatic failure (fulminant hepatitis, Reye syndrome, drug-induced hepatitis, and so on)
Inborn errors of metabolism
    Carbohydrates (glycogen storage disease, types I, III, IV, galactosemia, fructose intolerance, pyruvate carboxylase deficiency, phosphoenolpyruvate deficiency)
    Amino acids (maple syrup urine disease, methylmalonic aciduria, propionic acidemia, isovaleric acidemia)
    Fatty acids (carnitine deficiency and other abnormalities in fatty acid transport and oxidation such as hydroxymethylglutaryl coenzyme A lyase deficiency)

Drug-induced
Insulin, chlorpropamide, salicylates, acetaminophen, propanol, quinidine

Endocrine Causes
Hyperinsulinism (infants of diabetic mothers, erythroblastosis fetalis, Beckwith syndrome, nesidioblastosis, leucine-induced, islet cell adenoma)
Adrenal insufficiency
    Growth hormone deficiency
    Thyroid hormone deficiency
    Hypopituitarism
    Glucagon deficiency

life.[124, 125] The factors that contribute to make neonates and young infants more susceptible to hypoglycemia are summarized in Table 59–7.

Newborns have limited resources to provide for precursors of gluconeogenesis, as well as a limited reserve for glycogenolysis, which leads to hypoglycemia when glucose intake is limited or under conditions of stress with increased substrate requirements.

Etiology

Hypoglycemia in the pediatric intensive care unit often occurs as a result of systemic disorders in which the production and utilization of metabolic fuels is impaired (Table 59–8).

Table 59–8. DIAGNOSTIC APPROACH IN HYPOGLYCEMIA

History	Length of fasting Ingestion of galactose, fructose Availability of insulin and drugs
Physical examination	Short stature? Hepatomegaly? Small genitals? Pigmented skin?
Laboratory tests	Blood sample for insulin: glucose ratio, ketones, cortisol, growth hormone, C-peptide, pH, and bicarbonate, toxic screen Urine for reducing substances, ketones, toxic screens

Deficient Supply of Substrate

Abrupt discontinuation of a concentrated intravenous glucose infusion is a setting for hypoglycemia. Careful attention should be given to avoiding prolonged fasting before surgery or invasive procedures, particularly in small infants.

Endocrine Causes

Hypopituitarism, Adrenal Insufficiency, Hypothyroidism, and Glucagon Deficiency. Hypopituitarism or isolated growth hormone deficiency is associated with hypoglycemia. Approximately one third of the patients with adrenal insufficiency present with hypoglycemia, which may be unresponsive to exogenous glucagon and may lead to ketosis.[124, 145, 146, 148] The pathophysiology of these endocrine deficiencies is unclear. These hormones may increase the availability of substrates such as fatty acids and amino acids.[130] Hypothyroidism is a rare cause of hypoglycemia. A reduction of hepatic enzymatic activity and decreased availability of gluconeogenic substrates has accounted for hypoglycemia.[119] Glucagon deficiency has been reported as a cause of this rare entity is needed.[124, 157, 158]

Hyperinsulinemic States. Hyperinsulinemia induces hypoglycemia by increasing the rate of glucose utilization and decreasing the rate of glucose production. Hyperinsulinemic states are often seen in the newborn population. Transient neonatal hyperinsulinemia is seen in the following: infants with hemolytic disease secondary to isoimmunization;[136] infants of diabetic mothers;[137] and in the Beckwith-Wiedemann syndrome, manifested by umbilical hernia or omphalocele, visceromegaly, macrosomia, macroglossia, and hypoglycemia. The infusion of high-glucose concentrations into the pancreatic circulation, as occurs in neonates with an umbilical artery catheter placed at the level of the 11th thoracic vertebra (superior mesenteric and celiac arteries) will induce hyperinsulinism.[139] Abrupt discontinuation of intravenous concentrated glucose solutions may also result in hypoglycemia. In infants of diabetic mothers, decreased activity of gluconeogenic enzymes and lower secretion of glucagon has also been documented.[124]

Persistent hyperinsulinemic states in infants and older children are a cause of intractable hypoglycemia. Some of these children present with neoformation of pancreatic islet β cells arising from the exocrine pancreatic ducts. This entity was known as nesidioblastosis.[119] However, it was observed that the spread of β cells throughout the exocrine pancreatic tissue was a normal finding in children who did not present with hypoglycemia.[141, 142] Haymond has proposed a functional defect in insulin secretion in patients with so-called nesidioblastosis.[124] Islet cell adenomas have been reported in hypoglycemic children, either as an isolated finding or as part of multiple endocrine neoplasia syndrome.

A hyperinsulinemic state induced by drugs is sometimes seen in the pediatric intensive care setting. Ingestion of oral hypoglycemic agents such as sulfonylureas (glyburide and chlorpropamide) is a cause of sustained hypoglycemia.

Factitious hypoglycemia as a result of exogenous administration of insulin should be suspected as one more manifestation of child abuse in patients with persistent hypoglycemia of undetermined cause. An insulin:glucose ratio higher than 0.5 and an absence of plasma C peptide confirm the diagnosis.[143, 144]

Inborn Errors of Carbohydrate Amino Acids or Fatty Acids

Carbohydrate Metabolism. Glycogen storage diseases result from an inherited autosomal recessive enzymatic deficiency that prevents the release of glucose from glycogen. Not all glycogen storage diseases cause hypoglycemia; patients with type II (α-1,4-glucosidase deficiency) and type IV (amylo-1,4→1,6-transglucosilase deficiency) present with normal plasma glucose values. Inactivity of gluconeogenic enzymes such as fructose 1,6-diphosphatase, pyruvate carboxylase, or phosphoenol pyruvate carboxykinase are characterized by hypoglycemia and increased plasma lactate and pyruvate concentrations. Patients with these conditions may present with mental retardation, failure to thrive, and hepatomegaly.

Fructosemia and galactosemia present with hypoglycemia after the intake of fructose[151] or galactose.[150] Elimination of the offending sugar prevents the manifestations of this disease.

Lipid Metabolism. Carnitine deficiency has been described in association with a "Reye-like" syndrome[153] or with cardiomyopathy.[152] Carnitine allows long-chain fatty acid oxidation by transporting fatty acids through the mitochondrial membrane. Hypoglycemia in these children is thought to be secondary to increased rates of glucose utilization as a result of a decreased availability of ketone bodies.[153]

Amino Acid Metabolism. Maple syrup urine disease, a branched-chain and ketoacid dehydrogenase deficiency, is associated with hypoglycemia. The mechanism of hypoglycemia is unclear, but an enzymatic abnormality in the Krebs cycle has been suggested as being responsible.[156] Isovaleric acidemia, methyl malonic aciduria, and propionic acidemia are accompanied by hypoglycemia through an associated carnitine deficiency.[124, 155–157]

Drug-Induced Hypoglycemia

Salicylates, acetaminophen, propanol, quinine sulfonylureas, phenylbutazone, and ethanol have been associated with hypoglycemia. Large amounts of leucine induce release of insulin in normal children and adults.[159, 160] Intake of the unripe fruit of the ackee nut results in hypoglycemia and severe vomiting (Jamaican vomiting sickness) because of a metabolite identified as hypoglycin, which increases peripheral utilization of glucose by inhibiting the oxidation of fatty acids.[130, 161, 162]

Other Conditions. Hepatic diseases such as drug-induced hepatitis, Reye syndrome, or viral fulminant hepatitis are often accompanied by hypoglycemia. Altered gluconeogenesis and decreased glycogen stores are the probable mechanisms of low plasma glucose levels.

Ketotic hypoglycemia, also known as fasting functional hypoglycemia, appears to be an earlier manifestation of fasting. It occurs in underweight children after a period of fasting (usually overnight) and is treated with frequent high-carbohydrate meals.[130]

Hypoglycemia accompanies sepsis in both its very early and terminal stages. Hyperglycemia is present in the other stages of sepsis.

Clinical Manifestations

Manifestations of hypoglycemia include sweating, tachycardia, and weakness, and they reflect catecholamine release. If hypoglycemia persists, neuroglycopenia occurs and may become manifested by irritability, headaches, changes in consciousness, and seizures. Hypoglycemic newborns present with lethargy, cyanosis, feeding problems, and apnea.

Diagnosis

Whenever there are risk factors for hypoglycemia or when the clinical picture suggests this condition, the diagnosis needs to be confirmed by a plasma glucose measurement. At the same time that the diagnosis of hypoglycemia is confirmed, a blood sample for determination of insulin, cortisol, growth hormone (glucoregulatory hormones), ketone bodies, lactate, and alanine concentrations should be obtained. A urine sample for measurement of ketonuria should also be collected (Table 59–9).

Hypoglycemia without ketonemia indicates hyperinsulinism or a defect in ketogenesis. Hyperinsulinism is characterized by a high insulin:glucose ratio. Plasma insulin concentrations greater than 10 microunits/ml in the presence of glucose concentrations of 50 mg/dl or less are suggestive of hyperinsulinism. Increased serum insulin and C peptide levels with concomitant hypoglycemia indicate drug-induced hypoglycemia.[124, 129] However, high serum insulin levels without the presence of C peptide levels is indicative of factitious hypoglycemia.[124, 129, 132]

Abnormal ketogenesis (fatty acid oxidation) is associated with low values of plasma carnitine and with some organic acidurias. A urine sample for organic acid determination is necessary under these conditions. Fasting ketotic hypoglycemia is found in underweight infants older than 18 months of age. Hypoglycemia could also be associated with adrenal or pituitary deficiency. Non-glucose-reducing substances may be found in the urine of patients with galactosemia or fructosuria.

Treatment

As soon as the diagnosis of hypoglycemia has been established and the indicated diagnostic blood tests have been performed, an intravenous infusion of $D_{10}W$, 2.5 ml/kg (0.25 g glucose/kg) should be administered, followed by an increase in the maintenance glucose infusion

Table 59–9. TREATMENT OF HYPOGLYCEMIA

Newborns and Infants	Children	Adolescents
0.25 g glucose/kg IV* push (D$_{10}$W 2.5 ml/kg) followed by an increase to 1½ times maintenance glucose	0.25 glucose/kg (D$_{25}$W) followed by an increase in maintenance glucose (D$_{10}$W)	D$_{25}$, 25–50 ml IV followed by an increase in maintenance glucose (D$_{10}$W)
Confirm if glucose level is > 50 mg/dl after the glucose bolus	Confirm if glucose level is > 50 mg/dl after the glucose bolus	Confirm if glucose level is > 50 mg/dl after the glucose bolus
If hypoglycemia is persistent, repeat glucose bolus × 2	If hypoglycemia is persistent, repeat glucose bolus × 2	If hypoglycemia is persistent, repeat glucose bolus × 2
Hydrocortisone, 5 mg/kg/day; if adrenal insufficiency or hypopituitarism is suspected, the dose should be increased to 20–60 mg/m²/day divided in four doses	Hydrocortisone, 5 mg/kg/day IV up to 100 mg total dose	Hydrocortisone succinate, 100 mg IV
Glucagon, 0.03 mg/kg IV or IM† up to 1 mg if hyperinsulinemia or glucagon deficiency is suspected; if glycogen stores are depleted or there is an abnormality in the mobilization of glycogen, glucagon will not elicit an increase in glycogen	Glucagon, 0.03 mg/kg IV or IM up to 1 mg	Glucagon, 0.5–1 mg IV or IM
Diazoxide, 10–25 mg/kg/day PO or IV slowly (over 30 min) divided in three doses, should be used in hyperinsulinism	Diazoxide, 3–8 mg/kg/day PO‡ or IV slowly (over 30 min) divided in three doses	Diazoxide, 300 mg PO or IV slowly (over 30 min)

*IV = intravenous.
†IM = intramuscular.
‡PO = by mouth.

to 150% of the hepatic glucose production (3 to 5 mg/kg/min in infants and children and 5 to 8 mg/kg/min in neonates). After the initial intravenous glucose bolus, a plasma glucose determination should be repeated to ensure a steady concentration of greater than 50 mg/dl.[119] D$_{25}$W or D$_{50}$W is rarely indicated in infants because of the risk of rebound hypoglycemia and osmotic load; however, older children who present with coma secondary to hypoglycemia may require 25 to 50 ml of D$_{25}$W if central venous access is available. If the plasma glucose level cannot be sustained with this glucose concentration, hydrocortisone (5 mg/kg/day) should be used. If adrenal insufficiency or hypopituitarism is documented, hydrocortisone in doses of 20 to 60 mg/m²/day intravenously divided into four doses will increase blood glucose levels. Glucagon at doses of 0.1 to 0.3 mg/kg intravenously or intramuscularly[131] (maximal dose of 1 mg) may be tried if hypoglycemia persists. Note that glucagon's effect on blood glucose levels is through increased glycogenolysis; therefore, it will be ineffective in severe liver disease or glycogen storage diseases in which the availability of glycogen is limited.

If hyperinsulinism is considered, medical treatment with diazoxide (10 to 25 mg/kg/day administered orally in infants and children or 300 mg every 4 hours in adolescents) is indicated. Diazoxide inhibits the release of insulin and also induces hypotension. Therefore, the enteral route of administration is recommended, though it can be given slowly intravenously over 30 minutes (Table 59–10). If hyperinsulinism persists despite medical treatment, surgical intervention is warranted.[129]

THYROID DISORDERS

Hyperthyroidism

Hyperthyroidism is a rare condition in children, with an estimated incidence of 1 to 5 new cases/100,000/

year.[193] It can present as thyrotoxicosis, a life-threatening disease that needs to be considered in the differential diagnosis of critically ill patients who present with sudden multiple organ failure of unclear cause.

Etiology

Hyperthyroidism can occur as a result of an immunologic process similar to that in Graves disease, with production of antibodies against antigens in the thyroid hormone receptors,[166] the orbital tissues,[165] and the dermis;[167, 170] a chronic process as in chronic lymphocytic thyroiditis;[165, 166] or as a syndrome involving multiple endocrine abnormalities, café au lait pigmentation of the skin, and polyostotic fibrous dysplasia, as reported in the McCune-Albright syndrome. Hyperthyroidism in neonates has been reported as a result of transplacental passage of maternal thyroid-stimulating immunoglobins to the fetus.[169] These immunoglobulins play a major role in the pathogenesis of thyrotoxicosis.

Hyperthyroidism also occurs as a result of thyroid cancer, usually as a single adenoma or as papillary carcinoma.[171] Pituitary tumors can induce production of thyroid-stimulating hormone (TSH) and induce the excessive production of thyroid hormone.

Table 59–10. ETIOLOGY OF HYPERTHYROIDISM

Immune Causes	Tumors	Causes
Graves disease	Thyroid adenoma	Ingestion of thyroid hormone
Neonatal Graves disease	Thyroid papillary carcinoma	Ingestion of iodine
Hashimoto thyroiditis	Pituitary tumors	Ingestion of iodine-containing drugs
McCune-Albright syndrome		Exposure to iodine-containing radiocontrast materials or antiseptics

Hyperthyroidism can result as a manifestation of "central" (hypothalamic and pituitary) resistance, in which there is a loss of the feedback mechanism that regulates thyroid hormone production.[170, 172, 173]

Ingestion of thyroid hormone can also result in hyperthyroidism. There have been reported outbreaks of hyperthyroidism after intake of ground beef prepared from the untrimmed neck.[174, 175]

Iodine ingestion in the form of iodine-containing medications, such as amiodarone,[178] or as radiocontrast materials is another source of hyperthyroidism. Application of iodine-containing antiseptics has occasionally been associated with excessive thyroid hormone production (see Table 59–10).[170]

Thyrotoxicosis

Thyroid Hormone Physiology

Thyroid hormones are synthesized by the follicular cells of the thyroid gland. The synthetic process requires uptake and organification of iodide and incorporation into tyrosine to form iodotyrosine, which is stored in thyroglobulin. Triiodothyronine (T_3) and thyroxine (T_4) are the main thyroid hormones. T_4 is produced by the thyroid gland, but 80% of T_3 is produced by a deiodination of T_4 at the tissue level. Reverse T_3 (rT_3) is a biologically inactive form of T_3. The peripheral conversion of T_4 to T_3 or rT_3 is a regulatory mechanism of thyroid hormone activity.[177] Hypothalamic thyrotropin-releasing hormone stimulates pituitary synthesis and release of TSH, a hormone that induces synthesis and release of T_4 and T_3, which exert a negative feedback on the hypothalamic-pituitary axis. Hypothermia also induces release of TSH, whereas dopamine, somatostatin, fever, glucocorticoids, and T_4 and T_3 inhibit the release of TSH. Only the free fraction of thyroid hormone is biologically active. A large fraction of thyroid hormone is carried by thyroid-binding globulin and to a lesser extent by thyroxine-binding prealbumin.[177]

Thyroid hormone is a key element that regulates metabolic homeostasis (Table 59–11). It increases tissue sensitivity to catecholamines by inducing up-regulation of β-adrenergic receptors. Thyroid hormone increases thermogenesis by increasing synthesis of the sodium-potassium ATPase enzyme. The increased ATP hydrolysis requires further ATP production, with the resultant increase in O_2 consumption.[170] Thyroid hormone regulation depends on an intact hypothalamic-pituitary axis and on iodide supply.

Clinical Findings

Thyrotoxicosis occurs when there is excessive production of thyroid hormone, and it has been referred to as

Table 59–11. THYROID HORMONE ACTIONS

Regulation of metabolic homeostasis
Control of thermogenesis
Up-regulation of β-adrenergic receptors
Increases inotropic properties of cardiac muscle
Regulation of protein synthesis

Table 59–12. CLINICAL CHARACTERISTICS OF HYPERTHYROIDISM*

Nervous System	Cardiovascular	Ophthalmologic	Other
Tremor	Murmurs	Proptosis	Thin, fine hair
Anxiety	Palpitations	Lid retraction	
Irritability	Tachycardia	Lid lag	
Increased appetite	Atrial fibrillation	Diplopia	
Heat intolerance	Congestive heart failure	Eye pain	
Muscle weakness			
Hyperactive reflexes			

*Modified from Cooper DS: Which antithyroid drug? Am J Med 80:1165, 1986.

a hypermetabolic state.[177] Table 59–12 describes the clinical characteristics of hyperthyroidism. Often, there is previous knowledge of a hyperthyroid condition that suddenly worsens, but occasionally the history is of a previously healthy child who suddenly has vomiting, diarrhea, jaundice, and becomes pale and febrile with increased perspiration and dehydration. These patients present with sinus tachycardia (heart rate >200 bpm), or supraventricular arrhythmia may be present. Hypertension and a widened pulse pressure in a dehydrated, "shocked"-appearing patient should alert the clinician to the possibility of thyrotoxicosis. Often these patients present with central nervous system involvement such as lethargy, coma, dilated and unresponsive pupils, and seizures (Table 59–13). Extreme hyperthermia (41 to 42° C) and abnormal liver enzymes may be present. A physical examination may demonstrate proptosis and an enlarged thyroid gland. Abdominal tenderness and hepatomegaly are common and may mimic an acute abdomen. A hyperdynamic state with increased cardiac output and decreased peripheral vascular resistance is often found.

Diagnosis

Establishing the diagnosis of thyrotoxicosis relies on the finding of characteristic clinical signs and symptoms. Serum T_4 and T_3 concentrations may be increased, though on occasion T_4 levels may be normal and T_3 levels may be increased (T_3 thyrotoxicosis).[178] Total and free T_4 and T_3 determinations should be obtained. The protein binding capacity for thyroid hormone is estimated by the resin uptake test. This test indicates the free T_4 or T_3 index.[177]

The differential diagnosis should include septic shock, salicylate poisoning, anticholinergic poisoning, malignant hyperthermia, and any other entity that presents acutely with a hyperdynamic state and organ dysfunction (see Table 59–9).

Treatment

Specific and supportive treatments for the treatment of thyrotoxicosis are summarized in Table 59–14.

Table 59–13. CLINICAL CHARACTERISTICS OF THYROTOXICOSIS*

Cardiovascular	Central Nervous System	Abdominal	Other	Laboratory
Tachycardia > 200/min Arrythmias (supraventricular tachycardia) Increased cardiac output Decreased peripheral vascular resistance Hypertension Cyanosis Shock Wide pulse pressure	Irritability Tremor Agitation Coma Seizures Unresponsive pupils	Vomiting Diarrhea Hepatomegaly Jaundice Abdominal pain	Tachypnea Fever Metabolic acidosis Apnea Dehydration	Metabolic acidosis Hypoxemia Abnormal liver enzyme levels Abnormal BUN† and creatinine Hyperglycemia

*Modified from Emerson CM, Anderson AJ, and Howard WJ: Serum thyroxine and triiodothyronine concentrations during iodide treatment of hyperthyroidism. J Clin Endocrinol Metab 40:33, 1975. © The Endocrine Society.

†BUN = blood urea nitrogen.

Drugs that Reduce Synthesis and Release of Thyroid Hormones. For the critically ill patient with thyrotoxicosis, specific treatment includes the use of drugs that reduce the synthesis and release of thyroid hormones; propylthiouracil (PTU) and carbimazole are among the agents that inhibit the synthesis of iodothyronines by inhibiting organification of tyrosine residues.[180] PTU also inhibits peripheral conversion of T_4 to T_3 and for this reason is the preferred drug in the treatment of thyroid storm.[177, 178] An initial loading dose of 5 mg/kg followed by a maintenance dose of 10 to 20 mg/kg/day divided into four doses should be administered through a nasogastric tube. The side effects of these medications include agranulocytosis, a lupus-like syndrome, rash, and serum sickness. However, the use of these higher doses is indicated in these critically ill patients because of their high risk morbidity and mortality.[181] Older children and adolescents should receive an initial dose of 600 to 1200 mg of PTU followed by a daily maintenance dose of 200 to 300 mg every 6 hours.[182] Because of the large amount of stored thyroid hormone, treatment with drugs that only decrease the synthesis and release of thyroid hormones does not control the acute picture. Therefore, a drug with prompt inhibitory properties, such as iodide solution, should also be administered.

Iodide solutions that inhibit iodide organification and thyroid hormone release[177] are usually given as Lugol solution, 30 to 60 drops daily divided into three doses, or sodium or potassium iodide, 1.5 to 3 g/day. Sodium iodide may be given intravenously or orally.[178] Iodide solutions should be administered 1 hour after an inhibitor of thyroid hormone synthesis such as PTU or carbimazole has been given in order to avoid any accumulation of hormone stores within the gland.[177, 178, 180] Lithium salts have effects similar to iodide.

Glucocorticoids may also inhibit the release of thyroid hormone in patients with hyperthyroidism. Dexamethasone inhibits the peripheral conversion of T_4 to T_3[182] and may be used to help treat thyrotoxicosis.

In those patients in whom medical treatment fails, re-

Table 59–14. TREATMENT OF THYROTOXICOSIS

Specific Measures (Antithyroid therapy; drugs that inhibit synthesis and release of thyroid hormones)*

Drug	Newborn Infants	Children	Adolescents
Propylthiouracil	5–10 mg/kg PO† followed by 10 mg/kg/day divided every 8 hr	5–10 mg/kg PO followed by 20 mg/kg/day PO divided every 8 hr	800–1200 mg PO then 200–300 mg PO every 6 hr
Lugol solution or saturated solution of potassium iodide	1 drop every 8 hr	5 drops every 6 hr	4–5 drops every 8 hr
Sodium iodide	0.5 g IV every 12 hr	0.5 g IV every 12 hr	0.5 g IV every 12 hr
Dexamethasome	2 mg IV every 6 hr	2 mg IV every 6 hr	2 mg IV every 6 hr

Supportive Measures (ABCs; drugs that control clinical manifestations of thyrotoxicosis)

Drug	Newborn Infants	Children	Adolescents
Propanol	0.1 mg/kg IV slowly repeated to titrate heart rate < 200 bpm followed by 2 mg/kg/day PO divided every 6 hr	0.1 mg/kg/day IV slowly up to 1 mg, repeat to titrate heart rate < 150 bpm followed by 10 mg PO every 6 hr	1–3 mg IV over 10 min followed by 40 mg PO every 6 hr
Reserpine	0.02 mg/kg IM§	0.1 mg/kg PO	1–2.5 mg/day PO
Guanethidine	—	0.5–2 mg/kg PO	50–150 mg/day PO
Dantrolene if unable to control fever	—	2.5 mg/kg IV repeat PRN‖ up to cumulative dose of 10 mg/kg	2.5 mg/kg IV repeat PRN up to cumulative dose of 10 mg/kg

*Plasmapheresis in cases of thyroid hormone overdose or in life-threatening disease unresponsive to medical treatment.

†PO = by mouth.

‡IV = intravenous.

§IM = intramuscular.

‖PRN = as necessary.

moval of circulating thyroid hormones may be achieved by plasmapheresis or exchange transfusion;[184, 186] however, with current support measures and more aggressive medical management, this option is rarely considered.

Inhibition of Peripheral Effects of Thyroid Hormone

β-Adrenergic receptor–blockers, such as propranolol, improve the signs and symptoms of the hyperadrenergic state. Propranolol also inhibits peripheral conversion of T_4 to T_3.[178] However, propranolol has serious side effects in patients with reactive airways, and there is the potential for a worsening hemodynamic status by decreasing cardiac output when metabolic needs are increased. Newer β-blocker agents, such as esmolol, are now considered for the treatment of hyperadrenergic manifestations of thyrotoxicosis.[182-185] If β-blockers are contraindicated, as in the case of asthma, or if there is a poor response to these agents, other sympatholytic agents, such as guanethidine or reserpine, may rarely be considered.[177, 178, 182]

Supportive Measures

Supportive measures in these patients involve basic life support. If the patient presents in a lethargic or unconscious state, endotracheal intubation is indicated. Also, these critically ill, acidotic, hypermetabolic children often require mechanical ventilatory support. Despite hypertension, these patients frequently are dehydrated as a consequence of vomiting, diarrhea, high fever, and poor oral intake and present with a hyperdynamic pattern of shock. In these cases, fluid resuscitation is indicated to maintain an adequate central venous pressure. Further monitoring with a pulmonary artery catheter may be required to better assess oxygen consumption and delivery if the hyperdynamic state persists despite anti–thyroid hormone therapy. A nasogastric tube should be placed for gastric decompression and administration of medication.

High fever results in increased oxygen consumption, and every effort should be made to decrease the temperature. If, despite the use of a cooling blanket and acetaminophen, the fever persists, dantrolene sodium should be used.[188, 189] Seizure activity should be treated with diazepam, and if persistent seizure activity is observed, phenobarbital or phenytoin may be added.[190-192] Some patients may present with fixed, unresponsive pupils; decorticate or decerebrate posturing, and deep coma, which is suggestive of raised intracranial pressure; however, invasive monitoring with a subdural bolt in these patients has failed to prove increased intracranial pressure. Coagulopathy should be treated with fresh frozen plasma.

Treatment of the critically ill thyrotoxic child is a challenging experience that requires the expertise of the team in the intensive care unit.

Neonatal Thyrotoxicosis

Neonatal thyrotoxicosis has been described as a result of transplacental passage of maternal thyroid-stimulating immunoglobulin to the fetus,[170] but it has also has been described in infants born to euthyroid mothers.[194, 196] Neonatal hyperthyroidism may be manifested by growth retardation, fetal tachycardia, and premature birth. After birth, these infants present with irritability, microcephaly with ventriculomegaly, hyperphagia, poor weight gain, diarrhea, tachycardia, and heart murmur with bounding pulses that sometimes mislead one to the diagnosis of patent ductus arteriosus. Hepatosplenomegaly, jaundice, and liver dysfunction have also been described.[194, 195] Tachycardia (>200 bpm), cardiomegaly, cardiac failure, and supraventricular arrhythmias may be present. Advanced bone age is a frequent finding.

Diagnosis relies on increased concentrations of serum total and free T_4 and T_3 and low or undetectable TSH levels. The differential diagnosis includes sepsis; congenital heart diseases; toxoplasmosis, rubella, cytomegalovirus, and herpes simplex; and other causes of cholestasis.

Treatment includes PTU at doses of 5 to 10 mg/kg/day divided every 8 hours. In addition, Lugol iodine solution, one drop every 8 hours, should be given to prevent release of thyroid hormone. Propanol at doses of 1 to 2 mg/kg/day divided into four doses will help to control hyperadrenergic symptoms.

The Euthyroid Sick Syndrome

The euthyroid sick syndrome is seen in patients with a combination of clinical entities characterized by abnormal thyroid function with clinical euthyroidism.[197, 198, 201, 204, 207] It may occur as a consequence of an excess of T_4-binding proteins, such as globulins (as in the case of liver disease, estrogen therapy, or the intake of drugs [e.g., narcotics, fluoracil]), or abnormal T_4 binding to albumin or prealbumin. These conditions present with euthyroid hyperthyroxinemia. However, patients with euthyroid sick syndrome can also present with this thyroid "dysfunction" independent of T_4-binding proteins, as in critically ill or psychiatric patients and after exposure to some drugs like amiodarone, heparin, or iodinated contrast agents.[200, 204, 208]

Critically ill patients suffering from acute catabolic states; renal, liver, or multiple organ failure; and malnutrition exhibit a variety of abnormalities in thyroid function depending on the severity of the illness.[198, 201] Patients with mild to moderate illness have decreased conversion of T_4 to T_3 and inhibition of protein binding with a normal serum free T_4 value and normal function of the hypothalamic-pituitary axis.

Critically ill patients with severe euthyroid sick syndrome show the preceding characteristics, except that the serum free T_4 level is also low, together with evidence of hypothalamic-pituitary dysfunction.[198, 201, 212] This reduced TSH secretion may be induced by dopamine, opioid peptides, or release of cortisol triggered by stress.[198, 201, 210]

The mechanism of euthyroid sick syndrome is unclear, but a multifactorial cause is suspected. Cytokines, specifically tumor necrosis factor, have been associated with decreased thyrotropin-releasing hormone and TSH levels in laboratory animals.[214] Production of free radicals or release of an enzyme inhibitor may contribute to inhibit iodothyronine deiodinase enzymatic activity and reduce the conversion of T_4 to T_3.[198, 213, 214]

The severity of euthyroid sick syndrome correlates with delivery-dependent oxygen consumption[197] and is predictive of outcome in critically ill adult patients[202, 205, 206, 215] but not in children.[203] Concerns have been raised regarding the possibility of some degree of hypothyroidism in critically ill patients with euthyroid sick syndrome; however, as yet there is no evidence that patients with euthyroid sick syndrome require treatment with thyroid hormone. The abnormalities in thyroid function found in these patients improve when the patient recovers; therefore, treatment is aimed at the underlying conditions.[198]

ADRENAL FAILURE

Adrenal failure in children may present as an acute life-threatening event or as an ill-defined picture, which often leads to a delay in the diagnosis.

De novo adrenal failure is an unusual admitting diagnosis in the pediatric intensive care unit. However, the population in the intensive care unit is at a higher risk of presenting with this condition because of the prevalence of multiple factors that lead to multiple organ failure and the frequent use of glucocorticoid therapy in these patients.

Adrenal Cortex Physiology

Glucocorticoids

The adrenal cortex synthesizes three classes of hormones: glucocorticoids, mineralocorticoids, and sex steroids.[218]

Cortisol is the most potent glucocorticoid hormone and is produced in the zona fasciculata and in the zona reticularis (the innermost area of the adrenal cortex). The zona reticularis also produces androgenic sex hormones. Aldosterone, the most potent mineralocorticoid, is produced by the zona glomerulosa, which is the outer layer of the adrenal cortex.[218, 219]

After being released into the circulation, cortisol binds to specific cytoplasmic receptors. This cortisol-receptor complex migrates into the nucleus, allowing the expression of new proteins.[219, 220]

Cortisol regulates intermediary metabolism and is an important modulator of the stress response (Table 59–15).[221, 227] It increases the availability of glucose by promoting gluconeogenesis,[219, 221, 223] decreases the peripheral utilization of glucose, and increases the glucose blood level.[221, 224] Cortisol plays a major role in regulating glucose homeostasis in response to stress.[226]

It exerts a catabolic effect on protein metabolism, inducing proteolysis for gluconeogenic substrates and inhibiting protein synthesis.[221, 224, 225] It enhances lipolysis, releasing glycerol and lactate from adipose tissue for gluconeogenic purposes.[219, 221–224] Cortisol redistributes fat from peripheral deposits to centrally located areas.

Table 59–15. MAJOR EFFECTS OF CORTISOL

Regulates glucose metabolism in response to stress
Regulates glucose availability
    Increased gluconeogenesis
    Decreased peripheral glucose uptake
Increases protein breakdown and facilitates amino acid uptake by the liver
Increases lipolysis, redistributes fat
Anti-inflammatory properties:
    Induces expression of lipocortins
    Inhibits phospholipase A_2
    Blocks cytokines
Stimulates bone marrow release of polymorphonuclear leukocytes and decreases circulating eosinophils
Induces lymphopenia

The anti-inflammatory properties of cortisol are a major indication for its widespread use. These effects are carried out through the cortisol-mediated production of proteins that inhibit phospholipase A_2 preventing the activation of the arachidonic acid cascade and release of prostaglandins, and also by directly blocking the production of cytokines.[228–230, 233]

Cortisol stimulates bone marrow release of polymorphonuclear leukocytes and causes lymphopenia at pharmacologic doses.[229, 231]

Cortisol is regulated through corticotropin-releasing hormone, which through an adenylate cyclase mechanism stimulates the anterior pituitary to release adrenocorticotropic hormone (ACTH). ACTH, in turn, stimulates the adrenal cortex to produce cortisol. Cortisol exerts a negative feedback in the hypothalamic-hypophyseal-adrenocortical axis, resulting in decreased production of cortisol. The stress response and sleep-wake cycle also stimulate the hypothalamic-hypophyseal axis.

Mineralocorticoids

Aldosterone is the most potent mineralocorticoid and is involved in the maintenance of extracellular volume (Table 59–16) and the renal conservation of sodium in exchange for potassium and hydrogen ion, with resulting kaliuresis and proton loss. Aldosterone promotes sodium conservation and the loss of potassium by the distal renal tubule, alimentary tract, and the epithelial cells of sweat and salivary glands.[218, 219, 221, 222]

Aldosterone release is controlled by the response of the renin-angiotensin system to changes in volume, serum potassium level, and β-adrenergic stimulation. A decrease in the extracellular fluid induces changes in renal arterial blood flow and pressure, stimulating the juxtaglomerular cells and resulting in renin production. Renin acts on angiotensinogen (an octapeptide produced

Table 59–16. ALDOSTERONE EFFECTS

Maintenance of extracellular volume
Retention of sodium and water
Excretion of potassium
Excretion of H^+
Activation of Na^+, K^+-ATPase pump

Table 59–17. ETIOLOGY OF ADRENAL INSUFFICIENCY

Congenital
  Defective steroidogenesis
    20,22-Desmolase (incomplete masculinization in male, normal genitals in female, severe salt wasting)
    3β-Hydroxysteroid dehydrogenase (inadequate virilization in male, mild virilization in female, severe salt wasting)
    17α-Hydroxylase (delayed sexual development, hypertension, hypokalemic alkalosis)
    21-Hydroxylase (female virilization, normal genitals in male, salt wasting, pseudoprecocious puberty in non–salt wasting males)
    11β-Hydroxylase (female virilization, hypertension)
  Congenital adrenal hypoplasia
    X-linked (affects males)
    Autosomal recessive (associated with anencephaly)
  Some peroxisomal disorders
    Adrenoleukodystrophy (adrenal crisis with demyelinization of cerebral white matter and abnormal fatty acid metabolism)
    Adrenomyeloneuropathy (adrenal crisis with seizures, spasticity and abnormal fatty acid metabolism)
    Glycerol kinase deficiency (adrenal crisis, failure to thrive, mental retardation, muscular dystrophy)
    Refsum disease (sensorineural hearing loss, retinitis pigmentosa, adrenal failure in terminal stages)
  Others
    Wolman disease (familial xanthomatosis, hepatosplenomegaly, steatorrhea, and failure to thrive)
    Hereditary adrenocortical unresponsiveness to ACTH (recurrent hypoglycemia, seizures, coma; salt loss does not occur)
Acquired
  Polyglandular immune disorders
    Type I (adrenalitis, hypoparathyroidism, and chronic mucocutaneous candidiasis)
    Type II (adrenalitis and thyroiditis)
    Syndrome of adrenal insufficiency, achalasia, and alacrimia (AAA syndrome)
  Others
    Hypothalamic-pituitary tumors, radiation, surgery
    Hemorrhage
    Adrenal hemorrhage or infarcts
    Glucocorticoid therapy withdrawal
    Severe infection (Waterhouse-Friedericksen syndrome)
    Burns

*ACTH = adrenocorticotropic hormone.

by the liver) to form angiotensin I. Angiotensin-converting enzyme, which is produced by the lungs, converts angiotensin I to angiotensin II, a potent vasoconstrictor that induces aldosterone production. Aldosterone binds to cytoplasmic receptors that translocate to the nucleus and elicit protein synthesis. It may activate the Na^+, K^+-ATPase pump.[20, 221, 222, 229, 232]

Dopamine inhibits aldosterone secretion,[221] and, conversely, dopamine antagonists stimulate the release of aldosterone.[221]

Adrenal Insufficiency

Etiology

Adrenal insufficiency in the pediatric population occurs as a result of a congenital disorder in steroidogenesis, as in congenital adrenal hyperplasia, an autosomal recessive disorder with a wide range of manifestations depending upon the enzymatic defect[235, 236] (Table 59–17), or as a result of congenital adrenal hypoplasia inherited either as an x-linked or as an autosomal recessive defect.[236, 237] There is a group of miscellaneous disorders in which patients present with adrenal insufficiency, but the dominant clinical manifestations are extra-adrenal. Adrenoleukodystrophy, glycerol kinase deficiency, and other peroxisomal defects are included in this group.[235, 237–245, 248]

Other forms of congenital adrenal failure are represented by a hereditary adrenocortical unresponsiveness to ACTH, becoming manifested as recurrent hypoglycemia, seizures, and coma. Mineralocorticoid activity is not affected, and therefore there is no salt wasting. Wolman disease is a familial xanthomatosis characterized by hepatosplenomegaly, steatorrhea, and failure to thrive; the adrenal glands are also infiltrated with fat, leading to adrenal hypofunction.

Acquired adrenal insufficiency in children often presents as part of polyglandular immune disorders (type I: adrenalitis, hypoparathyroidism, and chronic mucocutaneous candidiasis or type II: adrenalitis and thyroiditis).[236, 246, 247, 249, 253, 254] An association between adrenal insufficiency achalasia and alacrimia (AAA syndrome) has been reported.[255]

Tumors, infarction, hemorrhage, surgery, or radiation of the hypothalamic-pituitary axis is an unusual cause of adrenal failure in children; however, perinatal adrenal hemorrhage may be seen as a result of traumatic birth. In these cases, a mass can be palpated in the flanks, and the differential diagnosis should be established with renal vein thrombosis.[236]

Adrenal insufficiency in the intensive care unit may

Table 59–18. CLINICAL CHARACTERISTICS OF ADRENAL INSUFFICIENCY

Hypotension	Anorexia
Poor perfusion	Abdominal pain
Shock	Hypoglycemia
Weakness	Hyponatremia
Nausea, vomiting	Eosinophilia
Encephalopathy	Elevated blood urea nitrogen
Behavioral changes	Hypercalcemia
Seizures	Metabolic acidosis
Hyperpigmentation	

Table 59–19. TREATMENT OF ACUTE ADRENAL CRISIS

	Neonates	Children	Adolescents
Specific			
Hydrocortisone	25–50 mg/m² day IV* divided in three doses	50–75 mg/m²/day IV divided in three doses	200 mg IV every 8 hr
Deoxycorticosterone acetate	1–2 mg IM† every day	1–3 mg IM every day	3 mg IM every day
Supportive	Intravenous normal saline with glucose; sodium polystyrene sulfonate (Kayexelate) if hyperkalemia present; close monitoring of hemodynamic status and laboratory values (glucose, sodium, potassium)		
	If stimulating ACTH test‡ is used, treatment should be initiated with dexamethasone, 10 mg/kg, and fluid support.		

*IV = intravenous.
†IM = intramuscular.
‡ACTH = adrenocorticotropic hormone.

be present in critically ill burn or septic patients, as in meningococcemia with Waterhouse-Friedericksen syndrome. Also, withdrawal of glucocorticoid therapy may lead to adrenal failure. As in adults, tuberculosis, autoimmune disease, and coumadin-induced adrenal hemorrhage may also cause adrenal insufficiency.

Clinical Manifestations

Adrenal insufficiency may become manifested by symptoms of primary glucocorticoid and mineralocorticoid deficiency.[221] It also can present with subtle, insidious manifestations or as a life-threatening episode. Table 59–18 describes common manifestations of adrenal insufficiency. Whenever cardiovascular collapse is unresponsive to fluids and catecholamines, adrenal failure should be suspected. Arrhythmias secondary to hyperkalemia are frequently a terminal event. Persistent hypoglycemia, metabolic acidosis, dehydration, vomiting, apathy, lethargy, behavioral changes, seizures, and encephalopathy are all manifestations of adrenal failure.[221, 222, 253, 256, 257] Frequently, clinical manifestations of adrenal insufficiency are covered by the aggressive therapeutic intervention given to these patients. In the newborn period, adrenal failure has been confounded with congenital heart disease in the setting of a dehydrated, cyanotic, poorly perfused, acidotic child with respiratory distress and hemodynamic instability.

Diagnosis

The diagnosis of adrenal insufficiency relies on measurement of plasma cortisol levels and the ACTH stimulation test. However, in the critically ill, stressed patient, an isolated cortisol level may not be conclusive of adrenal function, and stimulation tests are required. Under stress conditions, a serum cortisol level of 18 to 20 μg/dl is considered acceptable,[219, 221, 222, 258, 260] though cortisol levels in critically ill adult patients may vary from 15 to more than 400 μg/dl.[258] No correlation has been demonstrated between serum levels and the adequacy of the adrenal response to stress. In most cases, the ACTH stimulation test with 250 mg ACTH given intravenously and collection of blood samples at baseline (time 0) and 30 and 60 minutes after ACTH dosing will show at least an increase of more than 7 μg/dl from baseline at 60 minutes and a peak plasma cortisol level

of 18 μg/dl or less.[236] In the patient with adrenal insufficiency, collection of blood for ACTH determination at the time of the baseline sample will help to differentiate between primary adrenal insufficiency (high levels of ACTH) and secondary adrenal insufficiency (low levels of ACTH).[219, 221, 222] Stimulation tests with insulin and metyrapone are usually not recommended in the critically ill patient with decreased reserve and a potential for morbidity.

Treatment

Treatment of adrenal insufficiency is outlined in Table 59–19.

Specific therapy is aimed at replacement of the deficient hormones. In the case of critically ill, glucocorticoid-deficient children, a dose of 75 to 100 mg/m² of parenteral hydrocortisone should be administered. This accounts for a six- to eightfold increase in the basal secretory rate of cortisol, which is 12.5 ± 2.5 (SEM) mg/m²/day.[233, 263] Hydrocortisone has mineralocorticoid activity. Whenever possible, a blood sample should be obtained for cortisol determination, and a short ACTH stimulation test should be performed before therapy. If the patient requires immediate treatment, dexamethasone offers the advantage that it does not interfere with the plasma cortisol assay. Dexamethasone has minimal mineralocorticoid activity, and therefore support with parenteral normal saline solution is necessary.

If the patient shows manifestations of a salt-losing state, deoxycorticosterone acetate, 1 to 3 mg intramuscularly every day should be used. Once the patient is able to tolerate enteral feedings, fludrocortisone, 0.05 to 0.1 mg, every day should be started by mouth. As soon as the acute episode is under control, cortisol therapy should be decreased to maintenance cortisol rates in order to prevent poor growth. Supportive treatment is aimed at treating hypoglycemia, hypovolemia, hyponatremia, and hyperkalemia. These conditions should be aggressively treated at the same time that hormone replacement therapy is instituted.

References

1. Connell FA and Louden JM: Diabetes mortality in persons under 45 years of age. Am J Public Health 73:1174, 1983.

2. Sciblin J, Finegold D, and Dorman J: Why do children with diabetes die? Acta Endocrinol 279:326, 1986.

3. Tunbridge W: Factors contributing to deaths of diabetics under 50 years of age. Lancet 569:72, 1981.

4. Dorman J, Laporte R, and Kuller L: The Pittsburgh insulin-dependent diabetes mellitus morbidity and mortality study: Mortality results. Diabetes 33:271, 1984.

5. Faich GA, Fishbein HA, and Ellis SE: The epidemiology of diabetic acidosis: A population base study. Am J Epidemiol 117:551, 1983.

6. Czech MP: Molecular basis of insulin action. Ann Rev Biochem 46:359, 1977.

7. Tager H, Given B, and Baldwin I: A structurally abnormal insulin causing human diabetes. Nature 281:122, 1979.

8. Stryer L: Hormone action. *In*: Stryer L (ed): Biochemistry, 2nd ed. San Francisco, WH Freeman, 1981, pp. 840–859.

9. Foster DW and McGarry JD: The metabolic derangements and treatment of diabetic ketoacidosis. N Engl J Med 309:159, 1983.

10. Muller W, Faloona GR, and Unger RH: Hyperglucagonemia in diabetic ketoacidosis: Its prevalence and significance. Am J Med 54:52, 1973.

11. Gerich JE, Lorenzi M, and Bier, DM: Prevention of human diabetic ketoacidosis by somatostatin: Evidence for an essential role of glucagon. N Engl J Med 292:985, 1975.

12. Christenson MJ: Plasma catecholamines in juvenile diabetes. Scand J Endocrinol 76:165, 1987.

13. Schade DS and Eaton RP: The controversy concerning counter-regulatory hormone secretion: A hypothesis for the prevention of diabetic ketoacidosis. Diabetes 26:596, 1977.

14. MacGillivray MH, Bruck E, and Voorhees ML: Acute diabetic ketoacidosis in children: Role of stress hormone. Pediatr Res 15:99, 1981.

15. Harris GD, Fiordalisi I, and Finberg L: Safe management of diabetic ketoacidemia. J Pediatr 113:65, 1988.

16. Zerbe RL, Vinicor F, and Robertson GL: Plasma vasopressin in uncontrolled diabetes mellitus. Diabetes 28:503, 1979.

17. Tulassey T, Rascher W, and Körnet A: Atrial natriuretic peptide and other vasoactive hormones during treatment of severe diabetic ketoacidosis in children. J Pediatr 111:329, 1987.

18. Ataraski K, Mulroiv P, and Franco-Saenz R: Effects of atrial peptides on aldosterone production. J Clin Invest 76:1807, 1985.

19. Burnett JC, Granger J, and Opgenorth TJ: Effects of synthetic atrial natriuretic factors in renal function and renin release. Am J Physiol 247:F863, 1984.

20. Axelroad L, Shulman GI, and Blackshear P: Plasma level of 13,14-dihydro-15-keto-PGE$_2$ in patients with diabetic ketoacidosis and in normal fasting subjects. Diabetes 35:1004, 1986.

21. Mourits-Anderson T, Jensen I, and Mielsen GL: Plasma 6-keto PGF, alpha, thromboxane, B$_2$, and PGE$_2$ during diabetic ketoacidosis. Prostaglandins Leukot Essent Fatty Acids 40:39, 1990.

22. Chiavelli F, Verrotti A, and Tumini S: Fibronectin and thyroid hormones in children with diabetic ketoacidosis. Acta Pediatr Scand 76:665, 1987.

23. Foster DM and McGary JD: The metabolic derangements and treatment of diabetic ketoacidosis. N Engl J Med 309:159, 1983.

24. Richards CG and Vyeda K: Changes in the concentration of activation factor for phosphofructokinase in hepatocytes in response to glucose and glucagon. Biochem Biophys Res 97:1535, 1980.

25. Miles JM and Gerich JE: Glucose and ketone body kinetics in diabetic ketoacidosis. Clin Endocrinol Metab 12:303, 1983.

26. Richards CS and Vyeda K: Hormonal regulation of fructose-6-P$_1$-2-kinase and fructose-2, 6-P$_2$ by two mechanisms. J Biol Chem 257:8854, 1982.

27. Ishikawa S, Saito T, and Okada K: Prompt recovery of plasma arginine vasopressin in diabetic coma after intravenous infusion of a small dose of insulin and a large amount of fluid. Acta Endocrinol 122:455, 1990.

28. Cryer PE and Gerich JE: Glucose counterregulation, hypoglycemia and intensive insulin therapy in diabetes mellitus. N Engl J Med 313:232, 1985.

29. Malchoff CD, Pohl SL, and Kaiser N: Determinants of glucose and ketoacid concentrations in acutely hyperglycemic diabetic patients. Am J Med 77:275, 1984.

30. Kern E, Simmons D, and Martin D: Diabetic ketoacidosis and hyperglycemic nonketotic coma. *In*: Geelhoed G and Chernow

31. Hers HG and Van Schaftingen E: Fructose 2, 6-biphosphate two years after its discovery. Biochem J 206:1, 1982.

32. Foster DW: From glycogen to ketones and back. Diabetes 33:1188, 1984.

33. Owen OE, Block BS, and Patel M: Human splanchnic metabolism during diabetic ketoacidosis. Metabolism 38:289, 1989.

34. Cefalu WT: Diabetic ketoacidosis. Crit Care Clin 7:89, 1991.

35. Sanson TH and Levine SN: Management of diabetic ketoacidosis. Drugs 38:289, 1989.

36. Sperling MA: Diabetic ketoacidosis. Pediatr Clin North Am 31:591, 1984.

37. Owen OE, Trapp VE, and Skutches CL: Acetone metabolism during diabetic ketoacidosis. Diabetes 31:242, 1982.

38. McGang JD and Foster DV: Regulation of ketogenesis and clinical aspects of the ketotic state. Metabolism 21:471, 1972.

39. Evan LA, Davidson RJ, and Stowes JM: Alterations in erythrocytes in hyperosmolar diabetic decompensation: A pathophysiological basis for impaired blood flow and for an improved design of fluid therapy. Diabetologia 28:739, 1985.

40. Krane E: Diabetic ketoacidosis: Biochemistry, physiology, treatment, and prevention. Pediatr Clin North Am 34:935, 1987.

41. Duck SC and Wyatt DT: Factors associated with brain herniation in the treatment of diabetic ketoacidosis. J Pediatr 113:10, 1988.

42. Katz MA: Hyperglycemia-induced hyponatremia: Calculation of expected sodium depression. N Engl J Med 289:843, 1973.

43. Durr JA, Hoffman WH, and Hensen J: Osmoregulation of vasopressin in diabetic ketoacidosis. Am J Physiol 259:E723, 1990.

44. Chiarelli F, Tumini S, and Verroty A: Effects of ketoacidosis and puberty on basal and TRH-stimulated thyroid hormones and TSH in children with diabetes mellitus. Hormone Metab Res 21:494, 1989.

45. Turro J and Fulop M: Low serum triiodothyronine in diabetic ketoacidosis. NY State J Med 87:431, 1987.

46. Walker M, Marshall S, and Alberti K: Clinical aspects of diabetic ketoacidosis. Diabetes Metab Rev 5:651, 1989.

47. Ellis E: Concepts of fluid therapy in diabetic ketoacidosis and hyperosmolar hyperglycemic nonketotic coma. Pediatr Clin North Am 37:313, 1990.

48. Aubier M, Murciano D, and Lecocguia Y: Effect of hypophosphatemia on diaphragmatic contractility in patients with acute respiratory failure. N Engl J Med 313:420, 1985.

49. Tillman CR: Hypokalemic hypoventilation complicating severe diabetic ketoacidosis. South Med J 73:231, 1980.

50. Beigelman PM: Potassium in severe diabetic ketoacidosis. Am J Med 54:419, 1973.

51. Dorin R and Crapo L: Hypokalemic respiratory arrest in diabetic ketoacidosis. JAMA 257:1517, 1987.

52. Keller U and Berger W: Prevention of hypophosphatemia by phosphate infusion during treatment of diabetic ketoacidosis and hyperosmolar coma. Diabetes 29:87, 1980.

53. Knochell JP: The clinical status of hypophosphatemia: An update. N Engl J Med 313:447, 1988.

54. Kantes Y, Gerson A, and Beesman A: 2–3 Diphosphoglycerate, nucleotide phosphate, and organic and inorganic phosphate levels during the early phases of diabetic ketoacidosis. J Clin Endocrinol Metab 57:177, 1983.

55. Molitch ME, Rodman E, and Hirsch CA: Spurious serum creatinine elevations in ketoacidosis. Ann Intern Med 93:280, 1980.

56. Assali FK, John EG, and Fornell L: Falsely elevated serum creatinine concentration in ketoacidosis. J Pediatr 107:562, 1985.

57. Schrier BW, Berel T, and Anderson RJ: Osmotic and nonosmotic control of vasopressin release. Am J Physiol 236:F321, 1979.

58. Rascher W, Lang R, and Unger T: Vasopressin, cardiovascular regulation and hypertension. Curr Top Neuroendocrinol 4:101, 1985.

59. Franklin B, Liu J, and Ginsberg F: Cerebral edema and ophthalmoplegia reversed by mannitol in a new case of insulin dependent diabetes mellitus. Pediatrics 69:87, 1982.

60. Hoffman WH, Steinhart CM, and El-Gammal T: Cranial CT in children and adolescents with diabetic ketoacidosis. Am J Neuroradiol 9:733, 1987.

61. Shapiro HM: Intracranial hypertension: Therapeutic and anesthetic considerations. Anesthesiology 43:445, 1975.

62. Goldstein GW: The role of brain capillaries in the pathogenesis of hepatic encephalopathy. Hepatology 4:565, 1984.
63. Van Gelder NM and Barbeau A: The osmoregulatory function of taurine and glutamic acid. *In*: Oja SS, Ahtee L, and Kontro P (eds): Taurine: Biological Actions and Clinical Perspectives, Vol 179. New York, Alan R Liss, 1979, pp. 149–163.
64. Trachtinan H, Harbour R, and Sturman JA: Taurine and osmoregulation. Pediatr Res 23:35, 1988.
65. Uleck BW: Risk factors for cerebral edema associated with diabetic ketoacidosis. Ann Neurol 20:407, 1986.
66. Krane EJ: Cerebral edema in diabetic ketoacidosis. J Pediatr 114:166, 1989.
67. Harris GD, Fiordalisi I, and Harris WL: Minimizing the risk of brain herniation during treatment of diabetic ketoacidemia: A retrospective and prospective study. J Pediatr 117:22, 1990.
68. Harris GD, Firdalisi I, and Finberg L: Cerebral edema in diabetic ketoacidosis. J Pediatr 114:107, 1989.
69. Deitch EA: Does the gut protect us or injure us when ill in the ICU. *In*: Cerra FB (ed): Perspectives in Critical Care, Vol 1. St. Louis, QMP, 1988, pp. 1–24.
70. Fink MP: Leaky gut hypothesis: A historical perspective. Crit Care Med 18:579, 1990.
71. Sprung CL, Rackow EC, and Fein A: Pulmonary edema: A complication of diabetic ketoacidosis. Chest 68:253, 1975.
72. Rosenbloom AL and Schatz DA: Minimizing risk of brain herniation during treatment of diabetic ketoacidosis. J Pediatr 117:1009, 1990.
73. Reitano G: Diabetic ketoacidosis in children. J Endocrinol Invest 12:105, 1989.
74. Fisher JM and Kitabchi A: A randomized study of phosphate therapy in the treatment of diabetic ketoacidosis. J Clin Endocrinol Metab 57:177, 1983.
75. Ditzel J: Effect of plasma inorganic phosphate on tissue oxygenation during recovery from diabetic ketoacidosis. Adv Exp Med Biol 37:103, 1973.
76. Clerebaux T, Reynaert M, and Williams E: Effect of phosphate on oxygen-hemoglobin affinity, diphosphoglycerate, and blood gases during recovery from diabetic ketoacidosis. Intensive Care Med 15:495, 1989.
77. Wilson HK, Keuer SP, and Lu AS: Phosphate therapy in diabetic ketoacidosis. Arch Intern Med 142:517, 1982.
78. Sanson TH and Levine SN: Management of diabetic ketoacidosis. Drugs 38:289, 1989.
79. Edwards GA, Kohaut EC, and Wehring B: Effectiveness of low dose continuous intravenous insulin infusion in diabetic ketoacidosis: A prospective comparative study. J Pediatr 91:701, 1977.
80. Lightner ES, Kappy MS, and Revsin B: Low dose intravenous insulin infusion in patients with diabetic ketoacidosis: Biochemical effects in children. Pediatrics 60:681, 1977.
81. Lindsay R, and Bolte RG: The use of an insulin bolus in low dose insulin infusion for pediatric diabetic ketoacidosis. Pediatr Emerg Care 5:77, 1989.
82. Fort P, Waters SM, and Lifshitz F: Low dose insulin infusion in the treatment of diabetic ketoacidosis and hyperglycemic hyperosmolar nonketotic coma. Diabetes 5:78, 1982.
83. Luzi L, Barrett E, and Groop L: Metabolic effects of low dose insulin therapy on glucose metabolism in diabetic ketoacidosis. Diabetes 37:1470, 1988.
84. Jos J, Oberkampf B, and Couprie C: Comparison of 2 modes of treatment of diabetic ketoacidosis in children. Arch Fr Pediatr 45:15, 1988.
85. Keller U: Diabetic ketoacidosis: Current views on pathogenesis and treatment. Diabetologia 29:71, 1987.
86. De Fronzo RA and Lang R: Hypophosphatemia and glucose intolerance: Evidence for tissue insensitivity to insulin. N Engl J Med 303:1259, 1980.
87. Sheldon J, Hollis P, and Trafford J: Diabetic ketoacidosis due to insulin resistance treated by hemodialysis. Diabetic Med 2:59, 1985.
88. Migm L, Levy M, and Zuske H: Effects of changes of pH and of carbon dioxide tension on left ventricular performance. Am J Physiol 213:115, 1967.
89. Beierholm E, Grantham R, and O'Keefe D: Effect of acid-base changes, hypoxia, and catecholamines on ventricular performance. Am J Physiol 288:1555, 1975.
90. Samuelson RG and Magy G: Effects of respiratory alkatosis and

91. acidosis on myocardial excitation. Acta Physiol Scand 97:1581, 1976.
91. Lever E and Jasper JB: Sodium bicarbonate therapy in severe DKA. Am J Med 75:263, 1983.
92. Burear MA: Cerebral hypoxia from bicarbonate infusion in diabetic acidosis. J Pediatr 96:968, 1980.
93. Kaye R: Diabetic ketoacidosis: The bicarbonate therapy. J Pediatr 87:156, 1975.
94. McGarry JD: New perspectives in the regulation of ketogenesis. Diabetes 28:517, 1970.
95. Zimmet PZ, Taft P, and Ennis GC: Acid production in diabetic acidosis: A more rational approach to alkali replacement. Br Med J 3:610, 1970.
96. Munk P, Freedman MH, and Levison H: Effect of bicarbonate on oxygen transport in juvenile diabetes ketoacidosis. J Pediatr 91:706, 1977.
97. Ditzel J: Raised CSF pressure during treatment of diabetic ketosis. Lancet 2:730, 1971.
98. Assal JP, Aoki TT, and Manzano FM: Metabolic effects of sodium bicarbonate in management of diabetic ketoacidosis. Diabetes 23:405, 1974.
99. Morris LR, Murphy MB, and Kitbachi AE: Bicarbonate therapy in severe diabetic ketoacidosis. Ann Intern Med 105:836, 1986.
100. Hale PJ, Crase J, and Mattrass M: Metabolic effects of bicarbonate in the treatment of diabetic ketoacidosis. Br Med J 289:1035, 1984.
101. Rogers B, Sills I, and Cohen M: Diabetic ketoacidosis: Neurologic collapse during treatment followed by severe developmental morbidity. Clin Pediatr 29:451, 1990.
102. Greene SA, Jefferson IG, and Baum JD: Cerebral edema complicating diabetic ketoacidosis. Dev Med Child Neurol 32:633, 1990.
103. Bello FA: Cerebral edema in diabetic ketoacidosis in children. Lancet 336:64, 1990.
104. Rosenbloom A: Intracerebral crises during treatment of diabetic ketoacidosis. Diabetes Care 13:22, 1990.
105. Atluru VL: Spontaneous intracerebral hematomas in juvenile diabetic ketoacidosis. Pediatr Neurol 2:167, 1986.
106. Campbell RR, Foster NJ, and Sterling C: Paradoxical platelet behavior in diabetic ketoacidosis. Diabetic Med 3:161, 1986.
107. Matz R: Cerebral edema in diabetic ketoacidosis. Lancet 2:689, 1987.
108. Keller RJ, and Wolfsdorf JI: Isolated growth hormone deficiency after cerebral edema complicating diabetic ketoacidosis. N Engl J Med 316:857, 1987.
109. Chanson P, De Rohan CP, and Loirat P: Nontraumatic rhabdomyolysis during diabetic ketoacidosis. Diabetologia 29:674, 1986.
110. Garre M, Boles JM, and Garo B: Cerebral edema in diabetic ketoacidosis: Do we use too much insulin? Lancet 220, 1986.
111. Krane JE, Rockoff MA, and Wallman JK: Subclinical brain swelling in children during treatment of diabetic ketoacidosis. N Engl J Med 312:1147, 1985.
112. Carroll P and Matz R: Adult respiratory distress syndrome complicating severely uncontrolled diabetes mellitus: Report of nine cases and a review of the literature. Diabetes Care 5:574, 1982.
113. Mather HM: Management of hyperosmolar coma. J Soc Med 73:134, 1980.
114. Hoffman WH: Hyperglycemic hyperosmolar non-ketotic coma in a non-diabetic child. Diabetologia 25:531, 1983.
115. Casadevall I, Betremieux P, and Pladys P: Hyperosmolar coma in a premature newborn infant: Iatrogenic complication of parenteral feeding. Pediatrics 43:205, 1988.
116. Seki S: Clinical features of hyperosmolar hyperglycemic nonketotic diabetic coma associated with cardiac operations. J Thorac Cardiovasc Surg 91:867, 1986.
117. Pildes R, Cornblath M, and Warren I: A prospective controlled study of neonatal hypoglycemia. Pediatrics 54:5, 1974.
118. Grappuso PA and Schwartz R: Hypoglycemia in children. Pediatr Rev 11:117, 1989.
119. LaFranchi S: Hypoglycemia of infancy and childhood. Pediatr Clin North Am 34:961, 1987.
120. Koivisto M, Blanco-Sequeiros M, and Krause U: Neonatal symptomatic and asymptomatic hypoglycemia: A follow-up study of 151 children. Dev Med Child Neurol 14:603, 1972.

121. Cornblatt M and Schwartz R: Disorders of Carbohydrate Metabolism in Infancy, 2nd ed. Philadelphia, WB Saunders, 1976, p. 48.
122. Pagliara AS, Karl IE, and Haymond MW: Hypoglycemia in infancy and childhood. J Pediatr 83:694, 1973.
123. Ditchburn RK, Wilkinson RH, and Davis PA: Plasma glucose levels in infants 2,500 g and less fed immediately after birth with breast milk. Biol Neonate 11:29, 1967.
124. Haymond MW: Hypoglycemia in infants and children. Endocrinol Metab Clin North Am 18:211, 1989.
125. Greengard O: The developmental formation of enzymes in rat liver. In: Litwock G (ed): Biochemical Actions of Hormones. London, Academic Press, 1970 p. 53.
126. Frazer TE, Karl IE, and Hillman LS: Direct measurement of gluconeogenesis from $[2,3-^{13}C_2]$ alanine in the human neonate. Am J Physiol 83:E240, 1981.
127. Amiel SA, Sherwin RS, and Simonson DC: Effect of intensive insulin therapy on glycemic thresholds for counterregulatory hormone release. Diabetes 37:901, 1988.
128. Boden G, Reichard GA, and Hoeldike RD: Severe insulin-induced hypoglycemia of counterregulatory hormones. N Engl J Med 305:1200, 1981.
129. Shakir MK and Amin RM: Hypoglycemia. Crit Care Clin 7:75, 1991.
130. Senior B and Wolfsdorf JI: Hypoglycemia in children. Pediatr Clin North Am 26:171, 1979.
131. Sokoloff L: Circulation and energy metabolism of the brain. In: Albers RW, Siegel GJ, and Katzman R (eds): Basic Neurochemistry. Boston, Little, Brown, 1972, p. 299.
132. Grunberger G, Weiner JL, and Silverman R: Factitious hypoglycemia due to surreptitious administration of insulin: Diagnosis, treatment, and long-term follow-up. Ann Intern Med 108:252, 1988.
133. Fischer KF, Lees JA, and Newman JH: Hypoglycemia in hospitalized patients: Causes and outcomes. N Engl J Med 315:1245, 1986.
134. Susa JB, Cowett RM, and Oh W: Suppression of gluconeogenesis and endogenous glucose production by exogenous insulin administration in the newborn lamb. Pediatr Res 13:594, 1979.
135. Kalhan SC, Savin SM, and Adam PA: Attenuated glucose production rate in newborn infants of insulin-dependent diabetic mothers. N Engl J Med 296:375, 1977.
136. Barrett CT and Oliver TK: Hypoglycemia and hyperinsulinism in infants with erythroblastosis fetalis. N Engl J Med 278:1260, 1968.
137. Pildes RS: Infants of diabetic mothers. N Engl J Med 289:902, 1973.
138. Williams PR, Sperling MA, and Racasa Z: Blunting of spontaneous and amino-acid-stimulated glucagon secretion in infants of diabetic mothers. Diabetes 24:411, 1975.
139. Urbach J, Kaplan M, and Blondheim O: Neonatal hypoglycemia related to umbilical artery catheter malposition. J Pediatr 106:825, 1986.
140. Witte DP, Greider MH, and DeSchryver-Kecskemeti K: The juvenile human endocrine pancreas: Normal versus idiopathic hyperinsulinemic hypoglycemia. Semin Diag Pathol 1:30, 1984.
141. Haymond MW, Strauss AW, and Arnold KJ: Glucose homeostasis in children with severe cyanotic congenital heart disease. J Pediatr 95:220, 1979.
142. Jaffe R, Hashida Y, and Yunis E: Pancreatic pathology in hyperinsulinemic hypoglycemia of infancy. Lab Invest 42:356, 1980.
143. Scarlett JA, Mako ME, and Rubenstein AH: Factitious hypoglycemia: Diagnosis by measurement of serum C-peptide immunoreactivity and insulin binding antibodies. N Engl J Med 297:1029, 1977.
144. Bauman WA and Yalow RS: Child abuse: Parenteral insulin administration. J Pediatr 99:588, 1981.
145. Haymond MW, Karl IE, and Weldom VV: The role of growth hormone and cortisone on glucagon and gluconeogenic substrate regulation in fasted hypopituitary children. J Clin Endocrin Metab 42:846, 1976.
146. Samaan NA: Hypoglycemia secondary to endocrine deficiencies. Clin Endocrinol Metab 18:145, 1989.
147. Seltzer HS: Drug-induced hypoglycemia: A review of 1418 cases. Clin Endocrinol Metab 18: 163, 1989.
148. Artavia E, Chaussain PF, and Bougneres JC: Frequency of hypoglycemia in children with adrenal insufficiency. Acta Endocrinol (Suppl.) 279:275, 1986.
149. Hers HG, Van Hoof F, and de Basy T: Glycogen storage diseases. In: Stanbury JB, Wyngaarden JG, and Fredrickson DA (eds): The Metabolic Basis of Inherited Disease. New York, McGraw-Hill, 1989, p. 225.
150. Kliegman RM and Sparks JW: Perinatal galactose metabolism. J Pediatr 107:831, 1985.
151. Steinmann B and Gitzelmann R: The diagnosis of heredity fructose intolerance. Helv Paediatr Acta 36:297, 1981.
152. Waber LJ, Valle D, and Neil C: Carnitine deficiency presenting as familial cardiomyopathy: A treatable defect in carnitine transport. J Pediatr 101:700, 1982.
153. Slonim AE, Borum PR, and Mark RE: Non-ketotic hypoglycemia: An early indicator of systemic carnitine deficiency. Neurology 33:29, 1985.
154. Bougneres PF, Saudubray JM, and Marsac C: Fasting hypoglycemia resulting from hepatic carnitine palmitoyl transferase deficiency. J Pediatr 98:742, 1981.
155. Haymond MW, Ben-Galim E, and Strobel KE: Glucose and alanine metabolism in children with maple syrup disease. J Clin Invest 62:398, 1978.
156. Stanley CA, Berry GT, and Yudkoff M: Urine carnitine excretion in secondary carnitine deficiency. Pediatr Res 18:300A, 1984.
157. Roe CR, Millington DS, and Maltby DA: L-Carnitine enhances excretion of propionyl coenzyme A as propionyl carnitine in propionic acidemia. J Clin Invest 73:1785, 1984.
158. Vidnes J and Oyasaeter S: Glucagon deficiency causing severe neonatal hypoglycemia in a patient with normal insulin secretion. Pediatr Res 11:943, 1977.
159. Kollie LA, Monneus LA, and Cyka V: Persistent neonatal hypoglycemia due to glucagon deficiency. Arch Dis Child 53:422, 1978.
160. Loridon L, Sadeghi-Mejad A, and Senior B: Hypersecretion of insulin after the administration of L-leucine to obese children. J Pediatr 78:53, 1971.
161. Floyd J, Fajans S, and Knopf R: Evidence that insulin release is the mechanism for experimentally induced hypoglycemia in man. J Clin Invest 42:1714, 1963.
162. Tanaka K, Miller E, and Isselbacker K: Hypoglycin A: A specific inhibitor of isovaleryl CoA dehydrogenase. Proc Natl Acad Sci USA 68:20, 1971.
163. Sheroalt: Hypoglycin and related hypoglycemic compounds. Br Med Bull 25:250, 1969.
164. DeGroot L, Larson P, and Mefetoff S: The Thyroid and Its Diseases, 5th ed. New York, John Wiley, 1984 p. 62.
165. Hiromatsu Y, Fukazawa H, and Guinard F: A thyroid cytotoxic antibody that cross reacts with an eye muscle cell surface antigen may be the cause of thyroid-associated ophthalmopathy. J Clin Endocrinol Metab 69:622, 1989.
166. DeGroot LJ and Quintans J: The causes of autoimmune thyroid disease. Endocrinol Rev 10:5, 1989.
167. Bahn RS, Gorman CA, and Johnson CM: Presence of antibodies in the sera of patients with Grave's disease recognizing a 23 kilodalton fibroblast protein. J Clin Endocrinol Metab 69:622, 1989.
168. Samuel S, Gilman S, and Maurer HS: Hyperthyroidism in an infant with McCune-Albright syndrome: Report of a case with myeloid metaplasia. J Pediatr 80:275, 1976.
169. Smallridge RC, Wartofsky L, and Chopra I: Neonatal thyrotoxicosis: Alteration of serum concentrations of LATA-protector, T_4, T_3, reverse T_3, and $3,3^1T_2$. J Pediatr 93:118, 1978.
170. Zimmerman D and Gan-Gaisano M: Hyperthyroidism in children and adolescents. Pediatr Clin North Am 37:1273, 1990.
171. Gorlin J and Sallan S: Thyroid cancer in childhood. Pediatr Clin North Am 19:649, 1990.
172. Weintraub B, Gershengorn M, and Kourides I: Inappropriate secretion of thyroid stimulating hormone. Ann Intern Med 95:339, 1981.
173. Gershengorn M and Weintraub B: Thyrotropin-induced hyperthyroidism caused by selective pituitary resistance to thyroid hormone: A new syndrome of "inappropriate secretion of TSH." J Clin Invest 56:633, 1975.
174. Hedberg C, Fishbein D, and Janssen R: An outbreak of thyro-

toxicosis caused by the consumption of bovine thyroid gland in ground beef. N Engl J Med 316:993, 1987.

175. Cohen J, Ingbar S, and Braverman L: Thyrotoxicosis due to ingestion of excess thyroid hormone. Endocrinol Rev 10:113, 1989.

176. Martino E, Baschieri L, and Aghini-Lombardi F: Successful treatment of amiodarone associated thyrotoxicosis with KClO$_4$ and methinazole. Ann Endocrinol 45A:15, 1984.

177. Zaloga G and Chernow B: Thyroid function in acute illness. In: Geelhoed G and Chernow B (eds): Endocrine Aspects of Acute Illness. New York, Churchill Livingstone, 1985 pp. 67–96.

178. Hoffenberger R: Thyroid emergencies. Clin Endocrinol Metab 9:503, 1980.

179. Cooper DS: Which antithyroid drug? Am J Med 80:1165, 1986.

180. Emerson CM, Anderson AJ, and Howard WJ: Serum thyroxine and triiodothyronine concentrations during iodide treatment of hyperthyroidism. J Clin Endocrinol Metab 40:33, 1975.

181. Lee PW: Thyroiditis hyperthyroidism and tumors. Pediatr Clin North Am 26:53, 1979.

182. Reasner CH and Isley W: Thyrotoxicosis in the critically ill. Crit Care Clin 7:57, 1991.

183. Solomon DH: Treatment of Graves' hyperthyroidism. In: Ingbar SH and Braverman LE (eds): The Thyroid, 5th ed. Philadelphia, JB Lippincott, 1986, pp. 987.

184. Ashkar F, Katirns R, and Smoak W: Thyroid storm treatment with blood exchange and plasmapheresis. JAMA 214:1275, 1970.

185. Turlapaty P, Laddu A, and Shrinivas V: Esmolol: A titrable short-acting intravenous β-blocker for acute critical care settings. Clin Pharm 114:866, 1987.

186. May ME, Mintz PD, and Lowry P: Plasmapheresis in thyroxine overdose: A case report. J Toxicol Clin 20:517, 1984.

187. Galaburda M, Rosman P, and Haddoco J: Thyroid storm in a 11-year-old boy managed by propanolol. Pediatrics 53:920, 1974.

188. Stevens JJ: A case of thyrotoxic crisis that mimicked malignant hyperthermia. Anesthesiology 59:263, 1983.

189. Christensen P and Nissen L: Treatment of thyroid storm in a child with dantrolen. Br J Anaesth 59:523, 1987.

190. Aiello D, DuPlessis A, and Pattishall E: Thyroid storm presenting with coma and seizures in a 3-year-old girl. Clin Pediatr 29:571, 1989.

191. Wolfson B and Smith K: Cardiac arrest following minor surgery in unrecognized thyrotoxicosis. Anesth Analg 47:672, 1968.

192. Dahl I: Thyroid crisis in a 3-year-old girl. Acta Paediatr Scand 57:55, 1968.

193. Peter F: Juvenile thyrotoxicosis. Acta Endocrinol 279(Suppl):361, 1986.

194. Mandel S, Hanna CH, and LaFranchi S: Diminished thyroid-stimulating hormone secretion associated with neonatal thyrotoxicosis. J Pediatr 4:662, 1986.

195. Sheldon M and Gans B: Congenital thyrotoxicosis, hepatosplenomegaly, and jaundice in two infants of exophthalmic mothers. Arch Dis Child 30:460, 1955.

196. Hollingworth I, Maby C, and Echerd J: Hereditary aspects of Grave's disease in infancy and childhood. J Pediatr 81:446, 1972.

197. Palazzo M and Suter P: Thyroid hormone receptor expression in sick euthyroid syndrome. Lancet 335:662, 1990.

198. Fisher I: Euthyroid low thyroxine T$_4$ and triiodothyronine T$_3$ states in prematures and sick neonates. Pediatr Clin North Am 37:1297, 1990.

199. Ulartopky L and Burman K: Alterations in thyroid function in patients with systemic illness: The euthyroid sick syndrome. Endocrinol Rev 3:164, 1982.

200. Jackson J and Uerdonk C: Euthyroid hyperthyroxinemia and inappropriate secretion of thyrotropin. Arch Intern Med 147:1311, 1987.

201. Zaloga G and Chernow B: Thyroid function in acute illness. In: Geelhold G and Chernow B (eds): Endocrine Aspects of Acute Illness. New York, Churchill Livingstone, 1985, p. 67.

202. Zaloga G, Chernow B, and Smallridge B: A longitudinal evaluation of thyroid function in critically ill surgical patients. Ann Surg 201:456, 1985.

203. Zucker A, Chernow B, and Fields A: Thyroid function in critically ill children. J Pediatr 107:552, 1985.

204. Wartofsky L and Burman K: Alterations in thyroid function in critically ill patients with systemic illness: The "euthyroid sick syndrome." Endocrinol Rev 3:164, 1982.

205. Kapstein E, Weiner J, and Robinson W: Relationship of altered thyroid hormone indices to survival in nonthyroidal illness. Clin Endocrinol 16:565, 1982.

206. Silberman H, Eisenberg D, and Ryan J: The relationship of thyroid indices in the critically ill patient to prognosis and nutritional factors. Surg Gynecol Obstet 166:223, 1988.

207. Wise K and Zaritsky A: Endocrine manifestations of critical illness in the child. Pediatr Clin North Am 34:119, 1987.

208. Burger A, Dimichest D, and Micod P: Effect of amiodarone on serum triiodothyronine, reverse triiodothyronine, thyroxin, and thyrotropin. J Clin Invest 58:255, 1976.

209. Burman K: Thyroid hormones. In: Chernow B and Lake M (eds): The Pharmacologic Approach to the Critically Ill Patient. Baltimore, Williams & Wilkins, 1983, p. 586.

210. Morley JE: Neuroendocrine control of thyrotropin secretion. Endocrinol Rev 2:396, 1981.

211. Pang X, Hershman J, and Mirell C: Impairment of hypothalamic pituitary-thyroid functions in rats treated with human recombinant tumor necrosis factor. Endocrinology 125:76, 1989.

212. Lee H, Suhl J, and Pekong E: Secretions of thyrotropin with reduced concavalin-A binding activity in patients with severe nonthyroidal illness. J Clin Endocrinol Metab 65:942, 1987.

213. Chopra I, Huang T, and Beredo A: Conversion of thyroxine to 3,5,3'-triiodothyronine in sera of patients with nonthyroidal illness. J Clin Endocrinol Metab 60:66, 1985.

214. Delange R, Bourdoux P, and Ermans A: Transient disorders of thyroid function and regulation in pre-term infants. In: Delange R, Fisher D, and Malvaus P: Pediatric Thyroidology. Basel, S. Karger, 1985 p. 369.

215. Slag M, Morley J, and Elson M: Hypothyroxinemia in critically ill patients as a predictor of high mortality. JAMA 245:43, 1981.

216. Franklin R and O'Grady C: Neonatal thyroid function: Effects of nonthyroidal illness. Pediatrics 107:599, 1985.

217. Allan B, Dietrich A, and Zimmerman J: Thyroid hormone metabolism and level of illness severity in pediatric cardiac surgery patients. J Pediatr 114:59, 1989.

218. Nisser H: The adrenal cortex in childhood. Arch Dis Child 41:2, 1966.

219. Passmore J: Adrenal cortex. In: Geelhold G and Chernow B (eds): Endocrine Aspects of Acute Illness. New York, Churchill Livingstone, 1985, p. 97.

220. Williams B (ed): Textbook of Endocrinology, 6th ed. Philadelphia, WB Saunders, p. 128.

221. Chin R: Adrenal crisis. Crit Care Clin 7:23, 1991.

222. Chin R and Chernow B: Corticosteroids. In: Chernow B and Lake R: The Pharmacological Approach to the Critically Ill Patient. Baltimore, Williams & Wilkins, 1983, p. 510.

223. Stryer L: Hormone action. In: Stryer L (ed): Biochemistry, 2nd ed. San Francisco, WH Freeman, 1981, p. 476.

224. Baxter J and Tyrell J: The adrenal cortex. In: Felig P, Balter J, and Broads A (eds): Endocrinology and Metabolism. New York, McGraw-Hill, 1987, p. 511.

225. Axelroad J, and Reisine T: Stress hormones: Their interactions and regulation. Science 244:452, 1984.

226. Dallman M, Darlington D, and Suemaru S: Corticosteroids in homeostasis. Acta Physiol Scand 136:S 583:S27, 1989.

227. Feldman D: Mechanism of control. In: De Groot L, Besser G, and Cahill G: Endocrinology, 2nd ed. Philadelphia, WB Saunders, 1989, p. 1557.

228. Munck A, Guyre P, and Hoolbrook M: Physiological functions of glucocorticoids in stress and their relations to pharmacological actions. Endocrinol Rev 5:25, 1984.

229. Meyais S, Chekal M, and Jones W: Modulation of renal sodium-potassium-adenosine triphosphatase by aldosterone. J Clin Invest 76:170, 1980.

230. Munck A, Mendel D, and Smith L: Glucocorticoid receptors and actions. Am Rev Respir Dis 141:S2, 1990.

231. Fauci A, Dale D, and Balow J: Glucocorticoid therapy: Mechanisms of action and clinical considerations. Ann Intern Med 84:304, 1976.

232. Crabbe J: Mechanisms of action of aldosterone. In: De Groot L, Besser G, and Cahill G: Endocrinology, 2nd ed. Philadelphia, WB Saunders, 1989, p 1572.

233. Peers S and Flows N: The role of lipocortin in corticosteroid actions. Am Rev Respir Dis 141:S18, 1990.

234. Drucker S and New M: Disorders of adrenal steroidogenesis. Pediatr Clin North Am 34:1055, 1987.

235. Visser H: The adrenal cortex in childhood: Pathological aspects. Arch Dis Child 41:113, 1966.
236. Hughes I: Congenital and acquired disorders of the adrenal cortex. Clin Endocrinol Met 11:89, 1982.
237. Gutai J and Migen C: Adrenal insufficiency during the neonatal period. Clin Perinatol 2:163, 1975.
238. Moser H and Moser A: The adrenoleukodystrophies. Crit Rev Neurobiol 3:29, 1987.
239. Seltzer W, Firminger H, and Klein J: Adrenal dysfunction in glycerol kinase deficiency. Biochem Med 33:189, 1985.
240. Gumbinas M, Liu M, and Dawson G: Progressive spastic paraparesis and adrenal insufficiency. Arch Neurol 33:678, 1976.
241. Kolodny E and Cable W: Inborn errors of metabolism. Ann Neurol 11:221, 1982.
242. Wise J, Matalon R, and Morgan A: Phenotypic features of patients with congenital adrenal hypoplasia and glycerol kinase deficiency. Am J Dis Child 141:744, 1987.
243. Boles D, Craft D, and Padgett D: Clinical variation in X linked adrenoleukodystrophy: Fatty acid and lipid metabolism in cultured fibroblasts. Biochem Med Metab Biol 45:74, 1991.
244. Barness L, Chandras S, and Kling P: Progressive neurologic deterioration in a nine year old white male. Am J Med Genet 37:489, 1990.
245. Maider S, Moser A, and Moser H: Phenotypic and genotypic variability of generalized peroxisomal disorders. Pediatr Neurol 4:5, 1988.
246. Neufeld M, MacLaren M, and Blizzard B: Two types of autoimmune Addison's disease associated with different polyglandular autoimmune syndromes. Medicine 60:355, 1981.
247. Irvine W: Autoimmunity in endocrine disease. Recent Prog Horm Res 36:509, 1980.
248. Moser H, Mihalik S, and Watkins P: Adrenoleukodystrophy and other peroxisomal disorders that affect the nervous system, including new observations on L-pipecolic acid oxidase in primates. Brain Dev 11:80, 1989.
249. Rongen W, Drop S, and Van Der Anker J: Primary adrenocortical insufficiency in childhood. Acta Endocrinol 279(Suppl):279, 1986.
250. Rose C, and Goldsmith D: Childhood adrenal insufficiency, chorea and antiphospholipid antibodies. Ann Rheum Dis 49:421, 1990.
251. Russel G, Coulter J, and Isherwood D: Autoimmune Addison's disease and thyrotoxic thyroiditis presenting as encephalopathy in twins. Arch Dis Child 66:350, 1990.
252. Boles D, Craft D, and Padgett D: Clinical variation in x-linked adrenoleukodystrophy: Fatty acid and lipid metabolism in cultured fibroblasts. Biochem Med Metab Biol 45:74, 1991.
253. Eisenbarth GS: The immunoendocrinopathy syndromes. In: Wilson J and Foster D (eds): William's Textbook of Endocrinology. Philadelphia, WB Saunders, 1985, p. 1290.
254. Meivrich P: Addison's disease and thyrotoxicosis presenting simultaneously. Postgrad Med J 60:478, 1984.
255. Kalifa G, Silberman J, and Chaussian C: Addison's disease in children: Associated anomalies. Ann Radiol 29:327, 1986.
256. Zondek L and Zondek T: Congenital adrenal hypoplasia in two infants. Acta Paediatr Scand 57:250, 1968.
257. Favara B and Franciosi R: Idiopathic adrenal hypoplasia in children. Am J Clin Pathol 57:287, 1972.
258. Schein R, Sprung C, Marcial E, et al: Plasma cortisol levels in patients with septic shock. Crit Care Med 18:259, 1990.
259. Michaels D and Moore D: Serum cortisol response in febrile children. Pediatr Infect Dis 8:16, 1989.
260. Kaplan S: Disorders of the adrenal cortex. Pediatr Clin North Am 26:65, 1979.
261. Bongiovanni A: Disorders of the adrenal cortex. In: Kaplan SA (ed): Clinical and Adolescent Endocrinology. Philadelphia, WB Saunders, 1982, p. 172.
262. Job J and Chaussian J: The adrenals. In: Job J and Pierson M (eds): Pediatric Endocrinology. New York, John Wiley & Sons, 1981, p. 301.
263. Beisel WR: Metabolic response of host to infections. In: Feigin R and Cherry J (eds): Textbook of Pediatric Infectious Diseases, 2nd ed. Philadelphia, WB Saunders, 1987, p. 11.
264. Salem M, Chernow B, and Burke R: Bedside diagnostic blood testing. JAMA 266:38, 1991.

Disorders of Intermediary Metabolism

Paul S. Thornton, M.B., B.Ch., M.R.C.P.I.,
Gerard T. Berry, M.D., and Charles A. Stanley, M.D.

Coma, respiratory distress, vascular collapse, or intractable seizures in an infant or child are usually due to an acquired illness such as severe infection, cardiopulmonary disease, epilepsy, or drug ingestion. The same signs of critical illness, however, may also be caused by disorders in the intermediary metabolism of carbohydrates, fats, or proteins. The purpose of this chapter is to provide a framework for the pediatric critical care specialist to facilitate the recognition of these metabolic disorders, outline strategies for diagnosis, and discuss general as well as specific therapies.

It is not surprising that a wide variety of disorders in the metabolism of carbohydrates, fats, and proteins present in a similar fashion. Any profound disturbance in the use of these major fuels may interrupt energy metabolism severely enough to cause coma. In addition, in many cases there may be an accumulation of substrates, such as ammonium, that are toxic to the brain or other organs.

Most patients with disorders of intermediary metabolism present for the first time before 1 year of age. They often have symptoms out of proportion to the precipitating illness. Some of the disorders, such as the urea cycle defects, present in the immediate postnatal period when the first catabolic episode occurs. Others, such as the fatty acid oxidation defects, usually do not present until after 6 to 12 months of age. The family history may be helpful if it reveals consanguinity or a history in a sibling of sudden death, an acute life-threatening event, unexplained developmental delay, or seizures. A history of a birthweight that is large for gestational age is a useful indicator of hyperinsulinism in a newborn with intractable hypoglycemia. The physical examination is often not informative; however, the finding of hepatomegaly may indicate glycogen storage disease (GSD) or a disorder of fatty acid oxidation.

This chapter focuses on five groups of disorders of intermediary metabolism that present with a critical illness: disorders of carbohydrate metabolism, disorders of fatty acid oxidation, lactic acidoses, urea cycle enzyme defects, and the organic acidurias. Figure 60–1 shows how routine laboratory tests can be used to place a patient with one of these disorders in the appropriate group for further specific investigations. It should be emphasized that abnormalities in blood or urine that identify a specific disorder are usually most dramatic at the time of acute illness and, in some cases, may be completely absent when the patient is not sick. For this reason, it is very important to save a sample of serum or plasma (1 ml or more) and of urine (5 to 10 ml) from the time before, or simultaneous with, the start of treatment. This sample can be sent at a later time for specific assays to confirm a suspected diagnosis. These may be called the "critical" blood and urine specimens, not only because they are taken at the time of critical illness but also because having them can often be critical for making a diagnosis.

DISORDERS OF CARBOHYDRATE METABOLISM

This section discusses disorders of carbohydrate metabolism that are most likely to require that a patient be admitted to the intensive care unit. The common feature of these illnesses is hypoglycemia, which can cause permanent brain damage. Central nervous system (CNS) signs of hypoglycemia may include confusion, bizarre behavior, coma, and seizures. Adrenergic signs may include tachycardia, sweating, and pallor. In the neonate, signs of hypoglycemia are often nonspecific and easily missed but may include tremors, jitteriness, hypothermia, cyanosis, and apnea. The authors recommend using a plasma glucose value of 40 mg/dl (2.2 mmol/l) to define hypoglycemia in both neonates and older children. This simply reflects the experience that severe symptoms of hypoglycemia are not likely to be encountered at levels of plasma glucose above this value. Therapeutically, however, the goal is to maintain glucose concentrations above 65 to 75 mg/dl, because levels below 65 mg/dl are considered undesirable and possibly unsafe.

All of the hypoglycemic disorders in infants and children occur in the fasting state. Within 3 to 4 hours

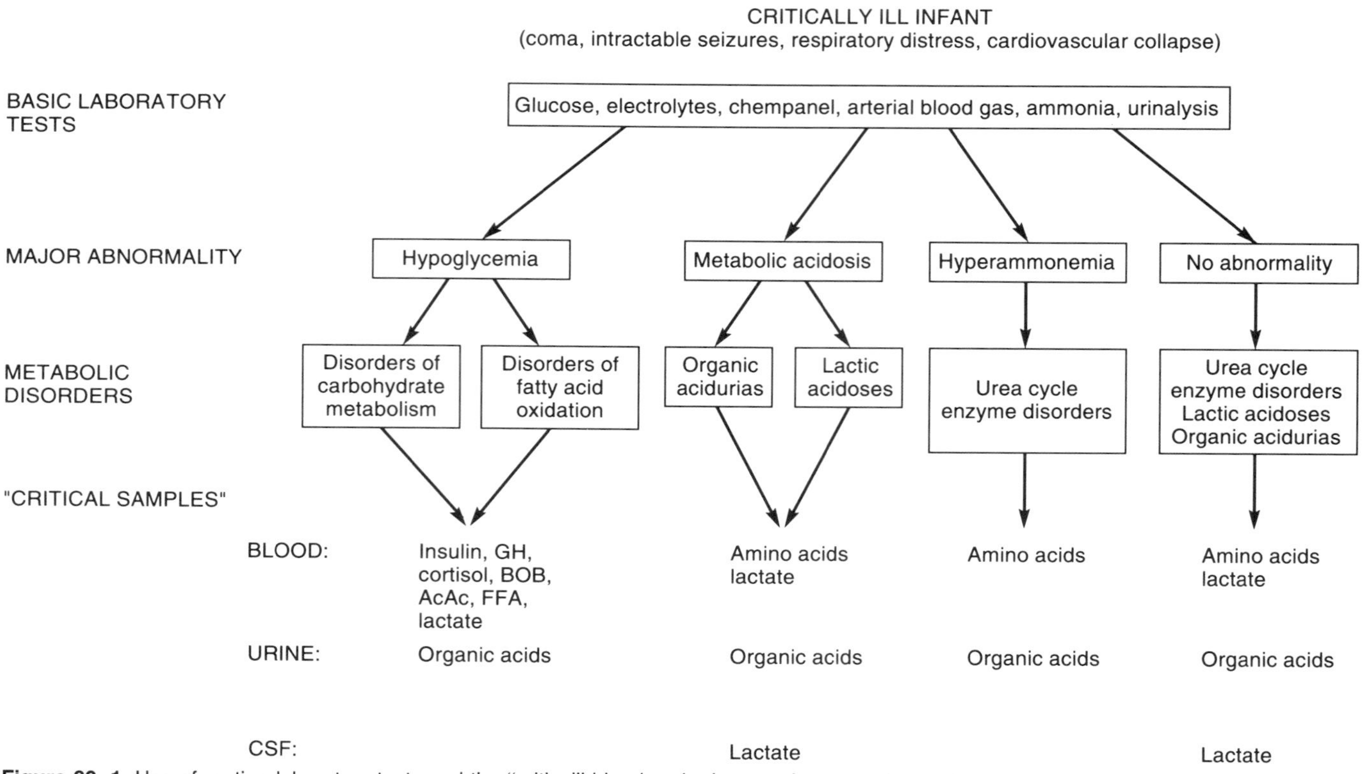

CRITICALLY ILL INFANT
(coma, intractable seizures, respiratory distress, cardiovascular collapse)

BASIC LABORATORY
TESTS

Glucose, electrolytes, chempanel, arterial blood gas, ammonia, urinalysis

MAJOR ABNORMALITY

| Hypoglycemia | Metabolic acidosis | Hyperammonemia | No abnormality |

METABOLIC
DISORDERS

| Disorders of carbohydrate metabolism | Disorders of fatty acid oxidation | Organic acidurias | Lactic acidoses | Urea cycle enzyme disorders | Urea cycle enzyme disorders / Lactic acidoses / Organic acidurias |

"CRITICAL SAMPLES"

BLOOD: Insulin, GH, cortisol, BOB, AcAc, FFA, lactate   Amino acids lactate   Amino acids   Amino acids lactate

URINE: Organic acids   Organic acids   Organic acids   Organic acids

CSF: Lactate   Lactate

Figure 60–1. Use of routine laboratory tests and the "critical" blood and urine specimens to detect disorders of intermediary metabolism in the critically ill infant or child.

after a meal, when the absorption of glucose from the gastrointestinal tract is complete, the maintenance of normoglycemia requires several specific biochemical systems (i.e., glycogenolysis, gluconeogenesis, and the utilization of fat as an alternative fuel). After a meal, the liver initially produces glucose by the breakdown of its glycogen stores (glycogenolysis). Within 3 hours in infants and 8 hours in older children, glycogen stores are depleted and the liver switches to gluconeogenesis, utilizing amino acids from muscle protein and glycerol that is released from adipose tissue by lipolysis. For fasting states beyond 12 hours, the body must conserve protein by utilizing free fatty acids, mobilized from adipose tissue triglyceride stores, as an alternative energy source. In tissues such as muscle, free fatty acids are directly oxidized for energy production, thus reducing the need for glucose and limiting gluconeogenesis from protein precursors. In the liver, fatty acids are partially oxidized to ketones, which are then released to serve as important fuels for the brain. By 18 hours of fasting, fat becomes the main fuel used, as reflected by the presence of ketones in the urine.[1] Figure 60–2 outlines the main steps in glycogenolysis and gluconeogenesis and highlights the enzyme deficiencies that may cause severe disruption of these pathways.

Hormonal regulation of fasting adaptation involves a decrease in secretion of insulin (which inhibits glycogenolysis, gluconeogenesis, lipolysis, and ketogenesis) and the availability of counter-regulatory hormones (e.g., growth hormone, cortisol, glucagon, and epinephrine).

Hyperinsulinism

Congenital hyperinsulinism is the most common cause of persistent hypoglycemia in the first year of life.[2] These infants are usually large for gestational age as a consequence of excess prenatal insulin. They may present within the first 48 hours of life or not until 2 to 4 months of age when feeding intervals stretch to beyond 4 hours. The rare child, who develops hyperinsulinism later in life, most often presents with a seizure or somnolence and coma on the first episode. Excessive glucose utilization is a striking and characteristic feature of hyperinsulinism; it may require glucose infusion rates of 20 mg/kg/min or more to maintain normoglycemia in these patients.[3]

The pathophysiology of hyperinsulinism reflects the widespread effects of insulin on fasting adaptation. Excess insulin inhibits all of the fasting systems outlined earlier. Therefore, there is not only increased glucose utilization but also decreased glucose production from glycogenolysis and gluconeogenesis as well as suppression of lipolysis and ketogenesis as alternate fuel sources. The pathologic changes in the pancreas may include normal or near-normal histology (nesidioblastosis), islet cell hyperplasia or hypertrophy, islet cell adenomatosis, or islet cell adenoma.[4] It has been postulated that many of the infants have diffuse pancreatic abnormalities of islet cell regulation, whereas older children, with onset of symptoms after 1 year of age, are more likely to have focal lesions, such as an ade-

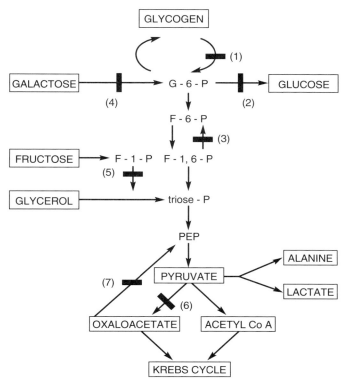

Figure 60–2. Enzyme defects in glucose metabolism that cause critical illnesses: (1) debrancher, (2) glucose-6-phosphatase, (3) fructose-1, 6-diphosphatase, (4) UDP-galactose transferase, (5) fructose-1-phosphate aldolase, (6) pyruvate carboxylase, (7) phosphoenolpyruvate-carboxykinase. (G-6-P = glucose-6-phosphate; F-6-P = fructose-6-phosphate; F-1,6 = fructose-1,6-diphosphate; F-1-P = fructose-1-phosphate; PEP = phosphoenolpyruvate.)

The goal of long-term treatment is to to maintain plasma glucose above 70 mg/dl on a regimen that can be continued at home. Diazoxide, the drug of first choice, should be given starting at the maximum dosage of 15 mg/kg/day by mouth, divided into two or three doses. Because diazoxide causes fluid retention, patients must be observed closely for signs of fluid overload. This may require the administration of a diuretic. If there is inadequate response by 1 to 3 days, a long-acting somatostatin analogue octreotide (Sandostatin) should be used starting at a dose of 5µg/kg subcutaneous (SC) every 6 hours and increased up to 30 µg/kg/24 hours until adequate response is achieved. If medical management is not successful, a 90 to 95% subtotal pancreatectomy should be undertaken. Surgical resection of a focal lesion may be curative; however, patients with normal histology may continue to have hypoglycemia and require medication (octreotide or diazoxide).[5] A gradual remission has been described in some patients, but only after medical treatment for periods of more than 5 years.

Transient and Exogenous Hyperinsulinism

Transient hyperinsulinism may occur in newborn infants secondary to maternal diabetes or, rarely, in association with hemolytic disease of the newborn. Hypoglycemia due to hyperinsulinism commonly occurs in diabetics, especially with attempts at tight control. Ingestion of oral hypoglycemics (e.g., sulfonylureas) cause stimulation of insulin release by the pancreas and, thus, hyperinsulinism. Acute treatment of hypoglycemia following ingestion of oral hypoglycemics is similar to that outlined earlier and is rarely required for longer than 1 to 2 days. Surreptitious insulin administration to a nondiabetic person may cause hypoglycemia (Munchausen syndrome or, in infants, Munchausen syndrome by proxy). Exogenous insulin administration may be distinguished from organic hyperinsulinism by the absence of elevated plasma C-peptide levels when insulin concentrations are high.

Disorders of Glycogenolysis

There are more than 10 different types of GSD,[6, 7] but only two types cause significant hypoglycemia: type III (debrancher deficiency) and type I (glucose-6-phosphatase deficiency). Type III GSD presents in infancy with hypoglycemia 3 to 6 hours after meals, massive hepatomegaly, and growth retardation. With increasing age, hypoglycemia become less of a problem, but cardiomyopathy and muscle weakness may develop. Deficiency of the debrancher enzyme, which is responsible for cleavage of the 1 to 6 branch points in the glycogen polymer, results in the inability to utilize any of the glucose stored interior to the outermost branch points of the multibranched glycogen tree. Hypoglycemia occurs 3 to 6 hours into fasting, because the other normal adaptive processes, gluconeogenesis, and the use of free fatty acids and ketones as an alternate fuels, cannot be switched on rapidly enough.

noma. There is no reliable method, either clinical or radiologic, to distinguish between a focal adenoma and any of the diffuse lesions that may be associated with hyperinsulinism.

The diagnosis of hyperinsulinism is made by demonstrating inappropriately high insulin levels ($>12\mu$U/ml) in the presence of hypoglycemia. Unfortunately, insulin levels fluctuate and this may not be high in the critical blood sample. In these cases, physiologic markers of excess insulin effects must be used for the diagnosis: excessive glucose utilization, suppressed plasma levels of free fatty acids and ketones, and an inappropriate glycemic response to glucagon (a rise of more than 30 mg/dl within 30 minutes) during hypoglycemia. This last feature also has therapeutic use in emergency situations when hypoglycemia is due to excess insulin.

Management consists of initial acute resuscitation and then maintenance of normoglycemia. The goal is to rapidly correct hypoglycemia in order to prevent permanent brain damage. An infusion of 0.5 g/kg of glucose (2 ml/kg of 25% dextrose) should be followed immediately by a constant infusion of sufficient glucose to maintain normoglycemia (65 to 75 mg/dl). Infusion rates of 8 to 20 mg/kg/min may be required. Glucagon (30 µg/kg, not exceeding 1 mg), intravenously (IV) or intramuscularly (IM), will rapidly elevate the blood glucose if IV access cannot immediately be achieved.

The diagnosis of type III GSD is suspected by a combination of the clinical findings outlined earlier, plus very high triglyceride levels and normal lactate levels. Liver transaminases are elevated. The response to IV or IM glucagon in the fed state will be normal (>30 mg/dl rise in plasma glucose) but will be minimal after more than 6 hours of fasting. Definitive diagnosis is made by demonstrating reduced enzyme activity in liver tissue (open biopsy preferred).

Treatment in the acute stage is correction of hypoglycemia by IV glucose, 0.5 g/kg, followed by an infusion of 8 mg/kg/min. Long-term treatment is to use a low-carbohydrate and high-protein diet in order to encourage continued gluconeogenesis and frequent feedings to avoid fasts of longer than 4 hours. Uncooked cornstarch or overnight continuous nasogastric glucose infusion is used to prevent nocturnal hypoglycemia.

Disorders of Gluconeogenesis

Type I GSD (Von Gierke disease) is caused by a deficiency of glucose-6-phosphatase. Although often classified as one of the GSDs, it is more appropriate to consider it as a disorder of gluconeogenesis since the enzyme defect blocks glucose production from lactate and amino acids as well as from glycogen. Type I GSD presents in the first year of life with hypoglycemia, massive hepatomegaly, and failure to thrive. These features are similar to type III GSD, but marked differences in their biochemical features make it possible to easily distinguish between the two disorders.

Glucose-6-phosphatase deficiency results in an inability to convert glucose-6-phosphate to glucose. This prevents the liver from generating glucose both from glycogen by glycogenolysis or from gluconeogenesis, utilizing amino acids, glycerol, fructose, or galactose. Patients with deficiency of glucose-6-phosphatase are characterized by the development of lactic acidosis as blood glucose falls (levels of lactic acid may be as high as 10 to 15 mmol/l). The brain is able to utilize lactate for energy production, and thus the neurologic symptoms of hypoglycemia may be less than expected. Hepatic ketogenesis is also impaired. Triglyceride levels are markedly increased. Liver function tests are usually normal; however, there may be mild elevation of transaminases. Hyperuricemia occurs secondary to accelerated degradation of adenosine, which occurs due to elevations of hepatic sugar-phosphate levels. In untreated patients, morbidity is primarily due to persistent acidosis. In treated patients, whose lactate levels are low, symptomatic hypoglycemia can occur with great rapidity and severity if glucose supplementation is suddenly interrupted.

The diagnosis is suspected based on the clinical findings of hepatomegaly and on failure to thrive, associated with hypoglycemia, lactic acidosis, hypertriglyceridemia, and hyperuricemia. The response to IV glucagon in both fed and fasting states produces no increase in blood glucose but does produce a marked increase in lactic acid.

Treatment in the acute stage is aimed at correcting the hypoglycemia by glucose IV, 0.5 g/kg, followed by an infusion of 10 mg/kg/min until the patient is fit for oral feeding. This will also correct the lactic acidosis, but if the pH is less than 7.1 and there is inadequate respiratory compensation, bicarbonate may be required. Long-term management combines frequent feeds, every 3 to 4 hours, overnight nasogastric tube feeding,[8] and the use of uncooked cornstarch as a "slow-release" glucose.[9] This maintains normoglycemia and ameliorates the lactic acidosis, hyperlipidemia, and hyperuricemia. Fructose (sucrose) and galactose (lactose) should be eliminated from the diet. It is important to remember that once treatment is begun, patients have a high risk of severe hypoglycemia if the overnight glucose infusion is abruptly discontinued or if meals are delayed.

Fructose-1,6-diphosphatase deficiency is the only other disorder of gluconeogenesis that causes hypoglycemia. Approximately 50% of patients present in the first week of life, and most of the remainder present within the first year. In the neonatal period, patients present with tachypnea, lethargy, hypotonia, and rapid progression to coma. The older infant or child may first present during an intercurrent illness with similar clinical signs. Physical examination reveals moderate hepatomegaly.

Deficiency of fructose-1,6-diphosphatase (see Fig. 60-2) results in impairment of gluconeogenesis utilizing amino acids, glycerol, pyruvate, and fructose as precursors, but not galactose. Because glycogenolysis is unaffected, glucose levels are maintained for 3 to 8 hours after a meal until glycogen stores have been depleted. As in type I GSD, lactate levels rise and acidosis develops as the glucose levels fall. Triglyceride levels are elevated and hyperuricemia and hypophosphatemia may occur, especially if large amounts of fructose are ingested.

The diagnosis is suspected in an infant with hepatomegaly, hypoglycemia, lactic acidosis, and raised urate levels. In contrast to patients with glucose-6-phosphatase deficiency, these patients have a normal glycemic response to glucagon in the fed state. The diagnosis is confirmed by demonstrating deficient enzyme activity in liver tissue or leukocytes.

Treatment of the acute phase of the illness involves correction of the hypoglycemia and lactic acidosis. IV infusion of 0.5 g/kg glucose as an initial dose, followed by continuous infusion of glucose (8 mg/kg/min), should be sufficient to correct hypoglycemia and maintain glucose above 65 to 75 mg/dl. Long-term treatment aims at avoiding fasts greater than 6 to 8 hours and the possible use of cornstarch or overnight dextrose infusions by nasogastric tube to prevent nocturnal hypoglycemia. The diet should be sucrose free, and IV infusions containing fructose should not be used.

Ketotic Hypoglycemia

Ketotic hypoglycemia is the most common cause of hypoglycemia in childhood.[2] This disorder presents in infants from 6 months of age up to 4 or 5 years of age. Affected children are usually less than the 25th percentile in weight. Ketotic hypoglycemia is characterized by hypoglycemia after 12 to 24 hours fasting, often triggered by a mild illness such as an upper respiratory tract infection or gastroenteritis. The normal mechanisms of fasting adaptation (i.e., glycogenolysis, gluconeogenesis, and the use of fatty acids as an alternate fuel for energy production) are intact. Hormonal regulation of fasting adaptation is also normal. Thus, children with ketotic hypoglycemia may be considered to have no specific defect, but instead to simply have accelerated fasting.

The diagnosis is made by demonstrating appropriately elevated levels of ketones in the urine and in the plasma at the time of hypoglycemia following a prolonged fast and by demonstrating normal hormonal responses of insulin, cortisol, and growth hormone (e.g., in the critical blood sample).

Treatment consists of preventing prolonged fasting (>12 hours), particularly during intercurrent illness. This condition usually resolves by 6 or 7 years of age. With treatment, symptomatic hypoglycemia should not recur; if it does, the diagnosis should be re-evaluated.

Failure of Hormonal Counter Regulation

Hypopituitarism, congenital or acquired, may cause hypoglycemia. Congenital hypopituitarism infrequently presents in the neonatal period with hypoglycemia. Clinical clues will be midline defects such as cleft lip or palate, absent septum pellucidum or corpus callosum, optic nerve hypoplasia (septo-optic dysplasia), encephalocele, hypertelorism, and, especially, micropenis. The hypoglycemia occurs because of impaired gluconeogenesis and lipolysis resulting from cortisol and growth hormone deficiency. The hypoglycemia is usually ketotic but may be hypoketotic similar to hyperinsulinism. Therefore insulin, cortisol, and growth hormone levels should be measured in the critical blood sample, and a glucagon stimulation test should be done. Further pituitary function tests are required if cortisol and growth hormone are not appropriately elevated in the critical blood sample.

Isolated growth hormone deficiency may present in first year of life with hypoglycemia alone, since growth rate is not significantly impaired by growth hormone deficiency in the first year of life Adrenal insufficiency may cause hypoglycemia during a concurrent illness or if hydrocortisone replacement medications have been omitted. With isolated deficiency of glucocorticoid, but not of mineralocorticoid, patients may have hypoglycemia and hyponatremia without hyperkalemia.

Sugar Toxicity Disorders

Hereditary fructose intolerance is a very rare inherited disorder manifested by vomiting, hypoglycemia, and the rapid development of renal tubular and hepatocellular damage that result from ingestion of fructose.[10] Fructose-1-phosphate aldolase enzyme activity is deficient, and patients are unable to convert fructose to glucose. The build-up of fructose-1-phosphate inhibits both glycogen-olysis and gluconeogenesis, resulting in hypoglycemia and a rapid depletion of adenosine triphosphate (ATP). The depletion of ATP is primarily responsible for the development of renal and hepatic dysfunction. The treatment is elimination of fructose from the diet and supportive care of renal and hepatic dysfunction.

Galactosemia usually presents in the neonatal period with jaundice, poor feeding, vomiting, diarrhea, and growth failure. These infants have a marked propensity for *E. coli* sepsis, which is often fatal. There is progressive liver disease, laboratory evidence of the renal Fanconi syndrome, and slit lamp examination usually reveals cataracts. The disorder is due to a deficiency of galactose-1-phosphate uridyl transferase. This enzymatic block ultimately impedes conversion of galactose to glucose. The diagnosis is suspected by finding galactose in urine and is confirmed by demonstrating deficient enzyme activity in red blood cells. The mainstay of treatment is dietary restriction of galactose.

DISORDERS OF FATTY ACID OXIDATION

Currently, 11 different defects in the pathway of mitochondrial fatty acid oxidation are known.[12-21] Most of these have only been recognized within the last decade.[22] One reason for the tardiness in identifying these disorders is that, with the exception of inappropriately low urinary ketones, routine laboratory tests do not provide many clues about the presence of a defect in fat metabolism. A second reason is that these patients may appear to be in good health until they suffer an attack of illness and, therefore, are easily misdiagnosed as having Reye syndrome, sudden infant death syndrome, and so forth.

As shown in Table 60–1, most of these defects present with acute episodes of hypoketotic hypoglycemia that are triggered by fasts of 12 hours or more. This reflects the fact that fatty acid oxidation becomes the dominant fuel for energy production only in the later stages of fasting adaptation.[23] In some of the disorders, cardiomyopathy and skeletal muscle weakness may occur. This relates to the important contribution that fatty acid oxidation makes to energy production in the heart and aerobically working muscle.

Fatty acids, derived from the diet or synthesized from surplus carbohydrate and protein, are stored as triglyceride in adipose tissue. The decline in insulin levels during fasting releases inhibition of lipolysis and triglycerides are broken down leading to increased plasma concentration of free (nonesterified) fatty acids. As shown in Figure 60–3, these free fatty acids are taken up by tissues, activated to their coenzyme-A esters, and then transported into mitochondria by a carnitine-dependent shuttle. Within the mitochondria, the fatty acids are degraded by repetitive cycles of the four-step β-oxidation sequence to acetyl-CoA with production of ATP via the electron transport chain. In most tissues, such as muscle, the acetyl-CoA is then further oxidized to CO_2 in the tricarboxylic acid cycle. However, in the liver, most of the acetyl-CoA is converted to the ketone

Table 60–1. CLINICAL FEATURES OF GENETIC DISORDERS OF MITOCHONDRIAL FATTY ACID OXIDATION

Episodes of hypoketotic hypoglycemia (most have secondary carnitine deficiency and dicarboxylic aciduria)

1. Carnitine palmityl transferase 1 (liver) (CPT-1)[12]	Elevated carnitine levels; minimal dicarboxylic aciduria
2. Carnitine palmityl transferase 2 (severe) (CPT-2)[13]	Rare; minimal dicarboxylic aciduria; cardiomyopathy and weakness
3. Medium-chain acyl-CoA dehydrogenase (MCAD)[14]	The most common defect; specific metabolites in urine and plasma
4. Long-chain acyl-CoA dehydrogenase (LCAD)[16]	Cardiomyopathy and weakness
5. Short-chain acyl-CoA dehydrogenase (SCAD)[16]	Very rare
6. Short-chain 3-hydroxyacyl-CoA dehydrogenase (SCHAD)[17]	Cardiomyopathy and weakness; urinary 3-hydroxydicarboxylic acids
7. Long-chain 3-hydroxyacyl-CoA dehydrogenase (LCHAD)[17]	Cardiomyopathy and weakness; urinary 3-hydroxydicarboxylic acids
8. Electron transfer flavoprotein (ETF)[18] or electron transfer flavoprotein dehydrogenase (ETF-DM)[18]	Specific metabolites in urine
9. 3-Hydroxy 3-methylglutaryl-CoA lyase (HMG-CoA lyase)[19]	Specific metabolites in urine

Chronic cardiomyopathy and muscle weakness (may also be seen in 2, 4, 5, 6, 7, 8 above)

1. Carnitine transport defect (CTD)[20]	Primary carnitine deficiency; occasional hypoglycemic coma

Episodes of rhabdomyolsis (may occur in 4, 5, 6, 7, 8 above)

1. Carnitine palmityl transferase 2 (mild) (CPT-2)[12, 21]	Rarely presents before 10 years of age; triggered by exercise or fasting; may cause acute renal failure.

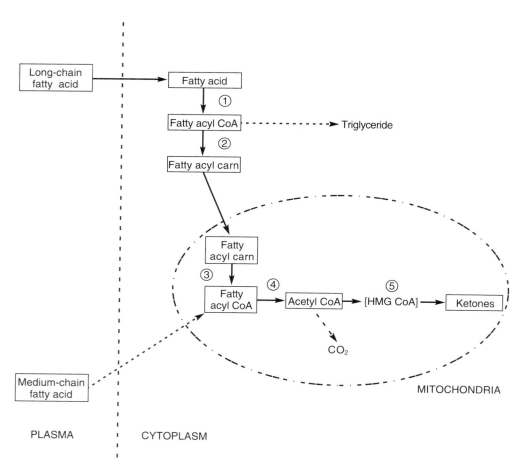

Figure 60–3. Pathway of mitochondrial fatty acid oxidation and hepatic ketogenesis. Major sequences include: (1) activation, (2) transfer to carnitine, (3) transfer back to coenzyme-A, (4) β-oxidation, and (5) ketone synthesis.

bodies, β-hydroxybutyrate (BOB) and acetoacetate (AcAc), via the 3-hydroxy-3-methylglutaryl-CoA pathway, and these are released into the circulation for oxidation by other organs, such as the brain. Since the blood-brain barrier prevents entry of fatty acids into the brain, hepatic ketogenesis serves to provide a fat-derived fuel for the brain and limits the need for converting essential body protein to glucose during prolonged starvation.[23]

The prototype of the genetic defects in fatty acid oxidation that present with episodes of fasting hypoglycemic coma is medium-chain acyl-CoA dehydrogenase (MCAD) deficiency.[14] This is both the most common and the mildest of these disorders. More than 100 cases of MCAD deficiency have been diagnosed since the defect was first described in 1983. The incidence of the disorder may be as high as 1 in every 10,000 live births. The usual age of first episode of illness in MCAD deficiency is between 1 and 2 years with a range from 3 months to more than 5 years.[24] Neonatal presentation is rare, since neonates are rarely exposed to fasts of more than 4 hours. Episodes of illness are precipitated by fasting for more than 10 to 12 hours, for example, if breakfast is missed or in association with an intercurrent infection. Commonly, there is lethargy and vomiting rapidly progressing to coma, seizures, and collapse. Up to 25% of patients have died during their first attack of illness. In some of the other more severe defects, cardiomyopathy and skeletal muscle weakness often complicate the illness.[22]

At the time of illness, hypoglycemia is usually found.[22] Because of the impaired oxidation of fatty acids by the liver, ketones remain inappropriately low, but the urine may show "trace," "small," or even "moderate" ketones. The liver may become moderately enlarged. Liver biopsy reveals fatty infiltration. Routine laboratory tests often show findings consistent with Reye syndrome: little or no acidosis, moderate elevations of transaminases, urea, uric acid, hyperammonemia, and prolonged prothrombin time (PT) and partial prothrombin time (PTT).

Blood and urine specimens obtained at the time of presentation before treatment is begun (the critical blood and urine samples, see Fig. 60–1) are particularly helpful in the diagnoses of the fatty acid oxidation defects, because abnormalities may not be present when patients are well. At times of hypoglycemia, plasma free fatty acid concentrations are quite high (>2mmol/l) and plasma ketones are inappropriately low (<1mmol/l). Urine ketones, by dipstick, will be lower than expected (less than "moderate" or "large"). The urinary organic acid profile will show low ketones and, in most of the disorders, marked increases in medium-chain dicarboxylic acids that are produced from microsomal oxidation of fatty acids. In a few defects, a specific diagnosis can be made by analyzing metabolites in urine or plasma: urinary 3-hydroxy-3-methylglutarate in 3-hydroxy 3-methylglutaryl-CoA lyase deficiency[19]; urinary glutarate, ethylmalonate, and isovalerylglycine in the severe forms of glutaric aciduria type II[20]; octanoylcarnitine, hexanoylglycine, and phenylpropionylglycine in urine and octanote and cis-4-decenoate in plasma in MCAD defi-

ciency.[24-26] In the carnitine transport defect, plasma and muscle carnitine levels are reduced to 1 to 3% of normal. In most of the other defects, plasma and tissue carnitine are moderately reduced to 25 to 50% of normal (secondary carnitine deficiency).[12]

Treatment of acute illnesses in these disorders is largely supportive.[12] Sufficient IV glucose must be given to elevate glucose and insulin levels and thus suppress lipolysis and any effort to oxidize fat (i.e., at least 10% dextrose at maintenance rates). In some of the disorders, hypertrophic or dilated cardiomyopathy may be found by echocardiography and may require supportive care. In rare instances, muscle weakness may be so profound that respiratory assistance is required. In the carnitine transport defect, carnitine replacement therapy (100 mg/kg/day, orally) is effective in reversing the cardiomyopathy within a few weeks to months.[20] In the defects associated with secondary carnitine deficiency, carnitine therapy can be considered, but its value has not yet been clearly demonstrated.[12]

Long-term treatment of these disorders consists primarily of limiting fasting stress. In MCAD deficiency, this means simply ensuring that the overnight fast never exceeds 10 to 12 hours. In more severely ill patients, continuous intragastric feedings using a high-carbohydrate, low-fat formula have been helpful.[12] In the carnitine transport defect, maintenance treatment with oral carnitine is required.[20]

DISORDERS OF INTERMEDIARY METABOLISM OF LACTATE

Lactic acid is the product of anaerobic oxidation of glucose. It is generated by anaerobically exercising muscle, red blood cells and, in times of severe hypoxia, by all tissues of the body. Lactate accumulates in the blood when there is a defect in the oxidation of pyruvate, its immediate precursor, when the cytosolic redox potential is elevated, or when the hepatic capacity for clearing lactate has been overwhelmed.[27] Secondary lactic acidosis is very common and is usually due to poor tissue oxygenation that occurs with shock or hypoxia. This section reviews the specific biochemical genetic disorders that are associated with primary lactic acidosis (PLA): pyruvate dehydrogenase complex (PDH) deficiency, pyruvate carboxylase (PC) deficiency, and disorders involving mitochondrial oxidative phosphorylation by the electron transfer chain (ETC) (Fig. 60–4). Other inherited disorders of intermediary metabolism may indirectly result in lactic acidosis either by interference with gluconeogenesis (e.g., glucose-6-phosphatase deficiency) or by mitochondrial energy metabolism (e.g., methylmalonic acidemia). These conditions are dealt with in other sections of this chapter.

The primary lactic acidoses are confusing in that a deficiency of a single enzyme may be associated with different clinical manifestations (e.g., encephalomyopathy, cardiomyopathy, or isolated myopathy[28]). The degree of residual enzyme activity provides one explanation for this variability; however, other factors may also play a role, such as tissue-specific isoenzymes and dif-

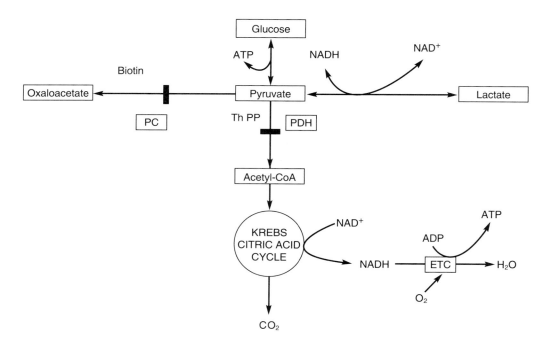

Figure 60–4. Sites of enzyme defects in the congenital lactic acidoses: pyruvate dehydrogenase complex (PDH), pyruvate carboxylase (PC), and electron transport chain (ETC). (ThPP = thiamine pyrophospate.)

ferences in tissue energy requirements. In some patients, congenital craniofacial and brain malformations are associated with the primary lactic acidosis.

One of the earliest descriptions of the pathologic changes that can occur in the brain in a primary lactic acidosis disorder was by Leigh.[29] His description, in 1951, of what is now known as subacute necrotizing encephalomyelopathy (SNE), was of a 7-month-old infant who presented with feeding difficulties, hypotonia, and lethargy. The child went on to develop blindness, deafness, rapidly progressive hypotonicity, abnormal respiratory patterns, drooling with an inability to swallow, and finally died 6 weeks later. Leigh described lesions in the brain that were bilateral and symmetric, involving the thalamus, basal ganglia, mid brain, and upper spinal cord. It is now known that the typical case of "Leigh syndrome" is associated with a more prolonged course beginning after 6 months of age and characterized by psychomotor regression, brain stem dysfunction, and abnormalities of respiratory control. Lactic acidosis may occur sporadically in these patients. Up to one quarter of cases of Leigh syndrome have a deficiency of PDH or mitochondrial respiratory chain enzyme defects, with no other apparent enzyme defect.[30] SNE is the prime example of a PLA associated with encephalopathy. However, there are other examples of PLA in which encephalopathy, cardiomyopthy, and myopathy coexist or in which there is only an isolated myopathy.

PDH Deficiency

PDH deficiency is the most common cause of PLA.[31] The PDH enzyme complex consists of three major subunits (E_1, E_2, E_3) and two regulatory subunits (phos-

phorylase and kinase) that regulate the E_1 subunit. The most severe form of deficiency of this complex presents in the newborn period with rapidly progressing lethargy, hypotonia, respiratory distress (secondary either to acidosis or to abnormal central respiratory control), seizures, and coma. Many of these infants are severely retarded and die by 6 months of age. They may have congenital malformations of the craniofacial structures. A less severe form of PDH deficiency is chacterized by the development of hypotonia, seizures, microcephaly, and mental retardation. It may present from 6 months of age onwards; 50% of these infants die before 3 years of age. These patients may demonstrate an illness compatible with ongoing neurodegenerative changes that suggest Leigh disease. Although some patients with PDH deficiency do manifest the characteristic neuropathology of SNE, a sizeable fraction and perhaps the majority do not. High carbohydrate loads may precipitate an attack of seizures and coma. Finally, PDH deficiency has been described in a group of male children with recurrent ataxia and mildly elevated lactate levels associated with the ingestion of large carbohydrate loads. These boys develop progressive neurologic degeneration. Magnetic resonace imaging (MRI) often shows agenesis of the corpus callosum or cystic lesions in the thalamus, basal ganglia, or brain stem in all of the aforementioned groups. "Cerebral lactic acidosis" has been described in patients who presented with progressive neurologic dysfunction and structural abnormalities of the brain.[32] The majority had normal or very slightly elevated serum lactate and pyruvate levels in the stable condition (as opposed to during acute deterioration) but had high CSF lactate (>3 mmol/l). Most of these patients had PDH deficiency. Thus, measurement of CSF lactate may be useful in patients with unexplained neurologic deterioration suggestive of a lactic acid disorder but who have normal blood lactate.

Disorders of the Mitochondrial Electron Transport Chain

These disorders constitute the second most common cause of primary lactic acidosis. They may actually be the most common cause, but delineation of these defects is difficult so that, in many patients, the site of defect remains unknown. These disorders are quite heterogeneous, but in general they have much more severe myopathy than do PDH and PC deficiencies. They may also have a severe cardiomyopathy that can present in the neonatal period or may not develop until much later in childhood or adulthood. The neonatal presentation is associated with severe lactic acidosis, malformations similar to those of PDH or PC deficiencies, cardiomyopathy, and renal Fanconi syndrome. The infantile form is a classic Leigh presentation with progressive neurologic deteroration over the first 1 to 3 years of life with death around 3 to 4 years of age. In some phenotypes, onset occurs in late childhood or early adulthood and is characterized by both myopathy and progressive encephalopathy. Distinctive patterns of illness include chronic progressive external ophthalmoplegia (CPEO), Kearns-Sayre syndrome (KSS), myoclonic epilepsy, ragged red fibers (MERRF), and myopathy, encephalopathy, lactic acidosis, and stroke-like episodes (MELAS).

Pyruvate Carboxylase (PC) Deficiency

This deficiency also presents with a spectrum of clinical phenotypes from acute neonatal onset to a chronic infantile relapsing course. These patients may present with severe lactic acidosis and hypotonia in the first week of life (type B PC deficiency). Some patients have brain and facial malformations. Patients with PC deficiency of this severity rarely live longer than 3 months. A milder form exists (type A) in which patients present after 3 to 6 months of age with mild or moderate lactic acidosis, developmental delay, and mild hypotonia. They also have intermittent episodes of severe lactic acidemia. Many die in the first year of life, and survivors have progressive neurologic deteroration. Although PC is involved in gluconeogenesis, it rarely causes hypoglycemia. Type B PC deficiency results in an inability to generate oxaloacetic acid (OAA) (see Fig. 60–4). Due to the shortage of OAA, aspartate levels fall. This causes (1) an interference with urea cycle function resulting in hyperammonemia and hypercitrullinemia and (2) opposing changes in the redox potential of the cytosol and the mitochondria resulting in an elevated lactate:pyruvate ratio (>35:1) and a decreased BOB:AcAc ratio (<2:1). This occurs because of failure of the aspartate shuttle that normally functions to transfer reducing equivalents between cytosol and mitochondria. In the milder type A deficiency, there are only minimal problems with ureagenesis and minor abnormalities of mitochondrial redox potential.

Differential Diagnosis

The critical blood and urine samples at the time of acute illness are very helpful in distinguishing primary from secondary lactic acidosis and may provide a clue about the site of defect. Blood saved at the time of initial presentation can be sent for testing of BOB, AcAc, and amino acids (see Fig. 60–1). Urine should be sent for organic acid quantitation. A fresh blood sample should be drawn for lactate and pyruvate and immediately deproteinized by adding 2 ml of 8% perchloric acid to block red blood cell glycolysis. If blood lactate is elevated or if clinical signs are very suggestive of a PLA, CSF lactate determination is indicated. It is important to remember that patients with substantial deficits in CNS energy metabolism due to a PLA may be obtunded even in the absence of a systemic disturbance in acid-base balance.

Abnormalities of urinary organic acids may identify cases of lactic acidosis secondary to defects in either fatty acid oxidation, biotinidase deficiency, or holocarboxylase synthetase deficiency. Methylmalonic aciduria and propionic acidemia cause lactic acidosis, as well as ketoacidosis, probably by altering CoA metabolism, secondarily interfering with mitochondrial enzymes or inhibiting the malate/aspartate shuttle. Hypoglycemia suggests either fatty acid oxidation defects or defects in gluconeogenesis.

The presence of a normal lactate:pyruvate ratio (<25:1) and normal blood glucose suggests type A PC deficiency or PDH deficiency. Type B PC deficiency presents with increased lactate:pyruvate ratio (>35:1), raised ammonium and citrulline, and decreased BOB:AcAc ratio (N<2:1). An increase in both the BOB:AcAc ratio (>2:1) and the lactate:pyruvate ratio (>35:1) suggests an electron transport chain disorder.

Treatment

The mainstay of treatment is to correct the metabolic acidosis and to remove lactic acid, because a pH<7.1 will impair cardiac output and further worsen the lactic acidosis.[33] Intravenous bicarbonate may be used initially. However, due to ongoing production of lactic acid, large amounts will be required that may cause hypernatremia, hyperosmolarity, and fluid overload. In addition, infusion of bicarbonate may cause paradoxic CSF acidosis and deepening of coma. An alternative therapy is bicarbonate-buffered peritoneal dialysis. This provides an unlimited supply of physiologic buffer without the problems of hypervolemia or hypernatremia[34] and directly removes lactic acid. Continuous arterial venous hemofiltration with dialysis (CAVHD) can remove lactate more rapidly and improve pH faster than peritoneal dialysis. However, experience with this therapy is limited. If the blood glucose is stable, IV fluids or dialysate should be low in glucose, because large carbohydrate loads may worsen lactic acidosis.

For PDH deficiency, thiamine (10 to 1,000 mg/day) may improve conversion of pyruvate to acetyl CoA. Dichloroacetate, which acts by stimulating a specific subunit of the PDH enzyme complex and increasing conversion of pyruvate to acetyl CoA,[35] is being evaluated in trials at doses of 50 mg/kg/day divided BID. Avoidance of high carbohydrate loads may prevent acute episodes of lactic acidosis. Aspartate supplementation has been suggested in PC deficiency in order to replenish levels in the brain for neuroregulation, to replenish OAA levels for the citric acid cycle, and to maintain the function of the malate-aspartate shuttle and urea cycle and thus reduce hyperammonemia.[36] Even with early treatment the prognosis for all of these disorders is poor with high risk of neurologic damage.

UREA CYCLE ENZYME DISORDERS

The urea cycle has two main functions. First, it is responsible for formation of urea, the water-soluble vehicle for waste nitrogen removal that is readily excreted by the kidneys. Second, it generates arginine. Defects in the urea cycle result in an accumulation of ammonium that is toxic to the brain. With the exception of argininase deficiency, the defects also result in deficient synthesis of arginine, which then becomes an essential amino acid.

The urea cycle and its enzymes are shown in Figure 60–5. The two nitrogen atoms in urea come from ammonium and aspartate. There are five enzyme defects: carbamyl phosphate synthase (CPS) deficiency, ornithine transcarbamylase (OTC) deficiency, argininosuccinic acid synthetase (AS) deficiency, argininosuccinate lyase (AL) deficiency, and arginase (A) deficiency. The first four of these enzyme deficiencies produce similar clinical features: either severe hyperammonemic coma of neonatal onset or a later onset form with episodic attacks of coma.[37] Arginase deficiency usually presents

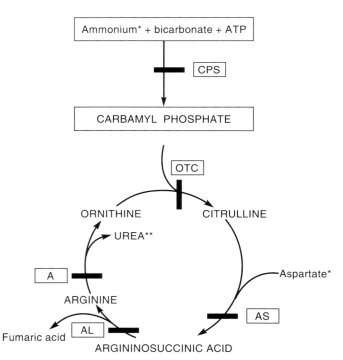

Figure 60–5. Sites of the urea cycle enzyme defects: carbamylphosphate synthetase (CPS), ornithine transcarbamylase (OTC), argininosuccinic acid synthetase (AS), argininosuccinic acid lyase (AL), and arginase (A). The asterisk denotes a waste nitrogen atom.

as a progressive neurodegenerative disorder. All of these disorders are inherited in an autosomal recessive fashion, except for OTC deficiency which is X-linked recessive. Hyperammonemia can also occur secondary to a variety of disorders that include severe liver disease and urinary tract obstruction complicated by infection with urea splitting organisms, as well as in the premature newborn with idiopathic respiratory distress syndrome (transient hyperammonemia of the newborn). Other inborn errors of intermediary metabolism may also cause hyperammonemia due to secondary inhibition of urea cycle enzyme function (e.g., the organic acidurias, PC deficiency, MCAD deficiency, and HMG CoA lyase deficiency).

Neonatal Onset Hyperammonemia

Newborn infants with severe urea cycle enzyme defects are usually well for the first 24 to 48 hours of life. They then develop poor feeding progressing to vomiting, hypothermia, tachypnea, lethargy, seizures, and coma. The accumulation of ammonium and glutamine are thought to be primarily responsible for the coma and other signs of CNS toxicity. Without specific therapy, these infants almost always die. The clinical presentation may resemble sepsis or intracranial hemorrhage. Many of these critically ill neonates develop the latter as a complication of their illness. Cerebral edema may be detected by a bulging fontanelle and is the usual cause of death. Laboratory studies reveal respiratory alkalosis, low blood urea, and very high plasma ammonium levels.

Diagnosis

Neonatal onset hyperammonemia is caused by deficiency of one of the following enzymes: OTC, CPS, AS, or AL. The common biochemical features of these enzyme deficiencies are elevations of ammonium and low levels of arginine. Differentiation among the four defects is based on measurement of plasma amino acids and urinary orotic acid. A plasma citrulline less than 5 μmol/l suggests either CPS or OTC deficiencies. In OTC deficiency urinary orotic acid is high, whereas it is low in CPS deficiency. A plasma citrulline of 1000 μmol/l or greater strongly suggests AS deficiency. Middle ranges of citrulline (100 to 300 μmol/l) and the presence of high levels of argininosuccinic acid suggest AL deficiency. The diagnosis of defects of the urea cycle can be confirmed by measuring enzyme activity in hepatic tissue or cultured fibroblasts.

The presence or absence of acidosis is important in distinguishing urea cycle enzyme defects from other causes of hyperammonemia in the newborn. Alkalosis is usually found in the urea cycle enzyme defects (Fig. 60–6). Acidosis suggests propionic acidemia, methylmalonic aciduria, glutaric aciduria type 2, pyruvate carboxylase, or pyruvate dehydrogenase deficiencies. Urinary organic acid quantitation and blood lactate help to identify these disorders.

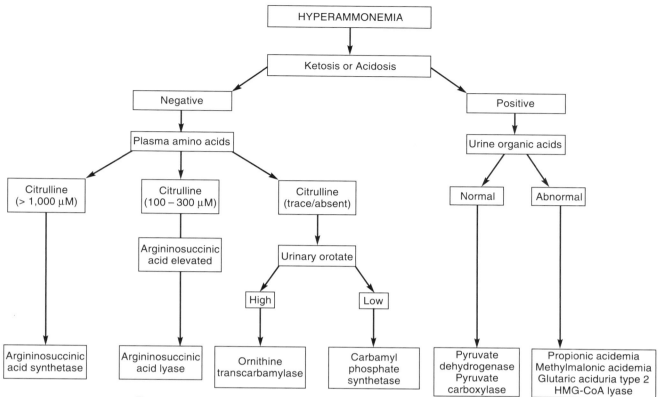

Figure 60–6. Differential diagnosis of enzyme defects causing hyperammonemia.

Treatment

Patients with neonatal hyperammonemic coma need early and aggressive intervention in order to survive. Treatment can be divided into two main areas: (1) nonspecific, supportive treatment of cerebral edema and respiratory failure and (2) specific treatment aimed at removing ammonium, glutamine, and other toxic metabolites and preventing further ammonium accumulation. The duration of hyperammonemic coma correlates with the extent of CNS damage. Therefore, therapy is aimed at rapid removal.[38]

For comatose patients with hyperammonemia, dialysis is the mainstay of treatment. There are three main forms of dialysis: continuous peritoneal dialysis, intermittent hemodialysis, and continuous hemofiltration with dialysis that may either be arteriovenous (CAVHD) or venovenous with pump assistance (CVVHD). Peritoneal dialysis has the advantage of not requiring vascular access. It removes not only ammonium but also glutamine, glutamate, and alanine (all of which contain waste nitrogen). If acidosis is present, a bicarbonate-buffered dialysate may be used. However, the clearance of ammonium is very slow with peritoneal dialysis (5 to 8 ml/min/m²).[39] Hemodialysis, on the other hand, provides a tenfold higher clearance of ammonium,[40] but vascular access is required. A major disadvantage is that the process is intermittent and catabolic; thus, rebound hyperammonemia usually occurs. Experience with the use of CAVHD or CVVHD is limited. However, advantages of these methods are that they are continuous, give faster clearance of ammonium and glutamine than peritoneal dialysis, are not catabolic so rebound hyperammonemia is less likely to occur, and have less risk of vascular instability than hemodialysis. Some authors suggest that the initial fall in ammonium is not as rapid as with hemodialysis. The efficacy of exchange transfusions is poor.[41] Thus, for the treatment of a critically ill infant with hyperammonemic coma, the patient must be transferred to a center where either intermittent hemodialysis, CAVHD, or CVVHD are available.

Attention must also be directed at eliminating catabolism and initiating anabolism. This is done by providing a high carbohydrate input (IV glucose of 8 to 12 mg/kg/min). Some authors recommend the use of insulin to maximize anabolic effects. Protein should be withheld until plasma ammonium and amino acids levels have normalized, but at that point becomes essential in order to prevent further catabolism.

Alternate pathway therapy must also be used to lower ammonium and to sustain the effect of dialysis. Sodium benzoate (250 mg/kg/24 hr) and sodium phenylacetate (250 mg/kg/24 hr) should be given by IV infusion. These compounds combine with glycine and glutamine to generate hippurate and phenylacetylglutamine, respectively, which remove nitrogen from the nitrogen pool and are easily excreted (Fig. 60–7).

Arginine levels are often low in affected patients, and these levels may fall lower with dialysis. It is important to replace arginine for two reasons. First, in OTC, CPS, AS, and AL deficiencies, arginine becomes an essential amino acid. Second, in both AS and AL deficiencies, infusion of arginine results in the formation of ornithine,

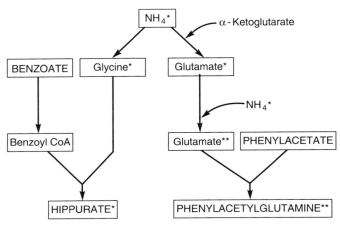

Figure 60–7. Alternate pathway therapy for hyperammonemia with benzoate or phenylacetate. The asterisk denotes a waste nitrogen atom.

which combines with carbamyl phosphate to form citrulline, which in turn is excreted in the urine with a clearance rate equal to 20% of the GFR.[37] In addition, in AL deficiency, citrulline can be converted to argininosuccinate, which is filtered by the kidneys but is not reabsorbed. Therefore, in AS and AL deficiencies, arginine helps to remove waste nitrogen. Patients with OTC or CPS deficiencies should receive arginine HCl, 1 mmol/kg, followed by an infusion of 1 mmol/kg/day; those with AL or AS deficiencies should be given 4 mmol/kg immediate dose followed by an infusion of 4 mmol/kg/day.

The prognosis for the neonatal onset group, even with early and aggressive intervention, is poor with survival rates of 68% in CPS deficiency, 28% in OTC deficiency, and 94% in AS deficiency. Almost all survivors are neurologically impaired.[37] Prospectively treated patients (i.e., when therapy is started before the onset of hyperammonemic coma) may undergo normal growth and development but are always prey to acute infection-induced metabolic crisis.

Late Onset Hyperammonemia

CPS, OTC, AS, and AL deficiencies may all also cause late onset of hyperammonemia at older ages ranging from infancy to adulthood. Episodes are triggered by concurrent illness that causes the patient to become catabolic or by ingestion of large protein loads (which patients seem to learn to avoid even if undiagnosed). Late onset hyperammonemic coma is especially common in female carriers of OTC deficiency. Depending on the lyonization of X chromosomes, there may be variable severity of this X-linked disorder in girls (boys tend to present with the severe neonatal form).

Clinical features are similar to the newborn with the onset of lethargy, confusion, and somnolence progressing to coma. Patients may also be irritable and develop ataxia. Often there will be unexplained developmental delay or seizures. Laboratory tests will demonstrate

respiratory alkalosis and hyperammonemia. The differential diagnosis is similar to neonatal hyperammonemia, but disorders of fatty acid metabolism are more common than the organic acidurias at this age.

Treatment of the acute hyperammonemic coma is similar to neonatal onset hyperammonemia. However, if the ammonium is less than 200 to 300 μmol/l and the patient is not comatose, sodium benzoate or sodium phenlyacetate and arginine may be sufficient treatment.[42]

Arginase Deficiency

Although arginase is one of the enzymes of the urea cycle, it presents in a manner completely different from the other defects outlined earlier. Arginase deficiency is a progressive neurologic disorder manifested by progressive spastic diplegia, seizures, and developmental delay. Coma is rare in these children. Hyperammonemia is present, but plasma levels are usually less than 200 μmol/l. In contrast to the other urea cycle enzyme defects, arginine levels are elevated. Urinary orotate is elevated. Acute intervention is not often required, and long-term management is based on protein restriction to reduce arginine intake.

ORGANIC ACIDURIAS

Inherited defects in oxidation of the branched-chain amino acids (BCAA), leucine, isoleucine and valine, are responsible for most of the disorders of organic acid metabolism.[43–48] Because of the enzymatic block, branched-chain organic acid metabolites accumulate in tissues, blood, cerebrospinal fluid and urine. The branched-chain organic acid pathways are outlined in Figure 60–8. Various inborn errors of organic acid metabolism are listed in Table 60–2 along with their characteristic clinical features, diagnostic urinary metabolites, and specific therapies. Most of the deficient enzymes are noted in Figure 60–8. All are inherited as autosomal recessive genetic diseases.

Patients with organicacidopathies often present with acute life-threatening problems including coma, seizures, and strokes. These episodes of acute metabolic decompensation are usually heralded by nonspecific but characteristic signs such as anorexia, vomiting, lethargy, and hyperventilation due to metabolic acidosis. Laboratory findings, particularly during an acute illness, may include decreased serum bicarbonate with an increased anion gap, increased plasma ammonium, increased ketone bodies in serum and urine, leukopenia and anemia, or thrombocytopenia. In some disorders, plasma and urine glycine levels may also be increased. Multiple secondary abnormalities in intermediary metabolism develop as a consequence of the accumulation of the branched-chain derivatives producing ketosis, lactic acidosis, hyperammonemia, hypoglycemia, and secondary carnitine deficiency. Poor intake and vomiting with dehydration and volume depletion may also be responsible for ketosis and lactic acidosis, respectively. High levels of some organic acids can affect the CNS, resulting

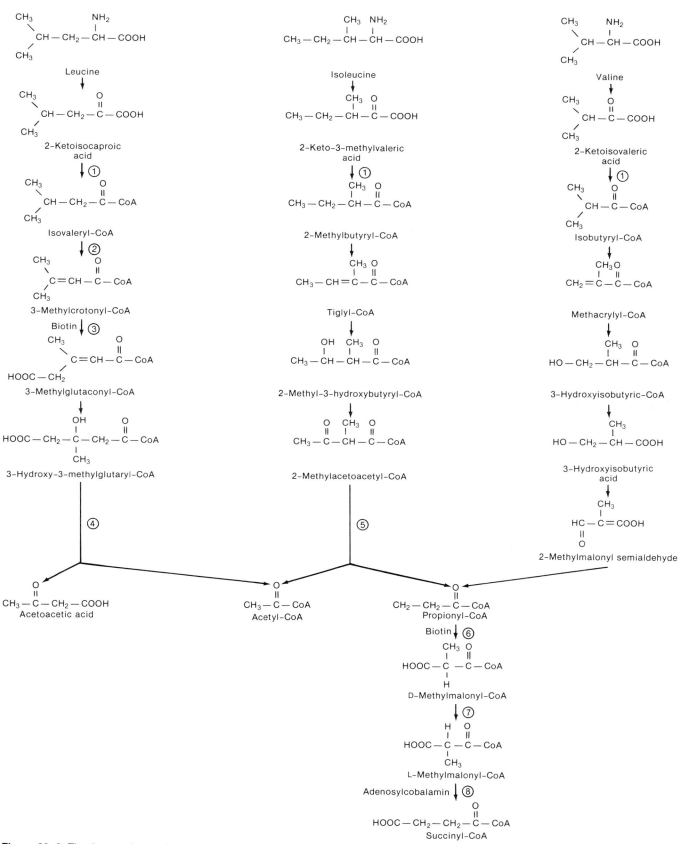

Figure 60–8. The three pathways for branched-chain amino acid catabolism. Enzyme defects identified numerically include: (1) branched-chain 2-keto acid dehydrogenase complex (MSUD), (2) isovaleryl-CoA dehydrogenase (IVA, also affected in GA, type 2), (3) 3-methylcrotonyl-CoA carboxylase (affected in MCD), (4) 3-hydroxy-3-methylglutaryl-CoA lyase, (5) 3-ketothiolase, (6) propionyl-CoA carboxylase (PA, also affected in MCD), (7) D-methylmalonyl-CoA racemase (MMA) and (8) L-methylmalonyl-CoA mutase (MMA).

Table 60–2. ORGANIC ACIDURIAS THAT ARE MOST LIKELY TO PRESENT WITH LIFE-THREATENING ILLNESS

Disease	Enzyme Defect	Diagnostic Urinary Metabolites	Characteristic Feature and Specific Therapy
Methylmalonic acidemia (MMA)[45, 48]	• Vitamin B$_{12}$ nonresponsive types: L-Methylmalonyl-CoA mutase, D-Methylmalonyl-CoA racemase and some defects in cobalamin metabolism • Vitamin B$_{12}$ responsive types: defects in cobalamin conversion to adenosylcobalamin	• Methylmalonate	• Most common organicacidopathy • Some defects respond to pharmacologic doses of cobalamin • Variable phenotypes (see text) • Restrict protein (ile[1], val, thr, met) intake • Empiric therapy with hydroxycobalamin (acute Rx, 1–2 mg/day) • Bowel sterilization, to reduce propionic acid formation • L-Carnitine[2]
Propionic acidemia (PA)[45, 48]	• Propionyl-CoA carboxylase	• 3-Hydroxypropionate, 2-methylglutaconate, propionylglycine, tiglylglycine, methylcitrate	• Phenotype usually severe • Metabolic acidosis and ketonuria may not be present with coma • Diet, bowel sterilization, as in MMA • L-Carnitine[2]
Multiple carboxylase deficiency (MCD)[45, 48, 53]	• Biotinidase or holocarboxylase synthetase deficiency (both cause deficiencies of propionyl-CoA carboxylase, 3-methylcrontonyl-CoA carboxylase, pyruvate carboxylase, and acetyl-CoA carboxylase)	• Lactate, 3-hydroxypropionate, 2-methylglutaconate, propionylglycine, tiglylglycine, methylcitrate, 3-hydroxyisovalerate, 3-methylcrotonylglycine	• Biotinidase deficiency more common, usually mild-moderate disease with developmental delay, hypotonia, alopecia, and rash • "Cerebral lactic acidosis" • Severe neonatal ketolactic acidosis and coma usual in synthetase deficiency • Biotin (10–20 mg/day) "curative" in biotinidase deficiency; usually beneficial in synthetase deficiency
Isovaleric acidemia (IVA)[44, 48, 52]	• Isovaleryl-CoA dehydrogenase	• Isovalerylglycine, 3-hydroxyisovalerate	• Severe neonatal-onset form • Chronic relapsing form • Sweaty feet odor • Restrict protein (leu) intake • Glycine (100–250 mg/kg/day) • L-Carnitine[2]
Glutaric aciduria, type 1[46, 48]	• Glutaryl-CoA dehydrogenase	• Glutarate episodic acidosis	• Presentation includes chronic basal ganglia signs, or stroke-like attacks • Restrict protein (lys, try) intake • Riboflavin (200–300 mg/day)[3] • L-Carnitine[3]
Glutaric aciduria, type 2[47, 48]	• Multiple acyl-CoA dehydrogenase deficiencies (isovaleryl-CoA, dehydrogenase, MCAD, LCAD, etc.) secondary to electron transfer flavoprotein (ETF), or ETF dehydrogenase deficiencies	• Isovalerylglycine, 3-hydroxyisovalerate, glutarate, adipate, suberate, sebacic, hexanolyglycine, suberylglycine, isobutyrylglycine, 2-methyl butyrylglycine, ethylmalonate	• Sweaty-feet odor • Restrict protein (leu, ile, val, lys, try) intake • Riboflavin (200–300 mg/day)[3] • L-Carnitine[2] • See Section B
HMG-CoA lyase deficiency[44, 48]	• 3-Hydroxy-3-methylglutaryl-CoA (HMG-CoA) lyase	• 3-Hydroxy-3-methylglutarate, 3-hydroxyisovalerate, 3-methylglutaconate	• Nonketotic hypoglycemia • No ↑ in plasma or urine ketones during fasting/hypoglycemia • Avoid fasting • See Section B
3-Ketothiolase deficiency[44, 48]	• Mitochondrial 2-methylacetoacetyl-CoA thiolase	• Isoleucine metabolites; 2-methylacetoacetate, 2-methyl-3-hydroxybutyrate, tiglylglycine	• Variable phenotype • May mimic ketotic hypoglycemia • Restrict protein (ile) intake • Avoid fasting
Maple syrup urine disease (MSUD)[43, 48]	• Branched-chain 2-keto acid dehydrogenase	• Branched-chain keto or hydroxyacids • ↑ Plasma leu, ile, val	• Severe neonatal-onset • Chronic and acute intermittent phenotypes • Maple syrup odor • Restrict protein (leu, ile, val) intake • Rarely, thiamine-responsive (5–20 mg/kg/day → 500 mg/day)

1. Amino acid code: ile-isoleucine; val-valine; thr-threonine; met-methionine; leu-leucine; lys-lysine; try-tryptophan.
2. Some workers suggest L-carnitine (50–150 mg/kg/day).
3. May be beneficial in rare cases.

in encephalopathy, and the differentiation of bone marrow hematopoietic precursors, producing diverse hematocytopenias.

Similar to the urea cycle enzyme defects phenotypic expression varies and is mainly dependent on severity of the enzyme deficiency. Major forms include a severe neonatal-onset, potentially fatal disease, a chronic type with failure to thrive, developmental delay or progressive psychomotor retardation with intermittent episodes of ketoacidosis, or a completely intermittent form in which disease expression is confined to acute eposides of metabolic decompensation. Clinical features variably include feeding difficulties, vomiting, poor growth, hypotonia, developmental delay, mental retardation, seizures, ataxia, lethargy, and coma. A specific and unique odor can usually be detected in a few select diseases such as the odor of maple syrup in maple syrup urine disease (MSUD) and the odor of sweaty feet in isovaleric acidemia and glutaric aciduria, type II. Vomiting may be pernicious during infancy and, unfortunately, several infants with these disorders such as isovaleric acidemia and propionic acidemia have undergone surgery for presumed pyloric stenosis. During episodes of acute metabolic decompensation associated with vomiting, dehydration and lethargy, hepatomegaly, as well as hyperammonemia, may develop. These patients not uncommonly are thought to be afflicted with Reye syndrome. With the exception of prominent ketoacidosis, this clinical picture may closely resemble that seen in the defects of fatty acid oxidation, exemplified by the medium-chain acyl-CoA dehydrogenase deficiency. The important point is that currently most patients who present with episodes that resemble Reye syndrome have inborn errors of organic acid or fatty acid metabolism or urea cycle enzyme defects.

The most common inborn error of organic acid metabolism is methylmalonic acidemia. Several enzymatic defects may be responsible including L-methylmalonyl-CoA mutase deficiency, D-methylmalonyl-CoA racemase deficiency, and several disorders of cobalamin metabolism. The combined incidence in newborns is approximately 1 in 10,000 to 1 in 40,000. Regardless of the enzyme defect, there is an accumulation of methylmalonyl-CoA and, secondarily, propionyl-CoA in tissues that in turn result in excess levels of methylmalonate and 3-hydroxypropionate, propionylglycine, propionylcarnitine, and methylcitrate due to excess propionyl-CoA build-up. In addition to the BCAA, isoleucine, and valine, other precursors of methylmalonic acid include methionine, threonine, thymine plus cholesterol, and odd-chain fatty acids via propionyl-CoA. Because of the effect of bowel sterilization on MMA levels, gut flora production of propionic acid from fatty acids may be an important source of MMA in some patients.[49]

Diagnosis

The diagnosis of the inherited defects of organic acid oxidation requires analysis of urinary organic acids. Any patient suspected of having such a disorder must have urine analyzed by gas chromatography-mass spectrometry (GC-MS). Plasma amino acid analysis by column chromatography is also required, particularly, for patients with MSUD. Definitive diagnosis of an enzyme deficiency can usually be performed using the patient's white blood cells or cultured skin fibroblasts.

Therapy

The acute management of patients suspected of an inborn error of organic acid metabolism is supportive care, IV fluids with glucose to eliminate hypoglycemia and suppress amino acid oxidation, and correction of acid-base disturbances. Large doses of water-soluble vitamins such as 1 to 2 mg of hydroxycobalamin, for methylmalonic acidemia, and 10 to 20 mg of biotin, for biotinidase and holocarboxylase synthetase deficiencies, may be administered even in the absence of a specific diagnosis, because these vitamin cofactors are inocuous and several disorders may be exquisitely responsive to megavitamin therapy. Specific therapy of an acute episode of metabolic decompensation requires elucidation of the enzymatic lesion. To prevent the development of acute strokes during acute metabolic decompensation, patients with MMA, and probably also PA, must be monitored very carefully because fluid, acid-base, and electrolyte balance should be restored to normal as quickly as possible.[50, 51] Chronic management involves the use of special diets restricted in certain amino acids; in some of the disorders specific agents may be used to enhance detoxification, such as glycine in isovaleric acidemia.[52] The prognosis for individual patients varies widely depending on the nature of the enzymatic deficiency, the delay in diagnosis, and the response to dietary, vitamin cofactor, or detoxificant therapy. For example, the prognosis is excellent for the biotin-responsive multiple carboxylase deficiencies with early treatment but is very poor for neonatal-onset cobalamin-unresponsive methylmalonic acidemia.[53–55]

References

1. Stanley CA and Baker, L: Hypoglcemia. *In*: Kaye R, Oski FA, and Barness LA (eds): Core Textbook of Pediatrics, 1st ed. Philadelphia, JB Lippincott, 1978, pp. 280–305.
2. Baker L and Stanley CA: Hyperinsulinism in Infancy: A pathophysiologic approach to the diagnosis and treatment. *In*: Chiumello G and Laron Z (eds): Recent Progress in Pediatric Endocrinology. London Academic Press, 1977, pp. 89–100.
3. Aynsley-Green A, Polak JM, Bloom SR, et al: Nesidioblastosis of the pancreas: Definition of the syndrome and management of the severe neonatal hyperinsulinaemic hypoglycaemia. Arch Dis Child 56:496, 1981.
4. Jaffe R, Hashida Y, and Yunis EJ: Pancreatic pathology in hyperinsulinemic hypoglycemia of infancy. Lab Invest 42:356, 1980.
5. Thomas CG, Jr, Cuenca RE, Azizkhan RG, et al: Changing concepts of islet cell dysplasia in neonatal and infantile hyperinsulinism. World J Surg 12:598, 1988.
6. Hers H-G, Van Hoof R, and de Barsy T: Glycogen storage diseases. *In*: Scriver CR, Beaudet AL, Sly WS, and Valle D (eds): The Metabolic Basis of Inherited Disease, 6th ed. New York, McGraw-Hill, 1989, pp. 425–452.
7. Hug G: Glycogen storage diseases. Birth Defects 12:145, 1976.
8. Stanley CA, Mills JL, and Baker L: Intragastric feeding in type I

glycogen storage disease: Factors affecting the control of lactic acidemia. Pediatr Res 15:104, 1981.

9. Chen Y-T, Cornblath M, and Sidbury JB: Cornstarch therapy in type I glycogen storage disease. N Engl J Med 310:171, 1984.

10. Gitzelmann R, Steinmann B, and van den Berghe G: Disorders of fructose metabolism. *In:* Scriver CR, Beaudet AV, Sly WS, and Valle D (eds): The Metabolic Basis of Inherited Disease, 6th ed. New York, McGraw-Hill, 1989, pp. 399–417.

11. Segal S: Disorders of galactose metabolism. *In:* Scriver CR, Beaudet AL, Sly WS, and Valle D (eds): The Metabolic Basis of Inherited Disease, 6th ed. New York, McGraw-Hill, 1989, pp. 453–472.

12. Demaurge F, Bonnefont JP, Mitchell G, et al: Hepatic and muscular presentation of carnitine palmitoyl transferase deficiency: Two distinct entities. Pediatr Res 24:308, 1988.

13. Bonnefont JP, Saudubray JM, Ragier D, et al: The hepatic presentations of carnitine palmitoyl transferase deficiency. Abstract No. 6, Meeting of the Society for Study of Inborn Errors of Metabolism, 1990.

14. Stanley CA, Hale DE, Coates PM, et al: Medium-chain acyl-CoA dehydrogenase deficiency in children with non-ketotic hypoglycemia and low carnitine levels. Pediatr Res 17:877, 1983.

15. Hale DE, Batshaw ML, Coates PM, et al: Long-chain acyl coenzyme A dehydrogenase deficiency: An inherited cause of nonketotic hypoglycemia. Pediatr Res 19:666, 1985.

16. Coates PM, Hale DE, Finochiarro G, et al: Genetic deficiency of short-chain acyl-CoA dehydrogenase in cultured fibroblasts from a patient with muscle carnitine deficiency and severe skeletal muscle weakness. J Clin Invest 81:171, 1988.

17. Hale DE: The L-3-hydroxy acyl-CoA dehydrogenase deficiency. *In:* Tanaka K and Coates PM (eds): Clinical, Biochemical, and Molecular Aspects of Fatty Acid Oxidation. New York, AR Liss, 1989, pp. 503–510.

18. Frerman FE and Goodman SI: Deficiency of electron transfer flavoprotein or electron transfer flavoprotein: Ubiquinone oxidoreductase in glutaric acidemia type II fibroblasts. Proc Nat Acad Sci USA 82:4517, 1985.

19. Robinson BH, Oei J, Sherwood WG, et al: Hydroxymethylglutaryl CoA lyase deficiency: Features resembling Reye syndrome. Neurology (NY) 30:714, 1980.

20. Treem WR, Stanley CA, Finegold DN, et al: Primary carnitine deficiency due to a failure of carnitine transport in kidney, muscle, and fibroblasts. N Engl J Med 319:1331, 1988.

21. DiMauro S and DiMauro PM: Muscle carnitine palmityltransferase deficiency and myoglobinuria. Science 182:929, 1973.

22. Stanley CA: New genetic defects in mitochondrial fatty acid oxidation and carnitine deficiency. Adv Pediatr 34:59, 1987.

23. Cahill GF: Starvation in man. N Engl J Med 282:668, 1970.

24. Roe CR and Coates, PM: Acyl-CoA dehydrogenase deficiencies. *In:* Scriver CR, Beaudet A, Sly WS, and Valle, D: The Metabolic Basis of Inherited Disease, 6th ed. New York, McGraw-Hill, 1989, pp. 889–914.

25. Rinaldo P, O'Shea JJ, Coates PM, et al: Medium-chain acyl-CoA dehydrogenase deficiency: Diagnosis by stable isotope dilution analysis of urinary *n*-hexanoyl glycine and 3-phenyl propionylglycine. N Engl J Med 319: 1308, 1988.

26. Duran M, Bruinvis L, Ketting D, et al: *cis*-4-Decenoic acid in plasma: A characteristic metabolite in medium-chain acyl-CoA dehydrogenase deficiency. Clin Chem 34:548, 1988.

27. Evans OB: Lactic acidosis in childhood, Part I. Pediatr Neurol 1: 325, 1985.

28. DeVivo DC and DiMauro S: Disorders of pyruvate metabolism, the citric acid cycle and the respiratory chain. *In:* Fernandes J, Sauderbray JM, and Tada K (eds): Inherited Metabolic Disease: Diagnosis and Treatment. Springer-Verlag, 1990, pp. 127–157.

29. Leigh D: Subacute necrotizing encephalomyelopathy in an infant. J Neurol Neurosurg Psychiatr 14:216, 1951.

30. DeVivo DC and DiMauro S: Cultured human skin fibroblasts and cerebral oxidative metabolic defects: Normative data and Leigh's syndrome. Ann Neurol 20:423, 1986.

31. Robinson BH: Lactic acidemia. Adv Hum Genet 18:151, 1989.

32. Brown GK, Hann, EA, Kirby DM, et al: "Cerebral" lactic acidosis: Defects in pyruvate metabolism with profound brain damage and minimal systemic acidosis. Eur J Pediatr 147:10, 1988.

33. Evans OB: Lactic acidosis in childhood, Part II. Pediatr-Neurol 2:5, 1986.

34. Vazinri DN, Ness R, Wellikson L, et al: Bicarbonate buffered peritoneal dialysis: An effective adjunct in the treatment of lactic acidosis. Am J Med 67:392, 1979.

35. Stacpoole PW: The pharmacology of dichloracetate. Metabolism 38:1124, 1989.

36. Baal MG, Gabreels FJM, Renier WO, et al: A patient with pyruvate carboxylase deficiency in the liver: Treatment with aspartic acid and thiamine. Develop Med Child Neurol 23:521, 1981.

37. Brusilow SW and Horwich AL: Urea cycle enzymes *In:* Scriver CR, Beaudet AL, Sly WS, and Valle D: (eds): The Metabolic Basis of Inherited Disease, 6th ed. New York, McGraw-Hill, 1989, pp. 629–663.

38. Msall M, Batshaw M, Suss R, et al: Neurologic outcome in children with inborn errors of urea synthesis. N Engl J Med 310:1500, 1984.

39. Wiegand C, Thompson T, Bock GH, et al: The management of life-threatening hyperammonemia: A comparison of several therapeutic modalities. J Pediatr 96:142, 1980.

40. Rutledge SL, Havens PL, Haymond MW, et al: Neonatal hemodialysis: Effective therapy for the encephalopathy of inborn errors of metabolism. J Pediatr 116:125, 1990.

41. Batshaw ML and Brusilow SW: Treatment of hyperammonemic coma caused by inborn errors of urea synthesis. J Pediatr 97:893, 1980.

42. Brusilow SW, Danney M, Waber LJ, et al: Treatment of episodic hyperammonemia in children with inborn errors of urea synthesis. N Engl J Med 310:1630, 1984.

43. Danner DJ and Elsas LJ: Disorders of branched chain amino acid and keto acid metabolism. *In:* Scriver CR, Beaudet AL, Sly WS, and Valle D (eds): The Metabolic Basis of Inherited Disease, 6th ed. New York, McGraw-Hill, 1989, pp. 671–692.

44. Sweetman L: Branched chain organic acidurias. *In:* Scriver CR, Beaudet AL, Sly WS, and Valle D (eds): The Metabolic Basis of Inherited Disease, 6th ed. New York, McGraw-Hill, pp. 791–819.

45. Rosenberg LE and Fenton WA: Disorders of propionate and methylmalonate metabolism. *In:* Scriver CR, Beaudet AL, Sly WS, and Valle D (eds): The Metabolic Basis of Inherited Disease, 6th ed. New York, McGraw-Hill, 1989, pp. 821–844.

46. Goodman SI and Frerman FE: Organic acidemias due to defects in lysine oxidation: 2-ketoadipic acidemia and glutaric acidemia. In: Scriver CR, Beaudet AL, Sly WS, and Valle D (eds): The Metabolic Basis of Inherited Disease, 6th ed. New York, McGraw-Hill, 1989, pp. 845–885.

47. Frerman FE and Goodman SI: Glutaric acidemia type II and defects of the mitochondrial respiratory chain. *In:* Scriver CR, Beaudet AL, Sly WS, and Valle D. (eds): The Metabolic Basis of Inherited Disease, 6th ed. New York, McGraw-Hill, 1989, pp. 915–931.

48. Nyhan WL and Sakati NA: Diagnostic Recognition of Genetic Disease. Philadelphia, Lea & Febiger, 1987.

49. Snyderman SE, Sansarico C, Norton P, and Phansalkar SV: The use of neomycin in the treatment of methylmalonic acidemia. Pediatrics 50:925, 1972.

50. Korf B, Wallman JK, and Levy HL: Bilateral lucency of the globus pallidus complicating methylmalonic acidemia. Ann Neurol 20:364, 1986.

51. Heidenreich R, Natowicz M, Hainline BE, et al: Acute extrapyramidal syndrome in methylmalonic acidemia: "Metabolic stroke" involving the globus pallidus. J Pediatr 113(6): 1022, 1988.

52. Berry GT, Yudkoff M, and Segal S: Isovaleric acidemia: Medical and neurodevelopmental effects of long-term therapy. J Pediatr 113:58, 1988.

53. Wallace SJ: Biotinidase deficiency: Presymptomatic treatment. Arch Dis Child 60:574, 1985.

54. Michalski AJ, Berry GT, and Segal S: Holocarboxylase synthetase deficiency: Nine year follow-up of a patient on chronic biotin therapy and a review of the literature. J Inher Metab Dis 12:312, 1989.

55. Matsui SM, Mahoney MJ, and Rosenberg LE: The natural history of the inherited methylmalonic acidemias. N Engl J Med 308:857, 1983.

Acid-Base Disorders

Peter R. Holbrook, M.D.

Acid-base disorders are very common in the care of pediatric critically ill patients. This chapter reviews the physiology, pathophysiology, and usual causes of acid-base disorders in the pediatric intensive care unit (ICU).

DEFINITIONS

An acid is a proton (H^+) donor. A base is a proton acceptor. *Acidosis* is a process that, if left uncorrected, leads to an accumulation of free hydrogen ion (H^+) in the blood. *Acidemia* is the condition of excess free H^+ in the blood. *Alkalosis* and *alkalemia* are the corresponding terms for a relative reduction of free hydrogen ion in the blood. Thus, acidoses and alkaloses are *processes*, whereas acidemia and alkalemia describe the state of the blood. All acidemias have an underlying acidosis, but not all acidoses result in an acidemia.

The normal expression of H^+ is pH:

$$pH = -\log (H^+)$$

This mathematical shorthand is utilized because of the extreme variability in H^+ concentration throughout the body and because many chemical reactions proceed logarithmically.

Acidoses and alkaloses are grouped into two types—respiratory and metabolic. The "respiratory" term is used to describe the status of carbon dioxide (CO_2). CO_2 is generated by the body as a byproduct of the breakdown of carbon-containing compounds and is then excreted by the body. Thus, an accumulation of CO_2 can result from either an overproduction or an underexcretion of CO_2. CO_2 is hydrated to form carbonic acid, which then enters the equilibrium:

$$CO_2 + H_2O \leftrightarrow H_2CO_3 \leftrightarrow H^+ + HCO_3^-$$

Operationally, respiratory acidosis is determined by measurement of the partial pressure of CO_2 (PCO_2). Thus, only one respiratory acidosis or alkalosis can exist at a time.

"Metabolic" acidosis refers to increased production or underexcretion of hydrogen ion, or from a loss of base. Although simply stated, this is more complex in reality because there are many processes that can lead to either an accumulation of H^+ (i.e., there are several different fixed acids that can be produced) or a loss of

(the several) fixed bases. Multiple metabolic acid-base disturbances can be occurring at the same time.

The other essential element in acid-base balance is the buffering system (Table 61–1). A buffer is a substance that reduces the change in concentration of free H^+ in a solution to which an acid or base has been added. Thus, for example, more hydrogen ion must be added to a buffered solution to result in a given increase in H^+ than would be true if the solution had no buffer. In a typical patient, there are 30 mEq/l of buffer base available to buffer hydrogen ion, 75% of which is bicarbonate (normal serum concentration of 23 mEq/l).*

HOMEOSTASIS

In the adult, there is a normal production and excretion of 24,000 nM/day of CO_2. There is also a turnover of hydrogen of 69 mEq/day. Thus, there is constant ongoing acid-base processing: CO_2 is exhaled, and bicarbonate is generated or excreted by the kidney, as necessary.

Despite the existence of approximately 105 mEq of hydrogen in the body, there is only 0.0021 mEq of free H^+ in body fluids. The remainder is buffered.

PATHOPHYSIOLOGY

If an acidosis occurs, hydrogen ion is buffered; some of the base is lost; and a base deficit appears. The maximum possible base deficit is 30. The base must be regenerated to return to normal. The addition of H^+ to the system generates more CO_2 and the respiratory rate increases. The lungs excrete CO_2 and thus affect pH through the Henderson-Hasselbalch relationship:

$$pH = pK + \log \frac{bicarbonate}{carbonic\ acid}$$

in which pK is the dissociation constant of the carbonic acid equation. Note, however, that although pH is

---

*This is practically but not theoretically correct. There are many additional chemicals in the body that may serve as proton acceptors. However, the dissociation constants of these reactions are such that clinical death will have occurred before they will accept protons.

Table 61–1. OPERATIVE BODY BUFFERS

HCO_3^-
Proteins (include hemoglobin)
NH_3
PO_4^{2-}
SO_4^{2-}

affected, no net loss of H^+ occurs. In other words, the respiratory system affects pH through modifications of the major body buffer system (carbonic acid) but can neither excrete H^+ nor regenerate HCO_3^-.

The kidneys control the hydrogen ion and bicarbonate concentrations by regulating bicarbonate reabsorption and by new bicarbonate generation. In addition, the kidneys synthesize ammonia in response to systemic acidosis.

METABOLIC ACIDOSIS

Metabolic acidosis is common in the pediatric ICU. If bicarbonate loss is the cause (e.g., diarrhea with HCO_3^- loss, or dilutional acidosis in which bicarbonate is diluted from infusion of non-bicarbonate–containing solutions), or if a precursor to hydrochloric acid (e.g., ammonium chloride) is added to the system (rare), the chloride will proportionately increase and the anion gap (major cations minus major anions) will be normal. Conversely, an increase in unmeasured cation will cause an increase in the anion gap. This can be caused by an accumulation of lactic acid, other organic acids, and exogenous acids (ethylene glycol, methanol, paralde-hyde, salicylic acid).

Metabolic acidemia causes decreased myocardial con-tractility, decreased peripheral resistance, and decreased adrenergic-receptor sensitivity and predisposes to myo-cardial irritability.

Much attention has been paid to the treatment of metabolic acidosis. Treatment of the underlying cause is paramount. Alkalinization of the body with bicarbon-ate ions has long been practiced. The intent of such therapy is to reverse the acidemia to allow a return to more normal organ function. This therapy has been criticized for a number of reasons: (1) there is a lack of data showing efficacy; (2) bicarbonate treatment has worsened blood pressure and cardiac output in certain experimental situations[2]; and (3) use of a systemic base reduces H^+ concentration extracellularly by generating CO_2. This CO_2 readily moves intracellularly and thus worsens intracellular acidosis. The sodium and osmotic load have also been of concern.

Despite these reservations, bicarbonate therapy is still used cautiously in the patient with severe metabolic acidosis. An alternative drug is tris-hydroxymethyl-amino-methane (THAM). Infusion of THAM consumes CO_2, does not have the sodium load, and may penetrate intracellularly more readily. It can cause respiratory depression, hyperkalemia, and hypoglycemia.

METABOLIC ALKALOSIS

Metabolic alkalosis in the ICU is most commonly due to iatrogenic fluid depletion resulting in concentration of HCO_3^-, increased tubular reabsorption of HCO_3^- due to chloride depletion, and loss of potassium thus obligating H^+ loss in the urine. It may also be found as the result of a loss of gastric secretions. Compensatory respiratory acidosis, which may delay weaning, is the major clinical effect. The treatment is to correct potas-sium deficiency and restore fluid volume if that is appro-priate. Alternatively, carbonic anhydrase inhibitors (acetazolamide) may be used. For severe cases (myo-cardial depression assumed to be due to severe meta-bolic alkalemia), 0.1 normal hydrochloric acid may be used.

RESPIRATORY ACIDOSIS

Respiratory acidosis is also common in the ICU. The cause is usually acute ventilatory failure. In patients with borderline ventilatory function, the effects of fever (13% increase in CO_2 production per degree centigrade above normal) and carbohydrate load from parenteral nutrition may become significant. The central nervous system (CNS) effects of hypercarbia are vasodilation and increased cerebral blood flow. At very high levels, CNS depression can occur. Cardiovascular changes in-clude depressed cardiac contractility and decreased sys-temic vascular resistance. Treatment is to improve ven-tilation.

RESPIRATORY ALKALOSIS

This condition is rarely encountered in the pediatric ICU. Mild cases may be due to pain or anxiety. Treat-ment involves reassurance or treatment of the underly-ing pain or anxiety state.

References

1. Elkington JR: Clinical disorders of acid-base regulation. Ann Intern Med 57:660, 1962.
2. Graft HW, Leach W, and Arieff AI: Evidence for a detrimental effect of bicarbonate therapy in hypoxic lactic acidosis. Science 227:754–756, 1984.

Hematologic Disorders

Frank E. Shafer, M.D., Nita L. Seibel, M.D., and Gregory H. Reaman, M.D.

When considering all the red blood cell abnormalities, anemia is the most commonly encountered problem in the pediatric intensive care unit. The treatment of anemia, in most cases, is easily accomplished by red blood cell transfusions. In specific situations, the treatment may be more complicated than a simple transfusion. This chapter will discuss the general approach to anemia in the pediatric critical care setting, focus on the life-threatening complications and treatment of patients with sickle cell disease, and briefly touch upon the other end of the spectrum from anemia, polycythemia. Other hematologic issues such as bleeding disorders, infections in immunocompromised hosts, hemolytic-uremic syndrome, and blood products will be discussed in other chapters of this book.

ANEMIA

Anemia is defined as a decrease in red blood cell mass or hemoglobin content to less than the level previously established as normal for age and sex. Differentiating anemic states from normal states is generally set at 2 standard deviations (SD) less than the mean hemoglobin value for the normal population (Table 62–1).[1] Hemoglobin content alone is inadequate to judge whether a patient is "functionally anemic." Other measures are needed in order to assess whether the body's oxygen metabolism and accompanying cardiovascular metabolism are being supplied adequately by the red blood cells.

Anemia can be classified on a physiologic as well as morphologic basis. A combination of both approaches may be helpful in making the diagnosis. Functional causes of anemia can be classified into three categories (Table 62–2):[2] (1) disorders of red blood cell proliferation, in which the rate of red blood cell production is less than expected for the degree of anemia; (2) disorders in erythrocyte maturation, in which erythropoiesis is largely ineffectual; and (3) disorders in which erythrocyte destruction or loss of red blood cell mass is primarily responsible for the anemia.

The size of the red blood cell can also provide a basis of classification for anemias. In Table 62–3, the anemias are divided into three groups: microcytic, macrocytic and normocytic, with further subdivisions.

Determining the cause of the anemia requires a detailed history and physical examination and a few essential laboratory tests. The history should try to elucidate symptoms of decreased oxygen delivery in relation to associated organ dysfunction. Specific questions should be asked about changes in behavior, appetite, fatiguability, onset of pallor or jaundice, dyspnea on exertion, palpitations, orthopnea, peripheral edema, headache, vertigo, faintness, tinnitus, cold sensitivity, decreased mental concentration, irregularity in menses, urinary frequency, and low-grade fever.

The clinical presentation of a patient with anemia depends on the timing of the occurrence. A patient who has experienced an acute onset is more likely to be symptomatic than will one who has been experiencing a

Table 62–1. VALUES (NORMAL MEAN AND LOWER LIMITS OF NORMAL) FOR HEMOGLOBIN, HEMATOCRIT, AND MCV DETERMINATIONS*

Age (yr)	Hemoglobin (g/dl) Mean	Lower Limit	Hematocrit (%) Mean	Lower Limit	MCV (μm) Mean	Lower Limit
0.5–1.9	12.5	11.0	37	33	77	70
2–4	12.5	11.0	38	34	79	73
5–7	13.0	11.5	39	35	81	75
8–11	13.5	12.0	40	36	83	76
12–14						
Female	13.5	12.0	41	36	85	78
Male	14.0	12.5	43	37	84	77
15–17						
Female	14.0	12.0	41	36	87	79
Male	15.0	13.0	46	38	86	78
18–49						
Female	14.0	12.0	42	37	90	80
Male	16.0	14.0	47	40	90	80

*From Oski FA: Differential diagnosis of anemia. *In*: Nathan DG and Oski FA (eds): Hematology of Infancy and Childhood, 3rd ed. Philadelphia, WB Saunder, 1988, p. 266.

Table 62–2. PHYSIOLOGIC CLASSIFICATION OF ANEMIA*

A. Disorders of red blood cell production in which the rate of red blood cell production is less than expected for the degree of anemia:
  1. Marrow failure:
    a. Aplastic anemia:
      Congenital
      Acquired
    b. Pure red blood cell aplasia:
      Congenital:
        Diamond-Blackfan syndrome
        Asse syndrome
      Acquired:
        Transient erythroblastopenia of childhood
        Other
    c. Marrow replacement:
      Malignancies
      Osteopetrosis
      Myelofibrosis:
        Chronic renal disease
        Vitamin D deficiency
    d. Pancreatic insufficiency-marrow hypoplasia syndrome
  2. Impaired erythropoietin production:
    a. Chronic renal disease
    b. Hypothyroidism, hypopituitarism
    c. Chronic inflammation
    d. Protein malnutrition
    e. Hemoglobin mutants with decreased affinity for oxygen
B. Disorders of erythroid maturation and ineffective erythropoiesis:
  1. Abnormalities of cytoplasmic maturation:
    a. Iron deficiency
    b. Thalassemia syndromes
    c. Sideroblastic anemias
    d. Lead poisoning
  2. Abnormalities of nuclear maturation:
    a. Vitamin B_{12} deficiency
    b. Folic acid deficiency
    c. Thiamine-responsive megaloblastic anemia
    d. Hereditary abnormalities in folate metabolism
    e. Orotic aciduria
  3. Primary dyserythropoietic anemia (types I, II, III, IV)
  4. Erythropoietic protoporphyria
  5. Refractory sideroblastic anemia with vacuolization of marrow precursors and pancreatic dysfunction
C. Hemolytic anemias:
  1. Defects of hemoglobin:
    a. Structural mutants
    b. Synthetic mutants (thalassemia syndromes)
  2. Defects of the red blood cell membrane
  3. Defects of red blood cell metabolism
  4. Antibody-mediated
  5. Mechanical injury to the erythrocyte
  6. Thermal injury to the erythrocyte
  7. Oxidant-induced red blood cell injury
  8. Infectious-agent-induced red blood cell injury
  9. Paroxysmal nocturnal hemoglobinuria
  10. Plasma-lipid-induced abnormalities of the red blood cell membrane

*From Oski FA: Differential diagnosis of anemia. *In*: Nathan DG and Oski FA (eds): Hematology of Infancy and Childhood, 3rd ed. Philadelphia, WB Saunders, 1988, p. 266.

chronic process in which the only symptoms and signs include fatigue and pallor. Specific abnormalities seen on physical examination in a child with anemia include pallor, jaundice, skin pigmentation, and pinkness of palmar creases, nail beds, conjunctivae, lips, and mucous membranes of the mouth. Eye ground changes may be present in patients with sickle cell anemia and include pallor of the retina and tortuous vessels with

microaneurysms. Retinal hemorrhages may be seen in severe anemia. Patients with thalassemia major have a characteristic facies. Frontal bossing, prominent malar eminences, and maxillary dental malocclusions are all prominent physical findings in patients with advanced and chronic hemolytic anemias. The cardiovascular examination may vary depending on the severity and duration of the anemia. Tachycardia, increased arterial and capillary pulsations, bruits, and an increased rate and depth of respirations may correlate with the anemia. The systolic blood pressure is usually normal when shock is not present, but the diastolic pressure is decreased. Cardiac enlargement and signs of cardiac failure may be present in addition to atrial and ventricular arrhythmias. An apical murmur may be heard, which usually disappears after transfusion.

The abdominal examination in infants and children with hereditary and acquired anemias may reveal splenomegaly, and rarely these patients may have hepatomegaly. Patients with congestive heart failure, as well as patients with sudden severe anemia, may also have enlargement of the liver. Secondary sexual maturation may be delayed in patients with hemosiderosis as a result of chronic blood transfusions. This is characterized by lack of facial, axillary, and pubic hair. Deepening of the voice may fail to occur, and underdevelopment of breasts and genitals is possible.[3]

Table 62–3. CLASSIFICATION OF ANEMIAS BASED ON RED BLOOD CELL SIZE*

Microcytic Anemias:
  1. Iron deficiency (nutritional, chronic blood loss)
  2. Chronic lead poisoning
  3. Thalassemia syndromes
  4. Sideroblastic anemias
  5. Chronic inflammation
  6. Some congenital hemolytic anemias

Macrocytic Anemias:
  1. With megaloblastic bone marrow:
    Vitamin B_{12} deficiency
    Folic acid deficiency
    Hereditary orotic aciduria
    Thiamine-responsive anemia
  2. Without megaloblastic bone marrow:
    Aplastic anemia
    Diamond-Blackfan syndrome
    Hypothyroidism
    Liver disease
    Bone marrow infiltration
    Dyserythropoietic anemias

Normocytic Anemias:
  1. Congenital hemolytic anemias:
    Hemoglobin mutants
    Red cell enzyme defects
    Disorders of the red cell membrane
  2. Acquired hemolytic anemias:
    Antibody-mediated
    Microangiopathic hemolytic anemias
    Secondary to acute infections
  3. Acute blood loss
  4. Splenic pooling
  5. Chronic renal disease (usually)

*From Oski FA: Differential diagnosis of anemia. *In*: Nathan DG and Oski FA (eds): Hematology of Infancy and Childhood, 3rd ed. Philadelphia, WB Saunders, 1988, p. 267.

Table 62–4. THE RELATIONSHIP OF RDW AND MCV IN A VARIETY OF DISEASE STATES*

RDW†	MCV‡ Low	MCV‡ Normal	MCV‡ High
Normal	Heterozygous α or β thalassemia		Aplastic anemia
High	Iron deficiency Hemoglobin H S-β-thalassemia	Chronic disease	Folate deficiency
		Liver disease Myelotoxic chemotherapy	Vitamin B_{12} deficiency
		Chronic lymphocytic or myelogenous leukemia Mixed deficiencies Sideroblastic hemoglobin SS or SC Myelofibrosis	Immune hemolytic anemia

*From Bessman JD, Gilmer PR Jr, et al: Improved classification of anemias by MCV and RDW. Am J Clin Pathol 80:322, 1983.
†RDW = red cell distribution width.
‡MCV = mean corpuscular volume.

The initial laboratory investigation should include a complete blood count (hemoglobin and hematocrit determinations, measurement of red cell indices, platelet count, white blood cell count, and differential count) and reticulocyte count. Most important in the initial evaluation of a patient with anemia is examination of the peripheral blood smear. Depending upon these results, other laboratory tests may be required. Red blood cell distribution width (RDW) is another useful measure for evaluating anemias. This is derived from the red blood cell histogram of electronic cell sizing that accompanies each analysis on electronic counting systems. The RDW is calculated from the histogram derived from the size of the red blood cells. The formula is expressed:

$$RDW = SD/MCV \times 100$$

where SD = standard deviation and MCV = mean corpuscular volume.

The normal range is from 11.5 to 14.5% but may vary depending on the model of electronic counter.[4] The RDW is an index of the variation of red blood cells and is useful in detecting anisocytosis. Anemias can be classified according to RDW and MCV (Table 62–4).[5]

Upon the completion of the history and physical examination, in combination with the results of laboratory tests, it is possible to categorize the patient's anemia according to the schema in Figure 62–1.

HEMOLYTIC ANEMIAS

Immune-mediated destruction of red blood cells constitutes a pathologic mechanism in which the survival of the erythrocytes is decreased secondary to the deposition of specific antibodies on the cell surface. They may be either autoantibodies or antibodies produced against antigens foreign to the host. Alloimmunization may be either passive or active (Table 62–5).

Autoimmune hemolytic anemia in children is commonly caused by an IgG antibody,[6] which is usually directed against the Rh erythrocyte antigens. Maximal activity of the antibody occurs at 37° C; hence, the term *warm antibody-induced hemolytic anemia*. Survival of the erythrocytes in children with autoimmune hemolytic anemia is usually proportional to the amount of antibody on the erythrocyte surface.

Autoimmune hemolytic anemias are most frequently a result of viral and respiratory infections. The anemias may vary between mild and severe, with the mild form being more prevalent. Other diseases associated with autoimmune hemolytic anemias are noted in Table 62–6. Red blood cells coated with IgG are cleared predominantly in the spleen by macrophages. These macrophages possess both IgG and C3b receptors that remove IgG-coated cells and IgG plus C3b-coated cells from the circulation. Hemolysis is almost always extravascular.[7]

Autoimmune hemolytic anemia occurs infrequently in children. The overall incidence is estimated to be 1 in 80,000 people, with the incidence in individuals less than 20 years of age slightly less than 0.2 in 100,000.[8] The peak age of occurrence in childhood is 4 years.[9-13]

The course of autoimmune hemolytic anemia is generally acute, with resolution of the disease within 3 months. The percentage of children who may have a more chronic course varies from 23 to 74%, depending on the series. The spectrum of chronic autoimmune hemolytic anemia in children ranges from full recovery to persistence of hemolysis or intermittant relapses.[9-13]

Children with autoimmune hemolytic anemias may present acutely with a sudden drop in the hemoglobin level over a period of hours to days. This is usually

Table 62–5. IMMUNE HEMOLYTIC ANEMIAS IN CHILDHOOD*

I. Autoimmune hemolytic anemia
  A. Idiopathic
  B. Secondary to underlying disorder
  C. Passive transfer of maternal antibodies
II. Alloimmune hemolytic anemias
  A. Passive transfer of antibody
    1. Hemolytic disease of the newborn
    2. Blood group incompatibility
  B. Active immunization
    1. Blood group incompatibility
III. Drug-induced hemolytic anemia
IV. Paroxysmal nocturnal hemoglobinuria

*From Schreiber AD and Gill FM: Autoimmune hemolytic anemia. In: Nathan DG and Oski FA (eds): Hematology of Infancy and Childhood, 3rd ed. Philadelphia, WB Saunders, 1988, p. 417.

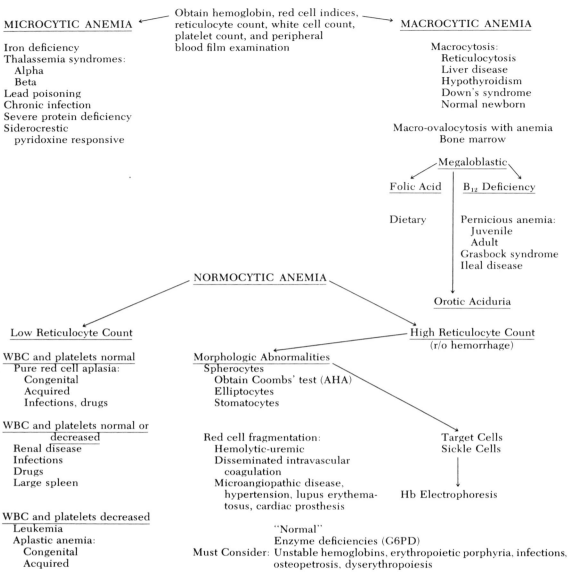

Figure 62–1. A diagnostic approach to anemia. (From Oski FA: Differential diagnosis of anemia. *In:* Nathan DG and Oski FA [eds]: Hematology of Infancy and Childhood, 3rd ed. Philadelphia, WB Saunders, 1988, p. 272.)

accompanied by pallor preceding the appearance of jaundice, tachycardia, fever, and hemoglobinuria. Depending on the rapidity of the drop in the hemoglobin level, symptoms may vary from fatigue to shock with tachycardia, tachypnea, and signs of hypoxia. Splenomegaly and hepatomegaly frequently are present. If intravascular hemolysis is present, renal failure may occur.

Children older than 10 years of age frequently will manifest the chronic form rather than the acute form. Often, the hemolytic anemia is not associated with a well-defined infection. The clinical course may be characterized by insidious onset of pallor, mild jaundice, and minimal to moderate splenomegaly. The disease may have episodes of increased erythrocyte destruction and aplastic crises. These crises may be life-threatening, depending on the rate of red blood cell destruction.[14]

Mortality in pediatric cases has been reported to be from 9 to 29%. Death during the acute phase can occur from severe anemia or bleeding from associated thrombocytopenia. Chronic cases have a higher mortality rate that is usually secondary to an underlying serious disorder.[9–13]

The diagnosis of autoimmune hemolytic anemia rests upon the presence of anemia, reticulocytosis, and a positive direct Coombs test. Peripheral blood examination may show spherocytes, tear drops, polychromasia, nucleated red blood cells, and erythrophagocytosis. Rarely, an associated leukopenia or thrombocytopenia, or both, may be present along with the autoimmune hemolytic anemia. In more than 20% of cases, reticulocytopenia may be present in the first few days of the anemia and, unlike the case in adults, it is not associated with a poor prognosis. The demonstration of immunoglobulin or complement components, or both, on the red blood cell surface establishes the diagnosis of au-

Table 62–6. DISEASES ASSOCIATED WITH AUTOIMMUNE HEMOLYTIC ANEMIA IN CHILDHOOD*

1. Infections
   a. Viral infections, especially respiratory infections
   b. Infectious mononucleosis and cytomegalovirus
   c. *Mycoplasma*, especially *pneumoniae*
   d. Tuberculosis
2. Disorders associated with autoantibody production
   a. Systemic lupus erythematosus
   b. Rheumatoid arthritis
   c. Thyroid disorders
   d. Ulcerative colitis
   e. Chronic active hepatitis
3. Immunodeficiency syndromes
   a. X-linked agammaglobulinemia
   b. Dysgammaglobulinemia
   c. Common variable hypogammaglobulinemia
   d. IgA deficiency
   e. Wiskott-Aldrich syndrome
4. Malignancies
   a. Non-Hodgkin lymphoma
   b. Hodgkin disease
   c. Acute lymphocytic leukemia
   d. Carcinoma
   e. Thymoma
   f. Ovarian cysts and tumors

*From Schreiber AD and Gill Fm: Autoimmune hemolytic anemia. *In:* Nathan DG and Oski FA (eds): Hematology of Infancy and Childhood, 3rd ed. Philadelphia, WB Saunders, 1988, p. 418.

toimmune hemolytic anemia and distinguishes it from other inborn or acquired abnormalities that can shorten red blood cell survival.

There is a population of patients with Coombs-negative hemolytic anemia. These patients have specific erythrocyte-bound antibody but negative results on the Coombs test. This reflects a limitation in the sensitivity of the antiglobulin test because a minimum of 250 to 500 molecules of IgG may be required for a positive result.[15]

Therapy for hemolytic anemia varies according to the severity. If the hemolysis is mild, no therapy may be required. When an underlying disease is present, treatment of the disease often will bring the hemolytic anemia under control. When the patient is having severe hemolysis, intervention is necessary. The goal of treatment is to decrease the rate of red blood cell destruction through a decrease in erythrophagocytosis and antibody synthesis and to support cardiovascular function.

Transfusion of red blood cells is necessary when there are objective signs of cardiovascular compromise or anoxia. Transfusions are more frequently used in the initial phase of the disease, before the effect of drugs can be seen. Transfusion therapy may be complicated by the fact that the blood bank cannot locate any "compatible" blood. This is based on the antibody specificity in warm hemolytic anemia being directed against an antigenic determinant basic to the Rh complex. The recommendation is to locate the "least incompatible" blood for transfusion as evidenced by the weakest in vitro reactivity when cross-matching the patient's serum with the red blood cells. Slow, small, periodic transfusions of packed red cells should be carried out, with the volume not to exceed 50 ml/m² because large transfusions could potentially increase the risk of cardiac

decompensation, and destruction of large quantities of red blood cells could lead to severe transfusion reactions.[14]

Drug therapy is generally instituted to reverse the pathophysiologic process mediated by specific antibody on the erythrocyte surface, to decrease phagocytosis, and to possibly decrease antibody synthesis.[16, 17] Corticosteroids have been the primary drug treatment for patients with IgG-induced immune hemolytic anemias.[18] The anemia generally responds to steroid dosages equal to 2 to 10 mg/kg of prednisone/day in three to four divided doses. Acutely ill patients should be given intravenous preparations such as methylprednisolone at a dose of 40 mg/m² for the first 24 to 48 hours or until an oral agent can be instituted. Steroids should be continued until a therapeutic response has been noted, which is often defined as a stabilization in the hemoglobin value at 10 g/dl or higher and a decrease in the reticulocyte production index. The steroids can be tapered slowly over a period of months. The success rate in children treated with steroids ranges from 32 to 77%. Only when steroids are unsuccessful initially or their administration is prolonged over several months or the effects are suboptimal should other therapeutic modalities be considered.[10–12, 18–20]

Alternative treatments that have had limited pediatric application include immunosuppressive agents (thiopurines or alkylating agents), the synthetic androgen danazol, intravenous gammaglobulin, plasmapheresis, and exchange transfusion and splenectomy.[21–26] Splenectomy is generally considered early in the rare patient who demonstrates little or no response to steroids and a continuing need for transfusions because of serious side effects of anemia experienced during 4 to 6 days of therapy. The increased risk of sepsis in splenectomized patients dictates that splenectomy not be considered until all other forms of acceptable therapy have been exhausted. The overall response rate to splenectomy varies between 50 and 70%, with the vast majority of responses being partial remissions.[27]

COLD AGGLUTININ DISEASE

Cold agglutinin disease is almost always caused by IgM antibody and is unusual in pediatrics. IgM-induced immune hemolytic anemia is most commonly associated with an underlying infection with *Mycoplasma pneumoniae*. These IgM antibodies have anti-I specificity. Cold agglutinin disease can occur with other infections, such as respiratory tract disease, infectious mononucleosis, cytomegalovirus infection, chickenpox, measles, and mumps.[28–30] When associated with an underlying infection, the cold agglutinin is polyclonal. The cause of the production of IgM cold agglutinins in patients with infection is not understood.

Erythrocyte survival is similar to that in warm autoimmune hemolytic anemia in that it is proportional to the amount of antibody on the erythrocyte surface. In the presence of cold temperatures in a patient with cold agglutinin disease, the IgM antibody interacts with the red blood cell surface and leads to activation of the classic complement pathway. Receptors capable of recognizing C3b-coated red blood cells are present on the macrophages. The macrophage C3b receptors bind the C3b-coated erythrocytes, resulting in phagocytosis of the red blood cell. Clearance of the erythrocytes takes place rapidly and primarily in the liver through hepatic macrophages.[7, 31, 32] Intravascular hemolysis may result from the presence of large numbers of IgM molecules on the red blood cell surface, which results in more extensive complement activation involving C8 and C9. The extent of hemolysis is the result of the cold agglutinin titer, the thermal amplitude of the IgM antibody, and the level of the circulating control proteins of the C3b inactivator system.[33] The activity of the IgM antibody is greatest between the temperatures of 0 and 30° C. Hemolysis may be precipitated by cold exposure in cold agglutinin disease. Patients may present as described for autoimmune hemolytic anemia. The skin of patients with severe cold agglutinin disease may display a livedo reticularis pattern when they are exposed to cold.[27]

The Donath-Landsteiner cold hemolysin, an unusual IgG antibody with anti-P specificity, is found, although infrequently, in children with viral infections. Hemolysis is usually mild and resolves with recovery from the infection. Intravascular hemolysis is seen with this antibody as a result of the unusual complement-activating efficiency of the IgG antibody.[34]

Diagnosis of cold agglutinin disease is made by detection of C3 on the red blood cell surface. The cold agglutinin titer is helpful in making the diagnosis, since this is the highest dilution at which the patient's serum will agglutinate normal ABO-compatible red blood cells containing the I antigen. Titers greater than 1:1,000 are seen in most patients with cold agglutinin disease.

Often, the hemolysis is mild in cold agglutinin disease. Recommendations for treatment include avoidance of cold and control of the underlying disease. Steroids are generally not effective except in a few patients having cold agglutinin disease with low titers of antibodies active up to temperatures of 37° C. The very few patients with IgG cold agglutinins seem to respond to steroids or splenectomy, or both.[17, 31] Splenectomy is not effective in cold agglutinin disease because the liver is the primary site of phagocytosis of IgM-coated erythrocytes. If the patient with cold agglutinin disease has such severe anemia that a transfusion is warranted, all intravenous infusions must be prewarmed to 37° C. This is to avoid the complication of a severe hemolytic reaction caused by the cold temperature locally in a vein, leading to enhancement of binding of the IgM antibodies to the red blood cells.[14] Plasmapheresis has been effective in reducing the level of IgM antibodies in IgM-induced hemolytic anemia, but on a short-term basis.[35]

ENZYME DEFECTS

Glucose-6-Phosphate Dehydrogenase Deficiency

The first enzyme in the pentose phosphate pathway of glucose metabolism is glucose-6-phosphate dehydrogenase (G6PD). It catalyzes the conversion of glucose-6-phosphate to 6-phosphogluconate and concomitantly reduces nicotinamide-adenine dinucleotide phosphate (NADP) to NADPH. A deficiency of this enzyme decreases the reductive energy of the red blood cell and results in erythrocyte hemolysis. The severity of the hemolysis depends upon the remaining quantity and type of G6PD and the nature of the associated hemolytic agent, which is usually an oxidation-reduction mediator.[36]

G6PD is transmitted in a sex-linked recessive mode of inheritance by a gene that is located on the X chromosome.[37] Thus, the disease may be fully expressed in the hemizygous male or the homozygous female. Heterozygous females may demonstrate variable intermediate expression because of the random deletion of the X chromosome according to the Lyon hypothesis. Three per cent of the general population is affected, with the highest frequency among individuals of Mediterranean countries and blacks. Several genetic variants have been described. The most common variants, B+ and *Mediterranean* are commonly observed among individuals in the southern Mediterranean area but are also present in individuals of Indian heritage and in peoples from southeast Asia. Two other abnormal variants, A− and A+, are observed in individuals from western and central Africa. A− is associated with markedly decreased activity (5 to 15% of normal), whereas A+ results in a mild decrease in activity (80 to 85% of normal).[38] Two other variants include *Canton*,[39] which is found in people from southern Asia, and *Debrousse*,[40] which is seen in individuals from North Africa.

In these individuals, the activity of G6PD falls rapidly and prematurely as the erythrocyte matures. There is reduced glucose metabolism and diminished reduction of NADP to NADPH. When exposed to oxidant agents, the red blood cell integrity is impaired and hemolysis is promoted. Episodes of hemolysis may occur upon exposure to numerous drugs (Table 62–7) in association with fever or infection.

Under normal conditions, the common types of G6PD deficiency are clinically silent. The hemolytic event usually occurs within a few hours to 3 days following the exposure to the precipitating oxidant agent. Many times, an offending agent is unidentifiable, and some other stress such as fever or infection may have precipitated the hemolytic crisis. Red blood cells in the newborn infant are particularly defective in the enzymatic machinery, and any added stress may result in a hemolytic crisis shortly after birth in the newborn with G6PD deficiency. Thus G6PD deficiency should be suspected in a newborn with hyperbilirubinemia occurring during the first several days of life in association with hemolytic anemia.[4]

These crises are characterized by intravascular hemolysis with red blood cell fragmentation, anemia, Heinz body formation, hemoglobinemia, hemoglobinuria, and hyperbilirubinemia. Pincer cells, which represent erythrocytes in which oxidized hemoglobin and membrane segments have been removed by splenic phagocytes, may be present on the peripheral smear. Reticulocytosis is the first indication that the marrow is

Table 62–7. AGENTS CAPABLE OF INDUCING HEMOLYSIS IN G6PD-DEFICIENT SUBJECTS*†

Clinically Significant Hemolysis	Usually Not Clinically Significant Hemolysis
Analgesics and Antipyretics	
Acetanilid	Acetophenetidin (phenacetin)
	Acetylsalicylic acid (large doses)
	Antipyrine†‡
	Aminopyrine‡
	p-Aminosalicylic acid
Antimalarial Agents	
Pentaquine	Quinacrine (Atabrine)
Pamaquine	Quinine‡
Primaquine	Chloroquine§
Quinocide	Pyrimethamine (Daraprim)
	Plasmoquine
Sulfonamides	
Sulfanilamide	Sulfadiazine
N-Acetylsulfanilamide	Sulfamerazine
Sulfapyridine	Sulfisoxazole (Gantrisin)§
Sulfamethoxypyridazine (Kynex)	Sulfathiazole
Salicylazosulfapyridine (Azulfidine)	Sulfacetamide
Nitrofurans	
Nitrofurazone (Furacin)	
Nitrofurantoin (Furadantin)	
Furaltadone (Altafur)	
Furazolidone (Furoxone)	
Sulfones	
Thiazolsulfone (Promizole)	Sulfoxone sodium (Diasone)
Diaminodiphenylsulfone (DDS, dapsone)	
Miscellaneous	
Naphthalene	Menadione
Phenylhydrazine	Dimercaprol (BAL)
Acetylphenylhydrazine	Methylene blue
Toluidine blue	Chloramphenicol†
Nalidixic acid (NegGram)	Probenecid (Benemid)
Neoarsphenamine (Neosalvarsan)	Quindine†
Infections	Fava beans†
Diabetic acidosis	

*From Lanzkowsky P: Hemolytic anemia. *In:* Manual of Pediatric Hematology and Oncology. New York, Churchill Livingstone, 1989, p. 100.
†Many other compounds have been tested but are free of hemolytic activity. Penicillin, the tetracyclines, and erythromycin, for example, will not cause hemolysis, and the incidence of allergic reactions in G6PD-deficient persons is not any greater than that observed in others. Any drug, therefore, not included in the list of those known to cause hemolysis may be given.
‡Hemolysis in whites only.
§Mild hemolysis in blacks, if given in large doses.

responding to the degree of hemolysis. Initially, the child may show more subtle signs of anemia, such as irritability, pallor, or lethargy. The hemolysis may rapidly progress with signs of jaundice, splenomegaly, and even tachycardia, tachypnea, and shock. A chronic, steady state of hemolysis is usually present; thus, these children may always have some degree of splenic enlargement. Because unconjugated bilirubin levels may remain elevated, gallstones are more common in these individuals.

Individuals, especially boys, who present with a hemolytic anemia and have a significant family history should be screened. Diagnosis is confirmed by a G6PD assay in the affected individual and comparing this value with that of a known normal individual. Since the G6PD level is higher in young red blood cells, the assay level may be falsely elevated during a period of brisk reticulocytosis.

In the child with confirmed G6PD deficiency, parental education regarding signs and symptoms of a hemolytic crisis should be undertaken when the diagnosis is initially made. A list of agents and drugs to be avoided should be given to the family and primary care provider. It should also be stressed that relatively common agents such as aspirin, sulfa-containing drugs, and naphthalene (moth balls) may result in life-threatening hemolytic anemia.

If the hemolytic event has already begun, initial treatment consists of removing the potential precipitating agent if this has not already been done. If the child is clinically symptomatic, with tachycardia and tachypnea along with a rapidly falling hemoglobin level and an elevated total serum bilirubin level, a packed red blood cell transfusion should be started emergently (see section on transfusion). A general guideline for transfusing packed red blood cells is to transfuse 10 ml/kg over 3 to 4 hours if the starting hemoglobin level is greater than 5 g/dl. If the starting hemoglobin level is lower than 5 g/dl, divide the transfusion into two 5-ml/kg transfusions. This lessens the risk of volume overload caused by an excessive transfusion rate. Signs of volume overload such as tachycardia, tachypnea, and hypertension should be monitored. The transfusion may be slowed or stopped, and furosemide should be given to aid in diuresis.

In the child with chronic splenomegaly and marked anemia, splenectomy may be beneficial in long-term management.[42]

Pyruvate Kinase Deficiency

Pyruvate kinase (PK) is the final enzyme active in the Embden-Meyerhof pathway. It is responsible for the conversion of phosphoenolpyruvate to pyruvate, which generates adenosine triphosphate (ATP) from adenosine diphosphate. A deficiency of this enzyme results in defective red blood cell glycolysis and decreased ATP formation. The end result is red blood cells that are deformed, rigid, and metabolically and physically vulnerable to intravascular hemolysis.

PK deficiency is inherited in an autosomal recessive manner. Severe and chronic hemolysis is seen in homozygotes.[43] The majority of the cases reported have been found in individuals of northern European extraction, although sporadic cases in other races have been observed.[44]

The diagnosis should be considered in any newborn or child with episodes of hemolysis and hyperbilirubinemia. Confirmation of the diagnosis is achieved by measuring enzyme levels and comparing them to known normal values.

Unconjugated hyperbilirubinemia is commonly encountered in PK-deficient newborns.[45] In the older child, the clinical abnormalities associated with chronic hemolysis include anemia, jaundice, and splenomegaly. The anemia may be profound, especially during a hemolytic crisis. Macrocytosis and spiculated erythrocytes may be seen on the blood smear. There is usually a compensatory reticulocytosis as well.

Unlike G6PD, hemolytic events are usually not precipitated by specific drugs. However, other stresses such as fever and infection may exacerbate acute hemolysis.[46] Late clinical features include chronic splenomegaly and cholelithiasis secondary to bilirubinate gallstone formation.

As described for G6PD deficiency, children with PK deficiency may also require regular packed red blood cell transfusions. Hyperbilirubinemia is frequently encountered in PK-deficient newborns and may require an exchange transfusion. Very brisk hemolysis may occur following stress such as fever or infection. During these episodes, the child may require emergent hospitalization and red blood cell transfusions.

In the long-term management of these children, splenectomy may decrease the transfusion requirements, result in a decrease in the serum bilirubin level, and increase the hemoglobin level, but a complete cure cannot be anticipated.[47]

Hexokinase Deficiency

Hexokinase deficiency is an uncommon cause of hemolytic anemia. The enzyme is responsible for the conversion of glucose to glucose-6-phosphate in the Embden-Meyerhof pathway. Deficiency of the enzyme results in red blood cells that have subnormal glucose metabolism and lactate production. Such erythrocytes may encounter a particularly unfavorable environment in the spleen, leading to increased hemolysis.[48] An autosomal mode of inheritance has been proposed for hexokinase deficiency.[49]

In mild cases of this deficiency, hemolysis and anemia may be fully compensated for by increased erythropoiesis; however, jaundice, reticulocytosis, and splenomegaly are usually present. Neonatal hyperbilirubinemia and intractable hemolytic anemia may be the presenting features in children with severe enzyme deficiency.[50] Because of a constant state of ongoing hemolysis, gallstones may be evident early in childhood.[51]

Consistent with reticulocytosis, macrocytosis and polychromasia are notable on examination of the blood smear; otherwise, the red blood cell morphologic appearance is usually unremarkable. The diagnosis is made by comparing the level of hexokinase with a known normal standard.

As in other forms of chronic hemolytic anemia, packed red blood cell transfusions are usually necessary on a regular basis. Episodes of brisk hemolysis may require emergent hospitalization, monitoring, and transfusion given judiciously, watching for evidence of volume overload.

Cholelithiasis may occur at a relatively young age during childhood. Experience with splenectomy is limited, but as in other forms of chronic hemolytic anemia resulting from enzyme deficiencies, transfusion requirements may be lessened following this procedure.[52]

MEMBRANE DEFECTS

Hereditary Spherocytosis

Hereditary spherocytosis (HS) is characterized by osmotically fragile, spherically shaped cells that are selectively sequestered by the spleen. HS is most common in individuals of northern European heritage. The prevalence in this population is approximately 1 in 5,000.[53] The disease is seen in other races as well, but less commonly. There are at least two inheritance patterns, with 75% of the families studied showing a classic autosomal dominant pattern of inheritance.[54, 55]

The cell membrane of the hereditary spherocytes are intrinsically defective. Spectrin is the major skeletal protein of the red blood cell membrane. This protein is highly flexible and has the ability to assume a variety of conformations, which is important for normal membrane pliancy.[56, 57] All patients with HS, including both the recessive and dominant forms of HS, are spectrin-deficient. But, in some patients with HS, ankyrin, the protein that anchors the spectrin-based skeleton to other transmembrane proteins, may also be deficient. The degree of deficiency correlates closely with the severity of the disease and the degree of spherocytosis.[58, 59] The resulting hemolysis is due to a number of factors, including reduced erythrocyte deformability leading to red blood cell entrapment in the spleen, loss of surface area relative to cell volume, increased influx and efflux of sodium, increased ATP utilization and glycolysis, and ultimately premature red blood cell destruction.

Clinically, the children have anemia, jaundice, and chronic splenomegaly. There may be much variability among patients, with some demonstrating a great deal of compensation and thus having only mild anemia. HS may present during the neonatal period with hyperbilirubinemia and anemia.[60] There is usually an accompanying reticulocytosis, spherocytosis, and increase in the number of nucleated red blood cells. Anemia is the most common presenting complaint in children, followed by jaundice and splenomegaly.

Hemolytic crises may occur in children with HS, precipitated by fever or infection. These episodes are marked by a rapid increase in the size of the spleen over baseline, as well as reticulocytosis and moderate anemia. Aplastic crises, however, can result in severe anemia. Parvovirus has been associated with this syndrome.[62] In the aplastic phase, the hemoglobin level drops precipitously and is not accompanied by reticulocytosis. Paradoxically, the serum bilirubin levels do not rise markedly because of the decline in the number of abnormal red blood cells that have to be destroyed.[63] Pallor, lethargy, and fatigue may progress rapidly to more serious symptoms of tachycardia, tachypnea, and cardiovascular shock.

Gallbladder disease is the most common long-term complication seen in HS.[64] Cholelithiasis may occur in young children, and gallbladder disease should be suspected in the child with HS who presents with a history of nausea, vomiting, and upper quadrant abdominal pain of biliary colic. Diagnosis may be aided by the demonstration of gallstones or gallbladder sludge on ultrasound.

Laboratory features include a normochromic, normocytic anemia that can be quite mild in compensated cases. However, in erythroblastopenic crises, the hemoglobin level may drop as low as 2 to 3 g/dl. The MCV and mean corpuscular hemoglobin are usually within normal limits, but the mean corpuscular hemoglobin concentration is usually increased (>36%). In most cases, there is a compensatory reticulocytosis (3 to 15%). The blood smear demonstrates a variable number of microspherocytes with polychromasia. The Coombs test is negative. Diagnostic confirmation is aided by demonstrating an increased osmotic fragility of the red blood cells; spherocytes lyse more readily in higher concentrations of saline when compared with known normal red blood cells. Other laboratory parameters include an increased serum bilirubin level, which is mainly unconjugated.

When an aplastic crisis or a severe hemolytic crisis is associated with HS, an emergent red blood cell transfusion is indicated in the face of marked anemia and splenomegaly, especially if there is little compensatory reticulocytosis. The newborn with hyperbilirubinemia and hemolysis may require an exchange transfusion.

Splenectomy is recommended for moderate to severe cases of HS. The major benefits include resolution of anemia and prevention of gallbladder disease. However, the risk of postsplenectomy sepsis must be considered.[65-67] Controversy exists regarding the performance of a simultaneous prophylactic cholecystectomy with the splenectomy.[68]

Hereditary Elliptocytosis

Hereditary elliptocytosis (HE) is a clinically and genetically heterogeneous disorder characterized by the presence of elliptically shaped cells in the peripheral blood. It is relatively common, affecting 1 in 25,000 individuals in the population. The disorder is inherited in an autosomal dominant pattern with variable penetrance. One of the elliptocytosis genes is linked to the Rh locus and is associated with mild anemia.[69] Another elliptocytosis gene is located near the Duffy blood group locus and is associated with a high incidence of severe anemia.[70] There are three main classifications of HE: common HE, spherocytic HE, and stomatocytic HE. All types have defects in the red blood cell membrane skeleton, which may be manifested by decreased thermal stability (as in hereditary pyropoikilocytosis) and decreased mechanical stability. Most commonly, there is a defect in the spectrin component of the cytoskeleton, but abnormalities of the other membrane proteins of ankyrin—protein 4.1, protein 3, and glycophorin C—have also been described.[71]

The disease has wide variability in clinical phenotypes, with some individuals showing little evidence of hemolysis, whereas others demonstrate bizarre erythrocyte morphologic features and chronic hemolytic anemia. Based on molecular characterization of the membrane skeletons, several subgroups have been identified.

In the common form of HE, 25 to 90% of the red blood cells have a characteristic elongated, oval, elliptocytic shape. Osmotic fragility is normal or increased. Patients with mild HE may experience transient uncompensated hemolytic anemia in response to a variety of stimuli that cause hyperplasia of the reticuloendothelial system. In the mild form of HE, most patients are asymptomatic.

Hereditary pyropoikilocytosis is a rare disease that is clinically manifested during infancy and early childhood and is characterized by marked erythrocyte thermal sensitivity resulting in intravascular red blood cell fragmentation, spherocyte and elliptocyte formation, and extreme anisocytosis with budding red blood cells. Fragmentation may occur at temperatures as low as 37° C. There is a chronic state of hemolysis manifested by anemia, reticulocytosis, and an elevated mean corpuscular hemoglobin concentration. The osmotic fragility is increased. Complications include growth failure, frontal bossing, splenomegaly, and gallbladder disease.[72]

In extreme cases of hemolysis, packed red blood cell transfusions are indicated (see section on hereditary spherocytosis). In patients with chronic hemolysis and splenomegaly, splenectomy may be indicated. The hemoglobin level may rise from a value of 4 to 6 g/dl to a value as high as 10 to 12 g/dl following splenectomy.[73] Of course, the postsplenectomy complications, including an increased risk of sepsis, must be kept in mind.

HEMOGLOBINOPATHIES AND RELATED SYNDROMES

Sickle Cell Disease

Sickle cell disease is a hemolytic anemia characterized clinically by vaso-occlusion resulting in acute and chronic ischemic tissue injury. The underlying defect is a single amino acid substitution of valine for glutamic acid at position 6 of the β-globin polypeptide. Hemoglobin S (Hb S) has a higher net electrical charge than does hemoglobin A (Hb A) and so has a separate electrophoretic mobility. In the deoxygenated state, Hb S is less soluble than is Hb A and forms polymers or aligned hemoglobin fibers that distort the erythrocyte and cause the cell to take on a characteristic sickled shape. These sickled cells are prematurely destroyed, resulting in a hemolytic anemia. Acute and chronic tissue damage results from impaired blood flow and thrombus formation in the microvasculature resulting from increased viscosity of the sickled cells.

In the homozygous state (sickle cell disease), there is no synthesis of normal Hb A, and the red blood cells contain 90 to 100% Hb S. In the heterozygous state (sickle cell trait), the red blood cells contain 20 to 30% Hb S.

Specific Problems

Aplastic Crisis. In the patient with sickle cell anemia, a normal steady state is achieved by balancing the rate of ongoing red blood cell hemolysis with a compensatory increase in bone marrow production by six- to eightfold when compared with normal marrow erythroid output.[74] Following an intercurrent viral or bacterial infection, temporary cessation of bone marrow activity may occur as clinically evidenced by a rapidly dropping hematocrit value with no compensatory reticulocytosis. Parvovirus has been linked to aplastic crisis in the patient with sickle cell disease.[75-77] Specifically, the maturation of the early red blood cell precursor, colony-forming units–erythrocyte (CFU-E), is retarded by the virus.[78, 79]

A spontaneous recovery occurs in most patients within 2 to 10 days. An increasing reticulocyte count and percentage of nucleated red blood cells indicates recovery of the erythroid units in the bone marrow. In the convalescent phase, hyperhemolysis may be assumed mistakenly because of the severe anemia and elevated reticulocyte count. Most aplastic episodes are short in duration with a minimal drop in the hemoglobin level. However, when the anemia is significant with evidence of clinical manifestations, especially tachypnea or tachycardia, or when recovery is delayed, a red blood cell transfusion is indicated.

Splenic Sequestration. In infants and young children whose spleens have not yet undergone multiple splenic infarctions, subsequent fibrosis, and eventual autoinfarction, acute and rapid engorgement of the splenic vasculature may occur. This emergent and potentially fatal situation is characterized by sudden and severe anemia, massive splenomegaly, and a clinical picture of hypovolemic shock.[80] This syndrome may also occur in older patients with Hb SC disease or Hb S thalassemia who have chronic splenomegaly. During severe sequestration events, trapping and pooling of a significant portion of the red blood cell volume may occur. In the child with sickle cell disease, these events are more common after the age of 5 months but are infrequently seen after 2 to 3 years of age.[81] Occasionally, a precipitating event such as a preceding viral illness may be identified; however, no precipitating cause is found in the majority of cases.

Minor episodes of sequestration are common. These events are characterized by moderate splenic enlargement and anemia with a hemoglobin value as low as 3 to 4 g/dl. Although these minor episodes may resolve by themselves, these infants should be identified as being more prone to further life-threatening events. Most centers instruct parents to seek immediate medical attention if they feel an enlarged spleen or note unusual weakness in the child.

During the more dramatic type of sequestration crisis, the spleen rapidly enlarges, often reaching the pelvic brim. Massive amounts of blood pool in the splenic vasculature, and the hemoglobin level drops precipitously. Hypovolemic shock rapidly ensues, and death occurs if appropriate medical management is not undertaken.[82]

The clinical history is characterized by an infant or young child noted to be initially fussy who quickly becomes weak and listless. Pallor, tachypnea, tachycardia, and abdominal fullness may be the first clinical indications of this crisis.

Treatment consists of emergent restoration of intravascular volume and oxygen-carrying capacity using packed red blood cells. By promptly reversing the hypovolemic shock, much of the blood that has pooled in the spleen can be remobilized, followed by dramatic regression of the splenomegaly and a rise in the hemoglobin level within a relatively short time.[83]

Because of the tendency toward recurrence of this potentially fatal event, splenectomy should be considered in children who have had two or more sequestration crises. Considering the fact that splenic autoinfarction renders the spleen nonfunctional after 6 to 9 months of age, the risk of postsplenectomy sepsis is not greatly increased. Another approach to prevent the chance of recurrence is the use of chronic simple transfusions. Decreasing the quantitative Hb S concentration maintains normal spleen size and prevents sequestration by decreasing the likelihood of splenic intravascular sickling. However, once transfusions are discontinued, the child is again at risk for sequestration.[84, 85]

Cerebrovascular Accident. Approximately 7% of children with sickle cell disease will experience a cerebrovascular accident (CVA) as a complication of an acute vaso-occlusive event in the brain. These localized neurologic events are due to an ischemic or hemorrhagic lesion in a specific vascular territory. Neurologic manifestations are usually focal and may include cranial nerve palsies, aphasia, hemiparesis, visual field defects, and hemianesthesia. Occasionally, seizures and coma may also be observed.

The term *transient ischemic attack* is used to describe

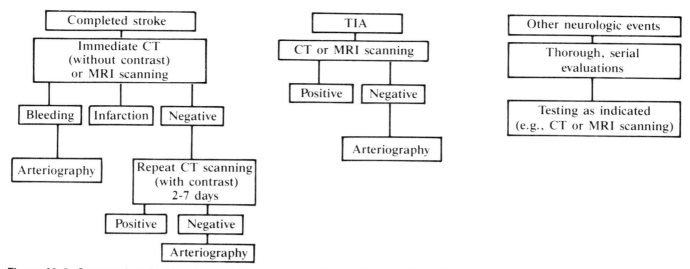

Figure 62–2. Suggested evaluation of neurologic events in sickle cell disease. (From Charache S, Lubin B, and Reid C: Acute splenic sequestration and aplastic crisis. *In:* Management and therapy of sickle cell disease. NIH Pub. No. 89-2117:23, 1989.)

a focal neurologic event that resolves within 24 to 48 hours and results in no residual deficits. Subarachnoid and intracerebral hemorrhages are more common in older children and adults, whereas cerebral infarction is the most common cause of stroke in children with sickle cell disease who are less than 10 years of age.[86]

The mortality rate following an untreated stroke in a patient with sickle cell disease is 20%, with approximately 70% of patients experiencing a recurrent neurologic event within 3 years. The abnormal neurologic signs may resolve completely or remain constant. Overall, however, more than 70% of patients are left with permanent motor and intelligence deficits.[87]

The pathologic presentation of the arterial lesion consists of proliferation of intimal fibroblasts and smooth muscles affecting mainly the large cerebral vessels.[88–90] The adherence of sickled red blood cells to the vascular endothelium is increased as a result of this intimal damage, which also serves as a focus for platelet adhesion and thrombus formation.[91] The most common abnormalities seen on angiography are narrowing or occlusion of the middle or anterior cerebral or internal carotid arteries, or both.[92] Vessel spasm or small emboli can cause transient neurologic symptoms. Intracranial hemorrhage is usually caused by rupture of an aneurysm in the circle of Willis. Bleeding can be either intracerebral or subarachnoid.

Infarctions are not surgically correctable; however, computed tomography (CT) scanning should be performed to rule out a treatable disorder such as a berry aneurysm, subdural hematoma, or other mass lesions of infectious or malignant nature. The CT scan may be normal immediately following the acute incident; however, rescanning in 2 to 7 days may show the infarcted area with surrounding edema. Obviously, if doubt remains regarding the correct diagnosis, other studies, including contrast-enhanced CT, magnetic resonance imaging (MRI), brain scan, perfusion study, Doppler study, electroencephalogram, and lumbar puncture (if no evidence of increased intracranial pressure is dem-

onstrated by CT scan), are indicated.[93] MRI has become a sensitive tool for the detection of intracranial bleeding or infarction and eliminates potential complications with the use of intravenous contrast material.[94, 95] Arteriography is not recommended until an exchange transfusion has been performed (see section on transfusion), since the hypertonic dye may potentiate further intracerebral sickling.[96] Confirmation of a cerebral infarction first seen by CT scan or MRI does not warrant exposing the patient with sickle cell disease to the potential complications of arteriography. However, arteriography is indicated for patients with subarachnoid hemorrhage or to detect a surgically correctable lesion.

CT scanning or MRI imaging, or both, is also indicated in the patient with transient neurologic symptoms. If doubt remains following these studies, underlying arterial disease must be ruled out by arteriography.[97]

Newer techniques, such as metabolic MRI or positron emission tomography, have not been standardized in patients with sickle cell disease. A schema for suggested evaluation and treatment of neurologic events in sickle cell disease is shown in Figure 62–2.

The ultimate treatment of the acute CVA with infarction includes emergent reduction in the concentration of Hb S to prevent further intravascular sickling and infarct progression.[98] Monitoring of changes in the neurologic status and treatment of the pediatric patient is best carried out in the intensive care setting. In order to control increasing intracranial pressure from cerebral edema, pharmacologic agents and assisted ventilation may be necessary. Pharmacologic seizure control and consultation with the pediatric neurology or neurosurgery departments, or both, should be employed as required.

Following or concurrent with the emergent basic life support techniques, a red blood cell transfusion should be initiated immediately.[99] As outlined in the section on transfusions, a partial exchange or a full-volume exchange should be used to decrease the quantitative level of Hb S to less than 30%.

Two thirds of patients who have one stroke resulting from infarction will experience similar recurrent events, with the risk greatest during the first 3 years following the initial event. Thus, it is recommended that this group of pediatric patients be placed on a regularly scheduled red blood cell transfusion protocol with the goal of maintaining the patient's Hb S level at less than 30%.[100, 101] There is no general concensus on the optimal duration of continued transfusion therapy.[102] Because of the risk of recurrence, most centers continue therapy for at least 3 years following the initial event.[103] The iron-chelating agent deferoxamine should be used to help prevent the unavoidable complication of iron overload. Patients who suffer stroke as a result of a hemorrhagic event have a mortality rate as high as 50%. A subarachnoid or intracerebral hemorrhage may present with focal findings, headache, clinical evidence of increased intracranial pressure, seizures, and coma. In this case, the CT or MRI scan should demonstrate a density consistent with a bleeding episode. In the case of a subarachnoid hemorrhage, a lumbar tap may be useful in confirming the diagnosis. Angiography, performed after appropriate transfusion preparation (see section on transfusion), will be needed to delineate a potentially surgically correctable lesion.

Another condition results from transient generalized arterial hypoxia secondary to sickling in the terminal arterial vessels of the cerebral vasculature. In this state, patients may initially show a clinical pattern of rapid, generalized lethargy and confusion with no localizing neurologic signs. Decorticate or decerebrate posturing may be observed. CT and MRI imaging shows no focal lesions. There is usually resolution of the neurologic findings over the following weeks to months. Again, the treatment involves increasing oxygen-carrying capacity and reducing the concentration of Hb S by performing an emergent exchange transfusion as described in detail in the section on transfusion. Treatment with hyperbaric oxygen (2 to 3 hours at 2 atmospheres [atm]/day) is suggested if available. Hypoxia should be aggressively controlled and should include the use of positive end-expiratory pressure if necessary.

Many new experimental therapies have been proposed for the treatment of both acute and chronic complications of sickle cell disease. Anticoagulation therapy using heparin or warfarin has not been shown in prospective studies to be effective in reducing the severity or number of subsequent strokes. The chronic use of antiplatelet therapy such as aspirin has no proven use in this group of patients.

Other experimental methods have been aimed at increasing the quantity of fetal hemoglobin. These therapies are based on the observation that patients with sickle cell disease who have an elevated percentage of fetal hemoglobin appear to be protected from many of the complications associated with intravascular sickling. This is because of the sparing effect of fetal hemoglobin on the polymerization of sickled hemoglobin.[104, 105] Current therapies under investigation include the use of various chemotherapeutic agents such as 5-azacytodine,[106] hydroxyurea,[107] hydroxybutyrate, and cytosine arabinoside. Several agents that act upon the red blood cell membrane have been proposed as potential antisickling agents. Cetiedil increases red blood cell filterability and prevents sickling by a direct effect on the red blood cell membrane.[108] Pentoxifylline modifies the rheologic features of Hb S cells and may ameliorate some symptoms associated with intravascular sickling.[109] Bone marrow transplantation using HLA-compatible allogenic donor marrow has been attempted in a small number of children with sickle cell disease.[110] Although the outcome was favorable, resulting in a decrease in clinical symptoms, prospective controlled studies are needed to confirm the efficacy of this treatment for sickle cell disease.

Acute Chest Syndrome. In the patient with sickle cell disease and hypoxia, fever, fatigue, and chest pain, it is often difficult to distinguish between pneumonia and pulmonary infarction as the underlying clinical cause. In many cases, a pulmonary infection may lead to focal hypoxia, sickling in the pulmonary vasculature, and areas of infarction. Depending on the degree of respiratory distress and the course of clinical deterioration, acute chest syndrome should be considered a medical emergency that may require management in the intensive care setting.

In children, the presenting symptoms may be as vague as cough and tachypnea. In the older child, a history of pleuritic chest pain may be elicited. Referred pain to the abdomen may indicate inflammation of the diaphragmatic pleura. If the source of the pain remains obscure, one should consider other causes, such as cholecystitis or sternal or rib infarction, or both.

Patients with sickle cell disease, particularly Hb SC disease may also experience a rare syndrome with similarity to the acute chest syndrome known as fat embolization syndrome. During a severe vaso-occlusive event, the pulmonary vessels may become embolized with liquified bone marrow fat. Symptoms associated with acute chest syndrome are more pronounced and may progress rapidly to include confusion, agitation, and coma. Acute renal failure, disseminated intravascular coagulation, and severe hemolytic anemia may also occur. Diagnosis may be difficult but may be aided by the presence of necrosis on bone marrow aspiration, refractile bodies on fundoscopic examination, fat globules in the urine, and petechiae of the head and neck.[111]

Laboratory evaluation should include a complete blood count and reticulocyte count with attention paid to the hemoglobin and hematocrit values and, if possible, comparison with the patient's normal baseline values. An increase in the total white blood cell count and shift toward the left may indicate an infection as the precipitating factor and thus help direct appropriate therapy. The chest radiograph may be normal and nondiagnostic during the first 2 to 3 days, especially if the patient is dehydrated. An infiltrate may be seen in one or more lobes, and a pleural effusion may be present. Lung scans are usually not useful in arriving at the diagnosis, nor do they often aid in directing the correct therapy. Because of the hypertonicity of contrast dye, pulmonary angiography carries the potential risk of potentiating further intravascular sickling and thus is rarely indicated. Specimens should be obtained for blood cultures. If possible, sputum and pleural effusion cultures should also be examined for an infectious pathogen. Based on the patient's history, *Mycoplasma, Chlamydia*, and viral cultures should also be indicated. A baseline room air arterial blood gas determination should be obtained. Ear or pulse oximetry as a measure of oxygen saturation has not been well established in the patient with sickle cell disease, and so simultaneous determination of arterial blood oxygen saturation is necessary.

Close observation is required for all patients with acute chest syndrome because of the high risk of rapid respiratory deterioration. Care in the intensive care unit may be indicated to closely monitor the rapidly changing clinical state. Oxygen is indicated for all patients with hypoxia and tachypnea. Monitoring the oxygen saturation requires frequent arterial blood gas sampling. Intravenous fluids should be delivered judiciously. Oral or parenteral analgesia is indicated, but sedation should be titered to avoid hypoventilation (see section on pain management).

Empirical antibiotic therapy is generally recommended because of the difficulty in differentiating an infarctive process from an underlying infectious cause. In 2 to 5% of cases of acute chest syndrome, a positive blood culture result is obtained. *Streptococcus pneumoniae* and *Haemophilus influenzae* are the most common isolates. Intravenous ampicillin (200 to 250 mg/kg/24 hr) should be given. If a β-lactamase–resistant organism such as *H. influenzae* is a possible pathogen, a cephalosporin such as cefuroxime (100 mg/kg/24 hr) is recommended. If no clinical improvement is noted after several days or if *Mycoplasma pneumoniae* is suspected, oral erythromycin should be added.

A red blood cell transfusion is indicated for any hypoxic patient with sickle cell disease.[112] The indications for an exchange transfusion include (1) rapidly progressive respiratory deterioration and insufficiency (Pao_2 less than 60 mm Hg in an adult or less than 70 mm Hg in a child while breathing oxygen), or (2) multiple pulmonary lobe involvement, or both (see section on transfusion).

Sepsis-Infection. The major cause of morbidity and mortality in the child with sickle cell disease is infection. Encapsulated bacteria pose the most serious problem during the first 5 to 7 years of life.[113–115] Infections due to *S. pneumoniae, Neisseria meningitis, H. influenzae, Staphylococcus aureus, S. pyogenes, Salmonella* sp, and *M. pneumoniae* are most common, with *S. pneumoniae* being the most significant cause of fatal septicemia and meningitis (Table 62–8). In children less than 5 years of age, the risk of sepsis or meningitis is estimated to be greater than 15%.[116] After the first decade of life, anaerobic and enteric organisms become important pathogens. In general, all infections, including bacterial, viral (cytomegalovirus and rubeola), parasitic (malaria), and granulomatous (histoplasmosis, tuberculosis, and coccidiomycosis), disseminate more rapidly, are more difficult to treat, and result in significantly more morbidity and higher mortality in the child with sickle cell disease than in normal children. Parvovirus has been implicated in aplastic crises in children with sickle cell anemia.

The major immunologic deficiencies responsible for this increased susceptibility to infection include splenic dysfunction from autoinfarction, reticuloendothelial blockage from increased stasis of sickled erythrocytes in the microvascular beds of the spleen and liver, and reduced serum opsonic activity. By the end of the first year of life "functional asplenia," the inability to clear particulate matter from the blood, develops in patients with sickle cell anemia. The presence of Howell-Jolly bodies marks this change in splenic function.[117] By 6 to 7 years of age, the spleen has become fibrotic, calcified and nonpalpable because of repeated microvascular infarctions.[118] Although the levels of serum immunoglobulins are normal in patients with sickle cell disease, there is a deficiency in the heat-labile opsonizing activity.[119] There are also functional abnormalities in cell-mediated immunity in these patients.[120]

The diagnosis and treatment of osteomyelitis deserves special attention in the discussion of infections in the patient with sickle cell disease. In the child with fever, localized bone pain and swelling, and leukocytosis, it is very difficult to fully differentiate between an infarction and an infection involving the bone. In one study, it was noted that acute long bone infarction was 50 times more common than osteomyelitis.[121] All patients with bony infarcts complained of localized tenderness, 85% were noted to have overlying swelling, 68% had joint complaints, and 65% had localized warmth. Fourteen per cent were described as appearing toxic, and 21% were febrile with temperatures greater than 39° C. The total white blood cell count ranged from 7,200 to 43,000/mm³. Various radionuclide scans have been used to distinguish between infarction and osteomyelitis. If the test is performed early in the course of the event by experienced personnel, the radiologist may be helpful in making this distinction.[122, 123]

Prevention of infection in the child with sickle cell disease involves two major therapeutic approaches: (1) the use of pneumococcal and *Haemophilus* B conjugate vaccines and (2) antibiotic prophylaxis. The pediatric immunizations of diphtheria, pertussis, tetanus, measles, mumps, rubella, and polio should be given as regularly scheduled. The pneumococcal polysaccharide vaccine (Pneumovax 23, Merck Sharp & Dohme; or Pnu-imune-23, Lederle) contains 23 polysaccharide antigens, representing 90% of the most common serotypes causing infection in the United States.[124] The *Haemophilus* B conjugate vaccine (ProHIBit) is a combined vaccine of *Haemophilus* B capsular polysaccharide covalently bound to diphtheria toxoid. The diphtheria toxoid serves as a carrier protein and serves to enhance antibody response.[125, 126] The recombinant hepatitis B vaccine (Recombivax HB, Merck Sharp & Dohme) is recommended for all HBsAb-negative patients of any age who require blood transfusions.

Eighty per cent of pneumococcal sepsis in children less than 5 years of age can be prevented with the use of oral prophylactic penicillin.[127] Oral penicillin VK (125 mg twice daily until the child is 3 years of age and then 250 mg twice daily) is mandatory for all children with sickle cell disease, Hb SC disease, and Hb Sβ-thalassemia starting at 2 months of age.

Table 62–8. INFECTIONS IN SICKLE CELL DISEASE*

Infection	Etiology	No. of Episodes	%
Pneumonia†	No bacterial confirmation	344	82
	Pneumococci	29	7
	Enteric gram-negative rods	17	4
	Staphylococcus aureus	6	1
	Mycoplasma	5	1
	Salmonella	4	1
	Haemophilus influenzae	3	<1
	Others (measles, chickenpox, *Herellea*, *Streptococcus*, partially treated)	12	3
		420 (total)	
Meningitis†	Pneumococci	35	57
	Partially treated	13	21
	Haemophilus influenzae	5	8
	Aseptic	4	6
	Others (*Escherichia coli, Staphylococcus aureus, Streptococcus,* meningococci)	4	6
		61 (total)	
Osteomyelitis†‡	*Salmonella*	14	70
	Staphylococcus aureus	3	15
	Pneumococci	3	15
		20 (total)	
Sepsis§	Pneumococci	12	40
	Haemophilus influenzae	3	11
	Gram-negative enterics	3	11
	Salmonella	3	11
	Staphylococcus aureus	2	8
	Anaerobic bacteria	2	8
	Staphylococcus pyogenes	1	4
		26 (total)	
Urinary Tract†‖	*Escherichia coli*	35	63
	Klebsiella	15	27
	Proteus	2	4
	Other (*Staphylococcus aureus, Herellea vaginicola,* paracoli)	4	8
		56 (total)	

*From Platt OS and Nathan DG: Sickle cell disease. *In*: Nathan DG and Oski FA (eds): Hematology of Infancy and Childhood, 3rd ed. Philadelphia, WB Saunders, 1988, p. 671.
†Data from two retrospective studies (Barrett-Connor, Robinson): 859 patients (728 SS, 74 SC, 57 S thalassemia) for 4133 patient years.
‡Data from Overturf GD, Powars D, et al: 422 patients (323 SS, 83 SC, 16 other) for 3442 patient years.
§Bacteriologically confirmed cases only.
‖Single organism culture cases only.

Fever in a child with sickle cell anemia should be considered an emergent medical problem and is an indication for prompt medical attention. A complete physical examination and history may be helpful in identifying the possible site of infection. Laboratory evaluation should include a complete blood count and reticulocyte count; cultures of the blood, urine, and throat; and examination and culture of the cerebrospinal fluid in the young child or in the child in whom there is clinical concern about the possibility of meningitis. A chest x-ray film should also be included in the initial evaluation.

Parenteral antibiotic therapy should be instituted immediately and not delayed pending laboratory studies. Because of the high incidence of β-lactamase–resistant *H. influenzae* in this age group, an appropriate antibiotic such as cefuroxime (100 mg/kg/24 hr) or ceftriaxone (50 to 75 mg/kg/24 hr) should be used. In the older child, or if a β-lactamase–resistant organism has been ruled out, ampicillin (200 to 250 mg/kg/24 hr) may be used. The duration of parenteral antibiotic therapy is based upon culture results and the patient's subsequent evolving clinical condition. In the patient with sepsis indicated by positive blood culture results, therapy should be continued for at least 7 days. The length of therapy for the patient with bacterial meningitis is based on his or her clinical condition and the infecting organism.

In regard to appropriate management of osteomyelitis, definitive diagnosis can be made only with a positive culture result. In order to isolate the organism, needle aspiration should be performed early in the course of the disease. It is often difficult to differentiate between an acute bone or bone marrow infarct and osteomyelitis. Imaging studies performed early in the course of the illness may be helpful.[128] Radiographic evaluation should include plain films of the bone or joint, as well as ^{99m}Tc radionuclide bone scans. Imaging and localization of acute bone infections using ^{111}In-labeled white blood cells may be helpful in detecting osteomyelitis in selected patients in whom ^{99m}Tc bone images and radiographs are difficult to interpret.[129] The most common cause of osteomyelitis in sickle cell disease is *Salmonella*.[130, 131] Thus, therapy should include an antibiotic such as ampicillin or an appropriate third-generation cephalosporin such as ceftriaxone or cefotaxime.

Transfusion of blood products should be used for specific indications in the treatment of patients with sickle cell disease, keeping in mind the specific goal to be accomplished with the transfusion.

Indications include the following:

1. Improvement of oxygen-carrying capacity, as in patients who are extremely anemic (usually with hemoglobin concentrations less than 5 g/dl and hematocrit values of 15% or lower). Hypoxia ($PO_2 \leq 65$ mm Hg) or symptoms of excessive fatigue, dyspnea, irritability, postural hypotension, angina, or cerebral dysfunction are other indications for an emergent red blood cell transfusion.

2. Improvement in microvascular perfusion by decreasing the percentage of Hb S-containing red blood cells is another indication. Acute medical conditions that can be relieved by an emergent partial exchange transfusion include (1) impending or suspected CVAs, including transient ischemic events; (2) acute splenic or hepatic sequestration, as evidenced by rapid spleen or liver enlargement accompanied by a marked decline in the hemoglobin and hematocrit values; (3) acute priapism that is unresponsive to analgesia and intravenous hydration after 6 hours of treatment; (4) life-threatening infectious events such as sepsis, meningitis, or severe pneumonia; (5) rapidly progressive acute chest syndrome; and (6) fat embolization syndrome.

Partial exchange transfusions are also used in the following less emergent clinical situations:

1. When general inhalation anesthesia is required for a surgical procedure, the preparation includes a partial exchange transfusion. Another indication for a partial exchange transfusion includes procedures in which a limb will be fitted with a tourniquet or for vitrectomy. Most procedures that can be performed using local anesthesia do not require a preparative transfusion method.

2. A partial exchange transfusion may aid in the resolution of symptoms and other pulmonary findings associated with acute chest syndrome that fail to subside within 4 to 5 days from the onset.

3. Intractable painful events that fail to subside after 7 days or more may be alleviated by a partial exchange transfusion.

4. When radiographic contrast material is to be injected intravenously, and especially when given intra-arterially, a partial exchange transfusion is indicated prior to the injection.

Several chronic conditions warrant the continued and regular use of red blood cell transfusions in order to maintain the percentage of sickled hemoglobin at less than 30%:

1. Transfusions should be continued for at least 3 years following a CVA.

2. Leg ulcers develop in 8 to 10% of patients with sickle cell disease. When the healing of these ulcers is delayed or they progress with persistent hyperpigmentation and induration of the surrounding skin, transfusions should be instituted for at least 6 months in order to aid in the healing process. Subsequent skin grafting may be avoided by a short period of transfusion therapy.

3. The role of chronic transfusion during pregnancy is controversial. The risks of prophylactic transfusion versus potential gain have yet to be examined in this clinical setting.[132, 133]

Transfusions are not indicated in sickle cell anemia for chronic steady state anemia in patients who are asymptomatic. There is no proven reason to transfuse for minor infections, uncomplicated painful episodes, or minor surgical procedures in which general anesthesia is not used.

Standard sickle cell–negative bank blood is appropriate for most patients with sickle cell anemia. All patients with a history of previous transfusions should be carefully screened for the presence of autoantibodies. In patients with a history of allergic reactions following prior red blood cell transfusions, washed or frozen reconstituted blood is indicated. Packed red blood cells is the product of choice, except when the elevated hematocrit level of the transfused blood could predispose the patient to increased blood viscosity.[134] In this situation, blood can be diluted with 0.9% normal saline in a closed system. When an immediate correction in the oxygen-carrying is necessary, exchange transfusion using blood less than 5 days old (less than 3 days old in the young infant) is recommended.

The simple transfusion is indicated in a patient on a chronic transfusion protocol, in preparation for surgery, or emergently when an acute hemolytic or aplastic event is suspected. A general rule is to transfuse packed red blood cells at 10 to 12 ml/kg over 2 to 3 hours, unless the hemoglobin level is lower than 5 g/dl. In this case, it is safer to infuse 5 ml/kg initially followed by close monitoring for cardiovascular overload. A second or third 5 ml/kg transfusion may be given subsequently. However, it is extremely important to avoid transfusing to a hemoglobin value over 12 g/dl as this degree of hyperviscosity may potentiate intravascular sickling.

The partial exchange transfusion is indicated in those clinical situations in which a rapid decrement in the percentage of sickled hemoglobin is needed. In some patients, whole blood can be removed from one arm at the same time that donor cells are transfused into the other arm. In the adult, 500-ml aliquots may be used, but in children automated methods using either continuous or discontinuous flow blood processors may be used more safely.[135] In very small children, less than 25 to 30 kg, an automated exchange transfusion may be complicated because of limitations of vessel size precluding the use of larger bore intravenous catheters, and in the case of discontinuous flow blood processors, by the excessive extracorporial blood volume.[136, 137]

The goal in using an exchange transfusion is to safely lower the sickle cell concentration to less than 30% while maintaining the hematocrit value at less than 36%. This is accomplished by using a total donor blood volume that is proportional to the patient's body weight and hematocrit value. The patient's total blood volume should remain constant throughout the procedure. The absolute amount of blood to be exchanged is a function of the patient's blood volume, which is approximated at 80 ml/kg body weight. The patient should be exposed to the least number of donor units given over the shortest, yet safest, period.[138] Different formulas are needed based on different initial hematocrit values and the desired final concentration of sickleable cells; the rate and type of exchange (continuous or discontinuous) are less important variables.[139, 140]

If the initial hematocrit value is lower than 15%, exchange should be performed with a packed red blood cell volume in amount equal to 4% of the patient's body weight. Thus, for a 25-kg child, the exchange transfusion should consist of 1,000 ml of donor packed red blood cells for 1,000 ml of whole blood removed from the patient.

When the hematocrit value is between 16 and 30%, the following exchange is recommended: First a donor packed red blood cell volume in an amount equal to 4% of the patient's body weight is transfused, as already described. This is then followed with an exchange transfusion using a donor whole blood volume in amount equal to 3% of the patient's body weight. Thus, for a 25-kg child, the first exchange consists of 1,000 ml of donor packed red blood cells for 1,000 ml of whole blood removed from the patient. The following exchange consists of 750 ml of donor whole blood for 750 ml of whole blood removed from the patient.

When the starting hematocrit value is greater than 30%, the patient's whole blood is removed first while replacing with a normal saline volume in amount equal to 0.8% of the patient's body weight. An exchange transfusion with a donor packed red blood cell volume in amount equal to 4% of the patient's body weight then takes place. This is followed with an exchange using a donor whole blood volume in amount equal to 4% of the patient's body weight. Thus, for a 25-kg child, 200 ml of the patient's whole blood is removed while 200 ml of normal saline is infused. The transfusion exchange of 1,000 ml of donor packed red blood cells for 1,000 ml of whole blood removed from the patient then takes place. This is followed with an exchange of 1,000 ml of donor whole blood for 1,000 ml of whole blood removed from the patient.[141]

The preceding calculations are based on the assumption that packed red blood cells usually have a hematocrit value near 70%, whereas the whole blood hematocrit value is close to 35%. Packed red blood cells may be diluted using normal saline to a hematocrit value of 35% and thus can be used instead of whole blood.[142]

A chronic transfusion program is used to maintain the percentage of Hb S at a constant value less than 30%. This regimen may be continued for a period of months to years and is primarily used for the patient who has suffered a CVA in order to prevent a recurrence. Once a sufficient level of normal cells (Hb A >70%) has been achieved, a simple transfusion of packed red blood cells infused at 3- to 4-week intervals will usually maintain the Hb S level at less than 30%.

The following complications must be considered in any patient receiving a red blood cell transfusion. For a more detailed discussion, the reader is referred to Chapter 63. Acutely, volume overload must be remembered in the patient receiving a large volume of blood given over a short period. As always, allergic reactions, including anaphylaxis, must be considered during the transfusion and immediately afterward. Other transfusion reactions, including delayed hemolysis, have also been described.[143, 144] In the patient who is receiving red blood cell transfusions on a chronic protocol, iron overload and alloimmunization to red blood cell antigens are two other complications.[145] Alloimmunization is a common and potentially serious problem in sickle cell anemia and is partially due to racial differences between the blood donor and recipient populations.[146–148] Hepatitis and other transmissible infectious diseases occur with the same frequency in patients with sickle cell disease as in the general population, yet the effects are far more severe in these patients.

Priapism is a persistent, sometimes painful, uncontrollable engorgement and erection of the penis. This distressing complication of sickle cell disease may occur at any age, with a median age of onset of 21 years. In one study, the frequency of priapism was estimated to be as high as 42%.[149]

Several distinct clinical patterns of priapism have been recognized.[150]

1. *Stuttering* priapism occurs with multiple, short, and reversible episodes of painful penile erections with detumescence within hours. Sexual dysfunction is less likely to occur with this pattern.[151] Episodes can be repetitive, are relatively short in duration, and are less painful than some of the other patterns.

2. *Severe* and *prolonged* (>24 hours) episodes may last for days to weeks. This pattern is usually accompanied by extreme pain, followed by impotence and complicated by urinary retention.[152]

3. Engorgement may persist for weeks to years. This pattern is often painless, may occur after a prolonged attack, and often results in complete or partial impotence.

The specific pathophysiologic mechanism precipitating priapism in men with sickle cell disease is not fully understood. Acute attacks may follow sexual activity, occur during sleep, or happen with no associated event. In general, the venous outflow from the corpora cavernosa is partially occluded, leading to a viscous sludge of deoxygenated and sickled erythrocytes. Further venous outflow continues, with resultant edema and inflammation.

Treatment follows the general management of a patient with sickle cell disease who suffers from a vasoocclusive event. With mild, repetitive, and self-limited episodes, patients may be managed on an outpatient basis. Oral hydration and analgesia should be encouraged. Some symptomatic relief may be achieved by emptying the bladder frequently, engaging in mild physical exercise, and taking tepid sitz baths. Extremes in temperature, especially the use of ice packs, are not recommended, as intravascular sludging may be exacerbated. If the episode does not resolve in 3 to 5 hours, medical attention should be sought.

The initial physical examination includes massage of the prostate, which may induce detumescence. If infection is suspected, prostatic fluid should be sent for culture to rule out prostatitis as an underlying cause for the priapism. A complete blood count and reticulocyte count should be obtained, as well as a blood culture specimen if the patient is febrile or infection is suspected.

With the acute and prolonged episodes, treatment should include intravenous hydration and analgesia using parenteral narcotics (as outlined previously in the section on management of the vaso-occlusive event.)[153] A Foley catheter may be needed to promote bladder emptying. A partial or complete exchange transfusion should be considered. By reducing the percentage of sickled red blood cells to less than 30% and the hematocrit value to less than 45%, the course of the episode may be greatly shortened.[154, 155] Usually, patients who respond to transfusion therapy will show improvement within a few days; however, complete detumescence may take months.

If detumescence has not begun 24 hours after a complete exchange transfusion, response to continued pheresis is unlikely, and surgical intervention should be undertaken. A Winter procedure (or a modification thereof) under local anesthesia should be performed by an experienced pediatric urologic surgeon.[156] Using a needle or scalpel, a corpus spongiosum shunt is achieved by creating a fistula between the glans and the corpora cavernosa.[157] Intermittent compression is applied to limit re-engorgement. Continuous drainage is promoted because a small communication at the skin closure site connecting to the newly created fistula remains patent. The shunt will spontaneously close over a period of weeks, or it can be closed surgically. In most cases, subsequent erectile function is unaltered. A larger corpus spongiosum shunt at the base of the penis may be placed under general anesthesia if the preceding procedure does not result in detumescence after 48 to 72 hours.

If no intervention is undertaken to treat severe, unrelenting episodes of priapism, it is estimated that partial to complete impotence will occur in more than 80% of cases. With judicious use of exchange transfusions and appropriate surgical intervention, the incidence can be reduced to 25 to 50%.[158]

In the chronic long-lasting form of priapism, sexual dysfunction is more common, though severe pain is less likely. Implantation of a prosthesis is recommended by some urologists in these cases; however, few cases have been described involving patients with sickle cell disease.

Pain Crisis. Intravascular erythrocyte sickling results in diminished blood flow, resulting in regional hypoxia and acidosis, which promotes further sickling and results in ischemic tissue damage.[159] The clinical manifestations often include acute, painful events. The organs most commonly involved include the bones, lungs, spleen, liver, brain, and penis. These episodes may persist from several days to weeks. Precipitating events include fever, infection, dehydration, acidosis, hypoxia, localized tissue injury, or exposure to temperature extremes.

Musculoskeletal discomfort is the most common type of pain. The underlying pathologic condition of acute bone pain is usually ischemia or infarction of the bone marrow.[160] In the infant, the first manifestation of sickle cell disease may be dactylitis.[161] This painful, fusiform swelling of the hands or feet, or both, may present with irritability and refusal to use the hands or bear weight. In the older child, vaso-occlusive events are more variable and are sometimes associated with localized warmth and swelling and low-grade fevers.[162] Often, it is extremely difficult to differentiate a painful bone crisis from an infectious cause such as osteomyelitis or septic arthritis (see section on sepsis-infection).

Abdominal pain is the second most common source of pain in the child with sickle cell disease. As with bone pain, it may be diagnostically difficult to distinguish ischemic pain resulting from an infarction from other infectious or surgical causes of an acute abdomen. The differential diagnosis should include other surgical causes, such as acute appendicitis or obstruction, as well as infectious causes, including urinary tract infections, pelvic inflammatory disease, severe gastroenteritis, pancreatitis, or cholecystitis.[163] Pneumonia may result in pain referred to the upper abdomen.

Evaluation of the patient with pain should include a complete blood count with reticulocyte count. An elevation of the total white blood cell count with a leftward shift should raise suspicion of an underlying or associated infectious cause of the pain crisis. Specimens of the blood, throat, and urine should be obtained for culture if a fever is present. If there are any respiratory symptoms present, a chest x-ray film and arterial blood gas determinations are indicated. Plain films of the affected limb or joint are not always helpful but are indicated if an infectious cause such as osteomyelitis or septic arthritis is suspected or if there has been a history of trauma. A radioisotope bone scan done early in the course of the event may help to make the distinction between a bone infarct and osteomyelitis. Serum electrolyte determinations are indicated in the dehydrated or acutely ill patient. Occasionally, the patient may present in pain, yet the history is unclear or there is no medical documentation available that the patient does indeed have sickle cell anemia versus sickle cell trait or another hematologic disorder. In this case, a blood sample should be obtained and sent for confirmation by hemoglobin electrophoresis. However, treatment should not be delayed pending these results.

In all painful crises, one should try to identify an underlying and precipitating illness. If sepsis or other infection is considered, appropriate antibiotic therapy should be instituted immediately.

General measures to help prevent pain crises include educating the patient and family to avoid hypoxia, dehydration, and extremes in temperature, especially cold. Patients should avoid flying in unpressurized aircraft, excessive physical activity at mountain altitudes, and swimming in frigid water.

Intravascular sickling is promoted by dehydration; thus, the child's hydration status should be closely assessed. Because of the frequency of hyposthenuria, one cannot rely on the urine specific gravity to assess hydration status. Fever and pain result in increased insensible water loss and decreased oral fluid intake. Oral hydration may successfully correct the condition in the child who is in mild pain, but intravenous fluids are recommended in the young child or when the child is experiencing a severe painful crisis. Following an appropriate intravenous fluid bolus, fluids should be continued at 1½ to 2 times maintenance levels (150 to 200 ml/kg/24 hr). Electrolyte values and the patient's hydration status will dictate the type of fluids, but in the uncomplicated case, D_5 1/4 NS or D_5 1/3 NS may be safely used. It

Table 62–9. RECOMMENDED DOSE AND INTERVAL OF ANALGESICS NECESSARY TO OBTAIN ADEQUATE PAIN CONTROL IN SICKLE CELL DISEASE*

	Dose-Rate	Comments
Severe-Moderate Pain		
1. Morphine	0.15 mg/kg/dose q 3–4 hr (IV, SC, IM PCA†) 0.6 mg/kg/dose q 4 hr (PO)	Drug of choice for pain; lower doses in aged, liver failure, and impaired ventilation.
2. Meperidine (Demerol)	1.5 mg/kg/dose q 2–4 hr (IM, IV) 1.5 mg/kg/dose q 4 hr (PO)	Increased incidence of seizures. Avoid in patients with renal or neurologic disease or who receive monoamine oxidase inhibitors.
3. Hydromorphone (Dilaudid)	0.02 mg/kg/dose (IM, IV) q 3–4 hr 0.04 mg/kg/dose q 4 hr (PO)	
4. Oxycodone	5–10 mg/dose q 4 hr (PO)	
Mild Pain		
1. Codeine	1.0 mg/kg/dose (PO) q 4 hr	Drug of choice for mild to moderate pain not relieved by aspirin or acetaminophen.
2. Propoxyphene	65 mg/dose (PO) q 4 hr (100 mg as napsylate)	Not recommended for children. A narcotic with addiction potential. Toxic metabolites accumulate with repetitive dosing.
Mild Pain‡		
3. Aspirin	0.3–0.6 g/dose (PO) q 4 hr (adults) 8 mg/kg/dose (children)	Often given with a narcotic to enhance analgesia. Can cause gastric irritation.
4. Acetaminophen (Tylenol)	0.3–0.6 g (PO) q 4 hr (adults) 8 mg/kg/dose (children)	Often given with a narcotic to enhance analgesia. Can cause gastric irritation.
5. Ibuprofen	300–400 mg/dose (PO) q 4 hr	Not FDA approved for children. Can cause gastric irritation.
6. Naproxen	250 mg/dose (PO) q 12 hr	Long duration of action. Can cause gastric irritation.
7. Indomethacin	25 mg/dose (PO) q 4–8 hr	Contraindicated in psychiatric, neurologic, renal diseases. Can cause gastric irritation. Useful in gout.
8. Tolmetin	400 mg (PO) q 8 hr	Approved for children.

*From Charache S, Lubin B, and Reid C: Acute splenic sequestration and aplastic crisis. *In*: Management and Therapy of Sickle Cell Disease. Washington, DC, NIH Publication No. 89–2117:17, 1989.

†Continuous intravenous infusion, patient-controlled analgesic (PCA) devices and continuous subcutaneous infusion are useful in pain control but should be performed only by institutions familiar with their use.

‡Other useful mild analgesics: piroxicam, sulindoc, tolmetin.

must be kept in mind that hyposthenuria, renal tubular dysfunction, papillary necrosis, and chronic renal failure are all common renal complications experienced by patients with sickle cell disease, and they begin early in the first decade of life. Serum electrolyte levels should be checked at least daily. Urine output and the subsequent hydration status should be closely monitored to avoid electrolyte imbalances or congestive heart failure as evidenced by clinical changes such as rales, tachypnea, tachycardia, gallop rhythm, hepatomegaly, or excessive weight gain.

The choice and route of administration of analgesic therapy should be guided by the drug's potency, mode of action, and side effects. Pain and patient anxiety can best be alleviated by administering the analgesics on a fixed time schedule and using a dosing interval that does not extend beyond the duration of the desired pharmacologic effect.[164] Although the oral route of administration avoids many complications associated with parenteral administration, the oral route is less than one-half as effective as the parenteral route. The side effects of narcotics must be considered. In general, they include respiratory depression, hypotension, altered seizure threshold, nausea, vomiting, and constipation. Synthetic narcotics such as pentazocine, butorphanol, and nalbuphine should not be used because of antagonistic induction of withdrawal symptoms or psychotomimetic effects.

Patient-controlled analgesia (PCA) has been used successfully in treating pain in sickle cell patients and can provide better analgesia than conventional IM or IV narcotic therapy and in general is associated with fewer side effects.

Non-narcotic analgesics should be tried first for the outpatient management of mild pain. Aspirin is not recommended for the pediatric age group because of its association with Reye syndrome. Acetaminophen is the oral analgesic of choice. The recommended dose of acetaminophen is 8 to 10 mg/kg/dose given every 4 to 6 hours. High doses can result in hepatic toxicity. Analgesia may be enhanced by combining with a narcotic such as codeine (elixer: 120 mg of acetaminophen and 12 mg of codeine/5 ml; tablets: 300 mg of acetaminophen with 7.5 mg of codeine (No. 1), with 15 mg of codeine (No. 2), with 30 mg of codeine (No. 3), or with 60 mg of codeine (No. 4). The recommended dose of codeine is 0.5 to 1 mg/kg/dose every 4 hours.[165]

Nonsteroidal anti-inflammatory oral agents such as ibuprofen and naproxen may also be useful. Ketorolac tromethamine is the first parenteral nonsteroidal anti-inflammatory drug successfully used in treating muscle pain in sickle cell disease.

If outpatient management has failed or if the patient presents with severe pain, parenteral narcotics should be started in the clinic or emergency room (Table 62–9). Hospitalization may be necessary. Pain medications should be given on a fixed schedule. Dosing and dosing intervals are based on the severity and type of pain.[166] Continuous infusion may be necessary initially until acute pain control is achieved. In the older child and adolescent, use of patient-controlled analgesia (PCA) is an alternative if appropriate medical expertise is available.[167] Other new techniques of analgesic medication delivery include subcutaneous opiate infusion[168] and epidural administration of morphine.[169, 170] There is limited experience using these techniques to control pain from sickle cell disease. Diazepam and chlorpromazine do not potentiate the analgesic effect of narcotics and should be avoided unless there is an additional need for a potent tranquilizer.

As adjunct therapies for pain management, alternative techniques include relaxation therapy, self-hypnosis, behavioral modification programs, and transcutaneous electrical nerve stimulation.[171] These approaches are obviously not indicated in the very young child. Oxygen therapy is not beneficial in the treatment of vaso-occlusive events unless hypoxia is present.

Sodium bicarbonate intravenous infusion is not indicated in the treatment of painful crises unless severe acidosis is present.

Gallbladder and Liver Disease. Because of the ongoing and constant state of red blood cell hemolysis, the total serum bilirubin level is chronically elevated in patients with sickle cell anemia. If the liver is functioning at maximum efficiency and is able to maintain a steady state of bilirubin metabolism, the total serum bilirubin level should not be more than 4 mg/dl and the conjugated fraction should not constitute more than 10% of the total bilirubin. Elevated serum alkaline phosphatase and lactic dehydrogenase levels are frequently caused by hemolysis and bone metabolism and do not necessarily reflect liver insufficiency. Because there is often a component of intrahepatic biliary obstruction associated with transient or chronic hepatic dysfunction, an elevation in total serum bilirubin levels may also be accompanied by an increase in the conjugated fraction.

Gallstones composed of bile or calcium bilirubinate are present in approximately 30% of children with sickle cell anemia and in 70% of patients by 30 years of age. Although gallstones may remain asymptomatic for years, acute complications include cholecystitis, episodes of extreme colicky pain associated with passage of stones, common bile duct obstruction, and acute pancreatitis.[172]

Symptoms associated with gallstones include nausea, vomiting, right upper quadrant pain, and bloating after eating. With episodes of biliary colic, the patient may complain of diffuse or localized central abdominal pain. Acute cholecystitis may be difficult to differentiate from pain caused by intrahepatic sickling. In the presence of gallstones, fever, nausea, vomiting, and abdominal pain are consistent with acute cholecystitis.

In sickle cell disease, only 50% of gallstones are radiopaque; thus, an oral cholecystogram or abdominal ultrasound is indicated.[173-175] A chest radiograph should be obtained because pneumonia should be entertained as a potential source in the child complaining of abdominal or chest pain.

An acute event similar to acute splenic sequestration may involve the liver. An intrahepatic vaso-occlusive crisis results in sudden, painful enlargement of the liver accompanied by a dramatic rise in the bilirubin and liver enzyme levels.[176]

Acute cholecystitis should be treated conservatively with hydration while monitoring for electrolyte imbalances. Appropriate antibiotic therapy and analgesia should be used. Elective cholecystectomy should be delayed until the acute attack has subsided but before adhesions can form around the gallbladder, usually about 6 weeks after the attack. Emergency surgery should be avoided unless there is evidence of obstruction.[177]

For asymptomatic gallstones, delaying surgery is generally recommended until symptoms occur and become chronic. For mild, vague right upper quadrant abdominal discomfort, avoiding fatty foods, along with administration of antispasmodic agents such as dicyclomine (Bentyl) may give some symptomatic relief.

The patient with suspected biliary obstruction as evidenced by right upper quadrant pain, unstable vital signs, and hyperbilirubinemia should be admitted for intravenous hydration and close observation. Deteriorating renal function and accompanying coagulopathy should be anticipated in the patient with progressive liver disease. Partial thromboplastin time, prothrombin time, platelet count, and fibrin split products should be monitored along with liver function studies and serum amylase determination.[178] Coagulation abnormalities and factor deficiencies should be treated with appropriate component therapy and platelet transfusion as indicated. An endoscopic retrograde cholangiopancreatoscopy may be useful for identifying a common bile duct obstruction. Pancreatitis should be considered in the differential diagnosis. Surgery should be involved in the management of these patients. If emergent cholecystectomy is indicated, the patient must receive an appropriate red blood cell transfusion or exchange transfusion in preparation for the surgery (see section on transfusion).

Sickle Cell Trait

Sickle cell trait is the condition in which an individual has one βS globin gene and a normal βA globin gene, thus resulting in the phenotypic expression of Hb AS. Eight per cent of the American black population carries the sickle cell trait. This condition is diagnosed by hemoglobin electrophoresis. These children have normal hemoglobin and hematocrit levels.

This condition does not result in anemia, nor do individuals experience vaso-occlusive events under normal physiologic conditions. Unlike patients with the homozygous condition, sickle cell disease, these children have a normal life expectancy. It has been observed that individuals with sickle cell trait may have hyposthenuria and benign hematuria. There is also an increased risk for urinary tract infections during pregnancy in these individuals.[179] Individuals with sickle cell trait do have an increased risk of elevated intraocular pressure associated with traumatic hyphemas and so require immediate ophthalmologic management for this condition.[180] A retrospective study of soldiers in basic training demonstrated that individuals with sickle cell trait had an increased risk of sudden death following extreme exertion when compared with soldiers with Hb A. The magnitude of the risk was quite small and was age-related.[181] There was no similar observation made for individuals who participate in strenuous athletic events. There is also no increased risk for individuals with sickle cell trait who undergo surgical procedures under general anesthesia. Splenic infarction has been reported as a result of flying in an unpressurized airplane at 15,000 feet.[182, 183]

Hemoglobin C Disease

Hemoglobin C (Hb C) is due to a single amino acid substitution at the same site of substitution as in Hb S but with lysine instead of valine substituted for glutamic acid at the β6 position. Homozygous Hb C disease is manifested by a mild hemolytic anemia with splenomegaly. The peripheral smear may demonstrate the presence of numerous target cells. Heterozygous individuals are clinically normal.

Hemoglobin SC Disease

Patients with Hb SC disease are double heterozygotes. These patients have a less severe hemolytic anemia and clinical course than do patients with classic sickle cell disease. However, patients with Hb SC disease are more likely to develop retinopathy and ischemic bone necrosis than are patients with homozygous Hb SS. Treatment for sickling manifestations and anemia should be carried out as outlined for patients with sickle cell disease.

UNSTABLE HEMOGLOBINS AND METHEMOGLOBINOPATHY

The general category of unstable hemoglobins (congenital Heinz body hemolytic anemia) refers to a heterogeneous group of anemias that result from structural changes in the amino acid composition of the globin chains. These hemolytic anemias have an autosomal dominant pattern of inheritance.[184] The majority of these mutations affect the β-globin chain and result in amino acid replacements within the heme cavity of the hemoglobin molecule. Substitutions in this region of heme attachment result in marked molecular instability of the globin-heme secondary structure. Once heme becomes displaced, the globin subunits dissociate from their tetrameric structure and aggregate to form intracellular precipitates referred to as Heinz bodies. These cells have decreased deformability characteristics and are trapped in the microcirculation, especially in the splenic sinusoids. More than 90 structural variants have been characterized.[185, 186]

The hereditary methemoglobinopathies are also due to globin amino acid substitutions in the region of heme attachment, but in this case the result is an increased susceptibility to oxidation of heme Fe^{2+} to Fe^{3+}. The consequence of this conversion is the accumulation of methemoglobin and clinical cyanosis rather than hemolysis. This condition is inherited in an autosomal recessive manner.

In congenital methemoglobinopathy and in many forms of unstable hemoglobinopathy, there is an increase in oxygen affinity, resulting in greater tissue anoxia and increased erythropoeitin stimulation. Thus, polycythemia may be a clinical manifestation, (e.g., Hb Chesapeake).

Because of the heterogeneity in the number of possible amino acid substitutions and deletions, there is a great deal of variability in the clinical features among the various types of unstable hemoglobinopathies. Usually these children present during the neonatal period or infancy with a nonspherocytic hemolytic anemia accompanied by jaundice and splenomegaly. Hemolysis may be aggravated by fever, infection, or an oxidant drug. During periods of brisk hemolysis, dark urine may be observed. Symptoms of lethargy, fatigue, jaundice, and paleness should alert the clinician of an acute episode of hemolysis. Red blood cell morphologic features may demonstrate microcytosis or hypochromia with prominent basophilic stippling. Upon incubation of red blood cells with brilliant blue or methyl violet, Heinz bodies and "bite" cells may become apparent.

Methemoglobinemia is clinically characterized by slate gray cyanosis, which is often initially mistaken as a sign of underlying pulmonary or cardiac disease. In this disease state, however, the degree of cyanosis is out of proportion to the hypoxic symptomatology.[187] The clinical sequalae of methemoglobinemia result from the reduced oxygen-carrying capacity and tissue hypoxia. Methemoglobin levels of 25 to 30% may be symptomatic, but with increasing concentrations to 35 to 40%, symptoms of exercise intolerence and headache are observed. Extreme fatigue and decreased levels of consciousness are observed with levels of 50 to 60%.[188] Levels greater than 70% are incompatible with life. Numerous drugs and chemical agents have the capacity to expose the susceptible erythrocyte to oxidant stress, resulting in an increased intracellular content of methemoglobin (Table 62–10).

Although anemia associated with unstable hemoglobinopathies is rarely severe enough to require red blood cell transfusions, episodes of brisk hemolysis or transient bone marrow aplasia may result in a significant drop in the hemoglobin value over a relatively short time. In these cases, red blood cell transfusions given judiciously are warranted. Prophylactic treatment with folic acid may be beneficial. Some benefit may be seen following splenectomy, but this procedure should be weighed against the risks of postsplenectomy sepsis and the fact that this procedure is curative for the underlying hemolytic anemia.

The management of methemoglobinemia, regardless of cause, is based on the degree of hypoxia (Table 62–11). Most patients require no therapy. For moderate methemoglobinemia, oral methylene blue is indicated. The oral dose is determined empirically. An average oral dose is 1.5 to 5 mg/kg/24 hr divided into four daily doses, to a maximum adult dose of 300 mg/24 hr.[189] For severe hypoxia, methylene blue is given intravenously at a dose of 1 to 2 mg/kg as a 1% solution in normal saline infused over 5 minutes. This will usually reduce the percentage of methemoglobin to less than 1% in less than 1 hour.[190] If further therapy is needed, it can usually be accomplished by continuing with oral dosing until the level of methemoglobin has decreased. Side

Table 62–10. METHEMOGLOBIN-GENERATING CHEMICALS*

Acetanilide	Hydroxylacetanilid	Phenols
Acetophenetidin	Hydroxylamine	Phenylazopyridine
Alloxans	Inks, marking	Phenylenediamine
α-Naphthylamine	Kiszka	Phenylhydrazine
Aminophenols	Lidocaine	Phenylhydroxylamine
Ammonium nitrate	Menthol	Phenytoin (Dilantin)
Amyl nitrite	Meta-chloraniline	Piperazine
Aniline dyes	Methylacetanilide	Plasmoquine
Anilinoethanol	Methylene blue	Prilocaine
Antipyrine	Monochloroaniline	Primaquine
Arsine	Moth balls	Propitocaine
Benzocaine	Naphthylamines	Pyridium
Bismuth subnitrate	Nitrates	Pyrogallol
Chlorates	Nitrites	Pyridine
Chloroanilines	Nitrobenzene	Quinones
Chlorobenzene	Nitrogen oxide	Resorcinol
Chloronitrobenzene	Nitrofurans	Shoe dye or polish
Cobalt preparations	Nitroglycerin	Spinach
Corning extract	Nitrophenol	Sulfonal
Crayons, wax (red or orange)†	Nitrosobenzene	Sulfonamides
Dapsone	Pamaquine	Sulfones
Diaminodiphenylsulfone	Para-aminopropiophenone	Tetranitromethane tetronal
Diesel fuel additives	Para-bromoaniline	Tetralin
Dimethylamine	Para-chloronaniline	Toluenediamine
Dimethylaniline	Para-nitroaniline	Toluidine
Dinitrobenzenes	Para-toluidine	Toluylhydroxylamine
Dinitrophenol	Pentaerythritol tetranitrate	Trichlorocarbanilide (TCC)
Dinitrotoluene	Phenacetin	Trinitrotoluene
Hydroquinone	Phenetidine	Trional

*From Feig S: Disorders of hemoglobin. *In*: Nathan DG and Oski FA (eds): Hematology of Infancy and Childhood, 3rd ed. Philadelphia, WB Saunders, 1988, p. 648; from Curry S: Methemoglobinemia. Ann Emerg Med 11:214, 1982. (Table untitled by original author.)
†No longer manufactured.

effects include nausea, vomiting, abdominal or precordial pain, headache, diaphoresis, and blue-green discoloration of the urine. Methylene blue is contraindicated in G6PD deficiency.[191]

An alternative for chronic therapy is ascorbic acid (5 to 8 mg/kg/24 hr divided into three or four doses daily). However, this is usually not as effective as methylene blue, and continued use has been associated with hyperoxaluria and nephrolithiasis.[192]

Thalassemia

The thalassemias are hereditary anemias resulting from a decrease in either α- or β-globin chain synthesis. The genetic defect may be either a point mutation or a larger deletion mutation involving the promoter, splicing, or polyadenylation elements of the gene.[193] Other

mutations that affect messenger ribonucleic acid (mRNA) translation or globin stability have also been described.[194] The result is a decrease in the expression of the globin chain at the protein level. The milder forms are among the most frequent genetic defects in humans, whereas the more severe forms, although less common, can result in chronic anemia with significant morbidity and mortality.

Two polypeptides, α and β, compose adult hemoglobin in equivalent ratios. In α thalassemia, there is a decrease or complete lack of α-globin synthesis, whereas in β-thalassemia, β-globin protein expression is diminished or lacking.

An imbalance in the α- and β-globin chain expression results in a decrease in the complementary pairs of tetrameric globin chains. These erythrocytes have a decreased amount of intracellular hemoglobin and thus appear hypochromic and microcytic. The severity of the

Table 62–11. CLINICAL APPROACH TO METHEMOGLOBINEMIA*

Severity (% Methemoglobin)	Symptoms	Treatment
10–30	Cyanosis	None
30–50	Headache, exercise intolerance	Methylene blue, oral; dose determined empirically
50–70	Altered consciousness	Methylene blue, 1–2 mg/kg IV push: (a) if improvement, oral methylene blue until oxidant stress eliminated; (b) if no improvement, exchange transfusion (consider hexose monophosphate shunt defect)
>70	May be rapidly fatal	

*From Feig S: Disorders of hemoglobin. *In*: Nathan DG and Oski FA (eds): Hematology of Infancy and Childhood, 3rd ed. Philadelphia, WB Saunders, 1988, p. 650.

anemia reflects the degree of α- or β-globin synthesis. The genetic mutation affecting either the α- or β-globin gene and whether the defect involves one (heterozygous) or both (homozygous) of the chromosomes determines the severity of the anemia.[195]

α-Thalassemia

α-Thalassemia is usually due to large deletions within the α-globin gene cluster on chromosome 16. These mutations result in the deletion of one (α⁺) or both (α⁰) globin genes. Less commonly, a single base pair point mutation may also result in α-thalassemia.[196] α-Thalassemia is more commonly observed in individuals of African, Malaysian, Indochinese, or Chinese ancestry.

Because of the diversity of potential deletions, there is a great deal of phenotypic heterogeneity displayed among individuals with α-thalassemia. The silent carrier has three rather than the usual complement of four functional α-globin genes. These individuals have a MCV that is slightly lower than in normal individuals. In infants with this genetic deletion, hemoglobin Bart (tetrameric structural formula of four γ-chains) may be slightly elevated in the newborn period. There is usually no significant amount of anemia noted, and these individuals remain asymptomatic.

When there is decreased expression of two of the four α-globin genes, this syndrome is referred to as α-thalassemia trait. This syndrome occurs with higher frequency in individuals of Asian origin and less frequently in American blacks and in individuals of African and Mediterranean ancestry. These individuals have a mild to moderate microcytic, hypochromic anemia and demonstrate a decreased α-chain:β-chain ratio. The diagnosis is often difficult to make, and this type of anemia is often incorrectly labeled as an anemia of iron deficiency.[197]

Hemoglobin H (Hb H) disease is due to a deletion of three of the usual four α-globin genes. These individuals demonstrate a hemolytic anemia of moderate severity. Erythrocytes have hypochromic, microcytic morphologic features with fragmentation. Hemoglobin electrophoresis or measurement of the α-chain:β-chain ratio may help with the diagnosis of this condition.[198]

Hydrops fetalis is a homozygous condition resulting in lack of production of α-globin. These infants are severely anemic, resulting in congestive heart failure, and are born grossly hydropic. Death usually occurs in utero or shortly after birth.[199]

The child who is a silent carrier or the individual with α-thalassemia trait rarely requires regular red blood cell transfusions. However, the patient with Hb H disease may require red blood cell transfusions on a chronic basis. Complications include growth failure, frontal bossing, splenomegaly, and bone changes due to marrow hyperplasia. Iron overload may be present secondary to the increased iron turnover and chronic transfusion therapy. Splenectomy may be considered in the child with hypersplenism, especially if the syndrome of splenic entrapment (leukopenia, thrombocytopenia, and progressive anemia) becomes an additional clinical problem.[200] Few children with hydrops fetalis have survived, but they require chronic transfusion therapy.[201]

β-Thalassemia

β-Thalassemia is caused by a deletional mutation of the β-globin gene cluster located on chromosome 11. Each normal diploid cell contains two β-globin genes, yet the degree of clinical heterogeneity of the β-thalassemias is explained by the great variability in protein expression specific for the position and extent of the deletion. Some mutations completely abolish any β-globin protein, whereas others merely result in a downregulation of protein expression.[202, 203] The symbol β⁰ is usually used to denote a lack of detectable β-chain synthesis because of the lack of β-chain mRNA. Decreased β-chain synthesis because of reduced or nonfunctional β-chain mRNA is denoted by β⁺.[204]

Like α-thalassemia, the resulting hemolytic anemia is caused by an imbalance in the α-chain:β-chain ratio. In most individuals with β-thalassemia, there is a coincident increase in the γ- and δ-globin chain expression, resulting in an increase in the fetal and Hb A2 components over the normal range.[205]

β-Thalassemia occurs more frequently in individuals of Mediterranean and African origin, but it is also prevalent in areas of India, the Middle East, Pakistan, and China.

The heterozygous states of β-thalassemia result from the multitude of potential deletion mutations in and near the β-globin gene locus. The common classification includes four clinical syndromes based on the degree of anemia.

The heterozygous forms, in which only one of the two β-globin chains is affected, are classified as silent trait (heterozygous β⁺ thalassemia) and thalassemia trait (heterozygous β⁰ thalassemia). In both of these syndromes, the patients are usually asymptomatic. The mild anemia may be discovered only on routine laboratory testing. The hemoglobin level is only slightly decreased, and the MCV is low. The RDW is normal. (The RDW may help distinguish between β-thalassemia and iron deficiency anemia, in which the RDW is usually elevated.) Close examination of the erythrocyte morphologic characteristics will demonstrate hypochromia with occasional basophilic stippling. Often the microcytic, hypochromic anemia of iron deficiency is confused with heterozygous β-thalassemia. The Hb A2 level may be slightly increased (>3 to 4%), and the Hb F level is also mildly elevated. Normal iron studies, normal RDW, and examination of the parental and family members' red blood cell parameters and erythrocyte morphologic features help make this diagnostic distinction. These children usually have normal physical examinations with normal growth and development.

The homozygous forms of β-thalassemia usually result in variable but more severe forms of hemolytic anemia. β-Thalassemia intermedia refers to the disease state in which both β-globin genes have some type of deletion, yet there is still a small amount of β-globin protein expression. β-Thalassemia major refers to the homozygous disease state in which there is no β-globin expression, thus resulting in a very severe form of microcytic anemia. In this form of hemolytic anemia, there is ineffective erythropoeisis with many red blood cell precursors prematurely destroyed because of unbalanced globin expression and α-globin chain excess. The life span of circulating red blood cells is markedly decreased, and there is splenic enlargement caused by sequestration.

A universal complication is hemosiderosis with iron deposition in the liver, pancreas, thyroid gland, parathyroid gland, adrenal zona glomerulosa, renal medulla, heart, bone marrow, and spleen. Iron overload results from the tremendous amount of iron absorption and turnover necessary to keep up with the shortened erythrocyte life span and reticulocytosis, as well as the fact that many of these children require chronic red blood cell transfusions. Thus, endocrinologic abnormalities such as growth retardation, delayed puberty, thyroid dysfunction, diabetes mellitus, and parathyroid dysfunction must be monitored closely. Cardiac hemosiderosis results in dilatation of the atrial and ventricular cavities and thickening of the muscle layers. Supraventricular tachycardia is a common complication. Chronic chelation therapy using parenteral deferoxamine is warranted in these children in order to slow the eventual progression of the many complications of iron overload.[206]

These children are transfusion-dependent, requiring red blood cell transfusion on the average of every 3 to 4 weeks. Occasionally, following a brisk and acute hemolytic event, a red blood cell transfusion may be needed emergently.[207]

A splenectomy is often necessary in the patient with severe β-thalassemia. Hypersplenism with leukopenia, thrombocytopenia, and worsening anemia is a progressive problem. Most patients have some improvement in the frequency of transfusion requirements following splenectomy. Of course one must be mindful of the risk of postsplenectomy sepsis.[208, 209]

As described previously, cardiac hemosiderosis and the resulting complications are the most common life-threatening problems faced by patients with thalassemia. Monitoring and treatment of these patients may best be carried out in the critical care setting. The most common abnormalities include left ventricular dilatation and wall thickening, decreased ejection fraction, and atrial and ventricular premature beats, often in pairs or runs.[210]

ANEMIAS OF UNDERPRODUCTION

As described at the beginning of this chapter, anemia in childhood should be classified according to the pathophysiologic causes. Specific causes will not be discussed again here, rather potential problems that may require care provided by the pediatric intensive care practitioner will be briefly mentioned.

Iron Deficiency Anemia and Vitamin B₁₂–Folate Deficiency

Although the most common nutrition-associated anemias—iron, vitamin B_{12}, and folate deficiency—may

result in markedly low hemoglobin values, rarely do children with these conditions require care and monitoring in the critical care setting. However, in very young children with clinical evidence of cardiovascular instability, a transfusion may be most safely carried out with the aid of cardiac monitoring. When treatment includes red blood cell transfusion, care should be taken to avoid restoring the patient's red blood cell mass too rapidly, resulting in volume overload. Specific guidelines for transfusion are outlined in Chapter 63.

Pure Red Blood Cell Aplasia

Bone marrow failure resulting in diminished or lack of development and maturation of the erythroid cellular components may be acquired or congenital. The anemia is usually normocytic with accompanying reticulocytopenia. Examination of the bone marrow confirms the maturational arrest or lack of red blood cell precursors. The congenital form (Diamond-Blackfan syndrome) most commonly presents during the first year of life. The inheritance pattern is not clear. The degree of anemia is variable and unremitting but may respond to steroid therapy.[211] Transient erythroblastopenia of childhood, in contrast, usually presents after the first year of life, may often be linked to a preceding viral infection, and usually resolves without treatment.[212] Acquired marrow failure syndromes have also been associated with drugs such as phenytoin and chloramphenicol, autoimmune diseases such as systemic lupus erythematosus and thymoma, and viral causes such as parvovirus and hepatitis.

Many chronic systemic diseases are associated with mild to moderate anemias of underproduction. Common causes include chronic renal failure, liver disease, chronic infection, or inflammation and malignancy.

In all forms of aplastic anemia, red blood cell transfusions may be indicated in the patient with marked anemia and impending cardiovascular instability. Care must be taken to avoid volume overload from restoring the red blood cell mass too rapidly.

Polycythemia

Polycythemia or erythrocytosis is defined as a pathologic state characterized by an elevated erythrocyte mass. Individuals with this condition who have an increased red blood cell count, hemoglobin level, or hematocrit value can be classified into three groups (see Table 62–1). Polycythemia rubra vera can be the result of increased proliferation of erythroid progenitors because of an intrinsic cellular defect or from altered regulation of erythropoietic activity.[213] Secondary polycythemia results from an excess of erythropoietin that is a manifestation of either decreased oxygenation (physiologically appropriate) or inappropriate erythropoietin secretion, as from a tumor. Both of these categories are characterized by an increased red blood cell mass. Relative polycythemia, also referred to as spurious or stress polycythemia (Gaisbocks syndrome), usually occurs almost exclusively in middle-aged men and is characterized by an elevated hematocrit value but normal erythrocyte mass. This does not represent true erythrocytosis.[214]

In secondary polycythemia, in which there is a physiologically inappropriate erythrocytosis, the elevated erythrocyte mass does not provide a compensatory mechanism. In physiologically appropriate erythrocytosis, the elevated erythrocyte mass increases the oxygen-carrying capacity and systemic oxygen transport. This may eliminate the deficit in tissue oxygenation and enable a new equilibrium to be established at a higher hematocrit value. However, an excessive rise in erythrocyte mass can also impair tissue oxygen delivery as a result of the increasing blood viscosity. Hyperviscosity compromises cardiac output and systemic oxygen transport and may lead to alterations in regional blood flow that can impair tissue oxygen delivery. The level of the erythrocyte mass at which the viscosity becomes a limiting factor for oxygen delivery depends on the total blood volume. Animal studies have shown that in a normovolemic state, systemic oxygen transport is optimal at a hematocrit value of 40 to 45%; however, in hypervolemia the optimal hematocrit value approaches 60%.[215, 216] Hematocrit values greater than 60% usually impair oxygen delivery even under hypervolemic conditions. An appropriate secondary erythrocytosis develops in patients with cyanotic congenital heart disease resulting from arterial hypoxemia. In many of these patients, the hematocrit value stabilizes at a higher level. However, in some patients, the hematocrit value may exceed 70%.[213]

Post-transplantation erythrocytosis has been reported in children and adults undergoing kidney transplantation. In adults, it has been associated with rejection, renal artery stenosis, and overproduction of erythropoietin by native kidneys.[217–219] Polycythemia with hypertension following transplantation in children may indicate the presence of arterial stenosis. It is not unusual, particularly in patients with cystinosis, and may indicate the presence of graft-artery stenosis.[220]

Familial polycythemias are rare.[221] Many patients previously classified in this group have been found to have high oxygen affinity hemoglobinopathies or congenital reduction in red blood cell 2,3 diphosphoglycerate (DPG), which leads to increased oxygen affinity or a hereditary elevated ATP content, which also results in a low DPG content. Several families have been described in which there were multiple siblings with polycythemia and hematologically normal parents.[222]

Polycythemia vera is a myeloproliferative disorder characterized by an abnormal proliferation of a multipotent stem cell. It is characterized by an increase in several hematopoietic cell lines with subnormal erythropoietin levels. The bone marrow contains unusual erythroid progenitor cells, which usually grow in culture without added erythropoietin. The incidence of polycythemia vera is approximately 1 in 100,000 individuals. It is rare in children, though childhood cases have been reported.[223–229] Less than 1% are younger than 25 years of age. The median age is 60 years. In the adult series, the male:female ratio is 1.2:1.[222] At diagnosis, all patients have increased red blood cell volumes. Approximately half of the patients have white blood cell counts greater than 12,000, platelet counts greater than 400,000, and reticulocyte count greater than 1.5%. The leukocyte alkaline phosphatase score is greater than 100 in 70% of patients and does not correlate with the white blood cell count. Bone marrow aspiration reveals increased megakaryocytes, hypercellularity, and a lack of stainable iron.[222] Clonal chromosome abnormalities have been described in 10 to 25% of patients at diagnosis. The changes are nonrandom and include trisomy 8, trisomy 9, and loss of part of either chromosome 5 or chromosome 22.[230]

The most common symptoms are headache, weakness, pruritis, and dizziness, which reflect the increased red blood cell mass, blood volume, hyperviscosity, and hypermetabolism. Most patients are plethoric on physical examination, have a palpable liver, an enlarged spleen, and an elevated diastolic pressure (more than 90 mm Hg noted in 32% of cases).[222]

Diagnosis and categorization of patients with elevated hematocrit values can be performed with a combination of history, physical examination, measurement of total red blood cell volume using radioactively labeled red blood cells, arterial blood gas oxygen saturation determination, measurement of oxygen pressure at which the hemoglobin is 50% saturated (P_{50}), and measurement of serum erythropoietin. A hematocrit value greater than 60% is pathognomonic for an increased red blood cell mass unless the patient is severely dehydrated.[231] Once true erythrocytosis has been confirmed, it is necessary to distinguish between polycythemia vera and secondary polycythemia. The diagnosis of polycythemia vera can be made by the criteria established by the Polycythemia Vera Study Group.[232] In most patients, the diagnosis of polycythemia vera is made after the major causes of secondary erythrocytosis have been excluded.

Treatment for patients with polycythemia consists predominantly of phlebotomy in patients who have uncomplicated erythrocytosis, erythrocytosis of uncertain cause, and erythrocytosis of any cause in young patients. Once the cause has been identified in patients with secondary erythrocytosis, all efforts should go toward eliminating the potential aggravating factors. The following formula may be employed to approximate the volume of exchange required to reduce the hematocrit reading to the desired level.[233]

$$V_e = V_b \frac{(Hct_o - Hct_d)}{Hct_o}$$

V_e = volume of exchange in milliliters
V_b = blood volume in milliliters
Hct_o = observed hematocrit reading
Hct_d = desired hematocrit reading

The end point of phlebotomy therapy would be maintenance of the hematocrit or hemoglobin concentration in the low normal range.

Specific treatment for patients with polycythemia vera has been guided by the results of a prospective trial designed to evaluate the effectiveness of controlling the disease with three arms of treatment. More than 400 patients were entered in the study and treated either by phlebotomy alone or myelosuppression with chemotherapy (chlorambucil or melphalan) or radioactive phosphorus (^{32}P). Analysis of the results did not reveal notable differences in the life expectancy among the three arms, the average life expectancy being between 9 and 12 years after initiation of treatment. Although acute leukemia may occur in patients with polycythemia vera, an increased frequency of leukemia was noted in patients treated with ^{32}P or chlorambucil. Based on the results of the study, the Polycythemia Vera Study Group recommends that no alkylating agent be used in this disorder.[213, 234] Phlebotomy alone is the treatment of choice initially in young patients. In the presence of complications such as splenomegaly or extreme thrombosis (platelet counts >1 million), the addition of hydroxyurea would be recommended.[235]

Patients with overcompensation from cyanotic congenital heart disease may benefit from a reduction of the erythrocyte mass by phlebotomy. The firmest indication for phlebotomy is significant hyperviscosity in patients with hematocrit values exceeding 65%. Clinical manifestations include lightheadedness, dizziness, headache, tinnitus, a congested sensation, and worsening of exercise capacity.[213] Symptoms of iron deficiency are generally indistinguishable from symptoms of hyperviscosity, but symptomatic hyperviscosity rarely occurs with hematocrit levels less than 65%.[236] In particular, if symptoms of hyperviscosity are present in a patient with a hematocrit value less than 65%, iron deficiency should be suspected. Iron deficiency leads to a significant increase in whole blood viscosity in patients with erythrocytosis, and the viscous effect rises with decreasing erythrocyte mean corpuscular hemoglobin.[237] In this situation, phlebotomy aggravates rather than alleviates the symptoms.[236] Cyanotic infants and young children less than 4 years of age who are iron-deficient are at greatest risk for cerebral infarction caused by thrombosis of intracranial veins and sinuses.[238, 239]

Phlebotomy without quantitative volume replacement is potentially dangerous, provoking a fall in systemic blood flow, oxygen delivery, and cerebral perfusion.[240] The volume removed should be replaced with an isovolemic crystalloid or colloid solution. Generally, in older children this can be accomplished with removal of 50-ml aliquots, followed by 50-ml volume replacement. Cuff blood pressure should be recorded in supine, sitting, and standing positions before and at 10- to 15-minute intervals after phlebotomy.[241] The total volume of blood removed in the phlebotomy should be the minimum volume required to achieve symptomatic relief. After phlebotomy, patients with erythrocytosis resulting from cyanotic congenital heart disease may have improved cardiac output, decreased arteriovenous oxygen content difference, decreased systemic vascular resistance, and increased systemic oxygen transport, as well as subjective improvement.[236] Patients who undergo repeated phlebotomies will become iron-deficient and require oral iron supplementation.

During cardiac operations for congenital heart disease involving a significant right-to-left shunt and polycythemia, special consideration should be given to lowering the hematocrit value to a level approximating that in a nonpolycythemic cardiopulmonary bypass patient. In patients with polycythemia who are undergoing cardiopulmonary bypass operations, sufficient reduction of hemoglobin and hematocrit values has proved effective in preventing postoperative coagulopathies.[242] Based on a study by Kawamura and associates, the safe limit for hemodilution for children with cyanotic congenital heart disease undergoing corrective procedures was 40%.[243]

In patients with cyanotic congenital heart disease, as well as in other patients with polycythemia, coagulation test results may be affected by the patient's state. Certain values of prothrombin time and activated partial thromboplastin time may be spuriously prolonged because of the reduced amount of plasma in the aliquot of blood and a relative excess of anticoagulant in the vacuum collection tube. Therefore, when the patient's hematocrit value is 60% or greater, the amount of anticoagulant should be reduced proportionally. The following formula should be used for adjusting the anticoagulant in patients with polycythemia:

$$X = \frac{0.5 \times (100 - \text{patient's hematocrit value})}{60}$$

where X = volume (in milliliters) of 3.8% sodium citrate for 4.5 ml of a patient's whole blood.[228]

In patients who have undergone renal transplantation and experience polycythemia, benefit may be derived from phlebotomy, depending upon the underlying cause.[220]

Iatrogenic infection with hookworms (*Ancyclostoma duodenale*) for the purpose of inducing continuous intestinal blood loss in congenital polycythemia has been reported to be successful; however, further evaluation is needed.[244]

References

1. Dallman PR and Siimes MA: Percentile curves for hemoglobin and red cell volume in infancy and childhood. J Pediatr 94:26, 1979.
2. Finch CA: Red Cell Manual. Washington, University of Washington, 1970.
3. Miller DR: Anemias: General considerations. Miller DR and Baehner RL (eds): *In*: Blood Diseases in Infancy and Childhood, 6th ed. St. Louis, C. V. Mosby, 1989, p. 108.
4. Oski FA, Sadowitz PD, and Helu B: Red cell volume distribution width (RDW) in the diagnosis of iron deficiency. Pediatr Res 19:265A, 1985.
5. Bessman JD, Gilmer PR Jr, and Gardner FH: Improved classification of anemias by MCV and RDW. Am J Clin Pathol 80:322, 1983.
6. Pirofsky B: Clinical aspects of autoimmune hemolytic anemia. Semin Hematol 13:251, 1976.
7. Schreiber AD and Frank MM: Role of antibody and complement in the immune clearance and destruction of erythrocytes. I: In vivo effects of the IgG and IgM complement-fixing sites. J Clin Invest 51:575, 1972.
8. Sokol RH, Hewitt S, Stamps BK, et al: Autoimmune haemolysis: An 18 year study of 865 cases referred to a regional transfusion center. Br Med J 282:2033, 1981.
9. Heisel MA and Ortega JA: Factors influencing prognosis in childhood autoimmune hemolytic anemia. Am J Pediatr Hematol Oncol 5:147, 1983.
10. Zuelzer WW, Mastrangelo R, Stulberg CS, et al: Autoimmune hemolytic anemia: Natural history and viral-immunologic interactions in childhood. Am J Med 49:80, 1970.

11. Buchanan GR, Boxer LA, and Nathan DG: The acute and transient nature of idiopathic immune hemolytic anemia in childhood. J Pediatr 88:780, 1976.

12. Zupanska B, Lawkowicz W, Gorska B, et al: Autoimmune haemolytic anemia in children. Br J Haematol 34:511, 1976.

13. Carapella deLuca E, Casadei AM, diPiero G, et al: Autoimmune haemolytic anaemia in childhood: Follow-up in 29 cases. Vox Sang 36:13, 1979.

14. Klemperer MR: Hemolytic anemias: Immune defects. In Blood Diseases of Infancy and Childhood, 6th ed. Miller DR and Baehner RL (eds): St. Louis, CV Mosby, 1989, pp. 233–244.

15. Dupuy ME, Elliott M, and Masouredis SP: Relationship between red cell bound antibody and agglutination in the antiglobulin reaction. Vox Sang 9:40, 1964.

16. Atkinson JP, Schreiber AD, Frank MM, et al: Effects of corticosteroids and splenectomy on the immune clearance and destruction of erythrocytes. J Clin Invest 52:1509, 1975.

17. Schreiber AD: Clinical immunology of the corticosteroids. Prog Clin Immunol 3:103, 1977.

18. Dameshek W, Rosenthal MC, and Schwartz LI: The treatment of acquired hemolytic anemia with adrenocorticotropic hormone (ACTH). N Engl J Med 244:117, 1951.

19. Sokol RJ, Hewitt S, Stamps BK, et al: Autoimmune haemolysis in childhood and adolescence. Acta Haematol 72:245, 1984.

20. Habibi B, Hombert JC, Schaison G, et al: Autoimmune hemolytic anemia in children: A review of 80 cases. Am J Med 56:61, 1974.

21. Johnson CA and Abilgaard CF: Treatment of idiopathic autoimmune hemolytic anemia in children: Review and report of two fatal cases in infancy. Acta Paediatr Scand 65:375, 1976.

22. Hitzig WH and Massimo L: Treatment of autoimmune hemolytic anemia in children with azathioprine (Imuran). Blood 28:840, 1966.

23. Ahn YS, Harrington WJ, Mylvaganam R, et al: Danazol therapy for autoimmune hemolytic anemia. Ann Intern Med 102:298, 1985.

24. Bussels J, Cunningham-Rundles C, Abraham C, et al: Intravenous treatment of autoimmune hemolytic anemia with very high dose gammaglobulin. Vox Sang 51:264, 1986.

25. McConnell ME, Atchison JA, Kohaut E, et al: Successful use of plasma exchange in a child with refractory immune hemolytic anemia. Am J Pediatr Hematol Oncol 9:158, 1987.

26. Feusner J, O'Leary M, and Beach B: Exchange transfusion for severe autoimmune hemolytic anemia. Am J Pediatr Hematol Oncol 9:302, 1987.

27. Schreiber AD and Gill FM: Autoimmune hemolytic anemia. In Nathan DG and Oski FA (eds): Hematology of infancy and childhood, 3rd ed. Philadephia, WB Saunders, 1988, pp. 413–426.

28. Calley EW: Paroxysmal cold haemoglobinuria after mumps. Br Med J 1:1552, 1964.

29. Nordhagen R, Stensvold K, Winsnes A, et al: Paroxysmal haemoglobinuria. The most frequent acute autoimmune hemolytic anemia in children. Acta Pediatr Scand 73:258, 1984.

30. O'Neill J and Marshall WC: Paroxysmal cold haemoglobinuria and measles. Arch Dis Child 42:183, 1967.

31. Schreiber AD, Herskovitz B, and Goldwein M: Low titer cold hemagglutinin disease: Mechanism of hemolysis and response to corticosteroids. N Engl J Med 296:1490, 1977.

32. Brown DL, Lochman PJ, and Dacie JV: The in vivo behavior of complement coated red cells: Studies in C6-deficient, C3-depleted and normal rabbits. Clin Exp Immunol 7:401, 1970.

33. Schreiber AD and Frank MM: Studies on the in vivo effects of antibody. Interactions of IgM antibody and complement in the immune clearance and destruction of erythrocytes in man. J Clin Invest 58:942, 1976.

34. Wolach B, Heddle N, Barr RD, et al: Transient Donath-Landsteiner hemolytic anaemia. Br J Haematol 48:425, 1981.

35. Brooks BD, Steane EA, Shuban RG, et al: Therapeutic plasma exchange in the immune hemolytic anemias and immunologic thrombocytopenia purpura. In: Tindall RSA (ed): Therapeutic apheresis and plasma perfusion. New York, Alan R Liss, 1982, pp. 317–329.

36. Kirkman HN: Glucose-6-phosphate variants and drug-induced hemolysis. Ann NY Acad Sci 151:753, 1968.

37. Kirkman HN: Glucose-6-phosphate dehydrogenase. Adv Hum Genet 2:1, 1971.

38. Long WK, Wilson SW, and Goldwein M: Associations between red cell glucose-6-phosphate dehydrogenase variants and vascular disease. Am J Hum Genet 19:35, 1967.

39. McCurdy PR, Kirkman HN, and Goldwein M: et al: A Chinese variant of glucose-6-phosphate dehydrogenase. J Lab Clin Med 67:374, 1966.

40. Kissin C, Dorche C, and Goldwein M: Le glucose-6-phosphate dehydrogenase type debrousse: Probleme d'un type enzymatique propre aux algerien de race Arabe. Bull Soc Chim Biol 52:1233, 1972.

41. Piomelli S: G6PD deficiency and related disorders of the pentose pathway. In: Nathan DG and Oski FA (eds): Hematology of Infancy and Childhood, 3rd ed. Philadelphia, WB Saunders, 1987, pp. 596–604.

42. Lanzkowsky P: Hemolytic anemia. In: Manual of Pediatric Hematology and Oncology. New York, Churchill Livingstone, 1989, pp. 96–97.

43. Oski FA, Nathan DG, et al: Extreme hemolysis and red-cell distortion in erythrocyte pyruvate kinase deficiency. I: Morphology, erythrokinetics, and family enzyme studies. N Engl J Med 270:1023, 1964.

44. Vives-Corrons JL, Marie J, et al: Hereditary erythrocyte pyruvate kinase deficiency and chronic hemolytic anemia: Clinical, genetic, and molecular studies in six new Spanish patients. Hum Genet 53:401, 1980.

45. Matthay KK and Mentzer WC: Erythrocyte enzymopathies in the newborn. Clin Haematol 10:31, 1981.

46. Duncan JR, Capellini MD, et al: Aplastic crisis due to parvovirus infection in pyruvate kinase deficiency. Lancet 2:14, 1983.

47. Mentzer WC: Pyruvate kinase deficiency and disorders of glycolysis. In: Nathan DG and Oski FA (eds): Hematology of Infancy and Childhood, 3rd ed. Philadelphia, WB Saunders, 1987, p. 568.

48. Keitt AS: Hemolytic anemia with impaired hexokinase activity. J Clin Invest 48:1997, 1969.

49. Gilsanz F, Meyer E, et al: Congenital hemolytic anemia due to hexokinase deficiency. Am J Dis Child 132:636, 1978.

50. Stocchi V, Magnani M, et al: Multiple forms of human red cell hexokinase: Preparation, characterization, and age dependence. J Biol Chem 275:2357, 1982.

51. Board PG, Trueworthy R, et al: Congenital nonspherocytic hemolytic anemia with an unstable hexokinase variant. Blood 51:111, 1978.

52. Rijksen G, Akkerman JWN, et al: Generalized hexokinase deficiency in the blood cells of a patient with nonspherocytic hemolytic anemia. Blood 61:12, 1983.

53. Spiegel JE, Beardsley DS, et al: An analogue of the erythroid skeletal protein 4.1 in nonerythroid cells. J Cell Biol 99:886, 1984.

54. Agre P, Orringer EP, et al: Deficient red cell spectrin in severe recessively inherited spherocytosis. N Engl J Med 306:1155, 1982.

55. Agre P, Casella JF, et al: Partial deficiency of erythrocyte spectrin in hereditary spherocytosis. Nature 314:380, 1985.

56. Speicher DW and Marchesi VT: Erythrocyte spectrin is composed of many homologous triple helical segments. Nature 311:177, 1984.

57. Speicher DW: Structural features of human erythrocyte spectrin: Functional and evolutionary implications. J Cell Biochem 9B(Suppl):4, 1985. (Abstract)

58. Lux SE: Disorders of the red cell membrane. In: Nathan DG and Oski FA (eds): Hematology of Infancy and Childhood, 3rd ed. Philadelphia, WB Saunders, 1987, p. 473.

59. Agre P, Casella JF, et al: Partial deficiency of erythrocyte spectrin in heriditary spherocytosis. Nature 314:380, 1985.

60. Trucco JI and Brown AK: Neonatal manifestations of heriditary spherocytosis. Am J Dis Child 113:263, 1967.

61. Krueger HC and Burgert EO: Hereditary spherocytosis in 100 children. Mayo Clin Proc 41:821, 1966.

62. Davidson RJ, Brown T, et al: Human parvovirus infection and aplastic crisis in hereditary spherocytosis. J Infect 9:298, 1984.

63. Koduri RPR, Patel AR, et al: Infection with parvovirus-like virus and aplastic crisis in chronic hemolytic anemia. Ann Intern Med 98:930, 1983.

64. MacKinney AA, Jr: Hereditary spherocytosis: Clinical family studies. Arch Intern Med 116:257, 1965.

65. Schwartz PE, Sterioff S, et al: Postsplenectomy sepsis and mortality in adults. JAMA 248:2279, 1982.
66. Krivit W: Overwhelming postsplenectomy infection. Am J Hematol 2:193, 1977.
67. Pederson FK: Postsplenectomy infection in Danish children splenectomized. Acta Paediatr Scand 72:589, 1983.
68. Mitchell A and Morris PJ: Surgery of the spleen. Clin Hematol 12:565, 1983.
69. Cook PJL, Noades JE, et al: On the orientation of the Rh:El₁ linkage group. Ann Hum Genet 41:157, 1977.
70. Keats BJB: Another elliptocytosis locus on chromosome 1? Hum Genet 50:227, 1979.
71. Lux SE: Disorders of the membrane skeleton: Hereditary spherocytosis and hereditary elliptocytosis. In: Stanbury JB, Wyngaarden JB, et al (eds): The Metabolic Basis of Inherited Disease, 5th ed. New York, McGraw-Hill, 1983, p. 1573.
72. Zarkowsky HS, Mohandas N, et al: A congenital haemolytic anemia with thermal sensitivity of the erythrocyte membrane. Br J Haematol 29:537, 1975.
73. Palek J: Hereditary elliptocytosis and related disorders. Clin Hematol 14:45, 1985.
74. Mac Iver JE and Parker-Williams EJ: Aplastic crisis in sickle cell anemia. Lancet 1:1086, 1961.
75. Serjeant GR, Manson K, et al: Outbreak of aplastic crisis in sickle cell anemia associated with parvoviruslike agent. Lancet 1:595, 1981.
76. Pattison JR, Jones SE, et al: Parvovirus infections and hypoplastic crises in sickle cell anemia. Lancet 1:644, 1981.
77. Conrad ME, Studdard H, and Anderson LJ: Aplastic crisis in sickle cell disorders; bone marrow necrosis and human parvovirus infection. Am J Med Sci 295:212, 1988.
78. Mortimer PP, Humphries RK, et al: A human parvovirus-like virus inhibits haematopoietic colony formation in vitro. Nature 302:426, 1983.
79. Saarinen UM, Chorba TL, et al: Human parvovirus B 19-induced epidemic acute red cell aplasia in patients with hereditary hemolytic anemia. Blood 67:1411, 1986.
80. Seeler RA: Deaths in children with sickle cell anemia. A clinical analysis of 19 fatal instances in Chicago. Clin Pediatr 11:634, 1972.
81. Topley AM, Rogers DW, Stevens CG, et al: Acute splenic sequestration and hypersplenism in the first five years in homozygous sickle cell disease. Arch Dis Child 56:765, 1981.
82. Seeler RA and Shwiaki MZ: Acute splenic sequestration crises in young children with sickle cell anemia. Clin Pediatr 1:701, 1972.
83. Rao S and Pang: Transfusion therapy for subacute splenic sequestration in sickle cell anemia. Blood 60(Suppl):489, 1982.
84. Charache S, Lubin B, and Reid C: Acute splenic sequestration and aplastic crisis. In: Management and Therapy of Sickle Cell Disease. NIH Publication No. 89–2117:29, 1989.
85. Kinney TR, Ware RE, Schultz WH, et al: Long term management of splenic sequestration in children with sickle cell disease. J Pediatr 117:194, 1990.
86. Portnoy B and Herion JC: Neurological manisfestations in sickle cell disease. Ann Intern Med 76:643, 1972.
87. Powars D, Wilson, et al: The natural history of stroke in sickle cell disease. Am J Med 65:461, 1978.
88. Merkel KH, Ginsberg PL, et al: Cerebrovascular disease in sickle cell anemia: A clinical, pathological and radiological correlation. Stroke 9(1):45, 1978.
89. Stockman JA, Nigro MA, et al: Occlusion of large cerebral vessels in sickle cell anemia. N Engl J Med 287:846, 1972.
90. Boros L, Thomas C, et al: Large cerebral vessel disease in sickle cell anemia. J Neurol Neurosurg Psychiatry 39:1236, 1976.
91. Hebbel RP, Yamada O, et al: Erythrocyte adherence to endothelium in sickle cell anemia. A possible determinant of disease severity. N Engl J Med 302:992, 1980.
92. Russell MO, Goldberg HL, et al: Effect of transfusion therapy on arteriographic abnormalities and on recurrence of stroke in sickle cell disease. Blood 63:162, 1984.
93. Hitchcock ER, Tsementizis SA, et al: Subarachnoid hemorrhage in sickle cell anemia. Surg Neurol 19:251, 1983.
94. Pavlakis SG, Bello J, Prohovnik I, et al: Brain infarction in sickle cell anemia; magnetic resonance imaging correlates. Ann Neurol 23:125, 1987.
95. Zimmerman RA, Gill F, Goldberg HI, et al: MRI of sickle cell cerebral infarction. Neuroradiology 29:232, 1987.
96. Platt OS and Nathan DG: Sickle cell disease. In: Nathan DG and Oski FA (eds): Hematology of Infancy and Childhood, 3rd ed. Philadelphia, WB Saunders, 1987, p. 673.
97. Charache S, Lubin B, and Reid C: Acute splenic sequestration and aplastic crisis. In: Management and Therapy of Sickle Cell Disease. NIH Publication No. 89–2117:22, 1989.
98. Prohovnik I, Pavlakis SG, Piomelli S, et al: Cerebral hyperemia, stroke and transfusion in sickle cell disease. Neurology 34:344, 1989.
99. Russell MO, Goldberg HI, Reis L, et al: Transfusion therapy for cerebro-vascular abnormalities in sickle cell disease. J Pediatr 88:383, 1976.
100. Sarnaik S, Soorya D, Kim J, et al: Periodic transfusion for sickle cell anemia and CNS infarction. Am J Dis Child 133:1254, 1979.
101. Lusher JM, Haghighat H, et al: A prophylactic transfusion program for children with sickle cell anemia complicated by CNS infarction. Am J Hematol 1:265, 1976.
102. Buchanan GR, Bowman WP, et al: Recurrent cerebral ischemia during transfusion therapy in sickle cell anemia. J Pediatr 103:921, 1983.
103. Wilimas J, Goff JR, Anderson HR Jr, et al: Efficacy of transfusion therapy for one to two years in patients with sickle cell disease and cerebrovascular accidents. J Pediatr 96:205, 1980.
104. Schechter AN, Noguchi CT, and Rodgers GP: Sickle cell anemia. In: Stamatoyannopoulos G, Nienhuis AW, Leder P, et al (eds): The Molecular Basis of Blood Diseases. Philadelphia, WB Saunders, 1987, pp. 179–218.
105. Noguchi CT, Rodgers GP, Serjeant G, et al: Levels of fetal hemoglobin necessary for treatment of sickle cell disease. N Engl J Med 318:96, 1988.
106. Ley TJ, DeSimone, Noguchi CT, et al: 5-Azacytodine increases gamma-globulin synthesis and reduces the proportion of dense cells in patients with sickle cell anemia. Blood 62:370, 1983.
107. Rodgers GP, Dover GJ, Noguchi CT, et al: Hematologic responses of patients with sickle cell disease to treatment with hydroxyurea. N Engl J Med 322:1037, 1990.
108. Benjamin LJ, Kokkini G, and Peterson CM: Cetiedyl: Its potential usefulness in sickle cell disease. Blood 55:265, 1980.
109. Chang H, Ewert SM, Bookchin RM, et al: Comparative evaluation of fifteen antisickling agents. Blood 61:693, 1983.
110. Vermulen C, Ninure J, Fernandez-Robles E, et al: Bone marrow transplantation in five patients with sickle cell anemia. Lancet 1:1427, 1988.
111. Shapiro MP and Hayes JA: Fat embolization in sickle cell disease. Report of a case with brief review of the literature. Arch Intern Med 144:181, 1984.
112. Mallouh AA and Asha M: Beneficial effect of blood transfusion in children with sickle cell chest syndrome. Am J Dis Child 142:178, 1988.
113. Pearson HA: Sickle cell anemia and severe infections due to encapsulated bacteria. J Infect Dis 136 (Suppl):525, 1977.
114. Zarkowsky HS, Gallagher D, Gill FM, et al: Bacteremia in sickle hemoglobinopathies. J Pediatr 109:579, 1986.
115. Dover GJ: Management of sickle cell anemia in children. MD Med J 39:371, 1990.
116. Overturf GD, Powars D, et al: Bacterial meningitis and septicemia in sickle cell disease. Am J Dis Child 131:784, 1977.
117. O'Brien RT, McIntosh S, et al: Prospective study of sickle cell anemia in infancy. J Pediatr. 89:205, 1976.
118. Fisher KC, Shapiro S, et al: Visualization of the spleen with a bone-seeking radionuclide in a child with sickle cell anemia. Radiology 122:398, 1977.
119. Winkelstein JA and Drachman RYH: Deficiency of pneumococcal serum opsonizing activity in sickle-cell disease. N Engl J Med 279:459, 1968.
120. Sanhadji K, Chout R, Gessain A, et al: Cell-mediated immunity in patients with sickle cell anemia. Thymus 12:203, 1989.
121. Keeley K and Buchanan GR: Acute infarction of long bones in children with sickle cell anemia. J Pediatr 101:170, 1982.
122. Sain A, Sham R, et al: Bone scan in sickle cell crisis. Clin Nucl Med 3(3):85, 1978.
123. Hammel CF, DeNardo SJ, et al: Bone marrow imaging in sickle cell disease: Diagnosis of infection. Semin Nucl Med 6:83, 1976.
124. Ammann AJ, Addiego J, et al: Polyvalent pneumococcal-poly-

saccharide immunization of patients with sickle cell anemia and patients with splenectomy. N Engl J Med 297:897, 1977.

125. Gigliotti F, Feldman S, Wang WC, et al: Immunization of young infants with sickle cell disease with a *Haemophilus influenzae* type b saccharide-diphtheria CRN 197 protein conjugate vaccine. J Pediatr 114:1006, 1989.

126. Rubin LG, Voulalas D, and Carmody L: Immunization of children with sickle cell disease with *Haemophilus influenzae* type b polysaccharide vaccine. Pediatrics 84:509, 1989.

127. Gaston MH and Verter JI: Prophylaxis with oral penicillin in children with sickle cell anemia. A randomized trial. N Engl J Med 314:1593, 1986.

128. Kim HC, Alavi A, Russell MO, et al: Differentiation of bone and bone marrow infarcts from osteomyelitis in sickle cell disorders. Clin Nucl Med 14:249, 1989.

129. Fernandez-Ulloa M, Vasavada PJ, and Black RR: Detection of acute osteomyelitis with indium-111 labeled white blood cells in a patient with sickle cell disease. Clin Nucl Med 14:97, 1989.

130. Bennett OM and Namnyak SS: Bone and joint manifestations of sickle cell anemia. J Bone Joint Surg 72:494, 1990.

131. Webb DK and Serjeant GR: Systemic *Salmonella* infections in sickle cell anaemia. Ann Trop Paediatr 9:169, 1989.

132. Miller JM, Horger EO III, and Key TC: Management of sickle hemoglobinopathies in pregnant patients. Am J Obstet Gynecol 144:237, 1981.

133. Morrison JC, Blake PG, and Reid CD: Therapy for the pregnant patient with sickle hemoglobinopathies: A national focus. Am J Obstet Gynecol 144:268, 1982.

134. Schmalzer EA, Lee JO, Brown AK, et al: Viscosity of mixtures of sickle and normal red cells at varying hematocrit levels. Implications for transfusions. Transfusion 27:228, 1987.

135. Kernoff LM, Botha MC, and Jacobs P: Exchange transfusion in sickle cell disease using a continuous flow blood cell separator. Transfusion 17:269, 1977.

136. Klein HG, Garner RJ, Miller DM, et al: Automated partial exchange transfusion in sickle cell anemia. Transfusion 20:578, 1980.

137. Morrison JC, Whybrew WD, and Bucovaz ET: Use of apartial exchange transfusion preoperatively in patients with sickle cell hemoglobinopathies. Am J Obstet Gynecol 132:59, 1978.

138. Piomelli S, Seaman C, Ackerman K, et al: Planning an exchange transfusion in patients with sickle cell syndromes. Am J Pediatr Hematol Oncol 12:268, 1990.

139. Fullerton V, Philippart AI, Sarnaik S, et al: Preoperative exchange transfusion in sickle cell anemia. J Pediatr Surg 16:297, 1981.

140. Lyday JG: Formulas to simplify partial red cell exchange. Plasma Ther 2:112, 1981.

141. Charache S, Lubin B, and Reid C: Acute splenic sequestration and aplastic crisis. *In*: Management and Therapy of Sickle Cell Disease. NIH Publication No. 89–2117:9, 1989.

142. McCullough J and Chopek M: Therapeutic plasma exchange. Lab Med 12:745, 1981.

143. Diamond WG, Brown FL, and Bitterman P: Delayed hemolytic transfusion reaction presenting as sickle cell crisis. Ann Intern Med 93:231, 1980.

144. Cox JV, Steane E, Cunningham G, et al: Risk of alloimmunization and delayed hemolytic transfusion reactions in patients with sickle cell disease. Arch Intern Med 148:2485, 1988.

145. Coles SB, Klein HG, and Holland PV: Alloimmunization in two multitransfused patient populations. Transfusion 21:462, 1981.

146. Luban NL: Variability in rates of alloimmunization in different groups of children with sickle cell disease: Effect of ethnic background. Am J Pediatr Hematol Oncol 11:314, 1989.

147. Vichinsky EP, Earles A, Johnson RA, et al: Alloimmunization in sickle cell anemia and transfusion of racially unmatched blood. N Engl J Med 322:1617, 1990.

148. Ofosu MD, Saunders DA, Dunston GM, et al: Association of HLA and autoantibody in transfused sickle cell disease patients. Am J Hematol 22:27, 1986.

149. Edmond AM, Holman R, et al: Priapism and impotence in homozygous sickle cell disease. Arch Intern Med 140(11):1434, 1980.

150. Sagalowsky AI: Priapism. Urol Clin North Am 9:225, 1982.

151. Seeler RA: Intensive transfusion therapy for priapism in boys with sickle cell anemia. J Urol 110:360, 1973.

152. Grace DA and Winter CC: Priapism: An appraisal of management of twenty-three patients. J Urol 99:301, 1968.

153. Karalyalcin G, Imran M, et al: Priapism in sickle cell disease: Report of five cases. Am J Med Sci 264:289, 1972.

154. Rifkind S, Waisman J, et al: RBC exchange pheresis for priapism in sickle cell disease. JAMA 242(21):2317, 1979.

155. Walker EM Jr, Mitchum EN, et al: Automated erythrocytopheresis for relief of priapism in sickle cell hemoglobinopathies. J Urol 130(5):912, 1983.

156. Nelson JR and Winter CC: Priapism: Evaluation of management in 48 patients in a 22-year series. J Urol 117:455, 1977.

157. Noe HN, Wilimas J, et al: Surgical management of priapism in children with sickle cell anemia. J Urol 126:770, 1981.

158. Charache S, Lubin B, and Reid C: Acute splenic sequestration and aplastic crisis. *In*: Management and Therapy of Sickle Cell Disease. NIH Publication No. 89–2117:45, 1989.

159. Baum FK, Dunn DT, Maude GH, et al: The painful crisis of homozygous sickle cell disease. A study of the risk factors. Arch Intern Med 47:1231, 1987.

160. Milner PF, Brown M, et al: Bone marrow infarction in sickle cell anemia: Correlation with hematologic profiles. Blood 60:1411, 1982.

161. Worrell VT and Batera V: Sickle cell dactylitis. J Bone Joint Surg 58:1161, 1976.

162. Keeley K and Buchanan GR: Acute infarction of long bones in children with sickle cell anemia. J Pediatr 101:170, 1982.

163. Bonadio WA: Clinical features of abdominal painful crisis in sickle cell anemia. J Pediatr Surg 25:301, 1990.

164. Shapiro BS: The management of pain in sickle cell disease. Pediatr Clin North Am 36:1029, 1989.

165. Benitz WE and Tatro DS: Drugs for symptomatic relief. *In*: The Pediatric Drug Handbook. Chicago, Year Book Medical Publishers, 1981, pp. 455–456.

166. Foley MK and Inturrisi EC: Analgesic drug therapy in cancer pain: Principles and practice. Med Clin North Am 71:207, 1987.

167. White PF: Use of patient-controlled analgesia for the management of acute pain. JAMA 259:243, 1988.

168. Campbell CF, Mason JB, and Weiler JM: Continuous subcutaneous infusion of morphine for the pain of terminal malignancy. Ann Intern Med 51:98, 1981.

169. Wang JK, Naus LA, and Thomas JE: Pain relief by intrathecally applied morphine in man. Anesthesiology 50:149, 1979.

170. Paice AJ: New delivery systems in pain management. Nurs Clin North Am 22:715, 1987.

171. Wang WC, George SL, and Wilimas JA: Transcutaneous electrical nerve stimulation treatment of sickle cell pain crises. Acta Haematol 80:99, 1988.

172. Rennels MB, Dunne MG, et al: Cholelithiasis in patients with major sickle hemoglobinopathies. Am J Dis Child 138:66, 1983.

173. Cunningham JJ, Houlihan SM, and Altray C: Cholecystectosonography in children with sickle cell disease. J Clin Ultrasound 9:231, 1981.

174. Sarnaik S, Slovis TL, et al: Incidence of cholelithiasis in sickle cell anemia using the ultrasonic gray-scale technique. J Pediatr 96:1005, 1980.

175. Nzeh DA, and Adedoyin MA: Sonographic pattern of gallbladder disease in children with sickle cell anemia. Pediatr Radiol 19:290, 1989.

176. Buchanan GR and Glader BE: Benign course of extreme hyperbilirubinemia in sickle cell anemia: Analysis of six cases. J Pediatr 91:21, 1977.

177. Webb DK, Darby JS, Dunn DT, et al: Gall stones in Jamaican children with homozygous sickle cell disease. Arch Dis Child 64:693, 1989.

178. Rosenblate HJ, Eisenstein R, and Holmes AW: The liver in sickle cell anemia. Arch Pathol 90:235, 1980.

179. McInnes BX III: The management of hematuria associated with sickle hemoglobinopathies. J Urol 124:171, 1980.

180. Deutsh TA, Weinreb RN, and Goldberg MF: Indications for surgical management of hyphema in patients with sickle cell trait. Arch Ophthalmol 102:566, 1984.

181. Kark JA, Posey DM, Schumaeker HR, et al: Sickle cell trait as a risk factor for sudden death in physical training. N Engl J Med 317:781, 1987.

182. Eichner ER: Sickle cell trait, exercise, and altitude. Phys Sports Med 14:144, 1986.

183. Lane PA and Githens JH: Splenic syndrome at mountain altitudes in sickle cell trait: Its occurrence in nonblack persons. JAMA 253:2251, 1985.

184. Bunn HF: Human hemoglobins: Normal and abnormal. *In*: Nathan DG and Oski FA (eds): Hematology of Infancy and Childhood, 3rd ed. Philadelphia, WB Saunders, 1987, p. 630.

185. Stamatoyannopoulos G, Nute PE, et al: De novo mutations producing unstable hemoglobins or hemoglobins M. Hum Genet 58:396, 1981.

186. White JM and Dacie JV: The unstable hemoglobins—molecular and clinical features. Progr Hematol 7:69, 1971.

187. Jaffe ER and Heller P: Methemoglobinemia in man. Progr Hematol 4:48, 1964.

188. Bodanansky O: Methemoglobinemia and methemoglobin producing compounds. Pharmacol Rev 3:144, 1951.

189. Benitz WE and Tatro DS: Drugs for symptomatic relief. *In*: The Pediatric Drug Handbook. Chicago, Year Book Medical Publishers, 1981, p 7.

190. Jaffe ER: Hereditary methemoglobinemias associated with abnormalities of erythrocytes. Am J Med 41:786, 1966.

191. Harvey JW and Keitt AS: Studies of the efficacy and potential hazards of methylene blue therapy in analine-induced methemoglobinemia. Br J Haematol 54:29, 1983.

192. Jaffe ER: Methaemoglobinaemia. *In*: Mentzer WC (ed): Clinics in Haematology, Vol 10. Philadelphia, WB Saunders, 1981, p 99.

193. Weatherall DJ, Clegg JB, et al: Linkage relationship between beta- and delta-structural loci in African forms of beta-thalassemia. J Med Genet 13:20, 1976.

194. Nienhuis AW and Maniatis T: Globin gene structure and expression. *In*: Stamatoyannopoulos G, Nienhuis AW, et al. (eds): Molecular Basis of Blood Diseases. Philadelphia, WB Saunders, 1986.

195. Orkin SH and Kazazian HH, Jr: Mutation and polymorphism of the human beta-globin gene and its surrounding DNA. Ann Rev Genet 18:131, 1984.

196. Higgs DR and Weatherall DJ: Alpha-thalassemia. Curr Top Hematol 4:37, 1983.

197. Pootrakul S, Sapprapa S, et al: Hemoglobin synthesis in 28 obligatory cases for alpha-thalassemia trait. Human Genet 29:121, 1975.

198. Kan YW, Schwartz E, et al: Globin chain synthesis in alpha-thalassemia syndromes. J Clin Invest 47:2515, 1968.

199. Weatherall DJ, Clegg JB, et al: The hemoglobin consitution of infants with haemoglobin Bart's hydrops foetalis syndrome. Br J Haematol 18:357, 1970.

200. Nienhuis AW, Wolfe L: The Thalassemias. *In*: Nathan DG and Oski FA (eds): Hematology of Infancy and Childhood, 3rd ed. Philadelphia, WB Saunders, 1987, p 732.

201. Yanofsky RA, Beaudry MA, et al: Survival of a hydropic infant with alpha-thalassemia. Blood 64(Suppl 1):60a, 1984.

202. Orkin SH and Kazazian HH Jr: Mutation and polymorphism of the human beta-globin gene and its surrounding DNA. Ann Rev Genet 18:131, 1984.

203. Nienhuis AW, Anagnou NP, et al: Advances in thalassemia research. Blood 63:738, 1984.

204. Lanzkowsky, P: Hemolytic anemia. *In*: Manual of Pediatric Hematology and Oncology. New York, Churchill Livingstone, 1989, p 115.

205. Wood WG, Weatherall DJ, et al: Interaction of heterocellular hereditary persistence of fetal hemoglobin with beta thalassemia and sickle cell anemia. Nature 264:247, 1976.

206. Graziano JH, Piomelli S, et al: Chelation therapy in beta-thalassemia major. III. The role of splenectomy in achieving iron balance. J Pediatr 99:695, 1981.

207. Cohen A, Markenson AL, et al: Transfusion requirements and splenectomy in thalassemia major. J Pediatr 97:100, 1980.

208. Engelhard D, Cividalli G, et al: Splenectomy in homozygous beta-thalassemia: A retrospective study of thirty patients. Br J Haematol 31:391, 1975.

209. Blendis LM, Modell CB, et al: Some effects of splenectomy in thalassemia major. Br J Haematol 28:77, 1974.

210. Nienhuis AW, Griffith P, et al: Evaluation of cardiac function in patients with thalassemia major. Ann NY Acad Sci 80:384, 1980.

211. Alter BP: Childhood red cell aplasia. Am J Pediatr Hematol Oncol 2:121, 1980.

212. Freedman MH and Saunders EF: Transient erythroblastopenia of childhood; varied pathogenesis. Am J Hematol 14:247, 1983.

213. Golde DW, Hicking WG, Koeffler HP, et al: Polycythemia: Mechanisms and management. Ann Intern Med 95:71, 1981.

214. Weinrib NJ and Shih CF: Spurious polycythemia. Semin Hematol 12:339, 1975.

215. Murray JF, Gold P, and Johnson BL Jr: The circulatory effect of hematocrit variations in normovolemic and hypervolemic dogs. J Clin Invest 42:1150, 1968.

216. Thorling EB and Erslev AJ: The tissue tension of oxygen in relation to hematocrit and erythropoiesis. Blood 32:332, 1968.

217. Nellans R, Otis P, and Martini DC: Polycythemias following renal transplantation. Urology 6:158, 1975.

218. Schramek A, Adler O, Hashmonai M, et al: Hypertensive crisis, erythrocytosis, and uremia due to renal artery stenosis of kidney transplants. Lancet 1:70, 1975.

219. Ianhez LE, Da fonseca JA, Chocair PR, et al: Polycythemia after kidney transplantation: Influence of the native kidneys on the production of hemoglobin. Urol Int 32:382, 1977.

220. Sinnassamy P and O'Regan S: Polycythemia in pediatric renal transplantation. Clin Nephrol 27:242, 1987.

221. Adamson J: Familial polycythemia. Semin Hematol 12:383, 1975.

222. Berlin NI: Diagnosis and classification of the polycythemias. Semin Hematol 12:339, 1975.

223. Modam B: The Polycythemia Disorders. Springfield, IL, Charles C Thomas, 1971.

224. Marlow AA and Fairbanks VF: Polycythemia vera in an eleven year old girl. N Engl J Med 263:950, 1960.

225. Dysktra OH and Halbertsma T: Polycythemia vera in childhood: Report of a case with changes in the skull. Am J Dis Child 60:907, 1940.

226. Marlow AA: Letter. Blood 45:463, 1975.

227. Aggeler PM, Pollycove M, Hoag S, et al: Polycythemia vera in childhood: Studies of iron kinetics with Fe-59 and blood clotting factors. Blood 17:345, 1961.

228. Hann HL, Festa RS, Rosenstock JG, et al: Polycythemia vera in a child with acute lymphocytic leukemia. Cancer 43:1862, 1979.

229. Danish EH, Rasch CA, and Harris JW: Polycythemia vera in childhood: Case report and review of the literature. Am J Hematol 9:421, 1980.

230. Wurgter-Hill D, Whang-Peng J, McIntyre OR, et al: Cytogenetic studies in polycythemia vera. Semin Hematol 13:13, 1976.

231. Grier HE: Chronic myeloproliferative disorders and myelodysplasia. *In:* Nathan DG and Oski FA (eds): Hematology of Infancy and Childhood. Philadelphia, WB Saunders, 1987, pp. 1070–1072.

232. Berlin NI: Diagnosis and classification of the polycythemias. Semin Hematol 12:339, 1975.

233. Rosenthal A, Nathan DG, Marty AT, et al: Acute hemodynamic effects of red cell volume reduction in polycythemia of cyanotic congenital heart disease. Circulation 42:297, 1970.

234. Berk PD, Goldberg JD, Silverstein MN, et al: Increased incidence of acute leukemia in polycythemia vera associated with chlorambucil therapy. N Engl J Med 304:441, 1981.

235. Grier HE: Chronic myeloproliferative disorders and myelodysplasia. *In:* Nathan DG and Oski FA (eds): Hematology of Infancy and Childhood. Philadelphia, WB Saunders, 1987, pp. 1070–1072.

236. Rosove MH, Perloff JK, Hocking WG, et al: Chronic hypoxaemia and decompensated erythrocytosis in cyanotic congenital heart disease. Lancet 2:313, 1968.

237. Linderkamp O, Klose HJ, Betke K, et al: Increased blood viscosity in patients with cyanotic congenital heart disease and iron deficiency. J Pediatr 95:567, 1979.

238. Phornphutkul C, Rosenthal A, Nadas AS, et al: Cerebrovascular accidents in infants and children with cyanotic congenital heart disease. Am J Cardiol 32:329, 1973.

239. Cottrill CM and Kaplan S: Cerebral vascular accidents in cyanotic congenital heart disease. Am J Dis Child 125:484, 1973.

240. Rosenthal A, Nathan DG, Marty AT, et al: Acute hemodynamic effects of red cell volume reduction in polycythemia of cyanotic congenital heart disease. Circulation 42:297, 1970.

241. Perloff JK, Rosove MH, Child JS, et al: Adults with cyanotic congenital heart disease: Hematologic management. Ann Intern Med 109:406, 1988.

242. Milam J, Austin SF, Nihill MR, et al: Use of sufficient hemodilution to prevent coagulopathies following surgical correction of cyanotic heart disease. J Thorac Cardiovasc Surg 89:623, 1985.

243. Kawamura M, Minamikawa O, Yokochi H, et al: Safe limit of hemodilution in cardiopulmonary bypass. Comparative analysis between cyanotic and acyanotic congenital heart disease. Jpn J Surg 10:206, 1980.

244. Walterspiel JN, Buchanan GR, Schad GA, et al: Erythropoietin-induced congenital erythrocytosis: Treatment with myelosuppressive agents and hookworm infestation. J Pediatr 107:575, 1985.

63

Transfusion Therapy in the Pediatric Intensive Care Unit

Naomi L.C. Luban, M.D., and Louis DePalma, M.D.

A wide range of medical conditions are encountered in patients admitted to the pediatric intensive care unit (PICU). The pediatric intensivist may treat the pediatric or adolescent trauma victim, children with malignancies who are pancytopenic, recipients of different transplanted organs, those with complex congenital heart disease who have undergone cardiopulmonary bypass, and other patients with multiple organ system failure from any number of causes. Such patients challenge the expertise of both the transfusion medicine specialist and the intensivist and their care requires a thorough knowledge of blood banking principles and transfusion practices. This chapter addresses the basic issues in transfusion medicine for the intensivist. The reader should use Table 63–1 as a summary of the types of blood components described in this chapter as well as their indications.

COMPONENTS AND DERIVATIVES

The use of blood components are preferable to the use of whole blood for several reasons. Most important,

component use conserves blood resources while providing specific therapy for specific deficiencies. If whole blood were always used in place of specific products, platelet concentrates, plasma, and albumin would not be available. Platelet function in whole blood stored for 24 hours is poor, and plasma coagulation factors (especially factors V and VIII) decrease throughout storage.[1, 2] Whole blood should be reserved for briskly bleeding patients who require both volume expansion as well as oxygen-carrying capacity. It is also indicated in the rare cases in which one or more blood volumes are to be exchanged and in selected cases of cardiovascular bypass pump priming, particularly in neonates.

Red Blood Cell Products

Red blood cells, commonly referred to as packed cells or packed red blood cells (PRBCs), are prepared from whole blood following centrifugation or sedimentation. PRBC units have a volume of 250 ml and a hematocrit of 70 to 80% and consist of 120 to 180 ml of PRBCs in 70 to 100 ml of plasma. Removal of much of the plasma

Table 63–1. BLOOD COMPONENTS AND INDICATIONS

Components	Major Indications	Precautions
Whole blood	Sympromatic anemia and hypovolemia	Must be ABO-identical
Red blood cells	Symptomatic anemia	Must be ABO-compatible
Red blood cells Leukocytes removed (centrifugation or filtration)	Symptomatic anemia, febrile reactions from leukocyte antibodies, prevention of CMV (?)	Must be ABO-compatible
Red blood cells, washed	Symptomatic anemia, febrile and/or allergic reactions, prevention of CMV (?)	Must be ABO-compatible, component expires 24 hours after washing procedure
Fresh frozen plasma	Deficit of labile and stable plasma coagulation factors	Should be ABO-compatible
Platelets, random	Bleeding of thrombocytopenia or platelet function abnormality	Should be ABO-compatible
Platelets, pheresis (HLA matched)	Same as above plus presence of anti-HLA or platelet specific antibodies	Should be ABO-compatible
Granulocytes	Neutropenia with infection	Must be ABO-compatible
Cryoprecipitate	von Willebrand's disease, hemophilia A, hypofibrinogenemia, factor XIII deficiency	Close laboratory monitoring of factor VIII, vWF as well as fibrinogen is necessary

773

during preparation reduces the amount of anticoagulant solution, lactic acid, and other plasma analytes and also reduces the isoagglutinins anti-A or anti-B present in the plasma of donors. When additive solutions such as Adsol, Nutricel, or Optisol are used as the anticoagulant, the hematocrit is reduced to 50 to 60%. It is important to know what type of anticoagulant has been used to assess the adequacy of the post-transfusion hematocrit increment; if additive anticoagulants are used, the post-transfusion hematocrit increment will be less than when PRBCs are used. Other red blood cells preparations include leukopoor, washed, and frozen deglycerolized red blood cells. Leukopoor PRBCs are prepared by a number of different techniques. Leukopoor products have been modified to remove at least 70% of the original leukocytes, although most of the currently used techniques remove more. The use of so-called third-generation in-line and bedside filters to produce leukopoor red blood cells has been reviewed[3]; such filters remove more than 70% of leukocytes. Cells may be washed in either an automated cell washer (Cobe 2991, Haemonetics V50) or by using manual techniques. Washing removes 70 to 90% of leukocytes as well as much of the original plasma, platelets, anticoagulant, and microaggregates. Red blood cells may be cryopreserved by using one of two methods using glycerol as a cryoprotectant. One method uses 20% weight per volume of glycerol and freezing in the gas phase of liquid nitrogen and maintenance at $-196°$ C. The second method uses 40% weight per volume of glycerol and a freezing temperature of $-80°$ C. Deglycerolization requires thawing and washing employing automated cell washers. Frozen, deglycerolized red blood cells are virtually free of white blood cells, platelets, plasma, anticoagulant solution, microaggregates and, if frozen within hours of collection, have high levels of 2,3-diphosphoglycerate (DPG) and adenosine triphosphate (ATP). As with washed red blood cells, deglycerolized cells have the disadvantage of a 24-hour expiration interval once they have been manipulated by washing. Deglycerolized, washed cells of rare red blood cell phenotype can be refrozen for future use, but with a loss of red blood cell number and decreased in vivo survival.

Occasionally, a massive transfusion recipient of unknown blood type may have received type O Rh-negative PRBCs during an acute resuscitation. When the group and type of the individual is known, it is advantageous to switch back to group- and type-compatible products to conserve type O Rh-negative blood resources. If the patient has received products containing plasma, such switching may be problematic due to the presence of naturally occurring anti-A and anti-B isoagglutinins present in group O donor plasma, which can cause hemolysis in the A, B, or AB recipient. If exclusively type O cells have been used, group A, B, or AB recipients receiving out-of-group plasma containing components should not receive their own blood group for 14 days or if anti-A or anti-B are still evident in the recipient's plasma. Use of equivalent formulas can be scaled down for the child's plasma volume by assuming 40 ml of plasma per kilogram of body weight.

PRBCs are indicated to restore blood volume and to prevent or treat shock. They are particularly useful when it is difficult to assess the rate of volume depletion, demands on oxygen delivery, and cardiopulmonary reserve of the patient. PRBCs are also indicated in patients with symptomatic anemia to increase oxygen delivery. They can be used with crystalloid solutions in surgical patients to replace operative losses of five to six units of blood. Specialized leukopoor PRBCs are indicated in patients who have recurrent or severe febrile transfusion reactions not prevented by pretransfusion antipyretics. These reactions develop secondary to the development of antileukocyte antibodies; these may be antineutrophil specific or anti-HLA specific either in previously pregnant females or in individuals who have had repeated transfusions. These specially prepared red blood cell products have several characteristics in common: they require more time to prepare, are more costly, must be transfused within 24 hours of preparation, and result in some red blood cell loss. Frozen deglycerolized PRBCs are indicated in patients with high-incidence red blood cell alloantibodies requiring blood of rare phenotype, in those who have IgA deficiency to avoid anaphylaxis secondary to recipient anti-IgA antibodies, and in those with recurrent febrile reactions to transfusion despite leukoreduction by more common methods.

Several formulas can be used to predict hemoglobin increments in transfused patients. In the setting of the PICU, hemoglobin and hematocrit frequently do not adequately reflect ongoing losses. On the other hand, the PICU setting permits close observation and quantitation of those physiologic mechanisms that compensate for blood loss, result in increased oxygen demands, and reflect oxygen delivery.

Red Blood Cell Transfusion Formulas

1. 6 ml of whole blood/kg of body weight increases the hemoglobin by 1 g/dl.
2. 3 ml of packed red blood cells/kg of body weight increases the hemoglobin by 1 g/dl.
3. Milliliters of blood to be transfused = (wt in kg)(blood volume in ml/kg)(desired Hb − actual Hb)/22 g/dl in which by 3 months of age an infant's blood volume is 70 to 75 ml/kg and in which 22 g/dl is the average hemoglobin of a PRBC unit

Platelets

A unit of random donor platelets is prepared by centrifugation of a whole blood unit within 8 hours of collection. The supernatant platelet-rich plasma undergoes a second centrifugation step at higher centrifugal force resulting in cell-free plasma components used in the manufacturing of plasma byproducts. When the platelet pellet is resuspended in 50 to 75 ml of residual plasma, it is called a platelet concentrate. Each platelet concentrate contains 0.7 to 0.9×10^{11} platelets (minimum 5.5×10^{10} in 50 to 75 ml of plasma). Platelets are stored at 22° C on a mechanical rotator to ensure their viability and may be stored for up to 5 days. Single donor platelets are obtained by thrombocytapheresis using any one of several automated blood cell processors. Depending on the number of blood volumes cycled through the apheresis machine, 6 to 12 units of platelet concentrate in 200 to 300 ml of plasma may be collected. Each thrombocytapheresis component contains at least 3×10^{11} platelets. Most are collected in sterile systems that permit 5-day storage, although occasionally thrombocytapheresis components with a 24-hour outdate may be provided; they are also stored at 22° C on a mechanical rotator. The degree of red blood cell and white blood cell contamination varies according to the technique and the machine used. Platelets have an in vivo survival of 9 to 10 days and are hemostatically effective for 3 to 5 days.

Platelets are indicated for quantitative and qualitative platelet disorders. They are used to prevent hemorrhage and to stop or attenuate ongoing bleeding. Clinical factors to be considered prior to platelet transfusion include the primary diagnosis of the child, the chance for marrow recovery and adequate platelet production, presence of fever, splenomegaly, sepsis, ongoing oozing, or bleeding that would increase consumption of platelets, and use of antibiotics or drugs that might induce platelet dysfunction. The decision to use platelets must be based on an assessment of these factors, because no prospective studies exist to guide the pediatric intensivist.

A platelet count of 50,000/mm³ appears to be adequate for hemostasis, as has been supported by the adult oncologic literature.[4] Even major abdominal surgery can be performed with platelet counts in this range, if there is no other coagulopathy.[5] Platelet counts between 20,000 and 30,000/mm³ are usually an indication for platelet transfusion, although many patients with platelets in this range will not bleed, especially if the marrow is recovering with young and active platelets.[6] However, clinical judgment must be used, especially in the patient with additional factors that might predispose to hemorrhage, those undergoing invasive neurosurgical or general surgical procedures such as liver biopsy, and in those who are septic or who have rapidly falling counts. Such individuals may or may not require transfusion to bring their platelet count to above 50,000/mm³. There are similarly no guidelines that help establish platelet counts above which it is safe to perform less invasive procedures like bone marrow aspiration, lumbar puncture, venous or arterial catheterization, or intubation.

Clinical judgment and knowledge of the cause for both the thrombocytopenia and the bleeding are essential. For example, antibody mediated idiopathic thrombocytopenic purpura (ITP) is frequently associated with profound thrombocytopenia (platelets < 10,000/mm³). Such patients will not benefit from platelet transfusions, because the transfused platelets are complexed with antibody and are rapidly removed from the circulation by the reticuloendothelial system, sometimes within minutes of transfusion.[6] Platelet transfusion in this case should be reserved only for life-threatening hemorrhage along with other therapeutic modalities.

The use of prophylactic platelet transfusions is very controversial, and few studies have been performed in children.[7, 8] Their use is limited to otherwise stable patients with leukemia, solid tumors, or bone marrow transplant recipients with severe thrombocytopenia (< 15,000 to 20,000/mm³), who are expected not to make platelets because of their therapy. If platelet counts are dropping rapidly, or if there is an increased risk of hemorrhage from concomitant illness, prophylactic transfusions might be indicated for a specific period of time.[9, 10]

Patients who have been massively transfused and in whom more than one blood volume has been replaced in a relatively short time may suffer from thrombocytopenia. In these patients, there is a combination of loss of endogenous platelets and dilution from use of both banked blood devoid of functioning platelets as well as crystalloid or colloid solutions. Studies in both adults[11] and children[12] demonstrate an inverse relationship between platelet counts and blood volume transfused, but the decrease in platelet count is less than predicted from published washout formulas. These studies suggest that there is mobilization of platelets from endogenous sources, most likely the spleen. In one study of massive trauma in children, the initial platelet count was a predictor of the need for platelet transfusion; only three of 26 patients had excessive bleeding requiring platelet transfusion, and each had an initial platelet count of less than 50,000 mm³. Some trauma transfusion algorithms recommend routine prophylactic use of platelets. One should not transfuse platelet concentrates based on number of units of red blood cells transfused, because many patients will not bleed despite low counts. Use of formulas may be helpful, however, in determining when platelet transfusion will be necessary based on the initial platelet count of the patient who has been massively transfused.[13]

Cardiopulmonary bypass induces platelet dysfunction and is associated with thrombocytopenia. Thrombocytopenia may develop because of platelet adhesion to the cardiotomy reservoir and plasticware, and by consumption at the surgical site. Platelet counts rarely fall below the number considered hemostatic, thus bleeding not considered to be "surgical" bleeding is more likely related to a functional defect or to fibrinolysis. Following bypass, the relationship between platelet count and bleeding time has been shown to be disparate, with prolonged bleeding times at platelet counts of greater than 100,000/mm³; this is likely due to release of α granules and dense bodies from the platelet.[14, 15] Platelet transfusions would be indicated in such circumstances in which platelet dysfunction was proved or suspected following a bypass procedure.

Platelet Transfusion Formulas

Most formulas have been developed for adults. The effective post-transfusion platelet count depends on the size of the patient, the number of platelets per unit, and complicating clinical factors. For these reasons, the corrected count increment (CCI) is more helpful in assessing post-transfusion effectiveness than the platelet count alone.[10]

$$CCI = \frac{\dfrac{\text{post-transfusion platelet count-pretransfusion platelet count}}{\text{No. of platelets in units} \times 10^{11}}}{} \times BSA$$

The CCI should be measured 1 hour after a platelet transfusion. Clinically stable patients have CCIs of 20,000 to 32,000/mm³ 1 hour after transfusion. Other formulas that may be useful are listed below:

$$\text{Expected increment} = \frac{2}{3} \frac{([0.7 \times 10^{11}] \times n)}{BV}$$

in which 2/3 = corrects for splenic sequestration
n = number of platelet units
BV = blood volume in μl

One unit of platelet concentrate per 10 kg of body weight should raise the platelet count by 100,000/mm³ and 1 unit of platelet concentrate per m² should raise the platelet count by 5,000 to 8,000/mm³. Poor CCIs may indicate the presence of anti-HLA as well as antiplatelet specific antibodies. Platelets from an HLA-matched donor (thrombocytapheresis) are indicated when anti-HLA antibodies are documented.

ABO antigens are present on platelets and may have relevance to the effectiveness of platelet transfusion. There are conflicting data concerning the survival of ABO-incompatible platelets. ABO matching can improve the response to platelet transfusions.[16, 17] Another concern in infants and young children is the transfusion of isoagglutinins A and B present in the plasma of the platelet concentrate. Sufficient anti-A or anti-B may be present in plasma to produce a positive direct Coombs test or hemolysis of recipient RBCs.[18] Rh antigens are not present on the platelet membrane, thus anti-Rh antibody should not affect platelet survival. However, red blood cells are present in platelet concentrates as a "contaminant" of the preparation of platelets and have caused Rh sensitization.

Whenever possible, ABO-compatible platelets should be administered. If ABO-incompatible platelets are to be administered and the blood group and transfusion needs of the patient are such that large volumes of incompatible plasma will be transfused, the platelets should be pooled; volume should be reduced; and platelets should be resuspended in a small volume.[19] However, the component must be transfused as soon as possible following plasma reduction as platelet viability deteriorates due to high platelet counts and the limited amount of buffering capacity of the residual plasma.

If Rh-positive platelet components are to be administered to Rh-negative females, Rh immunoglobulin should be used to prevent alloimmunization, secondary to the presence of Rh-positive red blood cells. The dose necessary can be calculated as follows:

Quantity of red blood cells in platelet concentrate =
volume (ml) × hematocrit of platelet concentrate =
volume of red blood cells (ml) per concentrate

Usual hematocrit of one platelet concentrate is 0.25%

Two other formulas that may be useful are:

No. of platelet concentrates transfused × 0.5 ml =
red blood cells transfused per transfusion episode

No. of vials needed =
$$\frac{\text{volume of blood component} \times \text{hematocrit of infused product}}{15}$$

A standard dose (300 μg) vial is protective for up to 15 ml of red blood cells, whereas a microdose vial (50 μg) can be used for 2.5 ml of red blood cells.

Plasma and Plasma Products

Plasma is prepared from whole blood during the preparation of either red blood cells or platelet concentrates. To be labelled as fresh frozen plasma (FFP), plasma must be separated from the red blood cells and stored at −18° C within 8 hours of collection. It may be stored frozen for 1 year, and once thawed it must be transfused within 24 hours. Single donor plasma is plasma that has been separated on or before the fifth day after the expiration date of a unit of whole blood. Alternatively, some blood banks stock frozen plasma that has been frozen up to 24 hours after collection; preliminary studies indicate that there is no appreciable difference in coagulation factors in plasma held before freezing for either 8 or 24 hours.[2]

Cryoprecipitated antihemophiliac factor (AHF) is the cold-insoluble portion of plasma remaining after FFP has been thawed between 1 and 6 degrees and then refrozen. It is most commonly known as cryoprecipitate. Each bag of 20 to 40 ml contains 80 units of factor VIII and between 100 and 350 mg of fibrinogen; these bags are frequently referred to as "units" of cryoprecipitate, confusing individuals trying to order units of factor VIII activity. Cryoprecipitate also contains factor VIII: von Willebrand factor and fibronectin, an opsonic protein that aids in phagocytosis of particulate debris. There are no standards for the quantity of either of these two proteins in the manufacture of cryoprecipitate. Once thawed, cryoprecipitate should be transfused within 4 hours.

A National Institutes of Health (NIH) Consensus Conference has evaluated the indications for use of FFP.[20] FFP is one of the most inappropriately used plasma components. FFP is indicated for deficiency of plasma proteins when no other more specific factor concentrates are available. Examples include congenital deficiencies of factors II, V, VII, IX, X, XI, and antithrombin III. Adequate replacement of factors II and XI may be difficult considering the volumes of plasma necessary to achieve greater than 50% concentration in homozygous deficiencies. FFP is used most commonly to treat multiple coagulation deficiencies that might occur in patients with liver disease, fat-soluble vitamin K deficiency due to malabsorption, biliary disease, starvation; when coumarin anticoagulants are used; or when disseminated intravascular coagulation (DIC) has developed. Other less common indications include provision of C1 esterase inhibitor in patients with hereditary angioedema and in patients with hemolytic uremic syndrome, and thrombotic thrombocytopenic purpura as a simple transfusion or as part of plasma exchange.[21] FFP should not be used as a volume expander, because the risk from transfusion transmitted diseases is as significant as with cellular products; use of albumin or plasma protein fractions that are pasteurized or crystalloid (which has no viral transmission risk) are preferable.

The appropriate volumes or FFP in milliliters for treatment of single coagulation deficiencies are easy to calculate. Calculations are based on the assumption that there is 1 ml of factor activity for each milliliter of FFP. For most factor deficiencies, 30% of factor activity is sufficient for hemostasis, but a higher percentage factor activity would be required for invasive surgical procedures. Factors VIII and IX deficiencies are most often treated with lyophilized factor concentrates that are heat-treated as well as solvent-detergent treated or monoclonally prepared. See Chapter 64 for more details.

The amount of factor V required for replacement in a factor V–deficient patient with 5% factor V who requires surgery at 30% can be calculated as follows:

1. Weight in kg $\times$ 70 ml/kg = blood volume in ml
2. Blood volume in ml $\times$ (1.0 − hematocrit) = plasma volume in ml
3. Plasma volume (ml) $\times$ (desired factor V units/ml − initial factor V units/ml) = units of factor V

Specifics:

35-kg child $\times$ 70 ml/kg = 2,450 ml of blood volume
2,450 $\times$ (1.0 − 0.4) = 1,470 ml of plasma volume
1,470 $\times$ (0.3 − 0.05) = 370 units of factor V
1 unit factor activity per ml of plasma
means that 370 ml of plasma would need
to be infused.

One also needs to know the half-life of transfused factor to plan the next infusion dose.[22] Measurement of the specific factor is helpful in monitoring transfusion frequency, because active consumption or ongoing blood loss will decrease the expected increment.

Cryoprecipitate

Cryoprecipitate is indicated in the treatment of von Willebrand disease and also for quantitative or qualitative deficiency of fibrinogen that may be congenital or acquired. The most likely causes of acquired deficiencies are DIC, severe liver disease, and dilutional hypofibrinogenemia.

Quantitative deficiencies of fibronectin are associated with massive trauma. Fibronectin replacement in the form of cryoprecipitate has been recommended by some intensivists, although randomized, controlled therapeutic trials are lacking to date.[23, 24] Fibronectin depletion may develop during starvation or sepsis, with burn injuries, and in fulminant hepatic failure,[25–27] but few studies have correlated administration of fibronectin in these settings with survival advantage.[25, 28]

For quantitative fibrinogen deficiency, the same formulas can be applied as for any factor deficiency, except that the normal fibrinogen should be estimated at 250 mg/dl in the child, with quantitatively lower estimates

in premature infants (150 to 200 mg/dl). The quantity of fibrinogen per milliliter of cryoprecipitate is approximately 2 mg/ml, with one bag of cryoprecipitate containing approximately 25 to 50 ml. For von Willebrand disease, one usually does not use formulas as von Willebrand factor is not quantitated. Replacement for major hemorrhage is usually based on increasing the factor VIII coagulant activity to between 80 and 100% and the bleeding time to normal. In practice, one to two bags of cryoprecipitate per kilogram of body weight are administered with additional doses at every 8- or 12-hour interval based on quantitative factor VIII coagulant levels and on the clinical status of the patient. There is 55 mg/ml of fibronectin of cryoprecipitate. Fibronectin is rarely quantitated, and there are no formulas that can replace fibronectin.

Other Issues on Use and Abuse

FFP and cryoprecipitate should be ABO-compatible with the recipient's red blood cells. Because there are no red blood cells, the Rh type is not considered. Compatibility testing (cross-match) is not required. When large volumes of FFP or cryoprecipitate are administered, the isoagglutinins A and B in the product may produce a positive result on an antiglobulin test and rarely hemolysis.[18] Adverse reactions to plasma are similar to those from cellular components, but there are disproportionately more anaphylactic and allergic reactions as well as cases of fluid overload. Large doses of cryoprecipitate in a patient with normal fibrinogen may also produce elevations of fibrinogen and precipitate acute thrombosis and DIC.

For complex coagulation factor deficiencies, FFP may be administered in combination with cryoprecipitate. No controlled studies support these practices. Therapy in DIC should be directed at correcting the underlying disease using antibiotics, volume expansion or, if applicable, the removal of the event that precipitated the episode (e.g., infarcted bowel). In the face of clinically apparent bleeding, 10 to 15 ml/kg of FFP may be administered every 12 to 24 hours with one bag of cryoprecipitate per 10 kg if quantitative fibrinogen is low. If the platelet count is less than 20,000/mm³, platelet concentrates are also indicated. Repeated use of coagulation tests are necessary to make sure that component therapy is appropriate. Component therapy should not be used prophylactically or empirically. Other conditions where the use of FFP is questionable include treatment of capillary leak syndromes, massive loss of lymph fluid, and nonbleeding patients with prolonged coagulation times (1.5 times normal) who are not candidates for invasive procedures.[20, 29]

Granulocyte Concentrates

Granulocyte concentrates are obtained by cytapheresis and contain 1×10^{10} cells in 200 to 400 ml. They are indicated in severely neutropenic patients who have a chance of marrow recovery and who have not responded to antibiotic therapy (see also Chapters 11, 12, 65, and 66). They are usually administered for 4 to 6 days. Because they have a hematocrit of 0.15%, they should be ABO and if possible Rh compatible with the recipient. Many adverse reactions to granulocyte transfusion have been reported including fever, rigors, and pulmonary reactions, including a respiratory distress syndrome and deoxygenation. In infants, their use has been advocated at 1×10^9 per kg. Products should be cytomegalovirus (CMV) negative and irradiated to prevent post-transfusion CMV and graft-versus-host disease (GVHD). A review of collection, storage, and indications for granulocyte concentrates has been made by Blajchman.[30]

SPECIALIZED BLOOD PRODUCTS

Occasionally, specialized blood products may be indicated for patients in the intensive care unit. Such components should be used only after consultation with a transfusion medicine physician and in consultation with the child's primary care physician.

Blood Products Prepared to Reduce the Risk of Cytomegalovirus

CMV is a ubiquitous virus of the herpes family that is harbored in white blood cells. A significant proportion of blood donors (30 to 70%) are CMV seropositive, although there are regional differences, which may in part be due to different donor demographics such as age, sex, race, and socioeconomic status. Older age, female sex, and lower socioeconomic strata predispose to higher seroprevalence rates.[31] Despite studies that confirm that seropositive donors can transmit CMV to seronegative recipients, only one study has been able to document viremia in blood donors.[32] This has led to the concept that both actively infected donors as well as latently infected donors can transmit CMV.

There are three types of CMV infections seen in the transfusion recipient. These types include primary infection and two kinds of secondary infections: reactivation and reinfection. Primary infection occurs in a seronegative recipient of blood from a donor who is actively or latently infected. It is frequently symptomatic with a mononucleosis-like syndrome that is heterophil-negative. Viremia, viruria, an IgM-specific and then IgG-specific anti-CMV antibody response can be demonstrated. Reactivation occurs when a CMV-seropositive recipient is transfused with blood from either a CMV-seropositive donor or a seronegative donor. The donor leukocytes trigger an allograft reaction that reactivates the recipient's latent CMV.[33] A rise in antibody titer and viral shedding may be found. Infections are usually asymptomatic, unless the patient is immunocompromised.[31] Reinfection or coinfection occurs in a CMV-seropositive recipient of blood with a strain of CMV that differs from the strain that initially infected the

recipient. An IgM and IgG response as well as viral shedding may be seen. The only way to distinguish reinfection is to use molecular markers specific for different strains of virus.

There is a wide clinical spectrum associated with post-transfusion CMV. CMV infection may be asymptomatic and may only be discovered because of serial serologic tests, or it may produce significant morbidity and mortality. The pediatric intensivist must be cognizant of certain select patient groups at risk for pneumonia, cytopenias, hepatopathy, graft rejection, unexplained fever, and increased risk of bacterial and fungal infections associated with post-transfusion CMV. These groups include low birthweight neonates, specifically those weighing less than 1,250 g who are seronegative and who required large amounts of blood. Bone marrow and solid organ transplant recipients and also infants who receive intrauterine transfusions are other patients at risk. Other immunocompromised patients, whether seronegative or seropositive, do not appear to be at increased risk for increased morbidity from CMV. To date, no studies have addressed the need for specialized CMV attenuated components for either seronegative or seropositive patients with human immunodeficiency virus (HIV) infection.

There are a number of different methods that can be used to prevent or lessen the chance of developing post-transfusion CMV. Because the virus is likely harbored in the white blood cells,[34] manipulations that can reduce or decrease white blood cell number should reduce the risk of transmission. These methods include washing and freezing followed by washing and filtration. Lower rates of CMV infection have been seen in open heart and neonatal patients receiving washed red blood cells.[35, 36] Use of frozen deglycerolized red blood cells, regardless of serostatus, is effective in preventing CMV in neonates[37, 38] and patients on dialysis.[39] Recently, third-generation leukocyte depletion filters have been developed for both platelets and red blood cell products and have been shown to be highly effective in preventing primary CMV infection in neonates[40] and in adult patients with hematologic malignancies.[41] Standard leukodepletion filters do not remove a sufficient leukocyte number to be as effective; the exact number of leukocytes that need to be removed is not known.

Some oncologists would argue that patients who *may* undergo bone marrow transplantation regardless of marrow donor serology should have blood and blood products manipulated to prevent reactivation of CMV or reinfection. No studies support this practice, although theoretically, infection with CMV may be as high is 51% in these patients, and clinical manifestations of newly acquired diseases are signficant. CMV pneumonia may develop in 10% of transplant patients, and 60 to 80% of these may be fatal.[42-44] More routine use of the third-generation filters may well be able to provide an acceptable product that does not depend on donor serostatus (see also Chapter 66).

Both prospective and retrospective studies have demonstrated that IgG-seronegative blood and blood products have a low to nonexistent risk of transmitting CMV. Donors with IgM-specific CMV antibody may be more able to transmit CMV because they are more likely to have acute viral infection and replication. Several abstracts and one published study[45] support this concept. IgM antibody assays, however, are not yet well standardized. Thus, use of IgG-seronegative blood is considered to be "gold standard," despite the fact that most IgG seropositive units are not infectious.

Gamma or cesium irradiation of blood to inhibit DNA replication (see later) does not prevent CMV infection.[46] Many patients undergoing chemotherapy (with or without transplantation) receive irradiated blood for prevention of GVHD. Similarly, many patients who receive blood that is CMV seronegative or mechanically leukodepleted receive CMV hyperimmune globulin or intravenous immunoglobulin with variable titers to CMV antibody and may also be receiving FFP for coagulopathy. They receive these plasma products to attenuate the development of graft-induced CMV or nosocomial acquisition of CMV.[47, 48] It may be very difficult to assess the serostatus of these individuals because of passive acquisition of CMV antibody. Tests for CMV early antigen or molecular markers will be necessary to establish post-transfusion CMV in these individuals but are not yet routinely available.

Irradiated Blood

Transfusion-associated graft-versus-host disease (TA-GVHD) occurs when an immunosuppressed or immunodeficient transfusion recipient receives immunologically competent donor lymphocytes. The transfused histoincompatible T lymphocytes proliferate and engraft in the immunocompromised host who is incapable of rejecting foreign cells. The degree of similarity between the HLA antigens of the blood donor and the recipient enhances the potential for engraftment. Once engraftment occurs, donor lymphocyte proliferation occurs and clinical symptoms begin, usually 4 to 30 days following transfusion. Clinical manifestations include fever, erythematous rash, anorexia, nausea, vomiting, and profuse watery diarrhea. The rash may progress to bullae and to desquamation (see also Chapter 67). Liver dysfunction from liver function test (LFT) elevations to fulminant hepatic coma can occur. Severe cytopenias occur and help differentiate TA-GVHD from that which occurs in bone marrow transplant recipients; in TA-GVHD, the bone marrow hematopoietic progenitors are particularly affected. TA-GVHD is fatal in 90% of reported cases in children.[49] Diagnosis is usually made post mortem but can be made premortem with biopsy of the skin or gastrointestinal tract, by looking for chimerism using DNA analysis (restriction fragment length polymorphisms), or differential typing of circulating lymphocytes and tissue.[50]

Patient groups at risk for TA-GVHD include bone marrow transplant recipients of any age and infants who received exchange or simple transfusion following intrauterine transfusion. Infants with unsuspected congenital immunodeficiency disease may also develop TA-GVHD, as well as older children with immunodeficiency acquired congenitally or through chemotherapy.

The incidence of TA-GVHD is not known. Estimates for patients with leukemia range from 0.1 to 1%[49] and 2% for lymphoma,[51] but such rates are impossible to verify. Most oncology units caring for children are part of large cooperative groups or specialized cancer hospitals and have been using irradiated products for several years. There are several reports of premature infants and one full-term infant developing TA-GVHD following exchange transfusion.[52] Some neonatal centers use irradiated blood for all premature infants on the basis of the known cellular and humoral immune dysfunction in these infants, but this practice is not agreed on by all.[53] It is likely that only the most severe cases of TA-GVHD are reported, or alternatively that many are missed because of the similarities between the clinical manifestations of TA-GVHD and chemotherapeutic and radiation-induced toxicities.

The incidence of TA-GVHD is further attenuated by its pathobiology. A certain number of viable lymphocytes, likely 1×10^7/kg, must be transfused to the recipient at a point when the recipient is maximally immunosuppressed. Therefore, certain malignancies or stages of a given malignancy are not associated with TA-GVHD, because the immunosuppression may be less intense at one point in the care of the same patient.[54] Other factors that may attenuate TA-GVHD are the kind of chemotherapy, concomitant use of radiotherapy, or other immunosuppressive regimens. The kind of product is also critical. Although TA-GVHD has been associated with whole blood, PRBC, frozen deglycerolized red blood cells, white blood cells, platelets, and fresh plasma, it has not been associated with frozen thawed plasma or frozen-thawed cryoprecipitate.

Because the lymphocyte is the most likely initiator of GVHD, the disease can be prevented by reducing the number of lymphocytes or by rendering them mitotically inactive. Since TA-GVHD has been reported following use of leukodepleted deglycerolized red blood cells, gamma irradiation is currently the only adequate method to prevent TA-GVHD. The appropriate dose should abrogate a mitogen or mixed lymphocyte culture response while producing no harm to the cellular components. Doses between 1,500 and 5,000 rads (15 to 50 Gy) have been used, with either cesium or cobalt source irradiators. ^{137}Cs blood irradiators are designed to hold blood bags and rotate during the process,[55] while ^{60}Co irradiators available in radiotherapy departments have not been as standardized.[56] Irradiation of platelet bags at 3,000 rads followed by storage does not alter platelet function.[57] The lack of adverse effect of irradiation of red blood cells[58] has come into question; several investigators have found that irradiation produces increases in plasma potassium and plasma hemoglobin when irradiated units are stored for periods of time that are still within their shelf-life.[59, 60] Red blood cell products transfused to fetuses, neonates, or children unable to tolerate potassium loads should be irradiated immediately prior to use and should not be stored[60] until additional data are available. Studies on the effect of irradiation of granulocyte products has produced variable results. While chemotaxis[61] and bactericidal killing[62] remain intact at 5,000 rads, superoxide production was adversely affected at 2,500 and 5,000 rads.[63, 64]

Parents as Donors

Fear over transfusion transmitted viruses has caused many parents to demand that their blood be used for their children. This practice has produced a new series of potential and real immunologic concerns. Although well recognized in Japan as postoperative erythroderma (POE), there are now several reports of GVHD occurring in nonimmunocompromised individuals following transfusion of blood donated by family members.[65–69] In these cases, a first-degree-relative donor, homozygous for their two HLA haplotypes, shares one HLA haplotype with the recipient. The recipient is incapable of eliminating the donor's lymphocytes because of the shared HLA haplotype. However, the donor recognizes the unshared recipient haplotype as "non-self" and may attack the host with a GVH type of reaction. Major U.S. blood collection agencies have recommended careful identification of units of blood and blood products obtained from first-degree relatives followed by irradiation of such units.[70, 71] This practice has many implications for small hospitals, where irradiation facilities may not be readily available. If blood centers irradiate for small hospitals, there are issues of storage and transportation. Serum potassium concentrations of 53 to 67 mmol/l have been reported in irradiated packed cells that were then stored for 7 days or more,[59] which might well cause significant elevations in patient potassium levels if blood is used for exchange transfusion or during cardiopulmonary bypass.

There are other concerns that are serologic in nature. Maternal plasma may contain alloantibodies directed toward paternal antigens; these may be red blood cell, granulocyte, or platelet specific or have HLA specificities. Transfusion of a maternal blood component containing plasma exposes the infant to these antibodies directed against paternally derived blood cell antigens. In utero, the placenta will not permit passage of these antibodies. In a study of 25 healthy women tested at the time of delivery, 16% had lymphocytotoxic and granulocytotoxic antibodies.[72] Although the clinical significance of these antibodies is as yet unknown, they are known to produce noncardiogenic pulmonary edema and purpura in adults.[73]

Use of the biologic father's blood also has possible consequences. Most maternal alloantibodies are directed toward paternally derived antigens. An infant may have passively acquired the maternal alloantibody that may be missed by standard pretransfusion testing, because the antibody may be directed toward a low incidence or "private" red blood cell antigen that is not present on the cells used for pretransfusion testing. Because most infants are not routinely cross-matched against donor units, an incompatibility might be easily missed. Therefore in cases in which a parent is to serve as a donor, a full major (parent cells and infant serum) and minor

cross-match (parent serum and infant's red blood cells) should be performed to prevent a possible hemolytic transfusion episode. Pretransfusion testing should include screening for possible HLA, platelet and granulocyte-specific antibodies, or plasma-containing components from mothers should be excluded.[74]

ALTERNATIVES TO THE USE OF BLOOD AND BLOOD PRODUCTS

Choice of Resuscitation Fluids

The primary treatment for a hemorrhaging patient should be nonsanguineous fluids such as crystalloid and colloid; such solutions are more readily available, more rapidly administered, and effective even at low hematocrits at improving microvascular flow.[75] As volume is restored, an assessment of extent of red blood cell loss can be made and red blood cells can be requested. In the emergency situation, type O positive or type O negative packed cells may be provided without compatibility testing, which must be completed at a later time. Type-specific blood can be available in 5 to 10 minutes, while full compatibility testing of donor and recipient requires 45 minutes to 1 hour. Only normal saline (0.9% sodium chloride) should be used in the same line as blood. Ringer's lactate contains calcium that chelates with the citrate anticoagulant and causes blood to clot in the bag, whereas 5% dextrose is hypotonic and causes red blood cells to lyse.

When red blood cells are transfused rapidly to a bleeding patient, several adverse reactions may occur. These reactions include hypothermia secondary to the cold blood and metabolic adverse effects including hypocalcemia, hyperkalemia, hypokalemia, hypernatremia, hypoglycemia, and hyperglycemia. Hypertension secondary to too rapid expansion of the intravascular space may also occur.

Hypothermia can produce a shift of the oxygen dissociation curve to the left, increased affinity, arrhythmia, low cardiac output, and DIC.[76] Hypothermia can be avoided by using commercially available blood warmers; however, these restrict flow rate and limit their usefulness. Modified warmers have been developed for red blood cells[77] and for FFP using a modified microwave.[78] Blood and blood products should never be heated in uncontrolled water baths or other warming devices, including standard microwave heaters.

Hypocalcemia is one of the most critical metabolic abnormalities to occur post-transfusion because of its association with depressed myocardial contractility. Studies on the extent of this problem are contradictory, but the liver transplant patient serves as the best model. Most transplant patients are anhepatic for a part of the procedure and therefore cannot metabolize citrate; they also receive large volumes of blood over a relatively short time. In such patients, rapid infusion is associated with decreased cardiac index, decreased ventricular function, and hypotension, and calcium infusion is indicated.[79, 80] Other massively transfused patients should be monitored but should not receive prophylactic calcium infusions. Hyperkalemia secondary to massive transfusion may also depress myocardial contractility and should also be monitored.[81] Because banked blood is acidic due to the initial anticoagulant and the production of lactic acid during storage, a metabolic acidosis is expected in the massively transfused recipient. It is more likely, however, that the acidosis is the result of hypoxemia and poor tissue perfusion.[82] Prophylactic administration of bicarbonate is not indicated, but pH should be monitored and metabolic defects should be treated as they are discovered.

Blood Salvage and Autologous Transfusion

The collection and reinfusion of a patient's own blood can decrease significantly the need for homologous blood transfusion. This may be accomplished by one or a combination of the following modalities: (1) preoperative blood donation with subsequent blood bank storage and reinfusion during or following surgery; (2) acute normovolemic hemodilution, by which blood is collected immediately preceding or following anesthetic induction and reinfused at the end of the surgical procedure; and (3) intraoperative and postoperative blood salvage, by which blood shed into the operative field or enclosed space is collected, washed, and reinfused during or after surgery. Although these procedures have been used frequently in adults, they are very useful in the pediatric population and are being utilized increasingly in many centers.[83]

The pediatric patient admitted to the intensive care unit following a surgical procedure by which any combination of the aforementioned methods may have been used may be at risk for the development of dilutional coagulopathy. Because these patients are receiving salvaged, washed PRBCs, coagulation factors as well as platelets may decrease to levels that place the patient at risk for hemorrhage. Laboratory monitoring of the platelet count as well as screening coagulation assays should be used to gauge the need for replacement therapy. Although some investigations advocate resuspension of the washed salvaged red blood cells with FFP, this may be unnecessary.[84] Only careful monitoring of both the clinical and laboratory data should dictate the need for additional blood components. When properly performed, blood salvage and autologous transfusion can decrease significantly the risk of transfusion transmitted diseases.[85, 86]

References

1. Baldini M, Costea N, and Dameshek W: The viability of stored human platelets. Blood 16:1969, 1960.
2. Nilsson L, Hedner U, Nilsson IM, and Robertson B: Shelf-life of bank blood and stored plasma with special reference to coagulation factors. Transfusion 23:377, 1983.
3. Wenz B: Leukocyte-free red cells: The evolution of a safer blood product I. In: McCarthy LJ and Baldwin ML (eds): Controversies of Leukocyte-Poor Blood and Components. Arlington, VA, AABB, 1989.
4. Dutcher JP, Schiffer CA, Aisner J, et al: Incidence of thrombocytopenia and serious hemorrhage among patients with solid tumors. Cancer 53:557, 1984.
5. Simpson MB: Platelet function and transfusion therapy in the surgical patient. In: Smith DM and Summers SH (eds): Platelets. Arlington, VA, American Association of Blood Banks, 1988.
6. Aster RH and Jandle JH: Platelet sequestration in man. II: Immunological and clinical studies. J Clin Invest 43:856, 1964.
7. Ilett SJ and Lilleyman JS: Platelet transfusion requirements of children with newly diagnosed lymphoblastic leukemia. Acta Haematol 62:86, 1979.
8. van Eyes J, Thomas D, and Olivos B: Platelet use in pediatric oncology: A review of 393 transfusions. Transfusion 18:169, 1978.
9. Schiffer CA and Aisner J: Platelet and granulocyte transfusion therapy for patients with cancer. In: Petz LD and Swisher SN (eds): Clinical Practice of Blood Transfusion. New York, NY, Churchill Livingstone, 1981.
10. Schiffer CA (ed): Platelet Physiology and Transfusion. Washington, DC, AABB, 1978.
11. Reed RL, Ciavarella D, Heimbach DM, et al: Prophylactic platelet administration during massive transfusion. Ann Surg 203:40, 1986.
12. Cote CJ, Liau LMP, Szyfelbein SK, et al: Changes in serial platelet counts following massive blood transfusion in pediatric patients. Anesthesiology 62:197, 1985.
13. Noe DA, Graham SM, Luff R, et al: Platelet counts during rapid massive transfusion. Transfusion 22:392, 1982.
14. Bick RL: Hemostasis defects associated with cardiac surgery, prosthetic devices and other extracorporeal circuits. Semin Thromb Hemost 2:249, 1985.
15. Harker LA, Malpass TW, Branson HE, et al: Mechanisms of abnormal bleeding in patients undergoing cardiopulmonary bypass: Acquired platelet dysfunction associated with α granule release. Blood 56:824, 1980.
16. Murphy S: ABO blood groups and platelet transfusion. Transfusion 28:401, 1988.
17. Skogen B, Rossebo-Hansen B, Husebekk A, et al: Minimal expression of blood group A antigen on thrombocytes from A_2 individuals. Transfusion 28:456, 1988.
18. Pierce RN, Reich LM, and Mayer K: Hemolysis following platelet transfusions from ABO incompatible donors. Transfusion 25:60, 1985.
19. Moroff G, Friedman A, Robkin-Kline L, et al: Reduction of the volume of stored platelet concentrates for neonatal use. Transfusion 24:144, 1984.
20. Consensus conference: Fresh frozen plasma: Indications and risks. JAMA 253:551, 1985.
21. Shepard KV and Bukowski RM: The treatment of thrombotic thrombocytopenic purpura with exchange transfusion, plasma infusions and plasma exchange. Semin Hematol 24:178, 1987.
22. Goldsmith JC: Plasma component therapy. In: Luban NLC (ed): Pediatric Transfusion Medicine. Baltimore, MD, Johns Hopkins Press, 1990.
23. Saba TM and Jaffe E: Plasma fibronectin: Its synthesis by vascular endothelial cells and its role in cardiopulmonary integrity following trauma as related to reticuloendothelial function. Am J Med 68:577, 1980.
24. Scovill WA, Saba TM, Blumenstock FA, et al: Opsonic alpha-2 surface binding glycoprotein therapy during sepsis. Ann Surg 188:521, 1978.
25. Hesselvic JF: Plasma fibronectin levels in sepsis: Influencing factors. Crit Care Med 15:1092, 1987.
26. Schena FP and Pertosa G: Fibronectin and the kidney. Nephron 48:177, 1988.
27. Yoder MC, Douglas SD, Gerdes J, et al: Plasma fibronectin in healthy newborn infants: Respiratoy distress syndrome and perinatal asphyxia. J Pediatr 102:777, 1983.
28. Fredell J, Takyi Y, Gwenigale W, et al: Fibronectin as a possible adjunct in the treatment of severe malnutrition. Lancet 2:962, 1987.
29. Snyder AJ, Gottschall JL, and Menitove JE: Why is fresh frozen plasma transfused? Transfusion 26:107, 1986.
30. Blajchman MA: Granulocyte transfusions. Transfusion Med Rev 4:1, 1990.
31. Tegtmeier GE: Posttransfusion cytomegalovirus infections. Arch Pathol Lab Med 113:236, 1989.

32. Diosi P, Moldovan E, and Tomescu N: Latent cytomegalovirus infection in blood donors. Br Med J 4:660, 1969.
33. Lang DJ: Cytomegalovirus infections in organ transplantation and posttransfusion: An hypothesis. Arch Gesamte Virusforsch 37:365, 1972.
34. Winston SJ, Ho WG, Howell CL, et al: Cytomegalovirus infections associated with leukocyte transfusions. Ann Intern Med 102:16, 1985.
35. Lang DJ, Ebert PA, Rogers BM, et al: Reduction of postperfusion cytomegalovirus infections following the use of leukocyte depleted blood. Transfusion 17:391, 1977.
36. Luban NLC, Williams AE, MacDonald MG, et al: Low incidence of acquired cytomegalovirus infections transfused with washed red blood cells. Am J Dis Child 141:416, 1987.
37. Brady MT, Milam JD, Anderson DC, et al: Use of deglycerolized red blood cells to prevent posttransfusion infection with cytomegalovirus in neonates. J Infect Dis 150:334, 1984.
38. Taylor BJ, Jacovs RF, Baker RL, et al: Frozen deglycerolized blood prevents transfusion acquired cytomegalovirus infection in neonates. Pediatr Infect Dis J 5:188, 1986.
39. Tolkoff-Rubin NE, Ruben RH, Keller EE, et al: Cytomegalovirus infection in dialysis patients and personnel. Ann Intern Med 89:625, 1978.
40. Gilbert GL, Hayes K, Hudson IL, et al: Prevention of transfusion-acquired cytomegalovirus infection in infants by blood filtration to remove leukocytes. Lancet 2:1228, 1989.
41. DeGraan-Hentzen YCE, Gratama JW, Mudde GC, et al: Prevention of primary cytomegalovirus infection in patients with hematologic malignancy by intensive white cell depletion of blood products. Transfusion 29:757, 1989.
42. Bowden RA, Sayers M, Flounoy N, et al: Cytomegalovirus immune globulin and seronegative blood products to prevent primary cytomegalovirus infection after marrow transplantation. N Engl J Med 314:1004, 1986.
43. Meyers JD, Flournoy N, and Thomas ED: Risk factors for cytomegalovirus infection after human marrow transplant. J Infect Dis 153:478, 1986.
44. Pecago R, Hill R, Applebaum FR, et al: Interstitial pneumonitis following autologous bone marrow transplant. Transplantation 42:515, 1986.
45. Lamberson HV, McMillan JA, Weiner LB, et al: Prevention of transfusion-associated cytomegalovirus (CMV) infection in neonates by screening donors for IgM for CMV. J Infect Dis 157:820, 1988.
46. Chou S, Kim DY, and Norman DJ: Transmission of cytomegalovirus by pretransplant leukocyte transfusions in renal transplant candidates. J Infect Dis 155:565, 1987.
47. Slichter SJ: Transfusion and bone marrow transplantation. Transfusion Med Rev 2:1, 1988.
48. Winston DJ, Ho WG, Lin C, et al: Intravenous immune globulin for prevention of cytomegalovirus infection and interstitial pneumonia after bone marrow transplantation. Ann Intern Med 106:12, 1987.
49. Von Fliedner V, Higby DJ, and Kim U: Graft-versus-host reaction following blood transfusion. Am J Med 72:951, 1982.
50. Dinsmore RE, Straus DJ, and Pollack MS: Fatal graft-versus-host disease following blood transfusion in Hodgkin's disease documented by HLA typing. Blood 55:831, 1980.
51. Stutzman L, Nisce L, Friedman M, et al: Increased toxicity of total nodal irradiation following combination chemotherapy. ASCO Abst C411:391, 1979.
52. Holland P: Prevention of transfusion-associated graft-versus-host disease. Arch Pathol Lab Med 113:285, 1989.
53. Sacher RA, Luban NLC, and Strauss RG: Current practice and guidelines for the transfusion of cellular blood components in the newborn. Transfusion Med Rev 3:39, 1989.
54. Holohan TV, Terasaki PI, and Deisseroth AB: Suppression of transfusion-related alloimmunization in intensively treated cancer patient. Blood 58:122, 1981.
55. Fearon TC and Luban NLC: Practical dosimetric aspects of blood and blood product irradiation. Transfusion 26:457, 1986.
56. McMican A, Luban NLC, Sacher RA, et al: Practical aspects of blood irradiation. Lab Med 18:299, 1987.
57. Read EJ, Kodis C, Carter CS, et al: Viability of platelets following storage in the irradiated state. Transfusion 28:446, 1988.
58. Moore GL and Ledford ME: Effects of 4000 rad irradiation on the in vitro storage properties of packed cells. Transfusion 25:583, 1985.
59. Ramirez AM, Woodfield DG, Scott R, et al: High potassium levels in stored irradiated blood. Transfusion 27:444, 1987.
60. Rivet C, Baxter A, and Rock G: Potassium levels in irradiation blood. Transfusion 29:185, 1989.
61. Valerius NH, Johansen KS, Nielson OS, et al: Effect of in vitro x-irradiation on lymphocyte and granulocyte function. Scand J Haematol 27:9, 1981.
62. Holley TR, Van Epps DE, and Harvey RL: Effect of high doses of radiation of human neutrophil chemotaxis, phagocytosis and morphology. Am J Pathol 75:61, 1974.
63. Buescher ES and Gallin JI: Radiation effects on cultured human monocytes and on monocyte-derived macrophages. Blood 63:1402, 1984.
64. Eastlund DT and Charbonneau TT: Superoxide generation and cytotoxic response of irradiated neutrophils. Transfusion 28:368, 1988.
65. Arsura EL, Bartelle A, Minkowitz S, et al: Transfusion-associated graft-versus-host disease in a presumed immunocompetent patient. Arch Intern Med 148:1941, 1988.
66. Juji T, Shibata Y, Ide H, et al: Host-transfusion graft-versus-host disease in immunocompetent patients after cardiac surgery in Japan. N Engl J Med 321:56, 1989.
67. Sakakibara T and Juji T: Post transfusion graft-versus-host disease after open heart surgery. Lancet 2:1099, 1986.
68. Sheehan T, McLaren KM, Brettle R, et al: Transfusion-induced graft-versus-host disease in pregnancy. Clin Lab Haematol 9:205, 1987.
69. Thaler M, Shamiss A, Orgad S, et al: The role of blood from HLA homozygous donors in fatal transfusion-associated graft-versus-host disease affects open heart surgery. N Engl J Med 321:25, 1989.
70. American Association of Blood Banks Memorandum to AABB Institution Members, November 6, 1989.
71. American Red Cross, Blood Services Letter No. 89–91, November 29, 1989.
72. Barrett F, Elbert C, Pittner B, et al: Are mothers dangerous directed donors for their infants? Transfusion 29:595, 1989.
73. Yomtovian R, Kline W, Press C, et al: Severe pulmonary hypersensitivity associated with passive transfusion of a neutrophil-specific antibody. Lancet 1:244, 1984.
74. Strauss RG and Sacher RA: Directed donations for pediatric patients. Transfusion Med Rev 2:58, 1988.
75. Isley MR, Kaley ER, Lucas WJ, et al: The hemodynamic and oxygen transport responses to automated acute normovolemic hemodilution. Anesth Analg 66:587, 1987.
76. Rueler JB: Hypothermia: Pathophysiology, clinical settings and management. Ann Intern Med 89:519, 1978.
77. Kruskall MS, Racini DG, Malynn ER, et al: Evaluation of a blood warmer that utilizes a 40° C heat exchanger. Transfusion 30:7, 1990.
78. Sohngen D, Kretschmer V, Franke K, et al: Thawing of fresh-frozen plasma with a new microwave oven. Transfusion 28:576, 1988.
79. Gray TA, Buckley BM, Sealey MM, et al: Plasma ionized calcium monitoring during liver transplantation. Transplantation 41:335, 1986.
80. Marquez J, Martin D, Virji MA, et al: Cardiovascular depression secondary to ionic hypocalcemia during hepatic transplantation in humans. Anesthesiology 65:457, 1986.
81. Linko K and Tigerstedt I: Hyperpotassemia during massive blood transfusion. Acta Anaesthiol Scand 28:220, 1984.
82. Collins JA, Simmons RL, James PM, et al: Acid-base status of seriously wounded combat casualties: Resuscitation with stored blood. Ann Surg 173:6, 1971.
83. DePalma L and Luban NLC: Autologous blood transfusion in pediatrics. Pediatrics 85:125, 1990.
84. Estrin JA, Belani KG, Karnavas AG, et al: A new approach to massive blood transfusion during pediatric liver resection. Surgery 99:664, 1986.
85. DePalma L and Luban NLC: Transfusion-transmitted diseases: AIDS and hepatitis. Contemp Pediatr 8:22, 1991.
86. DePalma L and Luban NLC: Transfusion-transmitted diseases: CMV to syphilis. Contemp Pediatr 8:87, 1991.

Inherited and Acquired Disorders of Hemostasis

Gordon L. Bray, M.D.

Excessive bleeding is a frequent complication in the management of critically ill infants and children. In most situations, the breakdown in hemostatic competence is precipitated by other underlying disease processes. This situation is exemplified by the relatively common occurrence of disseminated intravascular coagulation (DIC) from septic shock or by one of the other potential causes of this entity. However, it is not unusual for a patient with a pre-existing hemostatic disorder to present with a medical problem or bleeding complication that requires intensive care. An example of this situation is the patient with intracranial hemorrhage complicating either immune thrombocytopenic purpura (ITP) or hemophilia. This chapter discusses the diagnosis and management of several bleeding disorders that the clinician caring for critically ill children may confront in the emergency room or intensive care unit (ICU). Although less common than excessive bleeding, thrombosis is a problem that occasionally poses significant diagnostic and therapeutic challenges for the intensive care practitioner. Accordingly, the latter part of this chapter deals with several constitutional entities that predispose to abnormal clot formation.

CLASSIFICATION OF HEMOSTATIC DISORDERS

The majority of bleeding disorders in children can be categorized as resulting from abnormalities of primary hemostasis or secondary hemostasis, or both. *Primary hemostasis* refers to the events by which an effective platelet plug is formed as the initial response to vascular injury or insult. Abnormalities of primary hemostasis can result from decreased platelet number or function or abnormalities in the blood vessel wall. *Secondary hemostasis* refers to the series of biochemical reactions that ultimately lead to the formation of polymerized fibrin. Decreased concentration or function of one or more plasma coagulation proteins or accelerated degradation of fibrin (i.e., hyperfibrinolysis) can impair clot formation or stability (Fig. 64–1). From a physiologic standpoint, any differentiation between these two

groups of events is artificial since they are interdependent and occur simultaneously at sites of vascular disruption. Consider, for example, the role of thrombin in the overall hemostatic mechanism: It catalyzes the conversion of fibrinogen to monomeric fibrin; activates coagulation factor XIII (fibrin-stabilizing factor), factor VIII:C and factor V; and also is a potent agonist of platelet aggregation and secretion. Conversely, the coagulation protein interactions that result in the generation of both activated factor X and thrombin occur on the surface of platelets, vascular endothelial cells, and subendothelial protein matrix.[1]

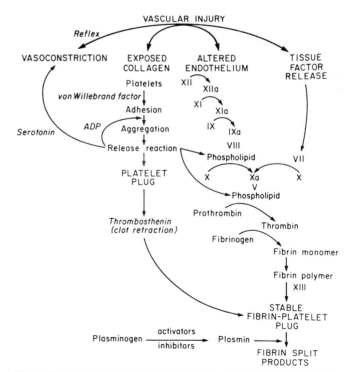

Figure 64–1. Diagrammatic representation of the hemostatic mechanism. (From Lusher JM: Diseases of coagulation: The fluid phase. *In*: Nathen DG and Oski FA [eds]: Hematology of Infancy and Childhood, 3rd ed. Philadelphia, WB Saunders, 1987, pp. 1293–1342.)

CONSTITUTIONAL DISORDERS OF PRIMARY HEMOSTASIS

Thrombocytopenias

Thrombocytopenia has been described in conjunction with a wide variety of syndromes on the basis of inheritance. In many cases, it either accompanies or is a harbinger of full-blown bone marrow failure (e.g., Fanconi aplastic anemia, amegakaryocytic thrombocytopenia). Several cytogenetic abnormalities, most notably trisomy 13 and trisomy 18, are associated with a high incidence of thrombocytopenia in the neonatal period.[2] Among the disorders that are associated with inherited thrombocytopenia in early infancy, the Wiskott-Aldrich syndrome (WAS) and thrombocytopenia absent radii (TAR) syndrome merit further discussion.

WAS is an X-linked recessive disorder characterized by eczema, progressive immunodeficiency, thrombocytopenia, and an increased predisposition to lymphoid malignancy[3] (see also Chapter 77). Patients may present at or shortly after birth with moderate to severe thrombocytopenia as well as hemorrhage of the skin and mucous membranes. On the peripheral blood smear, platelets appear abnormally small and the measured mean platelet volume is usually decreased. The combination of decreased platelet number and mass results in a bleeding risk that is virtually 100%. Although platelet transfusions are acutely effective in the control of bleeding, allosensitization to platelet antigens from repeated transfusions ultimately renders random donor platelet concentrates ineffective. Hemorrhage and overwhelming infection are the major causes of mortality in WAS.[3-5] In patients with a human leukocyte antigen (HLA)–compatible donor, bone marrow transplantation (BMT) is the treatment of choice to correct both the thrombocytopenia and immunodeficiency associated with this disorder.[5] Splenectomy has been shown to induce normalization of mean platelet volume and long-term remission of thrombocytopenia in patients who are not candidates for BMT.[4] For the occasional patient who either does not respond to splenectomy or for whom thrombocytopenia recurs post splenectomy, a pharmacologic approach that includes intravenous (IV) IgG, high-dose steroids, and vinca alkaloids may be useful.[6] Infants with X-linked thrombocytopenia who do not manifest the other features of WAS have been described, and their conditions are believed to represent variants of the disorder.[7]

TAR syndrome is an autosomal recessive disorder characterized by a lack or hypoplasia of the radii, the presence of cardiac malformations in as many as one third of cases, transient leukemoid reactions, and the development of severe thrombocytopenia, usually by 4 months of age.[7] The presence of thumbs in patients with TAR syndrome serves to distinguish patients with this disorder from those with Fanconi aplastic anemia in whom congenital anomalies of the forearms are associated with a lack of the thumbs.[2] The period of highest risk for bleeding is during the first year of life, and most deaths from hemorrhage occur during this time. Platelet transfusions are the only available therapy for bleeding associated with TAR syndrome, and they should be used judiciously in order to avoid allosensitization. The prognosis for patients who survive beyond the first year of life is good, and the majority exhibit a partial or complete resolution of the thrombocytopenia. TAR syndrome is not a precursor to the development of bone marrow aplasia or malignancy.[2]

Disorders of Platelet Function

Most inherited platelet function abnormalities are a consequence of (1) defects involving platelet membrane glycoprotein receptors that are integral to normal platelet-vessel wall or platelet-platelet interactions (e.g., Bernard-Soulier syndrome [BSS] and Glanzmann thrombasthenia [GT]), (2) quantitative or qualitative abnormalities in plasma protein ligands that mediate these interactions (e.g., von Willebrand disease [VWD], afibrinogenemia), (3) deficient platelet α or dense granule contents or release (e.g., gray platelet syndrome, storage pool deficiency), or (4) abnormalities in the biochemical pathways resulting in the generation of thromboxane A_2, the most potent in vivo agonist of platelet aggregation.[8]

Von Willebrand Disease

VWD is the most common inherited disorder of hemostasis: Prevalence estimates indicate that it may affect as many as 1.25 in 10,000 individuals. It is a paradigm of primary hemostatic disorders that result from abnormal platelet-vessel wall interaction. For the most part, VWD is inherited in an autosomal dominant fashion; only a small subset of patients with the most severe bleeding manifestations (i.e., type III VWD) exhibit autosomal recessive inheritance.[9] To understand the pathogenesis of VWD-related bleeding, it is necessary to have a basic understanding of von Willebrand factor (VWF) physiology, structure, and function.

VWF is synthesized in endothelial cells and megakaryocytes; it is one of the constituent proteins in platelet α-granules and is secreted following platelet activation. Secretion of VWF from endothelial cells occurs both constitutively and following stimulation; in the latter case, it is released from storage organelles known as Weibel-Palade bodies. Several biochemical stimuli—most notably thrombin, epinephrine, and vasopressin analogues—can induce the release of VWF from endothelial cell storage pools resulting in short-term increases in the plasma level of VWF as measured in both functional assays and immunoassays (see later). The function of VWF is to promote the binding of glycoprotein Ib-IX on the surface of platelets to collagen, which is exposed to the intravascular milieu at sites of vascular injury. Biochemically, VWF is a plasma protein ranging in size from 500 to more than 20,000 kDa. The basic subunit consists of two VWF molecules linked at their amino terminal ends, each with a molecular weight of 225 kDa. These dimers form higher-order oligomers and multimers that account for the wide range of molecular weights noted on analysis of the protein electrophoresed in SDS-agarose gels (see later). The highest molecular weight multimers are the most hemostatically effective; thus, impaired platelet adhesion can occur in situations in which these multimers are either lacking or are present in decreased concentrations.[9, 10]

Bleeding Manifestations

The bleeding tendency in most patients with VWD is mild, often escaping clinical recognition for years or even decades. There is a wide variability of phenotypic expression among affected family members and even in an affected individual at different times. It is not unusual to elicit a history of incapacitating bleeding symptoms in a patient during childhood that spontaneously remit during adolescence or adulthood. In my experience, several parents have been diagnosed with the condition only after their child presented with a VWD-related bleeding manifestation. Most symptomatic patients with VWD present with cutaneous or mucous membrane hemorrhage, or both, with recurrent epistaxis being the most common presenting bleeding manifestation. Bleeding from inflamed adenoidal or tonsillar tissue, from the mouth, or from other more distal points along the gastrointestinal tract also occurs commonly. In postpubescent girls, menorrhagia is a frequent and bothersome bleeding complication that often results in iron deficiency anemia owing to chronic blood loss. Excessive bleeding occurs, albeit inconsistently, following a major hemostatic challenge such as surgery, trauma, or dental procedures. Although rare, even relatively mild head injuries can result in intracranial hemorrhage and should prompt immediate neurologic evaluation and prophylactic therapy (see later). VWD-related bleeding and laboratory abnormalities frequently abate during pregnancy. Except in the most severely affected (i.e., type III) patients, musculoskeletal bleeding is not a common feature of VWD.[9, 11, 12]

Laboratory Diagnosis and Classification

The laboratory evaluation of a patient suspected of having VWD should include a platelet count and template bleeding time, assays of factor VIII coagulant activity (VIII:C) and factor VIII antigen, ristocetin-induced platelet aggregation (RIPA) and ristocetin cofactor (RCoF) activity,* and VWF multimeric analysis following electrophoresis in SDS-agarose gels.[9, 12] Multimeric analysis usually allows for an accurate assessment

---

*The difference between the RIPA assay and RCoF activity assay is a source of confusion to many clinicians who do not regularly care for patients with VWD. RIPA measures the ability of *platelets in patient, platelet-rich plasma* to aggregate in the presence of ristocetin (1.5–2.0 mg/ml). The aggregatory response is compared with that measured in a control platelet-rich plasma. It is a qualitative assay that is relatively insensitive in all patients with VWD except for those with types IIb or III. Decreased RIPA is observed in patients with Bernard-Soulier syndrome in addition to VWD; thus, it is somewhat lacking in specificity for the latter condition. RCoF activity measures the ability of *patient, platelet-poor plasma* to support agglutination of *control platelets*—that are either formalin fixed or freeze-dried—in the presence of ristocetin. Since the assay is performed on several patient dilutions and compared with a normal plasma pool control, results are expressed in quantitative fashion. Unlike the RIPA assay, decreased RCoF activity is specific for the diagnosis of VWD.

of VWD subtype, an important determinant of appropriate treatment and prevention of bleeding (see later). The results of laboratory studies in patients with the most common VWD subtypes are presented in Table 64–1.

Patients with type I VWD (the most common subtype) generally have the mildest bleeding symptoms and are frequently the most difficult to diagnose. Although plasma levels of VWF are borderline or below normal under baseline circumstances, hormonal and pharmacologic stimuli can raise levels into the normal range. Indeed, for patients in whom there is a high index of suspicion for VWD on the basis of bleeding history, it may be necessary to repeat some or all laboratory investigations on one or more occasions before confirmatory results are obtained. In contrast to type I patients, type III VWD is easy to diagnose. The bleeding diathesis is severe in these patients and is associated with virtually no detectable plasma VWF protein or RCoF activity. Since factor VIII coagulant protein depends on VWF for its in vivo stability, patients with severe VWD exhibit levels of factor VIII:C that are comparable with those seen in patients with hemophilia A (see later). In patients with type III VWD whose VWF genes have been evaluated by Southern blot analysis, gross deletions involving one or both VWF alleles have been noted.[13] Type IIb patients with VWD synthesize a qualitatively abnormal, high molecular weight (HMW) VWF that exhibits increased affinity for platelet membranes. Following secretion from endothelial cells, it spontaneously binds to platelet glycoprotein Ib-IX, which accounts for its decreased concentration or total absence in plasma assayed by multimeric analysis. Two laboratory abnormalities associated with type IIb disease are notable. First, some patients exhibit episodic borderline thrombocytopenia secondary to the formation of intravascular, VWF-mediated platelet aggregates. Mild thrombocytopenia has been reported via this mechanism as a presenting manifestation of type IIb disease in the newborn period.[14] Second, increased binding of type IIb VWF for platelet glycoprotein Ib-IX results in brisk aggregation in the RIPA assay at lower than normal concentrations of ristocetin.[9, 11, 12]

Treatment and Prevention of Bleeding

The approach to patients who present with or are at risk for bleeding is to acutely raise the level of functional VWF, either through infusion of an exogenously derived source or through stimulated secretion of endogenous storage pools. Cryoprecipitate is the most commonly employed and reliable source of exogenous VWF.[11, 12] While the amount of factor VIII:C activity per bag is relatively consistent (see section entitled "The Hemophilias"), there is great variability in the level of RCoF activity and bleeding time correcting ability. Furthermore, the degree to which either or both laboratory parameters are normalized by infusion of cryoprecipitate does not always correlate with clinical response. These considerations make it difficult to establish firm dosing guidelines in the treatment and prevention of bleeding

Table 64–1. RESULTS OF LABORATORY STUDIES IN PATIENTS WITH VON WILLEBRAND DISEASE

Laboratory Test	Type I	Type IIa	Type IIb	Type III
Bleeding time	Normal or prolonged	Usually prolonged	Usually prolonged	Always prolonged
Factor VIII:C	Normal or mildly decreased	Normal or mildly decreased	Usually normal	Always markedly decreased*
VWF antigen (Laurell assay)	Normal or mildly decreased	Normal or mildly decreased	Usually normal	Usually absent
Ristocetin-induced platelet aggregation (RIPA)	Usually normal	Usually decreased	Increased†	Markedly decreased to absent
Ristocetin cofactor activity	Normal or mildly to moderately decreased‡	Moderately to markedly decreased	Usually mildly to moderately decreased	Markedly decreased to absent
VWF multimeric analysis in SDS agarose gels	All MW multimers present and decreased proportionately	Absence of high and intermediate MW multimers; normal or increased low MW multimers	Absence of high MW multimers; normal or increased low and intermediate MW multimers	Lack of *all* MW multimers (high, intermediate, and low)

*Levels of factor VIII:C in most patients with type III VWD are comparable with those exhibited by patients with moderate to severe factor VIII deficiency.
†A diagnostic feature of type IIb VWD is the ability of low concentrations of ristocetin (0.2 to 0.3 mg/ml) to cause aggregation in platelet-rich plasma.
‡Patients with type I VWD usually have proportionate decreases in plasma levels of VIII:C, VWF antigen, and ristocetin cofactor activity.
MW = molecular weight; VWD = von Willebrand disease; VWF = von Willebrand factor.

and entail the need for an empirical approach to therapy.[11] In my experience, one bag of cryoprecipitate/5 kg of body weight (8 to 10 bags maximum) administered every 8 hours will provide adequate primary hemostasis in most acute circumstances. Consultation with a hematologist experienced in the care of VWD-related bleeding may help to determine the appropriate frequency and duration of replacement therapy. A pasteurized, freeze-dried factor VIII concentrate (Humate-P) has been shown to contain hemostatic levels of functional VWF. Anecdotal reports describe the use of this product in the successful treatment and prevention of bleeding in VWD, types I and IIa.[15, 16]

1-Desamino-(8-D-arginine)-vasopressin (DDAVP), a synthetic analogue of the antidiuretic hormone, arginine vasopressin, has been used for more than a decade to control non–life-threatening bleeding in patients with VWD and mild hemophilia.[17] Its major advantage lies in the fact that it is a hemostatically active agent which is not derived from blood. As a consequence of its ability to stimulate the release of factor VIII storage pools, IV DDAVP (0.3 µg/kg body weight) results in a transient, three to fivefold increase in all factor VIII-related functions (RCoF activity, factor VIII:C and VIII:Ag).[12, 17] Although DDAVP is effective in most patients with type I and in occasional patients with type IIa VWD, it is ineffective for patients with severe VWD and contraindicated in patients with type IIb disease. In the latter group of patients, DDAVP stimulates an outpouring of abnormal (type IIb) VWF resulting in the formation of intravascular platelet aggregates and mild-to-moderate thrombocytopenia.[9, 17] Even in patients with predictably good response to DDAVP, its effectiveness is limited by virtue of the tachyphylaxis that most patients exhibit with its continued use. Thus, DDAVP should be administered no more frequently than once every 24 hours. In some patients, DDAVP will be effective only if used once every 2 days.[12, 17] Frequent doses of IV DDAVP (i.e., more than once per day) can precipitate hyponatremia and seizures in critically ill children, particularly those receiving large volumes of IV fluids.[18] Thus, patients receiving daily doses of DDAVP over long periods should have close monitoring of serum and urine electrolytes. Data indicate that the biologic activity of DDAVP is comparable when given either by the IV or the subcutaneous route.[19, 20]

The administration of anovulatory medications and antifibrinolytic agents (e.g., ε-aminocaproic acid, tranexamic acid) are important adjunctive measures in the prevention and treatment of VWD-mediated menorrhagia and nasopharyngeal bleeding, respectively.[11]

Other Disorders of Platelet Function

BSS is a rare autosomal recessive disorder characterized by a lifelong bleeding tendency, prolonged bleeding time, the presence of large appearing platelets on peripheral smear, and mild-to-moderate thrombocytopenia. The molecular defect responsible for BSS is a severe deficiency or abnormal function of membrane glycoprotein Ib-IX, the platelet receptor for VWF that is necessary for normal platelet-vessel wall interaction. Thus,

Bernard-Soulier platelets do not adhere normally to subendothelial collagen, nor do they aggregate in the presence of ristocetin. In vitro aggregation in response to other platelet agonists such as adenosine diphosphate (ADP), epinephrine, and collagen is normal although aggregation in the presence of thrombin is decreased.[21–23] GT is also a rare, autosomal recessive disorder characterized by a prolonged bleeding time and moderate-to-severe bleeding symptoms. Platelets from patients with GT lack membrane glycoprotein IIb/IIIa, which, via the binding of fibrinogen, mediates normal platelet-platelet interaction. GT platelets do not aggregate in the presence of any of the agonists commonly used in platelet agglutination assays *except* ristocetin. In this respect, the defect in platelet function that characterizes GT is the mirror image of that observed in BSS, although the bleeding manifestations (i.e., epistaxis, cutaneous and mucosal bleeding, menorrhagia) and severity are comparable.[21, 23] It should be emphasized that patients with congenital afibrinogenemia exhibit bleeding time prolongation and in vitro platelet function abnormalities that are very similar to those of patients with GT, although the magnitude of the bleeding diathesis may not be as severe.[8]

Deficiency of either (or both) of the two major types of platelet secretory organelles, α- and dense granules, are associated with a bleeding diathesis of variable severity. The gray platelet syndrome is characterized by the lack or marked deficiency of platelet and megakaryocyte α-granules resulting in the characteristic gray appearance of platelets as noted on a Wright-Giemsa–stained blood film. Patients with the syndrome synthesize α-granule contents (β-thromboglobulin, platelet factor 4, platelet derived growth factor, VWF, fibrinogen, and others), as evidenced by their presence in platelet-poor plasma at normal or increased concentration. The primary defect is believed to be an inability to package these platelet proteins into developing α-granules in megakaryocytes. Prolongation of the bleeding time and abnormal aggregation and secretion in response to thrombin are the laboratory abnormalities noted most consistently in these patients. Storage pool deficiencies are a heterogeneous group of disorders characterized by mild-to-moderate bleeding and partial or complete deficiency of platelet dense granules; some patients with this condition also have an accompanying deficiency of α-granules. The most consistent in vitro platelet aggregation abnormalities noted in this group of patients are the absence of a second wave of aggregation in response to epinephrine and ADP and a complete or markedly impaired absence of aggregation in response to collagen.[8, 22]

ACQUIRED DISORDERS OF PRIMARY HEMOSTASIS

Like constitutional disorders, acquired disorders of primary hemostasis are generally attributable to decreased platelet number or function, or both. Acquired thrombocytopenias are a consequence of either immune or nonimmune mechanisms.

Immune Thrombocytopenias

In the immune thrombocytopenias, decreased platelet survival is related to the binding of IgG, IgM ($\pm$ complement), or immune complexes to the platelet surface resulting in their phagocytosis by cells of the reticuloendothelial system (RES).

Isoimmune Neonatal Thrombocytopenia

Maternal sensitization to paternally derived antigens on the surface of fetal platelets causes isoimmune neonatal thrombocytopenia. In most situations, maternal platelets lack a specific antigen, PL^{A1}, which is present on the platelets from 98% of the general population. Transplacental passage of PL^{A1}-positive fetal platelets into a PL^{A1}-negative mother results in the generation of anti-PL^{A1} antibodies that, upon passage into the fetal circulation, cause platelet destruction. In contrast to sensitization that occurs secondary to maternal-fetal red blood cell antigen incompatibility, a large percentage of infants born with isoimmune thrombocytopenia are the result of first pregnancies.[24, 25]

Neonates with isoimmune thrombocytopenia who do not present with life-threatening bleeding manifestations appear well. Signs of cutaneous hemorrhage are frequently present, and the complete blood count (CBC) is remarkable only for isolated thrombocytopenia; the mother's platelet count is normal. The latter observation helps to distinguish infants with isoimmune thrombocytopenia from those born to mothers with autoimmune thrombocytopenia in which there is usually some degree of maternal as well as neonatal thrombocytopenia. Since there is a significant risk of intracranial hemorrhage associated with isoimmune thrombocytopenia, definitive therapy should be instituted in the neonate who is either born with or acquires a platelet count less than 30,000/mm³ in the newborn period. The most consistently effective treatment is the transfusion of platelet concentrates from a PL^{A1}-negative donor, usually the infant's mother. Transfusion of random donor platelet concentrates is not helpful because of the extremely high prevalence of PL^{A1}-positive individuals in the donor pool. Similarly, there is no evidence to suggest any role for steroids or high-dose IV IgG in this disorder.[24]

Immune Thrombocytopenic Purpura

ITP is probably the most common cause of sporadic thrombocytopenia in pediatrics, occurring most commonly in children from 2 to 5 years of age. It probably occurs much more commonly than it is diagnosed, since many cases are mild and not associated with any symptoms. Typically, the child presents with the acute onset of petechiae and purpura and a history of recent, acute viral illness. Most patients exhibit platelet counts less than $40 \times 10^9/l$ at diagnosis; on peripheral blood smear, the platelets appear abnormally large. Coagulation screening studies (PT, PTT) are always normal. The diagnosis of ITP can be confirmed by examination of a bone marrow aspirate, which usually demonstrates normal to increased numbers of megakaryocytes. In addi-

tion to cutaneous hemorrhage, epistaxis and gastrointestinal bleeding are also presenting manifestations in approximately 30% and 5% of cases, respectively.[22] Intracranial hemorrhage complicates 0.5 to 1% of cases of ITP and is the major cause of long-term morbidity and mortality. While there are no definitive presenting features that identify patients at risk for intracranial hemorrhage, a history of head trauma, aspirin ingestion, or the presence of hypertension (e.g., induced by steroids, see later) in a child with severe thrombocytopenia may increase the likelihood of this potentially devastating complication.[22, 26, 27]

Natural History

The long-term outcome of children who present with ITP is depicted in Figure 64–2. Most patients have a self-limited disorder that resolves within a period of weeks to months. It is very likely that decreased platelet survival in this group of patients is due to the adsorption of viral antigen-antibody complexes to the platelet surface, resulting in their accelerated destruction in an "innocent bystander" fashion. Thus, acute ITP of childhood is probably more appropriately called acute postviral thrombocytopenia. ITP is considered chronic when the platelet count is decreased to less than 100,000/mm³ for a period of more than 6 months. Although chronic ITP may occur at any age, the likelihood is greater in children who present after 10 years of age. In contrast to acute ITP, decreased platelet survival in chronic ITP results from the binding of autoantibodies that are directed against platelet-specific surface antigens.[22] A subset of these patients will demonstrate other autoantibodies in serum at some time during their clinical course, and some ultimately develop a collagen-vascular disorder.[22]

Treatment

Infusions of platelet concentrates are contraindicated in the treatment of non–life-threatening hemorrhage secondary to ITP. Such infusions will not only fail to raise the patient's platelet count but pose a risk of allosensitization to foreign platelet antigens in the recipient.

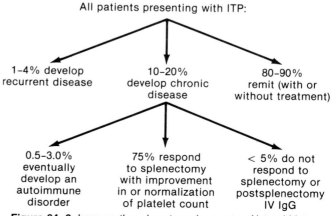

Figure 64–2. Immune thrombocytopenic purpura: Natural history.

Currently available treatment modalities for patients with new onset ITP are a short course of steroids or IV IgG. Disagreement exists among hematologists as to the best approach—and even if any treatment at all is indicated—for a disorder whose outcome is extremely favorable in 80 to 90% of cases with or without therapy.[28] Those clinicians who choose to institute some form of treatment do so out of concern for the risk of life-threatening hemorrhage (i.e., intracranial or severe gastrointestinal bleeding). The author's approach to the patient with new-onset ITP is dependent principally upon the platelet count and the nature of bleeding symptoms at presentation (Fig. 64–3). For patients who present with mucous membrane bleeding, extensive cutaneous purpura, or retinal hemorrhages, most would agree that IV IgG is the treatment of choice, in large part because of its rapid onset of action.[26] Most patients who respond to IV IgG exhibit significant increments in platelet count within days of its administration. The mechanism of action of IV IgG is incompletely understood; however, its effectiveness may be due in part to its ability to competitively block Fc receptors on the surface of RE cells, thus prolonging the survival of antibody-sensitized platelets.[26] Oral prednisone probably facilitates recovery of an adequate (if not normal) platelet count in patients with acute ITP.[22] In addition, electron microscopic evidence indicates that steroids improve the structural integrity of the microvasculature in acute thrombocytopenic states thus leading to decreased bleeding.[29] Therefore, for patients presenting with platelet counts of less than 20×10^9/l and mild or no bleeding symptoms, a 2- to 3-week course of pred-

nisone is recommended. If improvement in platelet count is not noted at the end of this period, steroids should be discontinued and alternative therapy with IV IgG should be considered.

For patients with chronic ITP, the most effective and best tolerated therapy options include IV IgG and splenectomy. IV IgG induces a partial or complete, albeit transient, normalization of the platelet count in most patients with chronic ITP. The effects of a course of IV IgG (400 mg/kg/day for 5 days or 1 g/kg/day for 1 to 3 days) generally last for several weeks to months. Some patients who initially respond to IV IgG will, at some point during their course, become refractory to its continued use. Splenectomy is the most effective long-term treatment for chronic ITP, resulting in either partial improvement or normalization of platelet count in approximately 75% of patients. In most cases, removal of the spleen results in the elimination of the major site of platelet destruction as well as a major focus of antiplatelet antibody production.[22, 27] Although splenectomy is an extremely effective treatment for most patients with chronic ITP, it carries a considerable risk of post splenectomy sepsis, especially in young children. Because of these considerations, we consider splenectomy only in patients with chronic ITP over 6 years of age and attempt the maintenance of an adequate platelet count (generally $\geq 30–40 \times 10^9$/l) in the younger child with periodic infusions of IV IgG. For patients who do not respond to this approach, an individualized therapy plan is necessary.

For patients who exhibit signs and symptoms consistent with an intracranial hemorrhage, an emergency

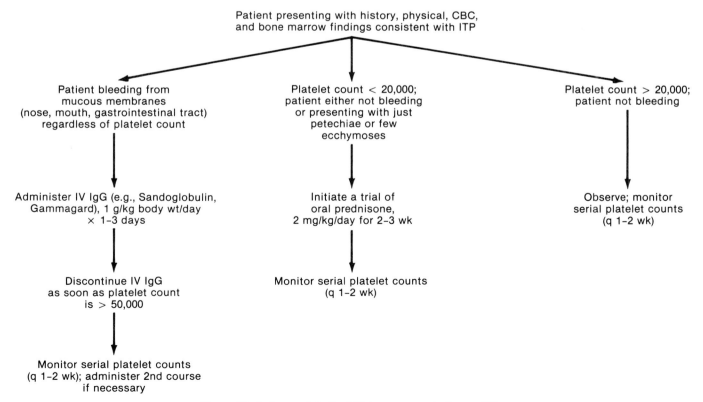

Figure 64–3. Approach to the initial management of acute ITP.

head computed tomography (CT) scan should be performed; consultation with a general surgeon and neurosurgeon should be obtained for findings consistent with a bleeding episode. Specific therapy for intracranial hemorrhage consists of emergency splenectomy and the infusion of platelet concentrates intraoperatively *after* the splenic pedicle is clamped. In many cases, the platelet count begins to rise shortly after blood flow to the spleen is interrupted. After the spleen is removed and an adequate platelet increment is documented, neurosurgical evacuation of some hematomas (particularly in the posterior fossa and in close proximity to the fourth ventricle) may be indicated.[22] Of course all of the requisite nonspecific measures to control intracranial hypertension should be instituted in the patient who is neurologically unstable.

Miscellaneous Causes of Thrombocytopenia

Other common causes of thrombocytopenia encountered in an ICU include systemic infection (bacterial, viral, malarial), infiltrative disorders of the bone marrow, and the effect of certain medications (in particular, heparin).

Thrombocytopenia has long been recognized as a complication of systemic bacterial and viral infections, although its pathogenesis is incompletely understood. It occurs more commonly when laboratory evidence of DIC is lacking than in its presence, indicating that its development is usually not a consequence of the consumptive effects of thrombin on platelets (see section on disseminated intravascular coagulation).[22] Decreased platelet survival, probably as a consequence of immune-mediated destruction, appears to be the operative mechanism in most cases of thrombocytopenia that accompany systemic infections. Elevated levels of platelet-associated immunoglobulin have been documented in thrombocytopenic patients at the onset of gram-positive and gram-negative septicemia as well as in systemic infections caused by viruses such as the Epstein-Barr virus. Infection-mediated damage to vascular endothelium and exposure of subendothelium may also increase platelet consumption, thus contributing to thrombocytopenia.[22]

Infiltrative disorders of the bone marrow are frequently associated with thrombocytopenia as a consequence of decreased platelet production. Leukemia and neuroblastoma are the most common malignant entities associated with thrombocytopenia, both at diagnosis and as a consequence of their treatment with myelosuppressive chemotherapy. Myeloproliferative and preleukemic conditions (e.g., chronic myelogenous leukemia, myelofibrosis, myelodysplastic syndromes) are also associated with thrombocytopenia and other features of bone marrow failure at presentation. In patients with systemic herpes virus infections, thrombocytopenia (and bone marrow failure) can occur as a consequence of histiocytic hyperplasia and hemophagocytosis in the bone marrow.[30]

In general, drugs induce thrombocytopenia either by decreasing platelet production or by decreasing survival (Table 64–2). In the former case, myelosuppressive chemotherapeutic agents are the most common class of medications causing thrombocytopenia, which occurs gradually, in fairly predictable fashion, and in the majority of patients treated in this manner. In situations in which drug-induced thrombocytopenia is a consequence of decreased platelet survival, it is idiosyncratic, generally sudden in onset, and usually immune in origin. Premature platelet destruction results from (1) the binding of immune complexes (consisting of the offending drug or drug-plasma protein complex and a specific antidrug antibody) to the platelet membrane; or (2) the binding of antibody directed against haptens created by drug-platelet interactions.[7, 22] The presence of co-morbid conditions that commonly cause decreased platelet counts (e.g., DIC, infection) and the concurrent administration of multiple medications can mask the diagnosis of idiosyncratic, drug-induced thrombocytopenia. Although any medication can cause thrombocytopenia on an idiosyncratic basis, perhaps the most commonly implicated of these drugs is heparin.

Thrombocytopenia occurs in approximately 1 to 5% of patients receiving heparin; it usually occurs between 8 and 11 days after initiation of heparin; and it appears more commonly in patients treated at the higher dosage ranges.[31] In most patients, thrombocytopenia is mild to moderate and paradoxically resolves with continued heparin therapy. In adult studies, a small subset of patients who develop heparin-induced thrombocytopenia have severe, often life-threatening thromboembolic phenomena resulting in ischemic gangrene of an extremity, stroke, or myocardial infarction.[22, 31] The occurrence of arterial thrombosis is an indication for the immediate cessation of heparin. In children whose thrombocytopenia is mild and in whom systemic anticoagulation is essential, it is reasonable to continue heparin therapy in conjunction with close monitoring of platelet counts with the expectation that the transition to an alternative anticoagulant (e.g., warfarin) will be made as soon as is possible.[22]

Platelet Dysfunction. Acquired platelet function defects can occur as a consequence of acute or chronic renal failure, extracorporeal circulation (e.g., "post-

---

Table 64–2. PATHOGENETIC MECHANISMS OF COMMON DRUG-INDUCED THROMBOCYTOPENIAS

Platelet Underproduction
 Myelotoxic chemotherapy agents
 Chloramphenicol

Decreased Platelet Survival
 Nonimmune-mediated
  Ristocetin
 Immune-mediated (idiosyncratic)
  Benzodiazepines (e.g., diazepam, lorazepam)
  Cimetidine
  Digoxin
  Penicillin, methicillin
  Quinidine
  Sulfa-containing antibiotics (e.g., sulfamethoxazole)
  Valproic acid
  Heparin

pump thrombocytopathy"), and the effects of medications. Each of these clinical situations is commonly associated with a prolonged bleeding time, and other abnormalities of platelet function that do not consistently correlate with bleeding risk.

The pathogenesis of bleeding secondary to acute or chronic renal failure is believed to be a consequence of the adverse effects of uremic retention products on normal platelet–vessel wall interactions. Specifically, both qualitative and quantitative abnormalities of plasma and platelet VWF have been noted in uremic patients.[32] The observation that both cryoprecipitate and DDAVP shorten the bleeding time as well as stop or prevent hemorrhage indicates that abnormalities in the concentration or functioning of VWF are contributing factors in uremic bleeding.[33] Likewise, increased plasma levels of prostacyclin (PGI$_2$), a potent antagonist of platelet aggregation that is secreted by endothelial cells, have been measured in uremic patients and may result in increased bleeding tendency. Correction of the anemia of chronic renal failure has also been shown to shorten the bleeding time and minimize bleeding in adults prior to renal biopsy or other surgical procedures. Thus, it appears that the bleeding time prolongation (and possibly the bleeding tendency) in uremia is, in part, a consequence of hematologic factors unrelated to platelet function per se.[33]

Hemodialysis or peritoneal dialysis three times/week and correction of the hematocrit to at least 25 to 30% are the modalities that are most consistently effective in the treatment or prevention of uremic bleeding.[33] Despite these measures, some patients with acute or chronic renal failure will continue to exhibit excessive bleeding even if confronted by minor hemostatic challenges. For these patients, infusions of cryoprecipitate or DDAVP can be quite effective in normalizing the bleeding time and minimizing hemorrhage. The effects of DDAVP and cryoprecipitate on bleeding tendency may outlast the short-lived (i.e., 4 to 8 hours) improvements in bleeding time that they induce.[17, 33]

Patients subjected to cardiopulmonary bypass (CPB) or extracorporeal membrane oxygenation (ECMO) exhibit a complex series of hemostatic alterations that predispose to excessive bleeding. Hemorrhage that complicates open heart surgery frequently results in the need for increased blood product support and, occasionally, surgical re-exploration. Factors that may contribute to excessive bleeding in this setting include: (1) inadequate neutralization of heparin that is required for systemic anticoagulation during the period of bypass; (2) mild thrombocytopenia; (3) transient (dilutional) decreases in the concentration of most coagulation factors; and (4) activation of the fibrinolytic mechanism.[34, 35] The most significant alteration from the standpoint of postoperative bleeding risk is an acquired defect in platelet function that occurs following passage of platelets through the oxygenator apparatus. The specific nature of this platelet defect is not fully understood; however, when platelets are recirculated through an oxygenator in vitro, alterations in platelet membrane receptors for fibrinogen and VWF occur that result in decreased binding of these plasma protein ligands. Additionally,

activation of platelets in the extracorporeal circuit results in the release (and partial deficiency) of α-granules that further impairs platelet function.[35] The magnitude of the defect increases with increasing duration of extracorporeal circulation.

The therapy for excessive hemorrhage secondary to postpump thrombocytopathy is transfusion of platelet concentrates. Prospective, randomized studies in adults undergoing CPB suggest that DDAVP and the serine protease inhibitor, aprotinin (Trasylol) may also decrease the severity of the platelet function defect in patients undergoing extracorporeal circulation.[34, 36]

Commonly used drugs that interfere with platelet function in vitro and that can contribute to a bleeding tendency are listed in Table 64–3.

INHERITED COAGULOPATHIES

Hemophilias

Hemophilia A (factor VIII deficiency) and hemophilia B (factor IX deficiency) are the most common inherited coagulopathies occurring at an incidence of 1 in 10,000 and 1 in 50,000 live male births, respectively. Both disorders are inherited in X-linked recessive fashion, and in approximately one third of newly diagnosed patients there is no history of a previously affected family member. Since hemophilia A and B are clinically indistinguishable, differentiation of these disorders from one another relies on the results of specific coagulation assays for factors VIII and IX. Patients with these disorders are characterized as mild, moderate, or severely affected depending on their baseline factor level. Bleeding severity correlates reasonably well with the degree of factor deficiency: mildly affected patients (> 5% of normal factor activity) tend to exhibit abnormal bleeding only in association with surgery, trauma, or

Table 64–3. COMMONLY USED DRUGS THAT PROLONG THE BLEEDING TIME OR DECREASE IN VITRO PLATELET AGGREGATION

Antiplatelet Agents
Aspirin
Dipyridamole
Sulfinpyrazone
Ticlopidine

Antibiotics
Semisynthetic penicillins
Cephalosporins

Nonsteroidal Anti-inflammatory Agents
Ibuprofen
Naproxen
Indomethacin
Phenylbutazone

Miscellaneous
Heparin
Dextran sulfate
Glyceryl guaiacolate
Ethyl alcohol
Valproic acid
ω$_3$-Polyunsaturated fatty acids
Phenothiazines

invasive dental procedures while severely affected patients ($<$ 1% of normal activity) experience frequent spontaneous hemorrhage without these predisposing conditions.[12]

Bleeding Manifestations

A common mode of presentation is the occurrence of excessive oozing following circumcision. Although excessive bleeding in this setting is very suggestive of hemophilia, the clinician should be aware that many newborns who are mildly or moderately affected may not bleed excessively. Beyond the first year of life, the most common sites of bleeding are the synovial membranes of the knees, ankles, and elbows, as well as major muscle groups of the extremities. The onset of bleeding into joints and muscles tends to coincide with the development of motor milestones such as walking, running, and climbing. Mucous membrane bleeding involving the nose and mouth also occurs commonly, the latter in association with tongue lacerations and the shedding of deciduous teeth. Clinical events that are acutely life-threatening to the individual with hemophilia include CNS, retropharyngeal, and retroperitoneal bleeding; surgery in the absence of effective factor replacement therapy; and multiple trauma.[12, 37, 38]

Results from two retrospective studies and one prospective study have documented an incidence of CNS bleeding in hemophilia of 2.6 to 13.8% with associated rates of mortality between 20% and 50%.[39] In approximately 40% of subjects in one large series, no history of head trauma or other precipitating factor could be discerned.[40] In patients for whom a history of antecedent head injury is elicited, symptom-free intervals lasting as long as several days can elapse between the traumatic episode and the diagnosis of the bleeding event. Intracranial bleeding is a well-described complication of vaginal delivery that requires the use of forceps.[39] A survey of 104 hemophilia treatment centers in the United States and Canada revealed that, of 1,070 infants who were born with hemophilia either vaginally or by cesarean section over a 5-year period, 1.8% experienced intracranial hemorrhage at or immediately following birth and an additional 1.9% had bleeding into the head after 1 month of age.[41]

Retropharyngeal hemorrhage poses a significant, immediate threat to the individual with hemophilia because even small bleeding episodes can cause extrinsic compression of the upper airway leading to obstruction and asphyxia. Typical presenting manifestations include sore throat, difficult or painful swallowing, change in voice quality, and signs and symptoms consistent with upper airway obstruction (e.g., nasal flaring, retractions, inspiratory stridor).[42] The diagnosis can be documented either by the presence of an abnormally widened retropharyngeal soft tissue shadow on lateral neck x-ray or an area of increased lucency in the retropharyngeal space on CT scan (Fig. 64–4A). Retroperitoneal hemorrhage can occur spontaneously but more commonly results from blunt injury to the abdomen or flank. Profound intravascular volume depletion can occur as a result of bleeding into the retroperitoneal space, typi-

cally over the course of hours to days. Presenting clinical manifestations include diffuse pain and tenderness involving the abdomen or back, or both, as well as signs and symptoms of impending shock (e.g., tachycardia, hypotension, decreased urinary output, poor peripheral perfusion). The diagnosis is confirmed by abdominal CT scan or by ultrasonography.[37, 38]

An expanding hematoma in an enclosed muscle bundle can compromise the functional integrity of peripheral nerves and blood vessels contained within. Compartment syndromes most commonly involve the iliopsoas muscle and the muscles of the forearm. Patients with iliopsoas muscle bleeding typically present with pain in the lower abdomen or groin, or both, and when it occurs on the right side, it is frequently confused with acute appendicitis. The hip involved is held in flexion and external rotation; any attempt to extent the hip causes exquisite pain as a consequence of reflex muscle spasm. Ischemic compression of the femoral nerve that runs through the iliopsoas muscle can result in paresthesias along the anterior aspect of the thigh, quadriceps muscle paresis, and loss of patellar reflexes. Diagnostic confirmation of iliopsoas muscle bleeding can be obtained by performing a retroperitoneal ultrasound that will allow visualization of the hematoma. Hemorrhage into the muscles of the forearm can lead ultimately to paralysis of the median and ulnar nerves and profound impairment of fine motor function in the hand.[37, 38]

Treatment of Hemophilia-Related Bleeding

Products that are currently available for the treatment of hemophilia A–related bleeding include cryoprecipitate and freeze-dried, factor VIII concentrates.[43] Cryoprecipitate is made from units of plasma that are tested for the presence of antibodies against HIV-1 and hepatitis B and hepatitis C (formerly non-A, non-B) viruses. In addition to factor VIII coagulant activity (VIII:C), cryoprecipitate is a rich source of fibrinogen and VWF and is thus the treatment of choice for bleeding secondary to hypofibrogenemia and afibrinogenemia and in some patients with VWD. For purposes of dose calculation, each bag contains 80 to 100 units of factor VIII:C.[43] Factor VIII concentrates are generally of intermediate or high purity. Intermediate purity concentrates contain variable quantities of fibrinogen, fibronectin, and VWF in addition to factor VIII, while high-purity products (manufactured by monoclonal antibody affinity chromatography) contain only factor VIII and pasteurized human albumin that is added as a stabilizer. Whether of intermediate or high purity, each lot of factor VIII concentrate is manufactured from between 2,000 and 30,000 units of donor plasma that are screened for evidence of infection with HIV-1 and then subjected to a viral inactivation process designed to destroy any residual virus that is not detected in the original screening process. Of the viral inactivation methods in use, pasteurization, exposure of the concentrate to a detergent-solvent suspension in the wet state or to very high temperatures (80° C) in the freeze-dried state also inactivate non-A, non-B hepatitis (NANBH) virus(es), a major cause of chronic liver disease in patients with

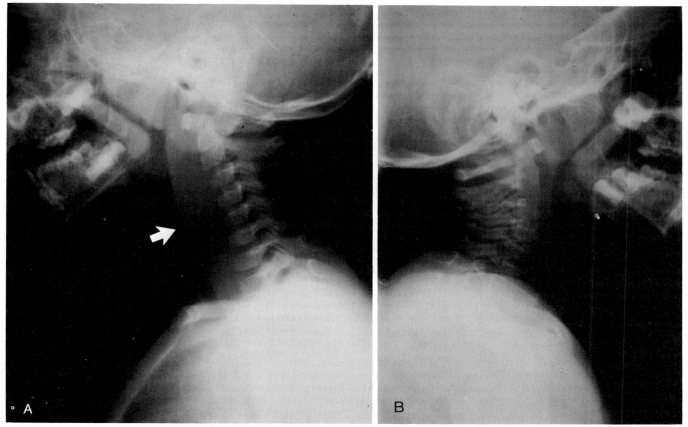

Figure 64–4. *A,* Lateral neck x-ray of a 3-year-old infant with severe factor IX deficiency (hemophilia B) with a spontaneous retropharyngeal hematoma. There is fusiform widening of the retropharyngeal soft tissue shadow that is most prominent at the level of the hyoid bone (*arrow*). *B,* Lateral neck radiograph on the same patient obtained after a 2-week course of daily factor replacement therapy. There is complete resolution of the retropharyngeal soft-tissue widening noted on the initial diagnostic film. (From Bray G and Nugent D: Hemorrhage involving the upper airway in hemophilia. Clin Pediatr 25:436, 1986.)

hemophilia.[44] The number of units of factor VIII activity in a bottle of concentrate is stated on the label of each vial. Large-scale production of factor VIII manufactured by recombinant DNA methods has recently become a reality; two commercially manufactured recombinant factor VIII products are currently in phase II/III clinical trials. The major theoretical advantage of such products is the elimination of infection risk by blood-borne viruses.[44]

Products that are available for the treatment of bleeding secondary to factor IX deficiency include fresh or fresh frozen plasma (FFP) and factor IX concentrates.[43] FFP contains 1 unit/ml of factor IX activity and thus is not a concentrated source of clotting protein. Constraints on the amount of fluid that can be administered—particularly in an ICU where the need to restrict fluid intake is commonplace—render FFP useful only in patients with mild factor IX deficiency who do not require very high plasma levels for the control of bleeding (e.g., for an invasive bedside procedure). In contrast, factor IX concentrates are the treatment of choice for patients who require plasma levels greater than 10 to 15% of their baseline.[12, 43] Since these products also contain appreciable amounts of factor II (prothrombin) and factor X, their use is appropriate in certain clinical situations involving congenital deficiency of these plasma proteins (see later). As with factor VIII concentrates, source plasma used in the manufacture of factor IX concentrates is screened for evidence of HIV-1 infection, and the final product is heat treated either in the freeze-dried or wet state.

The major complications associated with the use of factor IX concentrates are infection by NANBH virus(es) and the development of thrombosis.[12] The latter complication is believed to result from the in vitro activation of clotting proteins that may occur to a small extent during the purification process. The risk of thrombosis is greatest in patients who receive large quantities of factor IX concentrate over short periods of time, in those with underlying liver disease or polycythemia, and in those undergoing surgical procedures. For the prevention of this complication in patients with these risk factors, the addition of heparin, 5 IU/ml of concentrate, is recommended just prior to the infusion of the product.[12] The availability of more highly purified factor IX concentrates, which are currently under development, should also significantly decrease the risk of thrombosis.[45, 46]

The amount and frequency of factor replacement in a patient with hemophilia is a function of the degree of

Table 64–4. RECOMMENDED LEVELS OF FACTOR ACTIVITY CORRECTION IN THE TREATMENT OR PREVENTION OF HEMOPHILIA-RELATED BLEEDING

Bleeding Manifestation	Activity Level (%)	Comment
Acute hemarthrosis		
Early*	20–30	
Late†	40–50	Patient may require multiple infusions over several days for complete resolution of symptoms.
Muscle hematoma	50–60	For extensive hemorrhage involving large muscles (e.g., hamstring, quadriceps), twice per day infusions for several days to 1 week may be necessary for resolution of symptoms.
Hematuria	50	Treatment should include vigorous hydration via the intravenous route and avoidance of antifibrinolytic agents.
Mucous membrane bleeding/dental procedures	30–40	An antifibrinolytic agent (either ε-aminocaproic acid or tranexamic acid) should be used adjunctively to prevent rebleeding.
Life-threatening hemorrhage‡	80–100	
Preparation for surgery	80–100	Plasma *must* be screened for the presence of an inhibitor prior to any surgical procedure; prior to an elective procedure, determine the half-life of infused factor by measuring plasma levels 1, 2, 4, and 8 hours following a 50 unit/kg dose.

*Early hemarthroses are characterized by a subjective sense of pain or stiffness, or both, with little or no objective signs of bleeding.
†Late hemarthroses exhibit swelling, warmth, tenderness, and limited range of motion.
‡Includes intracranial, retroperitoneal, and retropharyngeal bleeding.

severity of the deficient clotting factor, the specific bleeding manifestation requiring treatment, the size of the patient, and the recovery and half-life of the infused coagulation factor. Recommendations for peak factor levels as a function of some specific bleeding manifestations are presented in Table 64–4. Factor VIII coagulant protein is a large molecule of approximately 300 kDa, which circulates in noncovalent association with VWF. Thus, approximately 80% of an infused dose of factor VIII remains in the intravascular compartment at 30 to 60 minutes after infusion. In contrast, factor IX is a smaller protein with a molecular weight of 56,000; its volume of distribution is significantly larger than that of factor VIII. Only about 40% of an infused dose of factor IX is recoverable intravascularly 30 to 60 minutes postinfusion. An infusion of 1 unit of factor VIII/kg of body weight generally results in a peak plasma factor VIII level of 2% in a patient with hemophilia A; 1 unit of factor IX/kg increases plasma factor IX activity by only 1% in a patient with hemophilia B. The biologic half-life of factor VIII is relatively short, 8 to 12 hours, whereas the half-life of factor IX is 18 to 24 hours.[12, 47]

Surgical measures aimed at treating life- or limb-threatening bleeding can be performed as in any other patient but only *after* appropriate factor replacement therapy. Neurosurgical evacuation of an intracranial hematoma can be performed safely as long as peak factor activity level has been corrected to 80 to 100% before surgery. Patients with retropharyngeal hemorrhage who are considered to be at significant risk of upper airway obstruction should have their airway protected either with endotracheal intubation or tracheostomy. Bleeding episodes that cause compartment syndromes in the forearm or other extremity muscle groups should be evaluated by an orthopedic surgeon in order to assess the need for decompressive fasciotomy.

Complications of Treatment

Inhibitor Formation

The formation of antibodies that inactivate factor VIII:C occurs in 10 to 15% of patients with severe hemophilia A; inhibitor formation complicates the management of severe hemophilia B in approximately 2% of patients.[12] In mild or moderately affected patients, inhibitor formation is rare. Patients with inhibitors are categorized as being high or low responders. High responders, which comprise the majority of individuals with inhibitors, predictably mount an anamnestic response to infusion of the deficient factor, whereas low responders do not increase their generally low level of inhibitor antibodies following factor infusion. Low responders may convert to high responders and vice versa. Factors that govern the development of inhibitors are unknown, although there is a high concordance among siblings, suggesting a genetic predisposition. There appears to be little relationship between cumulative factor VIII exposure and inhibitor formation, and some patients acquire antifactor VIII antibodies after just a few exposure-days of factor concentrate. Most patients destined to develop inhibitors do so by 20 years of age. Plasma should be screened for inhibitors routinely once per year, prior to any surgical procedure and in situations in which the response to appropriate doses of factor infusion is suboptimal.[44]

There are few universally accepted guidelines governing the management of bleeding in a patient with inhibitors. One's approach is usually influenced by the nature and extent of bleeding (life-threatening versus non–life-threatening), the type of inhibitor (high versus low responder), and the inhibitor titer at the time of the acute bleeding event. No approach will predictably stop (or prevent) bleeding in patients with high responder inhibitors.[12, 48] The management or prevention of bleeding in the critically ill patient with hemophilia with an inhibitor should always be carried out in close consultation with a hematologist (preferably in a hemophilia treatment center) who is familiar with currently available treatment modalities (see reference 48 for a detailed discussion of the management of inhibitor patients).[48]

Infection by Blood-Borne Viruses

The agents principally responsible for transfusion associated morbidity and mortality in hemophiliacs are

HIV-1 and the NANBH virus(es). Seventy-five to 90% of patients with severe hemophilia A and 50% of patients with severe hemophilia B exhibit serologic evidence of infection by human immunodeficiency virus (HIV)-1 as a consequence of contaminated factor concentrate usage during the early 1980s. As of 1990, the cumulative incidence of acquired immunodeficiency syndrome (AIDS) in the United States has reached 7 to 9%, and it has become the major cause of mortality in the hemophilia population.[44] The spectrum of opportunistic infections and malignancy seen in these patients is similar to other HIV-infected populations, although Kaposi sarcoma is rare. In one large series of prospectively followed patients whose HIV-1 seroconversion dates are known, the latency phase of infection was longer in patients infected with the virus prior to 18 years of age compared with those infected as adults. Regardless of the seemingly better prognosis of patients who were infected as children, the 8-year cumulative incidence of AIDS in this subset of patients is 13%.[49]

Infection by NANBH has been shown to be a major contributor to the development of chronic active hepatitis and cirrhosis among multiply transfused hemophiliacs.[44] Investigators have identified a single-stranded RNA virus (hepatitis C virus) that appears to be the cause of at least 80% of cases of NANBH; an immunoassay capable of detecting antibodies to this virus has also been developed. Use of this assay by blood banks and the plasma fractionation industry should decrease hepatitis C virus contamination of the blood supply.[50]

Other Coagulation Factor Deficiencies

Deficiency of contact activation factors XII, prekallikrein, or HMW kininogen are rare disorders that do not cause abnormal bleeding. Typically, they are identified after an isolated prolongation of the partial thromboplastin time (PTT) is observed as part of a routine preoperative coagulation screen.[12] Congenital deficiency of factor XI (below 30% of normal) occurs with relatively high frequency in individuals of Ashkenazi Jewish descent and is occasionally associated with excessive bleeding following surgery or major trauma.[12, 51]

Decreased concentration or function of factors X, V, and VII; prothrombin; fibrinogen; and factor XIII may all be associated with excessive bleeding, depending on the severity of the deficiency and on the extent of the hemostatic challenge to which the patient is subjected. Severe factor XIII deficiency is a rare autosomal recessive disorder. Patients with less than 5% of normal factor XIII activity typically present in infancy with prolonged oozing after shedding of the umbilical stump and they experience easy bruisability, mucous membrane bleeding, and poor wound healing later in life. The diagnosis is made in a patient with a normal PTT, prothrombin time (PT), and thrombin time (TT) whose fibrin clot demonstrates increased solubility in a solution of either 5M urea or 1% monochloracetic acid.[12, 47] Patients with hypofibrinogenemia or afibrinogenemia (<75mg/dl) may also exhibit excessive postsurgical bleeding and wound dehiscence. Patients with less than

15% of normal factor VII activity or less than 30 to 40% of normal prothrombin activity may bleed excessively following trauma or surgery.[43, 47]

ACQUIRED COAGULOPATHIES

Vitamin K Deficiency States

Vitamin K is a fat-soluble vitamin that is required by the liver for the normal post-translational, γ-carboxylation of coagulation factors II, VII, IX, and X. There are several clinical situations in which symptomatic vitamin K deficiency can occur in pediatrics. Classic hemorrhagic disease of the newborn (HDN) can occur as early as the first day of life in an infant exposed in utero to drugs that are known to interfere with vitamin K metabolism (e.g., warfarin, phenytoin, phenobarbital). These infants can present with spontaneous cephalohematomas, and some have exhibited intracranial hemorrhage in the immediate newborn period. More typically, HDN occurs in the second to fifth day postnatally in breast-fed infants in whom intramuscular vitamin K is not administered in the newborn period.[24] Even when vitamin K is given appropriately at birth, delayed HDN can occur as late as 3 months of age in infants who are breast-fed and who either develop a diarrheal illness or require prolonged treatment with broad-spectrum antibiotics. Common bleeding manifestations include the spontaneous appearance of ecchymoses, mucous membrane and gastrointestinal hemorrhage, and excessive oozing from venipuncture sites.[24, 52]

Clinically significant vitamin K deficiency can occur in older infants and children in association with fat malabsorption states (e.g., cystic fibrosis, biliary atresia) or in children who receive total parenteral nutrition that is not supplemented with vitamin K. Another important cause of vitamin K deficiency is the accidental or deliberate ingestion of large quantities of warfarin, which has a risk of bleeding for as long as 2 to 3 days after the ingestion.[12, 24]

Documented or suspected vitamin K deficiency is treated with parenterally administered vitamin K_1 (5 mg). Following vitamin K supplementation, amelioration of bleeding symptoms and correction of coagulation screening studies typically occur within 4 to 6 hours and 24 hours, respectively. For the patient who presents with life-threatening bleeding, the immediate infusion of FFP, 10 to 15 ml/kg, is indicated as well.[12]

Advanced Liver Disease

The major hemostatic abnormalities that have been observed in end-stage liver disease include: (1) mild thrombocytopenia secondary to accompanying hypersplenism; (2) decreased coagulation factor production and secretion; (3) low-grade DIC secondary to an inability on the part of the liver to metabolize activated coagulation proteins; (4) qualitative platelet function abnormalities secondary to increased concentrations of fibrin degradation products; and (5) increased fibrinolysis.[53]

The liver is the primary (if not exclusive) site of biosynthesis for all of the integral and regulatory proteins of the coagulation and fibrinolytic mechanisms. Thus, it is not surprising that coagulation factor deficiency of variable severity tends to dominate the clinical picture in both fulminant hepatic necrosis and advanced chronic liver disease. The only definitive therapy for patients in whom there is no chance of recovery of adequate protein synthesis is liver transplantation. Supportive therapy for coagulation factor deficiency can be provided in the form of FFP and cryoprecipitate. Infusions of prothrombin complex concentrates (particularly brands that contain large amounts of factor VII, such as Proplex-T, Baxter-Hyland Corp) are occasionally helpful in achieving hemostasis in the bleeding patient; however, their use is associated with considerable risk of DIC.[12, 53] Attempts to treat bleeding or to improve the results of coagulation screening studies with vitamin K are generally unsuccessful unless the liver disease is a consequence of biliary obstruction. Transient correction of the PTT and PT to less than 1.5 times the control with FFP and cryoprecipitate will usually allow for adequate hemostasis prior to the performance of minor invasive procedures (e.g., liver biopsy).

HEMOSTATIC DISORDERS INVOLVING BOTH PLATELETS AND CLOTTING FACTORS

Disseminated Intravascular Coagulation

DIC is probably the most common hemostatic disturbance encountered in an intensive care setting. When it is associated with an acute, fulminant illness (e.g., overwhelming sepsis, hypovolemic shock, multiple trauma), it is a serious thrombohemorrhagic complication with significant associated morbidity and mortality. In contrast, several illnesses (e.g., chronic liver or kidney disease) are associated with a steady-state, low-grade variety of DIC that is evident only upon laboratory evaluation. Disease entities that commonly precipitate DIC are listed in Table 64–5.

Pathophysiology. The development of DIC is a consequence of one or more of the following mechanisms: (1) extensive endothelial cell injury resulting in the release of tissue plasminogen activator (TPA) into the circulation and the exposure of subendothelial protein matrix to the intravascular compartment, triggering activation of factor XII; the latter results in activation of the intrinsic coagulation mechanism, prekallikrein, and plasminogen; (2) extensive tissue damage results in the exposure of blood to large amounts of tissue factor that leads to activation of factor X and factor IX by factor VIIa-tissue factor complex; and (3) certain snake venoms or other serine protease enzymes (e.g., pancreatic) can proteolytically activate factor X or prothrombin directly.[54] All of these mechanisms result in the generation of free plasma thrombin, which systemically cleaves fibrinogen to soluble fibrin; stimulates the aggregation and release of platelets; and activates factors V, VIII, and XIII. Free plasma kallikrein generated by the factor XIIa-mediated activation of prekallikrein results in the cleavage of bradykinin from HMW kininogen, which causes vasodilatation.[12] The release of TPA into the circulation, the cleavage of plasminogen to plasmin by factor XIIa and TPA and the generation of soluble fibrin results in secondary activation of the fibrinolytic mechanism. These multiple events result in hypotension, hypofibrinogenemia, thrombocytopenia, and the formation of platelet and fibrin thrombi in the lumina of small blood vessels with subsequent ischemic tissue damage.

Clinical Manifestations. Most patients with acute DIC exhibit varying degrees of bleeding and tissue ischemia resulting from thrombosis. Usually, one or the other dominates the clinical picture: ischemic organ damage tends to be more pervasive if reticuloendothelial system function is either impaired or overwhelmed or if there is relative inhibition of fibrinolysis.[54] The former condition results in suboptimal clearance of activated coagulation factors and soluble fibrin, whereas the latter allows for unopposed fibrin deposition and thrombosis. Intravascular fibrin deposition causes mechanical injury to red blood cells, which is manifested by the presence of microangiopathic changes on the peripheral blood smear.

Bleeding secondary to DIC is a consequence of platelet and coagulation factor consumption and secondary fibrinolysis. The skin is the most common site of hemorrhage; however, involvement of mucous membranes (epistaxis, hematuria, gastrointestinal bleeding) also occurs frequently. Hemorrhagic infarcts involving the central nervous system or the lungs also complicate the

Table 64–5. CONDITIONS THAT COMMONLY TRIGGER ACUTE DISSEMINATED INTRAVASCULAR COAGULATION IN PEDIATRICS

Neonatal Disorders
Intrauterine infections
Maternal toxemia
Abruptio placentae
Hyaline membrane disease, meconium aspiration
Necrotizing enterocolitis

Infectious Etiologies
Bacterial sepsis (either gram positive or gram negative)
Falciparum malaria
Rickettsial infections (e.g., Rocky Mountain spotted fever)
Disseminated fungal infections
Systemic viral infections (e.g., herpesvirus infections)

Other Illnesses
Hypovolemic shock
Acute (hypergranular) promyelocytic leukemia
Intravascular hemolytic transfusion reactions
Extensive burns or trauma
Intracranial injuries (e.g., gunshot wounds)
Hyperthermia or hypothermia
Proteolytic snake venoms (e.g., *Echis carinatus*)

Localized Consumptive Coagulopathy
Kasabach-Merritt syndrome (giant hemangioma, DIC*)
Hyperacute renal allograft rejection
Dead fetus syndrome

*DIC = disseminated intravascular coagulation.

most fulminant and severe cases of DIC. The skin, digits, and renal cortex are frequent sites of ischemic infarction in cases in which thrombosis predominates. Occlusion of cutaneous and digital blood vessels results in the formation of hemorrhagic bullae, the development of painful gangrene, and ultimately tissue sloughing (purpura fulminans); involvement of the hands and feet ultimately leads to autoamputation. Formation of platelet and fibrin thrombi within glomerular capillaries and afferent arterioles results in acute cortical necrosis and chronic renal failure.[12, 54]

Diagnosis and Treatment. Acute DIC is relatively easy to diagnose when it presents with moderate to severe manifestations; however, in patients with chronic, low-grade DIC, the diagnosis may be somewhat obscure. All patients with DIC exhibit some degree of thrombocytopenia and hypofibrinogenemia. Usually, the PT and PTT are prolonged and the concentration of fibrin degradation products (FDP) is increased to more than 10 ng/ml, reflecting generalized coagulation factor consumption and increased fibrinolysis, respectively. In addition to fibrinogen, the specific coagulation factors that are most consistently decreased are prothrombin, factor V, and factor VIII. Evaluation of a peripheral blood smear may reveal fragmentation of red blood cells. Performance of more sophisticated studies (e.g., radiolabeled platelet or fibrinogen survival studies, assays of fibrinolytic activity, antithrombin III levels) is rarely necessary and usually has limited value.

The mainstay of treatment for DIC is the elimination of its underlying cause or causes and high-quality supportive care until hemostasis can be normalized. Infusions of platelet concentrates for bleeding or severe thrombocytopenia ($<20,000/mm^3$) as well as FFP or cryoprecipitate for severe hypofibrinogenemia (<75 mg/dl) can prevent life-threatening bleeding complications until the underlying cause of DIC can be eliminated. Antiplatelet agents (e.g., aspirin, nonsteroidal anti-inflammatory drugs) and antifibrinolytic agents (ϵ-aminocaproic acid, tranexamic acid) have no role in the management of DIC. Anecdotal reports suggest that heparin can ameliorate the severity of purpura fulminans and may prevent DIC in patients with acute (hypergranular) promyelocytic leukemia, if instituted prior to beginning induction chemotherapy. In situations in which DIC is dominated by bleeding and not thrombotic manifestations, the benefits of heparin are more dubious. An increase in the fibrinogen concentration or platelet count within 24 to 48 hours of beginning heparin therapy (50 to 100 units/kg/hr via continuous infusion) is generally indicative of a beneficial effect and therefore justifies its continued use until the underlying cause of DIC can be eliminated and hemostasis can be normalized. In contrast, patients who do not exhibit an increased fibrinogen concentration or platelet count within 48 hours of its institution will probably not benefit from its continued use.

DIAGNOSTIC APPROACH TO THE BLEEDING PATIENT

An appropriate evaluation of the child who exhibits abnormal bleeding requires careful consideration of a focused personal and family history, appreciation of the significance of pertinent physical findings, and an accurate interpretation of common laboratory studies that are designed to assess the various facets of the hemostatic mechanism.

Certain aspects of the history can be very helpful in assessing the likelihood of a bleeding diathesis. Epistaxis that involves exclusively one nostril or that occurs only during periods of coryza or in low humidity environments is more likely caused by an anatomic problem rather than a predisposition to abnormal bleeding. Conversely, patients who require unusual measures to stop bleeding (e.g., silver nitrate cautery of nasal mucosa, packing of the nose, or suturing in a tooth socket following routine dental extraction) or patients who have a history of having received blood products in an effort to either stop bleeding or treat blood loss exhibit a relatively high probability of having a hemorrhagic diathesis. In postpubescent females, it is often helpful to determine if menorrhagia is present by ascertaining the total number of days in an average menstrual period and the number of days of heavy flow. If the former is more than 7 days and the latter is more than 3 days, the patient more than likely has menorrhagia and should therefore be evaluated for a bleeding problem (e.g., VWD).[11]

Whereas few bleeding manifestations are diagnostic of a specific hemostatic disorder, a few general principles can be helpful in directing a diagnostic evaluation: bleeding that involves primarily the skin (i.e., petechiae or purpura) or mucous membranes, or both, suggests a disorder of primary hemostasis (i.e., decreased platelet function or number), whereas deep hemorrhages involving muscles and joints and associated with swelling, warmth, and limited range of motion suggest a coagulation factor deficiency. Additionally, the onset of bleeding in infancy or early childhood (particularly in an otherwise well child) is more suggestive of an inherited rather than an acquired bleeding disorder.

The laboratory evaluation of a child with a suspected bleeding disorder should begin with a determination of the platelet count, bleeding time, PTT, PT, and TT tests. In assessing platelet count, it is important to inspect a well-prepared peripheral blood smear in order to confirm the accuracy of platelet enumeration by the electronic particle (e.g., Coulter) counter; evaluation of the blood film allows for identification of platelet aggregates as well as platelets that are either abnormally large (e.g., BSS, ITP, May-Hegglin anomaly) or abnormally small (e.g., WAS). The bleeding time, performed either with a template or spring-loaded device (e.g., Simplate), is the single best determinant of primary hemostasis in most circumstances; each laboratory must develop its own upper and lower limits of normal according to strict quality control standards of performance. In addition, bleeding time methodology and limits of normal differ substantially for newborns and young infants in comparison with older children and adults.[55] *Results of the bleeding time test must be interpreted with extreme caution in patients who have taken medications that can interfere with platelet function within a period of 2 weeks prior to its performance* (see Table 64–3).

The coagulation screening studies (PTT, PT, and TT) assess the functional integrity of various components of the coagulation cascade. The PTT measures the activity of coagulation proteins involved in the intrinsic pathway. Thus, an abnormal PTT occurs coincident with decreased concentration or function of any clotting factor(s) except factor VII. A prolongation of the PT in the face of a normal PTT and TT is indicative of factor VII deficiency. As with the bleeding time, interpretation of coagulation screening studies and factor activity assays must take into account the age of the patient. Normal newborns exhibit reduced plasma levels of all contact activation factors (factor XII, prekallikrein, HMW kininogen, factor XI) as well as all of the vitamin K–dependent coagulation proteins (factors II, VII, IX, and X), and these decreased levels are magnified in preterm infants. Conversely, the levels of VWF, factor VIII, and fibrinogen are equal to or higher than those noted in older children and adults.[56, 57] The most frequently encountered situation that confounds the interpretation of coagulation studies is heparin contamination of plasma samples. This is true especially in an intensive care setting in which critically ill patients have multiple indwelling lines that contain heparin. *No amount of blood and fluid aspirated from a heparin-containing catheter will consistently eliminate the anticoagulant from a specimen obtained for coagulation studies. Therefore, blood should be obtained via peripheral venipuncture whenever possible in order to optimize the chance of obtaining accurate results.* Although all of the coagulation screening studies are prolonged by heparin, the TT is the most sensitive to its presence. The effects of heparin in plasma obtained for coagulation studies can be assessed either by comparing TT and reptilase time assays or by heparin neutralization with protamine sulfate. Unlike thrombin, reptilase is not neutralized by AT III-heparin and thus will clot fibrinogen in the presence of heparin. Therefore, the combination of a normal reptilase time and a prolonged TT is very suggestive of heparin contamination. Likewise, shortening of even a couple of seconds in the TT following the addition of protamine sulfate to a plasma sample is highly suggestive of the presence of heparin.

An algorithmic approach to the evaluation of most types of bleeding disorders is presented in Figure 64–5.

DISORDERS PREDISPOSING TO THROMBOSIS

Plasma Anticoagulant Protein Deficiencies

Three plasma proteins—AT III, protein C, and protein S—are essential in the normal regulation of clot formation in vivo. Individuals with either decreased concentration or defective function of these anticoagulant proteins exhibit an increased risk of thrombosis, especially in clinical situations that predispose to abnormal clot formation (e.g., pregnancy, trauma, surgery, infection, prolonged immobility). In most instances, the pattern of inheritance for all three plasma protein defi-

ciencies is autosomal dominant with variable expressivity.

In vitro, antithrombin III (AT III) inhibits the activity of thrombin as well as factors Xa, IXa, XIa, and XIIa by formation of a 1:1 stoichiometric complex with each, a process that is increased approximately 1,000-fold in the presence of heparin. In vivo, AT III probably functions on endothelial cell surfaces where heparin-like glycosaminoglycans catalyze its inactivation of principally thrombin and factor Xa.[58, 59]

Typically, the first thrombotic event in individuals with AT III deficiency occurs between the ages of 10 and 30 years; the most common presenting clinical manifestations include superficial thrombophlebitis or deep vein thrombosis involving the lower extremities, pulmonary embolus, and mesenteric vein thrombosis. The diagnosis of AT III deficiency is made by documenting plasma levels of functional AT III that are below 50 to 60% of normal either with or without concomitantly decreased antigen levels. Since levels of AT III usually decline during acute thrombotic events—whether due to AT III deficiency or not—accurate determinations of baseline AT III activity may not be attainable until the patient is free of symptoms and is not receiving anticoagulant therapy.[59] Resolution of acute thrombosis in patients with mild AT III deficiency may occur with high-dose heparin alone. In patients with more profound deficiency, use of an exogenous source of AT III such as FFP in conjunction with heparin may be necessary. AT III concentrates manufactured from large plasma pools have been used successfully in the treatment of acute thrombosis for many years in Europe and have been licensed for use in the United States. Clinical trials of these concentrates have demonstrated their efficacy in the prevention of acute thrombosis in AT III-deficient patients subjected to high-risk clinical situations.[60] Long-term warfarin administration is recommended for the prevention of recurrent thrombotic events.

Protein C is a vitamin K–dependent plasma protein zymogen whose anticoagulant properties are a result of its ability to inactivate factors VIIIa and Va. Thrombin can proteolytically activate protein C in vitro, albeit too slowly to account for the latter's potent anticoagulant effects. This observation led investigators to hypothesize the presence of a cell surface receptor within the intravascular compartment that, in complex with thrombin, activates protein C rapidly and efficiently. Thrombomodulin, a high-density endothelial cell membrane protein that binds thrombin with high affinity, has since been identified as the ligand that participates in the in vivo activation of protein C. Upon formation of a 1:1 stoichiometric complex with thrombomodulin, thrombin loses its procoagulant function and assumes an anticoagulant role by rapidly activating protein C. The inactivation of factors VIIIa and Va by activated protein C (protein Ca) is facilitated by a cofactor protein, protein S (see later). In addition to its anticoagulant properties, protein Ca blocks the effects of a plasminogen activator inhibitor upon its natural substrate, TPA, thus increasing fibrinolysis (Fig. 64–6).[59, 61]

The onset of thrombosis in patients with heterozygous

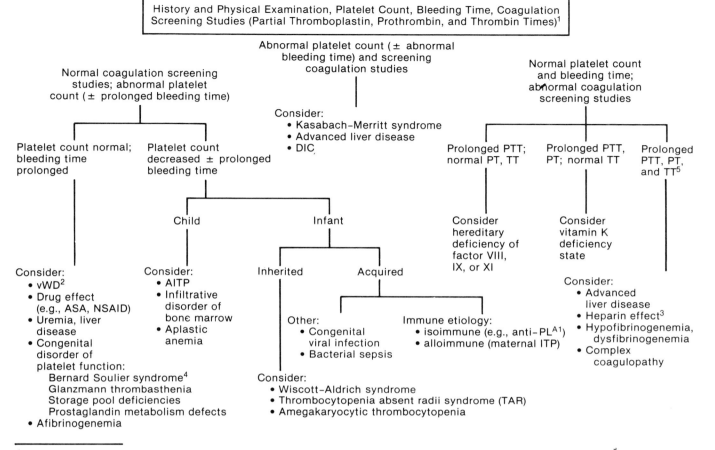

History and Physical Examination, Platelet Count, Bleeding Time, Coagulation Screening Studies (Partial Thromboplastin, Prothrombin, and Thrombin Times)[1]

[1]Consideration of age appropriate norms in the interpretation of results is essential. Consult references 55–57 for newborn normal values.
[2]Frequently associated with decreased factor VIII:C.
[3]Of the 3 screening coagulation studies, the TT is most prolonged in the presence of heparin.
[4]Associated with normal or decreased platelet count and giant platelets on peripheral smear.
[5]A rare but important bleeding disorder associated with a normal PT, PTT, and TT is factor XIII deficiency.

ASA = aspirin; NSAID = nonsteroidal anti-inflammatory drugs; AITP = autoimmune thrombocytopenic purpura; vWD = von Willebrand disease.

Figure 64–5. Algorithmic approach to the infant or child with a suspected bleeding disorder.

protein C deficiency generally occurs in late adolescence or early adulthood; thromboembolic manifestations are similar to those noted in patients with AT III deficiency. Affected individuals usually exhibit baseline protein C antigen levels that are below 50% of normal. As in the case of AT III deficiency, occasional protein C–deficient patients have normal antigen levels and depressed activity levels. Since a substantial number of patients with heterozygous protein C deficiency do not develop symptoms, institution of anticoagulant therapy is currently recommended only for patients with a history of thromboembolism or, without such a history, in patients acutely subjected to clinical situations known to predispose to thromboembolism.[59, 61]

Patients with homozygous protein C deficiency present in the neonatal period with extensive cutaneous and visceral thrombosis and laboratory abnormalities consistent with DIC. Both parents of affected infants demonstrate plasma levels of protein C consistent with heterozygous deficiency. This syndrome can rapidly progress to irreversible ischemic infarction of digits and whole extremities and subsequent fatality secondary to thrombosis within vital organs (purpura fulminans). Rapid institution of heparin and infusions of FFP (as a source of exogenous protein C) in patients suspected of this syndrome can reverse and prevent its fulminant thrombohemorrhagic manifestations. For infants who survive the acute presentation, purpura fulminans can be controlled on a long-term basis with warfarin therapy.[61, 62]

Protein S is a vitamin K–dependent plasma protein that catalyzes the rapid inactivation of factor Va and factor VIIIa by protein Ca in the presence of phospholipids or platelets. Unlike the other vitamin K–dependent coagulation proteins, protein S has no proteolytic activity of its own. It is also unique by virtue of its circulation in complex with C4b-binding protein, a regulatory protein of the complement cascade. Under normal circumstances, approximately 60% of the protein S in circulation is bound to C4b-binding protein, whereas 40% is unbound; only the latter possesses protein Ca cofactor activity. Thus, the level of functional protein S

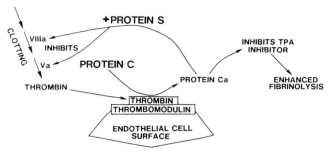

Figure 64–6. Protein C/protein S pathway. In this diagram, thrombin is generated by the clotting cascade and subsequently binds to thrombomodulin on the endothelial cell surface. When bound to thrombomodulin, thrombin rapidly converts protein C to activated protein C (protein C_a). Protein C_a then inhibits further clot formation by inactivating factors VIII_a and V_a with protein S serving as a cofactor for its action. Protein C_a promotes fibrinolysis by inhibiting tissue plasminogen activator inhibitor. This permits tissue plasminogen activator to generate plasmin, which in turn degrades the fibrin clot. (From Comp PC: Hereditary disorders predisposing to thrombosis. *In:* Coller BS [ed]: Progress in Hemostasis and Thrombosis. Orlando, Grune & Stratton, 1986, pp. 71–102.)

in plasma is dependent on the concentration of total protein S and C4b-binding protein as well as the binding characteristics of each for one another. Protein S–deficient individuals exhibit an increased thrombotic tendency with clinical manifestations and age of onset similar to protein C and AT III-deficient patient populations. Deficiency can be partial (autosomal dominant inheritance) or complete (autosomal recessive inheritance). In the latter case, both parents of a severe protein S–deficient propositus demonstrate mild-to-moderate deficiency. Unlike patients with homozygous protein C deficiency, homozygous protein S–deficient subjects do not acquire purpura fulminans.[59, 63]

References

1. Mann KG, Nesheim ME, Church WR, et al: Surface-dependent reactions of the vitamin K dependent enzyme complexes. Blood 76:1, 1990.
2. Alter BP: The bone marrow failure syndromes. *In:* Nathan DG and Oski FA (eds): Hematology of Infancy and Childhood, 3rd ed. Philadelphia, WB Saunders, 1987, pp. 159–241.
3. Perry III GS, Spector BD, Schuman LM, et al: The Wiskott-Aldrich syndrome in the United States and Canada (1892–1979). J Pediatr 97:72, 1980.
4. Lum LG, Tubergen DG, Corash L, et al: Splenectomy in the management of the thrombocytopenia of the Wiskott-Aldrich syndrome. N Engl J Med 302:892, 1980.
5. Corash L, Shafer B, and Blaese RM: Platelet-associated immunoglobulin, platelet size, and the effect of splenectomy in the Wiskott-Aldrich syndrome. Blood 65:1439, 1985.
6. Bray GL and Blaese RM: Unpublished observations.
7. Burstein SA, McMillan RM, and Harker LA: Quantitative platelet disorders. *In:* Bloom AL and Thomas DP (eds): Haemostasis and Thrombosis, 2nd ed. Edinburgh, Churchill Livingstone, 1987, pp. 333–364.
8. Rao AK: Congenital disorders of platelet function. Hematol/Oncol Clin 4(1):65, 1990.
9. Miller JL: von Willebrand's disease. Hematol/Oncol Clin 4:107, 1990.
10. Handin RI and Wagner DD: Molecular and cellular biology of von Willebrand factor. *In:* Coller BS (ed): Progress in Hemostasis and Thrombosis. Philadelphia, WB Saunders, 1989, pp. 233–259.
11. Coller BS: Von Willebrand's disease. *In:* Ratnoff OD and Forbes CD (eds): Disorders of Hemostasis. Orlando, Grune & Stratton, 1984, pp. 241–269.
12. Lusher JM: Diseases of coagulation: The fluid phase. *In:* Nathan DG and Oski FA (eds): Hematology of Infancy and Childhood, 3rd ed. Philadelphia, WB Saunders, 1987, pp. 1293–1342.
13. Ngo KY, Glotz VT, Koziol JA, et al: Homozygous and heterozygous deletions of the von Willebrand factor gene in patients and carriers of severe von Willebrand's disease. Proc Natl Acad Sci USA 85:2753, 1988.
14. Donner M, Holmberg L, and Nilsson IM: Type IIb von Willebrand's disease with probable autosomal recessive inheritance and presenting as thrombocytopenia in infancy. Br J Haematol 66:349, 1987.
15. Czapek EE, Gadarowski JJ Jr, Ontiveros JD, et al: Humate-P for treatment of von Willebrand's disease. Blood 72:110, 1988.
16. Fukui H, Nishino M, Terada S, et al: Hemostatic effect of a heat-treated factor VIII concentrate (Haemate P) in von Willebrand's disease. Blut 56:171, 1988.
17. Mannucci PM: Desmopressin: A nontransfusional form of treatment for congenital and acquired bleeding disorders. Blood 72:1449, 1988.
18. Weinstein RE, Bona RD, Altman AJ, et al: Severe hyponatremia after repeated intravenous administration of desmopressin. Am J Hematol 32:258, 1989.
19. Rocha E, Llorens R, Paramo JA, et al: Does desmopressin acetate reduce blood loss after surgery in patients on cardiopulmonary bypass? Circulation 77:1319, 1988.
20. Mannucci PM, Vicente V, Alberca I, et al: Intravenous and subcutaneous administration of desmopressin (DDAVP) to hemophiliacs: Pharmacokinetics and factor VIII responses. Thrombo Haemostas 58:1037, 1987.
21. Hardisty RM and Caen JP: Disorders of platelet function. *In:* Bloom AL and Thomas DP (eds): Haemostasis and Thrombosis, 2nd ed. Edinburgh, Churchill Livingstone, 1987, pp. 365–392.
22. Stuart MJ and Kelton JG: The platelet: Quantitative and qualitative abnormalities. *In:* Nathan DG and Oski FA (eds): Hematology of Infancy and Childhood, 3rd ed. Philadelphia, WB Saunders, 1987, pp. 1343–1478.
23. McEver RP: The clinical significance of platelet membrane glycoproteins. Hematol/Oncol Clin 4(1):87, 1990.
24. Buchanan GR: Hemorrhagic diseases. *In:* Nathan DG and Oski FA (eds): Hematology of Infancy and Childhood, 3rd ed. Philadelphia, WB Saunders, 1987, pp. 104–127.
25. Kunicki TJ and Beardsley DS: The alloimmune thrombocytopenias: Neonatal alloimmune thrombocytopenic purpura and post-transfusion purpura. *In:* Coller BS (ed): Progress in Hemostasis and Thrombosis. Philadelphia, WB Saunders, 1989, pp. 203–232.
26. Bussel JB: Intravenous immunoglobulin therapy for the treatment of idiopathic thrombocytopenic purpura. *In:* Coller BS (ed): Progress in Hemostasis and Thrombosis. Orlando, Grune & Stratton, 1986, pp. 103–125.
27. Bussel JB: Autoimmune thrombocytopenic purpura. Hematol/Oncol Clin 4(1):179, 1990.
28. Buchanan GR: The nontreatment of childhood idiopathic thrombocytopenic purpura. Eur J Pediatr 146:107, 1987.
29. Handin RI: Physiology of coagulation: The platelet. *In:* Nathan DG and Oski FA (eds): Hematology of Infancy and Childhood, 3rd ed. Philadelphia, WB Saunders, 1987, pp. 1271–1292.
30. McClain K, Gehrz R, Grierson H, et al: Virus-associated histiocytic proliferations in children. Am J Pediatr Hematol Oncol 10(3):196, 1988.
31. Warkentin TE and Kelton JG: Heparin and platelets. Hematol/Oncol Clin 4(1):243, 1990.
32. Gralnick HP, McKeown LP, Williams SB, et al: Plasma and platelet von Willebrand factor defects in uremia. Am J Med 85:806, 1988.
33. Carvalho AC: Acquired platelet dysfunction in patients with uremia. Hematol/Oncol Clin 4(1):129, 1990.
34. Salzman EW, Weinstein MJ, Weintraub RM, et al: Treatment with desmopressin acetate to reduce blood loss after cardiac surgery. N Engl J Med 314:1402, 1986.
35. Harker LA: Bleeding after cardiopulmonary bypass. N Engl J Med 314:1446, 1986.
36. Bidstrup BP, Royston D, Sapsford RN, et al: Reduction in blood loss and blood use after cardiopulmonary bypass with high dose aprotinin (Trasylol). J Thorac Cardiovasc Surg 97:364, 1989.

37. Levine PH: The clinical manifestations and therapy of hemophilias A and B. *In:* Colman RW, Hirsh J, Marder VJ, and Salzman EW (eds): Hemostasis and Thrombosis. Philadelphia, JB Lippincott, 1982, pp. 75–90.

38. Forbes CD: Clinical aspects of the hemophilias and their treatment. *In:* Ratnoff OD and Forbes CD (eds): Disorders of Hemostasis. Orlando, Grune & Stratton, 1984, pp. 177–239.

39. Bray GL and Luban NLC: Hemophilia presenting with intracranial hemorrhage. Am J Dis Child 141:1215, 1987.

40. Eyster ME, Gill FM, Blatt PM, et al: Central nervous system bleeding in hemophiliacs. Blood 51:1179, 1978.

41. Goldsmith JC and Kletzel M: Risk of birth related intracranial hemorrhage in hemophilic newborns: Results of a North American survey (Abstract). Blood 76(Suppl 1):1676a, 1990.

42. Bray G and Nugent D: Hemorrhage involving the upper airway in hemophilia. Clin Pediatr 25:436, 1986.

43. Buchanan GR: Coagulation factors. *In:* Nathan DG and Oski FA (eds): Hematology of Infancy and Childhood, 3rd ed. Philadelphia, WB Saunders, 1987, pp. 1606–1621.

44. Bray GL: Recent developments in the biotechnology of plasma-derived and recombinant coagulation factor VIII. J Pediatr 117:503–507, 1990.

45. Menache D, Behre HE, Orthner CL, et al: Coagulation factor IX concentrate: Method of preparation and assessment of potential in vivo thrombogenicity in animal models. Blood 64:1220, 1984.

46. Kim HC, McMillan CW, White GC, et al: Clinical experience of a new monoclonal antibody purified factor IX: Half-life, recovery and safety in patients with hemophilia B. Semin Hematol 27 (Suppl 2):30, 1990.

47. Rizza CR and Jones P: Management of patients with inherited blood coagulation defects. *In:* Bloom AL and Thomas DP (eds): Haemostasis and Thrombosis, 2nd ed. Edinburgh, Churchill Livingstone, 1987, pp. 465–493.

48. Kasper CK: Treatment of factor VIII inhibitors. *In:* Coller BS (ed): Progress in Hemostasis and Thrombosis. Philadelphia, WB Saunders, 1989, pp. 57–86.

49. Goedert JJ, Kessler CM, Aledort LM, et al: A prospective study of human immunodeficiency virus type 1 infection and the development of AIDS in subjects with hemophilia. N Engl J Med 321:1141, 1989.

50. Alter HJ, Purcell RH, Shih JW, et al: Detection of antibody to hepatitis C virus in prospectively followed transfusion recipients with acute and chronic non-A, non-B hepatitis. N Engl J Med 321:1494, 1989.

51. Seligsohn U: High gene frequency of factor XI (PTA) deficiency in Ashkenazi Jews. Blood 51:1223, 1978.

52. Hathaway WE: Haemostatic disorders in the newborn. *In:* Bloom AL and Thomas DP (eds): Haemostasis and Thrombosis, 2nd ed. Edinburgh, Churchill Livingstone, 1987, pp. 554–569.

53. Mannucci PM and Forman SP: Hemostasis and liver disease. *In:* Colman RW, Hirsh J, Marder VJ, and Salzman EW (eds): Hemostasis and Thrombosis. Philadelphia, JB Lippincott, 1982, pp. 595–601.

54. Brozovic M: Disseminated intravascular coagulation. *In:* Bloom AL and Thomas DP (eds): Haemostasis and Thrombosis, 2nd ed. Edinburgh, Churchill Livingstone, 1987, pp. 535–541.

55. Andrew M, Castle V, Mitchell L, et al: Modified bleeding time in the infant. Am J Hematol 30:190, 1989.

56. Corrigan JJ Jr: Neonatal thrombosis and the thrombolytic system: Pathophysiology and therapy. Am J Pediatr Hematol Oncol 10:83, 1988.

57. Andrew M, Paes B, Johnston M, et al: Development of the human coagulation system in the full-term infant. Blood 70:165, 1987.

58. Marcum JA, Reilly C, and Rosenberg RD: The role of specific forms of heparan sulfate in regulating blood vessel wall function. *In:* Coller BS (ed): Progress in Hemostasis and Thrombosis. Orlando, Grune & Stratton, 1986, pp. 185–215.

59. Comp PC: Hereditary disorders predisposing to thrombosis. *In:* Coller BS (ed): Progress in Hemostasis and Thrombosis. Orlando, Grune & Stratton, 1986, pp. 71–102.

60. Menache D, O'Malley JP, Schorr JB, et al: Evaluation of the safety, recovery, half-life, and clinical efficacy of antithrombin III (human) in patients with hereditary antithrombin III deficiency. Blood 75:33, 1990.

61. Clouse LH and Comp PC: The regulation of hemostasis: The protein C system. N Engl J Med 314:1298, 1986.

62. Marlar RA, Montgomery RR, and Broekmans AW: Diagnosis and treatment of homozygous protein C deficiency. J Pediatr 114:528, 1989.

63. Kamiya T, Sugihara T, Ogata K, et al: Inherited deficiency of protein S in a Japanese family with recurrent venous thrombosis: A study of three generations. Blood 67:406, 1986.

Oncologic Issues

Frederick P. Ognibene, M.D., and
Philip A. Pizzo, M.D.

Pediatric patients with oncologic problems may require an intensive care unit for one of three reasons. First, acute and life-threatening complications may develop from tumor-induced syndromes due to direct, local effects of the malignant process. As a consequence, emergent cytotoxic therapies may have to be administered in the intensive care unit. Second, there may be systemic manifestations of the tumor that produce critical illness. These manifestations typically involve metabolic or endocrine-induced side effects of the tumor. Third, the largest number of patients requires an intensive care unit because of complications of antineoplastic therapies. Critical care therapies range from hemodynamic and cardiovascular monitoring during the administration of potentially toxic chemotherapies to the management of life-threatening complications of these therapies, such as pulmonary failure and overwhelming infections with septic shock. Multiorgan failure, secondary to a variety of causes, may be seen after the initiation of these therapies.

In order to provide the highest level of care, intensivists must first fully understand the manifestations of the underlying disease. The patient's oncologist should continue to provide an active consultative role after the patient has been admitted to the intensive care unit. The comprehension of principles of both the effects and the toxicities of all chemotherapeutic agents is essential. Each agent may have peculiar local or systemic side effects, and the duration of these toxicities is frequently quite variable. Additionally, the consultative expertise of infectious disease specialists, nephrologists, and surgeons is frequently required to care for the critically ill oncology patient. As a consequence, a "team approach" is required for the optimal management of these patients.

PRIMARY TUMOR-INDUCED SYNDROMES—LOCAL EFFECTS

Cardiovascular

Local effects of malignant processes may be manifest because of either vascular disorders or direct cardiac involvement. One of the most common and most dramatic local effects of a tumor is extrinsic compression of the superior vena cava, commonly referred to as superior vena cava syndrome. This compression is usually caused by the mass effect of anterior mediastinal tumors. Most children with this syndrome have non-Hodgkin lymphoma with or without leukemic transformation.[1] The typical clinical presentation is plethora or facial cyanosis, cyanosis of the neck and upper chest, upper extremity edema, distended neck veins, and occasionally, evidence of venous collateralization on the chest and abdomen. Dyspnea can occur if there is an obstruction of the airway.[1-3] Because of increased intracranial pressure, there may be neurologic symptoms such as headache, stupor, coma, or seizures. This syndrome is life-threatening due to airway obstruction, cerebral edema, or cardiac compromise with shock, primarily due to decreased venous return and decreased ventricular volume.

A histopathologic diagnosis should be obtained as emergently as possible. Because most causes of this syndrome are due to hematologic malignancies, a bone marrow aspirate and biopsy should be performed first. Bone marrow assessment frequently provides a diagnosis. However, because the type of therapy is dependent of the histopathology of the tumor (e.g., Hodgkin versus non-Hodgkin lymphoma or another malignancy) and since the bone marrow biopsy may not yield a diagnosis, a biopsy of the tumor is important. Endotracheal intubation and mechanical ventilation may be especially hazardous in patients with mediastinal masses (see later), thus there should be special concern for the protection of the airway, and intubation should only be performed by those most proficient at airway control.

Therapy should be directed toward relief of respiratory symptoms and relief of the venous obstruction. Typically, multiagent chemotherapy regimens (frequently including corticosteroids) are used to treat these tumors. Radiation therapy is only rarely necessary for these malignancies.

Primary myocardial malignancies as well as metastatic disease with myocardial infiltration are rare in children. Tumors that can metastasize or invade the myocardium include osteogenic sarcoma, testicular carcinoma, Hodgkin disease, leukemia, and non-Hodgkin lymphomas.

When there is either a primary or metastatic myocardial neoplasm, it typically presents as a rhythm disturbance because of an invasion of the conducting system. Myocardial tumor may lead to irritable foci that can produce ventricular ectopy. In severe cases of myocardial tumor infiltration, complete heart block may occur. Invasive myocardial lesions rarely cause congestive heart failure or shock.

Pericardial involvement by tumor may occur from either metastases (e.g., Hodgkin disease or leukemia) or may occur after local invasion of a primary tumor.[4] Pericardial spread of tumor may lead to the development of a pericardial effusion with subsequent pericardial tamponade. Unlike tamponade secondary to trauma, tamponade due to pericardial tumor is usually more insidious in its onset.

As the pericardial fluid accumulates there is a gradual loss of compliance of the pericardium. Symptoms are typically due to this loss of compliance as well as due to right ventricular failure, which occurs partly because the right ventricle is thin walled and easily compressible. As a pericardial effusion increases in size and becomes more hemodynamically significant, the patient will complain of fatigue, shortness of breath, cough, abdominal distention, and abdominal pain (Table 65–1). Younger children will not be able to complain of these symptoms, but the signs will usually be apparent. Physical signs of right ventricular failure include distended neck veins due to elevation of central venous pressure, hepatomegaly, ascites, and lower extremity edema.

Pericardial tamponade should be considered in any patient with a malignancy and hemodynamic compromise. Initial diagnostic evaluation after the history and physical examination should include a chest roentgenogram that typically reveals cardiomegaly; however, with small, acute pericardial effusions the heart size may be normal on the roentgenogram. Comparison with previous chest roentgenograms is important to document the change in heart size. The diagnosis is supported when an echocardiogram reveals pericardial fluid. Pulmonary artery (right heart) catheterization shows equalization (within 2 to 3 mm Hg) of pressures in the right atrium, the right ventricle at end-diastole, the pulmonary artery at end-diastole, and the pulmonary artery

wedge pressure. Cardiac index is typically diminished (see also Chapter 35).

Echocardiographically guided pericardiocentesis, with a "pig-tailed" catheter, by an experienced cardiologist or intensivist is both therapeutic and diagnostic. Removal of even small amounts of fluid from the pericardial sac, which is under high pressure, results in the restoration of blood pressure and cardiac index because there is a drop in intrapericardial pressure with the removal of fluid. When able to be measured, the intrapericardial pressure is typically approximately equal to the other cardiac chamber pressures. Pericardiocentesis should remove as much fluid as is withdrawn easily, and the catheter can be left in place to monitor intrapericardial pressures and to facilitate the withdrawal of pericardial fluid if it should reaccumulate. This catheter can be safely left in place for up to 72 hours before the risk of infection becomes increasingly significant. The catheter is kept patent with intracatheter instillation of low concentration (100 units/ml) of heparin. The fluid removed should be assayed chemically (protein and glucose levels), hematologically (white and red blood cell counts and differential), microbiologically (Gram stain, routine bacterial, fungal, and mycobacterial cultures), and cytopathologically. Malignant effusions are confirmed by the presence of abnormal cells on cytology examination; however, positive results are seen in only about 50% of cytology examinations. The work-up for an infectious etiology for the pericardial effusion and tamponade is important because many of these patients are immunosuppressed secondary to either their underlying diseases or to therapy.

Therapies vary depending on the type of malignant process that causes the tamponade. In patients with hematologic malignancies, treatment of the underlying disease with systemic chemotherapy usually controls the pericardial effusion. However, when the effusion is due to a solid tumor, it is more difficult to treat and to limit reaccumulation of fluid. Local radiation to the mediastinum or instillation of sclerosing agents, such as nitrogen mustard, thiotepa, or tetracycline, may be used to palliate the reaccumulation of the malignant effusion.[5, 6] The formation of a pericardial window, using a limited approach thoracotomy, may also be considered as an initial palliative therapy. In situations in which the aforementioned maneuvers have failed to limit the reaccumulation of the pericardial fluid, a pericardiectomy may be considered. This should be considered only if there is associated constrictive pericardial disease or if a pericardial window was not technically possible because of extensive pericardial involvement with a tumor.

Nonbacterial thrombotic endocarditis (marantic endocarditis) is rarely seen in pediatric patients but may occur in the setting of a mucin-producing adenocarcinoma.[7] This noninfectious process is an example of a thromboembolic paraneoplastic syndrome and typically occurs because of a hypercoagulable state caused by the tumor. The valvular lesions are typically seen on left-sided heart valves and may be the source of systemic emboli to the central nervous system, kidneys, and so forth. Anticoagulation is typically used to limit repeat embolism; however, controversy exists over the role of

Table 65–1. CLINICAL SIGNS AND SYMPTOMS OF PERICARDIAL TAMPONADE

Symptoms
Fatigue
Dyspnea
Cough
Abdominal distention
Abdominal pain

Signs
Tachycardia
Hypotension with narrow pulse pressure
Distended neck veins (due to elevated central venous pressure)
Pulsus paradoxus
Hepatomegaly
Ascites
Lower extremity edema
Encephalopathy

anticoagulation in this disease process. Primary treatment should be directed toward the underlying malignancy.

Pulmonary

Disorders of the lungs commonly occur as primary manifestations of malignancies in children. The airways, mediastinum, lung parenchyma, and pleural spaces can all be involved as a local effect of the underlying tumor.

Airway problems may occur in any anatomic area, ranging from the proximal nasopharyngeal and tracheal portions of the airway to the terminal, bronchial portion of the airway. One of the most common problems is airway obstruction due to compression by mediastinal tumors. In addition to compressing vascular structures and invading the myocardium and pericardium (see earlier), mediastinal neoplasms can compress the trachea. The most common hematologic malignancies that cause tracheal obstruction include Hodgkin disease, non-Hodgkin lymphomas, and T cell acute lymphoblastic leukemias.[8] Both Hodgkin and non-Hodgkin lymphomas can present with the mediastinum as the primary site of involvement in up to 80% in some series.[9] Other airway-obstructing neoplasms include neuroblastomas and thymomas.

With tracheal compression, the signs of respiratory distress may be dramatic and include tachypnea, stridor, tachycardia, and in extreme cases lethargy and cyanosis. In less severe cases of compression, fever, cough, and mild shortness of breath may be the only presenting signs and symptoms.

Once an airway obstruction is suspected, the most urgent therapeutic goal should be to protect the child's airway. If necessary, the child should be electively intubated under controlled circumstances. Fiberoptic bronchoscopy guided intubation of the trachea may be required in situations of extreme airway compromise.

There is much controversy over the use of general anesthesia in patients with anterior mediastinal masses. Numerous reports document both cardiac and pulmonary catastrophes in these patients after general anesthesia.[2, 9–12] These complications are either due to tracheal and bronchial obstructions that may arise during intubation or positioning of the child after general anesthesia or may be due to compression of the superior vena cava, pulmonary artery, or other great vessels leading to an obstruction of blood flow and systemic hypotension. A series from Memorial Sloan-Kettering Cancer Center in New York reported the relative safety of general anesthesia in 44 pediatric patients with anterior mediastinal masses.[13] The authors reported that establishment of venous access in a lower extremity in order to allow delivery of pharmacologic agents in the event of superior vena cava obstruction, having a rigid bronchoscope available, and the induction of general anesthesia in either the semi-Fowler or sitting position, were helpful. Halothane and ketamine were the anesthetics of choice.[13] Despite those precautions, 15 to 20% of the patients in that series had life-threatening complications. As a result, other anesthesiologists have questioned the overall safety of general anesthesia in these patients because of the relatively high frequency of both airway and vascular complications.[14, 15] It would seem that the most reasonable approach is to consider alternatives to general anesthesia. If general anesthesia must be given, knowledge of and anticipation of the problems that can occur are essential.

Despite the risks of delay, an aggressive attempt should be made to establish a histopathologic diagnosis and to stage the extent of the malignant process prior to therapy. Many pathologists feel strongly that a pretherapy histopathologic diagnosis is essential, because even small doses of radiation therapy can convert a lymphomatous mass into "uncharacterizable" inflammation or fibrosis.[13] There have also been reports that empiric, antineoplastic high-dose corticosteroids can also obscure an accurate histopathologic diagnosis if they are given prior to a biopsy.[8] In addition, not all mediastinal masses are due to lymphomas, and specific therapies depend entirely on the histopathologic characteristics of the mass.[16]

Computed transaxial tomography (CTT) of the chest is a noninvasive adjunct that allows both characterization of the mass and delineation of the extent of the mass.[17, 18] Cine CT, which uses ultrashort scanning times yet still produces excellent images, eliminates some of the problems of conventional CTT scanning of the mediastinum in these patients, and it allows for effective high-quality mediastinal studies.[19]

It is important to note that even if a patient's airway is stable in the presence of a mediastinal mass, the initiation of therapy (radiation therapy in particular) may lead to local edema, which can then lead to stridor and airway compromise. Corticosteroids may limit some of the edema associated with radiation therapy. Because of this potential for respiratory deterioration associated with the onset of therapy, it is reasonable to admit these patients to an intensive care unit for aggressive monitoring of their respiratory status until the mediastinal mass has responded to therapy and the airway is no longer threatened.

In addition to mediastinal masses, paratracheal adenopathy may also be present and can potentially compromise the airway. It is important to note the presence and location of paratracheal disease on both chest roentgenograms and chest CTT. Occasionally, large nodes may cause tracheal deviation in either the lateral or the anteroposterior planes. If there is such tracheal deviation, intubation of the trachea with direct laryngoscopy may be difficult, and intubation guided by flexible fiberoptic bronchoscopy may be necessary. These paratracheal nodes can also produce hoarseness due to unilateral vocal cord paralysis if there is compression of the recurrent laryngeal nerve branches of the vagus nerve. Consideration must also be made of the ability of these children to protect their airways from aspiration if there is vocal cord paralysis.

Invasion of the parenchyma of the lung by leukemic or lymphomatous cells, albeit uncommon, can lead to respiratory compromise. It is frequently impossible to clinically distinguish patients with respiratory compromise due to leukemic or lymphomatous infiltration from those with an infectious cause of pulmonary infiltrates (see later). The patients typically have dyspnea or evidence of tachypnea on physical examination. Chest roentgenograms can vary from nodular densities or focal lobar infiltrates to diffuse interstitial infiltrates. As a result, the clinical and roentgenographic findings are indistinguishable from infectious pneumonias. Open lung biopsy or bronchoscopy (with transbronchial biopsy in older patients) should be performed early in order to establish the diagnosis of tumor infiltration and to effectively guide therapy and thus limit potentially toxic empiric therapies.[20, 21] In addition to the hematologic malignancies, pulmonary parenchymal disease may also be caused by metastases from Wilms' tumor, osteogenic sarcoma, rhabdomyosarcoma, Ewing sarcoma, and other soft tissue sarcomas. Typically, these present more insidiously, are noted on chest roentgenograms, and rarely cause respiratory failure or lead to admission to the intensive care unit.

In patients with acute leukemia and the blast phase of chronic myelogenous leukemia, circulating peripheral white blood cell counts of greater than 100,000 cells/mm^3 may occur and lead to leukostasis, which can have severe pulmonary manifestations of hypoxemia and respiratory failure (see later).[22, 23] Chest roentgenograms in these patients typically have diffuse interstitial infiltrates. In addition to pulmonary involvement, leukostasis can also cause symptoms in the cerebral, retinal, and peripheral vascular circulations, and thus it requires urgent intervention. Therapies aimed at cytoreduction include leukopheresis, plasma exchange, and chemotherapy. Leukopheresis produces the most acute drop in the number of circulating white blood cells, and it is typically the initial therapy pending the cytoreductive effects of chemotherapy.

Malignant pleural effusions in children are most commonly associated with underlying lymphomas, neuroblastoma, and sarcomas. Primary pleural tumors are rare in children. Unless pleural effusions are so large that lung volumes are reduced to the point of ineffective ventilation, pediatric patients with uncomplicated pleural effusions infrequently require intensive care units. If there is another reason for acute respiratory failure (e.g., infection, parenchymal metastases) and there is also a large pleural effusion, then the effusion may limit pulmonary recovery because of the reduction of lung volumes. In these situations, the effusion must be drained by either thoracentesis or by placement of a thoracostomy tube. At the time of drainage, pleural fluid should have a complete hematologic, biochemical, and cytopathologic analysis to confirm the presence of malignant cells. Malignant effusions typically recur after drainage unless definitive therapy to prevent reaccumulation of fluid is undertaken. Pleural obliteration by sclerosis and fibrosis can be achieved by the instillation of sclerosing agents into the thoracostomy tube. These agents include tetracycline as well as chemotherapeutic modalities, such as local nitrogen mustard, thiotepa, and bleomycin.[24] Pleural sclerosis is frequently a painful process, and because it is typically done for palliative purposes in the setting of advanced malignancy, the clinician must be sensitized to the pain control needs of the patient and should liberally administer analgesics. This pain may also be managed by intrapleural anesthesia using nerve blocks. Additional, more aggressive treatment modalities include intrapleural administration of talc, which can be extremely painful, and pleurectomy, which is performed as a last resort.

Gastrointestinal

Malignancies may directly involve the gastrointestinal tract or may involve it by extrinsic tumor compression. Abdominal neoplasms in children include lymphomas, neuroblastomas, hepatic tumors, sarcomas (e.g., rhabdomyosarcoma), and Wilms' tumor.[25, 26] Symptomatically, these children may have anorexia, changes in feeding or eating behaviors, weight loss, abdominal pain (with or without abdominal distention), and nausea with vomiting and constipation if the tumor has produced a gastrointestinal obstruction. Noninvasive techniques such as ultrasonography or CTT may establish the presence and location of the mass; however, surgical exploration is usually necessary to establish a histopathologic diagnosis. These patients are typically seen in intensive care units for fluid and electrolyte management if they present with intestinal obstruction or for postoperative management after an exploratory laparotomy.

In addition to obstructive symptoms from malignant masses, these patients may also present with gastrointestinal hemorrhage or bowel perforation secondary to the tumor involvement. These two complications occur more frequently after chemotherapy and its subsequent tumor lysis or may be due to associated mucositis, secondary gastrointestinal infections (e.g., *Candida* or cytomegalovirus), or secondary coagulopathies. If conservative management of hemorrhage fails, then surgical management of the bleeding may be required. This is necessary typically after significant transfusion of blood products and after interventional radiologic attempts to stop the hemorrhage with embolization to the bleeding site or with local, intra-arterial infusions of vasopressin. Perforations, obviously, require surgical interventions for resection or repair of the focus of perforation as well as for treatment of peritonitis. It is also important to note that certain hematologic malignancies have a predilection for different foci in the gastrointestinal tract. For example, nodular lymphomas typically involve the stomach,[27] whereas Burkitt lymphoma is most commonly found in the region of the distal ileum and proximal cecum.[28]

Although uncommon, children with leukemia may present with gastrointestinal symptoms due either to leukemic infiltration or to localized infections in the gastrointestinal tract. Symptomatically, both types of histopathologic processes may present with abdominal pain (with or without evidence of peritonitis). Frequently, these patients are receiving corticosteroid therapy, which may mask some signs of acute peritonitis. If these patients present with right lower quadrant pain, especially if they are receiving corticosteroids, then peritonitis must be considered. The main infectious causes of this pain are acute appendicitis and neutropenic enterocolitis (typhilitis), and they are discussed later in this chapter.[26, 29–31]

Primary hepatic tumors can occur in children. In addition, metastases to the liver from solid tumors as well as hepatic infiltration by leukemic or lymphomatous cells can be seen. These patients may present with hepatomegaly and have chemical evidence of intrahepatic cholestasis. Hepatic failure does not typically occur because of these lesions unless the entire liver parenchyma has been replaced by tumor. However, hepatic dysfunction can occur with infection, especially as a consequence of septic shock or in association with cytomegalovirus, herpes simplex virus, varicella zoster virus, or fungal disease (e.g., *Candida* or *Aspergillus*). A biopsy of liver via either the percutaneous approach (older children), laparoscopy, or exploratory laparotomy with direct visualization of the liver is necessary to establish the diagnosis of a malignant lesion.

Occasionally, either primary tumors of the biliary tree or large porta hepatis nodes, such as those seen with lymphoma, may cause extrahepatic biliary obstruction with jaundice. Biliary obstruction can also result from infection (e.g., bacterial or fungal). Visualization studies utilizing ultrasonography and CTT may provide anatomic delineation of these lesions and can guide an interventional radiologist, gastroenterologist, or surgeon who may decide to bypass or traverse those lesions with catheters in order to relieve the extrahepatic biliary obstruction.

Renal

Renal failure may occur because of two local tumor effects: renal parenchymal involvement by tumor and obstructive uropathy. Wilms' tumor, despite extensive renal parenchymal involvement, rarely produces renal failure but rather manifests primarily as abdominal pain and as an abdominal mass. Hematologic malignancies, however, such as leukemias and lymphomas, can infiltrate the kidney and produce organomegaly and can also cause renal failure.[32–34] Ultrasonography typically reveals renal enlargement in these patients, and, if possible, a biopsy should be performed for a histopathologic confirmation of this finding. Local irradiation as well as systemic chemotherapy have been effective in reversing the renal failure caused by the leukemic or lymphomatous infiltration.

Obstructive uropathy may occur because of tumor obstruction of the ureters or the bladder. In children, lymphomas are the most common causes of such obstructions. In addition, prior treatment with radiation therapy or chemotherapy with subsequent fibrosis or previous surgery with retroperitoneal adhesions may also cause an obstruction. If both ureters are blocked, then oliguria (anuria) and azotemia can occur. Unilateral obstruction does not produce renal failure; however, the hydronephrotic kidney will become nonfunctional unless the obstruction is relieved. In addition, the urinary tract proximal to the obstruction can serve as a nidus for systemic infection, which can be life-threatening. In effect, it is a loculated focus of infection, like

an abscess, that must be drained in order for the infection to respond to therapy. Renal ultrasonography can demonstrate the site(s) of obstruction as well as the hydroureter and hydronephrosis, and it is the most rapid method of establishing evidence of obstruction. Further localization of the obstruction(s) can be accomplished by CTT, without contrast dye, or retrograde pyelography.

Because these obstructions are slow to develop, many patients can be relatively free of symptoms, except for oliguria, until marked azotemia has occurred. When an obstruction is demonstrated, proximal percutaneous nephrostomy or ureterostomy drains can be placed. These drains will relieve the obstruction, leading to symptomatic and biochemical improvement of renal failure, and they are a temporizing measure pending the relief of the obstruction with radiation therapy or chemotherapy. If therapy is not effective, then more permanent relief of the obstruction can be achieved with either ureteral stents, or external drainage system, or other internal ureteral diversions. In some situations, the relief of the obstruction may result in a brisk, postobstruction diuresis. Accompanying the diuresis will be losses of critical electrolytes such as potassium, sodium, and magnesium. The clinician must pay particular attention to both the patient's volume status and electrolyte requirements as a result of this diuresis. An assessment of the electrolyte content of the urine is frequently helpful in determining the type of crystalloid replacement for the patient. As a consequence, an intensive care unit may be required in order to closely monitor the patient's intravascular volume status and electrolyte needs.

Occasionally, tumors of the urinary tract, especially primary bladder or ureter tumors, can produce hematuria, and, rarely, life-threatening hemorrhage. Although these tumors are not commonly seen in children, neoplasms of the urinary tract must be considered in the differential diagnosis of hematuria.

Central Nervous System

Brain tumors are the most common of the solid tumors in children and can produce a variety of primary syndromes that may require intensive care.[35] These syndromes include seizures and focal neurologic deficits due to intraparenchymal mass lesions, intracranial hypertension, alterations in the level of consciousness or coma, and paralysis due to either epidural or intraparenchymal spinal cord lesions.

Although most primary childhood brain tumors present infratentorially and thus should not cause seizures, astrocytomas, ependymomas, and malignant gliomas can occur in the cerebral hemispheres and produce seizures.[35] A variety of other tumors can metastasize to the brain and can lead to mass lesions that serve as seizure foci. These include lymphomas, retinoblastomas, and rhabdomyosarcomas, especially those occurring in the head and neck. In addition to seizures, other heralding signs may include headache, irritability or change in behavior, and vomiting. However, there may be many non–mass-related reasons for seizures in a child with neoplastic disease. These reasons are presented in Table 65–2.

If a child with a central nervous system mass lesion has a seizure, control of the seizure is the first priority. Prompt initiation of anticonvulsant therapy will decrease the morbidity and mortality of seizures that are related to the duration and degree of hypoxemia, metabolic acidosis, and hypoglycemia (see Chapter 23).[36]

Following pharmacologic control of the seizure, the next step is to sort through the differential reasons for the event. If infection is suspected, antibacterial agents should be started immediately. If a fungal lesion is suspected (e.g., the patient has evidence of necrotizing sinusitis, a mass lesion, or possible cryptococcal meningitis), then appropriate antifungal therapy should be started (i.e., amphotericin B or fluconazole). If a viral meningoencephalitis is suspected, acyclovir should be added to the regimen. If there is evidence of hemorrhage, and if there is an underlying bleeding diathesis, then that should be corrected. Therapy will most likely include transfusions of platelets and fresh frozen plasma or cryoprecipitate (in the setting of uremia). Follow-up head CTT studies may be necessary to indicate whether the hemorrhage has stabilized or progressed. If metabolic derangements are identified, they should be treated, and all potentially implicated pharmacologic agents should be stopped. If one is left with the primary tumor mass as the only cause of seizures, emergent radiotherapy, chemotherapy, or surgery is indicated depending on the location of the lesion and the type of neoplasia.

Elevation in intracranial pressure to herniation levels without seizure activity can occur with central nervous system masses. As noted with seizures, attempts to determine whether or not there is a superimposed reason for the rise in intracranial pressure (enlarging primary mass, hemorrhage, abscess, or infection) must be aggressively pursued by the intensivist. If signs of impending herniation are noted, a number of immediate ther-

Table 65–2. CAUSES OF SEIZURES IN PATIENTS WITH CENTRAL NERVOUS SYSTEM MASS LESIONS

Tumor
  Primary
  Metastatic
Intracranial hemorrhage
  Intraparenchymal secondary to thrombocytopenia within mass
Infection
  Meningitis
  Meningoencephalitis
  Brain abscess
Metabolic
  Hypoglycemia
  Hypocalcemia
  Hyponatremia
  Uremia
Drug induced
  Imipenem
  Lidocaine
  Intrathecal methotrexate
  L-Asparaginase
Fever
Idiopathic epilepsy

Table 65–3. THERAPIES FOR ELEVATION OF INTRACRANIAL PRESSURE/HERNIATION SYNDROME IN PATIENTS WITH NEOPLASTIC MASS LESIONS

Hyperventilation
  Bag-mask ventilation
  Intubation
Corticosteroids (dexamethasone)
Diuretics
  Mannitol/glycerol
  Furosemide
Platelets/fresh frozen plasma (if bleeding suspected)
Antiseizure treatment or prophylaxis
Computed transaxial tomography (to determine etiology)
Intracranial pressure monitoring (controversial)
Palliative therapy
  Whole brain irradiation
  Surgery

apies are indicated and are listed in Table 65–3 (see also Chapter 17).

Corticosteroids (typically dexamethasone) are administered if local or vasogenic edema is considered to be a contributing factor to the mass-related intracranial hypertension. However, the effect of corticosteroids is not noted for at least 4 to 6 hours after their administration. Once these therapies have been initiated and herniation has been avoided, as manifested by the return of pupillary reactivity and the improvement in other neurologic parameters, a CTT scan of the head should be performed. If bleeding is documented by head CTT, craniotomy with surgical decompression may be indicated. Surgery is probably also indicated for a solitary brain metastasis.[37]

There are limited clinical data concerning the use of intracranial pressure monitoring devices or ventricular drains in children with neoplastic mass lesions. However, these data contend that they may assist management.[38] Placement of a ventriculostomy or subdural bolt to monitor intracranial pressure is probably helpful after posterior fossa tumor resections as a method to detect unsuspected hemorrhage or marked cerebral edema and thus may decrease the need for cerebrospinal fluid shunts in these patients.[39] Infections complicating these devices are more likely to occur in patients who may have underlying or therapy-related immunosuppression.

Long-term palliative therapy for neoplastic mass lesions is limited to either whole-brain irradiation or to surgical resection, particularly of solitary metastatic lesions.[35, 37, 40] Therapeutic responses are based on the underlying histopathology, the extent of disease, previous therapy, and the patient's overall physical condition. If the overall prognosis is poor, with limited therapeutic options, and intracranial pressure elevation has produced herniation, then the level of therapeutic aggression should be based on this prognosis. It may be reasonable in these situations either to withdraw support or to limit therapy to comfort measures only.

In addition to the postictal state and increased intracranial pressure, there are other reasons for a patient with a neoplasm to develop obtundation or coma. These include hemorrhage into the central nervous system (parenchymal, epidural, or subdural) with or without an underlying mass lesion, infection (meningitis, meningoencephalitis, or abscess), metabolic derangements (hyponatremia, hypoglycemia, or uremia), and drug-related comas (chemotherapy, narcotics, sedatives). As in the work-up of seizures and intracranial hypertension, a central nervous system mass lesion (new or old) must be suspected in all patients with an underlying malignancy. After a physical assessment and acute therapeutic interventions have been performed, a head CTT scan is warranted before a lumbar puncture is done. If infection seems likely, it is not unreasonable to initiate antibiotics prior to the CTT scan.

If hypoglycemia is documented or suspected, then 50% dextrose, diluted to 25% dextrose with sterile water, is administered at a dose of 500 mg to 1 g/kg. It is especially important to consider glucose therapy in children with insulinomas or widespread hepatic metastases or in tumors with ectopic insulin production. If narcotic overdose is suspected, then naloxone can be given and the patient can be observed for an improvement in mental status. The standard dose of naloxone is 0.01 mg/kg. If a response is demonstrated, then repeated naloxone doses or a continuous naloxone infusion may be required because of the short half-life of this drug. The caregiver should exercise caution in administering naloxone to a patient who has been taking narcotics on a chronic basis. The drug should be given slowly and should be titrated to the response, because acute narcotic withdrawal can be precipitated by too rapid administration of naloxone.

Acute spinal cord compression is typically seen in children with lymphoma, neuroblastoma, or soft tissue sarcoma. The compression can be caused by either local extension or by tumor metastasis.[38, 41] Presenting symptoms include back pain, typically radicular in nature, and motor weakness. Sensory deficits are seen less frequently. Bladder and bowel dysfunction may also be noted with incontinence typical of lesions below the second lumbar vertebra. In addition to tumor, cord compression can also occur secondary to local hemorrhage in patients with thrombocytopenia or coagulopathy.

The diagnosis is based on demonstration of a vertebral lesion with dural compression. The imaging techniques that may be used include contrast myelography, spine CTT, or nuclear magnetic resonance imaging. Once documented, urgent therapy aimed at nerve decompression should be initiated. Acute therapy should include high-dose dexamethasone (50 mg/m² followed by 10 mg/m² every 6 hours) in an attempt to decrease tumor-associated edema.[41] This should be followed by radiation therapy if a tumor is causing the compression. Lymphomas and neuroblastomas are particularly radiosensitive. A laminectomy (surgical decompression) is indicated if hemorrhage is the etiology, if the tumor is not particularly radiosensitive, or if radiation therapy fails to produce neurologic improvement. Surgery is occasionally required in order to establish a diagnosis (i.e., spinal cord compression is the presenting manifestation of the malignancy) or if local hemorrhage needs to be evacuated (or ruled out).

The last neurologic emergency that the intensivist may encounter is carcinomatous meningitis. This complication in children is seen in the setting of leukemia or lymphoma, or when tumors have invaded the vertebral column or produced extradural compression. This noninfectious etiology of meningitis rarely causes signs of meningeal irritation or alterations in level of consciousness. Rather, it typically produces neurologic signs and symptoms at multiple foci, ranging from cranial nerves down to the cauda equina, because of multiple nerve root involvement. It must be distinguished from mycobacterial or fungal causes of meningitis. The diagnosis is established by the cytopathologic documentation of malignant cells in the cerebrospinal fluid. In some situations, the number of abnormal cells in the cerebrospinal fluid may be small or the cellular morphology may not be characteristic of a malignancy, and multiple lumbar punctures may need to be performed in order to establish a diagnosis.

Prognosis is generally poor in these patients, and therapy is generally palliative. However, patients with leukemic or lymphomatous meningitis tend to have better responses to therapy.[42] The palliative therapeutic options include craniospinal radiation and intrathecal chemotherapy. Short-term courses of corticosteroids may also be used in an attempt to decrease tumor-associated edema that may be causing symptoms.

SYSTEMIC EFFECTS OF TUMOR

Metabolic/Endocrine

A variety of metabolic emergencies may arise secondary to malignancies. These may be due to a large burden of malignant cells, primary or ectopic hormone production by tumor, or a variety of paraneoplastic processes.

Hypercalcemia is an infrequent complication of pediatric malignancies; however, it can be seen in patients with acute lymphoblastic leukemia, Hodgkin and non-Hodgkin lymphomas, primary bone tumors, or osteolytic metastatic tumors of bone.[41, 43–45] Most cases of hypercalcemia occur because of bone resorption due to a number of factors including increases in the amount of osteoclast-activating factor, ectopic parathyroid hormone production, and ectopic prostaglandin production.[45, 46]

Symptoms are usually seen when calcium levels are greater than 12 mg/dl and may involve a number of systems. Symptoms include anorexia, nausea, vomiting, constipation, bradycardias or other arrhythmias, fatigue, drowsiness, generalized weakness, stupor or coma, and polyuria. Hypercalcemia can be exacerbated by dehydration, thiazide diuretics, calcium-containing antacids, and immobilization. Levels of calcium greater than 20 mg/dl can be fatal.

The first step in treating hypercalcemia is to vigorously correct any dehydration in order to increase renal clearance of calcium. This is usually achieved with saline-containing crystalloids. Normal saline (0.9% sodium chloride) is the crystalloid preferred to replete sodium. Central venous or pulmonary artery catheters may be necessary to assess intravascular volume, especially if there is associated pulmonary or cardiac dysfunction. A

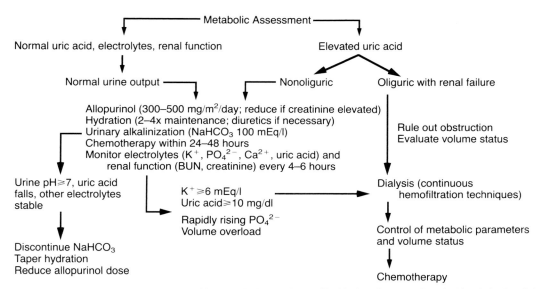

Figure 65–1. Management of patients with tumor lysis syndrome (Burkitt lymphoma or lymphoblastic leukemia).

forced diuresis with furosemide, after saline loading, usually leads to a drop in serum calcium within hours.[47] Patients must be followed very closely, preferably in the intensive care unit, because in addition to the monitoring of intravascular volume, there must be close attention paid to serum and urine electrolytes. Potassium and magnesium levels also fall during the forced saline diuresis with furosemide. If this therapy fails to stabilize or drop the serum calcium level in 12 to 24 hours, then more aggressive therapy is necessary.

An additional therapy is corticosteroids (2 mg/kg/day of prednisone) when hypercalcemia is considered to be due to osteoclast-activating factor or prostaglandin production by the tumor. They are also effective as direct antineoplastic therapy against hematologic malignancies. The onset of action of corticosteroids, however, is rarely seen before 3 days. Mithramycin, an antitumor antibiotic, effectively inhibits bone resorption. A dose of 25 μg/kg given intravenously can reduce serum calcium levels within 6 to 24 hours.[45] The dose can be repeated if there is no response in 48 hours. Mithramycin can cause marrow, renal, and hepatic toxicity. Diphosphonates, analogs of pyrophosphate, inhibit osteoclastic bone resorption. Etidronate disodium, which can be used in older children and adolescents, can be administered in a dosage of 7.5 mg/kg/day intravenously for up to 7 days.[45, 48] The oral preparation of etidronate has a limited effect. Intravenous phosphates should not be given because of the risk of metastatic calcification leading to renal failure and soft-tissue calcifications. Oral phosphorus, however, is effective for chronic hypercalcemia.

Hemodialysis or peritoneal dialysis can also effectively and rapidly treat hypercalcemia. However, these therapies are used only when patients present with renal failure and are unable to be volume loaded and to undergo a forced saline diuresis.

Tumor lysis syndrome is a metabolic derangement consisting of hyperkalemia, hyperuricemia, and hyperphosphatemia with secondary hypocalcemia and renal failure. This syndrome is typically seen in patients with rapidly proliferating tumors, such as Burkitt lymphoma and T cell leukemias and lymphomas, that undergo spontaneous cell lysis or after cytotoxic chemotherapy leads to a profound lysis of the malignant cells.[49, 50] In patients with Burkitt lymphoma, factors that predispose them to develop this syndrome include bulky abdominal tumors, elevations in serum uric acid and lactic dehydrogenase levels prior to chemotherapy, and oliguria.[49] Tumor lysis syndrome has been reported to occur occasionally in patients with other non-Hodgkin lymphomas, nonlymphoblastic leukemias, and some solid tumors.[45]

The tumor lysis syndrome occurs because there is malignant cellular degradation, and the intracellular metabolites that are released are present in quantities that overwhelm the ability of the kidneys to excrete them. In addition, uric acid, which is produced by the breakdown of nucleic acids, and phosphate also precipitate in the kidneys (collecting ducts and renal tubules), leading to renal failure and further impairment of renal excretion with additional increments in serum potassium, phosphorus, and uric acid levels. Oliguria is also important in the pathophysiology of this syndrome. Hypocalcemia occurs because of the formation and precipitation of calcium phosphate salts, due to the hyperphosphatemia. These salts can precipitate in the renal tubules, further limiting metabolite excretion and exacerbating the tumor lysis syndrome. Hyperkalemia, secondary to the tumor lysis syndrome, is the most worrisome metabolic derangement in this setting. It can occur rapidly and can lead to life-threatening cardiac arrhythmias and asystole.

The management of tumor lysis syndrome is shown in Figure 65–1. In our institution, the standard of care is that all pediatric patients with or at risk of developing tumor lysis syndrome are managed in the intensive care unit. As can be seen in Figure 65–1, the initial level of aggressiveness depends on the degree of metabolic derangement at presentation. If hyperuricemia is noted and the patient has oliguric renal failure, then dialysis should be initiated before chemotherapy is instituted. Once fluid and electrolyte management is achieved, then chemotherapy can be initiated. Hemodialysis is the preferred mode of dialysis for rapid control of volume overload and metabolic derangements. However, continuous arteriovenous hemofiltration (CAVH) with dialysis or continuous venovenous hemofiltration (CVVH) with dialysis are alternatives to conventional hemodialysis, if these methods can effectively control the serum electrolyte derangements.

The algorithm of management of other patients is aimed at preventing renal failure and limiting the metabolic and electrolyte derangements and is adapted from previously published recommendations.[49] Prevention of renal failure and metabolic control involves hydration, alkalinization of urine, and allopurinol.

Allopurinol inhibits xanthine oxidase and decreases the formation of uric acid from purine degradation products.[51, 52] The initial dose is typically 300 mg/m^2/day either orally or intravenously; however, up to 500 mg/m^2/day can be given. The dose should be lowered in the presence of renal failure, because allopurinol and its metabolites are excreted only in the urine, and approximately 3 to 4 days after chemotherapy has been initiated. Vigorous fluid therapy affects both adequate hydration and an adequate urinary flow rate that facilitates excretion of uric acid and phosphate. Volume replacement of two to four times the maintenance amount or 3,000 ml/m^2/day is recommended. Fluid therapy may have to be guided by hemodynamic monitoring using either a central venous catheter or a pulmonary artery catheter. This is especially true in the presence of renal failure or associated cardiac or pulmonary dysfunction. The type of crystalloid given is up to the caregiver, with 5% glucose/0.45 to 0.9% sodium chloride solutions being preferred. Supplemental potassium should not be added to the hydration. Sodium bicarbonate is added to the hydration fluid in order to increase urinary pH to at least 7 and thus limit or prevent uric acid precipitation in the collecting ducts, which occurs at an acidic pH. This should be done only until chemotherapy is started. Once chemotherapy begins, the bicarbonate should be discontinued to avoid the phosphates released during tumor lysis from precipitating as calcium phosphate salts in the kidneys.

The careful and frequent monitoring of serum and urine electrolytes, cardiac rhythm, and the patient's volume status is essential to this therapy. These patients usually have a central venous catheter or a pulmonary artery catheter placed to facilitate hemodynamic monitoring and an arterial line because of frequent phlebotomy. Serum electrolyte levels should be followed at least every 4 to 6 hours during the first 24 hours of therapy. If there are rapid rises in potassium, phosphorus, or uric acid levels, or if dialysis is required, these electrolytes should be monitored more frequently. Hyperkalemia is the most severe metabolic derangement of tumor lysis. If hyperkalemia (potassium $\geq$ 6 mEq/l) occurs, an electrocardiogram should be obtained to look for QRS widening, which is usually observed before the occurrence of malignant arrhythmias or asystole. Ther-

apy of hyperkalemia, including potassium-binding resins, glucose, and insulin should be given, and dialysis should be emergently started. This syndrome resolves once the tumor burden has been reduced by cytotoxic therapy, and metabolic and renal derangements should return to normal.

The syndrome of inappropriate secretion of antidiuretic hormone (SIADH) can occur with central nervous system tumors or injury, pulmonary malignancies, or other causes of pulmonary dysfunction (infection, inflammation, need for ventilatory support), and secondary to chemotherapeutic agents (vincristine and cyclophosphamide).[53] The most common tumor producing SIADH is small-cell carcinoma of the lung,[54] which is rarely seen in children. Antidiuretic hormone affects sodium and water balance by acting on the renal tubule and leads to sodium loss and water retention. The net metabolic results are hyponatremia and hypo-osmolality.

The clinical manifestations of the water intoxication and hyponatremia are primarily neurologic. In mild cases, fatigue, headaches, and nausea are the primary symptoms. When the serum sodium falls below 120 mEq/l, or the drop in serum sodium is precipitous, the neurologic symptoms become more severe, and confusion, coma, and seizures become more significant manifestations.[55]

Other causes of hyponatremia must be considered as the patient is evaluated. In the patient with malignancy, etiologies that one must consider include congestive heart failure, liver disease, renal failure, hypothyroidism, and glucocorticoid deficiency. In order to establish the diagnosis of SIADH, one must document a urine sodium concentration and urine osmolality that are inappropriately high for the degree of hyponatremia, and there must also be no renal, adrenal, or thyroid disease. In SIADH, urine osmolality is typically greater than 100 mOsm/g H$_2$O.[45]

The definitive treatment of SIADH is based on identifying the underlying cause (e.g., central nervous system metastasis, lung disease) and treating it. Pending a response to primary therapy, fluid restriction slowly increases the serum sodium and thus limits symptoms. If the degree of hyponatremia is severe enough to produce severe neurologic symptoms such as coma or seizures, then 3% (hypertonic) sodium chloride administered with furosemide will increase the serum sodium within hours.[56] This therapy must be undertaken cautiously and, ideally, in an intensive care unit, because fluid therapy and management must be monitored carefully, and serum electrolytes need to be checked at least every 2 hours. Volume overload leading to congestive heart failure may occur with 3% sodium chloride administration, especially in patients with underlying cardiac disease. In addition, the rate of correction of the hyponatremia should not exceed 1 to 2 mEq/hr in order to avoid neurologic deterioration, typically due to central pontine myelinolysis, and death.[57, 58]

Tumor-related hypoglycemia is another metabolic derangement that can be seen in patients with malignancies. It may occur secondary to insulin-secreting islet cell tumors, lymphomas, large mesenchymal tumors in the retroperitoneum or thorax, hepatomas, or adrenocortical tumors.[45, 59] Islet cell tumors excessively secrete insulin, whereas in nonislet cell tumors the etiology of hypoglycemia is less clear-cut and may be due to accelerated glucose metabolism by the tumor or to production of an insulin-like compound.[60] Symptomatically, patients may develop fatigue, confusion, lethargy, seizures, or coma as serum glucose levels fall. In some situations, the presentation of the hypoglycemia in children may be behavioral or emotional problems. Symptoms typically occur after fastings, and a fasting serum glucose level of 50 mg/dl or less is typically seen in patients with tumor-induced hypoglycemia.[45] It is important for the clinician to consider this metabolic problem in the workup of seizures or altered mental status in the pediatric patient with a malignancy.

Therapy should be primarily directed against the tumor in order to effect control of the hypoglycemia. The options include surgical resection, chemotherapy, or radiation therapy, depending on the histopathology, size, and location of the tumor. Additional therapeutic options include dietary modifications such that the patient is fed multiple times during the day and night in order to avoid periods of fasting and the use of high glucose-containing solutions (e.g., 10% dextrose or 20% dextrose) delivered via a central vein for either nutritional supplementation or total parenteral nutrition. The latter option is usually reserved for palliation.

Lactic acidosis in patients with neoplastic disorders without tissue hypoxia can cause a significant metabolic acidosis.[61-63] It has been associated primarily with Hodgkin disease, non-Hodgkin lymphomas, and leukemias. In most of these situations, the lactic acidosis is an indicator of a large tumor burden and active disease as well as a marker for a relapse of the tumor.[61] The etiology of the lactic acidosis is not clear but may be due to the inability of the liver to metabolize lactic acid, since this metabolic derangement is typically seen in patients with hepatic infiltration by leukemia or lymphoma or with significant hepatic metastases. Other possible etiologies include excessive production of lactic acid by neoplastic cells due to a high rate of glycolysis or microvascular aggregates of tumor cells that lead to poor tissue perfusion and hypoxemia with a shift toward anaerobic metabolism and lactate overproduction.[61, 62]

Therapy should be directed against the underlying process (i.e., chemotherapy against lymphoma).[63] As the tumor regresses and remission occurs, the lactic acidosis clears. Sodium bicarbonate is typically only needed acutely with severe lactic acidosis. This is controversial, thus it should be used with caution to avoid an iatrogenic metabolic alkalosis as well as hyperosmolality. The primary therapy should be chemotherapy.

Adrenal insufficiency of clinical significance requires the destruction of more than 90% of the adrenal glands. Bilateral adrenal hemorrhage may cause significant adrenal damage and may produce a loss of both mineralocorticoid and glucocorticoid secretion with marked adrenal insufficiency. This problem may occur in the setting of tumor-induced thrombocytopenia or disseminated intravascular coagulation (DIC) as well as in overwhelming infection.[64, 65] Another systemic effect of a tumor leading to adrenal insufficiency is the replacement of adrenal glands by significant adrenal metastases. Although rare in children, this condition can be caused by leukemic or lymphomatous infiltration of bilateral adrenal glands.

If adrenal insufficiency is suspected because of an appropriate clinical setting and because of shock unresponsiveness to volume replacement with or without the classic laboratory abnormalities of hyponatremia associated with hyperkalemia, then replacement therapy with hydrocortisone (which provides sufficient mineralocorticoid and glucocorticoid activity) should be initiated. An ACTH stimulation test with baseline, 30-minute, and 60-minute cortisol determinations should provide chemical evidence of hypoadrenalism and should be performed quickly, before hydrocortisone replacement therapy. An alternative is to give the patient dexamethasone as corticosteroid replacement therapy, and this will allow an ACTH stimulation test to be performed with interpretable results. Further work-up of hypoadrenalism is discussed elsewhere (see Chapter 59).

Hematologic

Hematologic derangements may also occur as systemic manifestations of malignancy. DIC may occur in association with a number of hematologic malignancies, most commonly with acute promyelocytic leukemia.[66, 67] Granules in the promyelocytes are thought to correlate with the occurrence of DIC. Treatment of DIC is based on chemotherapy directed against the underlying malignancy. Heparin may be used adjunctively to treat DIC, pending the onset of effects of the chemotherapy.[68] Heparin is given in order to control the consumptive coagulopathy, but it must be administered cautiously and, frequently, with platelet transfusions to maintain a platelet count of more than 50,000 platelets/mm³ in order to minimize the occurrence of secondary hemorrhage, especially intracranial bleeding. Once the chemotherapy has led to a measurable response against the leukemia and there is evidence that DIC is resolving, then heparin therapy can be discontinued (see also Chapter 64).

Another systemic manifestation of hematologic or other malignancies is marrow replacement by a tumor, leading to pancytopenia. A bone marrow aspirate and biopsy will confirm the replacement of normal bone marrow by tumor cells. Therapy should be directed against the primary malignancy. As the tumor burden in the marrow lessens, then the number of normal hematopoietic cells should increase and should produce adequate quantities of white blood cells, red blood cells, and platelets. Prior to that, transfusion support with red blood cells and platelets may be required.

Spontaneous hemorrhage of the mucous membranes and central nervous system typically occurs with platelet counts of less than 20,000/mm³, and that is an absolute platelet number on which we base the need for transfusions. For platelet counts in the range of 20,000 to 50,000/mm³, prophylactic transfusions are not necessary, except when there is evidence of bleeding or in the case of patients with central nervous system lesions. Platelet transfusions are indicated if there is evidence of active bleeding or oozing (e.g., epistaxis or gastrointestinal hemorrhage) or if an invasive procedure will be performed (e.g., central line placement, thoracentesis, or surgery). Vomiting, significant coughing (with or without the presence of an endotracheal tube), and retinal hemorrhage are additional indications for the prophylactic transfusion of platelets, because they may herald the potential for more significant hemorrhage.

Hyperleukocytosis with leukostasis occurs occasionally in children with acute lymphocytic leukemia and acute nonlymphocytic leukemia; however, it is a nearly universal occurrence in children with chronic myelogenous leukemia in the chronic phase.[22, 23, 69, 70] This is a medical emergency that can produce pulmonary leukostasis and respiratory failure (see earlier), central nervous system thrombosis or hemorrhage, peripheral vascular insufficiency, as well as the metabolic problems that accompany the tumor lysis syndrome (see earlier). Leukostasis typically occurs when peripheral white blood cell counts exceed 100,000 cells/mm^3, and it produces increased blood viscosity with secondary poor perfusion and anaerobic metabolism with lactic acidosis. In addition, significant leukostasis can result in direct damage to cerebral blood vessels and alveoli, respectively.[71]

The presenting symptoms of hyperleukocytosis with leukostasis may include confusion, blurred vision, and dyspnea secondary to the primary organ microcirculatory involvement. On physical examination, the patient may have cyanosis, retinal evidence of arterial and venous distention with papilledema, digital necrosis, and priapism.[69, 72, 73] A laboratory evaluation typically reveals hypoxemia and occasionally lactic acidosis. All patients with hyperleukocytosis and leukostasis should be monitored and treated in an intensive care unit.

Treatment requires rapid cytoreduction. Specific antileukemic therapy should begin immediately with the adjuncts of hydration, alkalinization, and allopurinol (see tumor lysis syndrome). Pending the tumor lytic effects of chemotherapy, leukopheresis or plasma exchange may be used to achieve cytoreduction. Leukopheresis can reduce the white blood cell count by 20 to 60%.[22, 69, 74] By doing so, it reduces both the systemic tumor burden and the metabolic requirements for the kidneys. Although effective, the procedure is not without risk because it requires both systemic anticoagulation and large catheters that may be difficult to place in the vasculature of small children.

Some investigators have suggested that emergency cranial irradiation can also be used as an adjunctive therapy in order to prevent intracranial hemorrhage[75]; however, this viewpoint is controversial. Special attention should also be given to the hyperviscosity associated with this syndrome. Transfusions of packed red blood cells or whole blood may increase viscosity, precipitate leukostasis, and lead to further organ dysfunction or death.[76] As a consequence, blood transfusions should be given cautiously only when the hemoglobin is less than 7 to 8 g/dl, until cytoreductive therapy has been effective.[23] During blood transfusions, the patient should be monitored closely for the development of hyperviscosity and leukostasis. Since platelets are less viscous and may be needed because of the risk of central nervous system hemorrhage, they may be transfused more liberally, especially if the platelet count falls below 20,000/mm^3.

COMPLICATIONS OF THERAPY

Cardiovascular

The therapies of neoplastic diseases may lead to cardiovascular dysfunction either in the form of cardiomyopathy, coronary artery disease, or pericardial disease. The most commonly recognized causes of a dose-related cardiomyopathy are the anthracycline antibiotics, daunorubicin (daunomycin) and doxorubicin (adriamycin). These drugs typically cause cardiomyopathy when the total dosage exceeds 550 mg/m^2.

Data from endomyocardial biopsy sampling indicate that the degree of endomyocardial injury is correlated statistically with the dosage and schedule of doxorubicin administration (i.e., less injury was associated with a lower cumulative dose and a weekly administration schedule).[77] In addition, the risk of development of congestive heart failure seems to increase in older patients who receive cumulative doses comparable with those in younger patients.[78] Others have variably reported an increased incidence in children, especially if they have received previous irradiation to the mediastinum or the heart.[79] In addition to total anthracycline dose and previous irradiation, other factors that may increase the incidence of anthracycline cardiomyopathy include the administration of other cytotoxic drugs (e.g., cyclophosphamide) and underlying cardiac disease.[80]

The mechanism of this cardiomyopathy is not entirely clear and may involve the generation of superoxide radicals by the anthracyclines with secondary myocardial cell damage and degeneration. Histopathologically, endomyocardial biopsies in these patients demonstrate loss of myofibrils and diffuse disorganization of myocytes. These drugs may also impair the growth of the ventricular myocardium, resulting in an inadequate ventricular mass that potentially leads to depressed left ventricular function.[81]

In addition to dose-related cardiomyopathy, doxorubicin can also cause acute left ventricular dysfunction with congestive heart failure after a single dose of the drug. This is an idiosyncratic toxicity and is not a dose-related phenomenon. A variety of supraventricular and ventricular arrhythmias have also been observed after anthracycline administration.

Cyclophosphamide has been reported to cause an acute cardiomyopathy when it is administered in high doses (i.e., > 220 mg/kg).[82, 83] Patients typically receive high-dose cyclophosphamide (albeit below the cardiotoxic level) before bone marrow transplantation or as part of experimental chemotherapeutic regimens. In one series, 25% of patients who received the drug in this dosage range developed congestive heart failure, although in our experience this is a much less common event.[82] The histopathologic characteristic of this type of cardiomyopathy is myocardial necrosis with hemorrhage.

Regardless of the etiology, patients with cardiomyopathy may present with historical and clinical evidence of congestive heart failure. If these children have been followed with serial cardiac assessments there may be objective evidence heralding myocardial dysfunction, such as decreased left ventricular ejection fraction as measured by radionuclide cineangiography or echocardiography. If followed prospectively, therapy consisting of diuretics, peripheral vasodilators, and digoxin may limit some of the clinical manifestations of congestive heart failure in these children. In other situations, these children may present acutely with either congestive heart failure or cardiogenic shock. With the latter, left ventricular ejection fractions in the range of 10% have been documented by echocardiograms or radionuclide studies.

Admission to the intensive care unit for management of shock is indicated, and peripheral artery and pulmonary artery catheters are frequently necessary for both hemodynamic monitoring and management. If cardiogenic shock is present, then inotropic and chronotropic therapy consisting of dopamine, dobutamine, and epinephrine, either alone or in combination, may be necessary to achieve an adequate blood pressure and cardiac index. Caution must be taken, however, because these chronotropic and inotropic agents may precipitate arrhythmias. With cardiogenic shock secondary to chemotherapeutic agents, cardiac indices may be less than 1.5 l/min/m². Attention must be paid to end-organ perfusion (central nervous system, liver, and kidneys) in the presence of cardiogenic shock. Additional pharmacologic therapy, consisting of digoxin and vasodilators, may be added for more chronic control of congestive heart failure after acute treatment of shock or refractory congestive heart failure. Cardiac transplantation may be considered as definitive therapy if the patient is either cured of the malignancy or shows no evidence of active malignant disease.

Radiation therapy can also produce a variety of cardiovascular complications. Acute pericarditis, secondary to acute inflammation, can occur during radiation therapy; however, more typically it may produce chronic pericarditis manifested by either constrictive pericarditis or pericardial effusion with tamponade (or both).[84] Symptoms of chronic radiation-induced pericardial disease may occur as early as 5 months after therapy and as late as 124 months after therapy.[85] Typically seen after high doses of radiation to the mediastinum (> 4,000 rads), this pericardial disease is also usually associated with some degree of myocardial or endomyocardial fibrosis.

A diagnosis of pericardial disease is based on a consistent history (previous radiation therapy) associated with clinical signs and symptoms of tamponade (see Table 65–1). Echocardiography will confirm the presence of a pericardial effusion; however, simultaneous right and left heart catheterization with volume loading and measurements of cardiac chamber pressures may be required to diagnose constrictive pericardial disease as well as restrictive cardiomyopathy. Pericardial tampon-

ade may also occur with large effusions. Management of tamponade has been presented earlier in the chapter. Definitive therapy for constrictive pericarditis is surgical removal of the pericardium; however, with less severe cases diuretic therapy, to treat the symptoms of venous congestion, may be all that is required.

Radiation therapy can also cause coronary vascular damage leading to premature coronary atherosclerosis with secondary angina or myocardial infarction.[86] Medical or surgical management of radiation-induced coronary artery disease may be necessary for symptomatic, critical coronary artery obstructions.

In the setting of chemotherapy-induced neutropenia, sepsis (with or without septic shock) is a common event. In a subset of adult patients with septic shock, significant, but reversible, right and left ventricular dysfunction manifested by a markedly decreased biventricular ejection fraction with associated biventricular dilatation has been described.[87, 88] Although similar clinical data have not yet been reported in children, the experience at our institution is that in some pediatric patients the same sepsis-induced cardiomyopathy occurs. In most situations, the cardiac index is maintained in a normal or elevated range, despite the decreased ventricular ejection fraction. In these situations, supportive therapy consists of fluids and vasopressors in order to maintain a blood pressure, primarily by increasing systemic vascular resistance, and to maintain adequate end-organ perfusion. In a few cases, this decreased ejection fraction is associated with a markedly decreased cardiac index. In those situations, inotropic support with epinephrine or dobutamine may be required to maintain both blood pressure and organ perfusion.

A variety of sepsis-induced vasoactive mediators and cytokines (e.g., interleukins, leukotrienes, prostaglandins) are hypothesized to cause this myocardial dysfunction. With the advent of immunotherapy strategies for the treatment of some neoplastic disorders, similar patterns of acute, reversible ventricular dysfunction and cardiomyopathy have been described. Interleukin-2, which is used for therapy of melanoma, renal cell carcinoma, and neuroblastoma, has been reported to produce transient left ventricular dysfunction and associated hemodynamic derangement that are indistinguishable from septic shock.[89, 90] As additional, innovative antineoplastic therapies using other cytokines are developed, clinicians will have to be aware of the potential for the occurrence of therapy-induced cardiomyopathy.

Pulmonary

The lungs of patients with malignancies can develop a number of significant clinical and roentgenographic abnormalities as complications of therapy against the underlying neoplasm. There is a broad spectrum of both noninfectious and infectious causes of these pulmonary complications, which typically are categorized as diffuse pulmonary infiltrates. Table 65–4 lists the most common etiologies of diffuse pulmonary infiltrates in these patients. Except for leukoagglutinin reactions and leukemic/lymphomatous infiltration, most of the etiologies

Table 65–4. DIFFERENTIAL DIAGNOSIS OF DIFFUSE PULMONARY INFILTRATES IN THE PEDIATRIC PATIENT WITH A MALIGNANCY

Noninfectious
  (Adult) respiratory distress syndrome
  Drug-induced pneumonitis
  Radiation pneumonitis
  Leukoagglutinin reactions and hyperleukocytosis
  Leukemic/lymphomatous infiltrates
  Hemorrhage (intra-alveolar)
  Congestive heart failure

Infectious
  Bacteria
  Fungi
  Parasites
  Viruses

listed are due to complications of therapy. In the immunosuppressed subgroup of pediatric patients with malignancies, the infectious pneumonias are probably the most common cause of morbidity and mortality.

History taking and physical examination are always important in evaluating these patients and may provide clues for the diagnosis; however, additional diagnostic tests are necessary to establish a definite diagnosis. Plain chest roentgenograms typically reveal diffuse alveolar or interstitial pulmonary infiltrates, thus chest x-ray pattern recognition rarely provides a definite diagnosis for the clinician. Pulmonary artery catheterization should be performed in any patient when there is a question of congestive heart failure or an elevated pulmonary artery wedge pressure, or if one would like to confirm a "noncardiogenic" cause of a pulmonary edema-like pattern on a chest roentgenogram. However, as is discussed later in this chapter and elsewhere in this textbook, many of these diagnoses either require bronchoalveolar lavage or histopathologic sections from transbronchial biopsy or open lung biopsy in order to make a diagnosis.

The adult respiratory distress syndrome (ARDS) typically occurs as a complication of sepsis in these patients. However, in oncology patients, it may also occur after multiple transfusions, diffuse lung infections, and with pancreatitis. In sepsis-induced ARDS, injury occurs to the pulmonary endothelium and leads to a diffuse "capillary leak" and noncardiogenic pulmonary edema. Pulmonary artery catheterization allows for measurement of intracardiac pressures to be obtained as well as for the assessment of the patient's hemodynamic profile. A cardiac index of more than 2.5 l/min/m² and a pulmonary artery wedge pressure of less than 18 mm Hg are consistent with normal left ventricular function and a noncardiogenic cause of clinical pulmonary edema or ARDS. The hallmark of therapy for ARDS is supportive care (primarily ventilatory and hemodynamic), whereas the underlying cause of ARDS (usually sepsis) is treated aggressively.

Drug-induced pneumonitis due to a chemotherapeutic agent is a diagnosis of exclusion. Importantly, there must be a prior history of exposure to a drug known to cause pulmonary disease, the histopathologic abnormalities must be consistent with drug toxicity, and other possible etiologies must be excluded. Table 65–5 lists the most common chemotherapeutic agents responsible for drug-induced pulmonary injury.

Bleomycin pulmonary toxicity has been well studied, and much is known about both acute and chronic side effects of this chemotherapeutic agent. The description of bleomycin pulmonary toxicity will serve as a model for the other chemotherapy-induced pulmonary toxicities. Bleomycin is only infrequently used as an active agent against a number of childhood malignancies. More commonly, it is used in the treatment of lymphoma and testicular cancer in adults.[91] Bleomycin-induced pneumonitis consists of an acute, reversible hypersensitivity type of pneumonitis with eosinophilia and a chronic, nonhypersensitivity type of pneumonitis that can be severe and can result in death.[91-93] The reported frequency of bleomycin pulmonary toxicity ranges from less than 5 to 50%, with an average incidence of 10%. Of this group approximately 10% of patients will die of progressive pulmonary fibrosis and respiratory failure attributable to bleomycin.[92]

Bleomycin toxicity typically occurs after a cumulative dose of more than 450 units of the drug; however, effects can be seen at much lower cumulative doses.[94] The pulmonary toxicity is aggravated by previous or concomitant oxygen or radiation therapy.[95-97] The intensive care physician must be aware of this synergistic toxicity when managing a patient who has received previous bleomycin therapy and who is also hypoxemic. The amount of supplemental oxygen delivered should be minimized—that is, aim for a partial pressure of oxygen (PaO_2) of about 60 mm Hg in order to limit or prevent bleomycin toxicity that is exacerbated by supplemental oxygen. The same care should be taken by anesthesiologists. When patients with previous bleomycin exposure have a surgical procedure performed, they should be exposed to the lowest intraoperative FiO_2 possible in order to provide adequate oxygenation without increasing the risk of oxygen toxicity. Postoperatively, the administration of oxygen must also be performed judiciously. Following supplemental oxygen therapy, bleomycin toxicity may occur between 1 and 14 days.

Acute bleomycin toxicity (hypersensitivity pneumonitis) manifests itself with the rapid onset of symptoms of cough, dyspnea, and fever. Chest roentgenograms typically reveal diffuse infiltrates. Histopathologically, there is evidence of eosinophilic infiltration in the pulmonary interstitium and alveolar spaces.[93] A peripheral eosinophilia may or may not be present. Therapy consists of the discontinuation of bleomycin and corticoste-

Table 65–5. CHEMOTHERAPEUTIC AGENTS MOST COMMONLY ASSOCIATED WITH DRUG-INDUCED PULMONARY INJURY

Bleomycin
Busulfan
Carmustine (BCNU)
Cyclophosphamide
Cytosine arabinoside
Methotrexate

roid administration, and a response is usually rapid. The chronic, fibrosing pneumonitis that occurs after higher cumulative doses of bleomycin also typically presents as cough, dyspnea, and fever; however, these symptoms may be more insidious than when they occur with acute toxicity. Hypoxemia may be significant. Chest roentgenograms reveal diffuse interstitial infiltrates, which may be associated occasionally with nodules. In some situations the appearance of nodules has led to the suspicion of metastatic disease; however, histopathologically, they have been due to bleomycin without evidence of associated metastases.[98] The typical pulmonary histopathologic abnormality is interstitial pneumonitis with a loss of type I pneumocytes and hyperplasia of type II pneumocytes.[99] Less invasive methods, such as bronchoalveolar lavage, have not yet provided consistent cellular data that would aid in the diagnosis. Treatment consists of the discontinuation of bleomycin and high-dose corticosteroids. Despite those interventions, the pulmonary fibrosis may be irreversible and progressive, and a percentage of patients die secondary to refractory hypoxemia and respiratory failure. Clinical and roentgenographic exacerbations have been described as corticosteroid therapy is tapered.[100] As a consequence, long courses of corticosteroids with slow tapering schedules and careful clinical follow-up are recommended.

Busulfan, an alkylating agent, also causes an interstitial fibrosis that is manifested in a manner similar to bleomycin (i.e., with cough, dyspnea, and occasionally fever).[101] Pleural effusions have also been noted with busulfan pulmonary toxicity. Discontinuation of the drug and corticosteroids are the recommended therapies.

Carmustine (BCNU) is a nitrosourea that can cause symptoms and histopathologic evidence of interstitial fibrosis that are indistinguishable from those caused by bleomycin and busulfan; however, a specific dose leading to pulmonary toxicity has not yet been identified.[102, 103] There may be an increased risk of pulmonary toxicity secondary to carmustine if it is used in combination with other chemotherapeutic agents known to produce pulmonary lesions.

Cyclophosphamide, an alkylating agent, has also been reported to cause interstitial pneumonitis and pulmonary fibrosis, and in children, it may also lead to a loss of lung volumes that are manifested during the rapid growth of adolescence.[104, 105] The true incidence of pulmonary side effects from cyclophosphamide is unknown. Symptoms consist of cough, dyspnea, and usually fever. Oxygen therapy and radiation therapy do not seem to increase the risk of cyclophosphamide pulmonary toxicity, and the response to corticosteroids is prompt.

Cytosine arabinoside (Ara-C) in high doses can cause noncardiogenic pulmonary edema (ARDS) either during or after therapy.[106, 107] The clinical picture is indistinguishable from other causes of ARDS and is associated with significant morbidity and mortality. Importantly, it has been described to occur either during or after cytosine arabinoside therapy. The standards of ARDS therapy should be followed during respiratory failure, and empiric corticosteroids should be considered.

Methotrexate, an antimetabolite, causes pulmonary toxicity that is typically a hypersensitivity pneumonitis rather than an interstitial pneumonitis with fibrosis. It has been observed in a number of children with acute lymphoblastic leukemia as well as with other malignancies.[108, 109] Methotrexate pneumonitis can also occur after intrathecal administration of the drug.[110] Histopathologic data consisting of eosinophils and granuloma formation in the lungs and bronchoalveolar lavage data demonstrating predominant T helper lymphocytes and an increased ratio of helper to suppressor cells support the hypothesis that methotrexate induces a hypersensitivity pneumonitis.[111, 112] After discontinuation of the drug, the outcome is generally favorable, and, interestingly, some patients who have been re-exposed to the drug have not redeveloped the pneumonitis.[108]

Radiation therapy to the thorax (i.e., mantle or chest wall) can include the lungs in the radiation treatment fields. As a consequence, radiation-induced pulmonary toxicity can occur and can manifest itself as acute pneumonitis that progresses to pulmonary fibrosis.[113, 114] It typically occurs after relatively high doses of radiation exposure to the lung. However, toxicity can also occur at lower doses of radiation, particularly if large volumes of the lung have been exposed (i.e., total lung irradiation prior to bone marrow transplantation).[115] It is also important to remember that synergy between radiation exposure and chemotherapeutic agents can lead to radiation changes at lower doses. The clinical presentation consists of cough, dyspnea on exertion, and occasionally fever. Hypoxemia and ventilatory failure may complicate the most severe cases. Chest roentgenograms typically reveal diffuse pulmonary infiltrates, similar to the pattern seen with drug-induced pulmonary toxicity. Depending on the time of histopathologic assessment, the histopathology of the lung will range from an early exudative phase with alveolar cellular damage to a final, fibrotic phase with interstitial fibrosis and chronic inflammatory changes.[116] Some data have emerged suggesting an immunologic mechanism, like a hypersensitivity reaction, as the cause of radiation pneumonitis.[117]

Because of the clinical and roentgenographic similarity of radiation pneumonitis to other noninfectious and infectious causes of diffuse pulmonary infiltrates, an aggressive diagnostic work-up should be undertaken, including bronchoscopy and open lung biopsy. The diagnosis of radiation pneumonitis should be made as an "exclusionary" diagnosis after infectious etiologies are ruled out. Once the diagnosis is established, and infections ruled out, corticosteroid therapy should be instituted in the setting of radiation pneumonitis and hypoxemia. They are frequently required for several weeks before symptoms begin to wane. At that point the corticosteroids should be tapered slowly because of the potential for radiation pneumonitis to recur or flare with the taper.[118] In addition, long courses of high-dose corticosteroids also make these patients susceptible to a superimposed opportunistic infection. If clinical deterioration or roentgenographic progression occurs, then an infectious pneumonia-complicating radiation pneumonitis should be considered, and additional diagnostic procedures should be performed.

The pulmonary manifestations of high-circulating

white blood cell counts (hyperleukocytosis) have been presented earlier in this chapter; however, respiratory failure may also occur due to leukoagglutinin reactions following the transfusion of blood products. Because oncologic patients frequently have their bone marrows ablated by chemotherapy or radiation therapy, there is usually a need for frequent and multiple transfusions of blood components. After massive transfusions, leukoagglutinin reactions manifested by acute dyspnea, hypoxemia, and diffuse infiltrates may occur. An urticarial rash may also accompany this reaction. The pathophysiology is not entirely clear; however, it is possibly due to an acute immunologic reaction between either donor or recipient antibodies and heterologous leukocytes. It is speculated that as a consequence either oxygen radical or leukocyte-derived enzymes damage the alveolar-capillary endothelium leading to an ARDS-like picture.[119, 120] The degree of respiratory failure can be quite severe with this process, such that ventilatory support with positive end-expiratory pressure may be required. The rapidity of its development and the temporal relationship to transfusions should aid in the diagnosis of this phenomenon; however, the other etiologies shown in Table 65–4 must always be considered as diagnostic possibilities.

Leukocyte transfusions were, until very recently, commonly used in the treatment of neutropenia-related, life-threatening gram-negative bacteremia with sepsis.[121] When given in close proximity to amphotericin B, frequently required for fungal infections in neutropenic patients with cancer, leukocyte transfusions have been associated with respiratory failure. This acute respiratory decompensation is manifested by dyspnea, hypoxemia, diffuse interstitial infiltrates, and occasionally hemoptysis.[122] Ventilatory support may be required, and death due to respiratory failure has also been reported with this syndrome. Leukocyte transfusions are, currently, used very rarely for the treatment of gram-negative sepsis in a neutropenic patient. However, if both leukocyte transfusions and amphotericin B are considered as therapy, it is recommended that the infusions be separated from each other by as much time as possible and that a careful assessment of the patient's respiratory status should be made.

Intra-alveolar hemorrhage with either hypoxemia or respiratory failure may occur in the setting of either thrombocytopenia or a coagulopathy.[123] Hemoptysis may or may not occur; however, chest roentgenograms typically show diffuse infiltrates that may be in an alveolar pattern. Hemorrhage may be aggravated by a coexisting infection or pneumonia. Infections due to *Pseudomonas aeruginosa* and *Aspergillus* sp. can invade pulmonary vascular structures and cause pulmonary infarction with secondary hemorrhage.[124, 125] Therapy is supportive and consists of supplemental oxygen, transfusions of platelets and red blood cells, and correction of any coagulopathies.

As noted earlier in this section, pulmonary infections account for most of the morbidity and mortality in oncology patients with diffuse pulmonary infiltrates. A full range of pathogens can lead to respiratory failure, and urgency exists in both establishing a diagnosis and

initiating therapy. Table 65–6 categorizes further the broad spectrum of possible infectious etiologies of pneumonia in these patients.

A routine examination of an expectorated or suctioned sputum specimen should be the first diagnostic step, since a characteristic Gram stain (i.e., plenty of polymorphonuclear leukocytes with a predominant organism) would guide initial antibiotic therapy. Hypertonic sodium chloride nebulization and special staining techniques have been utilized to reveal *Pneumocystis carinii* as the cause of pneumonia in a number of immunosuppressed pediatric patients, and more invasive procedures have been avoided.[126] In most situations, however, an examination of the sputum is not helpful in establishing a diagnosis in the pediatric patient with malignancy and diffuse pulmonary infiltrates.

Fiberoptic bronchoscopy with bronchoalveolar lavage can be performed in pediatric patients and may provide a diagnosis of the infection in these immunosuppressed patients.[127, 128] If technically feasible and there are no contraindications, such as refractory hypoxemia or a bleeding diathesis, then bronchoscopy should be considered as the initial diagnostic procedure. Bronchoscopy can also be performed in patients on mechanical ventilation, provided that an adequate PaO_2 can be achieved with supplemental oxygen and that the endotracheal tube can accommodate the bronchoscope without marked elevation of airway pressures or hypercarbia. Bronchoscopy with bronchoalveolar lavage can be effective in establishing the diagnosis of noninfectious causes of diffuse pulmonary infiltrates such as alveolar hemorrhage and neoplasia. There are diagnostic limitations with the lavage procedure, however, and the decision of when to proceed to a more invasive procedure is frequently a

Table 65–6. INFECTIOUS CAUSES OF DIFFUSE PULMONARY INFILTRATES IN THE IMMUNOSUPPRESSED PEDIATRIC PATIENT WITH A MALIGNANCY

Bacteria
  Gram-negative organisms
  Gram-positive organisms
  Mycobacterium sp.
  Legionella pneumophila

Fungi
  Aspergillus sp.
  Candida sp.
  Cryptococcus neoformans
  Histoplasma capsulatum
  Zygomycetes (*Mucor* sp., *Rhizopus* sp.)

Parasites
  Pneumocystis carinii
  Toxoplasma gondii

Viruses
  Cytomegalovirus
  Herpes simplex
  Influenza
  Measles
  Respiratory syncytial
  Varicella zoster

Other
  Chlamydia sp.
  Mycoplasma sp.

difficult one. In older pediatric and adolescent patients, bronchoscopy with transbronchial biopsy can be performed. In one small series, 12 patients (median age of 14.5 years) tolerated the biopsy procedure, and specific diagnoses were made in half of these patients.[129] Biopsies can be performed if the airway or endotracheal tube can accommodate the bronchoscope and still allow for effective oxygenation and ventilation. In addition, there should be no contraindications to biopsy, such as thrombocytopenia of less than 50,000 platelets/mm^3, bleeding diathesis, refractory hypoxemia, or mechanical ventilation with high levels of positive pressure. Biopsies, if positive, are helpful in establishing whether the pulmonary infiltrates are due to a malignancy, an invasive fungal infection (i.e., *Aspergillus*), or a viral pneumonitis.

If the child is too small to safely undergo bronchoscopy, has a contraindication to the procedure, or has had a nondiagnostic bronchoalveolar lavage or transbronchial biopsy, then an open lung biopsy should be considered in order to establish a diagnosis. Some controversy exists with regard to whether or not open lung biopsies add enough diagnostic information to sanction the procedure. It is our experience, and that of others, that early, aggressive diagnosis is essential and that increased durations of pulmonary symptoms and delays in diagnosis are associated with poor prognoses.[20, 130] In many series, open lung biopsy has been a valuable procedure that frequently provides a definite diagnosis, allows therapy to be modified such that the use of potentially toxic antimicrobial agents may be minimized, and also guides decision-making and prognosis.[131–133] An alternative approach is that the advent of trimethoprim-sulfamethoxazole as prophylaxis against *P. carinii* and empiric broad-spectrum antibiotics make open lung biopsy a less essential diagnostic procedure.[134] Our approach is to attempt to establish a diagnosis by the use of sputum induction techniques and bronchoscopy; however, if those procedures are unrevealing and the patient has progressive infiltrates despite empiric therapy, then we proceed to open lung biopsy in order to perform a complete microbiologic and histopathologic pulmonary work-up.

Renal

Tumor lysis syndrome has been discussed.

Hemorrhagic cystitis with hematuria and occasionally life-threatening blood loss may be a complication of the agents cyclophosphamide and (more recently) ifosfamide. The incidence of hemorrhagic cystitis complicating the use of cyclophosphamide has been reported to be as high as 40%.[135] This toxicity is dependent on both the dosage of the drug and the duration of bladder exposure to acrolein, the toxic metabolite of cyclophosphamide and ifosfamide that is implicated in the etiology of the hemorrhagic cystitis.[136]

In order to decrease the risk of hemorrhagic cystitis due to these drugs, aggressive attempts should be made to decrease their concentrations and that of their metabolites in the bladder. This is accomplished most readily by maintaining a brisk diuresis by using both aggressive hydration and diuretics. Occasionally, hemodynamic monitoring with a pulmonary artery catheter may be required for accurate volume management in patients with either significant cardiomyopathy with congestive heart failure or lung disease. 2-Mercaptoethane sulfonate sodium (Mesna), which can be administered parenterally during and after cyclophosphamide or ifosfamide infusions, has been demonstrated to be effective in limiting the incidence of hemorrhagic cystitis.[137, 138] Mesna functions as a regional detoxificant of the toxic metabolite, acrolein.

If these measures at prevention are unsuccessful and hemorrhagic cystitis occurs, then supportive therapy along with attempts at bladder drainage and irrigation are used. Thrombocytopenia and coagulopathies should be corrected, and red blood cells should be transfused to maintain an acceptable level of hemoglobin. Bladder lavage with local instillation of crystalloid should be aggressive in order to limit clot formation that may result in urinary tract obstruction. More aggressive attempts to control hemorrhage include bladder fulguration and bladder sclerosis with formaldehyde. In the most severe situations, when all other measures have failed, cystectomy may be required.

Nephrotoxicity with renal failure may occur after administration of some antineoplastic agents. Cisplatin (*cis*-platinum), which is used as treatment for some germinal tumors and solid tumors, may cause renal insufficiency, especially when there is pre-existing renal insufficiency or when used in conjunction with aminoglycoside antibiotics.[139, 140] In addition to azotemia, cisplatin may cause vasopressin-resistant polyuria and magnesium wasting with secondary hypokalemia and hypocalcemia.[139] Nephrotoxicity and renal failure due to cisplatin can be limited by maintaining adequate hydration and a forced diuresis, with mannitol if necessary.

High-dose methotrexate can also cause renal failure due possibly to renal tubular precipitation of methotrexate or its metabolites in the acidic environment of the distal renal tubules. Hydration and urinary alkalinization with sodium bicarbonate limit methotrexate-induced nephrotoxicity.[141]

Gastrointestinal

Several antineoplastic agents can cause hepatic or other gastrointestinal complications. High-dose methotrexate can cause an acute and marked chemical hepatitis manifested by a rise in serum transaminases.[142] The return of liver enzymes to normal occurs with the discontinuation of the drug, and there is usually no evidence of chronic liver disease as a sequela. Fulminant hepatic failure is rare. High-dose 6-mercaptopurine can also cause hepatocellular necrosis and occasionally causes intrahepatic cholestasis. These complications are rarely life-threatening.

L-Asparaginase, used very commonly in the treatment of childhood leukemias, can cause a chemical hepatitis as well as evidence of intrahepatic cholestasis.[143, 144] In addition, pancreatitis may complicate L-asparaginase therapy in more than 10% of patients with leukemia who receive the drug as part of combination chemotherapy.[145] Management consists of discontinuation of the drug as well as supportive therapy, primarily in the form of careful fluid and electrolyte management. Special attention must also be given to other organ function, such as the lungs and kidneys, because multiorgan failure (including ARDS) can occur as a complication of L-asparaginase-induced pancreatitis. In the most severe cases, hemorrhagic pancreatitis, pseudocyst formation, and death have been reported.

Infectious Diseases

Infections are a major cause of morbidity and mortality in patients with malignancies who are immunosuppressed. Alterations in neutrophil number and function, humoral and cell-mediated immunologic dysfunction, the presence of foreign bodies (i.e., indwelling catheters and monitoring devices), and immunosuppressive therapies all make the pediatric oncologic patient in the intensive care unit especially susceptible to infections and their complications. Early diagnosis of infection and prompt initiation of antibacterial therapy (frequently empiric) are important and may prevent the development of the sepsis syndrome and septic shock. We have a high index of suspicion and a low threshold for initiating therapy in these patients.

Granulocytopenia, which generally refers to an absolute total polymorphonuclear leukocyte count of less than 500 to 1,000 cells/mm^3, may be due to either the patient's underlying disease with bone marrow involvement or chemotherapy-related bone marrow failure. Neutropenia is probably the single most important risk factor for life-threatening infections in these patients. In addition, both the degree and the duration of the neutropenia are associated with the development of infectious complications.[146] Functional neutrophil defects, such as alterations in adhesion or chemotaxis, have also been reported to occur in patients with malignancies either as a primary defect or secondary to therapy. These factors may also render oncology patients more susceptible to bacterial infections.[147, 148]

Fever may be the only sign of infection in neutropenic patients and is an indication for empiric antibiotic therapy pending the identification of the offending microorganism and the localization of a focus for infection if it exists. A great deal has been written about the importance of early, empiric antimicrobial therapy in the neutropenic patient, and numerous, rational, empiric regimens exist.[149–154] The patient should be thoroughly examined, and sputum, urine, wounds, as well as all sterile fluids, should be cultured. Special attention should be given to whether the patient has oropharyngeal mucositis or a perirectal or intra-abdominal process, and in those situations anaerobic antimicrobial agents should be added as part of the initial, empiric regimen.

In febrile, neutropenic patients with indwelling, permanent venous access devices (e.g., Hickman catheter, Groshong catheter) or in patients already in an intensive care unit with catheters for invasive hemodynamic monitoring, gram-positive organisms must be added to the list of potential pathogens.[155, 156] As a result, empiric therapy in these patients should include vancomycin, which is first-line therapy against Staphylococcus epidermidis (the most likely agent for "line-related" bacterial infections).[155–158] If a patient with an indwelling catheter develops septic shock, which is not easily amenable to fluid resuscitation or short-term vasopressors, then those catheters should be suspected to be a nidus for infection, the reason for intractable shock, and therefore should be removed. In a patient in the intensive care unit with invasive hemodynamic monitoring devices (e.g., peripheral arterial catheter or pulmonary artery catheter) who develops shock, our policy is that catheters should be removed and placed in other vascular sites on the presumption that they may be the nidus for bacteremia and shock.

Guidelines for the use of antimicrobials in febrile, neutropenic patients have been developed to provide rational algorithms for therapy.[159] If fever persists for more than 3 days after empiric antibiotic therapy it may indicate that a resistant bacterial pathogen is the cause of the infection, or a new bacterial infection has developed, antibiotic levels are subtherapeutic, or there is a sequestered focus (i.e., catheter site or abscess) that is the source of the infection.[159] The patient should be thoroughly assessed, and the examination should include performing a chest and abdominal CTT in order to determine whether or not an abscess is present. Consideration should also be given to either modifying or broadening initial antibiotic coverage.

If fever persists in a neutropenic patient on broad-spectrum antibacterial therapy for 7 days or more, then fungemia or deep-seated fungal infections (e.g., Aspergillus or Candida sp. in the lung, liver, spleen) have to be suspected, and amphotericin B should be added to the antimicrobial regimen.[156, 159] Fungal infections are frequently difficult to diagnose, and if a clinician waits for either a positive result on a fungal culture or for evidence of a fungal infection from a histopathologic specimen before initiating amphotericin B therapy, then (frequently) antifungal therapy may be initiated too late. Every attempt to localize a deep-seated fungal infection (if it exists) should be undertaken, especially since documentation of such a fungal process will help to guide the duration of amphotericin B therapy.

In general, empiric antibacterial therapy can be discontinued 1 to 2 days after the absolute neutrophil count has been greater than 500 cells/mm^3 if no obvious infectious site or bacteremia was documented. In cases of culture-negative septic shock, antibiotic courses of 10 to 14 total days of therapy are reasonable. If there is a documented bacteremia, then therapy should continue for a total of 10 to 14 days. When the neutrophil count is greater than 500 cells/mm^3 in patients with a documented bacteremia, antibiotics can be tapered to organism-specific monotherapy. In situations of documented fungemia or with documented invasive organ involvement due to fungi, then at least 20 mg/kg of amphotericin B (total dose) should be administered. Higher doses and longer courses may be recommended for patients with hepatic candidiasis.

Neutropenic enterocolitis, typhilitis, is a particular infectious disease problem in the immunosuppressed oncologic or leukemic patient. It manifests as right lower quadrant pain indistinguishable from appendicitis.[26, 31] Since it may be difficult to distinguish from appendicitis, these patients frequently undergo an exploratory laparotomy because of their acute surgical abdomen. In one series of leukemic patients with right lower quadrant pain, approximately one half had evidence of neutropenic enterocolitis at surgery and the remaining one half had appendicitis.[31] With both disease processes in these immunosuppressed patients there is a high incidence of intestinal perforation and abscess formation, both of which significantly add to morbidity and mortality. It is the experience of most surgeons that emergency intra-abdominal surgery in patients with leukemia can have a mortality rate of more than 50%, with even higher mortality rates in patients who have leukemia and who are not in remission.[29, 30, 160]

The role of granulocyte transfusions in neutropenic patients with life-threatening infections is controversial. Data have emerged that indicate minimal or no survival benefit of these transfusions in the cancer patient with neutropenia.[161, 162] As consequence, their routine use is not recommended.[159]

References

1. Lampkin BC, Gruppo RA, Lobel JS, et al: Pediatric hematologic and oncologic emergencies. Emerg Med Clin North Am 1:63, 1983.
2. Northrip DR, Bohman BK, and Tsueda K: Total airway obstruction and superior vena cava syndrome in a child with an anterior mediastinal tumor. Anesth Analg 65:1079, 1986.
3. O'Brien RT, Matlak ME, Condon VR, et al: Superior vena cava syndrome in children. West J Med 135:143, 1981.
4. Theologies A: Neoplastic cardiac tamponade. Semin Oncol 5:181, 1978.
5. Flannery EP, Gregoratos C, and Corder MP: Pericardial effusions in patients with malignant disease. Arch Intern Med 135:976, 1975.
6. Davis S, Sharma SM, Blumberg ED, et al: Intrapericardial tetracycline for tamponade secondary to malignant effusion. N Engl J Med 299:1113, 1978.
7. Deppisch LM and Fayemi AO: Non-bacterial thrombotic endocarditis: Clinicopathologic correlations. Am Heart J 92:723, 1976.
8. King RM, Telander RL, Smithson WA, et al: Primary mediastinal tumors in children. J Pediatr Surg 17:512, 1982.
9. Halpern S, Chatlen J, Meadows T, et al: Anterior mediastinal masses: Anesthetic hazards and other problems. J Pediatr 102:407, 1983.
10. Bittar D: Respiratory obstruction associated with induction of general anesthesia in a patient with mediastinal Hodgkin's disease. Anesth Analg 54:399, 1975.
11. Levin H, Bursztein S, and Heifetz M: Cardiac arrest in a child with an anterior mediastinal mass. Anesth Analg 64:1129, 1985.
12. Azizkhan RG, Dudgeon DL, Buck JR, et al: Life-threatening airway obstruction as a complication to the management of mediastinal masses in children. J Pediatr Surg 20:816, 1985.
13. Ferrari LR and Bedford RF: General anesthesia prior to treatment of anterior mediastinal masses in pediatric cancer patients. Anesthesiology 72:991, 1990.
14. Tinker TD and Crane DL: Safety of anesthesia for patients with anterior mediastinal masses (Letter), Vol. 1. Anesthesiology 73:1060, 1990.
15. Zornow MH and Benumof JL: Safety of anesthesia for patients with anterior mediastinal masses (Letter), Vol. 2. Anesthesiology 73:1061, 1990.
16. Mullen B and Richardson J: Primary anterior mediastinal tumors in children and adults. Ann Thorac Surg 42:338, 1986.
17. Kirks DR and Korobkin M: Computed tomography of the chest in infants and children: Techniques and mediastinal evaluation. Radiol Clin North Am 19:405, 1981.
18. Siegel MJ, Sagel SS, and Reed K: The value of computed tomography in the diagnosis and management of pediatric mediastinal abnormalities. Radiology 142:149, 1982.
19. Frey EE, Sato Y, Smith WL, et al: Cine CT of the mediastinum in pediatric patients. Radiology 165:19, 1987.
20. Early GE, Williams TE, and Kilman JW: Open lung biopsy: Its effects on therapy in the pediatric patient. Chest 87:467, 1985.
21. Kovalski R, Hansen-Flaschen J, Lodato RF, et al: Localized leukemic pulmonary infiltrates: Diagnosis by bronchoscopy and resolution with therapy. Chest 97:674, 1990.
22. Karp DD, Beck JR, and Cornell CJ: Chronic granulocytic leukemia with respiratory distress. Arch Intern Med 141:1353, 1981.
23. Ablin AR: Managing the problem of hyperleukocytosis in acute leukemia. Am J Pediatr Hematol Oncol 6:287, 1984.
24. Austin EH and Flye MW: The treatment of recurrent malignant effusion. Ann Thorac Surg 28:190, 1979.
25. Osteen RT, Guyton S, Steele G, et al: Malignant intestinal obstruction. Surgery 87:611, 1980.
26. Stellato TA and Shenk RR: Gastrointestinal emergencies in the oncology patient. Semin Oncol 16:521, 1989.
27. Weingard DN, DeCosse JJ, Sherlock P, et al: Primary gastrointestinal lymphoma: A 30 year review. Cancer 49:1258, 1982.
28. Ziegler JL: Burkitt's lymphoma. Med Clin North Am 61:1073, 1977.
29. Sherman NJ, Williams K, and Wooley MM: Surgical complications in the patient with leukemia. J Pediatr Surg 8:235, 1973.
30. Schaller RT and Schaller JF: The acute abdomen in the immunologically compromised child. J Pediatr Surg 18:937, 1983.
31. Skibber JM, Matter GJ, Pizzo PA, et al: Right lower quadrant pain in young patients with leukemia. Ann Surg 206:711, 1987.
32. Kanfer A, Vanderwalle A, Morel-Maroger L, et al: Acute renal insufficiency due to lymphomatous infiltration of the kidneys. Cancer 38:2588, 1976.
33. Lundberg WB, Cadman ED, Finch SC, et al: Renal failure secondary to leukemic infiltration of the kidneys. Am J Med 62:636, 1977.
34. Laxter RM, deChadarevian JP, Anderson RJ, et al: Malignant lymphoma presenting with nonoliguric renal failure. Clin Pediatr 22:819, 1983.
35. Heideman RL, Packer RJ, Albright LA, et al: Tumors of the central nervous system. In: Pizzo PA and Poplack DG (eds): Principles and Practice of Pediatric Oncology. Philadelphia, JB Lippincott, 1989, pp. 505–553.
36. Pack B and Maria BL: Neurologic emergencies in pediatric oncology. J Assoc Pediatr Oncol Nurses 4:8, 1988.
37. Galicich JH, Sundaresan N, and Thaler HT: Surgical treatment of single brain metastases. J Neurosurg 53:63, 1980.
38. Carincross JG and Posner JB: Neurological complications of systemic cancer. In: Yabro JW and Bornstein RS (eds): Oncologic Emergencies. New York, Grune & Stratton, 1981, pp. 73–96.
39. Bruce DA, Berman WA, and Schut L: Cerebrospinal fluid pressure monitoring in children: Physiology, pathology and clinical usefulness. Adv Pediatr 24:233, 1977.
40. Borgett B, Gelber R, Kramer S, et al: The palliation of brain metastases: Final results of the first two studies by the Radiation Therapy Oncology Group. Int J Radiat Oncol Biol Phys 6:1, 1980.
41. Alegretta GJ, Weisman SJ, and Altman AJ: Oncologic emergencies. I: Metabolic and space-occupying consequences of cancer and cancer treatment. Pediatr Clin North Am 32:601, 1985.
42. Olson ME, Chernick NL, and Posner JB: Infiltration of the leptomeninges by systemic cancer. Arch Neurol 30:122, 1974.
43. Al-Rashid RA and Cress C: Hypercalcemia associated with neuroblastoma. Am J Dis Child 133:838, 1979.
44. Harquindey S, DeCastro L, Barcos M, et al: Hypercalcemia complicating childhood malignancies. Cancer 44:2280, 1979.
45. Silverman P and Distelhorst CW: Metabolic emergencies in clinical oncology. Semin Oncol 16:504, 1989.
46. Mundy GR, Ibbotson KH, D'Souza SM, et al: Hypercalcemia

of cancer: Clinical implications and pathogenic mechanisms. N Engl J Med 310:1718, 1984.

47. Suki WN, Yium JJ, Minden MV, et al: Acute treatment of hypercalcemia with furosemide. N Engl J Med 283:836, 1970.

48. Jacobs TP, Gordon AC, Silverberg SJ, et al: Neoplastic hypercalcemia: Physiologic response to intravenous etidronate disodium. Am J Med 82 (Suppl 2A):42, 1987.

49. Cohen LF, Balow JE, Magrath IT, et al: Acute tumor lysis syndrome: A review of 37 patients with Burkitt's lymphoma. Am J Med 68:486, 1980.

50. Stapleton FB, Strother DR, Roy S, et al: Acute renal failure at onset of therapy for advanced stage Burkitt lymphoma and B cell acute lymphoblastic lymphoma. Pediatrics 82:863, 1988.

51. DeConti RC and Calabresi P: Use of allopurinol for prevention and control of hyperuricemia in patients with neoplastic disease. N Engl J Med 274:481, 1966.

52. Spector T: Inhibition of urate production by allopurinol. Biochem Pharmacol 26:355, 1977.

53. Ebie N, Ryan W, and Harris J: Metabolic emergencies in cancer medicine. Med Clin North Am 70:1151, 1986.

54. Hainsworth JD, Workman R, and Greco FA: Management of the syndrome of inappropriate antidiuretic hormone secretion in small cell lung cancer. Cancer 50:161, 1983.

55. Anderson RJ, Chung H-M, Kluge R, et al: Hyponatremia: A prospective analysis of its epidemiology and the pathogenetic role of vasopressin. Ann Intern Med 102:164, 1985.

56. Hartman D, Rossier B, Zohlman R, et al: Rapid correction of hyponatremia in the syndrome of inappropriate secretion of antidiuretic hormone: An alternative treatment to hypertonic saline. Ann Intern Med 78:870, 1973.

57. Sterns RH: Severe symptomatic hyponatremia: Treatment and outcome. A study of 64 cases. Ann Intern Med 107:656, 1987.

58. Ayus JC, Krothapalli RK, and Arieff AL: Treatment of symptomatic hyponatremia and its relationship to brain damage: A prospective study. N Engl J Med 317:1190, 1987.

59. Blackman MR, Rosen SW, and Weintraub BD: Ectopic hormones. Adv Intern Med 23:85, 1978.

60. Kahn CR: The riddle of tumour hypoglycaemia revisited. Clin Endocrinol Metab 9:335, 1980.

61. Block JB: Lactic acidosis in malignancy and observations on its possible pathogenesis. Ann NY Acad Sci 230:94, 1974.

62. Mintz U, Sweet DL, Bitran JD, et al: Lactic acidosis and diffuse histiocytic lymphoma (DHL). Am J Hematol 4:359, 1978.

63. Nadiminti Y, Wang JC, Chou S-Y, et al: Lactic acidosis associated with Hodgkin's disease: Response to chemotherapy. N Engl J Med 303:15, 1980.

64. Irvine WJ and Barnes EW: Adrenocortical insufficiency. Clin Endocrinol Metab 1:549, 1972.

65. Margaretten W, Nakai H, and Landing BH: Septicemic adrenal hemorrhage. Am J Dis Child 105:346, 1963.

66. Pollack A: Acute promyelocytic leukemia with disseminated intravascular coagulation. Am J Clin Pathol 56:155, 1971.

67. Collins AJ, Bloomfield CD, Peterson BA, et al: Acute promyelocytic leukemia: Management of the coagulopathy during daunorubicin-prednisone remission induction. Arch Intern Med 138:1677, 1978.

68. Feinstein DI: Diagnosis and management of disseminated intravascular coagulation: The role of heparin therapy. Blood 60:284, 1982.

69. Lichtman MA and Rowe JM: Hyperleukocytic leukemias: Rheological, clinical, and therapeutic considerations. Blood 60:279, 1982.

70. Bunin NJ and Piu CH: Differing complications of hyperleukocytosis in children with acute lymphoblastic or acute nonlymphoblastic leukemia. J Clin Oncol 3:1590, 1985.

71. Tryka AF, Godleski JJ, and Fanta CK: Leukemic cell lysis pneumopathy: A complication of treated myeloblastic leukemia. Cancer 50:2763, 1982.

72. Rowe JM and Lichtman MA: Hyperleukocytosis: Common clinical features of childhood chronic myelogenous leukemia. Blood 63:1230, 1984.

73. Steinhardt GF and Steinhardt E: Priapism in children with leukemia. Urology 18:604, 1981.

74. Lane TA: Continuous flow leukopheresis for rapid cytoreduction in leukemia. Transfusion 20:455, 1980.

75. Gilchrist GS, Fountain KS, Dearth JC, et al: Cranial irradiation in the management of extreme leukemia leukocytosis complicating acute childhood lymphocytic leukemia. J Pediatr 98:257, 1981.

76. Harris AL: Leukostasis associated with blood transfusion in acute myeloid leukemia. Br Med J 2:1169, 1978.

77. Torti FM, Bristow MR, Howes AE, et al: Reduced cardiotoxicity of doxorubicin delivered on a weekly schedule. Ann Intern Med 99:745, 1983.

78. VanHoff DD, Layard MW, Basa P, et al: Risk factors for doxorubicin-induced congestive heart failure. Ann Intern Med 91:710, 1979.

79. Pinkel D, Camitta B, Kun L, et al: Doxorubicin cardiomyopathy in children with left-sided Wilms' tumor. Med Pediatr Oncol 10:483, 1982.

80. VanHoff DD, Rozencweig M, and Piccart M: The cardiotoxicity of anticancer agents. Semin Oncol 9:23, 1982.

81. Lipshultz SE, Colan SD, Gelber RD, et al: Late cardiac effects of doxorubicin therapy for acute lymphoblastic leukemia in childhood. N Engl J Med 324:808, 1991.

82. Goldberg MA, Antin JH, Guinan EC, et al: Cyclophosphamide cardiotoxicity: An analysis of dosing as a risk factor. Blood 68:1114, 1986.

83. Gottdiener JS, Applebaum FR, Ferrans VJ, et al: Cardiotoxicity associated with high-dose cyclophosphamide therapy. Arch Intern Med 141:758, 1981.

84. Stewart JR, Cohn KE, Fajardo LF, et al: Radiation-induced heart disease. Radiology 89:302, 1967.

85. Applefeld MM, Cole JF, Pollock SH, et al: The late appearance of chronic pericardial disease in patients treated by radiotherapy for Hodgkin's disease. Ann Intern Med 94:338, 1981.

86. Brosius FC, Waller BF, and Roberts WC: Radiation heart disease. Am J Med 70:519, 1981.

87. Parker MM, Shelhamer JH, Bacharach SL, et al: Profound but reversible myocardial depression in patients with septic shock. Ann Intern Med 100:483, 1984.

88. Parker MM, McCarthy KE, Ognibene FP, et al: Right ventricular dysfunction and dilatation, similar to left ventricular changes, characterize the cardiac depression of septic shock in humans. Chest 97:126, 1990.

89. Ognibene FP, Rosenberg SA, Lotze M, et al: Interleukin-2 administration causes reversible hemodynamic changes and left ventricular dysfunction similar to those seen in septic shock. Chest 94:750, 1988.

90. Lee RE, Lotze MT, Skibber JM, et al: Cardiorespiratory effects of immunotherapy with interleukin-2. J Clin Oncol 7:7, 1989.

91. Weiss RB and Muggia FM: Cytotoxic drug-induced pulmonary disease: Update 1980. Am J Med 68:259, 1980.

92. Bauer KA, Skarin AT, Balikian JP, et al: Pulmonary complications associated with combination chemotherapy programs containing bleomycin. Am J Med 74:557, 1983.

93. Yousem SA, Lifson JD, and Colby TV: Chemotherapy-induced eosinophilic pneumonia: Relation to bleomycin. Chest 88:103, 1985.

94. Bechard DE, Fairman RP, DeBlois GG, et al: Fatal pulmonary fibrosis from low-dose bleomycin therapy. South Med J 80:646, 1987.

95. Samuels ML, Johnson DE, Holoye PY, et al: Large-dose bleomycin therapy and pulmonary toxicity: A possible role of prior radiotherapy. JAMA 235:1117, 1976.

96. Goldiner PL, Carlon GC, Cvitkovic E, et al: Factors influencing postoperative morbidity and mortality in patients treated with bleomycin. Br Med J 1:1664, 1978.

97. Tryka AF, Skornik WA, Godleski JJ, et al: Potentiation of bleomycin-induced lung injury by exposure to 70% oxygen: Morphologic assessment. Am Rev Respir Dis 126:1074, 1982.

98. Scharstein R, Johnson JK, Cook BA, et al: Bleomycin nodules mimicking metastatic osteogenic sarcoma. Am J Pediatr Hematol Oncol 9:219, 1987.

99. Luna MA, Bedrossian CWM, Nightiger B, et al: Interstitial pneumonitis associated with bleomycin therapy. Am J Clin Pathol 58:501, 1972.

100. White DA and Stover DE: Severe bleomycin-induced pneumonitis: Clinical features and response to corticosteroids. Chest 86:723, 1984.

101. Oliner H, Schwartz R, Rubio F, et al: Interstitial pulmonary fibrosis following busulfan therapy. Am J Med 31:134, 1961.

102. Holoye PY, Jenkins DE, and Greenberg SD: Pulmonary toxicity in long term administration of BCNU. Cancer Treat Rep 60:1691, 1976.
103. Weiss RB, Shah S, and Shane SR: Pulmonary toxicity from carmustine (BCNU). Med Pediatr Oncol 6:255, 1979.
104. Alvarado CS, Boat TF, and Newman AJ: Late-onset pulmonary fibrosis and chest deformity in two children treated with cyclophosphamide. J Pediatr 92:443, 1978.
105. Spector JI, Zimbler H, and Ross JS: Cyclophosphamide and interstitial pneumonitis. JAMA 243:1133, 1980.
106. Haupt HM, Hutchins GM, and Moore GW: Ara-C lung: Non-cardiogenic pulmonary edema complicating cytosine arabinoside therapy of leukemia. Am J Med 70:256, 1981.
107. Kantarjian HM, Estey EH, Plunkett W, et al: Phase I-II clinical and pharmacologic studies of high-dose cytosine arabinoside in refractory leukemia. Am J Med 81:387, 1986.
108. Acute Leukemia Group B: Acute lymphocytic leukemia in children: Maintenance therapy with methotrexate administered intermittently. JAMA 207:923, 1969.
109. Sostman HD, Matthay RA, Putman CE, et al: Methotrexate-induced pneumonitis. Medicine 55:371, 1976.
110. Gutin PH, Green MR, Bleyer WA, et al: Methotrexate pneumonitis induced by intrathecal methotrexate therapy: A case report with pharmacokinetic data. Cancer 38:1529, 1976.
111. Sybert A and Butler TP: Sarcoidosis following adjuvant high-dose methotrexate therapy for osteosarcoma. Arch Intern Med 138:488, 1978.
112. White DA, Rankin JA, Stover DE, et al: Methotrexate pneumonitis: Bronchoalveolar lavage findings suggest an immunologic disorder. Am Rev Respir Dis 139:18, 1989.
113. Libshitz HI and Southard ME: Complications of radiation therapy: The thorax. Semin Roentgenol 9:41, 1974.
114. Gross NJ: Pulmonary effects of radiation therapy. Ann Intern Med 86:81, 1977.
115. Sullivan KM, Deeg HJ, Sanders JE, et al: Late complications after marrow transplantation. Semin Hematol 21:53, 1984.
116. Gross NJ: The pathogenesis of radiation-induced lung damage. Lung 159:115, 1981.
117. Gibson PG, Bryant DH, Morgan GW, et al: Radiation-induced lung injury: A hypersensitivity pneumonitis? Ann Intern Med 109:288, 1988.
118. Pezner RD, Bertrand M, and Cecchi GR: Steroid withdrawal radiation pneumonitis in cancer patients. Chest 85:816, 1984.
119. Popovsky MA, Abel MD, and Moore SB: Transfusion-related lung injury associated with passive transfer of antileukocyte antibodies. Am Rev Respir Dis 128:185, 1983.
120. Levy GJ, Shabot MM, Hart ME, et al: Transfusion-associated noncardiogenic pulmonary edema. Transfusion 26:278, 1986.
121. Schiffer CA: Principles of granulocyte transfusion therapy. Med Clin North Am 61:1119, 1977.
122. Wright DG, Robichaud KJ, Pizzo PA, et al: Lethal pulmonary reactions associated with the combined use of amphotericin B and leukocyte transfusions. N Engl J Med 304:1185, 1981.
123. Smith LJ and Katzenstein ALA: Pathogenesis of massive pulmonary hemorrhage in acute leukemia. Arch Intern Med 142:2149, 1982.
124. Soave R, Murray HW, and Litrenta MM: Bacterial invasion of pulmonary vessels: Pseudomonas bacteremia mimicking pulmonary thromboembolism with infarction. Am J Med 65:864, 1978.
125. Bennington JE: Aspergillus lung disease. Med Clin North Am 64:475, 1980.
126. Ognibene FP, Gill VJ, Pizzo PA, et al: Induced sputum to diagnose Pneumocystis carinii pneumonia in immunosuppressed pediatric patients. J Pediatr 115:430, 1989.
127. Leigh MW, Henshaw NG, and Wood RE: Diagnosis of Pneumocystis carinii pneumonia in pediatric patients using bronchoscopic bronchoalveolar lavage. Pediatr Infect Dis 4:408, 1985.
128. DeBlic J, McKelvie P, LeBourgeois M, et al: Value of bronchoalveolar lavage in the management of severe acute pneumonia and interstitial pneumonitis in the immunocompromised child. Thorax 42:759, 1987.
129. Fitzpatrick SB, Stokes DC, Marsh B, et al: Transbronchial lung biopsy in pediatric and adolescent patients. Am J Dis Child 139:46, 1985.
130. Wolff LJ, Bartlett MS, Baehner RL, et al: The causes of interstitial pneumonitis in immunocompromised children: An aggressive systematic approach. Pediatrics 60:41, 1977.
131. Imoke E, Dudgeon DL, Colombani P, et al: Open lung biopsy in the immunocompromised pediatric patient. J Pediatr Surg 18:816, 1983.
132. Prober CG, Whyte H, and Smith CR: Open lung biopsy in immunocompromised children with pulmonary infiltrates. Am J Dis Child 138:60, 1984.
133. Foglia RP, Shilyansky J, and Fonkalsrud EW: Emergency lung biopsy in immunocompromised pediatric patients. Ann Surg 210:90, 1989.
134. Doolin EJ, Luck SR, Sherman JO, et al: Emergency lung biopsy: Friend or foe of the immunosuppressed child? J Pediatr Surg 21:485, 1986.
135. Lodish JR and Boxer RJ: Urinary tract hemorrhage. In: Rieselbach RE and Garnick MD (eds): Cancer and the Kidney. Philadelphia, Lea & Febiger, 1982, pp. 625–661.
136. Cox PJ: Cyclophosphamide cystitis—identification of acrolein as the causative agent. Biochem Pharmacol 28:2045, 1979.
137. Hows JM, Mehta A, Ward L, et al: Comparison of mesna with forced diuresis to prevent cyclophosphamide induced haemorrhagic cystitis in marrow transplantation: A prospective randomized study. Br J Cancer 50:753, 1984.
138. Schoenike SE and Dana WJ: Ifosfamide and mesna. Clin Pharmacol 9:179, 1990.
139. Blachley JD and Hill JB: Renal and electrolyte disturbances associated with cisplatin. Ann Intern Med 95:628, 1981.
140. Loehrer PJ and Einhorn LH: Cisplatin. Ann Intern Med 100:704, 1984.
141. Pitman SW and Frei E: Weekly methotrexate-calcium leukovorin rescue: Effect of alkalinization on nephrotoxicity; pharmacokinetics in the CNS; and use in CNS non-Hodgkin's lymphoma. Cancer Treat Rep 61:695, 1977.
142. Weber BL, Tanyer G, Poplack DG, et al: Transient acute hepatotoxicity of high-dose methotrexate therapy during childhood. NCI Monogr 5:207, 1987.
143. Land VJ, Sutow WW, Fernbach DJ, et al: Toxicity of L-asparaginase in children with advanced leukemia. Cancer 30:339, 1972.
144. Cairo MS: Adverse reactions to L-asparaginase. Am J Pediatr Hematol Oncol 4:335, 1982.
145. Greenstein R, Nogiere C, Ohnuma T, et al: Management of asparaginase induced hemorrhagic pancreatitis complicated by pseudocyst. Cancer 43:718, 1979.
146. Bodey GP, Buckley M, Sathe YS, et al: Quantitative relationships between circulating leukocytes and infection in patients with acute leukemia. Ann Intern Med 46:328, 1966.
147. Baehner RL, Neiburger RG, Johnson DE, et al: Transient bactericidal defect of peripheral blood phagocytes from children with acute lymphoblastic leukemia receiving craniospinal irradiation. N Engl J Med 289:1209, 1973.
148. McCormack RT, Nelson RD, Bloomfield CD, et al: Neutrophil function in lymphoreticular malignancy. Cancer 44:920, 1979.
149. Bodey GP: Infections in cancer patients. Cancer Treat Rev 2:89, 1975.
150. Pizzo PA: Infectious complications in the child with cancer. I: Pathophysiology of the compromised host at the initial evaluation and management of the febrile cancer patient. J Pediatr 98:341, 1981.
151. Pizzo PA, Robichaud KJ, Wesley R, et al: Fever in the pediatric and adult patient with cancer: A prospective study of 1001 episodes. Medicine 61:153, 1982.
152. Winston DJ, Barnes RC, and Ito WG: Moxalactam plus piperacillin versus moxalactam plus amikacin in febrile granulocytopenic patients. Am J Med 77:442, 1984.
153. Pizzo PA, Hathorn JW, Hiemenz J, et al: A randomized trial comparing ceftazidime alone with combination antibiotic therapy in cancer patients with fever and neutropenia. N Engl J Med 315:552, 1986.
154. Shenep JL, Hughes WT, Roberson PK, et al: Vancomycin, ticarcillin, and amikacin compared with ticarcillin-clavulanate and amikacin in the empirical treatment of febrile, neutropenic children with cancer. N Engl J Med 319:1053, 1988.
155. Pizzo PA, Ladish S, Simon RM, et al: Increasing incidence of gram-positive sepsis in cancer patients. Med Pediatr Oncol 5:241, 1978.
156. Whimbey E, Kiehn TE, Brannon P, et al: Bacteremia and fungemia in patients with neoplastic disease. Am J Med 82:723, 1987.

157. Rubin M, Hathorn JW, Marshall D, et al: Gram-positive infections and the use of vancomycin in episodes of fever and neutropenia. Ann Intern Med 108:30, 1988.

158. Martin MA, Pfaller MA, and Wenzel RP: Coagulase-negative staphylococcal bacteremia: Mortality and hospital stay. Ann Intern Med 110:9, 1989.

159. Hughes WT, Armstrong D, Bodey GP, et al: Guidelines for use of antimicrobial agents in neutropenic patients with unexplained fever. J Infect Dis 161:381, 1990.

160. Koretz MJ and Neifeld JP: Emergency surgical treatment for patients with acute leukemia. Surg Gynecol Obstet 161:149, 1985.

161. Winston DJ, Ho WG, and Gale RP: Therapeutic granulocyte transfusions for documented infections. Ann Intern Med 97:509, 1982.

162. Wright DG: Leukocyte transfusions: Thinking twice. Am J Med 76:637, 1984.

Bone Marrow Transplantation

Karen L. Kaucic, M.D., and Ralph R. Quinones, M.D.

Bone marrow transplantation (BMT) is a therapeutic modality that is being used with increasing frequency in the treatment of hematologic and nonhematologic malignancies, complete or partial bone marrow failure, and disorders of cellular metabolic function. The process itself involves transplantation of the pluripotential bone marrow stem cell into a patient rendered immunoincompetent with high-dose chemotherapy or radiation. The complications of the transplantation process can result directly from the prolonged state of pancytopenia and immunodeficiency induced by marrow and lymphoid ablation, from the transplantation of immunocompetent tissue from an antigenically distinct donor, from the direct toxic effects of ablative therapy on nonhematologic and nonimmunologic tissues, or from the underlying disease itself. Many of the complications, especially those related to prolonged bone marrow aplasia, infections, and graft-versus-host disease (GVHD) can be life-threatening and may require intensive care management. This chapter presents a brief overview of the general principles of BMT that serves as the basis for a discussion of the complications of BMT relevant to the intensive care setting.

OVERVIEW

Role of Bone Marrow Transplantation

The pluripotential bone marrow stem cell is capable of self-renewal and terminal differentiation into mature T and B lymphocytes, red blood cells, platelets, granulocytes, and monocytes.[1] In addition, BMT has demonstrated that osteoclasts and microglial cells are specialized cells derived from the monocyte/macrophage lineage.

The transplantation of hematopoietic stem cells can be employed either as primary therapy for an intrinsic defect of bone marrow stem cell function or as a rescue modality after bone marrow ablative therapy for a primary malignancy (Table 66–1).

Primary Therapy. Intrinsic defects of bone marrow stem cell function include aplastic anemia, the severe

Table 66–1. ROLE OF BONE MARROW TRANSPLANTATION IN THE TREATMENT OF MALIGNANT AND NONMALIGNANT DISEASES IN THE PEDIATRIC POPULATION*

Primary Therapy
Hematopoietic stem cell defects
    Aplastic anemia
    Severe congenital immunodeficiencies
    Thalassemia major
    Osteopetrosis
Inborn errors of metabolism
    Mucopolysaccharidoses
    Metachromatic leukodystrophy

Rescue Therapy
Leukemias
    Acute lymphocytic leukemia
    Acute myelogenous leukemia
    Chronic myelogenous leukemia
Solid tumors
    Lymphoma
    Neuroblastoma
    Sarcomas ??
    Brain tumors ??

*Data from references 2 to 18.

congenital immunodeficiencies, osteopetrosis, and the inherited hemoglobinopathies. BMT as primary therapy for severe aplastic anemia and the severe congenital immunodeficiency syndromes is curative in more than 70% of cases.[2, 3] In the treatment of these disorders, BMT should be employed as early as possible after the diagnosis has been established in order to prevent morbidity and mortality from recurrent infections and blood product dependency and maximize the chance of successful transplantation.

BMT is the only successful therapy for malignant infantile osteopetrosis, a disorder characterized by insufficient bone resorption secondary to defective osteoclast activity. Bone encroachment on the marrow space leads to pancytopenia, and bone deposition at cranial nerve foramina results in blindness, deafness, and other cranial nerve deficits. Allogeneic BMT has resulted in histologic evidence of bone resorption and re-establishment of medullary hematopoiesis associated with clinical improvement in several patients.[4, 5]

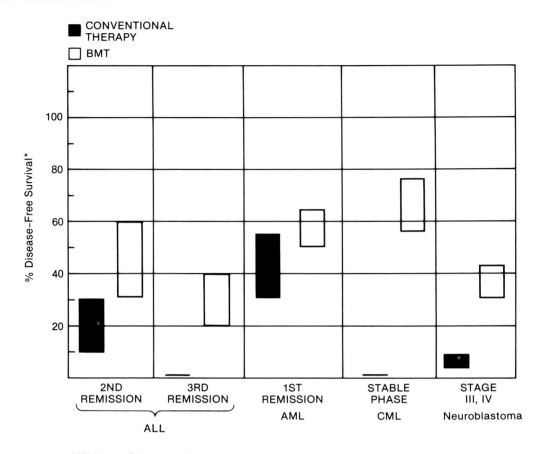

Figure 66-1. Comparison of disease recurrence among patients with ALL, AML, CML, and neuroblastoma: conventional therapy versus bone marrow transplantation. (Data from references 12 to 18.)

With respect to the hemoglobinopathies, BMT is used as primary therapy only in situations in which the natural history of the hemoglobinopathy is associated with greater morbidity than occurs with transplantation. Thalassemia major is characterized by profound anemia and extramedullary hematopoiesis and a life expectancy of approximately 30 years. BMT can replace conventional hypertransfusion therapy that is lifelong and associated with significant morbidity from infection and iron overload.[6] BMT is not employed as primary therapy for the sickle cell disease because of improved overall survival of these patients during the past 20 years with better anticipatory management and supportive care; however, transplantation may be of benefit in the subset of patients who experience severe complications.

BMT has been employed in the treatment of some of the inborn errors of metabolism, such as the mucopolysaccharidoses. Transplantation of bone marrow with hematopoietic stem cells possessing the missing host enzyme provides the entire organism with cells containing an enzyme source. In cases in which BMT has been employed, preliminary reports suggest at least partial reversal of clinical and tissue manifestations.[7]

Rescue Therapy. Historically, the therapy for many pediatric malignancies has been limited by the dose-related hematologic toxicity of a number of chemotherapeutic agents, as well as radiation therapy. BMT has provided a method of treating malignancies with very high doses of combination chemotherapy and radiation followed by restoration of hematopoietic function. This approach has been used with the most success in treating leukemia[8-13] and is being employed with increased frequency in the treatment of solid tumors such as neuroblastoma and lymphoma.[14-16] In general, the decision to utilize BMT in the treatment of any malignancy is based on the overall risks of BMT relative to those of conventional therapy, including comparison of the risks of disease recurrence between the two modalities (Fig. 66-1).[12, 13, 16-18]

The optimal timing of BMT in the treatment of pediatric malignancies cannot be absolutely defined, requiring continual re-evaluation with ongoing advances in both transplantation technology and conventional chemotherapeutic approaches. In addition, the development of recombinant hematopoietic growth factors and their use in combination with high-dose chemotherapy may abrogate the need for rescue of bone marrow function with BMT in some clinical situations.[19]

Types of Bone Marrow Transplantation

BMT can be divided into three major categories based on the source of donor bone marrow (Table 66-2).

Table 66–2. BONE MARROW TRANSPLANTATION CLASSIFIED BY THE SOURCE OF DONOR BONE MARROW

Type	Donor	Characteristics
Autologous	Self	Patient's own bone marrow; may require purging of residual tumor cells
Syngeneic	Identical twin	Identical at major and minor histocompatibility antigenic determinants
Allogeneic	Genotypic match (sibling)	HLA matched, MLC nonreactive; may be incompatible for minor determinants
	Phenotypic match (unrelated)	HLA matched, MLC nonreactive; will be incompatible for untyped major and minor determinants; may require T depletion
	Genotypic mismatch (parent)	Partially HLA matched (> haplotype); requires T cell depletion
	Phenotypic mismatch (registry)	Partially HLA matched; will be incompatible for untyped major and minor determinants; requires T cell depletion

HLA = human leukocyte antigen; MLC = Mixed lymphocyte culture.

Autologous Transplantation. Autologous BMT refers to the reinfusion of a patient's own bone marrow that has been harvested prior to the patient receiving cytoreductive therapy, depleted of red blood cells, and then cryopreserved until needed. Currently, autologous BMT cannot be employed to treat primary bone marrow dysfunction or metabolic deficiencies. It is used to provide rescue of hematopoietic function after treatment of a primary malignancy, especially in situations in which a human leukocyte antigen (HLA)-matched allogeneic bone marrow donor is not available. Autologous bone marrow can be infused in unaltered form if the underlying neoplasm does not involve the bone marrow. Malignancies that originate in or metastasize to bone marrow may necessitate treatment or "purging" of autologous bone marrow to remove microscopic residual malignant disease prior to infusion.[14, 20, 21] The role of bone marrow purging remains to be defined since (1) quantitation of contaminating malignant cells is limited by current methods of detection and (2) minimal allowable levels of microscopic residual tumor have not yet been established.

Syngeneic and Allogeneic Transplantation. Syngeneic bone marrow is obtained from an identical twin sibling, such that there is complete tissue identity between the donor and the recipient. Allogeneic bone marrow is obtained from any related or unrelated bone marrow donor other than an identical twin sibling. Both of these modalities can be employed as therapy for primary bone marrow dysfunction or as bone marrow rescue after marrow ablative therapy for a primary malignancy. Allogeneic (or syngeneic) bone marrow is usually harvested from the donor and infused into the patient on the same day. ABO red blood cell antigen incompatibility between a donor and a recipient is not a contraindication to transplantation, since bone marrow can be mechanically depleted of serum or red blood cells prior to infusion.

Donor Identification

As with other types of tissue transplantation, successful BMT is dependent on tissue histocompatibility between a donor and a recipient for antigens comprising the major histocompatibility complex (MHC), the HLA system.[22–24] MHC antigens are cell surface (classes I and II) and complement-associated (class III) proteins essential to immune recognition and regulation. Class I and II histocompatibility is crucial to tissue engraftment. HLA class I antigens (A, B, C) are expressed on most nucleated cells and platelets. Class II antigens (D, DR, DQ, DP) are expressed on lymphocytes, monocytes, and macrophages.

Serologic determination of HLA antigens (HLA typing) is utilized to identify donors who share common A, B, and DR determinants. Direct typing of the less immunologically polymorphic MHC antigens is not performed, and the minor histocompatibility antigens are not well defined in humans. Class II histocompatibility between donor-recipient pairs is confirmed by the absence of reactivity in mixed lymphocyte culture (MLC). Ideally, the bone marrow donor and recipient should be matched for the HLA A, B, and DR antigens and should be nonreactive in MLC. HLA-matched siblings are referred to as genotypic matches, implying identity of the undetermined MHC antigens.

In situations in which a matched sibling donor cannot be found, a related (parent) or unrelated partially mismatched donor may be utilized. In unrelated or phenotypic HLA-matched pairs (from a bone marrow donor registry), HLA identity is ensured only for the serologically determined A, B, and DR antigens. In the setting of HLA disparity, T lymphocyte depletion of donor bone marrow is necessary to minimize GVHD (see later) and may be warranted in some phenotypic HLA-matched transplantations as well.[23]

Transplantation Process

Identification and Evaluation. After a candidate for BMT has been identified, the process of preparation for transplantation begins with identification of a bone marrow source, followed by an evaluation of the donor for the presence of any underlying disease that might have an impact on the donation process. At the same time, the candidate for BMT is evaluated for any pre-existing medical conditions that might have an impact on the transplantation itself; infections and manifestations of the underlying disease or toxicity from previous therapy are especially significant.

Preparation. Patients are prepared for BMT with high-dose chemotherapy, with or without total body irradiation (TBI) or total lymphoid irradiation (TLI). The choice of preparative therapy depends on several factors including the age of the patient, pre-existing medical conditions, morbidity from previous therapy,

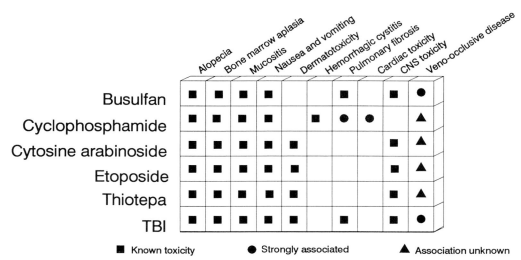

Figure 66–2. Typical components of BMT reparative regimens and their most frequently observed toxicities.

and, most important, the nature of the underlying disease. In general, more intensive doses of radiation and chemotherapy are required for the eradication of malignant disease, whereas less aggressive conditioning is possible in nonmalignant disorders in which ablative therapy is directed at the eradication of defective nonmalignant bone marrow precursors and host immunosuppression. The typical BMT regimen requires 5 to 10 days.

Transplantation. Following the ablative regimen, bone marrow is infused in the same manner as a standard blood transfusion. Peripheral pancytopenia begins 7 to 10 days following preparative therapy. In HLA-matched allogeneic transplantation, evidence of donor engraftment is observed in the peripheral blood with the appearance of leukocytes 10 to 21 days after bone marrow infusion. In general, lymphocytes and monocytes appear first, followed by the appearance of granulocytes. The peripheral absolute neutrophil count increases to 500 cells/m^3 or more by 21 to 30 days after transplantation. The recovery of the peripheral platelet count follows within 7 to 14 days after recovery of the peripheral neutrophil count. Reticulocytes appear at approximately the same time as platelets. Complete peripheral red blood cell recovery generally requires 4 to 6 weeks; however, recovery can be slightly delayed in ABO-incompatible transplants.

In contrast to newly engrafted platelets, erythrocytes, and neutrophils that are functionally near-normal, lymphocyte and monocyte function is significantly depressed in the early transplantation period. Recovery of peripheral T lymphocyte and B lymphocyte numbers may occur as early as 3 months after transplantation. Complete functional reconstitution is usually established within 12 months but can require 2 to 4 years in the setting of HLA disparity or GVHD.[25–27] The time to engraftment and complete immune reconstitution is somewhat shorter in autologous transplantations and somewhat longer in HLA-mismatched allogeneic transplantations. The absence of HLA disparity and GVHD accounts for the former observation. In contrast, HLA incompatibil-

ity and associated GVHD, which is characterized not only by intrinsic immune dysfunction but also by the need for exogenous immune suppression, contribute to delayed engraftment and immune reconstitution in the latter setting.[26]

COMPLICATIONS

The complications observed in BMT are often multifactorial but can be related pathophysiologically to at least one of the following: (1) the profound pancytopenia and alterations in cellular and humoral immunity resulting from the ablation of host hematopoietic and lymphoid tissue, (2) the transplantation of immunocompetent and immunologically distinct tissue, (3) the direct toxic effects of the bone marrow–ablative radiation and chemotherapy on nonhematopoietic tissues, and (4) the pathophysiologic characteristics of the underlying disease and previous therapy.

Preparative Regimen

A comprehensive review of the toxicities associated with radiation and the specific chemotherapeutic agents used to prepare patients for BMT is beyond the scope of this chapter. Figure 66–2 summarizes the most common therapeutic agents used in BMT conditioning regimens and their most frequently observed side effects, as well as those observed with TBI.[28, 29] Bone marrow aplasia, mucositis, and hepatic veno-occlusive disease (VOD) are discussed in detail later. Several specific toxicities warrant further comment.

Cyclophosphamide. This alkylating agent is the most commonly used chemotherapeutic modality used in preparative regimens. It is metabolized to acrolein, which binds to the transitional epithelium of the bladder and ureters and induces vasculitis, ulceration, and hemorrhage. Hemorrhagic cystitis can occur early during the administration of cyclophosphamide or at any time up to several months later. Its incidence is decreased substantially by vigorous hydration and by brisk diuresis at the time of cyclophosphamide infusion, which serves to decrease the transit time of acrolein through the bladder and ureters. In addition, the concomitant use of 2-mercaptoethanesulfonic acid (MESNA), which binds acrolein and prevents its attachment to bladder epithelium, has further decreased the incidence of hemorrhagic cystitis.[29] Cyclophosphamide also induces water retention and increased urinary sodium excretion as early as 4 hours after administration, necessitating meticulous attention to fluid status and sodium balance.[30] Cardiomyopathy and complete heart block have been observed in patients receiving high doses of cyclophosphamide.[31]

Total Body Irradiation. High-dose radiation is associated with the development of diffuse interstitial infiltrates occurring 2 to 3 months following radiation therapy.[32] The incidence of radiation-induced pneumonitis is related to the dose and rate of delivery of radiation. Some chemotherapeutic agents, such as bleomycin, busulfan, BCNU, CCNU, and cyclophosphamide, are themselves associated with the development of diffuse pulmonary disease. Past or concomitant exposure to these agents can potentiate radiation-induced pulmonary disease. Toxicity can be further exacerbated by mechanical ventilation with positive pressures and high oxygen tensions. Diffuse interstitial infiltrates are observed on a plain chest radiograph. A lung biopsy is required to definitively exclude other causes of interstitial pneumonitis (see Pulmonary Complications). In most cases, slow resolution of symptoms and radiographic findings occur over several weeks with corticosteroid therapy and supportive care. A few patients develop progressive pulmonary fibrosis and respiratory failure.

Cytosine Arabinoside. This nucleotide analogue is associated with the dose-related development of acute cerebellar ataxia, which is thought to be related to direct cytotoxic effects on Purkinje cells.[33] The degree of cerebellar dysfunction is variable both in severity and course, with some cases progressing to coma and death.

Dermatotoxicity. Erythema and desquamation are observed in patients receiving high doses of cytosine arabinoside, etoposide, and thiotepa. Care is symptomatic, consisting of meticulous hygiene, topical antibiotics, and surgical debridement in severe cases. Radiation can also induce mild-to-moderate skin erythema.

Hematologic Complications

During the prolonged period of pancytopenia constituting the first 4 to 6 weeks after bone marrow infusion, multiple transfusions of red blood cell and platelet components are required. In general, blood component support is intensive during the early period of pancytopenia and then gradually decreases as endogenous bone marrow production accelerates. Four aspects of transfusion therapy in the BMT setting deserve special emphasis.

Transfusion-Induced Graft-Versus-Host Disease. In profoundly immunocompromised patients, HLA-mismatched GVHD can result from the transfusion of blood components contaminated with immunocompetent donor lymphocytes. GVHD in this setting is severe and almost uniformly fatal. Inactivation of donor lymphocytes by gamma irradiation of cellular blood components prior to transfusion substantially reduces the risk of transfusion-induced GVHD.[34] Controversy exists regarding the need for irradiation of noncellular components such as fresh frozen plasma and cryoprecipitate given their minimal contamination with viable lymphocytes.

Alloimmunization. Leukocyte contamination of blood components provides a significant source of foreign HLA and platelet-specific antigens for multiply transfused patients. BMT patients who are extensively transfused prior to transplantation, or who require prolonged blood component support after transplantation, are at risk to become alloimmunized to HLA and platelet-specific antigens, and thus refractory to platelet transfusions.[35] Refractory patients often require HLA-matched platelet components obtained from individual donors by mechanical apheresis. Prevention of alloimmunization may be accomplished by routine leukocyte depletion of blood components or by the exclusive use of single donor apheresis platelet components.[35, 36]

Transfusion-Induced Cytomegalovirus Disease. Profoundly immunosuppressed patients are at risk for disseminated cytomegalovirus (CMV) infection. It has been shown definitively that the exclusive use of blood components from donors who are seronegative for IgG antibody to CMV significantly decreases the incidence of CMV infection among seronegative recipients of bone marrow from seronegative marrow donors.[37] Blood components from donors who are CMV-seronegative are therefore employed exclusively in transfusion therapy for this group of patients. Whether or not the exclusive use of CMV negative blood components for seropositive patients or seronegative recipients of bone marrow from seropositive marrow donors remains to be elucidated. Theoretically, it seems prudent to provide CMV seronegative blood components to BMT patients regardless of the CMV status of the BMT patient or the bone marrow donor, since (1) the seropositivity of the BMT donor does not necessarily reflect active infection, and (2) blood component transfusion may introduce new viral strains or induce reactivation of latent virus present in the recipient. Depending on the serologic status of the local blood donor population, however, the provision of CMV-negative blood components to all BMT patients may not be possible. Leukocyte depletion of blood components may decrease the risk of infection associated with the use of CMV-positive components (since the virus is latent in leukocytes); however, definitive benefit has not been shown.[38]

ABO Incompatibility. In major ABO incompatible BMTs, the graft recipient possesses antibodies against the marrow donor's ABO antigens. In minor ABO incompatible BMTs, the marrow donor produces antibodies against endogenous host ABO antigens. Although ABO incompatibility between bone marrow donor and recipient is not a barrier to allogeneic transplantation, modification of ABO transfusion guidelines is necessary during the period of transition between host and donor hematopoiesis in order to minimize hemolysis of donor red blood cells once engraftment has occurred. Blood components must be compatible with both the donor and the recipient until stable production of donor red blood cells has been documented (Table 66–3).[39]

Complications Involving Infection

Increased susceptibility to infection with bacteria, fungi, viruses, and protozoa poses the single greatest risk to BMT patients and accounts for most of the morbidity and mortality observed in transplantation (Fig. 66–3).[40–42] Although the risk of complications resulting from infection is greatest during the first 6 months following transplantation, patients are predisposed to infection until immune reconstitution is complete.

Every effort must be made to survey the BMT patient for risks of infection and bacterial and viral colonization before transplantation. During the transplantation process, infections can be minimized by appropriate antimicrobial prophylaxis (Table 66–4)[41, 43] and by maintenance of strict environmental infection control, including reverse isolation with high-efficiency air filtration of patient rooms and meticulous handwashing by caregivers and visitors. Other measures have theoretical benefit and are often used in an attempt to minimize infection. These measures include positive-pressure ventilation of patient rooms, strict screening of visitors, sterile drinking water, sterile water for bathing denuded mucosal surfaces, low-bacteria diet, and surveillance cultures of water and air to identify environmental pathogens (see also Chapters 71 and 72).

Bacteria. Susceptibility to bacterial infection is greatest during the period of granulocytopenia lasting for 2 to 4 weeks after transplantation. Profound neutropenia is the single most important risk factor. Host integrity is also compromised by the presence of indwelling central venous catheters and denuded oral and gastrointestinal epithelium secondary to mucositis. The risk of invasive bacterial disease decreases substantially once the peripheral neutrophil count is sustained above 500 cells/m³. Currently, with the early use of empiric anti-

Table 66–3. TRANSFUSION GUIDELINES IN ABO INCOMPATIBLE BONE MARROW TRANSPLANTATION

	Donor	Recipient	RBC and WBC	Platelets Plasma
Major ABO incompatibility	A	B	O	AB
	A	O	O	A,AB
	B	A	O	AB
	B	O	O	B,AB
	AB	A	A	AB
	AB	B	B	AB
	AB	O	O	AB
Minor ABO incompatibility	O	A	O	A,AB
	O	B	O	B,AB
	O	AB	O	AB
	A	AB	A	AB
	B	AB	B	AB

RBC = red blood cell; WBC = white blood cell.

Table 66–4. ANTIMICROBIAL PROPHYLAXIS AND ITS INDICATIONS IN BONE MARROW TRANSPLANTATION*

Prophylaxis	Target Organism	Patient Group
Trimethoprim/ sulfamethoxazole, pentamidine	*Pneumocystis carinii*	All patients
Acyclovir	HSV, VZV, CMV	All allogeneic; autologous if HSV, VZV, or CMV history or seropositivity
Intravenous immunoglobulin	CMV	All allogeneic; autologous if CMV culture or seropositive
Oral antifungal agent	*Candida* sp.	All patients
Penicillin	Encapsulated bacteria	Patients with chronic GVHD

*Data from references 40 to 43.
CMV = cytomegalovirus; GVHD = graft-versus-host disease; HSV = herpes simplex virus; VZV = varicella zoster virus.

biotic therapy in the febrile patient, approximately 15% of patients develop documented bacterial infections.[40] Prior to the widespread employment of this practice, bacterial disease occurred in 30% of patients. Sepsis and focal bacterial infections are most often due to gram-negative enteric organisms and *Pseudomonas* sp. during this early period; however, *Staphylococcus* sp. and anaerobic bacteria are also important pathogens. Focal infections are most often manifested as cellulitis, especially in the early post-transplantation period when production of neutrophils is inadequate for abscess formation. Invasive infection of the gut wall can be an insidious and fatal complication during this period of neutropenia.

An aggressive response to fever and other clinical signs of infection is crucial to the successful management of bacterial disease in these patients. A thorough physical examination and radiographic examination of all potential sites of infection, including the chest and sinuses, are essential. Bacterial cultures of blood, urine, and cerebrospinal fluid (if clinically indicated) should be obtained prior to the institution of antibiotic therapy. Abdominal ultrasound can be useful for the detection of edematous bowel wall suggestive of invasive infection. Empiric broad-spectrum antibiotic coverage must be instituted promptly. Antibiotic regimens should include adequate coverage for both gram-positive and gram-negative bacteria. In addition, consideration must be given to the antibiotic sensitivity patterns of pathogens known to colonize the patient, as well as those of nosocomial bacteria. Removal of indwelling devices is required in patients who remain persistently bacteremic despite appropriate antibiotic coverage. Focal abscesses require surgical drainage. White blood cell transfusions in neutropenic patients are limited to documented infections with gram-negative organisms. Their use remains controversial in light of the short-term viability of stored white blood cells (< 24 hours) and the association of white blood cell transfusion with severe respiratory compromise secondary to pulmonary leukoagglutination.[44]

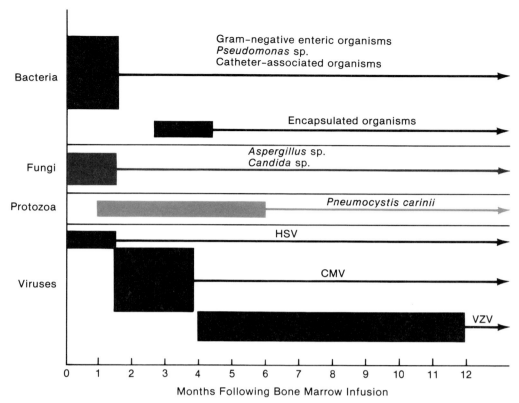

Figure 66–3. Chronology of infectious susceptibilities during BMT. (Adapted from Tutschka PJ: Infections and immunodeficiency in bone marrow transplantation. Pediatr Infect Dis J 7:522, 1988, and from Furman WL and Feldman S: Infectious complications. *In:* Johnson FL and Pochedly C [eds]: Bone Marrow Transplantation in Children. New York, Raven Press, 1990, pp. 427–450.)

Patients with chronic GVHD have prolonged immune dysfunction including defective humoral immunity and decreased or absent splenic function, resulting in infection with encapsulated bacteria in approximately 20% of patients, necessitating prolonged oral antibiotic prophylaxis with penicillin or erythromycin.[41]

Fungi. Like bacterial disease, fungal infections in the post-BMT period are most common during the initial period of granulocytopenia. Prolonged therapy with broad-spectrum antibiotics also contributes to increased susceptibility to invasive fungal disease by altering the host's endogenous composition of bacterial flora. Topical antifungal agents are used routinely to prevent or treat oral and gastrointestinal colonization with fungi. Early empiric use of antifungal therapy is employed in the neutropenic patient who remains persistently febrile despite broad-spectrum antibiotic therapy. The risk of fungal disease decreases dramatically with recovery of the peripheral neutrophil count but persists until T lymphocyte function has fully recovered.

Aspergillus sp. and *Candida* sp. are most commonly encountered. Infections with other fungi occur much less frequently. Fungemia; pneumonia; sinusitis; retinitis; and brain, renal, and hepatic abscesses have been described. *Candida* sp. frequently cause skin and mucous membrane infections (e.g., esophagitis) and catheter-related fungemia. Sinopulmonary and central nervous system infections occur more commonly as a result of invasive *Aspergillus* infection.

Extensive evaluation for potential sources of infec-

tion, including cardiac, renal, and hepatic ultrasonography; fundoscopy; and plain radiographs of chest and sinuses, is warranted in fungemic patients and in patients who remain persistently febrile despite broad-spectrum antibiotic coverage. Therapy consists of intravenous antifungal agents, such as amphotericin B. Aggressive surgical debridement of sites of focal infection is essential. Removal of colonized indwelling intravenous devices is often necessary. Despite appropriate management, recurrence of infection may follow the cessation of antifungal therapy as a consequence of inadequate cellular immunity.

Viruses. The decreased numbers and altered cellular function of T lymphocytes following BMT account for the increased susceptibility to viral infection observed among recipients of bone marrow grafts. Infection is most commonly due to herpesviruses (CMV, herpes simplex virus [HSV] types 1 and 2, varicella zoster virus [VZV], and Epstein-Barr virus [EBV]), adenoviruses, enteroviruses, paramyxoviruses (parainfluenzae), and influenzaviruses (influenza, respiratory syncytial virus [RSV]).[45]

HSV infection is encountered most often in the first 4 to 6 weeks after transplantation. Manifestations are usually mucocutaneous, but pneumonia, hepatitis, and meningoencephalitis can also occur. Morbidity and mortality from localized as well as disseminated HSV infection has been decreased substantially with the widespread use of intravenous acyclovir. The prophylactic use of acyclovir has also been shown to be effective in decreasing the incidence of HSV disease among seropositive patients.[46]

CMV infection occurs most commonly from 6 weeks to 4 months following transplantation and affects up to 50% of allogeneic BMTs. Its incidence is approximately 30% in patients with acute GVHD. Interstitial pneumonitis is the most common manifestation (see later). Other manifestations of CMV disease, such as chorioretinitis, hepatitis, gastroenteritis, bone marrow suppression, and a mononucleosis-like syndrome have also been observed. Seropositivity for IgG antibody to CMV and urinary shedding of virus should be documented before transplantation, because patients with evidence of current or previous CMV infection are more likely to develop serious CMV disease during the post-BMT period.[41] Acyclovir, the acyclovir analogue ganciclovir, intravenous immunoglobulin, trifluorothymidine, and foscarnet have been useful in the treatment of CMV disease in some patients; however, mortality remains high.[37, 41, 47–49] A decreased incidence of disseminated CMV disease has been observed in recipients of allogeneic BMTs treated prophylactically with intravenous immunoglobulin, in seropositive patients treated with acyclovir, and in seronegative patients transfused exclusively with blood components from seronegative blood donors.[49]

The cutaneous manifestations of VZV infection may be atypical in the BMT patient due to altered cell-mediated immunity. Pneumonitis, hepatitis, and widely disseminated disease have been reported. Most cases result from reactivation of latent virus rather than from primary infection. Rapid detection techniques utilizing fluorescent antibody technology can be useful in establishing an early diagnosis. Acyclovir has been shown to be effective in the treatment of and prophylaxis against VZV infection.[46] Empiric use of acyclovir is warranted in suspicious clinical situations. VZV immunoglobulin is administered within 96 hours of documented exposures.

EBV has been associated with both hepatitis and lymphoproliferative disorders in the post-transplantation period. The latter has been observed most commonly in the setting of HLA mismatch.[50] Successful therapy of EBV-related lymphoproliferative disorders with α-interferon has been reported.[51]

Pneumonitis associated with RSV and the parainfluenza and influenza viruses has also been observed.[45] Ribavirin has been shown to be efficacious in some cases of RSV, influenza, and parainfluenza–associated infections.[52] Pneumonitis, hepatitis, hemorrhagic gastroenteritis, and hemorrhagic cystitis have been reported in association with adenovirus.[53] Gastroenteritis has also been described in association with rotavirus and coxsackie virus.[54] No effective therapies currently exist.

Protozoa. Protozoal infections also occur in BMT patients as a result of deficient T lymphocyte function. Historically, *Pneumocystis carinii* was commonly observed as a cause of interstitial pneumonia in the period between 6 weeks and 4 months following transplantation (see later). The incidence of infection with this organism has decreased substantially with the widespread use of routine prophylaxis. Both trimethoprim-sulfamethoxazole and pentamidine are effective antiprotozoal agents for prophylaxis and therapy; however, mortality remains high.[55]

Toxoplasma gondii infections occur in fewer than 1% of BMT patients. Central nervous system disease and disseminated infection have been reported.[56]

Graft-Versus-Host Disease

Recipients of allogeneic BMTs are at risk to develop GVHD secondary to the reaction of immunocompetent donor T lymphocytes against the tissues of an immunocompromised host. Because host T lymphocyte function is deficient or absent, infused donor T lymphocytes are not destroyed, but rather proliferate in response to the antigenically distinct host. Tissue incompatibility between major (HLA) and minor (undefined) histocompatibility antigens may incite the donor T cell response, the former occurring in HLA-mismatched grafts and the latter occurring in HLA-matched grafts. HLA matching of donor-recipient pairs and the routine use of irradiated blood components decrease the incidence of GVHD secondary to major histo*in*compatibility; however, it is well established that without immunosuppressive chemoprophylaxis, the incidence of GVHD in genotypic HLA-matched BMTs alone is more than 90%.[57] Immunosuppressive regimens for GVHD prophylaxis include corticosteroids, methotrexate, cyclosporine A, or antithymocyte globulin used alone or in combination. T lymphocyte depletion of donor bone marrow prior to infusion is employed in HLA-mismatched transplantation.[58]

Even with the extensive prophylactic measures just outlined, GVHD occurs in more than 50% of HLA-matched allogeneic BMTs. The organs most frequently affected are the skin, liver, and gastrointestinal tract. Two distinct forms of GVHD exist, and these forms differ in their time of onset, clinical presentation, and pathologic findings.[42, 58–61]

Acute Graft-Versus-Host Disease. This form of GVHD occurs in 30 to 70% of HLA-matched BMTs. Onset is observed after bone marrow engraftment has occurred, but within the first 100 days after transplantation. One or more organ systems may be involved. Biopsy specimens from skin, liver, and gastrointestinal mucosa demonstrate lymphocytic infiltration and acute tissue damage with single cell necrosis.

Cutaneous manifestations include a diffuse, erythematous, maculopapular rash that typically involves the palms and soles. The rash is often initially evanescent and once established may remain limited or progress to involve variable areas of skin surface. Bullae formation and exfoliation can occur in severe cases.

Hepatic involvement is characterized initially by elevation of hepatic enzymes (aspartate aminotransferase, alanine aminotransferase, gamma glutamyltransferase, lactate dehydrogenase, and alkaline phosphatase), followed by clinical and laboratory evidence of cholestasis (jaundice and hyperbilirubinemia), hepatomegaly, and in severe cases decrease in hepatic protein synthesis as evidenced by hypoalbuminemia, and prolonged prothrombin and partial thromboplastin times. Clinical findings are sometimes indistinguishable from those associated with hepatitis and hepatic VOD; therefore, a liver biopsy is required to make a definitive diagnosis, especially in the absence of cutaneous manifestations. Hepatic dysfunction can progress to fulminant hepatic failure despite aggressive supportive care and immunosuppressive therapy.[62, 63]

Gastrointestinal acute GVHD typically affects the large and small bowel but has also been described in the esophagus and stomach. The most typical clinical symptoms are abdominal pain and secretory diarrhea, which is frequently bloody. Severe diarrhea can result in excessive loss of fluid, electrolytes, and protein. Fluid, electrolyte, and nutritional management are often required. Stool cultures are necessary to exclude bacterial, viral, and protozoal pathogens. A rectal biopsy is required for a definitive diagnosis.[62, 63]

Although patients with acute GVHD are predisposed to the development of diffuse interstitial pneumonitis and secondary pulmonary infections, the extent to which the bronchial mucosa is a primary target of acute GVHD is controversial. Lymphocytic infiltration of bronchial mucosa with destruction of mucosal and submucosal structures, called lymphocytic bronchitis, has been reported in association with acute GVHD.[32] Correlation between this entity and acute GVHD has not, however, been consistently documented clinically and has not been reproduced in animal models.

Clinical and pathologic grading systems have been devised to provide consistent assessment of the severity of acute GVHD for each of the three most often affected organ systems. Based on the degree of involvement of the skin, liver, and gastrointestinal tract in a particular patient, a clinical grade can be assigned, which is useful both in planning therapy and assessing clinical outcome (Table 66–5). Corticosteroids are the mainstay of acute GVHD therapy.[64] Topical steroids alone are often sufficient in the treatment of mild cutaneous acute GVHD. Systemic corticosteroid therapy is required for more extensive skin involvement or for mild to moderate involvement of multiple organ systems. Severe multisystem involvement often requires the addition of anti–T lymphocyte therapy with antithymocyte globulin, monoclonal antibodies, or monoclonal antibody-toxin conju-

Table 66–6. GRADING AND TREATMENT OF ACUTE GRAFT-VERSUS-HOST DISEASE

Grade	Type	Organ Involvement	Treatment
I	Mild GVHD	Skin stage 1–2	Topical steroids
II	Moderate GVHD	Skin stage 1–3 or liver stage 1–2 or GI stage 1–2	Systemic steroids; topical steroids if skin involved
III	Moderately severe GVHD	Skin stage 2–3 or liver stage 2–4 or GI stage 2–4	Systemic immunosuppression: high-dose steroids with or without anti-T cell therapy
IV	Severe GVHD	Same as grade III with extreme constitutional symptoms	As for grade III; may require ICU-level supportive care

GI = gastrointestinal; GVHD = graft-versus-host disease; ICU = intensive care unit.

gates (Table 66–6). Therapy is maintained until clinical symptoms resolve. Immunosuppressive therapy must be tapered slowly. Recurrence of clinical symptoms during the weaning process is not infrequent, often necessitating reinstitution of therapy at previous levels.

Chronic Graft-Versus-Host Disease. Chronic GVHD occurs between 100 days and 2 years following BMT. Patients with acute GVHD are at increased risk to develop chronic GVHD (either directly following acute GVHD or after a period of recovery), although chronic GVHD may occur de novo. Like acute GVHD, chronic GVHD may have limited clinical manifestations; however, the clinical findings associated with chronic GVHD are often more systemic, similar in nature to those observed in autoimmune disorders like scleroderma. In contrast to acute GVHD, the immune dysregulation associated with chronic GVHD, primarily T-helper cell dysfunction, affects mechanisms of humoral as well as cell-mediated immunity, as demonstrated by the development of a variety of autoantibodies. Histopathologically, chronic GVHD is characterized by a more marked inflammatory response and by more extensive destruction of both epithelial and mesenchymal tissue compared with acute GVHD. Fibrosis and loss of normal histologic architecture are also characteristic.

Cutaneous manifestations include lichen planus-like lesions, dyspigmentation, progressive dermal atrophy including loss of skin appendages, and poikiloderma. Contractures secondary to sclerodermatous changes are observed in severe cases.

Hepatic manifestations resemble those observed in other forms of chronic liver disease, with cholestatic jaundice, and decreased hepatic protein synthesis resulting in hypoalbuminemia and deficiencies in production of the coagulation factors.

Gastrointestinal chronic GVHD primarily affects the esophagus and small intestine. Esophageal manifestations include strictures, dysmotility, and reflux; vomiting and dysphagia are common complaints. Chronic diarrhea and steatorrhea result from small bowel involvement. Failure to thrive is not uncommonly observed as a result of inadequate oral intake and malabsorption.

Table 66–5. CLINICAL SKIN STAGING OF ACUTE GRAFT-VERSUS-HOST DISEASE

Stage	Skin	Liver	Intestinal Tract
1	Maculopapular rash less than 25% BSA*	Bilirubin, 2–3 mg/dl	Stool, 300–600 ml/m²/day
2	Maculopapular rash, 25–50% BSA	Bilirubin, 3–6 mg/dl	Stool, 600–1,000 ml/m²/day
3	Generalized erythroderma	Bilirubin, 6–15 mg/dl	Stool > 1,000 ml/m²/day
4	Generalized erythroderma/ bullae/ desquamation	Bilirubin > 15 mg/dl	Stool > 1,000 ml/m²/day; abdominal pain; ileus

*Body surface area, estimated from burn charts.

Chronic GVHD of the lungs primarily affects the lower airways. Bronchiolitis obliterans refers to the chronic obstructive pulmonary disease affecting patients with chronic GVHD, which is characterized by progressive dyspnea and nonproductive cough.[32] Plain chest radiograph may demonstrate mild hyperinflation but is otherwise unremarkable; however, pulmonary function testing reveals evidence of both restrictive and obstructive lung disease.

Sicca syndrome, oral involvement (with lichen planus-like lesions), polymyositis, polyserositis, electrocardiographic abnormalities, and renal involvement with associated histopathologic changes have also been described.

The management of chronic GVHD, not unlike that of autoimmune disease, involves primarily immunosuppressive therapy. High-dose corticosteroids in combination with anti-T lymphocyte therapy (antithymocyte globulin, monoclonal antibody, monoclonal antibody toxin conjugates) are used for initial induction therapy. Maintenance therapy consisting of corticosteroids with or without cyclosporine A, or azathioprine may be necessary for up to 3 years. Thalidomide may have some utility in the treatment of refractory disease.[65]

The profound immunodeficiency and immune dysregulation associated with GVHD predispose patients to infection with encapsulated bacteria and other opportunistic organisms for protracted periods. Antibiotic prophylaxis with oral penicillin or erythromycin and antiviral and antiprotozoal prophylaxis are warranted in these patients until adequate reconstitution of cell-mediated immunity has been established. Maintenance of meticulous mouth care, including oral antifungal therapy, is essential.

Graft Rejection

The persistence of host-alloreactive T lymphocytes following cytoreductive radiation and chemotherapy and their activation in response to donor bone marrow stem cells may result in marrow graft rejection by the BMT recipient. The incidence of rejection is highest in patients with aplastic anemia who have been extensively transfused prior to transplantation and in recipients of T lymphocyte–depleted bone marrow grafts.[24, 66-68] Sensitization to multiple HLA antigens and less intensive preparative regimens predisposes patients in the former setting to rejection. With T lymphocyte depletion of donor marrow, the elimination of residual host cell–mediated immunity by immunocompetent donor T lymphocytes is absent or decreased significantly compared with non-T lymphocyte–depleted grafts. It is thought that alloreactive donor T lymphocytes are effective in ablating residual host hematopoietic function following cytoreductive therapy. Early recognition of poor marrow engraftment or rejection, limited use of bone marrow–suppressive therapies, and early institution of immunosuppressive therapy such as corticosteroids, antithymocyte globulin, and cyclosporine A are the mainstays of therapy; however, success has been limited. Prophylactic immunosuppression has increased the rate of marrow engraftment in high-risk patients.

Pulmonary Complications

Interstitial pneumonitis is the most frequently observed pulmonary complication of BMT and is the causative factor in up to 40% of BMT-related deaths.[32] Peak incidence occurs between 6 weeks and 4 months after transplantation. Infection, GVHD, and toxicity from radiation or chemotherapy are the most common causes; however, in approximately 30% of cases no cause can be identified (Table 66–7). Both acute and chronic GVHD are associated with an increased risk of diffuse interstitial infiltrates and secondary pulmonary infections.

Viruses, bacteria, fungi, and protozoa have all been identified as causes of interstitial infiltrates. The most significant infectious agent is CMV, which accounts for approximately 50% of all cases of interstitial pneumonitis among recipients of allogeneic transplants. VZV and HSV are causative in up to 10% of cases.

The diffuse interstitial changes observed with radiation and chemotherapy-induced lung disease can result from inflammation or fibrosis. Specific offending agents are discussed in greater detail in Complications of the Preparative Regimen.

Interstitial pneumonitis can be rapidly progressive and is associated with a mortality rate of 50%. Rapid diagnosis and the institution of appropriate therapy are crucial. It is especially important in this setting to exclude infectious causes before instituting corticosteroid or other immunosuppressive therapy. Bronchoscopy, bronchoalveolar lavage, and transbronchial biopsy should be performed whenever feasible.[69, 70] It is essen-

Table 66–7. INTERSTITIAL PNEUMONITIS: DIFFERENTIAL DIAGNOSIS IN THE BONE MARROW TRANSPLANT PATIENT*

Infectious Agents
Viruses
    CMV, HSV, VZV
    RSV, parainfluenza
    Influenza
Protozoa
    Pneumocystis carinii
Bacteria
Fungi

Toxic Effects
Radiation
Chemotherapeutic agents
    Bleomycin
    Busulfan
    BCNU, CCNU
    Cyclophosphamide

Immunologic Effects
Associated with both acute
    GVHD and chronic GVHD

Idiopathic

*Data from references 32 to 42.
CMV = cytomegalovirus; HSV = herpes simplex virus; VZV = varicella zoster virus.

tial that material is obtained for bacterial, viral, and fungal cultures as well as for pathologic examination. Rapid fluorescent antibody examination for viral pathogens (VZV, CMV, HSV) may also be helpful. Although considerable morbidity is associated with open lung biopsy, it remains the definitive diagnostic modality in the setting of progressive respiratory deterioration despite maximal antimicrobial therapy, especially in patients who are too small to undergo bronchoscopy.

Gastrointestinal and Hepatic Complications

Mucositis. High-dose chemotherapy, used alone or in combination with TBI or TLI, effects ablation of malignant cells as well as cells of the hematopoietic and immune systems by interfering with some aspect of cell replication. They are effective modalities in part because of rapid cell turnover in these tissues. The toxic effects of these modalities can also be manifested in other tissues with similarly rapid rates of cell turnover, such as the oral and gastrointestinal mucosae. Preparative regimens containing thiotepa, melphalan, etoposide, and TBI are notable for the induction of especially severe mucosal breakdown. Onset of mucosal breakdown occurs 7 to 10 days after beginning cytoreductive therapy and can last for 2 to 4 weeks, coincident with recovery of the peripheral granulocyte count. Decreased mucosal integrity significantly increases the risk of bacterial and fungal infections in these patients by providing a portal of entry for microorganisms. Morbidity is decreased with meticulous mouth care aimed at minimizing bacterial and fungal colonization.[71] All successful mouth care regimens include the use of topical antibacterial and antifungal agents and, most important, mechanical debridement of devitalized tissue. Pain associated with oral mucositis may be severe and is exacerbated with mouth care. The liberal use of analgesia is essential for patient comfort and adequate debridement. Mouth care is more difficult and time-consuming in the intubated patient; however, morbidity is increased by the presence of a foreign body in close proximity to open oral mucosa, and strict adherence to repetitively performed mouth care is even more crucial.

Mucosal breakdown of the esophagus, stomach, and intestines can manifest as nausea, vomiting, diarrhea, hematochezia, melena, and abdominal or chest pain, depending on the location and extent of mucosal injury. Therapy consists of topical treatment with antacids or sucralfate. H_2-antagonists can be useful in decreasing mucosal irritation secondary to endogenous acid production. Oral intake should be tailored to patient tolerance. Suspension of oral intake and institution of hyperalimentation is usually necessary.

Veno-occlusive Disease (VOD). Hepatic VOD occurs in 15 to 20% of BMT patients. It is characterized histologically by hepatic centrolobular necrosis and by occlusion of hepatic venules by connective tissue.[72] It appears to be associated with extensive exposure to radiation and chemotherapy and has been observed outside the BMT setting in patients exposed to extensive antineoplastic therapy.

In general, VOD appears 1 to 4 weeks after transplantation. The onset is marked by sudden weight gain, right upper quadrant abdominal pain, hepatomegaly, jaundice, and ascites. Respiratory compromise may occur as a result of massive ascites or the accumulation of transudated pleural fluid or pulmonary edema. Hyperbilirubinemia, elevated hepatic transaminases, and prolonged prothrombin and partial thromboplastin times are observed in proportion to the extent of hepatic dysfunction.

Clinical and laboratory observations can be indistinguishable from infectious, drug-induced, or hyperalimentation-induced hepatitis, or hepatic GVHD. A liver biopsy is therefore required to make a definitive diagnosis. Decreased or reversed flow in the hepatic portal vein on an ultrasound examination and deficiency of natural anticoagulants (protein C, protein S, antithrombin III) have been reported in association with VOD; however, a clinical correlation has not been well established.[73, 74]

Management consists of fluid restriction, controlled diuresis, and supportive care. Thoracentesis or paracentesis may be required for symptomatic relief. Progressive hepatic dysfunction may lead to massive fluid overload and hepatorenal syndrome, requiring dialysis or ventilatory support. Irreversible hepatic failure, coma, and death occur in 7 to 50% of patients.

Bowel Wall Inflammation. Abdominal pain and distention, vomiting, diarrhea, and hematochezia are common symptoms of acute or chronic bowel inflammation. In the first 4 to 6 weeks after bone marrow ablation, these findings may be indicative of invasive bacterial or, less commonly, fungal infection. Rapid progression with bowel perforation and sepsis is not uncommonly observed. Gastroenteritis later in the post-transplantation period is more often the result of GVHD or viral infection.[62, 63] Pneumatosis intestinalis has been described in BMT patients in association with bowel inflammation, including both intestinal GVHD and infectious enteritis.[75]

Cardiovascular Complications

Cardiovascular collapse secondary to bacterial sepsis is the most common complication observed in pediatric BMT patients. Cardiovascular collapse secondary to sepsis is discussed in detail elsewhere in this text. Chemotherapy-related cardiac toxicity is associated with cyclophosphamide (as mentioned earlier). Adriamycin- and daunomycin-induced cardiomyopathies are observed in the pediatric age group with even greater frequency than that seen with cyclophosphamide. Although these agents are not widely used in BMT preparative regimens, they are commonly used in the treatment of many pediatric malignancies and are frequently part of the patient's pretransplantation therapy.

Renal Complications

Injury to the kidney secondary to sepsis and ischemia is discussed elsewhere in this text (see Chapters 12, 13, and 53). The chemotherapeutic agents used routinely in BMT are not associated with direct renal toxicity. Prolonged therapy with nephrotoxic antibiotics, cyclosporine A, methotrexate, and antifungal agents are major and often synergistic causes of the renal dysfunction and electrolyte wasting observed in transplantation.

Recurrence of Disease

Both malignant and nonmalignant diseases may recur after BMT. In the treatment of aplastic anemia, early post-transplantation bone marrow engraftment followed by subsequent loss of donor bone marrow function (occurring weeks to months after transplantation) and return to the pretransplantation state of dysfunctional host hematopoiesis has been described.[76] Inadequate pretransplantation conditioning and defects in the host bone marrow microenvironment have been postulated as potential causes.

The risk of malignant recurrence after BMT increases in proportion to the number of relapses occurring prior to transplantation. Recurrences of acute lymphocytic leukemia, acute monocytic leukemia, lymphoma, and neuroblastoma occur following both autologous and allogeneic BMT (see Fig. 66–3).[12, 13, 16] Relapse of malignant disease following transplantation results from incomplete in vivo ablation of microscopic residual malignant disease (allogeneic and autologous BMT) in the host. Intrinsic or acquired cellular resistance to antineoplastic agents, as well as dose limitation, account, at least in part, for inadequate ablation of malignant cells. It is now also well established that, at least with respect to the leukemias, in vivo ablation of microscopic malignant disease is also immunologically mediated.[77] Evidence for the destruction of malignant cells by immunocompetent donor lymphocytes, the so-called "graft versus leukemia" (GVL) effect has been demonstrated clinically in the decreased rate of leukemic relapse observed among patients who develop GVHD. Incomplete in vitro purging of microscopic residual neoplastic cells from autologous bone marrow prior to reinfusion may also increase the risk of relapse. Determination of the acceptable absolute minimal level of residual bone marrow disease and limitations in the detection of microscopic tumor remain major obstacles to better definition of the role of purging in autologous BMT.

References

1. Messner HA, Curtis JE, Minden MD, et al: Clonogenic hematopoietic precursors in bone marrow transplantation. Blood 70:1425, 1987.
2. McGlave PB, Haake R, Miller W, et al: Therapy of severe aplastic anemia in young adults and children with allogeneic bone marrow transplantation Blood 70:1325, 1987.
3. Vossen JM: Bone marrow transplantation in the treatment of primary immunodeficiencies. Ann Clin Res 19:285, 1987.
4. Sieff CA, Levinsky RJ, Rogers DW, et al: Allogeneic bone marrow transplantation in infantile malignant osteopetrosis. Lancet i:437, 1983.
5. Coccia PF, Krivit W, Cervenka J, et al: Successful bone marrow transplantation for infantile malignant osteopetrosis. N Engl J Med 302:701, 1980.
6. Lucarelli G, Galimberti M, Polchi P, et al: Bone marrow transplantation in patients with thalassemia. N Engl J Med 322:417, 1990.
7. Krivit W, Whitley CB, Chang PN, et al: Lysosomal storage diseases treated by bone marrow transplantation: Review of 21 patients. In: Johnson FL and Pochedly C (eds): Bone Marrow Transplantation in Children. New York, Raven Press, 1990, pp. 261–287.
8. Brochstein JA, Kernan NA, Groshen S, et al: Allogeneic bone marrow transplantation after hyperfractionated total-body irradiation and cyclophosphamide in children with acute leukemia. N Engl J Med 317:1618, 1987.
9. Coccia PF, Strandjord SE, Warkentin PI, et al: High-dose cytosine arabinoside and fractionated total-body irradiation: An improved preparative regimen for bone marrow transplantation of children with acute lymphoblastic leukemia in remission. Blood 71:888, 1988.
10. Tutschka PJ, Copelan EA, and Klein JP: Bone marrow transplantation for leukemia following a new busulfan and cyclophosphamide regimen. Blood 70:1382, 1987.
11. Champlin RE, Goldman JM, and Gale RP: Bone marrow transplantation in chronic myelogenous leukemia. Semin Hematol 25:74, 1988.
12. Poplack DG: Acute lymphoblastic leukemia. In: Pizzo PA and Poplack DG (eds): Pediatric Oncology. Philadelphia, JB Lippincott, 1989, pp. 323–366.
13. Grier HE and Weinstein HJ: Acute nonlymphocytic leukemia. In: Pizzo PA and Poplack DG (eds): Pediatric Oncology. Philadelphia, JB Lippincott, 1989, pp. 367–382.
14. Seeger RC, Lenarsky C, and Moss TJ: Bone marrow transplantation (BMT) for poor prognosis neuroblastoma. Am Soc Clin Oncol 6:221, 1987.
15. Armitage JO: Bone marrow transplantation in the treatment of patients with lymphoma. Blood 73:1749, 1989.
16. Williams TE and Safarimaryaki S: Bone marrow transplantation for treatment of solid tumors. In: Johnson FL and Pochedly C (eds): Bone Marrow Transplantation in Children. New York, Raven Press, 1990, pp. 221–242.
17. Ramsay NKC and Kersey JH: Indications for marrow transplantation in acute lymphoblastic leukemia. Blood 75:815, 1990.
18. Santos GW: Bone marrow transplantation in hematologic malignancies. Cancer 65:786, 1990.
19. Clark SC and Kamen K: The human hematopoietic colony-stimulating factors. Science 236:1229, 1987.
20. Kemshead JT, Trevleaven JG, Gibson FM, et al: Monoclonal antibodies and magnetic microspheres used for the depletion of malignant cells from bone marrow. Progr Clin Biol Res 175:413, 1985.
21. Yeager AM, Kaizer H, Santos GW, et al: Autologous bone marrow transplantation in patients with acute nonlymphocytic leukemia, using ex vivo marrow treatment with 4-hydroperoxycyclophosphamide. N Engl J Med 315:141, 1986.
22. Sachs DH: The major histocompatibility complex. In: Paul WE (ed): Fundamental Immunology. New York, Raven Press, 1984, pp. 303–346.
23. Filipovich AH: The histocompatibility barrier in bone marrow transplantation. In: Johnson FL and Pochedly C (eds): Bone Marrow Transplantation in Children. New York, Raven Press, 1990, pp. 27–52.
24. Anasetti C, Amos D, Beatty PG, et al: Effect of HLA compatibility on engraftment of bone marrow transplants in patients with leukemia or lymphoma. N Engl J Med 320:197, 1989.
25. Ma DDF: Hematopoietic reconstitution following bone marrow Transplantation. In: Johnson FL and Pochedly C (eds): Bone Marrow Transplantation in Children. New York, Raven Press, 1990, pp. 111–139.
26. Zander AR and Aksamit IA: Immune recovery following bone marrow transplantation. In: Johnson FL and Pochedly C (eds): Bone Marrow Transplantation in Children. New York, Raven Press, 1990, pp. 87–110.
27. Lum LG: The kinetics of immune reconstitution after human marrow transplantation. Blood 69:369, 1987.
28. Balis FM, Holcenberg JS, and Poplack DG: General principles of chemotherapy. In: Pizzo PA and Poplack DG (eds): Pediatric Oncology. Philadelphia, JB Lippincott, 1989, pp. 165–205.

29. Chabner BA and Myers CE: Clinical pharmacology of cancer chemotherapy. *In:* DeVita VT, Hellman S, and Rosenberg SA (eds): Cancer, Principles and Practice of Oncology, 3rd ed. Philadelphia, JB Lippincott, 1989, pp. 349–395.
30. Bode U, Seif SM, and Levine AS: Studies on the antidiuretic effect of cyclophosphamide; vasopressin release and sodium excretion. Med Pediatr Oncol 8:295, 1980.
31. Gottdiener JS, Appelbaum FR, Ferrans VJ, et al: Cardiotoxicity associated with high-dose cyclophosphamide therapy. Arch Intern Med 141:758, 1981.
32. Fort JA and Graham-Pole J: Pulmonary complications of bone marrow transplantation. *In:* Johnson FL and Pochedly C (eds): Bone Marrow Transplantation in Children. New York, Raven Press, 1990, pp. 397–411.
33. Lazarus HM, Herzig RH, Herzig GP, et al: Central nervous system toxicity of high-dose systemic cytosine arabinoside. Cancer 48:2577, 1983.
34. Anderson KC and Weinstein HJ: Transfusion-associated graft-versus-host disease. N Engl J Med 323:315, 1990.
35. Kickler TS: Management of alloimmunized patients with amega-karyocytic thrombocytopenia. *In:* Smith DM and Summers SH (eds): Platelets. Arlington, VA, American Association of Blood Banks, 1988, pp. 115–128.
36. Rodey G: Prevention of alloimmunization in thrombocytopenic patients. *In:* Smith DM and Summers SH (eds): Platelets. Arlington, VA, American Association of Blood Banks, 1988, pp. 93–113.
37. Bowden RA, Sayers M, Flournoy N, et al: Cytomegalovirus immune globulin and seronegative blood products to prevent primary cytomegalovirus infection after marrow transplantation. N Engl J Med 314:1006, 1986.
38. Tegtmeier GE: Transfusion-transmitted cytomegalovirus infections. Vox Sang 51 (Suppl):22, 1986.
39. Petz LD: Immunohematologic problems associated with bone marrow transplantation. Transfusion Med Rev 1:85, 1987.
40. Tutschka PJ: Infections and immunodeficiency in bone marrow transplantation. Pediatr Infect Dis J 7:S22, 1988.
41. Furman WL and Feldman S: Infectious complications. *In:* Johnson FL and Pochedly C (eds): Bone Marrow Transplantation in Children. New York, Raven Press, 1990, pp. 427–450.
42. Shannon KM, Cowan MJ, and Matthay KK: Pediatric bone marrow transplantation: Intensive care management. J Intens Care Med 2:328, 1987.
43. Sullivan KM, Kopecky KJ, Jocum J, et al: Immunomodulatory and antimicrobial efficacy of intravenous immunoglobulin in bone marrow transplantation. N Engl J Med 323:705, 1990.
44. Herzig RH: Granulocyte transfusion therapy: Past, present, and future. *In:* Garratty G (ed): Current Concepts in Transfusion Therapy. Arlington, VA, American Association of Blood Banks, 1985, pp. 267–290.
45. Wasserman R, August CS, and Plotkin SA: Viral infections in pediatric bone marrow transplant patients. Pediatr Infect Dis J 7:109, 1988.
46. Selby PJ, Powles RL, Easton D, et al: The prophylactic role of intravenous and long-term oral acyclovir after allogeneic bone marrow transplantation. Br J Cancer 59:434, 1989.
47. Kapoor N, Copelan EA, and Tutschka PJ: Cytomegalovirus infection in bone marrow transplant recipients: Use of intravenous gamma globulin as a prophylactic and therapeutic agent. Transplant Proc 21:3095, 1989.
48. Lungman P, Lonnqvist B, Ringden O, et al: A randomized trial of oral versus intravenous acyclovir for treatment of herpes zoster in bone marrow transplant recipients. Bone Marrow Transplant 4:613, 1989.
49. Meyers JD: Prevention of cytomegalovirus infection after marrow transplantation. Rev Infect Dis 11:S1691, 1989.
50. Zutter MM, Martin PJ, and Sale PG: Epstein-Barr virus lymphoproliferation after bone marrow transplantation. Blood 72:520, 1988.
51. Shapiro RS, Chauvenet A, McGuire W, et al: Treatment of B-cell lymphoproliferative disorders with interferon alpha and intravenous gamma globulin. N Engl J Med 318:1334, 1988.
52. Gilbert BE and Knight V: Biochemistry and clinical applications of ribavirin. Am Soc Micro 30:201, 1986.
53. Shields AF, Hackman RC, Fife KH, et al: Adenovirus infections in patients undergoing bone-marrow transplantation. J Med 312:529, 1985.
54. Yolken RH, Bishop CA, Townsend TR, et al: Infectious gastroenteritis in bone-marrow-transplant recipients. N Engl J Med 306:1010, 1982.
55. Davey RT and Masur H: Recent advances in the diagnosis, treatment, and prevention of *Pneumocystis carinii* pneumonia. Antimicrob Agents Chemother 34:499, 1990.
56. Hirsch R, Burke BA, and Kersey JH: Toxoplasmosis in bone marrow transplant recipients. J Pediatr 318:869, 1988.
57. Lazarus HM, Coccia PF, Herzig RH, et al: Incidence of acute graft-versus-host disease with and without methotrexate prophylaxis in bone marrow transplant patients. Blood 64:215, 1984.
58. Vega RA: Graft-vs.-host disease: Hepatic, gastrointestinal, and dermal toxicities. *In:* Johnson FL and Pochedly C (eds): Bone Marrow Transplantation in Children. New York, Raven Press, 1990, pp. 381–396.
59. Deeg HJ and Storb R: Graft-versus-host disease: Pathophysiological and clinical aspects. Annu Rev Med 35:11, 1984.
60. Wick MR, Moore SB, Gastineau DA, et al: Immunologic, clinical, and pathologic aspects of human graft-versus-host disease. Mayo Clin Proc 58:603, 1983.
61. Snover DC: Acute and chronic graft-versus-host disease: Histopathological evidence for two distinct pathogenetic mechanisms. Hum Pathol 15:202, 1984.
62. McDonald GB, Shulman HM, Sullivan KM, et al: Intestinal and hepatic complications of human bone marrow transplantation, Part I. Gastroenterology 90:460, 1986.
63. McDonald GB, Shulman HM, Sullivan KM, et al: Intestinal and hepatic complications of bone marrow transplantation, Part II. Gastroenterology 90:770, 1986.
64. Martin PJ, Schoch G, Fisher L, et al: A retrospective analysis of therapy for acute graft-versus-host disease: Initial treatment. Blood 76:1464, 1990.
65. Vogelsang GB, Taylor S, Gordon G, et al: Thalidomide, a potent agent for the treatment of graft-versus-host disease. Transplant Proc 18:904, 1986.
66. Pick TE: Graft rejection. *In:* Johnson FL and Pochedly C (eds): Bone Marrow Transplantation in Children. New York, Raven Press, 1990, pp. 341–348.
67. Champlin RE, Horowitz MM, van Bekkum DW, et al: Graft failure following bone marrow transplantation for severe aplastic anemia: Risk factors and treatment results. Blood 73:606, 1989.
68. Kernan NA, Flomenberg N, Dupont B, et al: Graft rejection in recipients of T-cell-depleted HLA-nonidentical marrow transplants for leukemia. Transplantation 43:842, 1987.
69. Cordonnier C, Bernaudin J, Fleury J, et al: Diagnostic yield of bronchoalveolar lavage in pneumonitis occurring after allogeneic bone marrow transplantation. Am Rev Respir Dis 132:1118, 1985.
70. Heurlin N, Lonnqvist B, Tollemar J, et al: Fiberoptic bronchoscopy for diagnosis of opportunistic pulmonary infections after bone marrow transplantation. Scand J Infect Dis 21:359, 1989.
71. Berkowitz RJ, Strandjord S, Jones P, et al: Stomatologic complications of bone marrow transplantation in a pediatric population. Pediatr Dent 9:105, 1987.
72. Rollins BJ: Hepatic veno-occlusive disease. Am J Med 81:297, 1986.
73. Brown BP, Abu-Yousef M, Farner R, et al: Doppler sonography: A noninvasive method for evaluation of hepatic veno-occlusive disease. Am J Roentgenol 154:721, 1990.
74. Harper PL, Jarvis J, Jennings I, et al: Changes in the natural anticoagulants following bone marrow transplantation. Bone Marrow Transplant 5:39, 1990.
75. Day DL, Ramsay NKC, and Letoureau JG: Pneumatosis intestinalis after bone marrow transplantation. AJR 151:85, 1988.
76. Sanders JE, Whitehead J, Storb R, et al: Bone marrow transplantation experience for children with aplastic anemia. Pediatrics 77:179, 1986.
77. Horowitz MM, Gale RP, Sondel PM, et al: Graft-versus-leukemia reactions after bone marrow transplantation. Blood 75:555, 1990.

Dermatologic Diseases

Neil S. Prose, M.D., and
Bernice R. Krafchik, M.B., Ch.B., F.R.C.P. (C)

TOXIC EPIDERMAL NECROLYSIS (STEVENS-JOHNSON SYNDROME)

Toxic epidermal necrolysis is a life-threatening dermatologic disorder that is characterized by the rapid exfoliation of large areas of the skin and mucous membranes. The relationship between this disorder and Stevens-Johnson syndrome, a severe form of erythema multiforme associated with fever and mucous membrane involvement, is controversial. Based on histologic and clinical criteria, however, these two disorders are probably part of a spectrum of disease severity.

Erythema multiforme may be caused by a variety of allergens and infectious agents (e.g., herpes simplex), but toxic epidermal necrolysis (TEN) almost always represents an adverse reaction to a medication. Most cases of TEN are due to either antibiotics (most commonly the sulfonamides), anticonvulsants (especially phenobarbital and carbamazepine), or nonsteroidal anti-inflammatory drugs.[1] The eruption begins 7 to 21 days after starting the drug. In patients with a previous history of TEN, cutaneous findings may develop within 48 hours of drug administration.[2]

The early clinical appearance of TEN is variable, and the course unpredictable in extent and time course. The earliest lesions are usually discrete erythematous macules with dusky centers (target lesions). These lesions may spread over a period of 2 to 15 days and become confluent (Fig. 67–1).

Oral involvement occurs in 81% of patients, and more than 50% have ocular and genital involvement.[2] Mucositis of the mouth, upper airway, and esophagus may cause significant discomfort and loss of function (Fig. 67–2). Most patients have fever and leukocytosis.

In the most severe and life-threatening form of the disease, a diffuse, deep red erythema is immediately followed by necrolysis. These patients may develop 100% skin involvement within 24 hours.[2]

Toxic epidermal necrolysis must be differentiated from other causes of diffuse erythema, fever, and exfoliation in children. Staphylococcal scalded skin syndrome (SSSS), toxic shock syndrome, and Kawasaki disease (KD) may all mimic TEN.

SSSS results from the effects of epidermolytic toxins produced by a staphylococcal infection. Blistering occurs superficially, and the skin beneath the peeled blister does not have the scalded appearance of TEN. Crusting around the mouth and eyes is particularly characteristic, and intraoral involvement is extremely rare.

The exanthem in toxic shock syndrome is erythematous and scarlatiniform, with prominent erythema of the palms and soles.[3] Bullae do not occur. The cutaneous manifestations of toxic shock syndrome are usually accompanied by vomiting, diarrhea, and hypotension.[4]

Generalized erythema and erythema multiforme–like lesions may occur in KD. However, erythema of the palms and soles, induration of the hands and feet, nonpurulent conjunctivitis, and lymphadenopathy help to distinguish this disorder. Large areas of denuded skin are not seen in KD.

In cases in which the diagnosis is in doubt, skin biopsy is helpful. Characteristic features of the histology of TEN are a perivascular lymphohistiocytic infiltrate in the superficial and deep dermis, necrotic keratinocytes scattered through the epidermis, and, in some cases, a clear separation between the dermis and epidermis.[5] When immediate diagnosis is required, a frozen section of denuded skin obtained from a fresh lesion will identify the level of splitting in the epidermis and will differentiate TEN from SSSS.[6]

TEN is associated with a high mortality (25 to 75%) and significant long-term morbidity. Refinements in the management of this disease have resulted in markedly improved survival and a lower incidence of ocular scarring.[7–9]

Children with severe disease are best managed in a pediatric intensive care unit or burn center. Reverse barrier isolation and careful management of fluid and electrolytes are critical. Cultures of blood, urine, eyes, and skin should be obtained regularly, and all catheters and intravenous lines should also be cultured after removal.

A number of different approaches to skin care have been used with success. In one center, which reported a mortality below 20%, patients with severe TEN were debrided in the operating room under general anes-

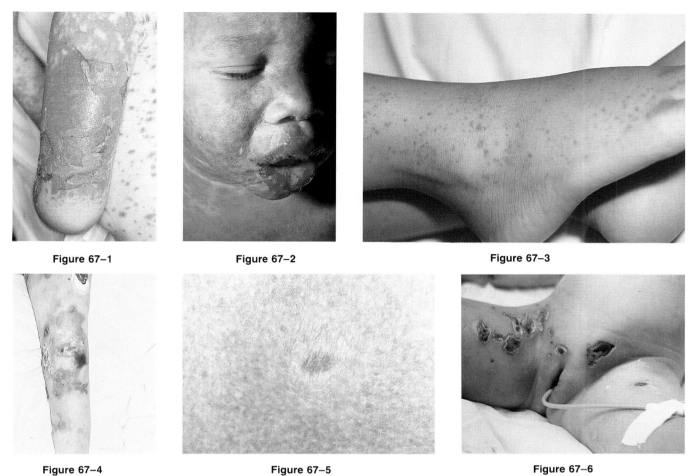

Figure 67–1.

Figure 67–2.

Figure 67–3.

Figure 67–4.

Figure 67–5.

Figure 67–6.

Figure 67–1. Toxic epidermal necrolysis. Discrete erythematous macules with areas of confluence and exfoliation are evident.

Figure 67–2. Toxic epidermal necrolysis. There is involvement of the oral mucous membranes.

Figure 67–3. Rocky Mountain spotted fever. Petechiae and palpable purpura are evident.

Figure 67–4. Meningococcemia. Necrosis and sloughing of large areas of skin are shown.

Figure 67–5. *Pseudomonas* septicemia. The earliest cutaneous lesion is a dusky red macule.

Figure 67–6. *Pseudomonas* septicemia. Fully developed ecthyma gangrenosum is evident.

thesia, and porcine xenografts were applied to all raw surfaces.[8] Other groups believe that debridement is unnecessary and that the roof of the bulla provides good coverage during re-epithelialization.[9] Silver nitrate solution 0.5% or polymyxin-bacitracin ointment may be applied to areas of involvement. Silver sulfadiazine may cause neutropenia and is not recommended.

Meticulous eye care may prevent scarring and visual loss. Daily separation of the eyelids and the bulbar and palpebral conjunctiva by an ophthalmologist allows inspection of the cornea. This manuever may be performed with a glass rod or a pair of Desmarres retractors.[8, 9]

The role of systemic steroids in TEN is controversial. Several studies have suggested that TEN does not respond to steroids and that therapy may mask or promote infection.[9] In one burn center, patients managed without corticosteroids had a 66% survival, compared with 33% in a group of historical controls who had been treated with systemic corticosteroids.[7]

ROCKY MOUNTAIN SPOTTED FEVER

Rocky Mountain spotted fever (RMSF), caused by *Rickettsia rickettsii* and transmitted by a number of dog and deer ticks, is most common in the South Atlantic states and in Oklahoma, Missouri, Arkansas, and Kansas.[10] Most cases occur during the spring and summer and in children under the age of 15. The mortality rate for children and young adults is 1.3%.

The severely ill child with RMSF is sometimes admitted to the intensive care unit prior to diagnosis. Because timely treatment may be lifesaving, the signs, symptoms, and laboratory findings of RMSF should be familiar to those specializing in pediatric intensive care.

Establishing the diagnosis of RMSF during the first 2 to 3 days of illness is extremely difficult, because the cutaneous findings may be absent. RMSF typically begins with a combination of fever, headache, myalgias, and abdominal pain with or without vomiting. In approximately 40% of patients, there is no history of known tick exposure.[11, 12]

During the next several days, the characteristic eruption of RMSF appears in most patients. The typical rash begins as blanching erythematous macules that are most evident on the wrists and ankles.[13] The lesions rapidly spread to involve the palms and soles, proximal extremities, and trunk. Soon after, petechiae, palpable purpura, and even ecchymoses develop in the areas of involvement (Fig. 67–3). Conjunctivitis and periorbital edema occur in a significant percentage of children.

Neurologic manifestations of RMSF are common and include meningismus, lethargy, seizures, and coma. The severe myalgia that may accompany RMSF has been misinterpreted as meningismus or an acute abdomen.[14]

In its early stages, RMSF may be difficult to differentiate from the numerous viral illnesses (especially enteroviruses) that commonly occur in the spring and summer. The fever and eruption of classical RMSF must be differentiated from bacterial septicemia (e.g., meningococcemia) and atypical measles.

Hyponatremia and thrombocytopenia are inconsistent findings in RMSF.[15] The total leukocyte count is usually normal, but there may be a marked polymorphonuclear leukocytosis.

The most rapid diagnostic procedure is the biopsy of a well-developed petechial lesion and direct immunofluorescent staining for rickettsial organisms.[16] Experienced microscopists can provide confirmation within 24 to 48 hours. This test is 100% specific, but a negative result does not rule out RMSF because the test has only a 70% sensitivity.[17] False-negative results are commonly seen after 48 hours of antirickettsial therapy.

Serologic tests do not become positive until the seventh day of illness and are therefore important only as a retrospective confirmation of the diagnosis. The indirect immunofluorescent antibody assay (IFA) is the most accurate serologic test available.[17] Latex agglutination (LA) has high sensitivity, is simple to perform, and is widely available. The Weil-Felix test, which detects antibody reactivity to certain strains of *Proteus* bacteria, is less sensitive and specific than the IFA and LA tests.

Rapid institution of therapy is recommended if the diagnosis of RMSF is considered possible or likely. In endemic areas, a significant number of children will be treated who do not have RMSF. In the intensive care setting, intravenous chloramphenicol (100 mg/kg/24 hr up to a total dose of 3 g) is the treatment of choice. As patients improve, the dose may be decreased to 50 mg/kg/24 hr orally. Patients who are less ill may be treated with oral tetracycline.

CUTANEOUS MANIFESTATIONS OF SEPSIS

Morbilliform, maculopapular, bullous, or vasculitic skin lesions may be observed in many forms of grampositive and gram-negative bacterial sepsis.[18] The cutaneous manifestations of meningococcemia and *Pseudomonas* septicemia are particularly distinctive, and their recognition may lead to rapid diagnosis and lifesaving therapy.

Meningococcemia

Acute meningococcemia typically presents with fever, myalgia, arthralgia, and signs of meningeal irritation. Two thirds of patients develop skin lesions.[19] These lesions may consist only of erythematous or violaceous macules and papules.[20, 21] Petechial lesions, which favor the trunk and lower extremities, are particularly suggestive of meningococcemia. They may also be noted on the oral mucous membranes and on the palms and soles. Large ecchymotic and purpuric lesions occur in 11% of childhood cases and may result in necrosis and sloughing of large areas of skin (purpura fulminans) (Fig. 67–4).[21] Patients with this severe form of involvement are susceptible to superinfection with other bacterial organisms and should be cultured regularly.

A skin biopsy shows evidence of acute vasculitis and thrombi in the dermal vessels. In many cases, meningococci can be visualized within the walls of vessels and in thrombi. Smears from petechial lesions often show gram-negative diplococci.[22] This is the most rapid method of establishing the diagnosis of meningococcemia.

Pseudomonas Septicemia

Systemic infection with *Pseudomonas aeruginosa* occurs most commonly in patients with significant immunosuppression (e.g., related to chemotherapy) or with severe burns. The early cutaneous lesions are multiple red macules that resemble the rose spots of typhoid fever (Fig. 67–5). Nodules and bullae may be the presenting cutaneous manifestation.[23]

The rapid enlargement of lesions with areas of necrosis and hemorrhage is particularly characteristic of systemic infection with *Pseudomonas*. The classic lesions of ecthyma gangrenosum, consisting of deep necrotic ulceration, are most commonly noted in the groin, legs, and axilla (Fig. 67–6). Multiple punched-out ulcers approximately 1 cm in diameter may occur.

Skin biopsy reveals a necrotizing vasculitis with bacilli in the walls of involved vessels. Tzanck smear of the base of a lesion often demonstrates the presence of gram-negative rods and allows for rapid diagnosis.

CUTANEOUS MANIFESTATIONS OF IMMUNOSUPPRESSION

Severe immune dysfunction in children may result from congenital immunodeficiencies, cancer chemotherapy, treatment associated with organ transplantation, and human immunodeficiency virus (HIV) infection. Cutaneous disease in this group of children is of great significance. In particular, the early recognition of the cutaneous manifestations of infection may prevent the rapid evolution of life-threatening illness. The task of differentiating these eruptions from the complications of multiple drug therapy can be particularly challenging.

Bacterial infections seen in the immunosuppressed child include furunculosis, cellulitis, and ecthyma. In addition, meningococcemia and *Pseudomonas* septicemia may evolve rapidly in children with defective humoral immunity. Rapid diagnosis, by means of Gram stain, culture, and skin biopsy, and the rapid institution of appropriate parenteral antibiotic therapy is mandatory.

Herpes simplex virus (HSV) and varicella-zoster virus infection are common viral infections in immunosuppressed patients. HSV infection may result in severe and progressive gingivostomatitis or ulcerative lesions in other locations. Primary varicella-zoster infection may lead to rapidly progressive chickenpox with necrotic skin lesions and severe visceral involvement. Herpes zoster (shingles), with clusters of vesicles in a zosteriform distribution, is also more common in children with defective cell-mediated immunity. Rarely, dissemination may occur. Tzanck smear of vesicular lesions is the most reliable method of rapid diagnosis; viral culture of fluid

from an intact vesicle is necessary, but, in the case of varicella-zoster, may take up to 1 week. In children with significant immunosuppression, antiviral therapy (usually with intravenous acyclovir) should be instituted pending confirmation of the diagnosis.

Candidiasis is the most common mucocutaneous manifestation of pediatric HIV infection and may also be seen in a number of immune disorders.[24] Oral thrush and recalcitrant monilial diaper dermatitis are particularly common; the development of dysphagia or loss of appetite may indicate the development of esophageal candidiasis.

Aspergillosis, which is most common in children receiving immunosuppressive therapy, presents in two discrete clinical contexts. Primary cutaneous *Aspergillus* infection consists of ulcerated nodules or plaques, occurring at sites of trauma or adhesive tape application (Fig. 67–7).[25] Disseminated aspergillosis results in multiple embolic lesions, usually clustered on the extremities. Treatment with amphotericin B should be instituted after a skin biopsy and cultures are obtained.

GRAFT-VERSUS-HOST DISEASE

Graft-versus-host disease (GVHD) most often occurs as a consequence of bone marrow transplantation (see Chapter 66). Acute GVHD presents within days, or as late as several months, after transplantation.[26] Principal target organs are the liver, intestine, and skin. A maculopapular or scarlatiniform eruption favors the face, palms, and soles. The rash of acute GVHD may become generalized and occasionally evolves to cause epidermal necrosis and blistering.[27] The early diagnosis of GVHD may sometimes be confirmed by the presence of satellite cell dyskeratosis on skin biopsy.

Chronic GVHD presents more than 100 days after bone marrow transplantation. The skin disease in this stage may mimic lichen planus or scleroderma.

ECZEMA HERPETICUM

Eczema herpeticum is a generalized cutaneous infection with herpes simplex virus, occurring in a patient with an existing skin disease. The pre-existing condition is usually atopic dermatitis but may also be Darier disease, seborrheic dermatitis, pemphigus, or a severe burn.

The term Kaposi varicelliform eruption has historically been used to encompass eczema herpeticum and eczema vaccinatum, which was due to disseminated infection with the vaccinia virus. The latter condition has not been observed since the eradication of smallpox and the discontinuation of smallpox vaccination.

Eczema herpeticum develops rapidly and is associated with significant morbidity and mortality. Visceral involvement occurs, and, more commonly, secondary cutaneous infection, usually with *Staphylococcus aureus*, may lead to overwhelming sepsis.

Eczema herpeticum most often occurs in active or recently healed atopic dermatitis.[28] The virus probably

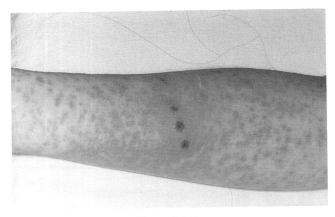

Figure 67–7

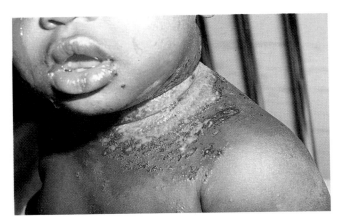

Figure 67–8

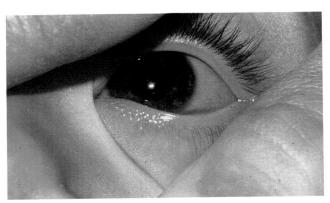

Figure 67–9

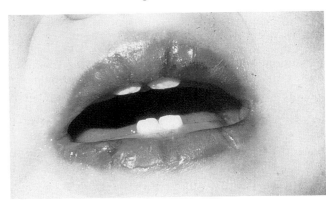

Figure 67–10

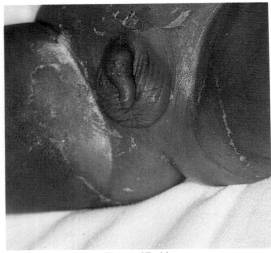

Figure 67–11

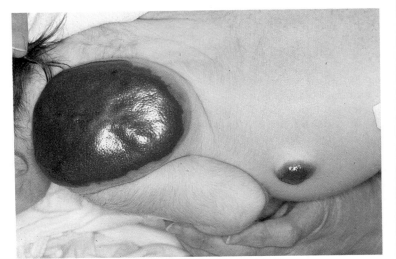

Figure 67–12

Figure 67–7. Primary cutaneous aspergillosis. Lesions noted under the site of the arm board.

Figure 67–8. Eczema herpeticum. Vesicles and erosions in skin previously involved with atopic dermatitis.

Figure 67–9. Kawasaki disease. Nonpurulent conjunctival injection.

Figure 67–10. Kawasaki disease. Erythema and fissuring of the lips.

Figure 67–11. Kawasaki disease. Perineal desquamation.

Figure 67–12. Giant hemangioma of the shoulder and back of an infant.

enters the skin during the viremic phase; autoinoculation is less common. Because eczema herpeticum is usually associated with a primary herpetic infection, it is mainly seen in infancy. However, it can occur at any age.

After an incubation period of 10 days, vesicles appear in crops. Involvement is confined initially to abnormal skin (Fig. 67–8), but tends to become generalized. The lesions, which are sometimes pustular, quickly crust and become hemorrhagic. Fever, malaise, and lymphadenopathy develop within a few days of the initial eruption. In recurrent cases, the constitutional symptoms are less severe.

Patients should be isolated from susceptible contacts and treated with intravenous acyclovir 250 mg/m²/dose, every 8 hours.[29, 30] Antibiotics may be needed to treat secondary infection.

KAWASAKI DISEASE

Mucocutaneous lymph node syndrome, widely known as KD, was first described by Kawasaki in Japanese children in 1967.[31] Although more prevalent in children of Asian descent, it has been reported worldwide.[32, 33] Young children and infants are predominantly affected, and 50% of cases occur in children under 2 years of age and 80% occur in children under 4 years of age. It rarely occurs in children after 12 years of age. There is a slight male predominance.

KD is an acute, febrile, multisystem disease and is the leading cause of childhood vasculitis. The characteristic clinical picture is important to recognize at an early stage, because the previously high cardiac morbidity (20%) and mortality (2%) have been significantly reduced with combination aspirin and intravenous gamma globulin therapy.[34, 35]

The etiology of KD is unknown. The peak occurrence in the spring and winter, and the occasional occurrence of epidemics, suggests an infectious etiology. A variety of bacterial and viral agents have been incriminated, but a causative organism has not been established.

Immune abnormalities consist of an absolute depression of suppressor T cells and an increase in T helper cells, stimulating polyclonal immunoglobulin production from increased circulating activated B cells. The T cell abnormality normalizes within 3 weeks.[34] Immune complexes are also increased during the acute phase.[36] C3 is raised, whereas C4 is normal.[37] The production of tumor necrosis factor and interleukin-1 by peripheral blood mononuclear cells during the acute phase of illness may be important in the pathogenesis of endothelial cell damage.[38, 39]

Six major clinical features aid in the diagnosis of KD (Table 67–1). Intermittent fever is the most consistent finding, and peak temperatures exceed 39.9° C. The fever is almost always associated with severe irritability. Without treatment, fever may persist for more than 10 days.[40]

In addition to fever, four out of the following five features are necessary for the diagnosis:

1. Conjunctival injection. Nonpurulent injection of

Table 67–1. PRINCIPAL DIAGNOSTIC CRITERIA FOR KAWASAKI DISEASE

Fever for more than 5 days and 4 out of 5 of the following:
1. Conjunctival injection
2. Changes in the mouth—erythema, fissuring and crusting of the lips, diffuse oropharyngeal erythema, strawberry tongue
3. Changes in the peripheral extremities—induration of the hands and feet, erythema of the palms and soles, desquamation of fingertips and toetips about 2 weeks after onset, transverse grooves across fingernails 2 to 3 months after onset
4. Rash—erythematous, morbilliform, or erythema multiforme–like eruption
5. Enlarged lymph node—measuring more than 1.5 cm in diameter

the conjunctivae occurs within the first week (Fig. 67–9). This tends to be more severe on the bulbar surface and typically spares the area around the limbus.[41]

2. Changes in the mouth. The oral mucous membranes are affected with fissuring, cracking, and bleeding of the lips (Fig. 67–10); strawberry tongue; and diffuse erythema of the oropharynx. The changes in the lips are characteristic and vary in severity.

3. Changes in the peripheral extremities. Involvement of the hands and feet constitute a distinctive feature. In the first week, they are indurated and swollen with nonpitting edema, while the palms and soles are erythematous. In the subacute phase, a distinctive pattern of epidermal desquamation occurs around the distal phalanges. After 2 to 3 months, transverse grooves of the fingernails may occur.

4. Cutaneous eruption. The eruption of KD, occurring early in the disease, is usually morbilliform but may have an erythema multiforme–like appearance. Ten per cent of children develop sterile pustules on their skin, and 10% have perineal desquamation (Fig. 67–11).

5. Lymphadenopathy. Lymph node involvement measuring more than 1.5 cm occurs in approximately 50% of patients. It is commonly unilateral in the anterior cervical chain, although it may also be widespread.

Other findings of KD occur with varying frequency. Sterile pyuria, due to urethritis, affects 75% of patients during the first week of illness. Arthralgias and arthritis of multiple joints (large and small) may be affected in the acute phase. Hydrops of the gallbladder, found in 5% of patients, is highly suggestive of KD, whereas the less distinctive features of abdominal pain, diarrhea, and nausea are more common. Central nervous system involvement, characterized by lethargy and aseptic meningitis, occurs in 25% of patients.

Patients who do not meet strict criteria for the diagnosis of KD may go on to develop some of the severe cardiac complications of this disorder. The clinician must have a high index of suspicion in order to correctly diagnose these "atypical" or "incomplete" forms of KD.[42]

The most important visceral manifestation of KD is cardiac involvement, which results in coronary artery aneurysm in 20% of untreated patients. Cardiac disease in KD presents clinically as a pericardial effusion, congestive heart failure, and arrhythmia.

In the early stages, the intima of the coronary vessels

is affected with acute inflammation and initial sparing of the media. This is associated with acute pancarditis. The acute polymorphonuclear infiltrate changes to a lymphocytic infiltrate from 2 to 12 weeks. Later, destruction of the media with multiple fractures of the internal elastic lumina occurs, causing aneurysmal dilatation. These findings are indistinguishable from infantile periarteritis nodosa. Acute thrombosis of inflamed arteries may lead to sudden death.[43] (For additional discussion of cardiac manifestations see Chapter 35).

The clinical features of KD may be divided into three main phases:

1. The acute febrile illness consists of fever, skin and mucous membrane involvement, and lymphadenopathy. This lasts 8 to 15 days without treatment.

2. The subacute phase lasts 3 to 4 weeks. The acute symptoms disappear, but the patient remains irritable. There is desquamation of the hands and feet and marked thrombocytosis. The major risk of acute coronary artery thrombosis and sudden death occurs during this phase.

3. In the convalescent phase, most symptoms and signs disappear. There remains a risk for death due to infarction or to chronic myocardial ischemia.

There is no diagnostic laboratory test for KD. The white blood cell count (especially polymorphonuclear leukocytes) and erythrocyte sedimentation rate (ESR) are elevated during the acute phase. Frequently, the platelet count is markedly elevated during the second and third week of illness. Even in an atypical case of KD, the ESR and platelet count are raised. These tests normalize over 8 to 12 weeks.

The child with KD should have an electrocardiogram and two-dimensional echocardiogram at the time of the child's admission to the hospital and at intervals in the acute and convalescent stage. Children with evidence of cardiac disease should be admitted to an intensive care unit and should be monitored carefully.

With the concurrent use of aspirin and intravenous gamma globulin, the rate of cardiac morbidity has been reduced from 20% to 5%. Treatment must be given within 10 days of the development of symptoms. There is no evidence that gamma globulin is of any value in patients who have already developed coronary artery disease.

Gamma globulin is given as an intravenous infusion over 10 to 12 hours in the dose of 2 g/kg.[44] This new treatment approach appears to be as effective as the previously recommended 4-day course of therapy (400 mg/kg/day).[45] A rapid decrease in irritability and fever occurs almost invariably. Doses below 1 g/kg are ineffective in reducing the incidence of coronary artery disease.[46]

Aspirin is used concurrently with gamma globulin. Because the optimal dose of this medication is not known, a variety of treatment schedules have been used. At present, a widely used dose is 100 mg/kg/day until the fever has subsided, followed by 5 mg/kg/day in a single daily dose until the ESR and platelet count are normal (approximately 3 months). In children with small aneurysms, aspirin should be continued indefinitely or until resolution takes place. In patients with giant aneurysms, anticoagulant therapy may be added to the aspirin therapy.

Although the overall risk for coronary aneurysms has been lowered with the concurrent use of aspirin and gamma globulin, 15% of infants under 1 year of age develop coronary abnormalities despite treatment.[47] If cardiac abnormalities are present, myocardial infarction, ischemia, and death may occur during the period at least 5 years after the acute illness. Cardiac evaluation should be performed every 6 months to 1 year depending on the severity of the aneurysms. Regression of coronary aneurysms has been noted to occur.

COMPLICATIONS OF HEMANGIOMA

Hemangiomas affect 4 to 10% of infants.[48] Most hemangiomas involute spontaneously: 50% by 5 years of age, 70% by 7 years of age, and 90% by 9 years of age.[49] However, a small percentage of hemangiomas, because of their size or location, may result in severe morbidity and may even be life-threatening. The management of patients with major complications of hemangioma is now discussed.

Hemangiomas in the subglottic area may cause obstruction of the trachea, with a mortality of up to 50%.[50] The infant usually presents between the ages of 6 weeks and 6 months with worsening stridor and dyspnea. At least 50% of subglottic hemangiomas are associated with superficial hemangiomas on the neck, and 8% of neck hemangiomas have an internal subglottic component.

The extent of airway involvement can be best assessed by direct laryngoscopy. If airway obstruction develops rapidly or is impending, an emergency tracheotomy is required.

In most cases, rapid reduction in the mass of the lesion can be achieved by administering systemic corticosteroids. Intravenous therapy, or oral prednisone in a dose of 2 to 4 mg/kg/day, are usually effective. Corticosteroid therapy should be maintained until the child is at least 1 year of age, and this therapy should be withdrawn slowly to avoid rebound growth of the hemangioma. Patients should be monitored carefully for the adverse effects of systemic steroids.[51] Excess weight gain and growth retardation are the most commonly seen side effects.

Treatment with the carbon dioxide laser has been used successfully in children with subglottic hemangioma.[52] The most significant adverse effect is subglottic scarring and stenosis, which occurs in approximately one fifth of patients.[53]

Children with large cutaneous hemangiomas (Fig. 67–12) or with associated visceral hemangiomas, especially in the liver, may develop high-output congestive heart failure. In addition to systemic corticosteroids, diuretics and digoxin may be required until the hemangioma is decreased in size.

Superficial ulceration and bleeding is not unusual in large cutaneous hemangiomas. Although significant blood loss is rare, children with bleeding should be monitored for the development of anemia. Oral iron supplementation may be required in some cases.

Table 67–2. STUDIES TO DETERMINE IF KASABACH-MERRITT SYNDROME IS PRESENT

Hemoglobin
Hematocrit
Smear for fragmented red blood cells
Platelet count
Prothrombin
Partial thromboplastin time
Fibrinogen level
Fibrin-split products
Coagulation factor levels II, V, and VIII
Soluble fibrin and fibrinopeptide A in plasma

One of the most serious complications arising in children with large hemangiomas is the Kasabach-Merritt syndrome, first described in 1940.[54] This disorder consists of a microangiopathic hemolytic anemia, an acute or chronic consumptive coagulopathy, and severe thrombocytopenia due to trapping, and increased destruction of platelets within the hemangioma.

Kasabach-Merritt syndrome usually occurs during the first 6 weeks of life in a child with a rapidly enlarging hemangioma, usually located on the extremity.[55] Bruising over the hemangioma is often the first sign. This is followed by generalized pallor and by petechiae and ecchymoses at areas distant from the hemangioma.

Without therapeutic intervention, the mortality rate of this disorder is 20 to 30%.[56] Death is most often due to severe bleeding.

The child with suspected Kasabach-Merritt syndrome should be evaluated for laboratory evidence of a consumptive coagulopathy (Table 67–2). Treatment depends on the severity of the disease. Systemic corticosteroids act by reducing the mass of vascular tissue, restoring the integrity of the clotting system, and increasing platelet survival time. Prednisone, at an initial dose of 2 mg/kg/day, usually decreases the size of the hemangioma and produces a rapid rise in the platelet count.[57, 58] The dose of prednisone should be increased to 4 mg/kg/day if there is no response in 1 week. Systemic corticosteroids should be administered for at least 2 weeks before alternative therapies are considered.

If corticosteroids fail, the addition of heparin is recommended in a dose of 100 μg/kg every 4 hours.[56, 59] Heparin has been shown to stabilize the platelet count, control the coagulopathy, and increase platelet, red blood cell, and fibrinogen levels. It also seems to enhance the angiostatic effect of corticosteroids.[60]

Other agents that have been successfully utilized in emergency situations are platelet concentrates, fresh frozen plasma, and cryoprecipitate (with or without aminocaproic acid).[61–63] These appear to be more effective when the patient is heparinized. Aspirin and dipyridamole, which are inhibitors of platelet function, have also been used effectively in Kasabach-Merritt syndrome.[64] In cases in which medical treatment fails, embolization and surgical removal have stabilized patients with this disorder.[55, 65, 66]

References

1. Guillaume J-C, Roujeau J-C, Revuz J, et al: The culprit drugs in 87 cases of toxic epidermal necrolysis (Lyell's syndrome). Arch Dermatol 123:1166, 1987.
2. Revuz J, Penso D, Roujeau J-C, et al: Toxic epidermal necrolysis: Clinical findings and prognosis factors in 87 patients. Arch Dermatol 123:1160, 1987.
3. Resnick SD: Toxic shock syndrome: Recent developments in pathogenesis. J Pediatr 116:321, 1990.
4. Wiesenthal AM and Todd JK: Toxic shock syndrome in children aged 10 years or less. Pediatrics 74:112, 1984.
5. Lever WJ and Schaumburg-Lever G: Histopathology of the Skin, 6th ed. Philadelphia, JB Lippincott, 1983, pp. 122–124.
6. Amon RB and Dimond RL: Toxic epidermal necrolysis: Rapid differentiation between staphylococcal- and drug-induced disease. Arch Dermatol 111:1433, 1975.
7. Halebian PJ, Madden MR, Finklestein JL, et al: Improved burn center survival of patients with toxic epidermal necrolysis managed without corticosteroids. Ann Surg 204:503, 1986.
8. Heimbach DM, Engrav LH, Mavin JA, et al: Toxic epidermal necrolysis: A step forward in treatment. JAMA 257:2171, 1987.
9. Prendiville JS, Hebert AA, Greenwald MJ, and Esterly NB: Management of Stevens-Johnson syndrome and toxic epidermal necrolysis in children. J Pediatr 115:881, 1989.
10. Centers for Disease Control: Rocky Mountain spotted fever—United States, 1987. MMWR 37:388, 1988.
11. Helmick CG, Bernard KW, and D'Angelo LJ: Rocky Mountain spotted fever: Clinical, laboratory, and epidemiological features of 262 cases. J Infect Dis 150:480, 1984.
12. Hattwick MAW, O'Brien RJ, and Hanson BF: Rocky Mountain spotted fever: Epidemiology of an increasing problem. Ann Intern Med 84:732, 1976.
13. Bradford WH and Hawkins HK: Rocky Mountain spotted fever in children. Am J Dis Child 131:1228, 1977.
14. Fischer JJ: Rocky Mountain spotted fever: When and why to consider the diagnosis. Postgrad Med 87:109, 1990.
15. Haynes RE, Sanders DY, and Cramblett HG: Rocky Mountain spotted fever in children. J Pediatr 76:685, 1970.
16. Walker DH, Cain BG, and Olmstead PM: Laboratory diagnosis of Rocky Mountain spotted fever by immunofluorescent demonstration of *Rickettsia rickettsii* in cutaneous lesions. Am J Clin Pathol 69:619, 1978.
17. Walker DH: Rocky Mountain spotted fever: A disease in need of microbiological concern. Clin Microbiol Rev 2:227, 1989.
18. Musher DM: Cutaneous and soft tissue manifestations of sepsis due to gram-negative enteric bacilli. Rev Infect Dis 2:854, 1980.
19. Hurwitz S: Clinical Pediatric Dermatology. Philadelphia, WB Saunders, 1981, pp. 220–221.
20. Rubenstein R and Esterly NB: Meningococcal meningitis with a benign skin rash. Pediatr Dermatol 3:414, 1986.
21. Toews WH and Bass JW: Skin manifestations of meningococcal infection. Am J Dis Child 127:173, 1974.
22. Bernhard SG and Jordan AC: Purpuric lesions in meningococcic infections. J Lab Clin Med 29:273, 1944.
23. Fleming MG, Milburn PB, and Prose NS: *Pseudomonas* septicemia with nodules and bullae. Pediatr Dermatol 4:18, 1987.
24. Prose NS: HIV infection in children. J Am Acad Dermatol 22:1223, 1990.
25. Estes SA, Hendricks AA, Merz WG, and Prystkowski FD: Primary cutaneous aspergillosis. J Am Acad Dermatol 3:397, 1980.
26. Ferrara JLM and Deeg HJ: Graft-versus-host disease. N Engl J Med 324:667, 1990.
27. Saurat JH: Cutaneous manifestations of graft-versus-host disease. Int J Dermatol 20:249, 1981.
28. Bohm C and Johne HO: Zur Kasuistik Des Eczema Herpeticum (Herpetiforme) Kaposi. Hautzart 7:216, 1956.
29. Swart RNJ: Treatment of eczema herpeticum with acyclovir. Arch Dermatol 13:19, 1983.
30. Woolfson H: Oral acyclovir in eczema herpeticum. Br Med J 288:531, 1984.
31. Kawasaki T: Acute febrile mucocutaneous syndrome with lymphoid children (Japanese). Arerugi 16:178–222, 1967.

32. Yanagawa H: Results of nationwide surveys on Kawasaki disease. *In*: Shigematsu I, Yanagawa H, and Kawasaki T (eds): Kawasaki Disease Epidemiological Data Book. Tokyo, Soft Science-sha Publications, 1986, pp. 37–51.
33. Dean AG, Melish ME, Hicks RV, and Palumbo NE: An epidemic of Kawasaki syndrome in Hawaii. J Pediatr 100:552–558, 1982.
34. Furosho K, Kamiya T, Nakano H, et al: High-dose intravenous gamma globulin for Kawasaki disease. Lancet 2:1055–1058, 1984.
35. Ogino H, Ogawa M, Harima Y, et al: Clinical evaluation of gamma globulin preparations for the treatment of Kawasaki disease. *In*: Shulman ST (ed): Kawasaki Disease. New York, AR Liss, 1987, pp. 555–556.
36. Leung DYM, Seigel RL, Grady S, et al: Immunoregulatory abnormalities in mucocutaneous lymph node syndrome. Clin Immunol Immunopathol 23:100–112, 1982.
37. Eluthesen K, Marchette N, and Melish ME: Immunoglobulins, complement circulating immune complexes in Kawasaki syndrome. Presented at the 21st Interscience Conference on Antimicrobial Agents and Chemotherapeutics, November 1985.
38. Leung DYM: Clinical and immunologic aspects of Kawasaki disease. Immunodef Rev 1:261–271, 1989.
39. Lang BA, Silverman ED, Laxer RM, and Lau AS: Spontaneous tumor necrosis factor in Kawasaki disease. J Pediatr 115:939–943, 1989.
40. Hicks RV and Melish ME: Kawasaki syndrome; rheumatic complaints and analysis of salicylate therapy. Arthritis Rheum 22:621–622, 1979.
41. Ohnos S, Miyajima T, Higuchi M, et al: Ocular manifestations of Kawasaki disease. Am J Ophthalmol 93:713–715, 1982.
42. Levy M and Koren G: Atypical Kawasaki disease: Analysis of clinical presentation and diagnostic clues. Pediatr Infec Dis J 9:122–126, 1990.
43. Fujiwar H and Hamashima Y: Pathology of the heart in Kawasaki disease. Pediatrics 61:100–107, 1978.
44. Newberger JW: For the United States Multicenter Kawasaki Study Group: Preliminary results of multicenter trial in IVGG treatment of Kawasaki disease with single infusion vs four-infusion regimen (Abstract). Pediatr Res 27:22A, 1990.
45. Newberger JW, Takahashi M, Beiser AS, et al: A single intravenous infusion of gamma globulin as compared with four infusions in the treatment of acute Kawasaki syndrome. N Engl J Med 324:1633–1639, 1991.
46. Okuni M, Harada K, and Yamaguchi H: Intravenous gamma globulin therapy in Kawasaki disease: Trial of low dose gamma globulin. *In*: Shulman ST (ed): Kawasaki Disease. New York, AR Liss, 1987, pp. 433–439.
47. Kato H, Ichinose E, and Kawasaki T: Myocardial infarction in Kawasaki disease. J Pediatr 108:923–928, 1986.
48. Holmdahl K: Cutaneous hemangiomas in premature and mature infants. Acta Paediatr Scand 44:370, 1955.
49. Bowers RE, Graham EA, and Tomlinson KA: The natural history of strawberry nevus. Arch Dermatol 82:667–680, 1960.
50. Shikhani AH, Marsh BR, Jones MM, and Holliday MJ: Infantile subglottic hemangiomas: An update. Ann Otol Rhinol Laryngol 95:336–345, 1986.
51. Lucky AW: Principles of the use of glucocorticosteroids in the growing child. Pediatr Dermatol 1:226, 1984.
52. Healy G, McGill T, and Friedman EM: Carbon dioxide laser in subglottic hemangioma: An update. Ann Otol Rhinol Laryngol 93:370, 1984.
53. Cotton RT and Tewfik TL: Laryngeal stenosis following carbon dioxide laser in subglottic hemangioma. Ann Otol Rhinol Laryngol 94:494, 1985.
54. Kasabach MM and Merritt KK: Capillary hemangioma with extensive purpura. Am J Dis Child 59:1063–1070, 1940.
55. Shim WKT: Hemangiomas of infancy complicated by thrombocytopenia. Am J Surg 116:896, 1968.
56. Lang PG and Dubin HV: Hemangioma-thrombocytopenia syndrome. Arch Dermatol 111:105, 1975.
57. Esterly NB: Kasabach-Merritt syndrome in infants. J Am Acad Dermatol 8:504, 1983.
58. Brown SH Jr, Neerhout RC, and Fonkalsrud EW: Prednisone therapy in the management of large hemangioma in infants and children. Surgery 71:186, 1972.
59. Staub PW, Kessler S, Schreiber A, et al: Chronic intravascular coagulation in Kasabach-Merritt syndrome. Arch Intern Med 129:475, 1972.
60. Folkman J, Weisz PB, Joullie MM, et al: Control of angiogenesis with synthetic heparin substitutes. Science 243:1490, 1989.
61. Corrigan JJ Jr: Disseminated intravascular coagulopathy. Pediatrics 64:37, 1979.
62. Bell R: Disseminated intravascular coagulation. Johns Hopkins Med J 146:289, 1980.
63. Neidhart JA and Roach RW: Successful treatment of skeletal hemangioma and Kasabach-Merritt syndrome with aminocaproic acid. Is fibrinolysis "defensive"? Am J Med 73:434–437, 1982.
64. Koerper MA, Addiego JE Jr, deLorimier AA, et al: Use of aspirin and dipyridamole in children with platelet trapping syndromes. J Pediatr 102:311, 1983.
65. Argenta LC, Bishop E, Cho KJ, et al: Complete resolution of life-threatening hemangioma by embolization and corticosteroids. Plast Reconstr Surg 70:739–742, 1982.
66. Martins AG: Hemangioma and thrombocytopenia. J Pediatr Surg 5:641, 1970.

Psychiatric Aspects of Critical Care

Thomas L. Walsh, M.D., and Rosemarie Scully, M.S.N.

EMOTIONAL RESPONSE TO THE INTENSIVE CARE UNIT

The Child

The child's adaptation to the intensive care environment may be characterized by behaviors as diverse as quiet, cooperative complacency or fearful, agitated resistance. The key to understanding the effect of the intensive care unit (ICU) on the child lies in looking beyond the observable behavior to the psychosocial/cognitive level of development, the child's understanding of his or her illness and the ICU experience, the child's temperament, stressors impinging on the child, and the support that the child receives from his or her family and caretakers. When all of these factors are considered together, meaning can be assigned to the behavior observed. For example, the complacent child may appear to be well adjusted to the ICU environment. However, if this child has a history of abuse, this "complacency" may be a maladaptive response to a sense of extreme anxiety. On the other hand, the extremely resistive child may seem to be poorly adjusted to the ICU environment. But if that child is a previously healthy toddler with a limited capacity to understand what is happening to him or her in the ICU, his or her resistance is quite healthy.

Cognitive and psychologic development is the first consideration in understanding a child's behavior in the ICU (Table 68–1). From birth to 2 years of age the child is in the sensorimotor phase of cognitive development and the trust phase of psychosocial development. During this time the child is learning that he or she is separate from the mother-figure and the environment. The child is also incorporating cues from the environment (e.g., pleasure in having needs satisfied, frustration in not having needs met) in developing a sense of self. This time is critical for developing a trust relationship with the mother and for the mother to bond to the child. At this point, the child is learning from a variety of sensory inputs—visual, olfactory, auditory, tactile, and

Table 68–1. ADJUSTMENT TO PHYSICAL ILLNESS

Age	Developmental Concerns	Intervention
0–1	Nurturance, comfort, relief of frustration	Liberal visitation by parents; provide frustration outlets; attention to pain and discomfort
1–3	Fears of separation	Provide transitional objects; liberal visitation by parents
3–7	Fear of bodily injury; concrete, egocentric thinking	Brief simple preparation for procedures; reassurance that the child is not "bad"; limited choices when possible; activity through play
7–12	Loss of control; fear of death	Explanations of procedures; involvement in care; reassurance
13–18	Independence, identity; fear of disfigurement, handicap, or death	Involvement in treatment decisions; opportunity to express fears; reassurance

oral. For a child at this level, the ICU threatens to interfere with the relationship with his or her primary caregiver and with his or her need for appropriate sensory stimulation.

From 2 to 7 years of age the child is in the preoperational period of cognitive development. This child develops language and the ability to express himself or herself, but his or her thoughts are concrete and egocentric. This child is focused on body integrity and will wish for bandages to be present to "keep his or her insides from falling out." At this age the child may also exhibit animistic thinking, attributing "life" to objects like monitors, pumps, and intravenous (IV) tubes. At the same time, children are attempting to establish a sense of autonomy from caregivers by asserting their will and by age-appropriate oppositional behavior. For a child at this age, limited choices to establish a sense of control will facilitate adaptation.

For the child aged 7 to 11, the capacity to understand cause and effect increases dramatically. This child's thinking begins to be somewhat abstract, and he or she is more able to generalize. The child begins to understand complex processes. This is the concrete operational period. Psychosocially, this child derives satisfaction from being able to master a situation, that is, to understand what is happening and to respond as he or she thinks is the expected response or at least in a way that "saves face." At this age, a child's involvement in his or her care and clear explanations are essential for adaptation.

The formal operations period begins at 12 years of age. At this time children can abstract quite well and thus can understand invisible body changes. At this age children can project a variety of possible outcomes and probably will worry about each one. The task at this age is to develop a sense of identity separate from parents. At this age the idealized body image becomes the all-important goal. Hospitalization in the ICU poses a threat to the child's independence, identity, and body image.

The child's understanding of his or her illness relates to his or her level of cognitive development and previous experience with illness/hospitalization. For the infant, pain is the primary attribute of illness, and if mother is not present, at least at regular intervals, it will be complicated by the absence of an important source of comfort. For the child aged 2 to 7, illness and hospitalization are likely to be interpreted as punishment for some wrongdoing. The child aged 7 to 11 may understand illness better, but he or she has also begun to formulate a concept of death and may reasonably fear his or her own demise. The adolescent can understand explanations about procedures or his or her illness, but often he or she fears disfigurement, handicap, or death as a result. These criteria provide guidelines, but individual assessment is necessary since hospital- or illness-related regression may cause the child to function at a lower level than chronologic age would imply.

Perceptions of the ICU can be variable, depending on the child's cognitive level. The child is exposed to confusing and potentially disturbing sights and sounds—children who are disfigured by bruises or swelling or attached to machines, and equipment that to the child may resemble torture devices. The child may also encounter children unclothed, children crying, and children struggling. In his or her attempt to make sense of the distressing sights and sounds, the child may assume blame for the "bad" or perplexing scenes that he or she witnesses, or the child may expect that what happened to a neighbor will also happen to him or her. The child may be frightened when he or she hears another child cry, or the child may assume that he or she cannot live without being connected to a monitor. Communication is the only way to discern these perceptions and to determine when further explanation or reassurance is necessary. The goal is for the child to integrate these experiences in a way that he or she can understand them so that resolution occurs. Mastery will then be accomplished, and the potential for emotional sequelae will be greatly reduced.

The child's temperament also plays a part in determining his or her adjustment to the ICU. Children enter this stressful situation with a pre-established pattern of dealing with difficulties, with certain sensitivities, and with certain strengths. For example, the child who usually copes by gathering information and retaining control will be more frustrated in the ICU than the child who usually copes by withdrawing or denying.

Stressors in the ICU in part determine the child's adjustment. The more stressors that are present, the greater will be the drain on the child's resources. Lack of diurnal variation, lack of familiar sensory stimulation (e.g., no window, no objects reminiscent of home, contact with multiple strangers, absence of parents), multiple intrusive procedures, inability to predict stressful events—all of these can consume a child's ability to cope. The specific developmental level may increase a child's vulnerability to certain stressors. The infant, for example, is extremely sensitive to separation from his or her mother or primary caregiver. The toddler is vulnerable to separation, lack of predictability, and intrusive procedures. The preschool and school-aged child is vulnerable to the lack of privacy, lack of sleep, and lack of connection with familiar people and surroundings. The adolescent is stressed by all of the preceding and by an understanding of the seriousness of the threat that the ICU poses.

The support offered by family and ICU staff can be factors that mediate the stress for the child and thus affect the child's adjustment to the ICU. In the best possible situation, parents are readily available and emotionally attuned to their child's needs and are capable of offering their child reassurance. Staff can also affect adaptation by giving age-appropriate information, preparing the child for procedures, involving the child in his or her care, and providing for normalizing experiences.

The Family

A child's admission to the ICU precipitates a crisis for the family. The parents initially feel shocked and numbed by the sudden overwhelming threat to their child's well-being. In this phase, parents' responses may be dulled, and questions may be absent or minimal while they try to comprehend what has happened to their child. They then begin a search for meaning and begin to question everything—"what could have caused this; what could have prevented this; why my child; why me; why now; what can I do; will my child die?" Parents may ask these questions of themselves and others over and over again as they attempt to make sense of the tragedy that has befallen them. Information that they begin to receive about their child's illness or injury may be so overwhelming that they need to deny the seriousness of the threat to their child. This denial may be frustrating to hospital staff who wish to help the family move toward acceptance of the situation; but this process of anticipatory grieving is one that must proceed at its own rate. Differences in rate and response may exist between the parents, and frequently these differences become a source of marital conflict during this period of heightened tensions. Parents may also develop a sense of guilt that they were unable to protect their child or that they are being punished for some prior transgression. While this guilt may help move the parent to the point of problem solving, excessive guilt may have the opposite effect, paralyzing the parents and impairing their ability to cope. Anger or depression may follow, resulting in distancing and emotional unavailability to the child.

Since parents are the most important source of comfort to the child in the ICU and because psychologic fallout from this ICU experience may affect families for years to come (separations and divorces are not uncommon after the family has undergone such a traumatic experience), attention must be given to the parents' coping. A social worker should meet with each family to provide support and guidance in their coping efforts, and medical staff must keep the family informed. Communication serves several important functions: (1) it is the foundation of the family's relationship with their child's physician; (2) it provides a link to the ICU system; (3) it can provide a stabilizing force for the family; and (4) it demonstrates to the family that their child's case is important. To be most effective, communication should be the responsibility of one physician. A primary nurse working with the child and family can alleviate anxiety and promote adaptation by providing consistency in care and information and, most important, by connecting with this family in an empathic relationship. Child life staff, chaplaincy staff, and psychiatric consultation liaison staff should also be available to assist the child and family with adjustment.

Siblings are also under stress during this time of crisis. They are often confused because no information or incomplete information is shared with them in attempt to "spare" them. In fact, they are quite aware of the tension in the household and the disrupted routines. Without information, siblings are left to imagine their own reality. They may begin to think that their sibling is dead, that they are somehow responsible, or that whatever happened to the sibling may soon happen to them. These fears arise at a time when parents are unavailable to reassure them. They may resent the parents' frequent absences and the special attention that the sick child is getting. All of these concerns must be dealt with sensitively. Efforts to help the parents cope will ultimately help siblings as well, but parents may need guidance and direct intervention for the siblings. Child life or psychiatry services can be helpful in these cases.

Some parents will come to the ICU with pre-existing psychopathology. The disorder may be clear with prior diagnosis and treatment or it may be latent and made manifest by the stress of the ICU admission. These parents can be especially draining to the ICU staff. In such cases, it is essential that staff remember that difficult behaviors are a parent's "best efforts" at coping, and they should not be taken personally. These behaviors may be contained by appointing one physician and one nurse as communication links, setting limits on abusive or out-of-control behavior, and using security support if the parent needs additional external restraint.

When available, other more healthy family members may be enlisted to help the disturbed parent seek psychiatric care. Ethically sound care also demands that this situation be handled nonjudgmentally.

A special consideration when dealing with parents with major psychiatric disorders is the concern that a child's illness or injury is caused by the parent. Although the issue of abuse is dealt with elsewhere (see Chapter 90), the specific entity of Munchhausen syndrome-by-proxy must be mentioned. In this disorder, physical illness in a child is induced or fabricated in order to give the parent access to and attention from medical professionals. Unfortunately, this parental disturbance may be difficult to recognize and difficult to treat.

Staff

For most staff, the ICU provides opportunity for excitement, stimulation, challenge, and status. Making judgments and interventions that save lives is a daily occurrence. But loss, disfigurement, and dehumanization are also inherent in the ICU experience and can take their toll on the staff. Staff members may respond with detachment, denial of feelings, overt depression, stress-related physical disorders, or impaired clinical judgment. These responses only serve to alienate them from colleagues who could offer support. In fact, staff members sometimes isolate themselves further by devaluing those around them to avoid further pain of loss. The environment is one of constant flux, thus detachment is perpetuated by the system. Occasionally, staff members go to the other extreme in that they become overinvested in a family or child, they take on an adversarial role in the name of "patient advocacy," or they disparage other staff to a family member.

As staff members become more isolated from each other, they also become targets for each other's frustrations. Latent tensions become open conflicts, and this interpersonal friction increases the general stress level and encourages a vicious cycle. Deviations from the norm can become the reason for group sanction and scapegoating. Subgroups split off and compete with other subgroups. The system can become totally dysfunctional and can impair the workings of the ICU. Interruption of this cycle occurs with repeated focused attempts at collaborative team effort and communication. Staff members need to have a personal plan for managing their stress as well.

The Environment

The ICU environment itself adds another variable to the issue of adjustment to a critical illness. Most ICUs are large, open, and quite busy with a multitude of stimuli. The child and family are exposed to an overwhelming array of technical equipment, an overload of information, and a variety of anxiety-provoking sights and sounds. At a time when a child and family are most vulnerable, the very setting that is meant to help unfortunately becomes a stressor.

While the need for humanization cannot take precedence over the need for the most efficient and functional clinical setting possible, it is important for ICU staff to remain aware of the specific problems that their workplace creates.

The sensory input that a child experiences can be both too great and too little. The sight of innumerable staff who are always busy, the possible view of other patients, and the sounds of equipment can all be overstimulating, while at the same time the child can feel isolated and alone. The multitude of intensive procedures, the constant care, the confusing language, and the limited availability of family members are all frightening. There is little to provide a sense of night and day with the constant activity, and often there are no orienting effects of daylight, meals, or sleep. Despite all the obstacles, recognition of the problems and an understanding of the child and family can help the staff to minimize the negative emotional effects of the ICU experience.

Psychosocial Care in the Intensive Care Unit

With the multitude of potential emotional problems the ICU is an ideal setting for an interdisciplinary approach to patient care. All members of the ICU staff as well as outside consultants can help to reduce the negative impact on the child and family.

Physicians and nurses can tailor their approaches to the patient once they are aware of the specific developmental issues and how a child perceives the hospital environment. An understanding of how to approach the child, what words will be understood, and what will support the family will help the physician to address emotional issues accompanying the medical problem.

Nurses, by nature of their ongoing presence with patients and family, are the ideal agents for helping the child to adapt by being available to educate and reassure, and by understanding important concerns and relaying them to other staff. The social worker, who is an integral part of the ICU staff, is necessary to provide support for parents and to help with concrete family-related problems that have an enormous negative impact on a family in crisis.

The child life specialist in the ICU can be instrumental in psychosocial care by providing the child with an outlet for feelings and concerns and can be seen by the child as a safe staff member who does not perform medical procedures. The child life worker can also help by providing therapeutic play and important age-appropriate distractions from the difficult medical experience.

The role of the child psychiatrist is an important one, and the psychiatrist can have a number of potential roles. Direct patient intervention includes an evaluation of patients and families for problems such as psychosis, behavioral disturbances, depression, and suicidal ideation as well as the provision of a variety of interventions

(e.g., pharmacologic or psychotherapeutic interventions). In addition, the psychiatrist can work closely with nursing, medical, child life, and social work staff to help address adjustment problems for the child and parents. In many cases the psychiatrist can work with the staff to help resolve difficult situations and to alleviate tension in the ICU.

Emotional Sequelae

Emotional behavioral responses may be manifested long after the patient is discharged from the ICU. Often, there is a delayed emotional reaction on the part of the child as the acute phase of an illness passes and the demands on adaptation to intensive medical care and procedures are no longer present. In the time immediately following the critical period, the child may be overly cautious and may fear a recurrence of his or her illness. The child may exhibit a variety of behavior and emotions not demonstrated earlier, based on generalized anxiety and specific confusion about the illness, its causes, and its effects. During this later period, the child is often more available to help in dealing with the emotional effects of a serious illness, thus providing the hospital and the child's family with an opportunity to achieve emotional adjustment.

In some cases, both short- and long-term adjustment are compromised, and the child may exhibit a post-traumatic stress disorder. In months after a serious emotional stressor, the child may manifest symptoms such as a preoccupation with illness or injury, recurrent nightmares, generalized anxiety, hypervigilance, irritability, and emotionality. The stimulus for this long-term problem with adjustment may be not only the illness or injury itself but also the unavoidably stressful experience of the ICU itself. It is often helpful to prepare parents for the possibility of these reactions and to help them to anticipate delayed reactions.

Parents, too, have the potential for long-term adjustment problems. The stress of the experience of having a critically ill child can stimulate anxiety and depression and can have a potentially negative effect on a marriage. Families often respond to the experience with guilt, and even in the absence of physical sequelae this can cause parents to unnecessarily view their child as one who is vulnerable and needs to be protected. The potential for a maladaptive parent-child relationship in this situation is great and needs to be anticipated and to receive appropriate intervention.

THE DYING CHILD

It is an unfortunate reality of critical care pediatrics that death is not a rare occurrence. The prospect of possible death presents the child, parents, and ICU staff with significant problems and challenges.

In order to deal effectively with these challenges it is important to understand the child's concept of death, which progresses somewhat predictably with increasing age. Before 6 years of age, children view death in a way that demonstrates their inability to understand its full impact. They believe that death is a temporary and reversible state, and they focus primarily on the thought of not being with their family. In addition, the fear of discomfort and pain are major concerns. Thus for the child under 6 years of age, anxiety about separation, pain, and bodily injury are paramount. The young child is also susceptible to parental anxiety and will react with more anxiety as parents do. Between 7 and 12 years of age, children begin to understand the reality and irreversibility of death but do not conceptualize it with complete abstract understanding. This child sees death as a final, permanent separation and may be able to begin to use cultural and religious concepts of life after death.

In general, discussions about death with children under 6 years of age meet with concrete responses, if any at all; talk about death tends to be nonproductive or to increase the anxiety of everyone involved. On the other hand, the older child or adolescent can benefit from talking about his or her thoughts and feelings about death. Even if the older child has not been told, he or she is alert to the reaction of the family and staff and is aware of changes in his or her treatment. Questions about death are never easy for family and staff, and invariably they come at the least opportune time. Medical staff must be able to approach the issue in a way that addresses the multitude of feelings that the child has and in a manner that is in keeping with parental wishes.

The dying child in the ICU is often not alert, and thus intervention is directed at the parents. However, frequently a child does hear discussions about his or her care when staff and family think that the child is not alert. Therefore, it should be assumed that a child can hear and understand what is said. When the child is alert and able to communicate, one must be aware of a number of issues related to death and be able to attend to questions about these issues. Questions often relate to a sense of being punished for perceived wrong-doing, concern about the experience of dying, concern for family, and discomfort with feelings of anger or depression.

The parent's response to the death of a child can vary dramatically depending on the length of the illness; the circumstances surrounding the illness; and multiple family factors, including parents' own personality characteristics, the support system available, and past experience with death. The ability to deal with the death of one's child is possibly the most difficult task that a parent can face. Some parents are so overwhelmed that they cannot accept the idea and thus have trouble being available to the dying child, spouse, and other children. Ideally, parents should be able to discuss death with their children; but if this is not possible and parents give permission, someone else may need to help the child directly.

At times, when death follows a long progressive illness, parents may gradually become more able to address the issue of death and engage in anticipatory grieving that allows the parent the time to progress at his or her own pace. In the case of a sudden illness or injury, the initial reactions may be more pronounced.

Upon learning the news of impending death, a parent will react with disbelief and shock, followed by denial and avoidance. Periods of depression and withdrawal are common. Many styles of coping with the extreme stress spring from guilt, anxiety, and frustration, producing withdrawal, intrusion, criticism, seeking of further medical opinions, and finally progress to a more workable regret and acceptance of the inevitable outcome. Some parents have extreme reactions in which they become physically unavailable or emotionally overwhelmed with panic or depression.

Whatever the reaction, it is necessary for ICU staff to remain nonjudgmental, to be available to support parents, and to understand the extreme assault on a person's psyche when presented with the death of a child. The ICU staff can thus attempt to understand underlying emotions rather than to react to behavior caused by those emotions. The majority of grieving is accomplished after the child's death and is therefore not a process that includes the ICU staff. It is important to ensure that someone will monitor the family's grieving process after the hospital experience. This can be done by a primary care physician, clergyman, or other family members. Some institutions have a follow-up protocol to monitor the adjustment of families and can intervene when necessary.

An often forgotten part of the family during this time of crisis is the dying child's sibling. The sibling often experiences confusion about the patient's hospitalization. He or she is unable to understand something that he or she cannot see and must cope with this uncertainty often in the absence of his or her parents. The sibling may feel a sense of guilt for the illness and hospitalization and often becomes depressed, wishing to take the place of the patient. There is a strange ambivalence between anger toward the sick child, envy of the attention that he or she receives, and sadness regarding the illness. When considering the acute and long-term adjustment of a family to the death of a child, there needs to be active consideration of psychosocial intervention to assure healthy adjustment of siblings.

The issue of allowing a sibling to visit the dying child is an important one that should be addressed by staff and parents. The wish to protect the child from the possibly overwhelming impact of the ICU needs to be balanced with the potential benefit of a visit to the child. In general, older children who can process the experience should be encouraged to visit if they themselves are truly willing and have family support to help them deal with the experience.

The response of the ICU staff should not be ignored when considering the dying child. Many other hospital staff think that the ICU staff become accustomed to dying children and thus forget that death takes its toll on all concerned. It is important for all caregivers to be alert to their own emotional response to this group of patients and to how these reactions can affect patient care. Impatience with parents, withdrawal from the patient, and conflict with other staff members can all occur during these difficult times. It is helpful for all staff to have a forum to process the complex reactions to the death of a patient, thus maintaining their usefulness to families and avoiding being overwhelmed personally by the experience.

DELIRIUM

Some children exhibit changes in behavior that go beyond the realm of adjustment to the intensive care experience, demonstrating abnormal or bizarre behavior often described as "ICU psychosis." The distorted thinking, hallucinations, delusions, disorientation, agitation, and panic are signs of delirium and need to be viewed as a transient derangement of cerebral function rather than as adjustment problems in the extreme, producing a psychotic state. The characteristic mental status changes in delirium need to be considered as an indication of an encephalopathic process and may be the earliest or most prominent sign of medical deterioration. If delirium is not recognized, this could prevent the timely identification and treatment of the underlying physiologic condition. In addition, an untreated delirium not only creates fear in the child and a sense of anxiety and frustration in parents and medical staff but also presents the possibility of the patient causing self-injury or interfering with medical care by such acts as self-extubation or other potentially dangerous behavior.

The diagnosis of delirium depends on a careful clinical evaluation. The symptoms vary with the age of the patient (Table 68–2). At all ages, symptoms tend to wax and wane, especially in the severe and less-pronounced cases. In young children, a lack of responsiveness to comfort measures or apathy can be the initial signs of delirium. Signs of distress such as irritability, crying, fearfulness, or hypervigilance may be early indicators of encephalopathy. The child may become preoccupied with fearful creatures and may also have accompanying visual hallucinations.

In older children, a more formal mental status examination may be combined with observations of other staff to elicit the more classic signs of delirium. Disordered thinking (including decreased attention; disorganization of speech; visual, auditory, or tactile hallucinations) and memory impairment may occur. Changes in

Table 68–3. POSSIBLE CONTRIBUTORS TO ORGANIC BRAIN SYNDROMES

Infection
Head trauma
Brain trauma
Metabolic imbalance
Fluid and electrolyte disturbance
Fever
Hypoxia and anoxia
Medication
General anesthesia
Sleep deprivation
Vasculitis

the level of consciousness or sleep disturbance and changes in motoric activity add to the concern about delirium. The child may also have increased autonomic activity, and an electroencephalogram will demonstrate diffuse slow-wave activity.

Once delirium is diagnosed, the primary intervention is the treatment of the underlying cause. Any medical disorder that can cause an encephalopathic process must be considered (Table 68–3). The most common causes are drug toxicity (Table 68–4), infection, metabolic or fluid and electrolyte disturbances, and hypoxia. Other causes such as head injury, space-occupying lesions, sleep deprivation, postoperative states, and drug withdrawal need also to be considered. Although not directly the cause of delirium, environmental factors may contribute to or exacerbate the condition. Symptoms of delirium may worsen with sleep deprivation inherent in the ICU; the sensory overstimulation resulting from sound and activity may also exacerbate the condition directly, as may the lack of orienting effects of day or night variation and the presence of familiar people.

The treatment of delirium is multidimensional. The primary goal is the correction of the underlying process. In addition to treating the cause, the symptoms of delirium can also be addressed. Environmental interventions that are commonly suggested as part of a psychiatric consultation are normalization of the environment with a decrease in stimulation, an increase in contact with staff and family, and a focus on continuous orientation. In addition, if there is a need to decrease

Table 68–2. CLINICAL ASPECTS OF DELIRIUM

Disordered thinking:	Visual, tactile, or auditory hallucinations, delusions of persecution, and extreme fears
Changes in cognition:	Misperceptions and distortions of environment, decreased attention, inability to focus, inability to understand, and memory impairment
Changes in consciousness:	Lethargy or agitation, somnolence or insomnia, and waxing and waning of consciousness
Presentation:	Worsens at night, develops over a short time, and varies with medical condition

Table 68–4. MEDICATIONS CAUSING PSYCHIATRIC SYMPTOMS

Psychosis:	Withdrawal of sedative-hypnotics and alcohol, antidepressants, CNS* stimulants, cimetidine, corticosteroids, indomethacin, anticonvulsants, aminophylline, hallucinogens, opiates, and ketamine
Anxiety/confusion:	Anticholinergics, anticonvulsants, CNS stimulants, drug withdrawal, cimetidine, corticosteroids, diazepam, digoxin, hydralazine, propranolol, sympathomimetics, thyroid hormones, tricyclic antidepressants, and anesthesia
Depression:	Cimetidine, corticosteroids, diazepam, digoxin, indomethacin, lidocaine, methyldopa, propranolol, and reserpine

*CNS = central nervous system.

agitation, and if sedation is necessary to facilitate medical care, psychotropic medication may be used. Benzodiazepines are often used; however, given the cortical effects of these agents, there is the potential for an exacerbation or prolongation of symptoms, especially with longer-acting agents such as diazepam. If hallucinations or delusions are present or in the case of severe agitation, neuroleptic agents such as haloperidol or chlorpromazine are effective in relatively low doses. Fortunately, in most cases acute confusional states are relatively short lived.

DEPRESSION

Many children in the ICU have a variety of emotional reactions that can include sadness related to pain, discomfort, worry about physical condition, fear of a frightening new environment, and separation from familiar surroundings and people. However, a child's change in mood can go beyond the expected sadness in response to a stressor and can become an exaggerated response that can be characterized as a clinical depression. As was described previously, the signs and symptoms of any emotional response depend on the child's age and developmental stage. In the infant and toddler the depression is characterized by irritability and crying, progressing to listlessness, withdrawal, and lack of response. Generally, these symptoms respond to environmental manipulation; when they do not respond, the possible pre-existence of developmental delays or a deprivation syndrome needs to be assessed.

Older children may manifest symptoms that are more clearly "depressive" (Table 68–5). With increasing age, children progress from primarily demonstrating depressive symptoms to gradually being nonverbal about depressing feelings. The evaluation of depression involves both careful observation by all staff members and thorough clinical psychiatric assessment. Important factors that should be considered in addition to observed symptoms and subjective reports by the child are a number of historical risk factors, such as prior emotional difficulties including depression, family dysfunction, developmental disorders (learning disabilities, mental retardation, attention deficit disorder), and a family history of psychiatric disturbance (depression, anxiety disorders, alcoholism, or psychosis). In addition, an assessment of the child's premorbid functioning and his or her ability to cope with prior hospitalization or other stressful events can be quite helpful.

Once a child is identified as being depressed, the decision of how and when to treat the child becomes important. The salient issue is not one of deciding between formal psychiatric consultation or no treatment at all but rather what level of intervention will be necessary at what time. As with any clinical problem, one must assess the level of subjective discomfort, the degree to which the symptoms interfere with medical care, and the possibility of recovery once the medical stressor is removed.

Treatment of the depressed child in the ICU can be challenging. The effect of physical illness on mood can be dramatic, and illness that involves the central nervous system can dramatically decrease coping skills based on higher mental functioning. The first step in treatment is manipulation of the environment when possible. Attempts to normalize the environment, such as increasing parental visits, the introduction of familiar objects from home, and an increase in activity, can be extremely helpful. In addition, successful treatment of the medical problem with a resultant decrease in stressful procedures and an increase in physical comfort will help. Direct intervention by mental health staff using play, art, and talking therapies can be of tremendous benefit. This intervention can be supportive and can help the child to express underlying concerns, often providing some relief of depressive symptoms. Supportive work with depressed, overwhelmed parents is also necessary in conjunction with direct psychotherapy with children.

The use of medication to treat depression in children in the ICU should come only after a careful evaluation and should be used in conjunction with psychotherapy. The decision to use medication is dependent on the severity of the symptoms (withdrawal and neurovegetative signs) and on the level of interference with medical care. Pharmacologic agents that can be used include tricyclic antidepressants and, less frequently, psychostimulants. The benefits of the psychostimulants can be the rapidity of their effect and their lack of some of the potentially serious side effects (anticholinergic and cardiovascular) of the tricyclic antidepressants. The use of pharmacologic agents in medically ill children is rare, and these agents should be used only after having a child psychiatric consultation.

SUICIDE

The issue of self-inflicted injury is not a foreign one in pediatric critical care. Although suicide attempts and completed suicides are certainly more common in adolescents, there are some preadolescent children who injure themselves intentionally. Children and adolescents who attempt suicide (especially those with more serious attempts) are cared for if only for a brief period in an intensive care setting. This is often the only opportunity for psychiatric attention, and thus the pediatrician's alertness to the issue is instrumental in obtaining a psychiatric consultation. The patient who

Table 68–5. SYMPTOMS OF DEPRESSION IN CHILDREN

Mood disturbance:	Sadness, crying spells, hopelessness, helplessness, loss of interest, self-deprecation, morbid preoccupations, and guilt feelings
Behavior disturbance:	Irritability, attention seeking, withdrawal, and decreased motivation
Neurovegetative symptoms:	Insomnia, hypersomnia, appetite disturbance, and diminished concentration
Suicidal ideation:	Preoccupation with death, suicidal thoughts, and self-injurious actions

makes a suicide attempt, no matter how benign medically, is at significantly increased risk for attempting a future successful suicide. As many as 10% of adolescent males admitted to psychiatric hospitals following a serious suicide attempt will subsequently die by suicide. This mandates both the skills to assess a patient's potential for suicide and to provide access to psychiatric consultation. In addition, a high index of suspicion for suicide attempts in injuries that are not presented as intentionally self-inflicted but that may be of a suspicious nature is necessary. The wish to deny or hide a suicide attempt by the patient or family needs to be resisted by medical caregivers. Thus, automobile accidents, falls, and "accidental" ingestions all need to be evaluated carefully.

The evaluation of the potential for suicide is as important as is the medical care of the patient with a self-inflicted injury. An inquiry about a patient's suicidal ideation does not stimulate suicidal thought where it did not exist but can be reassuring to the suicidal patient; this topic must be addressed directly. It is crucial to assess the intent behind the suicide attempt. The subjective intent is as important as the objective severity of the act. The details of the attempt, the potential for rescue, the degree of the wish to die, and the relief or resentment of survival are all important aspects of the evaluation.

During the patient's stay in the hospital, the intensive care medical and nursing staff have an important role in the psychiatric care as well as medical care of the patient. Observations about the patient's mood, cooperation, and interaction with staff and parents as well as observations about family functioning all provide valuable information to the psychiatric consultant. A supportive, available physician and nurse can help to make the patient more comfortable and open to psychiatric intervention.

While proceeding with medical care and a psychiatric assessment, the safety of the patient from other suicidal acts is imperative. Close observation is necessary until one can assess not only the severity of the attempt but also the degree of risk for further attempts.

Risk factors for suicidality that need to be identified are:

1. Depression
2. Psychosis
3. Substance abuse
4. Prior suicide attempts
5. Family history of suicidal behavior
6. Recent loss
7. Family discord
8. Delinquency
9. History of impulsivity

The presence of these factors must be assessed as part of a psychiatric evaluation. Most children and adolescents who need hospitalization in an intensive care setting following a suicide attempt will need a period of observation and evaluation in a psychiatric inpatient setting once they are medically stable. Only low-risk patients with clearly supportive families will be able to return home, and then only if clear plans are in place for follow-up within days of discharge from the hospital. The child and family must be able to make a contract for the patient's safety without doubt.

The critical care physician must be steadfast in his or her resolve to objectively recommend appropriate care once the patient is medically stable and should not be influenced by patient or parental denial or minimalization. Legal and social service support must be utilized when needed to obtain necessary care for the patient.

PAIN MANAGEMENT

Management of pain, though described elsewhere (see Chapter 81), deserves mention here because of its impact on the child's psychologic adaptation. The experience of pain is frightening to a child, and this trauma is one that practitioners can minimize. Health care professionals have moved beyond outdated beliefs that children do not feel pain, that children forget pain, or that children can tolerate pain better than adults. Better methods of assessing a child's pain and better techniques for controlling it are being developed. The ICU practitioner with IV access for each child has a wide variety of pharmacologic options and a mode of delivery that is both effective and inoffensive to the child. Liberal use of narcotics in the ICU setting is the humane approach, and tolerance is managed by increasing the dose or frequency of the medication. A child's physical dependency on the medication should not be a cause of concern, because it can be easily managed by gradually tapering the dose when narcotics are no longer needed.

Other supportive pain management interventions can alleviate the child's anxiety and promote mastery in the ICU setting. Anxiety can greatly increase pain perception; conversely, a decrease of anxiety can promote comfort by decreasing the subjective experience of pain. Anxiety management should never be a substitute for analgesia, but the wise practitioner uses it as an adjunct to analgesia. For the infant and toddler, kinesthetic interventions such as rocking or rhythmic rubbing of the affected part can provide a measure of comfort. Parental presence and provision for sucking can alleviate pain, as also can soothing music. For the preschool child, measures such as distraction during procedures and allowing the child some element of control can decrease pain perception. The school-aged child can use relaxation techniques and hypnosis to assist in managing pain; and the adolescent can use even more complex techniques, such as thought stoppage, to control pain and anxiety during procedures. Therefore, by blending pharmacologic and nonpharmacologic methods, medical staff can optimize pain relief and promote mastery and psychologic adaptation for the child in the ICU.

Bibliography

Behrman RE and Vaughan VC: Psychiatric considerations of central nervous system injury. In Behrman RE and Vaughan VC (eds): Nelson Textbook of Pediatrics, 13th ed. Philadelphia, WB Saunders, 1987, p. 55.

Biederman J and Jellinek MS: Psychopharmacology in children. N Engl J Med 310:968–972, 1984.

Green M and Solnit AJ: Reactions to the threatened loss of a child: A vulnerable child syndrome. Pediatrics 34:58, 1964.

Jellinek MS and Herzog D: Psychiatric Aspects of General Hospital Pediatrics. Chicago, Year Book Medical Publishers, 1990.

Jost E and Haase JE: At the time of death: Help for the child's parents. Children's Health Care 18(6):146–152, 1989.

Lipowski ZJ: Delirium (acute confusional states). JAMA 258:1789–1792, 1988.

McGrath P: Pain in Children and Adolescents. New York, Elsevier Science, 1987.

Perrin EC and Gerrity PS: There's a demon in your belly: Children's understanding of illness. Pediatrics 67(6):841–849, 1981.

Ross DM and Ross SA: Childhood Pain: Current Issues, Research and Management. Baltimore, Urban & Schwarzenberg, 1988.

Rutter M and Hersov L: Child and Adolescent Psychiatry. Oxford, Blackwell Scientific Publications, 1987.

Shaffer D, Garland A, Gould M, et al: Preventing teenage suicide: A critical review. J Am Acad Child Adolesc Psychiatry 27:675–687, 1988.

Tichy AM, Braam CM, Meyer TA, and Rattan NS: Stressors in pediatric intensive care units. Pediatr Nurs 14:40–42, 1988.

V Infectious Disease

69

Prevention of Nosocomial Infections

Nalini Singh-Naz, M.D., and
William J. Rodriguez, M.D., Ph.D.

Nosocomial infections result in increased morbidity and mortality, prolonged hospitalization, and increased direct and indirect patient care costs. Recent advances in critical care medicine ensure the survival of many critically ill patients. However, their recovery is frequently complicated by nosocomial infection. The incidence of infections in pediatric intensive care units (PICU) is second only to that in neonatal intensive care units (NICU). Infection rates in these units range from 6 to 20 per 100 patient discharges (mean of 13.1).[1-3] Even these figures may underestimate the true nosocomial infection rate, because the intensity and type of routine surveillance varies from one institution to another. Additionally, information may have been gathered only from chart reviews during hospitalization or from review of microbiologic reports of positive results on cultures. Many viral infections can go undiagnosed in the absence of full virology laboratory support; furthermore, extended follow-up of these patients after hospitalization may identify other nosocomial infections acquired at the end of the hospital stay. Nosocomial infection rates are influenced by the host, agent, and environmental factors. Host and agent factors are covered in detail in Chapter 70.

HOST AND AGENT FACTORS

The highest rate of infection occurs in infants younger than 24 months of age. This may be due, in part, to an immature immunologic status. Alternatively, host immunologic status may be impaired owing to primary disease processes or to therapeutic interventions that increase the risk of infection. Children with leukemia receiving immunosuppressive drugs or with bone marrow transplantation frequently acquire bacterial, fungal, and viral infections. Risk factors associated with infections in these patients include central venous catheters and intraventricular devices.

Another recently recognized host factor is severity of illness. In the context of the intensive care unit, severity of illness is usually considered as physiologic stability.[4] There is an association between high pediatric risk of mortality (PRISM) score with nosocomial infection.[5, 6] In a study of patients undergoing cardiovascular surgery, a major factor in the development of wound infection was a PRISM score equal to or more than 10. In this study, severity of illness as measured by a PRISM score was significantly associated with the future development of infection.

AGENT FACTORS

Data from the author's institution show that the pathogens most commonly involved in nosocomial infections in the PICU are gram-negative organisms (42%), followed by gram-positive organisms (32%), and fungal organisms (16%), clinical sepsis (7%) and viral pathogens (3%) (Fig. 69–1). The most prevalent gram-negative organisms are *Pseudomonas aeruginosa* and *Enterobacter* sp., which cause respiratory and genitourinary tract infections.

In patients with nosocomial sepsis, however, gram-positive organisms predominate (61%) (Fig. 69–2). Coagulase-negative organisms are predominantly responsible for systemic infections. These data are consistent with other PICUs.[2] These pathogens cause sepsis (29%), tracheitis (22%), urinary tract infection (18%), and pneumonia (8%). The remaining sites are divided (1 to 3%) among conjunctiva, gastrointestinal tract, middle ear, peritoneal cavity, sinuses, and soft tissue (Fig. 69–3). It is interesting that the distribution of organisms causing nosocomial infection in PICUs differs from that in NICUs. This may be due in part to different risk factors (e.g., age, birthweight, underlying disease, and duration of hospitalization) (Fig. 69–4).

ENVIRONMENTAL FACTORS

The risk of infection increases with increased length of stay, up to 10.9% after 2 weeks of hospitalization in

Gram + ☐ Gram − ☐ Fungal ☐ Cult. − ☐ Viral

☰ LRES ☐ OTHER ☒ PNEU ☒ SYS ☒ URES ☐ GU

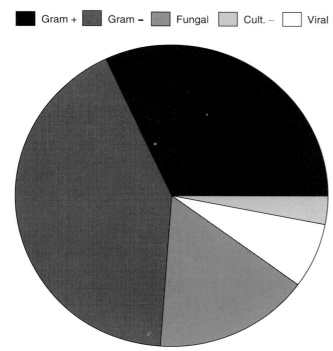

Figure 69–1. Distribution of organisms in the pediatric intensive care unit at Children's National Medical Center, Washington, DC, from 1989 to 1990 (Singh-Naz/Cantwell unpublished data). Gram negative 42%; gram positive 32%; fungal 16%; culture negative/clinical sepsis 7%; and viral 3%.

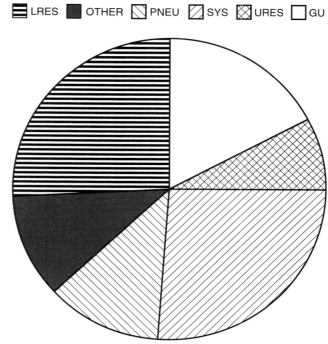

Figure 69–3. Distribution of infection by body site in PICU patients at Children's National Medical Center, Washington, DC, from 1989 to 1990 (Singh-Naz/Cantwell unpublished data). Sepsis (bloodstream) (SYS) 26%; lower respiratory tract/tracheitis (LRES) 26%; genitourinary (GU) 17%; pneumonia (PNEU) 12%; upper respiratory tract/sinusitis (URES) 8%. See text for the other 11%.

Gram + ☐ Gram − ☐ Fungal ☐ Cult. −

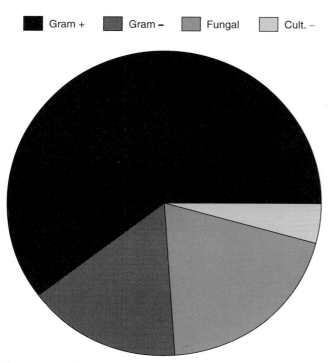

Figure 69–2. Distribution of organisms in sepsis at the pediatric intensive care unit in Children's National Medical Center, Washington, DC, from 1989 to 1990 (Singh-Naz/Cantwell unpublished data). Gram positive 61%; gram negative 16%; fungal 20%; and culture negative/clinical sepsis 3%.

Gram + ☐ Gram − ☐ Fungal ☐ Cult. − ☐ Viral

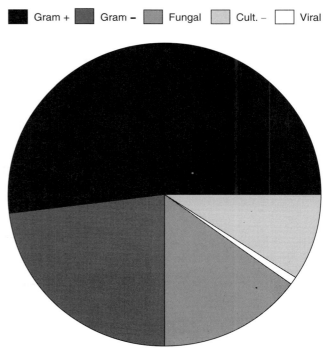

Figure 69–4. Distribution of organisms in NICU at Children's National Medical Center, Washington, DC, from 1989 to 1990 (Singh-Naz/Cantwell unpublished data). Gram positive 52%; gram negative 23%; fungal 15%; viral 1%; and culture negative/clinical sepsis 9%.

the ICU and 50% after 1 month.[3] While it is possible that severely ill patients require more invasive support and, therefore, are at higher risk of acquiring infection, it is also true that there is a longer exposure to the nosocomial milieu of the ICU. Guidelines for control of nosocomial infection have been developed and implemented by various infection control programs. The remainder of this chapter focuses on environmental controls designed to reduce nosocomial infection in patients as well as on policies designed to reduce the risk of transmission of infections to health care workers.

Infection Control Policies

Isolation Rooms

Patients infected with diseases in which air-borne transmission is likely (e.g., chicken pox and measles) should be in rooms with negative-pressure ventilation. Isolation precautions requiring a private room are often modified in the ICU when air-borne transmission is not likely (e.g., with respiratory syncytial virus or para influenza virus). Isolation areas for these patients can be demarcated by partitions, and appropriate isolation signs can be posted.

Immunosuppressed patients (e.g., bone marrow and cardiac transplants) requiring intensive care should be isolated in rooms with positive pressure and high-efficiency particulate air (HEPA) filters.

Construction has been associated with outbreaks of aspergillosis.[7] To decrease the risk of aspergillosis in immunocompromised patients, several control measures should be instituted at any construction site. Hospital construction activity should be coordinated with the infection control office. General measures should include construction of airtight plastic and drywall barriers at the construction site, use of negative-pressure ventilation in the work area, and decontamination of the work area with [8]Cu-quinolinolate.[7] Frequent cleaning of the work area is necessary if it is to be used for patients while the room's under construction. Patients who are immunocompromised should not go to areas under construction.

Universal and Isolation Precautions

Universal precautions for blood and body fluids must be used in the care of all patients to reduce the risk of transmission of blood-borne pathogens to health care workers.[8] Universal precautions supplement routine infection control practices (e.g., hand washing). Protective barriers (e.g., gloves, masks, and eye wear) reduce the risk of exposure to blood and body fluids. Some judgment must be exercised in clinical situations as to what type of barrier should be used.

In addition to universal precautions, specific isolation precautions (e.g., category/disease specific) must be used in patients with suspected or diagnosed communicable infections, whether community acquired or nosocomial.[8, 9] Protective isolation using disposable, polypropylene gowns, and latex gloves used in care of high-risk

children in the PICU has been shown to reduce the incidence of nosocomial infection without compromising patient care.[10]

Needle Stick Prevention Program

Needle stick injuries account for a large number of work-related accidents in hospitals. Such injuries continue to be a serious concern in transmission of blood-borne infections (e.g., hepatitis B and human immunodeficiency virus [HIV]). These injuries occur usually during manipulation or recapping of needles in the clinical setting. Support staff may sustain injuries as a result of improperly discarded needles. After use, needles should not be recapped, but should be placed in puncture-resistant units instead.

The American Hospital Association has developed several educational programs related to infection control, universal precautions, and needle stick prevention.[9, 11] Health care workers should receive appropriate training in infection control and universal precautions practices as mandated by Occupational Safety and Health Administration (OSHA) and Joint Commission Accreditation of Hospitals Organization (JCAHO). All health care workers should be cognizant of and adhere to employee health policies.

PREVENTION OF INTRAVASCULAR INFECTION

The length of time in situ of intravascular lines should be carefully monitored and managed with strict aseptic measures. There is a strong correlation between the overall nosocomial infection patient day rate and device use (e.g., central intravascular catheter).[12] The device use of an ICU may also serve as a marker for severity of illness of patients in the unit (i.e., patient's intrinsic susceptibility to infection) and the average length of time these patients are exposed to these devices (extrinsic risk factors). In general, the Centers for Disease Control (CDC) guidelines for the prevention and control of nosocomial infections/intravascular infection can be followed.[13] However, over the past decade, numerous developments have occurred in the area of intravenous infusion therapy, for example, for prolonged parenteral infusion of drugs and nutrition through Broviac/Hickman/implanted Port catheters. These catheters are at increased risk of colonization from the microorganisms on the skin, which are the principal pathogens in patients with catheter-related sepsis.[14, 15, 17] Topical application of antimicrobial agents, such as chlorhexidine gluconate, or use of silver impregnated cuffs, can decrease the cutaneous colonization or block the migration of microorganisms into the catheter.[18] These measures should decrease the incidence of catheter-related infection.[18] There are a few suggestive clinical predictors of catheter-related infection in patients receiving total parenteral nutrition, such as a positive result of a skin culture equal to or more than 50 colonies of organisms other than Staphylococcus epidermidis and an area of erythema 4 mm in diameter at the insertion site.[17]

Quantitative blood cultures should be obtained from central venous catheters; simultaneous culture from peripheral veins can help to diagnose catheter-related sepsis versus colonization.[18]

PREVENTION OF PNEUMONIA

Nosocomial pneumonia is a major infection control problem. In young children, it can occur with or without mechanical ventilation. The most common cause of pneumonia in children under 2 years of age is nosocomial viral respiratory infection, such as with respiratory syncytial virus, influenza viruses, and the parainfluenza viruses.[19] The epidemiology of hospital-acquired pneumonia parallels the respiratory tract disease in the community. What seems to be a mild viral respiratory infection in a visitor or staff can cause severe disease in hospitalized children, predominantly in the ICU.[20] The risk of pneumonia in a patient who is mechanically ventilated is higher than in nonventilated patients. With the use of an endotracheal tube the normal host defenses are bypassed and the risk of aspiration is higher in these patients.[21] CDC guidelines for the prevention and control of nosocomial infection are widely accepted.[22] Oropharyngeal and gastric colonization with aerobic gram-negative organisms is an important prerequisite to the development of nosocomial pneumonia.[21] To decrease the rate of colonization, systemic and local antibiotic prophylaxis of the oropharynx has been attempted with some success.[23] The selective decontamination with gentamicin, nystatin, and polymyxin of the oropharynx and gastrointestinal tract in patients in a cardiac ICU has lowered the incidence of pneumonia; however, it does not decrease the stay in ICU or the fatality rate.

Other key aspects in reducing nosocomial pneumonia include reducing the total number of ventilated days, (2) application of proper suctioning techniques, (3) the proper use of gloves, and (4) handwashing to prevent further transmission of infection. Above all, it appears that the status of the host is the key factor in prevention of nosocomial infections in the ICU.

References

1. Donowitz LG: High risk of nosocomial infection in the pediatric critical care patient. Crit Care Med 14:26, 1986.
2. Ford-Jones EL, Mindorff CM, Langles JM, et al: Epidemiologic study of 4684 hospital acquired infections in pediatric patients. Pediatr Infect 8:668, 1989.
3. Milliken J, Tait GA, Ford Jones EL, et al: Nosocomial infections in a pediatric intensive care unit. Crit Care Med 16:233, 1988.
4. Pollack MM, Ruttimann YE, Getson PR: Pediatric risk of mortality (PRISM) score. Crit Care Med 18:378, 1990.
5. Pollock EM, Ford-Jones EL, Rebeyka L, et al: Early nosocomial infection in pediatric cardiovascular surgery patients. Crit Care Med 18:378, 1990.
6. Singh-Naz N, Bramlett DG, Cantwell EG, et al: Association between admission severity of illness and subsequent development of nosocomial infections in critically ill children. Pediatr Res 29:557, 1991.
7. Opal SM, Asp AA, Cannudy PB, et al: Efficacy of infection control measures during a nosocomial outbreak of disseminated aspergillosis associated with hospital construction. J Infect Dis 153:634, 1986.
8. Recommendation for prevention of HIV transmission in health care setting. MMWR 36:2, 1987.
9. Pugliese G, Lynch P, and Jackson MM (eds): Universal precautions policies, procedures and resources. American Hospital Association 1–391, 1991.
10. Klein BS, Perloff WH, and Maki DG: Reduction of nosocomial infection during pediatric intensive care by protective isolation. N Engl J Med 320:1714, 1989.
11. American Hospital Association: Working Together: Needlestick Prevention Training Manual. San Francisco, American Hospital Association, 1989.
12. A report from National Noscomial Infection Surveillance (NNIS) system. Nosocomial infection rates for interhospital comparisons: limitations and possible solutions. Inf Cont and Hosp Epi 12:609–621, 1991.
13. Simmons BP: CDC guidelines for the prevention and control of nosocomial infections: Guidelines for prevention of intravascular infections. Am J Infect Control 11:183, 1983.
14. Maki DG, Weise CD, and Sarafin HW: A semiquantitative culture method for identifying intravenous catheter-related infection. N Engl J Med 296:1305, 1977.
15. Linares J, Sitges-Serra A, Garau J, et al: Pathogenesis of catheter sepsis: A prospective study with quantitative and semi-quantitative cultures of catheter hub and segments. J Clin Microbiol 21:357, 1985.
16. Maki DG, Cobb L, Garman JK, et al: An attachable silver-impregnated cuff for prevention of infection with central venous catheters: A prospective randomized multi-center trial. Am J Med 85:307, 1988.
17. Armstrong CW, Mayhall G, Miller KB, et al: Clinical predictors of infection of central venous catheters used for total parenteral nutrition. Infect Cont Hosp Epidemiol 11:71, 1990.
18. Raucher HS, Hyatt AC, Barzilai A, et al: Quantitative blood cultures in the evaluation of septicemia in children with Broviac catheters. J Pediatr 104:29, 1984.
19. Hall CB: Hospital-acquired pneumonia in children: The role of respiratory viruses. Semin Respir Infect 2(1):48, 1987.
20. Singh-Naz N, Willy M, and Riggs N: Outbreak of parainfluenza virus type 3 in a neonatal nursery. Pediatr Infect Dis J 9:31, 1990.
21. Craven DE and Steger KA: Nosocomial pneumonia in the intubated patient: New concepts of pathogenesis and prevention. Infect Dis Clin North Am 3(4):843, 1989.
22. Simmons BP and Wong ES: CDC guidelines for the prevention and control of nosocomial infections—guideline for prevention of nosocomial pneumonia. Am J Infect Control 11:230, 1983.
23. Flaherty J, Nathan C, Kabins A, et al: Nonabsorbable antibiotic versus sucralfate in preventing colonization and infection in a cardiac surgery intensive care unit. Abstracts from the 28th Interscience Conference on Antimicrobial Agents and Chemotherapy, 1988.

Nosocomial Infections in the Practice of Pediatric Critical Care*

J. Perren Cobb, M.D., and Robert L. Danner, M.D.

Nosocomial infection is defined as disease caused by bacteria, viruses, fungi, or parasites that is neither present nor incubating at the time of admission and develops (but is not necessarily manifest) during hospitalization. In this chapter, the impact of hospital-acquired infections in the pediatric intensive care unit (PICU) are discussed and their pathogenesis, diagnosis, control, and treatment are reviewed. Differences between adult and pediatric nosocomial infections are delineated to enable the reader to extrapolate appropriately from the more extensive adult literature. Potentially preventable nosocomial infections, such as those that are device- or procedure-related are emphasized.[1]

EPIDEMIOLOGY

Nosocomial infection is a major contributor to the morbidity, mortality, and cost of hospitalization.[2-7] It is estimated that 5 to 10% of the more than 38 million hospital admissions per year in the United States are complicated by a nosocomial infection.[2-4] This staggering figure equates nosocomial infections in magnitude with hospitalizations for accidents, cancer, and heart disease.[2] Hospital-acquired infection causes or contributes to death in 3.8% of all patients with this complication.[4] Nosocomial bacteremia alone occurs in approximately 200,000 patients per year in the United States and carries a high mortality.[7] Notably, pediatric patients with nosocomial infection have a very high incidence of secondary bacteremia (7.8%),[4] perhaps due to a reduced ability to localize infection as compared to adults.

Intensive care units (ICUs) are at the center of the nosocomial infection problem.[1, 8-12] Hospital-acquired infection rates are two- to five-fold higher in ICU patients than in the general hospital population.[8-12] In one surveillance study, 25% of all nosocomial infections and 33 to 45% of all nosocomial bacteremias occurred in ICU patients, who occupied only 8% of the total hospital beds.[10] ICU patients had bloodstream infection rates up to 24 times greater than ward patients.[10] Further, in a study of epidemics of hospital-acquired infection, 10 of 11 potentially preventable outbreaks occurred in ICUs (four of which were neonatal units).[10]

Nosocomial infections in pediatric patient populations have not been extensively studied. In general, infection rates vary with patient age. One study of pediatric patients reported hospital-acquired infection rates of 11.5% for patients 23 months old or younger, 3.6% for the 2- to 4-year old age group, and 2.6% for children older than 5 years.[11] Whether this variation is due to age-related differences in severity of illness, frequency of medical instrumentation, or immune system function is unclear.

Studies including all hospitalized patients regardless of age have shown that nosocomial infection rates appear to be lower on pediatric and newborn services than on adult wards.[4, 8, 10, 13] However, these large comparison studies were not designed to consider several aspects of pediatric nosocomial infections that differ from the adult experience, and these omissions may have skewed the results.[2-4] Nosocomial infections in children are frequently viral (23 to 27% of all identified etiologies[11, 12, 14] compared to less than 5% in adults) and hospital-acquired viral infections are often under-reported.[4] For example, the role of viral infections was not rigorously examined in either the Study on the Efficacy of Nosocomial Infection Control (SENIC) or the National Nosocomial Infection Surveillance (NNIS) survey, the two largest population-based studies in the United States.[2-4] Further, infants and children have fewer hospital-acquired urinary tract infections compared to adults, but more gastrointestinal infections, bacteremias, and upper respiratory infections.[11-13] Nosocomial gastrointestinal and upper respiratory infections were not reported by either SENIC or NNIS.[2-4] Interestingly, investigations conducted in large university pediatric hospitals that accounted for these epidemiologic differences found nosocomial infection rates of 4.1 to 6.0%[11, 12] which are similar to the overall rate of 4.1% reported by the NNIS survey for large teaching hospitals.[4] Another possible

---

Table 70–1. FREQUENCY OF PEDIATRIC NOSOCOMIAL INFECTIONS BY SITE IN GENERAL AND ICU POPULATIONS

Site	BCH*	HSC†	PICU 1A†	PICU 1B‡	PICU 1C§	PICU 2‖	PICU 3¶	PICU 4**
Gastrointestinal tract	16.3%	35%	9.2%	7.7%	1%	19.0%	13.3%	—
Blood	10.0%	21%	35.9%	39.6%	36%	12.1%	40.3%	8%
Respiratory tract								
Upper	23.9%	10%	2.6%	6.0%	6%	10.3%	26.7%	—
Lower		6%	12.2%	14.6%	10%	25.8%		21%
Surgical wound	8.4%	7%	5.6%	6.0%	15%	15.5%††	13.3%††	10%
Urinary tract	8.9%	6%	9.5%	7.7%	9%	17.2%	6.7%	15%
Skin	8.0%	5%	14.2%	6.9%	7%	—	—	—
Eye	7.9%	5%	9.8%	6.9%	5%	—	—	—
Central nervous system	—	3%	0.6%	—	—	—	—	—
Other	16.0%	2%	0.3%	4.2%	11%	—	—	46%

*Buffalo Children's Hospital (1980–1981).[12]
†Hospital for Sick Children, Toronto, Canada (1984–1987).[11]
‡Hospital for Sick Children, Toronto, Canada (1983–1985). Blood infections comprise primary and secondary bacteremias.[17]
§Hospital for Sick Children, Toronto, Canada (1987–1988). Blood infections comprise bacteremias and intravascular catheter–related infections.[20]
‖University of Wisconsin Hospital (1984–1987). Nonimmunosuppressed patients requiring mechanical ventilation.[19]
¶Porto Alegre, Brazil (1987–1988).[21]
**University of Virginia Hospital (1982–1983).[9]
††Includes nonwound infections of the skin.

reason for differences in both the types and the rates of infection between adult and pediatric studies is the small proportion of hospitalized children and newborns at high risk for infection, particularly at small hospitals.[4] High-risk interventions such as placement of transcutaneous medical devices, urinary catheterization, invasive procedures, and prolonged ventilatory support may be done less frequently in pediatric patients than in hospitalized adults.

These distinctions between general adult and pediatric hospital-acquired infections, however, may be blurred in the ICU environment where the severity of illness and need for medical instrumentation may be similar.[15] For example, conditions that predispose patients to nosocomial infection, such as major trauma or full-thickness burns,[1, 16] may be expected to put both children and adults at a similar high risk for infectious complications. A recent prospective study of PICU-acquired infections found that the risk of infection rose with increasing length of stay or duration of arterial or central venous catheterization, endotracheal intubation, mechanical ventilation, intracranial pressure monitoring, or neuromuscular blockade.[17] Clearly, the incidence of nosocomial infections in a particular PICU will depend on the mix of patients, their severity of illness, and the frequency with which different invasive medical devices or procedures are used.[18]

Four prospectively designed studies evaluating nosocomial infections in individual hospitals found PICU rates ranging from 6 to 13.7%.[9, 11–13] PICU patients had nosocomial infection rates that were two to three times higher than those in pediatric ward patients.[9, 11, 12] Three of these studies also collected data from the NICU in the same hospital.[11–13] PICU hospital-acquired infection rates were similar to the those in a hospital-matched NICU in one study (6.2 vs. 5.9%, respectively)[13] and half the NICU rate in two studies (6 vs. 14% and 11.0 vs. 22.2%, respectively).[11, 12] Another investigation demonstrated that within the PICU the youngest patients are at the highest risk for infection.[17] Nosocomial infection rates from the PICU in this study were shown to be two to three times higher for patients 1 month old or less compared with patients who were at least 2 years old.[17]

The PICU environment affects not only the incidence but also the types of infection that occur. Within the PICU, the relative contribution of gastrointestinal and upper respiratory tract infections decreases while the importance of bacteremia and lower respiratory tract infections increases compared to the general pediatric population (Table 70–1).[11, 12, 19–21] In a review of pediatric nosocomial infections by the Centers for Disease Control, Jarvis, noted that the distribution of infections by site in PICUs resembles that in adult ICUs.[15] This finding probably reflects the frequent use of certain high-risk interventions in PICUs, such as transcutaneous catheterization and mechanical ventilation.

MICROBIOLOGY

Table 70–2 summarizes the microorganisms most commonly isolated from pediatric nosocomial infections in the NNIS survey[4] and two university hospitals for children.[11, 12] This table excludes data on viral agents and does not consider some sites of infection, such as the gastrointestinal tract and the upper respiratory tract, that are important in general pediatric patients. As shown, *Staphylococcus aureus*, coagulase-negative staphylococci, *Escherichia coli*, and *Pseudomonas* species are major causes of pediatric nosocomial infections. Although the incidence of nosocomial gram-positive infections has been increasing recently on adult services,[22, 23] gram-positive bacteria are relatively more important than gram-negative bacteria as etiologies of hospital-acquired infection in children (Table 70–3) compared with adults.[4, 11, 12] This predominance of gram-positive organisms, however, may be less pronounced

Table 70–2. MOST COMMON ETIOLOGIC AGENTS OF PEDIATRIC NOSOCOMIAL INFECTIONS BY SITE

Site	NNIS (%)*	HSC (%)†	BCH (%)‡
Urinary Tract Infections			
Escherichia coli	30.4	33.3	40.3
Pseudomonas sp.	13.4	12.5	22.6
Enterococci	10.7	14.1	0.0
Klebsiella sp.	10.7	13.5	4.8
Candida sp.	10.7	5.4	4.8
Surgical Wound Infections			
Staphylococcus aureus	34.8	37.9	48.3
E. coli	10.6	9.6	27.6
Pseudomonas sp.	10.6	9.1	10.3
Coagulase-negative staphylococci	10.6	18.4	0.0
Enterococci	7.6	9.1	—
Lower Respiratory Infections			
Pseudomonas sp.	19.8	24.0	35.3
S. aureus	11.6	34.3	29.4
Klebsiella sp.	9.3	0.0	5.9
Enterobacter sp.	7.0	10.3	—
Candida sp.	3.5	13.7	0.0
Bacteremia			
Coagulase-negative staphylococci	29.0	59.1	42.2
S. aureus	14.0	12.4	24.1
E. coli	10.8	3.6	10.8
Klebsiella sp.	6.5	2.3	7.2
Candida sp.	6.5	4.0	7.2
Enterococci	—	3.6	—
Pseudomonas sp.	—	3.5	3.6
Skin and Soft Tissue			
S. aureus	40.3	34.0	93.9
Coagulase-negative staphylococci	19.4	18.4	0.0
E. coli	10.4	3.7	2.0
Candida sp.	7.5	8.5	0.0
Enterococci	4.5	8.2	—
Pseudomonas sp.	—	7.5	2.0

*National Nosocomial Infection Surveillance, 1984.[4]

†Hospital for Sick Children, Toronto, Canada (1984–1987). Data on lower respiratory tract infections were adapted from the reference by excluding viruses and *Asperigillus* sp.[11]

‡Buffalo Children's Hospital (1980–1981). Data on lower respiratory tract infections were adapted from the reference by excluding viruses.[12]

in the PICU environment (see Table 70–3).[19, 20] In one PICU study of nonimmunosuppressed, mechanically ventilated patients, gram-negative bacteria were the predominant cause of hospital-acquired infection (see Table 70–3).[19] This finding more closely mimics the adult experience with intubated patients and suggests that appropriately matched patients receiving the same medical interventions may have quite similar rates of infection, independent of age or hospital service.

In studies that specifically evaluated the role of viruses in nosocomial infections among general pediatric pa-

tients, viruses were a more common causative agent than gram-negative bacteria (see Table 70–3),[11, 12] and these infections prolonged hospitalization an average of 9.3 days.[14] Viral infections, however, appear to play only a small role in PICU-acquired infections, but this question has not been rigorously examined. One study found that nosocomial respiratory syncytial virus infection caused five cases of respiratory failure and one death out of a total of 372 hospital-acquired infections with known etiologies.[12] Further, a study of nosocomial infections from the Hospital for Sick Children in To-

Table 70–3. THE PROPORTION OF PEDIATRIC NOSOCOMIAL INFECTIONS CAUSED BY SPECIFIC CATEGORIES OF MICROORGANISMS

Microorganism	NNIS*	BCH†	HSC‡	PICU 1B§	PICU 1C‖	PICU 2¶
Gram-positive bacteria	36.0%	46.5%	49.7%	42.2%	42%	23.8%
Viruses	—	26.9%	22.9%	6.0%	—	—
Gram-negative bacteria	34.6%	23.7%	17.9%	36.2%	35%	47.6%
Fungi	8.8%	3.0%	4.4%	4.3%	19%	28.6%
Mixed or other	20.3%	—	5.1%	6.0%	—	—

*National Nosocomial Infection Surveillance, 1984.[4]
†Buffalo Children's Hospital (1980–1981).[12]
‡Hospital for Sick Children, Toronto, Canada (1984–1987).[11]
§Hospital for Sick Children, Toronto, Canada (1983–1985).[17]
‖Hospital for Sick Children, Toronto, Canada (1987–1988).[20]
¶University of Wisconsin Hospital (1984–1987). Nonimmunosuppressed, mechanically ventilated patients.[19]

ronto noted that "viral disease was occurring at a far lower incidence in the PICU than in other parts of the hospital."[20] An investigation of PICU-acquired infections from this same hospital found that viruses accounted for only 6% of the nosocomial pathogens isolated,[17] a rate much lower than that in the hospital as a whole (see Table 70–3).[11]

NOSOCOMIAL INFECTIONS CAUSED BY INTRAVASCULAR CATHETERS

Intravascular catheters are used in virtually every patient treated in an ICU. Although intravascular catheters are indispensable for fluid resuscitation, drug administration, transfusion therapy, blood drawing, and patient monitoring, infection is a common, serious, and potentially life-threatening complication of these devices. In a recent prospective study of nosocomial infections in the PICU, Pollock and colleagues identified central venous or arterial catheters as the cause of 24% of the nosocomial infections in their unit, affecting 3.6 patients per 100 admissions.[20]

The study of catheter-related infections is complicated by the lack of standardized, microbiologic definitions. The following definitions are used in this chapter. *Colonization* is the presence of microorganisms on a catheter as determined by an acceptable culture technique in the absence of any other signs of local or systemic infection. *Local infection* refers to catheter colonization accompanied by signs and symptoms of soft-tissue infection around the catheter insertion site, with or without systemic symptoms, which abate with removal of the catheter or the initiation of antibiotic therapy. Unequivocal *catheter-related sepsis* requires colonization of the catheter, systemic signs or symptoms of infection, positive blood cultures from a peripheral site for the same organism obtained from the catheter, no other identifiable source of infection, and resolution of symptoms with appropriate antibiotic therapy and removal of the catheter. The various types of catheters in common use are discussed together in regard to the pathogenesis, microbiology, diagnosis, and treatment of intravascular, catheter-related infection, followed by a discussion of device-specific considerations.

Pathogenesis

Catheter-related infection begins with catheter colonization, which can occur by one of three mechanisms: (1) entry of skin flora into the catheter insertion site and subsequent colonization of the subcutaneous or intravascular portion of the catheter; (2) hematogenous seeding of the catheter from a distant site of infection or colonization; or (3) contamination of the catheter interior or hub by organisms from the environment or fluid infusate.[24–28] The majority of evidence indicates that the first mechanism (colonization of the catheter exterior by skin flora) is the most common and important for all types of intravascular catheters (Table 70–4).[29, 30]

Catheter-related infections resulting from hematoge-

Table 70–4. PATHOGENESIS OF INTRAVASCULAR INFECTIONS*†

1. There is a strong correlation between organisms present on skin that surrounds the catheter wound and microorganisms recovered from catheters that produce septicemia.
2. Patients with burns experience a disproportionately high rate of catheter-related sepsis.
3. Coagulase-negative staphylococci, the predominant aerobic species on human skin, are the most frequently isolated organisms from cultures of intravascular catheters.
4. Heavy growth of bacteria on semiquantitative culture of the external surface of catheters is strongly associated with bacteremia caused by the catheter.
5. Hospitals with intravenous therapy teams that consistently adhere to recommended catheter care guidelines during insertion and maintenance have lower rates of catheter-related sepsis.

*Data that suggest that infection is secondary to bacterial invasion along the catheter insertion tract.[30]

†Adapted from Maki DG and Ringer M: Evaluation of dressing regimens for prevention of infection with peripheral intravenous catheters. JAMA 258:2396, 1987. Copyright 1987, American Medical Association.

nous seeding, the contamination of infusate, or colonization of in-line stopcocks, pressure transducer chamber-domes, continuous "flush" devices, and the catheter hub have been reported and occasionally lead to bacteremia.[31] In a study of adult patients, Band and Maki,[25] using a semiquantitative technique (discussed further on), found that only 14% of arterial catheters became colonized after documented exposure to bacteremia unrelated to the catheter. Similarly, Maki and others[32] found in adults that only 11% of peripheral venous catheters were colonized following exposure to bacteremia. Ducharme and colleagues[24] were unable to find any cases of colonization by the hematogenous route in a prospective study of 70 intravascular catheters in critically ill children. Likewise, catheter infection from intravenous fluid contamination is rare:[29, 30, 33] in a prospective study of peripheral venous catheters in adults, infusate contamination occurred in only 5 of 2,088 cases (0.25%).[30] The importance of hub and stopcock contamination as a cause of intralumenal catheter colonization and subsequent catheter-related infection or sepsis remains controversial. Some investigators have implicated this mechanism in the infection of pulmonary artery catheters and catheters used for parenteral nutrition (up to 70% of these catheter-related infections).[34] This mechanism appears to account for only a small percentage of all catheter-related infections[35] but may be significant in settings where infusion circuits are frequently interrupted or manipulated or aseptic technique is not strictly maintained.

The risk factors that have been associated with catheter-related infection are listed in Table 70–5 and support the basic pathogenic considerations discussed previously. The duration of catheterization is by far the most important and best established of these risk factors. The steep increase in the incidence of catheter-related infection after approximately 3 to 4 days has largely been determined from adult studies.[25, 29, 38] Damen and van der Tweel[36] made an attempt to define a safe duration for intravascular catheterization in pediatric patients receiving prophylactic antibiotics following car-

Table 70–5. RISK FACTORS FOR CATHETER-RELATED
INFECTION

Well-supported factors
Duration of catheterization[25, 30, 36–38]
Heavy bacterial contamination of skin around the catheter
    insertion site[29, 30, 37, 39]
Purulence at the catheter insertion site[40]
Immunosuppression[38, 41, 42]
Extremes of age[25, 36]
Loss of skin integrity at the insertion site (e.g., burn or
    "degloving" injury)[40]

Moderately supported or controversial factors
Femoral location (for[39]; against[43])
Local inflammation (for[25]; against[24, 39, 40, 43])
Need for inotropic cardiovascular support[36]
Visible moisture or blood under catheter dressing[30]
Multiple-lumen catheters[44, 45]
Surgical cutdown to vessel[25]
Emergency or difficult catheter insertion
Systemic antibiotics (may change flora responsible for infection[25];
    no effect[30, 39, 40, 46])

diac surgery. They found that for children less than 1 year of age the maximum duration of catheterization before a significant rise in the rate of catheter colonization was 3 days for peripheral, arterial, central venous, and pulmonary artery catheters. For children older than 1 year, some of these catheters could be left in place longer (4 days for arterial and 6 days for central venous catheters). Although this concept is well-supported by a number of studies, a recent prospective, controlled trial of frequent catheter changes (either "over wires" or to new sites) in adult surgical patients did not demonstrate a reduction in catheter infection rates.[47] Since catheter "rotation" is practiced in many ICUs, this intervention clearly requires further critical evaluation.

Microbiology

The microorganisms that have been recovered from cultures of intravascular catheters in three representative studies are shown in Table 70–6. Coagulase-negative staphylococci are the most common organisms recovered from cultures of those catheters considered colonized or infected (up to 77%).[30, 32, 36, 40, 43, 48–51] The study conducted by Damen and van der Tweel of peripheral, central venous, and systemic and pulmonary arterial catheter–related infections in almost 400 children undergoing cardiac surgery recovered coagulase-negative staphylococcal species from 60% of catheter-tip cultures.[36] Other gram-positive organisms commonly implicated include *S. aureus* and enterococcal species.[25, 32, 40, 43, 48–51] Gram-positive organisms as a group account for most episodes of catheter-related sepsis (45–70%).[25, 32, 49, 51] In general, gram-negative bacilli are implicated in 20 to 30% and *Candida* species in less than 10% of catheter-related infections, although these percentages may be higher in selected patient populations receiving antibiotics or immunosuppressive therapy. For example, Mirro and colleagues found that in children with cancer infections of "permanent" central venous catheters were

frequently caused by gram-negative bacilli (36%) or fungi (23%).[49]

Catheter-related infections are rarely polymicrobial. In a study of adult patients at high risk for infection, Moyer and associates found that 8 of 47 (17%) colonized intravenous catheters had more than one organism isolated using the semiquantitative culture technique (see Diagnosis below), although none of these resulted in polymicrobial bacteremia.[40] Another study, however, found that catheter-related sepsis was frequently polymicrobial during an unusual epidemic in an adult ICU. In this report, 6 of 73 patients admitted to an ICU over a 2-month period developed bacteremia and three of these episodes were polymicrobial.[52]

Diagnosis

The documentation of catheter colonization has been used to implicate the catheter as the possible source of an infection, and a number of culture techniques have been described for this purpose. The clinical relevance, however, of any "test" for catheter-related infection varies depending upon the chosen microbiologic technique and the criteria used to define a positive result. Principles common to all of the reported methods include an attempt to sterilize the skin around the site of insertion (usually using povidone-iodine and alcohol solutions) prior to removal of the catheter, followed by examination or culture of the catheter for the presence of bacteria. One early technique involved immersion of the catheter in trypticase-soy broth for culture.[26, 32] This method, however, did not distinguish colonization in vivo from contamination ex vivo.

Maki and coworkers[32] published a "semiquantitative" technique in 1977 in an attempt to overcome this deficiency of the broth culture method. His group directly compared semiquantitative cultures of intravenous catheters, obtained by rolling the catheter across a blood agar plate, with cultures obtained by the broth culture method. Of the 250 catheters cultured (13% of which were of the central venous type), 225 (90%) had "low-density" colonization (less than 15 colony-forming units [cfu] on semiquantitative culture) and were not associated with bacteremia. Twenty-five catheters had 15 or more colonies per plate, and four of these were associated with bacteremia.[32] Furthermore, catheters with 15 or more cfu were significantly associated with the presence of local imflammation.[32] Maki and colleagues therefore concluded that their semiquantitative culture method was sensitive and specific for the diagnosis of catheter-related infection. However, other investigators have not been able to demonstrate the superiority of the semiquantitative technique over traditional culture methods. Moyer and colleagues[40] in a prospective study of 101 intravenous catheters in patients at high risk for catheter-related infection found no significant difference between results of the broth and semiquantitative culture methods. Moreover, Colignon, Sitges-Serra, and their associates[53, 54] contend that the "arbitrary cut-off" of 15 cfu is too stringent, since it failed to detect up to 15% of the catheter-related infections in their studies,

Table 70–6. MICROBIOLOGY OF CATHETER-RELATED INFECTIONS

Organism	Adult Population Arterial Catheter (%)*	Pediatric Population Peripheral, Arterial, Central Venous, and Pulmonary Artery Catheters (%)†	Pediatric Population "Permanent" Central Venous Catheters (%)‡
Gram-Positive Bacteria	79	75	41
Staphylococcus epidermidis	50	61	28
Staphylococcus aureus	9	4	7
Streptococcus sp.	—	—	4
Enterococci	6	9	—
Micrococcus sp.	3	—	—
Other	11	1	2
Gram-Negative Bacteria	15	21	36
Pseudomonas sp.	3	—	13
Klebsiella sp.	3	3	—
Acinetobacter sp.	3	1	2
Serratia sp.	3	—	—
Escherichia coli	3	12	6
Enterobacter sp.	—	3	4
Other	—	2	5
Mycobacteria sp.	—	—	6
Fungi	6	4	23
Aspergillus sp.	—	—	2
Candida sp.	6	4	19
Other	—	—	2

*Thomas and associates.[43]
†Damen and van der Tweel.[36]
‡Mirro and associates.[49]

particularly when the infection originated from the catheter hub or lumen.

Because of such limitations, several investigators have sought to improve upon the semiquantitative technique. Cleri and colleagues[55] developed a semiquantitative technique using serial dilutions of cultures from catheter segments immersed and flushed in trypticase-soy broth to detect the presence of bacteria in the catheter lumen. Cooper and Hopkins[56] advocated a direct gram stain technique of whole catheter segments as an accurate and rapid test to document colonization. Catheter segments were stained using the conventional gram stain technique, then examined under an oil-immersion lens for the presence of bacteria on both internal and external surfaces and cultured using Maki's semiquantitative technique. Considering the presence of one organism per high-powered field as a positive result, they reported that their method was 100% sensitive and 97% specific compared with the results of semiquantitative culture from the same catheters. Similarly, another group gram stained "impression smears" made from intravascular catheters rolled on glass slides. The results were compared to those of the semiquantitative technique but the sensitivity and specificity were only 83 and 81%, respectively.[57] Both of these direct stain techniques have the advantage of assisting in the choice of empiric antibiotics by rapidly documenting the relative number and type of colonizing organisms, but they are technically cumbersome. Another reported technique evaluated the sensitivity of blood cultures drawn through the suspected catheter. Although this method does not require immediate catheter removal, it offers no advantage in the diagnosis of catheter-related infection.[39, 40]

Despite its limitations, the semiquantitative technique has been considered a major advance and has been widely adopted and used to define catheter-related infection in epidemiologic studies.* In clinical practice, however, this test is less useful. The semiquantitative technique documents catheter colonization but does not diagnose catheter infection, as is often asserted. In Maki's study, 32% of patients with a positive catheter culture had neither sepsis nor local inflammation.[32] Further, local inflammation was frequently found in association with catheters that were not colonized (65%), and other studies have found no correlation with the presence of catheter-related infection.[24, 39, 40, 43] This suggests that the positive predictive value of the semiquantitative technique is really less than the 68% calculated from Maki's data by combining the patients with sepsis and local inflammation.[32] Therefore, many patients with a positive semiquantitative culture are not infected. In addition, no test for catheter-related infection can immediately determine when the device is *not* the source, thereby sparing the febrile ICU patient the risk of catheter replacement and the consequences of (additional) antibiotic therapy.

Thus, there is no single microbiologic test for the diagnosis of catheter-related infection, and familiarity with the limitations and interpretation of catheter-culture methods is critical in order to apply them effectively to individual patients. The diagnosis can be complicated in ICU populations because (1) systemic signs of infection and bacteremia unrelated to intravascular catheters are common; (2) the presence of local inflammation of

*References 25, 29, 33, 36, 37, 39, 46, 50.

the catheter site is neither sensitive nor specific in predicting catheter-related infection or sepsis except in cases where frank purulence or cellulitis is present;[24, 39, 40, 43] and (3) the diagnosis of infection from the growth of organisms from catheter and blood cultures requires one to several days. These uncertainties frequently lead to empiric antibiotic therapy, unnecessary catheter replacement, and diagnostic confusion. The results of catheter cultures are useful, but only in retrospect, to support the clinical suspicion of catheter-related infection and to guide antibiotic therapy. The diagnosis of catheter infection is largely based on a preponderance of clinical evidence and careful exclusion of other sources.

Device-Specific Considerations

Peripheral Intravenous Catheters

The most common complication of these catheters is thrombophlebitis, with documented bacteremia occurring rarely. The incidence of phlebitis and bacteremia is believed to be lowest with the use of steel (butterfly-type, "scalp vein") needles; these catheters, however, are nonpliable and are usually in place for only a short time due to their often precarious position in small veins.[58] Recent advances in material science have resulted in catheters made of adhesion-resistant substances such as Teflon, which are associated with more infections than are steel needles but less than those associated with other types of plastic (polyethylene). Maki and Ringer[30] found the incidence of colonization of peripheral intravenous Teflon catheters in adults to be 8.7% using the semiquantitative technique and no instances of catheter-related bacteremia in 2,088 prospectively evaluated adult cases. Similarly, in a pediatric study of 286 peripheral Teflon catheters, Garland and colleagues found that only 10% were colonized and none caused either suppurative phlebitis or catheter-related sepsis.[59] A recent, multihospital, prospective study found an incidence of phlebitis in 3,094 patients using nonsteel intravenous catheters of 2.3% and a rate of associated bacteremia of only 0.08%.[38]

Central Venous Catheters

Central venous catheters are associated in adults with a relatively high rate of sepsis (1.0 to 2.4%).[50, 60] Similarly, in a recent prospective study, 1.8% of critically ill children developed a central venous catheter–related infection, which accounted for 12% of all PICU-acquired infections.[20] Damen and van der Tweel studied rates of catheter colonization in children using a modified semiquantitative method and found that central venous catheters (in place for a median time of 2 days) were colonized more frequently (6.9%) than either peripheral venous (1.1%) or arterial catheters (4.2%).[36] This tendency toward high rates of colonization and infection in central venous catheters has been attributed to the use of these catheters for blood drawing and multiple infusions, which result in frequent "breaks" in line integrity and sterility.[36]

Central venous catheters are also used for delivery of total parenteral nutrition (TPN), which because of its high nutrient content acts as a fertile medium for the growth of fungal and bacterial pathogens.[61] This along with length of the time that TPN catheters remain in place, resulted in septicemia rates as high as 27% in some early adult studies, with large percentages (up to 60%) caused by Candida species.[62] Routines for the prevention of catheter-related infection have been particularly successful at reducing this high incidence of TPN catheter infection in controlled studies.[31]

"Permanent" central venous catheters, either with externalized (Hickman or Broviac) or subcutaneous (Portacath) infusion ports, are often placed in children who require long-term access for hyperalimentation or chemotherapy. In patients with cancer or the acquired immunodeficiency syndrome, the incidence of bacteremia with these catheters is 0.15 to 0.68 episodes per 100 patient days and is associated with the degree of immunosupression.[49, 51, 63, 64] The duration of infection-free use appears to be longer for Portacaths than for other types of "permanent" catheters.[49] Because of the attendant patient discomfort, inconvenience, and risk associated with reinsertion, attempts have been made to treat infection without catheter removal. Acceptable success rates (80 to 90%) have been achieved with antibiotic therapy alone in patients with skin exit-wound infections or uncomplicated bacteremia.[42, 65, 66] Factors associated with treatment failure that would support early catheter removal include the presence of tunnel infection (70% failure rate), septic thrombophlebitis, and infection secondary to fungi or Bacillus species.[49, 51, 66-68] In addition, infected "permanent" catheters in patients who present with septic shock should be managed by immediate removal and empiric antibiotic therapy. Treatment failure necessitating catheter removal is indicated by persistent fever, bacteremia, or local inflammation for more than 48 hours after initiation of appropriate antimicrobial therapy.[68] A study in pediatric patients with "permanent" catheters suggested that ultrasonography is useful in children requiring catheter removal for persistent bacteremia to rule out the presence of central vein thrombosis; if thrombosis is documented, the authors advised 2 or more weeks of antimicrobial therapy after sterilization of the bloodstream.[69]

Arterial Lines

The incidence of arterial catheter colonization and catheter-related sepsis reported in the adult literature varies from 0 to 25% and 0 to 4%, respectively.[25, 26, 37, 39, 43, 70, 71] Moreover, Band and Maki[25] reported in adults that arterial catheters were responsible for 12% of all nosocomial bacteremias in their ICU population. Pollock and colleagues, reporting on a PICU population, found that 1.8% of their admissions acquired an arterial catheter–related infection, which represented 12% of all nosocomial infections in their unit.[20] Some investigators believe that arterial catheters are less frequently infected than venous catheters; possible reasons cited include faster arterial blood flow diminishing bacterial adherence, more stringent application of aseptic technique during insertion and dressing of the entry site, and the deeper location of cannulated arteries relative to peripheral veins.[24, 25, 72] Conflicting data exist regarding the potential for a higher incidence of infection when the femoral artery is cannulated compared to the radial artery.[24, 39, 43]

Arterial (including pulmonary artery) catheters have an added risk of infection from the pressure-transducer systems and continuous "flush" apparatus used with these devices. Maki and Hassemer[73] cultured fluid from the chamber-dome of 102 transducers and grew organisms from 12%, which resulted in four cases of bacteremia. In this study of adults, arterial infusate contamination was reduced significantly from 12 to 5.7% and documented bacteremia was reduced from 3.9 to 0% by changing continuous flush systems every 48 hours. However, after eliminating the static fluid column used in the foregoing study and replacing it with a continuous "flush" configuration, Shinozaki and coworkers found no instances of transducer fluid contamination in 117 arterial catheters (40% of which were in place ≥4 days).[70] Likewise, Ducharme and associates,[24] in a study of 70 arterial catheters in children found no cases of contaminated infusion fluid in patients with suspected catheter sepsis. Based on these data, some investigators believe that changing these pressure monitoring and "flush" devices every 48 hours is unwarranted because of the very low risk of infection and the increased cost.[24, 39, 40, 70] Although definitive recommendations for routine, prophylactic changes of this equipment await controlled clinical trials, for the present it is prudent to change these systems at least every 3 to 4 days given the frequency of "breaks" in line integrity associated with their use.[55]

Although many characteristics of arterial catheter-related infection are essentially indistinguishable from those of venous catheters,[25, 71] some of the complications that stem from these infections are unique. This difference between arterial and venous catheter-related infections is due to the high pressure found in arteries and their role in oxygen delivery. Complications of arterial catheter infections include delayed artery rupture and life-threatening hemorrhage, Osler's nodes, and ischemia secondary to thrombosis of end arteries.[41, 74]

Pulmonary Artery Catheters

The pulmonary artery (PA) catheter differs from the transcutaneous catheter types discussed in its extensive length and unique intravascular location. Further, the introducer catheter required for insertion acts as a "sleeve" that prevents the PA catheter from coming into direct contact with the subcutaneous tissue and skin. These features may explain why some investigators have shown an unusually poor correlation between catheter insertion site and PA catheter-tip cultures.[39, 46] More relevant data regarding colonization and infection might be obtained by culturing both the introducer and the PA catheter itself.

A relatively high incidence of catheter-related infection is reported with the use of PA catheters. In pediatric and adult series, the incidence of PA catheter-tip colo-

nization ranges from 5.8 to 16% using the semiquantitative culture method, and the rate of catheter-related sepsis is 2.7 to 3.5%.[36, 39, 46, 50] This high frequency of colonization and sepsis may be attributable to the multipurpose nature of these catheters (i.e., drug administration, fluid infusion, blood transfusion, pressure monitoring, and cardiac output determinations). Contamination of catheter hubs, stopcocks,[75] and infusion fluids may play a more dominant role in the pathogenesis of PA catheter–related infections compared with other types. The increased severity of illness[50] and frequent use of mechanical ventilation in patients with these catheters probably also contributes to the high incidence of infection.

Treatment

After a thorough evaluation to exclude other sources of infection has been made, management of patients with a suspected or diagnosed catheter–related infection includes removal and culture of the catheter (possibly including a direct gram stain of the catheter), changing the site of catheterization, drawing at least two blood cultures from different sites, and initiating empiric antibiotic therapy if indicated.[26, 40] Removal of the catheter is the single most important maneuver for either suspected or documented catheter–related infection as it eliminates the source of infection; this, however, may not always be desirable or possible.

Initial empiric antibiotic therapy for seriously ill patients with a suspected catheter–related infection in the absence of gram stain or culture results should be directed against methicillin-resistant *Staphylococcus* species,[25, 28] enteric gram-negative bacilli, and possibly *Pseudomonas aeruginosa* or other organisms (such as enterococci), depending on the most common isolates for a particular PICU (see Table 70–6). Regimens that include vancomycin[76] with either an aminoglycoside[65] or a third-generation cephalosporin usually provide effective, initial coverage. In patients with septic shock or immunosupression, "double" gram-negative coverage with two antimicrobial agents effective against *P. aeruginosa* should be considered. If the infection involves a "permanent" central venous catheter, antibiotics should be infused through the suspected catheter itself; if there is more than one lumen, antibiotic administration should be alternated between ports.[66] Prolonged immunosuppression with or without the prior use of antibiotics, other risk factors for invasive fungal disease, or retinal lesions consistent with *Candida* endophthalmitis are indications for the addition of amphotericin B. The duration and choice of antibiotic therapy will depend ultimately on culture results, the occurrence of complications, and the clinical response.

NOSOCOMIAL INFECTIONS ASSOCIATED WITH DEVICES USED FOR INTRACRANIAL PRESSURE MONITORING

A number of devices have been developed for monitoring intracranial pressure (ICP), and all have the

Table 70–7. RISK FACTORS FOR VENTRICULOSTOMY-
RELATED INFECTIONS*

Intravertebral hemorrhage with intraventricular hemorrhage
Neurosurgical operations
Intracranial pressure ≥20 mm Hg
Irrigation of the system
Ventricular catheterization for >5 days

*Adapted from information appearing in Mayhall CG, Archer NH, Lamb A, et al: Ventriculostomy-related infections: A prospective epidemiologic study. N Engl J Med 310:553, 1984.

potential to cause nosocomial infection. The risk varies depending on the type of device and its anatomic location with respect to the central nervous system (CNS). Of the methods available, the ventricular catheter has been in use the longest and has been the most extensively investigated regarding its potential to cause infection.

Ventriculostomy-related infections include simple wound infection at the catheter insertion site, osteomyelitis of the skull, and ventriculitis or meningitis. The incidence of ventriculitis or meningitis, the most serious infectious complications of ventriculostomy, ranges from 0 to 50% in published reports.[77–83] In one large series from a tertiary care center that included children and adults, 19 of 172 patients (11%) developed either ventriculitis or meningitis after a total of 213 ventriculostomies.[77] Table 70–7 shows the risk factors for ventriculostomy-related infection identified in this study.[77] As with many other transcutaneous devices, the risk of infection increased with the duration of catheterization, although one study conducted in a pediatric population actually found that the risk of infection diminished after the sixth day.[84] Factors that did not significantly alter the risk of developing a ventriculostomy-related infection included the use of prophylactic antibiotics, insertion of the ventricular catheter in the ICU, and diagnostic or therapeutic drainage of cerebrospinal fluid.[77]

Another study comparing three different techniques of ICP monitoring in pediatric and adult patients found that infection was associated with open trauma or hemorrhage, the use of a bacitracin-flush solution, and the use of steroids.[85] Subarachnoid screw devices (e.g., the Richmond bolt) had the lowest incidence of infection overall (7.5% with no cases of ventriculitis or meningitis), followed by the subdural-subarachnoid cup catheter (14.9% with a 4.1% incidence of ventriculitis or meningitis), and finally the ventricular catheter (26.8% with a 21.9% incidence of ventriculitis or meningitis).[85] The relatively high rate of ventriculostomy-related infections in this study was probably due to the fact that only patients undergoing craniotomy were included. The risk of infection from new fiberoptic pressure monitoring catheters* is unknown but is probably relatively low compared to ventricular and even subarachnoid cup catheters since they do not rely on fluid columns that may transport infection.[86]

The microbiology of transcutaneous intracranial catheter–related infection is summarized in Table 70–8. The

*Camino Laboratories, San Diego, CA.

findings are similar to those with other transcutaneous devices except that infection with *Candida* species is unusual. Gram-positive bacteria, including coagulase-negative staphylococci, cause a large proportion of the infections, though gram-negative organisms predominate in some studies.[77, 79, 84, 85]

The diagnosis of transcutaneous, transcranial device–related infection can be quite difficult. Impaired sensorium or meningismus may be absent or impossible to detect in infants or in patients with pre-existing CNS disease. Further, in patients with ventriculostomies, fever and peripheral leukocytosis are sometimes absent despite the presence of ventriculitis or meningitis and are frequently present in ICU patients without ventriculitis or meningitis.[77] Cerebrospinal fluid (CSF) pleocytosis is more predictive of infection but is absent in 22% of patients with positive CSF cultures and present in 23% of patients with negative CSF cultures.[77] Because of these diagnostic problems, some authors recommend routine cultures of the CSF three times per week in patients with ventriculostomies.[81] The culturing of intracranial pressure devices at the time of removal has not been found to be clinically useful.[85]

Treatment consists of device removal and the administration of appropriate antibiotics capable of penetrating the blood-brain barrier.[79, 81] Ventriculitis frequently requires a ventriculostomy for the administration of intrathecal antibiotics, particularly if the required antimicrobial agents penetrate into the CSF poorly.[79]

OTHER TRANSCUTANEOUS DEVICE–RELATED INFECTIONS

In addition to the devices already discussed, a wide variety of other catheters that breach the protective barrier of the skin are used in PICUs and place patients at risk for infection. A recent study of nosocomial infections in the PICU reported that one third of all documented infections were associated with transcutaneous devices,[20] and of these, 71% were central venous or arterial catheter–related. The remaining infections (29%) were associated with thoracostomy tubes in five cases, peritoneal drains in four, and a biliary T tube in one. Notably, nonintravascular devices resulted in a nosocomial infection rate of 1.4 infections per 100 admissions and accounted for 10% of all nosocomial infections in this particular PICU.[19] This investigation clearly demonstrates the substantial impact that a variety of medical devices used in the PICU can have on the acquisition of infection.

Transcutaneous, intravascular access for hemodialysis and continuous arteriovenous or venovenous hemofiltration in the PICU have not been extensively studied but probably have an infection risk and a microbial flora similar to those of other intravascular catheters.[87] Prolonged use of transhepatic-biliary drains,[88] biliary T tubes,[19] and nephrostomy tubes[89] frequently leads to colonization, usually with organisms known to infect the undiverted biliary tree or urinary tract, respectively, and may result in local infection or septicemia.

Peritoneal dialysis catheters deserve special mention

Table 70–8. MICROBIOLOGY OF CEREBROSPINAL FLUID IN PATIENTS WITH TRANSCUTANEOUS, INTRACRANIAL CATHETER–RELATED INFECTION

Isolate	Percentage of Patients			
	Mayhall et al[77]	Aucoin et al[85]*	Ohrstrom et al[79]	Kanter et al[84]
Gram-Positive	47	25	89	77
Coagulase-negative staphylococci	32	8	56	56
Staphylococcus aureus	5	17	33	0
Streptococcus faecalis	5	0	0	22
Other streptococci	5	0	0	0
Gram-Negative	53	58	11	22
Escherichia coli	5	8	0	0
Enterobacter aerogenes	11	0	0	0
Enterobacter cloacae	11	8	0	0
Klebsiella pneumoniae	5	33	7	0
Serratia marcescens	5	8	0	11
Providencia stuartii	5	0	0	0
Acinetobacter calcoaceticus	11	0	4	0
Polymicrobial (with at least one gram-negative isolate)	0	17	0	11

*Includes patients with subdural-subarchnoid catheters.

since infection of these devices in children has been extensively studied. Peritoneal dialysis is an attractive alternative to hemodialysis in some PICU patients, but as with other procedures that require a percutaneous catheter, it places the patient at increased risk for infection. In ambulatory pediatric populations[90–93] and neonates[94, 95] with renal failure treated with peritoneal dialysis, infection rates for peritonitis were one episode for every 6 to 16 patient-months. For patients receiving chronic dialysis, the majority develop exit site infections or peritonitis or both sometime during therapy.[96] The risk of infection in severely ill children with peritoneal dialysis catheters within the PICU environment is likely to be high, particularly in immunosuppressed patients. Peritoneal dialysis catheter–related infection is caused by gram-positive bacteria in 60 to 70% of the cases (usually *S. aureus* or *S. epidermidis*) and a variety of gram-negative bacteria in 20 to 30% of the cases.[90–98] Yeast are involved in less than 1% of the episodes, though fungal and gram-negative bacterial infections may be more common in immunosuppressed patients.

The diagnosis of peritoneal dialysis catheter–related infection may be difficult, particularly in critically ill infants and children who may not develop typical signs of peritonitis. Routine periodic peritoneal fluid cell counts and cultures may be warranted in patients at high risk for infection. Successful treatment may be accomplished by intravenous, oral,[99] or peritoneal dialysate–delivered antibiotics or combined routes of administration, and the dialysis catheter can frequently be left in place.[90] Treatment failure, manifested by persistent or recurrent peritonitis, is more common with *Pseudomonas, Serratia*, and fungal infections.[90, 96] Infection with these organisms, particularly *Candida* species, may require catheter removal.[90]

NOSOCOMIAL RESPIRATORY TRACT INFECTIONS

Respiratory tract infections comprise 15 to 36% of hospital-acquired infections in the PICU (see Table 70–

1) and affect up to 2 to 3% of all children admitted for intensive care.[9, 11, 15, 18–21] Unlike nosocomial respiratory infections on pediatric ward services where upper tract disease predominates, the majority of PICU-acquired infections are pneumonias, which are associated with a high morbidity and mortality.[9, 15, 18–21] Notably, more than 90% of newborn nosocomial pneumonias occur in the NICU, and over 50% of pediatric nosocomial pneumonias are acquired in the PICU.[100] The impact of these infections in the PICU can only be estimated from adult and neonatal studies. In one study of adult ICU patients, nosocomial pneumonia resulted in a duration of stay nearly three times longer and a mortality rate almost four times higher.[101] Similarly, a NICU study found that the occurrence of nosocomial pneumonia nearly doubled mortality compared with that in uninfected control patients.[102]

This section focuses on nosocomial pneumonias because of the relative importance of these infections in the PICU. Other lower tract diseases, including tracheitis, tracheobronchitis, and bronchiolitis, are acquired in the PICU by similar pathogenic mechanisms as pneumonia and are briefly mentioned mainly to distinguish them diagnostically. Sinusitis, a well-described complication of nasotracheal and nasogastric intubation, is an important upper respiratory tract infection in the PICU. These infections are frequently caused by aerobic gram-negative bacteria and aspiration of the involved sinus is recommended, whenever possible, for gram staining and culture.[103, 104] Moreover, nosocomial sinusitis should be remembered as a potential source of occult fever, leukocytosis, central nervous system infection, and bacteremia in the PICU.

Pathogenesis

Nosocomial pneumonia occurs by one of four mechanisms: aspiration, direct inoculation or aerosolization, hematogenous seeding, or contiguous extension (Table 70–9).[100] Hematogenous or contiguous spread of micro-

Table 70–9. MECHANISMS AND PREVENTION OF NOSOCOMIAL PNEUMONIA

Mechanism	Source of Microorganisms	Comment	Preventive Measures
Aspiration	*Endogenous:* Translocation or overgrowth of pathogenic organisms derived from the patient's own flora. *Exogenous:* Pathogenic organisms transferred to the patient from PICU personnel, respiratory equipment, food, or other fomites	The most frequent pathogenic mechanism leading to nosocomial pneumonia. Frequently preceded by colonization of the upper airway and gastrointestinal tract by pathogenic bacteria	Limit the use of antibiotics and immunosuppressive therapy Avoid therapy that raises gastric pH* Selective decontamination* Handwashing Protective isolation* Disposable devices Universal precautions Selective recolonization* Surveillance
Direct inoculation or aerosolization	*Endogenous or exogenous:* Microorganisms innoculated at the time of intubation. *Exogenous:* Microorganisms introduced via contaminated nebulizers, manual ventilation bags, spirometers, suctioning equipment, oxygen analyzers, nebulized medication, and ventilation tubing	Occasionally associated with outbreaks of nosocomial pneumonia in ICUs. Less frequent since the development of effective decontamination of equipment, disposable devices, and cascade humidifiers	Surveillance Decontamination and sterilization of equipment Disposable devices Change ventilator tubing every 48 hours Cascade humidifiers run at high temperatures (42° C)
Hematogenous seeding	*Endogenous or exogenous:* Septicemia from a distant site of infection	An infrequent cause of nosocomial pneumonia	Appropriate antibiotic therapy and management of the primary site of infection
Contiguous extension	*Endogenous or exogenous:* Direct extension from a contiguous site of infection	An infrequent cause of nosocomial pneumonia	Appropriate antibiotic therapy and management of the primary site of infection

*Investigational preventive measures.

organisms causes only a small proportion of hospital-acquired pneumonias but requires consideration in order to avoid missing occult sources of infection such as endocarditis or an abscess. Direct inoculation or aerosolization of pathogens into the respiratory tree is an important cause of procedure- or respiratory device–associated outbreaks of nosocomial pneumonia in ICUs.[105–108] Further, nebulized medication contaminated with bacteria has resulted in epidemics of nosocomial pneumonia.[100] Equipment that has been associated with the spread of respiratory pathogens includes nebulizers, manual ventilation bags, spirometers, suctioning equipment, oxygen analyzers, and ventilator tubing.[100, 109–111] This mechanism of infection is almost completely preventable and now occurs less frequently due to the development of effective methods for decontamination of equipment, the use of disposable devices and respiratory tubing, and the introduction of cascade-type humidifiers (Table 70–9).[105–111]

By far, aspiration is the pathogenic mechanism most frequently implicated in the development of nosocomial pneumonia. Huxley and colleagues demonstrated that oropharyngeal aspiration is a common event in both health and illness.[112] Using a sensitive ^{111}In chloride method they found that aspiration occurs in 45% of normal subjects during deep sleep and in 70% of patients with depressed consciousness. Other investigators have reported that 80% of intubated premature infants aspirate,[113] and that the risk of aspiration is seven times higher in young children with uncuffed (77%) compared with cuffed (11%) endotracheal tubes.[114]

The role of aspiration in this disease is supported by numerous other studies that have documented that colonization of the upper airway by pathogenic organisms frequently precedes the onset of pneumonia. In a prospective study, Johanson and coworkers demonstrated that the oropharynx of adult ICU patients frequently becomes colonized with gram-negative bacteria. Twenty-two percent of patients admitted to the ICU were colonized within 24 hours, and 45% within 4 days.[115] Notably, pneumonia occurred in 23% of colonized patients but in only 3.3% of noncolonized patients.[115] Other investigators have emphasized that colonization of the stomach by bacteria is an important pathogenic step leading to the development of hospital-acquired pneumonia.[116–118] Two prospective trials suggested that gastric colonization and possibly subsequent nosocomial pneumonia might be prevented in intubated patients by the use of sucralfate instead of antacids or H_2 antagonists, presumably because sucralfate does not alter the protective barrier provided by a low gastric pH.[119, 120] This hypothesis, however, remains controversial.[121–123] Finally, some studies have suggested that selective decontamination of the airway and gastrointestinal tract with nonabsorbable antibiotics prevents nosocomial pneumonia in mechanically ventilated patients.[124–126] Collectively, these data are consistent with the observation that colonization of the upper airway with pathogenic microorganisms followed by aspiration is the most frequent cause of pneumonia in hospitalized patients.

The events that control pathologic colonization of the airway and upper gastrointestinal tract, the first step in the development of most nosocomial pneumonias, are incompletely understood. In healthy adults, the prevalence of aerobic gram-negative bacilli in the oropharyngeal flora is low (2%),[127] although in normal infants it may reach 67%.[128] Factors that have been associated with pathologic colonization include hospitalization, airway instrumentation, chronic or acute illness, immunosuppression, coma, antibiotics, and viral infection.[105] The source of pathogenic bacteria may be either endogenous, due to translocation or overgrowth of pathogens from the normal flora, or exogenous, transferred from the hospital staff, equipment, or environment.[105] Most studies of nosocomial infection have focused on exogenous sources because they are potentially controllable. A recent prospective study by Klein and associates of mechanically ventilated, nonimmunosuppressed PICU patients underscores the potential importance of exogenously acquired pathogens in this population.[19] Protective isolation was found to delay the colonization of patients with pathogens by 5 days and increased the interval before the first infection from 8 to 20 days.[19] The respiratory tract was the most frequent site of infection in these patients. The authors concluded that the ICU environment and hospital personnel are significant sources of pathologic colonization and nosocomial infection.[19]

Identified factors that increase the risk of developing a nosocomial pneumonia and reflect the basic pathogenic considerations outlined previously are shown in Table 70–10.[108] In general, these risk factors promote pathologic colonization, increase the frequency of aspiration, or interfere with the ability of the host to clear the microorganisms that reach the airway. In the PICU, none of these factors is more important than endotracheal intubation and assisted ventilation. This single factor has been estimated to increase the risk of noso-

Table 70–10. RISK FACTORS FOR NOSOCOMIAL PNEUMONIA*

Alterations in host defenses
  Steroids
  Immunosuppressive therapy
Underlying conditions
  Bronchopulmonary dysplasia
  Severity of illness (hypotension, acidosis, azotemia)
  Nutritional status
  Prior viral infection
Increased risk of aspiration
  Altered consciousness
  Nasogastric intubation
Alterations in mechanical and mucociliary clearance
  Thoracic or upper abdominal surgery
  Diminished cough or gag reflexes
Abnormal colonization of the oropharynx and gastrointestinal tract
  Antibiotics
  Elevated gastric pH
Endotracheal intubation and assisted ventilation

*Adapted from Zucker JR and Goldmann DA: Nosocomial bacterial pneumonia. In: Shelhamer JA, Pizzo PA, Parillo JE, et al (eds): Respiratory Disease in the Immunosuppressed Host. Philadelphia, JB Lippincott, 1991, as adapted from Celis R, Torress A, Gatell JM, et al: Nosocomial pneumonia: A multivariate analysis of risk and prognosis. Chest 93:318, 1988; Hooton TM, Haley RW, Culver DH, et al: The joint associations of multiple risk factors with the occurrence of nosocomial infection. Am J Med 70:960, 1981; and Garibaldi RA, Britt MR, Coleman ML, et al: Risk factors for postoperative pneumonia. Am J Med 70:677, 1981.

Table 70–11. EFFECTS OF INTUBATION ON OROPHARYNGEAL COLONIZATION AND THE PATHOGENESIS OF PNEUMONIA*

Endotracheal tube
  Bypasses the nasopharynx
  Alters air temperature and humidity
  Acts as a foreign body
  Traumatizes pharyngeal and tracheal epithelium
  Impairs ciliary clearance
  Alters cough
  Causes retention of secretions
  Requires suctioning
  Impairs swallowing
  Changes oral flora
  Cuff may cause local trauma or leak contaminated secretions from the oropharynx

Nasotracheal tube
  May cause sinusitis

Nasogastric tube
  Acts as a foreign body
  May cause sinusitis
  Impairs swallowing
  Causes stagnation of oropharyngeal secretions
  Impairs lower esophageal sphincter
  Increases reflux
  Acts as a conduit for bacterial migration

*Adapted from Craven DE and Steger KA: Nosocomial pneumonia in the intubated patient: New concepts on pathogenesis and prevention. Infect Dis Clin North Am 3:843, 1989.

comial pneumonia between 7- and 21-fold.[3, 129, 130] Reasons for the association of intubation with nosocomial pneumonia are summarized in Table 70–11.[106] The risk of pneumonia after tracheostomy in children appears to be less than with endotracheal intubation but depends on the reason for the tracheostomy and the subsequent need for either mechanical ventilation or ICU support.[131] The overall incidence of pneumonia in children with tracheostomies is less than 5%,[132] although the incidence can be as high as 88% in some pediatric populations.[131] The risk of nosocomial pneumonia associated with immunosuppressive therapy is more difficult to assess but has been estimated to be increased by approximately five-fold.[3]

Microbiology

Table 70–2 lists the microorganisms most frequently isolated from pediatric patients with nosocomial pneumonia. *P. aeruginosa* and *S. aureus* are the most frequent etiologic agents.[4, 11, 12] The role of *Candida* species as a cause of nosocomial pneumonia is less clear, though it is reported frequently in pediatric series. *Candida* species often colonize the airway but rarely produce a significant pulmonary infection. Autopsies from cancer treatment centers have shown that less than 3% of patients had pulmonary candidiasis, and in less than 15% of these cases was *Candida* infection the most significant process on histopathologic examination.[133]

Viruses, the predominant cause of nosocomial respiratory tract infection on pediatric ward services, are a less frequent etiology of these infections in the PICU. In two separate studies from the Hospital for Sick

Children in Toronto, respiratory viruses accounted for less than 5% of infections acquired in the PICU.[18, 20] However, in certain hospitalized pediatric populations, such as children with immunosuppression or congenital heart disease, nosocomially acquired respiratory syncytial virus may be an important cause of PICU admission, respiratory failure, and death during the winter.[134–136]

Some opportunistic respiratory pathogens also cause nosocomial pneumonia during hospital-related outbreaks or in specific patient populations. *Legionella pneumophila,* for instance, may be spread to susceptible patients from air conditioning systems or water sources and has been linked to nosocomial epidemics on transplant services.[137] Further, hospital ventilaton systems and construction projects have been associated with episodes of pneumonia due to *Aspergillus* species in immunosuppressed patients.[133] Other opportunistic respiratory pathogens such as cytomegalovirus and *Pneumocystis carinii* may cause pneumonia in immunodeficient patients by either reactivation of latent infection or potentially through nosocomial acquisition, but the epidemiology of hospital transmission for these pathogens is not well established.[138–140]

Diagnosis

The diagnosis of nosocomial pneumonia is based on an increase in sputum production or purulence; the detection of pathogens by culture, microscopic examination, or special (viral) studies; a new and persistent infiltrate on chest radiograph; and systemic signs and symptoms consistent with infection. Use of these criteria in PICU patients, however, is hampered by their lack of specificity, since these findings are often present in patients without pneumonia. Microorganisms cultured from sputum may be the cause of a pneumonia or may merely represent oropharyngeal contamination, airway colonization, or tracheitis. Because of this, daily sputum examinations may be useful to identify changes in the quantity, character, Gram stain, or flora of respiratory secretions and thus aid in the detection of new episodes of infection.[141] Infiltrates on chest radiographs, although a sensitive test for pneumonia, lack specificity as they may be caused by congestive heart failure, diffuse lung injury, hemorrhage, atelectasis, or other noninfectious processes. Further, PICU patients may have many potential sources of fever unrelated to the lung. The difficulty in diagnosing nosocomial pneumonia in ICUs was clearly shown in a study of patients with the adult respiratory distress syndrome and suspected pneumonia. Using post mortem histology as the definitive test, the diagnosis of pneumonia by clinical criteria in this patient population was found to be incorrect 29% of the time.[142]

A number of methods have been advocated to improve the accuracy of diagnosing pneumonia in the intubated ICU patient, including use of the protected specimen brush and quantitative bronchoalveolar lavage.[143–146] In a well-controlled baboon study of pneumonia that compared bronchoalveolar lavage, the protected specimen brush, and transthoracic needle aspiration, 74%, 41%, and 56% of the bacterial species obtained from direct cultures of lung homogenate were recovered, respectively.[147] Thus, these methods reduce some of the diagnostic confusion created by sputum specimen contamination but do not always recover all of the pathogens involved in a pneumonitis. Notably, bronchoalveolar lavage recovered 100% of the bacterial species present in lung tissue at concentrations greater than 10^3 colony-forming units per gram compared to only 62% for the protected specimen brush.[147] Bronchoalveolar lavage and, when feasible, endobronchial biopsy may also be useful in the diagnosis of nosocomial pneumonia in immunocompromised hosts, although open lung biopsy is necessary in some of these patients for definitive diagnosis.

Treatment

The treatment of nosocomial pneumonia involves the use of antimicrobial agents directed at the identified pathogen or, if unknown, at the most likely etiologic agents based on the clinical setting, available diagnostic information, and the flora of the particular institution. Initial antibiotic therapy is frequently empirical, although it may be directed at either gram-negative or gram-positive organisms if the gram stain is sufficiently "diagnostic." Antimicrobial therapy is later tailored to the sensitivity patterns of the isolated microorganisms. Treatment is typically continued for 10 to 14 days, but certain pathogens such as *Legionella* species, *P. aeruginosa,* and *Candida* species usually require longer courses.

Empiric treatment regimens for gram-negative pneumonia often include a third-generation cephalosporin, such as cefotaxime or ceftriaxone for enteric gram-negative bacteria or ceftazidime if *P. aeruginosa* is suspected.[148, 149] Many authors prefer to treat gram-negative bacillary pneumonia with "double" antibiotic coverage, particularly pneumonia caused by *P. aeruginosa,* which carries a high mortality.[109, 150] Semisynthetic pencillins (mezlocillin, pipercillin, and others) may also be used but should always be combined with an aminoglycoside to prevent the emergence of resistance during therapy.[108] Further, combination therapy with two antibiotics directed against *P. aeruginosa* should be used if the patient is neutropenic or the pneumonia is severe.[108] Aminoglycosides should never be used as single agents to treat gram-negative pneumonia because this class of antibiotics has a narrow therapeutic index and poor penetration into bronchial secretions.[108]

Empiric gram-positive therapy should be directed primarily at *S. aureus* using antistaphylococcal penicillins or first-generation cephalosporins.[148, 149] At institutions where methicillin-resistant *S. aureus* or enterococci are prevalent, vancomycin should be used.[150] These antibiotics will also provide adequate initial coverage for group B streptococci, an important consideration, particularly in young infants.[150] Although, third-generation cephalosporins are effective against many gram-positive bacteria, none are considered to be a first-choice antibiotic for *S. aureus*. Ceftazidime should not be relied on as definitive therapy for any infection caused by gram-positive bacteria; this drug has been associated with treatment failures in neutropenic cancer patients infected with gram-positive bacteria including streptococci.[151] The presence of mixed flora on gram stain or a witnessed aspiration of oropharyngeal secretions suggests the need for antimicrobial therapy directed against anaerobic bacteria.[148]

Immunosuppressed patients with unrevealing routine evaluations for bacterial, viral, protozoal, and fungal pathogens are difficult to treat empirically and every effort should be made to arrive at a definitive diagnosis. For a full discussion of all of the diagnostic and therapeutic possibilities for this type of patient, the reader is referred to Chapter 73 and excellent reviews on this subject by Shelhamer and coworkers[152] and Ognibene and associates.[153]

NOSOCOMIAL URINARY TRACT INFECTIONS

Nosocomial urinary tract infection (UTI) is the most frequent hospital-acquired infection in the United States.[2-4] In the National Nosocomial Infection Surveillance survey the total UTI rate (cases per 1,000 discharges) for all patients and services was 12.9, and UTIs accounted for 38.5% of all nosocomial infections.[4] Among pediatric patients, however, the UTI rate was a mere 1.8 cases per 1,000 discharges and UTIs represented only a small fraction of all hospital-acquired infections (approximately 10%) in children.[4] Within the hospitalized pediatric population, however, the occurrence of UTIs is concentrated in children and infants who are critically ill. In the PICU environment, UTI rates as high as 20 cases per 1,000 admissions have been reported.[9] Fifteen to 25% of all nosocomial infections in some PICUs involve the urinary tract, a proportion second only to that for respiratory tract infections.[9, 15, 21]

Pathogenesis

The vast majority (80%) of all hospital-acquired UTIs are associated with the use of urethral catheters.[3, 154] Other urinary tract manipulations such as retrograde pyelography, cystoscopy, urethral dilation, and nephrostomy are responsible for about one half of the remaining cases (10%),[154, 155] with the rest occurring either spontaneously or secondarily to distant infections.[17] The incidence of UTIs in a particular PICU will depend on the frequency and duration of bladder catheterization and the proportion of patients requiring urologic procedures.

UTIs in catheterized patients occur by one of three mechanisms. First, infection may be caused by introduction of microorganisms into the bladder at the time of catheter insertion.[156] The risk of a UTI from a single "in and out" urethral catheterization is 1 to 3%.[3] In general, with the use of proper aseptic technique, this is not a major cause of UTIs in patients with indwelling urinary catheters.[156] Prolonged use of intermittent catheterization, however, results in a high incidence of bacteriuria

and symptomatic UTI that is only modestly lower than the rate seen with indwelling catheters and is probably caused by repeated urethral trauma and the direct inoculation of bacteria into the urinary bladder.[157-160] The second mechanism leading to UTIs in catheterized patients is the retrograde spread of microorganisms from the collection bag up the catheter intralumenally and into the bladder.[156, 161, 162] This was probably the major route of bladder colonization and subsequent infection prior to the introduction of aseptic "closed" drainage systems in the 1960s.[163] Microorganisms entered the urinary bladder by reflux of urine from the collection device or through the growth of bacteria up along the liquid biofilm that coated the lumen of the drainage system.[161, 164] Bladder colonization inevitably occurred in all patients after only 4 days of urethral catheterization.[165] The introduction of standardized aseptic techniques and "closed" drainage systems has delayed the onset of universal bladder colonization in catheterized patients to more than 30 days, but despite this advance, UTIs remain a frequent complication of indwelling urinary catheters.[163, 166] In patients with "closed" drainage systems, meatal and urethral colonization typically precedes the onset of bacteriuria, and a number of investigations support extralumenal migration of bacteria in the periurethral space as the most important pathogenic mechanism of bladder colonization from indwelling urinary catheters.[156, 167, 168] This mechanism, which results in urethral colonization or infection prior to involvement of the bladder, also explains the continued increased risk for the development of bacteriuria that has been seen following catheter removal.[169-172]

Microbiology

The microorganisms most frequently isolated from children with nosocomial UTIs are shown in Table 70-2. *E. coli* and *Pseudomonas* species (virtually all *P. aeruginosa*) are the most common pathogens, though outbreaks on particular wards or related to urologic instrumentation may briefly bring to prominence other organisms that are often antibiotic resistant.[155, 173] Therefore, it is important to be aware of up-to-date information on the local ecology when instituting empiric antibiotic treatment.

Diagnosis

The diagnosis of nosocomial UTIs may be difficult, particularly in infants and critically ill children who may be unable to communicate the presence of symptoms and who may have many potential reasons for a fever or abdominal pain. This task is further complicated in infants with UTIs who typically present with nonspecific findings such as "crankiness" or poor feeding.[174, 175] Diagnostic criteria for UTI, such as the presence of pyuria and bacteruria, may be unreliable in catheterized patients. Properly collected specimens from a catheterized patient should ideally be sterile. Any growth of pathogenic microorganisms should be regarded as colonization and raise suspicion of the presence of infection.[175] Although bacteriuria greater than 10^5 colony-forming units (cfu) of a single bacterial species per milliliter of urine remains a widely applied standard, it is important to remember that this definition is based on clean-catch specimens from symptomatic adult females.[175] Studies in infants and young children, using either a bag collection method or the midstream clean-catch technique (depending on the patient's age) and comparing the results to specimens obtained by suprapubic aspiration have found that the former have a high false-positive rate.[176] Further, the validity of the 10^5 cfu/ml cutoff has not been established in catheterized pediatric patients, and can be affected by nonspecific factors such as urine flow rate.

Treatment

The treatment of nosocomial UTI in the PICU includes the removal of any medical instrumentation (urethral, ureteral, or nephrostomy catheters) when feasible and the administration of appropriate antibiotics for 7 to 14 days depending on the severity of the infection and the presence or absence of pyelonephritis, bacteremia, or other complications. In general, infants and young children appear to be more prone to secondary bacteremia and renal damage than older children and adults.[175, 177] Single-dose antibiotics and "short course" treatment regimens have not been evaluated in the ICU setting and should not be used.

As with other nosocomial infections, the best treatment strategy remains prevention. Prophylactic antibiotics are routinely used for some urologic procedures and may be useful in decreasing the incidence of infection, though this is not without controversy.[178] Table 70–12 lists the risk factors that have been associated with urethral catheters using multivariate analysis.[179, 180] Above all other considerations, urethral catheters should be used sparingly and removed as soon as possible. Of note is a prospective study in adult patients that found that 36% of all catheter days were "medically" unnecessary.[181] When indwelling urinary catheters are used, the only interventions that have been proven to be effective in reducing infection are good aseptic insertion technique and the maintenance of a "closed"

Table 70–12. RISK FACTORS FOR NOSOCOMIAL URINARY TRACT INFECTIONS IN CATHETERIZED PATIENTS*

Duration of catheterization
Lack of systemic antibiotic during short catheter courses
Lack of urinometer drainage
Female sex
Diabetes mellitus
Microbial colonization of the drainage bag
Serum creatinine >2 mg/dl at time of catheterization
Catheterization for reasons other than surgery or urine output measurement
Unsatisfactory drainage system care

*Adapted from Platt R, Polk BF, Murdock B, et al: Risk factors for nosocomial urinary tract infection. Am J Epidemiol 124:977, 1986.

drainage system using sound nursing practices.[163, 179] Other innovations, including daily meatal care with povidone-iodine solution or antibiotic ointment,[182] surveillance cultures,[183] and antibiotic-impregnated catheters, appear not to be of value.[184] Although systemic antibiotics appear to have some impact on the incidence of catheter-related UTIs,[179, 185] this protective effect is short lived and the patient is more likely to become colonized with a resistant organism.[186, 187]

NOSOCOMIAL GASTROINTESTINAL TRACT INFECTIONS

Although an important site of nosocomial infection in the general pediatric population, the gastrointestinal tract is involved in less than 10% of PICU-acquired infections in most series (see Table 70–1).[11, 17, 20] Almost all nosocomial gastroenteritis in children is viral (70 to 100%),[11, 12, 14] and the most frequently isolated pathogen is rotavirus (approximately 33% of cases).[11, 12, 17] In a recent study of 116 nosocomial infections in PICU patients, enteric viruses were isolated from 5 of 9 patients with gastroenteritis.[17] Nonviral causes of gastrointestinal infection, if any, were not mentioned.[17]

The role of *Clostridium difficile*, the etiologic agent of pseudomembranous colitis, in PICU-acquired diarrhea is not clear. Healthy infants and young children are frequent carriers of toxin-producing *C. difficile* (up to 40%), and colonized infants have been found to have high stool titers of *C. difficile* toxin B in the absence of diarrhea.[188] Further, comparison studies between infants and children with and without antibiotic-associated diarrhea have failed to find differences in *C. difficile* colonization or toxin rates.[188] Thus, a causal relationship between this organism and simple antibiotic-associated diarrhea in children has not been established. Pseudomembranous colitis caused by *C. difficile*, however, has been documented in infants and children, though a recent review of the English literature uncovered only 44 cases, nine of which were fatal.[189] *C. difficile* has been found to persist in the hospital environment,[190, 191] and hospital epidemics, including one in an adult ICU, have been observed.[192–194]

A microbiologic diagnosis of *C. difficile*–induced diarrhea or colitis is based on the identification of *C. difficile* cytopathic toxin B in stool.[195] Treatment is usually with oral vancomycin or metronidazole.[196–199] Intravenous vancomycin or metronidazol has been used in patients with uncertain gastrointestinal tract function or ileus, but the efficacy of intravenously administered antibiotics has not been established.[189]

SURGICAL WOUND INFECTIONS

Surgical wound infections occur in approximately 0.085% of hospitalized pediatric patients in the United States[4] and account for 6 to 10% of nosocomial infections in children.[15] Among PICU patients, up to 2.2%[20] have been reported to acquire surgical wound infections and in some units this site represents 15% of all nosocomial infections (see Table 70–1).[15, 20] The incidence and importance of wound infections vary among different PICUs, depending in part on the number and types of surgical patients routinely admitted. Furthermore, it is known that surgical infection rates vary widely among institutions and surgeons and within the same institution over time, although the factors responsible for this variability are debated.[200, 201] Median sternotomy wound infection rates in children, for instance, have been found to be inversely related to the annual number of procedures that a hospital performs,[202] but exceptions to this relationship have been reported.[201]

Pathophysiology

Patient characteristics affecting the incidence of wound infections in children are also controversial. Wound infections in children appear to be independent of gender but may be affected by age. One study examining this issue found wound infection rates in neonates, infants, preschool-aged children, and school-aged children to be 14%, 6%, 4%, and 3%, respectively.[203] Other investigators, however, have not seen this trend toward higher infection rates in younger patients.[204, 205] Immunosuppression probably increases the risk of wound infection,[206] but there is inadequate information, especially for specific types of immunodeficiency, to make definite conclusions regarding the relative risk of infection in pediatric patients with abnormal immunity.[200] In addition, host factors that slow wound healing, such as steroids or malnutrition, probably increase the risk and incidence of infection by impairing capillary growth and tissue macrophage activity.[208] However, a recent study of surgical wound infections in pediatric patients found no relationship between incidence and nutritional status.[204] The same study also failed to find an increase in infections with longer hospital stays prior to surgery,[204] though another study in children demonstrated this association.[205] The additional risk of developing a surgical wound infection, if any, from admission to the PICU is difficult to determine because of the many confounding variables, and because no useful information is currently available.

The three basic factors that affect the risk of surgical wound infection are host resistance, the condition of the wound at closure, and the degree of bacterial contamination.[207, 208] The latter two considerations are by far the most important, as larger inocula of bacteria and severely traumatized wounds correlate with high rates of infection.[204, 209] Overall, local wound factors, including contamination, the presence of foreign material, tissue perfusion, and tissue manipulation during the procedure, appear to play a more important role than host-related factors such as age, nutrition, and resistance.[204] Table 70–13 summarizes the classification system devised by the National Research Council to grade operative wound contamination.[209] Stratification of cases using these surgical catagories is highly predictive of infection risk in both adult and pediatric patients (Table 70–14).[203–205, 210] Within catagories, other wound-related factors can become important. For instance, in a study

Table 70–13. NATIONAL RESEARCH COUNCIL CLASSIFICATION OF OPERATIVE WOUNDS IN RELATION TO CONTAMINATION AND INCREASING RISK OF INFECTION*

Clean
  Nontraumatic
  No inflammation encountered
  No break in technique
  Respiratory, alimentary, genitourinary tracts not entered

Clean-contaminated
  Gastrointestinal or respiratory tracts entered without significant spillage
  Appendectomy
  Oropharynx entered
  Vagina entered
  Genitourinary tract entered in absence of infected urine
  Biliary tract entered in absence of infected bile
  Minor break in technique

Contaminated
  Major break in technique
  Gross spillage from gastrointestinal tract
  Traumatic wound, fresh
  Entrance of genitourinary or biliary tracts in presence of infected urine or bile

Dirty and infected
  Acute bacterial inflammation encountered, without pus
  Transection of "clean" tissue for the purpose of surgical access to a collection of pus
  Traumatic wound with retained devitalized tissue, foreign bodies, fecal contamination, delayed treatment, or from dirty source

*Adapted from Cruse PJE: Wound infections. *In:* Howard RJ and Simmons RL (eds): Surgical Infectious Diseases, 2nd ed. Norwalk CT, Appleton and Lange, 1988, pp. 319–329, as adapted from Altemeier WA, Burke JF, Pruitt BA, et al (eds): *In:* Manual on Control of Infection in Surgical Patients. Philadelphia, JB Lippincott, 1976, p. 20.

of children undergoing "clean" cardiovascular surgery, the risk of wound infection was increased by pump bypass time in excess of 1 hour, excessive postoperative bleeding, low cardiac output for 24 hours or more, reexploration for control of bleeding, and inadequate antimicrobial prophylaxis.[202]

Microbiology

The most frequently isolated pathogens from wound infections are bacterial.[4] Fungal infections are infrequent (<5% of all surgical wound infections),[4, 203–205] though some studies in children have reported unusually high rates of infection with *Candida* species in certain patient subsets.[201, 202] Gram-positive aerobic organisms cause the majority of wound infections (50 to 70%) in children, and gram-negative bacilli account for most of the remaining episodes (see Table 70–2). Like incidence rates, the microbiology of surgical wound infections may show considerable variability over time within an institution and between institutions and types of operative procedures.[200, 201] This observation emphasizes the importance of knowing the current microbiologic data for specific procedures in one's own institution, especially during "epidemics" of wound infection. Further, the exact anatomy of a wound infection may influence its microbial flora, as shown in studies of patients undergoing median sternotomy.[202] Deep infections involving the

Table 70–14. INFECTION RATES STRATIFIED BY WOUND TYPE

	Foothills Hospital (adults) (1967–1977)[210]	University of New Mexico (pediatric) (1986–1988)[204]	Milwaukee Children's Hospital (pediatric) (1980–1981)[205]	Rohtak, India (pediatric) (1985)[203]
Overall	4.7%	2.5%	4.2%	5.4%
Clean	1.5%	1.0%	3.1%	1.8%
Clean-contaminated	7.7%	2.9%	7.8%	5.8%
Contaminated	15.2%	7.9%	17.0%	27.0%
Dirty or infected	40.0%	9.1%*	10.0%†	

*Excludes wounds that were not closed primarily.
†Includes wounds that were not closed primarily.

sternum and mediastinum, often characterized clinically by sternal instability, are more frequently caused by gram-negative bacteria and fungi than are superficial infections.[202]

Diagnosis

For epidemiologic purposes, the diagnosis of a wound infection requires purulent drainage. Other findings such as wound induration, erythema, and tenderness, with or without fever or leukocytosis may also indicate the presence of an infection and the need for antibiotic therapy. However, since these local characteristics are normal to some degree for all wounds as they heal, careful clinical correlation and consultation with the operating surgeon are critical to making the correct diagnosis. The diagnosis may be aided by knowledge of the type of surgical procedure that was performed and appreciation for the relative risk for subsequent infection; such categorization allows the intensivist to maintain a high degree of suspicion for infection in surgical cases classified as "contaminated" or "infected" (see Table 70–13).

Treatment

The treatment of wound infections involves drainage (opening) of the wound, removal of infected and devitalized tissues, and the initiation of an appropriate course of antibiotic therapy. Fortunately, infected material is often present for immediate gram stain and direct microscopic examination, allowing empiric antimicrobial therapy to be directed at a relatively specific group of pathogens. The final choice of agents, of course, will depend upon the results of culture. When cultures fail to yield the causative organisms, a therapeutic regimen is devised to cover the likely pathogens based on the type of surgery and the most recent experience within the hospital. Although mortality from surgical wound infections is usually low due to the ease and promptness of diagnosis and the generally rapid response to treatment, the morbidity may be considerable. Secondary bacteremia occurs in 4.9% of patients with surgical wound infections[4] and prolongation of hospitalization is often unavoidable.

TRANSFUSION-TRANSMITTED INFECTIONS

Transfusion-transmitted infections are infrequently considered with other nosocomial infections because they often become manifest months or even years after the administration of transfusion therapy. There are several reasons, however, for including them in a discussion of hospital-acquired infections in PICU patients. First, with the exception of the operating room, transfusion therapy is used more frequently in ICUs than in other areas of the hospital. The intensivist, therefore, should be well versed in the risks and complications of giving blood and blood products. Second, transfusion-related infection may produce acute symptomatic disease in the ICU that requires diagnosis and occasionally therapy. For example, failure to recognize cytomegalovirus infection as the cause of postoperative fever has led to inappropriate therapeutic intervention and potentially harmful diagnostic procedures including laparotomy.[213, 214] Rarely, infections transmitted by transfusion may result in significant morbidity and even mortality. Third, as discussed further on certain ICU patients require specially screened or processed blood to avoid potentially life-threatening infections. Finally, knowledge of blood-transmitted infections reinforces the need to strictly maintain universal precautions in the ICU environment where health care workers have a high risk for exposure to blood.

Transmission and Prevention

The prevention of transfusion-related infection starts with the screening of potential blood donors by history to eliminate those at high risk for harboring infection. Then, tests for infection are routinely performed on each donated unit of blood. Table 70–15 shows these tests along with the positive prevalance rates in the volunteer donor population.[257] Blood products that test positive for any of these markers, with the exception of anti-cytomegalovirus antibody (anti-CMV), are discarded.

Donation centers do not routinely test for anti-CMV antibody because its prevalance is so high and the consequences of its transmittal are usually trivial.[213–215] Some patients not already infected with CMV, however, are at high risk for serious acute CMV disease. Trans-

Table 70–15. TESTS FOR INFECTION ROUTINELY PERFORMED ON DONATED BLOOD

Infectious Agent	Marker(s) Tested*	Prevalance in Donor Blood†
Hepatitis viruses	HBsAg	0.035%
	Anti-HCV	0.75% (40% confirmed by recombinant immunoblot assay)
	Anti-HBc	1.8%
	ALT (elevation)	1.2% (2.5 times normal)
Retroviruses	HIV-1	0.010% (Western blot confirmed)
	HTLV-I/II	0.012%
Spirochetes	RPR	0.20% (35% confirmed by fluorescent antibody absorption test)
Herpesviruses	Anti-CMV (not routinely tested)	50%

*HBsAg = hepatitis B surface antigen; anti-HCV = antihepatis C virus; anti-HBc = antihepatitis B core; ALT = alanine aminotransferase; HIV-1 = human immunodeficiency virus-1; HTLV-I/II = human T cell leukemia virus I/II; RPR = rapid plasma reagin (screening test for syphilis); anti-CMV = anticytomegalovirus.
†Chyang Fang: Personal communication. American Red Cross, 1990.

mission of CMV can be eliminated by serotesting[215] or by using third-generation leukocyte removal filters.[216, 217] CMV-free products are indicated for uninfected patients who are pregnant,[213, 218] neonates weighing less than 1,200 g,[213, 214, 218–221] solid organ or marrow transplant recipients,[213–215, 222] and patients infected with human immunodeficiency virus[213–215, 223] or immunocompromised and receiving granulocyte transfusions.[213–215, 223] As shown in Table 70–16, CMV-seronegative recipients of blood have a high risk of acquiring CMV (5.0 to 24%).[213–217]

Like CMV, Epstein-Barr virus (EBV) can cause fever and hepatitis in PICU patients who have received transfusions. Although EBV is rarely transmitted by transfusion in adult patients (Table 70–16), transmittal may be more frequent in a susceptible pediatric population.[213, 214, 223] Parvovirus B19, the etiologic agent of erythema infectiosum, has been linked to aplastic crisis in patients with sickle cell disease.[213] Although the seroprevalance of this virus is high, the precise risk of transmittal via blood transfusion is unknown.[213]

Despite donor screening by history and a panel of specific and nonspecific laboratory tests (see Table 70–15), transfusion-related hepatitis remains a significant problem (see Table 70–16). Identification of cases by prospective screening of hepatic enzymes revealed that 5 to 10% of blood recipients contracted hepatitis although the majority of these episodes were not clinically apparent (see Table 70–16).[213, 214, 224] The recent introduction of screening for hepatitis C virus (HCV) will further reduce the incidence of hepatitis. One study, however, suggested that HCV screening may only exclude 60% of HCV infected donors.[225] Newer tests for HCV screening are expected to narrow the "window of time" during which newly infected HCV carriers can go undetected, and therefore the incidence of transfusion-related HCV-hepatitis should continue to fall. Less than 10% of transfusion-related hepatitis is still caused by HBV, and a similar percentage may be caused by non-A, non-B, non-C hepatitis agent(s).[213, 214, 223]

Screening for human immunodeficiency virus (HIV) (see Table 70–16), the etiologic agent of acquired immunodeficiency syndrome (AIDS), by both detailed histories and blood testing has been effective at reducing the risk of acquiring this virus by transfusion therapy (now <1:153,000 per unit of blood).[226–229] In addition to the long-term risk of developing AIDS, transmittal of HIV can cause an acute syndrome with fever, generalized rash, and lymphadenopathy. Case reports suggest that the incubation period for acute HIV disease in children may be as short as 1 week.[230–232] Human T cell leukemia virus (HTLV I/II) is also routinely tested for, though it has a very long latency and does not invariably cause overt disease.[213, 214, 223, 233]

Syphilis is rarely, if ever, transmitted by transfusion in modern industrialized nations due to the brief viability of *T. pallidum* in banked blood and the routine screening of all donated units, which also serves as a surrogate marker for high-risk sexual activities (see Table 70–16).[213, 223, 234] *Borrelia burgdorferi,* the spirochete responsible for Lyme disease, can remain viable in stored red cells and platelets, although there have been no reported cases of transfusion-transmitted Lyme disease.[235]

Parasites can also be transmitted by transfusion therapy, though this occurs rarely in the United States (see Table 70–16).[213, 223] Worldwide, malaria is the most frequent transfusion-related parasitic infection.[213] Other parasites that are rarely transmitted by transfusion in the United States include *Babesia microti,*[213, 223] *Trypanosoma cruzi* (Chagas disease),[213, 223, 235] and *Toxoplasma gondii*[213, 223]

Certain bacteria occasionally contaminate blood products and can cause severe reactions including septic shock and death (see Table 70–2).[213, 236] *P. fluorescens* and other nonaeruginosa species of *Pseudomonas*, probably introduced from contaminated iodophor-scrubbing solutions, can grow in whole blood and packed cells at 4° C and produce a septic shock syndrome.[237] In addition, *Yersinia enterocolitica* has been identified as the cause of over 20 cases of transfusion (red blood cell)-associated sepsis, many of which were fatal.[213, 238] Most of these cases were associated with an asymptomatic carrier state or recent recovery from gastroenteritis in the donor. Two other bacteria have been associated with contamination of platelets (see Table 70–15). *Salmonella* has been traced to donors with subclinical infections.[213, 239] *Staphylococcus* species, apparently picked up from donor skin during collection, grow exponentially at 22° C in platelet storage containers.[240] Other diseases such as brucellosis and rickettsiosis have rarely been transmitted by transfusion therapy.[213, 235]

In addition to the risk of the direct transmittal of

Table 70–16. INFECTIOUS DISEASES TRANSMITTED BY TRANSFUSIONS

Agent	Disease	Risk of Transmission with Current Screening Practices
Viruses		
Hepatitis B virus (HBV)	Hepatitis*	<5–10% overall (enzyme screening)
Hepatitis C virus (HCV)		<0.05 to 0.1% clinically relevant
Non-A, non-B, non-C Hepatitis (NANBNC)		<10% of total HBV
		<10% of total NANBNC
		HCV screening excludes only 60% of infectious units
Human immunodeficiency virus-1	AIDS	<1:153,000 per unit
Human immunodeficiency virus-2		No documented cases of HIV-2 transmitted by transfusion in US
Human T cell leukemia virus I	Adult T cell leukemia/lymphoma; tropical spastic paraparesis HTLV-I associated myelopathy	Low risk
		Highly cell-associated; no seroconversions with fresh frozen plasma cryoprecipitate or coagulation factors
Human T cell leukemia virus II	T cell variant hairy cell leukemia	
Cytomegalovirus (CMV)	Mononucleosis-like syndrome	High risk
	CMV pneumonitis	Transmitted to 5 to 24% of seronegative blood recipients; usually no sequelae. See text for special considerations.
	CMV hepatitis	
	CMV retinitis	
	CMV enteritis	
	CMV nephritis	
	CMV encephalitis	
Epstein-Barr virus (EBV)	Mononucleosis	Low risk
	EBV hepatitis	>90% of adults seropositive
Parvovirus B19	Erythema infectiosum	25% of blood donors have anti-B19 antibody. Precise transmission risk unknown.
	Aplastic crisis in sickle cell anemia	
Spirochetes		
Treponema pallidum	Syphilis	Very low risk
Borrelia burgdorferi	Lyme disease	No documented cases
Parasites		
Plasmodium sp. (particularly P. malariae)	Malaria	<1:4,000,000 per unit in USA. Most frequent parasite transmitted by transfusion in the world
Babesia microti	Babesiosis	<10 reported cases. May cause fatal disease in immunocompromised or splenectomized patients
Trypanosoma cruzi	Chagas disease	2 reported cases in USA. An important problem in South America
Toxoplasma gondii	Toxoplasmosis	<10 reported cases of transmission by granulocyte concentrates
Bacteria		
Pseudomonas fluorescens	Bacteremia/septic shock	>20 reported cases
Yersinia enterocolitica		>20 reported cases
Salmonella sp.		Very low risk, associated with platelet transfusions
Staphylococcus sp.		Very low risk, associated with platelet transfusions

*Risk given as per cent of blood recipients with this complication. On average each blood recipient receives blood from five different donors.

infection by transfusion therapy, there are animal and patient studies suggesting that blood products may cause a broad-spectrum immunosuppression and predispose patients to develop other nosocomial infections.[241–245] Although many of these studies are based on poorly controlled retrospective analyses of patient data, the question deserves further investigation.

The AIDS epidemic has led to a reappraisal of the clinical indications for transfusion therapy and a decline in the overall use of blood products.[246] Prevention of transfusion-related infections through blood screening and the avoidance of unnecessary transfusions needs to be stressed in the PICU, where transfusion therapy is frequently utilized. Above all, the infrequency of acute severe disease caused by transfusion-related infection requires a high degree of suspicion in order to arrive at the correct diagnosis.

CONCLUSION

Nosocomial infections cause more morbidity and mortality than all other PICU-related complications. Therefore, the prevention and control of hospital-acquired

Table 70–17. PREVENTION OF NOSOCOMIAL INFECTIONS

Established or Widely Accepted Practices
General practices
  Hand washing[106, 136, 249, 250]
  Cohort nursing[10, 19, 251]
  Intensive infection surveillance and control program[2, 247, 248]
  Limiting duration of use of medical devices[1]
  Limiting duration of use of systemic antimicrobial agents[1, 115]
  Isolation of patients with resistent or highly contagious
    organisms[2, 247, 248]
  Antimicrobial prophylaxis for selected patient populations
  Vaccination
For intravascular catheters
  Routine interval changes of disposable infusion sets and pressure
    transducer chambers[25, 247, 252, 253]
  Use of closed systems with as few "breaks" (stopcocks) and
    standing ("stagnant") fluid columns as possible[24, 70, 73, 76]
  Use of tunneled catheters (i.e., Hickman, Broviac, Portacath)
    when prolonged central-venous access is required[49, 51]
  Periodic replacement of intravascular devices[47]
    Reinsertion at new sites
    Change over guidewires
For mechanically ventilated patients
  Contact isolation for infection with respiratory syncytial virus or
    influenza virus[136]
  Routine ventilator circuit changes every 48 hours[106]

Potentially Useful or Investigational Practices
General practices
  Selective decontamination[124–126]
  Medical devices impregnated with antimicrobial agents[29, 184]
  Medical devices with antiadherent surfaces[29, 254]
For mechanically ventilated patients
  Maintenance of low gastric pH to prevent gastric colonization by
    pathogenic bacteria and subsequent nosocomial pneumonia[116–123]

Contact isolation (gown and gloves) for prevention of bacterial
  infection[19]
Selective oropharyngeal and tracheal decontamination[124–126]
For intravascular catheters
  Silver-impregnated intravenous catheter cuffs[29]
  Use of traditional gauze dressings (as opposed to new transparent-
    type dressings)[30]
For urinary catheters
  Silver oxide–coated urinary catheters[167, 185]
  Instillation of antimicrobial agents into bladder during intermittent
    catheterization[255, 256]

Abandoned Practices of No Proven Benefit[2, 247, 248, 252, 253]
General practices
  Routine culture surveillance of the environment, personnel, or
    ventilators
  General use of systemic antibiotic prophylaxis
  Tacky or aseptic floor mats
  Quarternary ammonium skin disinfection
  Environmental disinfection with ultraviolet light
For mechanically ventilated patients
  Routine changes of endotracheal tubes[129]
  Routine changes of nebulizers, humidifiers, or ventilator tubing
    more frequently than every 24 hours
  Routine sterilization of internal machinery of ventilators
For intravascular catheters
  Routine replacement of infusion tubing or in-line filters every 24
    hours
  Routine cultures of blood, infusion fluid, stopcocks, and
    catheters[2, 24]
  Use of antimicrobials, either topically or systemically[29, 30]
For urinary catheters
  Meatal care regimens[166, 182]

infections should be a major goal of every PICU in an effort to provide the safest environment possible for the care of critically ill children. Maximizing patient benefit entails balancing the risk of infection against the potential benefit that a medical device or intervention might provide. Precise delineation of the infection problem and the development of innovative prevention measures remain areas of active investigation. Table 70–17 summarizes many of the practices that are used, those that have been tried, and the interventions that have been abandoned in the struggle to prevent nosocomial infections and the harm they cause.

The most important means of minimizing nosocomial infections due to the placement or insertion of medical devices is the use of meticulous aseptic technique and removal of the device as soon as possible.[1] However, the modern ICU also requires an active infection control program to coordinate surveillance[2] and isolation procedures for patients with contagious or resistant pathogens[247, 248] and to promote sound ICU practices such as handwashing[249, 250] and cohort nursing.[10, 19, 251] Although handwashing is simple, inexpensive, and clearly beneficial, studies have documented its flagrant underutilization in the ICU setting.[249, 250] Emphasis of and adherence to standard practices must be the foundation on which to build new strategies. Some of the investigational practices listed in Table 70–17, if proven to be effective, could dramatically change the delivery of care in the ICU, from the materials that are used in medical devices to the basic ways by which care is given

to patients. The reader is referred to Chapter 73 and the references listed in Table 70–17 for additional information on this important topic.

References

1. Maki DG: Risk factors for nosocomial infection in intensive care: "Devices vs. nature" and goals for the next decade. Arch Intern Med 149:30, 1989.
2. Haley RW, Culver DH, White JW, et al: The nationwide nosocomial infection rate: A new need for vital statistics. Am J Epidemiol 121:159, 1985.
3. Haley RW, Hooton TM, Culver DH, et al: Nosocomial infections in US hospitals, 1975–1976. Estimated frequency by selected characteristics of patients. Am J Med 70:947, 1981.
4. Horan TC, White JW, Jarvis WR, et al: Nosocomial infection surveillance, 1984. Centers for Disease Control Surveillance Summaries 1986, 35:17SS.
5. Haley RW, Schaberg DR, and Crossley KB: Extra charges and prolongation of stay attributable to nosocomial infections: A perspective interhospital comparison. Am J Med 70:51, 1981.
6. Haley RW, Schaberg DR, Von Allmen SD, et al: Estimating the extra charges and prolongation of hospitalization due to nosocomial infections: A comparison of methods. J Infect Dis 141:248, 1980.
7. Maki DG: Nosocomial bacteremia: An epidemiologic overview. Am J Med 70:719, 1981.
8. Donowitz LG, Wenzel RP, and Hoyt JW: High risk of hospital-acquired infection in the ICU patient. Crit Care Med 10:355, 1982.
9. Donowitz LG: High risk of nosocomial infection in the pediatric critical care patient. Crit Care Med 14:26, 1986.
10. Wenzel RP, Thompson RL, Landry SM, et al: Hospital-acquired

infections in intensive care unit patients: An overview with emphasis on epidemics. Infect Control 4:371, 1983.

11. Ford-Jones EL, Mindorff CM, Langley JM, et al: Epidemiologic study of 4684 hospital-acquired infections in pediatric patients. Pediatr Infect Dis J 8:668, 1989.

12. Welliver RC and McLaughlin S: Unique epidemiology of nosocomial infection in a children's hospital. Am J Dis Child 138:131, 1984.

13. Brown RB, Hosmer D, Chen HC, et al: A comparison of infections in different ICUs within the same hospital. Crit Care Med 13:472, 1985.

14. Valenti WM, Menegus MA, Hall CB, et al: Nosocomial viral infections. I: Epidemiology and significance. Infect Control 1:33, 1980.

15. Jarvis WR: Epidemiology of nosocomial infections in pediatric patients. Pediatr Infect Dis J 6:344, 1987.

16. Caplan ES and Hoyt N: Infection surveillance and control in the severely traumatized patient. Am J Med 70:638, 1981.

17. Milliken J, Tait GA, Ford-Jones EL, et al: Nosocomial infections in a pediatric intensive care unit. Crit Care Med 16:233, 1988.

18. Hooton TM, Haley RW, Culver DH, et al: The joint associations of multiple risk factors with the occurrence of nosocomial infection. Am J Med 70:960, 1981.

19. Klein BS, Perloff WH, and Maki DG: Reduction of Nosocomial infection during pediatric intensive care by protective isolation. N Engl J Med 320:1714, 1989.

20. Pollock E, Ford-Jones EL, Corey M, et al: Use of the pediatric risk of mortality score to predict nosocomial infection in a pediatric intensive care unit. Crit Care Med 19:160, 1991.

21. Wagner MB, Petrillo V, Gay V, et al: A prevalence survey of nosocomial infection in a Brazilian hospital. J Hosp Infect 15:379, 1989.

22. Christensen GD, Bisno AL, Parisi JT, et al: Nosocomial septicemia due to multiply antibiotic-resistant Staphylococcus epidermidis. Ann Intern Med 96:1, 1982.

23. Mylotte JM, White D, McDermott C, et al: Nosocomial bloodstream infection at a Veterans Hospital; 1979 to 1987. Infect Control Hosp Epidemiol 10:455, 1989.

24. Ducharme FM, Gauthier M, Lacroix J, et al: Incidence of infection related to arterial catheterization in children: A prospective study. Crit Care Med 16:272, 1988.

25. Band JD and Maki DG: Infections caused by arterial catheters used for hemodynamic monitoring. Am J Med 67:735, 1979.

26. Thomas F, Orme JF, Clemmer TP, et al: A prospective comparison of arterial catheter blood and catheter-tip cultures in critically ill patients. Crit Care Med 12:860, 1984.

27. Ashkenazi S and Mirelman D: Adherence of bacteria to pediatric intravenous catheters and needles and its relation to phlebitis in animals. Pediatr Res 18:1361, 1984.

28. Eykyn SJ: Infection and intravenous catheters. J Antimicrob Chemother 14:203, 1984.

29. Maki DG, Cobb L, Garman JK, et al: An attachable silver-impregnated cuff for prevention of infection with central venous catheters: A prospective randomized multicenter trial. Am J Med 85:307, 1988.

30. Maki DG and Ringer M: Evaluation of dressing regimens for prevention of infection with peripheral intravenous catheters. JAMA 258:2396, 1987.

31. Henderson DK: Bacteremia due to percutaneous intravascular devices. In: Mandell GL, Douglas RG Jr, and Bennett JE (eds): Principles and Practice of Infectious Diseases, 3rd ed. New York, Churchill Livingstone, 1990, pp. 2189–2199.

32. Maki DG, Weise CE, and Sarafin HW: A semiquantitative culture method for identifying intravenous-catheter–related infection. N Engl J Med 296:1305, 1977.

33. Cercenado E, Ena J, Rodríguez-Créixems M, et al: A conservative procedure for the diagnosis of catheter-related infections. Arch Intern Med 150:1417, 1990.

34. Linares J, Sitges-Serra A, Garau J, et al: Pathogenesis of catheter sepsis: A prospective study with quantitative and semiquantitative cultures of catheter hub and segments. J Clin Microbiol 21:357, 1985.

35. Collignon P and Munro R: Limitations of semiquantitative method for catheter culture (Letter). J Clin Microbiol 26:1074, 1988.

36. Damen J and van der Tweel I: Positive tip cultures and related

37. Norwood SH, Cormier B, McMahon NG, et al: Prospective study of catheter-related infection during prolonged arterial catheterization. Crit Care Med 16:836, 1988.

38. Tager IB, Ginsberg MB, Ellis SE, et al: An epidemiologic study of the risks associated with peripheral intravenous catheters. Am J Epidemiol 118:839, 1983.

39. Singh S, Nelson N, Acosta I, et al: Catheter colonization and bacteremia with pulmonary and arterial catheters. Crit Care Med 10:736, 1982.

40. Moyer MA, Edwards LD, and Farley L: Comparative culture methods on 101 intravenous catheters: Routine, semiquantitative, and blood cultures. Arch Intern Med 143:66, 1983.

41. Maki DG, McCormick RD, Uman SJ, et al: Septic endarteritis due to intra-arterial catheters for cancer chemotherapy. I. Evaluation of an outbreak. II: Risk factors, clinical features and management. III: Guidelines for prevention. Cancer 44:1228, 1979.

42. Hartman GE and Shochat SJ: Management of septic complications associated with Silastic catheters in childhood malignancy. Pediatr Infect Dis J 6:1042, 1987.

43. Thomas F, Burke JP, Parker J, et al: The risk of infection related to radial vs femoral sites for arterial catheterization. Crit Care Med 11:807, 1983.

44. Early TF, Gregory RT, Wheeler JR, et al: Increased infection rate in double-lumen versus single-lumen Hickman catheters in cancer patients. South Med J 83:34, 1990.

45. Corona ML, Peters SG, Narr BJ, et al: Infections related to central venous catheters. Mayo Clin Proc 65:979, 1990.

46. Myers ML, Austin TW, and Sibbald WJ: Pulmonary artery catheter infections: A prospective study. Ann Surg 201:237, 1985.

47. Eyer S, Brummitt C, Crossley, K, et al: Catheter-related sepsis: Prospective, randomized study of three methods of long-term catheter maintenance. Crit Care Med 18:1073, 1990.

48. Miller JJ, Venus B, and Mathru, M: Comparison of the sterility of long-term central venous catheterization using single lumen, triple lumen, and pulmonary artery catheters. Crit Care Med 12:634, 1984.

49. Mirro J, Rao BN, Stokes DC, et al: A prospective study of Hickman/Broviac catheters and implantable ports in pediatric oncology patients. J Clin Oncol 7:214, 1989.

50. Pinilla JC, Ross DF, Martin T, et al: Study of the incidence of intravascular catheter infection and associated septicemia in critically ill patients. Crit Care Med 11:21, 1983.

51. Becton DL, Kletzel M, Golladay ES, et al: An experience with an implanted port system in 66 children with cancer. Cancer 61:376, 1988.

52. Ponce de Leon S, Critchley S, Wenzel RP: Polymicrobial bloodstream infections related to prolonged vascular catheterization. Crit Care Med 12:856, 1984.

53. Collignon PJ, Soni N, Pearson IY, et al: Is semiquantitative culture of central vein catheter tips useful in the diagnosis of catheter-associated bacteremia? J Clin Microbiol 24:532, 1986.

54. Sitges-Serra A and Linares J: Limitations of semiquantitative method for catheter culture (Letter). J Clin Microbiol 26:1074, 1988.

55. Cleri DJ, Corrado ML, Seligman SJ: Quantitative culture of intravenous catheters and other intravascular inserts. J Infect Dis 141:781, 1980.

56. Cooper GL and Hopkins CC: Rapid diagnosis of intravascular catheter–associated infection by direct staining of catheter segments. N Engl J Med 312:1142, 1985.

57. Collignon P, Chan R, and Munro R: Rapid diagnosis of intravascular catheter–related sepsis. Arch Intern Med 147:1609, 1987.

58. Peter G, Lloyd-Still JD, and Lovejoy FH: Local infection and bacteremia from scalp vein needles and polyethylene catheters in children. J Pediatr 80:78, 1972.

59. Garland JS, Nelson DB, Cheah TE, et al: Infectious complications during peripheral intravenous therapy with Teflon catheters: A prospective study. Pediatr Infect Dis J 6:918, 1987.

60. Collignon PJ, Munro R, and Sorrell TC: Systemic sepsis and intravenous devices: A prospective survey. Med J Aust 141:345, 1984.

61. Goldmann DA, Martin WT, and Worthington JW: Growth of bacteria and fungi in total parenteral nutrition solutions. Am J Surg 126:314, 1973.

62. Curry CR and Quie PG: Fungal septicemia in patients receiving parenteral hyperalimentation. N Engl J Med 285:1221, 1971.

63. Mirro J, Rao BN, Kumar M, et al: A comparison of placement techniques and complications of externalized catheters and implantable port use in children with cancer. J Pediatr Surg 25:120, 1990.

64. Gleason-Morgan D, Church JA, Bagnall-Reeb H, et al: Complications of central venous catheters in pediatric patients with acquired immunodeficiency syndrome. Pediatr Infect Dis J 10:11, 1991.

65. Wang EEL, Prober CG, Ford-Jones L, et al: The management of central intravenous catheter infections. Pediatr Infect Dis 3:110, 1984.

66. Hiemenz J, Skelton J, and Pizzo PA: Perspective on the management of catheter-related infections in cancer patients. Pediatr Infect Dis 5:6, 1986.

67. Eppes SC, Troutman JL, and Gutman LT: Outcome of treatment of candidemia in children whose central catheters were removed or retained. Pediatr Infect Dis J 8:99, 1989.

68. Press OW, Ramsey PG, Larson EB, et al: Hickman catheter infections in patients with malignancies. Medicine 63:189, 1984.

69. Rupar DG, Herzog KD, Fisher MC, et al: Prolonged bacteremia with catheter-related central venous thrombosis. Am J Dis Child 144:879, 1990.

70. Shinozaki T, Deane RS, Mazuzan JE, et al: Bacterial contamination of arterial lines: A prospective study. JAMA 249:223, 1983.

71. Gardner RM, Schwartz R, Wong HC, et al: Percutaneous indwelling radial-artery catheters for monitoring cardiovascular function: Prospective study of the risk of thrombosis and infection. N Engl J Med 290:1227, 1974.

72. Randel SN, Tsang BHL, Wung JT, et al: Experience with percutaneous indwelling peripheral arterial catheterization in neonates. Am J Dis Child 141:848, 1987.

73. Maki DG and Hassemer, CA: Endemic rate of fluid contamination and related septicemia in arterial pressure monitoring. Am J Med 70:733, 1981.

74. Arnow PM and Costas, CO: Delayed rupture of the radial artery caused by catheter-related sepsis. Rev Infect Dis 10:1035, 1988.

75. Crow S, Conrad SA, Chaney-Rowell C, et al: Microbial contamination of arterial infusions used for hemodynamic monitoring: A randomized trial of contamination with sampling through conventional stopcocks versus a novel closed system. Infect Control Hosp Epidemiol 10:557, 1989.

76. Scherer LR, West KW, Weber TR, et al: *Staphylococcus epidermidis* sepsis in pediatric patients: Clinical and therapeutic considerations. J Pediatr Surg 19:358, 1984.

77. Mayhall CG, Archer NH, Lamb A, et al: Ventriculostomy-related infections: A prospective epidemiologic study. N Engl J Med 310:553, 1984.

78. Chan KH and Mann KS: Prolonged therapeutic external ventricular drainage: A prospective study. Neurosurgery 23:436, 1988.

79. Ohrstrom JK, Skou JK, Ejlertsen T, et al: Infected ventriculostomy: Bacteriology and treatment. Acta Neurochir 100:67, 1989.

80. Stenager E, Gerner-Smidt P, and Kock-Jensen C: Ventriculostomy-related infections—an epidemiological study. Acta Neurochir 83:20, 1986.

81. Tenney JH: Bacterial infections of the central nervous system in neurosurgery. Neurol Clin 4:91, 1986.

82. van Ek B, Bakker FP, van Dulken H, et al: Infections after craniotomy: A retrospective study. J Infect 12:105, 1986.

83. Hasan D, Vermeulen M, Wijdicks EFM, et al: Management problems in acute hydrocephalus after subarachnoid hemorrhage. Stroke 20:747, 1989.

84. Kanter RK, Weiner LB, Patti AM, et al: Infectious complications and duration of intracranial pressure monitoring. Crit Care Med 13:837, 1985.

85. Aucoin PJ, Kotilainen HR, Gantz NM, et al: Intracranial pressure monitors: Epidemiologic study of risk factors and infections. Am J Med 80:369, 1986.

86. Ward JD: Intracranial pressure monitoring. *In:* Fuhrman BP and Shoemaker WC (eds): Critical Care: State of the Art. Fullerton, CA, Society of Critical Care Medicine, 1989, pp. 173–183.

87. Lally KP, Brennan LP, Sherman NJ, et al: Use of a subclavian venous catheter for short- and long-term hemodialysis in children. J Pediatr Surg 22:603, 1987.

88. Gleghorn EE, Rosenthal P, Vachon L, et al: Long-term external catheter biliary drainage for recurrent cholangitis after hepatoportoenterostomy. J Pediatr Gastroenterol Nutr 5:485, 1986.

89. Stanley P and Diament MJ: Pediatric percutaneous nephrostomy: Experience with 50 patients. J Urol 135:1223, 1986.

90. McClung MR: Peritonitis in children receiving continuous ambulatory peritoneal dialysis. Pediatr Infect Dis 2:328, 1983.

91. Alliapoulos JC, Salusky IB, Hall T, et al: Comparison of continuous cycling peritoneal dialysis with continuous ambulatory peritoneal dialysis in children. J Pediatr 105:721, 1984.

92. Brem AS and Toscano AM: Continuous-cycling peritoneal dialysis for children: An alternative to hemodialysis treatment. Pediatrics 74:254, 1984.

93. Levy M, Balfe JW, Geary DF, et al: Peritonitis in children undergoing dialysis: 10 years experience. Child Nephrol Urol 9:253, 1989.

94. Matthews DE, West KW, Rescorla FJ, et al: Peritoneal dialysis in the first 60 days of life. J Pediatr Surg 25:110, 1990.

95. Tapper D, Watkins S, Burns M, et al: Comprehensive management of renal failure in infants. Arch Surg 125:1276, 1990.

96. Stone MM, Fonkalsrud EW, Salusky IB, et al: Surgical management of peritoneal dialysis catheters in children: Five-year experience with 1,800 patient-month follow-up. J Pediatr Surg 21:1177, 1986.

97. Watson AR, Vigneux A, Bannatyne RM, et al: Peritonitis during continuous ambulatory peritoneal dialysis in children. Can Med Assoc J 134:1019, 1986.

98. Zaontz MR, Cohn RA, Moel DI, et al: Continuous ambulatory peritoneal dialysis: The pediatric experience. J Urol 138:353, 1987.

99. Shalit I, Greenwood RB, Marks MI, et al: Pharmacokinetics of single-dose oral ciprofloxacin in patients undergoing chronic ambulatory peritoneal dialysis. Antimicrob Agents Chemother 30:152, 1986.

100. Hughes JM: Epidemiology and prevention of nosocomial pneumonia. *In:* Remington JS and Swartz MN (eds): Current Clinical Topics in Infectious Diseases, Vol. 9. New York, McGraw-Hill, 1988, pp. 241–259.

101. Craig CP and Connelly S: Effect of intensive care unit nosocomial pneumonia on duration of stay and mortality. Am J Infect Control 12:233, 1984.

102. Hemming VG, Overall JC, and Britt MR: Nosocomial infections in a newborn intensive-care unit: Results of forty-one months of surveillance. N Engl J Med 294:1310, 1976.

103. Arens JF, LeJeune FE Jr, and Webre DR: Maxillary sinusitis, a complication of nasotracheal intubation. Anesthesiology 40:415, 1974.

104. Caplan ES and Hoyt NJ: Nosocomial sinusitis. JAMA 247:639, 1982.

105. Salata RA and Ellner JJ: Bacterial colonization of the tracheobronchial tree. Clin Chest Med 9:623, 1988.

106. Craven DE and Steger KA: Nosocomial pneumonia in the intubated patient: New concepts on pathogenesis and prevention. Infect Dis Clin North Am 3:843, 1989.

107. Pennington JE: Hospital-acquired pneumonia. *In:* Pennington JE (ed): Respiratory Infections: Diagnosis and Management, 2nd ed. New York, Raven Press, 1988, pp. 171–186.

108. Zucker JR and Goldmann DA: Nosocomial bacterial pneumonia. *In:* Shelhamer JA, Pizzo PA, Parrillo JE, et al (eds): Respiratory Disease in the Immunosuppressed Host. Philadelphia, JB Lippincott, 1991, pp. 255–276.

109. Reinarz JA, Pierce AK, Mays BB, et al: The potential role of inhalation therapy equipment in nosocomial pulmonary infection. J Clin Invest 44:831, 1965.

110. Weber DJ, Wilson MB, Rutala WA, et al: Manual ventilation bags as a source for bacterial colonization of intubated patients. Am Rev Respir Dis 142:892, 1990.

111. Craven DE, Goularte TA, and Make BJ: Contaminated condensate in mechanical ventilator circuits: A risk factor for nosocomial pneumonia? Am Rev Respir Dis 129:625, 1984.

112. Huxley EJ, Viroslav J, Gray WR, et al: Pharyngeal aspiration in normal adults and patients with depressed consciousness. Am J Med 64:564, 1978.

113. Goodwin SR, Graves SA, and Haberkern CM: Aspiration in intubated premature infants. Pediatrics 75:85, 1985.

114. Browning DH and Graves SA: Incidence of aspiration with endotracheal tubes in children. J Pediatr 102:582, 1983.

115. Johanson WG Jr, Pierce AK, Sanford JP, et al: Nosocomial respiratory infections with gram-negative bacilli: The significance of colonization of the respiratory tract. Ann Intern Med 77:701, 1972.

116. Atherton ST and White DJ: Stomach as source of bacteria colonising respiratory tract during artificial ventilation. Lancet 1:968, 1978.

117. Ruddell WSJ, Axon ATR, Findlay JM, et al: Effect of cimetidine on the gastric bacterial flora. Lancet 1:672, 1980.

118. Du Moulin GC, Paterson DG, Hedley-Whyte J, et al: Aspiration of gastric bacteria in antacid-treated patients: A frequent cause of postoperative colonisation of the airway. Lancet 1:242, 1982.

119. Driks MR, Craven DE, Celli BR, et al: Nosocomial pneumonia in intubated patients given sucralfate as compared with antacids or histamine type 2 blockers: The role of gastric colonization. N Engl J Med 317:1376, 1987.

120. Tryba M: Risk of acute stress bleeding and nosocomial pneumonia in ventilated intensive care unit patients: Sucralfate versus antacids. Am J Med 83:117, 1987.

121. Palmer RH: Nosocomial pneumonia in intubated patients (Letter). N Engl J Med 318:1465, 1988.

122. Gachot B, Jebrak G, Legras A, et al: Nosocomial pneumonia in intubated patients (Letter). N Engl J Med 318:1466, 1988.

123. Karlstadt RG and Palmer RH: Risk factors for nosocomial pneumonia in intensive care. Arch Intern Med 150:919, 1990.

124. Van Uffelen R, Rommes JH, and Van Saene HKF: Preventing lower airway colonization and infection in mechanically ventilated patients. Crit Care Med 15:99, 1987.

125. Clasener HAL, Vollaard EJ, and Van Saene HKF: Long-term prophylaxis of infection by selective decontamination in leukopenia and in mechanical ventilation. Rev Infect Dis 9:295, 1987.

126. Flaherty J, Nathan C, Kabins SA, et al: Pilot trial of selective decontamination for prevention of bacterial infection in an intensive care unit. J Infect Dis 162:1393, 1990.

127. Johanson WG, Pierce AK, and Sanford JP: Changing pharyngeal bacterial flora of hospitalized patients: Emergence of gram-negative bacilli. N Engl J Med 281:1137, 1969.

128. Baltimore RS, Duncan RL, Shapiro ED, et al: Epidemiology of pharyngeal colonization of infants with aerobic gram-negative rods. J Clin Microbiol 27:91, 1989.

129. Torres A, Aznar R, Gatell JM, et al: Incidence, risk, and prognosis factors of nosocomial pneumonia in mechanically ventilated patients. Am Rev Respir Dis 142:523, 1990.

130. Celis R, Torres A, Gatell JM, et al: Nosocomial pneumonia: A multivariate analysis of risk and prognosis. Chest 93:318, 1988.

131. Brook I: Bacterial colonization, tracheobronchitis, and pneumonia following tracheostomy and long-term intubation in pediatric patients. Chest 76:420, 1979.

132. Aass AS: Complications of tracheostomy and long term intubation: A follow-up study. Acta Anaesthesiol Scand 19:127, 1975.

133. Jones JM: Pneumonia due to *Candida, Aspergillus,* and *Mucorales* species. *In:* Shelhamer J, Pizzo PA, Parrillo JE, et al (eds): Respiratory Disease in the Immunosuppressed Host. Philadelphia, JB Lippincott, 1991, pp. 338–354.

134. Hall BC, Powell KR, MacDonald NE, et al: Respiratory syncytial viral infection in children with compromised immune function. N Engl J Med 315:77, 1986.

135. MacDonald NE, Hall BC, Suffin SC, et al: Respiratory syncytial viral infection in infants with congenital heart disease. N Engl J Med 307:397, 1982.

136. Hall BC: Hospital-acquired pneumonia in children: The role of respiratory viruses. Semin Respir Infect 2:48, 1987.

137. Kugler JW, Armitage JO, Helms CM, et al: Nosocomial Legionnaires' disease: Occurrence in recipients of bone marrow transplants. Am J Med 74:281, 1983.

138. Rawls WE, Wong CL, Blajchman M, et al: Neonatal cytomegalovirus infections: The relative role of neonatal blood transfusion and maternal exposure. Clin Invest Med 7:13, 1984.

139. Singer C, Armstrong D, Rosen PP, et al: *Pneumocystis carinii* pneumonia: A cluster of eleven cases. Ann Intern Med 82:772, 1975.

140. Ruebush TK, Weinstein RA, Baehner RL, et al: An outbreak of *Pneumocystis* pneumonia in children with acute lymphocytic leukemia. Am J Dis Child 132:143, 1978.

141. Salata RA, Lederman MM, Shlaes DM, et al: Diagnosis of nosocomial pneumonia in intubated, intensive care unit patients. Am Rev Respir Dis 135:426, 1987.

142. Andrews CP, Coalson JJ, and Smith JD: Diagnosis of nosocomial bacterial pneumonia in acute, diffuse lung injury. Chest 80:254, 1981.

143. Chastre J, Fagon JY, Soler P, et al: Diagnosis of nosocomial bacterial pneumonia in intubated patients undergoing ventilation: Comparison of the usefulness of bronchoalveolar lavage and the protected specimen brush. Am J Med 85:499, 1988.

144. Fagon JY, Chastre J, Hance AJ, et al: Detection of nosocomial lung infection in ventilated patients: Use of a protected specimen brush and quantitative culture techniques in 147 patients. Am Rev Respir Dis 138:110, 1988.

145. Tobin MJ and Grenvik A: Nosocomial lung infection and its diagnosis. Crit Care Med 12:191, 1984.

146. Faling LJ: New advances in diagnosing nosocomial pneumonia in intubated patients. Part I (editorial). Am Rev Respir Dis 137:253, 1988.

147. Johanson WG Jr., Seidenfeld JJ, Gomez P, et al: Bacteriologic diagnosis of nosocomial pneumonia following prolonged mechanical ventilation. Am Rev Respir Dis 137:259, 1988.

148. Pennington JE: New therapeutic approaches to hospital-acquired pneumonia. Semin Respir Infect 2:67, 1987.

149. LaForce FM: Systemic antimicrobial therapy of nosocomial pneumonia: Monotherapy versus combination therapy. Eur J Clin Microbiol Infect Dis 8:61, 1989.

150. Berk SL and Verghese A: Emerging pathogens in nosocomial pneumonia. Eur J Clin Microbiol Infect Dis 8:11, 1989.

151. Pizzo PA, Hathorn JW, Hiemenz J, et al: A randomized trial comparing ceftazidine alone with combination therapy in cancer patients with fever and neutropenia. N Engl J Med 315:552, 1986.

152. Shelhamer J, Pizzo PA, Parrillo JE, et al: Respiratory Disease in the Immunosuppressed Host. Philadelphia, JB Lippincott, 1991.

153. Ognibene FP, Pass HI, Roth JA, et al: The diagnosis and therapy of respiratory disease in the immunosuppressed host. *In:* Parrillo JE and Masur H (eds): The Critically Ill Immunosuppressed Patient: Diagnosis and Management. Rockville, MD, Aspen Publishers, 1987, pp. 39–80.

154. Stamm WE, Martin SM, and Bennett JV: Epidemiology of nosocomial infections due to gram-negative bacilli: Aspects relevant to development and use of vaccines. J Infect Dis 136:S151, 1977.

155. Echols RM, Palmer DL, King RM, et al: Multidrug-resistant *Serratia marcescens* bacteriuria related to urologic instrumentation. South Med J 77:173, 1984.

156. Kunin CM and Steele C: Culture of the surfaces of urinary catheters to sample urethral flora and study the effect of antimicrobial therapy. J Clin Microbiol 21:902, 1985.

157. Hardy AG: Experiences with intermittent catherization in acute paraplegia. Med Services J Can 22:538, 1966.

158. Perkash I: Intermittent catheterization and bladder rehabilitation in spinal cord injury patients. J Urol 114:230, 1975.

159. Pearman JW: Urological follow-up of 99 spinal cord injured patients initially managed by intermittent catheterization. Br J Urol 48:297, 1976.

160. Herr HW: Intermittent catheterization in neurogenic bladder dysfunction. J Urol 113:477, 1975.

161. Thornton GF and Andriole VT: Bacteriuria during indwelling catheter drainage. JAMA 214:339, 1970.

162. Blenkharn JJ: Prevention of bacteriuria during urinary catheterization of patients in an intensive care unit: Evaluation of the 'Ureofix 500' closed drainage system. J Hosp Infect 6:187, 1985.

163. Kunin CM, McCormack RC: Prevention of catheter-induced urinary-tract infections by sterile closed drainage. N Engl J Med 274:1155, 1966.

164. Nickel JC, Ruseska I, Wright JB, et al: Tobramycin resistance of *Pseudomonas* aeruginosa cells growing as a biofilm on urinary catheter material. Antimicrob Agents Chemother 27:619, 1985.

165. Kass EH: Asymptomatic infections of the urinary tract. Trans Assoc Am Physicians 69:56, 1956.

166. Schaeffer AJ, Story KO, and Johnson SM: Effect of silver

oxide/trichloroisocyanuric acid antimicrobial urinary drainage system on catheter-associated bacteriuria. J Urol 139:69, 1988.

167. Garibaldi RA, Burke JP, Britt MR, et al: Meatal colonization and catheter-associated bacteriuria. N Engl J Med 303:316, 1986.

168. Schaeffer AJ and Chmiel J: Urethral meatal colonization in the pathogenesis of catheter-associated bacteriuria. J Urol 130:1096, 1983.

169. Brehmer B and Madsen PO: Route and prophylaxis of ascending bladder infection in male patients with indwelling catheters. J Urol 108:719, 1972.

170. Britt MR, Garibaldi RA, Miller WA, et al: Antimicrobial prophylaxis for catheter-associated bacteriuria. Antimicrob Agents Chemother 11:240, 1977.

171. Butler HK and Kunin CM: Evaluation of specific systemic antimicrobial therapy in patients while on closed catheter drainage. J Urol 100:567, 1968.

172. Marple CD: The frequency and character of urinary tract infections in an unselected group of women. Ann Intern Med 14:2220, 1941.

173. Schaberg DR, Weinstein RA, and Stamm WE: Epidemics of nosocomial urinary tract infection caused by multiply resistant gram-negative bacilli: Epidemiology and control. J Infect Dis 133:363, 1976.

174. Spencer JR and Schaeffer AJ: Pediatric urinary tract infections. Urol Clin North Am 13:661, 1986.

175. Burns MW, Burns JL, and Krieger JN: Pediatric urinary tract infection: Diagnosis, classification, and significance. Pediatr Clin North Am 34:1111, 1987.

176. Aronson AS, Gustafson G, and Svenningsen NW: Combined suprapubic aspiration and clean-voided urine examination in infants and children. Acta Paediatr Scand 62:396, 1973.

177. Ginsburg CM and McCracken GH: Urinary tract infections in young infants. Pediatrics 69:409, 1982.

178. Chodak GW and Plaut ME: Systemic antibiotics for prophylaxis in urologic surgery: A critical review. J Urol 121:695, 1979.

179. Platt R, Polk BF, Murdock B, et al: Risk factors for nosocomial urinary tract infection. Am J Epidemiol 124:977, 1986.

180. Shapiro M, Simchen E, Izraeli, S, et al: A multivariate analysis of risk factors for acquiring bacteriuria in patients with indwelling urinary catheters for longer than 24 hours. Infect Control 5(11):525, 1984.

181. Hartstein AI, Garber SB, Ward TT, et al: Nosocomial urinary tract infection: A prospective evaluation of 108 catheterized patients. Infect Control 2(5):380, 1981.

182. Burke JP, Jacobson JA, Garibaldi RA, et al: Evaluation of daily meatal care with poly-antibiotic ointment in prevention of urinary catheter-associated bacteriuria. J Urol 129:331, 1983.

183. Garibaldi RA, Mooney BR, Epstein BJ, et al: An evaluation of daily bacteriologic monitoring to identify preventable episodes of catheter-associated urinary tract infection. Infect Control 3(6):466, 1982.

184. Johnson JR, Roberts PL, Olsen RJ, et al: Prevention of catheter-associated urinary tract infection with a silver oxide–coated urinary catheter: Clinical and microbiologic correlates. J Infect Dis 162:1145, 1990.

185. Garibaldi RA, Burke JP, Dickman ML, et al: Factors predisposing to bacteriuria during indwelling urethral catheterization. N Engl J Med 291:215, 1974.

186. Warren JW, Anthony WC, Hoopes JM, et al: Cephalexin for susceptible bacteriuria in afebrile, long-term catheterized patients. JAMA 248:454, 1982.

187. Mountokalakis T, Skounakis M, and Tselentis J: Short-term versus prolonged systemic antibiotic prophylaxis in patients treated with indwelling catheters. J Urol 134:506, 1985.

188. Cooperstock M: Clostridium difficile in infants and children. In: Rolfe RD and Finegold SM (eds): Clostridium Difficile: Its Role in Intestinal Disease. San Diego, Academic Press, 1988, pp 45–64.

189. Zwiener RJ, Belknap WM, and Quan R: Severe pseudomembranous enterocolitis in a child: Case report and literature review. Pediatr Infect Dis J 8:876, 1989.

190. Fekety R, Kim KH, Brown D, et al: Epidemiology of antibiotic-associated colitis: Isolation of Clostridium difficile from the hospital environment. Am J Med 70:906, 1981.

191. Kim KH, Fekety R, Batts DH, et al: Isolation of Clostridium difficile from the environment and contacts of patients with antibiotic-associated colitis. J Infect Dis 143:42, 1981.

192. Pierce PF Jr, Wilson R, Silva J Jr, et al: Antibiotic-associated pseudomembranous colitis: An epidemiologic investigation of a cluster of cases. J Infect Dis 145:269, 1982.

193. Wüst J, Sullivan NM, Hardegger U, et al: Investigation of an outbreak of antibiotic-associated colitis by various typing methods. J Clin Microbiol 16:1096, 1982.

194. Walter BAJ, Stafford R, Roberts RK, et al: Contamination and crossinfection with Clostridium difficile in an intensive care unit. Aust NZ J Med 12:255, 1982.

195. Bartlett JG, Moon N, Chang TW, et al: Role of Clostridium difficile in antibiotic-associated pseudomembranous colitis. Gastroenterology 75:778, 1978.

196. George WL, Rolfe RD, Finegold SM: Treatment and prevention of antimicrobial agent–induced colitis and diarrhea. Gastroenterology 79:366, 1980.

197. Cherry RD, Portnoy D, Jabbari M, et al: Metronidazole: An alternate therapy for antibiotic-associated colitis. Gastroenterology 82:849, 1982.

198. Tedesco FJ: Pseudomembranous colitis: Pathogenesis and therapy. Med Clin North Am 66:655, 1982.

199. Teasley DG, Gerding DN, Olson MM, et al: Prospective randomised trial of metronidazole versus vancomycin for Clostridium-difficile–associated diarrhoea and colitis. Lancet 1:1043, 1983.

200. Shenep JL: Antimicrobial prophylaxis of pediatric surgical wound infections. Adv Pediatr Infect Dis 5:157, 1990.

201. Pollock E, Ford-Jones EL, Rebeyka I, et al: Early nosocomial infections in pediatric cardiovascular surgery patients. Crit Care Med 18:378, 1990.

202. Edwards MS and Baker CJ: Median sternotomy wound infections in children. Pediatr Infect Dis 2:105, 1983.

203. Sharma LK and Sharma PK: Postoperative wound infection in a pediatric surgical service. J Pediatr Surg 21:889, 1986.

204. Bhattacharyya N and Kosloske AM: Postoperative wound infection in pediatric surgical patients: A study of 676 infants and children. J Pediatr Surg 25:125, 1990.

205. Davis SD, Sobocinski K, Hoffmann RG, et al: Postoperative wound infections in a children's hospital. Pediatr Infect Dis 3:114, 1984.

206. Goldman MH and Rose RC III: Complications of immunosuppression. In: Greenfield LJ (ed): Complications in Surgery and Trauma, 2nd ed. Philadelphia, JB Lippincott, 1990, pp. 216–230.

207. Nichols RE: Postoperative wound infection (editorial). N Engl J Med 307:1701, 1982.

208. Maki DG: Epidemiology of surgical wound infection. In: Condon RE and Gorbach SL (eds): Surgical Infection—Selective Antibiotic Therapy. Baltimore, Williams & Wilkins, 1981, pp. 166–176.

209. Cruse PJE: Wound infections: Epidemiology and clinical characteristics. In: Howard RJ and Simmons RL (eds): Surgical Infectious Diseases, 2nd ed. Norwalk, CT, Appleton & Lange, 1988, pp. 319–329.

210. Cruse PJE and Foord R: The epidemiology of wound infection: A 10 year prospective study of 62,939 wounds. Surg Clin North Am 60:27, 1980.

211. Siegman-Igra Y: Late postoperative fever—viral infection following multiple blood transfusion. Isr J Med Sci 19:267, 1983.

212. Lerner PI and Sampliner JE: Transfusion associated cytomegalovirus mononucleosis. Ann Surg 185:406, 1977.

213. Infectious agents transmitted by transfusion. In: Mollison PL, Engelfriet CP, Contreras M (eds): Blood Transfusion in Clinical Medicine. Oxford, Blackwell Scientific Publications, 1987, pp 764–807.

214. Transfusion-transmitted viruses. In: Walker RH (ed): Technical Manual of the American Association of Blood Banks. Arlington, VA, American Association of Blood Banks, 1989, pp. 59–90.

215. Forbes BA: Acquisition of cytomegalovirus infection: An update. Clin Microbiol Rev 2:204, 1989.

216. Murphy MF, Grint PCA, Hardiman AE, et al: Use of leucocyte-poor blood components to prevent primary cytomegalovirus (CMV) infection in patients with acute leukaemia (letter). Br J Haematol 70:253, 1988.

217. Gilbert GL, Hayes K, Hudson IL, et al: Prevention of transfusion-acquired cytomegalovirus infection in infants by blood filtration to remove leucocytes. Lancet 1:1228, 1989.

218. Adler SP: Neonatal cytomegalovirus infections due to blood. CRC Crit Rev Clin Lab Sci 23:1, 1986.

219. Adler SP, Chandrika T, Lawrence L, et al: Cytomegalovirus infections in neonates acquired by blood transfusions. Pediatr Infect Dis 2:114, 1983.

220. Griffin MP, O'Shea M, Brazy JE, et al: Cytomegalovirus infection in a neonatal intensive care unit: Blood transfusion practices and incidence of infection. Am J Dis Child 142:1188, 1988.

221. Griffin MP, O'Shea M, Brazy JE, et al: Cytomegalovirus infection in a neonatal intensive care unit: Subsequent morbidity and mortality of seropositive infants. J Perinatol 10:43, 1990.

222. Pollard RB: Cytomegalovirus infections in renal, heart, heart-lung and liver transplantation. Pediatr Infect Dis J 7:S97, 1988.

223. Bruce-Chwatt LJ: Infection, immunity, and blood transfusion. Br Med J 288:1782, 1984.

224. Bove JR: Transfusion-associated hepatitis and AIDS. N Engl J Med 317:242, 1987.

225. Esteban JI, Gonzalez A, Hernandez JM, et al: Evaluation of antibodies to hepatitis C virus in a study of transfusion-associated hepatitis. N Engl J Med 323:1107, 1990.

226. Cumming PD, Wallace EL, Schorr JB, et al: Exposure of patients to human immunodeficiency virus through the transfusion of blood components that test antibody-negative. N Engl J Med 321:941, 1989.

227. Leitman SF, Klein HG, Melpolder JJ, et al: Clinical implications of positive tests for antibodies to human immunodeficiency virus type 1 in asymptomatic blood donors. New Engl J Med 321:918, 1989.

228. Ward JW, Holmberg SD, Allen JR, et al: Transmission of human immunodeficiency virus (HIV) by blood transfusions screened as negative for HIV antibody. N Engl J Med 318:473, 1988.

229. Ward JW, Bush TJ, Perkins HA, et al: The natural history of transfusion-associated infection with human immunodeficiency virus: Factors influencing the rate of progression to disease. N Engl J Med 321:947, 1989.

230. Colebunders R, Greenberg AE, Francis H, et al: Acute HIV illness following blood transfusion in three African children. AIDS 2:125, 1988.

231. Shannon K, Ball E, Wasserman RL, et al: Transfusion-associated cytomegalovirus infection and acquired immune deficiency syndrome in an infant. J Pediatr 103:859, 1983.

232. Kalbfleisch JD and Lawless JF: Estimating the incubation time distribution and expected number of cases of transfusion-associated acquired immune deficiency syndrome. Transfusion 29:672, 1989.

233. Chen YC, Wang CH, Su IJ, et al: Infection of human T-cell leukemia virus type I and development of human T-cell leukemia/lymphoma in patients with hematologic neoplasms: A possible linkage to blood transfusion. Blood 74:388, 1989.

234. Seidl S: Syphilis screening in the 1990s. Transfusion 30:773, 1990.

235. Feldschuh J and Weber D: The risks of transfusion today. In: Safe Blood: Purifying the Nation's Blood Supply in the Age of AIDS. New York, The Free Press, 1990, pp. 71–95.

236. Tabor E, Rook AH, Quinnan GV Jr, et al: Bacterial infections transmitted by blood. In: Infectious Complications of Blood Transfusion. New York, Academic Press, 1982, pp. 147–165.

237. Scott J, Boulton FE, Govan JRW, et al: A fatal transfusion reaction associated with blood contaminated with *Pseudomonas fluorescens*. Vox Sang 54:201, 1988.

238. Tipple MA, Bland LA, Murphy JJ, et al: Sepsis associated with transfusion of red cells contaminated with *Yersinia enterocolitica*. Transfusion 30:207, 1990.

239. Heal JM, Jones ME, Forey J, et al: Fatal *Salmonella* septicemia after platelet transfusion. Transfusion 27:2, 1987.

240. Braine HG, Kickler TS, Charache P, et al: Bacterial sepsis secondary to platelet transfusion: An adverse effect of extended storage at room temperature (abstract). Transfusion 26:391, 1986.

241. Waymack JP: The effect of blood transfusions on resistance to bacterial infections. Transplant Proc 20:1105, 1988.

242. Tartter PI, Driefuss RM, Malon AM, et al: Relationship of postoperative septic complications and blood transfusions in patients with Crohn's disease. Am J Surg 155:43, 1988.

243. Tartter PI: Blood transfusion and postoperative infections. Transfusion 29:456, 1989.

244. Salo M: Immunosuppressive effects of blood transfusion in anaesthesia and surgery. Acta Anaesthesiol Scand 32S:26, 1988.

245. George CD and Morello PJ: Immunologic effects of blood transfusion upon renal transplantation, tumor operations, and bacterial infections. Am J Surg 152:329, 1986.

246. Surgenor DM, Wallace EL, Hao SHS, et al: Collection and transfusion of blood in the United States, 1982–1988. N Engl J Med 322:1646, 1990.

247. Simmons BP: CDC guidelines for the prevention and control of nosocomial infections: Guideline for prevention of intravascular infections. Am J Infect Control 11:183, 1983.

248. Simmons BP and Wong ES: CDC guidelines for the prevention and control of nosocomial infections: Guideline for prevention of nosocomial pneumonia. Am J Infect Control 11:230, 1983.

249. Knittle MA, Eitzman DV, and Baer H: Role of hand contamination of personnel in the epidemiology of gram-negative nosocomial infections. J Pediatr 86:433, 1975.

250. Preston GA, Larson EL, and Stamm WE: The effect of private isolation rooms on patient care practices, colonization and infection in an intensive care unit. Am J Med 70:641, 1981.

251. Goldmann DA, Durbin WA Jr, and Freeman J: Nosocomial infections in a neonatal intensive care unit. J Infect Dis 144:449, 1981.

252. Daschner F, Frank U, and Just H-M: Proven and unproven methods in hospital infection control in intensive care units. Chemioterapia 6:184, 1987.

253. Daschner FD: Useful and useless hygienic techniques in intensive care units. Intensive Care Med 11:280, 1985.

254. Gilsdorf JR, Wilson K, and Beals TF: Bacterial colonization of intravenous catheter materials in vitro and in vivo. Surgery 106:37, 1989.

255. Van den Broek PJ, Daha ThJ, and Mouton RP: Bladder irrigation with povidone-iodine in prevention of urinary-tract infections associated with intermittent urethral catheterisation. Lancet 1:563, 1985.

256. Haldorson AM, Keys TF, Maker MD, et al: Nonvalue of neomycin instillation after intermittent urinary catheterization. Antimicrob Agents Chemother 14:368, 1978.

257. Chyang Fang: Personal communication. Rockville, MD, American Red Cross.

258. Harvey J: Personal communication. Alter, Transfusion Medicine Department, National Institutes of Health, Bethesda, MD.

71

Principles of Antimicrobial Therapy

Henry Masur, M.D.

Infection is a frequent event among critically ill children, occurring either as a primary process that produces a life-threatening illness or as a complication of the disease, drug, or procedure that originally precipitated hospitalization. Management of an infection in a critically ill child differs markedly from management in other settings. By virtue of the need for the child to be in the critical care unit, there is an urgency to initiate appropriate therapy. It is a major priority to establish a specific diagnosis in critically ill patients to assure that the therapy is appropriate and effective and to eliminate the adverse effects caused by unnecessary antimicrobial agents. Despite this major priority to establish a specific diagnosis, critically ill patients may be unable to tolerate the definitive diagnostic procedure, or therapy may have to be initiated before the diagnostic procedure can be performed and analyzed. Thus, empirical therapy is necessary and appropriate much more often in the critical care setting than in other clinical situations.

When empirical therapy is initiated, it generally must also be more comprehensive and have a broader spectrum than empirical regimens used in other settings. Children sick enough to be in the critical care unit do not have a physiologic margin for error that can readily tolerate failure to treat the causative microorganism promptly. Thus, multiple-drug empirical regimens are often necessary. This increases the likelihood that the offending organism will be treated, but it also increases the likelihood that adverse effects and undesirable drug interactions will occur. Thus, establishing a definitive diagnosis is an important goal that may be difficult to achieve.

Another major issue in critically ill patients is the dosage and route of antimicrobial drug administration. Drugs must almost always be administered intravenously to assure delivery in a timely and predictable manner. Because critically ill patients often have altered renal function, hepatic function, and volumes of distribution, drug dosages must be carefully considered and reconsidered on at least a daily basis, and serum or plasma levels should be monitored regularly whenever possible. The capability to assay the levels of certain drugs, such as aminoglycosides, with rapid turnaround time, is a mandatory component of modern critical care.

The armamentarium of antimicrobial therapy has expanded rapidly during the past decade. Some of these new agents are potent and clinically effective drugs, which greatly enhance the likelihood that a patient can survive a bacterial, fungal, viral, or protozoal disease. Some of the newer agents, in contrast, offer only modest advantage or no advantage over older drugs, despite dramatically higher cost. It is important that, as responsible members of a health care community that is increasingly buffeted by cost considerations, intensive care practitioners refrain from using these expensive new agents unless there is a major advantage to be gained.

An important guideline for wisely choosing an antimicrobial armamentarium for an intensive care unit is to minimize the number of agents. It is difficult for physicians, nurses, and pharmacists to be knowledgeable about the antimicrobial spectrum, adverse effects, dosage, excretion, and distribution of a large number of drugs. Errors in drug selection, preparation, and administration are likely to be less frequent if the armamentarium is limited in terms of the number of agents included.

SELECTION OF ANTIMICROBIAL REGIMEN

The successful management of an infectious disease depends on a variety of factors, including not only the selection of an effective antimicrobial agent but also potentially prompt and accurate diagnosis, surgical drainage of pus, removal of necrotic tissue or foreign bodies, and consideration of unique host factors that might influence the efficacy, distribution, elimination, or tolerance of the drug.[1-3] For optimal therapy of an infectious process, a drug must reach the site of infection in an active form and attain a local concentration that is at least as high as the minimum inhibitory concentration of drug for the causative organism. Since antibiotic susceptibility data concerning the causative organism are seldom available when the antimicrobial regimen must be chosen, drug selection must be based on knowledge of the drug's activity against the presumed pathogen using data from both in vitro studies and clinical studies. It is important to recognize that some drugs have excellent in vitro activity against an organism but are clinically ineffective when assessed in human trials. The experience with colistin is a good example: In vitro activity against gram-negative aerobic bacilli is excellent, but clinical efficacy is dismal. Thus, antibiotic choice should not be based exclusively on in vitro data.

While waiting for final suspectibility data for the causative organism, clinicians must appreciate the importance of knowing the activity of a given drug against pathogens in the local community and in that hospital environment. Gentamicin may have excellent activity against virtually all strains of *Pseudomonas aeruginosa* in one hospital, but high-grade resistance may be encountered among many clinical isolates in another setting and thus amikacin may be more desirable. Similarly, *Staphylococcus aureus* may rarely be resistant to nafcillin in some hospitals, but resistance may occur in 20 to 50% of isolates in other hospitals, mandating the empirical use of vancomycin rather than nafcillin when *S. aureus* infection is suspected.

The mechanism of antimicrobial action is often considered in choosing an antimicrobial agent.[4-6] It is logical to use a drug that is bactericidal rather than bacteriostatic. In many situations in which host immune defenses are intact and the site of infection is neither intravascular nor neurologic, however, it is not at all certain that a drug's ability to kill microorganisms rather than inhibit them is crucial. However, endocarditis, meningitis, and infectious complications in neutropenic hosts are examples of situations in which bactericidal activity is a highly desirable feature that should influence the selection of an agent.

Combining drugs is a popular technique to achieve a variety of goals, including higher efficacy through additive or synergistic effects, reduced toxicity, a broader spectrum, or decreased emergence of resistance. The use of two or three agents against a gram-negative bacteremia in neutropenic patients or against a serious gram-negative bacillary pneumonia has been supported by clinical reviews even if the drugs are additive rather than synergistic.[7, 8] This seems justified, especially in neutropenic patients. Traditionally, there is considerable emphasis on attaining synergy. For the treatment of life-threatening *P. aeruginosa* infection, for example, the synergy between an aminoglycoside and an anti-*Pseudomonas* penicillin that can be demonstrated in vitro translates into heightened clinical efficacy.[6, 9] In most situations with other gram-negative bacilli, however, it is difficult to predict in advance which drug combinations will demonstrate synergy. In addition, in many of these situations it is not clear that synergy is clinically important. In most instances, a drug combination is more warranted by the need to have an extended spectrum of antimicrobial coverage than by a documented benefit produced by using two or three potentially synergistic agents in order to increase efficacy. There are situations, however, when the use of a drug combination permits the use of reduced doses of one agent, resulting in less toxicity with equivalent efficacy. The use of flucytosine with amphotericin B for the treatment of cryptococcal meningitis is a good example.[10]

Antagonism is often considered as a reason to avoid certain combinations of drugs. Antagonism between bacteriostatic and bactericidal drugs has been shown to be clinically relevant in a few situations: The combination of penicillin plus chlortetracycline is less effective for treating pneumococcal meningitis than is penicillin alone.[11] In most clinical settings, however, there is no documentation that in vitro antagonism has clinical implications, and thus antagonism rarely merits consideration when choosing drugs.

Drug toxicity is a vital factor in choosing the optimal antimicrobial agent. Critically ill children often have compromised renal, hepatic, or hematologic function. The use of nephrotoxic, hepatotoxic, or marrow-toxic agents can produce particularly undesirable consequences in the pediatric patient population. Thus, it may well be useful to avoid an aminoglycoside in children with hypotension and to choose an extended-spectrum monobactam, carbapenem, or cephalosporin instead. Similarly, flucytosine should probably be avoided for treatment of fungal disease in patients who are already neutropenic from cytotoxic chemotherapy, and imipenem should probably be avoided in children with structural brain lesions or seizures.

Since renal function, hepatic function, and volume of distribution are often abnormal in critically ill children, it is a major advantage to be able to measure drug concentration regularly. This allows the health care professional to maximize the likelihood that drug levels will be high enough to be effective but within a range that will reduce the likelihood of toxicity. Laboratory capability to measure levels is widely available for the aminoglycosides and vancomycin. The ability to be certain that desired drug concentrations are achieved is a major advantage that should encourage the use of these agents in preference to other drugs in a critical care setting. The ability to measure drug levels is far preferable to the use of nomograms, computer models, or other techniques that estimate drug levels and are useful but less reliable than direct clinical measurements. Drug levels may need to be monitored daily in very unstable patients. Measuring drug levels several times weekly may be expensive, but this approach is less expensive than dealing with the medical and legal consequences of renal impairment or permanent hearing loss.

How high should drug levels be to optimize efficacy? Clinicians often take solace in attaining levels that are much higher than the minimum inhibitory concentration or minimum bactericidal concentration of drug for the offending organism. Attaining peak serum concentrations at least eight times the minimum bactericidal concentration has been validated for endocarditis. In most other situations, however, attaining serum levels considerably higher than the minimum bactericidal concentration does not necessarily correlate with enhanced efficacy, though it is a logical approach to take.

The pharmacokinetics of an antibiotic are crucial in determining its suitability in a given clinical situation. Certain drugs penetrate to the site of infection, whereas other drugs are not well distributed beyond certain compartments. For the treatment of meningitis, for instance, aminoglycosides and first-generation cephalosporins do not penetrate reliably and adequately into the cerebrospinal fluid. Ceftazidime, piperacillin, imipenem, or aztreonam would be preferable choices. Knowledge of how the drug is eliminated and how thoroughly the host's renal or hepatic function has been compromised are also essential features of rational antibiotic selection, as previously indicated, especially if the drug has a low therapeutic:toxicity ratio.

Intensive care practitioners need to recognize that their choice of antibiotics, which they make on a regular basis, can have considerable epidemiologic and economic consequences for the hospital. Substantial antibiotic pressure in the intensive care unit can select out organisms that are multiply antibiotic-resistant. Even with excellent infection control practices, these organisms can rapidly spread throughout the hospital. The physician caring for a critically ill child has an obligation to use the most effective therapy possible but must consider epidemiologic factors as well.

The physician must introduce newer antibiotics rationally so that new drugs are not used indiscriminately but are available for unusual situations in which they might be uniquely useful. For instance, if a *P. aeruginosa* isolate is sensitive to both gentamicin and amikacin, there is generally no indication to use amikacin in preference to gentamicin. Amikacin, which generally has wider activity against aerobic gram-negative bacilli than does gentamicin should be reserved for those isolates that are gentamicin-resistant. Its indiscriminate use will increase the frequency of isolates that are both gentamicin- and amikacin-resistant. Similarly, there is no logical reason to regularly use a wide variety of broad-spectrum agents, such as parenteral quinolones, carbapenems, monobactams, third-generation cephalosporins, and β-lactam–β-lactamase inhibitor combinations in an intensive care unit: One or two drugs should be selected for regular use and the others reserved for unusual organisms with highly resistant susceptibility patterns.

Which drug should be selected for regular use depends on a given hospital's epidemiologic profile. At some institutions, for instance, the frequency of gentamicin- and tobramycin-resistant isolates may be so high that amikacin would have to be the aminoglycoside of choice. At some institutions, imipenem might be preferable to ceftazidime or timentin.

Antibiotics compromise a substantial portion of a pharmacy's drug acquisition costs. As already mentioned, newer drugs are usually more expensive than older, more conventional agents. Intensive care practitioners need to make sure that before introducing new drugs into their antimicrobial armamentarium, the increased cost of drug acquisition is warranted by well-documented advantages in terms of efficacy, toxicity, or ease of administration.

Finally, the selection of an antimicrobial agent should be influenced by the familiarity of the critical care team with the drug. The armamentarium of antibiotics is so extensive now that it is essentially impossible for health care providers to be knowledgeable about the necessary features of all of these agents, even if they carry handy pocket reference books with them.[12–14] The more antibiotics that are included in the antibiotic armamentarium, the higher the likelihood that errors will be made in drug selection, preparation, or administration. As already stated, it is preferable that physicians be highly knowledgeable about a reasonable number of antibiotics and reserve many of the newer, more expensive agents for unusual situations in which their unique properties are required. In these situations, consultants can be used to ensure the proper use of the unfamiliar agents.

SPECIFIC ANTIMICROBIAL AGENTS

In the 1990s, a hospital formulary could conceivably include many dozens of antibiotics that could be administered in a pediatric intensive care unit. As already mentioned, limiting the antimicrobial armamentarium used by an intensive care unit can have major epidemiologic and cost advantages and can maximize the likelihood that the health care staff will use the agents appropriately. Table 71–1 provides a list of 23 antibiotics that could provide therapy for most empirical and definitive uses that occur in a pediatric intensive care unit. Some choices of agents, such as those for specific extended-spectrum cephalosporins or for metronidazole in preference to clindamycin, are relatively arbitrary. In some hospitals, cost or epidemiologic considerations or staff familiarity might mandate other selections. A reasonable approach to antimicrobial therapy in a critical care setting, however, would be to emphasize knowledge and familiarity with about 2 dozen agents and to seek infectious disease consultation when other drugs are considered. Table 71–2 provides information about drug dosages and metabolism. Table 71–3 lists drugs of choice for life-threatening infections caused by specific organisms.

Table 71–1. TYPICAL ANTIBIOTIC ARMAMENTARIUM FOR PEDIATRIC CRITICAL CARE

Antibacterial Drugs

Penicillin	Aztreonam	Isoniazid
Nafcillin	Imipenem	Rifampin
Ampicillin	Vancomycin	
Piperacillin	Erythromycin	
Cefuroxime	Gentamicin	
Ceftriaxone	Metronidazole	
Ceftazidime		

Antifungal Drugs
Amphotericin
Fluconazole

Antiviral Drugs
Acyclovir
Ganciclovir
Ribavirin

Antiprotozoal Drugs
Pyrimethamine
Sulfadiazine

Antipneumocystic Drugs
Trimethoprim-sulfamethoxazole
Pentamidine

Table 71–2. ANTIMICROBIAL AGENTS FOR BACTERIAL, FUNGAL, AND VIRAL INFECTIONS IN CRITICALLY ILL CHILDREN

Drug	Usual Total Daily Dose* (Recommended Dose Interval)	Route of Administration	Peak Serum (μg/ml) Concentration (IV Dose)	Hepatic Metabolism-Excretion	Dose Alteration with Renal Dysfunction	Serum Concentration Altered by	
						Hemodialysis	*Peritoneal Dialysis*
Penicillins							
Aqueous crystalline penicillin G	100,000–250,000 units/kg/day (continuous–q 4 hr)	IV‡	18	No	Major	Yes	—
Ampicillin	100–400 mg/kg/day (q 4–6 hr)	IV	6	Yes	Major	Yes	No
Ampicillin-sulbactam	100–400 mg/kg/day	IV	6	Yes	Major	Yes	Yes
Carbenicillin	400–600 mg/kg/day (q 4 hr)	IV	150	Yes	Major	Yes	Yes
Ticarcillin	200–300 mg/kg/day (q 4 hr)	IV	140	Yes	Major	Yes	Yes
Timentin	200–300 mg/kg/day (q 4–6 hr)	IV		Yes	Major	Yes	Yes
Piperacillin	200–300 mg/kg/day (q 4 hr)	IV	320	Yes	Minor	Yes	No
Oxacillin	150–200 mg/kg/day (q 4–6 hr)	IV	50	No	Minor	No	No
Nafcillin	150 mg/kg/day (q 4 hr)	IV	11	Yes	Minor	No	
Cephalosporins and Cephamycins							
Cephalothin	75–125 mg/kg/day (q 4–6 hr)	IV	100	Yes	Minor	Yes	Yes
Cefazolin	50–100 mg/kg/day (q 8 hr)	IV	188	Yes	Major	Yes	No
Cefoxitin	80–160 mg/kg/day (q 4–6 hr)	IV	110	Yes	Major	Yes	—
Cefotaxime	100–200 mg/kg/day (q 6–8 hr)	IV	214	Yes	Minor	Yes	—
Ceftazidime	100–150 mg/kg/day (q 8 hr)	IV	130	No	Major	Yes	Yes
Ceftriaxone	50–100 mg/kg/day (q 12 hr)	IV	250	Yes	Minor	No	—
Other β-Lactams							
Imipenem-cilastatin	60–100 mg/kg/day (q 6–8 hr)	IV	70	No	Major	Yes	—
Aztreonam	90–120 mg/kg/day (q 6–8 hr)	IV	125	Yes	Major	Yes	Yes
Aminoglycosides							
Gentamicin	3–7.5 mg/kg/day (q 6–8 hr)	IV	3–6	No	Major	Yes	Yes
Tobramycin	3–6 mg/kg/day (q 6–8 hr)	IV	4–10	No	Major	Yes	Yes
Amikacin	15–20 mg/kg/day (q 8 hr)	IV	20	No	Major	Yes	Yes
Antimycobacterial Agents							
Isoniazid	10–20 mg/kg/day (q 24 hr)	PO§	1	Yes	Minor	Yes	Yes
Rifampin	10–20 mg/kg/day (q 24 hr)	PO	7	Yes	Minor	No	No
Ethambutol	15 mg/kg/day (q 24 hr)	PO		No	Major	Yes	No
Other Antibacterial Agents							
Vancomycin	40–60 mg/kg/day (q 6 hr or q 12 hr)	IV	20–40	No	Major	Yes	No
Erythromycin lactobionate	25–40 mg/kg/day (q 6 hr)	IV	9.90	Yes	No	No	No
Clindamycin	25–40 mg/kg/day (q 6 hr)	IV	14	Yes	Minor	No	No
Chloramphenicol	50–75 mg/kg/day (q 6 hr)	IV	11	Yes	Minor	No	No
Metronidazole	30 mg/kg/day (q 6–8 hr)	IV	26	Yes	Major	Yes	—
Tetracycline	20–30 mg/kg/day (q 6 hr)	IV	8.50	Yes	Avoid	Yes	No
Antiprotozoal Agents							
Pentamidine	4 mg/kg/day (q 24 hr)	IV	0.61		No	No	No
Trimethoprim-sulfamethoxazole	20 mg/kg/day (T)‖ and 100 mg/kg/day (S)** (q 6 hr)	IV, PO	100–150 (S)**	Yes	Major	Yes	Yes
Sulfadiazine	100 mg/kg/day (q 6 hr)	IV		Yes	Yes	Yes	Yes
Pyrimethamine	0.5–1.0 mg/kg/day (q 24 hr)	PO		No			
Antifungal Agents							
Amphotericin B	0.25–1.0 mg/kg/day (q 24 hr)	IV		No	Minor	No	No
Flucytosine	150 mg/kg/day (q 6 hr)	PO	75	No	Yes	Yes	Yes
Fluconazole	3–6 mg/kg/day (q 24 hr)	PO, IV	3.50			No	No
Antiviral Agents							
Acyclovir	25–50 mg/kg/day (q 8 hr)	IV	No	Yes	Yes	Yes	
Amantadine	5–8 mg/kg/day (q 12 hr)	PO	No	Yes			
Azidothymidine	(Consult literature)	PO, IV	Yes				
Ribavirin	1 vial (6 g) (q 24 hr)	Aerosol					
Ganciclovir	10 mg/kg/day (q 12 hr)	IV	No	Yes	Yes		—

*Doses for newborns may differ and should be checked in an appropriate source such as Nelson JD: Pocketbook of Pediatric Antimicrobial Therapy, 10th ed. Baltimore, Williams & Wilkins, 1991.
†q = every.
‡IV = intravenous.
§PO = by mouth.
‖T = trimethoprim.
**S = sulfamethoxazole.

Table 71–3. ANTIMICROBIAL DRUGS OF CHOICE FOR THE TREATMENT OF SPECIFIC INFECTIOUS AGENTS IN CRITICALLY ILL CHILDREN

Organism	Antimicrobial Agent of Choice*	Alternative Agents
Bacteria		
Gram-positive cocci (aerobic)		
Staphylococcus aureus		
Non–penicillinase-producing	Penicillin	Cephalothin, vancomycin
Penicillinase-producing	Nafcillin or vancomycin + aminoglycoside or rifampin	Cephalothin, oxacillin + rifampin, or oxacillin + aminoglycoside
Staphylococcus epidermidis	Vancomycin	Imipenem, trimethoprim-sulfamethoxazole
α-Streptococci (*Streptococcus viridans*)	Penicillin	Clindamycin, cephalothin, vancomycin
β-Streptococci (A,B,C,G)	Penicillin	Cephalothin, vancomycin
Enterococcus fecalis		
Serious infection	Ampicillin + aminoglycoside	Vancomycin + aminoglycoside
Uncomplicated urinary infection	Ampicillin, ciprofloxacin, norfloxacin	Vancomycin
Enterococcus bovis	Penicillin	Cephalothin, vancomycin
Streptococcus pneumoniae	Penicillin	Erythromycin, vancomycin, cephalothin
Gram-negative cocci (aerobic)		
Neisseria meningitidis	Penicillin	Ceftriaxone, chloramphenicol
Neisseria gonorrhoeae	Ceftriaxone	Ciprofloxacin
Branhamella catarrhalis	Ceftriaxone	Ceftazidime, ciprofloxacin, imipenem, aztreonem
Gram-positive bacilli (aerobic)		
Corynebacterium JK	Vancomycin	Ciprofloxacin
Gram-negative bacilli (aerobic)		
Acinetobacter sp.	Aminoglocoside + piperacillin	Imipenem, ciprofloxacin
Campylobacter jejuni	Erythromycin	Tetracycline
Campylobacter fetus	Aminoglycoside	Chloramphenicol, imipenem
Enterobacter sp.	Aminoglycoside	Ceftazidime, timentin, imipenem, aztreonam
Escherichia coli	Aminoglycoside	Cefuroxime, ceftriaxone
Haemophilus influenzae	Cefuroxime, ceftriaxone	Chloramphenicol
Klebsiella pneumoniae	Aminoglycoside	Aztreonam, ceftazidime, imipenem
Legionella sp.	Erythromycin + rifampin	Ciprofloxacin + rifampin
Listeria monocytogenes	Ampicillin + aminoglycoside	Chloramphenicol
Proteus mirabilis	Ampicillin	Aminoglycoside, cephalosporin
Other *Proteus* sp.	Aminoglycoside	Aztreonam, imipenem
Providencia sp.	Aminoglycoside	Aztreonam, imipenem
Pseudomonas aeruginosa	Aminoglycoside + piperacillin	Aztreonam, ceftazidime, timentin, imipenem
Other *Pseudomonas* spp.	Aminoglycoside + piperacillin	Aztreonam, ceftazidime, timentin, imipenem
Salmonella sp.	Ceftriaxone	Chloramphenicol, imipenem, ciproflexacin
Serratia marcescens	Aminoglycoside	Ceftazidime, ciproflaxocin, imipenem, aztreonam
Shigella sp.	Ceftriaxone	Chloramphenicol, ciprofloxacin
Anaerobes		
Anaerobic streptococci	Penicillin	Metronidazole, imipenem
Bacteroides sp.		
Oropharyngeal strains	Penicillin	Imipenem, timentin
Gastrointestinal strains	Metronidazole	Imipenem, timentin
Clostridium sp. (except *C. difficile*)	Penicillin	Imipenem, metronidazole
Clostridium difficile	Vancomycin (oral)	Metronidazole (IV or oral)
Other bacteria		
Actinomyces and *Arachnia*	Penicillin G	Tetracycline, clindamycin
Nocardia sp.	Trimethoprim-sulfamethoxazole	Minocycline, amikacin
Mycobacterium tuberculosis	Isoniazid (INH) + rifampin + pyrazinamide	Ethambutol, streptomycin
Fungi (Invasive)		
Aspergillus sp.	Amphotericin B	—
Blastomyces dermatitidis	Amphotericin B	—
Candida sp.	Amphotericin B	—
Coccidioides immitis	Amphotericin B	—
Cryptococcus neoformans	Amphotericin B + flucytosine	Fluconazole
Histoplasma capsulatum	Amphotericin B	Itraconazole†
Mucor-Absidia-Rhizopus	Amphotericin B	—
Protozoa		
Pneumocystis carinii	Trimethoprim-sulfamethoxazole	Pentamidine
Toxoplasma gondii	Sulfadiazine + pyrimethamine	Clindamycin + pyrimethamine
Viruses		
Herpes simplex	Acyclovir	Ganciclovir, foscarnet†
Influenza A	Amantadine	—
Herpes zoster	Acyclovir	Ganciclovir, foscarnet†
Cytomegalovirus	Ganciclovir	Foscarnet
Respiratory syncytial virus	Ribavirin	—
Human immunodeficiency virus	Azidothymidine (AZT)	Dideoxyinosine (ddI)†

Table continued on following page

Table 71–3. ANTIMICROBIAL DRUGS OF CHOICE FOR THE TREATMENT OF SPECIFIC INFECTIOUS AGENTS IN CRITICALLY ILL CHILDREN *Continued*

Organism	Antimicrobial Agent of Choice*	Alternative Agents
Other Organisms		
Borrelia burgdorferi	Tetracycline (early disease)	Penicillin G
	Ceftriaxone (late disease)	
Mycoplasma pneumoniae	Erythromycin	Tetracycline
Chlamydia (psittaci, trachomatis, pneumoniae)	Tetracycline	Chloramphenicol
Leptospira sp.	Penicillin G	Tetracycline
Rickettsia sp.	Tetracycline	Chloramphenicol

*Susceptibility testing of specific isolates must be considered in addition to these recommendations.
†Investigational.

Antibacterial Agents

Penicillin G (Benzylpenicillin)

Intravenous penicillin G has excellent activity against many, but not all, aerobic and anaerobic gram-positive and gram-negative cocci. Organisms that produce β-lactamase enzyme (such as many *S. aureus* or *Branhamella* sp.) will be resistant, as will organisms that have developed other mechanisms of resistance. In a pediatric critical care unit, its major use is for infections caused by β-hemolytic streptococci (such as group A streptococci), *Streptococcus pneumoniae*, *Neisseria meningitidis*, and *Listeria monocytogenes*. Penicillin resistance has been reported for some pneumococcal and neisserial isolates but is still an exceedingly rare occurrence. Penicillin G is no longer satisfactory therapy for most staphylococcal infections because most *S. aureus* and *S. epidermidis* isolates are penicillin-resistant.[15] Many anaerobic organisms are sensitive to penicillin G, though some isolates, such as *Bacteroides fragilis*, often elaborate β-lactamase and are therefore resistant. Penicillin is no longer a therapy of choice for most life-threatening anaerobic infections.

In the critical care unit, penicillin G is almost always given intravenously. It is widely distributed throughout the body but penetrates the cerebrospinal fluid well only when the meninges are inflamed. Interestingly, its penetration into the cerebrospinal fluid is quite unpredictable but is generally about 5% of concentrations attained in the plasma, which is adequate for most pathogens that are considered to be susceptible.

Penicillin is primarily excreted in the urine by tubular secretion. In adults, the half-life is 30 minutes, but in infants the half-life can be longer. In anuric patients, the half-life of penicillin G increases from 30 minutes to 10 hours, and the dose must be properly adjusted if dose-related toxicities are to be avoided.

Hypersensitivity is a major issue with penicillin G as with most other β-lactam antibiotics. Hypersensitivity reactions, in decreasing order of frequency, include maculopapular rash, urticarial rash, fever, bronchospasm, serum sickness, Stevens-Johnson syndrome, and anaphylaxis. These reactions occur in 0.7 to 10% of patients.[16, 17] Immediate hypersensitivity reactions such as anaphylaxis, laryngeal edema, or urticaria are usually indications to avoid cross-reacting β-lactam drugs in the future or to administer them in a desensitization proce-

dure under carefully controlled circumstances such as in a critical care unit. When there is a history of IgG-mediated reactions, such as nonurticarial maculopapular rashes, therapy with penicillins is usually not advised, but therapy with cephalosporins is generally well tolerated without serious sequelae. Management of hypersensitivity reactions requires considerable experience, especially if desensitization is being considered. The personnel, equipment, and drugs to treat anaphylaxis or laryngeal edema must be immediately available.

A variety of other adverse reactions, including granulocytopenia, hepatitis, hemolytic anemia, platelet dysfunction, lethargy, and seizures have been reported. Intensive care practitioners need to be aware that penicillin G and the other β-lactam drugs may be the cause. Lethargy, confusion, myoclonus, and seizures are especially likely to occur in patients receiving maximal doses of penicillin G and who either have not had the dose adjusted to compensate for renal failure or who have complicating neurologic disorders such as hyponatremia or structural lesions. Central nervous system dysfunction is common when cerebrospinal fluid levels exceed 10 μg/ml.

Nafcillin

Nafcillin is a semisynthetic penicillin that is highly resistant to penicillinase and is used almost exclusively to treat *S. aureus* infections.[18] Nafcillin-resistant strains of *S. aureus* are being seen with increasing frequency, especially among intravenous drug abusers. In some hospitals, a substantial percentage of isolates are resistant so that at these institutions vancomycin is the drug of choice when *S. aureus* infection is suspected and antibiotic sensitivity data are not yet available. Nafcillin is also not active against at least 40% of *S. epidermidis* isolates and is not the drug of choice for such infections.[19] Nafcillin has reasonable activity against some aerobic gram-positive cocci such as *S. pneumoniae* but has inadequate activity against group D streptococci and most anaerobes. Oxacillin and methicillin are closely related compounds with almost identical spectra of activity but somewhat different routes of excretion and toxicities. Most authorities prefer either nafcillin or oxacillin over methicillin because of a more favorable toxicity profile.

Nafcillin is widely distributed throughout the body and, like penicillin G, enters the cerebrospinal fluid only when the meninges are inflamed. It is excreted in the bile and to a limited extent in the urine. Adverse reactions are similar to those of penicillin G. Granulocytopenia is particularly common when high doses are used for at least several weeks. This effect is dose-dependent and rapidly reversible. Nephritis is more common with methicillin than with nafcillin or oxacillin.

Ampicillin and Ampicillin-Sulbactam

In the critical care unit, ampicillin is used primarily for coverage of group D streptococci such as *Enterococcus fecalis,* as well as for infections from *L. monocytogenes,* pneumococcal and meningococcal infection, and enteric gram-negative bacterial infections that are known to be susceptible. Ampicillin has good activity, similar to penicillin G, against most aerobic gram-positive cocci except staphylococci. It is active against many anaerobic bacteria and many enteric gram-negative bacilli but cannot be relied on for empirical treatment of these infections because of the high frequency of resistance, much of which is mediated by β-lactamase production. Ampicillin cannot be recommended for treatment of *Haemophilus influenzae* infections until drug susceptibility results are known because 20 to 30% of isolates from children with meningitis at many hospitals are highly resistant.[20] Ampicillin has no useful activity against most *Pseudomonas* sp.

The pharmacologic properties of and adverse reactions to ampicillin are similar to those of penicillin G. Maculopapular rashes are particularly common responses to ampicillin.

Sulbactam is a β-lactamase inhibitor (similar in structure to clavulanic acid) that has been combined with ampicillin to produce a drug that has an extended spectrum compared with ampicillin alone. Since the drug is effective against β-lactamase–producing *S. aureus, H. influenzae,* enteric gram-negative bacilli, and anaerobes, it can be used for presumed or documented polymicrobial infection. Ampicillin/sulbactam could be used as an alternative to imipenem, timentin, third-generation cephalosporins, or combination regimens in situations in which *Pseudomonas* sp. are not present.[21]

Piperacillin and other Anti-Pseudomonas Penicillins (Carboxypenicillins and Ureidopenicillins) plus Timentin

Piperacillin, ticarcillin, and carbenicillin are used primarily in critical care units in conjunction with aminoglycosides to treat *P. aeruginosa* infections. Although their antimicrobial spectra are similar to that of ampicillin (except that they are much more active against *P. aeruginosa* but less active against many group D streptococci such as *E. fecalis*), they are almost never used as single agents. *P. aeruginosa* has a predilection for developing in vivo resistance when these agents are used alone.

Piperacillin is preferred over carbenicillin and ticarcillin in some units because it is most active against *P. aeruginosa.* If a carboxypenicillin is to be used (i.e., carbenicillin or ticarcillin), ticarcillin is usually preferred

because it is more active than carbenicillin. These agents have pharmacologic and toxicity profiles that are similar to penicillin G. Carbenicillin administration results in a considerable sodium load and can produce hypokalemia when the carbenicillin anion is excreted. Carbenicillin also has an enhanced tendency to adversely affect platelet function.

Azlocillin and mezlocillin also have excellent anti-*Pseudomonas* activity and can be used instead of piperacillin.

Ticarcillin has been combined with the β-lactamase inhibitor clavulanate to produce an expanded-spectrum product, timentin.[22] The addition of clavulanate extends the spectrum of ticarcillin to include *S. aureus,* most anaerobes, and most aerobic gram-negative enteric bacilli but does not increase its activity against *Pseudomonas* sp. Timentin is a potent drug that can be used instead of imipenem, ceftazidime, or combination regimens including an aminoglycoside in some situations, especially when *P. aeruginosa* is suspected or documented to be the sole pathogen or part of a polymicrobial process.

Imipenem

Imipenem is a β-lactam drug with an extended spectrum of antibacterial activity. It is being used with increasing frequency in critical care units because of its excellent spectrum of activity, which includes activity against many *P. aeruginosa* sp.[23, 24] Imipenem is a bactericidal compound that is marketed in combination with cilastatin, a drug that inhibits degradation of imipenem by the renal tubular enzyme dipeptidase. Imipenem has outstanding activity against almost all anaerobic bacteria; against most aerobic gram-positive cocci, including methicillin-sensitive *S. aureus* (some strains of methicillin-resistant *S. aureus* are resistant); most pneumococci; β-hemolytic streptococci, *S. viridans;* most group D streptococci (though not all *E. fecium*); most Enterobacteriaceae; most *P. aeruginosa* but not certain other *Pseudomonas* sp. such as *P. maltophilia.*

Imipenem is well distributed throughout the body and crosses the blood-brain barrier. When administered in combination with cilastatin (which is the only preparation commercially available), 70% of imipenem is excreted in the urine. The toxicity profile of imipenem is similar to that of other β-lactam drugs. Nausea and vomiting are common. The drug cross-reacts with other β-lactam drugs. Seizures have been noted, especially in patients with renal insufficiency or structural central nervous system lesions. Many clinicians are reluctant to use this drug in patients who have had seizures or who have structural lesions of the central nervous system.

Imipenem has broad activity. As a β-lactam drug with activity against *P. aeruginosa,* imipenem could be used in many situations in which timentin would be used or when ceftazidime would be used (though ceftazidime has little activity against anaerobes). There is little rationale for having more than one (or possibly two) of these three agents on the formulary. A sound argument could be made for any one of them as long as they are used with a knowledge of the subtle differences among them.

Aztreonam

Aztreonam is a monobactam, a β-lactam drug that has a monocyclic structure.[25] In an intensive care unit, aztreonam is used for gram-negative bacillary infections in situations in which aminoglycosides are avoided because of their nephrotoxicity or ototoxicity.

The antimicrobial spectrum of aztreonam includes most aerobic gram-negative bacilli, including many *P. aeruginosa* sp. as well as *H. influenzae.* Aztreonam has no activity against gram-positive cocci or against any anaerobic organisms.

Aztreonam is well distributed throughout the body and crosses inflamed meninges. The drug is eliminated unaltered in the urine. The half-life for elimination is normally 1.7 hours; it is 6 hours in anuric patients, so the dosage must be altered in renal failure.

Aztreonam is generally well tolerated and has a unique property among the β-lactam drugs: It does not appear to cross-react with other drugs in this family.[26] Thus, patients with life-threatening immediate hypersensitivity reactions to other β-lactam drugs can be given aztreonam safely.

Cephalosporins

The most commonly used antibiotics in many pediatric critical care units are the cephalosporins.[27, 28] Alone or in combination with other agents, they have broad utility for diverse problems in both immunologically normal and immunologically compromised individuals—for example, meningitis and brain abscess, community acquired pneumonia, abdominal infections, severe soft tissue infections, and sepsis.

Understanding the cephalosporins (and related cephamycins) is becoming increasingly difficult as the number and diversity of agents increase. There is no reason for an intensive care practitioner to be familiar with a large number of these agents: Familiarity with several should be adequate to use this group of drugs to maximal advantage. Organization of cephalosporins into "generations" is arbitrary and leads to some historical and functional inconsistencies, yet such a scheme is the most practical approach to understanding these drugs.

First-generation cephalosporins include cephalothin and cefazolin. These agents have excellent activity against most aerobic gram-positive cocci, including most strains of *S. aureus,* but they are generally inactive against *E. fecalis, E. fecium, S. epidermidis,* and methicillin-resistant *S. aureus.* They have some activity against Enterobacteriaceae but that activity is modest compared with second- and third-generation cephalosporins. Their activity against anaerobic organisms is poor. They have little activity against *H. influenzae* or *P. aeruginosa.*

First-generation cephalosporins do not penetrate inflamed meninges. Cephalothin has a very short half-life (30 to 40 minutes) compared with cefazolin (1.8 hours). Both drugs are excreted to a substantial extent by the kidneys; thus the dosage of each must be adjusted in renal failure. Cefazolin is preferred over cephalothin in many critical care units because of its longer half-life.

First-generation cephalosporins are used primarily to treat methicillin-sensitive *S. aureus* infections in patients in whom nafcillin or vancomycin should not be used. First-generation cephalosporins can also be used to treat gram-negative bacillary infections not involving the central nervous system that are caused by isolates known to be susceptible.

Second-generation cephalosporins are being used less and less frequently in critical care units, being replaced by third-generation drugs that have additional useful properties. Cefamandole, cefuroxime, cefoxitin, and cefotetan can, however, be useful. Cefamandole and cefuroxime have somewhat more activity than first-generation cephalosporins against many gram-negative bacilli (but not *Pseudomonas* sp.). Their major strength is good activity against aerobic gram-positive cocci, such as *S. pneumoniae,* and good activity against *H. influenzae,* including those species that are β-lactamase producers. Thus, their major role is in respiratory infections, especially those in which anaerobic bacteria are not major considerations, although second-generation cephalosporins do have a moderate anaerobic spectrum of activity. Both cefuroxime and cefamandole cross the blood-brain barrier. Cefuroxime is often preferred to cefamandole because it has a longer half-life (1.7 hours compared with 0.8 hours) and it is more resistant to β-lactamases.

Cefoxitin and cefotetan are almost identical second-generation cephalosporins that have excellent anaerobic activity and excellent activity against *H. influenzae.* Like cefamandole and cefuroxime, they have better activity against many enteric gram-negative bacilli than do the first-generation agents but less activity than third-generation drugs. They have no activity against *P. aeruginosa.* They have good activity against aerobic gram-positive cocci, though somewhat less than cefamandole, cefuroxime, or first-generation cephalosporins. Both cross the blood-brain barrier. Cefotetan has a longer half-life (3.3 hours) than does cefoxitin (40 minutes), which may provide a modest practical advantage.

The role for cefoxitin or cefotetan in a pediatric critical care unit is limited. For lung abscess, pleural empyema, abdominal infections, or pelvic infections in which mixed aerobic and anaerobic organisms are present and the susceptibilities of the causative organisms are known, these drugs might be reasonable agents in an effort to use a drug with as narrow a spectrum as possible in these polymicrobial infections.

Third-generation cephalosporins generally have a very broad range of activity against aerobic gram-negative bacilli and adequate activity against aerobic gram-positive cocci. Some, but not all, have activity against *P. aeruginosa.*

Cefotaxime, ceftriaxone, and ceftizoxime are very similar third-generation cephalosporins that lack activity against *P. aeruginosa.* These drugs are quite resistant to β-lactamases and have better activity against several aerobic gram-positive cocci than do ceftazidime or cefoperazone. None has activity against *E. fecalis* or *E.*

fecium. These drugs are well distributed throughout the body, including the cerebrospinal fluid, and in many circumstances are the drugs of choice for treating meningitis. A major difference among these agents is their half-lives. Ceftriaxone has a very long half-life in plasma (8 hours) compared with cefotaxime (1 hour) or ceftizoxime (1.8 hours) and is therefore the preferred agent of this group in many critical care units.[29] About one-half dose of ceftriaxone can be recovered from the bile. The remainder is recovered in the urine, and thus dosage adjustment needs to be considered in severe renal failure.

Among the third-generation cephalosporins with activity against *P. aeruginosa,* ceftazidime is clearly the drug of choice. Cefoperazone has activity against *P. aeruginosa,* but its poor activity against many gram-positive cocci and many gram-negative bacilli restrict its utility to extremely unusual situations. Ceftazidime is widely used because of its extremely broad spectrum of activity.[30] It is important to keep in mind, however, that is does not have broad activity against anaerobes, and its activity against aerobic gram-positive cocci is substantially less than several other first-, second-, and third-generation cephalosporins. Thus, it must be used with caution as a single agent when there is high suspicion of infection caused by anaerobic bacteria or aerobic gram-positive cocci, especially with neutropenic patients, though some controversy surrounds this issue. Ceftazidime has a short half-life (1.5 hours) and is excreted unchanged in the urine, so the dosage must be adjusted in renal failure. Moxalactam should not be used except in very unusual circumstances, because it has no major advantage over other agents and it can be associated with significant hemostatic problems.

Cephalosporin drugs are generally well tolerated. They share many of the adverse effects of the penicillins. There is no conclusive evidence that any one cephalosporin is substantially more likely to produce hypersensitivity than the others. Immediate and delayed-type hypersensitivity reactions are observed.[17] As discussed previously, there can be cross-reactivity between cephalosporins and penicillins (though not aztreonam). Immunologic studies suggest cross-reactivity in 20% of patients, though clinical studies suggest a much lower rate (about 1%). A major problem is predicting hypersensitivity and cross-reactivity using commercially available reagents in a practical manner: Considerable expertise or an appropriate consultation is needed when a β-lactam drug is required in patients with penicillin allergies. In most situations, non–β-lactam alternatives are available.

The adverse reactions to cephalosporins that occur occasionally include granulocytopenia, development of a positive Coombs' test (rarely associated with hemolysis), and nephrotoxicity (acute tubular necrosis and interstitial nephritis). Cephalosporins in combination with aminoglycosides are somewhat more nephrotoxic than are aminoglycosides alone. Serious bleeding disorders have been reported in patients receiving cephalosporins with a *N*-methylthiotetrazole side chain (i.e., cefamandole, moxalactam, cefotetan, cefoperazone), but these instances are rarely clinically important except in association with moxalactam.[31]

Vancomycin

Vancomycin is an important drug in a critical care setting because of its excellent activity against aerobic gram-positive cocci, especially *S. aureus* (including species that are methicillin-resistant), *S. epidermidis,* group D streptococci (including *E. fecalis* and *E. fecium*), and other aerobic streptococci, including β-hemolytic streptococci and *S. pneumoniae.*[32] It is also very useful against most *Corynebacterium* sp. and *Clostridium* sp. Resistance among gram-positive cocci occurs but is still extraordinarily rare in North America. How soon resistance among these organisms, especially enterococci, will become a major problem remains to be seen.[33, 34] Vancomycin has only modest activity against anaerobic bacteria and no activity against gram-negative bacilli.

Vancomycin is well distributed and penetrates inflamed meninges. The drug has a half-life of 6 hours and is excreted almost totally by the kidneys. The dosage of this agent must be carefully adjusted in the face of renal dysfunction. With substantially impaired hepatic dysfunction, the dosage needs to be considered carefully.

Vancomycin has been associated with nephrotoxicity and ototoxicity, though the frequency of these adverse effects has fallen since the era of current manufacturing technique and careful serum concentration monitoring.[35] Concern about adverse effects should rarely be a valid reason to avoid this drug if serum concentrations can be monitored regularly. Maintaining peak serum concentrations of 30 to 45 µg/ml and trough concentrations of 5 to 10 µg/ml is often advocated. Nephrotoxicity and ototoxicity have been associated with levels greater than 80 to 100 µg/ml. Ototoxicity and nephrotoxicity may be somewhat more common when vancomycin is used in conjunction with aminoglycosides.[36, 37] When vancomycin is infused rapidly, shock can occur, probably because of histamine release (the "red man" or "red neck" syndrome).[38, 39] Infusion over 30 minutes or longer usually precludes this. Hypersensitivity reactions to vancomycin are unusual. Vancomycin can be irritating to veins. Central administration is often recommended.

Vancomycin is one of the few drugs that has a definite role as an oral agent in the critical care unit. Oral vancomycin is the drug of choice to treat colitis caused by *Clostridium difficile.* It is not clear that parenteral vancomycin is nearly as effective.

Clindamycin

Clindamycin is a macrolide that is used in critical care units primarily to treat anaerobic infections. Clindamycin has excellent activity against aerobic gram-positive cocci such as *S. pneumoniae, S. pyogenes,* and many (but not all) *S. aureus* strains. It is not active against *E. fecalis, E. fecium,* or many strains of *S. epidermidis,* nor does it have any activity against aerobic gram-negative bacilli. It has excellent activity against most anaerobic bacteria, although resistance does occur. Metronidazole, imipenem, and timentin have a broader spectrum of activity against anaerobes. Clindamycin in conjunction with pyrimethamine has a role in the treatment of

Toxoplasma gondii for patients who cannot tolerate sulfadiazine.

Although clindamycin is widely distributed, it does not reliably penetrate inflamed meninges. Excellent levels in bone are attained. Clindamycin is metabolized, and inactive metabolites are excreted in the urine and bile. Dosage adjustments must be made in patients with severe hepatic failure.

Diarrhea occurs commonly with clindamycin administration. Colitis from *C. difficile* has been associated with clindamycin use, though it is not clear that this complication is substantially more frequent in association with clindamycin compared with many other antibiotics. Hypersensitivity reactions to clindamycin occur but are uncommon. There are reports that clindamycin can potentiate neuromuscular blocking agents, but this does not need to be a deterrent to the use of this drug, except in extremely unusual situations.

Metronidazole

Metronidazole has broad activity against almost all obligate anaerobic bacteria, as well as *Giardia lamblia* and *Entamoeba histolytica*. Metronidazole is well distributed throughout the body, including the cerebrospinal fluid. It is thus a first-line agent for anaerobic infections. The drug has no activity against aerobic organisms, so it is almost always used in combination with other agents. The liver accounts for more than 50% of the clearance of metronidazole. Both metabolized and unmetabolized drug is excreted in the urine. Toxicity to metronidazole is rarely severe enough to require discontinuation. Nausea, vomiting, diarrhea, abdominal pain, and neurologic toxicity have been reported. The neurologic toxicity can include encephalopathy, ataxia, seizures, and paresthesias.

Erythromycin

In a critical care setting, parenteral erythromycin is primarily used to treat respiratory tract infection because it is active against *Mycoplasma pneumoniae*, *Legionella* sp., and *Chlamydia pneumoniae*, as well as *S. pneumoniae* and *S. pyogenes*. It has no activity against most gram-negative bacilli and should not be relied upon for treatment of life-threatening *H. influenzae* infections. *S. aureus* may be resistant to erythromycin or may become resistant during therapy.

Erythromycin does not penetrate the cerebrospinal fluid well. It is concentrated in the liver and is largely excreted in the bile, so dosage adjustment is usually not advocated in renal failure. Erythromycin is generally well tolerated, though high doses administered intravenously can cause considerable nausea and inflammation of veins. Central venous administration is often desirable. Hypersensitivity to erythromycin occurs only occasionally. Sensorineural hearing loss can occur, especially when high doses are given. Usually, this is quickly reversible.[40]

Chloramphenicol

There is rarely an indication to use chloramphenicol in the critical care unit. It has been a highly effective drug for pneumococcal or meningococcal meningitis, severe enteric infections, and anaerobic infections. Irreversible dose-independent aplastic anemia is a rare but potentially fatal complication of this drug.[41] Chloramphenicol can be used safely and effectively in older infants and children.[42, 43] Pediatricians continue to use it more frequently than other physicians. Given the fact that safer and equally effective alternatives usually exist, and given the unpleasant litigation often associated with chloramphenicol administration, this drug should be used with caution and only in well-defined situations.

Tetracycline

Tetracyclines have been used for many years for a wide variety of infections.[41] Their role in a modern pediatric critical care unit is limited to some relatively unusual but important situations such as rickettsial diseases (especially Rocky Mountain spotted fever), psittacosis, or as an alternative to erythromycin to treat *M. pneumoniae* infections. The tendency of intravenous tetracycline to cause phlebitis, and of tetracyclines in general to discolor the teeth of children (especially children between the ages of 2 months and 5 years), makes this category of drug an alternative of last resort in most situations.

Aminoglycosides

Aminoglycosides are commonly used in pediatric critical care units because of their outstanding spectrum of activity against aerobic gram-negative bacilli and their excellent record of clinical efficacy.[44–46] There is recurrent concern about their nephrotoxicity and ototoxicity, but this concern should rarely override the desirable features that these drugs have.

Gentamicin, tobramycin, amikacin, and netilmicin are the aminoglycosides most commonly used now for life-threatening aerobic gram-negative bacillary infections. These drugs have little useful activity against aerobic gram-positive cocci (except when used in combination with β-lactam drugs or vancomycin to achieve synergy) and no activity against anaerobic organisms. All four of these aminoglycosides are active against most aerobic gram-negative bacilli, although susceptibility patterns can vary dramatically among hospitals. It is important for the intensive care practitioner to know the recent susceptibility trends in the setting in which he or she practices. Tobramycin is usually more active against *P. aeruginosa* than is gentamicin. Amikacin is more likely to retain its activity than are the other three agents because of its relative resistance to the aminoglycoside-inactivating enzymes produced by some bacteria. Because of their broad aerobic gram-negative bacillary spectrum, aminoglycosides are excellent, and perhaps the best, empirical agents to treat life-threatening infections when aerobic gram-negative bacilli are possible pathogens.

Aminoglycosides do not penetrate the cerebrospinal fluid, and concentrations in many secretions, excretions, and tissues are low. Levels in respiratory secretions are low, although aminoglycosides can be used successfully to treat gram-negative bacillary pneumonias. High concentrations are, however, found in the renal cortex and in the endolymph and perilymph of the inner ear, a feature that is related to the capacity of these drugs to cause ototoxicity.

Aminoglycosides are almost entirely eliminated by glomerular filtration, and thus the dosage must be carefully adjusted in patients with renal insufficiency. The half-lives of the aminoglycosides are between 2 and 3 hours in patients with normal renal function.

Ototoxicity and nephrotoxicity are the major adverse effects of aminoglycosides.[47-50] The longer excessive serum levels persist, the more likely that these conditions will occur. Aminoglycosides accumulate in perilymph and otolymph of the inner ear. Accumulation is most likely to occur when serum levels are high: Back diffusion of aminoglycoside from the inner ear is a slow process. Ototoxicity is not entirely predictable based on drug levels and tends to be irreversible. Patients receiving other ototoxic drugs and patients with pre-existing impairment are more likely to manifest toxicity. Gentamicin has a predilection for damaging vestibular function, whereas amikacin preferentially damages auditory function. Tobramycin affects both equally. High-pitched tinnitus is often the first sign of cochlear toxicity. Although careful monitoring for ototoxicity is advocated, this is not easy to perform in children in a critical care unit. Tinnitus, auditory impairment, and vestibular dysfunction need to be monitored as much as feasible. Headache followed by nausea and vomiting may be early signs of vestibular toxicity.

Nephrotoxicity can occur in 8 to 26% of patients receiving aminoglycosides. Fortunately, when plasma levels of drug are monitored carefully, the renal dysfunction is usually not of major clinical importance and is reversible. Nephrotoxicity is usually manifested first by the excretion of renal tubular brush border enzymes followed by defective renal concentrating ability, mild proteinuria, the shedding of hyaline casts, and reduced glomerular filtration. There is then a mild rise in the plasma creatinine level. The damage is primarily to the proximal tubular cells, which can regenerate; thus, impairment is generally reversible. Acute tubular necrosis and severe dysfunction or anuria are rare complications. If there are real differences in the nephrotoxic potential of gentamicin, tobramycin, and amikacin, they are probably minor.

There is considerable debate about the optimal technique for minimizing renal toxicity or ototoxicity. Since children in intensive care units frequently have other physiologic and chemotherapeutic insults to their kidneys and ears, minimizing the toxic effects of aminoglycosides is obviously an important issue. The peak serum concentration of aminoglycosides clearly correlates with the likelihood of toxicity. Peak serum levels of gentamicin or tobramycin greater than 10 to 12 μg/ml and peak serum levels of amikacin greater than 30 to 40 μg/ml increase the likelihood of nephrotoxicity and ototoxicity. Maintaining trough levels of gentamicin and tobramycin less than 2 μg/ml (and probably maintaining amikacin levels less than 15 μg/ml) has been demonstrated in some studies to be useful and is advocated by many authorities. Regular monitoring of serum levels in critically ill children with unstable volumes of distribution and renal function is well warranted. Daily peak levels (drawn 30 minutes after a 30-minute infusion) and trough levels (drawn immediately before the next dose) are often appropriate. The use of nomograms or other formulas is not equally effective for assuring therapeutic doses but avoiding toxic levels.

Other untoward effects have been described in association with aminoglycoside administration. Neuromuscular blockade has been associated with aminoglycoside lavage of body cavities. Reports of this effect in association with parenteral administration are rare and have occurred in association with anesthesia, neuromuscular blocking agents, or myasthenia gravis. Hypersensitivity reactions occur but are very unusual.

Generally, intensive care practitioners faced with children having life-threatening infections should not be reluctant to use an aggressive loading dose of an aminoglycoside (i.e., 2.5 to 3 mg/kg of gentamicin or tobramycin), since patient survival is a more immediate issue than potential toxicity. At most hospitals, gentamicin is the aminoglycoside of choice because of its generally lower cost than the other agents. If the patient is known or suspected to be infected or colonized by organisms that are gentamicin-resistant but are sensitive to another aminoglycoside, or if the hospital has a high frequency of such isolates, tobramycin, or more likely amikacin, will be the aminoglycoside of choice.

Trimethoprim-Sulfamethoxazole

Trimethoprim-sulfamethoxazole is a fixed, often synergistic combination of a dihydrofolate reductase inhibitor and a sulfonamide. This combination product has broad activity against a variety of gram-positive and gram-negative bacteria. Its major use in pediatric critical care is to treat infections from *Nocardia* sp., *Pneumocystis*, and rare cases of exquisitely resistant gram-negative bacilli.[52]

Trimethoprim-sulfamethoxazole is widely distributed throughout the body, including the meninges. The majority of both drugs are excreted in the urine, so dosage must be adjusted in patients with renal dysfunction.

Untoward effects include hypersensitivity, nausea, vomiting, stomatitis, cholestatic jaundice, headache, fever, anemia, crystalluria, interstitial nephritis, and granulocytopenia. Patients infected with the human immunodeficiency virus (HIV) have a high frequency of hypersensitivity reactions. Folate deficiency is rarely caused by trimethoprim-sulfamethoxazole, but leucovorin is often given to granulocytopenic or thrombocytopenic patients receiving these antibiotics to preclude the possibility that folate deficiency is contributing to their cytopenia.

For the treatment of *Pneumocystis* pneumonia, peak serum levels of sulfamethoxazole should probably be maintained at 100 to 150 μg/ml; concurrent peak trimethoprim levels will be 3 to 5 μg/ml (drawn 30 minutes after a 30-minute infusion).

Ciprofloxin and Other Quinolones

Fluorinated 4-quinolones are relatively recent introductions to the available antimicrobial armamentarium.[53] They include ciprofloxin, norfloxacin, ofloxacin, temofloxacin, and a host of their compounds that inhibit the enzyme deoxyribonucleic acid (DNA) gyrase. In an outpatient setting, quinolones have found wide application for the therapy of urinary tract infections and diarrheal illnesses.

Ciprofloxacin is the only parenteral quinolone that is currently available. It has broad activity against many gram-negative bacilli, including *N. meningitidis, H. influenzae,* and many strains of *P. aeruginosa.* It is active against many strains of *S. aureus* (although resistant strains are quite common) and has some activity against *E. fecalis,* but it has poor activity against many strains of *S. pyogenes* and *S. pneumoniae* and no anaerobic activity. It has good activity against *Legionella* sp. and *M. pneumoniae.* In vivo resistance can develop during treatment of *Pseudomonas* infections. Thus, the only strong indication for quinolone use in an intensive care unit would be a severe gram-negative bacillus infection and probably one that is resistant to other agents. In children with cystic fibrosis, there may be some advantages in favor of the use of ciprofloxacin as well.

In postpubertal children, quinolones are well tolerated. Nausea is the major problem. Because quinolones are concentrated in bone plates and can cause arthropathies in immature animals, there is extreme reluctance to use them in prepubertal children except when there are no reasonable alternatives.

Antiviral Agents

Ribavirin

Ribavirin is a purine nucleoside analogue that inhibits a wide variety of ribonucleic acid (RNA) and DNA viruses. In a pediatric intensive care unit, its only use (with rare exception) is to treat respiratory syncytial virus infections. Even in this case, though, its clinical efficacy is controversial.[54-57]

For the therapy of respiratory syncytial virus pneumonia, ribavirin is administered as an aerosol using a specific nebulizer. In children who need mechanical ventilation, aerosol ribavirin can clog valves and create life-threatening mechanical difficulties if ventilator maintenance is not monitored with extraordinary care. Aerosolized ribavarin can cause conjunctival irritation, wheezing, and rash.

Zidovudine

Zidovudine is licensed for the treatment of HIV infection in certain settings.[59, 60] For children hospitalized in a critical care unit, careful consideration should be given to whether zidovudine should be continued (an investigational intravenous form is manufactured) or whether the adverse effects associated with zidovudine should warrant discontinuation while the more immediately life-threatening process is maintained.

Acyclovir

Acyclovir is a synthetic purine nucleoside analogue with excellent activity against herpes simplex and vari-

cella zoster but not against cytomegalovirus (CMV) or Epstein-Barr virus.[61-63] Its principal use in a pediatric intensive care unit is to treat herpes simplex encephalitis or life-threatening varicella in immunocompetent children and to treat herpes simplex stomatitis or disseminated herpes simplex or varicella zoster in immunologically abnormal children.[64-66]

Strains of herpes simplex and varicella zoster that are resistant to acyclovir have been described but are to date quite rare.[67] When resistance is suspected or documented, either ganciclovir or foscarnet are effective alternatives.

Acyclovir is well distributed throughout the body, although levels in cerebrospinal fluid and the aqueous humor are only one third of those in plasma. The plasma half-life is normally 4 hours. The drug is primarily excreted unchanged in the urine, and thus the dosage must be carefully adjusted for patients with impaired renal function.

Acyclovir infusions can cause local phlebitis. Excessively high levels can be associated with confusion or encephalopathy. The latter occurs most often in patients with renal failure. Crystalluria and obstructive nephropathy can also occur when high doses of acyclovir are used.[68, 69]

Ganciclovir

Ganciclovir is structurally similar to acyclovir, but its structural modification has provided it with activity against CMV, as well as herpes simplex and varicella zoster.[70-72] It has only limited activity against certain Epstein-Barr virus isolates. Resistance to ganciclovir is still extremely rare in herpes simplex, varicella zoster, and CMV.[73] Foscarnet is usually active against resistant strains. The major use of ganciclovir is to treat life-threatening CMV infections. Because of its toxicity, ganciclovir is less desirable for treating herpes simplex and varicella zoster infections unless viral resistance is an issue.

Ganciclovir is well distributed throughout the body, including the central nervous system. Its half-life in plasma is usually 3 to 4 hours. The drug is excreted unchanged in the urine, and the dosage must be substantially altered in renal failure.

Ganciclovir causes neutropenia and thrombocytopenia, especially during the second week of therapy. This feature can make the drug difficult to manage, especially in initially cytopenic patients in whom marrow recovery is expected imminently. Central nervous system toxicity includes headache and psychosis; seizures also occur when plasma levels are very high. Phlebitis at the infusion site occurs. Hypersensitivity to ganciclovir is unusual.

Ganciclovir has been used in conjunction with immune serum globulin or anti-CMV hyperimmune globulin to treat CMV pneumonia. The indications for combination therapy have not been well delineated with CMV disease, but for treating CMV pneumonia such combination therapy is probably desirable at this time.

Foscarnet

Foscarnet has excellent activity against CMV, which makes it a useful drug for patients who cannot tolerate ganciclovir.[67] It is also useful for patients with ganciclovir- and acyclovir-resistant herpes simplex or varicella zoster.

Foscarnet penetrates the central nervous system well. It is eliminated by the kidneys, and the dosage must be adjusted in renal failure. Patients receiving foscarnet need to be vigorously hydrated. Major toxicities include renal insufficiency, seizures, and hypocalcemia. Foscarnet does not have major bone marrow toxicity, although anemia occurs.

Antifungal Agents

Amphotericin B

Amphotericin B is the major drug for the treatment of life-threatening fungal infections.[74] In a critical care unit, there will rarely be indications to use other agents: Fluconazole, ketoconazole, and flucytosine will have only occasional utility. Antifungal therapy, unlike antibacterial therapy, is almost never selected on the basis of susceptibility testing from the hospital microbiology laboratory, since in vitro testing is unstandardized, controversial, and does not clearly lead to clinically useful information.

Amphotericin B is a polyene antibiotic with broad activity against most fungi. The drug is highly protein-bound. About 2 to 5% of the drug is excreted unchanged in the urine. The elimination of amphotericin B is not well understood, but severe hepatic or biliary disease is not known to alter its metabolism, nor is elimination changed by renal failure or hemodialysis. Little amphotericin B penetrates into the cerebrospinal fluid.

Amphotericin B is a toxic drug that is best administered by a standardized protocol. Initially, 1 mg is dissolved in 20 ml of 5% dextrose solution (not saline) and administered over 20 to 30 minutes. Fever, chills, dyspnea, and hypotension may result. The severity of these responses determines how rapidly the dose can be escalated. In a patient whose fungal infection is life-threatening and whose reaction is mild, the dose can be escalated immediately to 0.3 to 1 mg/kg infused over 2 to 6 hours. The infusing solution should not contain more than 0.1 mg amphotericin B/ml and may be mixed with 500 to 1,000 units of heparin to reduce phlebitis. Pretreatment with meperidine and acetaminophen may reduce the fever and chills.[75] If these pretreatments do not prevent severe systemic manifestations, hydrocortisone 0.7 mg/kg can be added to the infusion. If the patient has a severe reaction to the test dose, the amphotericin B doses should be escalated more gradually, for example, in 5 to 10 mg/day increments, until the desired or maximally tolerated daily dose is attained.

There is controversy over the optimal daily dose or total dose for treating fungal infections. Daily doses of 0.3 to 1.5 mg/kg are advocated by various authorities, depending on the gravity of the clinical situation and the patient's ability to tolerate the drug. Most prefer daily doses of 0.3 to 0.6 mg/kg. Total doses range from 100 mg for mucosal disease (e.g., Candida esophagitis) to 2 to 6 g for invasive aspergillosis: Decisions must be individualized when patients receiving long courses of amphotericin B become stable; amphotericin B can be administered every other day with double doses (up to 1 mg/kg in most situations).

Amphotericin B administration is associated with substantial toxicity. Fever and chills can last 2 to 4 hours and are more common at the beginning of therapy; they often decrease in severity later in the course of treatment. Bronchospasm and anaphylaxis rarely occur.

Azotemia occurs in most patients receiving amphotericin B. Renal tubular acidosis and wasting of potassium or magnesium are also seen. This toxicity is dose-dependent and is more likely to occur in patients receiving other nephrotoxic drugs. When less than 3 to 4 g of amphotericin B is given to adults; functional renal impairment is rarely permanent, though histologic changes may persist. Toxicity is caused by an increase in intrarenal vascular resistance. Sodium loading may reduce the likelihood of toxicity.[76] In adults, it is often the practice to give 0.5 l of normal saline prior to the infusion and again immediately after the infusion. Other adverse effects include anemia, headache, nausea, and vomiting.

Flucytosine

Flucytosine is a pyrimidine related to fluorouracil, which has activity against many yeasts. It is only available currently as an oral preparation. Resistance is an important cause of therapeutic failure. Flucytosine can cause cytopenia, nausea, vomiting, enterocolitis, and hepatitis, especially in patients with acquired immunodeficiency syndrome (AIDS) or azotemia or in patients with plasma levels greater than 100 μg/ml. Flucytosine is never used alone. In combination with amphotericin B, it may have a role in the treatment of cryptococcosis. The toxicities of the drug require that its use in critical care units be restricted to situations in which there are well-defined benefits to be gained and expertise available in managing its dosing schedule and toxicities.

Fluconazole

There are an expanding number of imidazoles and triazoles with excellent antifungal activity. Fluconazole is the agent most likely to be used in an intensive care unit because it is available in both oral and intravenous forms, has activity against Candida sp. and Cryptococcus, and penetrates the central nervous system.[77-79] Fluconazole has excellent efficacy for treating mucosal candidiasis, for example, oral candidiasis or Candida esophagitis. It is not yet clear, despite some favorable experience with AIDS patients who have cryptococcal meningitis, that is has a role for the acute treatment of candidemia or cryptococcosis, especially in patients sick enough to be in an intensive care unit. Species of candida other than C. albicans (e.g., C. Krusei) are more likely to be resistant.

Pentamidine Isethionate

In critically ill children in North America, the major indication for using parenteral pentamidine is the treatment of *Pneumocystis* pneumonia. Parenteral pentamidine is as effective as trimethoprim-sulfamethoxazole for this indication, but it is not the drug of choice because nephrotoxicity, dysglycemia (hypoglycemia followed by hyperglycemia), and leukopenia often occur. Fatalities from hypoglycemia have been reported both during therapy and many weeks after. Pentamidine should be administered only by slow intravenous infusion (60 minutes) at a dose of 4 mg/kg once daily. Intramuscular administration is no longer recommended. Inhaled pentamidine may still have a role for *Pneumocystis* prophylaxis in certain children, but it has no established role in acute therapy. Pentamidine has a very long half-life. Some of it is excreted in the urine, but the dosage schedule probably should not be altered in patients with renal insufficiency.

References

1. Pratt WB and Fekety R: The Antimicrobial Drugs. New York, Oxford University Press, 1986.
2. Kucers A and Bennett NMcK: The Use of Antibiotics. A Comprehensive Review with Clinical Emphasis, 4th ed. Philadelphia, JB Lippincott, 1987.
3. Moellering RC Jr: Principles of anti-infective therapy. *In:* Mandell GL, Douglas Jr RG, and Bennett JE (eds): Principles and Practice of Infectious Diseases, 2nd ed. New York, John Wiley & Sons, 1985, pp. 153–164.
4. Coleman DL, Horowitz RI, and Andriole VT: Association between serum inhibitory and bactericidal concentrations and therapeutic outcome in bacterial endocarditis. Am J Med 73:260, 1982.
5. Hackbarth CJ, Chambers HF, and Sande MA: Serum bactericidal titer as a predictor of outcome in endocarditis. Eur J Clin Microbiol 5:93, 1986.
6. Wolfson JS and Swartz MN: Serum bactericidal activity as a monitor of antibiotic therapy. N Engl J Med 312:968, 1985.
7. Klastersky J, Hensgens C, and Meunier-Carpentier F: Comparative effectiveness of combinations of amikacin with penicillin G and amikacin with carbenicillin in gram negative septicemia double blind clinical trial. J Infect Dis 134 (Suppl):433, 1976.
8. Lau WK, Young LS, Black RE, et al: Comparative efficacy and toxicity of amikacin/carbenicillin versus gentamicin/carbenicillin in leukopenic patients. Am J Med 62:659, 1977.
9. Rahal J Jr: Antibiotic combinations: The clinical relevance of synergy and antagonism. Medicine (Baltimore) 57:179, 1978.
10. Bennett JE, Dismukes WE, et al: A comparison of amphotericin B alone and combined with flucytosine in the treatment of cryptococcal meningitis. N Engl J Med 301:126–131, 1979.
11. Lepper MH and Dowling HF: Treatment of pneumococcic meningitis with penicillin plus aureomycin: Studies including observations on apparent antagonism between penicillin and aureomycin. Arch Intern Med 88:489, 1951.
12. Sanford JP: Guide to Antimicrobial Therapy 1991. Bethesda, Sanford, 1991.
13. Nelson JD: 1991–1992 Pocketbook of Pediatric Antimicrobial Therapy, 9th ed. Baltimore, Williams & Wilkins, 1991.
14. Bartlett JG: 1991 Pocketbook of Infectious Disease Therapy. Baltimore, Williams & Wilkins, 1991.
15. Peacock JE, Moorman DR, Wenzel RP, et al: Methicillin resistant *Staphylococcus aureus:* Microbiologic characteristics, antimicrobial susceptibility, and assessment of virulence of an epidemic strain. J Infect Dis 144:575, 1981.
16. Weiss ME and Adkinson NF. Beta-lactam allergy. *In:* Mandell GL, Douglas RG Jr, and Bennett JE (eds): Principles and Practice of Infectious Diseases, 3rd ed. New York, Churchill Livingstone, 1990, pp. 264–269.
17. Saxon A, Beall GN, Rohr AS, et al: Immediate hypersensitivity reactions to beta-lactam antibiotics. Ann Intern Med 107:204, 1987.
18. Neult C: Antistaphylococcal penicillins. Med Clin North Am 66:51, 1982.
19. Archer GL: Molecular epidemiology of multiresistant *Staphylococcus epidermidis.* J Antimicrob Chemother 21 (Suppl):133, 1988.
20. Doern GV, Jergensen JH, Thornsberry C, et al: National collaborative study of the prevalence of antimicrobial resistance among clinical isolates of *Hemophilus influenzae.* Antimicrob Agent Chemother 32:185, 1988.
21. Dajani AS: Sulbactam/ampicillin in pediatric infections. Drugs 35 (Suppl 7):35, 1988.
22. Leigh DA, Phillips I, and Wise R (eds): Timentin-ticarcillin plus clavulanic acid, a laboratory and clinical perspective. J Antimicrob Chemother 17(Suppl C):1, 1986.
23. Bodey GP, Alvarez ME, Jones PG, et al: Imipenem/colistin as initial therapy for ferule cancer patients. Antimicrob Agent Chemother 30:211, 1986.
24. Jones RN: Review of the in vitro spectrum of activity of imipenem. Am J Med 78:22, 1985.
25. Scully BE and Neu HC: Use of aztreonam in the treatment of serious infections due to multiresistant gram negative organisms including *Pseudomonas aeruginosa.* Am J Med 78:251, 1985.
26. Saxon A, Hassner A, Swabb EA, et al: Lack of cross-reactivity between aztreonam, a monobactam antibiotic, and penicillin in penicillin-allergic subjects. J Infect Dis 149:16, 1984.
27. Donowitz GR and Mandell GL: Cephalosporins. *In:* Mandell GL, Douglas RG Jr, and Bennett JE (eds): Principles and Practice of Infectious Diseases, 3rd ed. New York, Churchill Livingstone, 1990, pp. 716–721.
28. Donowitz GR and Mandell GL: Beta-lactam antibiotics. N Engl J Med 318:419, 490, 1988.
29. Brogden RN and Ward A: Ceftriaxone: A reappraisal of its antibacterial activity and pharmacokinetic properties, and an update on its therapeutic use with particular reference to once-daily administration. Drugs 35:604, 1988.
30. Pizzo PA, Hathorn JW, Heimenz J, et al: A randomized trial comparing ceftazidime alone with combination antibiotic therapy in cancer patients with fever and neutropenia. N Engl J Med 315:552, 1986.
31. Sattler FR, Weitekamp MR, and Ballard JO: Potential for bleeding with the new beta-lactam antibiotics. Ann Intern Med 105:924, 1986.
32. Cunha BA and Ristuccia AM: Clinical usefulness of vancomycin. Clin Pharm 2:417, 1983.
33. Schwalbe RS, Stapleton JT, and Gilligan PH: Emergence of vancomycin resistance in coagulase-negative staphylococci. N Engl J Med 316:927, 1987.
34. Uttley AHC, Collins CH, Naidodo J, et al: Vancomycin-resistant enterococci. Lancet 1:57, 1988.
35. Farber B and Moellering RC Jr: Retrospective study of the toxicity of preparations of vancomycin from 1974–1981. Antimicrob Agents Chemother 23:138, 1983.
36. Levine JF: Vancomycin: A review. Med Clin North Am 71:1135, 1987.
37. Woods CA, Kohlhepp SJ, Houghton DC, et al: Vancomycin enhancement of experimental tobramycin nephrotoxicity. Antimicrob Agents Chemother 30:20, 1986.
38. Davis RL, Smith AL, and Koup JR: The "redman's syndrome" and slow infusion of vancomycin. Ann Intern Med 104:285, 1986.
39. Newfield P and Roizen MF: Hazards of rapid administration of vancomycin. Ann Intern Med 91:581, 1979.
40. Karmody CS and Weinstein L: Reversible sensorineural hearing loss with intravenous erythromycin lactobionate. Ann Otol Rhinol Laryngol 86:9, 1977.
41. Standiford HC: Tetracyclines and chloramphenicol. *In:* Mandell GL, Douglas RG, Jr, and Bennett JE (eds): Principles and Practices of Infectious Diseases, 3rd ed. New York, John Wiley & Sons, 1990, pp. 284–295.
42. Craft AW, Brocklebank JT, Hey EN, et al: The "grey toddler": Chloramphenicol toxicity. Arch Dis Child 49:235, 1974.
43. Daum RS, Cohen DL, and Smith AL: Fatal aplastic anemia following apparent "dose-related" chloramphenicol toxicity. J Pediatr 94:403, 1979.
44. Kucers A and Bennett NMcK: Gentamicin. *In:* Kucers A and Bennett NMcK (eds): The Use of Antibiotics, 4th ed. Philadelphia, JB Lippincott, 1987, pp. 619–674.

45. Lietman PS: Aminoglycosides and spectinomycin: Aminocyclitos. *In:* Mandell GL, Douglas RG, Jr, and Bennett JE (eds): Principles and Practices of Infectious Diseases, 3rd ed. New York, Churchill Livingstone, 1990, pp. 269–284.

46. Yow MO: An overview of pediatric experience with amikacin. Am J Med 62:954, 1977.

47. Smith CR, Lipsky JJ, Laskin OL, et al: Double-blind comparison of the nephrotoxicity and auditory toxicity of gentamicin and tobramycin. N Engl J Med 302:1106, 1980.

48. Smith CR and Lietman PS: Effect of furosemide on aminoglycoside-induced nephrotoxicity and auditory toxicity in humans. Antimicrob Agents Chemother 23:133, 1983.

49. Smith CR, Bauthman KL, Edwards CQ, et al: Controlled comparison of amikacin and gentamicin. N Engl J Med 296:349, 1977.

50. Moore RD, Smith CR, Lipsky JJ, et al: Risk factors for nephrotoxicity in patients with aminoglycosides. Ann Intern Med 100:352, 1984.

51. Moore RD, Smith CR, and Lietman PS: Risk factors for the development of auditory toxicity in patients receiving aminoglycosides. J Infect Dis 149:23, 1984.

52. Ardati KO and Danjani AS: Intravenous trimethoprim-sulfamethoxazole in the treatment of serious infections in children. J Pediatr 95:801, 1979.

53. Hooper DC and Wolfson JS: Fluoroquinolone antimicrobial agents. N Engl J Med 324:384, 1991.

54. Connor JD, Hintz M, Van Dyke R, et al: Ribavirin pharmacokinetics in children and adults during therapeutic trials. *In:* Smith RA, Knight V, and Smith JAD (eds): Clinical Applications of Ribarivin. Orlando, FL, Academic Press, 1984, pp. 107–123.

55. Knight V, Yu CP, Gilbert BE, et al: Estimating the dosage of ribavirin aerosol according to age and other variables. J Infect Dis 158:443, 1988.

56. Hall CB, McBride JT, Walsh EE, et al: Aerosolized ribavirin treatment of infants with respiratory syncytial viral infection. N Engl J Med 308:1443, 1983.

57. Rodriguez WJ, Kim HW, Brandt CD, et al: Aerosolized ribavirin in the treatment of patients with respiratory syncytial virus disease. Pediatr Infect Dis J 6:159, 1987.

58. Fischl MA, Richman DD, Grieco MH, et al: The efficacy of azidothymidine (AZT) in the treatment of patients with AIDS and AIDS-related complex. N Engl J Med 317:185, 1987.

59. Volberding PA, Lagakos SW, Koch MA, et al: Zidovudine in asymptomatic human immunodeficiency virus infection—a controlled trial in persons with less than 500 CD4 positive cells. N Engl J Med 322:941, 1990.

60. Balis FM, Pizzo PA, Murphy RF, et al: The pharmacokinetics of zidovudine administered by continuous infusion in children. Ann Intern Med 110:279, 1989.

61. Blum RM, Liao SHT, and De Miranda P: Overview of acyclovir pharmacokinetic disposition in adults and children. Am J Med 73 (Suppl):186, 1982.

62. Dorsky DI and Crumpacker CS: Drugs five years later: Acyclovir. Ann Intern Med 107:859, 1987.

63. Wade JC, Newton B, McLaren C, et al: Intravenous acyclovir to treat mucocutaneous herpes simplex virus infection after marrow transplantation. Ann Intern Med 96:265, 1982.

64. Balfour HH Jr, Bean B, Laskin OL, et al: Burroughs Wellcome Collaborative Acyclovir Study Group. Acyclovir halts progression of herpes zoster in immunocompromised patients. N Engl J Med 308:1448, 1983.

65. Chatis PA, Miller CH, Schrager LE, et al: Successful treatment with foscarnet of an acyclovir-resistant mucocutaneous infection with herpes simplex virus in a patient with acquired immunodeficiency syndrome. N Engl J Med 320:297, 1989.

66. Feldman S and Lott L: Varicella in children with cancer: Impact of antiviral therapy and prophylaxis. Pediatrics 80:465, 1987.

67. Erlich KS, Facobson MA, Koehler JE, et al: Foscarnet therapy for severe acyclovir-resistant herpes simplex virus type-2 infections in patients with the acquired immunodeficiency syndrome (AIDS): An uncontrolled trial. Ann Intern Med 110:710, 1989.

68. Sawyer MH, Webb DE, Balow JE, et al: Acyclovir-induced renal failure: Clinical course and histology. Am J Med 84:1067, 1988.

69. Wade JC and Meyers JD: Neurologic symptoms associated with parenteral acyclovir treatment after marrow transplantation. Ann Intern Med 98:921, 1983.

70. Collaborative DHPG Treatment Study Group. Treatment of serious cytomegalovirus infections with 9-(1.3-dihydroxy-2-propoxymethyl) guanine in patients with AIDS and other immunodeficiencies. N Engl J Med 314:801, 1986.

71. Emanuel D, Cunningham I, Jules-Elysee K, et al: Cytomegalovirus pneumonia after bone marrow transplantation successfully treated with the combination of ganciclovir and high-dose intravenous immune globulin. Ann Intern Med 109:777, 1988.

72. Reed EC, Bowden RA, Dandliker PS, et al: Treatment of cytomegalovirus pneumonia with ganciclovir and intravenous cytomegalovirus immunoglobin in patients with bone marrow transplants. Ann Intern Med 109:783, 1988.

73. Erice A, Chou S, Biron KK, et al: Progressive disease due to ganciclovir-resistant cytomegalovirus in immunocompromised patients. N Engl J Med 320:289, 1989.

74. Bennett JE: Antifungal agents. *In:* Mandell GL, Douglas RG Jr, and Bennett JE (eds): Principles and Practice of Infectious Diseases, 3rd ed. New York, Churchill Livingstone, 1990, pp. 361–370.

75. Burks LC, Aisner J, Fortner CL, et al: Meperidine for the treatment of shaking chills and fever. Arch Intern Med 140:483, 1980.

76. Branch RA: Prevention of amphotericin B-induced renal impairment. Arch Intern Med 148:2389, 1988.

77. Grant SM and Clissold SP: Fluconazole—a review of its pharmacologic and pharmacokinetic properties, and therapeutic potential in superficial and systemic mycoses. Drugs 39:877, 1990.

78. Stern JJ, Hartman BJ, Sharkey P, et al: Oral fluconazole therapy for patients with acquired immunodeficiency syndrome. Am J Med 297:178, 1988.

79. Tucker RM, Williams PL, Arathoon RG, et al: Pharmacokinetics of fluconazole in cerebrospinal fluid and serum in human coccidioidal meningitis. Antimicrob Agent Chemother 32:369, 1988.

Characteristics of Pathogenic Microbes and Infectious Syndromes

Bernhard L. Wiedermann, M. D.

Clinical manifestations of infectious syndromes are determined by a wide range of variables in both the infecting agent and the host. In the practice of pediatrics, antimicrobial therapy is frequently begun on an empiric basis while awaiting culture results. The selection of a specific therapeutic agent is usually made with knowledge of the more common causes of a particular syndrome as well as the side effects of the drugs to be used, and coverage is often not intended to target every possible pathogen. However, in the critically ill child, these decisions are more important and more difficult. An error in coverage could have dire consequences in a critically ill individual, but overzealous use of broad-spectrum agents can result in more rapid selection of resistance as well as superinfection with opportunistic microbes. For example, broad coverage may result in successful treatment of an infection but also suppression of normal flora. With a critically ill individual, who usually has several foreign bodies in vascular sites and elsewhere, the potential for secondary infection and clinical deterioration is great. For these reasons, the critical care practitioner must have a thorough understanding of therapy for infectious syndromes in order to make the most logical treatment choices, weighing the crucial risk: benefit ratio involved.

This chapter addresses the management of infectious syndromes based on the particular microorganism involved. Emphasis is on the more serious manifestations of infections, rather than on minor and perhaps more common presentations. From a practical standpoint, the clinician may find this chapter useful when an initial identification of an organism is made from culture or serology. He or she can then refer to the appropriate section(s) to determine what types of serious syndromes are most commonly caused by the particular agent(s) and what modes of therapy are most likely to be effective. This approach has limitations, however. Most important, it should be recognized that virtually any microorganism can cause virtually any constellation of symptoms given the appropriate circumstances. The reader should appreciate that this chapter deals with the

more common scenarios, rather than listing every manifestation ever reported with a particular microbe. Second, the list of microorganisms discussed is lengthy but by no means complete. To address all pathogenic microbes would require a separate textbook, and several excellent sources are already available that contain a more complete discussion.[1-4]

Proper cultures and serologic studies are central to the management of infectious diseases and appropriate interpretation of laboratory tests. Where pertinent, methods of choice for laboratory diagnosis of the specific pathogens are discussed. However, as a general rule, the critical care practitioner should be aware of the problems associated with interpretation of laboratory studies in the face of prior therapy. Most commonly, this involves administration of antibacterial agents before cultures have been obtained. In many instances, this results from a need to institute therapy on an emergency basis in patients too unstable to allow safe performance of lumbar puncture or similar tests that may compromise cardiorespiratory status. Cultures obtained later may then contain antibiotics and result in falsely negative results. Similarly, administration of blood products can passively raise antibody levels to specific (especially common viral) pathogens, rendering serodiagnosis less useful.

Blood and urine specimens are almost always available in emergency situations, and it should be possible to obtain culture material at that time. When indicated, cerebrospinal fluid (CSF) analysis should be obtained when the patient's status permits, even if this means a delay of hours or days in performing lumbar puncture. In other cases, it is unlikely that a delay in several minutes in institution of antibiotic treatment will have an impact on eventual outcome, unlike true emergency measures such as intubation or administration of pressor agents. Therefore, antimicrobial therapy in critically ill children should be considered as urgent, rather than emergent, treatment, and one should take the extra few minutes necessary to obtain appropriate specimens for diagnostic tests. The alternative is to be faced with a child who improves after administration of broad-spectrum antimicrobial therapy but who does not have a specific diagnosis. In this situation, it is often necessary to continue this treatment for a poorly defined period, which places the patient at greater risk for colonization and infection with opportunistic or multiply drug-resistant organisms.

One final general caveat relates to duration of antimicrobial therapy. Many infectious syndromes require relatively specific treatment regimens for eradication of disease, but most commonly duration of therapy is relatively empiric. For example, uncomplicated bacterial meningitis may be treated for anywhere from 7 to 14 days without clear differences in outcome, and even shorter regimens may be effective for meningococcal meningitis. In general, the duration of therapy must be individualized and must take into account the patient's clinical course. A specific duration of therapy should be anticipated, then modified as clinical course and culture results dictate, and the drug should be discontinued when the specified period has elapsed.

BACTERIA

Gram-Positive Cocci

Staphylococci

Staphylococci are normal inhabitants of the skin and are noted for their relative hardiness. They are able to easily persist in the environment on fomites and are relatively resistant to the effects of drying and heat. They also have a great tendency to persist as pathogens and to seed distant sites in the body, resulting in metastatic foci of infection.

Staphylococcus aureus

Staphylococcus aureus, the major pathogen in this genus, is distinguished from other staphylococci by its positive coagulase reaction in laboratory testing. It is usually β-hemolytic on blood agar, whereas most coagulase-negative staphylocci are not, but this feature cannot be relied on to accurately identify *S. aureus*.

S. aureus usually gains entry into the body via skin structures, either from minor trauma such as an insect bite or from more serious injury. Locally, infections such as impetigo, furuncle, pyoderma, or pyomyositis may develop. Bacteremia may result in pneumonia with empyema or abscess formation, endocarditis, perinephric abscess (renal carbuncle), endocarditis, and many other syndromes. *S. aureus* is the most common cause of bone and joint infection, which usually develop by hematogenous seeding. However, this bacteremia can be transient, and evidence of bacteremia may be followed by a relatively quiescent period before signs and symptoms of bone and joint disease appear. In contrast to coagulase-negative staphylococci, *S. aureus* in culture of normally sterile body fluids is seldom a contaminant and should generally require specific therapy and a search for other foci of infection.

S. aureus strains can also produce several toxins that are important for disease production. Staphylococcal scalded skin syndrome occurs in infants with colonization of *S. aureus* strains producing an exfoliative toxin, and bullous impetigo is caused by a dermonecrotoxin of *S. aureus*. Several staphylococcal enterotoxins can produce a wide array of food poisoning syndromes. Foods most frequently implicated include ham, poultry, egg salad, and pastries with cream fillings. Some of these same enterotoxins (particularly enterotoxin B in nonmenstrual cases) are responsible along with toxic shock syndrome toxin 1, for the symptomatology of toxic shock syndrome. Some strains of *S. aureus* can produce erythrogenic toxins, which produce an illness similar to scarlet fever. Other toxins, such as α-hemolysin and leukocidin, are probably important virulence determinants.

In the early antibiotic era, strains of *S. aureus* were uniformly sensitive to penicillin, but with the widespread use of penicillin therapy, most strains have become resistant by means of penicillinase production. Still, in a given strain showing good in vitro susceptibility to penicillin (probably less than 10% of strains in most locales), penicillin therapy is adequate. However, most infections require treatment with a semisynthetic or isoxazoyl penicillin such as methicillin or oxacillin. Soon after these penicillinase-resistant antibiotics were developed, however, methicillin-resistant strains began to appear and are now a major problem in most medical centers, particularly as nosocomial infections, but increasingly in community-acquired infections as well. Vancomycin is the main type of therapy in these situations.

Coagulase-Negative Staphylococci

Coagulase-negative staphylococci (CN staph) infections are extremely common in intensive care settings, primarily because of their tendency to colonize intravascular lines. They are the leading cause of nosocomial bacteremias in most hospitals and the primary cause of infections of ventriculoperitoneal shunts. Administration of lipid emulsion may predispose to CN staph bacteremias in neonates.[5] Although they are generally thought to be less virulent than *S. aureus*, this distinction is not clear cut, and CN staph infections result in significant morbidity and mortality.[6] Members of this group include *S. epidermidis*, *S. hominis*, *S. haemolyticus*, and *S. warneri*. Production of an extracellular glycocalyx, or "slime," may aid in colonization but is not necessary for disease production. These organisms are also frequent contaminants of cultures, and it is difficult to distinguish contamination from true infection in many cases.[7] Isolation of the same species with the same antibiotic susceptibility pattern from multiple blood cultures, as well as high (>50 colony-forming units (cfu)/ml) colony counts from quantitative blood cultures, may help to document true infection, but many instances of infection may be represented by a single positive blood culture of low colony count.

Most CN staph intravenous line infections are easily cured by removal of the line, but this is not always the case.[8] In the critically ill individual, removal of the line and institution of appropriate antibiotic therapy is prudent, with continuation of therapy pending clinical response and further culture results.

Nosocomial CN staph isolates are usually resistant to multiple antibiotics, including methicillin and other penicillinase-resistant antibiotics, erythromycin, tetracycline, and clindamycin. Interpretation of susceptibility testing for cephalosporins and other β-lactam antibiotics may be misleading, and most authorities would consider staphylococci that test resistant to methicillin as also resistant to all β-lactams, even if in vitro testing appears to demonstrate susceptibility. Vancomycin is used in this situation, although there are rare reports of vancomycin resistance.

Streptococci

Streptococci are important causes of disease, and observations suggest they should be of increasing concern for critical care specialists. The nomenclature used to identify streptococci often causes confusion. Streptococci can be serogrouped based on antigenic content of the cell wall. Although there are at least 20 serogroups of streptococci, only five (groups A, B, C, D, and G) commonly cause human disease. Second, streptococci can be characterized by the appearance of hemolysis produced by growth on blood agar plates. β-Hemolysis refers to a clear zone of hemolysis around colonies, α-hemolysis is a greenish coloration, and γ-hemolytic organisms produce no zone of hemolysis around colonies. Finally, organisms are best identified by genus and species. The term *viridans streptococci*, or *Streptococcus viridans*, is confusing and should be considered a slang term for α-hemolytic streptococci. There is no "viridans" species of streptococci.

Streptococci can produce a variety of exotoxins. Streptolysin S is a hemolysin produced by most members of groups A, C, and G and is responsible for the hemolysis on blood agar. It has cytolytic activity but unclear significance for disease production. Streptolysin O is produced by most group A and G strains and most human strains of group C. It is cardiotoxic.

The erythrogenic toxins, or pyrogenic exotoxins, are the most important streptococcal toxins. The vast majority of group A strains produce these toxins, as do lesser numbers of groups B and C. In addition to causing the characteristic sandpaper-like rash of scarlet fever, these toxins can also cause tissue damage, especially to liver and myocardium, fever, and shock in experimental animals. Streptococcal pyrogenic exotoxin A is suspected to be the major cause of symptoms in the newly rediscovered "toxic strep syndrome" (see next section).[9] Other streptococcal exoenzymes, such as DNases, hyaluronidase, streptokinase, and NADase, all have some role in tissue invasion and abscess formation but are probably better known as antigenic substances that may permit serologic diagnosis of streptococcal (especially *S. pyogenes*) infection.

Streptococcus pyogenes

Virtually all strains of *Streptococcus pyogenes* exhibit β-hemolysis and are group A. These strains are the typical etiologic agents in streptococcal pharyngitis, tonsillitis, cervical adenitis, poststreptococcal glomerulonephritis, and acute rheumatic fever and may occasionally cause more serious disease such as bacteremia, osteomyelitis, and meningitis. The skin is the usual portal of invasion for these latter complications. Of major note for critical care specialists is the toxic strep syndrome.

In the early years of this century, *S. pyogenes* appeared to cause a relatively virulent form of infection, with some individuals with scarlet fever–like illnesses progressing rapidly to sepsis, shock, and death. In later years, scarlet fever and other group A streptococcal infections tended to be relatively mild, except for those with the nonsuppurative complications of rheumatic fever or glomerulonephritis. Although group A streptococcal infections still are relatively mild in most circumstances, there appears to have been a re-emergence of the more fulminant form of infection, first noted in adults and then in children. Affected individuals are usually previously healthy patients who develop a septic shock picture, usually with renal failure, adult respiratory distress syndrome, and often positive result on blood cultures for group A streptococcus. Other foci of infection, such as cellulitis or necrotizing fasciitis, may be present. Of interest is that these individuals tend to have group A streptococcal isolates with characteristics typical of strains seen 50 years ago but uncommonly seen in recent decades. In particular, pyrogenic exotoxin A is common to both the current strains from patients with toxic strep syndrome and to isolates prevalent in the past but not to scarlet fever and other isolates from the past 30 years. Based on epidemiologic and animal data, it now appears that a more virulent form of group A streptococci has reappeared, and increasing numbers of these patients are being seen in critical care units.

Fortunately, group A streptococci are still sensitive to penicillin, which is the drug of choice. Erythromycin is an alternative, but resistance to this agent is being seen. Other antibiotics with gram-positive activity are also suitable treatment alternatives. For the toxic strep syndrome, supportive care and aggressive debridement of abscesses and necrotic tissue may be as important as specific antibiotic therapy.

Streptococcus agalactiae

In pediatrics, *Streptococcus agalactiae*, or group B streptococcus, is a common cause of serious infection in the newborn and the leading cause of nonnosocomial sepsis and meningitis in this age group. In non-neonatal cases, this pathogen generally causes disease only in unusual circumstances, such as advanced age, diabetes mellitus, and pregnancy.

Carbohydrate antigens are used to subdivide strains into types Ia, Ib, II, and III, with other serotypes (Ia/c, IV, V) also recognized as distinct types based on different antigens. In early-onset disease (under 7 days of age) without meningitis, all three main serotypes are relatively equally represented; in late-onset disease and in patients with meningitis, most strains are type III. Newborns acquire infection during labor and delivery from mothers colonized with group B streptococcus in the birth canal, and factors such as prematurity, prolonged rupture of membranes, chorioamnionitis, and other traditional neonatal sepsis risk factors predispose to group B streptococcal infection of the newborn.

Although all group B streptococci are inhibited by penicillin, a small percentage of strains may exhibit the phenomenon of tolerance. In these cases, the growth of organisms is inhibited by low concentrations of penicillin, but bacterial killing does not occur as would be expected with a bactericidal agent such as penicillin. Mechanistically, such strains are defined as having a minimal bactericidal concentration for penicillin that is at least 32-fold higher than the minimal inhibitory concentration. It is unclear whether tolerant strains of group B streptococcus are more difficult to manage with penicillin therapy, but there are numerous reports of treatment failures in patients with meningitis caused by these strains. Therefore, some authorities recommend use of a synergistic agent, such as an aminoglycoside, with penicillin for the entire course of therapy for meningitis due to tolerant group B streptococci. This recommendation is based on theoretic grounds and some experimental data but remains controversial.[10] If tolerance is considered to be important clinically, the physician usually must request that the bacteriology laboratory perform specific testing (minimal bactericidal concentration for penicillin), because the routine susceptibility testing methods will only provide information about minimal inhibitory concentrations.

Streptococcus pneumoniae

Streptococcus pneumoniae, or the pneumococcus, is one of the most common causes of bacteremia, pneumonia, soft tissue infection, and meningitis in children and occasionally gives rise to bone and joint infection. It is the leading bacterial cause of acute otitis media. Although it is a common inhabitant of the respiratory tract, it should virtually never be considered a laboratory contaminant when isolated from normally sterile body sites. Pneumococcal meningitis has a higher rate of hearing loss and other neurologic sequelae than any other common form of childhood meningitis except group B streptococcal disease in the newborn. The capsular polysaccharide of the organism is probably its main virulence factor. Unfortunately, there are at least 84 distinct capsular serotypes of pneumococcus, making progress on effective vaccines for young children quite slow.

Most pneumococci are susceptible to penicillin, but resistance has been seen frequently in other countries and is starting to appear in the United States. Two different forms of resistance are noteworthy. Some isolates have intermediate susceptibility to penicillin, requiring 0.1 to 1.0 μg/ml to inhibit growth. This group is termed relatively resistant to penicillin, and the clinical significance of these strains is unclear. However, analogous to the observations with tolerant group B streptococci, meningitis caused by relatively resistant pneumococci has been anecdotally observed to respond poorly to penicillin therapy. Based on these observations

and on animal data, most authorities would choose either a third-generation cephalosporin, vancomycin, or chloramphenicol for treatment of meningitis caused by these relatively resistant strains.

Less common in this country are strains truly resistant to penicillin with minimal inhibitory concentrations >1 μg/ml. These strains are often resistant to multiple antibiotics, particularly tetracycline and chloramphenicol.[11] Isolates are usually seen in travelers from countries with higher rates of penicillin resistance, such as Spain, but have been observed in individuals who have never left the United States. Infections with resistant pneumococci will not respond to penicillin and require alternative therapy based on sensitivity results.

Enterococcus faecalis

Until recently, *Enterococcus faecalis* was classified as part of the genus *Streptococcus*. It serogroups as group D and may display any type of hemolysis on blood agar. Although *E. faecalis* is part of the normal intestinal flora, enterococcal infections are becoming increasingly common, both nosocomially and in newborns and other compromised hosts.[12] Enterococci are particularly common causes of secondary infections in patients receiving long-term third-generation cephalosporins or other broad-spectrum antibiotics. Principal clinical syndromes include sepsis (especially catheter related), endocarditis, meningitis, and urinary tract infection, but *E. faecalis* is not an uncommon laboratory contaminant, making interpretation of culture results somewhat difficult at times.

Antimicrobial therapy for enterococcal disease has always been complex, and trends in susceptibility patterns reported in the United States promise to cause further therapeutic problems. [13-15] For the past 30 years, enterococci have been uniformly susceptible to penicillin and ampicillin. Occasionally, and virtually always in the case of enterococcal endocarditis, a synergistic combination of ampicillin and gentamicin has seemed necessary for effective treatment. This synergy could be observed even in strains that were not susceptible to gentamicin or other aminoglycosides. Now, however, this picture is changing. First, resistance to ampicillin, mediated by β-lactamase or other mechanisms, was observed and is now present in at least 10% of all isolates. Second, a different type of aminoglycoside resistance, termed high-level resistance and demonstrable with concentrations of more than 2,000 μg/ml of gentamicin, has appeared. For these strains, it appears that synergistic effects with ampicillin therapy do not occur. Vancomycin is being used increasingly for therapy of enterococcal disease due to the advent of these newer, more resistant strains.

Viridans streptococci

As mentioned earlier, "viridans" is used merely as a descriptor for nonpneumococcal strains of streptococci displaying α, or green, hemolysis on blood agar. However, some may display β- or γ-hemolysis, and not all authorities agree on naming systems, further confusing the nomenclature. Members of the group include *S. mitis*, *S. sanguis*, *S. bovis*, *S. anginosus*, and others. Most are normal inhabitants of the mouth and are frequent laboratory contaminants. However, they represent the most common cause of bacterial endocarditis. The production of extracellular dextran by many of these strains may facilitate adhesion to cardiac valvular surfaces. Some possess unusual nutritional properties, such as dependence on large concentrations of vitamin B$_6$, that may make isolation in culture more difficult. Most are fully sensitive to penicillin, but relative and even full resistance has been observed. Synergistic therapy with aminoglycosides is utilized on an individual basis. Good communication among clinicians and laboratory personnel is necessary for optimal diagnosis and treatment of streptococcal endocarditis, particularly when dealing with nutritionally variant or multiply resistant strains.

Gram-Positive Bacilli

Listeria

Listeria monocytogenes is a relatively uncommon cause of disease in the pediatric age group, affecting principally newborns.[16] As with group B streptococcal infection, both early- and late-onset forms are seen. Early-onset disease typically is found in low-birthweight infants born to mothers with obstetric complications who present with pneumonia or sepsis. Classically, brown-stained amniotic fluid, placental granulomata, and pustular skin lesions are seen with more severely affected infants. Late-onset disease is more likely to present with meningitis in a term infant with normal delivery, and these children have a better prognosis than those with early-onset disease. Older children may occasionally develop listeriosis, particularly if immunocompromised or after ingestion of contaminated dairy products.

A CSF examination in children with meningitis usually shows a relatively low blood cell count with few organisms. Diagnosis is most often made by blood or spinal fluid culture. It is not uncommon for the organisms to show variable Gram staining properties, and positive results on cultures are occasionally dismissed as contaminants because of their morphologic similarity to diphtheroids, which seldom cause disease. Ampicillin, with or without gentamicin for possible synergy, is recommended for therapy.

Gram-Negative Cocci

Neisseria Species

Neisseria meningitidis

Neisseria meningitidis, or meningococcus, is probably best recognized as a cause of purpura fulminans and rapidly progressive sepsis. It is a frequent cause of bacterial meningitis and an occasional cause of pneumonia, endophthalmitis, and other infections. Sero-

group B is the most common, followed by serogroup C and then serogroup A. Serogroups W-135, Y, and Z are less common and more likely to cause pneumonia than fulminant sepsis or meningitis. Individuals with congenital deficiencies of complement components, particularly the terminal components, are at high risk for disseminated meningococcal disease and represent 10% of cases of sporadic meningococcal infection. Therefore, it is recommended that all patients with meningococcal disease be tested for complement component deficiency.

Although mortality from meningococcal disease has improved with better efforts at supportive care, it remains close to 10% overall. Poor prognostic factors for survival include presence of petechiae for less than 12 hours prior to admission, hypotension, absence of meningitis, normal or low peripheral white blood cell count, and normal erythrocyte sedimentation rate. Meningococcal myocarditis or pericarditis may complicate the early course of infection, and late-onset "allergic" manifestations such as reactive arthritis or cutaneous vasculitis may be a cause of prolonged fever in these patients.

Virtually all isolates are sensitive to penicillin, which is the drug of choice. Newer reports of relative resistance to penicillin bear watching but do not warrant modification of current therapeutic recommendations.[17] Many laboratories do not perform penicillin susceptibility testing of meningococcal isolates.

Secondary attack rates in household contacts are higher than 10% for small infants, and all age groups are at risk. Secondary cases may present soon after the primary case, thus institution of prophylactic measures should be undertaken as soon as the diagnosis of meningococcal disease is strongly suspected, rather than waiting 1 or 2 days for confirmation by culture. Sulfonamides have been effective for prophylaxis in the past but can no longer be considered reliable because of high rates of sulfa-resistant strains. Rifampin is probably effective for prophylaxis of meningococcal disease. Prophylaxis is generally indicated only for close, prolonged contact with the index case, such as occurs in households and day care centers, but usually not for relatively brief contact in classrooms and emergency rooms. Vaccination may be indicated for epidemic situations.

Neisseria gonorrhoeae

Disseminated gonococcal disease occurs infrequently but is usually manifested by fever, polyarthritis, and rash. Most patients are not critically ill, although complement deficiency states can predispose to disseminated disease. Penicillin resistance due to penicillinase production in gonococci is a serious and widespread problem, and usually a third-generation cephalosporin is the initial drug of choice for suspected gonococcal disease.

Moraxella catarrhalis

Although usually not a cause of serious, life-threatening illness, *Moraxella catarrhalis* (previously termed *Branhamella catarrhalis*) is commonly seen in critical care settings as an isolate from the respiratory tract. It is a normal inhabitant of the respiratory tract but can frequently cause otitis media and upper and lower respiratory tract infections in both normal and compromised hosts. Cases of septicemia or pneumonia are occasionally reported. Short of lung biopsy, it is difficult to prove a diagnosis of *M. catarrhalis* pneumonia in an intubated patient, but Gram staining of tracheal secretions showing many inflammatory cells and a predominance of gram-negative diplococci in a compatible clinical setting are usually sufficient for institution of therapy. Most isolates produce β-lactamase and are resistant to penicillins but are susceptible to second-and third-generation cephalosporins.

Gram-Negative Bacilli

Enterobacteriaceae

Escherichia, Klebsiella, Enterobacter, and Proteus

In the normal host, these organisms are part of the normal flora of the gastrointestinal tract, and most frequently appear as pathogens in the genitourinary tract. In the immunocompromised host, these organisms are relatively common causes of sepsis, meningitis, pneumonia, and other invasive infections. These bacteria are early colonizers of the upper and lower respiratory tract in the intensive care unit, particularly with the use of broad-spectrum antibiotics in the intubated patient. Paranasal sinuses may also become colonized, particularly if nasogastric or other tubes are in place for prolonged periods. Nosocomial, multiply resistant strains may overgrow normal flora. The stress of serious illness also appears to alter normal host resistance to colonization with these organisms, as these bacteria and others appear to increase their affinity for binding to epithelial cells of the respiratory tract. Detection of the change from harmless commensal to invasive infecting agent is difficult and is usually made on the basis of relatively nonspecific clinical and laboratory data. Again, gram-stained material showing evidence of inflammation and a predominance of bacteria with uniform morphology is corroborative evidence of clinical disease in the appropriate setting. Still, a diagnosis of tracheitis or pneumonia is usually clinical, with culture results serving to guide antibiotic selection. Serial cultures may be less helpful in following the course of disease, since many patients remain colonized with the same "infecting" strain after a course of antibiotic therapy. Persistence of the organism in culture or tracheal secretions or other nonsterile environment should not dissuade one from stopping antibiotics if the clinical response is adequate.

Salmonella

Salmonella species are common causes of bacterial enteritis and relatively uncommon causes of serious disease. In the newborn period or in immunodeficient states (particularly hemoglobinopathies), sepsis, meningitis, osteomyelitis, and other syndromes may be seen. Organisms more likely to cause bacteremic complica-

tions include *S. typhi*, *S. paratyphi* A, B, and C, and *S. choleraesuis*. Identification of these organisms should heighten concern for complications of disease. The organism is usually found in stool but may be present only intermittently. Shedding of organisms in stool may persist for months in young infants and does not indicate a need for treatment. Most cases of enteritis do not require treatment, but *S. typhi* infections, all infections in immunocompromised hosts, and all metastatic infections should be treated. Ampicillin, chloramphenicol, and third-generation cephalosporins are all appropriate agents for *Salmonella* infections, with choice based on susceptibility testing of the isolate.

S. typhi, the etiologic agent of typhoid fever, is the prototype for all gram-negative bacilli causing intracellular infections, which include other *Salmonella* species, *Brucella* species, *Francisella tularensis*, and *Yersinia* species. Gram-negative intracellular organisms can be considered as infections of the reticuloendothelial system. These organisms are able to survive and even replicate in monocytes, which provides them with a barrier to normal host defenses. All of these infections have bacteremic phases, and seeding of other organ systems can occur. With most *Salmonella* species, the bacteremia is transient and the reticuloendothelial system is able to clear the infection without therapy. With the more virulent organisms, such as *S. typhi*, or in compromised hosts, complications may develop.

Most patients with *S. typhi* infection acquired their infection either outside the United States or from individuals who acquired the disease in countries where this infection is endemic. Most do not have diarrhea, but present rather with fever and nonspecific complaints. Hepatosplenomegaly is common. At this time, organisms can usually be demonstrated in blood but are less commonly seen in stool, bone marrow, or urine. Complications can occur in untreated patients beginning by about the third week of illness, with intestinal ulceration, hemorrhage, and perforation the most feared manifestations. By this time, the results of blood, stool, and bone marrow cultures are usually positive, and the organism can occasionally (25%) be found in the urine. Manifestations of infection in other organ systems usually appear later, and almost any organ system can be involved. Stool cultures slowly become negative, with only about 10% positivity by 3 months following infection. Relapses occur in 10 to 20% of cases; there is controversy about relative frequencies of relapse with various antibiotic regimens, but no one regimen is clearly superior to another if the isolate is susceptible.

Shigella

Shigellosis is rarely associated with illness severe enough to require intensive care services, but one aspect of the disease deserves mention. Strains of *Shigella dysenteriae* produce an exotoxin with neurotoxic properties, and this may well be responsible for the clinical observation that many children with shigellosis develop altered mental status and seizures as an early presentation of their illness, sometimes preceding the gastrointestinal manifestations. This phenomenon also occurs with other *Shigella* infections but is generally not seen after 7 years of age. In the absence of diarrhea, some of these patients are thought to have viral encephalitis or other serious infections of the central nervous system. However, children with *Shigella* neurotoxicity usually improve rapidly with no long-term neurologic sequelae. It should also be remembered that hemolytic-uremic syndrome can follow shigellosis, as well as other bacterial diarrheas.

Pseudomonas and Xanthomonas

Pseudomonas aeruginosa

Pseudomonas aeruginosa is a ubiquitous organism found in a variety of ecologic settings, including the human gastrointestinal and respiratory tracts. It is relatively tolerant of variations in temperature and humidity and is therefore frequently isolated from nosocomial settings. Like the Enterobacteriaceae, it is an opportunist in most clinical settings, and the most serious morbidity is seen with pneumonia, sepsis, and occasionally meningitis or endophthalmitis in immunocompromised individuals such as burn patients and patients with neutropenia. It is well known as a primary pulmonary pathogen in cystic fibrosis, in which it causes a more indolent type of disease and virtually never disseminates beyond the respiratory tract. Urinary tract infections are relatively common in patients with long-term indwelling urinary catheters.

Treatment of *Pseudomonas* infections should reflect the ability of these organisms to develop resistance to therapy, particularly to β-lactam agents. Therefore, single drug therapy with ticarcillin, piperacillin, or similar agents is likely to be unsuccessful, and a second drug, such as an aminoglycoside, is used in combination to prevent development of resistance. Cystitis accompanying bladder catheterization can usually be treated merely by removing the catheter.

Pseudomonas cepacia and Xanthomonas maltophilia

Pseudomonas cepacia and *Xanthomonas* (formerly *Pseudomonas*) *maltophilia* are not commonly seen except in patients with cystic fibrosis. They tend to be multiply drug resistant and appear primarily as nosocomial pathogens. Clinical presentation is not distinguished from that of other bacterial infections.

Haemophilus influenzae

H. influenzae type b is the leading cause of bacterial meningitis in all ages, even though it seldom occurs after 4 years of age. The type b capsule appears to be the primary determinant of virulence, and animal data suggest less virulent properties for types a, c, d, e, and f as well as for nontypable strains. Nontypable strains rarely cause systemic disease but are a relatively common cause of otitis media. Other common manifestations of *H. influenzae* type b infection include sepsis, arthritis, epiglottitis, and pneumonia. Fulminant sepsis

similar to meningococcal disease may be seen. Recent approval and licensing of vaccines effective in prevention of *H. influenzae* type b infection in infants may dramatically change the epidemiology of this disease.

Antimicrobial therapy must take into account susceptibility testing. Approximately one third of *H. influenzae* type b strains produce β-lactamase and are resistant to ampicillin, the drug of choice for susceptible strains. A small number of strains are resistant to ampicillin by mechanisms other than β-lactamase production, and therefore a negative β-lactamase result should never be considered proof that the isolate is susceptible to ampicillin. For ampicillin-resistant strains, or for initial empiric therapy, third-generation cephalosporins are indicated in meningitis. Those agents or cefuroxime can be used for treatment of infection outside the central nervous system.

Rifampin prophylaxis for close contacts under the age of 4 years is recommended for prevention of secondary cases. Vaccination has no role in the prevention of disease acutely.

Legionella

The genus *Legionella* includes over 20 species of bacteria, but most clinical disease has been caused by *L. pneumophila*.

Legionella pneumophila

L. pneumophila is the cause of legionnaires' disease, named after the epidemic at an American Legion convention in Philadelphia in 1976. Since that time, much has been learned about the clinical syndromes produced by this organism. *L. pneumophila* is often found in moist environments, and outbreaks have been linked to contaminated water in air conditioning units and similar sources. The organism is probably acquired by aerosol inhalation, with subsequent production of disease in the upper and lower respiratory tracts. Other organ systems are rarely infected.

In the pediatric population, *L. pneumophila* is probably a rare cause of disease in otherwise healthy children, even though serosurveys have shown that antibody to this organism is relatively common in children. Most pediatric cases have occurred in immunocompromised patients, with fever, severe pneumonia with rapid progression, diarrhea, and headache being relatively common.[18] Neurologic abnormalities such as seizures have been noted.

Diagnosis is best made by growth of the organism from tracheal secretions, lung tissue, or other appropriate specimens. Specific processing and media are required, therefore the laboratory must be notified. Diagnosis can also be made by immunofluorescent microscopy of suitable specimens but requires experienced laboratory personnel for best results. The diagnosis can also be made retrospectively by acute and convalescent serology. Erythromycin is the drug of choice, and rifampin is often added for severe cases of the disease.

Legionella micdadei

Legionella micdadei, the Pittsburgh pneumonia agent, is known primarily for causing pneumonia in renal transplant recipients and other immunocompromised hosts. Clinical disease is not distinguishable from that caused by *L. pneumophila*, and diagnosis is again made by culture and specific immunofluorescence. Treatment with erythromycin with or without rifampin is recommended.

Anaerobic Bacteria

Suppurative Anaerobic Infections

Anaerobic bacteria outnumber aerobic bacteria as normal flora in humans and are frequently found in nature as well. Therefore, it is not surprising that anaerobic infections arise either endogenously, from spillage or overgrowth of intestinal, vaginal, or upper respiratory anaerobes, or exogenously from traumatic injuries, which may be contaminated by soil or animal or human bites. Anaerobic infections should be considered in any situation in which infection involves sites containing anaerobic bacteria as normal flora or in which signs of infection include a putrid odor, gas formation in tissues, or tissue necrosis. Abscess formation is also quite common. Table 72–1 lists common anaerobic bacteria causing disease in humans.

Serious anaerobic infections in children most commonly involve the oropharynx and the abdomen. Retropharyngeal or peritonsillar abscesses usually contain multiple anaerobic bacteria as primary pathogens. Brain abscesses secondary to sinusitis also frequently involve anaerobic bacteria. A ruptured abdominal viscus, most commonly due to appendicitis in children, may result in the formation of intra-abdominal abscesses with mixed aerobic and anaerobic bacteria. Animal models of ruptured abdominal visci suggest a biphasic process, by which aerobic bacteria are responsible for the early

Table 72–1. ANAEROBIC BACTERIA COMMONLY CAUSING DISEASE

Gram-Positive Nonsporulating Bacilli
  *Propionibacterium acnes**
  Eubacterium lentum
  Actinomyces species

Gram-Positive Cocci
  Peptostreptococcus species
  Peptococcus species

Gram-Negative Cocci
  Veillonella species

Gram-Positive Sporulating Bacilli
  Clostridium species

Gram-Negative Bacilli
  Bacteroides fragilis group (e.g., *B. fragilis*, *B. thetaiotamicron*, *B. distasonis*)
  Bacteroides melaninogenicus group
  Other *Bacteroides* species
  Fusobacterium necrophorium
  Fusobacterium nucleatum

*Also a common laboratory contaminant.

sepsis and mortality, while anaerobes are more prominently involved in late abscess formation. This is also seen clinically in humans. Septicemia commonly occurs in these situations, although aerobic organisms such as *E. coli* are more likely to be isolated from blood culture than any of the anaerobic bacteria present in the peritoneal space. Culture of the abscess material usually yields multiple aerobic and anaerobic bacteria.

Diagnosis of anaerobic infections requires a high index of suspicion based on the mode of presentation of illness as well as careful collection of specimens to support growth of anaerobic bacteria. Fortunately, most pathogenic anaerobes are tolerant of small amounts of oxygen and may even survive hours to days while exposed to oxygen. For optimal culture results, however, specimens from body fluid or abscesses should be collected with as little exposure to oxygen as possible and placed in an anaerobic transport container with prereduced media and taken for laboratory processing quickly.

Many antibiotics have some activity against anaerobes, but only a few can be considered adequate for treatment of anaerobic infections. Many isolates remain susceptible to penicillin and ampicillin, and most simple oropharyngeal infections, such as peritonsillar or retropharyngeal abscesses, can be treated with penicillin in combination with surgical drainage. Clinical success is usually seen even when some isolates are resistant to penicillin, such as with β-lactamase–producing *Bacteroides* species. For more serious anaerobic infections, such as anaerobic bacteremia, and for all intra-abdominal anaerobic infections, antibiotics active against these penicillin-resistant strains should be used. The combination of a β-lactam agent and a β-lactamase inhibitor, such as ticarcillin/clavulanic acid, is an alternative that can provide anaerobic, staphylococcal, *Pasteurella multocida*, and *Eikenella corrodens* coverage. Clindamycin (with other antibiotics active against gram-negative enteric organisms) and cefoxitin have been used frequently for intra-abdominal infections, but many centers are now reporting increasing resistance (approximately 10 to 20% of *B. fragilis* strains showing resistance) of anaerobes to these agents, and it appears that these drugs may eventually lose their utility in some situations. Metronidazole (for most anaerobes except *Propionibacterium* species) and chloramphenicol remain excellent drugs for use in the more serious anaerobic infections such as brain abscess, and imipenem-cilastatin also has activity against most anaerobes.

Clostridial Intoxication

Some clostridial species produce disease by elaboration of specific toxins. Although most of these clinical syndromes are relatively rare in the United States, individual cases may come to the attention of critical care practitioners and are easily misdiagnosed because nonspecific symptoms and laboratory findings may delay consideration of the diagnosis.

Clostridium botulinum

Clostridium botulinum produces at least seven toxins, of which three commonly produce disease in humans.

Infant botulism, the most common form of disease, is acquired primarily by ingestion of spores of *C. botulinum*, which then germinate in the intestinal tract and produce toxin. Rarely, this form is seen in adults. Constipation is often the first sign of disease, followed by slow progression to hypotonia, flaccid paresis of the extremities, and cranial nerve paresis over a few weeks. Respiratory arrest may occur. Supportive care is the primary form of therapy. Antitoxin is not helpful, probably due to the very small amounts of toxin elaborated, and the use of antibiotic therapy is controversial because of the theoretic possibility of releasing more toxin as bacteria in the gut are lysed.

Food-borne botulism usually follows ingestion of contaminated, commonly home-processed, foods. Onset is sudden, within hours of ingestion, and consists of paresis of extremities and cranial nerves. Gastrointestinal manifestations occur in fewer than half of cases. The clinical picture of wound botulism is similar to that in food-borne illness, but sensory changes may be seen near the site of the wound. Antitoxin is indicated for both of these forms of botulism, and surgical wound debridement and penicillin are used for wound botulism. Unfortunately, the antitoxin is of equine origin and may cause serum sickness or anaphylaxis.

Clostridium difficile

Clostridium difficile colitis is not rare in the setting of the intensive care unit, where patients frequently receive multiple antibiotic courses. Diagnosis usually is made by demonstration of the organism and the toxin in fecal samples from individuals with hemorrhagic colitis. Sigmoidoscopy may be helpful if the typical pseudomembranes are present. Asymptomatic carriage of the organisms and toxin is not uncommon, however, particularly in the newborn period. Also, some commercially available toxin assays lack specificity. Therefore, one should approach positive laboratory findings for *C. difficile* disease with some skepticism. Treatment consists of discontinuing prior antibiotics, if possible, and instituting oral vancomycin or metronidazole therapy.

Clostridium diphtheriae

Diphtheria is rarely seen in the United States. In nonimmune individuals, acquisition of the organism through the upper airway may be followed by tissue necrosis and formation of the characteristic white or gray adherent membrane, which is seen most commonly in the nose, tonsils, nasopharynx, and larynx, but may be found in other body sites as well. If the organism elaborates toxin, myocarditis and cranial nerve paresis and other neurologic abnormalities can develop. Occasionally, the membrane itself may occlude the airway, causing respiratory arrest.

Diagnosis depends on clinical findings with eventual isolation of the organism from the infected site. Penicillin and antitoxin are mainstays of treatment.

Clostridium perfringens

Clostridium perfringens, as well as other species of clostridia, may produce clostridial myonecrosis, or gas gangrene, when present in skin and subcutaneous tissues. α-Toxin, probably in combination with several other toxins produced by the organism, is primarily responsible for the rapidly progressive cellulitis that characteristically shows hemorrhagic bullae, tissue necrosis, and crepitus. Milder forms of cellulitis and necrotizing fasciitis may be seen. Both myonecrosis and necrotizing fasciitis require extensive surgical debridement as well as appropriate antibiotic therapy.

C. perfringens also produces a relatively mild form of food poisoning, which is commonly associated with meat ingestion and typically lasts 24 hours or less. A more uncommon form of necrotizing enteritis can also occur.

Clostridium tetani

Clostridium tetani is the etiologic agent of tetanus, and clinical manifestations are due to actions of the toxin tetanospasmin. The organism is usually introduced via trauma. Clinical disease in nonimmune individuals usually develops within 3 weeks, but longer incubation periods have been noted.

At present, minor wounds more commonly result in tetanus, probably because major wounds are more likely to come to medical attention and receive proper care and tetanus prophylaxis. Tetanospasmin acts on several areas of the peripheral and central nervous system to produce a distinctive clinical syndrome. Localized tetanus consists of painful muscular rigidity and spasms near the site of trauma. Generalized disease usually does not develop in this form, presumably because of some small amounts of antitoxin present, and recovery generally occurs over several weeks. Generalized tetanus, the more familiar form of disease, usually presents with trismus, followed by spasms and rigidity of multiple muscle groups. Risus sardonicus, the "smile" due to facial muscle involvement, and opisthotonic-like posture are seen. Fits of spasms may be precipitated by relatively minor noises or by touching the patient lightly. Fractures due to intense muscle activity can occur, and fever is common.

The diagnosis of tetanus can generally be suspected on the basis of the history and physical examination. The organism can occasionally be grown from wound exudate or tissue, but negative culture results should not preclude the diagnosis.

Treatment of all forms of tetanus consists of antitoxin administration, wound debridement, penicillin therapy, and, most important, supportive care. Many of these patients require intubation for airway protection, and sedatives, muscle relaxants, or even neuromuscular blocking agents are often necessary. Prevention is readily available via routine immunization and appropriate management of injuries with the use of vaccine or tetanus immune globulin as indicated.

Spirochete Infections

Lyme Disease

Borrelia burgdorferi is the etiologic agent of Lyme disease, which is most likely to come to the attention of intensivists due to its cardiac and central nervous system manifestations.[19] The organism is acquired from the bite of tick vectors. Although classically a disease occurring in Connecticut and Europe, clusters of cases in the United States have occurred along the mid and upper Atlantic coasts, the upper Midwest, and the western states. Early disease consists mainly of erythema chronicum migrans, and most serious complications occur within several weeks of the bite. Neurologic findings include meningitis, facial and other cranial nerve palsy, and transverse myelitis. Carditis usually manifests as myocarditis with conduction abnormalities, particularly atrioventricular block.

A history of tick bite in an endemic area followed by erythema chronicum migrans is helpful in making the diagnosis, as is a history of arthritis. Although the organism can be cultured under special conditions, diagnosis usually rests on a compatible clinical history and serologic evidence of disease. Unfortunately, the sensitivity and specificity of current serologic assays are suboptimal, and clinical findings should outweigh serologic testing in making the diagnosis of Lyme disease. Treatment of milder cardiac and nervous system findings may be accomplished with oral tetracycline or amoxicillin, but more serious disease should be treated parenterally with ceftriaxone or penicillin G.

Syphilis

Syphilis, caused by *Treponema pallidum*, has its most serious manifestations in the neonate, who may present with severe anemia, nonimmune hydrops fetalis, or nephrotic syndrome. Fetal infection may occur at any time during pregnancy and is more likely to happen early in maternal infection. Most infants have a positive serologic test for syphilis, unless infection occurred just prior to delivery. Specific antibody treponemal tests are used to verify the diagnosis, but unfortunately the currently available IgM tests for syphilis are unreliable in diagnosing congenital syphilis. Thus, IgG antibody tests are used with the knowledge that a positive result on a test may represent only passively acquired maternal antibody. Treatment is with penicillin G. The details of management of congenital syphilis are beyond the scope of this chapter but are readily available from other sources.[20]

Leptospirosis

Leptospirosis can be caused by many different species of *Leptospira*. The organisms are usually acquired from animals; in the United States, transmission from rodents to dogs may play a prominent role in transmission of disease to humans who come in contact with urine or blood from infected animals. If the organism penetrates mucous membranes or skin, infection results. The more serious form of leptospirosis is the icteric form, also known as Weil syndrome. In this form, a severe systemic vasculitis occurs that can result in clinical disease involving virtually any organ system. Classically, after an incubation period of 1 to 2 weeks, illness presents with fever for several days. There may be a brief period of quiescence followed by the second stage of illness, characterized by hepatitis with severe icterus, myocarditis, meningoencephalitis, renal failure, and hemorrhagic diathesis due to hypoprothrombinemia. Occasionally, the biphasic nature of the disease is not distinct. Mortality approaches 10% in the more severe form of the disease. Diagnosis is usually made serologically, and treatment is with penicillin or tetracycline in addition to supportive care.

Mycobacterial Disease

Tuberculosis

Tuberculosis, caused by *Mycobacterium tuberculosis*, is relatively common in the United States, particularly in major metropolitan areas. Disease usually occurs by respiratory transmission from adults with active pulmonary tuberculosis. Children with pulmonary tuberculosis are seldom contagious. Congenital infection occurs via placental infection. Following infection, lymphohematogenous dissemination occurs. Active disease may develop at that time, or latent infection may be established with disease presenting years later upon reactivation. The manifestations of tuberculosis are truly protean, but this discussion is limited to forms that are acutely life-threatening.

Tuberculous meningitis usually develops indolently over a period of a few weeks with symptoms of fever, anorexia, irritability, headache, and perhaps personality change (see also Chapter 20). This may progress to drowsiness, vomiting, cranial nerve palsies, and other signs of elevated intracranial pressure. Symptoms of meningeal irritation are usually not obtained by history. Tuberculous meningitis has a striking tendency to produce an intense basilar meningeal inflammation with subsequent interference with CSF flow, resulting in spinal block and hydrocephalus. This latter complication can develop relatively quickly and cause sudden deterioration and coma.

Use of contrast-enhanced cranial imaging may reveal the basilar exudate and inflammation and suggest the diagnosis. CSF examination usually shows a predominance of lymphocytes with a total cell count of less than 1,000, with depressed glucose and elevated protein. Very high protein levels are seen with spinal block. Tubercle bacilli are rare in CSF and are difficult to detect. Diagnosis is often made empirically, and questioning or examining family members for evidence of active disease such as pulmonary cavitary lesions may be helpful.

Tuberculous pericarditis and pleurisy can cause cardiorespiratory compromise due to the size of the effusions, which are characteristically lymphocytic and seldom reveal tubercle bacilli. Pleural or pericardial biopsy usually reveals typical caseating granulomas with visible acid-fast organisms. The effusions are considered to represent hypersensitivity reactions to organisms in tissue. Rarely, mediastinal adenopathy may be so large that superior vena caval syndrome or atelectasis may result.

Miliary tuberculosis is rare and can be difficult to diagnose. Some patients may be relatively asymptomatic, with diagnosis being made coincidentally by chest radiography. However, other patients may develop an indolent but downhill course and may even present with symptoms more suggestive of septic shock.

All of these entities may be indications for treatment with systemic corticosteroids, which are thought to decrease inflammation and may be lifesaving acutely. However, the role of steroid therapy has never been systematically analyzed. Above all, it should be noted that corticosteroids do not suppress the growth of mycobacteria and in fact may facilitate growth in the host. Therefore, this form of therapy should not be used without accompanying antituberculous therapy.

Treatment of active tuberculosis requires a minimum of two drugs because of the ability of drug-resistant subpopulations to develop when single drug therapy is used.[21] Drug resistance, primarily to isoniazid, is becoming more common around the world, so often three drugs are begun initially until susceptibility testing is performed. Also, more rapid elimination of bacilli may be accomplished with the use of multiple drugs with different mechanisms of activity against tuberculosis. In seriously ill individuals, such as those with tuberculous meningitis, a four-drug regimen is usually started, with at least one of the drugs given parenterally.

Isoniazid and rifampin are the mainstays of therapy, and pyrazinamide is commonly used as the third drug in pediatric cases. Streptomycin is still used for tuberculous meningitis. Usually two-drug therapy can be used after the first 2 months of treatment if susceptibility results are available. Total duration of therapy is 6 to 12 months, depending on the severity of disease and the dosage regimen being used.

Atypical Mycobacterial Disease

Disease due to mycobacteria other than tuberculosis is common and principally manifests as cervical adenitis that does not respond to common oral antibiotic therapy. However, some mycobacteria, particularly *M. avium-intracellulare* (MAI), are well known for causing disseminated disease in patients with the acquired immunodeficiency syndrome (AIDS) or other immunodeficiencies. In patients with AIDS, MAI most commonly causes prolonged fever and debilitation but is seldom a primary cause of death.

Diagnosis of disseminated MAI is usually made by blood culture: Mycobacterial culture should be specifically requested. Unfortunately, treatment is complex, requiring multiple drug therapy, and is seldom curative. Usually, however, one can see clinical improvement on therapy, and some authorities recommend attempting treatment.[22] Duration of therapy is indefinite, although drug side effects are usually limiting factors. Future

trials of combination drug regimens may result in a more effective, less toxic regimen for these individuals.

VIRUSES

DNA Viruses

Herpesviruses

Herpes Simplex Virus

Herpes simplex virus (HSV) is an extremely common viral infection that is most often seen clinically as gingivostomatitis (usually due to serotype 1) or as genital lesions (usually caused by type 2). Like other herpesviruses, HSV remains in a latent state after primary infection and may become reactivated in response to a variety of stressful or nonspecific stimuli. This is a particularly important point for HSV disease, because severe illness can often be the stressful event causing reactivation, and it is not uncommon for critically ill individuals to have HSV isolated from respiratory secretions. This finding is usually a sign of harmless reactivation rather than a true indication of HSV pneumonia or other illness.

HSV is most likely to cause serious illness in newborns with disseminated disease and in older children with HSV encephalitis. In the newborn period, disease may be limited to the skin, eyes, or mouth; may primarily involve the central nervous system; or may cause disseminated disease. In infants who do not present with skin lesions, diagnosis may be difficult because clinical findings are nonspecific and there may be no history of maternal genital lesions. Occasionally, postnatal transmission from family members with "fever blisters" has caused disease in the newborn, and this history should be sought. Severe pneumonia without obvious bacterial cause, and hepatitis with disseminated intravascular coagulation are clinical clues that one may be dealing with a severe viral rather than a bacterial illness in the newborn. Early use of viral cultures of mucous membranes and cutaneous surfaces can be helpful in diagnosis of neonatal HSV infection. Examination of epithelial cells from skin lesions by immunofluorescent techniques is quite helpful. HSV tends to grow rapidly in culture, with positive results evident within 24 to 48 hours in many cases.

Beyond the newborn period, meningoencephalitis is the most common serious manifestation of HSV infection, although forms of disseminated disease may occur also (see Chapter 20). Fever, focal seizures or neurologic deficits, and increased numbers of both red and white blood cells in the CSF are more common in HSV encephalitis than in other encephalitides, but differentiation is often difficult. Brain biopsy may be helpful in selected cases to rule out other treatable diseases and is mandatory in the immunocompromised patient with encephalitis, in whom these other treatable conditions are more likely to be present.

Treatment of serious HSV disease in the newborn can be accomplished with either vidarabine or acyclovir, although most authorities prefer acyclovir because of its ease of administration[23] and less frequent hematologic side effects. Acyclovir has been shown to be superior to vidarabine in the treatment of adult HSV encephalitis and is the preferred agent in older children and adults.

Cytomegalovirus

Cytomegalovirus (CMV) can cause severe disease in its congenital form, in which multiple organ system involvement can result in serious morbidity and mortality. In its most severe form, infants are small for gestational age, with chorioretinitis, intracranial calcifications and developmental delay, mild hepatitis, and hemolysis, among other findings. Although similar clinical manifestations and organ system involvement can be seen in older children who acquire CMV infection postnatally, it is most commonly a mild disease, producing few or no symptoms. In the immunocompromised host, however, CMV is often a life-threatening illness, and for that reason it is briefly mentioned here.

Transplant recipients are probably the group at greatest risk for development of severe CMV disease, particularly if seronegative for CMV prior to transplantation. Although a mild, mononucleosis-like syndrome similar to that in immunocompetent hosts may be seen, more serious disease with pneumonitis, leukopenia and thrombocytopenia, colitis, hepatitis, chorioretinitis, and meningoencephalitis can occur. Some patients have a rapid progression of disease with multisystem organ failure and death. Diagnosis is usually made from seroconversion and documentation of viremia or shedding of virus in saliva or urine. Some success in treating CMV disease in transplant patients has been achieved with a combination of ganciclovir and intravenous immunoglobulin.

Patients with AIDS represent the other immunocompromised group at high risk for complications from CMV disease, which most commonly manifest as a progressive chorioretinitis. Ganciclovir has been somewhat successful in preventing progression, but its long-term use is limited by side effects. The role of other antiviral agents and of immunoglobulin therapy is under investigation.

Epstein-Barr Virus

Epstein-Barr virus (EBV) infection typically produces a mild respiratory infection or mononucleosis-type syndrome. It is primarily an infection of the B cell and therefore is usually accompanied by a mild, transient deficiency in humoral antibody production. It is occasionally associated with unusual bacteremias, particularly if there is severe pharyngitis that may allow bloodstream invasion by mouth flora. The more severe manifestations of EBV infection include meningoencephalitis, aplastic anemia and other blood dyscrasias, hepatitis, and other organ system infection. Transplant patients and those with X-linked lymphoproliferative (Duncan) syndrome or severe combined or other serious T cell deficiencies are at risk for EBV-induced lymphoproliferative disorders. Diagnosis usually is made serologically and by detecting EBV nucleic acid sequences in tumor tissue. There is no known specific antiviral treatment for EBV disease, but ganciclovir does have

some EBV activity and may eventually prove beneficial in selected situations, including transplant patients who show evidence of recent EBV seroconversion.

Varicella Zoster Virus

Varicella zoster virus (VZV) produces chickenpox during primary infection and zoster in typical reactivation disease. In the normal host, these manifestations are usually not serious and are well tolerated; however, involvement of other organ systems occasionally occurs. Of principal importance to the intensivist is varicella encephalitis, which is usually quite easy to diagnose when it occurs with or soon after an episode of chickenpox. Rarely, encephalitis may be the presenting sign of varicella infection, with the rash appearing some days later. Varicella encephalitis occurring during active varicella infection probably represents viral invasion of the central nervous system, although the virus has been documented at this site only rarely. The encephalitis is usually generalized and is clinically indistinguishable from other viral encephalitides. Most postvaricella encephalitis is probably immune mediated, with cerebellar ataxia being the principal feature. Acyclovir treatment may be beneficial in the generalized form of varicella encephalitis, but no prospective randomized studies address this issue.

Varicella in the immunocompromised patient is likely to disseminate, causing nervous system, hepatic, and other organ system dysfunction, and mortality is high (20%) in these situations. Newborns lacking antibody to VZV (i.e., born at less than 28 weeks' gestation or to mothers who lack antibody) are also at high risk, principally when exposed within the first 2 days of life. Therapy with acyclovir at the onset of symptoms has improved outcome in disseminated varicella, and prophylaxis with varicella-zoster immune globulin within 96 hours of exposure to varicella can modify or prevent illness in this group. An effective VZV vaccine may be released soon.

Adenoviruses

The adenoviral group consists of a large number of DNA viruses of at least 41 serotypes. A wide variety of diseases are produced by this group of viruses, including both respiratory and enteric disease. Encephalitis, bronchiolitis obliterans, and myocarditis are rare but serious manifestations of adenoviral infection. Severe hepatitis and other organ system disease can occur in immunocompromised hosts. Diagnosis is usually made by culture, but electron microscopic examination of tracheal secretions has been beneficial in severe pneumonia. No specific antiviral therapy is available.

Hepatitis B Virus

Hepatitis B disease generally follows sexual or blood exposure to individuals carrying the hepatitis B antigen. Hepatitis B virus deserves special mention for two reasons. First, hepatitis due to hepatitis B is associated with a high rate of complications: 1% of those infected experience a fulminant course with hepatic necrosis, up to 10% develop chronic hepatitis, and 10% (up to 80% of those infected in the perinatal period) become chronic carriers with increased risk for hepatocellular carcinoma in later life. Hepatitis D infection can occur in individuals with hepatitis B surface antigen and cause progressive hepatic disease. Second, hepatitis B infection can produce atypical syndromes not generally recognized as being caused by this virus. Neurologic diseases such as Guillain-Barré syndrome or encephalitis, aplastic anemia, membranous glomerulonephritis, and a serum sickness–like illness due to immune complexes have all been observed. Diagnosis of hepatitis B infection is made serologically; current infection is best typified by the presence of hepatitis B surface antigen and IgM antibody to hepatitis B core antigen. Antibody to hepatitis B surface antigen appears within 1 to 2 months following clinical hepatitis in most cases and signifies clearance of surface antigen. A "window" period may occur between the time that surface antigen has decreased to undetectable levels but surface antibody has not yet appeared. Antibody to the core antigen is present during this period and can establish the diagnosis in the absence of positive results for surface antibody and antigen. IgG antibody to the hepatitis B core antigen may also be positive in cases of non-A, non-B hepatitis, including hepatitis C infection. No specific treatment for acute hepatitis B is available.

Human Parvovirus B19

B19 is the cause of erythema infectiosum (fifth disease), a common childhood disease. It can also cause acute illness with rash and arthropathy in older individuals and stillbirth after infection during pregnancy. Increasingly, it is being noted as a cause of aplastic crisis in patients with chronic hemolytic anemias, such as sickle cell disease, and in patients with AIDS. These patients appear capable of transmitting the disease for prolonged periods and require respiratory isolation. Diagnosis is made serologically. Intravenous immunoglobulin therapy appeared to be beneficial in at least one case.[24]

RNA Viruses

Arboviral Encephalitides

Arboviruses causing central nervous system infection are numerous, and the epidemiology of these diseases varies dramatically with geographic site (see also Chapter 20). Many occur in the United States but usually infrequently, and children are most often affected. Epidemics are common. Unfortunately, no specific treatment is available for any of these infections, but it is still important for clinicians to be aware of their principal features, however, because the differential diagnosis often includes treatable infections, such as bacterial meningitis and herpes simplex encephalitis. Also, early identification of cases may help to abort epidemics.

Table 72–2 lists the arboviral encephalitides that occur

Table 72–2. FEATURES OF COMMON ARBOVIRAL ENCEPHALITIDES IN THE UNITED STATES

Encephalitide	Vector	Geographic Site
St. Louis encephalitis	Mosquito	Entire U.S.
California encephalitis	Mosquito	Western U.S.
Western equine encephalitis	Mosquito	Western U.S.
Eastern equine encephalitis	Mosquito	Eastern U.S.
La Crosse encephalitis	Mosquito	Midwest and eastern U.S.
Powassan encephalitis	Tick	Northeastern U.S., Colorado
Venezuelan equine encephalitis	Mosquito or aerosol	Southern U.S., (especially Florida)

in the United States. The most common infections, St. Louis, California, western equine, and eastern equine encephalitis, account for most cases of arbovirus encephalitis. Illness peaks in summer months, when vectors are active. Clinical presentation is similar for all of the infections, with signs and symptoms usually including fever and ranging from headache and malaise to aseptic meningitis, meningoencephalitis, and encephalitis. It is usually not possible to distinguish one from the other on purely clinical grounds, although in general eastern equine encephalitis has the highest morbidity and mortality (50 to 70%) and CSF findings are more likely to mimic those of bacterial meningitis with high cell counts and a predominance of polymorphonuclear leukocytes. La Crosse encephalitis occurs almost exclusively in children.

Diagnosis is made serologically, and most laboratories offering arboviral serology will perform a panel of antibody testing for the most common arboviral infections. The reliance on serodiagnosis implies a retrospective diagnosis, but in some cases serum antibody is seen as early as 1 week after onset of illness.

Ortho- and Paramyxoviruses

Influenza Viruses

Influenza viruses A, B, and sometimes C are causes of febrile winter upper and lower respiratory diseases with varying degrees of myositis. Considerable morbidity occurs, and mortality is not uncommon in immunocompromised and debilitated individuals. Influenza infections most likely to come to the attention of intensivists include cases of severe pneumonia with respiratory failure and such complications as encephalitis, Guillain-Barré syndrome, myocarditis, myositis with rhabdomyolysis and renal failure, and bacterial superinfection, including necrotizing pneumonitis and toxic shock syndrome. Bacterial superinfection usually follows influenza infection, and a history of a biphasic illness with improvement after a flu-like illness followed by reappearance of fever and other symptoms is a common sequence for this complication.

Diagnosis is made by viral culture or by immunofluorescent microscopy of respiratory secretions. Amantadine is useful for prophylaxis and treatment of influenza A infections but has no significant activity against influenza B virus. Vaccine for high-risk individuals is effective but must be given yearly. Intensivists and other individuals commonly caring for high-risk patients should also be vaccinated to protect these patients.

Parainfluenza Viruses

Parainfluenza virus disease, due primarily to parainfluenza viruses types 1, 2, and 3, usually comes to the attention of the critical care specialist as viral croup. Parainfluenza type 1 is the most common of the three to cause croup. These viruses are also responsible for a number of other respiratory syndromes, including bronchiolitis, pneumonia, and mild upper respiratory infections. Epidemics are usually seen in the fall and spring, although these viruses are present to some degree at all times of the year. Disseminated disease is rare, even in immunocompromised individuals. No specific antiviral therapy is available.

Mumps Virus

Mumps, primarily a cause of parotitis, is seldom serious enough to come to the attention of the intensivist. The illness may often go unrecognized, yet central nervous system involvement is actually quite frequent, with CSF pleocytosis occurring in up to 50% of individuals. The meningoencephalitis of mumps is usually mild and may be present without parotitis. Spinal fluid abnormalities are characteristic of aseptic meningitis, although hypoglycorrhachia is more common in mumps than in other viral menigitides. Orchitis occurs in one quarter of post pubertal males and is the most common serious manifestation of disease. Generalized encephalitis, pancreatitis, and thrombocytopenia are among the relatively rare complications of mumps. No specific therapy is available.

Respiratory Syncytial Virus

Respiratory syncytial virus (RSV) is an extremely common infection of the upper and lower respiratory tracts that usually occurs in the winter and most often manifests in infants as bronchiolitis. In newborns under the age of 1 month and in infants with underlying cardiac or pulmonary disease, RSV bronchiolitis can be life-threatening. It is unclear whether rare reports of concomitant RSV infection and neurologic and myocarditic syndromes represent true cause and effect relationships, but RSV is neurotropic in animal models. Widespread dissemination of infection has not been a problem in immunocompromised individuals, although secondary bacterial infection may be more likely to occur.

Diagnosis is made by immunofluorescent microscopy or by antigen detection on nasal secretions and is readily available. Virus can also be grown in culture, which is the most sensitive method for diagnosis. Treatment with aerosolized ribavirin is effective in lessening shedding of the virus and in shortening the course of illness if given

early and is indicated in the treatment of high-risk infants and in those with more severe illness. It is unclear whether ribavirin results in lowered morbidity and mortality in more seriously ill infants, but it likely has some beneficial effects in the early stages of disease. When given via a ventilator, special care must be taken to avoid clogging of the system with crystallized drug.

Rubeola Virus

Rubeola virus is the cause of measles, which is resurgent in the United States. Typical disease is seen after an incubation period of about 10 days and commences with a prodromal period characterized by fever, malaise, and mild upper respiratory symptoms. Cough, coryza, conjunctivitis, and high fever develop over the course of a few days, with the appearance of pathognomonic Koplik spots (white specks on the buccal and lower labial mucosa). The erythematous morbilliform rash then develops, at which point the diagnosis is usually suspected. Most patients do not require hospitalization, but occasionally severe pneumonia, encephalitis, or myocarditis develops. In malnourished or immunocompromised individuals, measles is often fatal. Subacute sclerosing panencephalitis, a progressive degenerative disease, is a late, but fortunately rare, neurologic sequela of measles or measles vaccination.

Diagnosis of measles can usually be made clinically, but serology or viral culture may be helpful in unusual cases. No specific treatment is available. Measles is one of the most contagious infectious diseases known, and patients can become infected by the respiratory route simply by entering a room previously occupied by a patient with measles. Careful isolation of patients and adequate vaccination of contacts are essential. Immune globulin may be used for prophylaxis of young infants who have contact with measles cases.

Enteroviruses

The enteroviruses comprise more than 60 distinct viruses, which are generally grouped into polioviruses, coxsackieviruses, and echoviruses, but newly discovered enteroviruses are now being classified simply as enteroviruses, without assignment to one of these three groups. Enteroviruses are present year round but tend to produce epidemics in mid or late summer each year. The vast majority of infections are asymptomatic or minor nonspecific febrile illnesses. The term "enterovirus" refers to the primary site of viral replication rather than to any prominent intestinal symptoms from this group of viruses. It is only rarely that infection comes to medical attention, and even more rarely to the attention of the critical care practioner. Still, because these viruses are so prevalent in the community, serious disease is not uncommon in tertiary centers, and enteroviruses are the most common cause of viral meningitis. Newborns and immunocompromised individuals are at highest risk for serious complications.

Diagnosis of enteroviral disease is difficult, because there is no all-encompassing serologic test available. Also, shedding of virus from the intestinal tract may persist for weeks following clinical illness, so recovery of virus in stool is not proof of current infection. Usually, a combination of virus isolation from nasopharynx or stool and demonstration of fourfold change in serum neutralizing antibody to that specific isolate is needed for reasonable confirmation of diagnosis. Isolation of virus from the CSF is, of course, diagnostic, and the recently reported detection of virus in CSF with polymerase chain reaction is likely to be helpful for diagnosis of patients with viral meningitis.[25] No specific treatment is available for any of the enteroviral diseases.

Polioviruses

Infection with wild polioviruses has been virtually eliminated in the United States, and Central and South America are approaching this point. All paralytic polio disease seen in the United States recently has been due to vaccine strains of polio. Immunodeficient individuals are at high risk for development of disease following immunization or contact with an immunized individual. Paralytic poliomyelitis is primarily an inflammation of anterior horn cells that presents with fever and weakness in one or more extremities. There is progression to flaccid paresis that is usually asymmetric, and bulbar involvement may be present with spinal disease or as an isolated phenomenon. Guillain-Barré syndrome is similar to poliomyelitis, but tends to manifest as symmetric weakness in the absence of fever. CSF pleocytosis may be seen with polio but is generally not present in Guillain-Barré syndrome. Diagnosis by viral culture and serology is usually necessary, because the presence of vaccine strains of polio in fecal specimens is a common occurrence in highly vaccinated populations. Both oral live vaccine and parenteral killed vaccine appear highly effective in preventing infection with poliovirus types 1, 2, and 3.

Coxsackieviruses

Coxsackieviruses, discovered during a poliomyelitis outbreak in Coxsackie, New York, are perhaps the most virulent of commonly occurring enteroviruses. Two subgroups, A and B, have been described, and the six viruses in group B are most often associated with the serious manifestations of meningitis, meningoencephalitis, and myocarditis. They may also produce widespread organ involvement with hepatic failure and other serious manifestations. Up to 70% of patients with coxsackie B virus meningitis will have virus grown from CSF. Unfortunately, many coxsackie A viruses will not grow in tissue culture and therefore infection is virtually impossible to diagnose unless suckling mouse inoculation is performed.

Echoviruses

Echoviruses were named because, initially, they were viruses without a known disease, termed *enteric cytopathogenic human orphan* viruses. Clinical syndromes due to echoviruses are no different from those caused by other enteroviruses, but echovirus 11 is notorious as

a cause of fulminant hepatitis and disseminated intravascular coagulation in the newborn infant.

Rotaviruses

Human rotaviruses are common causes of gastroenteritis and may cause severe dehydration in young infants. They are particularly prevalent in the winter in temperate climates. Nosocomial infection with rotavirus is quite common on pediatric wards, and therefore should be suspected in patients with development of profuse watery diarrhea and vomiting while hospitalized for other problems, particularly during the winter. Diagnosis is made by demonstration of antigen by immunoassay or fluorescent microscopy, by visualization of viral particles on electron microscopy, or by culture. A number of vaccines are currently under investigation.

Hepatitis C Virus

Hepatitis C virus has recently been recognized as one of the non-A, non-B hepatitis viruses, and it is the most important cause of post-transfusion hepatitis. This prominence may diminish, however, now that serologic testing of donors is possible. Hepatitis C infection has a high rate of progression to chronic hepatitis, reaching 40 to 70% in some series, of whom 10 to 25% develop cirrhosis. Treatment of chronic disease with α-interferon has shown some transient beneficial effects.[26]

Rabies Virus

Human rabies is very uncommon in the United States, but animal rabies is quite prevalent. Skunks, raccoons, bats, and foxes are the most commonly infected animals in the United States. Unfortunately, up to one third of patients may have no history of bite or animal exposure, making diagnosis difficult. Rabies should be considered in the differential diagnosis of all encephalitides, and a careful history of exposure to or bites from potentially rabid animals should be obtained. Typically, rabies presents as paresthesia at the site of an animal bite, with hydrophobia and progressive obtundation and brain stem dysfunction. Hydrophobia is said to be pathognomonic, but there could be confusion with tetanus. One case of unsuspected human rabies resulted in an intensivist being bitten by the patient; diagnosis was made by brain biopsy for suspected HSV encephalitis.

Diagnosis is best made by fluorescent antibody stains of epithelial cells from the cornea or from the neck at the hairline, which are in close proximity to the brain and frequently have affected nerves. Serology does not become positive until late in the disease, although virus can be isolated from saliva early in disease. Pathognomic Negri bodies are seen in brain tissue in most, but not all, cases. Although survival has been reported rarely, rabies is generally a fatal disease. Intravenous ribavirin has been attempted for therapy. Rabies vaccine and rabies immune globulin are highly effective for prophylaxis if used properly.

FUNGI

Candida

Infections with *Candida* species occur commonly in intensive care settings as nosocomial septicemias, urinary tract infections, and meningitis. *Candida* organisms frequently colonize the oropharynx, intestinal tract, and skin of normal individuals, and immunocompromising diseases and drugs, broad-spectrum antibiotics, indwelling catheters, and parenteral nutrition all increase the risks of invasive disease due to these organisms. *C. albicans* is most frequently implicated, and *C. parapsilosis*, and *C. tropicalis* are also commonly seen. Other species, such as *C. guilliermondii* or *C. lusitaniae*, are seen occasionally.

Clinical presentations of invasive candidiasis are usually not distinctive enough to suggest the etiology, and a high index of suspicion must be maintained. An erythematous macronodular rash is seen in some cases of disseminated disease. The most common clinical predicament in the intensive care unit involves interpretation of a culture result showing growth of *Candida*. For blood cultures, any positive culture should be taken seriously. Infections of indwelling lines may be noticed in this manner, or this may be an indication of deep-seated or disseminated disease. Positive results of blood cultures for *Candida* should not be dismissed as contaminants, even though these yeasts are commonly present on skin.

Interpretation of urine culture positive for *Candida* species is more problematic, because low colony counts may reflect perineal or urethral colonization. Suprapubic aspiration of urine is helpful in eliminating this possibility. In general, the higher the colony count, the more likely the culture represents true infection, and levels of 10^4 to 10^5/ml are likely to be significant. Differentiation of upper from lower tract infection is difficult, although disappearance of organisms following removal of a urinary catheter is good evidence of lower tract infection. Rarely, large "fungus balls" involving the kidneys are evident on renal sonogram. Positive cultures from normally sterile sites, such as spinal fluid, peritoneal fluid, bones, or joints, are always indicative of disease.

Once a positive culture for *Candida* is noted, a thorough investigation should be undertaken to determine the extent of involvement. Fundoscopic examination to look for evidence of retinal exudates is necessary in all cases, although the yield is low. If present, this indicates widespread dissemination and merits prolonged therapy. *C. albicans* has a higher rate of ocular involvement than do other species. In cases of positive results on blood cultures with indwelling cardiac lines or repeated positive results on blood cultures, an echocardiogram should be done to look for valvular or mural vegetations. A sonogram may be useful in demonstrating fungal thrombosis of large veins in which deep lines have been placed. A urine culture should be obtained and, if the result is positive, renal sonography or other imaging study is performed. Other studies should be done as clinically indicated.

Common laboratory media, such as blood agar, will support the growth of *Candida* organisms, thus specialized fungal cultures are not necessary. This is not true of most other serious fungal infections, however. Serodiagnosis or antigen detection tests for candidiasis have not been promising to date.

Treatment for candidiasis varies with the extent of infection (see also Chapter 71). Unfortunately, there have been no systematic studies of candidiasis therapy, and most recommendations are based on prior experience. If the infection involves a foreign body (vascular line, urinary catheter, peritoneal dialysis catheter), it must be removed in nearly all situations. Heparin therapy for intravascular infections may be beneficial.[27] In the setting of bladder candidiasis with a Foley catheter, catheter removal may be sufficient to cure the infection if no other sites are involved and a renal sonogram is normal. For infection limited to the bladder but unassociated with indwelling catheters, bladder irrigation with amphotericin B is often curative. For bloodstream infections related to indwelling lines, a short course of parenteral amphotericin B (approximately 2 weeks) may be sufficient if the catheter is removed. For all deep-seated infections, a more prolonged course is probably indicated. A total amphotericin dose of approximately 30 mg/kg is administered for these situations. For central nervous system disease or for clinically unresponsive infections, flucytosine in addition to amphotericin B may be helpful. The role of fluconazole therapy in disseminated candidiasis is unclear, although it is quite helpful for less serious candidal infections.

Aspergillus

Aspergillosis is usually caused by *Aspergillus fumigatus* and *A. flavus*, although many other species are known to have caused invasive human disease. These molds are ubiquitous in the environment. Immunocompromised individuals, such as those with neutropenia from any cause or phagocytic disorders such as chronic granulomatous disease, are at highest risk. Exposure to construction activity in hospitals has resulted in epidemics in immunocompromised patients. The more common serious clinical manifestations include paranasal sinus disease with intracranial extension, invasive pulmonary aspergillosis, and widespread dissemination. *Aspergillus* has a tendency to invade vascular structures, causing infarct and tissue necrosis.

Diagnosis is made primarily by demonstration of invasive fungal elements on tissue biopsy. In the appropriate clinical setting, isolation of *A. flavus* or *A. fumigatus* from bronchial washings is suggestive of invasive pulmonary disease. The results of blood cultures are virtually never positive, even in disseminated disease, and serodiagnosis has been relatively unrewarding to date.

Treatment consists primarily of amphotericin B therapy, with surgical debridement of infected tissue in paranasal sinus disease or cerebral involvement. Itraconazole may be beneficial.

Mucor and Related Fungi

Mucormycosis is a serious disease of immunocompromised individuals with risk factors such as neutropenia, malignancy, and organ transplantation, as well as in diabetics, particularly those with diabetic ketoacidosis. The infectious agents are found in soil and isolated from moldy fruits and bread. Most serious infections are due to the genera *Rhizopus*, *Rhizomucor*, and *Absidia*, although many other genera have been reported to cause human disease. The most serious, and most common, form of disease is rhinocerebral mucormycosis, which presents with pain and swelling of the face and progresses to invade the sinuses and brain. Widespread disseminated disease is also seen, usually in immunocompromised individuals.

Because agents of mucormycosis are difficult to grow in culture and positive results on cultures from respiratory secretions may represent merely colonization, tissue diagnosis is usually necessary. Serodiagnosis is not helpful.

Treatment consists of administration of amphotericin B and aggressive surgical debridement in most cases. Still, mortality is approximately 50% for invasive forms of the disease.

Histoplasma

Histoplasma capsulatum is a yeast infecting humans primarily in the Ohio, Missouri, and Mississippi Valley regions of the United States. Exposure to bird or bat dung, caves, old buildings, and hollow trees has resulted in infection, because the organism prefers moist environments with high nitrogen content. The majority of infections with *H. capsulatum* are inapparent or occasionally nonspecific febrile respiratory infections; however, a few clinical forms may come to the attention of the intensivist.

In the normal host, massive mediastinal adenopathy may cause superior vena caval syndrome or respiratory compromise. Histoplasmosis is a rare cause of pericarditis. Disseminated disease occurs rarely in normal hosts. Acute disseminated histoplasmosis occurs in infancy, and a subacute form is sometimes seen in older children. Patients with AIDS and other immunodeficiencies are at higher risk for dissemination.

Diagnosis is usually made serologically, most commonly by complement fixation and immunodiffusion testing. Complement fixing antibodies develop within 4 to 6 weeks after infection, and the yeast phase test is more indicative of recent or active infection. However, many cases cannot be diagnosed by serologic methods, and biopsy is needed for confirmation. Skin testing is generally not useful for diagnosis and should be avoided, except as an epidemiologic tool.

Treatment of histoplasmosis is usually not necessary but must be employed in more severe cases. Amphotericin B has been the drug of choice, although ketoconazole may be helpful in less critical but symptomatic forms. Intraconazole may also be helpful. Surgical treatment is occasionally used for complications of medias-

tinal disease, such as tracheoesophageal fistula or hemoptysis.

Blastomyces

Infection due to *Blastomyces dermatitidis* is seen most commonly in the eastern part of the United States. The ecologic niche is probably soil.[28] Disease is usually mild, but rarely systemic blastomycosis can develop. This form of disease progresses slowly to involve not only the respiratory tract but also skin, bone and joints, genitourinary tract, central nervous system, and other sites. Over half of individuals die without treatment.

Diagnosis usually depends on growth of the organism in culture or demonstration of characteristic morphology on biopsy specimens. Treatment with ketoconazole is preferred for most forms of active disease, with amphotericin B used for life-threatening and central nervous system disease.

Coccidioides

Coccidioidomycosis, or San Joaquin Valley fever, is caused by the dimorphic fungus *Coccidioides immitis*.[29] Most cases in the United States originate in the Southwest, and the organism is usually found in soil. Although originally considered a serious infection, it is now appreciated that the vast majority of infected individuals have asymptomatic or self-limited disease requiring no therapy. More serious illness may occur in young infants who have disseminated disease or in those with infections of sites such as the central nervous system following penetrating trauma. Clinical findings are nonspecific, but the disease may be suspected in the appropriate geographic setting in patients with cavitary pulmonary disease, characteristic skin lesions, bone lesions, and other involvement. Diagnosis is made by culture or, especially for nervous system disease, by demonstration of coccidioidal antibody by precipitin assay.

In patients requiring treatment, amphotericin B is the standard therapy. Miconazole, ketoconazole, fluconazole, and itraconazole may also be beneficial. Fluconazole is particularly promising for central nervous system disease, which previously has required intrathecal amphotericin B administration.

PARASITES

Protozoa

Toxoplasma

With the exception of infants with congenital toxoplasmosis, most critically ill patients with *Toxoplasma gondii* infection are immunocompromised. Although the AIDS epidemic has resulted in an increasing incidence of toxoplasma encephalitis, retinitis, and disseminated disease, toxoplasmosis in pediatric AIDS is relatively uncommon. Diagnosis may be difficult. Serodiagnosis is commonly employed but may be misleading, particularly in immunocompromised patients who have blunted antibody responses. Organisms may be seen in tissue section in most but not all situations, and this is probably the most reliable form of diagnosis. Isolation of toxoplasma from blood or body fluids is possible in some laboratories and may be of benefit for immunodeficient patients. Treatment usually consists of pyramethamine plus sulfadiazine, with spiramycin, clindamycin, and trimethoprim-sulfamethoxazole employed occasionally for pediatric patients.

Plasmodium falciparum

Life-threatening malaria is caused by *Plasmodium falciparum*. *P. falciparum* is capable of infecting all ages of red cells and has a relatively short multiplication time, resulting in more rapidly progressive disease. *P. falciparum* infection is acquired outside the United States. The more severe forms are characterized by obtundation with cerebral malaria, due to massive hemolysis and sludging in blood vessels supplying the brain, and black-water fever, in which massive hemolysis results in hemoglobinuria and multiple organ system failure from a combination of factors. These scenarios can be rapidly fatal and require quick attention. Diagnosis of overwhelming disease is usually easy, since many trophozoites are evident on the peripheral blood smear, even to inexperienced observers. CSF examination may show a mild pleocytosis but is not particularly helpful.

Treatment for these more severe forms is usually undertaken with intravenous quinidine by continuous infusion, often supplemented by exchange transfusion.[30] Outcome in children is often good if treatment is begun before serious organ damage has occurred.

Pneumocystis carinii

Pneumocystis carinii is a cause of pneumonia and respiratory failure in patients with AIDS and other immunodeficiency disorders, as well as in malnourished infants. Clinical findings are nonspecific, with hypoxemia prominent. Diagnosis is made by bronchoalveolar lavage or lung biopsy, and treatment with trimethoprim-sulfamethoxazole is usually but not always effective. Corticosteroids are an effective adjunct to therapy, and pentamidine is used for patients unable to tolerate trimethoprim-sulfamethoxazole.

Entamoeba histolytica

Amebiasis is occasionally acquired in the United States and rarely causes severe manifestations such as fulminant colitis with ruptured abdominal viscus or toxic megacolon. Very young infants, malnourished individuals, pregnant women, and patients receiving corticosteroids are at particular risk for this complication. Diagnosis is made by visualization of the organism in fecal material. Metronidazole followed by iodoquinol is the preferred therapy, along with surgical repair if indicated.

Naegleria fowleri and Acanthamoeba

Free-living amebae include *Naegleria fowleri* and *Acanthamoeba* species. Primary amebic meningoencephalitis is caused by *N. fowleri*, while a more indolent encephalitis is seen with *Acanthamoeba*. *Acanthamoeba* can also cause a keratitis particularly associated with the use of soft contact lenses.

Most *N. fowleri* infections in the United States are acquired by swimming in fresh water in the central part of the country. Organisms gain access to the brain through the nose and olfactory tracts. Clinical presentation and laboratory findings often mimic bacterial meningitis, but CSF Gram stain and culture are negative. Examination of wet mounts of CSF allows visualization of motile organisms. The disease is usually fatal, although survival has been reported with the use of systemic and intrathecal amphotericin B, in one case in combination with miconazole, rifampin, and sulfisoxazole.

Other Parasites

Many other parasitic diseases can occasionally cause serious illness. For example, the roundworm, *Ascaris lumbricoides*, can cause intestinal obstruction due to massive intestinal infestation or respiratory arrest due to aspiration of worms migrating from the intestinal tract. *Strongyloides stercoralis* can cause a hyperinfection syndrome in immunodeficient patients. *Babesia microti* may produce a sepsis-like picture in asplenic individuals. It is beyond the scope of this chapter to cover all examples of serious parasitic disease, and the reader is referred to textbooks for detailed information.[1, 4]

RICKETTSIAE

Rickettsia rickettsii

Rocky Mountain Spotted Fever (RMSF) is a tick-borne illness caused by *Rickettsia rickettsii* that occurs principally in the mid-Atlantic states westward to the Midwest. In spite of its name, relatively few cases originate in the Rocky Mountain area. The peak season is from April to September. RMSF is a diffuse vasculitic illness, and patients usually present with fever, severe headache, and a petechial rash appearing on the wrists and ankles and spreading within hours to the rest of the body. The palms and soles are usually involved. There is a history of tick bite in about 60% of cases. The rash is quite useful in making the diagnosis but is unfortunately absent at the time of presentation in about one third of patients (see also Chapter 67). Seizures and other central nervous system manifestations, arrhythmias, congestive heart failure, and thrombocytopenia can complicate care. Mortality is approximately 25% in patients who do not have specific treatment.

Diagnosis can be made serologically, but antibody is usually not present early in the course of disease. Skin biopsy with immunofluorescent examination is helpful in atypical cases if the biopsy is done early in the course of disease. The Weil-Felix reaction is nonspecific and is probably of little use today with the increasing availability of specific serodiagnosis. Usually, treatment is begun when the disease is suspected, because of the risk of poor outcome in untreated cases. Tetracycline and chloramphenicol are both effective if given early.

Ehrlichia canis

Human ehrlichiosis, caused by *Ehrlichia canis*, is being increasingly recognized.[31] Previously thought to be only a disease prevalent in dogs, *E. canis* infection in humans has been seen in 18 states, predominantly in the South. The agent is tick-borne. The clinical illness ranges in severity and has been described as RMSF without a rash. However, some patients do develop a rash, which may be maculopapular or petechial. Serious illness has resulted in acute renal failure, coagulopathy, encephalitis, and pneumonia. Diagnosis is made serologically, but a high index of suspicion is needed to entertain the diagnosis. Optimal therapy has not been well defined, but tetracycline, doxycycline, and chloramphenicol seem to be effective.

MISCELLANEOUS ORGANISMS

Mycoplasmas

Mycoplasma pneumoniae, the most common mycoplasma infecting humans, usually produces mild upper respiratory symptoms or pneumonia. Rarely, the pneumonia is severe; this is particularly likely to occur in patients with sickle cell disease, in which pleural effusions and hypoxia may be seen in association with mycoplasmal pneumonia. Rare complications include hemolytic anemia, myocarditis, meningoencephalitis, and Guillain-Barré syndrome. *M. pneumoniae* may be grown with special media, but the organism can be excreted for prolonged periods following infection. Serodiagnosis with complement fixation is usually most helpful. Cold agglutinin testing is nonspecific and not likely to be helpful in evaluating serious illness. Therapy with erythromycin or tetracyclines may be helpful, although the benefit in serious cases is unclear because they are so rare.

M. hominis is an uncommon cause of sepsis and meningitis in the newborn period. It should be suspected in culture negative cases of disease. *Ureaplasma urealyticum* has likewise been reported as a rare cause of systemic illness in the newborn, but it is probably more important as a contributor to chronic lung disease in premature infants.

Chlamydia

Chlamydia trachomatis is a common cause of conjunctivitis and pneumonia in infants and of genital tract disease in older children and adolescents. Chlamydial pneumonia usually presents in afebrile infants with little or no oxygen requirement and seldom requires intensive care. Chlamydial myocarditis has been reported. Diagnosis is most accurately made by culture, but enzyme immunoassays or fluorescent microscopy can aid in diagnosis more quickly. Serologic diagnosis can also be helpful but is not widely available. Treatment with erythromycin is likely to shorten the course of illness.

References

1. Feigin RD, and Cherry JD: Textbook of Pediatric Infectious Diseases, 2nd ed. Philadelphia, WB Saunders, 1987.
2. Remington JS and Klein JO: Infectious Diseases of the Fetus and Newborn Infant, 3rd ed. Philadelphia, WB Saunders, 1990.
3. Committee on Infectious Diseases, American Academy of Pediatrics: Report of the Committee on Infectious Diseases, 22nd ed. Elk Grove Village, IL, American Academy of Pediatrics, 1991.
4. Mandell GL, Douglas RG Jr, and Bennett JE: Principles and Practice of Infectious Diseases, 3rd ed. New York, Churchill Livingstone, 1990.
5. Freeman J, Goldmann DA, Smith NE, et al: Association of intravenous lipid emulsion and coagulase-negative staphylococcal bacteremia in neonatal intensive care units. N Engl J Med 323:301, 1990.
6. Martin MA, Pfaller MA, and Wenzel RP: Coagulase-negative staphylococcal bacteremia: Mortality and hospital stay. Ann Intern Med 110:9, 1989.
7. St. Geme JW III, Bell LM, Baumgart S, et al: Distinguishing sepsis from blood culture contamination in young infants with blood cultures growing coagulase-negative staphylococci. Pediatrics 86:157, 1990.
8. Patrick CC, Kaplan SL, Baker CJ, et al: Persistent bacteremia due to coagulase-negative staphylococci in low birth weight neonates. Pediatrics 84:977, 1989.
9. Stevens DL, Tanner MH, Winship J, et al: Severe group A streptococcal infections associated with a toxic shock–like syndrome and scarlet fever toxin A. N Engl J Med 321:1, 1989.
10. Kim KS: Clinical perspectives on penicillin tolerance. J Pediatr 112:509, 1988.
11. Latorre C, Juncosa T, and Sanfeliu I: Antibiotic resistance and serotypes of 100 *Streptococcus pneumoniae* strains isolated in a children's hospital in Barcelona, Spain. Antimicrob Agents Chemother 28:357, 1985.
12. Dobson SRM and Baker CJ: Enterococcal sepsis in neonates: Features by age of onset and occurrence of focal infection. Pediatrics 85:165, 1990.
13. Rice LB, Calderwood SB, Eliopoulos GM, et al: Enterococcal endocarditis: A comparison of prosthetic and native valve disease. Rev Infect Dis 13:1, 1991.
14. Murray BE: The life and times of the enterococcus. Clin Microbiol Rev 3:46, 1990.
15. Oster SE, Chirurgi VA, Goldberg AA, et al: Ampicillin-resistant enterococcal species in an acute care hospital. Antimicrob Agents Chemother 34:1821, 1990.
16. Kessler SL and Dajani AS: *Listeria* meningitis in infants and children. Pediatr Infect Dis J 9:61, 1990.
17. Mendelman PM, Campos J, Chaffin DO, et al: Relative penicillin G resistance in *Neisseria meningitidis* and reduced affinity of penicillin-binding protein 3. Antimicrob Agents Chemother 32:706, 1988.
18. Brady MT: Nosocomial legionnaires' disease in a children's hospital. J Pediatr 115:46, 1989.
19. Stechenberg BW: Lyme disease: The latest great imitator. Pediatr Infect Dis J 7:402, 1988.
20. Centers for Disease Control: Guidelines for the prevention and control of congenital syphilis. MMWR 37(S-1):1, 1988.
21. Starke JR: Multidrug therapy for tuberculosis in children. Pediatr Infect Dis J 9:785, 1990.
22. Hoy J, Mijh A, Sandland M, et al: Quadruple-drug therapy for *Mycobacterium avium-intracellulare* bacteremia in AIDS patients. J Infect Dis 161:801, 1990.

23. Whitley R, Arvin A, Prober C, et al: A controlled trial comparing vidarabine with acyclovir in neonatal herpes simplex virus infection. N Engl J Med 324:444, 1991.
24. Kurtzman G, Frickhofen N, Kimball J, et al: Pure red -cell aplasia of 10 years' duration due to persistent parvovirus B19 infection and its cure with immunoglobulin therapy. N Engl J Med 321:519, 1989.
25. Rotbart HA: Diagnosis of enteroviral meningitis with the polymerase chain reaction. J Pediatr 117:85, 1990.
26. DiBisceglie AM, Martin P, Kassianides C, et al: Recombinant interferon alpha therapy for chronic hepatitis C: A randomized, double-blind, placebo-controlled trial. N Engl J Med 321:1506, 1989.
27. Ashkenazi S, Pickering LK, and Robinson LH: Diagnosis and management of septic thrombosis of the inferior vena cava caused by *Candida tropicalis*. Pediatr Infect Dis J 9:446, 1990.
28. Klein BS, Vergeront JM, Weeks RJ, et al: Isolation of *Blastomyces dermatitidis* in soil associated with a large outbreak of blastomycosis in Wisconsin. N Engl J Med 314:529, 1986.
29. Ampel NM, Wieden MA, and Galgiani JN: Coccidioidomycosis: Clinical update. Rev Infect Dis 11:897, 1989.
30. Miller KD, Greenberg AE, and Campbell CC: Treatment of severe malaria in the United States with a continuous infusion of quinidine gluconate and exchange transfusion. N Engl J Med 321:65, 1989.
31. Edwards MS, Jones JE, Leass DL, et al: Childhood infection caused by *Ehrlichia canis* or a closely related organism. Pediatr Infect Dis J 7:651, 1988.

Immunodeficient States in Children

Keith D. Herzog, M.D., and
Tamara A. Rakusan, M.D., Ph.D.

Serious localized or systemic infections, especially meningitis, pneumonia, and fulminant sepsis, are frequent causes for admission to pediatric intensive care units (ICUs). Although immunologically normal children do not escape such illnesses, the incidence of life-threatening bacterial and viral infections is greatly increased in the presence of either primary (congenital) or acquired immune defects. In addition, such patients are susceptible to unusual, opportunistic infections not seen in immunocompetent hosts. There are more than 50 congenital disorders that involve varying degrees of humoral or cellular immunodeficiency. Some of the more common, serious congenital immunodeficiency disorders will be discussed with reference to clinical presentation and appropriate intervention. Subsequent discussion will center on what has become the most common cause of intrinsic immunodeficiency in children, human immunodeficiency virus (HIV) infection. Secondary immunodeficiencies caused by malignancies and chemotherapy are discussed elsewhere.

A number of general observations are useful in understanding the clinical aspects of various immunodeficiency syndromes. Antibody or B cell defects tend to result in recurrent bacterial infections, whereas disorders of T cell function frequently are manifested by serious viral, fungal, or opportunistic infections. Disorders of phagocytic function often result in abscess formation in both cutaneous structures and internal organs. It should be noted, however, that humoral and cellular immune function are virtually inseparable, and a majority of immunodeficiency syndromes involve some degree of dysfunction of both limbs of the immune system.

In immunodeficiency states, the associated disorders are often as important as the immunodeficiency itself. A great many congenital immunodeficiency diseases are associated with other abnormalities, including anatomic (e.g., cardiac) anomalies and physiologic (e.g., endocrine) disorders. Although such conditions may have been diagnosed by the time a child presents to the ICU, proper management of these disorders may be critical to patient outcome.

Although nuances of management differ with each

disorder and with each patient, a number of general guidelines in patient care should be observed. Given the broad range of organisms that may be implicated in life-threatening illnesses in such patients, both routine and opportunistic pathogens should be aggressively sought through appropriate diagnostic procedures (e.g., bronchoalveolar lavage [BAL]). It should be remembered that serologic tests may be misleading, with false-negative results occurring because of intrinsic immunologic unresponsiveness and false-positive results found because of exogenously administered intravenous immunoglobulin (IVIG).

If the patient's illness is severe enough to require intensive care, it is prudent to initiate broad-spectrum antimicrobial therapy empirically. Such therapy may include an antistaphylococcal penicillin and a third-generation cephalosporin (ceftazidime should be used if *Pseudomonas* infection is suspected). If a central venous catheter (e.g., a Broviac catheter) is in place, vancomycin may be employed instead of the antistaphylococcal penicillin for better coverage of coagulase-negative staphylococci and enterococci. If *Pneumocystis carinii* pneumonia (PCP) is suspected, trimethoprim-sulfamethoxazole should be initiated pending BAL results. Once a pathogen is identified, therapy should usually be narrowed as much as possible to avoid predisposition to invasive fungal disease or emergence of highly resistant gram-negative pathogens.

Augmentation of the patient's immune system is frequently attempted by exogenous replacement of intrinsically deficient factors. IVIG is used frequently as prophylaxis and occasionally as a therapeutic modality for patients with B cell disorders, and granulocyte transfusions are occasionally employed for severely neutropenic patients. There are serious potential problems, inherent in the use of these products, however, and they should be used judiciously (see further on).

During acute illnesses, these children frequently require the administration of blood products. Careful thought should be given to the nature of the underlying disorder if potential adverse events are to be avoided. In patients with T cell defects, for example, transfusion-acquired cytomegalovirus (CMV) may cause severe disease; therefore, CMV-negative blood products should be employed if at all possible. Children with the most severe T cell defects (e.g., severe combined immunodeficiency disease [SCID]) may suffer graft versus host disease (GVH) secondary to contaminating white blood cells in blood products; therefore, such products should be irradiated before use.

B CELL DISORDERS

X-Linked Agammaglobulinemia

The prototypic B cell immunodeficiency disorder is X-linked agammaglobulinemia, a condition marked by drastically diminished or lacking serum immunoglobulins that results from a defect in pre–B cell differentiation. Transmitted in an X-linked recessive pattern, the disorder becomes manifested in affected boys by 6 to 12 months of age. Patients typically present with recurrent episodes of otitis media, sinusitis, and pneumonia caused by *Haemophilus influenzae*, *Staphylococcus aureus*, *Streptococcus pneumoniae*, and occasionally *Pseudomonas*. Gastroenteritis, pyoderma, arthritis, and meningitis are also common.

Although the response to most viral infections is generally adequate, episodes of complicated or prolonged cases of hepatitis and enteroviral meningoencephalitis[1] have been reported. Immunization with live viral vaccines should be avoided, as vaccine-associated disease (e.g., poliomyelitis) may occur.[2] Other unusual but often lethal complications of X-linked agammaglobulinemia include a severe form of dermatomyositis, progressive panencephalitis, and malignancies.

Laboratory findings primarily include markedly diminished or lacking immunoglobulins (Ig) and lack of peripheral B lymphocytes despite normal total leukocyte counts. T lymphocyte numbers and function are normal. Treatment involves replacement therapy with exogenous immunoglobulin. Although intramuscular (IM) injection has been used in the past, currently available IVIG preparations allow larger doses to be given in a less painful manner. The usual therapeutic regimen is 400 mg/kg (if given prophylactically, it may be given every 3 to 4 weeks). Although IVIG is usually well tolerated, serious reactions do occasionally occur. Infusions should be initiated slowly: 1 to 2 ml/kg/hr for the first 15 minutes, increasing the rate of infusion slowly, with completion over approximately 4 hours. IM preparations should never be given intravenously (IV) because of the risk of anaphylactoid reactions resulting from complement activation by protein aggregates.

Common Variable Immunodeficiency

A more frequent, though less severe, disorder is common variable immunodeficiency. This clinical entity actually encompasses a group of disorders in which the common denominators are markedly decreased serum immunoglobulin levels and deficient antibody response.

Given the number of intrinsic defects causing this disorder (e.g., antigenically unresponsive B lymphocytes, blocked antibody secretion), the age at presentation and the severity of clinical symptoms are variable. In most patients, however, the presenting symptoms are recurrent sinus and pulmonary infections, the latter often resulting in bronchiectasis. Gastrointestinal complaints are also common, and autoimmune disorders and autoantibodies are often found, reflecting yet another facet of B cell dysfunction.

Serum Ig levels are quite low, though they are usually higher than in X-linked agammaglobulinemia. There is also a defect in Ig class switching (IgM to IgG). The majority of patients have normal T cell function. Treatment, as in X-linked agammaglobulinemia, consists of replacement therapy with IVIG (see preceding discussion). The use of prophylactic antibiotics may also be useful.

Selective Immunoglobulin Deficiencies

Selective IgM and IgE deficiencies are rare. Conversely, IgA deficiency, defined as an IgA level less than 5 mg/dl, is the most common B cell disorder, occurring in 1 of every 400 to 800 individuals. Although selective or isolated IgA deficiency may occur in apparently healthy children and adults, numerous abnormalities have been noted in association with IgA deficiency, including pulmonary disease, gastrointestinal disorders (e.g., celiac sprue), central nervous system disease (ataxia-telangiectasia), and autoimmune disorders. Studies have also noted an association of IgA deficiency and allergy.[3] One of the most serious potential problems encountered in IgA-deficient patients involves sensitization to exogenous IgA with elaboration of anti-IgA antibodies. Administration of blood products (including IVIG, which contains trace amounts of IgA) may result in anaphylaxis. Gammagard immune globulin, with the lowest fraction of IgA should be used in IgA-deficient patients[4], and transfused red blood cells should be washed.

Clinical syndromes associated with IgG subclass deficiencies have been the subject of much recent research and debate. There are clearly patients who suffer recurrent bacterial infections, especially pulmonary infections, yet have normal total IgG determinations. Many such patients have been shown to have quantitative deficiencies in one or more of the IgG subclasses. Further investigation may also reveal defects in lymphokine production or neutrophil chemotaxis. As in other patients with primary antibody deficiencies, therapy consists of monthly IVIG administration.

Disorders of Complement

Disorders of the complement cascade may occasionally result in acute, life-threatening conditions. Invasive meningococcal disease has been noted in association with deficiencies of the terminal complement components C5 to C8.[5] It is important to note that many of these patients, especially the adults, have associated collagen vascular diseases. Some patients do have isolated complement deficiencies, however. Delineating such deficiencies in the index patient may reveal a familial condition that predisposes other family members to invasive meningococcal disease. An assay of total hemolytic complement activity, CH_{50}, serves as a screen for complement deficiencies by assessing the functional integrity of the classical pathway. Although useful, it is relatively insensitive, and individual assays may be required if complement deficiency is strongly suspected. Such assays should be performed after patient recovery, as complement levels are often altered because of acute bacterial illness.

Disorders of complement control are exemplified by the lack of C1 esterase inhibitor, resulting in hereditary angioedema. Uncontrolled C1 activation results in excessive release of vasoactive substances that induce localized edema. Episodes are not usually severe until later childhood or adolescence. Edema of the intestinal wall may cause severe abdominal pain, and when cutaneous signs are lacking, it may precipitate unnecessary laparotomy. Laryngeal edema is immediately life-threatening, and tracheostomy may be necessary in the face of airway obstruction. Prevention involves avoidance (if possible) of precipitating factors, including trauma, vigorous exercise, or emotional stress. The use of the semisynthetic androgen danazol has been associated with increased C1 inhibitor activity. ϵ-Aminocaproic acid may also be effective. Amelioration of acute episodes may be accomplished with epinephrine, and administration of fresh plasma may provide some inhibitor activity. Antihistamines and steroids are not effective.

T CELL DISORDERS

DiGeorge Syndrome

Although T cell disorders seldom occur in isolation, the DiGeorge syndrome is characterized by variable T cell dysfunction and normal or nearly normal B cell function. Disruption in embryogenesis of the first through the fourth and the sixth pharyngeal pouches results in clinical abnormalities of varying severity. Recognition of the syndrome may be based on characteristic dysmorphic features, including hypertelorism, an antimongoloid slant of the eyes, low set and abnormally formed ears, and micrognathia. Cardiovascular findings arise from conotruncal abnormalities; in fact it is not unusual for the DiGeorge syndrome to be suspected initially at the time of early cardiac surgery (e.g., for critical coarctation of the aorta) when hypoplasia or lack of the thymus is noted. Of critical importance is the occurrence of hypocalcemia and hyperphosphatemia in the first 24 to 48 hours of life caused by deficient parathyroid hormone production. Hypocalcemia may be severe enough to cause tetany or seizures, with resultant hypoxic cerebral injury. In addition, urologic abnormalities, including hydronephrosis, are common, so suspicion of the DiGeorge syndrome should lead to a full renal evaluation.

The severity of the immunodeficiency is variable. In general, infectious complications include recurrent pneumonias (including PCP), candidiasis, and gastroenteritis; therefore, opportunistic pathogens should be aggressively sought in any patient with the DiGeorge syndrome who presents with sepsis or respiratory distress.

Laboratory findings include hypocalcemia (<7 mg/dl), hyperphosphatemia, and low or lacking parathyroid hormone. Chest radiographs may reveal evidence of cardiac anomalies and no thymic shadow. Assays of immunologic function are variable. Total lymphocyte counts are often normal, though the percentage of T cells is usually reduced; mitogenic response may also be normal or reduced.

Therapy should include management of calcium and phosphorous balance and correction of cardiac anomalies. Although immunologic reconstitution has been achieved with fetal thymic implants, this is usually not necessary for less severely affected children. PCP prophylaxis should be employed and live viral vaccines avoided. As in other patients with cellular immunodeficiency, it is preferrable to avoid exposure to CMV-positive blood products. In addition, on rare occasion, GVH may result after transfusion in those patients with the most severe cellular deficiency; irradiated blood products should therefore be used.

Wiskott-Aldrich Syndrome

The Wiskott-Aldrich syndrome is an X-linked disorder manifested by recurrent infections along with eczema and thrombocytopenia. Although serious infections may not occur during the first few months of life because of protective maternal antibodies, hemostatic dysfunction may be apparent early, as evidenced by petechiae or frank bleeding. Although bleeding may sometimes be minor, intracranial hemorrhages do occur. Acute bleeding episodes respond to homologous platelet transfusions (irradiated to prevent GVH). Splenectomy reduces bleeding tendencies but increases the risk of sepsis (see also Chap. 68).

The cause of the progressive T and B cell defect in the Wiskott-Aldrich syndrome is unclear; it may be the result of defective antigen processing. The result is marked susceptibility to both common bacterial pathogens and opportunistic infections, including PCP and CMV. Laboratory findings include diminished T cell responsiveness and a characteristic Ig pattern: elevated IgA and IgE and diminished IgM levels. There is a marked inability to respond to polysaccharide antigens; in fact, polysaccharide vaccines (e.g., pneumococcal or *Haemophilus influenzae* type B) may cause worsening of some of the hematologic manifestations.

Ataxia-Telangiectasia

Ataxia-telangiectasia is manifested by progressive neurologic dysfunction, conjunctival and cutaneous telangiectasia, and frequent occurrence of malignancies.

In addition, endocrine dysfunction may exist, with some patients exhibiting relative insulin resistance that results in significant hyperglycemia.[6] The immunologic defect in ataxia-telangiectasia results in frequent viral and bacterial infections, especially pulmonary infection, but opportunistic infections are not common. The laboratory correlates of the immune deficiency are IgA deficiency (70%), reduced antibody responsiveness, and T cell dysfunction. There is no satisfactory therapy for ataxia-telangiectasia at this point.

X-Linked Lymphoproliferative Disorder

X-linked lymphoproliferative disorder (XLP) affects otherwise apparently healthy males upon exposure to the Epstein-Barr virus. Affected children initially appear normal and may have normal immunologic parameters. However, a severe aberrant response to the Epstein-Barr virus occurs, resulting in one or more of the following clinical entities: severe mononucleosis, malignant B cell lymphomas, aplastic anemia, or hypogammaglobulinemia. The only interventions available are acyclovir for infectious mononucleosis and IVIG for hypogammaglobulinemia.

COMBINED IMMUNODEFICIENCIES

Although the preceding disorders were classified under T cell deficiencies, as noted there is inevitably some degree of B cell dysfunction as well. Those disorders in which T cell and B cell function are both grossly impaired or even lacking are collectively termed combined immunodeficiency syndromes. The frequently used term SCID does not actually refer to a single pathologic state but rather describes a clinical entity resulting from stem cell, thymic, or intrinsic lymphocyte defects. Patients with SCID and adenosine deaminase deficiency, for example, refers to those children with severe compromise resulting from ADA deficiency.

Although B cell dysfunction results in frequent serious bacterial infections, T cell dysfunction is even more apparent, with refractory candidiasis, episodes of PCP, and overwhelming viral infections. In addition, these patients often have dermatitis (in some cases representing GVH) and severe malabsorptive problems that may cause wasting and even death.

The key in management of these patients is aggressive search for routine and opportunistic pathogens and prompt initiation of empirical therapy for any child with fever, clinical sepsis, or respiratory distress. In addition to antibacterial agents, the clinical scenario often mandates consideration of antiviral, antifungal, and antiparasitic therapy. All of these patients will be overtly hypogammaglobulinemic or will have poor or lacking antibody responses; therefore, IVIG is a mainstay of therapy (see section on B cell deficiencies). CMV-negative and irradiated blood products should be used—the latter to prevent GVH.

Definitive treatment for most of these disorders is bone marrow transplantation. For patients with specific enzyme defects (e.g. ADA), gene therapy may hold some promise for the future.

DISORDERS OF PHAGOCYTOSIS

Chronic Granulomatous Disease

Clinical disease resulting from deficient phagocytic function is clearly demonstrated in chronic granulomatous disease. This disorder involves an inability to achieve intracellular bacterial killing as a result of one or more molecular defects in the phagocytic oxidative burst. Affected patients suffer suppurative infections of skin, lymph nodes, lung, abdominal organs, bone, and occasionally brain. *S. aureus* is by far the most common offending pathogen, though infections with *Aspergillus, Nocardia,* and gram-negative rods also are common and severe. Complications may include gastrointestinal[7] or ureteral obstruction caused by granuloma formation. A presumptive diagnosis is easily established with the nitroblue tetrazolium dye reduction assay. Prolonged therapy with trimethoprim-sulfamethoxazole has been shown to reduce the frequency of severe infections in these patients.[8] In extreme circumstances, granulocyte transfusions may be of some benefit. However, extreme caution should be exercised in a number of situations involving granulocyte transfusions: When amphotericin B is given simultaneously with or following transfusion, respiratory decompensation with pulmonary infiltrates and intra-alveolar hemorrhage may occur.[9] In addition, individuals with the X-linked form of chronic granulomatous disease have rare K_0 erythrocytes and leukocytes and may have antibodies to Kell antigens.[10] Therefore, Kell status should be determined and transfusion avoided if possible if the patient is Kell-negative.

Chédiak-Higashi Syndrome

The Chédiak-Higashi syndrome is another disorder marked by defective leukocyte phagocytic function; these patients may be recognized by the presence of partial oculocutaneous albinism. The leukocyte deficiency is a result of defective degranulation after phagocytosis; intramedullary granulocyte destruction also results in peripheral neutropenia. The result is frequent, serious pyogenic infection. Although there is no standard therapy, ascorbate has been shown to decrease the number of infections in some patients.[11]

MISCELLANEOUS DISORDERS

Chronic mucocutaneous candidiasis results from a subtle defect in T cell responsiveness. Although infectious manifestations rarely result in illness severe enough to require intensive care, attention should be given to the frequent occurrence of associated endocrinopathies, including hypothyroidism, hypoparathyroidism, and Addison disease.

Hyper-IgE syndrome (in some cases referred to as

pl[...]

the Job syndrome) is a disorder characterized by an extraordinarily high IgE level and a poor humoral and cellular response to antigens. Despite a markedly high IgE level, patients do not typically manifest respiratory allergy symptoms. The clinical manifestation of the immune deficiency is recurrent pyogenic infections, predominantly cutaneous and pulmonary infection. By far, the most frequent pathogen is *S. aureus,* though *H. influenzae, S. pneumoniae,* group A streptococci, and fungal infections may occur. Pneumatocele formation is common, and superinfection with *Aspergillus* may result in life-threatening pulmonary hemorrhage. An unexplained observation in these patients is significant osteopenia, and recurrent fractures may occur.[12] Prevention of infection should be attempted with antistaphylococcal antibiotics.

Splenectomy

Many medical and surgical conditions result in either functional or anatomic asplenia. Although the resulting degree of immunodeficiency depends to some extent on the underlying disorder, asplenic patients have a greatly increased (>50-fold) incidence of serious bacterial sepsis, especially with *S. pneumoniae.* Caretakers should be cognizant not only of the increased incidence of serious bacterial infection but also of the frequently fulminant nature of such infections. It is therefore important to be aware of the presence of functional or anatomic asplenia in association with some forms of congenital heart disease as well as hemoglobinopathies.

PEDIATRIC HUMAN IMMUNODEFICIENCY VIRUS INFECTION

Acquired immunodeficiency syndrome (AIDS) was first recognized in adults in mid-1981. The number of reported cases of AIDS, representing those with the most advanced or severe manifestation of HIV infection, exceeded 140,000 in July 1990. Although the pediatric cases represent only 2% of the total reported cases, the projected number of children with AIDS within the next 2 to 3 years is between 6,000 and 20,000. At present, 80% of the pediatric cases are a result of vertical transmission from infected mothers.[13]

Diagnosis of HIV infection in young infants is problematic because of the passive acquisition of maternal antibodies during gestation. Thus, virtually all infants of HIV-seropositive women will be seropositive at birth. Although only about 30% of the infants will ultimately prove to be infected with HIV, those who are uninfected may retain maternal antibody for 15 to 18 months. Laboratory studies that help identify truly infected infants include viral culture and detection of HIV core antigen in serum. However, the former is costly, time-consuming, and not widely available, and the latter, though a specific technique for virus detection, has not been a sensitive technique for early detection of perinatal HIV infection. The technique that holds the most promise for early detection of perinatal infection is the polymerase chain reaction, which is capable of detecting minute amounts of HIV proviral deoxyribonucleic acid (DNA).[14]

The clinical picture of HIV infection in children differs in many ways from that in adults, particularly in the rate of disease progression. More than 50% of perinatally infected children will present with symptoms by 1 year of age, and 82% will be seen by 3 years of age. Lymphoid interstitial pneumonitis (LIP), which is rare in adults, is one of the most common AIDS-defining conditions in children, and HIV malignancies that are common in adults are unusual in children. In addition, because of higher normal values of CD4+ cells in young infants and children, the adult values cannot be used as prognostic markers of disease progression in children.[15]

Although some children with HIV infection present with nonspecific signs or symptoms (e.g., failure to thrive or chronic diarrhea), a significant number are hospitalized with life-threatening illnesses as their first presenting sign of HIV infection. In fact, a review of all children with AIDS admitted to a pediatric ICU in New York City revealed that the diagnosis of AIDS was made during the first ICU admission in 50% of the cases.[16]

The leading cause of admission to the ICU in children with HIV infection is acute respiratory failure (ARF), which is frequently secondary to PCP or severe bacterial pneumonia. Bacterial sepsis, with or without meningitis, is also a common presentation related to underlying immunodeficiency. Other infections that may be severe enough to require ICU management include infection with herpesviruses, rubeola, and respiratory viruses. HIV-related organ dysfunction (not involving secondary pathogens), including nephropathy, cardiomyopathy, hematologic and central nervous system abnormalities may be severe enough to require intensive care management (Table 73–1).[17] Many of these acute events may be superimposed on pre-existing medical problems, particularly those associated with premature birth (e.g., bronchopulmonary dysplasia, intraventricular hemorrhage).

Although the long-term prognosis of pediatric HIV infection remains poor, recent availability of antiretroviral therapy such as zidovudine (AZT) and other agents is likely to improve both the survival and the quality of

Table 73–1. INTENSIVE CARE UNIT ADMISSIONS IN CHILDREN LESS THAN 13 YEARS OF AGE WITH HUMAN IMMUNODEFICIENCY VIRUS INFECTION CHILDREN'S NATIONAL MEDICAL CENTER, WASHINGTON, DC 1989–1990 N = 19

Diagnosis	No. of Children
Pneumocystis carinii pneumonia	10
Bacterial sepsis	3
Candida pneumonia	1
Cardiomyopathy	1
Gastrointestinal bleeding	1
Necrotizing enterocolitis	1
Hypertension	1
Diabetes mellitus, diabetes insipidus	1

life of HIV-infected children. Aggressive management of acute illness is indicated, since many children may experience long, relatively asymptomatic periods.

This chapter will address major HIV-associated illnesses in children, with particular emphasis on infectious diseases and specifically on PCP, as this is one of the most common conditions prompting admission to the ICU. We will concentrate on disease presentation in young infants with vertical HIV infection, since they constitute the majority of pediatric AIDS patients and because their illness differs most from that of adults.

PNEUMOCYSTIS CARINII PNEUMONIA

In decades prior to the onset of the AIDS epidemic, PCP was an unusual disorder seen primarily in nutritionally deprived or congenitally immunodeficient infants. Although patients receiving chemotherapy for malignancies and organ transplant recipients also represent a significant at-risk population, in the 1980s patients with AIDS represented the vast majority of new cases of PCP. It is currently the most common opportunistic infection in pediatric AIDS patients[15] (Table 73-2), and it may be the first time that HIV-infected infants and children come to medical attention. The patients frequently require intensive care because of ARF; they present management problems both because of the natural history of the underlying disease and because of toxicities associated with antimicrobial therapy.

Microbiology and Epidemiology

Pneumocystis carinii (PC), recently classified among fungi, exists as a saprophyte in the lungs of humans and some animal species. Epidemiologic evidence suggests person to person transmission. Serologic studies indicate that most individuals are exposed to PC early in life.[17] This has led to the theory that overt clinical disease in immunosuppressed adults results from activation of latent infection; disease in young infants has generally been assumed to be a result of primary infection, which may account for its greater severity.

Table 73-2. AIDS DEFINING ILLNESS IN CHILDREN LESS THAN 13 YEARS OF AGE REPORTED BY CHILDREN'S NATIONAL MEDICAL CENTER, WASHINGTON, DC
(N = 50)

Diagnosis	No. of Cases (%)
Pneumocystis carinii pneumonia	22 (44)
Lymphoid interstitial pneumonitis	9 (18)
Bacterial infections	5 (10)
Encephalopathy	3 (6)
Mycobacterium avium, Mycobacterium intracellulare infection	3 (6)
Cytomegalovirus	2 (4)
Candida esophagitis	2 (4)
Cryptococcal infection	1 (2)
Kaposi sarcoma	1 (2)

Pathogenesis and Pathology

Although exposure to PC elicits an antibody response, humoral immunity is not protective. Cellular immunity appears to play a central role in resistance or susceptibility to this organism.

After gaining access to the lung, the organisms attach to the type 1 pneumocyte, propagate slowly, and gradually fill alveolar lumina. Diffuse alveolar damage occurs with a typical foamy exudate and interstitial edema, followed by interstitial inflammation and fibrosis.[18] The latter phenomenon may explain the beneficial effect of steroids as adjunctive therapy for PCP.

Clinical Features

Although in cancer patients PCP is often a rapidly progressive disease, the onset of symptoms in adult AIDS patients may be prolonged, occasionally as long as several days to weeks. Both ends of this spectrum are seen in pediatric AIDS patients. Typically, the history includes several days to weeks of cough and fever, followed by sudden rapid deterioration with increased hypoxia and severe respiratory distress. The median age at presentation in infants with vertical HIV infection is 5 months.[19] The patients typically manifest fever, tachypnea, dyspnea, and cough; flaring, retractions, and cyanosis may also be present. Lung auscultation is often unrevealing, especially early in the disease, with rales present in only one third of patients. Arterial blood gas determinations reveal hypoxemia with an elevated alveolar-arterial oxygen gradient; respiratory acidosis may ensue with progressive disease. Chest radiographs typically demonstrate bilateral diffuse alveolar disease beginning in the perihilar region and extending peripherally. However, the radiographic picture may vary from hyperinflation only (in early disease) to a "white out" compatible with adult respiratory distress syndrome. Peripheral leukocyte counts usually are not helpful; marked elevations of serum lactate dehydrogenase may occur, though this is not specific for pulmonary disease secondary to PC, nor does it occur in all infected children.

The differential diagnosis of diffuse bilateral pulmonary disease in HIV-infected children includes bacterial or mycobacterial disease; fungal, viral, chlamydial pneumonia; and LIP. The latter is a common cause of lung disease in pediatric AIDS patients and may be clinically distinguished by presentation at an older age, a more chronic course with minimal to mild hypoxemia, lack of fever, and the frequent presence of salivary gland enlargement, digital clubbing, and prominent lymphadenopathy. Chest radiographs in LIP reveal a reticulonodular rather than alveolar process, often accompanied by hilar lymphadenopathy.[20] Focal consolidation should suggest a bacterial process rather than PCP.

Diagnosis

Although in the past, open lung biopsy was often needed to confirm the diagnosis of PCP, the advent of fiberoptic bronchoscopy and BAL has allowed less invasive diagnostic methods.[21] The sensitivity of this procedure is on the order of 90%. In patients already intubated, comparable specimens may be obtained by passing a feeding tube through the endotracheal tube until it wedges in the small airways, followed by injection and aspiration of normal saline. Adequacy of such a specimen must be verified by the presence of alveolar macrophages on histologic examination. Obtaining induced sputum with nebulized hypertonic saline (3%) has been useful in uncomplicated cases of PCP in adults, with a sensitivity of 90%,[22] and has been reported to be effective in some pediatric patients.[23]

Specimens are stained by several methods, the most common of which is methenamine silver nitrate, which stains the cysts brownish black. This method will also stain fungal elements, which must be distinguished from PC organisms. Other stains include toluidine blue, which stains cysts blue, or Giemsa stain, which stains the trophozoite and sporozoite but not the cyst. Indirect fluorescent antibody staining may help increase sensitivity of detection, especially with induced sputum specimens.[17] Every attempt should be made to establish a definitive diagnosis of PCP.

Therapy

Treatment should be initiated at the first suspicion of PCP, even before BAL or other diagnostic procedures are performed, since a short course of treatment (up to 3 days) does not alter the diagnostic yield. If an adequate specimen obtained by BAL is negative for PCP, the therapy may be discontinued.

Trimethoprim-sulfamethoxazole is a first-line drug for treatment of PCP. The therapeutic dose is 20 mg of trimethoprim compound/kg/day, divided every 6 hours. The drug should be administered intravenously for at least the first 5 to 7 days at which time a change to the oral formulation may be considered in patients with rapid and complete response to therapy. The suggested length of therapy is 14 to 21 days (we use 21 days). It was recognized early in the AIDS epidemic that patients with PCP have a high rate of adverse reactions to trimethoprim-sulfamethoxazole. In our experience, the most frequent reactions necessitating discontinuation of therapy with trimethoprim-sulfamethoxazole in children are severe skin rash with fever, neutropenia, and hepatocellular damage.

Pentamidine is an alternate therapy to be used in children who do not respond to trimethoprim-sulfamethoxazole or who experience severe toxicity reactions. The recommended dose is 4 mg/kg/day administered once a day intravenously and given for 14 to 21 days. Pentamidine has its own potential life-threatening toxicity reactions, mainly hypotension, hypoglycemia (which usually occurs after repeated doses and may occur even after the therapy has been concluded), leukopenia, acute renal failure, and hypocalcemia. It is of note that two of our patients required admission to the ICU because of adverse reactions to pentamidine rather than because of PCP itself.

High mortality in acute episodes of PCP and high rates of adverse reactions to the available drugs indicate a need for the development of new therapies. There is only limited adult and virtually no pediatric experience with several newly tried drugs or drug combinations such as trimetrexate with leucovorin rescue, dapsone alone, or a dapsone-trimethoprim combination.[24]

It is typical for patients with PCP to show clinical progression with worsening hypoxemia for several days after hospitalization, despite appropriate antimicrobial therapy. Therefore, lack of response should not be considered a treatment failure until 4 to 5 days into therapy.

Recent evidence suggests that administration of steroids along with antimicrobial therapy may reduce morbidity and mortality, possibly by decreasing the host inflammatory response, as well as retarding the degradation of surfactant by phospholipase A_2. In several placebo-controlled trials, adult patients with moderate to severe PCP (defined as an alveolar-arterial oxygen gradient >35 mm Hg or PaO_2 less than 70 mm Hg on room air) who received steroids soon after initiation of antimicrobial therapy experienced significant decreases in both morbidity and mortality. These studies have led to the recommendation that adult patients with moderate to severe PCP, as defined, receive steroids within 72 hours of initiating anti-Pneumocystis therapy. The doses used in the largest trial were 40 mg of prednisone twice daily for 5 days, followed by 20 mg twice daily on days 6 to 10, and 20 mg/day until day 21. Adverse effects of steroid therapy included higher rates of thrush and herpes simplex virus (HSV) infection but no life-threatening events.[25] There is no comparable information about the efficacy of adjunctive steroid therapy in young children with PCP at this time. Concerns about steroid use in children include theoretical considerations regarding the pathogenesis of PCP in children (i.e., primary versus secondary infection) and fears of exacerbation of CMV pneumonia, as CMV is frequently a coexisting pathogen.

Secondary pathogens are frequent in children with ARF caused by PCP.[26] They include bacteria (S. pneumoniae, P. aeruginosa, Mycobacterium avium and M. intracellulare), viruses (CMV, parainfluenza virus), and fungi (Candida albicans). We have found the latter to be such a frequent complication in infants with PCP that we monitor the oral cavity closely and start ketoconazole (5 to 10 mg/kg/day in one oral dose) for thrush that is unresponsive to topical nystatin, particularly if there is obvious pharyngeal involvement. Ketoconazole is currently a drug of choice for Candida esophagitis or laryngitis. If the patient cannot be treated with an oral drug, if disease progression occurs, or if pulmonary candidiasis is diagnosed, amphotericin B (0.6 to 1 mg/kg/day administered intravenously over 4 to 6 hours) is indicated. There is no published pediatric experience with fluconazole, a new antifungal agent available in both oral and intravenous form. Vigorous attempts at diagnosis and therapy for secondary pathogens are necessary to further improve the prognosis of PCP in children.

In the ICU management of patients with PCP, careful

Table 73–3. MORTALITY IN CHILDREN WITH FIRST EPISODE OF *PNEUMOCYSTIS CARINII* PNEUMONIA

Reference	No. of Children with *Pneumocystis carinii* Pneumonia	No. of Deaths (%)	Comments
Bernstein, et al[27]	18	7 (39)	Children with perinatal HIV* infection (1983–1990)
Children's National Medical Center	25	6 (24)	Children with perinatal HIV infection (1986–1990)
	13	6 (46)	Children with acute respiratory failure (1986–1990)
Vernon et al[26]	13	11 (84)	Children with acute respiratory failure (1983–1986)
Bye, et al[56]	34	17 (50)	Children with acute respiratory failure (1985–1989)

*HIV = human immunodeficiency virus.

attention should be given to fluid management: Severely hypoxemic patients with PCP have global ST and T wave changes on electrocardiography, reflecting myocardial ischemia. Therefore, fluid overload may precipitate left ventricular failure. Respiratory support beyond mere administration of supplemental oxygen is often needed. The use of continuous positive airway pressure may obviate the need for mechanical ventilation in some less severely ill patients.

Prophylaxis

Availability of efficacious prophylaxis for PCP is crucial in view of the high morbidity and mortality associated with the disease. Prophylactic regimens previously established in cancer patients are effective in HIV-infected individuals as well. Regimens widely used in adults include intermittent oral trimethoprim-sulfamethoxazole or monthly aerosol pentamidine therapy.[24] Trimethoprim-sulfamethoxazole is effective for PCP prophylaxis in children and young infants. The recommended dose is 75 mg trimethoprim/m^2/dose administered twice daily by mouth on 3 consecutive days of the week. Dapsone (1 mg/kg/day in one or two doses given daily) is an alternative prophylactic regimen recently recommended in children. Pentamidine aerosol (300 to 400 mg monthly via nebulizer) is an alternative for children older than 5 years who do not tolerate trimethoprim-sulfamethoxazole. We and others have used pentamidine in the dose of 4 mg/kg administered intravenously once or twice a month in children who do not tolerate trimethoprim-sulfamethoxazole and are too young to cooperate with delivery via nebulizer. The most recent indications for initiation of PCP prophylaxis in HIV-infected or HIV-seropositive children are based on CD4+ cell counts.[28]

Prognosis

Although there are still limited data on the natural history of HIV infection in children, accumulating evidence suggests that those who present with opportunistic infections have particularly poor survival.[19] For example, those children presenting with their first episode of PCP

frequently have mortality rates much more than 30%.[27] In addition, patients who suffer respiratory failure have a particularly poor prognosis. Patients ventilated for reasons other than ARF (e.g., after surgical procedures) do not have extraordinary mortality rates.[54] However, pediatric ICU mortality rates for patients with HIV infection and ARF have been reported to be as high as 84%.[26] Although many of these patients had PCP alone, many had serious bacterial or viral infections or PCP with a copathogen. Although other studies have shown slightly better pediatric ICU survival (44%), as many as 50% of discharged patients died within 6 months.[55] The contribution of PCP alone to mortality is difficult to discern in these studies; one series reviewing only patients with ARF caused by PCP noted a 50% mortality rate.[56] Our experience is comparable, with a 46% mortality rate among children with ARF caused by PCP (Table 73–3). Although firm data are lacking, it is hoped that improved survival may be achieved with the greater use of antiretroviral agents and new adjunctive therapies—for example, steroids for PCP.

HUMAN HERPESVIRUS INFECTIONS

Herpesvirus infections, particularly those caused by HSV, varicella zoster virus (VZV), and CMV, are responsible for considerable morbidity and mortality in adults with HIV infection but are less frequent in young children, most likely because of a lack of exposure. However, in children who do become infected, the primary infection is often severe.

Herpes Simplex Virus

Severe disseminated HSV infection occurs in newborns and severely immunocompromised individuals and, rarely, in otherwise-normal immunocompetent children.[29] The clinical picture most frequently seen in HIV-infected children is a herpetic gingivostomatitis, which is often recurrent and is unlikely to lead to admission to the ICU. More serious illnesses such as HSV esophagitis, pneumonia, encephalitis, and disseminated disease are less frequent.

The diagnosis depends on a demonstration of HSV in

the involved organ by histologic examination, culture results, immunofluorescence, or nucleic acid hybridization. Recovery of HSV from the throat culture specimen of an immunocompromised patient does not constitute proof of its etiologic role in systemic infection.

Standard therapy for severe disease is parenteral acyclovir (10 mg/kg/dose, administered intravenously every 8 hours) given for 10 days. Less severe mucocutaneous manifestations may be managed with oral acyclovir, which has recently become available in a syrup formulation (doses 100 to 200 mg given five times a day).

Varicella Zoster Virus

Primary VZV infection may be life-threatening in immunocompromised individuals. It has been suggested by Jura and coworkers[30] that children infected with HIV are at risk for severe VZV infection as well. They described the outcome of chickenpox in eight children with severely symptomatic HIV infection. All eight children experienced a systemic dissemination of VZV infection. All were treated with acyclovir. Two children recovered, five children experienced chronic or recurrent VZV infection, or both, and one child died. Secondary bacterial infection with sepsis occurred in four children.

Diagnosis of VZV infection depends on a recognition of typical vesicular skin lesions, history of exposure and, when feasible, on the demonstration of the virus in the lesions.

Because of the potential severity of the disease, and because of diminished effectiveness of therapy started after systemic dissemination has occurred, we recommend that children with low CD4+ cell counts or severe HIV infection (i.e., AIDS), or both, be treated with parenteral acyclovir (500 mg/m^2/dose administered every 8 hours intravenously) as soon as the diagnosis of chickenpox is made. The usual course of therapy is 10 days, but longer treatment may be necessary if new lesions continue to form. In addition, considering the high reported incidence of bacterial superinfection, broad-spectrum antibiotic therapy must be considered, particularly in children who continue to be febrile while receiving acyclovir.

Severity and poor outcome of primary VZV disease in immunocompromised children argue in favor of prophylactic therapy. Passive immunization with varicella zoster immune globulin should be used in susceptible HIV-infected children after an exposure to chickenpox. The dose of 125 units/10 kg body weight (maximum 500 to 625 units) is administered IM as soon as possible after the exposure (i.e., within 72 hours, not later than 96 hours).

Cytomegalovirus

CMV disease is seen less frequently in HIV-infected young infants and children than in adults, but severe disseminated CMV infection with pancarditis,[31] CMV pneumonia,[29] chorioretinitis leading to blindness,[32] progressive encephalopathy,[33] and enterocolitis with gastrointestinal bleeding[34] or bowel obstruction[35] have all been described. CMV pneumonia and gastrointestinal involvement are most likely to result in admission to the ICU.

Diagnosis depends on recovery of the virus from the blood or the involved organs, demonstration of typical CMV-infected cells on histologic examination, or detection of CMV antigen or nucleic acid by immunofluorescence or nucleic acid hybridization, respectively. Diagnosis of CMV chorioretinitis can be established by ophthalmologic examination.[29] The recovery of CMV from cultures of throat and urine specimens, though suggestive, particularly in a child previously known not to be infected with CMV, is not by itself a proof of a causative role of CMV in systemic illness, and other causes of pneumonia, encephalitis, or hepatitis, or all of these, must be sought and excluded.

The treatment of CMV infection is not satisfactory. Ganciclovir is approved for use in adults and has been used in a limited number of children.[29] The initial dose for acute treatment of severe disease is 5 mg/kg/dose, administered twice a day for 14 to 21 days. Following induction treatment, maintenance therapy (5 mg/kg/dose once a day for 7 days or 6 mg/kg/dose once a day for 5 days of each week) is necessary. Relapses or progression of the CMV disease may occur while the patient is receiving maintenance therapy. The most frequent side effects are neutropenia and thrombocytopenia, which may present a problem particularly in children receiving other bone marrow–suppressive drugs such as AZT or trimethoprim-sulfamethoxazole. The role of other antiviral compounds, such as high-doses of acyclovir and foscarnet, and of high-titer anti-CMV immune globulins in the treatment of CMV disease in children with AIDS needs to be explored.

RESPIRATORY VIRUSES

The literature on the frequency and severity of respiratory viral infections in HIV-infected children is sparse. The immune mechanisms responsible for protection and recovery from viral infections are complex and poorly understood. In addition, there has been speculation that immune mechanisms may play a role in the pathogenesis of disease (e.g., respiratory syncytial virus [RSV]). Therefore, the response of HIV-infected patients to viral pathogens is difficult to predict. However, morbidity and mortality are increased in other immunocompromised children, and limited data suggest that extrapolation of this experience to HIV-infected children may be reasonable.

Respiratory Syncytial Virus

RSV is the most common cause of lower respiratory tract infection in infants and occurs in predictable yearly epidemics. Although mortality in otherwise normal infants is low, patients with underlying cardiac, pulmonary, or immunodeficiency disease suffer excessive morbidity and mortality. These patients also tend to demonstrate prolonged viral shedding.[36]

In a small series of 10 HIV-infected children with RSV, the frequency of pneumonia was no different from that in non–HIV-infected controls (50%).[37] However, the majority required therapy with ribavirin, and prolonged viral shedding (up to 90 days) was demonstrated. Bacterial superinfection was present more often than would be expected in immunocompetent children with RSV. Two of 10 patients died, though both of these patients also had PC infection. Interestingly, wheezing was unusual in the HIV-infected children as compared with the otherwise healthy controls with RSV. This raises the possibility, suggested in other studies, that immune mechanisms may be in part responsible for bronchiolar injury and hyperreactivity in RSV infection.

The only drug approved for the treatment of RSV infection is ribavirin. The American Academy of Pediatrics guidelines suggest considering ribavirin use in immunocompromised children.[38] The usual daily dose is 6 g administered via aerosol over 12 to 18 hours. Duration is based on clinical course, which is usually at least 3 days. Although problems may be encountered with administration in ventilated patients, proper use and maintenance of ventilator equipment and endotracheal tube suctioning should circumvent problems with blockage of valves or tubing.

Another therapeutic approach that has been investigated is the use of IVIG with high neutralizing antibody titers to RSV.[39] A larger multicenter trial is currently in progress in an attempt to verify these results.

Other Viruses

Parainfluenza viruses (PIVs) are the second most frequent cause of lower respiratory tract illness in infants and children. Prolonged excretion of PIV 3 has been documented in HIV-infected children and may be found in association with other pathogens, including *Pneumocystis*.[40] Severe disease caused by PIV 3 has been described in children with SCID,[41] and ribavirin has been used in other immunocompromised children.[42]

There is little information on the severity of influenza in HIV-infected children. However, they might be expected to do poorly because of both underlying lung disease (as already noted) and immunodeficiency. Patients who have pneumonia attributed to influenza may be treated with amantadine (for influenza A only) 4.4 to 8.8 mg/kg/day (max. of 200 mg/day) orally in two divided doses. Ribavirin is also efficacious in the treatment of both influenza A and influenza B. Although efficacy is uncertain, prevention of influenza should be attempted through yearly vaccination.

Measles

Although rubeola is not strictly a respiratory virus, some of its most severe manifestations are pulmonary because of either viral pneumonitis or bacterial super-

infection. Six cases of measles in HIV-infected children have been reported in the United States, and giant cell pneumonia occurred in five of these patients. Three patients had delayed, atypical, or no rash. Two patients died of pneumonia, emphasizing the risk of severe disease in HIV-infected children.[43] Ribavirin may be used for the treatment of viral pneumonitis, though its efficacy is unproved. Prevention is desirable through the use of live vaccine (measles, mumps, rubella) in HIV-infected patients, as well as passive immunoglobulin prophylaxis if exposure to rubeola occurs.

BACTERIAL INFECTIONS

Children with HIV infection experience an increased frequency of serious bacterial infections compared with children who are not infected with HIV.

Clinical Presentation and Microbiologic Features

Bacteremia is one of the most commonly encountered infections in HIV-infected children. Although a search for a focus of infection (including meningitis) is paramount, many patients have no obvious source.[44] *S. pneumoniae* is the most frequent isolate with or without a primary source. *H. influenzae* type b sepsis may also occur without a focus. Patients with *Salmonella* bacteremia generally manifest gastrointestinal symptoms. Relapse after antibiotic therapy is common in these patients. Although these are the most frequent pathogens in community-acquired bacteremia, HIV-infected patients who have indwelling catheters for hyperalimentation or administration of medications are at risk for infection from multiple opportunistic pathogens, including staphylococcal species, gram-negative organisms including *Pseudomonas*, and fungal agents. Prolonged use of oral antibiotics also predisposes the patient to superinfection with these agents.[45]

The most frequent focal bacterial infection identified in HIV-infected children is pneumonia. *S. pneumoniae* is again the most common agent, though *H. influenzae*, gram-negative enteric agents, and *Pseudomonas* are also frequently implicated. Although chest radiographs revealing lobar infiltrates are most compatible with bacterial pneumonia, these agents may also cause patchy or diffuse infiltrates. In the latter case, coexisting pathogens, especially *Pneumocystis* or viruses, should also be sought. In our experience, *Mycoplasma pneumoniae* is commonly isolated from throat swabs; there is very little data on the contribution of *Mycoplasma* to morbidity in these patients.

Urinary tract infections in HIV-infected children, as in otherwise normal children, are most frequently caused by *Escherichia coli*, followed by *Klebsiella*, *Enterobacter*, enterococci, and *Pseudomonas*.

Skin and soft tissue infections, especially cellulitis, lymphadenitis, and wound infections are most often caused by *S. aureus*.

Therapy

Because of the wide range of potential bacterial pathogens affecting HIV-infected children, the importance of aggressive pursuit of a definitive diagnosis and identification of the causative agent cannot be overemphasized. While cultures and diagnostic studies are pending, the initial presumptive antimicrobial therapy must be individualized according to the risk factor and severity of HIV-associated diseases. In cases of suspected bacteremia and pneumonia that are community acquired, empirical therapy for *Pneumococcus* and *Haemophilus* should be initiated. In a child with a central line or with fulminant sepsis suggesting gram-negative organisms, broad-spectrum therapy should be employed with vancomycin and either an aminoglycoside or third-generation cephalosporin. If *Pseudomonas* is suspected, ceftazidime should be used. Therapy for suspected urinary tract infections should be directed toward gram-negative organisms (aminoglycosides). Therapy for enterococci requires ampicillin or vancomycin. For skin and soft tissue infections, a semisynthetic penicillin (e.g., nafcillin or oxacillin) should be employed, though hospital-acquired wound infections may require more broad-spectrum therapy pending culture results.

Prevention

A multicenter trial of the efficacy of IVIG in prevention of bacterial infections in children with HIV infection has recently been concluded.[46] The study has clearly shown the beneficial effect of IVIG (400 mg/kg/dose, administered once a month IV) in decreasing the frequency of severe bacterial infections in children who entered the study with a CD4+ cell count greater than 200/mm^3. Vaccination may help to prevent some of the more common bacterial illnesses in these children. *H. influenzae*, type b conjugate vaccine is licensed for use beginning at 2 months of age with subsequent doses at 4, 6, and 15 months of age. Polyvalent pneumococcal vaccine elicits little response until the patient is 2 years of age but should be given as a single dose at that age.

CARDIOVASCULAR MANIFESTATIONS

Advances in noninvasive techniques of cardiac evaluation have allowed detection of cardiac abnormalities in a significant number of HIV-infected patients, though these abnormalities are not always clinically significant. Echocardiographic studies of children with HIV infection have demonstrated abnormalities in as many as 64[47] to 93%[48] of HIV-infected children. Evidence of left ventricular dysfunction is common, especially in patients with more symptomatic HIV disease.[48] Right ventricular dysfunction generally occurs only in association with left ventricular dysfunction and following repeated pulmonary infections.[49] Sterile pericardial effusions are present in as many as one quarter of patients, though tamponade is rare.[48] Electrocardiographic abnormalities are present in a large majority of patients. One series noted ventricular tachycardia in 10% of patients; the majority of these patients had hyperdynamic changes on the echocardiogram.[48] Cases of sudden unexpected death have occurred, implying the possibility of fatal dysrhythmias.

Clinical Considerations

Although rarely a presenting sign of HIV infection, cardiomyopathy with congestive heart failure (CHF) was eventually apparent in 14% of all patients in one retrospective review.[50] In another series, 20% of children with AIDS (and therefore those with the most advanced HIV disease) had CHF.[51] Symptomatic cardiac disease frequently presented at about 1½ years of age. Although the patients responded to medical management with inotropic support and diuretic therapy, long-term survival was poor.

Diagnosis of cardiac dysfunction without echocardiographic studies is often difficult. Hepatomegaly is a frequent pre-existing condition, adventitial breath sounds may be present because of pulmonary infections, and tachycardia may be a result of fever. In these circumstances, the emergence of an S3 gallop may be the only specific sign suggesting CHF. Chest radiographs also may be noncontributory, and creatine phosphokinase levels are usually normal.[51] Therefore, echocardiography becomes an important tool in the evaluation of any HIV-infected patient who presents with respiratory distress, and many centers consider serial cardiac evaluations (e.g., every 6 to 12 months) part of the routine care of HIV-infected children.

Treatment

At present, the management of HIV-related cardiac dysfunction centers primarily on symptomatic therapy with inotropic support (digoxin), diuretics, and occasionally afterload reduction with captopril. The rare instances of cardiac disease related to opportunistic pathogens may require specific antimicrobial therapy (e.g., ganciclovir for CMV). It is currently too early to gauge the role of antiretroviral therapy in the evolution of HIV-related cardiac disease.

HEMATOLOGIC MANIFESTATIONS

A number of hematologic abnormalities are seen in pediatric patients with HIV infection, both as a result of HIV infection per se and as a result of multiple medications, including antiretroviral therapy. Anemia associated with HIV infection is usually normocytic and normochromic. AZT therapy frequently causes a macrocytic anemia. Anemia is remediable with transfusion and does not require ICU management except in rare cases of severe hemolytic anemia. Neutropenia is also a frequent finding, and if severe (absolute neutrophil count less than 500/mm^3) may contribute to morbidity and mortality by increasing the risk of bacterial and fungal sepsis.

Coagulation defects are potentially the most dangerous of the hematologic disorders associated with HIV infection. Thrombocytopenia is common and in an acutely ill immunosuppressed child frequently represents bacterial sepsis with accompanying disseminated intravascular coagulation. Such children will have both thrombocytopenia and abnormal coagulation profiles, as well as fragmented red blood cells.

In contrast, isolated thrombocytopenia may be the initial manifestation of HIV disease in some children and ultimately occurs in at least 13% of children with symptomatic infection. Although severe bleeding is unusual in HIV-infected adults with isolated thrombocytopenia, life-threatening gastrointestinal and central nervous system hemorrhages were reported in 6 of 19 patients in one pediatric series.[52]

Treatment modalities for isolated thrombocytopenia have included the use of IVIG and steroids. A regimen of IVIG, 500 to 1,000 mg/kg on five consecutive days resulted in platelet increases in 40% of patients in one series.[52] Of those who failed to respond or those who relapsed, 71% responded to oral prednisone, 1.5 to 2 mg/kg/day for at least 2 weeks. With the availability of antiretroviral therapy, many patients respond to AZT therapy with increased platelet counts, emphasizing the primary role of HIV in this disorder.

In addition to quantitative defects, qualitative defects of platelets may be present as a result of immune complexes coating the membrane of platelets or secondary to any number of medications, such as β-lactam antibiotics and systemic H_2 antagonists. The functional defects are manifested by prolonged bleeding time in patients with normal platelet counts.

Abnormal coagulation profiles caused by circulating anticoagulant may be seen in pediatric patients with AIDS, usually manifested as normal prothrombin time with an activated partial thromboplastin time that is prolonged, sometimes as long as 50 to 60 seconds.[53] Although the presence of this anticoagulant and consequent prolongation of the activated partial thromboplastin time does not usually result in clinical bleeding, it is quite important to distinguish this profile from that caused by disseminated intravascular coagulation or coagulopathy from liver dysfunction.

Thrombocytopenia and functional platelet defects not only may cause spontaneous bleeding but also may exacerbate bleeding from trauma (especially mucosal bleeding) or infectious diseases—for example, CMV or antibiotic-associated colitis caused by Clostridium difficile. Therefore, patients who manifest severe bleeding should have a careful evaluation for coagulation defects.

Therapeutic Considerations

Management of coagulopathy and blood loss in HIV-infected patients involves the judicious use of replacement blood products. If possible, CMV-negative blood should be used in previously CMV-negative patients, inasmuch as transfusion-acquired CMV may cause significant disease in compromised hosts. Patients with significant HIV-related thrombocytopenia should receive AZT, and those who do not respond to antiretroviral therapy should receive a trial of IVIG, as outlined previously.

ANTIRETROVIRAL THERAPY

As in adults, the use of AZT has resulted in significant gains in the management of pediatric HIV infection. Clinical and laboratory improvement has been demonstrated in HIV-infected children receiving AZT.[57, 58] The standard dose at present is 180 mg/m²/dose given orally every 6 hours. In an ICU setting in which the use of oral medication may not be feasible, IV AZT can be given; because the bioavailability of oral AZT is 60 to 70%, roughly one half to two thirds of the oral dose may be given IV. Toxicity is primarily hematologic; anemia and neutropenia usually resolve with reduced dosage or temporary discontinuation. Myositis also occurs occasionally. It is important to carefully monitor hematologic parameters in patients receiving AZT who may also be receiving other marrow-suppressive drugs, such as trimethoprim-sulfamethoxazole or ganciclovir.

Dideoxyinosine has been investigated in children who are intolerant to AZT or whose disease is progressing while receiving AZT therapy. Again, clinical and laboratory improvement has been noted.[59] The major dose-limiting toxicity was pancreatitis, requiring drug discontinuation in two patients. Asymptomatic elevations in amylase may also be seen. Peripheral neuropathy has been seen in adults. Dideoxycytidine provides another alternative to AZT; children receiving a short trial of dideoxycytidine have shown improvement.[60] In adults, dose-limiting problems with dideoxycytidine have been painful peripheral neuropathy and occasional pancreatitis. Some children receiving this agent also had difficulty with oral ulcers and rashes. No definitive therapeutic dose for these agents has yet been established, but therapy is available at this point on protocol and compassionate release basis. Because the toxicities of dideoxycytidine and dideoxyinosine versus AZT do not overlap, it is hoped that alternating regimens will decrease overall toxicity and prolong clinical response, theoretically by retarding emergence of viral resistance.

References

1. Wilfert CM, Buckley RH, Mohanakumar T, et al: Persistent and fatal central nervous system echovirus infections in patients with agammaglobulinemia. N Engl J Med 296:1485, 1977.
2. Wright PF, Hatch MH, Kasselberg AG, et al: Vaccine-associated poliomyelitis in a child with sex-linked agammaglobulinemia. J Pediatr 91:408, 1977.
3. Buckley RH and Dees SC: Correlation of milk precipitins with IgA deficiency. N Engl J Med 281:465, 1969.
4. Apfelzweig R, Piszkiewicz D, and Hooper JA: Immunoglobulin A concentrations in commercial immunoglobulins. J Clin Immunol 7:46, 1987.
5. Ellison RT, Kohler PF, Curd JG, et al: Prevalence of congenital or acquired complement deficiency in patients with sporadic meningococcal disease. N Engl J Med 308:913, 1983.
6. Schalch DS, McFarlin DE, and Barlow MH: An unusual form of diabetes mellitus in ataxia-telangiectasia. N Engl J Med 282:1396, 1976.

7. Griscom NT, Kirkpatrick JA, Girdany BR, et al: Gastric antral narrowing in chronic granulomatous disease of childhood. Pediatrics 54:456, 1974.
8. Weening RS, Kabel P, Pizman P, et al: Continuous therapy with sulfamethoxazole-trimethoprim in patients with chronic granulomatous disease. J Pediatr 103:127, 1983.
9. Wright DG, Robichaud KJ, Pizzo PA, et al: Lethal pulmonary reactions associated with the combined use of amphotericin B and leukocyte transfusions. N Engl J Med 304:1185, 1981.
10. Giblett ER, Klebanoff SJ, Pincers SH, et al: Kell phenotypes in chronic granulomatous disease: A potential transfusion hazard. Lancet 1:1235, 1971.
11. Weening RS, Schoorel EP, van Schaik ML, et al: Effect of ascorbate on abnormal neutrophil, platelet, and lymphocyte function in a patient with Chédiak-Higashi syndrome. Blood 57:856, 1981.
12. Kirchner SG, Sivit CJ, and Wright PF: Hyperimmunoglobulin E syndrome: Association with osteoporosis and recurrent fractures. Radiology 156:362, 1985.
13. Oxtoby MJ: Perinatally acquired HIV infection. In: Pizzo PA and Wilfert CM (eds): Pediatric AIDS. Baltimore, Williams & Wilkins, 1991, pp. 3–21.
14. Rakusan TA, Parrott RH, and Sever JL: Limitations in the laboratory diagnosis of vertically acquired HIV infection. J AIDS 4:2, 1991.
15. Falloon J, Eddy J, Wiener L, et al: Human immunodeficiency virus infection in children. J Pediatr 114:1, 1989.
16. Wilkinson JD and Greenwald BM: The acquired immunodeficiency syndrome: Impact on the pediatric intensive care unit. Crit Care Clin 4:831, 1988.
17. Hughes WT: Pneumocystis carinii pneumonia. In: Pizzo PA and Wilfert CM (eds): Pediatric AIDS. Baltimore, Williams & Wilkins, 1991, pp. 288–298.
18. Joshi VV, Oleske JM, Minnefor AB, et al: Pathologic pulmonary findings in children with the acquired immunodeficiency syndrome: A study of ten cases. Hum Pathol 16:241, 1985.
19. Scott GB, Hutto C, Makuch RW, et al: Survival in children with perinatally acquired human immunodeficiency virus type 1 infection. N Engl J Med 321:1791, 1989.
20. Rubinstein A, Morecki R, Silverman B, et al: Pulmonary disease in children with acquired immunodeficiency syndrome and AIDS-related complex. J Pediatr 108:498, 1986.
21. Bye MR, Bernstein L, Shah K, et al: Diagnostic bronchoalveolar lavage in children with AIDS. Pediatr Pulmonol 3:425, 1987.
22. Leigh TR, Hume C, Gazzard B, et al: Sputum induction for diagnosis of Pneumocystis carinii pneumonia. Lancet 2:205, 1989.
23. Ognibene FP, Gill VJ, Pizzo PA, et al: Induced sputum to diagnose Pneumocystis carinii pneumonia in immunosuppressed pediatric patients. J Pediatr 115:430, 1989.
24. Fischl MA: Treatment and prophylaxis of Pneumocystis carinii pneumonia. AIDS 2 (Suppl 1):S143, 1988.
25. Consensus statement on the use of corticosteroids as adjunctive therapy for Pneumocystis pneumonia in the acquired immunodeficiency syndrome. N Engl J Med 323:1500, 1990.
26. Vernon DD, Holzman BH, Lewis F, et al: Respiratory failure in children with acquired immunodeficiency syndrome and acquired immunodeficiency syndrome–related complex. Pediatrics 82:223, 1988.
27. Bernstein L, Bye MR, and Rubinstein A: Prognostic factors and life expectancy in children with acquired immunodeficiency syndrome and Pneumocystis carinii pneumonia. Am J Dis Child 143:775, 1989.
28. Centers for Disease Control: Guidelines for prophylaxis of Pneumocystis pneumonia in children with HIV infection. MMWR 40, RR-2:1, 1991.
29. Bryson Y and Arvin A: Herpes group virus infections in HIV-1-infected infants, children and adolescents. In: Pizzo PA and Wilfert CM (eds): Pediatric AIDS. Baltimore, Williams & Wilkins, 1991, pp. 245–265.
30. Jura E, Chadiwick EG, Josephs SH, et al: Varicella-zoster virus infections in children infected with human immunodeficiency virus. Pediatr Infect Dis J 8:586, 1989.
31. Brady MT, Reinier CB, Singley C, et al: Unexpected death in an infant with AIDS: Disseminated cytomegalovirus infection with pancarditis. Pediatr Pathol 8:205, 1988.
32. Levin AV, Zeichner S, Duker JS, et al: Cytomegalovirus retinitis

33. Curless RG, Scott GB, Post MJ, et al: Progressive cytomegalovirus encephalopathy following congenital infection in an infant with acquired immunodeficiency syndrome. Child Nerv Syst 3:255, 1987.
34. Sivit CJ, Taylor GA, Patterson K, et al: Bowel obstruction in an infant with AIDS. Am J Radiol 154:803, 1990.
35. Schwartz DL, So HB, Bungarz WR, et al: A case of life-threatening gastrointestinal hemorrhage in an infant with AIDS. J Pediatr Surg 24:313, 1989.
36. Hall CB, Powell KR, MacDonald NE, et al: Respiratory syncytial virus infection in children with compromised immune function. N Engl J Med 315:77, 1986.
37. Chandwani S, Borkowsky W, Krasinsky K, et al: Respiratory syncytial virus infection in HIV-infected children. J Pediatr 117:251, 1990.
38. Committee on Infectious Diseases: Ribavirin therapy of respiratory syncytial virus. Pediatrics 79:475, 1987.
39. Hemming VG, Rodriguez W, Kim HW, et al: Intravenous immunoglobulin therapy of respiratory syncytial virus infection in infants and young children. Antimicrob Agents Chemother 31:1882, 1987.
40. Josephs S, Kim HW, Brandt CS, et al: Parainfluenza 3 virus and other common respiratory pathogens in children with human immunodeficiency virus infection. Pediatr Infect Dis J 7:207, 1988.
41. Jarvis WR, Middleton PJ, and Gelfand EW: Parainfluenza pneumonia in severe combined immunodeficiency. J Pediatr 94:423, 1979.
42. Herzog KD, Dunn SP, Langham MR, et al: Association of parainfluenza virus type 3 infection with allograft rejection in a liver transplant recipient. Pediatr Infect Dis J 8:534, 1989.
43. Krasinsky K and Borkowsky W: Measles and measles immunity in children infected with human immunodeficiency virus. JAMA 261:2512, 1989.
44. Krasinsky K, Borkowsky W, Bonk S, et al: Bacterial infections in human immunodeficiency virus infected children. Pediatr Infect Dis J 7:323, 1988.
45. Bernstein LJ, Krieger BZ, Novick B, et al: Bacterial infection in the acquired immunodeficiency syndrome of children. Pediatr Infect Dis J 4:472, 1985.
46. NICHD Intravenous Immunoglobulin Study Group: Efficacy of intravenous immunoglobulin for the prophylaxis of serious bacterial infections in symptomatic human immunodeficiency virus-infected children. N Engl J Med 325:73, 1991.
47. Isenberg HJ, Charytan M, and Rubinstein A: Cardiac involvement in children with acquired immune deficiency (Abstract). Am Heart J 110:710, 1985.
48. Lipschultz SE, Chanock S, Sanders SP, et al: Cardiovascular manifestations of human immunodeficiency virus infection in infants and children. Am J Cardiol 63:1489, 1989.
49. Sherron P, Pickoff AS, Ferrer PL, et al: Echocardiographic evaluation of myocardial function in pediatric AIDS patients. Am Heart J 110:710, 1985.
50. Stewart JM, Kaul A, Gromisch DS, et al: Symptomatic cardiac dysfunction in children with human immunodeficiency virus infection. Am Heart J 117:140, 1989.
51. Bharati S, Joshi V, Connor EM, et al: Conduction system in children with acquired immune deficiency syndrome. Chest 96:406, 1989.
52. Ellaurie M, Burns ER, Bernstein LJ, et al: Thrombocytopenia and human immunodeficiency virus in children. Pediatrics 82:905, 1988.
53. Burns ER, Krieger B, Bernstein L, et al: Acquired circulating anticoagulants in children with acquired immunodeficiency syndrome. Pediatrics 82:763, 1988.
54. Notterman DA, Greenwald BM, Di Majo-Hunter A, et al: Outcome after assisted ventilation in children with acquired immunodeficiency syndrome. Crit Care Med 18:18, 1990.
55. Marolda J, Pace B, Bonforte RJ, et al: Outcome of mechanical ventilation in children with acquired immunodeficiency syndrome. Pediatr Pulmonol 7:230, 1989.
56. Bye MR, Bernstein LJ, Glaser J, et al: Pneumocystis carinii pneumonia in young children with AIDS. Pediatr Pulmonol 9:251, 1990.

in an infant with acquired immunodeficiency syndrome. Pediatrics 84:683, 1989.

57. Pizzo PA, Eddy J, Falloon J, et al: Effect of continuous intravenous infusion of zidovudine (AZT) in children with symptomatic HIV infection. N Engl J Med 319:889, 1988.
58. McKinney RE, Pizzo PA, Scott GB, et al: Safety and tolerance of intermittent intravenous and oral zidovudine therapy in human immunodeficiency virus-infected pediatric patients. J Pediatr 116:640, 1990.
59. Butler KM, Husson RN, Balis FM, et al: Dideoxyinosine in children with symptomatic human immunodeficiency virus infection. N Engl J Med 324:137, 1991.
60. Pizzo PA, Butler K, Balis F, et al: Dideoxycytidine alone and in an alternating schedule with zidovudine in children with symptomatic human immunodeficiency virus infection. J Pediatr 117:799, 1990.

VI Pharmacology

74

Pharmacokinetics-Pharmacodynamics: Drug Delivery and Therapeutic Drug Monitoring

Gregory M. Susla, Pharm.D., and
Roger E. Dionne, Pharm.D.

This chapter is intended to provide an overview of developmental pharmacology in terms of the age-related changes in pharmacokinetics and pharmacodynamics seen in the pediatric patient. Clinical pharmacology and therapeutic principles governing the use of individual agents in treating various diseases will be covered in specific organ failure–related sections.

Applied clinical pharmacokinetics is concerned with a drug's concentration versus time relationship, occurring in an individual patient in a variety of disease-related conditions. Pharmacodynamics is, in turn, an examination of the resultant pharmacologic response achieved by various serum drug concentrations—in other words, the sensitivity, or lack thereof, of an individual patient to a drug at an observed serum concentration.

Both pharmacokinetic and pharmacodynamic responses are highly variable and are affected by the age and degree of maturation of the pediatric patient. In general, the youngest child will demonstrate the most significant alterations. However, a multiplicity of factors, all maturing at varying rates, results in a wide variety of potential responses. Subpopulations within the pediatric age group are essentially created, each with different dosing requirements. For the sake of clarity and uniformity, the definitions and terminology shown in Table 74–1 will be used throughout this chapter.

PHARMACOKINETIC ALTERATIONS

The absorption, distribution, metabolism, and elimination of any compound determines the drug concentration that reaches a targeted tissue or organ. Differences

in these factors in many compounds have been observed in preterm and full-term neonates, infants, and older children.

Kinetically, the combination of elimination half-life and volume of distribution is referred to as clearance and ultimately determines the steady state serum concentration achieved. The distribution pattern of a drug is determined primarily by body composition, protein binding, and a number of drug-specific characteristics such as molecular size, ionic charge, and hydro- and lipophilicity. Although related to distribution volume, the total body clearance of most drugs is determined by renal and hepatic function.

Absorption

Gastrointestinal Physiology

Most drugs are absorbed from the gastrointestinal (GI) tract by passive diffusion. The two most important

Table 74–1. PEDIATRIC TERMINOLOGY AND AGE RANGES

Premature: less than 38 weeks' gestation
Full term: between 38 and 42 weeks' gestation
Neonate: less than 1 mo of postnatal age
  Postnatal age: birth to present age
  Gestational age: duration of pregnancy
  Postconceptional age: time since conception (postnatal and gestational age)
Infant: less than 12 months of age
Child: less than 10 years of age
Adolescent: between 10 and 18 years of age
Adult: greater than 18 years of age

932

factors governing GI absorption are gastric pH and gastric and intestinal motility. Both are quite variable and undergo continuous maturational changes during the first several months of life. Other miscellaneous factors that influence the rate and extent of drug absorption include gastric contents, microbial bowel colonization, enzymatic activity, and biliary function.

Gastric pH. At birth, the gastric pH is close to neutral. Within minutes, acid secretion begins and gradually increases so that the gastric pH decreases to a level of 1 to 3 within hours. Gastric acidity then decreases within 24 to 48 hours and remains low during the first several weeks of life. Preterm newborns have impaired acid secretory mechanisms and may not demonstrate this early decrease in gastric pH.

In both preterm and full-term newborns, basal acid output (BAO) and maximal acid output (MAO) are approximately equal.[1, 2] Both are lower than seen in adults, being approximately one third to one half as active on a per-kilogram basis. Gastric acid secretion increases over the first 3 to 4 weeks of life, correlating with postnatal age rather than postconceptional age.[1] MAO improves slowly so that by 1 year of age, it is only twofold greater than BAO. During the second year of life, MAO increases more rapidly, and by 2 years of age is similar to adult values on a per kilogram basis, being about eightfold greater than BAO. Thereafter, gastric acid output increases in proportion to body weight.[3]

Gastric Emptying Time. Gastric motility is irregular in rate and rhythm in the newborn. Gastric emptying time is considerably prolonged at 6 to 8 hours, approaching adult values by 6 to 8 months of age. Likewise, intestinal transit time is prolonged. Both are characterized by irregular peristaltic contractions and are affected by gestational age, postnatal age, and the volume and composition of feedings.[4] Several neonatal diseases, such as gastroesophageal reflux, respiratory distress syndrome, and congenital heart disease, are associated with a prolonged gastric emptying time.

Biliary Function and Gastrointestinal Enzymes. Decreased amounts of bile acids are found in the duodenum for the first several weeks of life. The bile acid pool is reduced to approximately 50% of adult values in full-term newborns and to one third of adult values in preterm infants.[5, 6] Concentrations of both α-amylase and lipase activity are decreased in duodenal fluid of infants younger than 4 months of age.[4] The combination of low levels of bile acids and low lipase activity may result in poor absorption of lipid-soluble drugs and nutrients, such as vitamins D and E.[7, 8]

GI absorption is a function of ionization and aqueous solubility. With such a relatively high gastric pH, the absorption of weakly acidic drugs will be decreased and that of weakly basic drugs will be enhanced. Acid-labile drugs will likely demonstrate increased bioavailablility in neonates secondary to decreased destruction by gastric acid. Absorption may also be increased because of slower intestinal transit time, allowing prolonged mucosal contact. The relatively neutral pH of the GI tract explains, in part, the higher bioavailability reported for several β-lactam antibiotics, including penicillin,[9] ampi-

cillin,[10] and nafcillin,[11] as well as the reduced absorption of poorly soluble weak acids, such as phenobarbital,[12] phenytoin,[13] and acetaminophen.[14]

Jalling and coworkers[13] reported four infants, 22 to 78 days of age, who received oral phenytoin in doses of 8.2 to 18.8 mg/kg/day and failed to achieve serum concentrations greater than 4.8 mg/l. Painter and associates[15] reported nine newborns with undetectable serum concentrations of phenytoin despite oral maintenance doses of up to 12 mg/kg/day. When intravenous (IV) administration, 5 mg/kg/day, was substituted, serum levels of 26 ± 6 mg/l were achieved. Rapp and associates[16] reported two infants who required oral doses of 12.9 and 11 mg/kg/day, respectively, to achieve levels greater than 10 mg/l, whereas a third infant received 12 mg/kg/day without achieving detectable levels.

The absorption of chloramphenicol palmitate suspension has been shown to be erratic and inconsistent in premature and newborn infants. The palmitate suspension requires pancreatic enzymes for duodenal hydrolysis to free chloramphenicol. The bioavailability of the suspension in this population is only 25 to 50% of that seen in older children. Shankaran and Kauffman studied seven newborns (four preterm, three full-term) who weighed 680 to 3,580 g.[17] The bioavailability of chloramphenicol palmitate was significantly lower than IV chloramphenicol succinate. In three infants, the oral dose required to maintain equivalent serum levels was twice the IV dose. Peak serum concentrations with oral dosing occurred longer than 4 hours after dosing in four infants, and serum levels did not decline over the 6-hour dosing interval, demonstrating prolonged elimination. Prolonged and erratic absorption of chloramphenicol in newborns is consistent with immaturity of GI function in terms of decreased pancreatic lipase activity and prolonged gastric emptying time.

In contrast, Kauffman and colleagues evaluated the area under the curve (AUC) and urine excretion of IV and oral chloramphenicol in 18 children, 2 months to 14 years of age. The bioavailability of IV chloramphenicol succinate in this population was only 70% that of the oral palmitate salt. Approximately 36% of the IV dose was excreted as the inactive unhydrolyzed chloramphenicol succinate.[18] Therefore, in this age range, oral chloramphenicol suspension produced higher serum levels of active drug than did the IV succinate salt.

In summary, maturational differences can have dramatic and opposing effects on GI absorption. Both the rate and extent of absorption can be affected. Differences are primarily important during the first 2 weeks of life; however, the general finding is that for many drugs, the bioavailability remains low until 1 to 2 months of age. Although systematic data are lacking, the oral absorption rate of various drugs in infants follows an age-dependent relationship and is slower in newborns than in older children and adults.[12]

Rectal Absorption

The rectal route of administration is an effective alternative for patients who can have nothing by mouth and are without IV access. Especially in the pediatric patient, the rectal route of administration is associated with less pain and anxiety than are intramuscular (IM) or IV injections. Additionally, drugs administered into the lower rectum bypass first-pass hepatic elimination and are distributed directly into the systemic circulation. However, the use of suppositories is not optimal in a critical care setting because of slow and erratic absorption. Generally, drugs administered rectally as aqueous solutions are absorbed more quickly than are suppositories, and in certain cases they may be approximate to the serum levels achieved following IM administration.[19, 20] Lipophilic compounds such as benzodiazepines[19-23] and barbiturates[24] seem particularly suited for rectal administration.

The clinical efficacy of rectal diazepam solution in the prevention of recurrent febrile seizures has been demonstrated by Knudsen.[21] Rectal administration of diazepam in solution rather than suppository form resulted in faster and more predictable plasma levels and clinical effects.[20] Likewise, effective seizure control has been achieved with rectally administered sodium valproate solution.[25] Rectal midazolam has been shown to be an effective premedicant for alleviating the anxiety associated with the induction of anesthesia in children.[22, 23] No studies examining the clinical efficacy or kinetics of rectal drug administration specifically in the neonatal population are available.

Absorption from Extraintestinal Sites

Drug absorption from two extraintestinal sites deserves brief comment—that is, percutaneous drug absorption and IM injections. Absorption through the skin is inversely related to the thickness of the stratum corneum and directly proportional to skin hydration.[26] The absorption of topically applied medications is greater in newborns and infants because of a thinner stratum corneum. Additionally, because of the infant's larger ratio of body surface area:weight, greater absorption will occur in the infant than in the adult following the application of equal amounts of a substance. The systemic availability of such a dose has been estimated to be 2.7 times greater in the neonate.[27]

Systemic adverse reactions have been associated with the topical application of hexachlorophene[28, 29] and γ-benzene hexachloride solutions[30, 31] in infants. Both compounds have resulted in neurotoxicity and seizures when used in infants and therefore are not recommended for use in children less than 2 years of age. Viscous lidocaine has produced seizures following ingestion of oral doses intended for topical application to the oral mucosa.[32] Numerous other examples of inadvertent systemic absorption and toxicity have been reported.[33, 34] Therapeutic levels of theophylline, in the range of 4 to 12 mg/l, have been achieved in infants younger than 72 hours old following the use of a topically applied theophylline "gel."[35] Absorption rates decreased significantly after the first several days of life, but some infants continued to achieve therapeutic levels until up to 3 weeks of age.

IM injections are rarely used in newborns because skeletal muscle is decreased. However, neonates frequently have poor IV access, and IM injections then become a viable and effective alternative for many drugs. Table 74–2 lists agents that have been shown to be well absorbed following IM administration in neonates. Two factors that need to be considered and that may decrease drug absorption from an IM administration site are decreased peripheral perfusion resulting from compromised cardiac output and decreased muscle activity in a neuromuscularly paralyzed or otherwise critically ill infant.

Distribution

Body Composition

Body Water. Alterations in the size of body water compartments affect the distribution of drugs. As shown in Figure 74–1, total body water (TBW) and its distribution are different in the newborn versus the fully mature adult.[37] TBW accounts for 80% of total body weight in the neonate versus 60% in the adult. TBW decreases rapidly during intrauterine life, followed by a more gradual decline throughout childhood. Extracellular water (ECW) accounts for 45% of a newborn's body weight as compared with only 19% in adults. The proportion of body weight accounted for by intracellular water remains more constant and is 30% in neonates and 38% in adults (see also Chapter 58).

For drugs whose volume of distribution parallels TBW, the apparent volume of distribution is greater in newborns than in adults. Since most drugs are distributed throughout the ECW to reach their receptors, the

Table 74–2. DRUGS DEMONSTRATING EFFECTIVE SYSTEMIC ABSORPTION FOLLOWING INTRAMUSCULAR ADMINISTRATION IN NEONATES*

Antibacterial Agents	Sedatives-Tranquilizers
Amikacin	Chlorpromazine
Ampicillin	Promethazine
Carbenicillin	
Cefazolin	**Cardiovascular Drugs**
Cefotaxime	Hydralazine
Ceftazidime	Procainamide
Ceftriaxone	Pyridostigmine
Clindamycin	
Gentamicin	**Diuretic Agents**
Kanamycin	Acetazolamide
Methicillin	Bumetanide
Moxalactam	Furosemide
Nafcillin	
Oxacillin	**Endocrine**
Penicillin G benzathine	Corticotropin
Penicillin G	Cortisone
Piperacillin	Desoxycorticosterone
Ticarcillin	Glucagon
Tobramycin	
	Pituitary Agent
Antituberculous Agents	Vasopressin
Isoniazid	
Streptomycin	**Narcotics**
	Meperidine
	Morphine
Anticonvulsant Agents	
Diazepam	**Vitamins**
Phenobarbital	K
	D

*From Besunder JB, Reed MD, and Blumer JL: Principles of drug biodisposition in the neonate. A critical evaluation of the pharmacokinetic-pharmacodynamic interface, Part 1. Clin Pharmacokinetics 14:189, 1988.

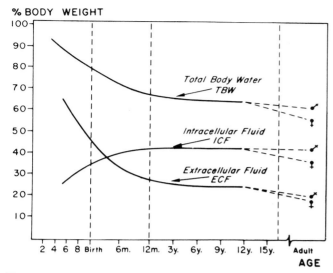

Figure 74–1. General patterns of changes in the volumes of total body water (TBW), extracellular fluid (ECF), and intracellular fluid (ICF) as a function of prenatal and postnatal age. (Data from Friis-Hansen B. *In*: Winter RW [ed]: The Body Fluids in Pediatrics, p. 100. Reprinted with permission from Little, Brown and Company, copyright 1973.)

size of the ECW compartment ultimately determines drug concentration, or apparent volume of distribution. Since infants have twice as much ECW as adults, administration of an equivalent milligram/kilogram dose of a water-soluble drug results in only one half as much serum concentration in the infant as in the adult. The volume of distribution of aminoglycosides, being approximately 0.48 l/kg in neonates and 0.2 l/kg in adults, demonstrates the application of body composition on initial drug distribution.[38, 39] Another example would be patients with cystic fibrosis who typically demonstrate a larger volume of distribution for aminoglycosides than does the population without cystic fibrosis.[40, 41] This is thought to result in part from a greater percentage of body weight being made up of lean body mass (muscle) with a decrease in percentage of body fat. Additionally, cor pulmonale results in an expanded intravascular volume in patients with cystic fibrosis and contributes to an increased apparent volume of distribution for water-soluble drugs.

Muscle Mass. This accounts for approximately 24% of total body weight in a full-term infant. The accretion of muscle mass is greater than the increase in the glomerular filtration rate (GFR) during childhood; therefore, serum creatinine levels increase gradually throughout childhood. Muscle mass accounts for 40% of total body weight by 11 to 13 years of age and between 40 and 50% of total body weight in adults.

Fat Content. A preterm infant at 6 months' gestation contains only 1 to 2% fat. A full-term newborn contains approximately 12 to 16% fat, which is still substantially less than in older infants and children.[37] One would anticipate smaller volumes of distribution for highly fat-soluble drugs in neonates. Fat content increases between 5 and 10 years of age in both sexes. Upon entering the period of adolescence, 13-year-old boys have a decrease

in fat content that continues through 17 years of age, whereas girls have a rapid increase in fat accumulation in association with puberty. Throughout the late teenage years and early adulthood, women have approximately twice as much body fat as do their male counterparts.

In summary, TBW content in the newborn and young infant is larger, the ratio of extracellular fluid:intracellular fluid is higher, fat tissue is relatively scarce, and skeletal muscle is reduced. These age-related differences cause drug distribution alterations that are primarily important during the first 10 to 12 months of life and give the neonate and infant a volume of distribution that is larger for polar drugs and smaller for lipid-soluble drugs. Examples of drugs with larger apparent volumes of distribution in infants include phenytoin, theophylline, aminoglycosides, salicylates, digoxin, and ampicillin. Diazepam has been shown to have a volume of distribution in neonates that is approximately one half of that in older children.[42]

Infants require larger loading and maintenance doses than do older children and adults (on a milligram/kilogram basis) to achieve comparable serum levels for many water-soluble compounds. As the child's age and weight increase, drug doses of relatively water-soluble drugs should be tapered downward to avoid exceeding normal adult doses.

Protein Binding. The degree of protein binding of drugs depends on several age-related factors, including the amount of protein available, the affinity between the drug and protein, the presence of endogenous interfering substances, and the existence of concurrent pathophysiologic conditions. Both "qualitative" and "quantitative" changes in the plasma proteins, albumin, globulin, and lipoproteins are important factors in reduced drug binding. Plasma protein binding of various drugs in the preterm and full-term infant is reduced. An increase in the free fraction of a drug increases the apparent volume of distribution or degree of tissue penetration and may, at least temporarily, accentuate both the therapeutic and adverse effects of a compound.

The concentrations of albumin, the primary drug-binding protein, and α_1–acid glycoprotein are lowest in the first 6 months of life and reach adult values by the end of the first year.[43] Globulin levels are low in both preterm and full-term neonates and do not reach adult levels until 7 to 12 years of age. Lipoprotein levels are low at birth but reach adult levels by 6 weeks of age.

In addition, the persistence of fetal albumin results in a lower drug-binding affinity. Acidic and neutral drugs bind primarily to albumin but may also bind to ligands such as fatty acids and bilirubin. Basic drugs bind to albumin, α_1–acid glycoprotein, and lipoprotein. During the neonatal period, high plasma concentrations of free fatty acids and unconjugated bilirubin compete with acidic drugs such as phenytoin and hexobarbital at albumin binding sites. At bilirubin concentrations of 15 to 20 mg/dl, the unbound fraction of phenytoin is twice that seen in normal adult serum.[44] The unbound fraction of phenytoin is related to the molar ratio of bilirubin:albumin concentration, suggesting competition for binding sites on the albumin molecule.[44]

In short, the overall binding of drugs to albumin, globulin, and α_1–acid glycoprotein is low early in life and increases with age. Differences in protein binding between adults and neonates favor a reduced quantity of plasma proteins, a reduced affinity of the proteins themselves, and the potential presence of compounds (bilirubin, free fatty acids) that may impair binding and further increase free drug concentrations. The rate at which protein binding matures varies, depending on the particular protein and drug in question. An understanding of the differences in protein binding and the resultant free drug concentration demonstrates the inappropriateness of using therapeutic "ranges" defined in adults to guide dosage titration in neonates and young infants. Table 74–3 lists a number of compounds that have been studied and demonstrates the extent of protein binding differences in adult and neonatal serum.[45, 46]

Metabolism-Biotransformation and Developmental Changes in Hepatic Function

The process of metabolism or biotransformation of a drug is intended to inactivate the parent compound and prepare it for excretion as a water-soluble polar compound. Age-related changes in hepatic metabolizing ability have been difficult to characterize because of the variety of enzymatic and chemical processes available. For many compounds, hepatic metabolizing ability is significantly reduced in the newborn period. The rate and extent to which drug metabolism is altered depends on the drug as well as the type of metabolic process involved. Since the final pathway of elimination of many drugs is via renal mechanisms, changes in the develop-

Table 74–3. PROTEIN BINDING OF VARIOUS DRUGS TO ADULT AND CORD PLASMA AS A PERCENTAGE OF TOTAL DRUG CONCENTRATION

| Drug | Binding $\bar{x} \pm S_{\bar{x}}$ | | |
	Adult Plasma	Cord Plasma	C:A
Isoniazid	0 ± 1.3	0 ± 0.3	1.0
Atropine	38.7 ± 1.1	21.1 ± 0.3	1.3
Morphine	42.1 ± 1.0	31.0 ± 1.0	1.2
Paracetamol	47.5 ± 0.6	36.8 ± 0.3	1.2
Phenobarbital	50.7 ± 1.3	32.4 ± 0.6	1.4
Phenacetin	52.6 ± 0.1	39.0 ± 0.9	1.3
Chloramphenicol	66.0 ± 0.9	45.9 ± 1.4	1.6
p-Aminosalicylic acid	67.4 ± 0.2	50.9 ± 0.6	1.5
Nitrofurantoin	74.2 ± 0.8	61.9 ± 0.6	1.2
Methicillin	74.2 ± 0.7	64.8 ± 0.9	1.4
Desipramine	82.7 ± 0.6	64.5 ± 1.9	2.1
Phenytoin	85.8 ± 1.0	74.4 ± 1.0	1.8
Promethazine	82.7 ± 0.2	69.8 ± 0.2	1.8
Sulfamethoxydiazine	90.1 ± 0.2	80.3 ± 0.6	2.0
Oxyphenbutazone	92.7 ± 0.3	89.6 ± 0.3	1.4
Thiopental	92.8 ± 0.2	87.0 ± 0.4	1.8
Digitoxin	93.4 ± 0.2	91.6 ± 0.3	1.3
Salicylic acid	96.4 ± 0.2	91.5 ± 0.6	2.4
Chlordiazepoxide	97.3 ± 0.2	94.0 ± 0.8	2.2
Sulfadimethoxine	97.5 ± 0.2	95.7 ± 0.3	1.8

*From Kurz H, Mauser-Ganshorn A, and Stickel HH: Differences in the binding of drugs to plasma proteins from newborn and adult man. I. Eur J Clin Pharmacol 11:463, 1977.
C:A is the ratio of unbound drug in cord (C) and adult (A) plasma. (N = 12 to 16, p <0.001).

ment of either hepatic or renal function significantly alter their elimination rates.

Reactions involved with drug metabolism can be broadly grouped into two major categories: phase I and phase II reactions. Phase I, also known as synthetic or preparative reactions, involves the transformation of the parent compound by molecular rearrangement to either inactivate the compound or prepare it for a phase II reaction, or both. Reactions such as oxidation, hydrolysis, hydroxylation, and reduction are considered phase I processes. Typically, byproducts of these reactions are cleared by renal elimination or biliary excretion or undergo further biotransformation. In some instances, metabolites are more active than the parent compound. Examples include theophylline to caffeine, chloramphenicol succinate to active chloramphenicol base, and azathioprine to 6-mercaptopurine.

Of the mixed-function oxidase systems, the cytochrome P_{450} system has been studied most extensively. The activity of the cytochrome P_{450} system in full-term and preterm neonates is markedly reduced at 20 to 70% of adult levels.[47] The activity increases rapidly with advancing postnatal age to reach or exceed adult levels within several months. In older children, the metabolism of theophylline, phenytoin, carbamazepine, quinidine, and procainamide is greater than in adults.[48]

Phase II reactions are known as synthetic or conjugative reactions and involve the addition of large endogenous polar compounds onto the drug molecule to make it more water soluble and hence excreted more easily. Glucuronide, sulfate, and glycine conjugates are the most common byproducts of these reactions. Typically, metabolites of these pathways are inactive and readily excreted by renal or biliary elimination. Glucuronide conjugation, the most common process, is catalyzed by a group of inducible microsomal transferases, whereas sulfate and glycine conjugation tends to be nonmicrosomal in nature. Drugs metabolized via glucuronidation include morphine, benzodiazepines, acetaminophen, salicylamide, chloramphenicol, phenobarbital, phenytoin, and steroids.

In general, oxidation and glucuronidation are among the most deficient processes at birth, whereas others such as dealkylation and sulfonation are well developed; however, much variability exists. The demethylation of mepivacaine and lidocaine is efficient in the neonate, whereas the rates of hydroxylation and demethylation of diazepam have been shown to be reduced in the newborn.[42] Similarly, the rates of oxidation and demethylation of theophylline are deficient in the newborn.[49]

Further confusing the issue is the possibility of in utero exposure to inducing agents such as phenytoin, carbamazepine, barbituates, ethanol, and tobacco tars. There is good evidence that induction in utero can occur, and various oxidative pathways may be increased or stimulated to varying extents.[50] How significant in utero induction is in terms of affecting neonatal drug metabolizing ability is controversial.

The insufficiency of one elimination pathway may lead to metabolism by alternative pathways. Age-related metabolic differences exist for both phase I and phase II processes. Because different metabolic processes ma-

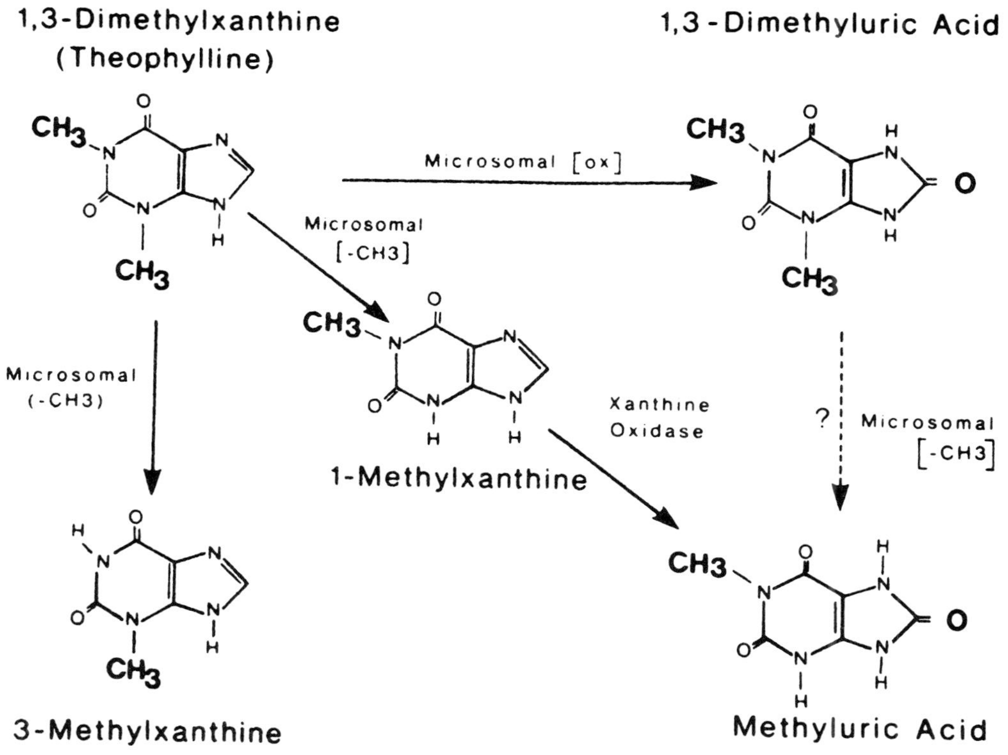

Figure 74–2. Metabolism of theophylline. (From Bukowshyj M, Nakatsu K, and Munt PW: Theophylline reassessed. Ann Intern Med 101:63, 1984.)

ture at varying rates, characterization is more difficult for compounds that follow more than one pathway. No flat rule exists, and each drug must be considered individually. The classic example of altered metabolic pathways in pediatrics is the conversion of theophylline to caffeine.

In adults and children older than 6 months of age, theophylline (1,3-dimethylxanthine) is eliminated almost completely by hepatic biotransformation into relatively inactive metabolites and is excreted in the urine.[51] The major metabolite (1,3-dimethyluric acid) is the result of C8 oxidation. Two other metabolites, 3-methylxanthine and 1-methylxanthine, result from N-demethylation (Fig. 74–2). Approximately 6% of theophylline is N-methylated to caffeine in adults. Although both phase I demethylation and oxidation processes are deficient in neonates, N-methylase activity is active. This combination favors the biotransformation of theophylline into caffeine (1,3,7-trimethylxanthine). During theophylline therapy in the newborn, 50% of theophylline is eliminated unchanged in the urine and 50% is converted to caffeine. Serum concentrations of caffeine will approximate 30 to 50% of the level of theophylline. Theophylline clearance increases dramatically during the first year of life (Fig. 74–3).[49] By 1 year of age, infants clear theophylline 100% more than do adults. Theophylline elimination then remains fairly constant until approximately 9 years of age when it progressively declines to adult values by 16 years of age.

The initial half-life of caffeine in the newborn is 100 hours (clearance = 9ml/kg/hr). Like theophylline, the ability to metabolize caffeine increases with age so that by 4 months of age, the clearance equals 105 ml/kg/hr,

with a half-life of 4 hours, which is less than the adult half-life of 6 hours.

Likewise, age-related differences in phase II metabolic pathways exists. Phase II sulfate conjugation is an efficient metabolic process in full-term newborns. The ability to metabolize acetaminophen through the normal adult pathway of glucuronide conjugation may not develop fully until 10 to 12 years of age.[14] Yet, infants and children with delayed glucuronide formation have an overall acetaminophen half-life that is similar to adult values. The compensating ability of sulfate conjugation is thought to explain, in part, the lower incidence of hepatotoxicity seen with acetaminophen use in children (see Chapter 80).

The assumption that alternative pathways are always available, however, is a dangerous one. The classic example of neonatal drug toxicity, the "gray baby syndrome," resulted from an accumulation of chloramphenicol because of a decreased capacity for glucuronidation and resulted in intracellular accumulation of free chloramphenicol and, ultimately, disruption of mitochondrial electron transport mechanisms. The gray baby syndrome was associated with chloramphenicol levels of 40 to 200 mg/l and a mortality rate of 40%.

A reduced capacity to dispose of drugs is consistently observed during the first 15 days of life in premature and full-term infants. In most cases, this stage of reduced metabolic degradation is followed by a dramatic increase in metabolic rate at approximately 2 weeks of age. The disposition rate may pass from one third to one fifth of the adult rate to two to three times faster than the adult rate. Therefore, a risk of overdosage is quickly converted to one of underdosing. Because of rapidly chang-

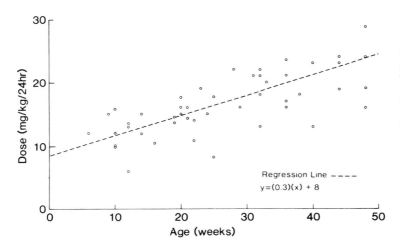

Figure 74–3. Relationship of age and dose required to achieve a steady-state peak serum theophylline concentration within the 10 to 20 μg/ml range among 50 infants 6 to 48 weeks old (r = 0.78; p < 0.001). The linear relationship between age and dose requirements is a function of progressively increasing clearance over the first year of life as the mixed function oxidative enzyme system slowly matures. (From Nassif EG, Weinberger MM, Shannon D, et al: Theophylline disposition in infancy. J Pediatr 98:158, 1981.)

ing parameters, the importance of individualizing therapy when using therapeutic drug monitoring is critical.

The increased metabolic rate is usually evident from 2 to 3 months of age until 2 to 3 years of age but is highly variable and can be much longer. Theophylline and quinidine are examples of compounds whose increased metabolic degradation can last up to 9 to 12 years of age before slowly decreasing to adult values by the midteens.

Elimination—Developmental Changes in Renal Function

Although renal function is only 20 to 40% of that seen in older children and adults, it usually maintains newborn homeostasis, and only during times of stress (infection, acid-base imbalance, dehydration, or fluid overload) does the immaturity of renal function become clinically apparent.

Although the ratio of kidney weight:body mass is twice that of adults, the organ is both anatomically and functionally immature at birth. Renal function is significantly lower in newborns even when normalized for body surface area. The three major aspects of renal function that deal with drug elimination—tubular secretion, tubular reabsorption, and glomerular filtration—are all decreased at birth and mature at varying rates during the first few months of life.

Tubular secretion is an energy-requiring process that involves the transport of drugs from the peritubular capillaries into the tubule lumen. Active tubular secretion increases the net excretion of drugs. Renal tubular secretory capacity increases over the first months of life to reach adult values (per unit of body surface area) at 6 to 7 months of age. Weak acids such as penicillins, sulfonamides, cephalosporins, and furosemide are initially cleared slowly by the neonate. The tubular functional capacity of glucose, phosphates, bicarbonates and *p*-aminohippurate is also reduced in the neonate.[52]

Despite the prolonged development of tubular transport pathways, pharmacokinetic studies with ampicillin,[53] ticarcillin,[54] and methicillin[55] have shown that their elimination varies inversely with gestational and postnatal age and decreases to 1 to 2 hours by 2 weeks of age. This enhanced elimination is thought to be due to substrate stimulation by repeated exposure to a drug and results in an overall clearance that is higher than that reported in older children.[56]

Tubular reabsorption is a passive concentration-dependent process in which compounds pass from the renal tubule lumen, back through peritubular cells, and into the vascular system, thereby decreasing net renal excretion. Since the reabsorption of some drugs is pH-dependent, the less acidic urine of an infant enhances the elimination of weak acids by increasing the degree of ionization and decreasing the amount available for renal tubular reabsorption, which may not reach full potential until 2 years of age.

The primary factor controlling the development of GFR is gestational age.[57] The preterm neonate who is born at less than 34 weeks' gestation has a deficient number of glomeruli and a GFR of 0.4 to 0.8 ml/min. A sudden increase in GFR is observed at 34 weeks of gestation (birth weight approximately 2,000 g) and corresponds to the cessation of glomerular formation and improved renal hemodynamics. Renal blood flow is reduced in the newborn and is characterized by a preferential intrarenal flow away from the cortex and toward the medullary areas. Newborns born at more than 34 weeks' gestation have a GFR ranging from 2 to 4 ml/min.

GFR increases after birth, but the adaptive increase is much greater in the full-term newborn than in the preterm infant.[58] The GFR increases two- to fourfold within 2 to 3 days of extrauterine life in the full-term infant to approximately 8 to 20 ml/min versus 2 to 3 ml/min in the preterm infant over the same period. GFR reaches levels comparable to adult values at 2½ to 5 months of age. The greater increase in GFR seen in full-term newborns during the first week of life is due to a greater increase in cardiac output, a decrease in pulmonary vascular resistance, and greater filtration surface area than in the preterm infant. When dealing with renal function measurements in any pediatric patient, one must be cognizant of the similarity of and, occasionally, lack of consistency in terminology (milliliters/minute, milliliters/minute/m², milliliters/minute/1.73 m²).

Many pediatric dosing references recommend lower doses and longer dosing intervals for renally eliminated medications in newborns, which are arbitrarily changed after the first week of life. Because of the differences already mentioned in the rates of improvement in GFR, this change in dose and dosing interval may be appropriate for full-term infants but not for premature newborns. Kasik and associates found a much stronger correlation between gentamicin half-life and postconceptional age versus postnatal age in newborns with postconceptional ages between 24 and 48 weeks.[59] Postconceptional age should be used for guiding empirical dosing requirements for compounds such as aminoglycosides[59] and vancomycin[60, 61] in neonates, and subsequent adjustment should be made on the basis of serum drug level monitoring.

The lower clearance rates and longer half-lives of drugs like aminoglycosides, which depend on GFR for elimination, or compounds like penicillins and sulfonamides, whose excretion depends on tubular secretion, are examples of how immature renal function modifies drug elimination.

Digoxin presents a unique example of developmental drug elimination mechanisms in the pediatric patient. Because of the immaturity of renal function, total body clearance of digoxin is initially low in the newborn period.[62] Renal clearance of digoxin increases with age to reach adult levels at 3 to 4 months of age.[48] Thereafter, total body clearance exceeds that seen in older children and adults but cannot be explained entirely by enhanced renal clearance alone. Nonrenal routes such as biliary excretion or metabolism have been proposed but not proved to be important. Tubular secretion is believed to play a significant role in digoxin elimination in infancy and childhood.[62] During the adolescent years, net tubular secretion and total renal clearance decrease toward adult values. It is of particular interest that renal tubular secretion of digoxin correlates better with full sexual maturity (Tanner stages 4 and 5) than with chronologic age.[63]

In general, the renal excretion of drugs is less in early postnatal life because of decreases in GFR and tubular secretion. Drug clearance improves as GFR matures. In infants (2 to 24 months), GFR and tubular secretion are more developed than tubular reabsorption; therefore, renal clearance of some compounds may be increased over values seen in older children and adults. Generally, the maturation of glomerular and tubular function is reached at 6 to 8 months of age. After 8 months of age, the renal excretion of most drugs is comparable with that of older children and adults.

Serum creatinine at birth, regardless of gestational age, represents maternal serum creatinine. Serum creatinine levels fall from 0.8 mg/dl at birth to 0.5 mg/dl at 5 to 7 days of age. After 8 to 9 days, a stable value of 0.4 mg/dl was observed between 1 and 52 weeks of life, indicating a simultaneous and proportional increase in muscle mass and renal function during infancy.[64] After 1 year of age, the accretion of muscle mass exceeds the increase in GFR; therefore, serum creatinine levels tend to increase slightly as the child grows to stabilize at 0.8 to 1 mg/dl. In both older infants and children, height and ideal body mass correlate with urinary creatinine concentrations. Several formulas for estimating creatinine clearance in children from 1 week to 21 years of age have been published.[64–66]

PHARMACODYNAMIC ALTERATIONS

As described earlier, pharmacodynamics is an examination of the pharmacologic response achieved by various serum drug concentrations in a given patient population. More specifically, it is concerned with the concentration of a free drug interacting with a specific receptor and the magnitude of the response produced. Children demonstrate unique pharmacologic responses to many medications in comparison with their mature adult counterparts. Pediatric patients may appear more or less sensitive to a particular drug by expressing either an enhanced or attenuated therapeutic response. In some instances, an entirely unexpected adverse effect may occur.

Although numerous examples of altered pharmacologic effects exist in the pediatric population, true differences in pharmacologic sensitivity between children and adults are not well documented by well-designed clinical trials. In order to establish true differences in sensitivity, a thorough and complete appreciation of pharmacokinetic differences of a given drug in the population in question needs to be considered. The recent examples of benzyl alcohol toxicity[68, 69] and the deaths associated with the E-Ferol emulsifiers polysorbates 80 and 20[70] represent unexpected adverse effects resulting from immaturity of metabolic and excretory pathways and not "true" pharmacodynamic differences. Accordingly, many instances of altered pharmacologic responses in children have a pharmacokinetic basis as their cause, resulting in higher than expected serum concentrations, impaired or altered metabolic pathways, or changes in the extent of tissue distribution. Theophylline, for example, is commonly quoted as having two therapeutic ranges. Serum concentrations of 6 to 13 µg/ml are desirable in treating apnea and bradycardia of prematurity, whereas concentrations of 10 to 20 µg/ml are used to achieve bronchodilating effects in older children and adults. If one examines the protein-binding differences that exist between the two populations and corrects for the amount of free drug available for receptor site interaction, the "therapeutic" range" of active free theophylline for both populations is very similar. Once again, this represents a pharmacokinetic alteration rather than a true difference in pharmacodynamic sensitivity.

Following is a brief discussion of the major classes of medications that have critical care applications and have been associated with unusual therapeutic responses in the pediatric population. In many instances, a definitive explanation of the mechanism involved is unknown. At present, many examples of pharmacodynamic differences exist based solely on clinical observations combined with data extrapolated from studies performed in other species.

Children are predisposed to unusual effects of medications throughout their growth and development. Analogous to teratogenic effects in the fetus, medications can adversely affect developing tissues postnatally. The effects of tetracyclines and corticosteroids on limiting bone growth are well known.[71, 72] More recently, the potential usefulness of the quinoline class of antibiotics in pediatrics has been severely limited by concerns raised by reports of cartilage malformations in weight-bearing joints of juvenile animals.[73] Trials in pediatric patients have therefore been delayed and have resulted in the recommendation that quinoline antibiotics not be used in children or pregnant women. Reversible arthropathy has been reported in adolescent patients with cystic fibrosis who received ciprofloxacin.[74]

Cardiovascular System

The newborn cardiovascular system responds differently to catecholamines and inotropic agents than does that of the older child and adult. Besides the structural changes associated with the transition from fetal to postnatal life, physiologic differences exist between the newborn infant and the older child or adult in terms of both adrenergic physiology and myocardial performance.[75, 76]

Research on age-related developmental differences in adrenergic receptor density, neurotransmitter quantity, and clinical response to endogenous or exogenous stimuli is limited by interspecies differences. The sympathetic innervation of the myocardium is incomplete at birth in many species[75, 77] and is associated with a reduced amount of presynaptic norepinephrine. Studies in young animals have demonstrated diminished contractile[78] and vascular responses[79] to exogenous catecholamines. These data suggest the human infant is also less responsive to exogenous catecholamines. Likewise, the development of cardiovascular adrenergic receptor density is believed to be age-related. The β-receptor density of polymorphonuclear leukocytes[80] and the α_2-receptor density of platelets[81] in human neonates have been shown to be reduced in comparison with adult values. Despite these findings, the fetal myocardium is more sensitive to exogenous norepinephrine than is the adult myocardium. This is thought to be related to reduced neuronal uptake of norepinephrine, which is normally the major inactivation mechanism. As a result, high concentrations are present at the postsynaptic receptor, rendering the infant myocardium more sensitive. This implies that infant myocardial adrenergic receptors are fully functional prior to complete maturation of the extrinsic nerve supply. There are no data available on cardiovascular adrenergic receptor development or on the timing of complete sympathetic innervation of the myocardium in the human neonate. The described difference in sensitivity between fetal and adult hearts decreases with age and appears to correspond with more efficient neuronal uptake and inactivation and, therefore, maturation of sympathetic innervation.[77]

Reflex responses to changes in blood pressure and hypoxia sensed by baroreceptors and chemoreceptors, respectively, are correspondingly immature at birth and may not produce the same magnitude of response as in an adult.[75] Concentrations of plasma catecholamines are lower in preterm than in full-term infants immediately after birth, suggesting that preterm infants have a limited ability to increase catecholamine release in response to stress.[82]

Important differences in myocardial function exist between the preterm and the newborn infant and the mature hearts of older children and adults. The neonatal myocardium contains relatively fewer muscle fibers with which to generate contractile force.[77] The greater percentage of noncontractile tissue results in less fiber shortening for any given preload; therefore, the infant myocardium derives less benefit from any degree of volume loading than does the mature myocardium. Additionally, the compliance of the infant's ventricular chamber is less.[83] Small increases in ventricular filling volume result in disproportionately large increases in myocardial wall tension, quickly reaching the limits of preload or diastolic reserve. The infant myocardium, therefore, operates on a relatively flat Starling curve and even without stress, functions near peak capacity to meet normal metabolic demands.

The infant has a limited ability to increase cardiac output. The combination of decreased compliance and reduced stroke volume augmentation limits the functional reserve capacity of the infant myocardium.[76] Additionally, because the baseline heart rate of the neonate is normally quite high, little additional improvement in cardiac output can be achieved by further increases in heart rate without significantly decreasing diastolic filling time and coronary perfusion. These age-related changes significantly limit the effectiveness of inotropic agents and catecholamines in the newborn infant. Considerable differences exist in both cardiovascular physiology and dose-response relationships between infants and adults. Reflex control of circulatory mechanisms and autonomic responses are not well developed in infants. Therefore, data from adult literature should not be extrapolated directly to the pediatric population (see also Chapter 29).

Catecholamines

Catecholamines such as dopamine and dobutamine are commonly used in infants and children with shock to raise cardiac output, increase blood pressure and urine output, and improve peripheral perfusion (see also Chapter 29). The response to these agents in any given patient is dependent on the interrelationships of blood pressure, heart rate, cardiac output, renal perfusion and systemic and pulmonary vascular resistance and is therefore susceptible to considerable variation. Age-related differences in response to endogenous catecholamines may result in alterations in vascular tone and myocardial function, which, in turn, influence the net effects of exogenous catecholamines.

There are extensive animal data demonstrating that the immature cardiovascular system responds differently to many of these agents. Puppies are more sensitive to the inotropic effects of propranolol than are adult dogs.[84] Animal studies suggest amrinone has a negative inotropic effect in the first 3 days of life, but between 4 and 10 days an increase in contractility occurs, which becomes progressively greater through 3 months of age.[85] Conversely, milrinone, a structural analogue of amrinone, was found to be inotropic at all ages from birth through 3 months of age in canine cardiac muscle.[86] The reason for these age-related differences in inotropic response to these agents is not understood. The results of animal trials such as these are unlikely to be clinically applicable because of interspecies differences. Further complicating their interpretation are the effects of anesthetic-induced suppression of hemodynamic reflexes and catecholamine responses. The use of exogenous catecholamines in the area of pediatric critical care has evolved based largely on the initial experience obtained in critically ill adult patients. Children may respond quite differently to these agents. Despite the wide use of dopamine and dobutamine in clinical practice, relatively little information is available concerning age-related responses to these agents.

A number of clinical trials have evaluated the use of dopamine and dobutamine in infants and children. These trials do not provide clear-cut evidence of a diminished response to exogenous catecholamines. Drummond and coworkers examined the usefulness of dopamine along with tolazoline and hyperventilation in the treatment of six infants with persistent pulmonary hypertension.[87] Dopamine was ineffective in doses of less than 6 µg/kg/min and frequently failed to increase systemic arterial pressure or urine output unless dosages of 20 to 125 µg/kg/min were infused. These infants were simultaneously receiving tolazoline infusions, which may have altered or antagonized the effects of dopamine. Lang and colleagues treated five children 1 to 24 months of age with dopamine following cardiovascular surgery.[88] Heart rate, blood pressure, and cardiac output did not increase significantly at infusion rates less than 15 µg/kg/min. The cardiovascular effects of low doses of dopamine were examined in 14 severely asphyxiated neonates in a randomized double-blind placebo-controlled trial.[89] After receiving volume expansion, patients were randomized to receive infusions of either dopamine 2.5 µg/kg/min or placebo. There was no significant change in heart rate when postinfusion values were compared with preinfusion values in either group. Myocardial contractility and systolic blood pressure, however, increased significantly in the dopamine-treated patients, without evidence of changes in systemic or pulmonary vascular resistances. Similarly, the effects of low doses of dopamine on blood pressure, urine output, and heart rate were studied in 18 hypotensive preterm infants with severe hyaline membrane disease.[90] Beneficial effects on blood pressure and urine output were observed at doses of 2, 4, and 8 µg/kg/min, whereas increases in heart rate were noted only with infusions of 8 µg/kg/min.

In perhaps the best-designed study to date, Padbury and associates compared the clinical responses of blood pressure, cardiac output, and heart rate with dopamine plasma concentrations to determine the minimal plasma concentrations that would produce discernible hemodynamic effects in 14 critically ill newborns.[91] Infusions of dopamine were administered in an increasing stepwise fashion at rates of 1, 2, 4, and 8 µg/kg/min in 40-minute intervals. The threshold value for increases in cardiac output was lower than the threshold for blood pressure, which was, in turn, lower than the threshold for heart rate. Serial echocardiography demonstrated dose-dependent increases in cardiac output and stroke volume without significant alterations in heart rate or systemic vascular resistance. A log-linear relationship between response and plasma dopamine concentration was observed. The investigators concluded that increases in blood pressure and cardiac output in newborn infants may be achieved at doses as low as 0.5 to 1 µg/kg/min. Although lower than commonly recommended, initiation of dopamine infusions at low dosages with incremental increases may be associated with positive inotropic effects and may avoid the tachycardia, arrhythmias, and excessive vasoconstriction noted at higher doses.

There was no correlation found between thresholds for increases in blood pressure or heart rate or dopamine plasma clearance and gestational age (27 to 42 weeks) or birth weight (0.9 to 4.3 kg). Infusions of dopamine at greater than 2 to 3 µg/kg/min were associated with increasing heart rate. In adults, dopamine infusions of less than 10 µg/kg/min increase cardiac output with little change in mean arterial pressure or heart rate.

These findings demonstrate that a marked difference exists in the dose-response relationship between adult and pediatric patients. Newborns appear to demonstrate a lower threshold and increased sensitivity to dopamine, rather than a decreased sensitivity as previously proposed.

In this study,[91] no changes in plasma norepinephrine concentrations were observed, suggesting that reflex sympathetic activation and release of endogenous norepinephrine did not occur. In older children and adults, dopamine is thought to produce positive inotropic effects by releasing norepinephrine from sympathetic nerve terminals. The results of this trial support the concept of immaturity of myocardial sympathetic innervation and demonstrate that the beneficial response to dopamine in newborns results from direct stimulation of myocardial β-adrenergic receptors.

Dobutamine is a direct β_1 agonist whose effects are independent of endogenous norepinephrine stores. In older patients, it augments cardiac output by increasing myocardial contractility with minimal effects on heart rate. It has only modest α and β_2 effects and lacks the selective dopaminergic increases in renal and mesenteric blood flow of dopamine. Available data on its use in infants and children are limited.

Perkin and coworkers studied the hemodynamic effect of dobutamine in 33 infants and children (mean age of 5.1 years) with cardiogenic and septic shock.[92] Ten patients were 12 months of age or younger. Dobutamine infusions of 2.5, 5, 7.5, and 10 µg/kg/min significantly increased cardiac index and left ventricular stroke work index. No significant changes in heart rate, mean systemic arterial pressure, or right atrial pressure occurred. Increases in pulmonary capillary wedge pressure occurred with increasing doses of dobutamine and were significantly increased at infusions of 10 μg/kg/min. Twenty-six per cent of dobutamine infusions were complicated by adverse reactions and included dysrhythmias, systemic hypertension, elevated pulmonary capillary wedge pressure, and symptomatic chest pain. Children less than 12 months of age showed a trend toward an attenuated response to the inotropic effects of dobutamine, which appeared to be more efficacious in the treatment of cardiogenic shock. When used in patients with septic shock, it appeared much less effective with only temporary beneficial effects.

Dobutamine was administered in doses of 2 or 7.75 μg/kg/min to 12 children with congenital heart disease undergoing cardiac catheterization. No change in heart rate or pulmonary or systemic vascular resistance occurred, whereas cardiac output, stroke volume, and mean systemic blood pressure increased significantly.[93]

Dobutamine was given to 12 children ranging in age from 1 day to 14 years with low-output cardiac failure in doses of 7.5 to 10 μg/kg/min.[94] Cardiac output increased significantly with only minor changes in heart rate. This was felt to suggest that increases in cardiac output resulted primarily from increased contractility and stroke volume.

Further work is needed to characterize the pharmacokinetics and pharmacodynamics of these agents in children in different age groups and with various underlying diseases. Age-specific dosage recommendations for these agents cannot be made. In critically ill infants, it is difficult to predict the cardiovascular effects of these agents in a specific patient, and their use requires individual titration with continuous hemodynamic monitoring.

Digoxin

During the 1950s, digoxin emerged as the cardiac glycoside of choice, and it was appreciated that children required larger doses than adults when based on a milligram/kilogram basis of body weight. It is of historical interest that the fact that maintenance doses of digoxin given to infants in the 1950s ranged from 30 to 120 μg/kg/day.[95, 96] Despite the magnitude of these doses, symptoms of toxicity were noted in only one third to one fourth of patients and were generally felt to be minor in nature and readily reversible. The practice of using large doses of cardiac glycosides in infants evolved on the basis of the infant's ability to tolerate large doses rather than on the basis of the degree of functional response achieved. This led to the belief that infants were less sensitive to the inotropic effects of digitalis glycosides.

Lacking a reliable and convenient measure of myocardial effect, most early studies of digitalis glycosides used toxicity as the end point. With the advent of noninvasive echocardiography and systolic time measurements, along with the ability to measure digoxin serum concentrations using radioimmunoassay technology, much insight has been gained over the past 2 decades concerning both the pharmacokinetic and pharmacodynamic effects of digoxin. Despite these advances, however, many controversies still exist.[97] Attempts at determining whether the immature myocardium is less sensitive to the effects of digitalis glycosides than is the adult myocardium have resulted in numerous conflicting reports. The three mechanisms by which an altered end organ response to digitalis would be mediated are altered sensitivity to the inhibition of myocardial Na^+, K^+-ATPase, altered inotropic response to a given concentration, or altered uptake and binding within the infant myocardium.[97]

In an attempt to demonstrate decreased Na^+, K^+-ATPase receptor sensitivity, Kearin and coworkers found that the dissociation constant for digoxin in newborn erythrocytes was twice that measured in adult erythrocytes.[98] This would imply that a twofold higher concentration of digoxin was necessary in the neonate to produce an equivalent effect if one assumes myocardial and red blood cell Na^+, K^+-ATPase sites behave in similar fashion. However, in fetal and adult hearts in both animal and human trials, other investigators have found no difference in the sensitivity of the Na^+, K^+-ATPase enzyme to ouabain.[99, 100]

The sensitivity of newborn atrial and ventricular tissues to the inotropic actions of ouabain is equal to that of adult tissue.[101] Sandor and colleagues found similar degrees of improvement in systolic time intervals between patients with high (3.6 ± 0.95 ng/ml) and low (1.9 ± 0.35 ng/ml) serum digoxin concentrations.[102] Other investigators have found no improvement in left ventricular performance with high serum digoxin concentrations (3.5 ng/ml, range 1.4 to 7.5 ng/ml) when compared with low (1.73 ng/ml, range 1.2 to 3 ng/ml) concentrations.[103]

The myocardium in infants and children is thought to bind more digoxin than does adult myocardial tissue. Several studies have shown an age-dependent relationship to myocardial tissue binding of digoxin.[104, 105] Park and colleagues found that the mean myocardial:serum ratio was 149:1 in infants and 28:1 in adults, a greater than fivefold increase. Serum concentrations of digoxin were not different between infants and adults, though adults had received daily milligram/kilogram doses that were one third of those used in infants.[104] In a group of children whose mean age was 5 years, Krasula and associates found a myocardial:serum digoxin ratio of 52:1.[105] The reason for the increased myocardial digoxin concentrations in infants is unknown, and it remains unclear as to what percentage of digoxin is bound to Na^+, K^+-ATPase receptors versus nonspecific tissue binding. The rate at which this binding changes with advancing age and the age at which it approximates adult values is also unclear. Wagner and colleagues have disputed these findings and attributed more of the observed variability in tissue binding of digoxin to the dose, height, weight, and renal function of the individual patient, rather than to age alone.[106]

Although not completely resolved, the present data do not support any significant age-related difference in the sensitivity of the Na$^+$, K$^+$-ATPase enzyme system nor of the myocardium to the inotropic action of digoxin. The significance of increased tissue binding is unclear at present. When normalized for weight, the dose of digoxin needed to achieve a given serum concentration in children is larger than it is in adults. This is due to a "true" pharmacokinetic difference reflected in an increased total body clearance.[26, 97, 104]

The incidence of digoxin toxicity in the pediatric population is not well established but is generally felt to be a relatively uncommon occurrence.[103, 107] The reason why higher serum concentrations of digoxin are better tolerated by infants is unknown. Proposed theories include incomplete sympathetic innervation of the infant myocardium, decreased sensitivity of the conduction system, lower susceptibility to arrhythmias because of less atherosclerotic coronary arteries and a less ischemic myocardium, and immaturity or imbalance of the central nervous system (CNS) sympathetic and parasympathetic nerves that mediate digoxin-induced arrhythmias.[97, 103]

The diagnosis of digoxin toxicity rests on the assessment of electrocardiographic determinations, electrolyte and metabolic imbalances, serum digoxin concentrations, and clinical symptoms. The detection of digoxin toxicity is made more difficult by subjective symptoms such as anorexia (poor feeding), nausea, vomiting, diarrhea (feeding intolerance), blurring of vision, and fatigue, which are nonspecific and difficult to assess in infants and children. As in adults, digoxin toxicity may not correlate well with serum concentrations, and the overlap between therapeutic and toxic serum levels in children appears to be at least as wide as that seen in adults.[107] Serum digoxin concentrations less than 3.5 ng/ml are unlikely to be associated with significant signs and symptoms of toxicity in children.[108]

There are important differences in the electrocardiographic effects of digoxin between infants and adults.[97, 107] The electrocardiographic signs of toxic and nontoxic effects are summarized in Table 74–4. Pediatric patients are more likely to develop atrioventricular (AV) conduction impairment than arrhythmias, which are more common and are earlier signs of toxicity in adults.

Table 74–4. ECG CHANGES ASSOCIATED WITH DIGITALIS*

Nontoxic Signs
Shortening of QT interval (corrected for heart rate, QTc), earliest manifestation of digitalis effect
Sagging ST segment and diminished amplitude of T wave (T vector usually does not change)
Lowering of heart rate

Toxic Signs
Prolongation of PR interval (first-degree AV block)—this may be therapeutic in certain tachyarrhythmias; prolongation may progress to second- or third-degree block
Profound sinus bradycardia or sinoatrial block
Atrial or nodal ectopic beats and tachycardia, particularly when accompanied by AV block
Ventricular arrhythmias such as ventricular bigeminy or trigeminy (extremely rare)

*From Park MK: Use of digoxin in infants and children with specific emphasis on dosage. J Pediatr 108:871, 1986.

Table 74–5. ARRHYTHMIAS OBSERVED IN DIGOXIN-TOXIC PATIENTS*

Rhythm	Children (no. = 125)	Adults (no. = 134)
Sinus bradycardia	37	21
Second-degree block	20	7
Third-degree block	11	9
Ventricular ectopic activity	9	29
Supraventricular tachycardia	11	42
Ventricular tachycardia	2	14
Ventricular fibrillation	7	8
Death	4	7

*Hougen TJ: Use of digoxin in the young. *In:* Smith TW (ed): Digitalis Glycosides. Orlando, Grune & Stratton, 1986, p. 196.

This same trend is reported in adult patients with healthy myocardium versus those with cardiac disease.[109] In pediatric patients, first-degree AV block is a more reliable and earlier sign of toxicity, whereas ventricular arrhythmias are relatively late-onset signs of toxicity.[107] Hougen compared 125 cases of digoxin toxicity in infants and children with 134 adult cases reported in the literature.[107] As shown in Table 74–5, there were 37 instances of sinus bradycardia in children versus 21 cases in adults. Combined first-, second-, and third-degree AV block occurred in 68 pediatric cases versus 37 adults—1.8 times as frequently. Supraventricular tachycardia, ventricular ectopic activity, and ventricular tachycardias were three to four times more common in adults. Serious arrhythmias and death, however, occurred with similar frequency in both groups.

The fact that children and infants tolerate higher digoxin levels does not mean they gain a greater benefit from such levels. No therapeutic advantage of digoxin serum levels greater than the therapeutic range of 0.8 to 2 ng/ml occurs in infants.[102] Table 74–6 shows current pediatric dosage recommendations of digoxin.

The recent detection of digoxin-like immunoreactive substances that cross-react with many digoxin assays casts doubt on the validity and meaning of earlier pharmacokinetic work done in infants.[110] Newborns not receiving digoxin have been reported as having digoxin serum concentrations within and occasionally greater than, the therapeutic range. The concentrations of digoxin-like immunoreactive substances detected varies, depending both on the assay used and on day-to-day variations in the same infant.[111] Although Pudek and

Table 74–6. RECOMMENDED ORAL DIGOXIN DOSAGE IN CONGESTIVE HEART FAILURE*

	Digitalizing Dose (μg/kg)	Maintenance Dose (μg/kg)
Premature infant	20	5
Full-term neonate (up to 2 months of age)	30	8–10
Infant (<2 years)	40–50	10–12
Child (>2 years)	30–40	8–10

*Park MK: Use of digoxin in infants and children with specific emphasis on dosage. J Pediatr 108:871, 1986.
Intravenous dose = 75% of oral dose.
Dose for supraventricular tachycardia may be higher.

associates[110] reported a decreasing incidence and concentration of digoxin-like immunoreactive substances after 2 months of age in full-term infants, others found persistent interference in older infants and children.[111, 112] Phelps and coworkers found that 100 of 374 (27%) pediatric patients from 0 to 6 years of age tested positive for digoxin-like immunoreactive substances. Concentrations of these substances ranged from 0.2 to 1.37 ng/ml and averaged 0.39 ± 0.18 ng/ml. Although an inverse relationship between the presence of digoxin-like immunoreactive substances and age existed, when present the concentration of these substances did not correlate with age. Twenty-seven per cent of patients who tested positive for digoxin-like immunoreactive substances had concentrations within the therapeutic range of 0.8 to 2 ng/ml. Therefore, clinicians need to be aware of the potential for falsely elevated concentrations when interpreting digoxin serum concentrations in younger patients and adjust doses based on clinical response.

Verapamil

Verapamil is an effective agent for the treatment of supraventricular tachyarrhythmias in both adult and pediatric patients. Several reports of severe cardiac decompensation and arrest have been reported following the use of intravenous verapamil in infants.[113-116] The mechanism involved may include immaturity of the sympathetic innervation of the infant myocardium and a dependence of cardiac output on heart rate rather than stroke volume. The combined effects of the negative inotropic and chronotropic actions of a decreased myocardial calcium influx result in depressed cardiac output that cannot be adequately compensated for by reflex increases in circulating catecholamines. For this reason, the use of verapamil in neonates and young infants is not recommended. If used in older infants and children, extreme caution is recommended, and IV calcium should be readily available to counteract adverse effects.[116]

Central Nervous System

Dopamine Blockade

Medications that block dopamine receptors appear to produce extrapyramidal reactions more commonly in pediatric patients than in adults. Using data from the United Kingdom's Adverse Reaction Register program, acute dystonic and dyskinetic reactions were the most frequently reported extrapyramidal side effects associated with the use of prochlorperazine and haloperidol. Reactions varied significantly with age and were more common in younger patients.[117] Metoclopramide in doses of 2 mg/kg has been shown to be a well-tolerated effective antiemetic in adults, with mild sedation as the predominant adverse effect.[118] The use of metoclopramide as an antiemetic in children and adolescents, however, has been limited by both an age- and dose-related occurrence of extrapyramidal side effects.[119, 120] In one study, the incidence of extrapyramidal reactions during

the first 24 hours of therapy, using 8 mg/kg/day administered as four doses of 2 mg/kg every 2 hours, was 14%. Two doses of diphenhydramine, 0.5 mg/kg given 4 hours apart, were administered prophylactically along with metoclopramide in this trial. Akathisia occurred primarily with high doses and was noted in 9 of 27 (33%) patients receiving doses greater than 2 mg/kg. The incidence of extrapyramidal reactions increased to 50% on the second consecutive day of metoclopramide administration despite continued use of diphenhydramine.[119] Terrin and associates reported 13 adverse reactions in seven of eight (88%) patients treated with metoclopramide as an antiemetic in doses of 0.5 to 2 mg/kg. Prophylactic diphenhydramine was not used in these patients. Twelve of the 13 adverse reactions were extrapyramidal in nature, and in seven cases, patients had received 1 mg/kg or less of metoclopramide.[121]

There appears to be a true age-related increase in sensitivity to the CNS effects of dopamine antagonists. Bateman and colleagues found no difference in pharmacokinetic variables or plasma levels of metoclopramide between children suffering dystonic reactions and those not experiencing adverse effects.[122] The reason for the increased sensitivity is unknown. It has been proposed that the penetration of metoclopramide into the CNS may be higher in pediatric patients.[122] Dopamine-blocking agents may induce an increase in synthesis and release of dopamine within the CNS, resulting in stimulation of unblocked or hypersensitive receptors.[123] A greater concentration of dopamine-2 receptors has been documented in the substantia nigra of younger subjects.[124] Also, an age-related decrease in both dopamine-2 and serotonin-2 receptors has been demonstrated in subjects between the ages of 19 and 73 years.[124]

Theophylline Toxicity

Severe and potentially life-threatening adverse effects of theophylline toxicity include seizures and cardiac arrhythmias. In adults, these effects appear to be dose-related, occurring with increasing frequency as levels rise to greater than the therapeutic range.[51] Generalized seizures are the major cause of morbidity and mortality in the pediatric age group.[125] Although theophylline concentrations greater than 40 μg/ml are associated with an increasing frequency of seizures in adults, refractory seizures have been reported with levels as low as 25 μg/ml.[126] Some evidence exists that children and adolescents are less likely to experience severe complications following acute theophylline ingestion.[127] Arrhythmias and seizures were uncommon and no deaths occurred in one report of 28 pediatric and adolescent patients with theophylline serum concentrations less than 80 μg/ml.[127]

However, the clinical presentation of acute versus chronic theophylline toxicity differs significantly.[128] Seizures are more commonly the presenting symptom in cases of chronic toxicity and may occur with serum levels less than 40 μg/ml. Richards reported four cases of pediatric patients on chronic therapy who experienced seizures with theophylline serum levels in the mildly toxic range of 21 to 32 μg/ml.[129] In 27 of 28 patients included in the report by Gaudreault and associates, theophylline was ingested as a suicide gesture. Whether any of these patients had been receiving prior chronic[127] theophylline therapy was not reported. The adult patients reported by Zwillich and associates[126] all had underlying cardiopulmonary disease and were receiving IV aminophylline therapy at the time they experienced seizure activity.

These observations have been incorporated into guidelines for the management of acute and chronic theophylline overdoses.[125] In acute theophylline ingestion, aggressive intervention using hemodialysis or hemoperfusion is not recommended unless theophylline levels are greater than 100 μg/ml, or unless "severe clinical complications" such as seizures or arrhythmias have been noted. Vigorous GI tract decontamination and supportive care are the primary treatments for the majority of these patients. This is in contrast to the more aggressive measures used in cases of chronic toxicity associated with levels of only 40 to 60 μg/ml. Therefore, whether children and adolescents are actually less sensitive to the CNS effects of theophylline is unclear. It appears that the incidence of seizures may be more a function of acute versus chronic exposure to theophylline rather than a true age-related sensitivity.

Liver

Acetaminophen

Young children appear to have a lower incidence of hepatotoxicity following acute ingestion of acetaminophen than do adolescents and adults (see also Chapter 80). Acute ingestion of acetaminophen in doses equal to or greater than 7.5 g in adults or 150 mg/kg in children is considered hepatotoxic.[130] Fifty-five of 417 children (13.2%) 5 years of age or younger who had ingested potentially serious amounts of acetaminophen included in a national multicenter open trial had acetaminophen plasma levels in the potentially toxic range. Only three (5.2%) experienced serum glutamic-oxaloacetic transaminase values greater than 1,000 international units/l, a value normally considered indicative of hepatotoxicity. As shown in Table 74–7, this is in comparison to a 29% incidence seen in adolescent and adult patients with similar plasma concentrations of acetaminophen.[130]

The reason for this reduced effect is unknown but may be due to age-related differences in acetaminophen metabolism associated with either a larger sulfate pool or greater glutathione stores.[131] Acetaminophen is metabolized primarily to acetaminophen sulfate and acetaminophen glucuronide, with a small fraction undergoing oxidation via the cytochrome P_{450} mixed-function oxidase system to ultimately form conjugates of cysteine and N-acetylcysteine. It is the cytochrome P_{450} pathway that produces potentially toxic intermediate metabolites in an overdose situation.

There are age-related differences in excretion of glucuronide and sulfate conjugates. As discussed in the section on developmental kinetics and shown in Figure 74–4, children less than 9 to 12 years of age metabolize

Table 74–7. COMPARISON OF ADULT AND PEDIATRIC DATA FOR ACETAMINOPHEN OVERDOSE*†

Plasma Acetaminophen Level	Pediatric Cases‡ (no. = 17)	Adult Cases§ (no. = 639)
Toxic		
No. (%) of cases	55 (13.2)	148 (23.2)
No. (%) with SGOT >1,000 international units	3 (5.5)	43 (29.0)
Nontoxic		
No. (%) of cases	276 (66.2)	297 (46.5)
No. (%) with SGOT >1,000 international units	0	1 (0.4)

*From Rumack BH: Acetaminophen overdose in young children. Treatment and effects of alcohol and other additional ingestants in 417 cases. Am J Dis Child 138:428, 1984. Copyright 1984, American Medical Association.
†For purposes of analysis, "adult" = patients >12 years of age, "pediatric" = patients 12 years of age or less.
‡Patients in current study (not all patients had plasma levels determined).
§Data from Rumack BH, Peterson RC, Koch G, et al: Acetaminophen overdose: 662 cases with evaluation of oral acetylcysteine treatment. Arch Intern Med 141:380, 1981. Patients younger than 13 years were subtracted from 662 cases in this study. Toxic plasma level of acetaminophen considered probable risk group only for comparison. Hepatotoxic reaction was defined by an SGOT level of 1,000 international units/l.

a larger portion of acetaminophen via the sulfate conjugation pathway rather than by glucuronidation.[131] At what age a child metabolizes acetaminophen like an adult is unclear, but some data suggest that a transition occurs between 9 and 12 years of age. The mean urinary glucuronide:sulfate excretion ratio is 0.34 in neonates and infants, 0.75 in children 3 to 9 years of age, and 1.8 in adults receiving therapeutic doses of acetaminophen.[132] This demonstrates the younger child's dependence on the sulfate pathway for the primary metabolism of acetaminophen versus that of the older child or adult. The alternate pathway of sulfate conjugation may result in a lower incidence of hepatotoxicity by providing a smaller amount of metabolites available for the mixed-function oxidase pathway, thereby generating fewer free radicals.[133] This theory is supported by the observed differences in toxicity seen in children less than 6 years of age versus older children, adolescents, and adults.

The cytochrome P_{450} mechanism is responsible for the production of toxic intermediate metabolites normally inactivated by glutathione. In an overdose situation, however, hepatic glutathione becomes depleted and the toxic intermediates accumulate. A threefold increase in cytochrome P_{450} reactive metabolites has been found in the urine of adult patients following the ingestion of toxic doses of acetaminophen.[134] This is thought to be a result of saturation of the sulfate and glucuronide conjugation pathways. Similar data are unavailable in the pediatric population.

It has also been proposed that children possess a higher amount of available glutathione for acetaminophen metabolism.[135] A fourfold higher rate of glutathione turnover has been noted in young animals, suggesting that the immature liver provides a mechanism for increased rates of detoxification.[136] Higher median lethal dose values (LD50) of acetaminophen in younger animals have been reported, adding further support to this theory.[137]

Despite a lower trend of hepatotoxicity associated

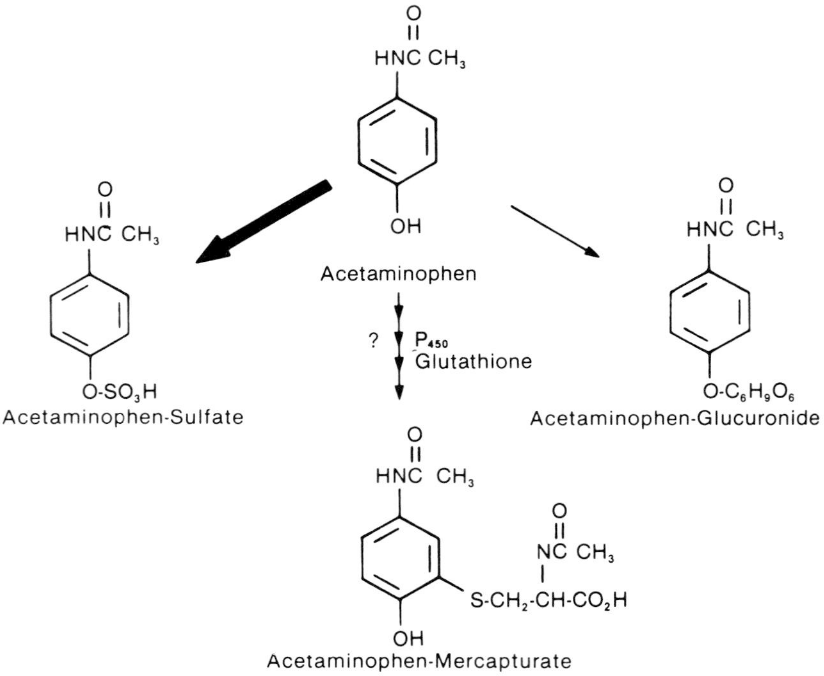

Figure 74–4. Proposed metabolic pathways for acetaminophen metabolism in children. The central pathway (P_{450}) in the diagram has not yet been characterized in children. (From Peterson RG and Rumack BH: Age as a variable in acetaminophen overdose. Arch Intern Med 141:390, 1981. Copyright 1981, American Medical Association.)

with acetaminophen ingestion in infants and children, cases of severe liver damage and death have occurred;[135, 138, 139] therefore, all potential ingestions of acetaminophen regardless of age need to be investigated fully and treated aggressively with standard protocols, including the use of *N*-acetylcysteine if serum acetaminophen levels are elevated.[130]

Isoniazid

Isoniazid is associated with asymptomatic increases in liver function tests (serum glutamic-oxaloacetic transaminase, serum glutamic-pyruvic transaminase) in 10 to 20% of adult recipients.[140] Similarly, 41 of 239 children (17.1%) 9 to 14 years of age receiving prophylactic isoniazid had increases of at least one transaminase level to greater than the normal range during the initial 12 weeks of therapy.[141] These abnormalities resolved completely within 4 to 8 weeks in the majority of patients despite continued therapy. In only two children (0.8%) did enzyme values greater than 100 units occur, necessitating discontinuation of therapy. Routine monitoring of liver function tests, therefore, in patients younger than 35 years of age, including children, is not recommended.[142]

A smaller percentage of patients experience a more significant liver involvement referred to as isoniazid-associated hepatitis. The risk of the development of isoniazid-associated hepatitis increases with age. The rates quoted most often follow: less than 20 years of age, 0%; 20 to 34 years of age, 0.3%; 35 to 49 years of age, 1.2%; 50 to 64 years of age, 2.3%; and older than 64 years of age, 0.8%.[143] These incidence numbers are from a U.S. Public Health Service study involving more than 13,000 patients, 18% of whom were less than 20 years of age. The extremely low incidence rates quoted in the young age group are, therefore, felt to accurately represent the true incidence.

The pathogenesis of isoniazid-induced liver damage is thought to be related to the formation of hepatotoxic metabolites. Isoniazid is metabolized by acetylation to acetylhydrazine, which is, in turn, converted to hepatotoxic acylating compounds by hepatic microsomal enzymes.[140] Although a patient's acetylator phenotype has been proposed as a risk factor, other investigators have found no correlation between rapid and slow acetylator status and the development of hepatotoxicity.[144, 145]

The production of chemically reactive metabolites may be enhanced by concurrent therapy with enzyme-inducing compounds such as phenobarbital or rifampin.[140] Of concern are several reports of severe hepatotoxicity in children treated with combinations of rifampin and isoniazid.[146, 147] The frequency of hepatotoxic reactions to combinations of rifampin and isoniazid in children has been reported to be 3.2%, similar to that occurring in adults.[148] Hepatotoxic reactions were six times more frequent among children receiving rifampin as part of their treatment regimen, and the majority who experienced hepatotoxicity had received doses of isoniazid greater than 10 mg/kg or rifampin greater than 15 mg/kg, or both.[149] In another recent report, 37% of 73 children receiving isoniazid and rifampin experienced biochemical evidence of hepatotoxicity.[145] Five patients (7%) experienced clinical signs and symptoms of hepatitis, and these investigators found a higher incidence of liver involvement in infants less than 18 months of age. Although not a consistent finding, a dose-related hepatotoxicity has been suggested; therefore, daily doses of 15 mg/kg of rifampin and 10 mg/kg of isoniazid should not be exceeded.[148]

Kidney

Aminoglycoside nephrotoxicity and ototoxicity appear to be relatively infrequent occurrences in infants and children.[150] Although aminoglycosides are widely used in children of all ages, there is a relative lack of well-designed, controlled studies assessing the toxicities of these agents in this population. The incidence and severity of both nephrotoxicity and ototoxicity are generally assumed to be lower than in adults and related to long duration of therapy or higher than recommended dosage regimens, or both.[150] Animal studies support the impression that the immature or young kidney is more tolerant of the effects of aminoglycosides.[151, 152] Young animals experience less severe impairment of renal function than do older animals when given equivalent milligram/kilogram doses of aminoglycosides.

The low incidence of nephrotoxicity in the newborn period may be related to a decrease in renal accumulation of aminoglycosides and to the relative protection of cortical nephrons during the newborn period when renal blood flow is directed primarily toward the medullary region.[150, 153] Several factors complicate the assessment of nephrotoxicity in the newborn period. The use of serum creatinine determinations in newborns is limited by the interference of maternal creatinine. Small changes of 0.3 to 0.5 mg/dl may be difficult to distinguish from laboratory variation yet represent significant changes in renal function. Any rise in serum creatinine levels during the first week of life may be masked as maternal creatinine is excreted and the infant's serum creatinine level falls. Renal injury may also be the result of non–drug related factors commonly seen in the neonatal period, such as hypoxia and sepsis.

A highly sensitive index of renal tubular damage is the measurement of urinary alanine aminopeptidase, N-acetyl-β-D-glucosaminidase, and urinary β_2-microglobulin. Several investigators have found increased urinary concentrations of these enzymes and microglobulin following aminoglycoside use in neonates.[154, 155] Although enzymuria may have predictive value in older patient groups, Adelman and coworkers found that these substances were not helpful in predicting the development of nephrotoxicity in newborns.[153] Measurements of urinary enzyme activity varied markedly from day to day and bore little relationship to changes in serum creatinine levels or creatinine clearance in the 112 infants studied. Initial and final urinary enzyme activities were no different in infants with nephrotoxicity from those without nephrotoxicity. Peak and trough amikacin levels also did not differ between infants with and without nephrotoxicity. Despite these findings, amikacin use was associated with a delayed postnatal maturation of GFR and a significant fall in creatinine clearance of greater than 25% in 40% of the treated patients. Therefore, the clinical predictive value of enzymuria remains to be determined. Tessin and associates found similar increases in urinary activity of alanine aminopeptidase and N-acetyl-β-D-glucosaminidase in 66 neonates after only 2 days of antibiotic therapy with either ceftazidime or tobramycin.[156] The possibility that enzymuria may be caused by non–drug related factors or other drugs used concurrently in the neonatal period (i.e., ampicillin) needs to be investigated.

Many years of clinical experience with aminoglycosides indicate that nephrotoxicity in terms of elevated serum creatinine and blood urea nitrogen values or proteinuria is uncommon in newborn infants. The frequency with which aminoglycosides are used and the rarity of proven nephrotoxicity implies a high degree of safety when given in recommended doses for 5 to 10 days in this age group.[150]

Similarly, the incidence of vestibular and cochlear damage associated with aminoglycoside therapy in pediatric patients appears no greater than that seen in a control population. Finitzo-Hieber and coworkers, using auditory brain stem response audiometry in a longitudinal assessment of 150 newborn infants given an aminoglycoside antibiotic, found no significant difference in hearing impairment when compared with age- and sex-matched controls.[157]

There have been few well-controlled studies evaluating the toxicity of aminoglycoside antibiotics in older children and adolescents, and this also may be due to the belief that toxicities are uncommon in this age group.[150]

The exact mechanism by which aminoglycosides cause ototoxicity and nephrotoxicity is not known. Tissue accumulation related to an enhanced affinity for specific cellular binding sites is believed responsible.[150] It is unclear whether the lower incidence of toxicity is due to developmental differences in tissue binding or altered perfusion and distribution of renal blood flow during the newborn period. This would not explain, however, the lower incidence of toxicity seen in older pediatric patients.

High doses of aminoglycoside antibiotics are often recommended for treating pulmonary infections in patients with cystic fibrosis.[40, 41] These large dosage requirements have been attributed to a larger apparent volume of distribution and higher total body clearance in patients with cystic fibrosis.[40, 41] These observations, however, have not been a consistent finding. Other investigators have found that the volume of distribution and total body clearance of aminoglycosides in patients with cystic fibrosis do not differ from those seen in a comparable pediatric population without the disease.[158–161] The larger dose requirements in patients with cystic fibrosis are thought to be related more to the selection of high target peak serum concentrations (8 to 12 μg/ml) than to altered drug disposition.[158] Despite the large doses, high peak serum concentrations, long courses of therapy, and repeated exposures used in patients with cystic fibrosis, permanent hearing impairment and renal toxicity are extremely uncommon in this population.[150]

The use of vancomycin in combination with an aminoglycoside appears to increase the nephrotoxic potential of both drugs significantly. Farber and Moellering in a retrospective analysis found evidence of nephrotoxicity in 12 of 34 (35%) adult patients receiving vancomycin and an aminoglycoside, compared with a 5% incidence (3 of 60 cases) in patients given vancomycin alone.[162] Dean and colleagues reported a similar incidence of nephrotoxicity in pediatric patients.[163] Two of 345 (0.6%) patients receiving an aminoglycoside alone, 2 of 19 (11%) patients receiving vancomycin alone, and 2 of 9 (22%) patients receiving combination therapy for 1 week had significant increases in serum creatinine values, defined as elevations greater than or equal to 0.5 mg dl. In all six patients, trough serum concentrations of vancomycin or the aminoglycoside, or both, rose prior to elevations in the serum creatinine value. Therefore, close monitoring of trough concentrations may correspond with tissue accumulation and aid in the early detection of nephrotoxicity.[164] Odio and associates reported four pediatric patients who experienced nephrotoxicity, defined as a twofold increase in serum creatinine concentrations, during combined vancomycin-aminoglycoside therapy.[165] Patients included in this report ranged in age from 3 to 13 years and had received combination therapy for periods of 3 to 31 days. Although the exact incidence of toxicity in pediatric patients is unknown, serum creatinine and serum drug concentrations should be monitored closely during combined therapy with these or other potentially nephrotoxic agents.

DRUG DELIVERY

Pediatric patients are often admitted to intensive care units with complicated medical problems. The multiplicity of disease states can result in complicated medication regimens. Aranda and coworkers evaluated 293 patients admitted to a newborn intensive care unit and showed that 76.1% of neonates received between 1 and 26 medications.[166] The average number of medications administered was 6.19/patient. Fifty-four per cent of all babies received four different medications. Medications were administered intravenously (57.35%) and orally (19.12%). Intramuscular, topical, and rectal routes of administration were used less frequently. Antibiotics were among the most commonly prescribed agents. Comparable data for pediatric intensive care units are not available.

The goal of drug delivery is to administer medications completely and consistently. Failure to accurately deliver medications may result in under- or overdelivery of medications, leading to therapeutic failure or toxicity.

Oral Administration

Medications are frequently administered orally or through nasogastric or feeding tubes. Oral administration of medication is limited by several factors. Many medications are not available in pediatric dosage forms or concentrations. Solid adult dosage forms must be crushed and formulated into solutions or suspensions prior to administration. Little information is available on the proper formulation, stability, sterility, and bioavailability of these preparations. Liquid dosage forms may contain undesirable or unlabeled ingredients that can produce adverse effects. These ingredients include dyes, preservatives, or flavoring agents.

Oral medications can have osmolalities severalfold higher than parenteral products of the same concentration. The high osmolalities are usually due to the secondary additives such as diluents and preservatives.[167]

The high osmolality of liquid medications can be a common cause of diarrhea in patients.[168]

Caution should be used when administering medications through nasogastric or feeding tubes. Antiepileptic medications have been shown to bind to the inside of feeding tubes, resulting in incomplete drug delivery.[169, 170] This binding may be a function of pH, dilution of the dose, or fluid used to flush the tube.[170, 171] Several studies have documented drug incompatibilities with enteral feedings.[172, 173] Medications may form a complex with the enteral product, resulting in decreased amounts of drug available for absorption.[174, 175] Also, medications added to enteral formulas may increase the osmolality of the formula. The osmolality of drug-formula mixtures can increase by 300% over that of the formula alone.[176] Necrotizing enterocolitis has been reported in premature infants receiving hyperosmolar enteral formulas.[177] White and Harkavy recommend that if oral medications must be administered with enteral feedings, IV preparations be administered through the feeding tube to avoid increasing the osmolality of the formula.[176]

In summary, the absorption of oral medications depends on the age of the child, underlying pathophysiology, dosage formulation, and method of administration. Medications administered by the oral route may be erratically absorbed, resulting in variable clinical responses and erratic serum drug concentrations. Table 74–8 summarizes the limitations of administering oral medications to critically ill pediatric patients.

Parenteral Administration

The IV route of administration has been thought to provide rapid, complete, and consistent drug delivery. In vitro and in vivo studies have shown that this may not be true in pediatric patients. The IV infusion system, injection site, IV fluid flow rate, and internal diameter of the IV tubing can influence the completeness of drug delivery. A typical IV infusion system is shown in Figure 74–5.

In vitro studies have shown that the completeness of gentamicin, aminophylline, and chloramphenicol delivery was dependent on the IV flow rate and on the site of drug injection into the IV system.[178, 179] Using varying IV flow rates and injecting into the flashball, y site, and buretrol, it was noted that there was a delay in the time

Table 74–8. FACTORS AFFECTING DRUG DELIVERY TO PEDIATRIC PATIENTS

Oral Administration
Limited pediatric dosage forms and concentrations
Osmolality of liquid dosage forms
Medication binding to feeding tubes
Medication interaction with enteral feeding solutions

Parenteral Administration
Intravenous infusion system
Medication injection site
Intravenous fluid flow rate
Intravenous tubing internal diameter and length
In-line filters
Medication specific gravity

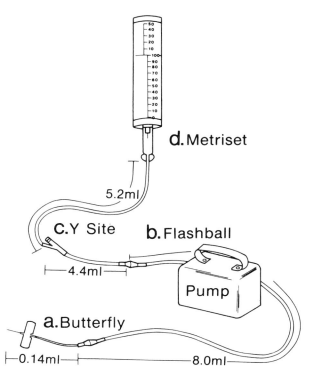

Figure 74–5. Intravenous infusion system commonly used in pediatric patients. (Adapted from Gould T and Roberts RJ: Therapeutic problems arising from the intravenous route for drug administration. J Pediatr 95:465, 1979.)

required for the drug to begin to infuse into the patient. The time for complete infusion of the drug was also prolonged. This was especially true for drugs injected into the distal injection sites and infused at slow infusion rates. In vivo, peak chloramphenicol and chloramphenicol succinate levels were higher and occurred earlier after the IV infusion when the dose was injected into the flashball versus the buretrol.[179]

The type of infusion system used can affect drug delivery and serum drug concentrations. Nahata and coworkers showed that a syringe pump delivery system delivered tobramycin over a more predictable period compared with standard delivery systems. This resulted in higher and earlier tobramycin peak concentrations.[180, 181]

The IV tubing lumen can also affect drug delivery. Complete drug administration can be delayed with larger bore tubing compared with smaller bore tubing.[182–184] The mechanism to explain this is unclear but may be due to the specific gravity of the medication, volume of fluid contained within the IV tubing, and laminar flow characteristics.[182, 183] This may be important because residual drug in the tubing may lead to significant amounts of drug being discarded with routine changing of the IV tubing. Also, residual drug may interact with other drugs, leading to inactivation of one of the agents.[185]

In addition to flow rate and injection site, other factors such as y site "dead space" and in-line filters can affect drug delivery. Small volumes of drug injected into large injection ports with insufficient flushing may lead to

drug retained in the injection port. Injecting drug past the end of the injection port with thorough flushing after the drug is injected should prevent medication from being retained in the injection port. Increased velocity from fast-running IV fluids or small-diameter IV tubing may create enough turbulence to pull medication retained in the injection port and allow mixing in the IV tubing.

The design and position of in-line filters can affect drug delivery, depending on the IV flow rate and drug specific gravity.[186, 187] When a filter is positioned with the fluid exit above (inverted) the filter, drug delivery is enhanced for drugs with specific gravities less than the primary IV fluid and is delayed for drugs with specific gravities greater than the primary IV fluid. The reverse is true when the fluid exits below (upright) the filter. Drugs with specific gravities less than the IV fluid move away from dependent portions of the filter, whereas drugs with specific gravities greater than the IV fluid move toward these portions of the filter. Drug retention results from inadequate mixing in the fluid chamber of the filter.

The specific gravity of a drug also plays a role when in-line filters are not used. Dye studies have shown that with slow infusion rates and drugs with specific gravities less than the IV fluid, back diffusion occurs and retards drug delivery. The opposite is true with drugs that have specific gravities greater than the IV fluid.[186]

Retrograde Administration

Fluid administration is often limited in pediatric patients. Patients receiving multiple IV medications can meet or exceed their daily fluid allotment using normal IV drug delivery methods. Benzing and Loggie first described an alternate drug delivery system to reduce fluid administration to pediatric patients.[188] This method was known as the retrograde method.

The system consists of two three-way stopcocks with a length of IV tubing between them (Fig. 74–6). When the drug is administered, the stopcocks are turned off to prevent flow to the patient and from the primary IV line. The drug is injected in a retrograde fashion into the IV tubing through the stopcock closest to the patient. A second syringe is placed in the stopcock nearest the IV pump to accept the displaced IV fluid from the IV tubing. After the drug is injected, the stopcocks are opened to allow fluid to flow to the patient. The IV infusion rate is adjusted, depending on the volume of drug injected and the desired infusion time. The volume of drug injected is usually limited to less than or equal to one half of the volume in the IV tubing. Volumes greater than this may cause drug to be expelled into the "discard syringe."[189] Figure 74–7 outlines a scheme based on IV flow rate and dosage volume that can be used to determine whether a medication should be administered using the retrograde system or a syringe pump infusion system.

Controlling drug delivery with the retrograde method can result in reliable and consistent serum drug levels.[190] However, delayed drug delivery can still occur using

A

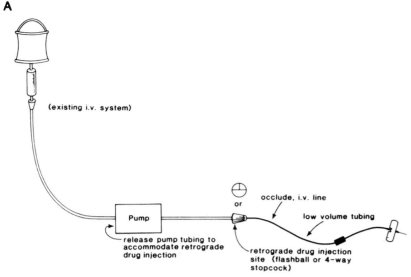

(existing i.v. system)

occlude, i.v. line

low volume tubing

Pump

release pump tubing to accommodate retrograde drug injection

retrograde drug injection site (flashball or 4-way stopcock)

B

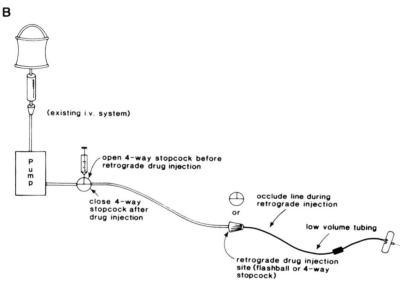

(existing i.v. system)

open 4-way stopcock before retrograde drug injection

P u m p

close 4-way stopcock after drug injection

occlude line during retrograde injection

low volume tubing

retrograde drug injection site (flashball or 4-way stopcock)

Figure 74–6. *A*, Construction of an intravenous (IV) system for manual retrograde injection. An injection site (flashball or stopcock) and low-volume extension tubing are located at the distal end of the existing IV set-up. *B*, Construction of IV system for retrograde injection modified for a volume infusion pump device unable to accept retrograde injections. System consists of existing IV to which is attached an extension set with a proximal four-way stopcock and distal flashball injection site. A large-volume syringe is attached to the four-way stopcock and acts as an overflow reservoir for the IV fluid displaced by the dosage volume. (Adapted from Leff RD and Roberts RJ: Methods for intravenous drug administration in the pediatric patient. J Pediatr 98:632, 1981.)

this system.[183, 191] The delay in drug delivery may be due to the injected drug volume, tubing internal diameter, IV tubing length, and the IV flow rate.[183, 191–193]

The retrograde method may allow the sequential administration of several medications. Several authors have investigated whether incompatible medications could be administered sequentially if separated by a fluid barrier.[194–196] Using different barrier fluids, barrier volumes, and IV flow rates has resulted in contradictory results. Although immediate precipitation may not occur with some drug combinations in the IV tubing, it may occur in the stopcock because of incomplete flushing of the stopcock or in the catheter between the patient and the retrograde system. This would indicate that a delayed interaction can occur. Therefore, only one medication at a time should be administered using the retrograde system.

In summary, various components of the IV infusion system can influence the completeness of drug delivery to a patient. Medications should be administered into injection ports as close to the patient as possible. All medications should be followed by a sufficient volume of flushing solution to ensure that residual drug does not remain in the IV tubing. Erratic serum drug concentrations or variable pharmacologic responses may be attributable to incomplete drug delivery. Efforts should be made to evaluate the method of drug delivery prior to attributing erratic results to underlying patient pathophysiology.

THERAPEUTIC DRUG MONITORING

Therapeutic drug monitoring may be defined as the process of using drug concentrations, pharmacokinetic principles, and pharmacodynamic criteria to optimize drug therapy.[197] The goal of therapeutic drug monitoring is to maximize the therapeutic effect while avoiding toxicity. Therapeutic drug monitoring is not applicable to all drugs. Drugs that do not produce toxicity at serum

Steps

#1. On admission establish only a "basic" I.V. set-up which includes I.V. fluid container, volume control device (Metriset) and associated I.V. tubing connected directly to venous catheter (butterfly, abocath, etc.).

#2. On the basis of **I.V. FLOW RATE** and **DOSE VOLUME** select the appropriate system (retrograde or syringe infusion).

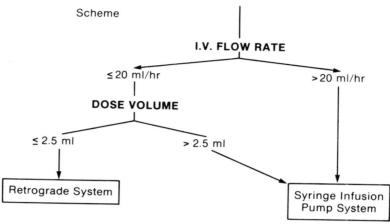

Figure 74–7. Selection of an appropriate method (retrograde versus syringe infusion pump system) for intravenous drug administration based on intravenous flow rate and dose volume. (Adapted from Roberts RJ: Intravenous administration of medication in pediatric patients: Problems and solutions. Pediatr Clin North Am 28:23, 1981.)

concentrations close to those required for therapeutic efficacy usually do not require monitoring (i.e., penicillins, β-blockers, and so forth). Drugs that can produce toxicity at serum concentrations close to those required for therapeutic effect are the drugs most commonly monitored. These agents are said to have a narrow therapeutic index—that is, the ratio of effective concentration:toxic concentration is low. The indications for therapeutic drug monitoring include (1) narrow therapeutic range, (2) no clinically observable end point, (3) unpredictable dose-response relationship, (4) serious consequences of toxicity or lack of effectiveness, (5) correlation between serum concentration and efficacy and toxicity, and (6) serum drug concentrations are available.[198] The medications commonly administered in a pediatric intensive care unit that require therapeutic drug monitoring are listed in Table 74–9.

There are multiple indications for obtaining serum drug concentrations. It is important in that it will affect the timing of the sample. The time the sample is obtained depends on the question being asked. The common indications for obtaining serum drug concentrations are listed in Table 74–10.

The timing of the serum drug concentration is critical to the interpretation of the result. The timing of peak serum drug concentration is dependent on the route of administration and the drug product. Peak serum drug concentration occurs soon after an IV bolus dose, whereas it is usually delayed after an IM, subcutaneous, or oral dose. Oral medications can be administered as either (1) liquid or (2) rapid- or slow-release solid dosage forms (e.g., theophylline). The absorption and distribution phases must be considered when obtaining a peak serum drug concentration. The peak level may be much higher and occur earlier after a liquid or rapid-release solid dosage form compared with a sustained-release dosage form. Trough concentrations are usually obtained just prior to the next dose. Drugs with long half-lives (e.g., phenobarbital) or sustained-dosage forms (e.g., theophylline) may have minimal variation in their peak and trough serum drug concentrations. The timing of the determination of serum drug concentrations may be less critical in patients taking these dosage forms. If toxicity is suspected, serum drug concentrations can be obtained any time during the dosing interval.

Appropriate interpretation of the serum drug concentration is the step that requires an understanding of the relevant patient factors, pharmacokinetics of the drug

Table 74–9. COMMONLY ADMINISTERED MEDICATIONS THAT REQUIRE THERAPEUTIC DRUG MONITORING

Antiarrhythmic agents	Digoxin
Antibiotics	Aminoglycosides
	Chloramphenicol
	Sulfamethoxazole
	Vancomycin
Anticonvulsant agents	Phenobarbital
	Phenytoin
Bronchodilators	Theophylline

Table 74–10. CLINICAL INDICATIONS FOR THERAPEUTIC DRUG MONITORING IN THE PEDIATRIC INTENSIVE CARE UNIT

Therapeutic confirmation
Limited objective monitoring parameters available
Poor patient response
Suspected toxicity
Identification of drug interactions
Determination of individual pharmacokinetic parameters
Changes in patient pathophysiology or disease state

being monitored, and dosing regimen. Misinterpretation of the serum drug concentration can result in ineffective and, at worst, harmful dosage regimen adjustments.

Understanding the patient factors that can affect the interpretation of serum drug concentrations in children is especially important. Plasma protein binding may be reduced or altered in children. This can result in an increased free fraction of drugs. Drugs that have been shown to have increased free fractions in neonates include salicylates, digoxin, phenytoin, and diazepam.[199] An increased free fraction of drug may account for the increased responsiveness or toxicity seen in a patient.

The metabolite pattern of a drug may be different in a pediatric patient, accounting for increased efficacy or toxicity. Neonates metabolize theophylline to caffeine. Caffeine may explain the responsiveness to lower serum concentrations of theophylline in the treatment of neonatal apnea.[200] Other agents that show differences in metabolite production include acetaminophen and chloramphenicol.

Endogenous interfering substances can also cause misinterpretation of a serum drug concentration. The digoxin-like immunoreactive substance that has been identified in neonates and infants has been shown to falsely elevate digoxin assay results.[110] The cross-reactivity may be due to structurally similar serum steroid compounds, and the degree of interference may depend on the assay used.[201] Medications administered by other routes can interfere with the determination of the same medication administered systemically. Significant absorption of aerosolized aminoglycosides can interfere with the determination of serum aminoglycoside levels.[202]

Technical information required to interpret serum drug concentrations must not be overlooked. The dosage information required to interpret a serum drug concentration includes the dose, route of administration, duration of therapy, and site of administration. The starting and stopping times for intermittent infusions and the rate of infusion for continuous infusions must be recorded. The exact sampling times in relation to the dose are critical.

Pediatric blood drawing tubes should be used to minimize volumes of blood drawn. Most assays require less than 0.1 ml of serum or plasma.[202] If samples are collected by skin puncture, multiple samples can lead to tissue trauma. Artificial dilution of the sample can occur with tissue fluid if vigorous squeezing is used.[202]

Drug interactions can affect serum drug concentrations. Aminoglycosides can be inactivated by extended-spectrum penicillins in vitro.[185] This interaction is time-, temperature-, and concentration-dependent and can result in lower than expected aminoglycoside levels. Patients receiving aminoglycosides and extended-spectrum penicillins should have their aminoglycoside levels assayed immediately after blood is drawn. If this is not possible, the samples should be centrifuged, separated, and frozen until the assay is performed.

The serum drug concentration should be interpreted within the context of the patient's condition. Therapeutic ranges serve as initial guidelines for each patient. Doses should not be adjusted on the basis of the result

Table 74–11. GUIDELINES FOR INTERPRETATION OF SERUM DRUG CONCENTRATIONS

Determine if the patient is being given an appropriate dose
Determine if the patient is at steady state
Determine the exact time of the blood samples
Determine if timing of blood samples is appropriate for indication for samples
Evaluate the method of drug delivery to assess the completeness of delivery

alone. Individual dosage ranges should be developed for each patient because various patients may experience therapeutic efficacy, failure, or toxicity within a given therapeutic range. Guidelines for interpreting serum drug concentrations are listed in Table 74–11.

References

1. Hyman PE, Clarke DD, Everett SL, et al: Gastric acid secretory function in preterm infants. J Pediatr 106:467, 1985.
2. Euler AR, Byrne WJ, Meis PJ, et al: Basal and pentagastrin-stimulated acid secretion in newborn human infants. Pediatr Res 13:36, 1979.
3. Deren JS: Development of structure and function of the fetal and newborn stomach. Am J Clin Nutr 24:144, 1971.
4. Lebenthal E, Lee PC, and Heitlinger LA: Impact of development of the gastrointestinal tract on infant feeding. J Pediatr 102:1, 1983.
5. Watkins JB, Ingall D, Szczepanik P, et al: Bile salt metabolism in the newborn; measurement of pool size and synthesis by stable isotope technique. N Engl J Med 288:431, 1973.
6. deBelle RC, Vaupshas V, Vitullo BB, et al: Intestinal absorption of bile salts: Immature development in the neonate. J Pediatr 94:472, 1979.
7. Dallman PR: Iron, vitamin E and folate in the preterm infant. J Pediatr 85:742, 1974.
8. Hillman LS, Martin LA, and Haddad JG: Absorption and maintenance dosage of 25-hydroxycholecalciferol (25-HCC) in premature infants. Pediatr Res 13:400, 1979.
9. Huang NN and High RH: Comparison of serum levels following the administration of oral and parenteral preparations of penicillin to infants and children of various age groups. J Pediatr 42:657, 1953.
10. Silverio J and Poole JW: Serum concentrations of ampicillin in newborn infants after oral administration. Pediatrics 51:578, 1973.
11. O'Connor WJ, Warren GH, Edrada LS, et al: Serum concentrations of sodium nafcillin in infants during the perinatal period. Antimicrob Agent Chemother 5:220, 1965.
12. Heimann G: Enteral absorption and bioavailability in children in relation to age. Eur J Clin Pharmacol 18:43, 1980.
13. Jalling B, Boreus LO, Rane A, et al: Plasma concentrations of diphenylhydantoin in young infants. Pharmacol Clin 2:200, 1970.
14. Levy G, Khanna NN, Soda DM, et al: Pharmacokinetics of acetaminophen in the human neonate: Formation of acetaminophen glucuronide and sulfate in relation to plasma bilirubin concentrations and d-glucaric acid excretion. Pediatrics 55:818, 1975.
15. Painter MJ, Pippenger C, MacDonald H, et al: Phenobarbital and diphenylhydantoin levels in neonates with seizures. J Pediatr 92:315, 1978.
16. Rapp RP, Young B, Perrier D, et al: Phenytoin dosing in infants. Drug Intel Clin Pharm 11:462, 1977.
17. Shankaran S and Kauffman RE: Use of chloramphenicol palmitate in neonates. J Pediatr 105:113, 1984.
18. Kauffman RE, Thirumoorthi MB, Buckley JA, et al: Relative bioavailability of intravenous chloramphenicol succinate and oral chloramphenicol palmitate in infants and children. J Pediatr 99:963, 1981.

19. Agurell S, Berlin A, Ferngren HG, et al: Plasma levels of diazepam after parenteral and rectal administration to children. Epilepsia 16:277, 1975.

20. Knudsen FU: Plasma-diazepam in infants after rectal administration in solution and by suppository. Acta Paediatr Scand 66:563, 1977.

21. Knudsen FU: Effective short-term diazepam prophylaxis in febrile convulsions. J Pediatr 106:487, 1985.

22. Govaerts MJ and Capouet V: Rectal benzodiazepines for premedication in children. Review and personal experience. Acta Anaesth Belg 38(Suppl)1:53, 1987.

23. DeJong PC and Verburg MP: Comparison of rectal to intramuscular administration of midazolam and atropine for premedication of children. Acta Anaesthesiol Scand 32:485, 1988.

24. Burckart GJ, White TJ, Siegle RL, et al: Rectal thiopental versus an intramuscular cocktail for sedating children before computerized tomography. Am J Hosp Pharm 37:222, 1980.

25. Snead OC and Miles MV: Treatment of status epilepticus in children with rectal sodium valproate. J Pediatr 106:323, 1985.

26. Morselli PL, Franco-Morselli R, and Bossi L: Clinical pharmacokinetics in newborns and infants: Age-related differences and therapeutic implications. Clin Pharmacokinet 5:485, 1980.

27. Lester RS: Topical formulary for the pediatrician. Pediatr Clin North Am 30:749, 1983.

28. James LS: Hexachlorophene. Pediatrics 49:492, 1972.

29. Tyrala EE, Hillman LS, Hillman RE, et al: Clinical pharmacology of hexachlorophene in newborn infants. J Pediatr 91:481, 1977.

30. Pramanik AK and Hansen RC: Transcutaneous gamma benzene hexachloride absorption and toxicity in infants and children. Arch Dermatol 115:1224, 1979.

31. Davies JE, Dedhia HV, Morgade C, et al: Lindane poisonings. Arch Dermatol 119:142, 1983.

32. Rothstein P, Dornbusch J, and Shaywitz BA: Prolonged seizures associated with the use of viscous lidocaine. J Pediatr 101:461, 1982.

33. Filloux F: Toxic encephalopathy caused by topically applied diphenhydramine. J Pediatr 108:1018, 1986.

34. Shawn DH and McGuigan MA: Poisoning from dermal absorption of promethazine. Can Med Assoc J 130:1460, 1984.

35. Evans NJ, Rutter N, Hadgraft J, et al: Percutaneous administration of theophylline in the preterm infant. J Pediatr 107:307, 1985.

36. Blumer JL: Therapeutic agents. In: Fanaroff and Martin (eds): Neonatal-Perinatal Medicine: Diseases of the Fetus and Infant, 4th ed. St. Louis, CV Mosby, 1987, p. 1248 (Appendix B).

37. Friis-Hansen B: Water distribution in the fetus and newborn infant. Acta Paediatr Scand 305(Suppl):7, 1983.

38. Haughey DB, Hilligoss DM, Grassi A, et al: Two-compartment gentamicin pharmacokinetics in premature neonates: A comparison to adults with decreased glomerular filtration rates. J Pediatr 96:325, 1980.

39. Thomson AH, Way S, Bryson SM, et al: Population pharmacokinetics of gentamicin in neonates. Dev Pharmacol Ther 11:173, 1988.

40. Kearns GL, Hilman BC, and Wilson JT: Dosing implications of altered gentamicin disposition in patients with cystic fibrosis. J Pediatr 100:312, 1982.

41. Kelly HB, Menendez R, Fan L, et al: Pharmacokinetics of tobramycin in cystic fibrosis. J Pediatr 100:318, 1982.

42. Morselli PL, Principi N, Tognoni G, et al: Diazepam elimination in premature and full term infants and children. J Perinat Med 1:133, 1973.

43. Pacifici GM, Viani A, Taddeucci BG, et al: Effects of development, aging and renal and hepatic insufficiency as well as hemodialysis on the plasma concentrations of albumin and a1-acid glycoprotein: Implications for binding of drugs. Ther Drug Monit 8:259, 1986.

44. Rane A, Perknut ML, Jalling B, et al: Plasma protein binding of diphenylhydantoin in normal and hyperbilirubinemic infants. J Pediatr 78:877, 1971.

45. Kurz H, Mauser-Ganshorn A, and Stickel HH: Differences in the binding of drugs to plasma proteins from newborn and adult man. I. Eur J Clin Pharmacol 11:463, 1977.

46. Kurz H, Michels H, and Stickel HH: Differences in the binding of drugs to plasma proteins from newborn and adult man. II. Eur J Clin Pharmacol 11:469, 1977.

47. Nitowsky HM, Matz L, and Berzofsky JA: Studies on oxidative drug metabolism in the full term newborn infant. J Pediatr 69:1139, 1966.

48. Milsap RL and Szefler SJ: Special pharmacokinetic considerations in children. In: Evans WE, Schentag JJ, and Jusko WJ (eds): Applied Pharmacokinetics—Principles of Therapeutic Drug Monitoring, 2nd ed. Spokane, Applied Therapeutics, 1986, pp. 294–330.

49. Nassif EG, Weinberger MM, Shannon D, et al: Theophylline disposition in infancy. J Pediatr 98:158, 1981.

50. Gelehrter TD: Enzyme induction. N Engl J Med 294:522, 589, 646, 1976.

51. Bukowshyj M, Nakatsu K, and Munt PW: Theophylline reassessed. Ann Intern Med 101:63, 1984.

52. Arant BS: Developmental patterns of renal functional maturation compared in the human neonate. J Pediatr 92:705, 1978.

53. Kaplan JM, McCracken GH, Horton LJ, et al: Pharmacologic studies in neonates given large doses of ampicillin. J Pediatr 84:571, 1974.

54. Nelson JD, Shelton S, and Kusmiesz H: Clinical pharmacology of ticarcillin in the newborn infant: Relation to age, gestational age and weight. J Pediatr 87:474, 1975.

55. McCracken GH, Ginsberg C, Chrane DF, et al: Clinical pharmacology of penicillin in newborn infants. J Pediatr 82:692, 1973.

56. Schwartz GJ, Hegyi T, and Spitzer A: Subtherapeutic dicloxacillin levels in a neonate: Possible mechanisms. J Pediatr 89:310, 1976.

57. Leake RD, Trygstad CW, and Oh W: Inulin clearance in the newborn infant: Relationship to gestational and postnatal age. Pediatr Res 10:759, 1976.

58. Aperia A, Broberger O, Elinder G, et al: Postnatal development of renal function in pre-term and full term infants. Acta Paediatr Scand 70:183, 1981.

59. Kasik JW, Jenkins S, Leuschen MP, et al: Postconceptional age and gentamicin elimination half life. J Pediatr 106:502, 1985.

60. James A, Koren G, Milliken J, et al: Vancomycin pharmacokinetics and dose recommendations for preterm infants. Antimicrob Agent Chemother 31:52, 1987.

61. Koren G and James A: Vancomycin dosing in preterm infants: Prospective verification of new recommendations. J Pediatr 110:797, 1987.

62. Halkin H, Radomsky M, Millman P, et al: Steady-state serum concentrations and renal clearance of digoxin in neonates, infants, and children. Eur J Clin Pharmacol 13:113, 1978.

63. Linday LA, Drayer DE, Ali Khan MA, et al: Pubertal changes in net renal tubular secretion of digoxin. Clin Pharmacol Ther 35:438, 1984.

64. Schwartz GJ, Feld FG, and Langford DJ: A simple estimate of glomerular filtration rate in full term infants during the first year of life. J Pediatr 104:849, 1984.

65. Traub SL and Johnson CE: Comparison of methods of estimating creatinine clearance in children. Am J Hosp Pharm 37:195, 1980.

66. Schwartz GJ and Gauthier B: A simple estimate of glomerular filtration rate in adolescent boys. J Pediatr 106:522, 1985.

67. Friis-Hansen B and Winter RW: Regulation of normal water and electrolyte metabolism. In: Winter RW (ed): The Body Fluids in Pediatrics. Boston, Little, Brown, 1973, p. 100.

68. Lovejoy FH Jr: Fatal benzyl alcohol poisoning in neonatal intensive care units. Am J Dis Child 136:974, 1982.

69. LeBel M, Ferron L, Masson M, et al: Benzyl alcohol metabolism and elimination in neonates. Dev Pharmacol Ther 11:347, 1988.

70. Arrowsmith JB, Faich GA, Tomita DK, et al: Morbidity and mortality among low birth weight infants exposed to an intravenous vitamin E product, E-Ferol. Pediatrics 83:244, 1989.

71. Yaffe SJ, Bierman CW, Cann HM, et al: Requiem for tetracyclines. Pediatrics 55:142, 1975.

72. Loeb JN: Corticosteroids and growth. N Engl J Med 295:547, 1976.

73. Schluter G: Ciprofloxacin: Review of potential toxicologic effects. Am J Med 82(Suppl 4A):91, 1987.

74. Alfaham M, Holt ME, and Goodchild MC: Arthropathy in a patient with cystic fibrosis taking ciprofloxacin. Br Med J 295:699, 1987.

75. Zaritsky A and Chernow B: Use of catecholamines in pediatrics. J Pediatr 105:341, 1984.

76. Friedman WF and George BL: Treatment of congestive heart

failure by altering loading conditions of the heart. J Pediatr 106:697, 1985.

77. Friedman WF: The intrinsic physiologic properties of the developing heart. Prog Cardiovasc Dis 15:87, 1972.

78. Buckley NM, Gootman PM, Yellin EL, et al: Age-related cardiovascular effects of catecholamines in anesthetized piglets. Circ Res 45:282, 1979.

79. Manders WT, Pagani M, and Vatner SF: Depressed responsiveness to vasoconstrictor and dilator agents and baroreflex sensitivity in conscious newborn lambs. Circulation 60:945, 1979.

80. Roan Y and Galant SP: Decreased neutrophil beta adrenergic receptors in the neonate. Pediatr Res 16:591, 1982.

81. Corby DG and O'Barr TP: Decreased alpha adrenergic receptors in newborn platelets: Cause of abnormal response to epinephrine. Dev Pharmacol Ther 2:215, 1981.

82. Lagercrantz H and Bistoletti P: Catecholamine release in the newborn infant at birth. Pediatr Res 11:889, 1973.

83. Romero TE and Friedman WF: Limited left ventricular response to volume overload in the neonatal period: A comparative study with the adult animal. Pediatr Res 13:910, 1979.

84. Driscoll DJ, Fukushige J, Lewis RM, et al: The comparative hemodynamic effects of propranolol in chronically instrumented puppies and adult dogs. Biol Neonate 41:8, 1982.

85. Binah O, Legato MJ, Danilo P Jr, et al: Developmental changes in the cardiac effects of amrinone in the dog. Circ Res 52:747, 1983.

86. Binah O, Sodowick B, Vulliemoz Y, et al: The inotropic effects of amrinone and milrinone on neonatal and young canine cardiac muscle. Circulation 73 (Suppl III):III-46, 1986.

87. Drummond WH, Gregory GA, Heymann MA, et al: The independent effects of hyperventilation, tolazoline, and dopamine on infants with persistent pulmonary hypertension. J Pediatr 98:603, 1981.

88. Lang P, Williams RG, Norwood WI, et al: The hemodynamic effects of dopamine in infants after corrective cardiac surgery. J Pediatr 96:630, 1980.

89. DiSessa TG, Leitner M, Ti CC, et al: The cardiovascular effects of dopamine in the severely asphyxiated neonate. J Pediatr 99:772, 1981.

90. Seri I, Tulassay T, Kiszel J, et al: Cardiovascular response to dopamine in hypotensive preterm neonates with severe hyaline membrane disease. Eur J Pediatr 142:3, 1984.

91. Padbury JF, Agata Y, Baylen BG, et al: Dopamine pharmacokinetics in critically ill newborn infants. J Pediatr 110:293, 1986.

92. Perkin RM, Levin DL, Webb R, et al: Dobutamine: A hemodynamic evaluation in children with shock. J Pediatr 100:977, 1982.

93. Driscoll D, Gillette PC, Duff DF, et al; Hemodynamic effects of dobutamine in children. Am J Cardiol 43:581, 1979.

94. Schranz D, Stopfkuchen H, Jungst BK, et al: Hemodynamic effects of dobutamine in children with cardiovascular failure. Eur J Pediatr 139:4, 1982.

95. Sapin SO, Donoso E, and Blumenthal S: Digoxin dosage in infants. Pediatrics 18:730, 1956.

96. Hauck AJ, Ongley PA, and Nadas AS: The use of digoxin in infants and children. Am Heart J 56:443, 1958.

97. Park MK: Use of digoxin in infants and children with specific emphasis on dosage. J Pediatr 108:871, 1986.

98. Kearin M, Kelly JG, and O'Malley K: Digoxin "receptors" in neonates: An explanation of less sensitivity to digoxin than in adults. Clin Pharmacol Ther 28:346, 1980.

99. Marsh AJ, Lloyd BL, and Taylor RR: Age-dependence of myocardial Na+-K+-ATPase activity and digitalis intoxication in the dog and guinea pig. Circ Res 48:329, 1981.

100. Inturrisi CE and Papaconstantinou MC: Ouabain sensitivity of Na-K-ATPase from rat neonatal and human fetal and adult heart. In: Askari A (ed): Properties and functions of (Na-K)-activated adenosine triphosphate. Ann NY Acad Sci 242:710, 1974.

101. Park MK: Ouabain-induced inotropism of isolated newborn and adult rabbit myocardium. Dev Pharmacol Ther 2:201, 1981.

102. Sandor GGS, Bloom KR, Izukawa T, et al: Noninvasive assessment of left ventricular function related to serum digoxin levels in neonates. Pediatrics 65:541, 1980.

103. Pinsky WW, Jacobsen JR, Gillette PC, et al: Dosage of digoxin in premature infants. J Pediatr 96:639, 1979.

104. Park MK, Ludden T, Arom KV, et al: Myocardial vs serum digoxin concentrations in infants and adults. Am J Dis Child 136:418, 1982.

105. Krasula RW, Hastreiter RA, Levitsky S, et al: Serum, atrial and urinary digoxin levels during cardiopulmonary bypass in children. Circulation 49:1047, 1974.

106. Wagner JG, Dick M II, Behrendt DM, et al: Determination of myocardial and serum digoxin concentrations in children by specific and nonspecific assay methods. Clin Pharmacol Ther 33:577, 1983.

107. Hougen TJ: Use of digoxin in the young. In: Smith TW (ed): Digitalis Glycosides. Orlando, Grune & Stratton, 1986, pp. 169–207.

108. Hastreiter AR, van der Horst RL, and Chow-Tung E: Digitalis toxicity in infants and children. Pediatr Cardiol 5:131, 1984.

109. Smith TW and Willerson JT: Suicidal and accidental digoxin ingestion: Report of five cases with serum digoxin level correlations. Circulation 44:29, 1971.

110. Pudek MR, Seccombe DW, and Whitfield MF: Digoxin-like immunoreactivity in premature and full-term infants not receiving digoxin therapy. N Engl J Med 308:904, 1983.

111. Valdes R Jr, Graves SW, Brown BA, et al: Endogenous substance in newborn infants causing false positive digoxin measurements. J Pediatr 102:947, 1983.

112. Phelps SJ, Kamper CA, Bottorff MB, et al: Effect of age and serum creatinine on endogenous digoxin-like substances in infants and children. J Pediatr 110:136, 1987.

113. Porter CJ, Gillette PC, Garson A Jr, et al: Effects of verapamil on supraventricular tachycardia in children. Am J Cardiol 48:487, 1981.

114. Radford D: Side effects of verapamil in infants. Arch Dis Child 58:465, 1983.

115. Garson A Jr: Medicolegal problems in the management of cardiac arrhythmias in children. Pediatrics 79:84, 1987.

116. Epstein ML, Kiel EA, and Victorica BE: Cardiac decompensation following verapamil therapy in infants with supraventricular tachycardia. Pediatrics 75:737, 1985.

117. Bateman DN, Rawlins MD, and Simpson JM. Extrapyramidal reactions to prochlorperazine and haloperidol in the United Kingdom. Q J Med 59:549, 1986.

118. Gralla RJ, Itri LM, Pisko SE, et al: Antiemetic efficacy of high dose metoclopramide: Randomized trials with placebo and prochlorperazine in patients with chemotherapy-induced nausea and vomiting. N Engl J Med 305:905, 1981.

119. Allen JC, Gralla R, Reilly L, et al: Metoclopramide: Dose-related toxicity and preliminary antiemetic studies in children receiving cancer chemotherapy. J Clin Oncol 3:1136, 1985.

120. Kris MG, Tyson LB, Gralla RJ, et al: Extrapyramidal reactions with high-dose metoclopramide. N Engl J Med 309:433, 1983.

121. Terrin BN, McWilliams NB, and Maurer HM: Side effects of metoclopramide as an antiemetic in childhood cancer chemotherapy. J Pediatr 104:138, 1984.

122. Bateman DN, Craft AW, Nicholson E, et al: Dystonic reactions and the pharmacokinetics of metoclopramide in children. Br J Clin Pharmacol 15:557, 1983.

123. Marsden CD and Jenner P: The pathophysiology of extrapyramidal side effects of neuroleptic drugs. Psychol Med 10:55, 1980.

124. Wong DF, Wagner HN, Dannals RF, et al: Effects of age on dopamine and serotonin receptors measured by positron tomography of the living human brain. Science 226:1393, 1984.

125. Albert S: Aminophylline toxicity. Pediatr Clin North Am 34:61, 1987.

126. Zwillich CW, Sutton FD, Neff TA, et al: Theophylline-induced seizures in adults—correlation with serum concentrations. Ann Intern Med 82:784, 1975.

127. Gaudreault P, Wason S, and Lovejoy FH: Acute pediatric theophylline overdose: A summary of 28 cases. J Pediatr 102:474, 1983.

128. Olson KR, Benowitz N, Woo O, et al: Theophylline overdose: Acute single ingestion versus chronic repeated overmedication. Am J Emerg Med 3:386, 1985.

129. Richards W, Church JA, and Brent DK: Theophylline-associated seizures in children. Ann Allergy 54:276, 1985.

130. Rumack BH: Acetaminophen overdose in young children. Treatment and effects of alcohol and other additional ingestants in 417 cases. Am J Dis Child 138:428, 1984.

131. Peterson RG and Rumack BH: Age as a variable in acetaminophen overdose. Arch Intern Med 141:390, 1981.
132. Miller RP, Roberts RJ, and Fischer LF: Acetaminophen elimination kinetics in neonates, children, and adults. Clin Pharmacol Ther 19:284, 1976.
133. Lieh-Lai MW, Sarnaik AP, Newton JF, et al: Metabolism and pharmacokinetics of acetaminophen in a severly poisoned young child. J Pediatr 105:125, 1984.
134. Davis M, Labadanis D, and Williams R: Metabolism of paracetamol after therapeutic and hepatotoxic doses in man. J Intern Med Res 4:40, 1976.
135. Rumack BH, Peterson RC, Koch G, et al: Acetaminophen overdose: 662 cases with evaluation of oral acetylcysteine treatment. Arch Intern Med 141:380, 1981.
136. Lauterburg BH, Vaishnav Y, Stillwell WG, et al: The effects of age and glutathione depletion in hepatic glutathione turnover in vivo determined by acetaminophen probe analysis. J Pharmacol Exp Ther 213:54, 1980.
137. Mancini RE, Sonaware BR, and Yaffe SJ: Developmental susceptibility to acetaminophen toxicity. Res Commun Chem Pathol Pharmacol 27:603, 1980.
138. Nogen AG and Bremner JE: Acetaminophen overdosage in a young child. J Pediatr 92:832, 1978.
139. Greene JW, Craft L, and Ghishan F: Acetaminophen poisoning in infancy. Am J Dis Child 137:386, 1983.
140. Mitchell JR, Zimmerman HJ, and Ishak KG: Isoniazid liver injury: Clinical spectrum, pathology, and probable pathogenesis. Ann Intern Med 84:181, 1976.
141. Spyridis P, Sinaniotis C, Papadea I, et al: Isoniazid liver injury during chemoprophylaxis in children. Arch Dis Child 54:65, 1979.
142. Bass JB Jr, Farer LS, Hopewell PC, et al: Treatment of tuberculosis and tuberculosis infection in adults and children. Am Rev Respir Dis 134:355, 1986.
143. Kopanoff DE, Snider DE, and Caras GJ: Isoniazid related hepatitis. Am Rev Respir Dis 117:991, 1978.
144. Gurumurthy P, Krishnamurthy MS, Nazareth O, et al: Lack of relationship between toxicity and acetylator phenotype in three thousand South Indian patients during treatment with isoniazid for tuberculosis. Am Rev Respir Dis 129:58, 1984.
145. Martinez-Roig A, Cami J, Llorens-Terol J, et al: Acetylation phenotype and hepatotoxicity in the treatment of tuberculosis in children. Pediatrics 77:912, 1986.
146. Casteels-Van Daele M, Igodt-Ameye L, Corbeel L, et al: Hepatotoxicity of rifampin and isoniazid in children. J Pediatr 86:739, 1975.
147. Bistritzer T, Barzilay Z, and Jonas A: Isoniazid-rifampin-induced fulminant liver disease in an infant. J Pediatr 97:480, 1980.
148. O'Brien RJ, Long MW, Cross FS, et al: Hepatotoxicity from isoniazid and rifampin among children treated for tuberculosis. Pediatrics 72:491, 1983.
149. Adverse drug reactions among children treated for tuberculosis. Morbid Mortal Week Rep 29:589, 1980.
150. McCracken GH: Aminoglycoside toxicity in infants and children. Am J Med 80 (Suppl 6B):172, 1986.
151. Cowan RH, Jukkola AF, and Arant BS Jr: Pathophysiologic evidence of gentamicin nephrotoxicity in neonatal puppies. Pediatr Res 14:1204, 1980.
152. Provoost AP, Adejuyigbe O, and Wolff ED: Nephrotoxicity of aminoglycosides in young and adult rats. Pediatr Res 19:1191, 1985.
153. Adelman RD, Wirth F, and Rubio T: A controlled study of the nephrotoxicity of mezlocillin and amikacin in the neonate. Am J Dis Child 141:1175, 1987.
154. Rajchgot P, Prober CG, Soldin S, et al: Aminoglycoside-related nephrotoxicity in the premature newborn. Clin Pharmacol Ther 35:394, 1984.
155. Tessin I, Trollfors B, Bergmark J, et al: Enzymuria in neonates during treatment with gentamicin or tobramycin. Pediatr Infect Dis 6:870, 1987.
156. Tessin I, Trollfors B, Bergmark J, et al: Enzymuria in neonates during treatment with tobramycin or ceftazidime. Pediatr Infect Dis 7:142, 1988.
157. Finitzo-Hieber T, McCracken GH, and Brown KC: Prospective controlled evaluation of auditory function in neonates given netilmicin or amikacin. J Pediatr 106:129, 1985.

158. Hendeles L, Iafrate RP, and Stillwell PC: Individualizing gentamicin dosage in patients with cystic fibrosis: Limitations to pharmacokinetic approach. J Pediatr 110:303, 1987.
159. Levy J, Smith AL, Koup JR, et al: Disposition of tobramyin in patients with cystic fibrosis: A prospective controlled study. J Pediatr 105:117, 1984.
160. MacDonald NE, Anas NG, Peterson RG, et al: Renal clearance of gentamicin in cystic fibrosis. J Pediatr 103:985, 1983.
161. Kildoo CW, Harralson AF, Folli HL, et al: Direct determination of tobramycin clearance in patients with mild-to-moderate cystic fibrosis. Drug Intel Clin Pharm 21:639, 1987.
162. Farber BF, and Moellering RC: Retrospective study of the toxicity of preparations of vancomycin from 1974 to 1981. Antimicrob Agent Chemother 23:138, 1983.
163. Dean RP, Wagner DJ, and Tolpin MD: Vancomycin/aminoglycoside nephrotoxicity. J Pediatr 106:861, 1985.
164. Schentag JJ, Cerra FB, and Plaut ME: Clinical and pharmacokinetic characteristics of aminoglycoside nephrotoxicity in 201 critically ill patients. Antimicrob Agent Chemother 21:721, 1982.
165. Odio C, McCracken GH, and Nelson JD: Nephrotoxicity associated with vancomycin-aminoglycoside therapy in four children. J Pediatr 105:491, 1984.
166. Aranda JV, Collinge JM, and Clarkson S: Epidemiologic aspects of drug utilization in a newborn intensive care unit. Semin Perinatol 6:148, 1982.
167. Ernst JA, Williams JM, Glick MR, et al: Osmolality of substances used in the intensive care nursery. Pediatrics 72:347, 1983.
168. Edes TE, Walk BE, and Austin JL: Diarrhea in tube fed patients: Feeding formula not necessarily the cause. Am J Med 88:91, 1990.
169. Cacek AT, DeVito JM, and Koonce JR: In vitro evaluation of nasogastric administration methods for phenytoin. Am J Hosp Pharm 43:689, 1986.
170. Clark-Schmidt AL, Garnett WR, Lowe DR, et al: Loss of carbamazepine suspension through nasogastric feeding tubes. Am J Hosp Pharm 47:2034, 1990.
171. Fleisher D, Sheth N, and Kou JH: Phenytoin interaction with enteral feedings administered through nasogastric tubes. JPEN 14:513, 1990.
172. Cutie AJ and Altman E: Compatibility of enteral products with commonly employed drug additives. JPEN 7:186, 1983.
173. Bauer LA: Interference of oral phenytoin absorption by continuous nasogastric feedings. Neurology 32:570, 1982.
174. Miller SW and Strom JG: Stability of phenytoin in three enteral nutrient formulas. Am J Hosp Pharm 45:2529, 1988.
175. Kuhn TA, Garnett WR, Wells BK, et al: Recovery of warfarin from an enteral nutrient formula. Am J Hosp Pharm 46:1395, 1989.
176. White KC and Harkavy KL: Hypertonic formula resulting from added oral medications. Am J Dis Child 136:931, 1982.
177. Book LS, Herbst JJ, Atherton SO, et al: Necrotizing enterocolitis in low-birth-weight infants fed an enteral formula. J Pediatr 87:602, 1975.
178. Gould T and Roberts RJ: Therapeutic problems arising from the use of the intravenous route for drug administration. J Pediatr 95:465, 1979.
179. Nahata MC, Powell DA, Glazer JP, et al: Effect of intravenous flow rate and injection site on in-vitro delivery of chloramphenicol succinate and in-vivo kinetics. Pediatrics 99:463, 1981.
180. Nahata MC, Powell DA, Durrell DE, et al: Effect of infusion methods on tobramycin serum concentrations in newborn infants. Pediatrics 104:136, 1984.
181. Nahata MC, Powell DA, Durrell D, et al: Delivery of tobramycin by three infusion systems. Chemotherapy 30:84, 1984.
182. Arwood LL, Cordero L, and Visconti JA: Effect of intravenous tubing lumen diameter on drug delivery. Dev Pharmacol Ther 7:259, 1984.
183. McCormack JP, Pleasants RA, and O'Neal W: The accuracy of vancomycin delivery with retrograde administration at low flow rates. Hosp Pharm 25:933, 1990.
184. Kubajak CAM, Leff RD, and Roberts RJ: Influence of physical characteristics of intravenous systems on drug delivery. Dev Pharmacol Ther 11:189, 1988.
185. Pickering LK and Rutherford I: Effect of concentration and time upon inactivation of tobramycin, gentamicin, netilmicin and

amikacin by azlocillin, carbenicillin, mecillinam, mezlocillin and piperacillin. J Pharmacol Exp Ther 217:345, 1981.

186. Rajchgot P, Radde IC, and MacLeod SM: Influence of specific gravity on intravenous drug delivery. J Pediatr 99:658, 1981.

187. Nazeravich DR and Otten NHH: Effect of inline filtration on delivery of gentamicin at a slow infusion rate. Am J Hosp Pharm 40:1961, 1983.

188. Benzing G and Loggie J: A new retrograde method for administering drugs intravenously. Pediatrics 52:420, 1973.

189. Gauger LJ and Cary JD: The theory and practice of retrograde infusion: Influence of tube diameter on drug delivery. Drug Intel Clin Pharm 20:616, 1986.

190. Massey KL, Hendeles L, and Neims A: Identification of children for whom routine monitoring of aminoglycoside serum concentrations is not cost effective. J Pediatr 109:897, 1986.

191. Nahata MC: Delayed delivery of antibiotics by retrograde intravenous infusion. Am J Hosp Pharm 43:2237, 1986.

192. Berro MS, Edwards DL, Khalidi N, et al: Factors affecting drug delivery by retrograde infusion. Am J Hosp Pharm 44:1412, 1987.

193. Leff RD and Roberts RJ: Methods for intravenous drug administration in the pediatric patient. J Pediatr 98:631, 1981.

194. Garner SS and Wiest DB: Compatibility of drugs separated by a fluid barrier in a retrograde intravenous system. Am J Hosp Pharm 47:640, 1990.

195. Kirkpatrick AE, Holcolmbe BJ, and Sawyer WT: Effect of retrograde aminophylline administration on calcium and phosphate solubility in neonatal total parenteral nutrient solutions. Am J Hosp Pharm 46:2496, 1989.

196. Johnson CE, Roesner MP, Berman JR, et al: Administrating incompatible drugs by a retrograde intravenous infusion system. Am J Hosp Pharm 42:109, 1985.

197. Evans WE: General principles of applied pharmacokinetics. *In:* Evans WE, Schentag JJ, and Jusko WJ (eds): Applied Pharmacokinetics-Principles of Therapeutic Drug Monitoring, 2nd ed. San Francisco, Applied Therapeutics, 1986, pp. 1–8.

198. Robinson JD and Taylor WJ: Interpretation of serum drug concentrations. *In:* Taylor WJ and Caviness MHD (eds): A Textbook for the Clinical Application of Therapeutic Drug Monitoring. Irving, CA, Abbott Laboratories, Diagnostics Division, 1986, pp. 31–45.

199. Stewart CF and Hampton EM: Effect of maturation on drug disposition in pediatric patients. Clin Pharm 6:548, 1987.

200. Bory C, Baltassat P, Porthault M, et al: Metabolism of theophylline to caffeine in premature newborn infants. J Pediatr 94:988, 1979.

201. Gilman JT: Therapeutic drug monitoring in the neonate and paediatric age group problems and clinical pharmacokinetic implications. Clin Pharmacokinet 19:1, 1990.

202. Walson PD, Edwards R, and Cox S: Neonatal therapeutic drug monitoring—its clinical relevance. Ther Drug Monit 11:425, 1989.

Receptor Physiology

Kathryn Weise, M.D.

Metabolism in the healthy organism is regulated by endocrine and neural regulatory systems that interact in an ongoing manner to allow maintenance of a stable physiologic balance in the face of changing demands of the environment. Illness places greater demands on these regulatory systems to maintain physiologic stability and may result in insults to the patient that are severe enough to warrant further support in the form of medical intervention. Many interventions performed by the critical care physician involve the use of pharmacologic agents that influence these control systems until the patient can once again achieve physiologic stability without support.

Both endogenous and exogenously imposed regulation of interacting physiologic systems is achieved through communication between and within organ systems, as well as between and within cells. Active research in the fields of cell and molecular biology, pharmacology, genetics, and physiology have begun to describe a wide range of signal transduction systems; these systems have been discussed in detail in Chapter 3. Many of these systems function through initial binding of specific molecules to cell surface or intracellular receptors, followed by activation of postreceptor messenger systems that direct the final cellular event. Alterations in signal transduction at the receptor or postreceptor level may occur as a homeostatic mechanism, or through pharmacologic or physiologic manipulation, and may occur at numerous specific points in signal transduction pathways. Clinical effects of altering signal transduction may include modulation of mechanical or secretory functions of specific organs, alteration in growth and development, change in metabolic rate or functions, and alteration of specific pharmacologic actions. A number of disease states seen in the pediatric critical care population are caused by receptor defects or by altered receptor responsiveness secondary to a disease process.

This chapter addresses clinical aspects of basic receptor physiology, including receptor terminology, an overview of clinically relevant signal transduction mechanisms, developmental aspects of receptor systems, the influence of critical illness on receptor systems, and a discussion of several receptor-associated diseases that frequently need the intervention of the pediatric intensivist.

PRINCIPLES OF RECEPTOR PHYSIOLOGY

Receptors and Ligands: Definitions

Receptors are molecular structures, localized to cell membrane or intracellular sites, with which other molecules, termed ligands, bind to produce a specific effect. Ligands may be endogenous substances such as hormones or neurotransmitters or may be exogenous substances such as toxins or drugs. An agonist is a ligand whose binding to a receptor results in the expected effect, whereas an antagonist is a ligand whose binding to a receptor results in a decrease in or termination of an agonist-induced activity. The action of a competitive antagonist may be overcome by increasing the concentration of an agonist at the same receptor, while a noncompetitive antagonist prevents an agonist effect either by irreversible binding of an antagonist to a receptor or by preventing formation of the receptor-agonist compound.[1] A partial agonist binds to a receptor but has less capacity to produce a response than does a full agonist.

A molecule may be identified as a receptor if its binding to an appropriate agonist is specific, saturable, reversible, of high affinity, and produces a measurable response. Specificity implies that a given receptor binds only one or a number of structurally similar ligands, thus ensuring that the final effect will be seen only in response to defined stimuli in the normal setting. Pharmacologic agents that act at receptors for endogenous compounds may have even greater specificity for receptor subtypes than a related endogenous compound, allowing intentional manipulation of physiologic parameters. Specificity is used to advantage in the clinical setting by using agents that have been developed to avoid side effects of pharmacologic doses of endogenous compounds of lesser specificity. Examples include the use of dobutamine as a relatively specific β_1-adrenergic agonist for support of cardiac output and the use of selective β_2-agonists for the treatment of reactive airway disease. Such agents avoid the α-adrenergic effects seen with the major endogenous circulating catecholamine, epinephrine, while allowing the desired β-adrenergic effect appropriate for the treatment of a given disease state.

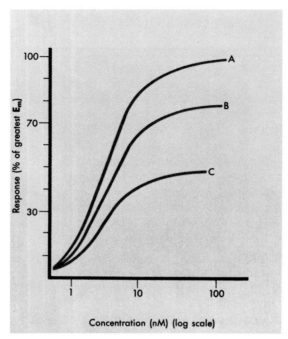

Figure 75–1. Series of agonists that vary in efficacy (E_m) at essentially constant potency. Drug A is the most efficacious, and drug C is the least efficacious. Concentrations are arbitrary but in the therapeutic plasma concentration range for many drugs. (From Wingard LB, Brody TM, Larner J, and Schwartz A: Human Pharmacology: Molecular-to-Clinical. St. Louis, Mosby Year Book, 1991.)

Saturable binding of ligand to receptor implies the presence of a limited number of receptor sites, thus distinguishing receptors from other abundant molecules that may bind a large number of ligands nonspecifically. Early theories of receptor-mediated response held that the magnitude of response was proportional to the percentage of receptors occupied by ligand,[2] allowing prediction of the degree of measured response to ligand if the extent of receptor occupancy is known. It has since been recognized that a group of ligands all with high specificity and affinity for the same receptor may induce different maximal degrees of the measured response; such agents are described as having different intrinsic activity or efficacy with respect to that receptor (Fig. 75–1). Partial agonists may be agents which, by virtue of their structure, have low intrinsic activity for a particular receptor. The magnitude of response of any agent at a given drug concentration is now recognized as being related to both its intrinsic activity and to the extent of receptor occupancy, resulting in different dose-response relationships for different agonists.[1] A series of agonists for the same receptor subtype may exhibit different potencies, that is, produce the same maximal effect at different concentrations of drug (Fig. 75–2).

Receptor Location and Structure

Functional receptors are located at specific sites on or within cells, although the site may change during the signal transduction process or as a regulatory mechanism (Table 75–1). For example, adrenergic receptors are in

a functional state while part of the cell membrane but may move to an intracellular site during receptor down-regulation (see later). Glucocorticoid hormone receptors, on the other hand, first bind to ligand within target cell cytoplasm, then move to an intranuclear location in a form that has a high affinity for sites on nuclear chromatin. After binding of the activated ligand-receptor complex to chromatin, mRNA transcription is regulated.[3] Specific receptors and receptor subtypes may be found only on particular tissues, leading to responsiveness of that tissue to a receptor-ligand interaction, and the concentration of receptor may be specific to the area of an organ in which it is being measured.

Receptor structures have not been defined in all cases. Conceptually, most receptors are thought of as having two main structural components, or domains, which correspond to two functional aspects, binding of ligand and production of an effect. Growing sophistication in molecular biologic techniques, such as amino acid sequencing, photoaffinity probes, and site-directed mutagenesis studies, has led to the identification of probable ligand binding and effector domains for several receptor types, including adrenergic and insulin receptors.[4–6]

Cell surface receptors are classically complex protein molecules whose primary, secondary, and tertiary chemical structure determines its ultimate three-dimensional shape. This final form allows its appropriate positioning within the lipid bilayer of the cell membrane and determines to which ligands it will bind and what the resultant effect (agonist or antagonist action) will be.

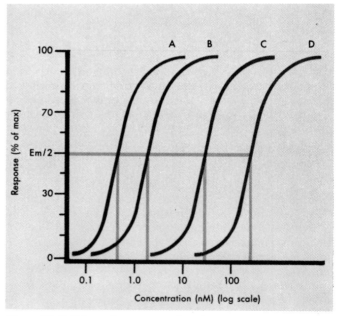

Figure 75–2. Schematic representation of log concentration-response curves for a series of agonists (A, B, C, and D). Note that all of the drugs are shown as having the same maximum response. The most potent drug produces half-maximal efficacy ($E_m/2$) at the lowest concentration; thus, drug A is the most potent. The concentration of each drug needed to produce 50% of the maximum response is also shown. Concentration values are arbitrary. (From Wingard LB, Brody TM, Larner J, and Schwartz A: Human Pharmacology: Molecular-to-Clinical. St. Louis, Mosby Year Book, 1991.)

Table 75–1. RECEPTOR LOCATION AND FUNCTION

Receptor	Location	Messenger Transduction System
Adrenergic	Cell membrane	Adenylate cyclase (stimulation or inhibition) or phospholipase C pathway activation
Insulin	Cell membrane	Tyrosine phosphorylation
Thyroid hormone	Intranuclear	Induction of gene expression
	Cell membrane	Direct actions
	Mitochondrial membrane	Direct actions
Glucocorticoid	Cytosol	Induction of gene expression
Muscarinic acetylcholine	Cell membrane	Adenylate cyclase inhibition
Nicotinic acetylcholine	Cell membrane	Sodium channel activation
Histamine (H_1)	Cell membrane	Phospholipase C activation
Adenosine (A_1)	Cell membrane	Adenylate cyclase inhibition
Opiate	Cell membrane	Adenylate cyclase inhibition

Receptor Classification

The placement of receptors in categories is useful for purposes of predicting the response to agonists and antagonists, and in order to define functional similarities that may relate to mechanisms of postreceptor regulation. Classically, receptors have been categorized by defining their affinity for and response to specific agonists and antagonists, such as in the case of adrenergic receptors. It is now known that receptor subtypes within a broad category, such as the adrenergic receptor family, may perform message transduction by coupling to different second messenger systems, providing another means of classification.[4] Interestingly, while information defining the diversity of receptors, receptor subtypes, and postreceptor events accumulates, ongoing research has begun to identify structural relationships between receptor groups that may reflect the evolution of message transduction systems. Molecular genetic techniques have demonstrated close structural homology among a number of steroid hormone receptors (glucocorticoid, mineralocorticoid, progesterone, estrogen, and vitamin D), two subtypes of thyroid hormone receptors, and retinoic acid receptors and have shown that these structural similarities cross species boundaries. While ligands for these receptor systems are structurally diverse, all are involved in regulation of morphologic development, suggesting that mechanisms responsible for development and homeostasis may be more universal than has been previously appreciated.[7]

Regulation of Receptor Function

Receptor activation is an initiating event in a number of signal transduction pathways that allow responsiveness of an organism to its environment. Since environmental influences are not static, the organism must be able to adjust to changing influences in the internal and external environment; on the cellular level, this is achieved through modulation of signalling mechanisms. Signal transduction mechanisms may become either more or less responsive to a given stimulus, teleologically seeming to work to maintain a baseline level of measured effect by the cell in the face of a changing level of stimulus. Mechanisms of receptor regulation include changes of receptor concentration at the cell surface or intracellularly, attenuation of receptor activity through phosphorylation or through alteration of affinity for ligand, or postreceptor modulation of agonist action (Table 75–2).

Downregulation refers to a decrease in receptor concentration, usually in response to the continuous presence of an agonist.[8] Cell surface receptor number may be decreased rapidly through receptor sequestration or through internalization.[9] This process has been described for β-adrenergic receptors, which may be transiently stored in cytoplasmic vesicles, then either returned to the cell membrane after agonist stimulation has decreased, or destroyed if stimulation continues. Downregulation classically refers to a decrease in total cellular receptor concentration through degradation and reduced production of receptors. This process is responsible for tachyphylaxis, or decreased responsiveness to prolonged agonist stimulation, as seen in the case of gradual decrease in effectiveness of exogenous catecholamine infusions after prolonged administration. Reversal of pharmacologically induced downregulation usually requires cessation or decrease in agonist administration, with subsequent production of new receptors. Clinically, exogenously administered agonists may need to be weaned gradually to allow the production of an adequate number of new receptors to maintain cell or organ function, a process that may occur over hours to days.

Rapid desensitization of receptors to the agonist may also occur through phosphorylation, which has been described for β-adrenergic, insulin, and nicotinic acetylcholine (ACh) receptors.[4, 10] Phosphorylation alters the ability of the receptor to induce a second messenger response, without a decrease in receptor concentration.

Table 75–2. MECHANISMS OF RECEPTOR REGULATION

Mechanisms that Decrease Receptor Action	
Rapid:	Receptor internalization
	Phosphorylation
	Pharmacologic postreceptor modulation
Slow:	Downregulation
	Altered affinity of receptor for ligand

Mechanisms that Increase Receptor Action	
Rapid:	Receptor externalization
	Pharmacologic postreceptor modulation
Slow:	Upregulation

Table 75–3. ADRENERGIC RECEPTORS: LOCATION AND PHYSIOLOGIC RESPONSES

Receptor		Physiologic Responses
α_1		Stimulation of smooth muscle contraction in blood vessels and genitourinary tract
α_2	Stimulation of:	1. Smooth muscle relaxation, gastrointestinal tract 2. Smooth muscle contraction in certain vascular beds (e.g., renal) 3. Potassium and water secretion by salivary glands 4. Gluconeogenesis and glycogenolysis
	Inhibition of:	1. Norepinephrine release from sympathetic nerve terminals 2. Lipolysis 3. Renin and insulin release
β_1	Stimulation of:	1. Rate and force of myocardial contraction 2. Lipolysis 3. Amylase secretion by salivary glands
β_2	Stimulation of:	1. Smooth muscle relaxation in bronchi, blood vessels, gastrointestinal and genitourinary tracts 2. Facilitation of norepinephrine release 3. Muscle glycogenolysis 4. Insulin and glucagon secretion by pancreatic cells 5. Renin release 6. Cellular uptake of potassium
Dopamine	Stimulation of:	1. Renal and mesenteric vasodilatation (low doses) 2. Increase in glomerular filtration rate, renal blood flow, and sodium excretion (low doses) 3. β-Adrenergic receptor responses (intermediate doses) 4. α-Adrenergic receptor responses—vasoconstrictive (high doses)

Homologous desensitization refers to a decrease in responsiveness to a single agonist after exposure to that agent, whereas heterologous desensitization implies decreased responsiveness to a number of agonists after exposure to a single related agonist.

In the continued presence of an antagonist or in the case of a lack of agonist stimulation, receptor concentration may increase. This upregulation allows enhanced responsiveness in the face of a decreased basal level of stimulation. The classic example of upregulation is an increase in β-adrenergic receptor concentration after the administration of a β-antagonist such as propranolol. While these receptors are blocked, cell function does not reflect the increased number of β-receptors present. This phenomenon may result in rebound hypertension after the abrupt withdrawal of β-blocker therapy, since a greater than normal number of β-receptors are now available for stimulation by endogenous agonists.[11]

CLINICAL ASPECTS OF RECEPTOR PHYSIOLOGY

Types of Signal Transduction Mechanisms

A wide range of mechanisms of initiating and regulating message transduction have been defined, including passive diffusion, ion channels, receptor endocytosis, second messenger systems, and induction of gene expression. These systems have been discussed in detail in Chapter 3. The critical care physician may manipulate signal transduction through a variety of pharmacologic interventions. The major receptor systems that are known to be affected by critical illness or by treatment are the adrenergic and thyroid hormone receptor sys-

tems; insulin, steroid, opiate, and muscarinic receptors have also been shown to be important regulators of function during stress.

Adrenergic Receptors

Catecholamines are frequently administered to the critically ill patient in an attempt to improve cardiovascular function. While specific effects may be achievable through the use of drugs specific to receptor subtypes, endogenous catecholamines have wide-ranging effects in a number of organ systems. These include positive myocardial inotropy and chronotropy, peripheral vasodilatation or vasoconstriction, bronchial smooth muscle relaxation, and modulation of metabolic processes such as glycogenolysis, lipolysis, amylase secretion, insulin release, and water and electrolyte balance (Table 75–3).[8, 12] Specific physiologic responses to catecholamines are determined by the location of the target receptor, the intrinsic activity of the administered agonist or antagonist, and all factors that modulate receptor responsiveness at each point in time.

Effects of Adrenergic Receptor Manipulation

Specific effects of adrenergic agonists and antagonists are achieved by stimulation or inhibition of particular receptor subtypes. The overall physiologic response to the administration of a pharmacologic agent will be a function of the location of the target receptors, the specificity and intrinsic activity of the agent for receptor subtypes, and the combination of all factors modulating receptor responsiveness at the time of drug administration. Consideration of these principles often allows the choice of a drug that will achieve the therapeutic goal without undesirable effects due to stimulation of other adrenergic receptor subtypes.

Adrenergic receptor regulation is responsible not only for alteration of myocardial and vascular smooth muscle function but also for modulation of several morphologic and metabolic effects. Myocardial hypertrophy is recognized as a long-term effect of catecholamine administration in animals, at doses below those that induce myocardial necrosis.[13-16] Exposure of infants to ritodrine in utero has been shown by echocardiography to result in myocardial hypertrophy.[17] The degree of functional significance of catecholamine-induced myocardial hypertrophy, its severity relative to the inducing agent in humans, or the ability to regress after removal of excess catecholamine is unclear at this time.

Metabolic effects of catecholamine infusions include regulation of lipolysis, renin release, insulin release, gluconeogenesis, glycogenolysis, amylase secretion, and potassium flux across cell membranes (see Table 75–3). The insulin-antagonistic effects of epinephrine are thought to be mediated by β_2-stimulation.[18] Epinephrine infusion in normal adult women leads to an increased metabolic rate, increased carbohydrate oxidation, and decreased lipid oxidation.[19] Plasma potassium levels are acutely regulated in part by α- and β-adrenergic receptors. β_2-Agonists enhance cAMP-mediated activation of sodium-potassium ATPase,[20] promoting cellular uptake of potassium, thus decreasing plasma potassium levels.[21-25] The converse appears to be true through α-adrenergic receptor stimulation, since agonists such as phenylephrine impair the extrarenal disposal of acute potassium loads and this effect can be blocked by phentolamine.[26-28]

Adrenergic Receptor Regulation

Downregulation, which clinically results in decreased responsiveness of target cells over time to the same dose of an administered pharmacologic agent, may be a significant clinical problem after prolonged use of catecholamine infusions. Chronic use of β-agonists for augmentation of cardiac output or for bronchodilatation leads to a decrease in measured concentrations of β_2-receptors in tissues available for study.[29-32] Unfortunately, target tissues are rarely available for study of receptor regulation in vivo. Consequently, most research in humans has used easily available tissues such as circulating lymphocytes or polymorphonuclear cells. Human lymphocytes have been shown to reflect receptor density and function on myocardial tissue from the same patient[33] and thus are thought to be reasonable models of receptor physiology on other tissues. This has not been demonstrated, however, for most other tissue types.

Downregulation of α-adrenergic effects also occurs. Chronic exposure of cultured neuronal cells to norepinephrine results in a biphasic pattern of desensitization, during which long-term exposure results in decreased α-receptor concentration,[34] while early (<2 hour) ex-

posure causes a decrease in phosphoinositide hydrolysis. Chronic exposure of platelets, which carry α_2-receptors, to α-agonists results in decreased receptor affinity and decreased agonist-induced platelet aggregation.[35, 36]

A return to normal number of receptors after downregulation requires the removal of excessive agonist stimulation and the formation of new receptors. This process may take up to several days.[29, 34] In the case of β_2-receptor downregulation in asthmatic patients secondary to β_2-agonist administration, the process of upregulation may be accelerated by the administration of glucocorticoids after the removal of agonist.[29, 37]

Upregulation is commonly seen after administration of β-receptor–blocking agents such as propranolol and may be responsible for rebound hypertension seen after abrupt withdrawal of this drug.[11, 38] Baseline lymphocyte β_2-receptor concentrations in adults with essential hypertension are greater than those in normotensive controls. If presynaptic β_2-receptors are also present in elevated concentrations in hypertensive patients, hypertension may result from increased presynaptic norepinephrine release in response to epinephrine.[39]

Other Influences on Adrenergic Receptor Activity

Adrenergic receptor activity is modulated through hormonal and nonhormonal influences, which may themselves be altered during critical illness (Table 75–4). The most clinically relevant noncatecholamine hormonal influences on adrenergic receptor activity are exerted by thyroid hormones and glucocorticoids.

Since hyperthyroid patients display many symptoms clinically associated with a hyperadrenergic state, whereas hypothyroid patients display the reverse, many investigators have sought correlations between circulating thyroid hormone levels and concentrations of α- or β-receptors. Unfortunately, no unifying pattern relating thyroid hormone levels with tissue responsiveness to

Table 75–4. NONADRENERGIC INFLUENCES ON ADRENERGIC RECEPTOR ACTIVITY

Effector	Response
Thyroid hormone	Altered adrenergic receptor concentration and postreceptor mechanisms; tissue variable
Glucocorticoids	Generally enhanced adrenergic responses but also tissue variable
Hypokalemia	Decrease in β-receptor and increase in α-receptor concentration
Uremia	Decrease in myocardial α-receptor density and affinity
Acidosis	Attenuated α_1 and α_2-mediated vasoconstriction
Chronic hypoxia	Blunted cardiac response to β-adrenergic stimuli Increase in β_2-receptors in lung tissue
Phosphodiesterase inhibitors	Potentiation of cAMP–mediated adrenergic responses

catecholamines has been found, because different tissue types from humans and from animal studies yield conflicting results.[40] Thyroid hormone modulation of adrenergic responsiveness appears to occur both by altering the receptor concentration and by postreceptor mechanisms.[41]

As in the case of thyroid hormone, glucocorticoid modulation of adrenergic receptor may vary between tissue types. Generally, one measures enhancement of adrenergic activity in the presence of agonist after treatment with glucocorticoids. Regulatory effects include increase[42-44] or decrease[45] in β-adrenergic receptor concentration on tissues, possibly through induction of receptor synthesis or by post-transcriptional mechanisms.[44] Adrenergic responses may be augmented at the postreceptor level through enhanced coupling of β-adrenergic receptors to cAMP production,[46] increase in cAMP concentrations through inhibition of cyclic nucleotide phosphodiesterase activity,[47] and enhancement of coupling of receptors to G proteins in some tissues.[48] These regulatory functions may have an impact on acute management of down-regulation of β-receptors in, for example, asthmatic patients treated with β-agonist therapy.[29, 37] Other uses, such as attempted augmentation of catecholamine response in shock by receptor or postreceptor modulation, remain to be justified.

Other factors influencing adrenergic receptor responsiveness include electrolytes, uremia, acidosis, hypoxia, and certain drugs. As seen with hormonal modulation of receptor activity, modulation by these nonhormonal factors may occur at a number of levels in the signal transduction cascade. Hypokalemia may decrease the concentration of β-receptors on muscle cells and cause the appearance of new α_1-receptors.[49] The reduced baroreceptor sensitivity and attenuated pressor dose-response curves seen in end-stage renal disease may be explained by a decrease in both myocardial α_1-receptor density and affinity of receptor for ligand, which has been shown in animal models of uremia.[50] Pure acidosis in the absence of hypoxia attenuates α_1- and α_2-mediated vasoconstriction. Mild alkalosis potentiates or has no effect on α_1-adrenoreceptor–mediated pressor responses yet attenuates or has no effect on α_2-mediated pressor responses.[51, 52] Animal studies of chronic hypoxia show a blunted cardiovascular response to β-adrenergic stimuli, associated with either a decrease[53] or no change in myocardial β-adrenergic receptor number, and a concomitant selective increase in β_2-adrenergic receptors in lung tissue.[54] Methylxanthines, such as aminophylline, and other structurally different phosphodiesterase inhibitors, such as amrinone,[55, 56] may potentiate adrenergic responsiveness through postreceptor modulation.

Developmental Changes in Adrenergic Receptors

Since target tissues are seldom available for study and correlations between circulating blood cell receptors and cardiovascular tissue receptors have not been made in children, little is known about the developmental changes in adrenergic receptor density and responsiveness in humans. Ontogeny of receptors is tissue specific in animals.[57] Studies comparing density and responsiveness of neonatal and adult leukocyte β-receptors and platelet α-receptors have yielded conflicting results,[44, 58-61] making the prediction of pharmacologic response or relative toxicities of catecholamines based on receptor concentrations unreliable at this time.

Adenosine Receptors

Adenosine and certain adenine nucleotides have been recognized as having effects on a wide variety of tissue types through binding with cell membrane purinergic receptors. Adenosine demonstrates greater potency at P_1 receptors, while adenosine triphosphate (ATP) and adenosine monophosphate (AMP) show greater potency at P_2 receptors. Since their initial identification, adenosine receptors have been classified into A_1 and A_2 receptors with further subclassification based on their apparent second messenger systems and cellular effects.[62, 63]

While adenosine receptors have been identified on most tissues studied, adenosine effects on neurotransmitter systems and cardiovascular tissue are of special interest to the field of critical care. Adenosine concentrations in myocardial interstitium increase when an unfavorable oxygen supply/demand ratio exists, resulting in coronary vasodilatation, increased coronary blood flow, and improvement in energy supply.[64] Adenosine also decreases the release of many neurotransmitters, which is consistent with its role of modulating the rate of energy consumption in response to energy supply in tissues.[65] Effects of adenosine on cardiac tissue include depression of sinoatrial and atrioventricular nodal activity, reduction in atrial contractility, attenuation of the stimulatory actions of catecholamines in ventricular myocardium, and depression of ventricular automaticity.[63]

A_1-receptor–mediated responses are coupled through multiple G proteins to a large number of different effectors in different tissues. These include adenylyl cyclase, potassium channels, phospholipase C, and sodium-calcium exchange (Table 75–5). In general, this results in depression of excitable tissues by reduction of ionized calcium concentrations. Although cardiovascular responsiveness to adenosine has been shown to decrease during development in animal models, it is not yet clear at what level(s) in the signal transduction pathway this ontogenetic change in responsiveness is determined.[64, 66]

Insulin Receptors

The insulin receptor, a cell membrane tetramer, is a protein kinase that is capable of phosphorylating itself and other substrates that contain tyrosine.[67] After binding of insulin to its receptor, a number of immediate cellular events occur, including stimulation of glucose transport and phospholipid turnover, changes in ion flux, and activation of specific intracellular enzymes. Other events that occur hours after receptor activation

Table 75–5. EFFECTORS OF A₁ ADENOSINE
RECEPTORS IN VARIOUS TISSUES*

Effect of A₁ Agonists	Tissue
Inhibition of adenylyl cyclase	Fat Heart Pituitary
Activation of K_{ACh}† channels	Atria Striatal neurons
Activation of K_{ATP}‡ channels	Heart
Inactivation of Ca^{2+} channels	Dorsal root ganglia Mouse sensory neurons
Stimulation of Cl^- conductance	Hippocampal dendrites
Inhibition of Cl^- transport	Shark rectal gland
Enhanced glucose transport	Adipose tissue Cardiac muscle
Activation of low K_m PDE§	3T3-L1 cells
Increased inositol phosphates	Guinea pig cortex FRTL-5 thyroid cells Vas deferens
Decreased inositol phosphates	Mouse cortex Brown fat GH₃ pituitary cells
Inactivation of phospholipase A_2 Decreased Ca^{2+} sensitivity	Brown fat Frog motor nerves
Activation of Na^+/Ca^{2+} exchange	Heart

*Adapted with permission from Linden J: Structure and function of A₁
adenosine receptors. FASEB J 5:12, 1991.
†These channels appear to be identical to the K^+ channels that are activated
by acetylcholine (ACh) via muscarinic receptors.
‡These channels are activated by a decrease in intracellular ATP and are
blocked by sulfonylureas such as tolbutamide and glybenclamide.
§Particulate cyclic AMP phosphodiesterase (PDE).

include stimulation of protein, lipid, RNA, and DNA
synthesis[5]; these mediate events affecting growth and
development. Receptor responsiveness to insulin is regulated by hormonal influences. Downregulation occurs
in adults in response to prolonged hyperinsulinemia.[68]
Glucocorticoid administration results in variable effects
on receptor responsiveness depending on the glucocorticoid used and on the tissue studied.[69–71] The physiologic
impact in the critically ill patient remains unclear.

Thyroid Hormone Receptors

Thyroid hormone controls a wide range of cellular
processes in a tissue-specific manner, resulting in profound effects on growth, development, and regulation
of metabolic functions. While many cellular responses
to thyroid hormones occur through thyroid hormone's
nuclear receptor-mediated regulation of gene expression, several forms of thyroid hormone receptor may
exist, each responsible for different functions. Cell membrane receptors for thyroid hormone may mediate endocytosis of hormone.[72, 73] These binding sites are
thought to mediate both hormone internalization and
the initiation of early hormonal responses to thyroid
hormone, including increased uptake of amino acids,

nucleosides, and glucose and stimulation of certain
ATPases.[74] Mitochondrial thyroid hormone-binding sites
have also been found and may be identical with the
carrier protein adenine nucleotide translocase, which
transports ADP into and ATP out of the mitochondrion.[74] These non-nuclear thyroid hormone receptor
sites appear to be involved in actions of thyroid hormone
that are rapid in onset.

Binding of thyroid hormone with the nuclear thyroid
hormone receptor, which is related to the c-erb-A oncogene superfamily of receptors, results in delayed and
presumably less transient metabolic effects of thyroid
hormone. The thyroid hormone-receptor complex induces tissue-specific increases in mRNA; regulation of
mRNA appearance may occur at both transcriptional
and post-transcriptional levels.[74, 75]

During severe illness, measured levels of circulating
thyroid hormones are often altered in a pattern called
the "euthyroid sick syndrome."[76] In this setting free
thyroxine and thyroid-stimulating hormone levels are
usually normal, and little evidence supports the presence
of tissue hypothyroidism,[76] despite abnormally low levels
of triiodothyronine concentrations. Studies have shown
an association between the administration of the mediator tumor necrosis factor α and the development of
serum patterns of thyroid hormone levels consistent with
the euthyroid sick syndrome in humans[78]; a cause and
effect relationship has not yet been defined. The production of certain mRNAs induced by the nuclear thyroid hormone-receptor complex is increased in patients
with the euthyroid sick syndrome, possibly in order to
maintain specific cellular functions in the face of reduced
levels of triiodothyronine.[79] Whether or not reduced
thyroid hormone levels affect the rapid, short-term
effects of triiodothyronine is unknown but could conceivably play a role in altered homeostasis during critical
illness.

Opiate and Muscarinic Receptors

Opiate receptors play important roles in mediation of
pain impulses, inhibition of reflex responses of certain
motor neurons, production of stress-induced analgesia,
and attenuation of the baroreceptor response, especially
in the presence of anesthetic agents. Subtypes of opiate
receptors with varying affinity for different endorphins
and drugs have now been described.[80]

Several subtypes of muscarinic ACh receptors are
found in neural, cardiac, smooth muscle, and exocrine
glandular tissue; all appear to be structurally related to
α₂-, β₁-, and β₂-receptors, and use a G_i protein second
messenger system.[77] Strength and rate of contraction of
cardiac myocytes are decreased after ACh administration. Smooth muscles that contain muscarinic receptors,
including bronchial smooth muscle, demonstrate increased tone in the presence of ACh; this effect may
antagonize the smooth muscle relaxation seen after
β-adrenergic stimulation. This is a clinically important
interaction of receptor-mediated events in patients with
reactive airway disease.

Structural and functional characteristics of many other

receptors have been described, including steroid hormone and histamine receptors. However, this information has not yet become useful in the care of critically ill patients, since their diverse effects on different tissues precludes one from ensuring specificity of action in response to currently available drugs. For example, while the positive inotropic effects of histamine administration would be useful in augmenting cardiac output if this were the only histamine response that affects hemodynamics, simultaneous stimulation of other vasoactive and secretory responses by histamine lead to numerous unwanted side effects in an unstable patient.

Receptor-Associated Diseases

Several diseases seen in critically ill children are related to structural receptor abnormalities or specific receptor dysfunction. This category includes myasthenia gravis, types I and II diabetes mellitus, and perhaps asthma. In many disease states, such as septic shock or cardiac failure, pathophysiology directs therapies toward one or more sites in specific message transduction systems.

Three forms of myasthenia gravis are seen in children, all of which result from reduced function of nicotinic ACh receptors at the motor end plate. Congenital myasthenia gravis may be caused by an autosomal recessive condition characterized by progressive decrease in ACh release with repeated stimulation, by abnormalities in either receptor structure or number, or by absence of acetylcholinesterase. Transient neonatal myasthenia gravis is characterized by a reduction of ACh receptors at the motor end plate secondary to the presence of ACh receptor antibodies derived from the maternal circulation. Juvenile onset myasthenia gravis is an autoimmune disease that also results from ACh autoantibodies at the motor end plate.[81–83] Resultant muscle weakness may complicate the clinical assessment of respiratory muscle fatigue, impede ventilator weaning efforts, and necessitate the use of either smaller increments of nondepolarizing relaxants or larger doses of depolarizing agents than are needed in normal children.[84, 85]

Insulin receptor responsiveness is decreased in obese patients through a variety of mechanisms, including decreased receptor number, decreased receptor affinity for insulin, and defects of insulin action at postreceptor sites. Insulin resistance in type II diabetes is associated with lower numbers of high-affinity receptors in some tissues as well as postreceptor effects. Type I diabetes may also be associated with insulin resistance due to postreceptor unresponsiveness; this may be reversible with insulin therapy.[86]

Receptor-mediated pathophysiologic mechanisms of asthma have been reviewed by Barnes.[87] A major thrust of pharmacologic therapy of acute asthma is directed at relaxation of bronchial smooth muscle through stimulation of β_2-adrenergic receptors. Resting bronchomotor tone, however, may not be determined by sympathetic nerve fibers, since there seem to be few sympathetic nerves innervating human lung, and β-antagonists have no influence on bronchomotor tone in normal subjects. Instead, bronchoconstricting cholinergic neurotransmission, which appears hyperresponsive in asthmatics, may be indirectly moderated by endogenous β-agonists. Although cholinergic hyperresponsiveness alone is not thought to be responsible for asthma, anticholinergic agents have a major role in the treatment of this condition. β-Agonist therapy may directly improve pulmonary mechanics in asthma through decreased release of inflammatory mediators from mast cells, reduced mucosal edema and extravasation of plasma, release of a relaxant from airway epithelial cells, and increased clearance of airway mucus.[87]

References

1. Ross EM and Gilman AG: Pharmacodynamics: Mechanisms of drug action and the relationship between drug concentration and effect. *In*: Gilman AG and Goodman LS (eds): The Pharmacological Basis of Therapeutics, 7th ed. New York, Macmillan, 1985, pp. 35–48.
2. Clark AJ: The Mode of Action of Drugs on Cells. London, Edward Arnold, 1933.
3. Catt KJ: Molecular mechanisms of hormone action: Control of target cell function by peptide, steroid, and thyroid hormones. *In*: Felig P, Baxter JD, Broadus AE, et al (eds): Endocrinology and Metabolism, 2nd ed. New York, McGraw-Hill, 1987, pp. 82–165.
4. Raymond JR, Hinatowich M, Lefkowitz RJ, et al: Adrenergic receptors: Models for regulation of signal transduction processes. Hypertension 15:119, 1990.
5. Kahn CR: The molecular mechanism of insulin action. Ann Revu Med 36:429, 1985.
6. Rosen OM: After insulin binds. Science 237:1452, 1987.
7. Evans RM: The steroids and thyroid hormone receptor superfamily. Science 240:889, 1988.
8. Lefkowitz RJ, Caron MC, and Stiles GL: Mechanisms of membrane-receptor regulation: Biochemical, physiological and clinical insights derived from studies of the adrenergic receptors. N Engl J Med 310:1570, 1984.
9. Motulsky JH, Cunningham EMS, DeBlasi A, et al: Agonists promote rapid desensitization and redistribution of beta-adrenergic receptors on intact human mononuclear leukocytes. Am J Physiol 250:E583, 1986.
10. Bouvier M, Leeb-Lundberg LMF, Benovic JL, et al: Regulation of adrenergic receptor function by phosphorylation. J Biol Chem 262:3106, 1987.
11. Aarons RD, Nies AS, Gal J, et al: Elevation of beta-adrenergic receptor density in human lymphocytes after propranolol administration. J Clin Invest 65:949, 1980.
12. Zaritsky A and Chernow A: Medical progress: Use of catecholamines in pediatrics. J Pediatr 105:341, 1984.
13. Alderman EL and Harrison DC: Myocardial hypertrophy resulting from low dosage isoproterenol administration in rats. Proc Soc Exp Biol Med 136:268, 1971.
14. Bartolome JV, Trepanier PA, Chait LA, et al: Role of polyamines in isoproterenol-induced cardiac hypertrophy: Effects of L-diflouromethyl-ornithine, an irreversible inhibitor of ornithine decarboxylase. J Mol Cell Cardiol 14:461, 1982.
15. Laks MM and Morady F: Norepinephrine–the myocardial hypertrophy hormone? Am Heart J 91:674, 1976.
16. Middleton KM: Catecholamine-induced necrosis and hypertrophy: Hemodynamic factors. Adv Myocardiol 6:339, 1985.
17. Nuchpuckdee P, Brodsky N, Porat R, et al: Ventricular septal thickness and cardiac function in neonates after in utero ritodrine exposure. J Pediatr 109:687, 1986.
18. Lager I, Attvall S, Eriksson BM, et al: Studies on the insulin-antagonistic effect of catecholamines in normal man: Evidence for the importance of β_2-receptors. Diabetologia 29:409, 1986.
19. Sjostrom L, Schutz Y, Gudinchet F, et al: Epinephrine sensitivity

with respect to metabolic rate and other variables in women. Am J Physiol 245:E431, 1983.

20. Clausen T: Adrenergic control of Na$^+$ - K$^+$ homeostasis. Acta Med Scand 672(Suppl.):111, 1983.

21. Lockwood RH and Lum BKB: Effects of adrenergic agonists and antagonists on K$^+$ metabolism. J Pharmacol Exp Rev 189:119, 1974.

22. Ollson AM, Persson S, and Schroder R: Effects of terbutaline and isoproterenol on hyperkalemia in nephrectomized rabbits. Scand J Urol Nephrol 12:35, 1978.

23. Reis JL, Whyte KF, and Struthers AD: Epinephrine-induced hypokalemia: The role of beta adrenoceptors. Am J Cardiol 57(12):23F, 1986.

24. Struthers AD and Reid JL: The role of adrenal medullary catecholamines in K$^+$ homeostasis. Clin Sci 66:377, 1984.

25. Todd EP and Vick RL: Kalemotropic effect of epinephrine: Analysis with adrenergic agonists and antagonists. Am J Physiol 220:1963, 1971.

26. Brown RS: Extrarenal potassium homeostasis. Kidney Int 30:116, 1986.

27. Williams ME, Gervino EV, and Rosa RM: Catecholamine modulation of rapid potassium shifts during exercise. N Engl J Med 312:823, 1985.

28. Williams ME, Rosa RM, Silva P, et al: Impairment of extrarenal potassium disposal by alpha-adrenergic stimulation. N Engl J Med 311:145, 1984.

29. Brodde O-E, Brinkmann M, Schemuth R, et al: Terbutaline-induced desensitization of human lymphocyte β-2 adrenoceptors: Accelerated restoration of β-adrenoceptor responsiveness by prednisone and ketotifen. J Clin Invest 76:1096, 1985.

30. Galant SP, Duriseti L, Underwood S, et al: Beta-adrenergic receptors of polymorphonuclear particulates in bronchial asthma. J Clin Invest 65:577, 1980.

31. Neve KA and Molinoff PB: Effects of chronic administration of agonists and antagonists on the density of beta-adrenergic receptors. Am J Cardiol 57:17F, 1986.

32. Tashkin DP, Conolly ME, Duetsch RI, et al: Subsensitization of beta-adrenoceptors in airways and lymphocytes of healthy and asthmatic subjects. Am Rev Respir Dis 125:195, 1982.

33. Brodde O-E, Kretsch R, Ikezono K, et al: Human beta-adrenoceptors: Relation of myocardial and lymphocyte beta-adrenoceptor density. Science 231:1584, 1986.

34. Gonzales R, Crews FT, Sumners C, et al: Norepinephrine regulation of alpha-1 receptors and alpha-1 stimulated phosphoinositide hydrolysis in primary neuronal cultures. J Pharmacol Exper Ther 242(3):764, 1987.

35. Hollister AS, FitzGerald GA, Nadeau JHJ, et al: Acute reduction in human platelet alpha-2 adrenoreceptor affinity for agonist by endogenous and exogenous catecholamines. J Clin Invest 72:1498, 1983.

36. Cooper B, Handen RI, Young LH, et al: Agonist regulation of the human platelet α-adrenergic receptor. Nature 274:703, 1978.

37. Sertl K, Paietta E, Meryn S, et al: Effects of prednisolone on beta-adrenergic desensitization of normal peripheral lymphocytes: An in vitro model for steroid-controlled tachyphylaxis. Wein Klin Wochenschr 98:445, 1986.

38. Aarons RD and Molinoff PB: Changes in density of β-adrenergic receptors in rat lymphocytes, heart, and lung after chronic treatment with propranolol. J Pharmacol Exp Ther 221:439, 1982.

39. Brodde O-E, Prywarra A, Daul A, et al: Correlation between lymphocyte beta-2 adrenoceptor density and mean arterial blood pressure: Elevated beta-adrenoceptors in essential hypertension. J Cardiovasc Pharmacol 6:678, 1984.

40. Bilezikian JP and Loeb JN: The influence of hyperthyroidism and hypothyroidism on α- and β-adrenergic receptor systems and adrenergic responsiveness. Endocr Rev 4:378, 1983.

41. Cryer PE: Adrenergic receptors in endocrine and metabolic diseases. In: Insel PA (ed): Adrenergic Receptors in Man. New York, Marcel Dekker, 1987, pp. 285–301.

42. Cotecchia S and DeBlasi A: Glucocorticoids increase beta adrenoceptors on human intact lymphocytes in vitro. Life Sci 35:2359, 1984.

43. Fraser CM and Venter JC: The synthesis of β-adrenergic receptors in cultured human lung cells: Induction by glucocorticoids. Biochem Biophys Res Commun 94:390, 1980.

44. Insel PA and Motulsky JH: Physiological and pharmacologic regulation of adrenergic receptors. In: Insel PA (ed): Adrenergic Receptors in Man. New York, Marcel Dekker, 1987, pp. 201–235.

45. Smith TJ, Dana R, Krichevsky A, et al: Inhibition of β-adrenergic responsiveness in muscle cell cultures by dexamethasone. Endocrinology 109:2110, 1981.

46. Marone G, Lichtenstein LM, and Plant M: Hydrocortisone and human lymphocytes: Increases in cyclic adenosine 3′:5′-monophosphate and potentiation of adenylate cyclase-activating agents. J Pharmacol Exp Ther 215:469, 1980.

47. Lee TP and Reed CE: Effects of steroids on the regulation of the levels of cyclic AMP in human lymphoctyes. Biochem Biophys Res Commun 78:998, 1977.

48. Davies AO and Lefkowitz RJ: Agonist-promoted high affinity state of the beta-adrenergic receptor in human neutrophils: Modulation by corticosteroids. J Clin Endocrinol Metab 53:703, 1981.

49. Hirata A, Yoshida H, Oyama Y, et al: Hypokalemia modulates alpha- and beta-adrenoceptor bindings in rat skeletal muscle. Cell Mol Neurobiol 6:255, 1986.

50. Meggs LG, Ben-Ari J, Gammon D, et al: Effect of chronic uremia on the cardiovascular alpha-1 receptor. Life Sci 39:169, 1986.

51. Grant TL, McGrath JC, and O'Brien JW: The influence of blood gases on alpha-1-and alpha-2-adrenoceptor-mediated pressor responses in the pithed rat. Br J Pharmacol 86:69, 1985.

52. Korstanje C, Mathy M-J, van Charldorp K, et al: Influence of respiratory acidosis or alkalosis on pressor responses mediated by alpha-1- and alpha-2-adrenoceptors in pithed normotensive rats. Naunyn-Schmeideberg's Arch Pharmacol 330:187, 1985.

53. Voelkel NF, Hegstrand L, Reeves JT, et al: Effects of hypoxia on density of beta-adrenergic receptors. J Appl Physiol 50:363, 1981.

54. Winter RJD, Dickinson KEJ, Rudd RM, et al: Tissue specific modulation of beta-adrenoceptor number in rats with chronic hypoxia with an attenuated response to down-regulation by salbutamol. Clin Sci 70:159, 1986.

55. Colucci WS, Wright RF, and Braunwald E: New positive inotropic agents in the treatment of congestive heart failure: Mechanisms of action and recent clinical developments (First of two parts). N Engl J Med 314:290, 1986.

56. Colucci WS, Wright RF, and Braunwald E: New positive inotropic agents in the treatment of congestive heart failure: Mechanism of action and recent clinical developments (Second of two parts). N Engl J Med 314:349, 1986.

57. Whitsett JA, Noguchi A, and Moore JJ: Developmental aspects of α- and β-adrenergic receptors. Semin Perinatol 6(2):125, 1982.

58. Boreus LO, Hjemdahl P, and Lagercrantz H: Beta-adrenoceptor function in white blood cells from newborn infants: No relation to plasma catecholamine levels. Pediatr Res 20:1152, 1986.

59. Foged N, Bertelsen H, and Johansen T: Beta-adrenoceptor responsiveness in intact leukocytes from adults and newborn infants: Effect of phosphodiesterase inhibitors. Scand J Clin Lab Invest 50:169, 1990.

60. Reinhardt D, Zehmisch T, Becke B, et al: Age-dependency of alpha and beta adrenoreceptor on thrombocytes and lymphocytes of asthmatic and nonasthmatic children. Eur J Pediatr 142:111, 1984.

61. Roan Y and Galant SP: Decreased neutrophil beta adrenergic receptors in the neonate. Pediatr Res 16:591, 1982.

62. Linden J: Structure and function of A$_1$ adenosine receptors. FASEB J 5:12, 1991.

63. Belardinelli L, Linden J, and Berne RM: The cardiac effects of adenosine. Prog Cardiovasc Dis 32:73, 1989.

64. Matherne GP, Headrick JP, Coleman S, and Berne RM: Interstitial transudate purines in normoxic and hypoxic immature and mature rabbit hearts. Pediatr Res 28:348, 1990.

65. Fredholm BB and Dunwiddie TV: How does adenosine inhibit transmitter release? TIPS 9:130, 1988.

66. Matherne GP, Headrick JP, and Berne RM: Ontogeny of adenosine response in guinea pig heart and aorta. Am J Physiol 259 (Heart Circ Physiol 28):H1637, 1990.

67. Kahn CR and White MF: The insulin receptor and the molecular mechanism of insulin action. J Clin Invest 82:1151, 1988.

68. Bar RS, Harrison LC, Muggeo M, et al: Regulation of insulin receptors in normal and abnormal physiology in humans. Adv Intern Med 24:23, 1979.

69. Beck-Nielsen H, DePirro R, and Pedersen O: Prednisone in-

creases the number of insulin receptors on monocytes from normal subjects. J Clin Endocrinol Metab 50:1, 1980.

70. Carter-Su C and Okamoto K: Effect of insulin and glucocorticoids on glucose transporters in rat adipocytes. Am J Physiol (Endocrinol/Metab) 5:E441, 1987.

71. DePirro R, Bertoili A, Fusco A, et al: Effect of dexamethasone and cortisone on insulin receptors in normal human male. J Clin Endocrinol Metab 51:503, 1980.

72. Cheng SW, Maxfield FR Robbins J, et al: Receptor-mediated uptake of 3,3'5'-triiodo-L-thyronine by cultured fibroblasts. Soc Nat Acad Sci 77:3425, 1980.

73. Hioruchi R, Chang SW, Willingham MC, et al: Inhibition of the nuclear entry of 3,3',5'-triiodo-L-thyronine by monodansylcadaverine in GH₃ cells. J Biol Chem 257:3139, 1982.

74. DiLiegro F, Savettieri G, and Cestelli A: Cellular mechanism of action of thyroid hormones. Differentiation 35:165, 1987.

75. Samuels HH, Forman BM, Horowitz Z, et al: Regulation of gene expression by thyroid hormone. J Clin Invest 81:957, 1988.

76. Wartofsky L and Burman KD: Alterations in thyroid function in patients with systemic illness: The "euthyroid sick syndrome." Endocr Rev 3:164, 1982.

77. Goyol RK: Muscarinic receptor subtypes: Physiology and clinical implications. N Engl J Med 321:1022, 1989.

78. van der Poll I, Komijn JA, Wiersinga WM, et al: Tumor necrosis factor: A putative mediator of the sick euthyroid syndrome in man. J Clin Endocrinol Metab 71:1567, 1990.

79. Williams ME, Franklyn JA, Neuberger JM, et al: Thyroid hormone receptor expression in the "sick euthyroid" syndrome. Lancet 2:(8678–8679)1477, 1989.

80. Carmody JT: Opiate receptors: An introduction. Anaesth Intensive Care 15:27, 1987.

81. Lisak RP: Myasthenia gravis: Mechanisms and management. Hosp Pract 18(3):101, 1983.

82. Perlo VP: Treatment of the critically ill patient with myasthenia. In: Ropper AH and Kennedy SF (eds): Neurological and Neurosurgical Intensive Care, 2nd ed. Rockville, MD, Aspen Publishers, 1988.

83. Snead OC, Benton JW, Dwyer D, et al: Juvenile myasthenia gravis. Neurology 30:732, 1980.

84. Brown TCK, Gebert R, Meretoja OA, et al: Myasthenia gravis in children and its anaesthetic implications. Anaesth Intensive Care 18:466, 1990.

85. Weise KL: Myasthenia gravis. In: Blumer JL (ed): A Practical Guide to Pediatric Intensive Care, 3rd ed. St. Louis, Mosby Year Book, 1990.

86. Shafrir E, Bergman M, and Felig P: The endocrine pancreas and diabetes mellitus. In: Felig P, Baxter JD, Broadus AE, et al (eds): Endocrinology and Metabolism, 2nd ed. New York, McGraw-Hill, 1987.

87. Barnes PJ: Neural control of human airways in health and disease. Ann Rev Respir Dis 134:1289, 1986.

76

Anesthetic Agents—Actions and Toxicity

Constance S. Houck, M.D.

Many anesthetic agents have moved from the operating suite into the pediatric intensive care unit not only to aid in sedation and analgesia but also as life-saving treatments. This chapter will discuss the local and systemic anesthetic agents that are used in the operating room and are then continued in the intensive care unit. In addition, agents that have found specific therapeutic utility will be covered. Specific examples of these include ketamine and halothane for refractory status asthmaticus, thiopental and lidocaine for intubation and treatment of increased intracranial pressure in head trauma patients, and propofol for rapid sequence induction and anesthesia for short procedures. Sedative agents and analgesics are discussed in Chapter 77.

LOCAL ANESTHETICS

Continuous Epidural Anesthesia

Regional anesthesia is rapidly becoming an important part of complete anesthesia for major pediatric surgical cases. Many patients are returning to the intensive care unit with catheters placed in the epidural space in the caudal, lumbar, or thoracic regions. These catheters are used to administer intermittent or continuous infusions of local anesthetics alone, narcotics alone, or combinations of these agents. It is important for the pediatric intensive care practitioner to understand the mechanism of action, complications, and side effects of epidural local anesthetics and their administration.

The epidural space is a space between the ligamentum flavum and the dural sac. It can be reached from various approaches in order to place local anesthetics for anesthesia and analgesia during surgery. In adults and older children, this space is most easily approached by placing a needle just through the ligamentum flavum in the lumbar region between L1 and L5 (Fig. 76–1). In infants and young children, the caudal epidural space is often the most easily accessed because of its relatively large size and the ease of locating the landmarks for proper needle placement (Fig. 76–2). A "one-shot"

(single injection through the needle) technique can be used, or a catheter can be placed for continuous or intermittent drug administration.

The local anesthetics most often used for continuous epidural anesthesia are bupivacaine in 0.125% and 0.25% strengths and 1% or 2% lidocaine. The pharmacology of these drugs is shown in Table 76–1. Bupivacaine is the more commonly used because of its longer duration of action. In the 0.125% strength it causes minimal motor blockade but provides enough sensory blockade for adequate postoperative pain relief.[1]

When local anesthetics are administered into the epidural space, they gradually diffuse through the dura into the subarachnoid space and affect conduction along the nerves in the region. The epidural space is filled with fat, epidural veins, lymphatics, and traversing nerves. There is gradual absorption of the local anesthetic by these epidural blood vessels, and serum blood levels are obtained. The systemic effects of local anesthetics are dependent on both the total amount of drug administered and the rapidity of absorption into the blood. Therefore, inadvertent intravascular injection of local anesthetics leads to the most common complications noted with epidural anesthesia. It is important to be aware that even a well-placed catheter has the potential to migrate into an epidural vein. Periodic aspiration of the catheter to observe for evidence of blood is essential.

Complications of intravascular injection into an epidural vein include both central nervous system and cardiovascular toxicity. The symptoms of central nervous system toxicity usually begin with numbness of the highly vascular tissues of the tongue and circumoral region. As plasma concentrations rise, restlessness, vertigo, tinnitus, and difficulty in focusing are noted. Slurred speech and skeletal muscle twitching, most notably of the face and extremities, may then signal the onset of tonic-clonic seizures. Seizures are classically followed by profound central nervous system depression with accompanying hypotension and apnea.[2] In infants and young children who cannot verbalize these more vague manifestations of central nervous system toxicity, restlessness and agitation may be the only indications of

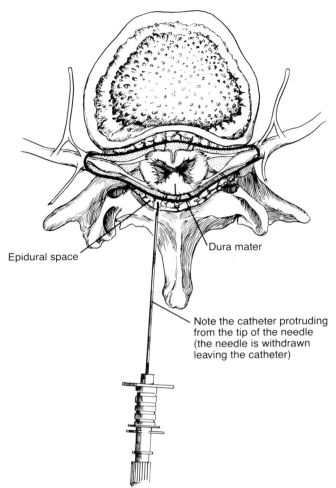

Epidural space

Dura mater

Note the catheter protruding from the tip of the needle (the needle is withdrawn leaving the catheter)

Figure 76–1. Cross-section of the spinal canal revealing the location of the epidural space just posterior to the dural sac. As illustrated, the dura mater is not punctured.

toxic blood levels of local anesthetics, and seizures may be the first recognizable outward manifestation.

The cardiovascular system tends to be more resistant to the effects of high plasma concentrations of most local anesthetics. However, profound hypotension may result from drug-induced relaxation of arteriolar smooth muscle and direct myocardial depressant effects.[2] Bupivacaine, specifically, may have selective cardiac toxicity and has been implicated in cases of severe cardiac collapse at levels lower than those causing central nervous system toxicity.[3, 4] Inadvertent injection of this drug directly into an epidural vein may cause precipitous hypotension, cardiac dysrhythmias, and atrioventricular heart block.[3] In recent years, the use of concentrations no greater than 0.5% has minimized this complication significantly.[1]

Initial treatment of toxicity resulting from local anesthetics focuses on the maintenance of adequate oxygenation, ventilation, and cardiac support. Rapid control of seizures is also important, as even brief convulsions can lead to hypercarbia, acidosis, and increased brain uptake of local anesthetic agents.[5] Benzodiazepines are effective in suppressing local anesthetic-induced seizures because of their ability to facilitate the inhibitory neurotransmitter γ-aminobutyric acid.[6] Cardiac depression caused by high plasma levels of bupivacaine can be reversed with bretyllium (20 mg/kg), which will also elevate the threshold for ventricular tachycardia.[7]

Inadvertent intrathecal injection of large amounts of local anesthetic can lead to profound respiratory and cardiovascular collapse. The amount of local anesthetic needed to achieve regional block through the epidural route is approximately 10 times that needed for spinal blockade. Overdosage of local anesthetic through the subarachnoid route leads to maximal dilatation of the venous system and blockade of the cardiac accelerator fibers (T_1 to T_4), resulting in decreased venous return, decreased cardiac output, and bradycardia.[2] Respiratory arrest results from the ischemic paralysis of the medullary ventilatory centers that develops with profound hypotension.

Although the occurrence is rare, migration of the catheter into the intrathecal space does occur and can be life-threatening if not detected and treated early. The sudden inability of a patient who is receiving a continuous infusion of local anesthetics to move his or her legs may be an indication that too much local anesthetic

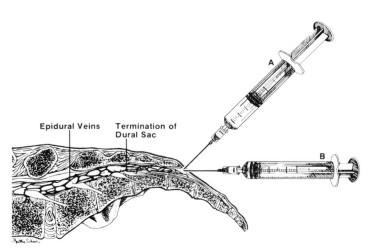

Epidural Veins   Termination of Dural Sac

Figure 76–2. The caudal epidural space is often used for the administration of local anesthetics in children because the space is large and the external landmarks are easily located even in small children. (From Broadman LM: Regional anesthesia for the pediatric outpatient. Anesthesiol Clin North Am 5:60, 1987.)

Table 76–1. PHARMACOLOGY OF THE MOST COMMONLY USED LOCAL ANESTHETICS FOR CONTINUOUS EPIDURAL ANESTHESIA*

Agent	Relative Potency	Onset (min)	Duration after Infiltration (min)	Maximum Dose in Children (mg/ml)	Protein Binding (%)	Lipid Solubility	Clearance (l/min)	Elimination Half-time (min)
Lidocaine	1	Rapid	60–120	5 (10 with epinephrine)	70	2.9	0.95	96
Bupivacaine	4	Slow	240–280	3	95	28	0.47	210

*Data from Stoelting RK: Local anesthetics. *In*: Pharmacology and Physiology in Anesthetic Practice. Philadelphia, JB Lippincott, 1987.

is reaching the subarachnoid space and that migration of the catheter may have occurred.

Intravenous and Intratracheal Local Anesthetics

Specific utility has been found for intravenous and intratracheal administration of lidocaine (1.5 mg/kg) in the intensive care unit to prevent coughing caused by irritation from the endotracheal tube. It also ameliorates the reflex-induced bronchoconstriction that occurs during suctioning. Patients with increased intracranial pressure who are exquisitely sensitive to cough-induced increases in intracranial pressure may benefit from the antitussive and anesthetic actions of this local anesthetic prior to suctioning.[8] In addition, lidocaine has direct effects on intracranial pressure by drug-induced cerebral vasoconstriction and has been used as an adjunctive agent in the control of intracranial hypertension.[9]

After cardiovascular surgery, routine suctioning of the patient postoperatively has been associated with abrupt symptomatic rises in pulmonary vascular resistance. Intravenous and intratracheal lidocaine has been found to attenuate reflex-induced bronchospasm and is used to ameliorate this adverse effect of suctioning.[10–12] Caution must be used when intravenous lidocaine is administered to patients with right-to-left intracardiac shunts, however, since venous blood enters directly into the systemic circulation through the defect, bypassing the lungs. Peak concentrations of lidocaine would therefore be expected to occur more rapidly and reach higher levels.[1] A study in lambs, in which a right-to-left intracardiac shunt was created, appeared to confirm this speculation, as peak lidocaine levels in the treated animals were double those of normal controls.[13]

Topical Anesthetics

Transdermal administration of local anesthetics has become much more popular in recent years with the development of eutectic mixtures of local anesthetics (EMLA). These are mixtures of lidocaine and prilocaine base in a weight ratio of 1:1. The crystalline powders of the two anesthetics melt at a lesser temperature than they do separately and as a result constitute a liquid at room temperature. This increases the concentration of the anesthetics in the emulsion droplets from approximately 20% for lidocaine alone to 80% for the combi-

nation of lidocaine and prilocaine.[14] The usefulness of EMLA cream for the placement of intravenous lines in the pediatric population has been demonstrated in several studies.[15–17] Its use in the intensive care unit is limited by the fact that the cream must be placed on the intended puncture site and covered with an occlusive dressing for a minimum of 60 minutes prior to the procedure. In addition, the duration of the effect is usually less than 1 hour. It still holds value, however, for routine central and arterial line changes and elective procedures. Caution must be observed in the use of EMLA in infants less than 3 months of age because the metabolism of prilocaine results in the production of oxidants that can lead to the development of methemoglobinemia. Neonates are especially at risk, not only because they have decreased levels of methemoglobin reductase but also because fetal hemoglobin is more easily oxidized to methemoglobin.[1] Because of this concern, EMLA is not currently approved for use in the United States though it is used extensively in Europe for the placement of intravenous catheters in children. Newer and more lipophilic preparations of topical local anesthetics, such as amethocaine, have been studied in Europe and have been found to provide excellent anesthesia in approximately 30 minutes with a duration of effect of more than 3 hours.[18]

INTRAVENOUS ANESTHETICS

Ketamine, thiopental, and the new short-acting intravenous anesthetic agent propofol have all been found clinically useful in the intensive care unit for anesthesia in short, often painful procedures such as endotracheal intubation. In addition, thiopental has also been found to significantly reduce intracranial pressure and has been found to be particularly useful in the intubation of patients who have sustained head injuries and in the treatment of acute spikes in intracranial pressure. Because of the short half-life and apparent lack of cumulative effect with propofol, it has been suggested as an excellent agent for patients in the intensive care unit who must undergo procedures in which general anesthesia is needed but in whom monitoring of the level of consciousness is imperative.

Ketamine

Ketamine has been used most extensively in the intensive care unit as an anesthetic for endotracheal intubation in asthmatic and hemodynamically unstable patients. It has also been used as a therapeutic agent for refractory status asthmaticus. Its unique ability to increase catecholamine levels makes it an excellent anesthetic choice for patients prone to bronchoconstriction and those with hemodynamic instability secondary to blood loss or vasodilatation.

Ketamine is a phencyclidine (PCP) derivative that has profound effects on the central nervous system. Its anesthetic properties are induced by a functional dissociation between the cortical thalamic and limbic systems, preventing the higher centers from perceiving visual, auditory, or painful stimuli.[20] In addition, it inhibits the reuptake of catecholamines into postganglionic sympathetic nerve endings of the central nervous system.[21] This latter effect results in a centrally mediated increase in heart rate, cardiac index, and mean aortic, pulmonary artery, and central venous pressures.[22] Ketamine has also been shown to have an effect at the level of the sympathetic ganglia, inhibiting the intraneuronal uptake of catecholamines (i.e., a cocaine-like effect).

Use of this agent in a dose of 1 to 2 mg/kg as an anesthetic for intubation of hypovolemic patients causes either no change or a slight increase in blood pressure and heart rate.[23] Ketamine has shown to have proven efficacy as an anesthetic for the intubation of patients with pericardial tamponade, constrictive pericarditis, and cardiogenic shock. However, in patients with more long-standing cardiovascular depression who may have depleted catecholamine levels, an unmasking of the direct myocardial depressant effects of this drug may occur. This has led to profound cardiovascular depression in this group of patients.[24]

There have been several case reports in the literature describing the dramatic effects of single-dose and continuous infusions of ketamine for the treatment of status asthmaticus.[25, 26] In one report, intubation was averted by the use of this drug.[25] Ketamine directly relaxes bronchial smooth muscle in vitro, though the bronchodilatation in vivo appears to be related only to its effects on β-receptors.[22] Continuous infusions of 1 to 2.5 mg/kg/hr have been used for 1 to 3 days with sustained, and at times dramatic, improvement without apparent sequelae. However, the use of this agent in the presence of other β-agonist drugs can lead to very high levels of circulating catecholamines and an increased risk for arrhythmias. Therefore, it has been recommended that isoproterenol infusions be decreased or stopped during continuous administration of this drug.[25] Emergence reactions characterized by hallucinations and vivid dreams have been reported in 24 to 34% of patients older than 16 years of age and approximately 10% of children less than 16 years of age receiving intravenous ketamine.[27] Concomitant administration of benzodiazepines has been shown to significantly decrease the incidence of these emergence phenomena but may prolong the sedative effects of this drug.[22]

Ketamine's bronchodilating properties make it the preferred anesthetic for the intubation of patients with bronchospastic disease.[28] Muscle relaxants should be administered when airway manipulation of this type is planned, however, as ketamine has been reported to exaggerate laryngeal reflexes and may precipitate laryngospasm.[29] Most authors recommend that this drug be avoided in patients with increased intracranial pressure or head injury because ketamine dilates the cerebral vasculature and can increase intracranial pressure by as much as 60%.[30]

Thiopental

Thiopental has long been the drug of choice for the induction of anesthesia and intubation of patients with increased intracranial pressure. Thiopental is a derivative of barbituric acid with a sulfur substitution at the carbon in the number 5 position. This change gives it greater hypnotic potency, a more rapid onset, and a shorter duration of action than the less lipid-soluble derivatives phenobarbital and pentobarbital. It is, therefore, an excellent agent for the rapid induction of unconsciousness. Barbiturates as a group rapidly decrease intracranial pressure by two mechanisms: (1) vasoconstriction of cerebral blood vessels with a resultant decrease in cerebral blood volume and (2) pronounced drug-induced lowering of cerebral oxygen consumption.[31] In patients with intracranial hypertension who had intracranial pressure monitoring devices in place, studies have demonstrated a reduction in intracranial pressure and an increase in cerebral perfusion pressure when this drug is administered prior to endotracheal intubation.[32]

Thiopental has long been used as an adjunct to control increased intracranial pressure in patients with head injuries. Attempts to confer cerebral protection by intravenous drips of barbiturates and prophylactic pentobarbital coma have been disappointing,[33, 34] but many authors still advocate their use in intermittent boluses to acutely decrease intracranial pressure prior to noxious stimuli such as endotracheal suctioning.[35] Barbiturates also appear to be protective when there is focal ischemia in the nondominant areas of the brain, and metabolic suppression of the normal brain may decrease subsequent secondary injury.[36] Patients who are refractory to the more standard treatment with hyperventilation and osmotic therapy may benefit from acute reduction in intracranial pressure when herniation seems imminent. No improvement in neurologic outcome has ever been proved, however.

Caution must be exercised in the use of thiopental in the unstable patient because this drug may have profound depressant effects on mean arterial pressure. Barbiturates depress the medullary vasomotor center, thereby decreasing central nervous system sympathetic outflow and inducing peripheral vasodilatation. Direct myocardial depressant effects are also noted, but they are usually offset by baroreceptor-induced increases in heart rate if the compensatory responses remain intact.[31] Profound hypotension may result when hypovolemia follows the treatment of increased intracranial pressure with osmotic diuretics and fluid restriction. Peripheral pooling of blood in this instance can lead to sustained reductions in venous return and cardiac output.

Thiopental has been advocated as a therapy for refractory status epilepticus that is unresponsive to standard treatment with benzodiazepines, phenobarbital, phenytoin, and paraldehyde. Termination of intractable seizures has been achieved with good neurologic recovery in several series.[37–40] A loading dose of 15 to 30 mg/kg has been suggested, followed by an infusion of 5 mg/kg/hr with continuous or frequent electroencephalographic monitoring. Infusion rates of up to 55 mg/kg/hr were used in one series in order to achieve burst suppression on the electroencephalogram and possibly some degree of cerebral protection.[37] Most authors would advocate using a dose that suppresses epileptiform activity on a consistent basis for a 24- to 48-hour period.[38, 39] Good neurologic recovery was reported in patients whose seizures were rapidly controlled in this manner. Conversely, a rather dismal prognosis for complete neurologic recovery has been reported in several large series when the seizures could not be controlled and the duration of convulsive activity was prolonged.[41, 42] Dopamine and volume infusions were often needed in order to maintain adequate blood pressure and support cardiac output.

Propofol

The use of propofol has recently been proposed as an additional and possibly better agent for sedation and anesthesia in the intensive care unit.[19, 43–45] Propofol is a short-acting nonbarbiturate anesthetic agent that has just recently been approved for use in the United States. It is one of a series of alkyl phenols found to have anesthetic properties in humans. Propofol is rapidly redistributed, has a high plasma clearance, and a short elimination half-life, which makes it a good anesthetic agent for patients in whom close monitoring of neurologic function is essential.[46] Patients who are anesthetized with this drug recover very rapidly without the drowsiness normally experienced with other anesthetic agents.[46]

Propofol has been investigated for use as an adjunct to other therapies for the reduction of intracranial pressure in head trauma patients. A significant reduction in intracranial pressure was demonstrated when these patients were given a dose of 2 mg/kg.[47] However, unlike barbiturates, it also concurrently decreased mean arterial pressure and cerebral perfusion pressure. In addition, propofol did not appear to favorably affect cerebral metabolic rate, and its effects on cerebral vascular resistance were not consistent.[47] Further studies have been proposed to determine if propofol in lower doses (e.g., 1 mg/kg, which did not decrease mean arterial pressure in previous studies) will lower intracranial pressure without the hemodynamic effects noted at the higher dose.[47] Despite this, it remains an appealing agent for sedation and anesthesia of patients with brain trauma because of its intracranial pressure lowering effects and the patient's rapid return to an alert state after discontinuation of the drug.

The hemodynamic effects of propofol are still being elucidated in pediatric patients, but studies in adults have demonstrated a dose-related reduction in systemic vascular resistance with resultant hypotension.[46] The cardiac index is not consistently affected. Propofol may also lower heart rate because of a resetting of baroreceptor reflexes, allowing lower heart rates despite a decrease in arterial blood pressure. In addition, it is a profound respiratory depressant and may significantly decrease minute volume and central CO_2 responsiveness when given as a bolus infusion.[46]

Propofol is an oil at room temperature; an emulsion must be formed with 10% soybean oil, 2.25% glycerol, and 1.2% purified egg phosphatide in order to make an aqueous solution. Pain on injection is a common feature (58% in one series)[48] when this agent is injected into the dorsum of the hand. When given in the antecubital fossa, pain was reported in less than 10% of patients.[49] Less common side effects of this drug include the potential for coagulation abnormalities, as the emulsion is similar to intralipid, which has been associated with alterations in blood coagulation. Propofol also interacts with fentanyl, leading to a rise in blood propofol concentrations when these drugs are given together. In addition, a greenish discoloration of the urine has been reported during continuous infusions of this drug, possibly secondary to metabolites of this phenolic compound accumulating in the urine.

INHALATIONAL ANESTHETICS

Halothane

Inhalational anesthetics are rarely used in the intensive care unit because of the difficulties associated with scavenging of exhaled gases and the necessity of trained personnel to administer them. However, halothane and isoflurane have both been useful in the intensive care unit for treatment of severe bronchospasm.

Inhalational anesthetics have been used for more than 50 years as a treatment for intractable asthma.[50] More recently, halothane has been used as a treatment of last resort in patients who cannot be adequately ventilated despite maximal medical therapy. Halothane administration results in dose-dependent bronchodilatation. Its mechanism of action is not entirely clear but most authors feel the primary mechanism is due to β_2-receptor stimulation. There is some evidence, however, that halothane also causes direct bronchodilatation that is unrelated to β-adrenergic pathways.[51]

Halothane has many side effects that limit its use, including myocardial depression, arrhythmias, and loss of hypoxic pulmonary vasoconstriction resulting from its vasodilatory effects.[52] Hepatic toxicity has also been reported in a small subset of patients because of the production of fluoride ion as a metabolite.[53]

Halothane is a negative inotrope and therefore decreases cardiac output, stroke volume, and mean arterial pressure. This is felt to be secondary to drug-induced left ventricular depression.[54] The addition of hypoxia and hypercarbia, which are often seen in the ventilated asthmatic patient, further compounds the myocardial depression and may contraindicate the administration of this agent. However, clinical experience with halothane in patients with refractory bronchospasm has not shown an association with significant cardiovascular side effects.[52, 57] In an experimental dog model, halothane (1.25 to 1.5%) induced cardiac arrest in severely hypoxic animals (PaO$_2$ <30 mm Hg) on controlled ventilation.[55] This response was felt to be secondary to a potentiation of the depressant effects of hypoxia and acidosis by halothane rather than to the induction of arrhythmias. Careful titration to effect and close hemodynamic monitoring are imperative with the use of this drug.

Halothane also lowers the threshold for catecholamine-induced cardiac arrhythmias. This may be especially important with the concomitant administration of intravenous and inhaled β-agonists. The combined administration of halothane, aminophylline, and isoproterenol has been studied, and though the results were inconsistent, arrhythmias did appear to occur more frequently when the three drugs were administered together.[56]

There have been several case reports since the 1970s showing dramatic response with this agent after only a short period of administration.[52, 57] Whether this response is due to more profound bronchodilatation than can be achieved by other β$_2$-agonists is not entirely clear. It does appear that halothane can break the "cycle" of bronchoconstriction, since improvement in ventilation continues even after the halothane is discontinued.

Isoflurane

To minimize the risk of cardiovascular side effects during treatment of life-threatening bronchospasm, isoflurane has been advocated as an efficacious and possibly safer agent than halothane.[58-61] A recent report by Johnston and colleagues described its use in two adults and two children with refractory status asthmaticus.[61] No significant complications were noted with this treatment over 1 to 2 days. Although no major side effects have been noted with either halothane or isoflurane, isoflurane has the advantage of being less arrhythmogenic[62] than halothane in equipotent doses. In addition, it does not have the potential for hepatic toxicity that halothane does. It is also the least fat-soluble of the anesthetic vapors, and the time to recovery is shorter despite prolonged use.[63]

CONCLUSION

Many anesthetic agents have proved to be invaluable in the pediatric intensive care unit to treat life-threatening symptoms. In addition, increased comfort and lack of recall of painful events can be provided by these agents. Further studies are under way to provide better and safer agents that can be used not only to relieve pain and anxiety but also to provide therapeutic intervention for difficult to treat entities such as intracranial hypertension and intractable seizures. Critical care medicine has been enhanced by the development of newer and safer anesthetic agents and should continue to be in the future.

References

1. Yaster M and Maxwell LG: Pediatric regional anesthesia. Anesthesiology 70:323, 1989.
2. Stoelting RK: Local anesthetics. In: Pharmacology and Physiology in Anesthetic Practice. Philadelphia, JB Lippincott, 1987.
3. Albright GA: Cardiac arrest following regional anesthesia with etidocaine or bupivacaine (Editorial). Anesthesiology 51:285, 1979.
4. Reiz S and Nath S: Cardiotoxicity of local anesthetic agents. Br J Anaesth 58:736, 1986.
5. Simon RP, Benowitz NL, Bonstein J, et al: Increased brain uptake of lidocaine during bicuculline-induced status epilepticus in rats. Neurology 34:384, 1984.
6. deJong RH and Heavner JE: Diazepam prevents and aborts lidocaine convulsions in monkeys. Anesthesiology 41:226, 1974.
7. Kasten GW and Martin ST: Bupivacaine cardiovascular toxicity: Comparison of treatment with bretylium and lidocaine. Anesth Analg 64:911, 1985.
8. Donegan M, Bedford RF, and Dacey R: IV lidocaine for prevention of intracranial hypertension. Anesthesiology 51:S201, 1979.
9. Sakabe T, Maekawa T, Ishikawa T, et al: The effects of lidocaine on canine cerebral metabolism and circulation related to the electroencephalogram. Anesthesiology 40:433, 1974.
10. McNally JF, Enright P, Hirsch JE, et al: The attenuation of exercise-induced bronchoconstriction by oropharyngeal anesthesia. Am Rev Respir Dis 119:247, 1979.
11. Fish JE and Peterman VI: Effects of inhaled lidocaine on airway function in asthmatic subjects. Respiration 37:201, 1979.
12. Downes H, Gerber N, and Hirshman CA: I.V. lignocaine in reflex and allergic bronchoconstriction. Br J Anaesth 52:873, 1980.
13. Bokesch PM, Castaneda AR, Ziemer G, et al: The influence of right-to-left shunt on lidocaine pharmacokinetics. Anesthesiology 67:739, 1987.
14. Bodin A, Nyqvist-Mayer A, Wadsten T, et al: Phase diagram and aqueous solubility of the lidocaine-prilocaine binary system. J Pharm Sci 73:481, 1984.
15. Halperin DL, Koren G, Attias D, et al: Topical skin anesthesia for venous, subcutaneous drug reservoir and lumbar punctures in children. Pediatrics 84:281, 1989.
16. Soliman IE, Broadman LM, Hannallah RS, et al: Comparison of the analgesic effects of EMLA (eutectic mixture of local anesthetics) to intradermal lidocaine infiltration prior to venous cannulation in unpremedicated children. Anesthesiology 68:804, 1988.
17. Maunuksela EL and Korpela R: Double-blind evaluation of a lignocaine-prilocaine cream (EMLA) in children: Effect on the pain associated with venous cannulation. Br J Anaesth 58:1242, 1986.
18. McCafferty DF, Woolfson AD, and Boston V: In vivo assessment of percutaneous local anaesthetic preparations. Br J Anaesth 62:17, 1989.
19. Norreslet J and Wahlgreen C: Propofol infusion for sedation of children. Crit Care Med 18:890, 1990.
20. Corssen G, Miyasaka M, and Domino EF: Changing concepts in pain control during surgery: Dissociative anesthesia with CI-581. Anesth Analg 47:746, 1968.
21. Chodoff P: Evidence for central adrenergic action of ketamine. Anesth Analg 51:247, 1972.
22. White PR, Way WL, and Trevor AJ: Ketamine—its pharmacology and therapeutic uses. Anesthesiology 56:119, 1982.
23. Reich DL and Silvay G: Ketamine: An update on the first twenty-five years of clinical experience. Can J Anaesth 36:186, 1989.
24. Waxman K, Shoemaker WC, and Lippmann M: Cardiovascular effects of anesthetic induction with ketamine. Anesth Analg 59:355, 1980.
25. Rock MJ, Reyes de la Rocha S, L'Hommedieu CS, et al: Use of ketamine in asthmatic children to treat respiratory failure refractory to conventional therapy. Crit Care Med 14:514, 1986.
26. Strube PJ and Hallam PL: Ketamine by continuous infusion in status asthmaticus. Anaesthesia 41:1017, 1986.

27. Sussman DR: A comparative evaluation of ketamine anesthesia in children and adults. Anesthesiology 40:459, 1974.

28. Corssen G, Gutierrez J, Reves JC, et al: Ketamine in the anesthetic management of asthmatic patients. Anesth Analg 51:588, 1972.

29. Sears BE: Complications of ketamine. Anesthesiology 35:231, 1971.

30. Takeshita H, Okuda Y, and Sari A: The effects of ketamine on cerebral circulation and metabolism in man. Anesthesiology 36:69, 1972.

31. Stoelting RK: Barbiturates. In: Pharmacology and Physiology in Anesthetic Practice. Philadelphia, JB Lippincott, 1987.

32. Shapiro HR, Galindo A, Whyte SR, et al: Rapid intraoperative reduction of intracranial pressure with thiopentone. Br J Anaesth 45:1057, 1973.

33. Ward JD, Becker DP, Miller JD, et al: Failure of prophylactic barbiturate coma in the treatment of severe head injury. J Neurosurg 62:383, 1985.

34. Trauner DA: Barbiturate therapy in acute brain injury. J Pediatr 109:742, 1986.

35. Bedford RF, Persing JA, Pobereskin L, et al: Lidocaine or thiopental for rapid control of intracranial hypertension. Anesth Analg 59:435, 1980.

36. Todd MM, Chadwick HS, Shapiro HM, et al: The neurological effects of thiopental therapy following experimental cardiac arrest in cats. Anesthesiology 57:76, 1982.

37. Orlowski JP, Erenberg G, Lueders H, et al: Hypothermia and barbiturate coma for refractory status epilepticus. Crit Care Med 12:367, 1984.

38. Partinen M, Kovanen J, and Nilsson E: Status epilepticus treated by barbiturate anaesthesia with continuous monitoring of cerebral function. Br Med J 282:520, 1981.

39. Feneck RO: A case of status epilepticus: Use of thiopentone and IPPV to control otherwise refractory convulsions. Anaesthesia 36:691, 1981.

40. Brown AS and Horton JM: Status epilepticus treated by intravenous infusions of thiopentone sodium. Br Med J 1:27, 1967.

41. Aminoff MJ and Simon RP: Status epilepticus: Causes, clinical features, and consequences in 98 patients. Am J Med 69:657, 1980.

42. Aicardi J and Chevrie JJ: Convulsive status epilepticus in infants and children: A study of 239 cases. Epilepsia 11:187, 1970.

43. Harris CE, Grounds RM, Murray AM, et al: Propofol for long-term sedation in the intensive care unit: A comparison with papaveretum and midazolam. Anaesthesia 45:366, 1990.

44. Albanese J, Martin C, Lacarelle B, et al: Pharmacokinetics of long-term propofol infusion used for sedation in ICU patients. Anesthesiology 73:214, 1990.

45. Beller JP, Pottecher T, Lugnier A, et al: Prolonged sedation with propofol in ICU patients: Recovery and blood concentration changes during periodic interruptions in infusion. Br J Anaesth 61:583, 1988.

46. Sebel PS and Lowdon JD: Propofol: A new intravenous anesthetic. Anesthesiology 71:260, 1989.

47. Herregods L, Verbeke J, Rolly G, et al: Effect of propofol on elevated intracranial pressure: Preliminary results. Anaesthesia 43(Suppl):107, 1988.

48. Valanne J and Korttila K: Comparison of methohexitone and propofol (Diprivan) for induction of enflurane anesthesia in outpatients. Postgrad Med J 61(Suppl):138, 1985.

49. Nightingale P, Healy TEJ, Hargreaves J, et al: Propofol in emulsion form: Induction characteristics and venous sequelae. Eur J Anaesthesiol 2:361, 1985.

50. Meyer NE and Schotz S: Relief of severe intractable bronchial asthma with cyclopropane anesthesia: Report of case. J Allergy 10:239, 1939.

51. Hirshman CA and Bergman NA: Halothane and enflurane protect against bronchospasm in an asthma dog model. Anesth Analg 57:619, 1978.

52. O'Rourke PP and Crone RK: Halothane in status asthmaticus. Crit Care Med 10:341, 1982.

53. Stoelting RK: Inhaled anesthetics. In: Pharmacology and Physiology in Anesthetic Practice. Philadelphia, JB Lippincott, 1987.

54. Merin R, Kumazawa T, and Luka N: Myocardial function and metabolism in the conscious dog and during halothane anesthesia. Anesthesiology 44:402, 1976.

55. Cullen DJ and Eger EI: The effects of halothane on respiratory and cardiovascular responses to hypoxia in dogs. Anesthesiology 33:487, 1970.

56. Takaori M and Loehning RW: Ventricular arrhythmias during halothane anaesthesia: Effect of isoproterenol, aminophylline, and ephedrine. Can Anaesth Soc J 12:275, 1965.

57. Schwartz SH: Treatment of status asthmaticus with halothane. JAMA 251:2688, 1984.

58. Bierman MI, Brown M, Muren O, et al: Prolonged isoflurane anesthesia in status asthmaticus. Crit Care Med 14:832, 1986.

59. Parnass SM, Feld JM, Chamberlin WH, et al: Status asthmaticus treated with isoflurane and enflurane. Anesth Analg 66:193, 1987.

60. Revell S, Greenhalgh D, Absalom SR, et al: Isoflurane in the treatment of asthma. Anesthesia 43:477, 1988.

61. Johnston RG, Noseworthy TW, Friesen EG, et al: Isoflurane therapy for status asthmaticus in children and adults. Chest 97:698, 1990.

62. Joas TA and Stevens WC: Comparison of the arrhythmic doses of epinephrine during forane, halothane and fluroxane anesthesia in dogs. Anesthesiology 35:48, 1971.

63. Pearson J: Prolonged anesthesia with isoflurane. Anesth Analg 64:92, 1985.

77

Sedatives and Analgesics

William Keyes, M.D., Ph.D.

Children suffering with pain, fear, and anxiety remain an all too common sight in today's pediatric intensive care unit. Providing relief for these symptoms remains one of the most difficult challenges facing the pediatric intensive care practitioner. Oftentimes the introduction of an agent to provide relief of these discomforts precipitates physiologic instability and serious side effects that cause the novice to avoid these agents or to use them only when symptoms are severe. Conversely, delivery of drugs by protocol or rigid schedule can lead to unnecessary and excessive medication. The clinician needs to be aware that the perception of and reaction to pain is an individual, subjective, and dynamic process. Similarly, the response to a specific agent can vary dramatically among patients and temporally in the same patient.

Pain has been described as "an unpleasant sensory and emotional experience associated with actual or potential tissue damage, or described in terms of such damage."[1] The mechanisms of the production of and the physiologic response to pain in infants and children have been reviewed elsewhere.[2] Suffice it to say that pain may cause significant changes in cardiovascular, endocrine, metabolic, immunologic, and stress responses. The issue of pain in the fetus and newborn has also been thoroughly addressed, and current knowledge suggests that humane considerations should apply as forcefully to the care of neonates and young, nonverbal infants as they do to children and adults in similar painful and stressful situations.[3] In adult patients, the relief of pain has been associated with improved outcome. These effects mandate that clinicians critically address pain issues.

ANALGESICS

"Analgesic Ladder"

The concept of an "analgesic ladder"[4] has been employed in the management of both adult and pediatric pain associated with cancer and may be helpful in understanding and using analgesics in the pediatric intensive care unit. It involves a stepwise approach to the management of pain, tailoring the medication or medications to the specific current needs of the patient. To minimize side effects, the clinician usually begins with less potent analgesics and gradually adds or replaces agents until the desired amount of analgesia is achieved. Obviously, circumstances will often dictate advancing or descending the analgesic ladder more rapidly than usual or skipping several steps on the ladder as conditions require.

Nonpharmacologic approaches can often either obviate the need for medication or lessen the amount or number of agents employed. Cognitive-behavioral techniques, such as increased (or in some cases decreased) parental presence, behavioral modification, and child life programs can have enormous impact on the need for analgesia and sedation and should be considered.

Local Anesthesia

Local anesthetics are underused in the pediatric intensive care unit. Currently, the typical patient does not receive pain control for "minor" procedures such as venipuncture or intravenous catheter insertion. Many minor and some more involved procedures can be performed with local anesthesia alone or in combination with a smaller than usual dose of an anxiolytic or opioid drug. Even one of the most frequently performed procedures, venipuncture, can be made less painful by the topical application of a cream containing a mixture of lidocaine and prilocaine.[5] The application of such a cream necessitates additional delay before venipuncture can be performed and is an unfortunate, but obligatory, effect of the attempting of good pain control.

Regional Anesthesia

Over the last 5 to 10 years, techniques and agents have been developed and refined for the administration of regional anesthesia to children and even infants.[6] Regional anesthesia has the advantage of providing unparalleled postoperative pain relief while preserving consciousness and normal ventilatory control. When prolonged anesthesia is required, a catheter can be inserted for intermittent or continuous administration of drug locally. Unfortunately, these techniques require extra time and specialized training to perform. Regional

974

anesthesia may also offer an alternative to opioids in the patient with ventilatory or central nervous system disease. Regional anesthesia is contraindicated in patients with a coagulopathy, infection, or tumor at the site of block or ongoing degenerative axonal disease.

Nonopioid Analgesics

The term *opioid* was coined to refer, in a generic sense, to all drugs, natural and synthetic, with morphine-like action. With the increasing use of the term *narcotic* in a legal context to refer to any drug that can cause dependence, it is no longer useful in a pharmacologic context.

Nonsteroidal Anti-inflammatory Agents

Aspirin and acetaminophen are the most widely known nonopioid analgesics and are useful in the management of mild pain. Because the use of aspirin frequently causes or exacerbates pre-existing gastritis and because of its suspected role in the pathogenesis of Reye syndrome, it has fallen into disfavor. Because concerns for hemostasis are common in children in intensive care units, indications for aspirin and nonsteroidal anti-inflammatory agents are quite narrow. In pediatrics, acetaminophen and not aspirin should be considered the nonopioid analgesic of choice. Agents used occasionally in children include ibuprofen, indomethacin, naproxen, and tolmetin. Usual preparations are administered orally, a route that is often inappropriate for the patient in an intensive care unit. In one study, however, prophylactic continuous infusion of indomethacin was shown to result in better postoperative pain relief than did intramuscular morphine alone, and it was not associated with clinically important side effects.[7]

Ketamine

Ketamine came into use in the 1970s and was touted as an agent that produced good somatic analgesia, excellent cardiovascular stability, and preserved protective airway mechanisms and normal respiratory drive. Ketamine produces dissociation of the cortex from the limbic system. It appears to block afferent impulses in the diencephalon and associated pathways of the cortex but spares the reticular formation of the brain stem. Thus, ketamine produces a dissociative, catatonic state of analgesia in which the eyes may remain open, often with blinking, nystagmus, and sometimes intact corneal reflexes. Occasional nonpurposeful movements or vocalization may occur. The advantages of ketamine include excellent somatic analgesia, preservation of CO_2 responsiveness and airway protective reflexes, and a decrease in airway reactivity and bronchospasm. Unfortunately, ketamine has been found to have a number of undesirable side effects that limit its usefulness. Ketamine is sialagogic, a poor visceral analgesic, and a cerebrovascular vasodilator. It is a direct myocardial depressant and markedly increases myocardial oxygen consumption. However, it usually increases heart rate

and blood pressure through direct stimulation of central nervous system sympathomimetic pathways.

Ketamine is most useful in providing sedation for short procedures (burn débridement, cardiac catheterization) or for inducing anesthesia in an uncooperative child. Unfortunately, ketamine frequently produces emergence phenomena, including nightmares and hallucinations. They can be minimized by the concurrent use of benzodiazepines. Ketamine is also useful for the induction of anesthesia in patients with hypovolemia or septic or hemorrhagic shock and in the patient prone to reactive airway disease. For reasons previously outlined, ketamine is best avoided in patients with intracranial or systemic hypertension.

Opiate Analgesics

Opiate analgesics remain the backbone of pain relief in the intensive care unit. In the last decade, there has been an explosion of knowledge related to the opiates and their effects. The discovery of classes of opiate receptors and the agonist and antagonist effects at each receptor has greatly aided our understanding of appropriate pharmacotherapy. The primary indication for the use of opiates is their effect on the central nervous system. None of the agents, however, is a pure agonist or antagonist at any of the receptor sites. In addition to their action on the central nervous system, opiates act to varying degrees on the respiratory, cardiovascular, genitourinary, and gastrointestinal systems. The usual desired effect on the central nervous system is analgesia; however, side effects on the central nervous system and other body systems are numerous (Table 77–1).

Morphine

Morphine is probably the most frequently used analgesic in the intensive care unit. It is a potent, moderately long-acting opioid. Morphine has the most respiratory and cardiovascular side effects; however, it also provides nearly the longest period of analgesia. Hypotension is common after administration of morphine and results from increased venous capacitance and arterial vasodil-

Table 77–1. NONSPECIFIC SIDE EFFECTS OF OPIATE ANALGESICS

Central nervous system
  Dysphoria, loss of consciousness
  Nausea and vomiting
  Miosis
  Physical dependence
Respiratory system
  Respiratory depression (decreased CO_2 responsiveness, apnea, hypoxia)
  Blunted airway reflexes (cough)
Gastrointestinal system
  Constipation
  Delayed gastric emptying
  Biliary tract spasm
Genitourinary system
  Urinary bladder spasm
  Urinary retention

atation as a direct consequence of histamine release. The histamine release may also initiate or exacerbate bronchospasm in susceptible patients. In high doses morphine can elicit seizures, and with rapid infusion it can lead to nausea and profound dysphoria. All the opioids are metabolized by the liver and should be used with caution in patients with hepatic disease. Allergic phenomena can occur but are usually limited to pruritus and urticaria and can often be relieved with histamine antagonists. Infants, especially those with a history of apnea, are particularly sensitive to the respiratory depression induced by morphine.

Fentanyl

Fentanyl is a synthetic opioid that differs from morphine in several respects. It is more lipophilic, more potent, and shorter acting when administered as a bolus. Perhaps the most useful benefit of the short half-life of fentanyl is that it lends itself to the use of continuous intravenous infusion, as well as its attendant advantages over bolus intermittent administration. The relative potencies of commonly used opioids are outlined in Table 77–2. Fentanyl produces less histamine release than does morphine and may be a useful alternative to morphine in the patient with severe pruritus that is refractory to treatment with antihistamines. Many intensive care practitioners prefer fentanyl over morphine because of its rapid onset, shorter duration of action, lower likelihood of producing histamine release, and minimal cardiovascular side effects. Fentanyl, however, has a predilection for causing a dose-related bradycardia and also chest wall rigidity.

Sufentanil and Alfentanil

Sufentanil and alfentanil are newer fentanyl derivatives that are primarily used in the operative setting. Sufentanil is about ten times more potent than fentanyl and is most often used for cardiovascular surgery. Alfentanil has a shorter duration of action and faster onset that fentanyl and may be useful for short procedures in the intensive care unit.

Meperidine

Meperidine is similar to morphine except that it is much less likely to cause histamine release and can be given orally with excellent absorption from the gastrointestinal tract. At high levels, a meperidine metabolite, normeperidine, can produce central nervous system excitation, leading to tremors, muscle twitches, and even seizures. Since normeperidine is eliminated by both the kidney and the liver, decreased renal or hepatic function increases the likelihood of toxic side effects. Meperidine is most commonly used for postoperative analgesia.

Methadone

Consistent, prolonged analgesia can be obtained with methadone. Methadone is essentially as potent as morphine, but unlike morphine, methadone is consistently well absorbed from the gut and can provide analgesia after a single dose for periods up to 24 hours. Methadone also produces less sedation, less euphoria (perceived as dysphoria in many children), and less constipation than does morphine. It may prove most useful in the intensive care patient with chronic pain requiring prolonged analgesia.

Although short-term use of opioid analgesia in the intensive care setting is generally safe, prolonged use can lead to physical or psychologic dependence, or both. Abrupt withdrawal of opioids in such a patient can lead to acute withdrawal symptoms and may occur much more often than most intensive care practitioners suspect. Methadone administration has been shown to be a safe and effective method of treating infants with iatrogenic drug dependency.[8]

Combinations of Opiates and other Agents

Lytic cocktail, also known as DPT cocktail or cardiac cocktail, is a mixture of a fixed combination of meperidine, promethazine, and chlorpromazine and was originally designed as a premedication for children prior to cardiac catheterization. Over the years its use broadened to include premedication for many noxious pediatric procedures. Although still occasionally employed, this particular regimen can no longer be recommended because of the frequency of untoward side effects and the development of more sophisticated and safer methods of achieving sedation and analgesia for pediatric procedures.[9] Ideally, one would like a drug regimen that was safe, easy to administer, predictable, and reversible. To this end, the combination of intravenous midazolam and fentanyl has become more frequently used to achieve these goals and is now commonly employed in many pediatric intensive care units. Although not without its own hazards, the use of this combination with proper monitoring can provide the benefits of analgesia and sedation for most painful intensive care procedures with minimal risk.[10]

SEDATIVES AND ANXIOLYTICS

Anxiety and fear are routinely encountered in the pediatric intensive care unit. Despite the large amount of attention these problems have received in the adult literature, disappointingly little has been written on the pharmacologic management of anxiety and fear in children. Short-acting anxiolytic-sedative agents are gaining more widespread acceptance in the pediatric intensive care unit and may substitute for more dangerous drugs.

Table 77–2. EQUIPOTENT DOSES OF VARIOUS OPIOIDS

Agent	Dose (mg)
Sufentanil	0.002
Fentanyl	0.01
Morphine	1.0
Methadone	1.0
Meperidine	7.5

A similar stepwise approach as was proposed for analgesics would likely prove useful with sedatives and anxiolytics.

Chloral Hydrate

Chloral hydrate has been the mainstay of sedation for pediatricians for many years. It has minimal cardiovascular and respiratory effects and provides a duration of sedation useful for many pediatric diagnostic procedures. It provides mild sedation but, as with benzodiazepines and barbiturates, provides no analgesia. Chloral hydrate is generally regarded as nontoxic by pediatricians; however, this has recently been brought into question. It is now clear that chloral hydrate can produce direct hyperbilirubinemia in the newborn, and metabolites of chloral hydrate can accumulate in infants and lead to encephalopathy. Despite these problems, chloral hydrate continues to be employed frequently as a sedative for many diagnostic procedures and to facilitate sleep.

Barbiturates

Barbiturates are commonly administered to pediatric patients for sedation, premedication for endotracheal intubation, and treatment of seizures. Commonly used barbiturates include thiopental, pentobarbital, and methohexital. They are all rapidly absorbed and have a rapid onset of action that is terminated by redistribution of the drug to other body compartments. Upon saturation of these compartments, recovery can become extremely prolonged. These medications can cause myocardial depression, leading to hypotension, especially in the face of hypovolemia. Administration of barbiturates can lead to dysphoria in patients with pain. It is important to remember that long-term administration can lead to tolerance and dependence. Barbiturates are contraindicated in patients with porphyria and may induce bronchospasm in patients with reactive airway disease. Apnea is common in children following the administration of thiopental, and a dose-related depression of respiratory drive is common to all barbiturates. These agents reduce cerebral metabolic blood flow and can lower intracranial pressure, making them useful for intubation of patients with elevated intracranial pressure.

Benzodiazepines

Benzodiazepines, which commonly include diazepam, lorazepam, and midazolam, are frequently employed to relieve symptoms of anxiety and fear. Another useful effect of benzodiazepines is that they provide varying degrees of amnesia. However, they produce no analgesia. Diazepam has a fairly rapid onset of action and a prolonged duration of action, occasionally as long as 6 to 8 hours. It is irritating to veins, painful when admin-

istered, and can lead to phlebitis. Lorazepam has a longer duration of action than does diazepam and is not irritating to veins. It is a potent anticonvulsant. A newer benzodiazepine, midazolam, has a short duration of action and rapid onset, properties that make it ideal for administration by continuous intravenous infusion. The use of midazolam infusions for long-term sedation in the intensive care unit is gaining in popularity, particularly in pediatric patients.[11] However, initial enthusiasm for this agent and method of administration has been tempered by reports of acute benzodiazepine withdrawal syndrome in children upon discontinuation of midazolam infusions.[12]

Neuroleptic Agents

Neuroleptic agents, such as haloperidol or droperidol, though common in adult intensive care units, are infrequently used in the pediatric intensive care setting. They are occasionally used in the older pediatric patient or as an adjunct to opiates or benzodiazepines in the younger child. Despite a large body of knowledge regarding their use in pediatric patients with psychiatric disorders, little or nothing has been reported concerning their use in the management of agitated or delirious patients in the intensive care setting. Long-term use of these agents can lead to tardive dyskinesia and is not recommended. Occasionally, one will encounter dystonic reactions after administration of neuroleptic agents, which can usually be managed with antihistamines.

References

1. International Association for the Study of Pain Subcommittee on Taxonomy: Pain terms: A list with definitions and notes on usage. Pain 6:249, 1979.
2. Anand KJS and Carr DB: The neuroanatomy, neurophysiology, and neurochemistry of pain, stress, and analgesia in newborns and children. Pediatr Clin North Am 36:795, 1989.
3. Anand KJS and Hickey PR: Pain and its effects in the human neonate and fetus. N Engl J Med 317:1321, 1987.
4. Berde C, Ablin A, Glazer J, et al: Report of the subcommittee on disease-related pain in childhood cancer. Pediatrics 86:818, 1990.
5. Hopkins CS, Buckley CJ, and Bush GH: Pain-free injection in infants. Anaesthesia 43:198, 1988.
6. Yaster M and Maxwell LG: Pediatric regional anesthesia. Anesthesiology 70:324, 1989.
7. Maunuksela E, Olkkola KT, and Korpela R: Does prophylactic intravenous infusion of indomethacin improve management of postoperative pain in children? Can J Anaesth 35:123, 1988.
8. Tobias JD, Schleien CL, and Haun SE: Methadone as treatment for iatrogenic narcotic dependency in pediatric intensive care unit patients. Crit Care Med 18:1292, 1990.
9. Snodgrass WR and Dodge WF: Lytic/"DPT" cocktail: Time for rational and safe alternatives. Pediatr Clin North Am 36:1285, 1989.
10. Yaster M, Nichols DG, Deshpande JK, et al: Midazolam-fentanyl intravenous sedation in children: Case report of respiratory arrest. Pediatrics 86:463, 1990.
11. Silvasi DL, Rosen DA, and Rosen KR: Continuous intravenous midazolam infusion for sedation in the pediatric intensive care unit. Anesth Analg 67:286, 1988.
12. Sury MRJ, Billingham I, Russell GN, et al: Acute benzodiazepine withdrawal syndrome after midazolam infusions in children. Crit Care Med 17:301, 1989.

78

Neuromuscular Blockers

William Keyes, M.D., Ph.D.

Neuromuscular blocking agents play a crucial role in the treatment of many of the disease entities that are encountered by the pediatric intensivist. Neuromuscular blocking agents are most frequently used to facilitate mechanical ventilation. However, these drugs are also commonly employed to assist in the treatment of intracranial hypertension, to facilitate endotracheal intubation, and as muscle relaxants for various surgical procedures. At the dawn of pediatric critical care medicine, few agents were available to the practitioner, and those that were available (primarily succinylcholine, d-tubocurare, and pancuronium) had numerous side effects and contraindications that limited their use. Today, however, more sophisticated drugs are available with fewer side effects and fewer limitations to their use. Because they are so frequently employed under a variety of circumstances and because their misuse can have such serious consequences for the patient, the intensivist needs to be acquainted not only with the agents themselves but also with their mechanism of action and potential hazards.[1]

PHYSIOLOGY OF THE NEUROMUSCULAR JUNCTION

A complete understanding of the physiology of the neuromuscular junction is essential to the safe use of this class of drugs (see also Chapter 24). When an action potential reaches the neuromuscular junction (or synapse), it causes the release of a specific neurotransmitter, acetylcholine, from the presynaptic nerve terminal. The acetylcholine travels across the synaptic cleft to bind to receptors on the postsynaptic membrane, or neuromuscular endplate. There, the acetylcholine binds to acetylcholine receptors. Binding allows for the movement of small cations (Na^+, K^+, Ca^{2+}) across the neuromuscular endplate, the propagation of the action potential, and the release of Ca^{2+} from the sarcoplasmic reticulum with subsequent muscle contraction. Acetylcholine is rapidly hydrolyzed by plasma cholinesterase and rendered ineffective, thus terminating the muscle contraction.

TYPES OF NEUROMUSCULAR BLOCKERS

On the basis of their mechanism of action, neuromuscular blockers can be classified as either *depolarizing* or *nondepolarizing* agents. Depolarizing agents, of which succinylcholine is the prototypical agent, bind to the postsynaptic cholinergic receptors. Their initial action is similar to that of acetylcholine; that is, they act as competitive cholinergic agonists and cause muscle depolarization. This accounts for the usual clinical observation of brief muscle fasciculation with the initial dose of these agents. However, unlike acetylcholine, succinylcholine is not susceptible to rapid enzymatic degradation by cholinesterase, and muscle depolarization is prolonged, effectively increasing the refractory period and prohibiting further muscle stimulation. Eventually, this is manifested clinically by the onset of flaccid paralysis. Only with sufficient time for diffusion away from the receptor and competition with acetylcholine can sufficient succinylcholine be removed for reversal of paralysis to occur.

Nondepolarizing agents prevent neuromuscular transmission by acting as competitive antagonists at the postsynaptic cholinergic receptor and effectively blocking the unoccupied receptors to acetylcholine; hence the name "neuromuscular blocker." Binding by this class of drugs is reversible and competitive; that is, if a sufficient number of molecules of neuromuscular blocking agent are present at the postsynaptic receptor, depolarization will not occur. However, because binding is reversible, if sufficient acetylcholine is available the receptor blockade can be overwhelmed (by mass action) and membrane depolarization can again occur. It becomes obvious then that drugs that cause excess accumulation of acetylcholine at the postsynaptic membrane (physostigmine, neostigmine, etc.) can cause acetylcholine to accumulate in sufficient quantity to overwhelm the blockade and restore neuromuscular integrity.

There are many locations along these pathways where specific physiologic perturbations can either augment or interfere with the action of neuromuscular blockers (Table 78–1). In addition, considerations regarding developmental pharmacology can become important. Infants have a larger volume of distribution (on a per

Table 78–1. FACTORS AFFECTING NEUROMUSCULAR BLOCKADE

Enhancing Factors
  Renal failure (with certain agents)
  Hepatic failure (with certain agents)
  Hypothermia
  Respiratory acidosis
  Electrolyte abnormalities (hypokalemia, hypermagnesemia, hypocalcemia, hyponatremia)
  Certain antibiotics (aminoglycosides, polymyxin)
  Certain cardiovascular drugs (diphenylhydantoin, propranolol, procainamide, quinidine)
  Neuromotor diseases (myasthenia gravis, muscular dystrophy)
  Local anesthetics
  Furosemide
  Malnutrition
  Prolonged immobilization

Inhibiting Factors
  Theophylline, caffeine
  Azathioprine
  Hyperkalemia
  Hemiparesis (affected side is inhibited)
  Burn injuries
  Respiratory alkalosis

kilogram basis) and generally require higher initial dosages (mg/kg) of many of the neuromuscular blockers.[2] Equally as important, maturational changes in the neuromuscular junction can affect the time to onset of action, intensity of effect, and duration of effect.

MONITORING NEUROMUSCULAR BLOCKADE

There is great individual variability in response to neuromuscular blockers. Furthermore, the changing physiologic milieu of the patient can dramatically alter response to a given dose. Therefore, use of these agents mandates some means of assessment of degree of blockade. In the past, crude clinical evaluation has sufficed and may still be adequate under some circumstances. Unfortunately, many of these clinical signs require voluntary action (head lift, leg lift) on the part of the patient and may not be applicable to the infant or small child. Common methods for clinically monitoring the degree of neuromuscular blockade are outlined in Table 78–2.

A more precise method of assessing degree of blockade is by myoneural monitoring using a transcutaneous nerve stimulator.[3] In brief, this monitoring method requires stimulation of the ulnar nerve at the wrist using a peripheral nerve stimulator delivering a train-of-four* stimulus. A level of approximately 90% neuromuscular blockade can be achieved and maintained by adjusting the dose or infusion rate of neuromuscular blocker to provide one response (muscle twitch) to the train-of-four stimulus. By frequently testing the train-of-four response, one can easily adjust infusion rates or dosages to maintain a satisfactory level of neuromuscular blockade and simultaneously avoid overaccumulation, which

*"Train-of-four" refers to four equal electrical impulses delivered approximately ½ second apart.

can lead to prolonged recovery times. It is important to allow the muscle sufficient time to recover between tests, as repetitive stimulation can lead to muscle fatigue and erroneous interpretation.

It should be remembered that peripheral neuromuscular function is being tested by the train-of-four method. To extrapolate from these data an assessment of breathing function assumes that information obtained from testing skeletal muscles accurately reflects the status of the muscles of the diaphragm. In the case of pancuronium, it has been shown that the diaphragm appears to be more resistant to neuromuscular blockade than peripheral skeletal muscle.[4]

METHODS OF ADMINISTRATION

One of the characteristics of modern critical care medicine is careful tailoring of therapy to meet the patient's individual and changing needs. Although bolus administration of neuromuscular blockers remains the most commonly employed technique of administration, it is probably not the best because of wide variation of drug levels in the blood and subsequently at the receptor site. Clinically this leads to wide swings in effect varying from the underrelaxed patient who is suddenly thrashing in bed to the "overdosed" patient with inadvertently prolonged recovery time. Continuous infusion of the newer shorter acting agents offers several advantages over intermittent bolus administration. First, by using myoneural monitoring the caretaker can carefully titrate the infusion rate to meet the patient's minute-to-minute needs. Massive over- or undermedication is avoided, preventing unintended movement and possible dislodgement of various medical appliances. Second, there is a relatively short time interval from cessation of drug infusion to full recovery, allowing for rapid and frequent neurologic assessment and rapid extubation.

Unfortunately, drugs administered by constant infusion frequently require a "committed" intravenous line to avoid incompatibility issues. In infants and small children, vascular access is often limited and in addition the volume of mandatory vehicle is often also limited. Multilumen vascular catheters and microinfusion pumps have helped to circumvent some of these problems.

Priming Doses

Occasionally one may wish to achieve rapid paralysis, but the use of a rapidly acting depolarizing agent is

Table 78–2. CLINICAL SIGNS OF DEGREE OF NEUROMUSCULAR BLOCKADE

Sign	% Receptors Occupied
Decrease in:	
Tidal volume	80
Vital capacity	70–75
Leg lift	70
Inspiratory force	50
Sustained head lift	33

contraindicated. Although the use of "priming" doses remains controversial, especially in pediatric patients, it probably has its place in the intensive care setting.[5] The technique involves administering one tenth the normal dose of relaxant 3 to 4 minutes before giving the full dose. The neuromuscular junction has a large margin of safety—even when 70 to 80% of the receptors are occupied, neuromuscular transmission can still occur. Since the initial dose is subtherapeutic and binds to less that 75% of the receptors, little clinical effect is seen. Because the second dose is required to act on only the remaining available receptors, the onset of neuromuscular blockade occurs much faster. By presaturating the receptors the onset of action with the full dose is shortened. Because patients requiring muscle relaxation frequently have some degree of pre-existing respiratory compromise and because of the unpredictable response of the individual patient to neuromuscular blockers, the intensivist should have all the equipment and medications necessary to control the airway and ventilation when the priming dose is given.

Another technique that is often combined with a priming dose to achieve rapid paralysis is to give a relative overdose of neuromuscular blocker (usually two times the normal dose) to overwhelm the receptor and shorten the time to onset of action.

REVERSAL OF NEUROMUSCULAR BLOCKADE

Under certain circumstances it may be desirable to hasten the eventual spontaneous reversal of neuromuscular blockade. Pharmacologic reversal is not possible with depolarizing agents, and only the passage of time allows for recovery. However, nondepolarizing agents can be "reversed." Reversal agents are more commonly employed in the operating room than in the intensive care setting; nevertheless, the intensivist should be familiar with this technique. The pharmacologic reversal of nondepolarizing agents is obtained by increasing the concentration of acetylcholine at the neuromuscular junction. This is achieved by the use of anticholinesterases, which act by inhibiting acetylcholinesterase, the enzyme that degrades acetylcholine, thus allowing the accumulation of acetylcholine at the neuromuscular junction. As acetylcholine accumulates it displaces the neuromuscular blocker from the postsynaptic receptors and allows for restoration of neuromuscular junction integrity. The anticholinesterases most commonly employed are neostigmine, edrophonium, physostigmine, and pyridostigmine. The receptor for acetylcholine at the neuromuscular junction is classified as *nicotinic*; however, acetylcholine also binds to *muscarinic* receptors at sites other than the neuromuscular junction. Because of this, side effects due to muscarinic receptor stimulation may be seen when anticholinesterase inhibitors are used; these include bradycardia, miosis, excessive secretions, and bronchospasm. It is therefore also necessary to use specific muscarinic anticholinergics such as atropine or glycopyrollate to block these effects.

Attempting reversal shortly after administering a neuromuscular blocker or when no twitch can be elicited is usually not successful as the neuromuscular blockade is too intense for pharmacologic reversal. More time, rather than more reversal agent, is necessary before reversal is attempted again. Careful monitoring of the patient is required after pharmacologic reversal as occasionally sufficient neuromuscular blocker can reaccumulate to compromise the patient.

SPECIFIC AGENTS

Short-Acting Agents

Succinylcholine

Succinylcholine, the only depolarizing neuromuscular blocking agent available for use in the United States, is composed of two joined acetylcholine molecules. Its small molecular size allows rapid distribution throughout the extracellular fluid, which accounts for its rapid onset of action. It acts by binding to the acetylcholine receptor at the neuromuscular junction, causing sustained depolarization. Its action is terminated by hydrolysis by plasma cholinesterase (pseudocholinesterase). Because succinylcholine is hydrolyzed much more slower than acetylcholine, its presence in the neuromuscular junction is prolonged. A small percentage of the population have abnormal pseudocholinesterase activity and very prolonged muscle relaxation after a dose of succinylcholine.

The advantages of succinylcholine include its rapid onset of action (usually within 1 minute) and its short duration of action (5 to 10 minutes). These characteristics make it useful for induction of anesthesia and for use during rapid sequence intubation. Succinylcholine also stimulates muscarinic receptors, and in infants and children in whom parasympathetic tone predominates, this stimulation can lead to severe bradycardia. For this reason atropine is usually administered along with succinylcholine.

The disadvantages of succinylcholine are numerous and have to a certain degree limited its use. Succinylcholine increases serum potassium levels by 0.5 to 1 mEq/l in normal patients. Strong muscle fasciculations are not necessary to produce hyperkalemia in susceptible patients, and preadministration of small defasciculating doses of nondepolarizing neuromuscular blockers does not prevent the rise in serum potassium. Alarmingly high levels of serum potassium and associated cardiovascular collapse have been reported in a variety of situations that have in common either massive tissue destruction or central nervous system injury with muscle wasting. Clinical situations in which this has been encountered include burns, massive trauma (especially crush injuries), stroke, myotonias, muscular dystrophies, Guillain-Barré syndrome, and spinal cord injury. It is believed to be due to the proliferation of extrajunctional acetylcholine receptors. This increased sensitivity to succinylcholine usually appears 5 to 15 days after the injury and persists for 2 to 3 months in burn and trauma patients and for 3 to 6 months in patients with neuromotor diseases. It is generally safer to paralyze such patients with a nondepolarizing agent.

Other untoward effects of succinylcholine include elevations of serum myoglobin and creatine phosphokinase, especially in children. Succinylcholine increases intragastric pressure in direct relation to the degree of muscle fasiculations, which can potentially lead to regurgitation and subsequent pulmonary aspiration. Administration of succinylcholine increases intraocular pressure due to contraction of extraocular muscles. In the patient with a penetrating injury to the globe, administration of succinylcholine can lead to extrusion of the vitreous and permanent visual impairment. Masseter spasm (inability to open the mouth) can occur when succinylcholine is administered. Succinylcholine is also a well-known trigger for malignant hyperthermia in susceptible patients.

Intermediate-Acting Agents

Atracurium

The many contraindictions and side effects of succinylcholine and the long duration and slow onset of action of many of the older nondepolarizing neuromuscular blockers has led to the development of newer agents with fewer of these drawbacks.[6] Atracurium is an intermediate-acting neuromuscular blocker with a benzylisoquinolium ester structure that is degraded by ester hydrolysis and Hofmann elimination. Temperature and pH affect both processes. Atracurium is unique among the nondepolarizing neuromuscular blocking agents because it was designed to be independent of either renal or hepatic function for its elimination. At physiologic temperature and pH, atracurium is degraded by a nonenzymatic process, Hofmann elimination, that results in the formation of laudanosine. With prolonged administration, laudanosine can accumulate and toxic levels can be epileptogenic. The major route of elimination, however, is mainly by ester hydrolysis in the liver. Despite this, fulminant hepatic or renal failure does not seem to affect elimination pharmacokinetics.

The onset of blockade occurs in approximately 4 minutes in children. The ED50 (the dose required to produce a specified intensity of effect in 50% of individuals) of atracurium varies with age and is lowest in neonates, next lowest in children, and highest in adolescents. Recovery from atracurium blockade occurs in 20 to 30 minutes and is the same in all age groups. Atracurium releases histamine in adults, but this does not appear to be as serious a problem in children, even with massive overdosage.[7] Because of its short duration of action, atracurium can be administered by continuous infusion in infants and children.[8, 9]

Vecuronium

Vecuronium is a steroidal neuromuscular blocker related to pancuronium; it has a similar potency but a shorter duration of action. Vecuronium has an onset of action of 1.5 to 3 minutes and a duration of action of 25 to 35 minutes. Vecuronium lacks any vagolytic effect and does not cause the release of histamine, which makes it more useful in cardiovascularly compromised patients.

Elimination of vecuronium occurs primarily in the liver, making it useful in patients with renal failure. The duration of action is generally prolonged in patients with hepatic failure. Most of the drug is excreted unchanged by the hepatobiliary system. Like atracurium, vecuronium can be administered to infants and children by continuous infusion due to its short duration of action.[10]

Long-Acting Agents

Pancuronium

Pancuronium is a long-acting steroidal, nondepolarizing agent with an onset of action of 0.5 to 3 minutes and a duration of action of 45 to 60 minutes. Because pancuronium blocks muscarinic cholinergic receptors, tachycardia and hypertension can result. The majority of a dose is eliminated by the kidneys; thus renal failure can markedly prolong its effect.

References

1. Cook DR: Muscle relaxants in infants and children. Anesth Analg 60:335, 1981.
2. Costarino AT and Polin RA: Neuromuscular relaxants in the neonate. Clin Perinatol 14:965, 1987.
3. Lee C and Katz RL: Neuromuscular pharmacology: A clinical update and commentary. Br J Anaesth 52:173, 1980.
4. Laycock JRD, Baxter MK, Bevan JC, et al: The potency of pancuronium at the adductor pollicis and diaphragm in infants and children. Anesthesiology 68:908, 1988.
5. Cook DR and Davis PJ: Pharmacology of pediatric anesthesia. In: Motoyama EK and Davis PJ (eds): Smith's Anesthesia for Infants and Children, 5th ed. St. Louis, CV Mosby, 1990, pp. 157–197.
6. Miller RD, Rupp SM, Fisher DM, et al: Clinical pharmacology of vecuronium and atracurium. Anesthesiology 61:444, 1984.
7. Charlton AJ, Harper NJN, Edwards D, et al: Atracurium overdose in a small infant. Anaesthesia 44:485, 1989.
8. Goudsouzian N, Martyn J, Rudd GD, et al: Continuous infusion of atracurium in children. Anesthesiology 64:171, 1986.
9. Goudsouzian NG: Atracurium infusion in infants. Anesthesiology 68:267, 1988.
10. Meeretoja OZ, Wirtavuori K, and Neuvonen PJ: Age-dependence of the dose-response curve of vecuronium in pediatric patients during balanced anesthesia. Anesth Analg 67:21, 1988.

VII Poisoning and Environmental Hazards

79

Evaluation of the Poisoned Child

Anthony L. Pearson-Shaver, M.D., and
Curt M. Steinhart, M.D.

Poisoning continues to be a major health problem in this country. In 1989, the American Association of Poison Control Centers reported a total of 1,581,540 poison exposures and 590 poisoning fatalities in people of all ages.[1] While fatalities represent less than 1% of the total exposures, the number of exposures increased from 1988 by 15.5%. These data suggest that physicians providing care for acutely ill patients must continue to consider poisoning as an etiology for unusual or otherwise unexplained acute illness. Though recent advances in poison prevention have decreased fatalities, poisoning remains an important problem. The Poison Prevention Packaging Act (PPPA), child-resistant containers, the availability of poison control centers, and home use of ipecac have clearly reduced the number of these preventable deaths but unfortunately have not eliminated them entirely.

EPIDEMIOLOGY OF CHILDHOOD POISONING

In 1989, approximately 1,000,000 poison exposures occurred in children less than 13 years old,[1] the largest number in those less than 6 years old. The under-13 age group accounted for 61% of all exposures, with children younger than 3 years accounting for 46.3%. Children 6 to 13 years of age and adolescents 13 to 17 years of age accounted for 5.5 and 4.4% of all poison exposures, respectively. There was a male predominance in children less than 13, but a female predominance in adolescent poisonings.[1]

Most reported poisonings occurred at the patient's

residence.[1] Those patients who were not poisoned at home were most frequently poisoned in another household,[3] commonly those of babysitters or grandparents. Interestingly, grandparents were usually less prepared to administer first aid for poisoning than babysitters.[3]

In the same 1989 report, 43 children less than 17 years of age died as a result of poisonings.[1] These childhood deaths represented only 12% of all poisoning deaths in 1989. Four per cent of all poisoning deaths occurred in children less than 6 years old, 1% occurred in children between 6 and 12 years old, and 7% occurred in adolescents less than 17 years old. In a 4-year study, Trinkoff and Baker[4] noted 24 deaths in 4,271 pediatric patients admitted to hospitals for poisoning. Four deaths were in children under 5 years old and 20 were in adolescents 13 to 19 years old. In Maryland between 1979 and 1982, adolescent poisoning deaths accounted for 80% of all poisoning deaths.[4] Trinkoff and Baker found that childhood hospital admissions for poisoning in children younger than 5 years occurred with a prevalence of 110 per 100,000 members of the population.[4] They also noted that the prevalence of adolescent admissions for poisoning was twice that of the younger age group. Despite the fact that young children were more frequently involved in poisoning exposures than adolescents, adolescents were involved in more serious exposures.

When children require hospitalization for poisoning, a significant number require physiologic monitoring or observation. In a 2-year study by Fazen and associates, poisoning accounted for 1% of all general ward admissions and 4.5% of medical intensive care unit (MICU) admissions.[5] In the same study, 64% of the poisoned patients were admitted directly to the MICU either for suicide precautions or for significant toxicity. Of those admitted to the MICU, 64% had some degree of central nervous system (CNS) depression and 43% required artificial ventilation.

Despite the large number of pediatric poisonings, most poisoned children fare quite well.[1] Moderate effects occurred in 0.7%, while major effects occurred in less than 0.1% of all poisoned children,[1] and only 12% of all children exposed to poisons had even minor effects from the poisoning agent.

Important factors leading to childhood poisoning are availability of substances, patient mobility, and family stress.[4, 6, 7] Poisoning in infants less than 6 months old commonly is due to inappropriate drug administration by caregivers.[8] Older children tend to poison themselves with whatever they find in their immediate environment.[4, 6, 7] This "poisoning environment" is determined by the child's mobility. Infants and toddlers ingest agents "available" at ground level, frequently nondrug toxic agents.[8, 9] Children in walkers (6- to 9-month-olds) find bushy plants and mushrooms within their reach.[8] Infants who are mobile without the use of walkers are able to reach plants, tobacco, cleaning products, and cosmetics.[8, 9]

Family stress is a common factor in childhood poisoning.[6, 10] Stress disrupts normal family routines and results in lax observation of children. Pregnancy, a recent family move, single-parent households, parental anxiety, parental depression, and unemployment all can contribute to family stress. Social discord and limited or detached family relationships are common features of households with repeat ingestors.[6, 10] Disruptions in family or peer relationships are important contributing factors among adolescents who poison themselves.[7, 11]

Ninety per cent of all self-poisoned children ingest the first substance they find.[4] In one study, ingested tablets were found in the poisoned patient's own home in 88% of cases.[7] In a report by Calnan and colleagues, the ingested poison was being utilized for its intended use just prior to the poisoning incident in 91% of cases.[12]

Although fewer than 15% of all reported poisonings are due to analgesics, sedatives, hypnotics, and antipsychotics, this group accounted for more than half of all poisoning deaths.[1] Children and adolescents are poisoned with these agents because they have ready access to them. In a 1986 study, Trinkoff and Baker found that 70% of ingestions in young children and 95% of adolescent ingestions were of medicinal products.[4] Recent data suggest that only 38% of pediatric poisonings (children less than 17 years of age) are due to medications that one might commonly find in most households[1] (Table 79–1). In 1989, only 40.9% of childhood poisonings were due to agents normally found around the house such as cleaning substances, analgesics, cosmetics, plants, and cough and cold preparations.[1] These findings seem to indicate that a large percentage of poisonings are due to medications brought into households for specific illnesses rather than to items commonly used in the home. The child or adolescent finds the medicinal agent and the poisoning occurs.

Poisonings can be divided into two groups, accidental and intentional. Intentional poisonings involve the inges-

Table 79–1. POISON EXPOSURES TO COMMON HOUSEHOLD MEDICATIONS, 1989*

	Patient Ages	
	<6 yr	6–17 yr
Analgesics	85,507	24,774
Anticonvulsants	2,704	1,210
Antidepressants	3,284	2,797
Antihistamines	11,805	3,697
Antimicrobials	32,296	5,818
Asthma preparations	6,579	2,593
Cardiovascular drugs	9,981	1,466
Cough and cold remedies	68,916	9,528
Diuretics	2,486	475
Electrolytes and minerals	10,657	1,211
GI preparations	26,314	2,020
Hormones	15,822	1,346
Muscle relaxants	906	579
Sedatives/hypnotics/antipsychotics	7,965	4,545
Topicals	45,742	2,713
Vitamins	34,147	3,669
Total number of exposures	964,573	156,082

*Adapted from Litovitz TL, Schmitz BF, and Bailey KM: 1989 Annual Report of the American Association of Poison Control Centers National Data Collection System. Am J Emerg Med 8:394, 1990, with permission.

tion of harmful substances for recreational use, in suicide attempts, and from inappropriate self-treatment. Accidental poisonings were responsible for 88.3% of all reported poisonings in 1989.[1] Sixty per cent of all accidental poisonings occurred in children less than 6 years old and Fazen and coworkers noted that most accidental poisonings occurred in children less than 4 years old.[5] Ten per cent of children admitted to the hospital for poisoning in Fazen's study were less than 1 year old.

Accidental poisonings usually involve ingestion of a single agent (90%) and rapid solicitation of help (within 2 hours).[5] Intentional poisonings are more complex and involve many psychosocial issues. Intentional poisonings in older children and adolescents often involve multiple agents[4] and delayed initiation of therapy.[5] Substance abuse involving recreational drugs and steroids is an important causes of intentional poisoning.[2, 4, 13, 14] In 1989, 30% of high school seniors who completed the National High School Senior Survey reported having used marijuana during the previous year and 3% admitted to daily use.[2] Cocaine use was reported in 8.5% of high school seniors, with 4.7% using cocaine in the form of "crack." Sixty per cent of the respondents admitted to having used alcohol (ethanol) within the previous 30 days, and 33% had experienced a drinking binge in the 2 weeks preceding completion of the survey. Risk factors for adolescent substance abuse include parental drug use or indifference to it, drug use by peers, and individual personal characteristics including rebelliousness, alienation, sensation seeking, anxiety, and depression.[2]

The incidence of steroid use among high school athletes has been reported to range from 6.6%[13] to 11%.[14] Most steroid users report a desire to improve athletic performance or strength. The fact that 22% of those using steroids were unable to identify any possible risks and many were unable to accurately identify purported benefits[14] is indicative of the naiveté exhibited by adolescent drug abusers. Among steroid users, peer pressure was an important influence: 10% of steroid users reportedly did so because friends were using them.[14] Johnson and colleagues suggested that "black market" tactics used to distribute and obtain steroids may put adolescents at risk for using other illicit drugs merely because they become knowledgeable about acquiring drugs.[14]

Intentional poisoning frequently constitutes a suicide attempt among older children and adolescents. Thirteen- to 17-year-old females accounted for 2.2% of poisonings.[1] One study has indicated an increasing number of admissions for deliberate self-poisonings in patients between the ages of 7 and 15 years.[7] In this group, those who deliberately poisoned themselves took whatever agent was available. Apparently because they were so universally available, analgesics were the most common class of drugs ingested.[7] In the same study, the author noted that a suicide attempt did not suggest true intent.[7] He found that very few of these children aged 7 to 15 years old took measures to avoid being discovered, and approximately 70% contacted a family member following the ingestion. Interviews conducted during hospitalizations for intentional poisoning among adolescents revealed that only 6% actually intended to kill themselves.[7] While some expressed ambivalence concerning the outcome of their poisoning, the majority stated that they intended to harm but not kill themselves. Taylor and Stansfield believe that childhood suicide attempts by poisoning do not represent psychiatrically trivial events.[11] Children (8 to 17 years old) who attempted suicide by poisoning displayed more psychiatric symptoms than children referred for psychiatric evaluation for other reasons. A strong association was noted between self-injury and depressive disorders. Family disruptions and poor peer relationships were important contributing factors.[7, 11]

The number of poisoning fatalities decreased between 1963 and 1989,[1, 15] a time when several prevention programs were introduced to limit the access of children to various poisons. These efforts resulted in a decrease in fatalities in children less than 5 years from 454 children in 1963 to 149 in 1973, and the number of poisoning fatalities due to medications in this same age group for the same 2 years decreased from 216 to 102. These numbers have further decreased to a total of 24 deaths in children younger than 6 years during 1989 with only 14 being due to medications.

The Poisoning Prevention Packaging Act of 1973[15] requires child-resistant containers for toxic, corrosive, irritant, and strong sensitizing products.[15] Child-resistant containers are designed to take a child less than 5 years old at least 5 minutes to open,[16] thus giving caretakers time to reach the child before the toxin is ingested. Since the PPPA was enacted, inappropriate ingestions of regulated drugs fell from 95,000 in 1973 to 52,000 in 1978, a decrease of 45%.

By providing advice and often directing the early institution of medical care,[17] regional poison centers have reduced the need for emergency room treatment.[18] In 1989, only 25% of all poison control center contacts resulted in treatment being obtained in a health care facility.[1]

INITIAL EVALUATION

History

The value of historical data should not be underestimated as toxic agents are frequently identified by history. Fazen and coworkers reported that historical data identified as many as 90% of the agents ingested by children admitted to the hospital for poisoning.[5] In a study examining 265 adolescent and adult poisoning admissions, drug information was collected by history at admission and from toxicologic screening: 86% of the agents ingested were identified by history alone and little additional information was gained from extensive toxicologic screening.[19]

Interviewing witnesses or caretakers is particularly important when evaluating childhood poisonings. The following questions must be asked:

1. What medication/agent was found in the vicinity of the patient?
2. What medications are in the home?
3. How much of the suspected agent did the patient likely take?
4. How much of the agent was available before the ingestion?
5. How much was left after the ingestion?
6. When did the ingestion occur? How much time has passed since the ingestion?
7. Were any characteristic odors found at the scene?
8. How alert was the patient when found?
9. What has the patient's level of consciousness been since?
10. How has the patient behaved since the ingestion?
11. Does the patient have a history of substance abuse?

The clinician must maintain a high index of suspicion for any possible trauma as central nervous system (CNS) depression is a frequent presenting symptom in both trauma and poisoning. Even if the primary problem is clearly poisoning, this does not completely eliminate trauma as a contributing factor in CNS depression.

Physical Examination

As with any resuscitation, a systems management–oriented physical examination must be performed. Resuscitation should proceed in an orderly manner with attention paid to airway patency, ventilation, and perfusion. Airway obstruction may occur as a result of relaxation of pharyngeal muscles as might be seen with ingestion of opioids, barbiturates, or other sedatives. If the ingested agent causes emesis, the patient's airway may become obstructed by gastric contents regurgitated into the mouth or hypopharynx. This is a particular risk if the patient ingested large particulate material or if a meal was recently taken.

As many ingestants can cause respiratory depression or respiratory failure, the clinician must be mindful of each patient's ventilatory status. Respiratory depression can occur as a result of central respiratory depression.

Uncoordinated muscular function may also be a cause of respiratory failure, as can occur during seizures and with intercostal muscle rigidity caused by fentanyl.

A number of frequently ingested medications and poisons cause significant circulatory compromise. The tricyclic antidepressants are particularly dangerous as they produce both dysrhythmias and hypotension. Agents that cause significant emesis (e.g., salicylates and iron) can cause hypovolemia and circulatory embarrassment.

Symptoms may present as "complexes" and depend on the particular poison ingested. Several symptom complexes or "toxidromes" are listed in Table 79-2.[20]

CNS depression is a common presentation in the poisoned patient. Therefore, physicians providing care for poisoned patients must develop an organized approach to the evaluation of the comatose patient.

EVALUATION OF THE UNRESPONSIVE CHILD

All unresponsive patients should be evaluated for trauma and cervical spine injury. Witnesses should be interviewed and questioned, and evidence of physical trauma should be collected. If trauma is suspected, flexion and extension of the neck must be avoided until cervical spine injury is ruled out by radiography.

Table 79-2. TOXIDROMES OR SYMPTOM COMPLEXES*

Toxidrome or Complex	Consciousness	Respirations	Pupils	Other	Possible Toxic Agent
Cholinergic	Coma	↑ ↓	Pinpoint	Fasciculations Incontinence Salivation, wheezing Lacrimation Bradycardia	Organophosphate insecticides, carbamates, nicotine
Anticholinergic	Agitated, hallucinating	↑	Dilated	Fever, flushing Dry skin and mucous membranes Urinary retention	Anticholinergics (Atropine, Jimson weed) (Antihistamines)
Opioid	Coma	↓	Pinpoint	Tracks Hypothermia Hypotension	Opiates, Lomotil, Pentazocine, Darvon
Structural	Coma	Apneustic	Pinpoint	Decerebrate Babinski sign	Pontine (brain stem) structural lesions
Extrapyramidal	Awake	↑	—	Torsion head/neck	Phenothiazines, haloperidol
Phenothiazine	Coma	↓	Pinpoint	Cardiac arrhythmia Orthostatic hypotension, anticholinergic findings	Phenothiazines
Tricyclic antidepressant	Coma (initially agitated)	↓	Dilated	Cardiac arrhythmia Convulsions Hypotension QT interval prolongation Cardiac conduction defect Myoclonus, hyperreflexia	Tricyclic antidepressants
Uremia	Coma	↑	—	Uremic frost Detectable shunt Hyperkalemia Acidosis	(Uremia)
Sedative/hypnotic	Coma	↓	Dilated	Hypothermia Decreases reflexes Hypotension	Sedatives, barbiturates
Salicylates	Semicoma, agitation	↑	—	Diaphoresis Tinnitus Agitation Alkalosis (early) Acidosis (late) Fever	Salicylates Oil of wintergreen
Sympathomimetic	Agitated, hallucinations	↑	Dilated	Seizures Tachycardia Hypertension Diaphoresis Metabolic acidosis Tremor Hyperreflexia	Cocaine Theophylline Amphetamines Caffeine

*From Haddad LM, Roberts JR: A general approach to the emergency management of poisoning. *In:* Haddad LM and Winchester JF (eds): Clinical Management of Poisoning and Drug Overdose, 2nd ed. Philadelphia, WB Saunders, 1990, p. 7, with permission.

Table 79–3. SYMPTOMS DUE TO SPECIFIC DRUGS CAUSING DELIRIUM, STUPOR, OR COMA*

Drug	Chemical Diagnosis	Behavior	Physical Signs
Amphetamine	Blood or urine	Hypertension; aggressive, sometimes paranoid, repetitive behavior progressing into agitated paranoid delirium, auditory and visual hallucinations.	Hyperthermia, hypertension, tachycardia, arrhythmia. Pupils dilated. Tremor, dystonia, occasionally convulsions.
Cocaine	None available	Similar to above but more euphoric, less paranoid.	
Psychedelics (LSD, mescaline, STP, PCP)	Blood or urine	Confused, disoriented, perceptual distortions, distractable, withdrawn or eruptive. Can lead to accidents or violence.	Hypertension and tachycardia. Pupils small, nystagmus. Movements hyperactive; myoclonus or dystonia.
Atropine-scopolamine (Sominex)	None available	Delirium; often agitated; responding to visual hallucinations. Drowsiness: delirium, agitation; rarely coma.	Fever, flushed face; dilated pupils; sinus or supraventricular tachycardia; hot dry skin.
Tricyclic antidepressants Imipramine (Tofranil) Amitriptyline (Elavil)	Blood or urine	Drowsiness; delirium, agitation; rarely coma.	Fever; supraventricular tachycardia; conduction defects; ventricular tachycardia or fibrillation. Hypotension. Dystonia.
Phenothiazines	Blood	Somnolence; coma rare.	Arrhythmias, hypotension, dystonia.
Lithium	Blood	Lethargic confusion, mute state, eventually coma. Multifocal seizures can occur. Onset can be delayed by hours or days after overdose.	Appearance of distraction; roving conjugate eye movement; pupils intact; paratonic resistance; tremors, akathisia.
Benzodiazepines (Valium, Librium, Dalmane)	Blood or urine	Stupor, rarely unarousable.	Essentially no cardiovascular or respiratory depression.
Methaqualone (Quaalude)	Blood or urine	Hallucinations and agitation blend into depressant drug coma.	Mild: resembles barbiturate intoxication. Severe: increased tendon reflexes, myoclonus, dystonia, convulsions. Tachycardia and heart failure.
Glutethimide (Doriden)	Blood	Stupor or coma fluctuating over hours or days.	Resembles barbiturate coma but pupils midposition, often unequal, and sometimes fixed.
Barbiturate	Blood or urine	Stupor or coma.	Hypothermia; skin cool and dry. Pupils reactive; doll's eyes absent; hyporeflexia; flaccid hypotension; apnea.
Alcohol	Blood or breath	Dysarthria, ataxia, stupor. Rapidly changing level of alertness with stimulation.	With stupor: hypothermia, skin cold and moist; pupils reactive, midposition to wide; tachycardia.
Opiates	Blood or urine	Stupor or coma.	Needle marks; hypothermia; skin cool and moist; pupils symmetrically pinpoint reactive; bradycardia; hypotension; hypoventilation; pulmonary edema.

*From Plum F and Posner JB (eds): The Diagnosis of Stupor and Coma, 3rd ed. Philadelphia, FA Davis, 1982, p. 242, with permission.

Poisoned patients can present with a wide variety of CNS findings. Not all will be obtunded or somnolent; some are easily aroused while others may be agitated or violent. Presenting signs and symptoms provide the clinician with clues as to the causative agent or agents. Clouding of consciousness, obtundation, stupor, and delirium should be recognized as degrees of CNS depression. On the other hand, psychosis is a mental disorder that does not reflect CNS depression. The distinction between delirium and psychosis is important as its recognition may suggest a class of toxic agents when the particular poison is in doubt.[21] Delirium is characterized by extreme motor and mental excitation, defective perception, impaired memory, and a rapid succession of confused and unconnected ideas. Delirious patients are disoriented, confused, and have visual hallucinations. Psychotic patients present with auditory hallucinations and paranoia. Unlike delirious patients, psychotic patients display an intact sensorium. Chronic use of certain stimulants such as amphetamines and cocaine can cause psychosis.[21]

Patients who have ingested CNS depressants present with predictable findings.[22] Vestibular and cerebellar functions become depressed before cerebral function is affected. Therefore, these patients appear inebriated and present with nystagmus, ataxia, and dysarthria. While impaired consciousness will ultimately develop, cerebral dysfunction is not an early feature. Reflex function and muscle tone are depressed. The oculocephalic reflex, oculovestibular (cold caloric) responses, and stretch reflexes are all affected to some extent by CNS depressants. Muscle tone can be depressed to such a degree that flaccidity results. When a poisoning is due to a CNS depressant, neurologic depression is symmetrical. In contrast, patients with trauma or structural disease often present with focal signs and symptoms (Table 79–3).

Because areas of the brain stem that control consciousness are anatomically close to those that control pupillary function, pupillary responses assist in localization of brain stem lesions. Pupillary light reflexes tend to be resistant to metabolic (poisoning) injury. As such, pupillary light reflexes are preserved along with ciliospinal reflexes. Absence or sluggishness of pupillary responses indicates injury to the brain stem. Pupillary dilation occurs with lesions in the midbrain, ipsilateral third nerve damage, and drugs such as atropine and scopolamine. Pupillary constriction is seen with lesions in the pontine, medullary, spinal, or hypothalamic area and with opioid or barbiturate intoxication. CNS depressants commonly cause small yet reactive pupils unless the patient ingested a fatal amount in which case the pupils may become nonreactive.[23] Midpoint nonreactive pupils or unilateral changes suggest structural lesions[20] (Table 79–4).

Poisons can cause respiratory failure either by depressing central respiratory activity or by reducing ventilatory muscle function. Opioids, barbiturates, and benzodiazepines depress brain stem respiratory center and reticular activating system function. Central depressants tend to cause coma before respiratory depression. Therefore, CNS depressant–poisoned patients may be unresponsive but still breathe normally. Ventilatory muscle dysfunction can be caused by neuromuscular blocking agents, organophosphates, and rapid administration of fentanyl. Organophosphates cause nicotinic receptor blockade while fentanyl causes intercostal muscle rigidity when administered rapidly.

Some toxic agents cause respiratory stimulation either from direct respiratory center stimulation or from a metabolic acidosis with respiratory compensation. Salicylates, amphetamines, cocaine, and caffeine are central respiratory stimulants. Central stimulants affect the medullary respiratory center and cause an increase in respiratory rate and depth.[21] Carbon monoxide and cyanide interfere with oxygen uptake and oxidative phosphorylation, respectively. As a result, anaerobic metabolism occurs and lactic acidosis develops, and the resulting metabolic acidosis can lead to respiratory stimulation.

Evaluating the character of motor movements is essential in the poisoned and unresponsive child. Poisoned patients may present with muscular weakness, flaccidity, hyperkinesis, or seizures. Muscle movement should be observed for symmetry, quantity, control, and strength. Poisoned patients and those with metabolic disorders display symmetry of muscle movements, whereas trauma

Table 79–4. PUPILLARY CHANGES CAUSED BY CENTRAL NERVOUS SYSTEM LESIONS AND DRUGS

Lesion	Size	Reactive Versus Nonreactive
Midbrain (tectal)	Dilation	Nonreactive
Ipsilateral third nerve	Dilation	Nonreactive
Atropine	Dilation	Nonreactive
Scopolamine	Dilation	Nonreactive
Pons	Constriction	Reactive
Medulla	Constriction	Reactive
Spinal cord	Constriction	Reactive
Hypothalamus	Constriction	Reactive
Opiates	Constriction	Reactive
Barbiturates	Constriction	Nonreactive
Glutethimide	Midpoint frequently unequal	Fixed pupils

victims or those with other CNS lesions may have asymmetric movements.

Seizures often occur in poisoned patients, particularly young children. Common causative agents include theophylline, tricyclic antidepressents, isoniazid, amphetamines, phencyclidine, and cocaine.[24, 25] Seizures caused by tricyclic antidepressants are frequently preceded by widening of the QRS complex on the electrocardiogram.[26] Seizures in poisoned patients have serious consequences and should be treated aggressively. Respiratory failure, hyperthermia, and rhabdomyolysis can result from prolonged seizures if not treated. Routine anticonvulsants are generally appropriate, but several exceptions warrant further discussion.

Theophylline-induced seizures are frequently difficult to control.[27] Reducing the theophylline level is the most effective measure. Repeated doses of activated charcoal and charcoal hemoperfusion are both effective methods of reducing the serum theophylline level. Isoniazid-induced seizures require pyridoxine[28] for control. Cyanide, fluoride, and organphosphate poisonings each require specific antidotes to reduce symptoms and to control seizures.

Hyperkinetic activity can be caused by either central- or peripheral-acting drugs. As is the case with seizures, prolonged activity can result in hyperthermia and rhabdomyolysis. Hyperkinesis presents as rigidity, dyskinesia, myoclonus, or chorea. Ironically, some drugs used to treat dystonic reactions (anticholinergics and antihistiminics) can also cause dyskinesia.[29] Hyperkinetic activity often results from an imbalance between central dopaminergic and central cholinergic activity.[29] Dopaminergic blockade results in rigidity, bradykinesia, and parkinsonian posturing. Antipsychotic agents, metoclopramide, and 1-methyl-4-phenyl-1,2,5,6-tetra-hydropyridine (MPTP) cause dopaminergic blockade. MPTP, a contaminant of illegal opioids, causes permanent parkinsonism by destroying cells in the substantia nigra.[30] Increased dopaminergic activity can present as hyperkinetic dyskinesia with myoclonic jerks, twitching, facial grimacing, head tossing, and rapid tongue movements. Dopaminergic activity is increased by levodopa, amphetamines, tricyclic antidepressants, anticholinergics, and antihistaminics.[21]

Muscular activity can be either increased or decreased as a result of certain poisons. Muscular rigidity and hyperactivity both result from overstimulation of muscle receptors. Muscular rigidity can be noted with black widow spider bites and strychnine ingestion. Black widow spider bites cause increased neurotransmitter release, persistent muscular contraction, and localized, painful rigidity.[21] Strychnine interferes with inhibitory neurons in the spinal cord, resulting in muscular rigidity without CNS toxicity.[31] Muscular hyperactivity also results from stimulation of peripheral cholinergic receptors as is seen with the nicotinic effects of organophosphate intoxication, which manifests as fasciculations.

Muscular weakness is seen with CNS depressants (barbiturates, sedatives, hypnotics, and opioids), hypokalemia, and hypermagnesemia. Muscle weakness, hypokalemia, and hypophosphatemia have been noted in toluene abusers.[21]

Anticholinergic poisoning presents as a toxidrome that results from inhibition of acetylcholine activity at post-synaptic receptors. In toxic doses, tricyclic antidepressants, phenothiazines, antihistamines, and antiparkinson agents can cause anticholinergic symptoms. The degree to which these drugs affect postsynaptic receptors determines whether patients will present with specific anticholinergic symptoms or the toxidrome associated with anticholinergic poisoning, which includes psychosis, tachycardia, mydriasis, vasodilation, hyperpyrexia, ileus, urinary retention, decreased salivation, decreased sweating, amnesia, agitation, and seizures. Anticholinergic poisoning can also occur during atropine treatment for organophosphate poisoning.

Therapy for anticholinergic poisoning is usually supportive; however, physostigmine salicylate can be used to treat patients with serious CNS involvement.[32] Pediatric doses of 0.5 mg over 2 minutes intravenously are recommended. Doses of 1 to 2 mg can be used in adolescents and young adults. Treatment can be repeated every 20 to 30 minutes until symptoms resolve. Physostigmine is contraindicated if bradycardia, asthma, or mechanical gastrointestinal obstruction is present. Adverse reactions are common and include nausea and vomiting, epigastric pain, miosis, salivation, lacrimation, dyspnea, bronchospasm, CNS stimulation, seizures, and muscle fasciculations.

LABORATORY EVALUATION

Toxicologic and routine laboratory tests are useful adjuncts in the evaluation of the poisoned patient. In addition to toxicologic laboratory tests, evaluation of electrolytes, serum glucose, arterial blood gases, serum osmolarity, and serum creatine phosphokinase (CPK) can also be helpful.

Serum potassium levels are useful in determining the degree of autonomic stimulation in patients poisoned by autonomic agents and in determining the significance of acid-base derangements. Alkalosis and β_2-adrenergic stimulation increase cellular uptake of potassium, thus decreasing serum potassium levels.[21, 33] Therefore, in theophylline and caffeine toxicity, epinephrine released from the adrenal medulla can cause hypokalemia.[21, 34] Alternately, serum potassium levels can reflect the degree of α-adrenergic stimulation or β_2-adrenergic antagonism as both cause hyperkalemia.[35] Muscle activity increases potassium release from myocytes, and seizure-inducing drugs, nonsteroidal anti-inflammatory agents, and cardiac glycosides may increase serum potassium levels.

The serum glucose concentration can provide important etiologic clues in certain intoxications. Hyperglycemia can indicate a catecholamine-mediated stress response secondary to β_2-adrenergic stimulants, caffeine, theophylline, and iron. Serum glucose concentrations greater than 150 mg/dl have been shown to be predictive of toxicity following acute iron ingestion.[36] Hypoglycemia may follow ingestion of hypoglycemic (antidiabetic) agents, ethanol (in patients with insufficient glycogen stores), and drugs or toxins that induce hepatic failure.

Arterial blood gas and oxygen saturation measurements aid in the determination of respiratory status. Respiratory acidosis results from agents that depress CNS function such as opioids, barbiturates, and benzodiazepines. Following aspiration, hydrocarbons cause pneumonitis and pulmonary edema. Pulmonary edema can also be seen following ingestion of salicylates, iron, or paraquat. Blood gas evaluations help to determine the severity of such ingestions as well as the need for certain therapeutic interventions.

Respiratory alkalosis may be noted with salicylate toxicity as a result of CNS respiratory stimulation. In addition, discrepancies between measured and calculated (from PO_2) oxygen saturations occur with methemoglobinemia, sulfhemoglobinemia, and carbon monoxide poisoning.

Metabolic acidosis is a feature of many poisonings. It can occur secondary to lactic acid production or from metabolism of parent compounds to acidic byproducts. The anion gap is an important index in treating poisoned patients who are acidotic because agents that cause lactic acidosis and those that cause nonlactate acidosis both increase the anion gap. Lactic acidosis can develop from disturbances in oxygen transport (carbon monoxide) or oxygen delivery (iron, tricyclic antidepressants, digoxin, and anticholinergics), or inhibition of oxidative phosphorylation (cyanide, salicylates). Salicylates can also cause nonlactate anion gap acidosis, as can methanol, ethylene glycol, and iron.

Serum osmolarity can be affected by osmotically active agents; these increase measured but not "calculated" serum osmolarity.[38, 39] The osmolar gap is defined as the difference between the measured serum osmolarity and the calculated serum osmolarity. The presence of an osmotic gap and an increased anion gap strongly suggest methanol or ethylene glycol poisoning.[39]

In patients with increased muscular activity, CPK and creatinine should be monitored. Significant elevations of CPK suggest rhabdomyolysis. Should rhabdomyolysis be suspected, serum myoglobin and renal function tests should be obtained.

Dysrhythmias are often indicative of certain poisonings (Table 79–5). Supraventricular tachycardia, ventricular tachycardias, conduction delays, and bradycardia have all been described in poisoned patients. Increased sympathetic tone, inhibition of cholinergic tone, enhanced ventricular irritability, and re-entry phenomena can all lead to tachydysrhythmias. Bradydysrhythmias are seen when toxic agents cause decreased sympathetic tone, increased cholinergic tone, or decreased ventricular automaticity.

RADIOLOGIC EVALUATION

Radiologic evaluation of the CNS should be individualized. An unresponsive patient may require radiologic evaluation to assess the possibility of trauma, intracranial hemorrhage, or tumor. If there is any suspicion of trauma, the cervical spine requires radiographic assessment along with a thorough neurologic examination.

Computed tomographic (CT) scans, electroencepha-

Table 79–5. DYSRHYTHMIAS IN POISONED PATIENTS

Symptom	Reason	Toxic Agents
Tachydysrhythmias	Increased sympathetic tone	Methylxanthines
		Caffeine
		Theophylline
	Inhibition of cholinergic tone	Anticholinergics
	Enhanced ventricular irritability	Amphetamines
		Cocaine
	Re-entry phenomena	Tricyclic antidepressants
		Digoxin
Conduction delays	Prolongation of the QRS complex	Tricyclic antidepressants
		Phenothiazines
		Quinidine
		Procainamide
	Prolongation of the QT interval	Tricyclic antidepressants
		Type I antidysrhythmics
		Phenothiazines
		Digoxin
Bradycardia	Decreased sympathetic tone	β-Blockers
	Increased cholinergic tone	Organophosphates
		Physostigmine
		Digoxin
	Decreased ventricular automaticity	Lidocaine

lograms (EEGs) and transcranial Doppler studies have no special significance in poisonings. CT scans allow evaluation of structural lesions greater than 5 mm in cross-sectional diameter and assist the evaluation of progressive lesions, but they are not useful if poisoning is the sole cause of CNS dysfunction. If a poisoned patient undergoes neurologic deterioration following cardiopulmonary arrest, prolonged hypotension, or hypoxia, CT scanning and transcranial Doppler studies may indicate development of cerebral edema and the presence of increased intracranial pressure.

The mnemonic CHIPS (Chloral Hydrate, Heavy metals, Iron, Phenothiazines, and Slow-release enteric-coated medications) has been used to describe pills that can be seen on the routine abdominal films. Savitt and associates[40] found 312 pills to be radiopaque in 15 cm water, and of these, 23 were found to be radiopaque in cadaver stomachs (Table 79–6). Their results suggest that the CHIPS mnemonic is incomplete. Routine radiographs have limited value in confirming the presence of pills or pill fragments when the patient is unable to give a history.

Fast-growing areas of bone fail to calcify cartilage following exposure to lead, which results in hypodense areas on long bone radiographs known as "lead lines." The proximal fibula is very sensitive to lead owing to its rapid growth. Blickman and coworkers suggest that lead bands can be noted with serum lead levels as low as 40 μg/dl.[41]

Toxicology Laboratory Evaluation

Brett[42] reported that as many as 95% of poisons in episodes leading to hospital admission can be identified by history alone. In his study of 209 patients admitted for poisoning, 95% had toxicologic laboratory studies.[42] Though there was a significant rate of disagreement between the results of these studies and the initial clinical impressions of the medical staff, discovery of an unexpected agent rarely led to changes in therapy. Important unsuspected drugs were found infrequently and clinical characteristics with unexpected drugs were no different than those with known drugs. In a different study, the actual toxic agent was identified in 86% of 265 self-poisonings by history and routine laboratory tests.[19] Experience in children's hospitals agrees with adult data that the history was the single most important identification factor in 90% of patients seen.[5]

These data suggest that toxicologic screening is not a diagnostic panacea in poisoned patients. Prior to ordering a battery of assays, the physician should determine which toxic agents are the most likely etiologic agents. History, prevalence of drugs in the community, and physical examination will be most helpful in guiding this selection. Toxicologic assays may require large sample volumes, may be very time consuming, may be delayed, and may be expensive. The narrower the spectrum of assays ordered by the clinician, the greater the likelihood such tests will be fruitful.

Evaluating toxicology results requires consideration of the accuracy, sensitivity, specificity, and precision of the tests ordered. Accuracy refers to how close to the true value the assay's results actually are.[43] Sensitivity is the assay's ability to determine the true positive cases in the face of all possible positive results (false negatives and true positives). Screening tests require good sensitivity to detect test conditions in low prevalence situations.[33] Specificity is the ability of the assay to determine true negative results in the face of all possible negative results (false positives and true negatives). Diagnostic tests require good specificity to detect the absence of the test conditions in a situation of high probability. Precision refers to the reproducibility of the technique within the same laboratory and among different laboratories. Precision helps to determine the reliability of the assay, which in turn depends on several characteristics of the laboratory performing the assay, including

Table 79–6. RADIOPACITY OF INGESTED MEDICATIONS*

Compound	Radiopacity
Potassium chloride (2 preparations)	S†
Ferrous sulfate	S
Calcium carbonate	S
Multivitamin with iron	M‡
Tranylcypromine	W§
Perphenazine/amitriptyline	W
Chloral hydrate	W
Zinc sulfate	W
Trifluoperazine	W
Brompheniramine/phenylephrine/ phenylpropanolamine	W
Pseudoephedrine/dexbrompheniramine	W
Ferrous gluconate	W
Acetazolamide	W
Busulfan	W
Sodium chloride	W
Phosphorus	W
Meclizine	W
Prochlorperazine	W
Liothyronine	W
Trimeprazine	W
Calcium lactate	O‖
Chlorpromazine	O
Protriptyline	O
Lithium carbonate	O
Aluminum/magnesium hydroxide	O
Niacin	O
Oxytriphylline	O
Hydroxyzine	O
Nafcillin	O
Neostigmine	O
Penicillin V potassium	O
Thioridazine	O
Berocca	O

*From Savitt DL, Hawkins HH, and Roberts JR: The radiopacity of ingested medications. Ann Emerg Med 16:333, 1987, with permission.
†S = strongly visible.
‡M = moderately visible.
§W = weakly visible.
‖O = not visible.

appropriate manpower, sample workload, timeliness, and difficulty of the assay itself.

Chemical spot tests can provide a quick, initial screen with limited utility.[33] These tests depend on chemical reactivity between the toxic agent and specific reactants. Chemical spot tests are excellent for urine screening in the emergency department. Urine is a good sampling medium owing to high drug/metabolite concentrations. Table 79–7 lists those drugs that can be detected using chemical spot tests, the required reagents, and their sensitivities.

Light absorbance techniques depend on a chemical reaction to convert the target drug into a light-absorbing species.[34] Colorimetry is used to identify the unknown. Light absorbance assays are still used to identify some toxins (carboxyhemoglobin, methemoglobin, cyanide, salicylates, boric acid, and acetaminophen). In simple cases, light absorbance provides an accurate assay for quantifying appropriate chemicals. The greatest disadvantage of light absorbance is that it is prone to interference and requires an extremely pure sample for accuracy.

Chromatography separates unknown drugs by their interaction with a stationary, chromatographic phase.[33, 43] Agents migrate at different rates and over different distances. Migration depends on the purity of the mobile phase and the reactivity between the unknown drug in the mobile phase and the stationary phase. Highly reactive mobile phase unknowns do not migrate as far as those with low reactivity. Unknown drugs are detected by several different techniques, including chemical reactions between a known reagent and unknowns on the chromatography plate, ultraviolet light absorption, refractometry, conductivity, oxidation-reduction reactions, and mass spectrometry. Chromatography is widely used in emergency toxicology because a large number of drugs can be detected on a single chromatogram. Sensitivity is adequate for many common drugs; however, prior to performance of the assay unknown drugs must be extracted from the specimen.

Thin-layer chromatography (TLC) is a chromatographic separation technique that allows specimen extraction to occur by drying the unknown on a chromatographic plate.[33, 43] Solutions are eluted onto a silica gel medium (stationary phase) and allowed to migrate. Detection is accomplished by "staining," in which a chemical reaction between a known reagent and an unknown substance occurs on the chromatographic plate. TLC is operator dependent, and operator variability limits reproducibility of this assay technique; however, standardization of certain aspects of TLC has decreased interoperator variability. TLC is simple, inexpensive, and reasonably reliable. It has high specificity but low sensitivity. Detection is generally limited to concentrations of 0.5 to 1 µg/ml, but even this varies depending upon the particular drug, the detection method used, and the amount of unknown in the sample.

High-performance liquid chromatography (HPLC) is a chromatographic separation technique similar to TLC.[33, 43] As with TLC, either an unknown solution is eluted onto a silica gel or a nonpolar phase is bonded to small particles. HPLC differs from TLC in that the solution is eluted under pressure to achieve greater separation of unknown compounds. Compounds are identified by the time required to elute them past one of several types of detectors, including those utilizing ultraviolet absorbance, refractometers, and conductivity sensing detectors. Only a narrow range of polarity can

Table 79–7. SPOT TESTS FOR UNKNOWN TOXIC AGENTS*

Drug	Reagent	Sensitivity
Salicylate	Trinder's	td,†od‡
Acetaminophen	Ortho-cresol	td,od
Phenothiazines	Forrest	td,od
	Ferric-perchlorate-nitric	
Ethchlorvynol	Diphenylamine	od
Phencyclidine	Tetrabromophenolphthalein	od
Methadone		
Tricyclics		
Chloral hydrate	Fujiwara	od

*From Osterloh JD: Utility and reliability of emergency toxicologic testing. Emerg Med Clin North Am 8:693, 1990, with permission.
†td = therapeutic dose.
‡od = overdose.

be used on each run, which limits HPLC's value as a drug screening method. Its high degree of resolution makes it useful in screening for various classes of toxic substances. HPLC can also be used to reliably quantify drug levels by comparing the size of peaks of unknowns with those of known concentrations.

Gas chromatography (GC) is a chromatographic technique that separates volatile gases on a stationary phase.[33, 43] Samples are heated from 80 to 300° C, and the resultant volatile gases are exposed to the stationary phase and separated. Several properties of elemental reactions make GC a highly specific technique, including unique melting points and different polarities, which cause each compound to migrate a different distance in the stationary medium. GC can be made extremely specific if mass spectrometry is used to detect unknowns. For these reasons, GC is regarded as the best available method for toxicologic screening.

Immunoassays can be performed to detect unknown substances in solution.[33, 43] Drug-specific antibodies bind to unknown free drug in the solution. The drug-antibody complexes cause chemical reactions that result in a color change. Light absorbance readings are taken and compared with those determined by linear regression graphs of known concentrations. Immunoassays require specific assays for each drug and usually have analytic sensitivity in excess of that needed. These immunoassays are rapid, easy to perform, and can be performed reliably by medical personnel. Enzyme multiplied immunotechniques (EMITs) are the most common immunoassays. EMIT uses enzymes to enhance the reaction between antibody and unknown.

No single analytic technique can test for all possible toxic agents. As mentioned earlier, local laboratories must decide which agents are most prevalent in their community and develop batteries of tests to screen for them. This is particularly important for illicit drugs being used recreationally.

A logical approach to testing must be employed. Historical data should be obtained and a physical examination performed, and this information should then be used to determine what substances are to be analyzed and what samples are required. Tables 79–8 and 79–9 list laboratory tests useful in the evaluation of the poisoned patient.

Sample selection may be as important as the test itself.[43] Blood sampling allows measurement of concentrations that reflect tissue exposure, but this can be misleading with many substances as very few drugs distribute uniformly between the cellular and the fluid compartments. A disadvantage of blood samples is that drug concentrations tend to be extremely low and difficult to detect.

Urine offers certain advantages, including possible high concentrations of agents or metabolites, but sample purity is a problem. Unfortunately, there is no correlation between the concentration of urinary metabolites and the serum concentration of an agent. Gastric aspirates are helpful in confirming the presence of suspected toxins, but as with urine, no correlation exists between gastric concentrations and serum concentrations.

GENERAL MANAGEMENT MEASURES

A useful precept in managing the poisoned patient is, "It is more important to treat the patient than the poison." Airway patency, ventilation, and perfusion must be addressed prior to using any specific drug therapy or antidotes. Supportive care depends on characteristics of the ingested agent, symptoms, severity of illness, and available therapies.

Table 79–8. USEFUL LABORATORY TESTS IN TOXICOLOGIC DIAGNOSIS*

Classes of Drugs	Clinical and Laboratory Tests	Toxicologic Procedures for Identification
Narcotics	IV Narcan, ABGs	IA, TLC, GC, GC-MS
Alcohols	Breath odor, osmolar gap	GC, EZ, IA
Sedatives	Calorics, ABGs	IA, TLC, HPLC, GC, GC-MS
Anticholinergics	EKG, CPK, K	TLC, GC, HPLC, GC-MS
Stimulants	CPK,	IA, TLC, GC, GC-MS
Antipsychotics	EKG, ABGs	Spot, TLC, GC, HPLC, GC-MS
Tricyclics	EKG, ABGs	Spot, IA, TLC, GC, HPLC, GC-MS
β-blockers	EKG	TLC, GC, HPLC
Oral hypoglycemics	Serum glucose	TLC, HPLC, GC
SPECIFIC TOXINS		
Salicylates†	Anion gap, HCO₃ gap	Spot, SM, IA, HPLC, GC
Theophylline†	K, glucose	IA, HPLC, SM
Acetaminophen†	ALT, AST	TLC, IA, SM, HPLC
Methanol†	Anion and osmolar gaps	GLC
Ethylene glycol†	Anion and osmolar gaps	GLC
Lithium†	Serum creatinine	Flame, ISE
Iron†	Deferoxamine challenge, serum iron, TIBC	SM
Carbon monoxide	O₂ saturation gap	Co-oximeter, SM
Cyanide	A-V O₂ difference	SM
Nitrites	Brown blood	Co-oximeter, SM

*From Osterloh JD: Utility and reliability of emergency toxicologic testing. Emerg Med Clin North Am 8:693, 1990, with permission.
†Requires quantitation for effective therapy. Concentration-effect relationships are known. EZ = enzymatic; SM = spectrometric; spot = chemical test; ISE = ion-selective electrode; flame = flame emission spectrometry; ABGs = arterial blood gases; K = potassium; CPK = creatine phosphokinase; HCO₃ = bicarbonate; IA = immunoassay; TLC = thin-layer chromatography; GC = gas chromatography; HPLC = high-performance liquid chromatography; GC-MS = gas chromatography-mass spectrometry; GLC = gas liquid chromatography; TIBC = total iron-binding capacity.

Table 79–9. COMPARISON OF GENERIC TOXICOLOGIC METHODS*

Method†	Specificity	Sensitivity	Multidrug Drug Detection Possible	Quantitative Ability	Turnaround Time (Hr)	Labor Intensive	Technical Expertise	Initial Capital Costs ($)
Chemical spot	+	+	No	No	<0.5	+	0	500
Spectrometric	+	+	No	Yes	<2	+ +	+ +	10,000
IA	+ +	+ +	Some	Some	<1	+	+	7,000
TLC	+ +	+	Yes	No	2–4	+ + +	+ + +	1,500
GC	+ +	+ +	Yes	Yes	<4	+ +	+ +	15,000
HPLC	+ +	+ +	Yes	Yes	<4	+ +	+ +	20,000
GC-MS	+ + +	+ + +	Yes	Yes	<8	+ + +	+ + + +	65,000

*From Osterloh JD: Utility and reliability of emergency toxicologic testing. Emerg Med Clin North Am 8:693, 1990, with permission.

†IA = immunoassay; TLC = thin-layer chromatography; GC = gas chromatography; HPLC = high-performance liquid chromatography; GC-MS = gas chromatography-mass spectrometry.

The goals of treatment for any poisoning are to limit toxin absorption, enhance toxin elimination, and provide supportive care until the toxic effects of the substance abate.[44] Emetics, gastric lavage, activated charcoal, and cathartics can be used to remove toxic agents from the gastrointestinal tract and limit absorption. Forced diuresis, alkaline diuresis, administration of an absorbing resin, hemodialysis, peritoneal dialysis, and hemoperfusion are currently accepted methods of enhancing elimination. Antidotes are available for some toxic agents. As these are specific for each toxin, they are discussed with the specific agents in Chapter 80.

Removal of Gastric Contents

Although gastric emptying can be accomplished by emesis (spontaneous or forced) or gastric lavage, it is not universally required. Over the past several years, the use of emetics in poisonings has decreased while that of activated charcoal has increased.[1] A number of factors appear to account for this trend: Emesis occurs spontaneously following many childhood ingestions;[45] children frequently ingest nontoxic substances; children frequently ingest nontoxic amounts of toxic substances; and use of emetics frequently delays use of activated charcoal. Emesis is contraindicated when certain hydrocarbons are ingested, when rapid onset of CNS depression is likely, and for infants younger than 6 months old.[45]

The efficacy of gastric emptying has recently been called into question. Kulig and coworkers[46] suggested that gastric emptying does not significantly alter the clinical course if the exposure occurred more than 1 hour before gastric emptying. These authors also indicated that gastric lavage was only slightly more effective than ipecac if performed within the first hour. However, the fact that most children present for treatment within 2 hours of ingestion[5] and that many poisons delay gastric motility, the case for using ipecac in children remains strong.

Ipecac, the most frequently employed emetic agent, is a mixture of alkaloids derived from the *Cephaelis ipecacuanha* and the *Cephaelis acuminata* plants. Emetine and cephalin[45] appear to be the active components, which possess a local irritant effect on the stomach and a central effect on the chemoreceptor trigger zone (CTZ).[45, 47] Once the CTZ is activated, the vomiting center in the reticular formation causes coordination of muscular activity in the stomach and small intestine, which results in emesis.

Ipecac is currently available only as a syrup. It was previously available as a potent extract, but due to the increased risk of toxicity this form is no longer recommended for human use.[45, 48, 49] Efficacy and dose-response relationships have been studied.[50–52] One 10-ml dose in infants older than 6 months of age[50] or a 30-ml dose in children older than 1 year[51, 52] produced significant success rates. With an additional dose, success rates approached 100%. Vomiting episodes are often multiple, and vomiting usually occurs within 30 minutes of administration.[53]

In children, forced emesis with ipecac appears to be a more effective means of gastric emptying than gastric lavage.[54] Adult data suggest that gastric lavage is the most effective means of gastric emptying in adults within the first hour after ingestion.[46] Results of animal experiments also suggest that ipecac is less efficacious than gastric lavage. This information along with trends toward alternative therapy suggests that ipecac may not continue to enjoy widespread use.

Diarrhea, drowsiness, irritability or hyperactivity, diaphoresis, flushing, and fever have been noted in varying degrees in infants and younger children following ipecac administration.[50] These side effects are infrequent and usually minor. Deaths from overdose and improper use have been reported[55, 56] but are extremely rare. Esophageal tears (Mallory-Weiss syndrome) have been reported in adults,[57, 58] and an esophageal stricture was reported in a single child.[59]

The pediatric literature suggests that there are benefits to keeping ipecac in the home and that these benefits outweigh the risks. Home administration of ipecac is regarded as both safe and cost effective. When ipecac is administered at home, an overall decrease in the time from ingestion to therapy improved efficacy,[50] and fewer emergency room visits from ingestions were reported.[60] Concerns about inappropriate home administration appear to be unfounded. Mothers from various socioeconomic backgrounds were found capable of utilizing ipecac appropriately[61, 62] and of seeking professional supervision prior to its use.[63]

Ipecac has an impressive safety record[45] and its availability in all households with children should be encouraged. One study noted that 78% of practicing pediatricians in a major metropolitan area supported the availability of ipecac in the home, but only 3% actually distributed ipecac to families.[63] This same study reported that ipecac was available in only 24% of households.

Apomorphine is a centrally acting emetic that induces CNS depression, respiratory depression, and hypotension.[45] It is available only in intravenous form and is effective in inducing emesis in up to 92% of pediatric patients.[65, 66] Apomorphine offers no clear advantage over ipecac,[65] and indeed, the requirement of an intravenous line with its potential side effects makes apomorphine a poor choice in the management of childhood poisonings.

Though difficult to swallow, liquid dish detergent is an effective emetic in dogs and humans.[67-69] As a result of direct gastric irritation liquid dish detergents induce emesis in 5 to 25 minutes and have no toxic effects in dogs.[67] No human toxicity has been noted and liquid dish detergents have been 90% successful in inducing emesis in humans when diluted with water.[68] Compared with ipecac, liquid dish detergents are slightly less effective. Ninety-seven per cent of those who received ipecac and 83% of those who received liquid dish detergent had emesis successfully induced, but the elapsed time before emesis was shorter for the detergent.

Only liquid dish detergents are suggested for use as emetics. Laundry and dishwasher detergents have components that may be toxic. A mixture of 30 to 45 ml of liquid detergent diluted with 8 oz of water appears to be useful[68, 69] for those able to swallow the concoction despite its taste. Other emetics such as mechanical stimulation, sodium chloride, and copper sulfate have been advocated in the past but have proven unreliable, unsafe, or both.[70-73]

Gastric lavage accomplishes gastric emptying by instillation of a liquid through an orogastric or nasogastric tube with subsequent drainage. Lavage is indicated if the patient has a depressed sensorium, cannot protect the airway, or is actively convulsing. If the patient has ingested an agent that might rapidly lead to convulsions or CNS depression,[74] gastric lavage should be considered. In addition, gastric lavage can alter a toxin's bioavailability.[74] As previously stated, lavage is most effective in adults if performed within an hour of the ingestion.

The gag reflex should be checked to determine the patient's ability to maintain or protect the airway. A significant portion of the normal population has a hypoactive gag reflex. Therefore, gastric lavage should not be avoided in patients who are neurologically normal but have hypoactive gag reflexes.

Lavage is contraindicated when there is a reliable history of an insignificant ingestion,[74] in alkali or acid ingestions, in hydrocarbons ingestion, or when ingested particles exceed the luminal size of the largest orogastric tube that can be placed.[45] It should be noted that gastric lavage is more difficult in very young children and that these children less frequently present with clear indications for gastric lavage.

Any delay in treatment significantly diminishes the usefulness of gastric lavage. One[46] to three[74] hours post ingestion is the limit of its effectiveness. This time period is extended when the ingested substance delays gastric emptying or is neurotoxic.

Once the airway is secured and the largest possible orogastric or nasogastric tube is placed, patients should be positioned with the left side down.[74] Lavage should be started with warm normal saline in small aliquots. The lavage fluid should be a warm isotonic solution; hyponatremia and hypothermia have been noted with improper lavage fluids.[74] In addition, warm fluid may delay gastric emptying and improve yield.[74] Lavage is most safely performed via gravity drainage, but manual lavage is more commonly employed. Forceful instillation and large volumes of fluid can push material through the pylorus and aid absorption. The procedure should be continued until the lavage fluid is clear and particulate matter is no longer noted. Caution must be exercised during placement of the lavage tube as esophageal and gastric perforations due to improper tube passage or placement have been reported.

Activated Charcoal

Activated charcoal is a product of the pyrolysis of various organic compounds. "Activation" is achieved by exposing the residue to oxidizing agents and high temperatures.[45, 76] Activation increases the adsorptive capacity of the residue by removing impurities and increasing surface area. It essentially places a number of depressions on the particle's surface similar to the "dimples" on a golf ball. Charcoal preparations vary in their source of base material, surface area, binding capacity, binding affinity, and binding avidity.[76] Total adsorptive capability may vary up to 50-fold.[77] Petroleum charcoals demonstrate the greatest binding capacity.[78]

Charcoal is at least as effective as gastric emptying, and some studies suggest that it is more effective. Several studies have shown that charcoal was more effective than ipecac in reducing the absorption of certain drugs.[79-81] Another study suggested that patients had similar clinical outcomes whether treated with emesis or lavage followed by activated charcoal and a cathartic or by activated charcoal and a cathartic.[46]

Activated charcoal can be given either in single or multiple doses. Multiple doses of activated charcoal have been noted to reduce the half-life of carbamazepine,[82] phenylbutazone,[82] phenobarbital,[83] theophylline,[84] digoxin,[85] digitoxin,[85] desmethyldoxepin,[86] nadolol,[87] and sotalol.[88] Drug elimination is enhanced for compounds that undergo enterohepatic recirculation. Activated charcoal in the gastrointestinal tract adsorbs the portion of the compound that is secreted or passively diffused back into the gastric or intestinal lumen.[83, 84, 89, 90]

Nonionized particles bind more readily to charcoal than ionized particles.[45] For this reason, both gastric pH and the pKa of the toxin are important variables when considering the efficacy of activated charcoal. Gastric motility determines whether any toxin will be available for adsorption.[82] If gastric motility is depressed, more toxin will be available. Delays in charcoal administration beyond 60 minutes diminish its usefulness;[91, 92] nertheless, charcoal should not be withheld even if there has been a significant delay. Many toxins slow gastric emptying, thus preserving charcoal's beneficial effects.[76]

Doses of 15 to 30 g for small children and 50 to 100 g for larger children and adolescents are recommended. Alternatively, a dose of 1 to 2 g/kg body weight may be used. The charcoal can be given as a slurry with water but is often combined with the cathartic sorbitol. Cherry syrup, chocolate syrup, saccharin, fructose, and sucrose have all been used as flavoring agents without compromising charcoal's adsorptive capacity.[93-95]

Food can either hinder or enhance the effect of charcoal depending on when the food and charcoal mix. Except for the flavoring agents mentioned, mixing charcoal with foods prior to administration will decrease charcoal's adsorptive capacity and thus its effectiveness.[76] Interestingly, if food is already present in the stomach prior to charcoal administration, gastric emptying is slowed and the effectiveness of charcoal seems to be enhanced.[76, 96]

Activated charcoal is contraindicated for ingestion of highly ionized molecules (mineral acid, alkali, boric acid, cyanide, iron, and lithium ingestions). Complications include gagging and vomiting.[45] Aspiration of activated charcoal has been reported.[82]

Cathartics

Cathartics (Table 79–10) are frequently used in conjunction with activated charcoal.[97] Saline cathartics are poorly absorbed osmotic laxatives that cause diarrhea. This group of compounds includes magnesium sulfate, magnesium phosphate, and the tartrate salts of sodium and potassium. Saline cathartics decrease gastrointestinal transit time and thus the duration of time over which drugs are available for absorption. When used alone, cathartics are not effective gastric decontamination agents.[47] Magnesium citrate and sodium sulfate do not enhance the effect of activated charcoal in salicylate ingestion.[98, 99]

Sorbitol, a nonabsorbable sugar, acts as an osmotic cathartic. When given with activated charcoal, it has been shown to increase charcoal adsorption of aspirin, pentobarbital, chloroquine, and chlorpheniramine.[100] Oil cathartics are not recommended owing to the risk of aspiration.[99]

Cathartics are contraindicated following caustic ingestions, when bowel sounds are absent, or when there is a history of recent bowel surgery.[45] Since additional sodium is poorly tolerated in patients with congestive heart failure or hypertension, such individuals should not be given sodium cathartics. Similarly those with chronic renal failure or those who ingest nephrotoxic agents should not be given magnesium-containing cathartics.[45]

Diuresis

Forced diuresis and alkaline diuresis effectively eliminate water-soluble toxins that are cleared by the kid-

Table 79–10. CATHARTIC DOSES*

Drug	Dose
Magnesium sulfate	250 mg/kg
Sodium sulfate	250 mg/kg
Magnesium citrate	4 ml/kg

*From Steinhart CM and Pearson-Shaver AL: Poisoning. Crit Care Clin 4:845, 1988, with permission.
Sorbitol is given as 70% (w/v) solution in an activated charcoal suspension with the appropriate dose of charcoal.

neys. Prior to initiation of diuresis, an adequate circulating blood volume must be assured. Forced diuresis is accomplished using a loop or osmotic diuretic to increase urine output. Alkaline diuresis can increase the ionized fractions of certain water-soluble toxins with low pKa. Alkalinization of the urine increases the ionized portion of the agent and thereby renders it unsuitable for reabsorption by renal cells. Alkalinization is best accomplished in the presence of an adequate circulating blood volume and normal electrolytes. Sodium bicarbonate (1 to 2 mEq/kg) is given every 1 to 2 hours to raise the serum pH to 7.5 or a continuous infusion of sodium bicarbonate (appropriately diluted) may be used.

Extracorporeal Therapy and Peritoneal Dialysis

Extracorporeal therapy (hemodialysis, hemoperfusion) removes drugs across a membrane via a concen-

Table 79–11. PHARMACOKINETIC PROPERTIES IMPORTANT TO EXTRACORPOREAL THERAPY*

Will passive diffusion through a membrane be possible?	Most drugs are eliminated by passive diffusion, therefore a concentration gradient and molecular size are important.
Is the drug lipid soluble?	Lipid-soluble drugs accumulate in lipid-rich tissues and are not accessible for elimination.
Does the drug ionize at physiologic pH?	Ionization inhibits drug transport across body membranes. This can aid in elimination by trapping the ionized form of the drug on one side of the membrane. Drugs that ionize remain in the serum and are more available for elimination.
Is the drug highly protein bound?	Only the unbound form of the drug participates in the diffusion equilibrium.
What is the drug's volume of distribution?	A high volume of distribution is consistent with high tissue concentrations, therefore less drug is accessible to extracorporeal removal.
Is there a high degree of variability in equilibrum for various tissues?	If there is, changes in one compartment may not accurately reflect changes in other compartments. Serum levels may fall quickly but if tissue levels lag behind, the clinical effect of the intoxication will continue.

*From Steinhart CM and Pearson-Shaver AL: Poisoning. Crit Care Clin 4:845, 1988, with permission.

Table 79–12. INDICATIONS FOR EXTRACORPOREAL
THERAPY*

Progressive deterioration despite intensive supportive therapy
Severe intoxication with hypoventilation, hypothermia, or
hypotension
Impairment of normal excretory function due to hepatic, cardiac, or
renal insufficiency
Development of coma or other complications during therapy (e.g.,
pneumonia or sepsis) or the existence of conditions predisposing
to such complications (e.g., obstructive airway disease)
Potentially lethal ingestion and probable absorption of the intoxicant
Toxin metabolized to more toxic substances (methanol, ethylene
glycol)
Poisoning by agents with delayed toxicity (e.g., paraquat)

*From Steinhart CM and Pearson-Shaver AL: Poisoning. Crit Care Clin
4:845, 1988, with permission.

tration gradient (hemodialysis) or by direct exposure of
the blood to adsorbant particles (hemoperfusion). Not
all substances are effectively removed by extracorporeal
therapy (Table 79–11), and not all patients are sick
enough to require it (Table 79–12). Effectiveness of
extracorporeal therapy depends largely on several pharmacokinetic properties including molecular size, lipid
solubility, pKa, protein binding, volume of distribution,
and degree of variability in equilibrium between various
tissues.[101] Hemodialysis is effective if substances can
diffuse across a membrane down a concentration gradient, have a small volume of distribution, are minimally
bound to protein, and have a small molecular size.[101]

Hemoperfusion involves percolating blood through a
cartridge containing an "adsorbant" (usually a preparation containing activated charcoal).[101] Hemoperfusion
is preferred over hemodialysis for substances that are
highly protein bound. Hemodialysis may be preferable
when the toxin is distributed in extracellular water and
when electrolyte abnormalities already exist. Indications
for extracorporeal therapy are listed in Table 79–12.

The principles that govern peritoneal dialysis are
similar to those that govern hemodialysis.[101] Peritoneal
dialysis is of limited use because mesenteric blood flow
cannot be adjusted. Since the clearance of toxins depends upon both the blood flow rate and the dialysate
flow rate, hemodialysis is a more rapid and efficient
means of dialyzing the poisoned patient.

Recent experience with continuous arteriovenous hemofiltration with dialysis suggests that this method may
be helpful in situations in which hemodialysis is desirable
but difficult to perform.[102] Criteria for efficacy with this
technique are similar to those for hemodialysis.

References

1. Litovitz TL, Schmitz BF, and Bailey KM: 1989 Annual Report
of the American Association of Poison Control Centers National
Data Collection System. Am J Emerg Med 8:394, 1990.
2. Slap GB: Substance abuse by adolescents. Hosp Prac 25(4A):19–
20, 23, 26–30, 1990.
3. Polakoff JM, Lacouture PG, and Lovejoy FH: The environment
away from home as a source of potential poisoning. Am J Dis
Child 138:1014, 1984.
4. Trinkoff AM and Baker SP: Poisoning hospitalizations and
deaths from solids and liquids among children and teenagers.
Am J Public Health 76:657, 1986.
5. Fazen LE, Lovejoy FH, and Crone RK: Acute poisoning in a
children's hospital: A 2-year experience. Pediatrics 77:144, 1986.
6. Rogers J: Recurrent childhood poisonings as a family problem.
J Fam Pract 13:337, 1981.
7. Kerfoot M: Deliberate self-poisoning in childhood and early
adolescence. J Child Psychol Psychiatry 29:335, 1988.
8. Gaudreault P, McCormick MA, Lacouture PG, et al: Poisoning
exposures and use of ipecac in children less than 1 year old. Ann
Emerg Med 15:880, 1985.
9. Litovitz TL, Klein-Schwartz W, Oberda BM, et al: Ipecac
administration in children younger than one year of age. Pediatrics 76:761, 1985.
10. Sibert R: Stress in families of children who have ingested poisons.
Br Med J 3:87, 1975.
11. Taylor EA and Stansfield SA: Children who poison themselves.
I: A clinical comparison with psychiatric controls. Br J Psychiatry
145:127, 1984.
12. Calnan NW, Dale JW, and Fonseka CP: Suspected poisoning in
children. Arch Dis Child 51:180, 1976.
13. Johnson MD: Anabolic steroid use in adolescent athletes. Pediatr
Clin North Am 37:1111, 1990.
14. Johnson MD, Jay MS, Shoup B, et al: Anabolic steroid use by
male adolescents. Pediatrics 83:921, 1989.
15. Walton WW: An evaluation of the poison prevention packaging
act. Pediatrics 69:363, 1982.
16. Woolf A and Lovejoy FH: Prevention of childhood poisonings.
In: Haddad LM and Winchester JF (eds): Clinical Management
of Poisoning and Drug Overdose, 2nd ed. Philadelphia, WB
Saunders, 1990, pp. 465–482.
17. Thompson DF, Trammel HL, Robertson NJ, et al: Evaluation
of regional and nonregional poison centers. N Engl J Med
308:191, 1983.
18. Marcus SM, Chafee-Bahamon C, Arnold VW, et al: A regional
poison control system: Effect on response of hypothetical poisonings. Am J Dis Child 138:1010, 1984.
19. Rygnestad T and Berg KJ: Evaluation of benefits of drug analysis
in the routine clinical management of acute self poisoning. Clin
Toxicol 22:51, 1984.
20. Haddad LM and Roberts JR: A general approach to the emergency management of poisoning. In: Haddad LM and Winchester
JF (eds): Clinical Management of Poisoning and Drug Overdose,
2nd ed. Philadelphia, WB Saunders, 1990 pp. 2–22.
21. Olson KR, Pentel PR, and Kelley MT: Physical assessment and
differential diagnosis of the poisoned patient. Med Toxicol 2:52,
1987.
22. Plum F and Posner JB: Multifocal, diffuse and metabolic brain
diseases causing stupor or coma. In: Plum F and Posner JB
(eds): The Diagnosis of Stupor and Coma, 3rd ed. Philadelphia,
FA Davis, 1982, pp. 177–304.
23. Plum F and Posner JB: The pathologic physiology of signs and
symptoms of coma. In: Plum F and Posner JB (eds): The
Diagnosis of Stupor and Coma, 3rd ed. Philadelphia, FA Davis,
1982, pp. 1–87.
24. Messing RO, Closson RG, and Simon RP: Drug-induced seizures: A 10-year experience. Neurology 34:1582, 1984.
25. Olson KR, Benowitz NL, and Pentel PR: Survey of the causes
and consequences of seizures during drug intoxication (Abstract).
Vet Human Toxicol 24:268, 1982.
26. Boehnert MT and Lovejoy FH: Value of the QRS duration
versus the serum drug level in predicting seizures and ventricular
arrhythmias after an acute overdose of tricyclic antidepressants.
N Engl J Med 313:474, 1985.
27. Olson KR and Becker CE: Poisoning. In: Mills J, Ho MT,
Trunkey DD, et al (eds): Current Emergency Diagnosis and
Treatment, 2nd ed. Los Altos, CA, Lange Medical Publication,
1985, pp. 451–482.
28. Wason S, Lacoutre PG, and Lovejoy FH: Single high-dose
pyridoxine treatment for isoniazid overdose. JAMA 246:1102,
1981.
29. Bianchine JR: Drugs for Parkinson's disease, spasticity and acute
muscle spasms. In: Gillman AG, Goodman LS, Rall TW, et al
(eds): The Pharmacological Basis of Therapeutics, 7th ed. New
York, MacMillan, 1985, pp. 473–490.
30. Ballard PA, Tetrud JW, and Langston JW: Permanent human

parkinsonism due to 1-methyl 4-phenyl-1, 2, 3, 6-tetrahydropyr-idine (MPTP). Neurology 35:949, 1985.

31. Weiner N and Taylor P: Neurohumoral transmission: The autonomic and somatic motor nervous systems. *In:* Gilman AG, Goodman LS, Rall TW, et al (eds): The Pharmacological Basis of Therapeutics, 7th ed. New York, MacMillan, 1985, pp. 66–99.

32. Goldfrank, L, Flomenbaum N, and Lewin N: Anticholinergic poisoning. J Toxicol Clin Toxicol 19:17, 1982.

33. Osterloh JD: Utility and reliability of emergency toxicologic testing. Emerg Med Clin North Am 8:693, 1990.

34. Brown MJ: Hypokalemia from beta-2-receptor stimulation by circulating epinephrine. Am J Cardiol 56:3D, 1985.

35. Williams ME, Rosa RM, Silva P, et al: Impairment of extrarenal potassium disposal by alpha-adrenergic stimulation. N Engl J Med 33:145, 1984.

36. Lacoutre PG, Wason S, Abrams A, et al: Acute isopropyl alcohol intoxication: Diagnosis and management. Am J Med 75:680, 1983.

37. Gennari FJ: Serum osmoality—use and limitations. N Engl J Med 310:102, 1984.

38. Cadnapaphornchai P, Taher S, Bhathena D, et al: Ethylene glycol poisoning: Diagnosis based on high osmoal and anion gaps and crystalluria. Ann Emerg Med 10:94, 1981.

39. Jacobsen D and McMartin KE: Methanol and ethylene glycol poisonings: Mechanism of toxicity, clinical course, diagnosis and treatment. Med Toxicol 1:309, 1986.

40. Savitt DL, Hawkins HH, and Roberts JR: The radiopacity of ingested medications. Ann Emerg Med 16:331, 1987.

41. Blickman JG, Wilkinson RH, and Graef JW: The radiologic "lead band" revisited. AJR 146:245, 1986.

42. Brett AS: Implications of discordance between clinical impression and toxicology analysis in drug overdose. Arch Intern Med 148:427, 1988.

43. Tilstone WJ and Deutsch DG: Laboratory diagnosis and drug testing. *In:* Haddad LM and Winchester JF (eds): Clinical Management of Poisoning and Drug Overdose, 2nd ed. Philadelphia, WB Saunders, 1990, pp. 46–64.

44. Steinhart CM and Pearson-Shaver AL: Poisoning. Crit Care Clin 4:845, 1988.

45. Rodgers GC and Matyunas NJ: Gastrointestinal decontamination for acute poisoning. Pediatr Clin North Am 33:261, 1986.

46. Kulig K, Bar-Or D, Cantrill SV, et al: Management of acutely poisoned patients without gastric emptying. Ann Emerg Med 14:562, 1985.

47. Steward JJ: Effects of emetic and cathartic agents on the gastrointestinal tract and the treatment of toxic ingestion. J Toxicol Clin Toxicol 20:199, 1983.

48. Manno BR and Manno JE: Toxicology of ipecac: A review. Clin Toxicol 10:221, 1987.

49. Smith RP and Smith DM: Acute ipecac poisoning: Report of a fatal case and review of the literature. N Engl J Med 256:523, 1961.

50. Litovitz TL, Klein-Schwartz W, Oderda GM, et al: Ipecac administration in children younger than one year of age. Pediatrics 76:761, 1985.

51. Gaudreault P, Lewander WJ, Parent M, et al: Ipecac syrup: Lack of dose-response effect (Abstract). Vet Hum Toxicol 26:403, 1984.

52. Krenzelok EP and Dean BS: Syrup of ipecac in children less than one year of age (Abstract). Vet Hum Toxicol 26:413, 1984.

53. Rauber AP and Marocelli RD: The duration of emetic effect of ipecac: Duration and frequency of vomiting. Vet Hum Toxicol 24:281, 1982.

54. Boxer L, Anderson FP, and Rowe DS: Comparison of ipecac-induced emesis with gastric lavage in the treatment of acute salicylate ingestion. J Pediatr 74:800, 1969.

55. Dershewitz RA and Niederman LG: Ipecac at home—a health hazard? Clin Toxicol 18:969, 1981.

56. Robertson WO: Syrup of ipecac associated fatality: A case report. Vet Hum Toxicol 21:87, 1979.

57. Tandberg D, Lischty EJ, and Fishbein DO: Mallory-Weiss syndrome: An unusual complication of ipecac induced emesis. Ann Emerg Med 10:521, 1981.

58. Tenenbein M: Two interesting button battery ingestions (Abstract). Vet Hum Toxicol 25:281, 1984.

59. Allport RB: Ipecac is not innocuous. Am J Dis Child 98:786, 1954.

60. Mofenson HC, Greensher J, and Caraccio TR: Ingestions considered non toxic. Emerg Clin North Am 2:159, 1984.

61. Dershewitz RA, Posner MK, and Parchel W: The effectiveness of health education on home use of ipecac. Clin Pediatr 22:268, 1983.

62. Dershewitz RA and Parchel W: Effectiveness of a health education program in a lower socioeconomic population. Clin Pediatr 23:686, 1984.

63. Chaefee-Bahamon C, Lacouture PG, and Lovejoy FH: Risk assessment of ipecac in the home. Pediatrics 75:1105, 1985.

64. Mallory MH and Rhoads GG: Syrup of ipecac. Am J Dis Child 142:640, 1988.

65. Corby DG, Decker WJ, and Moron MJ, et al: Clinical comparison of pharmacological emetics in children. Pediatrics 42:154, 1968.

66. MacLean WC Jr: A comparison of ipecac syrup and apomorphine in the immediate treatment of ingestion of poisons. J Pediatr 82:121, 1973.

67. Weaver JE: A fast-acting oral liquid emetic agent. *In:* Rumack BH and Temple AR (eds): Management of the Poisoned Patient. Princeton, NJ, City Science Press, 1977, pp. 175–179.

68. Gieseker DR and Trautman WG: Emergency induction of emesis using liquid detergent products: A report of 15 cases. Clin Toxicol 18:277, 1981.

69. Rogers GC and Fort P: Use of liquid dishwashing detergent as an emetic in the outpatient management of poisonings—an update (Abstract). Vet Hum Toxicol 28:321, 1985.

70. Barer W, Hill LL, Hill RM, et al: Fatal poisoning from salt used as an emetic. Am J Dis Child 125:889, 1973.

71. Karlsson B and Norein L: Ipecacuanha and copper sulfate as emetics in intoxications in children. Acta Pediatr Scand 54:331, 1965.

72. Lundkaer-Jensen S and Nellemanm-Sorensen P: Inhibition of salicylate and lithium absorption in the human intestine by copper sulfate. Toxicology 35:175, 1976.

73. Mellenchamp F: Copper sulfate as an emetic. Lancet 1:233, 1966.

74. Lanphear WF: Gastric lavage. J Emerg Med 4:43, 1986.

75. Kulig KW, Rumack BH, and Rosen P: Clinical use of the gag reflex (Abstract). Vet Hum Toxicol 23:353, 1983.

76. Watson WA: Factors influencing the clinical efficacy of activated charcoal. Drug Intell Clin Pharmacol 21:160, 1987.

77. Holt LE and Holtz PH: The black bottle—a consideration of the role of charcoal in the treatment of poisoning in children. J Pediatr 63:306, 1963.

78. Van De Graaf WB, Thompson WL, Sunshine I, et al: Adsorbent and cathartic inhibition of enteral drug absorption. J Pharmacol Exp Ther 221:656, 1982.

79. Curtis RA, Barone J, and Geacona N: Efficacy of ipecac and activated charcoal cathartic: Prevention of salicylate absorption in a simulated overdose. Arch Intern Med 144:48, 1984.

80. Neuvonen PJ, Tokala O, and Vartiauien M: Comparison of activated charcoal and ipecac syrup in prevention of drug absorption. Eur J Clin Pharmacol 24:557, 1983.

81. Tenebein M, Cohen S, and Sitar DS: Efficacy of ipecac induced emesis, orogastric lavage and activated charcoal for acute drug overdose (Abstract). Vet Hum Toxicol 28:321.

82. Neuvonen PH and Elonen E: Effect of activated charcoal on absorption and elimination of phenobarbitone, carbamazepine and phenylbutazone in man. Eur J Clin Pharmacol 17:51, 1980.

83. Bert KJ, Berlinger WG, Goldberg MJ, et al: Acceleration of the body clearance of phenobarbital by oral activated charcoal. N Engl J Med 307:642, 1982.

84. Berlinger WG, Spector R, Goldberg MJ, et al: Enhancement of theophylline clearance by oral activated charcoal. Clin Pharmacol Ther 33:351, 1983.

85. Park GD, Goldberg KJ, Spector R, et al: The effects of activated charcoal on digoxin and digitoxin clearance. Drug Intell Clin Pharmacol 19:937, 1985.

86. Scheinen M, Virtanen R, and Ilsalo RP: Effect of single and repeated doses of activated charcoal on pharmacokinetics of doxepin. Int J Clin Pharmacol Ther 37:367, 1985.

87. DuSovich P, Caille G, and Larchelle P: Enhancement of nadolol elimination by activated charcoal and antibiotics. Clin Pharmacol Ther 33:585, 1983.

88. Karkkainen S and Neuvonen PJ: Effect of oral charcoal and urine pH on sotalol pharmacokinetics. Int J Clin Pharmacol Ther Toxicol 22:441, 1984.
89. Levy G: Gastrointestinal clearance of drugs with activated charcoal. N Engl J Med 307:676, 1982.
90. Reissell P and Manninen V: Effect of administration of activated charcoal and fibre on absorption, excretion and steady state blood levels of digoxin and digitoxin: Evidence of intestinal secretion of the glycosides. Act Med Scand 668 (Suppl):88, 1982.
91. Decker WJ, Corby DG, and Ibanez JD: Aspirin absorption with activated charcoal. Lancet 1:754, 1968.
92. Decker WJ, Shall RA, Corby DG, et al: Inhibition of aspirin absorption by activated charcoal and apomorphine. Clin Pharmacol Ther 10:710, 1969.
93. Chung DC, Murphy JE, and Taylor TW: In vivo comparison of the absorption capacity of "superactive charcoal" and fructose with activated charcoal and fructose. J Toxicol Clin Toxicol 19:319, 1982.
94. Scholtz EC, Joffe JM, and Coliayzi JL: Evaluation of five activated charcoal formulations for inhibition of aspirin absorption and palatability in man. Am Hosp Pharmacol 35:1335, 1978.
95. Yancy RE, O'Barr TP, and Cosby DG: In vitro and in vivo evaluation of the effect of cherry flavoring on the absorptive capacity of activated charcoal for salicylic acid. Vet Hum Toxicol 19:163, 1977.
96. Olkkala KT and Neuvonen PJ: Do gastric contents modify the antidotal efficacy of oral activated charcoal? Br J Clin Pharmacol 18:663, 1984.
97. Reigel JM and Becker CE: Use of cathartics in toxic ingestion. Ann Emerg Med 10:254, 1979.
98. Easom JM and Lovejoy FH: Efficacy and safety of gastrointestinal decontamination in the treatment of oral poisoning. Pediatr Clin North Am 25:827, 1979.
99. Sketres IS, Mowry JB, Czajka PA, et al: Saline cathartics: Effect on aspirin bioavailability in combination with activated charcoal. J Clin Pharmacol 22:59, 1982.
100. Picchioni AL, Chin L, and Gillespie T: Evaluation of activated charcoal-sorbitol suspension as an antidote. J Toxicol Clin Toxicol 19:433, 1982.
101. Blye E, Larch J, and Cartell S: Extracorporeal therapy in the treatment of intoxication. Am J Kidney Dis 11:321, 1984.
102. Assadi FK: Treatment of acute renal failure in an infant by continuous arteriovenous hemodialysis. Pediatr Nephrol 2:320, 1988.

80

Specific Poisoning Agents

Curt M. Steinhart, M.D., and
Anthony L. Pearson-Shaver, M.D.

In this chapter, specific poisoning agents that commonly cause pediatric intensive care unit admission are discussed. Certain agents such as clonidine and the tricyclic antidepressants almost universally require cardiac monitoring and close observation. Others, such as marijuana and LSD, only rarely cause life-threatening symptoms but are discussed because they have features in common with more dangerous substances. The list of agents is not exhaustive nor does it include all known causes of major pediatric intoxications. However, the discussion does cover pharmacologic agents, drugs of abuse, and nonmedicinal poisons.

PHARMACOLOGIC AGENTS

Acetaminophen

Concerns about the relationship between aspirin and Reye syndrome have resulted in the increased use of acetaminophen as an analgesic and antipyretic in the pediatric population. Advertisements in television and other media espousing the efficacy and safety of acetaminophen presumably have increased its use even more. However, in these advertisements, little is mentioned about the potential toxicity of this substance.

As in nearly all pediatric intoxications, patients at risk for acetaminophen poisoning are "exploring" toddlers and suicidal adolescents.[1] Interestingly, toxic blood levels are noted twice as commonly in adolescents than in toddlers, and hepatotoxicity occurs six times more often in the older age group.[1] Fortunately, pediatric deaths from acetaminophen are very uncommon; most mortality occurs in adults.[2]

Acetaminophen is an effective antipyretic and analgesic that it is usually dispensed as an oral preparation either in liquid, tablet, or "caplet" forms. Rectal suppositories are also available over the counter. Acetaminophen is a component of numerous combination preparations containing codeine, hydrocodone, antihistaminics, or decongestants. The wide availability of many of these preparations makes acetaminophen toxicity quite common.[3]

Following oral ingestion, peak serum levels are reached within 30 to 60 minutes.[4] With massive ingestions, gastrointestinal absorption is delayed, which in turn results in delayed peak serum levels of up to 4 hours. The volume of distribution is slightly greater than the total body water volume, suggesting that high tissue levels are achieved.[4]

Metabolism is nearly entirely hepatic with just 2% excreted renally in the unchanged form.[4] Adults and adolescents convert about 94% to glucuronide or sulfate conjugates, with the remaining 4% undergoing cytochrome-P_{450} oxidase metabolism to mercapturic acid. Evidence exists that infants and young children have increased sulfonation capacity with less reliance on the cytochrome P_{450} oxidase system.[5, 6]

Toxicity occurs because metabolism via the cytochrome P_{450} pathways results in production of the toxic intermediate N-acetyl-p-benzoquinonimine. When there is insufficient glucuronidation and sulfonation to handle a given acetaminophen load, cytochrome P_{450} oxidation increases with resulting increased N-acetyl-p-benzoquinonimine levels.[4] This substance binds to hepatocellular proteins and centrilobular-type hepatocellular necrosis develops.[7] Reticular collapse may follow.[8] Hepatic transaminases increase as does unconjugated bilirubin. Prothrombin times may become markedly elevated.

Renal and cardiac toxicity can also develop. N-acetyl-p-benzoquinonimine apparently binds to renal tubular cells, creating acute tubular necrosis and renal failure.[9, 10] Fatty changes in the myocardium may also be noted.[11] Clinically, dysrhythmias and nonspecific electrocardiographic (ECG) changes may develop. Although renal injury may occasionally be found in the absence of hepatic injury, myocardial dysfunction has been noted only when hepatic insults are present.

Acetaminophen intoxication occurs in four stages[12] (Table 80–1). When a patient initially presents with altered consciousness, another toxic cause should be sought (e.g., codeine or hydrocodone).

Plasma levels should be drawn upon initial presentation and 4 hours after ingestion. Assays should be performed by radioimmunoassay or chromatographic methods. Colorimetric test kits may be inaccurate.[4] Plasma levels should be plotted using the Rumack-Matthew nomogram[13] (Fig. 80–1) to determine the need for N-acetylcysteine therapy.

Table 80–1. STAGES OF ACETAMINOPHEN INTOXICATION*

Stage 1
Nausea, vomiting, malaise, and diaphoresis develop within 12 to 24 hours after ingestion, Children younger than 6 years old usually vomit earlier and rarely demonstrate diaphoresis. Patients with toxic levels all develop symptoms by 14 hours. Transaminases, bilirubin, and prothrombin times are normal at this stage.

Stage 2
24 to 48 hours postingestion the patient usually feels better. If therapy is delayed, transaminases, bilirubin, and prothrombin times increase.

Stage 3
Peak hepatotoxicity is noted 72 to 96 hours postingestion. SGOT is elevated (usually greater than 1000 IU/l, occasionally with dramatic elevations of 20,000 to 30,000 IU/l). Even with this degree of toxicity, less than 1% of patients in stage 3 develop fulminant hepatotoxicity.

Stage 4
Resolution begins to occur 7 to 8 days after ingestion. At this time, the SGOT begins to normalize.

*From Steinhart CM and Pearson-Shaver AL: Poisoning. Crit Care Clin 4:848, 1988, with permission as adapted from Rumack B: Acetaminophen overdose. Am J Med 75:106, 1983, with permission.

Induced emesis should not be delayed by blood drawing. Gastric lavage should be used when indicated or when induced emesis is not successful. Activated charcoal should be given if definitive therapy with *N*-acetylcysteine is to be withheld or if a decision to use *N*-acetylcysteine is pending. Activated charcoal should be withheld if *N*-acetylcysteine is to be given. If already administered, activated charcoal should be removed prior to instituting *N*-acetylcysteine as it is bound by activated charcoal.

The precise mechanism of action of *N*-acetylcysteine is uncertain. Possibilities include direct binding of *N*-

acetyl-*p*-benzoquinonimine, which then prevents hepatocellular binding; decreased *N*-acetyl-*p*-benzoquinonimine production; prevention of sulfonation pathway saturation; and regeneration of glutathione, which binds mercapturic acid thus allowing greater conversion of *N*-acetyl-*p*-benzoquinonimine to mercapturic acid.[14]

N-Acetylcysteine should be used when the plotted plasma level is in either the "possible" or "probable" hepatic toxicity ranges noted on the nomogram, when ingestion occurred within 24 hours, or when the history suggests that more than 140 mg/kg was ingested (7.5 g in adolescents).[4, 12] It is administered orally as a 5% solution diluted with citrus juice, carbonated beverages, or water. An initial dose of 140 mg/kg should be followed by 17 additional doses of 70 mg/kg. Intravenous therapy remains investigational in the United States but is used in Great Britain in the same dosages as in oral administration. With intravenous use, only 12 maintenance doses, rather than 17, are recommended. The efficacy of *N*-acetylcysteine in decreasing both morbidity and mortality is well documented.[4]

If hepatic failure develops, therapy is supportive. Vitamin K, lactulose, neomycin, intravenous dextrose, fresh frozen plasma, or cryoprecipitate may be needed to avert bleeding, encephalopathy, hyperammonemia, or hypoglycemia.

Salicylates

While the decline in salicylate poisoning has been a welcome development, it has reduced the opportunities for students of toxicology to assess clinical information about this fascinating poisoning. There are several reasons for this reduced incidence in salicylate intoxications. First, product safety packaging has vastly improved since the early 1970s. Second, concomitant with improved packaging came the voluntary reduction in tablet strength agreed to by aspirin manufacturers. Third, a strong statistical relationship between aspirin use in children with acute febrile illnesses and Reye syndrome was established, and warnings to that effect by manufacturers, physicians, and public health officials have markedly reduced aspirin use in children. Finally, gastrointestinal irritation from aspirin has limited its use in some patients. Acetaminophen and ibuprofen preparations have increased in popularity as over-the-counter (OTC) analgesic/antipyretics.

Aspirin (acetylsalicylic acid) is the most common cause of salicylate intoxication. Poisoning may also occur from salicylic acid ointments, from methyl salicylate (oil of wintergreen), and from teething gels that contain salicylic acid.

Following oral intake, aspirin is readily absorbed in the upper small intestine and to a lesser extent in the stomach. Food in the stomach delays absorption as does massive overdose, perhaps due to pylorospasm.[15, 16] A more important factor might be the preparation itself. Disintegration and dissolution rates vary greatly among preparations, especially enteric-coated formulations. High luminal pH along absorptive mucosal surfaces also slows absorption.

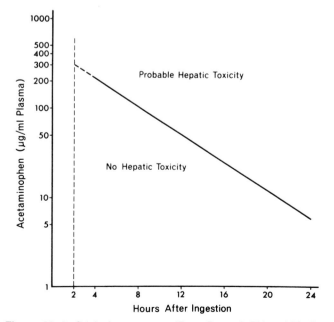

Figure 80–1. Original nomogram. (From Rumack BH and Matthew H: Acetaminophen poisoning and toxicity. Reproduced by permission of Pediatrics Vol. 55, p. 873. Copyright 1975.)

Aspirin is distributed throughout most body tissues and fluids including the brain and cerebrospinal fluid (CSF).[16] Peak plasma concentrations generally occur within 8 to 12 hours after ingestion but may peak as late as 24 hours.[17] Salicylates are highly protein bound to albumin at both high and low affinity sites, and great individual variation in protein binding has been reported.[18]

Metabolism is primarily hepatic via three pathways: (1) conjugation with glycine to form salicyluric acid, (2) glucuronidation to either acyl glucuronides or glucuronide esters, and (3) oxidation to gentisic acid, 2,3-dihydroxybenzoic acid, and 2,3,5-trihydroxybenzoic acid. These metabolites are then excreted renally. Approximately 10% of an ingested dose is excreted in the urine as unchanged compound. If the urine is alkalinized, this percentage may increase up to 30%, but when the urine is acidic it decreases to 2%.[16]

With therapeutic doses, elimination is by first-order kinetics with a half-life of 2 to 3 hours; with large overdoses, elimination is by zero-order kinetics and half-life may increase to 30 hours.[19] Dose-dependent elimination rates appear to be due to limited hepatic ability to form salicyluric acid and glucuronide metabolites. Increased potential for toxicity occurs as protein-binding sites become saturated and tissue levels rise.

Pathophysiologic derangements following salicylate overdose are complex and variable. Classically, adults develop an initial respiratory alkalosis followed by a metabolic acidosis,[20] while children more commonly present with metabolic acidosis as the foremost acid-base disorder.[21] Mechanisms proposed to explain the initial respiratory alkalosis include increased CSF hydrogen ion concentration and increased basal metabolic rate.

Salicylates produce their pharmacologic activity by inhibiting cyclooxygenase, an important enzyme in arachidonic acid metabolism. Production of certain prostaglandins, including thromboxane and prostacyclin, is blocked by cyclooxygenase inhibitors. Traditional thinking held that salicylates in high amounts uncoupled oxidative phosphorylation, resulting in increased heat production, basal metabolic rate, oxygen consumption and cardiac output and hyperpyrexia, but the role of oxidative phosphorylation uncoupling has been recently questioned.[22, 23]

Metabolic acidosis can develop from a variety of causes. Although salicylates are weak acids, it is unlikely that significant acidosis results from the compound itself due to the high degree of protein binding. Increased ketosis and organic acid formation may contribute, but solid evidence for this is lacking. Lactic acidosis may develop from circulatory derangements or perhaps from uncoupling of oxidative phosphorylation.[15, 24] Precise mechanisms to account for the acid-base abnormalities have not been worked out.

Vomiting is a common clinical symptom that may originate from direct CNS stimulation or from gastric irritation. Increased respiratory fluid losses from hyperventilation and increased heat production can exacerbate fluid deficits brought about by vomiting, and electrolyte abnormalities including hypokalemia can occur.

Hyperglycemia, often followed by hypoglycemia, warrants careful attention.

Tinnitus is commonly encountered in adults and older children. Young children and infants may have difficulty verbally communicating this malady. CNS findings include agitation, lethargy, and confusion. Unconsciousness in the absence of another intoxicant is uncommon but may occur. Seizures and coma may be late manifestations. Respiratory depression can also develop as might an encephalopathy indistinguishable clinically from that seen with Reye syndrome. The presence of an elevated plasma salicylate level rules out the latter. Other symptoms of salicylism include fluid retention, noncardiogenic pulmonary edema, oliguria, purpura, and hypoprothrombinemia.[25]

Significant toxicity develops with ingestions greater than 240 mg/kg. Plasma levels correlate poorly with symptoms but are useful for following the course of the illness. CNS symptoms are a better indicator of severity. Mortality is unusual with doses less than 480 mg/kg.

Treatment of alert patients should begin with induced emesis. Obtunded patients should undergo lavage using a nasogastric tube and tepid saline. Immediately afterwards, repetitive doses of activated charcoal should be administered. The role of cathartics is minimal.

Forced alkaline diuresis remains a mainstay of therapy. A urine pH of 7.5 or higher is desirable. Care must be maintained to avoid fluid overload and exacerbation of any pulmonary edema. Volume expansion may be hazardous in the face of altered CNS function. Caution must be exercised during fluid replacement due to the potential for cerebral edema. Potassium homeostasis may be altered by vomiting, fluid losses, diuretics, and bicarbonate.

Hemodialysis and charcoal hemoperfusion are effective methods of enhancing salicylate elimination, but they should be reserved for only the most severe intoxications. Although we have not found any relevant reports, continuous arteriovenous hemofiltration with dialysis (CAVHD) would also likely be effective. It is easier and safer than either hemodialysis or charcoal hemoperfusion and smaller intravascular devices can be utilized.

Tricyclic Antidepressants

Tricyclic antidepressants (TCAs) are frequently prescribed for symptomatic treatment of depressive disorders in adults and adolescents as well as for hyperkinesis, school phobia, sleep disorders, and enuresis.[26] As such, these compounds are readily available to the suicidal adolescent or the unsuspecting toddler. Their narrow therapeutic margin and potential for lethal toxicity make them an important cause of poisoning, and fatal outcomes have been frequently reported.[27, 28]

The name "tricyclics" derives from the basic structure of these compounds, which contain a seven-membered central ring bounded by two benzene rings. Numerous possibilities for structural changes and substitutions account for the multitude of agents sharing this basic chemical makeup (Table 80–2).

Table 80–2. GENERIC AND TRADE NAMES OF TRICYCLIC ANTIDEPRESSANTS

Amines	Trade Names
Tertiary Amines	
Amitriptyline	Elavil, Triavil, Limbitrol
Butriptyline†	
Clomipramine HCL†	
Doxepin	Sinequan, Adapin
Imipramine	Tofranil, Janimine, Berkomine
Trimipramine	Surmontil
Secondary Amines	
Desipramine	Norpramin, Pertofrane
Nortriptyline	Pamelor, Allegron
Protriptyline	Vivactil, Concordin

*Adapted from Pentel PR, Keyler DE, and Haddad LM: Tricyclic and newer antidepressants. *In:* Haddad LM and Winchester JF (eds): Clinical Management of Poisoning and Drug Overdose, 2nd ed. Philadelphia, WB Saunders, 1990, pp. 636–655.
†Not available in the United States as of December 1989.

These compounds block presynaptic uptake of neurotransmitters in both the central and the peripheral nervous systems.[29] Norepinephrine and serotonin reuptake in the CNS is inhibited, and down-regulation of presynaptic receptors and enhanced neurotransmitter release develops.[30] The autonomic nervous system is altered by TCAs. They block sympathetically mediated α-adrenergic receptors as well as the muscarinic receptors of the parasympathetic nervous system.[31]

Following oral ingestion, TCAs are well absorbed, and anticholinergic slowing of gastrointestinal motility may further enhance absorption.[32] Tissue binding is affected by pH, with an acidic milieu favoring less tissue binding and more free drug.[33] The drug is hepatically metabolized via demethylation, oxidation, glucuronidation, and hydroxylation,[34] with the latter being the metabolic pathway that renders these agents nontoxic. Many metabolites retain the pharmacologic properties of the parent compounds.

In addition to being readily bound to tissues, these substances are highly lipid soluble and protein bound,[32] properties that increase the toxicologic propensity of TCAs, which are readily taken up by the CNS, are virtually nondialyzable, and are not readily excreted in the urine. These characteristics also make plasma level determinations less helpful than with other intoxicants. The elimination half-life is extremely variable and can range from 10 to more than 80 hours.[35]

Initial symptoms are usually related to the anticholinergic activity of TCAs. Flushing, dry mouth, mydriasis, fever, and urinary retention may occur, and tachycardia and CNS excitation, including seizures, may develop. Myoclonus or tremors may also be noted. Central nervous system depression may follow the initial excitation or may be the initial CNS derangement. Respiratory depression, unconsciousness, or coma can occur without warning.

Despite the severe CNS alterations that TCAs may create, greater potential for death probably comes from their quinidine-like actions on the cardiovascular system.[27, 32] Sudden cardiovascular collapse can occur from dysrhythmias, decreased cardiac output, or periph-eral vasodilatation. More worrisome is the fact that all three of these cardiovascular alterations can be present in the same patient at the same time. Sinus tachycardia may be due initially to cholinergic blockade. Malignant ventricular dysrhythmias, including ventricular tachycardia and ventricular fibrillation, may develop in the absence of prior sinus tachycardia.[36] Altered conduction is best evidenced by a widened QRS complex, but prolonged PR and QT intervals as well as nonspecific ST changes may be seen on the ECG.[37, 38]

Hypotension may precede cardiac arrest and should be considered an ominous sign. Along with seizures, hypotension may exacerbate any acidemia present and lead to increased tissue release of drug, which can further aggravate symptoms.

Treatment is made difficult by both the pharmacokinetic properties cited and the sudden life-threatening changes that can occur following TCA overdose. Immediate attention to the ABCs of basic life support (i.e., *A*irway, *B*reathing, and *C*irculation) is paramount. Patients with unstable clinical or vital signs should be intubated early to avoid having to undergo the procedure after cardiac or respiratory arrest ensues. Some asymptomatic patients may safely be given ipecac to induce emesis, but several authors suggest that it be withheld because alterations in consciousness may precede emesis.[32, 39] If concerns about inducing emesis are substantial, gastric lavage should be performed followed by repeated small doses of activated charcoal along with a cathartic. TCAs do undergo some enterohepatic circulation, which supports the use of repetitive activated charcoal instillation.

Seizures should be aggressively treated as they can aggravate any metabolic acidosis. Diazepam (0.2 to 0.4 mg/kg IV) or lorazepam (0.05 to 0.2 mg/kg IV) can be given although both will enhance respiratory depression; some evidence exists that lorazepam may do so less than diazepam. Phenytoin can be given for persistent seizures or as "maintenance" therapy but should be administered very slowly (10 to 15 mg/kg IV over 15 to 20 minutes). In addition to its anticonvulsant effects, phenytoin can also ameliorate some concomitant conduction disturbances by increasing conduction time through myocardial tissues.[32] It must be remembered that phenytoin can enhance the negative inotropic effects of TCAs in conjunction with acidemia and, when coupled with α-adrenergic blockade, can cause profound hypotension. If prolonged seizure control is needed, we advocate endotracheal intubation and phenobarbital (10 to 20 mg/kg IV). Whether hepatic metabolism is improved by phenobarbital in this setting is unknown, but it represents a potential advantage in using phenobarbital.

Cardiovascular effects should be treated with crystalloid volume expansion and sodium bicarbonate.[32, 39, 40] The latter is used to reduce free TCA and thus combat some toxic manifestations. We recommend frequent arterial blood gas measurements with titration of the pH to between 7.45 and 7.50 using a combination of mild hyperventilation (arterial P_{CO_2} 28 to 32 mm Hg) and a continuous infusion of sodium bicarbonate. Ventricular dysrhythmias can also be treated initially with lidocaine by continuous infusion (5 to 30 μg/kg/min).

Lidocaine is a negative inotropic agent that can further reduce blood pressure but when used carefully can be helpful.

As noted, phenytoin can enhance conduction through the His-Purkinje system, which may ameliorate some symptoms. Bretylium tosylate, β-blockers,[41] and atropine have limited usefulness. Isoproterenol may ameliorate bradydysrhythmias but will not sufficiently improve blood pressure in hypotensive patients.

Norepinephrine by continuous infusion (0.1 to 2.0 µg/kg/min) has the advantage of having both β- and α-adrenergic activity. This allows it to combat both conduction disturbances and hypotension, making it the agent of choice. Hypotension may also respond to phenylephrine (0.1 to 1.0 µg/kg/min). Because it is an indirect acting catecholamine, dopamine is unlikely to be helpful in increasing either heart rate or blood pressure.

Physostigmine, once touted as the drug of choice for CNS manifestations of TCA intoxication, has numerous cardiovascular side effects including asystole and heart block. For these reasons, anticholinergic symptoms other than bradycardia (discussed earlier) should probably not be specifically treated.

Clonidine

Clonidine is an oral antihypertensive commonly prescribed as a single drug or in combination with other agents to control hypertension in adults. Like most medications, clonidine is a potential toxin in the pediatric age group. Toddlers can inadvertently take the medication prescribed for someone else (often a grandparent),[42] and it may be purposely ingested by a suicidal adolescent.

Clonidine has become a popular antihypertensive agent for use in adults because of its wide therapeutic margin and moderately long duration of action. Pharmacologic effects can be seen within 30 to 60 minutes after oral ingestion.[43] Maximum blood pressure reduction occurs within 2 to 3 hours and often lasts 8 hours or longer.[44] The drug has a large volume of distribution due to its high lipid solubility. With a half-life of about 12 hours, it can be prescribed in twice-a-day regimens.[45] Clearance is mostly renal with about 50% removal occurring daily.[46] Other metabolic pathways are poorly defined.

The antihypertensive effects of clonidine are quite interesting in that the drug is an α-adrenergic agonist. This suggests that peripheral vascular constriction would occur,[47] but actually, clonidine exerts its effects primarily through CNS α-adrenergic stimulation, which is inhibitory to the cardiovascular control centers in the medulla oblongata.[43, 48, 49] The result is a reduction in centrally mediated sympathetic tone, which "overwhelms" the mild peripheral α-adrenergic vasoconstriction. Only with massive overdose or intravenous injection is hypertension noted.[50-52]

In addition to its cardiovascular effects, clonidine has several other CNS actions. In infants and children, lethargy and somnolence are common,[53, 54] which may

be due to clonidine's interaction with the endogenous opioid system. Decreased norepinephrine outflow in the CNS may result.[55] In addition, clonidine increases central dopamine turnover.[56] Precisely how these actions lead to a depressed level of consciousness is unclear.

Clonidine can also cause hypothermia through CNS mechanisms.[57] Stimulation of CNS α-adrenergic receptors can alter serotonin-acetylcholine receptors in such a way as to decrease metabolic heat production and increase heat loss.[58] Other effects include decreased ACTH levels, increased antidiuretic hormone (ADH) secretion, decreased gut peristalsis, and reduced anxiety in certain depressed patients.[58]

The signs and symptoms of clonidine intoxication are listed in Table 80-3. Depressed consciousness, respiratory depression, and hypotension are the most common findings in children.[53, 54] Bradycardia, hypotonia, hypothermia, and miosis are also often seen. Hypertension is infrequent as are seizures.

Treatment consists of general supportive care and correction of any life-threatening abnormalities. Recent ingestions should be treated with induced emesis unless severe lethargy or unconsciousness has developed, in which case gastric tube placement and lavage are indicated. Activated charcoal and cathartics should be used unless otherwise contraindicated.[12]

If respiratory depression is significant, endotracheal intubation may be necessary. Numerous reports of naloxone reversal of clonidine's depressant effects exist,[59, 60] but more recent and larger surveys strongly suggest that naloxone is unpredictable and should not be relied upon to reverse clonidine-induced symptomatology.[54, 61]

Hypotension may not be present initially and may follow a period of initial hypertension. Frequent monitoring of blood pressure is absolutely essential, and in moderate or severe ingestions, intra-arterial continuous monitoring is indicated. When present, hypertension that merits treatment should be controlled with short-acting intravenous agents such as sodium nitroprusside (0.5 to 5.0 µg/kg/min) by continuous infusion or tolazoline (1 to 2 mg/kg IV followed by 1 to 2 mg/kg/hr). These agents must be used with extreme caution as hypotension may soon follow. If hypotension is the initial blood pressure derangement or if it develops after

Table 80-3. SIGNS AND SYMPTOMS OF CLONIDINE OVERDOSE*

Signs or Symptoms	Children (%)	Adults (%)
Cardiovascular		
Bradycardia	30–40	50–60
Hypotension	50	40–50
Hypertension	5–10	15–25
Neurologic		
Coma/depressed mental status	80–85	75–80
Hyporeflexia/hypotonia	30–40	30–40
Seizures	5	5
Miosis	30–40	30–40
Respiratory depression	50–60	20–30
Hypothermia	50	10–20

*Adapted from Roberts JR and Zink BJ: Clonidine. In: Haddad LM and Winchester JF (eds): Clinical Management of Poisoning and Drug Overdose, 2nd ed. Philadelphia, WB Saunders, 1990, pp. 1351–1359.

a period of hypertension, rapid volume expansion with intravenous crystalloids should be used. If rapid improvement with crystalloid infusion is not noted, or if bradycardia is present, a continuous infusion of dopamine (5 to 20 μg/kg/min) or epinephrine (0.1 to 1.0 μg/kg/min) should increase both heart rate and blood pressure.

Hypothermia can be managed with cloth blankets or a warming blanket. Heating lamps or radiant warmers can create rapid warming and vasodilatation, which may reduce blood pressure further. Observation is often an effective conservative approach.

Iron

Iron intoxication is one of the more common pediatric poisonings. In 1986, as many as 16,000 pediatric cases occurred, mostly in the toddler age group.[62, 63] The common use of iron-containing preparations as hematinics and in multivitamins makes them highly accessible to the exploring youngster, and nearly all pregnant women receive oral iron supplements. In addition, the potential toxicity of iron-containing compounds is underappreciated, particularly when they are formulated as "cartoon characters."

Iron poisonings almost always occur from oral ingestions. When consumed orally, iron is readily absorbed by the duodenal and jejunal mucosa in the ferrous form.[63] It is then oxidized to the ferric state and complexed to ferritin, the chief iron storage protein. Next, it is released from ferritin into plasma where it is bound to transferrin. This bound form attaches to the reticuloendothelial cells in bone marrow where transfer of the ferric molecule allows erythropoiesis to occur.[63] Additional iron is stored as ferritin or hemosiderin in the liver or spleen.

The total iron-binding capacity (TIBC) indicates the total available binding potential by plasma transferrin. When the TIBC is exceeded, a small amount of iron is bound by albumin, but the remainder circulates as free iron. Virtually no excretory metabolism for iron is available, with only very small amounts (1 to 2 mg/day) eliminated by gastrointestinal desquamation or menstrual loss.[63]

With toxic ingestions, the TIBC is overwhelmed and free iron circulates. The free iron can cause postarteriolar vasodilatation, increased capillary permeability, metabolic acidosis, and mitochondrial dysfunction. Postarteriolar dilatation may be due directly to ferric ion release from ferritin, serotonin/histamine release, or both.[63, 64] Altered capillary permeability appears to be due to iron's direct effects. Metabolic acidosis may be caused by direct hydrogen ion release during conversion of ferrous iron to the ferric state and/or to subsequent hydration of the ferric ion.[64–67]

Mitochondrial poisoning occurs primarily in hepatocytes. Iron serves as a potent catalyst of lipid peroxidation, which may alter mitochondrial membranes.[64] Iron may also shunt electrons away from the electron transport system.[64]

Clinically, iron poisoning is divided into five phases.[12, 67] The initial phase occurs in the first several hours after ingestion, when gastrointestinal disturbances including vomiting, diarrhea, hematochezia, and abdominal pain may be present. In severe cases, bleeding and fluid losses can lead to hypotension, tachycardia, and metabolic acidosis. Fever, lethargy, or coma may develop. In the absence of a severe ingestion, most patients develop only the gastrointestinal symptoms of the first phase.

The second phase is a quiescent period lasting from 4 to 48 hours during which the patient appears well. In this second phase, subtle hemodynamic changes may indicate the onset of the third phase.

The third phase is characterized by circulatory derangements including overt shock. Metabolic acidosis may be severe and cardiac output exceedingly low. A coagulopathy may develop from inadequate formation of clotting factors, from consumption of clotting factors during earlier bleeding, or from the effects of acidosis and hypoperfusion on coagulation.[12, 67] Further bleeding may aggravate the compromised cardiovascular system.

The fourth phase is infrequently seen but is noted by hepatic necrosis and fulminant hepatic failure. Mortality is somewhat common in this phase.[65, 68, 69]

The final phase occurs 2 to 6 weeks after the original ingestion. In this phase, gastrointestinal scarring may occur, and gastric outlet or proximal small bowel stenosis may be severe enough to cause acute obstruction. Patients may develop the sequelae of the fifth phase without having entered the fourth phase or having only minimal signs of the third phase.

Gastric decontamination should be performed in all recent iron intoxications. Forced emesis or gastric lavage should be used as with other ingestions. Although lavage with phosphate-containing compounds has been advocated frequently,[70] evidence exists that bicarbonate lavage[71] or even normal saline is as effective, avoiding the problem of potential phosphate toxicity.[72] We recommend either 5% sodium bicarbonate or normal saline as the lavage fluid. The former has the advantage of converting some iron to poorly absorbed ferrous carbonate, and for that reason, a small amount of bicarbonate solution should be left in the stomach after lavage.

Activated charcoal does not complex iron and therefore is not indicated. Oral deferoxamine remains controversial as the iron-deferoxamine complex can be absorbed.

Some authors advocate abdominal radiographs to help determine both the presence of ingested iron and the amount.[73, 74] Although helpful in determining adequacy of gastric removal when the iron is in a radiopaque formulation or when an iron-containing bezoar is present, such studies are not universally indicated.

A serum iron level should be performed immediately, although peak levels may not be seen until 2 to 4 hours after ingestion. It seems prudent to measure an initial and then a 4-hour level. Serum iron levels greater than 300 mg/dl should be considered toxic and patients whose levels exceed that number should receive intramuscular deferoxamine at a dose of 40 mg/kg unless hypotension is already present.

Hypotensive patients should have a secure intravenous line placed and volume expansion with crystalloid solutions (20 ml/kg as an initial bolus) should be started. Intravenous deferoxamine should then be initiated via continuous infusion at a rate of 15 mg/kg/hr. Hypotensive patients will require direct monitoring of arterial blood pressure and continuous electrocardiographic assessment. The placement of a central venous line will help guide further volume therapy. Those with serum iron levels greater than 500 mg/dl, even if normotensive, should also receive intravenous deferoxamine at 15 mg/kg/hr. In either group, deferoxamine infusion should be continued until the "vin rose" urine color (indicative of the iron-deferoxamine complex) clears. Serum iron levels should also be repeated to help guide therapy.

If hepatic failure develops, therapy should be supportive and should consist of measures to control bleeding, correct blood volume deficits, maintain normoglycemia, and decrease ammonia levels. CNS injury may occur from hypotension and inadequate perfusion or from hepatic encephalopathy.

Surgical gastrotomy to remove iron,[75] hemodialysis,[69] and total body exchange transfusion[76] have been helpful in rare reported cases but must be approached with caution as these procedures are extremely hazardous in unstable patients. Fortunately, they are usually unnecessary.

Digoxin

The pattern of digoxin intoxication differs from that seen with many other agents in that many cases result from inadvertent intoxication in the course of prescribed therapy.[77, 78] Additionally, acute digoxin ingestions from accidents and suicide attempts are not uncommon.

The precise incidence of pediatric digoxin intoxication is not known. In 1980, digitalis-containing preparations were the eighth most commonly prescribed medications.[79] Fortunately, the availability of serum concentrations, first utilized in the 1970s, has reduced the likelihood of toxicity from inadvertant therapeutic intake. A retrospective review from three large children's hospitals found only 46 cases over a 10-year period.[80] The potential for catastrophic consequences from massive acute digoxin ingestion remains. A variety of extraordinary case reports, the availability of a specific antidote, and the frequent use of digoxin in the pediatric ICU make an understanding of digoxin toxicology pertinent in pediatric critical care.

The pharmacologic actions of the cardiac glycosides are quite similar but complex. The various preparations differ primarily in their bioavailability and pharmacokinetics. As a class of drugs, these agents have pharmacologic and toxicologic effects on both the cardiovascular system and CNS.

Digitalis-containing compounds are dispensed for their myocardial action, either inotropic, electrophysiologic, or both. These actions result from inhibitory actions on the Na^+-K^+ ATPase pump, which maintains Na^+ extracellularly and K^+ intracellularly.[81] When the pump is inhibited, excess sodium remains in the intracellular space, which causes increased intracellular calcium and ultimately creates a positive inotropic response.[78]

High concentrations of glycosides reduce the resting potential (phase IV), which brings the cell close to the threshold for depolarization, resulting in increased rhythmicity and ectopic impulse activity.[79] A reduced rate of rapid depolarization (phase 0) lowers the electrical conduction velocity, which may produce dysrhythmias from conduction velocity slowing. Ectopic activity may also result from the same mechanism.[78, 82] Digitalis preparations also exert negative chronotropy partly via vagal mediation and partly from direct sinoatrial node effects.

Due to its low lipid solubility, very little digoxin normally enters the central nervous system.[79] CNS entry can occur through either the vitreous humor with diffusion along the optic nerve or via concentration in the fourth ventricle choroid plexus. In toxic amounts, digoxin is found in the brain stem chemoreceptor trigger zone and the vagus nerve nucleus.[83] These finding may help explain the nausea, vomiting, and visual disturbances found with digoxin toxicity.

Proper dosing in infants and children requires the prescribing physician to assess the patient's age, renal function, other medications, and serum concentrations during administration. Young infants with immature renal function and older infants and children with renal dysfunction require reduced dosages.

Electrolyte abnormalities, most importantly hypokalemia and hyperkalemia, markedly alter digoxin's toxicity.[78, 79] Hypokalemia, which is frequently due to concomitant diuretic therapy, can cause signs of digitalis toxicity even in the presence of therapeutic levels. Hypomagnesemia and hypercalcemia are also known to aggravate digitalis toxicity.[78]

The gastrointestinal manifestations of digitalis toxicity include nausea, vomiting, anorexia, and abdominal pain. Nausea and vomiting may be protracted and increase the likelihood of electrolyte derangements. Central nervous system symptoms include lethargy, drowsiness, weakness, and behavioral disturbances. Color vision changes are also described.[84]

Cardiovascular manifestations include dysrhythmias of virtually any type, some of which can occur in combination. Supraventricular tachydysrhythmias (atrial or atrioventricular [AV] nodal) may be paroxysmal and are sometimes seen in conjunction with varying degrees of AV block.[77-79, 85, 86] Ventricular ectopy does occur in children but less prominently than in adults. Older children and adolescents may be more prone to first-degree and Mobitz type I (Wenckebach) second-degree block, whereas sinus bradycardia appears more often in infants and young children.[79, 87] A shortened QT interval is often noted and is related to the serum concentration of the glycoside.[79]

Multiple reviews seem to indicate that nearly all symptomatic patients have plasma digoxin levels greater than 2.0 ng/ml. Evidence exists that infants and young children rarely develop symptoms until plasma levels exceed 3.5 ng/ml.[80]

Initial treatment should follow standard approaches

to toxic ingestions. Those receiving the drug for therapeutic use should have the medication withdrawn, and in many cases, further therapy is unnecessary. Accidental overdoses in those with prescribed medication, acute accidental toxic ingestions, and suicide attempts can be handled similarly.

Removal of gastric contents is indicated if the preparation was ingested within the past 6 hours. Forced emesis or gastric lavage should be performed, as in other poisonings. Following gastric emptying, cathartics are indicated. Several reports lend credence to repetitive instillation of activated charcoal.[88, 89]

Monitoring cardiac status is essential. Serial ECGs are useful to follow conduction changes. Continuous monitoring of cardiac rhythm is also necessary. Maintaining adequate circulating volume is essential as is monitoring and correcting electrolyte abnormalities. Potassium infusion without close monitoring of serum potassium levels is fraught with danger. Continued use of diuretics during digoxin toxicity may exacerbate any electrolyte abnormalities present.

Chronotropic agents to combat bradydysrhythmias can be tried but will likely be unsuccessful in severe intoxications. Atropine and isoproterenol are the most frequently used. The risk of generating ectopic beats with isoproterenol makes caution mandatory. Transvenous pacing may be required in refractory bradydysrhythmias or to provide overdrive pacing for ventricular or junctional tachycardias. Cardioversion may be necessary for refractory ventricular tachycardias but can result in ventricular fibrillation if ectopy is also present. Cardioversion energy levels should be kept as low as possible (0.1 to 0.5 joules/kg) and increased gradually only if necessary. Some advocate placing a transvenous pacemaker prior to cardioversion or use of antidysrhythmic agents.[78, 79]

Intravenous lidocaine is the drug of choice for ventricular ectopy and for ventricular tachycardia in the presence of adequate blood pressure. Cardioversion is indicated for ventricular tachycardia with unstable blood pressure. Intravenous potassium may correct certain cases of ventricular tachycardia, AV junctional tachycardia, and frequent multifocal premature ventricular contractions. Supraventricular ectopic rhythms can be treated with phenytoin, propranolol, or both. For ventricular fibrillation, phenytoin is the drug of choice as an alternative or in combination with lidocaine, bretylium, and potassium also indicated. Epinephrine is also indicated with ventricular fibrillation as is electrical defibrillation using standard advanced life support techniques.

Antidote therapy using digoxin-specific antibodies provides a unique form of treatment. Developed from sheep IgG formed in response to digoxin, purified antigen-binding fragments (Fab) are indicated in any life-threatening digoxin (or digitoxin) intoxication.[90, 91] Several characteristics make immunotherapy highly efficacious. First, the Fab fragments bind equimolar amounts of free digoxin in the serum. Binding occurs rapidly following intravenous administration leading to an abrupt decrease in the extracellular free drug level. Intracellular free drug which is in equilibrium with extracellular free drug then moves to the extracellular compartment, which in turn promotes intracellular release of receptor-bound drug with reversal of receptor-mediated toxicity.[90, 91] Second, the lower molecular weight of the Fab, as compared to the entire IgG molecule, readily allows for renal clearance of formed Fab-digoxin complexes. Third, since Fab lacks the immunogenicity of the parent IgG, anaphylactic reactions are extremely rare.

A number of case reports[91–93] and several series[94–96] indicate that therapy with digoxin-specific Fab is extremely helpful in managing critically ill patients. Doses are given intravenously for 30 minutes, and dosage is based on either the amount ingested or on the serum digoxin level. The package insert provides several tables for proper dosing, including one specifically for infants and children. The few complications reported with digoxin-specific Fab include hypokalemia, allergic reactions, and emergence of dysrhythmias previously inhibited by digoxin.

Thyroid Hormones

Thyroid hormone preparations are among the most widely prescribed medications: annually more than 400 million tablets containing some form of thyroid preparation are dispensed.[97] The incidence of thyroid hormone ingestion is uncertain. Nationally as many as 5,600 suicidal or accidental ingestions were noted in one report,[98] while in another only 2,231 thyroid hormone ingestions were reported in 1986.[62] The number of pediatric patients in these studies was not specified.

Despite the potential for major end-organ system dysfunction from thyroid hormone excess, children often remain asymptomatic even in the face of massive ingestions.[99–101] When symptoms develop, they are usually delayed and frequently are minor. Serious toxicity is infrequent. In a series of 22 thyroxine ingestions in one study, only 20% of patients developed any symptoms.[102] In a brief review of 78 cases by another group, only 3 patients required hospital admission.[98] A review of annual cases from a well-known Poison Control Center reported that only 27% of documented ingestions ever became symptomatic.[100]

L-Thyroxine (T_4) is the most commonly prescribed form of thyroid hormone, but desiccated thyroid, thyroglobulin, liothyronine (T_3), and liotrix (T_3 and T_4) are also available. These products stimulate intracellular mRNA and protein synthesis, increase mitochondrial oxidative phosphorylation, and enhance certain membrane transport functions in all tissues except brain, spleen, and testes.[97]

Although both thyroxine (T_4) and triiodothyronine (T_3) are readily absorbed from the gut, those who ingest T_4 and do not undergo gastrointestinal removal often will not develop symptoms for several days.[100, 103] Massive doses have been associated with earlier onset of symptoms.[102]

Under physiologic conditions, the T_4 half-life in children is 3 to 5 days and the T_3 half-life is 1 day.[104] Lewander and colleagues found that with acute intoxications, the half-life of T_4 actually decreased (2.8 days) while that of T_3 increased (6 days).[102] Their explanation was that T_3 half-life lengthened due to the continual conversion of excess T_4 to T_3 and that T_4 half-life was reduced via reduced TSH activity in response to T_4 excess.

Clinical symptoms include cardiovascular, neurologic, and gastrointestinal manifestations.[97] Tachycardia, palpitations, cutaneous vasodilatation, hypertension, and dysrhythmias can occur. Gastrointestinal disturbances include vomiting, diarrhea, and abdominal pain. Anxiety, mydriasis, diaphoresis, and agitation may be noted. In severe cases, seizures, acute psychosis, and coma can develop.[105]

Treatment depends on the time of ingestion, the amount ingested, the preparation, the child's previous condition, and symptoms noted. Care should be taken to obtain an accurate history of the amount ingested. If less than 0.5 mg of thyroxine was ingested, no treatment is indicated.[102] Children ingesting more than 0.5 mg within the previous 6 hours should undergo gastric decontamination including ipecac and/or activated charcoal and a cathartic.[102] It has been suggested that those ingesting more than 4 mg of L-thyroxine should have a serum T_4 level drawn 2 to 6 hours after ingestion. Admission should be limited to those with serum T_4 levels greater than 75 μg/dl or those with symptoms.[102]

Treatment recommendations vary, but trends favor a conservative approach.[98–100, 102] Earlier recommendations included acetaminophen for fever, propranolol for prevention of tachydysrhythmias, propylthiouracil for blocking uptake, prednisone to decrease conversion of T_4 to T_3, and cholestyramine to decrease enterohepatic circulation.[106, 107]

Little evidence exists that therapy to prevent adverse effects is beneficial. Reviews suggest that only symptomatic patients be treated.[98, 100, 102] Regimens limited to acetaminophen for fever and propranolol for tachydysrhythmias seem most appropriate. In severe cases with seizures or cardiovascular collapse, standard intensive supportive care including fluid replacement, establishing an adequate circulating volume, and anticonvulsants may be necessary. Extracorporeal removal via charcoal hemoperfusion or plasmapheresis appears to be unnecessary and potentially risky.

DRUGS OF ABUSE

Cocaine

Concomitant with the dramatic increase in cocaine use over the past two decades has been an increase in cocaine-related deaths. In 1987, more than 1,500 deaths were reported to the National Institute on Drug Abuse.[108] Although the number of pediatric patients dying annually from cocaine intoxication is unknown, adolescent use of this dangerous drug has paralleled adult use. Additionally, numerous reports of intoxication occurring in infants and small children make knowledge of the pharmacologic effects of cocaine an essential part of the critical care physician's armamentarium.[109–114]

Cocaine is the crystalline alkaloid found in the leaves of *Erythroxylon coca*, a bush that thrives in the Andes Mountains of South America. Its nonmedicinal use was outlawed in the United States in 1914, but it is still used medicinally as a topical anesthetic by otolaryngologists and anesthesiologists.

The water-soluble crystalline salt, cocaine hydrochloride, is 89% cocaine by weight and has a melting point of 195°C. It can be easily converted chemically to the non–water soluble "freebase" alkaloid, which melts at 98°C and vaporizes at high temperatures. The crystalline salt form is usually mixed with other substances known as adulterants[115] and "snorted" intranasally or injected intravenously. The "freebase" form, also known as "crack," is heated and then smoked, creating an immediate "rush" quite similar to that following intravenous use and increasing its capacity to cause addiction.[116]

Cocaine is rapidly and extensively metabolized via several methods.[117] Plasma and hepatic cholinesterases hydrolyze it to ecgonine methyl ester, while nonenzymatic hydrolysis to benzylecgonine also occurs. Additionally, small amounts of cocaine are converted to norcocaine by demethylation. Following inhalation or intravenous injection, the plasma half-life is about 60 to 90 minutes. A longer half-life is seen with intranasal or gastrointestinal intake due to variable absorption rates.[117]

The clinical manifestations of cocaine intoxication are multiple and involve numerous organ systems. The predominant effects result from stimulation of the autonomic nervous system, which may be mild or quite severe. Common cardiovascular effects include hypertension, tachycardia, palpitations, and chest pain. Major complications include ventricular tachydysrhythmias, myocardial ischemia, myocardial infarction, myocarditis, shock, and end-organ ischemia. Hypertension and tachycardia result from sympathetic nervous system stimulation. Increased systemic vascular resistance and increased cardiac output each contribute to the hypertension. Intracranial hemorrhage[118] and acute aortic dissection have both been related to cocaine intoxication.[119]

Dysrhythmias are quite common and may be due to sympathetic stimulation, myocardial ischemia, or myocarditis. Tachydysrhythmias predominate, especially sinus tachycardia, and supraventricular tachycardia or ventricular tachycardia can also develop. Other dysrhythmias reported include atrial fibrillation, complete heart block, ventricular fibrillation, and asystole.[120]

Myocardial infarction in those with and without coronary artery disease is well described.[121, 122] It may be due to increased myocardial workload, coronary vasospasm, or coronary artery thrombosis.[123, 124] Intense sympathetic activity can markedly increase myocardial oxygen demand. Because vasoconstriction can affect coronary blood flow and tachycardia can inhibit coronary filling, coronary blood flow may be unable to meet myocardial tissue demand, resulting in ischemia or infarction. Coronary vasospasm has also been noted and can cause myocardial infarction.[124] Cocaine-induced coronary vasospasm and platelet aggregation can lead to coronary artery thrombosis. New infarcts have been noted as long as several days after the last cocaine use.[117]

Intense catecholamine stimulation can also result in myocarditis and myonecrosis in a manner similar to that seen with pheochromocytoma.[117, 125] Myocardial ischemia or brain stem dysfunction can lead to hypotension and overt shock. This low cardiac output state may be enhanced further by tachydysrhythmias. Ischemic renal failure may develop or hypotension may exacerbate any renal insult occurring from rhabdomyolysis.[126]

In addition to cardiovascular effects, central nervous systems effects are also common[127, 128]; these range from mild headache, dizziness, anxiety, and confusion to hyperexcitability, hallucinations, depression, suicidal ideation, seizures, stroke, encephalopathy, and coma. Headaches may be due to hypertension, cocaine-induced migraine, or even subarachnoid or intracranial hemorrhage.[117]

Seizures from cocaine are likely due to its local anesthetic properties, which reduce the seizure threshold, but may be further stimulated by hyperthermia and/or acidosis.[117] Pascual-Leone and colleagues reported seizures within 90 minutes of cocaine use as the primary diagnosis in 7.9 percent of patients with cocaine intoxication.[129] Generalized tonic-clonic seizures were the most common type which is consistent with other reports. Cocaine intoxication should be considered in the differential diagnosis of infants and children presenting with seizures.[109, 111, 112]

Pulmonary complications are generally due to smoking "crack" and include pneumothorax, bronchospasm, and pulmonary edema.[130] Pulmonary edema may develop from direct lung injury or may be secondary to cardiac failure.

Severe hyperthermia and rhabdomyolysis are two other major life-threatening manifestations of cocaine intoxication. Rhabdomyolysis may lead to renal injury and progressive renal failure. In a study of 39 patients reported by Roth and associates with cocaine-induced rhabdomyolysis, 13 (33%) developed acute renal failure and six of those patients died.[126]

Diagnosing cocaine intoxication requires a careful history and physical assessment. Laboratory screening will often find cocaine in plasma or one of its metabolites in urine. Screening is also necessary to test for other drug use. Radiographic studies looking for drug-filled packets or condoms may be necessary with certain adolescents.[131]

Treatment begins with the basic ABCs. Those with sufficient respiratory or cardiovascular compromise will require endotracheal intubation. Intravenous naloxone may be utilized to ameliorate effects caused by other intoxicants. Agitation can be treated with benzodiazepines. Midazolam (0.05 to 0.10 mg/kg IV) and diazepam (0.1 to 0.4 mg/kg IV) are both quite useful. When seizures are present, diazepam is preferred. Haloperidol (0.1 to 0.3 mg/kg IM) is also beneficial but may reduce the seizure threshold. Benzodiazepines can create CNS depression or enhance CNS depressant effects of other drugs, so their use requires constant attention to the airway and respiratory effort.

Hyperthermia can be treated with tepid sponging. In severe cases, external cooling and neuromuscular blockade using vecuronium (0.05 to 0.2 mg/kg IV or pancu-

ronium 0.1 mg/kg IV) may be necessary. With neuromuscular blockade, seizure activity will be inapparent. In such cases, bedside electroencephalographic (EEG) monitoring or allowing the blockade to wear off intermittently seems warranted.

Gastrointestinal decontamination via standard methods should be employed, but concerns about sudden onset of seizures make induced emesis potentially dangerous. When the route of intake is intranasal, inhalation, or intravenous there is no role for induced emesis, lavage, or catharsis. Oral ingestions including packet swallowing will benefit from catharsis. Isosmotic bowel preparations have been advocated.[117]

Seizures are often self limited but may persist or recur. Management with diazepam (0.2 to 0.4 mg/kg IV) followed by phenytoin (10 to 20 mg/kg IV over 10 to 20 minutes) will usually suffice. Alternatively, lorazepam (0.05 to 0.1 mg/kg IV) followed by phenobarbital (10 to 20 mg/kg IV) is equally effective.

Hypertension can be treated initially with sedation. If significant elevations in blood pressure exist, β blockade with propranolol (0.01 to 0.05 mg/kg IV) or labetalol (0.25 mg/kg IV over 2 to 3 minutes or 25 µg/kg/min via continuous infusion). Esmolol by continuous infusion (50 µg/kg loading dose followed by 50 to 200 µg/kg/min) or sodium nitroprusside (0.5 to 5.0 µg/kg/min) are each effective as is α-adrenergic blockade with phentolamine (0.05 to 0.10 mg/kg IV).

Dysrhythmias can also be treated with β-adrenergic blockers such as propranolol. A recent study in rats showed enhanced cocaine toxicity manifesting as seizures with administration of the calcium antagonists verapamil, diltiazem, and nifedipine.[132] Their use appears to be controversial.

Myocardial ischemia and infarction can be treated with nitrates, calcium antagonists, or both. Thrombolytic therapy is recommended for severe injuries or those not responding to more conservative treatment.[133]

Rhabdomyolysis should be verified by checking for heme pigment in the urine in the absence of red cells and by testing for urine myoglobin. Adequate intravenous fluids should be administered to ensure high urine flow, and alkalinization with sodium bicarbonate should be utilized to reduce myoglobin toxicity.

Deaths from cocaine intoxication are due to dysrhythmias, myocardial infarction, seizures, or respiratory failure.[117, 128] Myoglobin-induced renal failure can result in death later in the course of hospitalization.[126]

Other Stimulants

Medical indications for amphetamines and chemically related compounds (the sympathomimetics) include narcolepsy, attention deficit disorders in children, and obesity.[134] Because of limited clinical uses for these agents, potential for pediatric patients to become intoxicated is comparatively small. Still, toddlers may accidentally ingest methylphenidate prescribed for a sibling or amphetamines being abused by a parent. Still widely available as a "diet pill," phenylpropanolamine is potentially available to the wandering toddler. Since all drugs of this type have great abuse potential, adolescents involved with drug abuse more than likely will have the opportunity to use these drugs.[135]

Each substance in this group of agents chemically resembles the parent compound phenylethylamine and each has similarities with the endogenous catecholamines dopamine, norepinephrine, and epinephrine. Minor structural alterations of the parent compound create a variety of different agents, including some with hallucinogenic properties.

Sympathomimetics can be taken orally, intranasally, intravenously, subcutaneously, or by smoking and inhaling.[134] The onset of action is shortest (within minutes) with smoking and intravenous intake. Snorting and subcutaneous administration result in symptoms in about 30 minutes, while the effects of oral ingestion may not develop for 1 to 2 hours.[134] The duration of action is extremely variable and depends on the route of administration, the dose taken, and the pharmacokinetic properties of the agent itself.

In the periphery, stimulants cause release of neurotransmitters responsible for α- and β-adrenergic effects. In addition, amphetamines appear to block reuptake of catecholamines in presynaptic neurons and to inhibit monoamine oxidase,[134, 136] resulting in increased neurotransmitter concentration in the synapse.

In the CNS, these compounds increase neurotransmitter release, causing increased CNS activity in both the dopaminergic and the adrenergic pathways. Stimulation of the reticular activating system causes increased alertness, and stimulation of the reward center in the median forebrain bundle accounts for the feelings of euphoria and increased libido. Dopaminergic stimulation may explain the acute psychosis frequently associated with amphetamine use.[137]

As noted, amphetamines are readily absorbed from a variety of mucosal surfaces. Most undergo hepatic degradation with urinary excretion of metabolites. In the presence of an acidic urine, urinary excretion of unchanged drug increases significantly.[134, 136] Methylphenidate differs from other amphetamines in that it undergoes nearly complete ester hydrolysis with virtually no urinary excretion of unchanged drug.[134, 136]

Clinical effects involve stimulation of the CNS and the cardiovascular system and increased neuromuscular activity. CNS symptoms include agitation, irritability, anxiety, hallucinations, delusions, and paranoia. Seizures are not uncommon. Rarely, cerebral ischemic stroke, intracranial hemorrhage, or encephalopathy may develop.

Cardiovascular signs and symptoms include palpitations, chest pain, tachycardia, hypertension, and dysrhythmias. Hypertension may be severe and, along with tachycardia, may lead to marked increases in myocardial work and oxygen demand, which can cause worsening dysrhythmias or myocardial ischemia. Congestive heart failure and cardiomyopathy can develop.

Neuromuscular hyperactivity may produce mydriasis, tremor, and hyperthermia and in severe cases, rhabdomyolysis may develop.[138] Other complications include abdominal pain, diarrhea, nausea, and vomiting. De-

hydration due to decreased oral intake can cause hypotension, especially when coupled with myocardial failure. Myoglobinuric renal failure may result from rhabdomyolysis. Death can occur from seizures, intracranial hemorrhage, hypertensive crisis, myocardial failure, or myoglobinuric renal failure.[134]

Treatment is supportive and nonspecific. No antidote exists. Gastrointestinal decontamination should follow the same rules as for other ingestions. Seizures can be ablated with lorazepam (0.05 to 0.1 mg/kg IV) or diazepam (0.2 to 0.4 mg/kg IV) and control maintained with phenytoin (10 to 15 mg/kg IV over 10 to 20 minutes) or phenobarbital (10 to 20 mg/kg IV). We prefer the combination of lorazepam and phenobarbital in this setting over diazepam and phenytoin as avoidance of cardiovascular effects of phenytoin seems desirable. We usually avoid diazepam and phenobarbital in combination because of their respiratory depressant synergy. If endotracheal intubation has been performed, however, diazepam and phenobarbital are extremely effective in controlling seizures.

Agitation should not be treated unless severe. Benzodiazepines such as midazolam (0.05 to 0.2 mg/kg IV) or diazepam (0.1 to 0.2 mg/kg IV) are helpful. Alternatively, haloperidol (0.1 to 0.3 mg/kg IM) may be used. Phenothiazines should be avoided as they lower the seizure threshold.

Control of hypertension is essential to avoid development of encephalopathy, intracranial hemorrhage, or myocardial failure. Sodium nitroprusside by continuous intravenous infusion in doses ranging from 0.5 to 5.0 μg/kg/min will allow for careful titration of the blood pressure. Its short duration of action also allows for immediate discontinuation should that be necessary.

Supraventicular tachycardia (SVT) can be treated with digoxin loading using 30 to 40 μg/kg as the total digitalizing dose. Half of the total dose should be given initially with subsequent one-fourth of the total dose given at 4- to 8-hour intervals followed by a daily dose of 10 μg/kg/day in two divided doses. If continuous intravenous infusion is desired for SVT control, esmolol as a 50 μg/kg IV bolus followed by a continuous infusion at 50 to 200 μg/kg/minute may prove effective and have the convenience of rapid discontinuation. Although verapamil is useful, numerous cautions for its use in pediatric patients have been reported. Ventricular dysrhythmias can be treated with esmolol or intravenous lidocaine at doses of 1 mg/kg bolus followed by a continuous infusion of 5 to 30 μg/kg/min. Should myocardial failure develop, inotropic agents such as dopamine or dobutamine may be required. Myocardial ischemia should be treated with nitrates. Thrombolytic therapy has not been used.

Hyperthermia without muscle rigidity should be treated with tepid sponging, antipyretics, and perhaps a cooling blanket. If muscle rigidity is present or if hyperthermia is severe, aggressive external cooling and neuromuscular blockade may be necessary. Intravenous dantrolene sodium used as in the malignant hyperthermia syndrome may be lifesaving.

Marijuana

Marijuana remains the most commonly used illicit drug in the United States. In 1978, marijuana use peaked at an estimated 20 million users, but diminished by 40% to 12 million by 1988.[139] Continued significant declines in adolescent and childhood use are equally encouraging, but as many as 5% of high school seniors may still use marijuana regularly.[140] As such, it remains a major health problem.

Acute marijuana intoxication rarely results in critical illness; however, a recent report of three children who developed coma from marijuana intoxication requires us to reconsider previous beliefs that marijuana intoxication is entirely benign.[141]

Marijuana is derived from the flowering tops, leaves, stems, and seeds of *Cannibis sativa*. The plant grows in temperate and subtropical climates as a rather hearty "weed." Sinsemilla, the seedless flowering tops from female plants; hashish, the dried resin made from flowering tops; and hash oil, a dark liquid obtained by nonpolar extraction of plant material, have higher concentrations of the active compound, δ-9-tetrahydrocannabinol (δ-9-THC), than combinations of ground leaves, stems, and seeds.

In most instances, marijuana is smoked in rolled papers (joints) or in pipes. To enhance uptake, the smoke is held in the lungs for 15 to 30 seconds prior to exhaling. Active ingredients pass immediately into the blood stream. Oral ingestion is well known, with marijuana baked into cookies or brownies being the preferred "agents." Gastrointestinal absorption is somewhat erratic, and clinical findings may be less obvious than with inhalation.[145]

Being highly lipophilic, δ-9-THC is taken into all lipoid tissues, resulting in a large volume of distribution.[142] High lipid solubility explains why serum levels of δ-9-THC do not correlate with clinical findings and why quantities of metabolites can be found in the urine for several weeks following use. Excretion is about 65% fecal and 20% urinary, but remaining cannabinoid may persist for several weeks presumably due to its slow release from fatty tissues. Metabolism is almost completely hepatic.[143, 144]

δ-9-THC appears to bind to certain CNS receptors to produce changes unique to cannabinoids.[146] Membrane alterations occur at high drug levels in a manner similar to that with highly lipophilic anesthetics. Noradrenergic, dopaminergic, serotonergic, cholinergic, and GABAergic neurotransmitter functions are affected.[147] Tolerance can develop with chronic use, but addiction does not appear to occur.[148, 149]

Clinically, most findings are usually nonspecific, short lived and fortunately benign. Confusion, short-term memory loss, conjunctival inflammation, slight pupillary constriction, tachycardia, and increased appetite are the most reproducible findings. Decreased coordination and dimished ability to perform complex motor functions are also quite common.[144, 150] In pediatric patients, hypothermia, ataxia, nystagmus, tremor, and pallor were reported in at least one of three young siblings who accidentally ingested marijuana-containing cookies.[151]

Recently, coma was reported in three of six children with proven cannabinoid intoxication.[141]

For the intensivist, severe marijuana intoxication will most likely present as a nonspecific poisoning. Because street preparations may be combined with amphetamines or phencyclidine, clinical presentations may reflect intoxication with these agents rather than marijuana.[150] Previous concerns about toxic effects of paraquat sprayed into fields have not resulted in any literature reports.

Since marijuana poisoning is nearly always benign, treatment is entirely supportive. Severe anxiety reactions can be treated with midazolam (0.05 to 0.2 mg/kg IV), diazepam (0.1 to 0.2 mg/kg IV), or haloperidol (0.1 to 0.3 mg/kg IM). Care must be taken to test for other agents including alcohol or more dangerous compounds such as phencyclidine.

Opioids

Opioids are naturally occurring or synthetic compounds with morphine-like activity. The term "opioid" is preferred to the term "narcotic," which connotes only the potential to induce sleep. The more specific term "opiate" refers only to agents derived from opium.

This group of drugs has been known about for thousands of years. In the 19th century, opium began to be employed for modern medicinal use primarily as an analgesic. Morphine, the major alkaloid analogue derived from opium, steadily increased in popularity, but as understanding of the agent grew, its untoward side effects became more troublesome. Once its potential for physical and psychologic dependence was recognized, a search for natural analogues and synthesized compounds was undertaken to produce nonaddicting, potent alternatives to morphine. Heroin was one of the earliest semisynthetic analogues produced. Unfortunately, it was soon discovered that it had the same addicting properties as morphine, primarily due to the fact that it is converted to morphine in vivo. Numerous other compounds have also been manufactured, many of which are extremely useful when properly prescribed. Some of these agents and their trade names and indications are listed in Table 80–4.

The pharmacologic actions of the opioids are now well understood. They appear to interact with specific CNS receptors to inhibit pain fiber activity[152] by decreasing neurotransmitter release[153] or altering transmembrane polarization.[154] This results in pain perception but relative indifference to it.[155]

Five different opioid receptors have been identified; mu, kappa, delta, sigma, and epsilon.[155] μ, κ, and δ receptors mediate analgesia above the spinal cord with μ being the most important.[156] Spinal analgesia is mediated by κ and δ receptors, while sigma receptors affect dysphoria or psychomimetic responses.[156] Subgroups of the μ receptors (labeled 1 and 2) have been differentiated. $μ_1$-receptors appear to be responsible for analgesia, while $μ_2$-receptors may mediate respiratory, gastrointestinal and cardiovascular manifestations.[155, 156]

Paralleling the understanding of opioid receptors

Table 80–4. OPIOIDS: NAMES AND INDICATIONS

Generic Name	Trade Name	Uses
Alfentanil	Alfenta	Analgesic, anesthetic
Apomorphine		Emetic
Codeine		Analgesic, antitussive
Diphenoxylate	Lomotil	Antidiarrheal, antispasmodic
Fentanyl	Sublimaze	Analgesic, anesthetic
Heroin		Abuse
Hydromorphone	Dilaudid	Analgesic
Loperamide	Imodium	Antidiarrheal, antispasmodic
Meperidine	Demerol	Analgesic
Methadone	Dolophine	Opioid withdrawal
Morphine		Analgesic
Oxycodone	Percodan	Analgesic
Oxymorphone	Numorphan	Analgesic
Paregoric		Antidiarrheal, antispasmodic
Pentazocine	Talwin	Analgesic
Propoxyphene	Darvon	Analgesic
Sufentanyl	Sufenta	Analgesic, anesthetic

has been an increased knowledge of the endogenous opioid molecules, namely enkephalins, endorphins, and dynorphins.[157, 158] These peptides function either as short-acting neurotransmitters or as long-acting hormones. They may interact at one or several different receptors.[159] The importance of these compounds in critical care is beyond the scope of this chapter, but excellent reviews exist[156, 158, 159] and the subject is discussed in Chapters 76 and 77.

Opioids produce a characteristic clinical triad of CNS depression, respiratory depression, and miosis. CNS depression can follow an initial period of excitation, which in adult heroin users may present as a "rush." Nausea and vomiting may develop early. Infants and children may present with seizures, which are usually generalized.[157] Soon after, CNS depression intervenes, with drowsiness or lethargy that can progress to unresponsiveness and coma. An impaired gag reflex may predispose the patient to aspiration of oral or gastric contents, especially during vomiting.

Respiratory depression may be heralded by a decreased respiratory rate or reduction in tidal volume. As hypoventilation worsens, hypercarbia develops followed by hypoxia. Complete cessation of respirations is not uncommon and is the leading cause of death from opioids.[157] Pulmonary edema has been noted with both intravenous and orally administered opioids, but only with intoxicating doses.[160] The cause of pulmonary edema remains controversial but may relate to hypoxic-mediated pulmonary vasoconstriction and transcapillary fluid leak. With intravenous street drugs, adulterants such as talc and impurities have been implicated. Bronchospasm may also develop.[161]

Miosis develops from effects on the Edinger-Westphal nucleus. Despite their small size, pupils often remain reactive. Under certain circumstances, pupillary size may be normal or even mydriatic such as with meperidine overdose, in the early stages of Lomotil intoxication when the atropine effects predominate, with hypoxia, and after naloxone administration.[155] Other complications such as rhabdomyolysis,[162] severe myocardial depression, and hypotension[163] may develop but are rare in pediatric patients.

Clinical pharmacology and toxicology will vary depending on the agent and its mode of intoxication (medicinal, accidental, or abuse). Because certain opioids are extremely uncommon causes of pediatric intoxication, only those compounds encountered with some frequency are discussed.

Lomotil

Although virtually nontoxic in adults and older children, Lomotil (2.5 mg of diphenoxylate hydrochloride and 0.025 mg of atropine sulfate per tablet or 5 ml of liquid) has caused severe toxicity and even deaths in infants and toddlers.[164–166] Manufacturer's warnings prohibit dispensing to this age group, but accidental ingestions and misuse still occur.

Early signs of Lomotil intoxication are predominately due to atropine effects. Hyperpyrexia, flushing, tachypnea, and lethargy are common. Tachycardia may be present, but pupillary dilatation is usually not because of the opioid present. Seizures can also develop early during an intoxication. Clinical signs may change suddenly with the onset of hypothermia, loss of flush, CNS depression, and respiratory depression. Seizures may also begin at this point. Several deaths from Lomotil intoxication have been reported.[164, 165]

Treatment is supportive and specific. For recent ingestions (within 1 hour) and with a responsive patient, emesis may be induced. However, if lethargy has developed, emesis is probably not safe. Lavage via a large orogastric tube may be helpful in removing retained tablets. Because of the antiperistaltic action of both agents found in Lomotil, ememis or lavage is nearly always indicated. Activated charcoal binds most opioids, and although no studies show that it binds diphenoxylate, it most likely does. Saline cathartics or glycerol should be copiously provided until charcoal is apparent in stools. There does not appear to be any role for forced diuresis.

Naloxone should not be withheld in any suspected opioid intoxication including Lomotil.[166] Dosing recommendations have changed recently, with 0.1 mg/kg now suggested for those less than 5 years of age and 2.0 mg for those weighing more than 20 kg or older than 5 years.[167] These new recommendations are based on numerous reports demonstrating reversal of opioid intoxication with this higher dose after the previously recommended dose[166] (one tenth the presently recommended dose) failed to reverse symptoms. No severe side effects from massive doses of naloxone have been reported in either healthy volunteers or in episodic case reports.[155, 157]

Signs and symptoms of Lomotil intoxication may persist for more than 12 hours. When repeated dosing of naloxone is necessary, the agent can be administered by continuous intravenous infusion.[168] Doses of 0.4 mg/hr have been suggested, but it seems more prudent to use the drug on a per-kilogram basis. We suggest doses in the range of 20 to 40 µg/kg/hr titrated to clinical effect based in part on the findings reported by Lewis and associates.[168]

If given promptly, naloxone may obviate the need for

endotracheal intubation should respiratory failure develop. Naloxone may also ameliorate Lomotil-induced seizures, obviating administration of anticonvulsants that could further depress respirations.

Morphine and Meperidine

Morphine and meperidine overdoses usually occur when errors in dosing occur in hospital or clinic settings. Meperidine frequently causes seizures, and pupillary changes may not be present. Many centers employ meperidine as part of a sedative "cocktail" mixed with promethazine and chlorpromazine (DPT cocktail). Potential for overdosage with this combination seems high. Inadvertent overdose with morphine in a 1-month-old infant being sedated for a CT scan led to apnea and cardiac arrest,[169] but successful resuscitation with administration of naloxone resulted in an uneventful recovery.

Propoxyphene

Propoxyphene poisoning[170, 171] was somewhat common in the 1970s, but evidence that its analgesic strength is not superior to that of acetaminophen or aspirin has decreased its use.

Dextromethorphan

A common ingredient in over-the-counter cough preparations, dextromethorphan is often ingested by young children. Signs and symptoms of dextromethorphan intoxication apparently are reversed by naloxone.[172] Although the opioid potency of this agent is comparatively mild, the availability of a specific antidote should be recognized in case of a severe intoxication.

Therapy for All Opioid Intoxications

Adolescents who may be addicted to opioids and who present with acute intoxication should not have naloxone withheld. Concerns about precipitating withdrawal appear only partly justified. Although withdrawal reactions may develop, they are generally short-lived and always nonfatal, unlike with alcohol withdrawal. Withdrawal symptoms can be easily managed with good supportive care.[155, 157]

Phencyclidine and Other Hallucinogens

This group of compounds is discussed together because each of these agents are drugs of abuse with no demonstrable therapeutic value. They are loosely termed hallucinogens but more often cause illusions and altered perceptions rather than true hallucinations. Other monikers for this group include psychomimetics, psychedelics, pseudohallucinogens, and dysleptics.

Phencyclidine piperidine (PCP) is the most commonly abused drug in this group. It has numerous street names including "angel dust," "Sherman," "peace pill," "crystal," and "hog." A stable white crystalline solid, it is usually smoked either sprinkled on tobacco or marijuana leaves and rolled into a cigarette or coated onto a cigarette by dipping. It can be taken orally (by dusting it onto food), intranasally, or intravenously,[173] and percutaneous absorption also occurs.

Once absorbed, the drug is highly lipid soluble and accumulates in adipose tissue and brain tissue.[173] It is metabolized by hepatic hydroxylation with subsequent urinary excretion of metabolites. Its very high lipid solubility accounts for its prolonged half-life of from 7 to 72 hours. The substance has a pKa of 8.5, making it susceptible to ion trapping in an acid environment.[173, 174]

PCP has complex mechanisms of action. It interacts with virtually all neurotransmitters.[173] By inhibiting gamma-aminobutyric acid (GABA), it may induce dopaminergic symptoms. PCP also has centrally mediated anticholinergic effects via acetylcholine receptor blockade as well as sympathomimetic effects.[175] Anticholinergic drugs (e.g., atropine) can aggravate symptoms while physostigmine can reverse some symptoms such as tremor, nystagmus, agitation, and panic. In addition, PCP produces cocaine-like sympathetic stimulation and some opiate receptor activity. Finally, PCP is capable of causing vasospasm in a variety of vascular beds.

The hallmark of PCP intoxication is unpredictability. Common findings in adults include hypertension, nystagmus, tachycardia, diaphoresis, miosis or mydriasis, and altered consciousness.[173] Patients may be entirely alert, extremely agitated, and violent, then suddenly unresponsive and comatose. Mental status changes include confusion, disorientation, delusions, and sometimes visual or auditory hallucinations. An acute psychosis mimicking schizophrenia has been described. Abnormal movements including choreoathetosis, dystonic posturing, and opisthotonus have been reported. Patients presenting with self-mutilation should lead caregivers to consider PCP use as the cause. With extremely high doses, seizures may develop. During emergence from severe, acute PCP intoxication, symptoms more characteristic of mild intoxication then appear in a waxing and waning fashion. Rhabdomyolysis, often associated with severe agitation, can result in renal failure and represents a major cause of morbidity in older patients.[173]

Interestingly, children have a somewhat different clinical presentation with lethargy being the most common symptom. Staring episodes, intermittent agitation, ataxia, opisthotonus, and nystagmus are also frequently noted.[176, 177] Seizures, hypertension, and coma are less likely, and aggressive behavior is notably absent.

Treatment involves the ABCs of life support along with supportive measures. Extremely agitated adolescents should be placed in a quiet environment. "Pharmacologic" restraint with benzodiazepines such as midazolam (0.05 to 0.2 mg/kg IV) or diazepam (0.1 to 0.4 mg/kg IV) or with haloperidol (0.1 to 0.3 mg/kg IM) is preferred to physical restraint because of the concern that isometric muscle contractions against restraining devices may precipitate or accentuate rhabdomyolysis. Phenothiazines are contraindicated because they lower the seizure threshold. When present, dystonia can be treated with diphenhydramine (1.0 to 2.0 mg/kg IV). Although physostigmine may reverse some of the symptoms associated with PCP intoxication[178] (e.g., tremors, nystagmus, agitation), it is not recommended for use because it may accentuate cholinergic symptoms.

Seizures are treated with lorazepam (0.05 to 0.2 mg/kg IV) or diazepam (0.2 to 0.4 mg/kg IV), but most seizures are brief and will resolve without therapy. To our knowledge, young children have not been reported to develop rhabdomyolysis, but adolescent patients may, and urine and serum tests for myoglobin should be performed. As mentioned, phencyclidine clearance may be enhanced by acidification of gastrointestinal contents to prevent further absorption and by acidification of urine. Ascorbic acid and ammonium chloride have been utilized for this purpose.[177, 179] Concerns about aggravating renal deposition of myoglobin and the fact that less than 15% of PCP is renally cleared make urinary acidification controversial. It is probably more prudent to simply use forced diuresis with IV hydration and diuretics and avoid urinary acidification.

Deaths from PCP intoxication appear to be related to simultaneous use of other drugs, traffic accidents, drownings, and homicide.[173]

Lysergic acid diethylamide (LSD) is a water-soluble compound that is tasteless, odorless, and colorless. Intoxication usually follows oral intake of foods previously "treated" with the agent or paper containing blots of the chemical. It can also be insufflated, smoked, or injected. It is produced by chemical synthesis combining lysergic acid with diethylamine. Related compounds are found naturally in morning glory plants such as *Rivea corynbosa* and *Ipomoea violacea*.

Symptoms generally begin within 30 to 60 minutes following oral ingestion. The drug has a half-life of 100 to 175 minutes and is excreted primarily in stool after biliary concentration.[173]

The precise mechanism of action of LSD is unknown. One theory is that it inhibits serotonin with resultant disinhibition of sensory and higher cortical functions which in turn produces distortions of perception and thought. Alternatively, LSD may alter postsynaptic dopaminergic receptors, perhaps explaining LSD-induced psychosis. More than likely, both serotonergic and dopaminergic neurotransmission are altered.[180, 181]

Signs and symptoms of LSD use include nausea, flushing, chills, tachycardia, hypertension, and tremor. These may be followed by altered affect, time distortion, illusions (both visual and auditory), and synesthesia (feeling colors or seeing sounds). Altered perception may frighten users or they may become "philosophical" and expound on thoughts and ideas. Symptoms generally resolve in 6 to 12 hours. "Flashbacks" in which symptoms recur without repeat usage are not uncommon and appear to be related to increased use.[182]

Treatment is entirely supportive and seldom involves major invasive modalities. Verbal reassurance is often effective to counteract fear. As with other intoxications marked by agitation or acute psychosis, benzodiazepines and/or haloperidol are useful (see discussion under phencyclidine). Hospitalization is often unnecessary, but infants and small children probably should be observed for 24 hours as convulsions have been reported.[183, 184] No deaths have been reported from LSD intoxication in any age group.

Other agents in the broad category of hallucinogens include the *phenylalkylamines* and the *indolealkylamines*. DMT is the prototype indolealkylamine. It produces visual distortions similar to LSD but has a very short onset of action and half-life. The phenylalkylamines are subdivided into the phenylethylamines (e.g., mescaline) and the phenylisopropylamines (e.g., 4-methyl-2,5-dimethoxyamphetamine). These substances rarely cause pediatric intoxication. Excellent reviews are available elsewhere.[173, 185]

NON-MEDICINAL POISONINGS

Organophosphates

Organophosphate intoxications are the most common of all pesticide poisonings. This appears to be due to their wide use as agricultural, animal, household, and golf course insecticides. They are ideal for agricultural use because they have an unstable chemical structure[186] that allows them to disintegrate into harmless compounds several days after application.[187]

Despite their rapid disappearance from the environment, they are highly toxic substances capable of being rapidly absorbed from the respiratory, gastrointestinal, ocular, and dermal routes. They have been classified as having high, intermediate, or low toxicity.[187] Parathion appears to be the most important human toxin.

Following absorption from one or several of the aforementioned routes, organophosphates bind to cholinesterase enzymes, resulting in excess acetylcholine activity. The two major human cholinesterases are acetylcholinesterase (true cholinesterase) found in nervous tissue and red blood cells and pseudocholinesterase, which is found in the liver and in the serum. When organophosphates bind to cholinesterases, the resultant complex inactivates the cholinesterase, and, if not reversed, the binding may become virtually irreversible.[188]

Clinically, most of the toxicologic effects of the organophosphates are due to acetylcholinesterase inhibition. Therefore, red blood cell (true) cholinesterase levels more accurately reflect the significance of organophosphate poisoning. Unfortunately, most hospital laboratories measure pseudocholinesterase levels. The value of pseudocholinesterase measurements is due to the fact that levels fall more rapidly and return to normal more rapidly than red cell (acetyl-) cholinesterase levels.[189, 190] Thus, pseudocholinesterase levels aid in both the differential diagnosis and monitoring of organophosphate poisonings.

For symptoms to develop, a greater than 50% reduction in cholinesterase enzyme activity must occur. This can take place rapidly or over many hours, depending upon the type of exposure and the exact compound. Initial symptoms include headache, dizziness, weakness, sweating, hypersalivation, lacrimation, abdominal cramps, wheezing, and diarrhea. The propensity for gastrointestinal symptoms has caused organophosphate poisoning to be mistaken for acute gastroenteritis.[191] Miosis, muscle fasciculations, bronchorrhea, and bradycardia may also be seen. In severe intoxications, respiratory muscle paralysis, pulmonary edema, and convulsions can develop.[187] Other severe manifestations include coma, pancreatitis,[192] and dysrhythmias.[193]

Proper emergency management is required for even mildly symptomatic patients. Aggressive removal of any cutaneous agent must be performed with copious amounts of soap and water. Health care workers must wear gloves and other protective garments to prevent their accidental exposure. We believe induced emesis for oral ingestions in alert children is indicated even if the organophosphate was contained in a hydrocarbon carrier. Indications for gastric lavage are similar to those for most other poisonings. Activated charcoal and a cathartic should also be used.

A secure airway is vital, particularly when bronchorrhea or pulmonary edema is present. Endotracheal intubation should be handled expectantly rather than emergently. Respiratory compromise may be due to bronchorrhea, excess salivation, pulmonary edema, aspiration, muscle paralysis, or even the adult respiratory distress syndrome. Theophylline-like preparations are not indicated for wheezing.[187]

Cardiac monitoring should be started upon presentation as dysrhythmias have been reported. Bradydysrhythmias are the most common, but ventricular tachycardia and QT-interval prolongation have also been reported.[194]

Atropine sulfate in high doses can be used both diagnostically and therapeutically. An initial dose of 0.05 mg/kg IV should be followed by maintenance doses of 0.02 mg/kg IV every 15 to 30 minutes in an effort to "atropinize" the patient. Signs of adequate "atropinization" include flushing, dry mouth, and dilated pupils. Tachycardia is not a reliable sign, as cholinesterase inhibition is capable of producing tachycardia.[195] Atropine will reverse central and muscarinic effects, but not nicotinic effects (muscle weakness, fasciculations, paralysis). It should be continued for at least 24 hours in severe poisonings. If atropine toxicity occurs, marked by fever, muscle fasciculations, and delirium, atropine should be withheld. If cholinergic symptoms recur, atropine must then be reinstituted.

Fortunately, specific antidote therapy is available. Pralidoxime iodide (PAM, 2-PAM) and pralidoxime chloride (Protopam) can be used interchangeably. These oximes reactivate cholinesterases by cleaving the phosphorylated bond between the organophosphate and acetylcholinesterase, by directly detoxifying the organophosphate, and by its own anticholinergic effects.[196] Delays in therapy must be avoided to prevent irreversible organophosphate-acetylcholinesterase binding. Waiting for cholinesterase levels in symptomatic patients is inappropriate.

Pralidoxime preparations should be placed in 5% dextrose with 0.45 normal saline solution in doses of 25 to 50 mg/kg and should be administered over 10 to 30 minutes. Older children and adolescents should receive 0.5 to 1.0 g over the same time period. One to two hours after the initial dose, a second equal dose should be infused followed by a third dose 12 hours later if cholinergic signs persist or recur. Side effects include nausea, headache, dizziness, diplopia, hypertension, and respiratory depression. Treatment for more than 24 hours is seldom necessary. Additional therapy is supportive and depends on associated findings.[12]

Hydrocarbons

Hydrocarbons are derived from crude oil (petroleum distillates) or pine oil. This group is chemically very heterogeneous but clinically quite similar. Hydrocarbons are found around most households, often placed in containers meant for other uses such as soft drink bottles, making them accessible to toddlers.[197-199]

Hydrocarbon ingestions occur more than 28,000 times per year in children under age 5.[200, 201] They account for a comparatively high mortality with reports ranging from 5 to 25 percent. The most commonly ingested substances in decreasing order are gasoline, turpentine and pine oil, mineral spirits, kerosene, lubricating oils, and lighter fluid.[202] Kerosene ingestion is particularly common in the southeastern United States. Seasonal differences in incidence also exist.

Three important physical properties of hydrocarbons help determine their toxic potential: viscosity, the resistance to flow or change in form; surface tension, the molecular cohesiveness at air-liquid interfaces; and volatility, the tendency of liquids to become gases. Low viscosity favors easy spread along contacted surfaces, particularly the oropharyngeal, tracheal, and bronchial mucosae. Low surface tension also favors spreading of the toxic agent, while high volatility increases aspiration potential. Contact with warm mucosal surfaces increases volatility, resulting in cough and aspiration.

We prefer to divide these compounds into only two groups based upon their potential for extensive injury beyond the respiratory system. The aromatic hydrocarbons, primarily benzene, toluene, and xylene, make up one group. Benzene is the prototype aromatic hydrocarbon and perhaps the most toxic.[203] It is rapidly absorbed from the gastrointestinal tract and is taken up readily in neural tissue. Following an early excitatory phase, benzene and its derivatives can cause CNS depression. Respiratory depression and overt respiratory failure may ensue. Benzene also can cause renal injury,[204] hepatic injury,[205] hematopoietic abnormalities,[205] pulmonary edema,[203] and myocardial sensitization to catecholamines.[206]

Aliphatic hydrocarbons including turpentine comprise the second group, which primarily cause only pulmonary injuries, although pine oil and turpentine can cause gastrointestinal and CNS changes. Pulmonary injury occurs secondary to aspiration and often occurs with minimal or no actual ingestion. Although some gastrointestinal absorption does occur, it is minimal. Numerous animal studies have demonstrated the minimal importance of gastrointestinal absorption in most hydrocarbon intoxications.[199, 207]

Despite the pleasant scent of many hydrocarbons, their taste is generally foul and a burning sensation occurs quickly following contact with oral mucous membranes. Initial CNS symptoms are primarily related to hypoxia from either displacement of oxygen from alveoli (such as with gasoline sniffing) or from the rapid onset of pulmonary injury.

Pulmonary abnormalities are the crucial derangements caused by hydrocarbons. An early, acute alveolitis peaks around 3 days after aspiration that is characterized by inflammation, necrosis, edema formation, and hemorrhage.[208] A chronic, proliferative alveolitis develops at around 10 days, marked by alveolar thickening or hyaline membrane formation.[208] Complications can include pneumothorax, pneumatocele formation, bacterial pneumonia, bronchiectasis, and small airways disease.[202] Ventilation-perfusion abnormalities include intrapulmonary shunting and increased dead space ventilation.[208] Bronchospasm can develop early or can be delayed.

Other organ system involvement can occur but is somewhat uncommon and often of no major clinical significance. These include fatty infiltration of the liver, gastrointestinal ulceration, intravascular hemolysis,[209] myocardial degeneration, and renal tubular dysfunction.[210]

Vomiting is often the initial clinical symptom. Coughing, choking, gagging, and dyspnea may be present early. Tachypnea with or without cyanosis may ensue. Fever, leukocytosis, and pulmonary infiltrates can develop in the first 6 hours.[211] Auscultation may reveal rales, rhonchi, and wheezing, alone or in any combination. Patients who remain asymptomatic for 6 hours are unlikely to develop clinically important findings.[211] It seems prudent to observe asymptomatic patients for 6 hours and then discharge them. We advocate hospitalization for all symptomatic patients.

Gastric emptying remains controversial, but our review of the literature leads us to advocate induced emesis with ipecac for ingestion of aromatic hydrocarbons or when the hydrocarbon is in a mixture with another highly toxic substance such as an organophosphate, heavy metal, or camphor. We previously advocated induced emesis for large volume (>1 ml/kg) ingestions[12] but determining the actual volume ingested is fraught with many uncertainties, and we now hesitate to advocate emesis in such situations. It should be obvious that obtunded patients should never undergo induced emesis, especially with hydrocarbon ingestions. Nasogastric lavage is dangerous, as dilatation of the gastroesophageal junction by the lavage tube may increase the likelihood of aspiration. We discourage this therapeutic measure.

Administration of oils such as mineral oil or olive oil in an effort to alter the hydrocarbon's viscosity is contraindicated. These agents can themselves be aspirated, compounding pulmonary injury.

There appears to be no role for either corticosteroids or prophylactic antibiotics in this form of aspiration pneumonia.[198, 212] Antibiotic use should follow infectious symptoms such as leukocytosis and fever, but these symptoms may appear before actual infection. It is therefore more prudent to obtain tracheobronchial aspirates or washings at least 48 hours after presentation and then let Gram stain and culture findings determine the need for antibiotics. Corticosteroids appear to play no definitive role in preventing an adult respiratory distress syndrome-type injury but may have a limited role later by altering potential for pulmonary fibrosis.

Respiratory support should initially be with supplemental oxygen. Measuring arterial oxygenation by either pulse oximetry or repeated arterial blood gas measurement is indicated if significant pulmonary involvement develops.

Endotracheal intubation and mechanical ventilation will be necessary for those unable to maintain adequate arterial oxygen saturation in 60% inspired oxygen. Intubation should be via rapid sequence induction to minimize the likelihood of further aspiration. Positive end-expiratory pressure (PEEP) may improve arterial oxygenation but must be used cautiously as pneumothorax and cardiovascular compromise are ever-present dangers. Sedation with opioids or benzodiazepines along with neuromuscular blockade may lessen the risk of pneumothorax.

Newer methods of respiratory support, including high-frequency ventilation and extracorporeal lung support may be helpful. The former offers the opportunity to effectuate adequate gas exchange at relatively lower mean airway pressures, thus reducing the risk of pneumothorax. Extracorporeal support via arteriovenous ECMO (extracorporeal membrane oxygenation) or venovenous $ECCO_2R$ (extracorporeal carbon dioxide removal) provides adequate oxygen and removes carbon dioxide with minimal or no lung support.

In addition to pulmonary support, the cardiovascular and renal systems may require attention. Experiments using plasmapheresis to decrease extravascular lung water by limiting intravascular hydrostatic pressure suggest that circulating volume should be kept to minimal levels with provision of just enough circulating volume to avoid compromising cardiovascular or renal integrity.[213] Although plasmapheresis is impractical in most clinical settings, monitoring and controlling filling pressures can be achieved with central venous or pulmonary arterial catheterization. We believe there may also be a role for continuous arteriovenous hemofiltration (CAVH) in lowering transcapillary hydrostatic pressure.

Caustics

Caustic ingestions are of interest to the critical care physician because of their potential for acute upper airway problems, esophageal perforation, mediastinitis, lower respiratory tract injury, gastric perforation, and intestinal perforation. The incidence of caustic substance ingestion is unknown, but conservative estimates suggest as many as 15,000 cases per year with many occurring in pediatric patients.[214] Like most other pediatric poisonings, caustic ingestions involve a bimodal age distribution with the majority occurring in those less than 5 years of age.[215] In children, caustic burns of the esophagus involve sodium hydroxide or lye 75% of the time with 83% of such cases occurring in those less than 3 years of age.[216]

The most common caustic substances ingested are alkalis, including liquid drain cleaners, paste oven cleaners, Clinitest tablets, ammonia and ammonium hydroxide, disc batteries, detergents, and household bleach.[214, 216–218] Of these, only household-strength detergents and household bleach (sodium hypochlorite) appear to be relatively benign. Sodium hypochlorite has a pH of 6 and appears to cause only mucosal inflammation and edema without necrosis.[219] As such, stricture formation does not occur.

On the other hand, sodium hydroxide is extremely caustic. Although household products are now available only in dilute forms (liquids less than 10% sodium hydroxide), industrial-strength liquids may contain up to 30% and crystals and pellets may be pure sodium hydroxide. The liquid agents are tasteless and odorless. The lack of taste and absence of burning prevent the activation of protective reflexes, and the substance generally proceeds to the posterior pharynx and esophagus where the major injury occurs. Liquid products have a high specific gravity, making injury to the lower esophagus and stomach possible. Soft tissues of the upper airway may be involved, with rapid onset of inflammation and edema.[217, 220, 221]

In the esophagus, strong alkali produces liquefaction necrosis with severe injuries extending through the muscular layers and into the mediastinum.[217, 220, 221] Bacteria may then pass through the denuded mucosa or directly through a perforation to create an inflammatory and infectious mediastinitis. Extension to the pleural and pericardial spaces may develop. In the absence of perforation and mediastinitis, esophageal strictures resulting from fibrous healing of the injured sites are the major cause of morbidity.[214, 217, 220–224]

Ammonia and ammonium hydroxide have associated vapor production, and pulmonary injury can occur in addition to, or independent of, mucosal injuries and esophageal burns.[225] Clinitest tablets also contain strong alkaline agents capable of producing caustic and thermal injuries to the esophagus. Stricture formation following ingestion of these tablets is quite common.[226]

Disc batteries that pass through the esophagus and stomach into the intestine are generally not a clinical problem. Stools should be checked for several days to ensure passage from the gastrointestinal tract, and serial radiographs are helpful in following their course. Those that lodge in the esophagus require immediate removal prior to leakage of any contents.[214, 218] These devices contain heavy metals such as mercury, zinc, silver, nickel, and cadmium in concentrated alkaline solutions, and injury from the caustic alkali can be compounded by heavy metal intoxication.

Corrosive acids, such as sulfuric, hydrochloric, and phosphoric acids, are found in toilet bowl cleaners, battery fluids, swimming pool cleaners, soldering fluxes, and antirust compounds. They cause immediate burning and have a bitter taste and are therefore expectorated quickly and very little is usually swallowed. Upon contact with mucosal surfaces and the esophagus, strong acids cause coagulation necrosis rather than liquefaction necrosis. The resulting injuries seldom extend beyond the mucosa and strictures are rare.[214]

As acidic corrosives pass along the lesser curvature of the stomach, they reach the pylorus and create pylorospasm. This leads to pooling of the acid in the prepyloric area, which can cause deep ulceration or perforation in this area.[214]

Regardless of whether the caustic agent is alkaline or acidic, emesis is contraindicated as is placement of a lavage tube. Initial care may include administration of a small amount of water to dilute any residual agent remaining on oral or esophageal mucosal surfaces. Neutralizing agents are generally not recommended as mixing alkaline and acidic materials results in an exothermic reaction that may exacerbate the injury.[214]

When an ingestion occurs, effort should be made to determine the precise content of the substance and the amount ingested. Although references disagree over exactly who should undergo esophagascopy,[214, 222, 224] we believe all those ingesting a sufficiently caustic agent should undergo esophagoscopy within 12 hours of ingestion. The endoscope should be passed only as far as the initial esophageal lesion encountered as deeper passage greatly increases the likelihood of traumatic perforation. Grading of lesions at esophagoscopy has therapeutic as well as prognostic value.[221, 222]

Most authors recommend corticosteroids in doses of 2 mg/kg/day of methylprednisolone for up to 21 days with gradual tapering over 2 to 3 weeks.[214, 217, 220, 221] The use of antimicrobials is more controversial. On an empiric basis, the advantages of using prophylactic antibiotics seem to outweigh the risks, but no carefully designed studies on the efficacy of corticosteroids or antibiotics exist. When prescribed, coverage for gram-positive organisms found in oral flora should be obtained.

For those sustaining injuries to the lower esophagus or stomach, antacid therapy with either an H_2-receptor antagonist or therapeutic doses of antacids should be used for 6 to 8 weeks as the original injury may be exacerbated by excess stomach acid.

Contrast esophagrams are utilized to document the presence of strictures and their location, number, and length.[224] Early use of water-soluble agents is helpful to determine severity or the presence of perforation.

The likelihood of stricture formation in those without documented esophageal burns is slight, occurring in one report in only 2 of 330 cases.[227] Patients with ulceration have been reported to have an incidence of eventual stricture formation in the 2 to 4% range.[221, 222] Patients developing strictures will require either antegrade or retrograde dilatation, some for the rest of their lives. Those failing to benefit from dilatation may require colon interposition to obtain satisfactory esophageal function.[217]

Experiments in animals have involved placing "stents" in the esophagus so that scar formation will result in a functional lumen.[228] "Lathyrogen" compounds have been used successfully in animals to interfere with collagen crosslinkage, thus reducing scar formation.[229] These techniques are not yet available for human use.

Finally, there appears to be a clear predisposition to esophageal carcinoma in those ingesting caustic materials. As many as 5% of patients with esophageal carcinoma have a history of caustic substance ingestion.[230]

Mushroom Poisoning

The toxic properties of mushrooms have been known for thousands of years. Over the centuries these properties have been differentiated into adverse and beneficial effects. Desirable effects have been ascribed to those mushrooms causing euphoria followed by hallucinations. They are intentionally used in some cultures during religious ceremonies and in others as drugs of abuse.

Psychotropic changes occur in response to the central nervous system effects of the indoles found in the *Psilocybe* genus, which contains more than 100 species.[231] Clinically, those ingesting these mushrooms develop symptoms 30 to 60 minutes after ingestion.[231, 232] Euphoria followed by hallucinations are noted; tachycardia, mydriasis, and paresthesias may develop and seizures have been reported. Therapy involves supportive care, often in the form of gentle reassurance. Occasionally, mild anxiolysis or sedation with agents such as midazolam may be necessary. Flashbacks are known to occur.

Life-threatening mushroom intoxications are limited to ingestions of certain members of the *Amanita* genus, but the *Gyromitra* genus also has several dangerous species. The deadliest of all mushrooms is clearly *Amanita phylloides*. It contains two groups of toxins, the amatoxins and the phallotoxins. Cooking may fail to denature these toxins and ingestion of one mushroom cap can be fatal to an adult.[233] Toxic effects appear to be related primarily to the amatoxins, of which α-amanitin is the principal agent. This substance causes nucleolar destruction in hepatocytes with inhibition of RNA polymerase II, resulting in interference with DNA transcription.[231, 234–238] Although extremely potent, the phallotoxins are very poorly absorbed and appear to play only a minor role in symptomatology.[231]

A. phylloides poisoning can be clinically divided into three stages.[233, 239] The first stage is characterized by abdominal pain, cramps, nausea, vomiting, and diarrhea 6 to 14 hours after ingestion. There is usually resolution of this stage within 24 to 36 hours. The second stage is a quiescent period with few or no clinical symptoms, but with laboratory evidence of ensuing hepatocellular and renal damage characterized by elevations in serum transaminases, urea nitrogen, and creatinine. The third stage is marked by massive hepatocellular dysfunction and acute renal failure noted 2 to 4 days after ingestion. Bleeding, hypoglycemia, sepsis, and coma can occur.

Treatment is generally supportive with more intensive therapy based upon the severity of hepatic and renal dysfunction. Initial care consists of gastric emptying and prevention of gastrointestinal absorption. For recent ingestions, emesis should be induced. Once the first clinical stage begins, replacement of fluids and electrolytes is essential. Monitoring of hepatic and renal function should also be started at this time, and surveillance of visceral organ function should continue through the second stage. As hepatic and renal failure ensue, intensive supportive care with maintenance of circulating volume, control of bleeding, prevention of hypoglycemia, and reduction of serum ammonia levels are required as with any case involving hepatic failure.

A variety of other therapeutic modalities have been utilized. Thioctic acid, a Krebs cycle coenzyme, in doses of 300 mg/kg/day intravenously has been reported to be useful in several studies.[236, 240, 241] Its precise mechanism of action remains unclear and its efficacy has not been substantiated in controlled trials.[242] Penicillin in doses of 300,000 to 1,000,000 units/kg/day has been advocated based upon in vitro evidence that it reduces or inhibits hepatic uptake of amatoxins.[239, 243, 244] Silymarin (silibinin), a compound extracted from the milk thistle, also appears to diminish hepatic uptake of amatoxins.[238, 244, 245] Corticosteroids have also been advocated, but no evidence for efficacy is available.[232]

Recently in a murine model of *Amanita* poisoning, the H_2-receptor antagonist cimetidine was shown to protect against hepatocellular destruction caused by intraperitoneal injection of α-amatoxin.[246] Its potential beneficial effects may be due to competitive inhibition of cytochrome P_{450} and/or reducing hepatic blood flow and thereby decreasing amatoxin hepatic uptake.

Several recent case reports of successful liver transplantation following *Amanita* poisoning indicate that this therapy may allow survival in otherwise terminal cases.[244, 247]

As stated earlier, mushrooms of the *Gyromitra* genus may be highly poisonous if sufficient toxin is absorbed.[231, 232, 234, 239] These mushrooms contain monomethylhydrazine, which causes clinical manifestations similar to those in isoniazid poisoning by inhibiting CNS formation of GABA. Vomiting, diarrhea, dizziness, and muscle cramps may be seen, and delirium, coma, and convulsions can occur in severe cases. Methemoglobinemia and hemolysis have also been reported.[231] Intravenous pyridoxine is used for seizures as it is a cofactor for GABA synthesis. It may also act as an antidote by complexing with monomethylhydrazine. Doses of 10 to 100 mg/kg/dose with a maximum dose of 5 g seem appropriate.[239]

Ingestion of other types of mushrooms can also cause clinical manifestations, many of which occur shortly after ingestion. Anticholineric effects are seen 30 to 120 minutes following ingestion of *A. muscarina* and *A. pantherina*.[231, 232] Despite the presence of muscarine in *A. muscarina*, anticholinergic rather than cholinergic effects predominate. The presence of muscimol and ibotenic acid in these mushrooms can produce ataxia, euphoria, and hallucinations, and seizures, psychotic reactions, and coma can develop with large ingestions. Physostigmine may reverse the CNS symptoms, but extreme caution should be used with this potentially dangerous agent. Additional therapy is entirely supportive.

Cholinergic symptoms are noticed within 30 to 60 minutes following the ingestion of *Inocybe* and *Clitocybe* species, but they are usually mild and self limited. In severe cases, atropine in doses of 0.01 mg/kg (minimum 0.10 mg/dose) should be given and repeated as often as is necessary to reverse the major symptoms.

Severe disulfiram-like reactions can be seen following the ingestion of *Coprinus atramentarius* with ethanol. Flushing, palpitations, dyspnea, chest pain, and diaphoresis have been seen even with ethanol intake after as much as 5 days or more.[231, 232] As with disulfiram, the coprine found in this mushroom appears to inhibit ethanol metabolism with acetaldehyde accumulation. Treatment requires only adequate fluid replacement, and symptoms usually resolve after several hours.

Finally, mushrooms of the *Cortinarius* genus can contain the bipyridyl toxins orelline and orellanine.[231] Gastritis, chills, headaches, and myalgias can develop the day after ingestion. A small percentage of afflicted patients will then develop acute renal failure characterized by tubulointerstitial nephritis with fibrosis. The delayed onset of symptoms prohibits gastrointestinal decontamination. Therefore, therapy is directed toward detection and then treatment of any resulting renal failure.

References

1. Rumack BH: Acetaminophen overdose in young children—treatment and effects of alcohol and other additional ingestants in 417 cases. Am J Dis Child 138:428, 1984.
2. Wilson JT, Kasantikul V, Harbison R, et al: Death in an adolescent following an overdose of acetaminophen and phenobarbital. Am J Dis Child 132:466, 1978.
3. Mitchell AA, Lovejoy FH, Slone D, et al: Acetaminophen and aspirin: Prescription, use and accidental ingestion among children. Am J Dis Child 136:976, 1982.
4. Rumack BH: Acetaminophen overdose in children and adolescents. Pediatr Clin North Am 33:691, 1986.
5. Lieh-Lai MW, Sarnaik AP, Newton JF, et al: Metabolism and pharmacokinetics of acetaminophen in a severely poisoned young child. J Pediatr 105:125, 1984.
6. Miller RP, Robert RJ, and Fischer LF: Acetaminophen elimination kinetics in neonates, children and adults. Clin Pharmacol Ther 19:284, 1976.
7. Davis MG, Valla Briffa D, and Greaves M: Systemic toxicity for topically applied salicylic acid. Br Med J 1:661, 1979.
8. Portman B, Talbot IC, Day DW, et al: Histopathological changes in the liver following a paracetamol overdose: Correlation with clinical and biochemical parameters. J Pathol 117:169, 1975.
9. Boyd JA and Eling TE: Prostaglandin endoperoxide synthetase–dependent cooxidation of acetaminophen to intermediates which covalently bind in vitro to rabbit renal medullary microsomes. J Pharmacol Exp Ther 219:659, 1981.
10. Mohandas J, Duggin G, Horvath J, et al: Metabolic oxidation of acetaminophen (paracetamol) mediated by cytochrome P 450 mixed function oxidase and prostaglandin endoperoxide synthetase in rabbit kidney. Toxicol Appl Pharmacol 61:252, 1981.
11. Hamlyn AN, Douglas AP, and James O: The spectrum of paracetamol (acetaminophen) overdose: Clinical and epidemiological studies. Postgrad Med J 54:400, 1978.
12. Steinhart CM and Pearson-Shaver AL: Poisoning. Crit Care Clin 4:845, 1988.
13. Rumack BH and Matthew H: Acetaminophen poisoning and toxicity. Pediatrics 55:871, 1975.
14. Strubelt O, Siegers CP, and Schutt A: The curative effects of cysteamine, cysteine, and dithiocarb in experimental paracetamol poisoning. Arch Toxicol (Berl) 33:55, 1974.
15. Snodgrass WR: Salicylate toxicity. Pediatr Clin North Am 33:381, 1986.
16. Flower RJ, Moncada S, and Vane JR: Analgesics-antipyretics and antiinflammatory agents: Drugs employed in the treatment of gout. In: Goodman-Gilman A, Goodman LS, and Murad F (eds): The Pharmacologic Basis of Therapeutics, 7th ed. New York, Macmillan, 1985, pp. 680–689.
17. Ferguson RK and Boutros AR: Death following self-poisoning in a children's hospital: A 2-year experience, Pediatrics 77:144, 1986.
18. Levy G and Yaffe SF: Relationship between dose and apparent volume of distribution of salicylates in children. Pediatrics 54:713, 1974.
19. Hartwig-Otto H: Pharmacokinetic considerations of common analgesics and antipyretics. Am J Med 75(Suppl):9, 1980.
20. Gabow PA, Anderson RJ, Potts DE, et al: Acid-base disturbances in the salicylate-intoxicated adult. Arch Intern Med 138:1481, 1978.
21. Temple AR: Pathophysiology of aspirin overdosage toxicity, with implications for management. Pediatrics 62(Suppl):873, 1978.
22. Bartels PD and Lund-Jacobsen H: Blood lactate and ketone body concentrations in salicylate intoxication. Human Toxicol 5:363, 1986.
23. Proudfoot AT: Salicylates and salicylamide. In: Haddad LM and Winchester JF (eds): Clinical Management of Poisoning and Drug Overdose, 2nd ed. Philadelphia, WB Saunders, 1990, pp. 909–920.
24. Meredith TJ and Vale JA: Non-narcotic analgesics. Problems of overdose. Drugs 32(Suppl 4):177, 1986.
25. Proudfoot AT: Toxicity of salicylates. Am J Med 75(Suppl):99, 1983.
26. Pettit JM and Biggs JT: Tricyclic antidepressant overdoses in adolescent patients. Pediatrics 59:283, 1977.
27. Callahan M: Epidemiology of fatal tricyclic antidepressant ingestion: Implications for management. Ann Emerg Med 14:1, 1985.
28. Crome P and Newman B: The problem of tricyclic antidepressant poisoning. Postgrad Med J 55:528, 1979.
29. Hollister L: Tricyclic antidepressants. N Engl J Med 299, 1106, 1978.
30. Horn AS: The mode of action of tricyclic antidepressants. A brief review of recent progress. Postgrad Med J 56(Suppl):30, 1983.
31. Pentel P, Keyler DE, and Haddad LM: Tricyclics and newer antidepressants. In: Haddad LM and Winchester JF (eds): Clinical Management of Poisoning and Drug Overdose, 2nd ed. Philadelphia, WB Saunders, 1990, pp. 636–655.
32. Frommer DA, Kulig KW, Marx JA, et al: Tricyclic antidepressant overdose: A review. JAMA 257:521, 1987.
33. Sullivan J, Peterson R, and Rumack B: The plasma protein binding of amitriptyline with pH. Presented to the American Academy of Toxicology, Minneapolis, MN, August 15, 1980.
34. Baldessarini RJ: Drugs and the treatment of psychiatric disorders. In: Goodman-Gilman A, Goodman LS, and Murad F (eds): The Pharmacological Basis of Therapeutics, 7th ed. New York, Macmillan, 1985, pp. 413–423.
35. Spiker DG, Biggs JT: Tricyclic antidepressants: Prolonged plasma levels after overdose. JAMA 236:1711, 1976.
36. Nicotra MB, Rivera M, Pool JL, et al: Tricyclic antidepressant overdose: Clinical and pharmacologic observations. Clin Toxicol 18:599, 1981.
37. Rudorfer MV: Cardiovascular changes and plasma drug levels after amitriptyline overdose. J Toxicol 19:67, 1982.
38. Smith RK and O'Mara K: Tricyclic antidepressant overdose. J Fam Pract 15:247, 1982.
39. Mack RB: Imipramine overdose—prejudiced and proud. Contemp Pediatrics 5:93, 1988.
40. Braden NJ, Jackson JE, and Walson PD: Tricyclic antidepressant overdose. Pediatr Clin North Am 33:287, 1986.
41. Roberts MJ, Mueller S, and Laver RM: Propranolol in the treatment of cardiac arrhythmias associated with amitriptyline intoxication. J Pediatr 82:65, 1973.
42. Stein B and Volans GN: Dixarit overdose: The problem of attractive tablets. Br Med J 2:667, 1978.
43. Conner CS and Watanabe AS: Clonidine overdose: A review. Am J Hosp Pharm 36:906, 1979.
44. Dollery CT, Davies DS, Draffan GH, et al: Clinical pharmacology and pharmacokinetics of clonidine. Clin Pharmacol Ther 19:11, 1976.
45. Jain AK, Ryan JR, Vargas R, et al: Efficacy and acceptability of different dosage schedules of clonidine. Clin Pharmacol Ther 21:382, 1977.
46. Davis DS, Wing LMH, Reid JL, et al: Pharmacokinetics and pharmacological studies with clonidine in normal subjects. Clin Sci Mol Med 51:6395, 1976.
47. Mroczek WJ, Davidov M, and Finnerty FA: Intravenous clonidine in hypertensive patients. Clin Pharmacol Ther 14:847, 1971.
48. Naylor, WG, Rosenbaum M, McInnes I, et al: Effect of a new hypotensive drug, ST-155, on the systemic circulation. Am Heart J 72:764, 1966.
49. Onesti G, Bock KD, Heimsoth B, et al: Clonidine: A new antihypertensive agent. Am J Cardiol 28:74, 1971.
50. Anderson RJ, Hart GR, Crumpler CP, et al: Clonidine overdose: Report of six cases and review of the literature. Ann Emerg Med 10:107, 1981.

51. Hunyor SN, Bradstock K, Sommerville PJ, et al: Clonidine overdose. Br Med J 4:23, 1975.
52. Marruecos L, Roglan A, Frat MW, et al: Clonidine overdose. Crit Care Med 11:959, 1983.
53. Heidemann SM and Sarnaik AP: Clonidine poisoning in children. Crit Care Med 18:618, 1990.
54. Wiley JF, Wiley CC, Torrey SB, et al: Clonidine poisoning in young children. J Pediatr 116:654, 1990.
55. Gold MS and Pottash AC: The neurobiological implications of clonidine HCl. Ann NY Acad Sci 362:191, 1981.
56. Martin PR, Ebert MH, Gordon EK, et al: Effects of clonidine on central and peripheral catecholamine metabolism. Clin Pharmacol Ther 35:322, 1984.
57. Pai GA and Lipsitz DJ: Clonidine poisoning. Pediatrics 58:749, 1976.
58. Roberts, JR and Zink, BJ: Clonidine. In: Haddad LM and Winchester JF (eds): Clinical Management of Poisoning and Drug Overdose, 2nd ed. Philadelphia, WB Saunders, 1990, pp. 1351–1359.
59. North OS, Wieland MJ, Peterson CD, et al: Naloxone administration in clonidine overdosage. Ann Emerg Med 10:317, 1981.
60. Kulig K, Duffy J, and Rumack BH: Naloxone for treatment of clonidine overdose. JAMA 247:1697, 1982.
61. Banner W, Lund ME, and Clawson L: Failure of naloxone to reverse clonidine toxic effect. Am J Dis Child 137:170, 1983.
62. Litovitz TL, Martin TG, and Schmitz B: 1986 Annual Report of the American Association of Poison Control Centers National Data Collection System. Am J Emerg Med 5:405, 1987.
63. Eisen TF, Lacouture PG, and Lovejoy FH: Iron. In: Haddad LM and Winchester JF (eds): Clinical Management of Poisoning and Drug Overdose, 2nd ed. Philadelphia, WB Saunders, 1990, pp. 1010–1017.
64. Robotham JL and Leitman PS: Acute iron poisoning—a review. Am J Dis Child 134:876, 1980.
65. Reynolds LG and Klein M: Iron poisoning—preventable hazard of childhood. S Afr Med J 67:680, 1985.
66. Reissman KR and Coleman TJ: Acute intestinal iron intoxication. II: Metabolic, respiratory and circulatory effects of absorbed iron salts. Blood 10:46, 1955.
67. Banner W and Tong TG: Iron poisoning. Pediatr Clin North Am 33:392, 1986.
68. Gleason WA, deMello DE, Castro FJ, et al: Acute hepatic failure in severe iron poisoning. J Pediatr 95:138, 1979.
69. Doolin EJ and Drueck C: Fatal iron intoxication in an adult. J Trauma 20:518, 1980.
70. Stein M, Blayney D, Feit T, et al: Acute iron poisoning in children. West J Med 125:289, 1976.
71. Czajka PA, Konrad JD, and Duffy JP: Iron poisoning: An in vitro comparison of bicarbonate and phosphate lavage solution. J Pediatr 98:491, 1981.
72. Geffner ME and Opas LM: Phosphate poisoning complicating treatment for iron ingestion. Am J Dis Child 134:509, 1980.
73. Hosking CS: Radiology in the management of acute iron poisoning. Med J Aust 1:576, 1969.
74. Lacouture PG, Wason S, Temple AR, et al: Emergency assessment of severity in iron overdose by clinical and laboratory methods. J Pediatr 99:89, 1981.
75. Foxford R and Goldfrank L: Gastrotomy—a surgical approach to iron overdose. Ann Emerg Med 14:1223, 1985.
76. Movassaghi N, Purugganan MD, and Leikin S: Comparison of exchange transfusion and deferoxamine in the treatment of acute iron poisoning. J Pediatr 75:604, 1969.
77. Aronson JK: Digitalis intoxication. Clin Science 64:253, 1983.
78. Goodman LS: Digitalis. In: Haddad LM and Winchester JF (eds): Clinical Management of Poisoning and Drug Overdose, 2nd ed. Philadelphia, WB Saunders, 1990, pp. 1293–1314.
79. Hastreiter AR, van der Horst RL, and Chow-Tung E: Digitalis toxicity in infants and children. Pediatr Cardiol 5:131, 1984.
80. Lewander WJ, Gaudreault P, Einhorn A, et al: Acute pediatric digoxin ingestion: A ten-year experience. Am J Dis Child 140:770, 1986.
81. Smith TW, Antman EM, Friedman PL, et al: Digitalis glycosides: Mechanisms and manifestations of toxicity (in three parts). Prog Cardiovasc Dis, Part I 26:413, 1984; Part II 26:495, 1984; Part III 27:26, 1984.
82. Rosen MR: Cellular mechanisms of cardiac arrhythmias. In: Harrison DC (ed): Cardiac Arrhythmias: A Decade of Progress. Boston, GK Hall, 1981, pp. 25–38.
83. Spiehler VR, Sedgwick BS, and Richards RG: The use of brain digoxin concentrations to confirm blood digoxin concentrations. J Forensic Sci 26:645, 1981.
84. Rietbrock N and Aeiken RG: Color vision deficiencies: A common sign of intoxication in chronically digoxin-treated patients. J Cardiovasc Pharmacol 2:93, 1980.
85. Pick A: Digitalis and the electrocardiogram. Circulation 15:603, 1967.
86. Fisch C: Digitalis intoxication. JAMA 216:1770, 1971.
87. Krasula R, Yanagi R, Hastreiter AR, et al: Digoxin intoxication in infants and children: Correlation with serum levels. J Pediatr 84:265, 1974.
88. Jones J, McMullen MJ, Dougherty J, et al: Repetitive doses of activated charcoal in the treatment of poisoning. Am J Emerg Med 5:305, 1987.
89. Boldy DAR, Smart V, and Vale JA: Multiple doses of charcoal in digoxin poisoning. Lancet 2:1076, 1985.
90. Hursting MJ, Raisys VA, and Opheim KE: Drug-specific Fab therapy in drug overdose. Arch Pathol Lab Med 111:693, 1987.
91. Rollins DE and Brizgys M: Immunological approach to poisoning. Ann Emerg Med 15:1046, 1986.
92. Leikin J, Vogel A, Graft J, et al: Use of Fab fragments of digoxin-specific antibodies in the therapy of massive digoxin poisoning. Ann Emerg Med 14:175, 1985.
93. Zucker AR, Lacina SJ, DasGupta DS, et al: Fab fragments of digoxin-specific antibodies used to reverse ventricular fibrillation induced by digoxin ingestion in a child. Pediatrics 70:468, 1982.
94. Kaufman J, Leilein J, Kendzierski D, et al: Use of digoxin Fab immune fragments in a seven-day-old infant. Pediatr Emerg Care 6:118, 1990.
95. Wenger TL, Butler VP, Haber E, et al: Treatment of 63 severely digitalis-toxic patients with digoxin-specific antibody fragments, abstracted. J Am Coll Cardiol 5:118A, 1985.
96. Smolarz A, Roesch E, Lenz E, et al: Digoxin-specific antibody (Fab) fragments in 34 cases of severe digitalis intoxication. J Toxicol Clin Toxicol 23:327, 1985.
97. Ladenson PW and White JD: Thyroid. In: Haddad LM and Winchester JF (eds): Clinical Management of Poisoning and Drug Overdose, 2nd ed. Philadelphia, WB Saunders, 1990, pp. 1431–1440.
98. White JD and Livovitz TL: Levothyroxine poisoning. Pediatrics 75:129, 1985.
99. Gorman RL, Chamberlain JM, Rose SR, et al: Massive levothyroxine overdose: High anxiety—low toxicity. Pediatrics 4:666, 1988.
100. Golightly LK, Smolinske SC, Kulig KW, et al: Clinical effects of accidental levothyroxine ingestion in children. Am J Dis Child 141:1025, 1987.
101. Mandel SH, Magnusson R, Buton BT, et al: Massive levothyroxine ingestion. Clin Pediatr 28:374, 1989.
102. Lewander WJ, Lacouture PG, Silva JE, et al: Acute thyroxine ingestion in pediatric patients. Pediatrics 84:262, 1989.
103. Kulig K, Golightly LK, and Romack BH: Levothroxine overdose associated with seizures in a young child. JAMA 254:2109, 1985.
104. Haddad HM: Rates of I-labelled thyroxine metabolism in euthyroid children. J Clin Invest 39:1590, 1960.
105. Roberts JA: Correct use of thyroxine. Med J Aust 2:650, 1975.
106. Lehrner MC and Wesr MR: Acute ingestions of thyroid hormones. Pediatrics 73:313, 1984.
107. Roesch C, Becker PG, and Sklar S: Management of a child with acute thyroxine ingestion. Ann Emerg Med 14:1114, 1985.
108. National Institute on Drug Abuse. 1987 Annual data report statistical service. Rockville, MD, National Institute on Drug Abuse, 1987, NIDA publication No. (ADM) 88–1684.
109. Garland JS, Smith DS, Rice TB, et al: Accidental cocaine intoxication in a nine-month-old infant: Presentation and treatment. Pediatr Emerg Care 5:245, 1989.
110. Kharasch S, Vinci R, and Reece R: Esophagitis, epiglottitis and cocaine alkaloid ("crack"): "Accidental" poisoning or child abuse? Pediatrics 86:117, 1990.
111. Bateman DA and Heagarty MC: Passive freebase cocaine ("crack") inhalation by infants and toddlers. Am J Dis Child 143:25, 1989.
112. Ernst AA and Sanders WM: Unexpected cocaine intoxication presenting as seizures in children. Ann Emerg Med 18:774, 1989.

113. Chasnoff IJ, Lewis DE, and Squires L: Cocaine intoxication in a breast-fed infant. Pediatrics 80:836, 1987.
114. Riggs D and Weibley RE: Acute toxicity from oral ingestion of crack cocaine: A report of four cases. Pediatr Emerg Care 6:24, 1990.
115. Shannon M: Clinical toxicity of cocaine adulterants. Ann Emerg Med 17:1243, 1988.
116. Peterson RC: Childhood and Adolescent Drug Abuse: A Physician's Guide to Office Practice. Rockville, MD, American Council for Drug Education, 1987, pp. 39–43.
117. Mueller PD, Benowitz NL, and Olson KR: Cocaine. Emerg Med Clin North Am 8:481, 1990.
118. Tardiff K, Gross E, Wu J, et al: Analysis of cocaine positive fatalities. J Forensic Sci 34:53, 1989.
119. Barth CW, Bray M, and Roberts WC: Rupture of the ascending aorta during cocaine intoxication. Am J Cardiol 57:496, 1986.
120. Nanji AA and Filipenko JD: Asystole and ventricular fibrillation associated with cocaine intoxication. Chest 85:132, 1984.
121. Schachne JS, Roberts BH, and Thompson PD: Coronary artery spasm and myocardial infarction associated with cocaine use. N Engl J Med 310:165, 1984.
122. Cregler LL and Mark H: Relation of acute myocardial infarction to cocaine abuse. Am J Cardiol 56:794, 1985.
123. Lange RA, Cigarrva RG, Yancy CW, et al: Cocaine-induced coronary vasoconstriction. N Engl J Med 321:1557, 1989.
124. Zimmerman FH, Gustafson GM, and Kemp HG: Recurrent myocardial infarction associated with cocaine abuse in a young man with normal coronary arteries: Evidence for coronary vasospasm culminating in thrombosis. J Am Coll Cardiol 9:964, 1987.
125. Peng SK, Franks WJ, and Pelikan PCD: Direct cocaine cardiotoxicity demonstrated by endomyocardial biopsy. Arch Pathol Lab Med 113:842, 1989.
126. Roth D, Alarcon FJ, Fernandez JA, et al: Acute rhabdomyolysis associated with cocaine intoxication. N Engl J Med 319:673, 1987.
127. Lowenstein DH, Masso SM, Rowbotham MC, et al: Acute neurologic and psychiatric complications associated with cocaine abuse. Am J Med 83:841, 1987.
128. Haddad LM: Cocaine. In: Haddad LM and Winchester JF (eds): Clinical Management of Poisoning and Drug Overdose, 2nd ed. Philadelphia, WB Saunders, 1990, pp. 730–737.
129. Pasqual-Leone A, Shuna A, Ahafullah I, et al: Cocaine-induced seizures. Neurology 40:404, 1990.
130. Shesser R, Davis C, and Edelstein S.: Pneumomediastinum and pneumothorax after inhaling alkaloid cocaine. Ann Emerg Med 10:213, 1981.
131. McCarron MM and Wood JD: The cocaine "body packer" syndrome: Diagnosis and management. JAMA 250:1417, 1983.
132. Derlet RW and Albertson TE: Potentiation of cocaine toxicity with calcium channel blockers. Am J Emerg Med 7:464, 1989.
133. Smith HWB, Liberman HA, Brady SC, et al: Acute myocardial infarction temporally related to cocaine use: Clinical, angiographic and pathophysiologic observations. Ann Intern Med 107:13, 1987.
134. Shields RO: Designer drugs and amphetamines. Part B. Amphetamines. In: Haddad LM and Winchester JF (eds): Clinical Management of Poisoning and Drug Overdose, 2nd ed. Philadelphia, WB Saunders, 1990, pp. 771–780.
135. Nicholi AM: The non-therapeutic use of psychoactive drugs. N Engl J Med 308:928, 1983.
136. Caldwell J: Amphetamines and Related Stimulants: Chemical, Biological, Clinical, and Sociological Aspects. Boca Raton, FL, CRC Press, 1980.
137. Linden CH, Kulig KW, and Rumack BH: Amphetamines. Trends Emerg Med 7:18, 1985.
138. Scandling J and Spital A: Amphetamine-associated myoglobinuric renal failure. South Med J 75:237, 1982.
139. National Institute on Drug Abuse: Highlights of the 1988 National Household Survey on Drug Abuse. Rockville, MD, Press Office of NIDA, August, 1989.
140. Secretary, Department of Health and Human Sciences: Drug Abuse and Drug Abuse Research. Second Triennial Report to Congress. DHHS Publ. No. (ADM) 87-1486, Rockville, MD, 1987.
141. MacNab A, Anderson E, and Susak L: Ingestion of cannabis: A cause of coma in children. Pediatr Emerg Care 5:238, 1989.
142. Wall ME, Sadler BM, Brine D, et al: Metabolism, disposition, and kinetics of delta-9-tetrahydrocannabinol in men and women. Clin Pharmacol Ther 34:352, 1983.
143. Hawks RL: The constituents of cannabis and the disposition and metabolism of cannabionoids. In: Haws RL (ed): Analysis of Cannabinoids. NIDA Research Monograph 42. Rockville, MD, NIDA, 1982, pp. 125–137.
144. Selden BS, Clark RF, and Curry SC: Marijuana. Emerg Med Clin North Am 8:527, 1990.
145. Ohlsson A, Lindgren JE, Wahlen A, et al: Plasma delta-9-tetrahydrocannabinol concentrations and clinical effects after oral and intravenous administration and smoking. Clin Pharmacol Ther 28:409, 1980.
146. Martin BR: Cellular effects of cannabinoids. Pharmacol Rev 38:45, 1986.
147. Nahas GG: Cannabis: Toxicological properties and epidemiological aspects. Med J Anest 145:82, 1986.
148. Peterson RC: Childhood and Adolescent Drug Abuse: A Physician's Guide to Office Practice. Rockville, MD, American Council for Drug Education, 1987, pp. 29–38.
149. Tennant FS: The clinical syndrome of marijuana dependence. Psychiatr Ann 16:225, 1986.
150. Szara S: Marijuana. In: Haddad LM and Winchester JF (eds): Clinical Management of Poisoning and Drug Overdose, 2nd ed. Philadelphia, WB Saunders, 1990, pp. 727–748.
151. Weinberg D, Lande A, and Holton N: Intoxication from accidental marijuana ingestion. Pediatrics 72:948, 1983.
152. Jaffe JH and Martin WR: Opioid analgesics and antagonists. In: Gilman AG, Goodman LS, Rall TW, et al (eds): The Pharmacological Basis of Therapeutics, 7th ed. New York, MacMillan, 1985.
153. Wouters W and van den Bercken J: Hyperpolarisation and depression of slow synaptic inhibition enkephalin in frog sympathetic ganglion. Nature 277:53, 1979.
154. Henderson G: Electrophysiological analysis of opioid actions in the central nervous system. Br Med Bull 39:59, 1983.
155. Ford M, Hoffman RS, Goldfrank LR: Opioids and designer drugs. Emerg Med Clin North Am 8:495, 1990.
156. Pasternak GW: Multiple morphine and enkephalin receptors and the relief of pain. JAMA 2591362, 1988.
157. Hubbell KC: Opiates and narcotics. In: Haddad LM and Winchester JF (eds): Clinical Management of Poisoning and Drug Overdose, 2nd ed. Philadelphia, WB Saunders, 1985, pp. 706–717.
158. Patterson SJ, Robson LE, and Kosterlitz, HW: Classification of opioid receptors. Br Med Bull 39:31, 1983.
159. Thompson JW: Opioid peptides. Br Med J 288:259, 1984.
160. Katz S, Aberman A, Frank UI, et al: Heroin pulmonary edema: Evidence for increased pulmonary capillary permeability. Am Rev Respir Dis 106:472, 1972.
161. Oliver RLM: Bronchospasm and heroin inhalation. Lancet 1:915, 1986.
162. D'Agostino RS and Arnett EN: Acute myoglobinuria and heroin snorting. JAMA 241:277, 1979.
163. Lowenstein E, Howell P, Levine FH, et al: Cardiovascular response to large doses of intravenous morphine in man. N Engl J Med 281:1389, 1969.
164. Curtis JA and Goel KM: Lomotil poisoning in children. Arch Dis Child 54:222, 1979.
165. Rumack BN and Temple AR: Lomotil poisoning. Pediatrics 53:495, 1974.
166. Moore RA, Rumack BH, Conner CS, et al: Naloxone: Underdosage after narcotic poisoning. Am J Dis Child 134:156, 1980.
167. Committee on Drugs: Naloxone dosage and route of administration for infants and children: Addendum to emergency drug doses for infants and children. Pediatrics 86:484, 1990.
168. Lewis JM, Klein-Schwartz W, Benson BE, et al: Continuous naloxone infusion in pediatric narcotic overdose. Am J Dis Child 138:944, 1984.
169. Gober AE, Kearns GL, Yokel RA, et al: Repeated naloxone administration for morphine overdose in a 1-month-old infant. Pediatrics 63:606, 1979.
170. Lovejoy FH, Mitchell AA, and Goldman P: The management of propoxyphene poisoning. J Pediatr 85:98, 1974.
171. Mitchell AA, Lovejoy FH, and Goldman P: Drug ingestions associated with miosis in comatose children. J Pediatr 89:303, 1976.

172. Shaul WL, Wandell M, and Robertson WO: Dextromethorphan toxicity: Reversal by naloxone. Pediatrics 59:117, 1977.

173. Shepherd SM and Jagoda AS: Phencyclidine and the hallucinogens. *In:* Haddad LM and Winchester JF (eds): Clinical Management of Poisoning and Drug Overdose, 2nd ed. Philadelphia, WB Saunders, 1990, pp. 749–769.

174. Cook CE, Brine DR, Jeffcoat AR, et al: Phencyclidine disposition after intravenous and oral doses. Clin Pharmacol Ther 31:625, 1982.

175. Aniline O and Pitts FN: Phencyclidine (PCP): A review and perspectives. CRC Crit Rev Toxicol 10:145, 1982.

176. Karp HN, Kaufman ND, and Anand SK: Phencyclidine poisoning in young children. J Pediatr 97:1006, 1980.

177. Welch MJ and Correa GA: PCP intoxication in young children and infants. Clin Pediatr 19:510, 1980.

178. Castellani S, Giannini AJ, and Boering JA: Physostigmine treatment of acute phencyclidine intoxication. J Clin Psychiatr 43:10, 1982.

179. Aronow R and Dore AK: Phencyclidine overdose: An emerging concept of management. Am Coll Emerg Physicians 7:56, 1978.

180. Glennon R, Titeler M, and McKenney J: Evidence for 5HT2 involvement in the mechanism of action of hallucinogenic agents. Life Sci 35:2505, 1984.

181. Mokler D, Stoudt K, and Rech R: The 5HT2 antagonist pirenperone reverses disruption of FR-40 by hallucinogenic drugs. Pharamacol Biochem Behav 22:677, 1985.

182. Roy A: LSD and onset of schizophrenia. Can J Psychiatr 26:64, 1981.

183. Ianzito BM, Liskow B, and Steward MN: Reaction to LSD in a two-year old child. J Pediatr 80:643, 1972.

184. Samuelsson BO: LSD intoxication in a two-year-old child. Acta Pediatr Scand 63:797, 1974.

185. Shulgin AT: Chemistry of phenylethylamines related to mescaline. J Psychedel Drugs 11:41, 1979.

186. Milby TH: Prevention and management of organophosphate poisoning. JAMA 216:2131, 1971.

187. Haddad JM: Organophosphates and other insecticides. *In:* Haddad LM and Winchester JF (eds): Clinical Management of Poisoning and Drug Overdose, 2nd ed. Philadelphia, WB Saunders, 1990, pp. 1076–1087.

188. Smith PW: Bulletin: Medical Problems in Aerial Applications. Washington, DC, Office of Aviation, Federal Aviation Administration, Department of Transportation, 1977.

189. Moss DW, Henderson AR, Kachmar JF: 5-Enzymes. *In:* Tietz NW (ed): Textbook of Clinical Chemistry. Philadelphia, WB Saunders, 1986, pp. 746–749.

190. Coye MJ, Barnett PJ, Midtling JE, et al: Clinical confirmation of organophosphate poisoning by serial cholinesterase levels. Arch Intern Med 147:438, 1987.

191. Zwiener RJ and Ginsburg CM: Organophosphate and carbamate poisoning in infants and children. Pediatrics 81:121, 1988.

192. Moore PG and James OF: Acute pancreatitis induced by acute organophosphate poisoning. Postgrad Med J 57:660, 1981.

193. Namba T, Nolte CT, Jackson J, et al: Poisoning due to organophosphate insecticides. Am J Med 50:475, 1971.

194. Ludomirski A, Klein HO, Sarelli P, et al: Q-T prolongation and polymorphous ("torsades de pointes") ventricular arrhythmias associated with organophosphorous insecticide poisoning. Am J Cardiol 49:1654, 1982.

195. Mortensen ML: Management of childhood poisoning caused by selected insecticides and herbicides. Pediatr Clin North Am 33:421, 1986.

196. Hayes WJ: Toxicology of Pesticides. Baltimore, Williams & Wilkins, 1975.

197. Tinker TD: Hydrocarbon ingestion in children: Its sequelae and management. Ok State Med Assoc J February 79:95, 1986.

198. Klein BL and Simon JE: Hydrocarbon poisoning. Pediatr Clin North Am 33:441, 1986.

199. Truemper EJ, Reyes dela Rocha S, and Atkinson SD: Clinical characteristics, pathophysiology and management of hydrocarbon ingestion: Case report and review of the literature. Pediatr Emerg Care 3:187, 1987.

200. Press E: Co-operative kerosene poisoning study: Evaluation of gastric lavage and other factors in the treatment of accidental ingestion of petroleum distillate products. Pediatrics 29:648, 1962.

201. Steele RW, Conkline RH, and Mark HM: Corticosteroids and antibiotics for the treatment of fulminant hydrocarbon aspiration. JAMA 219:1434, 1972.

202. Ervin ME and Manske MG: Petroleum distillates and turpentine. *In:* Haddad LM and Winchester JF (eds): Clinical Management of Poisoning and Drug Overdose, 2nd ed. Philadelphia, WB Saunders, 1990, pp. 1177–1186.

203. Browning E: Toxicity and Metabolism of Industrial Solvents. London, Elsevier, 1965.

204. Taher A, Anderson R, McCortney R, et al: Renal tubular acidosis associated with toluene "sniffing." N Engl J Med 290:765, 1974.

205. Laskin S and Goldstein B: Benzene Toxicity, A Critical Care Evaluation. Washington, DC, Hemisphere Publishing, 1977.

206. Geehr E: Management of hydrocarbon ingestion. Top Emerg Med 1:97, 1979.

207. Wolfe BM, Brodeur AE, and Shields JB: The role of gastrointestinal absorption of kerosene in producing pneumonitis in dogs. J Pediatr 76:867, 1970.

208. Gross P, McNerney JM, and Babyak MA: Kerosene pneumonitis: An experimental study with small doses. Am Rev Respir Dis 88:656, 1963.

209. Stockman, JA: More on hydrocarbon-induced hemolysis. J Pediatr 90:848, 1977.

210. Ashkenazi AE and Berman SE: Experimental kerosene poisoning in rats. Pediatrics 28:642, 1961.

211. Anas N, Namasonthi V, and Ginsburg CM: Criteria for hospitalizing children who have ingested products containing hydrocarbon. JAMA 246:840, 1981.

212. Marks MI, Chicaine I, Legare G, et al: Adrenocorticosteroid treatment of hydrocarbon pneumonia in children—a cooperative study. J Pediatr 81:366, 1972.

213. Zucker AR, Sznajder JI, Becker CJ, et al: The pathophysiology and treatment of canine kerosene pulmonary injury: Effect of plasmapheresis and positive end-expiratory pressure. J Crit Care 4:184, 1989.

214. Rothstein FC: Caustic injuries to the esophagus in children. Pediatr Clin North Am 33:665, 1986.

215. Leape LL, Ashcroft KW, Scarpelli DG, et al: Hazard to health—liquid lye. N Engl J Med 284:578, 1971.

216. Buntain WL and Cain WC: Caustic injuries to the esophagus: A pediatric overview. South Med J 74:590, 1981.

217. Anderson KD: Alkali Injury. *In:* Haddad LM and Winchester JF (eds): Clinical Management of Poisoning and Drug Overdose, 2nd ed. Philadelphia, WB Saunders, 1990, pp. 1056–1062.

218. Litovitz T: Alkali Injury. *In:* Haddad LM and Winchester JF (eds): Clinical Management of Poisoning and Drug Overdose, 2nd ed. Philadelphia, WB Saunders, 1990, pp. 1062–1065.

219. Landau G and Saunders W: The effect of chlorine bleach on the esophagus. Laryngol Rhinol Otol (Stuttg) 92:499, 1978.

220. Wasserman RL and Ginsburg CM: Caustic substance injuries. J Pediatr 107:169, 1985.

221. Haller JA, Andrews, HG, White JJ, et al: Pathophysiology and management of acute corrosive burn of the esophagus: Results of treatment of 285 children. J Pediatr Surg 6:578, 1971.

222. Gaudreault P, Parent M, McGuigan MA, et al: Predictability of esophageal injury from signs and symptoms: A study of caustic ingestion in 378 children. Pediatrics 71:767, 1983.

223. Crain, EF, Gershel JC, and Mezey AP: Caustic ingestions: Symptoms as predictors of esophageal injury. Am J Dis Child 138:863, 1984.

224. Stannard MW: Corrosive esophagitis in children: Assessment by the esophagogram. Am J Dis Child 132:596, 1978.

225. Hawkins DB, Demeter MJ, and Barnett TE: Caustic ingestion: Controversies in management: A review of 214 cases. Laryngoscope 90:98, 1980.

226. Genieser NB and Becker MH: Clinitest strictures of the esophagus. Clin Pediatr 8:17, 1969.

227. Adam JJ and Brick HG: Pediatric caustic ingestion. Ann Otol Rhinol Laryngol 91:656, 1982.

228. Mills LJ, Estrera AS, and Platt MR: Avoidance of esophageal stricture following severe caustic burns by use of an intraluminal stent. Ann Thorac Cardiovasc Surg 28:60, 1979.

229. David WM, Madden JW, and Peacock EE: A new approach to the control of esophageal stenosis. Ann Surg 176:469, 1972.

230. Appleqvist P and Salno M: Lye corrosion carcinoma of the esophagus—a review of 63 cases. Cancer 45:2655, 1980.

231. Brent J, Kulig K, and Rumack BH: Mushrooms. *In:* Haddad LM and Winchester JF (eds): Clinical Management of Poisoning and Drug Overdose, 2nd ed. Philadelphia, WB Saunders, 1990, pp. 581–590.
232. Lampe KF and McCann MA: Differential diagnosis of poisoning by North American mushrooms, with particular emphasis on *Amanita phylloides*–like intoxication. Ann Emerg Med 16:956, 1987.
233. Mack RB: Poisonous mushrooms—nature's iscariot. Contemp Pediatr 3:59, 1986.
234. Bivins HG, Knopp R, Maners R., et al: Mushroom ingestion. Ann Emerg Med 14:1099, 1985.
235. Fiume L and Wieland T: Amanitins: Chemistry and action. FEBS Lett 8:1, 1970.
236. Vesconi S, Langer M, Iapichino G et al: Therapy of cytotoxic mushroom intoxication. Crit Care Med 13:402, 1985.
237. Lindell TJ, Weinberg F, Morris PW, et al: Specific inhibition of nuclear RNA polymerase by alpha-amanitin. Science 170:447, 1970.
238. Kroncke DK, Fricker G, Meier PJ, et al: Alpha-amanitin uptake into hepatocytes. J Biol Chem 261:12562, 1986.
239. Hanrahan JP and Gordon MA: Mushroom poisoning: Case report and a review of therapy. JAMA 251:1057, 1984.
240. Finestone AJ, Berman R, Widmer B, et al: Thioctic acid treatment of acute mushroom poisoning. Pa Med 75:49, 1972.
241. Culliton BJ: The destroying angel: A story of a search for an antidote. Science 185:600, 1974.
242. Floersheim GL: Treatment of mushroom poisoning. JAMA 253:3252, 1985.
243. Floersheim GL: Treatment of human amanitin mushroom poisoning: Myths and advances in therapy. Med Toxicol Adverse Drug Exp 2:1, 1987.
244. Klein AS, Hart J, Bruns, JJ, et al: *Amanita* poisoning: Treatment and the role of liver transplantation. Am J Med 86:187, 1989.
245. Floersheim GL, Eberhard M, Tschumi P, et al: Effects of penicillin and silymarin on liver enzymes and blood clotting factors in dogs given a boiled preparation of *Amanita phylloides*. Toxicol Appl Pharmacol 46:455, 1978.
246. Scheider SM, Borochowitz, D, and Krenzelok EP: Cimetidine protection against alpha-amanitin hepatotoxicity in mice: A potential model for the treatment of *Amanita phylloides* poisoning. Ann Emerg Med 16:1136, 1987.
247. Woodle ES, Moody RR, Cox KL, et al: Orthotopic liver transplantation in a patient with *Amanita* poisoning. JAMA 253:69, 1985.

81

Envenomation

Muriel D. Wolf, M.D.

This chapter focuses on the recognition and management of bites and stings by venomous animals, particularly bites that are severe enough to cause a person's admission to an intensive care unit. Envenomation by both terrestrial and marine animals is addressed with emphasis on envenomation by animals in the continental United States. Reference, however, is made to several particularly severe life-threatening envenomations by snakes outside the continental United States.

Venomous Terrestrial Animals

Arthropoda
  Spiders
  Scorpions
Vertebrae—Venomous
  Reptilia
    Viperidae
    Crotalidae
    Elapidae
    Colubridae

Venomous Marine Animals

Phylum Coelenterata
  Hydrozoa
    Portuguese man-o-war
    Blue Bottle
  Scyphozoa
    Jellyfish
    Sea nettles
    Sea wasps
Subphylum Vertebrae
  Chondrichythes
    Stingrays
  Reptilia
    Hydrophiidae (sea snakes) (discussed under
      other reptiles)

ARTHROPOD ENVENOMATION

There are more than one and one half million members of the phylum Arthropoda, joint-footed members of the animal kingdom with an exoskeleton. The classes of arthropods of medical importance include the arachnids with spiders and scorpions, the chelopods including centipedes, the diplopods or millipedes, and the insects. This discussion concentrates on envenomation by spiders and scorpions, whose bites may be severe enough to cause a patient's admission to a critical care unit.

Arachnids

The arachnids of medical importance include the widow spiders, the brown spiders, scorpions, ticks, and mites.

Widow Spider

The widow spider, *Latrodectus* genus, is named because the female may destroy the male after insemination. These arachnids are found all over the world: the commonest ones in the United States are the black widow or *Latrodectus mactans* and the *L. hesperus*, which is found in the Western states; the *L. bishopi*, the brown widow, found in the South; and the red widow, *L. geometricus*, found in Florida. Parish reported 63 deaths in the United States between 1950 and 1959 due to Latrodectus bites. The *Latrodectus* genus is found throughout the temperate and tropical zones of the earth and includes the *L. tredecimguttatus* (found in Europe), which has 17 red spots distributed over its abdomen and the widow spider, *L. hasselti*, the redback spider, which is found in Australia. The *L. mactans*, the black widow spider of North America, is shiny black; on its central under surface it has red markings consisting of two triangles arranged apex to apex, appearing as an hourglass.

Spiders of the genus *Latrodectus* are not aggressive and bite only in self-defense. Bites are more common in the warm months of the year, reflecting the greater activity of the spider and more contact with humans. There is also evidence to suggest that the spider venom may be more toxic at higher temperatures. Bites on the buttocks and genitalia were not uncommon when the outdoor privy was a necessity. These arachnida prefer obscure corners. The *Latrodectus* venom is considered one of the most potent toxins, more poisonous than many snake venoms, but it is available in smaller amounts. The venom is stored in glands in the thorax and injected through fangs by the female spider. The male black widow spider is not considered dangerous because it is much smaller and also has a much smaller store of venom. The venom causes release of neurotransmitters at the synaptic junctions by inducing exocytosis of synapatic vesicles; noradrenaline and acetylcholine are released.

Latrodectus bites may not be noticed, or there may be a slight sensation of a pinprick at the site of the bite. In most situations any systemic reaction is delayed for 30 minutes to even several hours. The more the systemic symptoms, the more severe will be the envenomation. Cramping pain develops in the chest, abdomen, and lumbar regions and extends to the extremities; muscle rigidity develops. There may be sweating, intense salivation, lacrimation, and increased bronchial secretions. Restlessness, nausea, vomiting, hypertension, respiratory compromise, and convulsions may occur. Major manifestations occur within the first 24 to 48 hours and, if untreated, may persist for 7 days. Muscle weakness and pain may persist for weeks.

Treatment includes the use of intravenous calcium and muscle relaxants. Diazepam has been used with some success. Methocarbamol (Robaxin) has been found to be less effective than calcium gluconate intravenously (a 10% solution, 0.1 ml/kg per dose, up to 10 ml for an adult), which is given slowly while monitoring the heart rate and rhythm. An antivenin, which is manufactured from horse serum, may be used after skin testing for sensitivity to horse serum; one to two vials of antivenin reverse the effects of the venom. This antivenin should be used for young children or elderly patients or for anyone with respiratory difficulty or marked hypertension; usually one vial (2.5 ml of antivenin Lactrodectus mactans, made by Merck, Sharpe & Dohme) is sufficient to treat most patients. Even though there is a chance for hypersensitivity to the horse serum from the antivenin, the reaction is unlikely to be fatal because of the small amount of antivenin used.

Brown Spiders

Brown spiders or *Loxosceles* are found all over the Western Hemisphere. In South America the *Loxosceles laeta* and in the Middle and Eastern United States the *L. reclusa* (brown recluse spider) present particular problems. The brown recluse spider has a violin configuration on its head. These spiders live both indoors and outdoors in temperatures from 8°C to 43°C; they can live up to 6 months without food or water. Their coloration is from light to dark brown; they range in size from 1 to 4 cm leg to leg; the legs are long and thin with rows of black hairs.

The clinical response to brown recluse envenomation ranges from a mild, local reaction to a severe systemic response. The bite may be relatively painless and go unrecognized; within 2 to 6 hours, pain and itching develop at the site of the bite. Within 24 hours a blister develops that is then followed by an erythematous ring. This ring becomes dark blue in color as necrosis begins;

this necrosis may extend into the deeper layers of the skin over the next several days causing a necrotic ulcer. An eschar forms and subsequently sloughs, leaving an ulcer that varies in size from 1 to 30 cm in diameter. Healing may take several months, and skin grafting may be necessary.

Systemic involvement occurs usually within 24 to 72 hours after the bite. Weakness, nausea, vomiting, fever, malaise, chills, arthralgia, myalgia, and convulsions develop. Disseminated intravascular coagulopathy, thrombocytopenia, and hemolytic anemia have also been noted. Severe hemolysis may result in hemoglobinemia and hemoglobinuria with resultant renal failure and death. Fatal cases have been more common in young children.

Hyaluronidase and other enzyme proteins have been reported in the venom. A phospholipase enzyme sphingomyelinase D acts on cell membranes and is considered to be an important dermonecrotic substance that causes the release of polymorphonuclear leukocytes. Prostaglandins, thromboxane, and leukotrienes contribute to the inflammatory reaction that, along with platelet aggregation and vascular thrombosis, may lead to ischemia and tissue injury.

The diagnosis of brown recluse spider envenomation is usually a presumptive one because this spider is rarely captured. Other species of spider in the United States are capable of producing similar lesions including the Atrax, the *Lycosa* (the wolf species), the *Phidippus* (jumping spiders), the *Argiope* (the orb spider), and the *Chiracanthium* (the running spider).

Laboratory findings in patients with systemic effects of envenomation include hematuria, hemoglobinuria, hemolytic anemia, leukocytosis, hypofibrinogenemia, and thrombocytopenia.

Treatment includes management of the local and systemic effects of the venom. Skin lesions should be managed with good care of the wound; tetanus prophylaxis should be administered; antibiotics may be indicated. Some authors have suggested early wide surgical excision, but this is controversial. Dapsone, a polymorphonuclear leukocyte inhibitor, has been used in some situations to decrease the pain, erythema, and duration of the lesion; this drug, however, can cause serious side effects including toxic hepatitis and hemolytic anemia in patients with glucose-6-phosphate dehydrogenase deficiency.

These patients require close observation since envenomation can be life-threatening. Steroids have been noted to produce a protective effect against red blood cell hemolysis; however, a coagulopathy may occur necessitating treatment with platelet and packed red blood cell transfusions. If renal failure occurs, hemodialysis or peritoneal dialysis may be indicated. Currently there is no proven widely available antivenin for brown recluse spider envenomation in the United States. There is an antivenin for the South American species (*L. laeta*).

Scorpions

There are over 600 species of scorpions that are also members of the class Arachnida; they are capable of stinging their victims and causing severe envenomation. These animals live in warm climates; in Arizona alone, there are approximately 20 species of scorpions. Scorpions are nocturnal creatures who hide in dark places, including shoe boxes or clothing or under debris; they only sting when disturbed in that quiet habitat. The bark scorpion, *Centruroides sculpturatus,* found in Arizona and neighboring states, is the most important medically because it can cause serious envenomation. This animal has a stinger on the end of a long tail. The venom is released from two venom glands and may cause severe neurotoxic effects; in fact, the bark scorpion causes the most severe venomous bite of the scorpion species.

Envenomation may be graded according to its severity. Grade 1 envenomation causes only local discomfort and paresthesias. In grade 2 envenomation, pain and paresthesias extend up along the extremity. With grade 3 envenomation, there is early motor hyperkinesis and cranial nerve dysfunction with evidence of dysphagia, roving eyes, facial paresthesias, and restlessness. In grade 4 envenomation, marked cranial nerve dysfunction develops with drooling, uncontrollable eye movements, fasciculations of both facial and distal muscles, and neuromuscular hyperactivity progressing to opisthotonus. Convulsions, wheezing, hyperthermia, and cyanosis may develop (Table 81–1).

Treatment includes supportive care while the patient recovers over several hours or days; the patient may be extremely uncomfortable. In grades 3 and 4 scorpion envenomation, a specific antivenin derived from goat serum has been used in Arizona and has greatly reduced the death rate; this antivenin can be obtained through the Antivenin Production Laboratory at Arizona State University in Tempe, Arizona, 85287, telephone (602) 965-1457. Phenobarbitol has been used in an attempt to treat the hyperactivity and seizures, and calcium gluconate (0.1 ml/kg of the 10% solution) has been used to reduce muscle contractions; neither of these medications, however, has been definitely proven efficacious.

VENOMOUS SNAKES

Worldwide, there are over 2,500 to 3,000 species of snakes, of which 375 species are considered venomous.

Table 81–1. SCORPION ENVENOMATION

Grade 1: Local discomfort and paresthesias
Grade 2: Pain and paresthesia extend up the extremity
Grade 3: Motor hyperkinesis
        Cranial nerve dysfunction
        Dysphagia
        Roving eyes
        Facial paresthesias
        Restlessness
Grade 4: Cranial nerve dysfunction
        Drooling, uncontrollable eye movements
        Fasciculations, facial and distal muscles
        Neuromuscular hyperactivity
        Opisthotonus
        Convulsions
        Wheezing
        Hyperthermia
        Cyanosis

Table 81–2. FAMILIES OF VENOMOUS SNAKES*

1. Viperidae—Old World Vipers		
	Bitis	: Adders, vipers, asps
	Bothrops	
	Cerastes	
	Echis	
	Vipera	
2. Crotalidae—Pit Vipers		
	Agkistrodon	: Copperhead
		Cottonmouth
		Malayan pit viper
		Mamushi
	Bothrops	: American lanceheads
	Crotalus	: Rattlesnakes
	Lachesis	: Bushmaster
	Sistrurus	: Massasaugas
		Pygmy rattlesnakes
	Trimeresurus	: Asian lanceheads, habu
3. Elapidae		
	Micrurus	: Coral snakes
	Naja	: Cobras
	Ophiophagus	
	Bungaraus	: Kraits
	Dendroaspis	: Mambas
	Pseudechis	: Brown and black snakes
4. Colubridae		
	Dispholidus	: Boomslang
	Thelotornis	: Bird snake
5. Hydrophiidae		
	Hydrophis	: Sea snakes
	Lapemis	
	Pelamis	

*Including some common snakes.

These venomous snakes belong to one of five families: (1) the Viperidae or Old World Vipers, which include asps and adders; (2) the Crotalidae or pit vipers, including the genus *Agkistrodon* with the copperhead and cottonmouth snakes and the Asian pit vipers, the genus *Crotalus* with over 32 species of rattlesnakes, the genus *Bothrops* with American lanceheads, the genus *Trimeresurus* with Asian lanceheads, and the genus *Sistrurus* that includes the massasaugas and pygmy rattlesnakes; (3) the family Elapidae, which includes coral snakes, cobras, kraits, mambas, and brown and black snakes from Asia and Australia; (4) the family Colubridae, including boomslangs and bird snakes; (5) the family Hydrophiidae or sea snakes (Table 81–2).

In the United States 8,000 of the 40,000 snakebites are caused each year by venomous snakes, accounting for 10 to 15 deaths per year. The largest number of deaths occur in North Carolina, Arizona, Texas, Georgia, and Florida. Most snakebites are by members of the Crotalidae family with the Elapidae family accounting for approximately 2% of snakebites and a lesser number by the Colubridae. Children are common victims of snakebites because of their inquisitiveness and adventuresome nature.

Crotalidae

The family Crotalidae or pit vipers usually have a triangular-shaped head with an elliptical pupil. They have hollow fangs, maxillary teeth, and a tail with a long row of single scales on the undersurface. The pit, which is localized between the eye and the nostril, is a heat-sensitive receptor that allows the snake to localize objects with a higher temperature than the surrounding environment. These poisonous snakes deliver their venom through a venom apparatus that includes two glands situated in the maxilla, two venom ducts, and two maxillary teeth that are hollow. The fangs in this viper are directed posteriorly. When the mouth is closed, the fangs rest against the maxilla; when the mouth is open, the fangs move forward. The rattlesnake, which is an important member of this family, takes its name from the loosely attached horny rings extending from the button at the end of the tail (rattle).

Rattlesnakes, all members of the Crotalidae family, are divided into two genera, *Crotalus* and *Sistrurus;* they are all venomous (Table 81–3). They are generally readily identifiable because of the rattle; however, in young rattlesnakes, the rattle may be small and not readily seen. In other rattlesnakes, the rattle may be lost through injury or may break off when the rattle becomes too long. The genus *Crotalus* includes the diamondback rattlesnake, which is particularly aggressive and can cause a lethal bite; the Eastern diamondback rattlesnake, which is found in an area extending south from North Carolina to Florida and west from Florida to Louisiana; and the Western diamondback rattlesnake, which is found in an area extending east from Southern California, through Oklahoma, to Arkansas (Fig. 81–1). Other rattlesnakes that cause severe bites include the sidewinder, the timber rattlesnake, and the Pacific rattlesnake. The sidewinder is found in California, Nevada, Arizona, and Utah. The timber rattler has a wide distribution from New England south to Florida and westward to Texas; it is also found in the Midwest in Minnesota, Wisconsin, Nebraska, and Iowa (Fig. 81–2). The *Crotalus* genus accounts for approximately 60% of all pit viper attacks.

The genus *Sistrurus* includes the massasauga and the pygmy rattlesnake that inflicts a less toxic bite than other rattlesnakes. The desert massasauga inhabits a region in New Mexico and Western Texas; the Western massasauga extends from mid-Texas north through Oklahoma into Iowa, whereas the Eastern massasauga inhabits an area around the Great Lakes.

The genus *Agkistrodon* includes the copperhead and cottonmouth snakes in the United States, and the mamushi and Malayan pit viper in Asia. Copperheads, *Agkistrodon contortrix,* are pit vipers that inhabit a large area extending from New England south to Florida, west toward Texas, and then north in the Midwest into Nebraska and Iowa (Fig. 81–3). These snakes account for approximately one third of all venomous snakebites in the continental United States; rarely are these bites lethal. The snakes measure approximately 3 ft in length and are usually not aggressive unless threatened. Water mocasins, or cottonmouths, *Agkistrodon piscivorus,* live in the southeastern United States in an area extending south from Virginia to Florida, westward through Kentucky, Illinois, and Tennessee to Texas (Fig. 81–4). These snakes, which prefer a fresh water environment,

Table 81–3. POISONOUS SNAKES OF THE UNITED STATES

Pit Vipers

Agkistrodon contortrix contortrix	Southern copperhead
Agkistrodon contortrix laticinetus	Broad-banded copperhead
Agkistrodon contortrix mokeson	Northern copperhead
Agkistrodon contortrix phaeogaster	Osage copperhead
Agkistrodon contortrix pictigaster	Trans-Pecos copperhead
Agkistrodon piscivorus conanti	Florida cottonmouth
Agkistrodon piscivorus piscivorus	Eastern cottonmouth
Agkistrodon piscivorus leucostoma	Western cottonmouth

Rattlesnakes

Crotalus adamanteus	Eastern diamondback
Crotalus atrox	Western diamondback
Crotalus cerastes cerastes	Mojave Desert sidewinder
Crotalus cerastes cercobombus	Sonoran Desert sidewinder
Crotalus cerastes laterorepens	Colorado Desert sidewinder
Crotalus enyo enyo	Lower California rattlesnake
Crotalus horridus horridus	Timber rattlesnake
Crotalus horridus atricaudatus	Canebrake rattlesnake
Crotalus lepidus lepidus	Mottled rock rattlesnake
Crotalus lepidus klauberi	Banded rock rattlesnake
Crotalus mitchelli pyrrhus	Southwestern speckled rattlesnake
Crotalus molossus molossus	Northern blacktail rattlesnake
Crotalus pricei pricei	Twin-spotted rattlesnake
Crotalus ruber ruber	Red diamond rattlesnake
Crotalus scutulatus scutulatus	Mojave rattlesnake
Crotalus tigris	Tiger rattlesnake
Crotalus vipidis abyssus	Grand Canyon rattlesnake
Crotalus vipidis cerberus	Arizona black rattlesnake
Crotalus vipidis helleri	South Pacific rattlesnake
Crotalus vipidis lutosus	Great Basin rattlesnake
Crotalus vipidis nuntius	Hopi rattlesnake
Crotalus vipidis oreganus	North Pacific rattlesnake
Crotalus viridis viridis	Prairie rattlesnake
Crotalus willardi willardi	Arizona ridgenose rattlesnake
Sistrurus catenatus catenatus	Eastern massasauga
Sistrurus catenatus edwardsi	Desert massasauga
Sistrurus catenatus tergeminus	Western massasauga
Sistrurus miliarius barbouri	Southeastern pigmy rattlesnake
Sistrurus miliarius miliarius	Carolina pigmy rattlesnake
Sistrurus miliarius streckeri	Western pigmy rattlesnake

Elapids

Micruroides euryxanthus	Sonoran coral snake
Micrurus fulvius fulvius	Eastern coral snake
Micrurus fulvius tenere	Texas coral snake

Colubrids

Dispholidus typhus	Boomslang

are moderately belligerent animals; they take their name from the distinctive white color of the open mouth, seen as the animal prepares to strike.

Crotalid Envenomation

Classically two fang marks are seen at the site of the snakebite; the distance between the fang marks gives some indication as to the size of the snake; this is particularly helpful if the snake has not been brought to the medical facility. Frequently, however, only one fang mark will be present since the second fang may not have

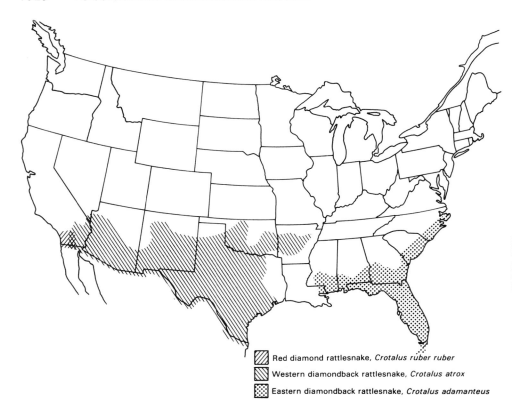

Figure 81–1. Distribution of diamond-back rattlesnakes in the United States. (Used by permission of the American Map Co., Inc. [© American Map Co., Inc., New York, No. 18435].)

Red diamond rattlesnake, *Crotalus ruber ruber*

Western diamondback rattlesnake, *Crotalus atrox*

Eastern diamondback rattlesnake, *Crotalus adamanteus*

Figure 81–2. Distribution of common rattlesnakes in the United States. (Used by permission of the American Map Co., Inc. [© American Map Co., Inc., New York, No. 18435].)

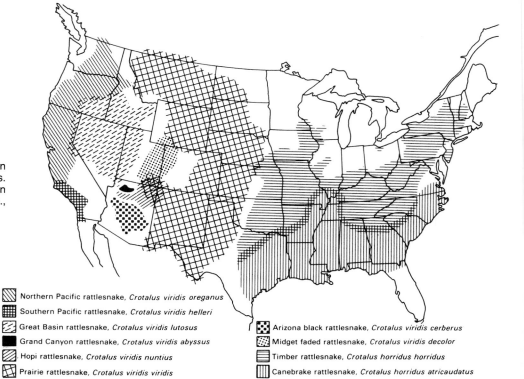

Northern Pacific rattlesnake, *Crotalus viridis oreganus*

Southern Pacific rattlesnake, *Crotalus viridis helleri*

Great Basin rattlesnake, *Crotalus viridis lutosus*

Grand Canyon rattlesnake, *Crotalus viridis abyssus*

Hopi rattlesnake, *Crotalus viridis nuntius*

Prairie rattlesnake, *Crotalus viridis viridis*

Arizona black rattlesnake, *Crotalus viridis cerberus*

Midget faded rattlesnake, *Crotalus viridis decolor*

Timber rattlesnake, *Crotalus horridus horridus*

Canebrake rattlesnake, *Crotalus horridus atricaudatus*

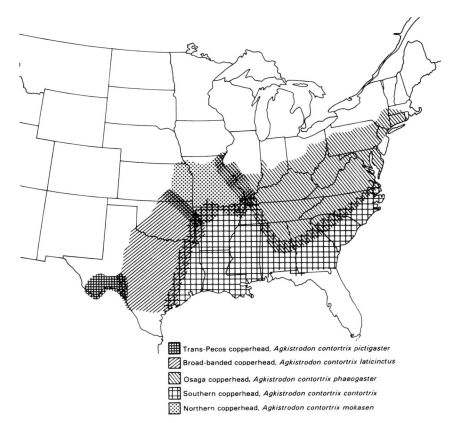

Figure 81–3. Distribution of common copperheads in the United States. (Used by permission of the American Map Co., Inc. [© American Map Co., Inc., New York, No. 18435].)

Trans-Pecos copperhead, *Agkistrodon contortrix pictigaster*

Broad-banded copperhead, *Agkistrodon contortrix laticinctus*

Osaga copperhead, *Agkistrodon contortrix phaeogaster*

Southern copperhead, *Agkistrodon contortrix contortrix*

Northern copperhead, *Agkistrodon contortrix mokasen*

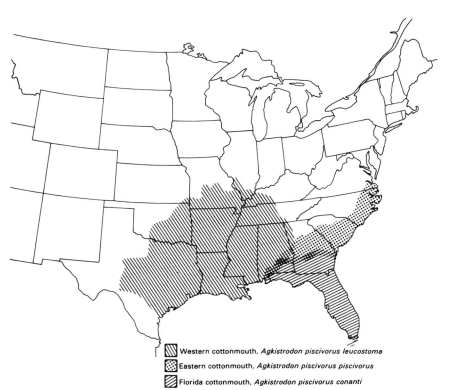

Figure 81–4. Distribution of common cottonmouth snakes in the United States. (Used by permission of the American Map Co., Inc. [© American Map Co., Inc., New York, No. 18435].)

Western cottonmouth, *Agkistrodon piscivorus leucostoma*

Eastern cottonmouth, *Agkistrodon piscivorus piscivorus*

Florida cottonmouth, *Agkistrodon piscivorus conanti*

actually embedded in the patient's skin. Usually with pit viper envenomation the site will begin to swell and become ecchymotic within 15 minutes, and the area will become exquisitely tender (Fig. 81–5A and B). In the absence of swelling and ecchymosis, one should consider whether venom has actually been injected. Approximately 30 to 40% of snakebites may actually be dry; in this situation, use of antivenin would be contraindicated. The snake may occasionally strike more than once, and more than two fang marks may be present. Bites by the copperhead and Mojave rattlesnake may appear less severe initially, because there is little pain at the site of the bite, but swelling will occur with envenomation.

Other rattlesnake bites cause severe pain as well as ecchymoses and swelling. Nonvenomous snakes may leave a row of teeth marks although venom will not be injected. In some venomous snakebites, there may also be a row of small teeth marks; however, the presence of pain and swelling at the site of the bite will help to decide that envenomation has actually occurred.

In severe rattlesnake envenomation, but not normally with copperhead bites, vesiculation may be noted over the back and the neck. Swelling may rapidly progress proximally as vesicles develop at the site of envenomation. The patient may feel cold and develop chills; fever, headache, nausea, vomiting, and finally hypotension may occur. In severe rattlesnake envenomation, there may be blurred vision, difficulty swallowing, and the feeling of thirst as hypotension develops. Serious bleeding from sites other than the envenomation site begins, and hematuria, hemoptysis, and bloody diarrhea occur.

Treatment

The goals for treatment of venomous snakebites are: (1) to stabilize the patient, (2) to interfere with the effects of the venom by preventing further absorption of venom from local sites and by binding any free circulating venom, and (3) to treat the local and systemic effects of the venom.

On initiating treatment, blood studies should be obtained immediately, including a complete blood count, platelet count, blood for type and cross-match, prothrombin time, partial thromboplastin time, plasma fibrinogen, creatinine, electrolytes, arterial blood gases, and urinalysis (Table 81–4).

The Scientific Review Subcommittee of the American Association of Poison Control Centers has established a grading system for evaluating pit viper bites (Table 81–5). In *mild* envenomation, there is severe pain, swelling, erythema, and ecchymoses occurring within 10 to 15 cm of the bite. There is no systemic reaction nor are there any abnormalities in the laboratory data. In *moderate* envenomation, the local signs of pain and swelling extend beyond the wound site; systemic symptoms include weakness, nausea and vomiting, paresthesia of the face and scalp, a metallic taste, tachycardia, pallor, and mild hypotension. Laboratory studies may show hemoconcentration, hypofibrinogenemia, and thrombocytopenia. In *severe* envenomation, the entire extremity is involved; systemic findings include hypotension and shock. There may be a severe bleeding diathesis and respiratory distress. Laboratory studies show severe anemia, prolongation of clotting time, and metabolic acidosis.

Elapidae

Coral snakes account for approximately 1 to 2% of venomous snakebites in the United States. They are not aggressive animals; in fact, it is unusual for them to bite

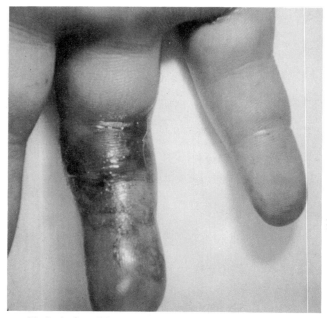 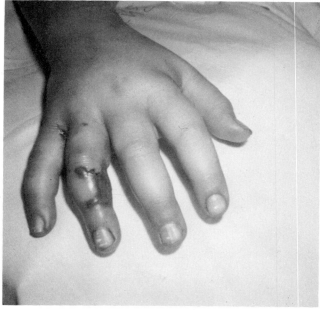

Figure 81–5. *A,* Crotalid envenomation, photograph taken 60 minutes after bite. Marked swelling and ecchymosis are apparent. Fang marks are barely visible. *B,* In the same patient, the back of the hand shows extensive swelling.

Table 81–4. INITIAL LABORATORY STUDIES

Complete blood count	Blood urea nitrogen
Platelet count	Creatinine
Type and cross-match	Electrolytes
Prothrombin time	Arterial blood gas
Partial thromboplastin time	Urinalysis
Plasma fibrinogen	

Table 81–5. GUIDELINES FOR GRADING PIT VIPER ENVENOMATION*

Grade	Local Reaction	Systemic Reaction	Abnormal Laboratory Data
Mild	Severe pain Swelling Erythema Ecchymoses within 10–15 cm of bite	None	None
Moderate	Pain and swelling beyond wound site	Weakness Nausea Vomiting Paresthesias Metallic taste Tachycardia Hypotension	Hemoconcentration Decreased fibrinogen Thrombocytopenia
Severe	Entire extremity involved	Hypotension Shock Bleeding Respiratory distress	Anemia Prolonged clotting time Metabolic acidosis

*As established by the Scientific Review Subcommittee of the American Association of Poison Control Centers.

unless they are handled roughly. The genus includes the Eastern coral snake, *Micrurus fulvius fulvius,* the Texas coral snake, *Micrurus fulvius tenere,* and the Arizona or Sonoran coral snake, *Micruroides euryxanthus* (Fig. 81–6). These snakes have small black heads and thin bodies with bright rings of red coloration next to yellow or white bands. In the nonvenomous snakes resembling the coral snake, the red and yellow are separated by black. Thus, the line

Red on yellow, kill a fellow
Red on black, good for Jack.

The Eastern coral snake is 20 to 44 inches in length, whereas the Arizona coral snake is even smaller and measures 20 inches in length.

Elapidae Envenomation

The coral snake has two venom glands that are connected by venom ducts to stationary anterior axillary teeth. The Eastern coral snake can open its mouth widely, grab firmly onto its victim, and, by using a chewing motion, inject the venom teeth deep into the tissue. There may be one or two puncture wounds approximately 8 mm apart or small teeth marks; usually, there is minimal local reaction with minimal swelling. In other bites, however, pain may radiate up the extremity and onto the chest on the side of the involved extremity. Coral snakes account for approximately 2% of snakebites in the United States; a few deaths may be due to the *Micrurus* species. The Sonoran coral snake,

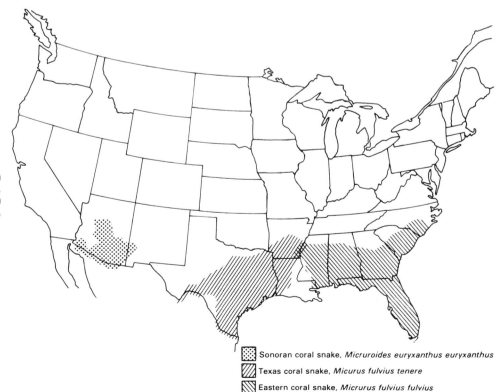

Figure 81–6. Distribution of common coral snakes in the United States. (Used by permission of the American Map Co., Inc. [© American Map Co., Inc., New York, No. 18435].)

Sonoran coral snake, *Micruroides euryxanthus euryxanthus*
Texas coral snake, *Micrurus fulvius tenere*
Eastern coral snake, *Micrurus fulvius fulvius*

because of its small jaw and head, has more difficulty with biting and with severe envenomation; no deaths have been documented as being caused by this species. As coral snake envenomation occurs into the deeper tissues, incision and suctioning are contraindicated. Within 2 hours of coral snake envenomation, the extremity may feel weak and numb. Systemic symptoms, which are initially delayed for several hours, then begin to progress rapidly. The patient can have feelings of drowsiness, tension, nausea and vomiting, tremor of the tongue, and difficulty in swallowing, speaking, or handling secretions. Diplopia may develop with paresis of the extraocular muscles. There may be ptosis, blurring of vision, and pinpoint pupils. Breathing difficulties may develop along with paralysis of the limbs. With severe envenomation hypotension may occur in association with a weak irregular pulse, and finally death may ensue within 24 hours from respiratory distress and failure from shock leading to complete cardiovascular collapse.

Treatment

As with patients with Crotalid envenomation, on arrival at the medical facility the patient who has been bitten by a coral snake should be quickly evaluated for the degree of envenomation; intravenous access should be established immediately. The prehospital care should be quickly evaluated.

Local reactions to the bite may be mild or may not be present at all; once envenomation has been recognized, it is important to proceed with treatment before systemic signs and symptoms develop. Skin testing is performed immediately, and then a minimum of three vials of specific antivenin for *Micrurus fulvius* (Wyeth) is administered intravenously; with severe pain locally, 5 units of antivenin may be indicated. With the appearance of any symptoms such as drowsiness, weakness, dysphasia, difficulty in swallowing, or respiratory distress, an additional 3 to 5 units of antivenin are indicated. There is no antivenin for the Sonoran coral snake; treatment is mainly supportive, however the envenomation is usually not severe. Unlike the situation with pit viper envenomation, since coral snake envenomation is into deeper tissues, suction and local drainage are not indicated because these local measures will not retard absorption of the venom.

Respiratory embarrassment may be severe enough to necessitate intubation and ventilation. In patients with difficulty in handling secretions, a tracheostomy may be indicated. Once the patient has been stabilized, the site of the constricting band should be evaluated to ensure that there has been no local tissue injury. If, indeed, there has been venous or arterial obstruction, after the patient has been treated with adequate fluids, a constricting band should be placed proximal to the tourniquet. The tourniquet is then slowly released, and the physician must watch carefully for signs of hypotension. Measurements should be made at the site of the envenomation and at the most proximal site of swelling; the time of evaluation should be recorded. These measurements will be important for evaluating the speed of

spread of swelling proximally when determining whether more antivenin is indicated.

As with patients with crotalid envenomation, once the patient is stable, the wound should be cleaned and the patient should be given appropriate tetanus prophylaxis. Eventually, the site of the wound may require debridement.

Colubridae

Colubrids are indigenous to the southwestern desert area. They include the nightsnake, the Texas lyre snake, the Sonora lyre snake, and the Mexican vine snake. All of these snakes may cause envenomation.

Exotic Snakes

Bites by exotic snakes have become an increasing problem; personnel may need to contact a poison control center or local zoo for help with identification of the snake and for advice on treatment and acquisition of antivenin. Several centers are available to provide information, including the Oklahoma Poison Control Center (405) 271-5454; the Regional Poison Center Office (the number can be found in the yellow pages of the phone book), 1-800-525-9083, in New Jersey, 1-800-962-1253; or the Antivenin Index in Tucson, Arizona (602) 626-6016. When evaluating a bite by a venomous snake, it is important to know which species of snake is indigenous to the region. For some snakes an immune diagnostic assay for venom or antibodies to venom by Enzyme-Linked Immuno Sorbent Assay (ELISA) test may be helpful in differentiating the envenomating snake. Table 81–6 lists some poisonous snakes that cause serious envenomation in areas outside the continental United States, including some major systemic effects of these envenomations.

Hydrophiidae (Venomous Sea Snakes)

Venomous sea snakes, members of the family Hydrophiidae, are found in the tropical Pacific and Indian Oceans, from Japan to the Persian Gulf and along the coast of Asia, extending to Australia throughout the Indo-Australian Sea. The *Pelamis planturus*, the yellow-bellied sea snake, has the widest distribution in the Indo-Pacific area, extending from the Soviet Union to Australia and from the West Coast of Central America to the East Coast of Africa.

Sea snakes have large, flat bodies with a paddle-shaped tail. Many are docile creatures who will envenomate only if stepped on while swimming or wading. The *Enhydrina schistosa*, however, is a more aggressive animal and will attack humans.

Sea snakebites can be painless and inapparent, and not all bites result in envenomation. When envenomation occurs, however, generalized symptoms may develop within 5 minutes to hours after the bite. The patient may present with malaise, anxiety, muscle stiffness, or a thick tongue. Ptosis and difficulty with swallowing and speaking may develop; muscle weakness progresses to paralysis of the legs and spreads proximally to involve the trunk, the arms, and the neck with death resulting from respiratory failure. The venom is also myotoxic and causes muscle pain, spasm, trismus, and myoglobinuria, which can cause renal tubular damage and renal failure.

Sea snake envenomation is a medical emergency that requires emergency supportive measures. After appropriate sensitivity testing, antivenin should be injected intravenously. The antivenin is made by the Commonwealth Serum Laboratories of Melbourne, Australia, and the Snake and Venom Research Laboratories of Penang, Malaysia. If neither of these antivenins is available, a polyvalant antiserum containing a krait (elapidae) fraction can be used.

Pathophysiology of Snakebites

Snake venoms vary significantly in composition, and some venoms have as many as 20 different components. A venom may contain peptides, polypeptides, enzymes, glycoproteins, and organic substances including minerals or metals. Enzymes that play an important role in venomous snakebites include proteolytic enzymes, hyaluronidase, phospholipase A-2, B, C, lactate dehydrogenase, phosphodiesterase, RNase, and acetylcholinesterase. Most snake venoms contain at least 10 of these enzymes in common; the other enzymes are scattered throughout the venom of the five families and seem to be characteristic for certain families or genera. Elapid and sea snake venoms are rich in acetylcholinesterase; crotalid and viperid venoms lack this enzyme but are rich in endopeptidase. Other venoms are rich in proteinase activity that produces marked tissue destruction. Arginine ester hydrolase is found in the crotalids and viperids and in some sea snakes, but it is not usually present in the elapids. The bradykinin-releasing and clotting activities of some venoms may be related to this esterase activity. Collagenase has been noted in the venom of a number of species of crotalids and viperids. Hyaluronidase has been noted to decrease the viscosity of connective tissue, thus allowing other factors of venom to penetrate the tissues. Phospholipase A, present in all five families of venomous snakes, is thought to catalyze the hydrolysis of fatty ester linkages and cause disruption of cell membranes by releasing histamines, kinins, serotonin, and acetylcholine. Hemolysis may be caused indirectly by the liberation of lysophosphatidase. These enzymes, by causing increased vascular permeability to plasma protein and red blood cells, may cause significant hypotension, lactic acidemia, hemoconcentration, and hypoproteinemia. Phosphodiasterase, which attacks DNA and RNA, has also been found in the venoms of all five families of venomous snakes.

The venom polypeptides, which are low molecular weight proteins, have no enzyme activity but have been shown to have neurotoxic, hemolytic, and smooth muscle–stimulating properties. These polypeptides have been shown to cause a transient increase in vascular permeability to plasma proteins, which with other proteins can cause a loss of red blood cells. The venoms also contain procoagulant and anticoagulant activity that can result in thrombocytopenia, hemolysis, and activation of plasminogen resulting in severe bleeding and death.

Crotalid venom contains proteases, which break down tissue and protein, and phosphorylases, which alter membrane integrity. Both enzymes affect coagulation. Death can occur within 1 hour and commonly within 18 to 32 hours in serious envenomation for which there is no treatment. Death can result from extensive hemorrhage and from changes in the pulmonary vasculature with pulmonary edema and hemorrhage or from cardiac or renal failure. The Mohavi rattlesnake, unlike other Crotalids, produces a venom that interferes with neuromuscular transmission.

Elapid venom causes changes in neuromuscular transmission, causing an interference with conduction and central nervous system symptomatology. In some snakes there are also enzymes that will cause local tissue destruction with bleeding and renal changes.

First Aid for Venomous Snakebites

The guidelines of the American Association of Poison Control Centers and the American College of Emergency Medicine should be followed. These guidelines include:

1. Put the patient at rest and attempt to ease his or her anxiety. Keep the patient warm; constricting clothing should be removed from the affected area, and the injured part should be kept below heart level.
2. In Crotalid envenomation of an extremity, place a constricting band ¾ to 1½ inches in width above the site of the bite to interfere with lymphatic but not venous or arterial drainage. This band may be applied several inches above the bite or above the closest proximal joint. As swelling progresses, the constricting band should be reapplied proximally above this reaction. The band should not be placed over the joint itself.
3. If transport to a hospital will take several hours, then, in pit viper envenomation, incision and suctioning from the involved area may be attempted. A 1 cm long by 0.5 cm deep incision is made through or between the fang marks along the long axis of the extremity. Suctioning using the suction cup from a snakebite kit is safest; if such a kit is not available, venom can be removed by oral suction, however this should only be done when the companion has no open oral lesions, since envenomation can occur through these lesions. To be effective, suctioning should be initiated within 10 minutes of the bite as 10 to 40% of the venom may be removed from the envenomated site early on.

Since Elapid envenomation is into deeper tissues, incision and suctioning is contraindicated. If transportation to a medical facility will take more than 1 hour, a tourniquet may be applied, but it should be released for 1 minute every 10 minutes to prevent tissue damage from the constriction. The tourniquet should continue

Table 81–6. SELECTED DANGEROUS SNAKES OF THE WORLD

Name	Common Name (Including Distribution)	Effect of Envenomation
Mexico and Central America		
Elapidae		
Micruroides euryxanthus	Arizona coral (New Mexico)	See text
Crotalidae		
Agkistrodon bilineatos	Cantil	Severe local lesion, rarely death
Bothrops atrox	Barba amarilla	Dangerous, local pain and bleeding, toxic venom
		Neurotoxic, myotoxic, causes apnea, dangerous
Crotalus durissus	Cascabel	Toxic venom, but nocturnal snake
Lachesis mutus	Bushmaster	
South America		
Elapidae		
Leptomicrurus narducci	Amazon slender coral	Neurotoxic, snakes are nocturnal
Micrurus sp.	Coral snake	Multiple sp., neurotoxic
Crotalidae		
Bothrops atrox	Barba amarilla	Local pain and bleeding
Bothrops alternatus	Urutu	Severe local effects
Bothrops jararaca	Jararaca	Deadly
Bothrops jararacussu	Jararacussu	Blindness, deadly, neurotoxic
Crotalus durissus terrificus	Cascabel	Neurotoxic, myotoxic, causes apnea
Lachesis mutus	Bushmaster	See under Central America
Europe		
Viperidae		
Vipera berus	European viper (Northern Europe to North Korea)	Bite not usually lethal, local swelling, some systemic effects
Vipera aspis	Asp viper (Southern Europe)	Not usually lethal
Vipera ammodytes	Long-nosed viper (S.E. Europe and Asia Minor)	Dangerous, toxic venom
Vipera xanthina	Ottoman viper (Istanbul)	Local swelling, hemolysis, lethal
Vipera lebetina	Levantine viper (Eastern Mediterranean islands)	Local swelling, hemolysis, serious, like Russell viper
Crotalidae		
Agkistrodon halys intermedius	Pallas' vipera (Southeast Europe and Asia)	Nocturnal snake; fatalities rare
North Africa		
Elapidae		
Naja haje	Egyptian cobra	Venom toxic like Indian cobra venom
Naja nigricollis	Spitting cobra	Local swelling, neurotoxic, deadly like Indian cobra venom
Walterinnesia aegyptia	Desert black snake	Neurotoxic
Viperidae		
Bitis arietans	Puff adder	Severe local tissue destruction, death from internal hemorrhage
Echis carinatus	Saw-scaled viper, carpet viper	Local necrosis, severe hemorrhage, many fatalities
Echis coloratus	Saw-scaled viper (Eastern Egypt)	Local pain and swelling, alteration of clotting mechanism
Central and South Africa		
Colubridae		
Dispholidus typus	Boomslang	Severe internal bleeding
Elapidae		
Dendroaspis polylepsis	Black mamba	Neurotoxin causes apnea, tachycardia, death
Hemachatus haemachatus	Ringhals	Spits, causing blindness, neurotoxic, deadly
Naja nigricollis	Spitting cobra	See under North Africa
Naja nivea	Yellow cobra (Cape cobra)	Most toxic African cobra, neurotoxic
Viperidae		
Bitis arietans	Puff adder	Tissue destruction, systemic bleeding, lethal potential
Bitis caudalis	Horned puff adder	Tissue destruction, bleeding
Bitis gabonica	Gaboon viper	Local effect, systemic hemorrhage, deadly
Echis carinatus	Saw-scaled viper	See under North Africa
Near and Middle East		
Elapidae		
Naja haje	Egyptian cobra (Jordan, Saudi Arabia, Yemen)	See under North Africa
Naja naja oxiana	Asiatic cobra (Iran, Afghanistan, South USSR)	Neurotoxic, myotoxic
Walterinnesia aegyptia	Desert black snake	See under North Africa
Viperidae		
Bitis arietans	Puff adder	See under Central and South Africa
Echis carinatus	Saw-scaled viper	See under North Africa
Echis coloratus	Saw-scaled viper	See under North Africa
Pseudocerastes persicus	False-horned viper	Little local reaction, highly toxic
Vipera lebetina	Levantine viper	See under Europe
Vipera xanthina palaestinae	Near East viper	See under Europe

Table 81–6. SELECTED DANGEROUS SNAKES OF THE WORLD *Continued*

Name	Common Name (Including Distribution)	Effect of Envenomation
Southeast Asia		
Elapidae		
Bungarus caerulus	Indian krait	Very toxic, lethal
B. candidus	Malayan krait	Lethal
Naja naja naja	Indian cobra	Necrotizing, neurotoxic
Naja naja oxiana	Oxus cobra (West Pakistan to Eastern Iran and Southern Russia)	See under Near and Middle East
Naja naja kaouthia	Monocellate cobra (West Bengal, East Pakistan, Burma, Thailand, Malaya, West China)	Neurotoxic
Naja naja atra	Chinese cobra (Thailand, South China east to Viet Nam, Taiwan)	Neurotoxic
Naja naja sputatrix	Malay cobra (Malay Peninsula and larger islands of Indonesia)	Neurotoxic
Naja naja miolepis	Borneo cobra (Borneo, Phillipines)	Neurotoxic
Naja naja philippinensis	Phillipine cobra (Luzon and Mindoro, Phillipines)	Neurotoxic
Ophiophagus hannah	King cobra, hamadryad (Peninsular India across eastern China, Phillipines, Indonesia)	Neurotoxic extending to apnea, less toxic than naja, but dangerous
Viperidae		
Echis carinatus	Saw-scaled viper	See under North Africa
Pseudocerastes persicus	False-horned viper (West Pakistan)	See under Near and Middle East
Vipera lebetina	Levantine viper (West Pakistan)	See under Europe
Vipera russelii	Russell's viper (Eastern West Pakistan, India, Burma, Thailand, South East China, Taiwan, Indonesia)	Leading cause of snakebite, local swelling, coagulapathy, neurotoxic, rhabdomyolysis
Crotalidae		
Agkistrodon acutus	Sharp-nosed pit viper (South China, North Viet Nam, Taiwan)	Dangerous, internal bleeding
Agkistrodon rhodostoma (Calloselasma rhodostoma)	Malayan pit viper (Thailand, Malaysia, Cambodia, Laos, Viet Nam, Java)	Dangerous, bleeding
Trimeresurus gramineus	Indian green tree viper (Peninsular India)	Leading cause snakebite, not usually fatal, bleeding
Trimeresurus stejnegeri	Chinese green tree viper (Central and South China, Taiwan)	
The Far East		
Elapidae		
Bungarus multicinctus	Krait (Taiwan)	Neurotoxic
Naja naja	Cobra (Philippines, Taiwan)	See under Southeast Asia
Ophiophagus hannah	King cobra (Philippines)	See under Southeast Asia
Viperidae		
Vipera russelii	Russell's viper (Taiwan)	See under Southeast Asia
Crotalidae		
Agkistrodon acutus	Sharp-nosed pit viper (Taiwan, South and East China, North Viet Nam)	See under Southeast Asia
Agkistrodon halys	Mamushi (Japan, Korea, East and North China) Okinawa habu (Amami and Okinawa)	Less severe envenomation
Trimeresurus flavoviridis	Chinese habu (Taiwan, South China, to North Viet Nam, Laos, Burma)	Venom, low toxicity
T. mucrosquamatus		Low toxicity, few fatalities
Australia and Pacific Islands		
Elapidae		
Acanthophis antarcticus	Death adder (Australia, except desert, New Guinea)	Neurotoxic, hemolytic, dangerous (without treatment 50% mortality)
Demansia textilis (pseudo naja nuchelis)	Australian brown snake	Toxic venom, neurotoxic, hemolytic, coagulopathy
Denisunia superba (Austrelaps)	Australian copperhead (South East Australia)	Dangerous, neurotoxic, hemolytic
Notechis scutatus	Australian tiger snake (Southern Australia)	Most dangerous snake of Australia, neurotoxic, coagulopathy, hemolytic, myotoxic
Oxyuranus scutellatus	Taipan (North Australia, South East New Guinea)	Dangerous, local reaction, hemolytic, coagulopathy, neurotoxic, myotoxic
Pseudechis australis	Australian mulga snake (North and Mid Australia, South New Guinea, Melville I.)	Very dangerous, neurotoxic, myotoxic, hemolytic, coagulopathy
Pseudechis papuanus	Papuan black snake (South East New Guinea, Yale Island)	Very dangerous
Pseudechis porphyriacus	Red bellied black snake (South East Australia)	Only 1% deadly, hemolytic, coagulopathy

to be applied until 3 minutes after the first dose of intravenous antivenin.

4. If possible, the snake should be killed and brought to the medical facility along with the patient. Care should be taken in handling the snake since a second person could be envenomated by reflex action from the head of the killed snake even up to several hours after the original snakebite. The snake should be carried on a stick sufficiently far away from the second person to prevent envenomation.

5. Cryotherapy should not be initiated, since the application of ice can cause further damage at the envenomated site and can cause the enzymes in the venom to be diverted into deeper layers of the extremity.

On arrival at the medical facility, the patient should be quickly evaluated for systemic toxicity. Vital signs should be recorded, and an intravenous line should be established immediately. The site of the snakebite should be quickly examined and determination should be made whether envenomation has actually occurred.

HOSPITAL TREATMENT OF SNAKEBITES

Treatment of Hypovolemia

In moderate to severe pit viper envenomation, there will be continued leakage of intravenous fluids and plasma proteins into the tissues. As much as one volume of body fluid can extravasate into the tissues of an envenomated extremity. Pulmonary edema from damaged lungs may occur within the first hour or may not occur for 6 to 24 hours. Hypovolemia as manifested by capillary hypoperfusion, oliguria, anemia, tachycardia, and hypotension may occur.

A separate intravenous line must be established to maintain volume replacement using normal saline or lactated Ringer's solution, 20 ml/kg initially; fresh whole blood or blood components, including 5% albumin, may be necessary. Patients require constant intravascular monitoring and measurements of urinary output. Vasopressors such as dobutamine may be required to maintain the blood pressure until adequate volume replacement has been obtained (see Chapter 12).

Treatment of Blood Loss

Severe hemolysis and systemic bleeding may occur due to the coagulopathy caused by the venom. Blood replacement with either fresh whole blood or blood components, including packed red blood cells (10 ml/kg) and fresh frozen plasma (10 ml/kg) will be necessary. With continued severe bleeding, platelets (0.2 units/kg) and fibrinogen as cryoprecipitate (one bag per 5 kg body weight) may also be indicated. Laboratory monitoring includes complete blood counts, platelet counts, fibrinogen levels, and partial thromboplastin times.

Treatment with Antivenin

Antivenin has been considered the cornerstone of treatment for snakebite envenomation. First one must be certain that the individual has actually been envenomated, because 25 to 40% of patients are not envenomated and another 15% of bites are so mild that they do not require antivenin. In those patients, it is important to cleanse the wound, to administer tetanus toxoid or antitoxin, and to start antibiotics to prevent local and systemic infections.

Since one aim of treatment is to bind the circulating free venom, to be most effective the antivenin should be administered within 4 to 6 hours of envenomation. A reasonable response will be obtained with antivenin that is administered within 12 hours of envenomation; after 24 hours, the antivenin is ineffective except in cases in which there is a severe coagulopathy.

Since the antivenin is a horse serum extract, skin testing is required before administering a therapeutic dose. Because even the skin testing can precipitate an anaphylactoid reaction, this testing should be done with intravenous epinephrine (1 to 10,000), antihistamines, steroids, and resuscitative equipment readily available. The package insert has directions for administering this skin testing, but usually an intradermal injection of 0.02 ml of a 1:10 dilution of the reconstituted antivenin is used. If there is a question of potential reaction, a 1:100 dilution can be used instead. A saline control is usually administered in the opposite extremity. Usually within 15 minutes any reaction will be apparent. If the result of the skin test is negative, one then can proceed with diluting the reconstituted antivenin in saline in either a 1:1 or 1:10 dilution and slowly infusing the antivenin intravenously. If there is no allergic reaction in the first 10 to 20 minutes, the infusion can be increased to up to 5 vials/hr.

Fortunately, in the United States the antivenin against pit viper envenomation (Wyeth) contains antivenin against all pit vipers of North America. If the patient is mildly sensitive to the antivenin, as illustrated by skin testing, intravenous diphenhydramine can be given 15 minutes before giving the antivenin. If the result of the test is strongly positive, the antivenin should be given only for life-threatening envenomation or when the actual limb is threatened. The antivenin package suggests desensitizing for allergic reactions; since this procedure would require at least 3 hours to complete, in situations of severe envenomation this is not practical. In this situation intravenous epinephrine, diphenhydramine, and steroids must be administered through a separate intravenous access line at the same time that antivenin is being given.

The amount of antivenin to be administered intravenously varies somewhat with the type and severity of snakebite being treated. Russell recommends starting with 5 to 8 vials of antivenin for minimal envenomation, 9 to 12 vials for moderate envenomation, and at least 13 vials to as many as 40 vials for severe envenomation. Since copperhead and cottonmouth envenomation may be less severe, one may start with 3 to 5 vials for a mild envenomation and 6 to 8 vials for a moderate envenomation. Russell further recommends that if the swelling is confined to the site of the snakebite at 30 minutes to 1 hour after envenomation, and if there is no evidence of paresthesias, fasciculations, ecchymoses, or bleb formation and only minor local pain, these patients may not need any antivenin. I have personally seen patients referred to our institution 8 to 12 hours after copperhead envenomation where there was moderate swelling beyond the snakebite wound and local pain and ecchymoses at the bite site; these patients recovered uneventfully without the use of antivenin. In Mohave rattlesnake envenomation, in which there may be less local edema but more systemic reaction, the amount of antivenin used may be twice the amount that one would usually use for other rattlesnake envenomations.

Although local infiltration of antivenin is usually not necessary, some medical personnel prefer to give one third of a vial of antivenin locally, while initiating systemic treatment. In situations in which antivenin is infiltrated locally, it should never be given into a digit; this may increase local swelling and cause vascular compromise. Once the antivenin has been given systemically, the local constricting band may be removed; this should be done cautiously to prevent rapid infusion centrally of venom that has been trapped distal to the band.

After initiating intravenous treatment with antivenin, the circumference of the involved extremities should be measured at 15-minute intervals to determine the progression of swelling, and the patient should be observed for systemic reactions. The initial dose of the antivenin should be repeated as long as there is continuing progression of pain and swelling locally and systemic symptomatology. Once the rate of swelling has slowed, the involved extremity can be measured every 30 to 60 minutes for the next 48 hours. The patient should continue to be monitored carefully for systemic symptomatology, and antivenin should be readministered as necessary.

Allergic Reactions

Despite a negative result on a skin test, acute allergic reactions to antivenin can occur. This may be due to too rapid infusion of the antivenin; when the infusion is stopped and subsequently restarted, at a slower rate, the antivenin may be tolerated. Of patients with a negative result on a skin test, however, 3 to 5% will still have a systemic reaction unrelated to a rapid antivenin infusion. These patients may present with hypotension, malaise, facial swelling, and angioneurotic edema. They may develop tachypnea, tachycardia, and shock.

The continued use of intravenous antivenin at the time of a systemic allergic reaction is determined by the severity of the allergic reaction and by the severity of the envenomation. Consultation with a regional poison control center or with a medical herpetologist may be necessary. Discussion with the family members is important when the patient is in such a serious situation.

In mild allergic reactions, after interrupting the antivenin infusion, diphenhydramine, 1 to 2 mg/kg, should be given intravenously. Once the allergic symptoms have resolved, the antivenin infusion may be reinstituted at a slower rate. In cases of severe envenomation it may be necessary to continue with the antivenin infusion while also infusing epinephrine intravenously at 0.1 μg/kg/min at another site. At the same time steroids, methylprednisolone 2 mg/kg every 6 hours, should be initiated.

Delayed Allergic Reactions

Delayed allergic reactions including serum sickness have been reported in more than half the patients treated with horse serum antivenin. Currently antivenin is being developed using sheep serum rather than horse serum, and this may reduce the problem of delayed allergic reactions.

Other Systemic Involvement

Because of damage to the capillary endothelium, pulmonary edema may develop with associated respiratory failure. The patient may require oxygen and respiratory assistance. Damage to the myocardium may cause cardiac failure; ECG monitoring is important, and treatment with diuretics and digoxin may be indicated. Renal failure from hypotension or secondary to massive hemoglobinuria and myoglobinuria may develop, necessitating frequent monitoring of urinary output and in severe situations renal dialysis.

Treatment of Pain

Once respiratory embarrassment is no longer an issue, codeine may be used to alleviate the pain of the snakebite; morphine may occasionally be required. Diazepam may also be indicated for sedation.

Wound and Follow-up Care

After the patient has been stabilized and is no longer in severe danger, the wound should be cleaned with thorough irrigation. A loose dressing should be applied. Tetanus prophylaxis should be instituted either in the form of tetanus toxoid or antitoxin, depending on whether the patient has been previously immunized. Initially, the involved extremity should be placed below the level of the heart in a position of function. Cotton padding should be placed between the swollen digits to prevent skin maceration. Surgical debridement of bloody vesicles and superficial necrosis may be necessary 3 to 5 days after the injury, and the debrided area should be treated like a superficial burn. Surgical intervention with fasciotomy for swelling of the extremity is contraindicated unless there is evidence for a compartment syndrome with the venous pressure remaining above 40 mm Hg, and unless there is evidence of severe vascular embarrassment. To prevent bacterial infection from the

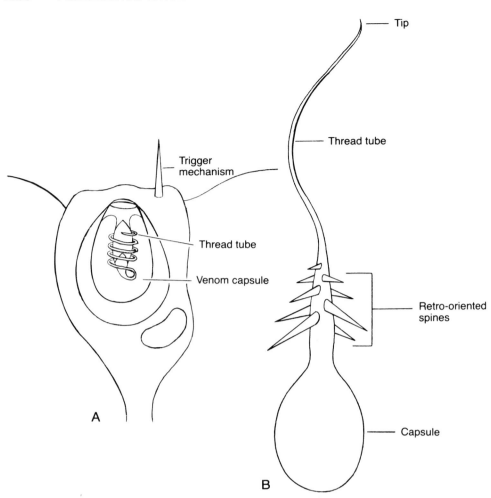

Figure 81–7. Typical nematocyst. Stimulation of trigger mechanism causes ejection of venom capsule. Retro-oriented spines hold thread tube in place while venom passes down the thread tube into the victim. *A,* Undischarged. *B,* Discharged. (Adapted from Kreuzinger R. *In:* Halstead BW: Poisonous and Venomous Marine Animals of the World. Princeton, NJ, The Darwin Press, 1978.)

contaminated snakebite, systemic antibiotics should be administered.

When the patient is stable, he or she should be evaluated for joint mobility, muscle strength, and sensation. Early initiation of physical therapy including whirlpool baths may be indicated to prevent contractures. Ongoing physical therapy, even after discharge from the hospital, is indicated to prevent loss of function and to prevent contractures in the involved extremities. Some patients may experience paresthesias for months after envenomation.

PHYLUM COELENTERATA, HYDROIDS, AND JELLYFISH

The phylum Coelenterata includes marine animals with simple bodies composed of two epithelial layers covering an internal cavity that opens to the outside through a mouth; these animals have tentacles with nematocysts. There are three classes: (1) the Hydrozoa, which includes the orange-striped jellyfish and the Portuguese man-o-war; (2) the Scyphozoa, which includes jellyfish, sea nettles, and sea wasps; and (3) the Anthosoa, which includes sea anemones and corals.

Envenomation by these animals can cause a mild reaction with erythema and local discomfort to an overwhelming systemic reaction with instant death. The tentacles are equipped with the nematocyst apparatus that contains the venom (Fig. 81–7). When stimulated, the coiled tubule is ejected from the cyst, the venom is released through the tubule and into the tissue of the victim. The severity of envenomation is affected by the species of the animal, the number of nematocysts involved, the potency of the venom, the depth of skin penetration, and the sensitivity of the victim to the venom.

Hydrozoan stings may be mild, as with the hydroid, to extremely severe as with the *Physalia*, which includes the Portuguese man-o-war and the bluebottle. One species occurs in the tropical Atlantic, occasionally as far north as the Bay of Fundy, and in the Mediterranean; the other species is found in the Indo-Pacific, as far north as Southern Japan, and near Hawaii. There may be severe pain over the involved extremity, extending along the area of lymphatic drainage, with associated malaise, headache, fever and chills, muscle cramps, collapse, and death.

As with the Hydrozoa, the Scyphozoa sting may be mild with local pain and erythema, occasionally with numbness, urticaria, and even some facial flushing, sneezing, or rhinitis.

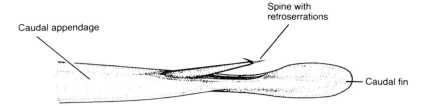

Figure 81–8. Venomous apparatus of the stingray. Venom is stored in acini below the skin of the caudal appendage and is released after puncture by the spine. (Adapted from Kreuzinger R. *In:* Halstead BW: Poisonous and Venomous Marine Animals of the World. Princeton, NJ, The Darwin Press, 1978.)

More severe reactions may occur with the *Cyanea capillata*, the sea nettle or lion's mane, which is found in the North Atlantic and Pacific, from New England to the Arctic Ocean, from Alaska to the Puget Sound, along the coast of Japan, China, and Australia, from France to North Russia, and in the Baltic Sea; and with the *Chrysaora quinquecirrha*, the sea nettle, found in New England to the tropics, in West Africa, in the Indian Ocean, and from the Malayan Archipelago to Japan in the Western Pacific Ocean, and also along the coast of the Philippines. Generalized symptoms may be more severe with muscle cramps, coughing, urticaria, mental depression, respiratory distress, and loss of consciousness. If the victim is in the water, drowning may occur.

Even more severe reactions occur with *Chironex fleckeri*, the sea wasp found off the coast of Australia, and with *Chiropsalmus*, sea wasps found in the Atlantic Ocean from North Carolina to Brazil, and off the coast of Northern Australia, in the Indian Ocean, and in the Philippines. Victims of sea wasp stings develop painful muscular spasms, respiratory distress, tachycardia, and cardiovascular collapse; death can occur within 15 minutes to 2 hours after envenomation.

Toxicology

Coelenterate venoms cause pain, paralysis, and an urticarial-type reaction. It has been suggested that the pain is caused by 5-hydroxytryptamine, a known pain producer and a releaser of histamine. Tetramine has been implicated in the paralyzing effects of the venom, and the urticarial effects of the venom are due to histamine released by 5-hydroxytryptamine and other histamine releasers. Studies on the venom suggest a musculotoxic effect of the toxins that prevent uptake of calcium ions in skeletal muscles.

Treatment

The goals of treatment include relieving pain, alleviating the neurotoxic and urticarial effects of the venom, and controlling shock.

Jellyfish tentacles must be removed immediately using sand, towels, or other materials, since the nematocysts will continue to discharge venom until they are removed. Alcohol, dilute ammonia, suntan lotion, or suntan oil can also be used to inhibit further release of venom by the nematocysts. Care should be taken in removing the

tentacles because the rescuer can also become envenomated.

Oral antihistamines may be used to alleviate the urticarial reaction, and morphine may be necessary to alleviate pain. Intravenous calcium gluconate (10 ml of a 10% solution) may relieve muscle spasms. Supportive measures including plasma expanders may be necessary to treat systemic hypotension; oxygen and cardiac and respiratory stimulants may be necessary.

For severe envenomation by *Chironex fleckeri*, an antivenin is available through the Commonwealth Serum Laboratories in Melbourne, Australia. One vial of antivenin should be administered intravenously; however, if on the scene of the envenomation an emergency exists and there is no one to introduce the antivenin intravenously, then three vials of antivenin can be given intramuscularly.

Prevention

Care should be taken to prevent envenomation, especially by *Physalia* and by the cubomedusae Chiropsalmus. Since the tentacles are long, care should be taken when swimming in an area where these animals exist. After storms, particular care should be taken when swimming in jellyfish-infested waters since pieces of tentacles can still envenomate. Even jellyfish appearing dead on a beach can cause envenomation as stimulated nematocysts discharge their venom on unsuspecting victims.

VENOMOUS STINGRAYS

Venomous stingrays are members of the Vertebrate subphylum, class *Chondrichythes;* they have highly developed jaws and fins and also a cartilaginous skeleton. They can usually be found buried in sand or mud, and they envenomate their victims who unknowingly step on them.

The venom apparatus is a caudal appendage with a retroserrated dentinal spine, covered by thick skin containing venom-producing glandular acini (Fig. 81–8). The stinger penetrates flesh easily, but it is difficult to remove because of the retroserrations; severe lacerations may result from the sting itself or from removal of the stinger.

Sharp stabbing pain from envenomation occurs within 10 minutes, becomes more severe within 30 minutes, and may last up to 48 hours. The venom causes systemic symptoms of hypotension, nausea, vomiting, arrhythmia, muscular paralysis, respiratory embarrassment, and death.

Prompt treatment should be aimed at alleviating pain, counteracting the venom, and preventing infection. The wound should be irrigated with cold, salt water that will cause vasoconstriction and decrease the venom absorption. In severe envenomation, a tourniquet may be placed on the extremity but must be briefly released every few minutes. Surgical exploration of the wound is necessary for removal of all stinger integument to prevent further envenomation. Hot water soaks should then be initiated, followed by further debridement. Systemic antibiotics are indicated.

Narcotics may be necessary for relief of pain. Supportive measures should be instituted since shock and cardiovascular collapse can occur.

Toxicology

Crude extracts of the stingray venom have contained serotonin, 5-nucleotidase, and phosphodiesterase, which may cause peripheral vasodilatation, although peripheral vasoconstriction and cardiac arrhythmias are more usual. Respiratory compromise and seizures may occur.

Bibliography

Halstead BW: Poisonous and Venomous Marine Animals of the World. Princeton, Darwin Press, 1978.
Hobbs GD and Harrell RE: Brown recluse spider bites: A common cause of necrotic arachnidism. Am J Emerg Med 7(3):309–312, 1989.
Kunkel DB: The sting of the arthropod. Emerg Med 20:41–48, 1988.
Rauber A: Black widow spider bites. J Toxicol Clin Toxicol 21 (4 and 5):473–485, 1983–1984.
Russell FE: Snake Venom Poisoning. Great Neck, Scholium International, 1983.

82

Heat Syndromes

Carl B. Ramsey, M.D., and Peter R. Holbrook, M.D.

HISTORY

Heat stroke was originally described over 2,500 years ago in a pediatric patient.[1] Another report of heat stroke dates back over 2,000 years to 24 B.C., when a Roman army was virtually destroyed by heatstroke in Arabia.[2] The defeat of King Edward's crusaders in the final battle for the Holy Land was as much by "heat and fever" as by a well-acclimatized army of Arabs.[3] In World War I, heat-related casualties severely hindered a British campaign against the Turks in Mesopotamia.[4] The largest numbers of casualties lost to heat stroke currently comes from religious pilgrimages to Mecca. This results in hundreds of fatalities from heat stroke each year.[5, 6]

The military has a long history of experience with heat illnesses. During World War II, military recruits were exposed to conditioning and training in hot and humid environments in order to prepare them for duty in tropical or desert environments. There is one report of 125 cases of heat stroke–related deaths associated with this training.[7] Athletes often encounter similar heat exposure during training, and heat stroke is a leading cause of death among athletes, second only to head and spinal injuries.[8] During summer training, there is significant morbidity and mortality associated with the intense exertion in activities such as twice-daily football practices and distance running.[8, 9]

Even so, the nonathletic civilian population has suffered from heat stroke and related illnesses more than the younger and better-conditioned athlete or military personnel. This was observed during 5 "heat wave" years (1952 to 1955 and 1966) and was reported in a review of heat-related illnesses.[10] This study found 820 heat stroke deaths occurring during "heat wave" years, compared with 179 deaths/yr during "non-heat wave" years. It is interesting that this same report estimates that ten heat-precipitated deaths occur, predominantly from cardiovascular events (e.g., cerebrovascular accidents, myocardial infarction, congestive heart failure) for each isolated case of heat stroke–induced death. The role of elevated environmental temperature is difficult to prove in illness and death that is not obviously associated with the full-blown syndrome of heat stroke. Due to this, it is difficult to define the effect of environmental heat on patient populations by routine epidemiologic or demographic studies.

Although heat stroke has been described in infants and children,[11–16] the morbidity and mortality from heat-related illnesses in pediatrics is probably underestimated. This may be due to confusion of heat-related illnesses with the more common infectious causes of hyperpyrexia. The diagnosis may also be thwarted by euthermic or only mildly hyperthermic presentation of an infant who has cooled before an assessment of core temperature is made.

The recently described syndrome of "hemorrhagic (or hyperpyrexic) shock and encephalopathy" (HSE) may represent a pediatric form of heat shock. The clinical course and autopsy findings of patients with HSE are remarkably similar to those of older patients with exertional heat stroke.

In this chapter we discuss thermoregulation, acclimatization, and the different heat syndromes. Emphasis is placed on the pathophysiology, diagnosis, and management of those syndromes that are likely to come to the attention of the practitioners of pediatric critical care and emergency medicine.

THERMOREGULATION

Humans are homeothermic animals and as such must maintain a core body temperature within a very narrow range around 37° C. This is essential to ensure adequate function of temperature-dependent enzyme systems that provide physiologic and biochemical homeostasis. Under basal metabolic conditions that are controlled by catecholamines and thyroid hormone, an adult produces 60 to 70 kcal of heat per hour.[17] Radiation from the sun can cause a gain of up to 150 kcal/hr.[18] Intense physical work can produce as much as 1,000 kcal/hr for brief periods.[19]

In the basal metabolic state, a normal person attains thermal equilibrium with the environment and maintains a core temperature of 37°C when the ambient temperature is 29°C or 84.2°F.[20] When ambient temperature exceeds this value and the humidity is maximal, in the absence of thermoregulation, an obligatory rise in body temperature occurs. Under these conditions, at basal metabolic rate, the progressive rise in body temperature is predicted to be 1.1°C or 2°F/hr.[17] In a similar environment, the temperature rise under a work load expenditure of only 300 kcal/hr will exceed 5°C or 9°F/hr.[19] This highlights the need for dissipation of heat from the body to the environment through radiation, conduction, and convection with vaporization of sweat.

If ambient temperature is lower than the surface temperature of the body, heat will be conducted down its gradient to the surrounding air. Conduction is aided by convection. By convection, body heat is transferred to another substance, such as sweat or exhaled air, and is carried (convected) away.[21] In hot weather, neither conduction nor convection are very effective. Therefore, when ambient temperature exceeds 35°C or 95°F, there is minimal dissipation of heat by conduction or convection. Warming of blood causes the reflex that initiates sweating. The hypothalamus, in a reflexive response to elevated blood temperature, dilates skin blood vessels and stimulates sweat production by skin sweat glands. This is known as the Benzinger reflex.[22] Each 1.7 ml of sweat vaporized eliminates 1 kcal of heat load.[17] In ideal conditions, an acclimatized person can sweat at rates of more than 3.5 l/hr.[23]

A more typical situation involves the unacclimatized person who can yield a maximal sweat rate of 1.5 l/hr. This volume of sweat provides dissipation of 900 kcal/hr of heat. This efficiency is never attained however, since 20% or more of sweat may be lost by dripping.[24] In addition to this, high sweat rates cannot be maintained indefinitely and ideal conditions are rarely encountered. In warm humid conditions that prevent efficient loss of heat by usual mechanisms, the limits of heat dissipation are approached at caloric expenditures of 650 kcal/hr.[25] Cutaneous blood flow decreases dramatically as exhaustion occurs during exercise in heat.[26] Due to this, removal of heat from the blood to the body surface is impaired. Diminished sweat production occurs, and hyperpyrexia follows if work is continued.[27, 28]

ACCLIMATIZATION

Acclimatization to heat is defined as the physiologic process by which an individual becomes tolerant to heat stress safely and relatively comfortably. The adaptation mostly involves the cardiovascular, endocrine, and exocrine systems. While a great deal of acclimatization can occur within 5 days, 2 weeks or more are required for maximal acclimatization.[17, 21] The status of physical training is critical to tolerance of heat stress and physical work in heat. Physical conditioning produces prolonged elevation of body temperature and physiologic changes very similar to those seen in the heat-acclimatized state. An unacclimatized person who is in excellent physical condition can withstand much more heat stress than a person who is not conditioned. Work or exercise that does not elevate body temperature does not produce acclimatization.[29]

NONACCLIMATIZED RESPONSES TO ACUTE HEAT STRESS

Muscular work in heat causes vasodilation in the skin and skeletal muscles. Shunting of blood to muscle can be massive and can produce what is called *exercise hyperemia*. Blood flow to muscle varies proportionately to the degree of muscular work and ranges from 1 ml/100 g/min at rest to 20 to 40 times this value during intense exercise.[30] A significant loss of plasma volume into muscular tissue occurs as glycogen and other substrates are broken down into smaller molecules that have high osmotic activity. The loss of plasma volume to the extravascular space can amount to as much as 10% or more of the inflowing arterial volume.[31] In addition to this there is loss of fluid via sweating. Without compensatory mechanisms, these losses could quickly produce hypotension. In response to this loss of effective blood volume, the splanchnic circulation vascular resistance increases by as much as 120%.[31] Decreased splanchnic blood flow is paralleled by decreased urine sodium concentration and oliguria as the renin-angiotensin axis is activated and aldosterone levels increase. The decrease in splanchnic blood flow alone is not sufficient to compensate for the loss of intravascular volume to skeletal muscle and sweat, along with the complicating factor of decreased vascular tone in skin and muscle beds. A two-fold increase in cardiac output may be necessary to meet the demands of acute exercise hyperemia.[31] It is the unconditioned or unacclimatized person who has difficulty meeting these demands. The central circulatory response to decreased intravascular volume and decreased venous return is tachycardia and decreased stroke volume. If heart rate and venous return are adequate, cardiac output may remain the same or may rise slightly. If hyperthermia progresses, the cardiac output and stroke volume falls.

ACCLIMATIZATION TO HEAT STRESS

A characteristic of the heat-acclimatized individual is a smaller incremental rise in core temperature in response to any given work load. In the acclimatized and physically conditioned person's muscle, there is a greater metabolic efficiency and less heat production due to increased myoglobin content and mitochondrial density.[33, 34] The decreased plasma volume seen in response to acute heat exposure causes stimulation of the renin-angiotensin system and elevation of plasma aldosterone. In the acute situation, vasoconstriction helps to maintain blood pressure. In the acclimatized state, aldosterone levels remain high.[35] In response to this, urinary sodium falls, and plasma volume as well as extracellular fluid volume and total body water expands. These fluid stores are available to replenish intravascular volume losses during muscular work in heat. This provides greater venous return and preload to the heart during heat stress. There is subsequent elevation of stroke volume and cardiac output with a lower peak heart rate. These cardiovascular responses are characteristic of the acclimatized and well-conditioned individual.

Serum potassium concentrations are effected by acclimatization and physical training.[17] With heat exposure, hyperventilation occurs causing respiratory alkalosis. The serum potassium may drop by as much as 1 mEq/l, probably due to the respiratory alkalosis.[36] However, if body temperature reaches 39° C serum potassium may rise instead of falling.[37] The febrile hyperkalemia persists, even in the face of a progressive alkalosis. The cause of this is not known.

Acclimatized individuals, as well as distance runners and the person who has physically trained may have a low normal serum potassium. In some cases, there is hypokalemia at rest.[38] This occurs without total body potassium deficiency.[35] Severe hypokalemia may occur in the unacclimatized or untrained person who works or exercises to the point of exhaustion.[39] Severe hypokalemia increases the risk for several heat-related injuries,[40] including exercise-induced rhabdomyolysis. Despite the possibility of hypokalemia, potassium supplements should not be given prophylactically due to the possibility of hyperkalemia with rhabdomyolysis occurring during exhaustive work or exercise.[21]

CLINICAL SPECTRUM OF ENVIRONMENTAL HEAT ILLNESS

Heat Syncope

Heat syncope is loss of consciousness or orthostatic dizziness after exposure to high environmental temperatures, with other causes ruled out. Heat-induced vasodilation, postural pooling of blood, and diminished venous return to the heart cause low cardiac output and transient cerebral ischemia. Transient ischemia and syncope may be aggravated by hyperventilation and hypocapneic alkalosis, which is commonly seen in the heat-stressed individual.[41] Heat syncope seems to occur more often in persons with heart disease (impaired cardiac response to heat stress) and in individuals taking diuretics (decreased effective circulating blood volume). With the volume expansion that occurs with acclimatization, syncope and dizziness should resolve.

Heat Edema

Heat edema is mild dependent edema that occurs in the unacclimatized within a couple of days of exposure to a hot climate. It may be due to increased aldosterone or growth hormone production, or both.

Heat Tetany

Heat tetany occurs when normal persons are exposed to hot climates or breath-heated air. In response to this, there is hyperventilation and acute respiratory alkalosis.[41] The patients complain of the usual effects of hyperventilation, such as acral and circumoral paresthesias, and occasionally frank tetany.[42] Alkalosis reduces cerebral blood flow; therefore, while hyperventilation causes tetany, it may also be involved with heat syncope.

Heat Cramps

Heat cramps are intense spasmodic contractions that usually affect the muscles involved with work, although they occasionally affect the abdominal muscles. Heat cramps are not associated with elevated body temperature. They usually develop in acclimatized and well-trained individuals who can produce large volumes of sweat. Acclimatized sweat has a lower sodium concentration than nonacclimatized sweat (75 mEg/l versus 100 mEq/l) due to higher aldosterone levels in individuals chronically exposed to work in heat. The volume of sweat that an acclimatized individual can produce is so much higher than an unacclimatized person (2.5 l/hr versus 1.5 l/hr) that the acclimatized person may actually lose more sodium.[2] The replacement of sweat volume with free water results in a modest hyponatremia.[43] This hyponatremia may enhance cytosolic calcium concentration to a level sufficient to initiate muscular contraction.[44] Salt-containing fluids taken orally, or intravenous saline, will rapidly reverse cramping.

Heat Exhaustion

Heat exhaustion is usually a mixed disorder of water and sodium deficiency, although isolated water or salt deficiencies can precipitate heat exhaustion. Heat exhaustion usually develops over several days and affects those who are unacclimatized in epidemic patterns that parallel heat waves.

Heat Exhaustion from Sodium Depletion

Heat exhaustion from sodium depletion occurs in unacclimatized individuals who replace sweat losses with free water. The affected person is usually afebrile, tachycardic, and mildly hypotensive. The person's skin is cool and clammy, and urine output as well as sweat volume is normal. Laboratory evaluation reveals hyponatremia. If the patient is communicative, he or she usually does not complain of severe thirst but will often have muscle cramps, weakness, fatigue, myalgias, headache, or altered mental status as signs of hyponatremia.[45] Gastrointestinal upset manifested as nausea, vomiting, or diarrhea is seen in adults as well as in children and infants and may tempt the practitioner to diagnose gastrointestinal infection. A high index of suspicion and a thorough history should aid in the diagnosis of heat exhaustion. Hyponatremia is usually mild, and the clinical syndrome is usually corrected easily by administration of salted fluids orally or by intravenous saline.

Water Depletion Heat Exhaustion

This form of heat exhaustion usually occurs when the water supply is limited to those subjected to heat stress. It occurs in athletes or workers who ingest salt without adequate water intake and in infants and older patients who cannot express or control alleviation of their thirst. This is the more serious form of heat exhaustion, and lack of prompt recognition and treatment opens the way for progression to heat stroke. If circulatory failure progresses or seizures occur, the rise in body temperature accelerates and the patient rapidly develops heat stroke.

The patient with water depletion heat exhaustion shows signs of hypernatremic dehydration with tachycardia and hypotension and is invariably febrile. If communicative, the patient will complain of intense thirst and anxiety. These patients often show agitation and confusion that can, in severe cases, progress to hysterical or overtly psychotic behavior. They exhibit muscular fatigue, discomfort, and incoordination. There may be heat-induced hyperventilation with complaints of paresthesias and dizziness. Sweating continues, although its volume decreases. The patient exhibits oliguria and urinary concentration with low urine sodium.

This form of heat exhaustion can be treated by judicious replacement of free water. An easy way to approximate the free water deficit is to assume that the total body water (TBW) has been reduced in reverse proportion to the elevation of serum sodium. For example, a patient whose normal weight is 40 kg presents with a serum sodium of 160 mEq/l. The child's normal TBW can be estimated as 60% of body weight or 24 l.

(Normal serum sodium ×
        normal TBW) / actual serum sodium = actual TBW
        or, (140 × 24) / 160 = 21 l actual TBW.
    (24 l normal TBW − 21 l actual TBW) = 3 l deficit

If fluid boluses are needed for acute stabilization, normal saline may be used to correct hypotension without fear of lowering serum sodium too rapidly. Once the patient is stabilized, the remainder of the free water deficit may be replaced over 48 hours (in addition to normal maintenance fluids) at a rate that should not exceed ½ to 1 mEq/hr of sodium. Frequent assessment of serum and urine sodium is important for guiding therapy. Regardless of the method chosen to normalize intravascular volume and serum sodium, care should be taken to avoid rapid correction of serum sodium. Any syndrome of serum hypertonicity is theoretically associated with development of "ideogenic" osmoles in brain cells. It is hypothesized that this is done in an attempt to maintain intracellular volume. A rapid correction of serum sodium after the development of these "idiogenic" osmoles in brain cells creates an osmotic imbalance favoring flow of free water into brain cells, which produces cerebral edema. Due to this, it is considered to be prudent to lower serum sodium slowly.

HEAT STROKE

Heat stroke is a medical emergency that is defined as a body temperature above 40.6°C (105°F) and a functional disturbance of the central nervous system.[17, 21, 46, 47] Heat stroke is usually divided into two forms: classic and exertional. The differences between the two forms are contrasted in the following pages. In addition to the usual classifications, we describe infant heat stroke and hemorrhagic (hyperpyrexic) shock and encephalopathy (HSE) as similar entities, representing a fairly recent recognition of a separate form of pediatric heat syndrome.

Emphasis is placed on exertional stroke and HSE, because these heat syndromes are seen most often in pediatric critical care and emergency medicine.

Classic Heat Stroke

Classic heat stroke involves hyperthermia, central nervous system dysfunction, and anhidrosis. It affects the very old or the infirm and often occurs in epidemics during heat waves. It usually causes irreversible central nervous system impairment, yet it is associated with less severe impairment of muscular, renal, and hematologic systems than is seen in infant or exertional heat stroke. The usual metabolic findings are respiratory alkalosis and hypokalemia. There may be a metabolic acidosis that is partially compensated. Hyperkalemia is rarely seen. In general, patients who die of classic heat stroke show much less tissue damage than do patients with exertional heat stroke. This does not seem to be due to higher core temperatures in exertional heat stroke. Indeed, there are patients who recover fully from classic heat stroke, having exhibited core temperatures of 43.7°C (110°F).[48] One patient with classic heat stroke survived without sequelae after exhibiting a rectal temperature of 46.5°C (115.7°F), measured by a reliable instrument.[49] In comparison, almost total body destruction has been observed in patients with exertional heat stroke whose core temperature did not exceed 40.6°C (105°F).[17]

Only 5% of patients with classic heat stroke develop renal insufficiency, compared with a 25% incidence in patients with exertional heat stroke. The likely explanation for this is the very low incidence of significant rhabdomyolysis in patients who have classic heat stroke.[50]

Exertional Heat Stroke

This is a syndrome of hyperthermia in which heat is produced by muscular work at a rate that exceeds the body's capacity to dissipate the heat produced. Approximately 50% of patients with exertional heat stroke retain the capacity to sweat, compared with the anhydrosis of classic heat stroke. Fatal exertional heat stroke can occur in healthy acclimatized and physically conditioned individuals when the ability to dissipate heat is exceeded by endogenous heat production. This usually occurs in competitive distance runners, football players, and military recruits. Hyperpyrexia and rhabdomyolysis are also seen in some cases of amphetamine and cocaine overdoses,[17] as well as in LSD and phencyclidine overdose.[51–53]

Cardiovascular complications are severe in exertional heat stroke. Hemodynamic studies reveal two main patterns.[54, 55] One group of patients exhibit high cardiac output with low peripheral vascular resistance, an elevated central venous pressure, and moderately low arterial blood pressure. These hemodynamic changes are corrected by cooling.

A second group of patients present with low cardiac output, marked elevation of central venous pressure, hypotension, and cyanosis. If cooling does not restore hemodynamic normality, these patients should respond to inotropic support. Prudent fluid resuscitation is important in this syndrome, because patients with exertional heat stroke are predisposed to the development of ischemic, and nonischemic myocardial dysfunction, as well as cardiogenic, and noncardiogenic pulmonary edema.[56–58, 101, 102]

Myocardial damage is common in victims of heat stroke.[56] Subendocardial hemorrhages may occur in the area of the interventricular septum along with diffuse fragmentation and rupture of muscle fibers. Transmural myocardial infarction has been reported in a young man with exertional heat stroke.[57] Autopsy revealed no evidence of occlusive coronary artery disease. There is another report of hemorrhagic infarction of an anterior papillary muscle in a healthy young football player who had exertional heat stroke.[58] The mechanism for myocardial infarction and patchy areas of myocardial necrosis in heat stroke victims is not known. It is not uncommon for heat stroke victims to exhibit electrocardiogram (ECG) abnormalities, seen most often during the rapid cooling portion of their resuscitation.[21] These abnormalities include diffuse T wave and ST segment changes, Q waves, conduction defects, as well as ventricular ectopy and atrial dysrhythmias. Peaked T waves are an early indication of hyperkalemia. These patients should have their electrical cardiac activity monitored carefully throughout treatment. This important issue is often neglected as well-meaning practitioners become narrowly focused on cooling measures.

The central nervous system is affected in all patients with heat stroke. They are either markedly disoriented, psychotic, or comatose on presentation. Psychosis may precede the hyperthermia. The pupils may be fixed and dilated on presentation and return to normal after treatment of the heat stroke. Coma should reverse rapidly with cooling. Prolonged coma indicates a poor prognosis.[59] If seizures occur, it is usually during the rapid cooling phase of the treatment. While elderly patients are more likely to have central nervous system sequelae, hemiparesis and cerebellar dysfunction (e.g., ataxia, nystagmus, dysarthria, dysmetria) are occasionally seen in younger patients.[60] Peripheral neuropathies may also be seen.

Renal injury is a common complication of exertional heat stroke. Mild proteinuria and modest abnormalities of the urinary sediment are found in almost all patients, and acute renal insufficiency occurs in approximately 30% of all cases. Rhabdomyolysis contributes to renal injury in several ways. The patient is, by definition, dehydrated and has a concentrated acidic urine. Muscle injury precipitates myoglobinemia and hyperuricemia and deposition of these nephrotoxins into the concentrated acidic urine. Acute tubular damage can occur.[61, 62] In addition, potassium deficiency may suppress renal

plasma flow and glomerular filtration rate (GFR).[63] Patients with renal failure may recover full renal function.

Pulmonary injury may occur as a result of disseminated intravascular coagulation (DIC) with pulmonary hemorrhage or infarction. Pulmonary edema may present as a complication of impaired myocardial function and overly zealous fluid resuscitation. Noncardiogenic pulmonary edema (acquired respiratory distress syndrome [ARDS]) may also occur as a result of the shock state and is sometimes complicated by aspiration occurring around the time of a seizure or by tracheal intubation for airway control.

Liver damage is also common in exertional heat stroke[64, 65] and often causes jaundice and decreased synthesis of clotting factors. Histologic findings include perisinusoidal edema and patchy necrosis that may be predominantly centrilobular.[17] Aspartate amino transferase (AST) levels of greater than 1,000 IU within the first 24 hours after cooling are associated with a poor prognosis. Patients who survive usually show no chronic impairment of liver function.

Almost all patients with exertional heat stroke exhibit DIC. It occurs almost without exception in fatal cases of heat stroke.[66] Exposure to heat may promote fibrinolytic activity without lowering plasma fibrinogen concentration.[67] Heat activation of the fibrinolytic system is less marked with acclimatization.[68] Thrombocytopenia is usually evident within the first 24 hours. This resolves by the fifth to seventh day. Severe cases show thrombocytopenia that is worse by the second to third day and is associated with hypofibrinogenemia and elevated fibrin degradation products. Hemorrhage associated with DIC is a common cause of death in patients with severe heat stroke who survive the initial period of hyperthermia. It is very common in exertional heat stroke.[65]

There are reports of abnormal neutrophil nuclear morphology in as many as 90% of patients presenting with heat stroke.[69] The abnormalities include nuclear hypersegmentation, budding, and chromatin condensation. These findings, as well as spherocytosis, can be seen on admission blood smears and occur in the presence of normal serum folate and vitamin B_{12} levels. Similar findings are not seen in heat exhaustion.

Profound hypocalcemia (< 3 mg/dl) has been observed in patients with heat stroke. It is usually observed on the second or third day and precedes frank azotemia. This same level of hypocalcemia is seen in other rhabdomyolysis syndromes and is considered to be due to calcium deposition in damaged skeletal muscle.[71, 72] Hypercalcemia may occur during the second week after rhabdomyolysis.[73] It is speculated that the profound hypocalcemia during the early phase of rhabdomyolysis and renal failure may provide a powerful stimulus to parathyroid hyperplasia and excessive production of parathyroid hormone causing a transient state of hyperparathyroidism.[17]

Hypophosphatemia may be seen transiently in patients with heat stroke. It is usually seen early in the course and may reflect altered serum levels due to the respiratory alkalosis seen in early phases of heat stroke.

It may not indicate a phosphorous deficiency, as total muscle phosphorous has been shown to be normal in at least one patient who had heat stroke and respiratory alkalosis with a serum phosphorous of 0.9 mg/dl.[74]

Up to 50% of patients with exertional heat stroke exhibit hypoglycemia early in their illness.[75] The precise cause of this is unknown.

Infant Heat Stroke

Infant heat stroke is a syndrome characterized by sudden onset of shock, seizures, hepatopathy, and renal and respiratory insufficiency, with DIC.[11-16] This occurs in the absence of viral or bacterial growth from blood cultures. These patients are usually less than 1 year of age and may exhibit a core temperature of less than 40.5°C (105°F), which is required to make the diagnosis in older patients. Other findings may include leukocytosis and loose watery stools. While cases may parallel heat waves, many are seen during the winter with the history of excessive bundling or wrapping and occasionally with other evidence of environmental overheating. The syndrome is probably underdiagnosed due to the tendency of infants, with their larger surface area to body mass ratio, to cool quickly. This tendency may preclude a markedly febrile presentation and thus hinder the diagnosis of heat stroke. An infant or child who presents with the typical findings of shock and encephalopathy should prompt the clinician to consider the possibility of heat stroke, regardless of the presenting temperature.

The clinician should anticipate cerebral edema, acute renal failure, and DIC in the patient with this history or constellation of findings.

Hemorrhagic Shock and Encephalopathy

As mentioned earlier, there is a striking similarity between the syndrome of HSE, infant heat stroke, and exercise-induced heat stroke. HSE was first described in the British literature by Levin and associates.[76] It was considered to be a new syndrome with a significant incidence and grave prognosis, and it was thought to possibly be the cause of some cases of sudden infant death syndrome (SIDS). Due to this, the United Kingdom set up a surveillance system to study the possible link between heat stroke, HSE, and SIDS.[77]

The term "hemorrhagic" was used initially to describe the bleeding from DIC that is a prominent component of this syndrome. The syndrome may actually be "hyperpyrexic shock and encephalopathy," as hemorrhage secondary to DIC is almost expected in the degree of organ system dysfunction. Hyperpyrexia has been linked to the syndrome.[78] The cause of shock in this syndrome is probably endotoxin mediated and perhaps as a result of hyperpyrexia. Endotoxin, also known as lipopolysaccharide (LPS), exists in high concentrations in the gut, approximately 1 mg LPS/g of feces. LPS is capable of causing many of the changes seen in HSE, including

shock and DIC.[78, 79] While endotoxin is usually impermeable to the gut wall, interruption of the gut wall barrier promotes leakage of LPS into the blood stream and causes shock. There is evidence in nonhuman primates that during heat stress, there is intense splanchnic arterial constriction that diverts blood flow from the viscera to the skin, in order to dissipate heat.[17, 21] This splanchnic constriction is associated with leakage of endotoxin into the blood stream[80, 81] and all the clinical hemodynamic findings of septic (endotoxic) shock, despite negative cultures. Treatment with antibody to LPS improves mortality in these heat-stressed primates,[82] as does gut decontamination.[83]

The apparent rarity of HSE in patients less than 6 weeks of age could be explained by the presence of maternal antibodies to LPS in the infants' blood stream until that age. It is also interesting to note that while most patients reported to have HSE have high mortality or severe neurologic impairment as a residual finding, there are reports of some patients who have volume resuscitation, including fresh frozen plasma (FFP), never require inotropic support and have a good outcome.[84] It is thought that antibody to endotoxin, contained in the FFP, may alleviate endotoxemia and therefore improve the outcome.[85]

To date, there are no reports of endotoxemia in patients with HSE. Further research is needed in this area and should include studies of LPS, tumor necrosis factor, and lymphokines. Epidemiologic studies should be undertaken to investigate the possibility of environmental overheating as an inciting stimulus in the cascade of events.

Treatment of infant heat stroke and HSE is supportive and is aimed at correction of any elevated core temperature. It is important to obtain a true core temperature, as opposed to a rectal temperature, because the two are often discrepant in heat syndromes. A deep rectal thermister should be used liberally if there is any question of a heat syndrome. Hyperthermia can be treated by iced gastric lavage, by enemas, or by vaporization of water from the body surface.

Treatment with FFP along with fluid resuscitation has resulted in better than usual outcome in a small series of patients.[84] These patients may also benefit from antibody to LPS, if it is available clinically. It is also important to remember that the typical patient with HSE or heat stroke can be expected to progress to cerebral edema, DIC, renal insufficiency, and seizures. Treatment should be given with these problems anticipated.

Malignant Hyperthermia

Malignant hyperthermia (MH) is a rare hereditary disorder of acidosis, muscular rigidity, and hyperpyrexia in patients who have had depolarizing neuromuscular blockade or general anesthesia with one or more of a variety of anesthetic agents.[86] The most common offenders are halothane and succinylcholine. MH may also occur with the use of local anesthetics that depolarize muscle cells, such as xylocaine.[17] In approximately 70%

of cases, muscle rigidity precedes hyperpyrexia. A rapidly rising end-tidal carbon dioxide may be one of the first clues to MH in the paralyzed patient. Body temperatures rise rapidly in MH and have been reported to reach values as high as 46°C (114.8°F) by the time the diagnosis is suspected.[88] Mortality in MH varies from approximately 30 to 70%.[86, 88]

MH causes profound metabolic and respiratory acidosis. Elevation of serum glucose, phosphate, calcium, magnesium, and potassium are early findings. As rhabdomyolysis occurs, serum calcium falls and creative phosphokinase rises and severe DIC may develop.

The precise cause of MH is not known, although it appears to be a disorder of cytosolic calcium regulation, allowing elevation of cellular calcium. There is evidence that the sarcoplasmic reticulum of affected patients' skeletal muscle is unstable and inappropriately releases calcium in response to a number of triggering stimuli.[89]

The treatment for MH is dantrolene, given at a dosage of 2 mg/kg intravenously. Dantrolene is functional therapeutically and prophylactically in MH. Additionally, mechanical ventilation to control oxygenation and carbon dioxide removal may be necessary. Buffering of the marked acidosis may also be required.

Neuroleptic Malignant Syndrome

Neuroleptic malignant syndrome (NMS) is another drug-induced disorder involving hyperpyrexia and rigidity. Most cases involve the use of haloperidol alone or with other drugs, especially lithium.[90] Thioxanthenes and phenothiazines have also been proposed as inciting agents.[91, 92] Metabolic derangements are essentially the same as those seen in MH but are usually less severe, as is indicated by the lower fatality rate of 10 to 20%.[95] The cause of NMS is not known. The similarity between NMS and MH has prompted the use of dantrolene in the treatment of NMS, with some success.[93, 94]

NMS should be distinguished from neuroleptic-related heat stroke (NRHS). The patient taking phenothiazines, or the butyrophenone haloperidol, is at increased risk for environmental heat syndromes due to suppression of sweating or (possibly) to altered hypothalamic temperature regulation, respectively.[17]

The patient with NRHS presents with the usual findings of typical heat stroke, confused or agitated, with dry skin, and without muscular rigidity. The environmental temperature is usually high. The patient with NMS is alert and mute, as opposed to the agitation and confusion seen in the patient with NRHS. In addition, the patient with NMS exhibits muscular rigidity and usually has moist skin.[95]

Additional drugs that increase the risk of environmental heat injury include diuretics that cause dehydration and salt depletion. Anticholinergics, antiparkinsonians, and antihistamines suppress sweating and thus alter appropriate dissipation of heat. Sympathomimetic amines and tricyclic antidepressants increase motor activity and heat production.

Treatment of Heat Stroke

Treatment is centered initially around efforts to cool the patient. Delay in cooling is probably the single most important factor leading to death and serious residual deficits in patients who survive.[17] Delay in cooling occurs when the diagnosis is delayed or there is a lack of proper cooling facilities. There is much evidence indicating the value of early diagnosis and cooling of patients with exertional heat stroke.[96, 97] In these reports of military recruits, all survived. Even in elderly high-risk patients with classic heat stroke, there is a high survival rate if cooling measures are performed rapidly.[48]

General resuscitation measures should include venous (and eventually arterial) access, obtained as rapidly as possible. If this is prevented by severe peripheral vasoconstriction, central venous or intraosseous lines should be placed. If the patient is comatose, the next procedure is removal of gastric contents, and rapid-sequence tracheal intubation (see Chapter 39). This is done in part to protect the patient from aspiration of vomitus that typically occurs during the seizures associated with rapid cooling.

A rectal thermistor should be placed deep within the rectum to allow measurement of true core temperature. Standard thermometers measure anal temperature, which may not accurately reflect core temperature.

Efforts to cool the patient can be made while these necessary procedures are being performed. Cooling by immersion in iced water and massaging of the skin to facilitate exchange of heat is the conventional method of cooling in the adult literature. Another method involves placing the patient in an air-conditioned room, in front of a large fan, and rubbing the wet body with plastic bags that contain ice. While these methods are commonly used, cold-induced vasoconstriction may impair heat loss and aggravate hyperthermia. Due to these concerns, a fairly novel unit has been designed to cool the patient without using ice.[98] With this unit, the patient is placed on a mesh sling in the path of warm air flow containing atomized water. The patient is cooled by vaporization of the atomized water from the warm skin. This method of cooling allows a heat loss of 0.06° C/min. Studies of this method in 1,119 patients show a survival rate of 90 to 95%.[99] These rates are approximately equal to those achieved by conventional methods.[45, 75, 97, 100]

When core temperature reaches values around 38.9° C (102° F), cooling measures should be stopped because the body will continue to cool on its own once the temperature is lowered to this level. The clinician should be aware of the possibility of recurrent hyperthermia if seizures occur during cooling. Close monitoring of core temperature should provide early recognition of this phenomenon. Spontaneous hyperthermia may occur 3 to 4 hours after cooling in the absence of seizures. This usually indicates impaired ability to sweat. This is not an unusual finding in patients recovering from heat stroke, and recovery of normal sweating mechanisms may take several weeks.

Many patients exhibit hypotension on initial presentation. Cooling will promote movement of blood volume from dilated superficial vessels and muscles back to the central circulation, and this is often all that is required to restore blood pressure to normal values. Myocardial depression is occasionally involved in the hypotension, and treatment by inotropic support should restore blood pressure if cooling does not. Hemodynamic and fluid therapy may be guided more effectively by the use of a pulmonary arterial (Swan-Ganz) catheter. This consideration is important because it is desirable to maintain an adequate intravascular volume and blood pressure for renal perfusion and urine output in the face of hyperuricemia and myoglobinuria. Yet it is prudent to avoid overhydration in this syndrome in which there is potential for impaired myocardial function and the development of cardiogenic and noncardiogenic pulmonary edema (ARDS).

Other therapy is supportive and involves treatment of electrolyte abnormalities, hypoglycemia, and occasionally hyperglycemia. Nonketotic hyperosmolar coma is seen occasionally in some patients with heat stroke who survive for several days. It may be related to excessive administration of glucose in conjunction with renal insufficiency or the pancreatic insufficiency that is seen occasionally in victims of heat stroke.

References

1. II Kings 4:18–20.
2. Jarcho S: A Roman experience with heatstroke in 24 B.C. Bull NY Acad Med 43:767, 1967.
3. Lindsay P: Kings of Merry England. London, Ivor Nicholson and Watson, 1936.
4. Wilcox WH: The nature, prevention and treatment of heat hyperexia. Br Med J 1:392, 1920.
5. El Halawani AW: Heat illness during the Mecca pilgrimage. WHO Chron 18:283, 1964.
6. Ralston R: Heat stroke. Minn Med 59:411, 1976.
7. Malamud N, Hatmaker W, and Custer RP: Heat stroke: A clinicopathologic study of 125 fatal cases. Milit Surg 99:397, 1946.
8. Knochel JP: Dog days and siriasis: How to kill a football player. JAMA 233:513, 1979.
9. Hanson PG and Zimmerman SW: Exertional heat stroke in novice runners. JAMA 242:154, 1979.
10. Ellis FP: Mortality from heat illness and heat aggravated illness in the United States. Environ Res 5:1, 1972.
11. Bacon CJ and Bellman MH: Heat stroke as a possible cause of encephalopathy in infants. Br Med J 287:328, 1983.
12. Bacon C, Scott D, and Jones P: Heatstroke in well-wrapped infants. Lancet 24:422, 1979.
13. Goodyear JE: Heat hyperpyrexia in an infant (a case report). Med Sci Law 19 (3):208, 1979.
14. Monteleone JA and Keefe DM: Transient hyperglycemia and aketotic hyperosmolar acidosis with heat stroke. Pediatrics 44:737, 1969.
15. Danks DM, Webb DW, and Allen J: Heat illness in infants and young children: A study of 47 cases. Br Med J 2:287, 1962.
16. Wadlington WB, Tucker AL, and Fly F: Heat stroke in infancy. Am J Dis Child 130:1250, 1976.
17. Knochel, JP: Heat stroke and related heat stress disorders. Dis Mon 35(5):301, 1989.
18. Leonard AL and Nelms RJ Jr: Hypercalcemia in the diuretic phase of acute failure. Ann Intern Med 73:137, 1970.
19. Passmore R and Durnin JVGA: Human energy expenditure. Physiol Rev 35:801, 1955.
20. Hardy JD: Body temperature regulation. In: Mountcastle VB (ed): Medical Physiology, 14th ed. St. Louis, CV Mosby, 1980, p. 1430.
21. Anderson RJ, Reed G , and Knochel J: Heatstroke. Dallas, TX, Year Book Medical Publishers, 1980.
22. Benzinger TH: On physical heat regulation and the sense of temperature in man. Proc Natl Acad Sci U.S.A. 46:645, 1959.
23. Bean WB and Eichna LW: Performance in relation to environmental temperature: Reactions of normal young men to simulated desert environment. Fed Proc 2:144, 1943.
24. Consalazio CF, Johnson RE, and Pecora LJ: Physiological Measurements of Metabolic Function in Man. New York, McGraw-Hill International Book Co., 1963.
25. Adolph EF and Dill DB: Observations on water metabolism in the desert. Am J Physiol 123:369, 1938.
26. Barger AC, et al: Venous pressure and cutaneous reactive hyperemia in exhaustive exercise and certain circulatory stresses. J Appl Physiol 2:81, 1949.
27. Thysen JH and Schwartz IL: Fatigue of sweat glands. J Clin Invest 34:1719, 1955.
28. Schwartz IL and Thaysen JH: Excretion of sodium and potassium in human sweat. J Clin Invest 35:144, 1956.
29. Avellini BA, Shapiro Y, Fortney SM, et al: Effects of heat tolerance of physical training in water and on land. J Appl Physiol 53:1291, 1982.
30. Barcroft H: Circulation in skeletal muscle. In: Handbook of Physiology: A Critical Comprehensive Presentation of Physiologic Knowledge and Concepts. Baltimore, Williams & Wilkins, 1963, pp. 1353–1386.
31. Schlein EM, Jensen D, and Knochel JP: The effect of plasma water loss on assessment of muscle metabolism during exercise. J Appl Physiol 34:568, 1973.
32. Rowell LB, et al: Reductions in cardiac output, central blood volume and stroke volume with thermal stress in normal men during exercise. J Clin Invest 45:1801, 1966.
33. Pattengale PK and Halloszy JO: Augmentation of skeletal muscle myoglobin by a program of treadmill running. Am J Physiol 213:783, 1967.
34. Gollnick PD and King DW: Effect of exercise and training on mitochondria of rat skeletal muscle. Am J Physiol 16:1502, 1969.
35. Knochel JP, Dotin LN, and Hamburger RJ: Pathophysiology of intense physical condition in a hot climate. I: Mechanisms of potassium depletion. J Clin Invest 51:242, 1972.
36. Burnell JM, et al: The effect in humans of extracellur pH change on the relationship between serum potassium concentration and extracellular potassium. J Clin Invest 35:935, 1956.
37. Coburn JW, Reba RC, and Craig FN: Effect of potassium depletion on response to acute heat exposure in unacclimatized man. Am J Physiol 211:117, 1966.
38. Rose KD: Warning for million: Intense exercise can deplete potassium. Physician Sportsmed 3:67, 1975.
39. Rai UC and Ambwany P: Cardiovascular changes during varied thermal stress. Indian J Physiol Pharmacol 2:119, 1980.
40. Finberg JPM, Katz M, Gazit H, et al: Plasma renin activity after acute heat exposure in nonacclimatized and naturally acclimatized man. J Appl Physiol 36:519, 1974.
41. Sprung CL, Portocarrero CJ, Fernanine AV, et al: The metabolic and respiratory alterations of heat stroke. Arch Intern Med 140:665, 1980.
42. Iampietro PR: Heat-induced tetany. Fed Proc 22:884, 1963.
43. Talbot JH: Heat cramps. Medicine 14:232, 1955.
44. Balaustein MP: Sodium ions, calcium ions, blood pressure regulation, and hypertension: A reassessment and hypothesis. Am J Physiol 232:C165, 1977.
45. McCance RA: Medical problems in mineral metabolism. III: Experimental salt deficiency. Lancet 1:823, 1936.
46. Leithhead CS and Lind AR: Heat Stress and Heat Disorders. Philadelphia, FA Davis, 1964, p. 129.
47. Knochel JP: Clinical physiology of heat exposure. In: Maxwell MH and Kleeman CR (eds): Disorders of Fluid and Electrolyte Metabolism. New York, McGraw-Hill, 1980.
48. Hart GR, Anderson RJ, Crumpler CP, et al: Epidemic classical heat stroke: Clinical characteristics and course of 28 patients. Medicine 61:189, 1982.
49. Francesconia RP and Mager M: Heat-injured rats: Pathochemical indices and survival time. J Appl Physiol 45:1, 1978.
50. Knochel JP: Environmental heat illness. Arch Intern Med 133:841, 1974.
51. Klock JC, Boerner U, and Becker CE: Coma, hyperthermia, and bleeding associated with massive LSD overdose: A report of eight cases. Clin Toxicol 8(2):191, 1975.

52. Barton CH, Sterling ML, and Vaziri ND: Rhabdomyolysis and acute renal failure associated with phencyclidine intoxication. Arch Intern Med 140:568, 1980.
53. Patel R, Maloy D, Palazzalo M, et al: Myoglobinuric acute renal failure in phencyclidine overdose: Report of observations in eight cases. Ann Emerg Med 9(11):549, 1980.
54. O'Donnell TF and Clowes GHA: The circulatory abnormalities of heatstroke. N Engl J Med 287:734, 1972.
55. O'Donnell TF: The hemodynamic and metabolic alterations associated with acute heat stress injury in marathon runners. Ann NY Acad Sci 301:262, 1977.
56. Kew MC, Tucker BK, Bersohn I, et al: The heart in heat stroke. Am Heart J 77:324, 1969.
57. Knochel JP, Beisel WR, Herndon EG, et al: The renal cardiovascular, hematologic and serum electrolyte abnormalities of heat stroke. Am J Med 30:299, 1961.
58. Barcenas C, Hoeffer HP, and Lie JT: CPC obesity, football, dog days and siriasis: A deadly combination. Am Heart J 92:237, 1976.
59. Shibolet S, Coll R, Gilat T, et al: Heat stroke: Its clinical picture and mechanism in 36 cases. Q J Med 525, 1967.
60. Mehta AC and Baker RN: Persistent neurological deficits in heatstroke. Neurology 20:336, 1970.
61. Schrier RW, et al: Nephropathy associated with heat stress and exercise. Ann Intern Med 67:356, 1967.
62. Knochel JP, Dotin LN, and Hamburger RJ: Heat stress exercise, and muscle injury: Effects of urate metabolism and renal function. Ann Intern Med 81:321, 1974.
63. Rubini ME: Water excretion in potassium-deficient man. Clin Res 8:2215, 1960.
64. Herman RH and Sullivan BH Jr: Heat stroke and jaundice. Am J Med 27:154, 1959.
65. Chao TC, Sinniah R, and Pakiam JE: Acute heat stroke deaths. Pathology 13:145, 1981.
66. Selye H and Bajusz E: Conditioning by corticoids for the production of cardiac lesions with noradrenaline. Acta Endocrinol 30:183, 1959.
67. Bedrak E, Beer G, and Fuhrman KI: Fibrinolytic activity and heat stress. Isr J Exp Med 11:1, 1963.
68. Bedrak E, Beer G, and Fuhrman KI: Fibrinolytic activity and muscular exercise in heat. J Appl Physiol 19:469, 1964.
69. Navari RM, Sheehy TW, and McLean BK: The peripheral blood smear in heat stroke: An aid to diagnosis. Alabama Med Sci 20:138, 1983.
70. Friedman EW, Williams JC, and Prendergast E: Polymorphonuclear leukocyte hypersegmentation in heat stroke. Br J Haematol 50:169, 1982.
71. Knochel JP: Biochemical, electrolyte and acid-base disturbances in acute renal failure. In: Brenner BM and Lazarus JM (eds): Acute Renal Failure, 2nd ed. New York, Churchill Livingstone, 1988, pp. 685–688.
72. Knochel JP: Rhabdomyolysis and myoglobinuria. Annu Rev Med 33:435, 1982.
73. Leonard A and Nelms RJ Jr: Hypercalcemia in diuretic phase of acute renal failure. Ann Intern Med 73:137, 1970.
74. Knochel JP: The mechanism of hypophosphatemia in acute heat stroke. JAMA 238:425, 1977.
75. Costrini AM, Pitt HA, Gustafson AB, et al: Cardiovascular and metabolic manifestations of heat stroke and severe heat exhaustion. Am J Med 66:296, 1979.
76. Levin MC, Kay JDS, Gould JG, et al: Hemorrhagic shock and encephalopathy: A new syndrome with a high mortality in young children. Lancet 2:64, 1983.
77. Joint Paediatric Association and Communicable Disease Surveillance Centre surveillance scheme for hemorrhagic shock encephalopathy syndrome: Surveillance report for 1982–4. Br Med J 290:1578, 1985.

78. Sofer S, Phillip M, Hershkowits J, and Bennett H: Hemorrhagic shock and encephalopathy syndrome: Its association with hyperthermia. Am J Dis Child 140:1252, 1986.
79. Pinsky MR and Matuschak GM: Multiple systems organ failure: Failure of host defense homeostasis. Crit Care Clin 5:199, 1989.
80. McCabe WR: Endotoxin: Microbiological, chemical, pathophysiological, and clinical correlations. In: Weinstein L and Fields BN (eds): Seminars in Infectious Diseases, Vol. 3. New York, Thieme-Stratton, 1980, pp. 38–88.
81. Gathiram P, Wells MT, and Raidoo JG: Portal and systemic plasma lipopolysaccharide concentrations in heat-stressed primates. Circ Shock 25:223, 1988.
82. Gathiram P, Gaffin SL, and Brock-Utne JG: Time course of endotoxemia and cardiovascular changes in heat-stressed primates. Aviat Space Environ Med 58:1071, 1987.
83. Gathiram P, Wells MT, and Brock-Utne JG: Antilipopolysaccharide improves survival in primates subjected to heat stroke. 23:157, 1987.
84. Gathiram P, Wells MT, and Brock-Utne JG: Prevention of endotoxemia by non-absorbable antibiotics in heat stress. J Clin Pathol 40:1364, 1987.
85. Conway EE, Varlotta L, and Singer LP: Hemorrhagic shock and encephalopathy: Is it really a new entity? Crit Care Med 6:131, 1990.
86. Conway EE and Singer LP: Letters to the editor. Crit Care Med 18:792, 1990.
87. Britt BA: Etiology and pathophysiology of malignant hyperthermia. Fed Proc 38:44, 1979.
88. Leonard DC and Eichner ER: Acute renal failure and transient hypercalcemia in idiopathic rhabdomyolysis. JAMA 211:1539, 1970.
89. Gronert GA: Malignant hyperthermia. Anesthesiology 53:395, 1980.
90. Nelson TD and Bee DE: Temperature perturbation studies of sarcoplasmic reticulum from malignant hyperthermia pig muscle. J Clin Invest 64:895, 1979.
91. Cohen WJ and Cohen NH: Lithium carbonate, haloperidol, and irreversible brain damage. JAMA 230:1283, 1974.
92. Henderson VW and Wooten FD: Neuroleptic malignant syndrome: A pathogenetic role for dopamine receptor blockage? Neurology (NY) 31:132, 1981.
93. Caroff SN: The neuroleptic malignant syndrome. J Clin Psychiatry 41:3, 1980.
94. Coons DJ, Hillman FJ, and Marshall RW: Treatment of neuroleptic syndrome with dantrolene sodium: A case report. Am J Psychiatry 139:944, 1982.
95. May DC, Morris SW, Stewart RM, et al: Neuroleptic malignant syndromes response to dantrolene sodium. Ann Intern Med 98:183, 1983.
96. Lazarus A: Differentiating neuroleptic-related heatstroke from neuroleptic malignant syndrome. Academy of Psychosomatic Medicine 30(4), 1989.
97. O'Donnell TF Jr: Acute heat stress: Epidemiologic, biochemical, renal and coagulation studies. JAMA 234:824, 1975.
98. Beller FA and Boyd AE: Heat stoke: A report of 113 consecutive cases without mortality despite severe hyperpyrexia and neurologic dysfunction. Milit Med 140:464, 1975.
99. Weiner JS and Khogali M: A physiological body-cooling unit for treatment of heat stroke. Lancet 1:507, 1980.
100. Khogali M: The Makkah body cooling unit. In: Khogali M and Hales JRS (eds): Heat Stroke and Temperature Regulation. New York, Academic Press, 1983, pp. 139–148.
101. Sofer S and Eliezer S: Myocardial infarction in hemorrhagic shock and encephalopathy syndrome. Pediatr Emerg Care 5:99, 1989.
102. Zahger D, Moses A, and Weiss A: Evidence of prolonged myocardial dysfunction in heat stroke. Chest 95:1089, 1989.

83

Cold Syndromes

Peter R. Holbrook, M.D.

Homeothermic humans must maintain a core temperature within narrow limits for optimal physiologic and metabolic functioning. Considerable resources are committed to and much energy is consumed in maintaining a normothermic state. Although isolated cold syndromes are uncommonly encountered in most pediatric intensive care units (ICUs), the risk of heat loss is common both in and out of the hospital.

PHYSIOLOGY

Normothermia is generally considered to be a core temperature of 36 to 37.9° C. Heat loss occurs through the normal physical processes of radiation, convection, conduction, and evaporation (see Chapter 82). In the normal situation, heat loss is counterbalanced by endogenous heat production. As heat loss becomes excessive, physiologic mechanisms are activated. At the simplest level regional vasoconstriction occurs, reducing further heat loss. Local conditions cause local responses, and the exposed area may drop in temperature to that approaching the ambient temperature. Vasoconstriction can persist to temperatures as low as 10° C, at which time vasomotor paralysis occurs.[1] Further cold stress activates the anterior hypothalamus, which induces avoidance behavior (in patients who are able) and thermogenesis. The latter normally takes the form of productive or nonproductive (shivering) muscular activity.

In very young children, nonshivering thermogenesis is induced by the oxidation of brown fat. Brown fat—so-called because it contains iron-containing cytochrome—is located strategically around the core of the body. This tissue is highly vascular and is innervated by sympathetic nervous system fibers that are controlled by the temperature of the anterior hypothalamus. When metabolically active, brown fat produces heat via lipase stimulation of triglycerol breakdown-liberating free fatty acids. Some of these are further broken down to CO_2 and H_2O, and others are resynthesized to triglyceride. These processes are highly exothermic: brown fat temperature may be 2 to 3° C higher than core temperature in animals.[2, 3] The effect is dual: heat is produced and, in animals, shivering is apparently suppressed through

warming of the low cervical/high thoracic spinal cord near the ventral spinothalamic tracts.[1]*

PATHOPHYSIOLOGY

If the temperature control mechanisms fail, hypothermia begins and each organ system is affected. The brain shows decreased cerebral blood flow (approximately 6 to 7%/° C decrease). Cerebral metabolic rate is transiently increased and then decreases. The level of consciousness is maintained early, although responses are sluggish. Lethargy and confusion are noted in adults at approximately 30° C. Dysarthria is common at these levels. Peripheral deep tendon reflexes are depressed, and sluggish pupillary reaction leading to anisocoria may be noted. At approximately 25 to 27° C, the patient loses all clinical neurologic findings. The electroencephalogram (EEG) may not go flat until 18° C. During hypothermia there is a reduced seizure threshold.

Initial cardiovascular responses are vasoconstriction with an increase in systemic vascular resistance, increased oxygen consumption, and increased pulse and stroke volume resulting in increased cardiac output and blood pressure. Later, the heart rate and cardiac output decrease while mean arterial pressure remains elevated. Systemic vascular resistance and blood pressure fall by approximately 25° C. The electrocardiogram shows generalized slowing with bradycardia, T wave inversions, and the appearance of the Osborne or J wave, an acute elevation of the ST segment. This latter phenomenon occurs at about 32 to 33° C. Below 30° C ventricular fibrillation increases in incidence.

Respiratory responses include initial tachypnea with later bradypnea and decreased tidal volume. A mild respiratory acidosis is common. This leads to a shift of the oxyhemoglobin dissociation curve to the right with reduced oxygen unloading at the tissues. Airway protective reflexes are progressively lost, thus aspiration is an increased risk.

---

*Brown fat is essential in hibernating animals. It is present in large quantities and insulates the central organs. Virtually all peripheral blood passes through an area of brown fat concentration prior to getting to the central core organs. In addition, it is involved in arousal from hibernation. Shivering is suppressed, a factor that allows smooth emergence from hibernation as the body temperature rises.

Renal effects include a "cold diuresis" secondary to the peripheral vasoconstriction. Later, depression of tubular reabsorption enzymes leads to continued diuresis. Acute tubular necrosis may follow.

Hemoconcentration occurs secondary to diuresis. White blood cell numbers and function may be depressed. Thrombocytopenia can occur and disseminated intravascular coagulation is common.

Ileus occurs below 34° C. Liver function may be depressed. Insulin secretion is depressed, and hypothermia blocks insulin action at the tissues.[4, 5] The older patient develops hyperglycemia. In contrast, hypoglycemia may be a late finding in neonates.

Sodium drops due to loss into the interstitial space, and potassium increases.

SPECIFIC SYNDROMES

Neonatal cold injury is a commonly encountered condition in regions of the world where home heating is less than optimal. The infant shows neonatal manifestations of the aforementioned effects (apathy, poor appetite, diuresis followed by oliguria, and, commonly, an edema and erythema of the exposed or peripheral parts of the body). The edema may be indurated and nonpitting (sclerema neonatorum) and may immobilize the joint. Hypoglycemia is prominent. Hemorrhage is common. Treatment is gradual warming with close attention to hypoglycemia and metabolic disturbances. This is a severe condition of multiple organ system failure and carries a mortality of at least 25%.

Isolated accidental hypothermia in children is not commonly encountered. More frequently, in the near-drowning patient, hypoxia/ischemia is superimposed on hypothermia. If the patient is fortunate, rapid cooling may have occurred, blunting the effects of the hypoxia. Ice is normally found in the water if a child is submersed for a long period but makes a good recovery.[6]

Induced hypothermia is practiced daily in pediatric cardiac surgical centers. The depth of hypothermia varies depending on the case being done but can extend to as low as 16° C. The usual technique is to combine surface cooling with cooling via the extracorporeal circuit and anaesthetic management that promotes smooth gradual shifts in temperature. In addition, a cardioplegia solution that rests the heart in diastole thus decreasing myocardial oxygen requirements is utilized. Total circulatory arrest of up to 60 minutes under these circumstances is considered safe, although subtle findings have been noted,[7-10] and these correlate with length and depth of hypothermia.

The cardiac surgery experience has led to further understanding on two issues. The first is rewarming techniques (discussed later), and the second is the changes in blood gases in the hypothermic patient. Since metabolism decreases and there is increased solubility of CO_2 in colder blood, the $Paco_2$ may drop significantly. Should the $Paco_2$ be artificially elevated or left where it is using conventional ventilation techniques? Consensus thinking now is that the target blood gases should be normal when the blood is warmed to 37° C (as is done automatically in most blood gas machines).[5, 11]

Frostbite is occasionally encountered in the patient admitted to the ICU for more severe hypothermia or other injuries. The hallmarks of frostbite are extreme pallor of the skin and insensitivity to touch. Thawing and refreezing are lethal to the tissue. Thus, rewarming must be undertaken only when there is no risk of further cold exposure. The frostbitten tissue must never be rubbed; solid ice crystals can physically damage tissue. Rewarming is usually undertaken by immersion in water slightly above body temperature, 38 to 40°C. Following rewarming, the affected area may manifest skin and deeper injury ranging from an increased sensation to cold to gangrene. Superficial skin slough is common.

TREATMENT OF HYPOTHERMIA

How long should the accidental hypothermia patient be resuscitated? Ventricular fibrillation may be irreversible if there is a greater than 1° C transmyocardial difference.[5, 12] Thus, inability to defibrillate a cold patient should not call for discontinuation of efforts. Similarly, the protective effect of hypothermia may be present. On the other hand, elevation of potassium has been used as a prognostic factor.[13, 14]

In the nonarrested patient, initial management consists of an accurate assessment of the patient's status. The child may be hypovolemic and hyperkalemic, and, with rewarming, may become progressively more acidemic. Thus, rewarming should proceed under careful monitoring and at a speed consistent with the clinical situation. If the child has ventricular irritability, rapid warming is essential. Techniques of rewarming are listed in Table 83–1. Common to all is a concern that the liquid or gas that comes into contact with the patient must not burn the tissue, and gradual rewarming at approximately 1° C/hr is appropriate.

Appropriate intravascular monitoring should be undertaken to guide fluid balance. Because of cardiac irritability, insertion of a pulmonary artery catheter should be done only with the strongest indication.

The patient's condition should gradually improve. Deterioration suggests paradoxic core cooling with surface rewarming as cold fluid is shunted to the core, or cerebral edema.

Table 83–1. REWARMING TECHNIQUES

Passive
    Eliminate ongoing heat loss while providing
        gradually increasing ambient temperature
Active
    Surface warming
    Core rewarming
        Extracorporeal techniques
        Peritoneal lavage
        Inhalation
        Gastric/colonic irrigation
        Microwave rewarming

OUTCOME

The underlying disease status of the patient, concurrent or superimposed disease states (e.g., hypoxic ischemic encephalopathy), and the effects of the hypothermia itself all comprise prognosis. It can be expected that defibrillation will be difficult at temperatures below 30°C. The adage that "No one is dead until he or she is warm and dead" has been called into question,[14] and clinical judgment will have to be exercised.

References

1. Keating WR: Direct effects of temperature on blood vessels: Their role in cold vasodilation. *In*: Hardy JD, Gagge AP, and Stolwijk JAJ (eds): Physiological and Behavior Temperature Regulation. Springfield, IL, Charles C Thomas, 1970, pp. 231–236.
2. Dawkins MJR, and Hull D: Brown fat and the response of the newborn rabbit to cold. J Physiol (Lond) 169:101, 1963.
3. Ahern W, and Hull D: Brown adipose tissue and heat production in the newborn infant. J Pathol 91:223, 1966.
4. Curry DL, and Curry KP: Hypothermia and insulin secretion. Endocrinology 87:750, 1970.
5. Elder P: Accidental hypothermia. *In*: Shoemaker WWC et al: Textbook of Critical Care. Philadelphia, WB Saunders, 1989.
6. Orlowski JP: Drowning, near-drowning, and ice-water submersions. Pediatr Clin North Am 34:75, 1987.
7. Weiss M, Weiss CJ, Nocolas F, et al: A study of the electroencephalogram during surgery with deep hypothermia and circulatory arrest. J Thorac Cardiovasc Surg 70:316, 1975.
8. Coles JG, Taylor MJ, Pearce JM, et al: Cerebral monitoring of somatosensory evoked potentials during profoundly hypothermic circulatory arrest. Circulation 70:96, 1984.
9. Anderson K, Waaben J, Husum B, et al: Non-pulsatile cardiopulmonary bypass disrupts the flow-metabolism couple in the brain. J Thorac Cardiovasc Surg 90:570, 1985.
10. Rebeyka IM, Coles JG, Wilson GJ, et al: The effect of low flow cardiopulmonary bypass on cerebral function: An experimental and clinical study. Ann Thorac Surg 43:394, 1987.
11. Prough DS, Stump DA, Roy RC, et al: Response of cerebral blood flow to changes in carbon dioxide tension during hypothermic cardiopulmonary bypass. Anesthesiology 64:576, 1986.
12. Mouritzen CV and Anderson MV: Myocardial temperature gradients and ventricular fibrillation during hypothermia. J Thorac Cardiovasc Surg 49:937, 1965.
13. Hauty MG, Esrig BC, Hill JG, and Long WB: Prognostic factors in severe accidental hypothermia: Experience from the Mt. Hood tragedy. J Trauma 27:1107, 1987.
14. Schaller MD, Fisher A, and Ferret CL: Hyperkalemia: A prognostic factor during acute severe hypothermia. JAMA 264:1842, 1990.

VIII Trauma and Burns

84

Intensive Care Management of the Traumatized Child

Kristan M. Outwater, M.D.

Prehospital care and initial resuscitation techniques have improved survival in the multiply injured child. Survivors often present complex management problems and may develop life-threatening complications. Many benefit from intensive supportive care and lifesaving interventions. The intensive care management of these traumatized children requires a multidisciplinary approach that combines the efforts of pediatric or trauma surgeons, pediatric intensivists, and critical care nurses. In addition, subspecialties such as neurosurgery, orthopedics, neurology, and family support services are also required. Debate as to how this care should be coordinated continues. Because of the potential need for surgical intervention and the desire to provide continuity of care following the patient's discharge from the hospital, the attending trauma or pediatric surgeon is often the physician responsible for coordinating the care of the patient. The critical care team, although sometimes not involved in the initial resuscitative efforts, and rarely involved in operative care, provides the 24-hour coverage and minute-to-minute bedside management that the surgical team, because of demands outside of the intensive care unit, is often unable to provide.

Even if children survive the initial traumatic incident, their mortality rates remain unacceptably high. Complications that lead to death include sepsis and multiple organ system failure—conditions that are worsened by the presence of an increased metabolic rate and inadequate nutrition. Reducing the number of these late deaths in the intensive care unit remains a challenge today.

ASSESSMENT AND STABILIZATION AFTER RESUSCITATION

After successful resuscitation has been accomplished and hemodynamic stability is re-established, assessment is continued, missed or evolving injuries are sought, and basic patient needs are attended to. Frequent reassess-

ment of the patient is mandatory to ensure stability and to diagnose and treat developing problems in their early stages.

Respiratory Assessment and Stabilization (Table 84–1)

When the patient arrives in the intensive care unit the initial assessment includes an evaluation of the patient's "airway, breathing, and circulation"—the ABCs of resuscitation—to note any instability present and to de-

Table 84–1. INITIAL INTENSIVE CARE UNIT EVALUATION: CLINICAL ASSESSMENT

Airway	Airway patency, including need for artificial airway
	Airway trauma, including inhalation injury
	Endotracheal tube placement, patency, size, stability
	Tracheostomy tube placement, patency, size, stability
Breathing	Rate
	Chest wall excursion, asymmetry, splinting
	Accessory muscle use
	Retractions, grunting
	Altered breath sounds
	Color
Circulation	Heart rate
	Skin color and temperature
	Capillary refill
	Peripheral pulses
	Blood pressure
	Urine output
	Hematocrit
Neurologic	Level of consciousness
	Eye opening
	Pupillary response
	Motor response to stimulation
	Verbal response to stimulation

termine immediate therapeutic needs. Airway patency is checked. If the patient does not have an artificial airway in place, the need for such an airway is assessed. Has there been clinical deterioration in the patient's mental status or in the ability to maintain an airway? What is the potential for airway deterioration? Is there a need for hyperventilation to control increased intracranial pressure? In an intubated patient, endotracheal tube placement is checked because of the risks of tube dislodgement during transport. The need for suctioning is checked, and blood or gastric secretions in the endotracheal tube are noted. Any difficulties in the initial placement of the airway in the emergency room are noted, and tube size and taping position are documented. Continued need for the endotracheal tube is determined. If a surgical tracheostomy is in place, stability is checked. Replacement endotracheal or tracheostomy tubes of the appropriate size are made available at the bedside.

Airway assessment should be followed by observation of the patient's breathing effort, chest wall excursion, use of accessory muscles, presence of retractions, and grunting or altered breath sounds on auscultation.

Initial ventilator settings should be set, and the response of the patient should be determined clinically (Table 84–2). Using a volume-cycled ventilator, a tidal volume of 10 to 15 ml/kg and a respiratory rate of 15 to 25 breaths/min usually produce adequate chest wall excursion and minute ventilation. A rate of 25 to 30 breaths/min might be chosen if hyperventilation is required for therapy of increased intracranial pressure. In children weighing less than 10 to 15 kg, a pressure-limited time-cycled ventilator is often chosen. A peak inspiratory pressure of 20 to 30 cm H_2O and a respiratory rate of 15 to 25 breaths/min are usually required for adequate chest expansion and ventilation. Inspiratory time is set between 0.6 second and 1 second. The initial Fio_2 of 1.00 can be reduced after adequate oxygenation

Table 84–3. MAINTENANCE FLUID OR CALORIC REQUIREMENTS

Weight	Fluid (ml) or Calories (kCal)/day
≤ 10 kg	100 × body weight (kg)
11–20 kg	1,000 + 50/kg for each kilogram above 10
> 20 kg	1,500 + 20/kg for each kilogram above 20

has been ensured. The need for positive end-expiratory pressure (PEEP) is based on the presence of lung disease and on the vulnerability of the patient to develop atelectasis. A small amount of PEEP (3 to 5 cm H_2O) may help to prevent atelectasis. In a patient at risk for intracranial hypertension, the lowest amount of PEEP possible should be set to minimize the potential adverse affects of PEEP on intracranial pressure. Ideally, all children should be monitored with pulse oximetry and end-tidal CO_2 monitoring (see also Chapters 38 and 40).

Trauma patients require frequent reassessment of adequacy of oxygenation and ventilation in the evolving situation. Respiratory insufficiency may be caused by several factors. Decreasing level of consciousness from head injury or medication leading to vasodilatation and hypovolemia, aspiration of gastric contents, pulmonary edema from fluid overload, missed spinal cord injury, or a lung contusion may alter oxygenation and ventilation. Symptoms from a pulmonary contusion may develop slowly and include tachypnea, respiratory distress, tachycardia, altered breath sounds, and hypoxemia. A chest radiograph obtained 12 to 18 hours after the injury may show dense infiltrates. Fluid resuscitation may contribute to pulmonary congestion in the noninjured lung as well, secondary to increasing capillary pressure from augmented blood flow and vasodilatation in the noninjured lung.

Circulatory Assessment and Stabilization

"Circulation" is also rapidly assessed when the patient is admitted to the intensive care unit (see Table 84–1). Although vigorous fluid therapy may result in an adequate blood pressure and normal heart rate, resuscitation is not complete until the patient is warm and well perfused, has adequate peripheral pulses, good urine output, and a reasonable hematocrit. Inadequate perfusion is most often due to inadequate resuscitation or continued bleeding. Use of inotropic or vasopressor support to maintain blood pressure is usually not necessary if an adequate amount of fluid has been administered.

After resuscitation is complete, D5 ¼ normal saline with potassium 20 mEq/l is usually adequate for maintenance fluid therapy. Maintenance fluid (and caloric) requirements for children can be calculated using a standard formula (Table 84–3). Excess losses (nasogastric drainage, stools, chest tube drainage, or third-space fluid losses) should be replaced with the appropriate crystalloid or colloid solution.

Table 84–2. INITIAL INTENSIVE CARE UNIT EVALUATION: VENTILATOR SETTINGS

Fio_2* is 1.00 until saturation can be monitored.

Volume-cycled ventilator:	TV† 10–15 ml/kg Rate 15–25 breaths/min 　25–30 breaths/min for hyperventilation therapy PEEP‡ 3–5 cm H_2O 　0 if intracranial hypertension present
Time-cycled pressure-limited ventilator (children less than 10–15 kg):	PIP§ 20–30 cm H_2O Rate 15–25 breaths/min 　25–30 breaths/min for hyperventilation therapy IT ‖ 0.6–1 sec PEEP 3–5 cm H_2O 　0 if intracranial hypertension present

*Fio_2 = fraction of inspired oxygen.
†TV = tidal volume.
‡PEEP = positive end-expiratory pressure.
§PIP = peak inspiratory pressure.
‖IT = inspiratory time.

The patient should remain under surveillance in the intensive care unit until stability has been maintained for at least 24 hours. Reassessment is the continued theme of this period. Any recurrence of signs of circulatory failure, however mild, should prompt an aggressive investigation. Hypovolemia due to hemorrhage or plasma loss should be immediately suspected. Children can maintain a normal blood pressure in the face of hypovolemia by increasing systemic vascular resistance and heart rate. Therefore, any alteration in peripheral perfusion or pulses, a rising heart rate, or a drop in urine output should prompt a therapeutic challenge of a crystalloid solution while an evaluation for hypovolemia is undertaken. Lack of response to repeated fluid challenges or a drop in hematocrit may suggest the need for exploration in the operating room.

Hemorrhagic shock may precipitate myocardial dysfunction.[1] Possible mechanisms include hypoxic/ischemic damage or the release of myocardial depressant factors. Data from echocardiography or pulmonary artery catheterization will help to distinguish myocardial failure from hypovolemia or a mechanical cause such as tamponade or pneumothorax. Inotropic support may be necessary.

Chest trauma may cause a myocardial contusion, resulting in chest pain and an abnormal electrocardiogram (ECG) and echocardiogram. Myocardial enzymes may be elevated. Patients need to be monitored closely for arrhythmias.

Neurologic Assessment

Neurologic status is assessed next. Level of consciousness, eye opening, pupillary response, motor response to painful stimulation, and responses to verbal commands are noted. Neurologic assessment includes a determination of the need for therapeutic measures to control intracranial hypertension, including mannitol, fluid restriction, and hyperventilation. Head trauma may have been missed in the hypotensive child with obvious intra-abdominal or intrathoracic bleeding. Patients may deteriorate as adequate hemodynamic resuscitation increases intracranial pressure. In addition, inhalation anesthetics used in the operating room may have cerebral vasodilating effects. Medications used in the operating room may also cause central nervous system (CNS) depression, complicating neurologic assessment.

Additional Assessment

After the initial evaluation has been completed and therapeutic priorities have been set, a more careful assessment of the patient may document undiagnosed or evolving problems. A complete skeletal examination should include an evaluation of facial bones as well as extremity fractures. Pulmonary, myocardial, or renal contusions or a bowel injury may become apparent at this time. An examination of the patient's skin should include an assessment of any undressed abrasion or lacerations that require attention.

Monitoring

Patient monitoring should include continuous ECG recording, respiratory rate, intermittent blood pressure measurement, temperature assessment, and a Foley catheter for quantitative measurement of urine output (Table 84–4). Temperature assessment is important in patients whose initial injury may have included exposure or in patients who have undergone massive transfusions. Small children are especially susceptible to hypothermia following resuscitative efforts in the emergency room or operating theater. Oximetry and end-tidal CO_2 monitoring complete the standard noninvasive monitoring that is usually available.

The need for invasive monitoring is determined by the clinical status of the patient and known injuries. An indwelling arterial catheter will provide continuous blood pressure monitoring and access to arterial blood sampling in patients with hemodynamic or pulmonary instability.

Central venous catheters can be inserted via the femoral, antecubital, subclavian, or jugular vein and placed in the superior or inferior vena cava or right atrium. Right atrial pressure is monitored as a reflection of right ventricular preload. Patients who require invasive hemodynamic monitoring include those who have not responded rapidly to fluid resuscitation, those who have responded but deteriorate despite adequate resuscitation, children who require careful fluid management for treatment of intracranial hypertension, and patients who have developed multiple organ system failure.

If the aforementioned monitoring techniques do not provide an accurate means of assessing hemodynamic status and guiding therapy, a pulmonary artery catheter allows for accurate assessment of ventricular function, volume status, and adequacy of oxygen delivery.[2] Placement of a pulmonary artery catheter should be considered in children with compromised ventricular function (e.g., from direct myocardial trauma, effects of hypo-

Table 84–4. INITIAL INTENSIVE CARE UNIT EVALUATION: MONITORING

Bedside	Electrocardiogram
	Respiratory rate
	Blood pressure
	Temperature
	Urine output
	Pulse oximetry
	Capnography
	Consider: Arterial catheter
	Central venous catheter
	Pulmonary artery catheter
Laboratory	Chest x-ray
	Complete blood count
	Electrolytes
	Glucose
	Calcium
	Magnesium
	Blood urea nitrogen
	Creatinine
	Arterial blood gas
	Coagulation studies
	Urinalysis

tension or hypoxia prior to adequate resuscitation, or cardiac dysfunction as a part of multiple organ system failure), complicated fluid resuscitation (e.g., balancing shock and intracranial pressure treatment) or when oxygen supply:demand ratios are in question.[3]

Measurements of cardiac output and filling pressures from the right and left heart guide inotropic and volume support, while minimizing the potential for fluid overload and edema. In addition, adequacy of oxygen delivery to meet demands of the body can be assessed. Hemodynamic and pulmonary effects of high PEEP (>10 to 15 cm H_2O) can also be determined and used as a guide to appropriate therapy.[3]

Initial and ongoing laboratory assessment of the trauma patient include measurement of the complete blood count (CBC), blood chemistries including serum electrolytes, glucose, calcium, magnesium, blood urea nitrogen (BUN), creatinine, arterial blood gas monitoring, coagulation studies, and urinalysis.

Complications of Massive Transfusion

If resuscitation has included the use of massive transfusion of blood products, defined as a transfusion greater than one blood volume in a 24-hour period, complications may ensue. An initial coagulopathy seems to be dilutional, is usually transient, and is related to the amount of fluid used for resuscitation. A more profound coagulopathy follows and is related to the duration of hypotension, and therefore to the adequacy of resuscitation. Clotting factors and platelets are consumed as clot formation occurs in injured vessels. Disseminated intravascular coagulation may occur as large amounts of fibrinolytic products are released. Several studies have demonstrated a lack of correlation between coagulation factor concentrations and the occurrence of bleeding complications.[4] These data suggest that bleeding may result from platelet consumption, circulation of fibrinolytic products, or other variables rather than from decreased coagulation factor concentrations. Therefore, routine use of fresh frozen plasma in massively transfused patients may not be necessary. On the other hand, aggressive treatment of hypotension, hypothermia, hypoxia, and acidosis should be beneficial.

Massive transfusion increases the risk of hypothermia. This risk is compounded in small patients in whom exposure to the ambient temperature of the emergency room was necessary for access during resuscitative efforts. Patients may need to be actively rewarmed in the pediatric intensive care unit with increased ambient temperature, heating lamps, blankets, warmed intravenous solutions, and heated humidified inspired gases for patients requiring mechanical ventilation.

Massively transfused patients are also susceptible to pulmonary dysfunction thought to result from activated neutrophils and metabolites of the prostaglandin pathway.[4]

Although hyperkalemia occurs when transfusions are rapidly administered, hypokalemia occurs more commonly during massive transfusions. Metabolic alkalosis, release of catecholamines, and hormones such as aldosterone, antidiuretic hormone, and corticosteroids all contribute to hypokalemia. Hypocalcemia may also occur because stored blood is anticoagulated with citrate, which binds calcium. The decreased ventricular contractility and low peripheral vascular resistance caused by low serum calcium are exacerbated by hypothermia, decreased liver function, or hypovolemia. Hypomagnesemia occurs in situations similar to those causing hypocalcemia. Patients who are symptomatic but do not respond to the administration of calcium may require magnesium.

Metabolic alkalosis may occur as citrate in transfused blood is metabolized to bicarbonate. Metabolic acidosis results from persistent hypoperfusion and should be treated by more aggressive resuscitative efforts. Massive transfusions may also contribute to the suppression of the immune system that occurs following resuscitation from multiple trauma, increasing the risk of septic complications.

NUTRITIONAL SUPPORT

Nutritional support of the pediatric trauma victim is imperative to speed wound healing and recovery of the injury and also to reduce the likelihood that patients will develop septic complications and multiple organ system failure. Even if such complications develop, nutritional therapy remains an important component of management (see also Chapters 14 and 15).

Three phases of the metabolic response to injury have been defined.[5] The first phase is the immediate sympathetic response to the injury and includes tachycardia, fever, and hypoglycemia. Beginning within minutes and lasting for 1 or 2 days is the second, or "ebb" phase, associated with hypovolemia; decreased cardiac output and metabolic rate; and decreased blood flow to the liver, kidney, and small intestine. Recovery from this phase clearly depends on adequate fluid resuscitation. The "flow" or hypermetabolic phase is the inflammatory and reparative period. This phase is marked by fever, increased resting energy expenditure, tachypnea, tachycardia, a local inflammatory response, and increased oxygen consumption and CO_2 production. Neuroendocrinologic mediators include catecholamines, glucagon, cortisol, and growth hormone.

Carbohydrate, fat, and protein metabolism are altered.[5] Carbohydrate metabolism is marked by an increase in glycogenolysis and gluconeogenesis, which cannot be suppressed by the administration of glucose or insulin. In fact, glucose tolerance is abnormal despite elevated insulin levels seen in post-traumatic patients. Fat metabolism is characterized by increased lipolysis and decreased lipogenesis. Endogenous fat is the principle energy source in the trauma patient. Protein catabolism is related to the severity of the injury. Amino acids are used in wound healing, the cellular inflammatory process, hepatic gluconeogenesis, and hepatic protein synthesis. Branch chain amino acids are used as a fuel source for skeletal muscle. Urine nitrogen loss increases with the catabolism of amino acids. If unchecked, protein catabolism leads to a decrease in skeletal muscle mass. Subsequently, visceral proteins are used, increasing susceptibility to infection and multiple organ system failure.[6]

Nutritional therapy is tailored to the needs of the patient in order to achieve nitrogen balance and to provide adequate energy while avoiding complications of overly aggressive therapy. Some form of nutrition should be initiated immediately after hemodynamic stability has been achieved. Delays in nutritional intervention result in negative nitrogen balance and increased risk of sepsis.[6]

Feeding Mode

The enteral route is used, if possible. Enteral feedings may result in a lower rate of infection by preserving gut mucosal integrity and decreasing the likelihood of bacterial translocation.[6] Nasogastric feedings are the simplest way to begin enteral feeding. Continuous infusions are preferred rather than bolus feedings, to reduce the risk of aspiration or gastric distention. A nasojejunal feeding catheter provides access for continuously infused solutions without the risk of aspiration that nasogastric feedings present, but this catheter is more difficult to position correctly. A soft Silastic feeding tube with a weighted tip may be passed nasogastrically, and continuous feeding can be begun at a low rate, allowing gastric motility and peristalsis to carry the tube into the jejunum. In infants under 1 year of age, a standard infant formula is used. In older children, an isotonic, low residual formula is used. An elemental formula may be tried if standard formulas are not tolerated.

Unfortunately, the presence of abdominal injury or an ileus often prevents use of the enteral route for nutritional support in patients with trauma. Parenteral nutrition may be delivered via a peripheral vein, although the calories supplied by this route are limited by the tonicity of the solution. The central route is preferred for the infusion of optimal calories.

Caloric Requirements

Caloric requirements for the severely injured child have not been determined. Although these patients are thought to be "hypermetabolic," severely injured children are confined to bed, mechanically ventilated, and occasionally receive neuromuscular relaxing agents, all of which reduce energy needs. Formulas have been devised to calculate caloric requirements in the critically ill trauma patient that are based on basal metabolic rate (BMR, defined as energy expenditure at rest in the fasting state), or, more appropriately in the patient in the intensive care unit receiving glucose-containing intravenous fluids, resting energy expenditure (BMR and the specific dynamic action of food). When measured in mechanically ventilated children (primarily trauma victims), resting energy expenditure (REE) was found to be 1.5 times the predicted basal energy expenditure.[7] Others have suggested multiplying BMR by factors accounting for stress and activity. None of these for-

mulas has been verified in larger series in critically ill children. A reasonable approach to estimating caloric needs is to start with 1.5 × BMR (or approximately the standard caloric needs calculated for a healthy child of the same age), since this accounts for increased needs due to stress, but decreased requirements while mechanically ventilated and bed-ridden. Provision of adequate calories is often hindered by limits of fluid management in patients on other necessary infusions, and compromises are required.

Nonprotein Calories

The ideal composition of the parenteral solution for the pediatric trauma patient is not known. In adult patients glucose infusion rates above 5 mg/kg/min increase the respiratory quotient (V_{CO_2}/V_{O_2}), which increases the risk of CO_2 retention in patients who are unable to compensate for increased CO_2 production.[8] A glucose infusion rate of greater than 7 mg/kg/min does not increase glucose oxidation rates and may result in increased hepatic fat synthesis. In normal newborns, a glucose infusion rate of 10 mg/kg/min increases the respiratory quotient to 1.08, compared with 0.96 while receiving 7 mg/kg/min of glucose.[9] Transcutaneous P_{CO_2} was not affected at the higher glucose infusion rate but minute ventilation increased, suggesting that respiratory compensation occurred. These data suggest that newborns may be able to tolerate higher glucose infusion rates compared with adults without an adverse effect on respiratory rate or CO_2 retention. Comparable studies in children out of the newborn period have not been done.

Endogenous fat is the principal form of energy used by the trauma patient. Lipid emulsions are provided to reduce nitrogen losses, to prevent essential fatty acid deficiencies, and to provide calories while reducing the risk of high carbohydrate loads and hyperosmolar infusions. Excessive fat administration may produce adverse effects on the pulmonary circulation, with pulmonary hypertension and hypoxemia, and a platelet inhibitory effect.[10] In a study comparing a high-fat (2.8 g/kg/day) versus a low-fat (1.0 g/kg/day) regimen in newborns receiving total parenteral nutrition, respiratory quotient, and CO_2 production were lower during the high-fat regimen, but P_{O_2} was also lower, suggesting that pulmonary diffusing capacity decreased.[9] The mechanism for this alteration is uncertain.

Protein

One of the most important goals of nutritional therapy following a traumatic insult is the attenuation of protein catabolism and the reversal of negative nitrogen balance. However, nitrogen requirements in critically ill children have not been well defined. Studies in adults suggest a protein requirement of approximately 1.5 g/kg/day.[5] Nitrogen excretion data in critically ill children also indicate that 1.5 g/kg/day is an appropriate amount of protein.[7] Others recommend 2 to 3 g/kg/day for infants and 1.5 to 2 g/kg/day for children. In burned children, 4 g/kg/day of protein produced better survival and fewer bacteremic days than did a lower protein intake.[11] If verified, these data will have important implications for nutritional management of pediatric patients in the intensive care unit.

Nitrogen balance monitoring at the patient's bedside to guide success of therapy is not available in most institutions. A rising BUN:creatinine ratio, or an elevated BUN in a well-hydrated patient may suggest excessive protein intake or decreased nitrogen utilization.

Specific Recommendations for Nutritional Support

Initial caloric intake should approximate that recommended for healthy children of the same weight or age (see Table 84–3). Nonprotein caloric needs may be divided equally between carbohydrate and fat sources. An initial glucose infusion rate of 5 mg/kg/min may be increased slowly to 10 mg/kg/min while monitoring for glucose intolerance and CO_2 retention (Table 84–5). A lipid infusion of 1 g/kg/day may be increased to 2 to 3 g/kg/day while monitoring serum triglyceride levels. Patients with severe lung disease should receive less lipids because of the potential for interference with oxygen diffusion. Protein intake should be 2 g/kg/day and may be advanced while monitoring the BUN:creatinine ratio. The protein:energy ratio should be approximately 15 to 20%. Intravenous amino acid intake should not exceed 3 g/kg/day. Adequate vitamins and minerals are also added to the parenteral nutritional solution.

PAIN CONTROL AND SEDATION

The need for adequate pain control and sedation in the post resuscitation phase must be carefully balanced against ongoing attempts to establish and maintain hemodynamic stability. Side effects of analgesic and sedative agents, most notably respiratory depression, hypotension, decreased gastrointestinal motility, depressed mental status, and altered response to noxious stimuli may interfere with cardiopulmonary, neurologic, and nutritional resuscitation efforts. However, in addition to the obviously beneficial effects of pain relief, anxiolysis, and sedation, analgesic and sedative agents may facili-

Table 84–5. RECOMMENDATIONS FOR PARENTERAL NUTRITIONAL SUPPORT

Initial Infusion Rates		Final Infusion Rate*	Monitor
Glucose	5 mg/kg/min	10 mg/kg/min	Serum glucose, P_{CO_2}, respiratory rate
Lipids	1 g/kg/day	2–3 g/kg/day	Serum triglyceride levels
Protein	1.5–2 g/kg/day	3 g/kg/day	BUN†:creatinine ratio

*Infusion rate may be increased to the amounts given.
†BUN = blood urea nitrogen.

tate wound care and dressing changes, aid in control of intracranial hypertension in patients with closed head injury, restore ventilatory function in patients with chest trauma, and help in re-establishing normal sleep cycles in patients in the intensive care unit.[12]

More important, analgesic and sedative agents alter the response to stress.[13] In adults, reduction of the stress response by various anesthetic techniques during major surgery has produced lower morbidity and mortality rates postoperatively. In neonates undergoing surgery, narcotics blunt the hormonal response to stress and reduce postoperative endogenous protein breakdown and perioperative complications. Clinical outcome is improved using high-dose narcotic techniques. These data suggest that aggressive treatment of pain and anxiety in trauma patients attenuates the metabolic response to injury and may improve clinical outcome. Whether the desired response can be obtained using narcotic doses sufficient for analgesia, or will require the high-dose techniques used in the operating room, has not been determined.

Despite the appropriateness of providing pain relief for patients with trauma, analgesics may mask physical signs of underlying illness or injury. The initial physical examination and diagnostic studies should be done keeping in mind the need for analgesics and careful follow-up.

In the pediatric intensive care unit, no ideal regimen for analgesia, anxiolysis, and sedation exists (see also Chapter 77). Benzodiazepines and opiates are most commonly used to achieve these effects. Morphine is the least expensive opiate, but its use may be limited by cardiovascular instability induced by vasodilatation and by histamine release. Fentanyl has less potential for cardiovascular instability, but, as with morphine, accumulation and a need for increasing doses may occur with prolonged use. All opiates affect gastrointestinal motility and may interfere with enteral feedings.

Benzodiazepines are often used as adjuncts to the opiates to potentiate sedation and relieve anxiety. Diazepam is the least expensive benzodiazepine, but active metabolites accumulate and produce excessive sedation and delay in return to consciousness. Lorazepam does not have active metabolites, but excessive sedation may still occur. Midazolam can be administered by continuous infusion and provides a steady level of sedation; however, prolonged sedation may occur and the cost is high. The pharmacokinetics of midazolam in critically ill children have not been well studied.

We use a combination of morphine or fentanyl and valium or midazolam (Table 84–6). Continuous infusions of morphine or fentanyl provide optimal relief from pain if adequate intravenous access is available, and diazepam or lorazepam is added intermittently to blunt awareness and relieve anxiety. If adequate sedation cannot be achieved with this regimen by adjusting doses, the benzodiazepine is changed to midazolam by constant infusion. In agitated patients, the possibilities of hypercarbia, hypoxia, or missed injury resulting in persistent hemorrhage or pain, need to be explored before additional sedation is administered.

Table 84–6. INITIAL DOSES OF OPIATES AND BENZODIAZEPINES IN THE CRITICALLY ILL CHILD

Drug	Route	Dose
Morphine	Intermittent IV*	0.1 mg/kg q 2–3 hr
	Continuous IV	0.05 mg/kg/hr
Fentanyl	Continuous IV	2–4 µg/kg/hr
Diazepam	Intermittent IV	0.1 mg/kg every 2–4 hr
Lorazepam	Intermittent IV	0.05 mg/kg every 6–8 hr
Midazolam	Continuous IV	0.025–0.05 mg/kg/hr

*IV = intravenous.

ADULT RESPIRATORY DISTRESS SYNDROME

Adult respiratory distress syndrome (ARDS), or perhaps more appropriately in children, acute hypoxemic respiratory failure (AHRF), is a complication in the severely injured trauma patient (see also Chapter 47). ARDS is characterized by severe hypoxemia and hypercarbia, poor lung compliance, increased work of breathing, bilateral diffuse pulmonary infiltrates, and normal left ventricular filling pressure. Precipitating events in children include sepsis, shock, and near-drowning. Pulmonary aspiration of gastric contents, massive blood transfusions, pneumonia, and pulmonary contusions commonly precipitate ARDS in adults and may initiate ARDS in children as well. The prevalence of ARDS in pediatric patients with trauma is not known, but milder forms of the disease that resolve with oxygen and supportive care may occur frequently.[14] Mortality rates range from 30 to 90%, comparable with those in adults.[15] Sepsis rather than respiratory failure is the leading cause of death in adult patients with ARDS.[16]

The inciting event triggers diffuse alveolar damage with disruption of the alveolar capillary membrane. Edema fluid, white blood cells, and other intravascular substances leak into the interstitium and alveoli. White blood cells may release granular contents and oxygen-derived free radicals that may further damage the lungs. The destruction of alveolar type 1 and type 2 pneumocytes in the early stages of ARDS halts production of surfactant and leads to atelectasis. During the final proliferative phase, fibroblasts appear, and severe fibrosis and restrictive lung disease may occur.[17]

Interstitial edema leads to intrapulmonary shunting that does not improve with oxygen therapy. Arteriocapillary obstruction (secondary to interstitial edema, fibrosis, thrombosis, and destruction by bacteria) and pulmonary vasoconstriction increase pulmonary vascular resistance. Pulmonary artery hypertension occurs despite normal capillary wedge pressures. Mechanical ventilation can accelerate the process of ARDS. Toxic levels of oxygen and increased airway pressures may cause further lung damage or can directly initiate ARDS.

Therapy for ARDS is supportive. Augmentation of cardiac output and aggressive ventilator support and correction of the inciting event will improve oxygen delivery. Inotropic agents are used to increase cardiac output, since volume expansion beyond the euvolemic state may worsen gas exchange by increasing pulmonary hydrostatic pressure and edema. Diuretics reduce lung water and improve ventilation-perfusion relationships allowing oxygen levels and airway pressures to be lowered, thus reducing risks from barotrauma and oxygen toxicity. Diuretics do not directly alter lung injury, although evidence suggests that fluid restriction and lower pulmonary capillary wedge pressures may improve the patient's survival.[18, 19]

Ventilator support includes the use of volume-cycled or pressure-limited modes of "conventional" ventilator management, along with the application of PEEP. PEEP improves lung compliance and gas exchange and relocates edema fluid from the alveoli to the interstitium. The redistribution of pulmonary blood flow may improve shunting. PEEP does not prevent ARDS nor does it alter the course of the lung damage. It may lead to barotrauma and decreased cardiac output by reducing preload and the compliance of the left ventricle. Low cardiac output may be treated with inotropic agents as well as judicious use of fluids.

Other forms of artificial ventilation have been attempted with varying degrees of success. High-frequency ventilation does not improve outcome when compared with conventional ventilation.[20] Pressure-controlled inverse ratio ventilation (I:E ratio of 2:1 or greater) has been used to improve oxygenation at lower peak airway pressures.[21] Although inverse ratio ventilation did not improve oxygen saturation or delivery in adult patients with ARDS, this approach maintained oxygenation and adequate ventilation at lower peak airway pressures, without altering hemodynamic parameters. However, the elevated mean airway pressures and high PEEP from the prolonged inspiration and lack of complete expiration increase the risk of barotrauma.

Extracorporeal membrane oxygenation (ECMO) is currently being re-evaluated as a therapy for ARDS. Although a multicenter study showed that ECMO and conventional ventilation each produced mortality rates of 90%,[22] improved technology and less invasive methods may reduce morbidity of ECMO. In adult patients undergoing venovenous bypass for extracorporeal CO_2 removal in conjunction with low-frequency conventional ventilation, the mortality rate was 50%.[23] In a smaller series of patients with venovenous bypass, high extracorporeal flows to support oxygenation as well as CO_2 removal produced a similar mortality rate.[24] Partial extracorporeal support, used earlier in the disease course, and allowing percutaneous cannulation, may prove efficacious in selected patients.[23] In pediatric patients, no generally accepted selection criteria exist, and no controlled trials of ECMO for ARDS have been published. Studies of ECMO and of an intravenous capillary membrane lung (IVOX) are underway.

Attempts to control the systemic inflammatory response that perpetuates the lung injury of ARDS may provide therapeutic alternatives.[17] Steroids do not improve disease course or outcome. Prostaglandin E_1 has anti-inflammatory, antiplatelet and antithromboxane effects, and stabilizes lysosomes. Theoretically these effects should be beneficial to patients with ARDS. However, a multicenter randomized clinical trial of PGE_1

failed to demonstrate improved survival. Beneficial effects on oxygen transport suggest that PGE_1 may have a role as an adjunct to treatment.[25] Although indomethacin provides short-term improvement in oxygenation, longer term use of nonsteroidal anti-inflammatory agents has not been studied.[26] Another agent that antagonizes inflammatory mediators, pentoxifylline, may also help to attenuate the inflammatory response in ARDS.

MULTIPLE ORGAN SYSTEM FAILURE

Multiple organ system failure (MOSF) is a syndrome of survival and high technology. Technology allows patients who survive their initial trauma to die of the effects of pulmonary, hepatic, renal, and eventually cardiac failure. Factors that predispose patients to MOSF include a persistent perfusion deficit, with or without sepsis, and persistent infection or an inflammatory focus. MOSF is a leading cause of late death after trauma in adult and pediatric patients.

Pathophysiology

Development of MOSF proceeds in four stages (Table 84–7).[27] (1) Circulatory failure and poor perfusion secondary to hemorrhage, sepsis, tissue damage, or an inflammatory reaction, is followed by a period of hemodynamic stability after (2) resuscitation. Patients may then become (3) hypermetabolic and develop acute lung injury. The final phase (4) of MOSF starts with the onset of hepatitis and renal failure. The brain, hematologic and immune systems, and the gastrointestinal tract may also be failing organs. The overall mortality rate in pediatric patients is 54%.[28] Mortality may be related to the number of failed organs ranging from 26% for two failed organs, up to 88% for four failed organs.[29]

During the phase of relative or absolute circulatory failure, decreased perfusion results in endothelial injury, platelet aggregation, neutrophil infiltration, and activation of vasoactive mediators. Increased capillary permeability decreases intravascular volume and increases the perfusion defect. Reperfusion may release inflammatory mediators into the systemic circulation to damage distant organs and reperfused tissue. Hypoxia, acidosis, formation of microthrombi, and direct tissue injury all contribute.

Table 84–7. MULTIPLE ORGAN SYSTEM FAILURE

Stages	Treatment
1. Circulatory failure and direct tissue damage	Prevention of original traumatic event
2. Resuscitation	Aggressive resuscitation to minimize organ damage, improve oxygen delivery to tissues
3. Hypermetabolism and development of acute lung injury	Control of inciting event, respiratory support, nutritional support
4. Multiple organ failure	Support of failing organs

Following the initial phases of circulatory failure and resuscitation, the patient may become hypermetabolic. Fever, tachypnea, tachycardia, and elevated white blood cell count are followed by a picture of diffuse infiltrates on chest radiograph, progressive hypoxia, and inadequate ventilation.[17] Pulmonary disease usually manifests as ARDS, although primary lung damage from pneumonia or contusion may initiate the hypermetabolic phase. Increased cardiac output and oxygen consumption, lactic acidosis, and reduced systemic vascular resistance are present. Skeletal muscle proteolysis provides a carbon source for increased hepatic ureagenesis and gluconeogenesis. Fat and protein metabolism are also altered. The macrophage appears to be involved in the hypermetabolic phase. Systemic hormones released during this phase include hydrocortisone, glucagon, epinephrine, and possibly growth and thyroid hormones. Although hormone release may initially be adaptive, later these hormones help to mediate MOSF.

Gastrointestinal hypoxic, ischemic, or reperfusion injury during shock and resuscitation may initiate or perpetuate the hypermetabolic phase. Gut bacteria may seed the respiratory tract or traverse the gut wall and enter the adjacent tissue or systemic circulation. MOSF proceeds with the development of hepatitis and renal failure. Bleeding with stress ulceration, ileus, and diarrhea are signals of gastrointestinal failure. Pancreatic injury or ischemia and pancreatitis stimulate release of free oxygen radicals and activated protease enzymes leading to activation of various coagulation cascades that contribute to the ongoing MOSF process.

Cardiac function becomes impaired. Encephalopathy, disseminated intravascular coagulation, and a suppressed immune system may also occur. If infection was not the inciting event, it will almost certainly occur during MOSF.

Treatment

Treatment of MOSF should be aimed at supporting individual organs to restore microcirculatory perfusion and to prevent further deterioration. Elimination of the process that activates organ failure is equally important.

Clinical criteria to assess the adequacy of resuscitation include heart rate, blood pressure, skin perfusion, peripheral pulses, and urine output. These criteria may not reflect the point at which oxygen delivery is equal to oxygen demand. Invasive monitoring to measure and improve the relationships between oxygen delivery and oxygen consumption may improve outcome. Treatment should improve oxygen-carrying capacity and cardiac output, even to supranormal levels. The increased blood volume required to improve microcirculatory perfusion should be balanced against the risks of increasing interstitial edema in the lungs. Respiratory support, treatment to prevent gastric ulceration and bleeding, treatment of hematologic abnormalities, and medical and dialysis support of renal function should also be aggressively applied.

Malnutrition may contribute to morbidity and mortality in MOSF, and control of malnutrition appears to improve outcome.[30] Goals of nutritional therapy are to achieve nitrogen balance with amino acid infusions while avoiding complications of excessive caloric, glucose, and fat infusions. Although exogenous amino acids, fat, or glucose do not effectively suppress protein catabolism, protein synthesis will respond to amino acid infusions and nitrogen balance can be achieved.[27]

Early and aggressive action to drain infection, debride necrotic tissue, control hemorrhage, and stabilize fractures may remove the inciting cause of MOSF. Signs of ARDS and persistent fever indicate a secondary infection until proven otherwise and suggest the need for re-exploration of the surgical site. If MOSF progresses, surgical intervention may be ineffective, as the infected patient becomes more debilitated and local defense mechanisms fail to prevent bacterial or fungal dissemination. The ongoing secondary infections may sustain organ failure despite adequate control of original factors inciting MOSF.

Because of excessive mortality and lack of specific therapy to control the onset and progression of MOSF, new therapies are being explored.[17, 27] Attempts have been made to alter immune function and augment the ability of the patient to contain microbes and to prevent dissemination. Altering gastrointestinal flora to prevent colonization of the respiratory tract from the gastrointestinal tract, or translocation of gut flora, does not appear to alter the progression of MOSF or mortality. The effects of oxygen free radicals or prostaglandin inhibition are being studied.

Nutritional manipulation has been suggested to alter inflammatory mediators or to support specific metabolic pathways.[27] Specific lipid emulsions may alter the synthesis of inflammatory mediators such as prostaglandins, leukotrienes, tumor necrosis factor, and interleukin-1. These effects have not been well studied clinically. Administration of specific proteins may improve gut mucosal integrity. Efforts to attenuate the effects of shock, hypermetabolism, and organ failure have also been attempted. Inhibitors of prostaglandins and leukotrienes, platelet activating factors, tumor necrosis factor, and antioxidant therapies are being tested clinically.

References

1. Alyono D, Ring S, and Chao RYN: Characteristics of ventricular function in severe hemorrhagic shock. Surgery 94:250, 1983.
2. Goldenheim PD and Kazemi H: Cardiopulmonary monitoring of critically ill patients. N Engl J Med 311:717, 1984.
3. Pollack MM, Reed TP, Holbrook PR, et al: Bedside pulmonary artery catheterization in pediatrics. J Pediatr 96:274, 1980.
4. Rutledge R, Sheldon GF, and Collins ML: Massive transfusion. Crit Care Clin 2:791, 1986.
5. Kien CL: Nutrition in burn and trauma patients. In: Grand RJ, Sutphen JL, and Dietz WH (eds): Pediatric Nutrition. Boston, Butterworths, 1987, pp. 549–570.
6. Moore EE: Nutritional considerations in critical care medicine: Observations from postinjury total enteral nutrition versus total parenteral nutrition. In: Lumb PD and Shoemaker WC (eds): Critical Care: State of the Art, Vol. II. Fullerton, CA, Society of Critical Care Medicine, 1990, pp. 33–57.
7. Tilden SJ, Watkins S, Tong TK, et al: Measured energy expenditure in pediatric intensive care patients. Am J Dis Child 143:490, 1989.
8. Wolfe RR, O'Donnell TF Jr, Stone MD, et al: Investigation of factors determining the optimal glucose infusion rate in total parenteral nutrition. Metabolism 29:892, 1980.
9. Piedboeuf B, Chessex P, Hazan J, et al: Total parenteral nutrition in the newborn infant: Energy substrates and respiratory gas exchange. J Pediatr 118:97, 1990.
10. Venus B, Smith RA, Patel C, et al: Hemodynamic and gas exchange alterations during intralipid infusion in patients with adult respiratory distress syndrome. Chest 95:1278, 1989.
11. Alexander W, MacMillan BG, Stinnett JD, et al: Beneficial effects of aggressive protein feeding in severely burned children. Ann Surg 192:505, 1980.
12. Mackersie RC and Karagianes TG: Pain management following trauma and burns. Crit Care Clin 6:433, 1990.
13. Anand KJ and Carr DB: The neuroanatomy, neurophysiology, and neurochemistry of pain, stress, and analgesia in newborns and children. Pediatr Clin North Am 36:795, 1989.
14. Rinaldo JE: The prognosis of the adult respiratory distress syndrome. Chest 90:470, 1986.
15. Zucker AR: Therapeutic strategies for acute hypoxemic respiratory failure. Crit Care Clin 4:813, 1988.
16. Montgomery AB, Stager MA, Carrico CJ, et al: Causes of mortality in patients with adult respiratory distress syndrome. Am Rev Respir Dis 132:485, 1985.
17. Demling RH: Current concepts on the adult respiratory distress syndrome. Circ Shock 30:297, 1990.
18. Simmon RS, Berdine GG, Seidenfeld JJ, et al: Fluid balance and the adult respiratory distress syndrome. Am Rev Respir Dis 135:924, 1987.
19. Humphrey H, Hall J, Sznajder I, et al: Improved survival in ARDS patients associated with a reduction in pulmonary capillary wedge pressure. Chest 97:1176, 1990.
20. Hurst JM, Branson RD, David K, et al: Comparison of conventional mechanical ventilation and high-frequency ventilation. Ann Surg 211:486, 1990.
21. Abraham E and Yoshihara G: Cardiorespiratory effects of pressure controlled inverse ratio ventilation in severe respiratory failure. Chest 96:1356, 1989.
22. Zapol WM, Snider MT, Hill JD, et al: Extracorporeal membrane oxygenation in severe acute respiratory failure: A randomized prospective study. JAMA 242:2193, 1979.
23. Pesenti A, Kolobow T, and Gattinoni L: Extracorporeal respiratory support in the adult. Trans Am Soc Artif Intern Organs 34:1006, 1988.
24. Snider MT, Campbell DB, Kofke WA, et al: Venovenous perfusion of adults and children with severe acute respiratory distress syndrome. Trans Am Soc Artif Intern Organs 34:1014, 1988.
25. Silverman HJ, Slotman G, Bone RC, et al: Effects of prostaglandin E$_1$ on oxygen delivery and consumption in patients with the adult respiratory distress syndrome. Chest 98:405, 1990.
26. Steinberg SM, Rodriguez JL, Bitzer LG, et al: Indomethacin treatment of human adult respiratory distress syndrome. Circ Shock 30:375, 1990.
27. Barton R and Cerra FB: The hypermetabolism-multiple organ failure syndrome. Chest 96:1153, 1989.
28. Wilkinson JD, Pollack MM, Ruttimann UE, et al: Outcome of pediatric patients with multiple organ system failure. Crit Care Med 14:271, 1986.
29. Wilkinson JD, Pollack MN, and Glass NL: Mortality associated with multiple organ system failure and sepsis in pediatric intensive care unit. J Pediatr 111:324, 1987.
30. Cerra FB: The multiple organ failure syndrome. In: Gallagher TJ and Shoemaker WC (eds): Critical Care, State of the Art, Vol 9. Fullerton, CA, Society of Critical Care Medicine, 1988, pp. 107–128.

Critical Management of Chest, Abdomen, and Extremity Trauma

Arthur Cooper, M.D.

The critical care of the injured child presents a unique challenge to the pediatric critical care physicians and surgeons entrusted with this responsibility. Although the initial phases of resuscitation have the most direct impact upon outcome (inadequate resuscitation remains the leading cause of preventable death)[1, 2] competent, compassionate management in the intensive care unit (ICU) is essential to optimal recovery, both somatic[3] and psychic.[4] Fortunately, most pediatric trauma victims admitted to the ICU have been previously stabilized. Conversely, the fact that most serious childhood injuries—including those to the chest, abdomen, and extremities—are now managed nonoperatively, mandates the need for intensive observation and nursing care, as well as timely and appropriate critical medical and surgical intervention as needed.

It is not the purpose of this chapter to focus solely on the early phases of pediatric trauma resuscitation (see Chapter 8), though the same principles that apply to the management of traumatic cardiopulmonary failure prior to arrival at the hospital and in the emergency department obviously apply to injured children who experience respiratory failure or shock during their stay in the ICU. Rather, it also aims to focus on the critical aspects of care following resuscitation and the postoperative management of the child with injuries of the chest, abdomen, and extremities that are commonly encountered by the pediatric critical care physician or surgeon. However, a brief review of the clinical spectrum, as well as the relevant anatomy and physiology, will first be undertaken to provide both a context and a rationale for therapy. The chapter concludes with a short description of the organization and function of the pediatric trauma system, the smooth operation of which is vital to the optimal recovery of the pediatric multiple trauma victim, and a discussion of systems for chest drainage and suction.

SPECTRUM OF CHEST, ABDOMEN, AND EXTREMITY INJURIES IN CHILDREN

Trauma is the leading cause of death and permanent disability in children aged 1 to 14 years in the United States, killing almost 10,000 annually nationwide.[5] It affects boys twice as frequently as girls, but all age groups are affected more or less equally.[6] It is responsible for some 10% of all pediatric hospitalizations nationwide,[7] about 15% of all pediatric ICU admissions,[8] approximately 25% of pediatric emergency department visits,[9] and 50% or more of all pediatric ambulance runs.[10] Blunt injuries predominate by a ratio of 6:1, of which motor vehicle and bicycle injuries account for less than half, though they cause most of the deaths (Table 85–1). Unfortunately, however, penetrating injuries, which generally are more lethal, are on the rise, especially in urban areas.[11–16]

Most blunt trauma in childhood is sustained unintentionally, though 7% of serious injuries are due to physical assault and 3% to physical abuse.[6] The mechanism of trauma determines the pattern of injuries that may occur. Motor vehicle trauma gives rise to two distinct syndromes: (1) pedestrian injuries, in which fracture of the midshaft of the femur is coupled with closed head and torso injuries (i.e., "the Waddell triad")[17] and (2) occupant injuries, in which closed head and cervical spine injuries predominate,[18] unless the child is properly restrained in an infant car seat or child safety seat. Injuries due to forward-facing car seats (i.e., isolated cervical spine injuries)[19–22] and lap belts (i.e., lumbar spine, intestinal, hepatic, and diaphragmatic injuries)[23–28] all have recently been described, however. Falls from extreme heights also result in head, torso, and long bone injuries, their severity being directly related to the magnitude of vertical displacement.[29, 30] Bicycles, too, are notoriously associated with serious

Table 85–1. INCIDENCE AND MORTALITY OF PEDIATRIC TRAUMA*

	Incidence	Mortality
By Injury Mechanism		
Blunt	85%	3%
Motor vehicle	35%	5%
Occupant	18%	4%
Pedestrian	17%	5%
Fall	26%	1%
Less than 8 ft	21%	<1%
More than 8 ft	5%	2%
Bicycle	8%	2%
Sports	5%	<1%
Struck	4%	1%
Beating	3%	5%
Motorcycle	1%	2%
Recreational vehicle	1%	2%
Other blunt	1%	22%
Penetrating	13%	5%
Gunshot	6%	10%
Stab	5%	<1%
Animal bite	1%	0%
Other penetrating	1%	0%
Other	2%	8%
By Body Region		
Multiple†	44%	5%
Extremities	19%	0%
Head and neck	17%	6%
External	13%	0%
Abdomen	3%	2%
Face	2%	0%
Thorax	1%	3%
By Anatomic Diagnosis		
Head injury	28%	10%
Fracture	21%	4%
Open wound	17%	3%
Superficial wound	11%	3%
Contusion	9%	3%
Intrathoracic intra-abdominal injury	7%	14%
Spine injury	2%	9%
Other	5%	9%

*From DiScala C, Gans BM, Barlow B, et al: National Pediatric Trauma Registry Biannual Report. Boston, Tufts University Rehabilitation and Childhood Trauma Research and Training Center, 1990.
†More than one body region affected.

trauma in children, particularly (1) closed head injury following an unprotected fall from a moving bicycle and (2) splenic, hepatic, or gastrointestinal injury caused by a fall against the handlebar.[31, 32]

The true incidence of traumatic injury in children is unknown; however, the incidence of *serious* traumatic injury—using hospitalization as the indicator of injury severity—is 420 in 100,000.[16] The in-hospital mortality rate (case fatality ratio) in this group is 0.57% (2.4:100,000). This contrasts with a population-based mortality ratio of 11.8:100,000, indicating that some 82% of children die before they reach the hospital. The mortality rate for injuries serious enough to require pediatric trauma center care is approximately 3%[6] and mainly results from intracranial trauma (see Table 85–1).[6, 33] Intrathoracic and intra-abdominal injuries are associated with a fatal outcome in 14% of all cases of serious childhood trauma but are rarely the immediate cause of death, unless irreversible hemorrhagic shock caused by severe lacerations of the spleen or liver, or both, are also present.[33, 34] Axial skeletal trauma virtually never causes death unless it is associated with a severe

comminuted pelvic fracture or cervical spinal cord injury.

Serious intrathoracic injuries occur in about 6% of pediatric blunt trauma victims and rarely require thoracotomy, but chest tubes are needed in about 50% of cases.[6, 34–41] Although thoracic injury is the proximate cause of death in less than 1% of all pediatric blunt trauma, that associated with major intrathoracic injury is nearly 10 times more deadly than blunt trauma not associated with this type of injury; thus, the presence of major intrathoracic injury serves as an indicator of the severity of the injury.[41] Both pulmonary contusions and rib fractures are present in greater numbers than is generally appreciated[40]; the former occurs in about one half of all blunt trauma cases, and the latter occurs in about one third of cases (Table 85–2).[34] In contrast, pneumothorax occurs in about 25% of serious blunt thoracic injury, and significant hemothorax occurs in about 15% of cases. Injuries to the heart, large airways, great vessels, diaphragm, and esophagus are rare.

The child's ability to compensate for respiratory derangements associated with serious thoracic injury is limited by (1) larger oxygen consumption but smaller functional reserve capacity, which makes the child more susceptible to hypoxia; (2) lesser pulmonary compliance yet greater chest wall compliance, which dictates chiefly a tachypneic response to hypoxia; and (3) horizontally aligned ribs and rudimentary intercostal musculature, which makes the small child a diaphragmatic breather. The thorax of the child usually escapes major harm because the pliable nature of the cartilaginous ribs allows the kinetic energy associated with even forceful impact to be absorbed without significant injury. Pulmonary contusions are a frequent concomitant of this type of injury, but they seldom cause physiologic derangements that are truly life-threatening. Conversely, blows that are sharp enough to cause rib fractures are indicative of severe injury and are commonly associated with tension pneumothorax or hemothorax, or both, because of lacerations of the lung parenchyma or intercostal vessels,

Table 85–2. INCIDENCE AND MORTALITY OF INJURIES TO THORACOABDOMINAL ORGANS*

	Incidence	Mortality
Chest		
Lung	52%	18%
Pneumothorax-hemothorax	42%	17%
Ribs-sternum	32%	11%
Heart	6%	40%
Diaphragm	4%	16%
Great vessels	2%	51%
Bronchi	<1%	20%
Esophagus	<1%	43%
Abdomen		
Liver	27%	13%
Spleen	27%	11%
Kidneys	25%	13%
Gastrointestinal tract	21%	11%
Great vessels	5%	47%
Genitourinary tract	5%	3%
Pancreas	4%	7%
Pelvis	<1%	7%

*From Cooper A, Barlow B, DiScala C, et al: Mortality and thoracoabdominal injury: The pediatric perspective. J Trauma, in press.

placing the child in grave danger of sudden, marked ventilatory and circulatory compromise as the mediastinum shifts.

Serious intra-abdominal injuries occur in about 8% of pediatric blunt trauma victims and can usually be managed nonoperatively.[6] They may be caused by any or all of the following biomechanical events: (1) crushing of solid upper abdominal viscera against the vertebral column, (2) sudden compression and bursting of hollow upper abdominal viscera against the vertebral column, and (3) shearing of the posterior attachments or vascular supply of the upper abdominal viscera following rapid deceleration.[42] Injuries to the solid viscera of the upper abdomen (i.e., the liver and spleen) are most common and account for the overwhelming majority of deaths, which invariably are due to irreversible hemorrhagic shock. Other types of solid organ injuries (i.e., renal and pancreatic) generally are less debilitating, seldom require operation, and rarely cause death (see Table 85–2).[34] The same is true of most hollow organ injuries, particularly intramural and mesenteric hematomas; however, perforated or obstructed bowel segments always require prompt surgical repair but rarely are associated with fatal outcome unless they are overlooked.

The abdomen of the child is vulnerable to injury for several reasons. Flexible ribs cover only the uppermost portion of the abdomen, whereas thin layers of muscle, fat, and fascia provide little protection for the large solid viscera. Moreover, the overall small size of the abdomen predisposes the child to multiple rather than single injuries as energy is dissipated from the impacting force. Finally, gastric dilatation from the swallowing of air, which often confounds abdominal examination by simulating peritonitis, may also lead to ventilatory or circulatory compromise, or both, by (1) limiting diaphragmatic motion, (2) increasing risk of aspiration, and (3) causing vagally mediated dampening of the normal tachycardic response to hypovolemia.

By contrast, serious extremity injuries (i.e., fractures) are rarely, if ever, the immediate cause of death in blunt trauma, though they are the leading cause of disability; however, they are present in some 21% of serious blunt injury cases and constitute the principal anatomic diagnosis in 19% of cases.[6] Overall, upper extremity fractures outnumber lower extremity fractures by 7:1, though in serious blunt trauma this ratio is 2:3. Again, the mechanism of injury determines the pattern of fractures that will be encountered. The most common long bone fractures sustained during childhood pedestrian motor vehicle accidents, for example, are fractures of the femur and tibia, whereas falls typically are associated with both upper and lower extremity fractures— but only if the height of the fall is significant—for example, from the top of a bunk bed[43] or the window of a high-rise dwelling,[29, 30] not from falls from beds[44, 45] or down stairs.[46] Significantly, isolated long bone fractures are rarely, if ever, associated with significant hemorrhage;[47] thus, if signs of shock are observed, a search must be made for another source of bleeding, which usually will be found in the abdomen.

The pediatric skeleton is susceptible to fractures because cortical bone in childhood is highly porous and is therefore easily disrupted. The periosteum, however, is more resilient, elastic, and vascular. Although this re-

sults in higher percentages both of incomplete fractures (i.e., torus and greenstick fractures) and complete but nondisplaced fractures, it makes their diagnosis less straightforward.[48] Indeed, nuclear scans are sometimes needed to rule in fractures initially undetected by plain x-ray films. There are other factors that make skeletal trauma in children unique: (1) a rapid rate of healing and freedom from nonunion; (2) a tendency to remodel in the plane of the fracture; (3) a high incidence of ischemic vascular injuries, particularly around the elbow, which, even if they do not immediately threaten the limb, may cause disfiguring contracture; and (4) a low incidence of associated ligamentous injuries. However, the most important feature of children's fractures relates to long-term growth disturbances: Diaphyseal fractures of the long bones are associated with overgrowth of some 1 to 3 cm in the 2- to 10-year-old age group, whereas fractures involving the physeal growth plate, particularly if the injury is severe (i.e., Salter-Harris types 3 and 4), may be associated with significant undergrowth.[49]

INITIAL RESUSCITATION IN CHEST, ABDOMEN, AND EXTREMITY INJURIES

The critical care of the child with chest, abdomen, and extremity injuries begins in the field and continues in the emergency department. The fact that the full extent and consequences of serious injury often are not immediately recognized clearly mandates a physiologic approach to resuscitation. Rapid clinical assessment of ventilation, oxygenation, and perfusion is fundamental to this process, the purpose of which is to identify and treat any condition that may lead imminently to cardiopulmonary failure. Thus, priority attention is directed not only to the airway, breathing, and circulation[50] but also to a "primary survey," the purpose of which is to rule out thoracoabdominal conditions that pose an immediate threat to life (e.g., tension pneumothorax, massive hemothorax, flail chest, cardiac tamponade, and, rarely, gastric dilatation). Several protocols have been published that describe these principles in great detail.[51–56] Since the major iatrogenic cause of mortality in pediatric trauma has been the failure to recognize and stop internal bleeding in a timely manner,[1, 2] a surgeon should be involved as early as possible in the course of the resuscitation—particularly since the limited circulatory reserves of the child demand immediate relief from uncontrolled hemorrhage, if present (see also Chapter 8).[57]

Any child who presents with major trauma to the chest, abdomen, or extremities must receive high concentrations of oxygen by the most appropriate means. This therapy is needed to treat the mixed venous oxygen desaturation that invariably accompanies significant hemorrhage, though patients with thoracic injuries may also need oxygen to correct the arterial hypoxemia associated with ventilation-perfusion abnormalities (i.e., arteriovenous shunting) caused by damage to pulmonary parenchyma. For the child who presents with simple respiratory distress, a nonrebreathing mask normally will suffice provided that the airway is open and breathing is spontaneous. For the child who presents with frank respiratory failure (i.e., apnea, cyanosis, progressive fatigue), assisted ventilation with a bag-valve device attached to a face mask or endotracheal tube will be required. Orotracheal intubation and hyperventilation are mandatory in traumatic arrest and near-arrest to correct the profound respiratory and metabolic acidosis that accompany these conditions, as well as in coma to mitigate the effects of cerebral swelling. Once airway control is established, however, a nasal or oral gastric tube must be inserted for gastric decompression, unless there are specific contraindications to its use (e.g., severe craniofacial trauma).

The child who presents with major trauma to the chest, abdomen, or extremities also requires volume resuscitation. This is best carried out by means of short, fat peripheral lines placed percutaneously in the median cubital veins at the elbow or saphenous veins at the ankle or by cutdown in the saphenous veins at the ankle or groin. Urinary output should be measured in all seriously injured children as an indirect indicator of splanchnic perfusion. If blood is seen at the urinary meatus, or pelvic fracture is suspected, bedside retrograde urethrography should be performed prior to insertion of a urinary catheter to exclude the possibility of urethral damage.

Any child with chest, abdomen, or extremity injuries whose circulation cannot be stabilized by rapid infusion of 40 to 60 ml/kg of lactated Ringer solution probably has internal bleeding and likely needs emergency operation. Since oxygen-carrying capacity, as well as intravascular volume, will be jeopardized by continued hemorrhage, additional volume resuscitation mandates the use of type-specific blood if available (type O, preferably Rh-negative blood if type-specific blood is not available) in rapidly infused aliquots of 10 to 20 ml/kg of packed red blood cells or 20 to 40 ml/kg of whole blood. If a child with chest, abdomen, or extremity injuries presents in shock and has no signs of intrathoracic, intra-abdominal, or intrapelvic bleeding but fails to improve despite seemingly adequate volume resuscitation, other forms of shock (i.e., obstructive, cardiogenic, distributive) must be considered and the following questions asked: (1) Has tension pneumothorax or cardiac tamponade developed? (2) Is there an unrecognized myocardial contusion? (3) Is there a possible spinal cord injury—either spinal shock or frank neurogenic shock due to a partial or complete transection that was missed on the initial physical examination?[58] These conditions obviously must be treated if found; however, it must be emphasized again that *most children in hypotensive shock are victims of unrecognized hemorrhage* that can only be reversed if promptly recognized and appropriately treated by means of rapid transfusion and immediate surgical intervention.

If surgical intervention is not readily available, use of an appropriate-sized pneumatic antishock garment (PASG) (i.e., military or medical antishock trousers) may "buy time" until the surgeon arrives. Care must be taken to avoid using the abdominal compartment if it impedes ventilation. Aside from evisceration and impaled objects, the only absolute contraindication to the use of the PASG is major arterial disruption in the thorax or upper abdomen.[59] In this type of injury, increasing the afterload—the mechanism by which the device appears to work—may seriously accelerate blood loss. The PASG is of added benefit in splinting fractures of the lower extremities and is of proven utility in helping to contain the often massive retroperitoneal hemorrhage resulting from severe comminuted pelvic fractures.[60] However, the device must *never* be used in such a way as to delay needed volume resuscitation, which is the definitive treatment of hypovolemic shock and the only one that effectively reverses the tissue hypoxia and systemic acidosis associated with severe hemorrhage.[61] Obtaining venous access in the upper extremities sometimes is facilitated by PASG application.

Any child with chest, abdomen, or extremity injuries who presents with respiratory insufficiency or shock or requires resuscitation in an emergency department, or both, should be admitted to a critical care unit for further treatment, whether or not operation is ultimately performed. Children who are less ill but have sustained injuries serious enough to warrant resuscitation require definitive assessment of the physiologic risk of injury to ensure that potentially life-threatening injuries are not overlooked. Children should be considered for triage or transfer to a regional trauma center with pediatric expertise if the mechanism of injury suggests that this level of care may be required (Table 85–3)[62] or if the Pediatric Trauma Score,[63] Champion Trauma Score,[64] or Revised[65] Trauma Score (Table 85–4) suggests that the injuries sustained are of sufficient magnitude to have caused serious physiologic derangement. As a general rule, it is probably safe to proceed with "routine" admission and work-up if the chosen index falls within the low-risk category.[66]

DEFINITIVE EVALUATION OF CHEST, ABDOMEN, AND EXTREMITY INJURIES

Once the primary survey has been performed and stabilization has been achieved, a secondary survey is undertaken for definitive evaluation of the injured child. The cornerstone of this next phase of the trauma response is a careful head-to-toe examination, addressing all organ systems, including the central and peripheral nervous systems and the musculoskeletal system. To be sure no injuries are missed, complete exposure of the patient and "log-rolling," especially in penetrating trauma, must be included; however, care must be taken to avoid the subsequent development of hypothermia. The attention of the examiner should be directed specifically to the chest if there is a history of chest pain, noisy or rapid breathing, respiratory insufficiency, or hemoptysis. In like manner, a history of abdominal pain, bruising or tenderness, distention, or vomiting, particularly if the emesis is stained with blood or bile, mandates a thorough abdominal examination.

In examining the chest, the physician's first responsibility is to identify life-threatening injuries that may have been overlooked during the primary survey. The combination of unilaterally decreased breath sounds with hyperresonance to percussion and contralateral

Table 85–3. POSSIBLE INDICATIONS FOR TRANSFER TO A PEDIATRIC TRAUMA CENTER*

History of Injury
Patient thrown from a moving vehicle
Falls from >15 feet
Extrication time >20 minutes
Passenger cabin invaded >12 inches
Death of another passenger
Accident in a hostile environment (heat, cold water, etc)

Anatomic Injuries
Combined system injury
Penetrating injury of the groin or neck
Three or more long bone fractures
Fractures of the axial skeleton
Amputation (other than digits)
Persistent hypotension
Severe head trauma
Maxillofacial or upper airway injury
Central nervous system injury with prolonged loss of
    consciousness, posturing, or paralysis
Spinal cord injury with neurologic deficit
Unstable chest injury
Blunt or penetrating trauma to the chest or abdomen
Burns, flame or inhalation

System Considerations
Necessary service or specialist not available
No beds available
Need for pediatric intensive care
Multiple casualties
Family request
Paramedic judgment
Severity scores:
    Trauma Score 12 or less; or
    Revised Trauma Score 11 or less; or
    Pediatric Trauma Score 8 or less

*From Harris BH, Barlow BA, Ballantine TV, et al: American Pediatric Surgical Association: Principles of pediatric trauma care. J Pediatr Surg 27:423–426, 1992.

tracheal shift suggests the development of tension pneumothorax, whereas the same auscultatory findings in tandem with dullness to percussion and a midline trachea indicate massive hemothorax. Both conditions should be treated immediately. The sufficiency of gas exchange is then assessed by inspecting and auscultating bilaterally for adequate chest rise and air entry. The presence of point tenderness, palpable bony deformity, crepitus, or subcutaneous emphysema suggests the presence of rib fracture.

In examining the abdomen, the physician must first be aware of the extent to which gastric dilatation may confound evaluation: In addition to its deleterious effects upon ventilation and circulation, it can mimic or mask life-threatening intra-abdominal hemorrhage. It may also cause sufficient abdominal tenderness to simulate peritonitis. Thus, the first step in examining the abdomen, if it has not already been done, is to pass a nasal or oral gastric tube to empty the stomach and to simultaneously look for blood or bile. An abdomen that remains distended following gastric decompression is strongly suggestive of intra-abdominal bleeding, most often from the spleen or liver. However, if there is fever, marked tenderness or involuntary guarding, or both, together with abdominal distention (particularly if the gastric aspirate is stained with blood or bile) or if bowel sounds cannot be auscultated, acute peritonitis caused by enteric disruption should be suspected instead.

In examining the pelvis and extremities, all axial skeletal components should be palpated for evidence of instability and discontinuity, especially bone prominences such as the anterior superior iliac spines, which commonly are injured in major blunt trauma. When no such obvious deformities are present, fractures should be suspected if there is point tenderness, whether or not it is associated with laceration or hematoma, or both. This is particularly true of pelvic fractures. If this type of fracture is clinically suspected on the basis of perineal swelling or discoloration, examination should include a careful search for concomitant genitourinary trauma to the bladder, bladder neck, prostate gland, and urethra. The integrity of the pelvic ring may be tested in two ways: (1) by auscultating over one anterior superior iliac spine while gently tapping over the other to see if bone conduction is preserved (which will be the case only if the ring is intact) and (2) by pressing simultaneously on the anterior superior iliac spines to see if the pelvic wings "spring" apart from separation of the pubic symphysis. Most long bone fractures, of course, will be self-evident; however, such injuries are occasionally missed during the secondary survey, emphasizing the need to (1) assume a fracture is present on the basis of history alone (even if there is no obvious deformity) until it is proved otherwise and (2) perform ongoing evaluation of all injured extremities for evidence of *pain, pallor, pulselessness, paresthesias,* and *paralysis* (the classic signs of associated neurovascular trauma) so that they may be identified at the earliest possible moment following injury.

Laboratory evaluation is part of the secondary survey. Arterial blood gas determinations are of importance in determining the adequacy of ventilation and oxygenation. However, it must be remembered that the *critically important determinant of blood oxygen content, and hence tissue oxygen delivery, is the blood hemoglobin concentration. Serial* hematocrit determinations offer a better clue to the extent of blood loss than does the initial value, which most often is of limited utility because there generally has not been adequate time for equilibration to have occurred.[67] However, if physical and vital signs indicate the presence of shock, an initial hematocrit value of 30% or less is suggestive of significant hemorrhage, and one of 25% or less indicates massive hemorrhage.[68]

Elevations of the serum concentrations of hepatic transaminases suggest injury to the liver.[69] Elevation in the serum concentration of amylase indicates the presence of injury to the pancreas and possibly the spleen, which is contiguous with the tail of the pancreas.[70] Urine that is grossly bloody or is positive for blood by dipstick or microscopy (20 or more red blood cells/high-power field), or both, suggests renal damage and, indirectly, damage to adjacent organs.[71] It should be noted that myoglobin also may yield positive results on dipstick evaluation of the urine.[72] If this should occur or if significant crush injury is present or suspected, creatine phosphokinase levels should be measured to see if the skeletal muscle fraction is elevated.

Radiologic examination of the child with chest, abdomen, or extremity injuries also constitutes a vitally important part of the secondary survey. The specific

Table 85–4. PEDIATRIC ASSESSMENT OF THE PHYSIOLOGIC RISK OF INJURY

Pediatric Trauma Score[63]*	+2	+1	−1
Size (kg)	>20	10–20	<10
Airway	Normal	Maintained	Unmaintained
Systolic blood pressure (mm Hg)	>90	50—90	<50
Central nervous system	Awake	Obtunded	Coma
Open wound	None	Minor	Major
Skeletal trauma	None	Closed	Open-multiple

Champion Trauma Score[64]

Glasgow Coma Scale Score	Systolic Blood Pressure (mm Hg)	Respiratory Rate (breaths/min)	Respiratory Effort	Capillary Refill	Coded Value
14–15	>89	10–24			5
11–13	70–89	25–34			4
8–10	50–69	>34			3
5–7	0–49	1–9		Normal	2
3–4	Pulse	None	Normal	Delayed	1
			Retractive	None	0

Revised Trauma Score[65]

Glasgow Coma Scale Score	Systolic Blood Pressure (mm Hg)	Respiratory Rate (breaths/min)	Coded Value
13–15	>89	10–29	4
9–12	76–89	>29	3
6–8	50–75	6–9	2
4–5	1–49	1–5	1
3	0	0	0

*Data from Tepas JJ, Mollitt DL, Talbert JL, et al: The pediatric trauma score as a prediction of injury severity in the injured child. J Pediatr Surg 22:14–18, 1987.

trauma x-ray series obtained in every seriously injured child includes supine chest and combined (when possible) supine abdominal and pelvic roentgenograms. Other x-ray films may be taken as indicated by clinical findings (e.g., painful, tender, bruised, swollen, or obviously deformed, disfigured extremities). At no time should x-ray studies take precedence over resuscitation or whatever immediate therapy may be required for treatment of life-threatening injuries; only hemodynamically stable patients should be taken to the radiology department and then only if the physician accompanies and continuously monitors the child.

A few points must be emphasized regarding interpretation of plain x-ray films of the chest in seriously injured children.

1. Geometry and gravity both dictate that small amounts of blood or air, or both, will "layer out" anteriorly and posteriorly, respectively, when a supine anteroposterior chest x-ray film is obtained—a fact that can make detection extremely difficult. Thus, after physiologic stability has been achieved, a posteroanterior chest x-ray film should be obtained in the upright position in any child for whom the history or physical examination suggests chest injury may have been sustained.

2. The supine chest x-ray film will often show a widened mediastinum suggestive of aortic rupture, which is extremely rare in children.[73] If there is no other radiographic indication of aortic disruption, the child is hemodynamically stable, there are no signs of cervical spine injury, the lateral cervical spine x-ray film is normal, and there are no physical signs of cervical spine injury, a repeat chest x-ray film (preferably a posteroanterior view obtained in a semiupright or sitting position *while carefully maintaining the cervical spine in a neutral position*) may obviate the need for aortography. Computed tomography of the aortic arch, even if ob-

tained immediately following intravenous contrast administration, is rarely definitive.

3. Although the diagnosis of isolated rib fracture may be missed on as many as 50% of initial radiographs, roentgen diagnosis by means of rib x-ray studies is expensive and time-consuming and requires frequent painful repositioning, whereas adding little information vital to therapy.

Diagnosis of abdominal injuries by plain films also deserves special comment.

1. Although abdominal films are frequently normal, the most common roentgen signs of solid visceral injury in the child on supine radiography are (A) a ground-glass appearance of the abdominal cavity as a whole, suggesting the presence of intraperitoneal fluid (i.e., blood or urine); (B) medial displacement of the lateral border of the stomach (marked by the nasogastric tube) by the spleen, suggesting splenic laceration or hematoma, or both[74]; and (C) scoliosis, obliteration of the renal outline and psoas shadows, and fractures of the lower ribs, suggesting renal injury.

2. Signs of hollow visceral injuries are subtle. Short of contrast studies, the only clue to duodenal or proximal jejunal hematoma may be the relative lack of gas in the distal small intestine. Similarly, disruptions of the duodenum or proximal jejunum may be heralded only by tiny retroperitoneal gas shadows on the right side of the abdomen, adjacent to and slightly below the liver or ileus. Computed tomography or radiopaque contrast studies *may or may not* demonstrate the injury. The chance that pneumoperitoneum will be detected therefore will be maximized if air injected via the nasogastric tube is used as a radiolucent contrast agent when an upright or left lateral decubitus view is obtained.

The introduction of sophisticated imaging modalities to the diagnostic armamentarium has revolutionized the management of pediatric trauma.[75-79] In general, ultrasonography is best for evaluation of pancreatic injuries[80] and detection of intraperitoneal fluid (i.e., blood), particularly in the splenic and pelvic fossae. Computed tomography is best for evaluation of liver, kidney, and spleen injuries and, to a lesser extent, gastrointestinal injuries,[81] particularly in comatose patients.[82, 83] Moreover, computed tomography appears more sensitive than routine supine anteroposterior chest radiography in detecting both subtle airway abnormalities[84] and minor chest injuries.[85] It seems wise therefore to insist that the uppermost "cuts" of the abdominal scan visualize the lower part of the thoracic cavity. The utility of computed tomography is dependent upon both the use of oral and intravenous contrast agents and the patient's lying still, which may require the use of sedation or neuromuscular blockade, or both.

Computed tomography of the abdomen should be performed whenever there are signs of internal bleeding such as abdominal tenderness, distention, bruising, or gross hematuria.[86] It should also be performed if there is a pattern that suggests significant intra-abdominal injury may have occurred. Computed tomography cannot be used to predict the need for laparotomy because this is a clinical decision that is based not upon test results but upon physiologic status.[87, 88] Ultrasonography generally is reserved for those cases in which intra-abdominal injury is suspected and computed tomography cannot be performed though it has been successfully used in screening for intra-abdominal injuries.[89, 90] Nuclear scans, which remain the "gold standard" for detection of splenic and hepatic injuries,[91, 92] are now reserved for follow-up of solid visceral injuries and in cases in which these injuries are strongly suspected but computed tomography cannot be performed and ultrasonography results are normal.

The radiographic diagnosis of blunt renal injury has undergone especially rapid evolution in recent years. Ultrasonography has become the elective diagnostic study of choice when information is sought regarding the structural integrity of the kidneys, whereas nuclear renal perfusion scans have become the first-line nonemergent test of renal function. Nonetheless, computed tomography of the abdomen will serve to rule in or out major abnormalities.[93, 94] Finally, although intravenous urography has been largely supplanted by these techniques, it is still used in situations in which isolated blunt renal injury is suspected and urinalysis reveals microscopic hematuria.[95-98] Arteriography is required only for the diagnosis of renal pedicle injury in which specific information regarding vascular anatomy is desired in preparation for urgent operation; such injuries are rare and hematuria may not be present.[99, 100]

Diagnostic peritoneal lavage was for many years the procedure of choice for early detection of intra-abdominal bleeding in children, as well as in adults. However, the decision to operate upon patients with hepatic or splenic lacerations, most of which heal spontaneously in children, is now based not upon the presence or lack of intraperitoneal blood but upon the ongoing transfusion requirement.[101, 102] It is, therefore, reserved for patients in whom the usual diagnostic modalities of serial physical, laboratory, and radiologic evaluation are unavailable or unreliable—for example, in patients who are unconscious or who must undergo immediate general anesthesia for repair of life-threatening intracranial or axial skeletal injuries. If performed, diagnostic peritoneal lavage is considered abnormal if the effluent obtained through the instillation of 10 ml of 0.9% normal saline or lactated Ringer solution/kg of body weight into the peritoneal cavity (via a catheter inserted through the lower peritoneal midline under direct visualization, preferably by the operating surgeon) contains 100 or more red blood cells/mm³.

There may be a role for diagnostic peritoneal lavage in children who have sustained blunt or penetrating injuries in which the integrity of the bowel possibly has been violated. However, frequent, careful serial examination of the child for signs of peritoneal irritation is probably the more sensitive test. It certainly avoids the complications associated with diagnostic peritoneal lavage. It also negates the possibility that later physical examinations will be confounded by tenderness resulting from blood or air introduced at the time of the procedure.

CRITICAL MANAGEMENT OF CHEST, ABDOMEN, AND EXTREMITY INJURIES

Acute management of the child with chest, abdomen, and extremity injuries depends upon the type, extent, and severity of these injuries. In the unstable patient, immediate surgical treatment generally will be required. In the stable patient, definitive therapy will be directed by the appropriate specialists. Regardless, any child requiring resuscitation (i.e., anything more than simple evaluation or wound care) should be admitted to the hospital under the care of a surgeon experienced in the management of childhood injuries.[103, 104]

With the single exception of the hypopharyngeal soft tissue upper airway obstruction that accompanies head injury severe enough to alter consciousness, virtually all respiratory insufficiency results from serious injuries of the upper airway or chest, or both. Similarly, virtually all instances of shock observed in children result from serious intra-abdominal or *multiple* long bone fractures, or both, since shock resulting from intrathoracic or *isolated* axial skeletal injuries[47] is uncommon. The specific diagnosis and critical management of these injuries are outlined further on.

Chest Injuries

Most intrathoracic injuries in childhood can be managed expectantly or by means of simple tube thoracostomy. Few such injuries require urgent thoracotomy—excepting penetrating trauma. Indeed, the outcome of emergency department thoracotomy in children who present in traumatic cardiac arrest from blunt trauma has been dismal.[105, 106] The treatment of life-threatening conditions is outlined further on.

Upper airway obstruction caused by laryngotracheal contusion or fracture is an unusual event in the child trauma victim. Far more commonly, passive closure results from loss of the pharyngeal muscle tone associated with coma.[107, 108] The diagnosis is made solely on clinical grounds: In its partial form, it is recognized by inspiratory gurgling or snoring, and in its complete form, it is recognized by severe rocking chest motions (i.e., marked intercostal and substernal retractions associated with complete cessation of gas exchange). Treatment consists of a modified jaw thrust maneuver, oropharyngeal suctioning and, if foreign body obstruction is suspected, laryngoscopically guided retrieval while simultaneously stabilizing the cervical spine in a neutral position. Intubation may be attempted if the airway remains obstructed. Only when intubation fails should a surgical airway be created. Needle cricothyroidotomy in anticipation of urgent tracheostomy in the controlled environment of the operating room is the preferred approach, as emergency tracheostomy is challenging under the best circumstances.

Tension pneumothorax is caused by accumulation of air behind a one-way, "flap-valve" type of defect in the lung or airway and usually results from the barotrauma sustained when the chest is exposed to a severe compressive force as the glottis is held tightly closed, but sometimes it is caused by a fractured rib. It also is observed in cases of penetrating trauma, particularly stab wounds, in which the chest wall defect is not large enough to allow the free bidirectional exchange of gas between the atmosphere and the pleural space. The diagnosis should be made on clinical grounds. Examination reveals profound respiratory distress, distended neck veins, contralateral tracheal deviation, ipsilateral hyperresonance to percussion and decreased breath sounds and, ultimately, circulatory collapse as the mediastinum shifts. The condition is treated by means of tube thoracostomy; however, immediate decompression by means of an over-the-needle catheter placed percutaneously through the second intercostal space on the midclavicular line just above the third rib should first be performed if respiratory failure or shock is present.

Open pneumothorax (sucking chest wound) cannot occur without penetration sufficient to result in loss of at least a small portion of the chest wall; hence, it is rare in childhood. It is most often caused by a shotgun or blast injury and results in nearly complete cessation of ventilation resulting from equilibration of intra- and extrathoracic pressure. Treatment consists of assisted positive-pressure ventilation until direct occlusion of the defect with gauze impregnated with petroleum jelly and tube thoracostomy can be accomplished, followed in most cases by thoracotomy for repair of the chest wall.

Massive hemothorax is typically associated with bleeding from a major artery, which is encountered infrequently in blunt trauma. As in tension pneumothorax, examination reveals respiratory distress and, occasionally, contralateral tracheal deviation. In contrast to tension pneumothorax, however, neck veins are flat, the chest sounds dull on percussion, and the development of shock precedes the development of respiratory failure rather than the reverse. This injury requires urgent treatment by means of posteriorly directed lateral tube thoracostomy. Thoracotomy for control of bleeding will be required only if the volume of the blood initially evacuated from the hemithorax exceeds 25% of the total blood volume or if ongoing blood loss exceeds 2% of the total blood volume/hr.

Cardiac tamponade is an extremely rare sequela of blunt childhood trauma; it is usually seen in stab wounds because gunshot wound victims typically die at the scene or in transport to the hospital. Examination reveals muffled heart tones, distended neck veins, a narrowed pulse pressure, and pulsus paradoxus. Sudden hypotensive deterioration will ensue once enough blood is contained within the pericardial sac to compromise venous return. The diagnosis generally is obvious on physical examination in penetrating trauma, although in blunt trauma it is a diagnosis of exclusion. Echocardiography is a useful noninvasive means of establishing the diagnosis at the bedside in questionable cases. Definitive treatment requires emergency thoracotomy, pericardiotomy, and direct myocardial repair.

Flail chest is caused by major trauma or crush injury that is sufficient to result in parallel double fractures of two or more adjacent ribs and concomitant loss of bony continuity with the remainder of the chest wall.[109] Small flail segments are often overlooked during the primary survey because of the associated muscle spasm; however, large flail segments, particularly in the posterolateral aspect of the chest wall, are especially poorly tolerated by children because of the small size of the chest cavity. Examination usually reveals asymmetric, "paradoxic" chest wall motion and crepitus at the fracture sites. Immediate treatment is supportive and is aimed at prevention of the arterial hypoxemia that is due as much if not more to the underlying pulmonary contusion as to the flail segment itself, but which in severe cases may require "splinting" by means of positive-pressure ventilation, including positive end-expiratory pressure (PEEP) and, occasionally, neuromuscular blockade. Intercostal nerve blocks are preferable to parenteral narcotics if long-term pain control is required.

Pulmonary contusion refers to the indirect, forceful disruption of pulmonary parenchyma; it typically results from direct transmission of the kinetic energy associated with a severe blunt impact from the overlying chest wall to underlying lung tissue in the form of a shock wave.[110] Although the leaky capillary membranes of injured lung tissue readily permit passage and hence sequestration of fluid in the interstitial space, the contracted state of the circulation in the child with multiple injuries may retard accumulation of this fluid. For the same reason, an increased $PAO_2 - PaO_2$ is a poor early indicator of pulmonary contusion. The treatment of pulmonary contusion is expectant. The goals are (1) to prevent clinically significant arterial hypoxemia using the least possible amount of artificial respiratory support, (2) to restore lost functional residual capacity and prevent oxygen toxicity, and (3) to forestall progression to post-traumatic pulmonary insufficiency (PTPI)—that is, adult respiratory distress syndrome (ARDS). Thus, PEEP should be used whenever the FIO_2 required to maintain a PaO_2 of 70 to 80 mm Hg exceeds 40%, whereas excessive administration of crystalloid fluids should be avoided. Truly life-threatening pulmonary contusions are encountered infrequently, but they are significantly worsened if there has been concomitant aspiration of gastric contents. Although the role of corticosteroids in PTPI (ARDS) remains unproved,[111] use of these drugs is probably harmful in cases of pure acid pneumonitis.[112]

Myocardial contusion also results from a concussive force applied to the chest, though the impact typically is directed centrally and anteroposteriorly instead of laterally or obliquely.[113–116] The symptoms and signs are nonspecific, consisting chiefly of poorly localized chest pain; thus, the diagnosis rests upon a battery of specific tests (electrocardiography, echocardiography, radionuclide angiography, and serial determination of myocardial enzymes). However, neither specific clinical nor electrocardiographic abnormalities are common in children and sudden life-threatening dysrhythmias are rare. Thus, echocardiography and radionuclide angiography, which are exquisitely sensitive in detecting subtle myocardial dysfunction, do not seem sufficiently specific to justify routine clinical use. Nevertheless, if myocardial contusion is suspected, the child should be observed in a fully monitored environment, and baseline myocardial enzyme determinations should be obtained. Further tests may then be undertaken as necessary.

Traumatic bronchial disruption results either from direct shearing, if associated with crushing injuries or, more often, from severe compression of the chest during expiration against a closed glottis (the Valsalva maneuver). When it occurs, it nearly always is located adjacent to the carina.[117] It is often a lethal injury, particularly if undetected: As many as one half of these patients are said to die within the first hour following injury. When there is no hemoptysis (the characteristic presenting sign), clues to the diagnosis are failure to re-expand the lung or persistence of a large air leak despite tube thoracostomy, or both. Bronchoscopy is diagnostic. Mild bronchial disruptions may require nothing more than tube thoracostomy and supportive care until effective healing occurs. Uncontrollable bleeding or massive air leak, seen as an inability to ventilate the patient once an adequate airway has been established, consititute the indications for emergency thoracotomy for repair of bronchial injury.

Traumatic diaphragmatic hernia due to blunt injury, once considered rare in childhood, is being identified with increasing frequency in association with automobile lap belt injuries and penetrating trauma. It is more common on the left side than on the right side.[118–122] The immediate pathophysiologic effects of this condition are not due to the diaphragmatic injury per se but to the subsequent herniation of abdominal contents into the chest. Thus, the time to onset of symptoms and signs usually varies inversely with the size of the rent in the diaphragm. In left-sided blunt injury, the impacting force typically produces immediate herniation, whereas in right-sided blunt injury and penetrating trauma, presentation is often delayed. This often results in confusing radiologic findings—for example, (1) unexplained elevation of the hemidiaphragm, (2) unrelieved acute gastric dilatation, and (3) loculated subpulmonic hemopneumothorax. The diagnosis is confirmed fluoroscopically using a water-soluble contrast agent. Direct surgical repair is indicated as soon as feasible.

Traumatic rupture of the aorta following blunt injury, usually at the level of the ligamentum arteriosum, is extremely rare in childhood,[123, 124] and the majority of such injuries are likely to be fatal at the scene.[125, 126] The lesion is suspected clinically when there is a murmur that radiates to the back, particularly if the mechanism of injury involves severe deceleration—for example, high-speed motor vehicle accidents and falls from extreme heights. However, as this murmur is infrequently heard, the diagnosis rests upon certain radiologic criteria: (1) a widened mediastinum with obliteration of the aortic knob, (2) deviation of the trachea (endotracheal tube) to the right or of the esophagus (nasogastric tube) to the left and, especially, (3) the presence of an apical pleural cap, particularly if associated with fractures of the first or second ribs. The most commonly encountered of these signs is a widened mediastinum; however, this is rarely due to aortic disruption in a child and should not mandate aortography unless other signs of mediastinal hemorrhage are present. If necessary, aortography should be performed in an appropriate clinical setting. Immediate repair must be undertaken if the lesion is demonstrated. Intraoperative cardiopulmonary bypass occasionally may be required.

Traumatic esophageal rupture due to blunt injury is virtually unknown in childhood; it is believed to result from a blow to the upper abdomen forceful enough to inject gastric contents into the lower esophagus under extremely high pressure as the cricopharyngeus muscle is held tightly closed in anticipation of the impact. The resulting injury is similar to that observed in the Boerhaave syndrome—that is, postemetic esophageal rupture, which progresses rapidly to mediastinitis, sepsis, and death if unrecognized. It should be suspected if there is pain or shock out of proportion to the apparent severity of the injury, or if a chest tube inserted for treatment of pneumothorax drains food or saliva or bubbles equally and continuously throughout the respiratory cycle. "Mediastinal crunch," or the Hamman sign, is rarely heard in the child; thus, the only clue to the diagnosis may be the presence of mediastinal emphysema on chest x-ray film, as the small volume of gas entrapped is unlikely to dissect superiorly as far as the neck at which point it can be palpated subcutaneously. If present, the diagnosis is easily confirmed fluoroscopically using a water-soluble contrast agent. Direct transthoracic repair and wide mediastinal drainage is the treatment of choice, although total exclusion by means of cervical esophagostomy and gastrostomy may be necessary if the esophagus is irreparably damaged.

Simple pneumothorax may result from a tear in the parietal and visceral pleural membranes caused by the sharp end of a fractured rib or by a pointed instrument. Either way, the injury results from a transpleural laceration of peripheral lung tissue. Unless the wound is large, it is usually self-sealing because of the high concentration of tissue thromboplastins in lung tissue and the low pressure within the pulmonary circulation. Because pneumothorax and hemothorax so often coexist in victims of serious chest trauma, however, treatment consists of upright positioning and placement of a posteriorly directed lateral chest tube, even for simple pneumothorax. Indeed, observation or aspiration, or both, of small intrapleural air collections—even if they are not becoming larger—is dangerous in the patient with multiple injuries and is frankly contraindicated for the child who requires positive-pressure ventilation, general anesthesia, or emergency transport. This is particularly true for patients who must be evacuated by air ambulance.

Simple hemothorax may result from the same mechanisms of injury that cause simple pneumothorax; however, the intercostal or intramammary vessels may be injured as well as the pulmonary parenchyma. Unfortunately, this injury can rarely be safely diagnosed at the time of initial presentation, as it is impossible to know just how fast the patient is bleeding without the benefit of tube thoracostomy. Occasionally, however, patients present late enough after their injuries (several hours or days) that it can be safely assumed that bleeding has stopped. Although small collections of blood can be reabsorbed by the body, and at worst will result in mild basilar pleural scarring, collections of blood that *appear* small on chest x-ray studies taken in an upright position may be significant: To be identified radiographically, their volumes must approach about 10 ml/kg of body weight. For this reason, even "small" traumatic collections should be drained by means of large-caliber, posteriorly directed chest tubes placed through the midaxillary line at nipple level to minimize the chance of subsequent pulmonary restriction due to "trapped lung."

Rib fractures are uncommon sequelae of all but the most severe types of pediatric blunt trauma in young children.[127, 128] First-rib fractures are particularly ominous in terms of prognosis.[129] The posterolateral aspects of the middle and lower ribs sustain most of the injuries, as these are the areas most commonly struck by a moving vehicle or affected after a fall; however, they are also the areas most accessible to assailants during child battering, a diagnosis that should be considered whenever a clear-cut history of severe trauma is lacking in an infant or young child with rib fractures,[130] particularly if they are multiple and in various stages of healing (see also Chapter 86). Greenstick fractures and costochondral separations will not normally be seen on the chest x-ray film but may be suspected if there are obvious deformities or areas of exquisite point tenderness or crepitus directly over a rib or costochondral junction. No specific treatment is indicated for rib fractures beyond that provided for associated injuries, as they rarely cause enough discomfort in children to result in splinting or atelectasis. As such, there is no role for splints or analgesics in the acute treatment of pediatric rib fractures, and their use is not recommended, though intercostal nerve blocks have been used in selected cases for long-term pain control.

Traumatic asphyxia is a rare but striking phenomenon that may be associated with severe blunt injury to the chest. It results when a sudden increase in intrathoracic pressure associated with a massive compressive force to the chest is transmitted to the venules of the head, neck, and upper body via the valveless great veins of the thoracic inlet.[131] The resultant acute increase in extrathoracic venous pressure causes the fragile capillaries feeding these venules to rupture, resulting in petechial hemorrhage in the areas adjacent to the damage. The diagnosis is made when petechiae are identified in the

conjunctivae, sclerae, scalp, and integument of the upper body. Unfortunately, the same type of petechial hemorrhages visible on external body surfaces also occur internally, particularly within the brain. As a result, when traumatic asphyxia is severe, it may be associated with transient neurologic findings.[132] Although the condition requires no specific treatment other than supportive care, since the effects of the suffusion injury usually resolve over the course of several days as hemorrhages are resorbed and capillaries are repaired, its presence serves to indicate the extreme severity of blunt force applied to the chest and mandates an especially thorough search for intrathoracic injury.

Abdominal Injuries

The treatment of serious intra-abdominal injuries has undergone rapid change in recent years. This evolution has largely been driven by the extraordinary power of current imaging technologies. Indeed, the definitive therapy is frequently nonoperative, especially with respect to lacerations, hematomas, and extravasations of the spleen, kidneys, and liver. However, the term *nonoperative* does not mean *nonsurgical,* for, as with appendicitis, mature surgical judgment is needed to determine whether or when surgical intervention will be required and, if so, what type of operation should be performed.[104] The specific management of major intra-abdominal injuries will be described.

Liver

Since the advent of computed tomography, the liver has been recognized as the solid organ most commonly injured in cases of blunt trauma. Clinical presentation is dependent upon the extent of damage to the organ and ranges from nonspecific abdominal pain to post-traumatic cardiac arrest; however, the majority of hepatic injuries encountered in children are minor and will remain undetected unless liver enzyme[69] determinations or imaging studies,[133] or both, are obtained. Although the nonoperative management of small capsular lacerations that have ceased actively bleeding, as well as self-contained subcapsular hematomas in children, is now widely accepted as safe,[134–137] large stellate lacerations and subcapsular hematomas that have eroded through the Glisson capsule rarely stop bleeding without surgical intervention.[138] Nevertheless, children with hepatic injuries who do not present in hypotensive shock and who respond promptly to volume resuscitation will not require laparotomy for control of bleeding unless the ongoing transfusion requirement exceeds 50% of estimated circulating blood volume (40 ml/kg during the 24 hours immediately following injury).[139, 140] Hemobilia, of course, is a recognized late complication of nonoperative management.[141, 142]

Most hepatic lacerations that require laparotomy for active bleeding can be managed by means of direct suture repair and drainage, regardless of size. Liver resection is rarely indicated, unless it simply completes removal of a nearly transected lobe or segment. Prophylactic drainage of the biliary tree is neither necessary nor desirable. Management of retrohepatic venous injuries usually presents the greatest challenge, as bleeding from tears in these extremely short veins, which may extend into the retrohepatic vena cava, is often massive and difficult to control. Therefore, the surgeon is well advised to insist that, insofar as possible, circulating blood volume be restored prior to incising the peritoneum, and certainly before disturbing whatever clot may form in the areas adjacent to these injuries. On rare occasions, direct suturing of these vessels may prove so difficult that it becomes necessary to use a thoracic catheter as a temporary intracaval shunt until vascular repair is accomplished. The use of gauze packs for primary hemostasis occasionally may be successful if all else fails, but this method is regarded as a temporizing measure that should be used only as a last resort.

Spleen

The spleen is the solid organ most liable to be seriously injured in childhood. It typically is associated with left upper quadrant pain that radiates to the left shoulder and left upper quadrant tenderness, though the diagnosis should also be suspected if there is persistent unexplained leukocytosis or hyperamylasemia. Nonoperative management is somewhat more successful than it is for hepatic injuries because the transverse orientation of most splenic parenchymal lacerations (parallel to the blood vessels) and the thicker, more elastic nature of the splenic capsule in childhood promote the spontaneous cessation of bleeding.[143] Nevertheless, the same caveats that apply to blunt hepatic injury concerning presentation in decompensated shock are also true for blunt splenic injury.[144, 145] The fact that the overwhelming majority of splenic injuries will heal spontaneously on a regimen of limited activity, beginning with 7 to 10 days of strict bed rest, must not lull the surgeon into a false sense of security: Splenic lacerations that have ceased actively bleeding and previously contained subcapsular hematomas may subsequently leak or rupture, classically on the third to fifth day following injury. Thus, the surgeon who selects a nonoperative course of management must be prepared for an extended period of careful observation, including frequent re-examination.

In the rare instance that operation is required, active splenic bleeding is found, and control of hemorrhage proves impossible, a splenic salvage procedure is used if at all feasible because the incidence of overwhelming postsplenectomy infection in childhood (particularly those caused by the encapsulated bacterial organisms *Streptococcus pneumoniae*, *Haemophilus influenzae*, *Neisseria meningitidis*, *Staphylococcus aureus*, and *Escherichia coli*) remains considerable. Fortunately, the results of splenorrhaphy, or partial splenectomy if either the superior or inferior pole of the spleen has been shattered beyond repair, have been as good as with nonoperative management.[146–148] However, care must be taken to ensure that sufficient splenic mass (approximately 50%) is left behind to perform the functions of the organ.[149–152] Most important, of course, is the recognition that splenic salvage procedures should be undertaken only if there is no untoward risk to the life of the child; if splenectomy must be performed, it should be accompanied by omental implantation (autotrans-

plantation) of splenic remnants, fashioned into thin "wafers."[153, 154] Finally, when splenectomy, partial or complete, is anticipated or has been performed, the patient should receive antipneumococcal vaccine as soon as possible before or after operation, even though the antibody response may be both inconsistent and impermanent.[155, 156]

Kidneys

After the liver and spleen, the kidneys are the solid organs most commonly injured in blunt childhood trauma. The fact that they are well protected by the paraspinous muscles and are embedded in fat pads enclosed by tough fascial envelopes means that substantial force is required to injure them. It is therefore hardly surprising that injuries to adjacent, less well protected organs occur in as many as 80% of the cases in which renal injury is present. Since the classic findings of renal injury—flank pain, tenderness, and a mass—are difficult if not impossible to elicit in the child, the lack of these symptoms and signs in no way excludes the diagnosis of renal trauma. The diagnosis of significant renal injury therefore is heralded by the presence of significant hematuria.[71, 95–98] Unfortunately, there appears to be no direct correlation between the degree of hematuria and the severity of injury. Thus, any child who presents with significant hematuria must be assumed to have sustained serious injury until it is proved otherwise.

Although the long-term results of surgical intervention in the acute stage are good,[157] blunt renal injuries do not require operative management[98, 158–162] unless (1) the injury is so severe that direct communication exists between the renal arterioles and the renal calyx, resulting in the presence of bright red hematuria and shock or (2) the renal pedicle is injured, resulting in the occasional development of hypertension or hematuria, or both.[99, 100] With the single exception of the former, in which exsanguination via the urinary tract can be swift, the tight fascial compartment within which the kidney is situated causes prompt tamponade of renal parenchymal hemorrhage, effectively limiting the amount of blood lost to no more than about 25% of circulating blood volume—within the normal range of compensated shock.[74] Most renal injuries, of course, are much less severe. Contusions and small capsular lacerations predominate; rarely, retroperitoneal extravasation may develop when communication exists between the renal calyx and the perinephric space (usually at the pelvocalyceal junction) and leaks through a rent in the Gerota fascia. Although this injury may ultimately require surgical repair, it is rarely necessary in the acute stage, unless there is major disruption or frank transection of a portion of the main collecting system. Indeed, most small urinary leaks are self-sealing, particularly if they are parenchymal in origin, though direct surgical attack will be necessary if the "urinoma" persists or becomes infected.

Pancreas

The pancreas is rarely seriously injured in blunt trauma. Its location deep in the upper abdomen accounts for this relative invulnerability, though its fixed position directly anterior to the vertebral column suggests that when the impact is of sufficient force, it will not be displaced out of harm's way but will absorb the full dose of kinetic energy applied to it. As a result, serious injuries to the pancreas tend to be central and consist mainly of moderate to severe pancreatic hematomas and in severe cases transection.[163] Disruption of the pancreatic duct is obviously a constant feature of the latter condition but may also occur in the former; in these instances, unless the injury is self-sealing or there is free communication with the lesser peritoneal sac, a pancreatic pseudocyst will begin to develop within 3 to 5 days, in contrast to the chemical peritonitis that results immediately upon leakage of pancreatic fluid into the peritoneal sac, causing pancreatic ascites.

Although severe pancreatic injury is rare, traumatic pancreatitis is not infrequently observed in cases of blunt trauma.[70, 164] The condition is suspected if there is deep epigastric pain radiating to the back or deep tenderness on palpation of the upper abdomen, or both. It is confirmed by the presence of elevated serum levels of amylase or lipase, or both. These enzymes, together with other activated pancreatic enzymes, are responsible for both the inflammation and the erosive, necrotizing pancreatic autolysis or chemical peritonitis associated with the more localized, and more generalized, forms of the disease, respectively. The treatment of simple traumatic pancreatitis is expectant and consists of bed and bowel rest, nasogastric decompression as tolerated, intravenous fluids as necessary and, if pain persists for more than a few days, total parenteral nutrition. Refeeding with clear liquids, followed by a low-fat diet, is allowed when pain and tenderness subside, and the serum amylase level falls into the normal range. By contrast, patients with severe pancreatic injury—that is, a large, tender, epigastric mass complicated by acute peritonitis or pancreatic ascites, or both—are candidates for external surgical drainage of the lesser peritoneal sac or partial resection or repair of lacerated pancreatic ducts.[163] Patients in whom a pancreatic pseudocyst develops require 6 to 8 weeks of complete bowel rest and total parenteral nutrition in preparation for an external or internal drainage procedure (cystogastrostomy, or a Roux-en-Y cystojejunostomy.)[165, 166]

Alimentary Tract

As a group, solid visceral injuries are far more common than hollow visceral injuries in blunt trauma; however, the latter occur with some frequency, particularly injuries to the duodenum and proximal jejunum.[167–169] "Blowout" injuries are the type most frequently encountered. They are best detected by means of frequent serial physical examinations, looking particularly for signs of parietal peritoneal irritation, which invariably will develop within 6 to 12 hours of injury.[68] Treatment of gastrointestinal perforations, once they are recognized, is relatively straightforward and consists of primary suture repair and nasogastric decompression. Colonic perforations, however, require diversion (i.e., colostomy) if the degree of contamination and inflammation is so great that suture repair cannot be performed

safely. By contrast, obstructing hematomas of the duodenum or jejunum, or both, rarely require operative management. Treatment consists of nasogastric decompression, as well as the administration of intravenous fluids and electrolytes appropriate for the level of obstruction.[170–172]

Retroperitoneum

Significant injuries to upper retroperitoneal structures other than the kidneys, duodenum, and pancreas are confined nearly exclusively to the blood vessels. Fortunately, they are quite rare except in severe deceleration injuries and massive physical abuse.[68, 74] They are caused by the shearing effect associated with such injuries and therefore affect the junctions of great veins with smaller feeding branches (e.g., lumbocaval anastamoses), though larger vessels may also be involved, namely, the cavomesenteric and cavohepatic venous junctions. In the former case, hemorrhage usually proves to be confined to the upper retroperitoneal space and, if seen at laparotomy, will present as small areas of retroperitoneal bruising, which are sometimes best left undisturbed because the increased pressure within the retroperitoneal space effectively tamponades further venous bleeding. However, if the great veins themselves are involved, a large upper retroperitoneal hematoma will be present, and the overlying peritoneal membrane will usually have been disrupted, resulting in massive intraperitoneal hemorrhage. In these instances, prompt control of bleeding and repair of damaged vessels is necessary, though ligation of great veins that are damaged beyond repair is not incompatible with life, given the abundant collateral vessels generally available.

Pelvis

Despite the fact that pedestrian motor vehicle trauma—a mechanism of injury involving substantial force—accounts for the great majority of pelvic fractures, more than half of such injuries may be classified as stable. Among the remainder, unstable injuries predominate, most of which are undisplaced, whereas crush injuries are rare.[173–178] Nonetheless, crush injuries and unstable fractures, particularly if fragments are displaced, are responsible for most of the complications: Retroperitoneal hematoma is present in nearly all such injuries, though associated genitourinary and arterial injuries are uncommon. Pelvic hemorrhage and serious associated injuries (e.g., severe closed head trauma), which are present in 80% of pelvic fractures, cause most of the deaths. These occur infrequently—that is, in 2 to 5% of all patients with pelvic fractures—though secondary infection also results in significant mortality. Treatment is chiefly nonoperative, even in high-risk cases, because the associated hematoma, which is most often due to venous oozing, will usually be contained by the peritoneal membrane. Although transfusion is universally required in children who sustain severe pelvic fractures, operation is required only when hemorrhage is ongoing and cannot be controlled using PASG[60] or selective pelvic angiography with embolization, or both.[179]

Genitourinary Tract

Injury to the genitourinary tract, other than renal trauma, is extremely rare in children and is associated with only severe blunt or penetrating injury to the abdomen or pelvis. Intraperitoneal rupture of the dome of the bladder,[180, 181] which is an intra-abdominal organ in the child when distended, and ureteropelvic junction avulsion[182, 183] are associated with severe blunt abdominal trauma, whereas extraperitoneal vesical and urethral injuries are associated with severe blunt pelvic trauma (i.e., unstable fractures or crush injuries). Because intraperitoneal extravasation of urine causes little, if any, peritoneal reaction, the diagnosis of intraperitoneal rupture of the bladder may be missed—especially in child abuse—until self-dialysis across the peritoneal membrane causes hypochloremic, hyperkalemic metabolic acidosis and azotemia.[184, 185] Extraperitoneal vesical disruption resulting from bone spicules or ligamentous shear should be suspected in any pelvic fracture involving the pubic bones or rami, as is also the case in urethral injuries, which typically are associated with bloody urethral discharge, inability to void, and a boggy, high-riding prostate gland on rectal examination. The diagnosis of ureteral and bladder injuries is made by excretory urography. Direct operative repair is required, with the exception of extraperitoneal vesical rupture, which should be managed by suprapubic or Foley catheter drainage plus intravenous antibiotics until the associated hematoma is resorbed and complete healing occurs, usually in 2 to 3 weeks. Urethral injuries, which in severe pelvic fractures typically occur at or below the urogenital diaphragm and therefore are diagnosed by retrograde cystography,[186] are preferentially treated by means of suprapubic catheter drainage because of their proximity to the bladder neck. This is because treatment of urethral disruption by means of Foley catheter drainage, which usually is impossible because the severed urethral ends usually are separated by several centimeters, is associated with both a higher rate of intractable stricture and impotence in a substantial percentage of cases. Moreover, most pelvic fracture–related posterior urethral strictures in children whose urethral injuries are managed conservatively are amenable to straightforward transpubic or transperineal repair.[187, 188]

Extremity Injuries

The orthopedic management of the numerous types of extremity fractures that may be encountered in childhood is beyond the scope of this chapter but is described extensively elsewhere.[17, 48] Nonetheless, a few comments are in order. Since long bone fractures in and of themselves are rarely life-threatening, the general care of the patient always takes precedence. However, early stabilization will serve both to decrease patient discomfort and limit the amount of blood loss. Closed treatment predominates for the clavicle, upper extremity, tibia, and femur. Skeletal traction may be required for fractures of the femur, particularly in the older child. Open treatment is required for open fractures (for débridement and irrigation), displaced supracondylar fractures (because of their association with ischemic vascular injury), and major or displaced physeal fractures (which must be reduced anatomically). Fortunately, reductions of diaphyseal fractures need not be perfectly anatomic because of the ability of most long bone fractures in children to remodel. Indeed, these fractures may require "bayonet" (overlapping) approximation if overgrowth is a significant possibility. However, remodeling is generally poor in "plastic bowing deformities" such as torus and greenstick fractures because the hyperemia typical of complete fractures is less likely to occur.

Traumatic fat embolism[189, 190] is a rare complication of long bone fracture in childhood. It also has been reported in association with massive soft tissue injury alone.[191] Signs include fever, hypoxemia, abnormalities in blood coagulation and lipid metabolism, and excretion of fat in urine and sputum.[192] Treatment is supportive but heparin use may be required if the associated coagulopathy is severe. The critical care physician or surgeon must also be aware that rhabdomyolysis frequently accompanies massive soft tissue trauma, particularly crush injury, whether or not associated skeletal injury is present. It is confirmed by the presence of myoglobinuria or elevation in the plasma concentration of creatine phosphokinase, or both. Again, treatment is supportive and is aimed at the prevention of acute renal failure from precipitation of myoglobin in the proximal renal tubules. It consists of aggressive hydration at two or more times the maintenance rate, a therapy that must be balanced against the need for fluid restriction in patients with concomitant head injuries.

Penetrating Injuries

Penetrating injuries in children are being encountered in greater numbers than ever before.[193–195] Because management by experienced surgeons obviously is required, all such children should be referred to a trauma center with pediatric capabilities. All penetrating wounds are contaminated and must be treated as infected by means of aggressive débridement and intravenous administration of antibiotics. Accessible missile fragments should be removed once swelling has subsided to prevent the subsequent development of lead poisoning.[196] Early notification of responsible law enforcement is mandatory in most jurisdictions; early involvement of child welfare agencies is advisable for all but clearly accidental cases of penetrating trauma in childhood. The initial history is rarely accurate when injuries are not accidental.

The usual problem in penetrating chest injury is hemopneumothorax caused by lung injury. Although expeditious treatment by means of tube thoracostomy obviously is required, few such injuries will require thoracotomy for control of bleeding. If this proves to be necessary, however, the usual cause will be injury to the intercostal vessels, as most parenchymal injuries are self-sealing. Fortunately, violation of other thoracic viscera, vessels, and airways is uncommon following gunshot and stab wounds in children. If present, however, all require immediate surgical repair and should be excluded by means of appropriate radiographic or endoscopic studies if the location and direction of penetration or missile tract suggest that such an injury could have occurred. Finally, thoracoabdominal injury should be suspected (1) if the chest is penetrated at or below the level of the sixth rib; (2) if abdominal findings (tenderness or peritonitis) develop following thoracic penetration or in association with hemopneumothorax (even without a coexisting abdominal wound); (3) if food, chyme, or saliva is recovered from the chest tube; or (4) if the injury trajectory or noninvasive studies (computerized tomography, ultrasonography, fluoroscopy) indicate the possibility of penetrating diaphragmatic injury.

Immediate exploration is warranted for all gunshot wounds and most stab wounds of the abdomen. Selective management of the latter type of injury may be practiced if (1) there are no signs of shock or peritonitis and none occurs during the ensuing 12 to 24 hours, (2) there is no blood in the stomach, rectum, or urine, and (3) there is no evidence of free or retroperitoneal air on plain x-ray films of the abdomen. Exploration, however, is mandated if there is evidence or a history of evisceration. In the former case, exposed bowel should be kept moist with saline-soaked gauze sponges and must not be allowed to assume a dependent position, (i.e., below the level of the anterior abdominal wall). Again, the possibility of thoracoabdominal injury must be kept in mind whenever there is penetration of the upper abdomen, particularly if it caused by a missile. If such injury is strongly suspected, laparotomy should be undertaken even when there are no other indications.

Penetrating thoracoabdominal injuries, when present, require a special approach. In addition to the tube thoracostomy that is mandatory for all such injuries, laparotomy must be performed for diaphragmatic closure as well as evaluation and possible repair of intra-abdominal organs. Thoracotomy is required as indicated but precedes laparotomy only for life-threatening chest injury. Otherwise, laparotomy for closure of lacerated viscera precedes the "cleansing" thoracotomy, which will be necessary only if intestinal contents are found in the chest.

INTENSIVE CARE OF CHEST, ABDOMEN, AND EXTREMITY INJURIES

Because most childhood injuries are self-limited, and pediatric trauma care is therefore nonoperative, ICU management is vital to optimal patient outcome. Avoidance of further deterioration, once physiologic stability has been achieved, is of paramount importance because the child's limited physiologic reserves may not withstand a second insult unless fully replenished. Thus, monitoring must be designed to warn the critical care physician or surgeon responsible for the injured child of impending respiratory failure or shock while the child is still in the compensated phase so that treatment can be instituted well in advance of deterioration. In the child with potential respiratory insufficiency, this should include frequent determination of vital signs, continuous measurement of arterial oxygen saturation, and measurement of arterial blood gases as needed. In the child with potential circulatory embarrassment, it should include frequent examination for signs of tissue hypoperfusion; ongoing measurement of systolic, diastolic, and mean blood pressure by means of Doppler ultrasonography or an indwelling arterial catheter; and, when necessary, determination of central venous pressure. Finally, urinary output and the volume of external losses of blood or fluid, or both, particularly from the chest, should be recorded hourly. Similarly, abdominal girth at the level of the umbilicus should be recorded hourly if there is any question of intra-abdominal hemorrhage.

Definitive management of the respiratory insufficiency that accompanies severe chest injury is expectant. In general, the least amount of artificial respiratory support necessary to maintain the PaO_2 at 70 to 80 mm Hg should be employed to minimize the effects of oxygen toxicity and retard the development of resorption atelectasis. Continuous positive airway pressure or PEEP is therefore used for maintenance of arterial oxygen tension and functional residual capacity whenever the required FiO_2 exceeds 40%. Adverse effects of PEEP on the required circulation should be avoided. If fresh bronchial or pulmonary suture lines or pneumothoraces are present, special effort should be made to keep the peak inspiratory pressure less than 20 to 25 cm H_2O when positive-pressure ventilation must be used. Naturally, spontaneous ventilation is preferred, and extubation should be accomplished as soon as feasible.

Much has been made of the many similarities between pulmonary contusion, or "traumatic wet lung," and PTPI, or "shock lung." Aside from a much shorter interval to disease onset (6 to 12 hours versus 12 to 24 hours), a key difference is the elaboration of tissue factors as well as endothelial factors from damaged pulmonary elements at the time of injury. These differences obviously alter the nature of the lung's putatively "nonspecific" response to injury, for the natural history of pulmonary contusion is to resolve spontaneously within 7 to 10 days unless PTPI supervenes. The specific management of PTPI, which is one manifestation of ARDS, is described elsewhere in this volume (see Chapter 47). It should be noted, however, that great care should be taken to avoid the use of therapies known to be associated with the development of this condition, particularly excessive administration of crystalloid fluids.

Indications for early thoracotomy in the ICU include the rapid reaccumulation of blood or air, or both (i.e., blood loss that exceeds 2 to 4 ml/kg of body weight/hr) or massive air leak, particularly if full pulmonary reexpansion cannot be achieved despite maximum therapy. Indications for late thoracotomy—2 to 3 weeks following injury—include (1) trapped lung resulting from clotted hemothorax or, rarely, empyema, and (2) a persistent air leak. Bedside thoracotomy in the ICU is rarely, if ever, indicated following blunt trauma, in contrast to the situation following open heart surgery. Although there is no contraindication to open-chest cardiac massage in blunt trauma, and there is some evidence that more effective compressions can be achieved with this technique in euvolemic patients,[197] the uniformly fatal outcome of similar resuscitative measures in the emergency department[105, 106] suggest that, when indicated, cardiopulmonary resuscitation by means of external chest compressions is a wiser choice for this group of patients. Proper management of systems for chest drainage and suction[198] is discussed further on.

Nonoperative management of children with lacerations of the solid viscera of the upper abdomen requires a minimum of 7 to 10 days of strict bed rest, the first 2 to 3 days of which should be spent in a fully monitored environment. If respiratory care is required, incentive spirometry is preferred, as clots that are organizing may be disturbed by vigorous chest physiotherapy. During this interval, excessive palpation of the abdomen should also be avoided. Additionally, in cases of splenic laceration or hematoma, or both, the stomach should be kept empty to prevent reactivation of splenic bleeding from tension on the gastrosplenic ligament, which accompanies gastric dilatation. Although most hepatic and splenic bleeding is self-limited, laparotomy is generally required for repair of hepatic or splenic injuries if the transfusion requirement exceeds 40 ml/kg of body weight—that is, half the circulating blood volume—within 24 hours of injury. However, laparotomy for management of renal, pancreatic, gastrointestinal, or genitourinary injuries is performed only as indicated by the development of the appropriate physical signs. It need not be anticipated if damage is not detected by computed tomography or ultrasonography.

Life-threatening hemorrhage from dilutional coagulopathy may occur in patients with near-fatal intra-abdominal hemorrhage that requires massive transfusion. These patients typically will also have severe anemia in the preoperative and intraoperative phases of management. This can be prevented to some extent through the intraoperative use of the autotransfusion device, when feasible.[199] The best treatment, however, is prevention. Therefore, in cases of massive blunt or penetrating trauma in which significant intraoperative hemorrhage is expected, it is wise to assign a member of the critical care team to the operating room with the sole responsibility of closely and continuously monitoring blood loss and ensuring ongoing replacement of blood components warmed to body temperature (including platelet concentrates, especially if the transfusion requirement exceeds the calculated circulating blood volume) sufficient to maintain the hematocrit value just greater than 30%.[200, 201] This responsibility passes to the pediatric critical care physician or surgeon in charge once the patient is moved to the ICU. Administration of fresh frozen plasma and intravenous calcium supplements should be guided by the results of the partial thromboplastin time and the ionized calcium level. The latter will be especially labile if the rate of transfusion exceeds 5 to 10 ml/kg/min, but the former generally will be ineffective until all surgical bleeding has been properly controlled.

The long-term ICU management of children with intra-abdominal injuries also deserves special comment. Because deficient gastric mucosal energy production has been associated with the pathogenesis of stress ulcers,[202] all children who require more than 24 to 48 hours of bowel rest should receive nutritional support[203, 204] as well as hourly antacid therapy sufficient to maintain gastric pH at 4 or greater[205] to prevent the development of these lesions, cimetidine being ineffective when used alone.[206] Antacids are also useful in stopping stress ulcer bleeding if the pH is kept at greater than 7,[207] thus obviating the need for more invasive therapies such as selective intra-arterial vasopressin[208] or direct surgical attack by means of total gastrectomy,[209] vagotomy, and antrectomy,[210] or gastric devascularization,[211] in the great majority of cases (see also Chapter 57). Children with hematomas of the liver, spleen, or pelvis may experience slight fever, no higher than about 37.5° C, as the hematomas are resorbed. However, high fever, particularly if associated with spiking temperatures, should occasion a search for intrahepatic or splenic abscess, infected sympathetic pulmonary effusions, or pelvic osteomyelitis. Children with large retroperitoneal hematomas resulting from pelvic fractures may also experience hypertension on rare occasions, presumably caused by pressure on the renal vessels. The condition may require the temporary use of antihypertensive agents but invariably resolves without the need for surgical decompression.

Although multiple organ system failure is not uncommon among the broad range of critically ill pediatric surgical patients,[212] it is a relatively rare complication of serious childhood trauma. Indeed, patients who are successfully resuscitated by and large will remain hemodynamically stable and recover other vital functions quickly. Sepsis rarely supervenes unless devitalized or infected tissues (e.g., dirty wounds, open fractures) are inadequately treated. However, patients with indwelling tubes or catheters (chest tubes, urinary catheters) are at risk for systemic infection and hence multiple organ system failure, and should receive prophylactic or suppressive antibiotics as long as the tube is required. Likewise, patients with gastrointestinal injuries should be fed as quickly as possible by the enteral route to obviate the need for a central venous catheter, especially if a tracheostomy is present, and to avoid the breakdown of the gut mucosal barrier. Nutritional support of the critically injured child is discussed elsewhere in this volume (see Chapter 14); however, it appears that the added dietary requirements of the pediatric trauma victim are for nitrogen rather than energy and are not related directly to injury severity.[213, 214]

The initial ICU care of extremity injuries consists chiefly of careful observation for signs of neurovascular compromise. Although fracture-associated arterial insufficiency usually will be obvious at the time of fracture diagnosis because of the presence of a pulse deficit, detection of subtler forms of ischemic injury (i.e., compartment syndromes) is much more difficult.[215, 216] However, if swelling is sufficient to obscure the pulse, and tissue pulp pressure as measured by the Whitesides device or other such instrument exceeds 40 cm H_2O,[217, 218] fasciotomy is indicated.[219, 220] By contrast, the ongoing ICU care of extremity injuries should focus on preventing the complications of long-term immobilization, such as friction burns and bed sores. Children in skeletal traction should therefore be nursed on "eggcrate" or similar mattresses and provided with a trapeze to permit limited freedom of movement. Likewise, the importance of providing early rehabilitative services to children with extremity injuries cannot be understated. Physiatric consultation should be routine for such patients and should be ordered as soon as physiologic stability has been assured and fractures have been immobilized.

Finally, every effort must be made to attend to the emotional needs of the healing child and his or her family. In addition to the disempowerment experienced by parents of all critically ill children, parents of seriously injured children may also feel enormous guilt about their child's injuries, even though these feelings are most often unwarranted. Every effort should therefore be made to create as normal an environment as possible for the child and to allow parents to participate meaningfully in the ICU care of their child—both to restore their sense of control over their child's destiny and to mitigate the child's natural fears of abandonment and of what may lie ahead. In this way, the provision of critical medical and nursing care is facilitated, as the child rightly perceives that critical caretakers are working together with his or her parents to assure an optimal recovery.

PEDIATRIC TRAUMA SYSTEM

The early care of the injured child is an extraordinarily complex undertaking that requires the active and cohesive participation of a large number of professionals—those the patient sees before arriving at the hospital, as well as medical, nursing, and allied health professionals. It truly is a team endeavor that requires the best efforts of all members of that team if optimal recovery of the child is to be assured. Overall direction should be the responsibility of the most qualified and experienced physician available—usually a trauma surgeon with extensive experience in the management of childhood injuries.[104] The seriously injured child is best cared for in a hospital that has made a strong institutional, financial, and moral commitment to priority comprehensive care of the injured child.[62] Most full-service general, university, or children's hospitals will meet these criteria and, to the extent possible, seriously injured children should be preferentially transported to these facilities by properly trained and equipped personnel in accordance with regional emergency medical services system policies and protocols and formally established interinstitutional transfer agreements. Indeed, there is now good evidence that children who are once seriously injured do, in fact, fare better in organized trauma systems in which there is emphasis upon the special needs of children, both in the prehospital sector and in the trauma center itself,[221–223] particularly the ICU.[224] The requirements for establishing and maintaining such systems have been widely disseminated.[225–228]

A key responsibility of the pediatric critical care physician or surgeon is to understand the capabilities and limitations of the emergency medical and trauma care system responsible for field stabilization, emergency transport, and initial evaluation and resuscitation of the pediatric trauma victim. The fact that some 80% of pediatric trauma deaths occur before admission to the hospital,[16] and that emergency medical services system personnel are called to assist in resuscitating most of them,[229] suggests that reducing the toll of what has been called "the neglected disease of modern society"[230] will require particular emphasis on prehospital care. Several excellent teaching programs for providers who care for patients before arrival at the hospital have now been developed and are available for nationwide distribution and designed to meet the needs of a variety of environments, both urban and rural.[231–234] Unfortunately, although great strides have been made toward specific incorporation of protocols and equipment for pediatric trauma in prehospital emergency care systems nationwide during the last several years, only 27 states now have active programs in emergency medical services for children.

Trauma scores are a vitally important tool in pediatric trauma care and serve three important functions: (1) field triage, (2) quality assurance, and (3) epidemiologic surveillance. To be useful, however, a score must be valid, reliable, and practical. Anatomic scores such as the Abbreviated Injury Scale[235] and the Injury Severity Score[236] are used primarily for quality assurance and epidemiologic surveillance, whereas physiologic scores such as the Champion Trauma Score[64] and Revised Trauma Score[65] are more frequently used for field triage. Although both of these physiologic scoring systems have been shown to be valid and reliable in children,[237] neither is ideal. For this reason, two scoring systems that attempt to combine the best features of both types of indices have been developed: the Modified Injury Severity Score[238] and the Pediatric Trauma Score.[63] Both have been prospectively validated.[239–241] Of the two, the Pediatric Trauma Score appears somewhat easier to use. Moreover, although it may result in slight overtriage when compared with the Revised Trauma Score,[242] it has been prospectively validated for field use as well as outcome assessment and carries the endorsement of both the American Pediatric Surgical Association Committee on Trauma[62] and the American College of Surgeons Committee on Trauma.[52, 65]

Assuring high-quality care is the most important reason for establishing an organized pediatric trauma system[243]; however, optimal results cannot be realized without a regular case review conference, in which all team members participate, to focus upon detailed evaluation of system as well as human error.[244] Trauma registries also constitute a unique and powerful tool for quality assurance, particularly when the data are pooled in national or regional banks, thus allowing results to be compared with those of other centers. The National Pediatric Trauma Registry, which focuses on long-term disability as well as short-term outcome, has been especially successful in this regard.[245] The aim of both types of efforts is to improve the *effectiveness*[246] of trauma care—that is, to reduce the rates of preventable death and disability. Use of objective criteria such as the Pediatric *Trauma Score*, the Modified *Injury Severity Score*, the Abbreviated Injury Scale or the "TRISS" methodology—all of which have been successfully used in children—is necessary for this purpose,[240, 247–250] though no consensus has yet emerged as to the ideal method. Whatever index is chosen, however, the quality assurance process must take place within the context of the trauma system as a whole. Trauma center care, by and large, is excellent, yet is of little use to the patient who needs it but is not transported to a hospital capable of providing the special needs of the critically injured child.

MANAGEMENT OF SYSTEMS FOR CHEST DRAINAGE AND SUCTION
(Fig. 85–1)

The critical management of children with multiple trauma requires a working knowledge of the systems for chest drainage and suction commonly used in managing patients with intrathoracic injuries.[198] Although a number of commercial devices are available, all are based upon the "three-bottle" system of drainage in use since the time of Evarts Graham. The three "bottles" consist of (in order from chest tube to wall suction) (1) an underwater seal apparatus (the purpose of which is delineated further on); (2) a vacuum-breaking (i.e., suction-regulating) device, which limits negative pressure by allowing air to be entrained from the atmosphere whenever the force of the vacuum is sufficient to overcome the weight of a water column set at a predetermined height in centimeters; and (3) a trap to prevent water or other fluid from entering the vacuum source. The third of these "bottles" obviously is not necessary for the overall function of the chest drainage system itself and is not part of most currently marketed products. However, an additional "bottle" is now interposed

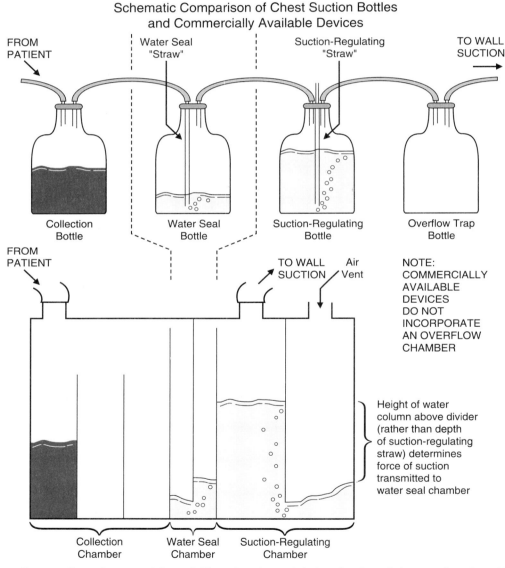

Schematic Comparison of Chest Suction Bottles and Commercially Available Devices

Figure 85–1. Schematic comparison of commercially available underwater seal devices for chest drainage and suction with the time-honored three-bottle system (see text). Note that despite the apparent complexity of the modern, one-piece, disposable units, each of their self-contained chambers is analogous to a "bottle" in the traditional method. In the former, however, the force of the suction applied to the water seal chamber—which, normally, is initially set at 10 cm H_2O—is determined by the height of the water column in the suction-regulating chamber above the divider, whereas in the latter, it is determined by the depth of the suction-regulating "straw" beneath the surface of the water column contained within the suctioning-regulating bottle. In like manner, the underwater seal itself—which is conventionally set at 2 cm H_2O—is maintained by the height of a water column instead of the depth of the water seal "straw." Moreover, while the commercially available devices universally include an additional, separate collection chamber for shed blood and fluid—omitted in the traditional three-bottle system, which utilizes the first bottle both for drainage, and maintenance of the underwater seal—they do not typically interpose a "trap," or overflow chamber, immediately proximal to the vacuum source.

between the chest tube and the underwater seal apparatus by most manufacturers, the purpose of which is to serve as a "collection" chamber for thoracic drainage.

Unfortunately, although these commercially produced chest drainage units have greatly facilitated postinjury and postoperative nursing care of patients with intrathoracic trauma by providing fully enclosed disposable receptacles for shed blood and fluid, they have also served to obscure the relatively simple applied physics upon which adequate chest drainage and suction depend. In this regard, it is important to realize that only the underwater seal apparatus itself—the first bottle in the traditional "three-bottle" system—is actually necessary for preservation of normal respiratory mechanics, except when large air leaks are present. The underwater seal apparatus serves two important functions: (1) it provides a one-way valve for escape of air entrapped within the pleural cavity, thus preventing the development of tension pneumothorax and (2) through the use of a water column siphon in the "water seal straw," it maintains the normal negative intrathoracic pressure gradient with respect to the surrounding atmosphere, thus ensuring that air, which always enters the lung passively via the path of least resistance, will travel via the natural airways rather than a hole in the chest wall, avoiding "paradoxic" respiration. Because air is both compressible and expansible, an excessively large collection chamber interposed between the chest tube and the underwater seal apparatus produces an "air lock," which can dampen the effectiveness of the water column siphon rising in the water seal straw during inspiration, thereby decreasing the transpleural pressure gradient upon which normal spontaneous ventilation depends. By allowing pressure to build during expiration, however, the air lock that results from an excessively large collection chamber may also lead to the development of intrathoracic tension, with all of its complications, which are far more dangerous. Indeed, it is precisely for this reason that commercially produced chest drainage units are sold in infant-, child-, and adult-sized versions and *must* be limited to the use for which they are intended.

Because of this risk of tension pneumothorax, commercially produced chest drainage units that include a separate "collection" chamber generally *also* require the use of constant suction, even when a strict medical indication is lacking. In fact, maintenance of the normal negative transpleural pressure gradient by means of the simple underwater seal apparatus, plus an occasional cough, is all that is required to maintain full lung expansion, hence expulsion of unwanted air and fluid from the pleural space (the very purpose for which chest drainage and suction are needed in the first place)—unless a major air leak is present. In such a circumstance, exceptionally high-pressure suction (-40 to -60 cm H_2O) is sometimes required to achieve full lung expansion. Unfortunately, most commercially produced chest drainage units limit suction to no more than -25 to -30 cm H_2O, in which case an Emerson-type pump (an air turbine attached to a simple vacuum cleaner–type motor) must be used. Failing this, a Wangensteen suction device, which also uses a water siphon to maintain high-pressure suction, must be used.

Air leaks are identified by telltale bubbling at the tip of the water seal straw of the underwater seal chamber during normal negative-pressure inspiration or assisted positive-pressure inspiration. The more vigorous the bubbling, the larger is the leak. However, care must be taken to ensure that the entire chest drainage and suction system, from pleural space to vacuum source, is intact before concluding that a pulmonary air leak is present: (1) Does the chest tube lie completely within the chest (i.e., are all side holes internal to the parietal pleura on chest x-ray film) and is the tube thoracostomy site properly sealed with petroleum jelly–impregnated gauze? (2) Are all connections secure and airtight? (3) Is the chest drainage unit itself defective or did it crack when it fell on its side? All of these questions must be answered appropriately before it can be assumed that an air leak may be present. In doing so, it is often helpful to obtain the advice of a surgeon skilled in the management of thoracic problems of infants and children. Indeed, chest drainage devices are notoriously "fussy" and require a great deal of attention if they are to perform their function properly and efficiently.

A word is also in order about proper use of the chest tubes. All acute collections of blood or air, or both, regardless of amount, requires immediate drainage by means of posterolateral tube thoracostomy. This alone will prove sufficient treatment for the vast majority of hemothoraces and pneumothoraces, as most such drainage will stop shortly after the lungs fully re-expand. In general, it is best to avoid using the site of injury for tube insertion in penetrating trauma, as placement through a contaminated tract may introduce infection into the chest.

Once inserted, a chest tube should *never* be clamped, unless (1) it has stopped draining, (2) removal is imminent, and (3) the sugeon managing the tube assumes direct responsibility for doing so. It should be noted, in this regard, that the narrow-gauge thoracic catheters used for chest drainage in infants and children, the diameter of which should approximate the width of the intercostal space, are easily kinked as the child wanders about the bed; this has the same effect as if they were clamped. It must also be noted that although children with chest tubes should be nursed in a semiupright position to promote dependent drainage, fluid should not be allowed to collect in dependent loops of tubing, as the fluid column within the tube may serve to prevent egress of trapped air, predisposing the child to the development of tension pneumothorax. Tubing should therefore be arranged on the bed to discourage the formation of dependent loops because "stripping" the tube too frequently allows (1) transmission of dangerously high negative pressure to the thoracic cavity because of the large volume of the tubing relative to the pleural space and (2) potential reflux of stagnant fluid into the thoracic cavity as this pressure is released. Finally, chest tubes inserted for drainage of traumatic collections of blood or air, or both, are best left in place for a minimum of 5 days provided that (1) drainage has stopped and (2) complete obliteration of the pleural space has been achieved—unless, of course, they are no longer functioning, as indicated by the lack of regular, cyclic respiratory oscillation of the fluid column in the water seal straw.

References

1. McKoy C and Bell MJ: Preventable traumatic deaths in children. J Pediatr Surg 18:505, 1983.
2. Dykes EH, Spence LJ, Young JG, et al: Preventable pediatric trauma deaths in a metropolitan region. J Pediatr Surg 24:107, 1989.
3. Wesson DE, Williams JI, Spence LJ, et al: Functional outcome in pediatric trauma. J Trauma 29:589, 1989.
4. Harris BH, Schwaitzberg SD, Serman TM, et al: The hidden morbidity of pediatric trauma. J Pediatr Surg 24:103, 1989.
5. Rice DP, MacKenzie EJ, et al: Cost of Injury in the United States: A Report to Congress. Atlanta, Centers for Disease Control, 1989.
6. DiScala C, Gans BM, Barlow B, et al: National Pediatric Trauma Registry Biannual Report. Boston, Tufts University Rehabilitation and Childhood Trauma Research and Training Center, 1990.
7. Graves EJ: Detailed Diagnoses and Procedures: National Hospital Discharge Survey, 1989. Hyattsville, National Center for Health Statistics, Vital Health Stat 13(108), 1991.
8. Klem SA, Pollack MM, Glass NL, et al: Resource use, efficiency, and outcome prediction in pediatric intensive care of trauma patients. J Trauma 30:32, 1990.
9. Krauss BS, Harakal T, and Fleisher GR: The spectrum and frequency of illness presenting to a pediatric emergency department. Pediatr Emerg Care 7:67–71, 1991.
10. Tsai A and Kallsen G: Epidemiology of pediatric prehospital care. Ann Emerg Med 16:284, 1987.
11. Mayer T, Walker ML, Johnson DG, et al: Causes of morbidity and mortality in severe pediatric trauma. JAMA 245:719, 1981.
12. Peclet MH, Newman KD, Eichelberger MR, et al: Patterns of injury in children. J Pediatr Surg 25:85, 1990.
13. Velcek FT, Weiss A, DiMaio D, et al: Traumatic death in urban children. J Pediatr Surg 12:375, 1977.
14. Holmes MJ and Reyes HM: A critical review of urban pediatric trauma. J Trauma 24:253, 1984.
15. Vane D, Shedd FG, Grosfeld JL, et al: An analysis of pediatric trauma deaths in Indiana. J Pediatr Surg 25:955, 1990.
16. Cooper A, Barlow B, Davidson L, et al: Epidemiology of pediatric trauma: Importance of population-based statistics. J Pediatr Surg 27:149–154, 1992.
17. Rang M: Children's Fractures, 2nd ed. Philadelphia, JB Lippincott, 1983.
18. Cristoffel KK and Ranz R: Motor vehicle injury in childhood. Pediatr Rev 4:247, 1983.
19. Neville BG: Hyperflexion cervical cord injury in a children's car seat. Lancet 2:103, 1981.
20. Conry BG and Hall CM: Cervical spine fractures and rear car seat restraints. Arch Dis Child 62:1267, 1987.
21. Fuchs S, Barthel MJ, Flannery AM, et al: Cervical spine fractures sustained by young children in forward-facing car seats. Pediatrics 84:348, 1989.
22. Keller LJ and Mosdal C: Traumatic odontoid epiphysiolysis in an infant fixed in a child's car seat. Injury 21:191, 1990.
23. Agran PF, Dunkle DE, and Winn DG: Injuries to a sample of seatbelted children evaluated and treated in a hospital emergency department. J Trauma 27:58, 1987.
24. Hoffman MA, Spence LJ, Wesson DE, et al: The pediatric passenger: Trends in seatbelt use and injury patterns. J Trauma 27:974, 1987.
25. Stylianos S, terMeulen DC, Latchaw LA, et al: Seatbelt injuries in children. Ann Emerg Med 20:169, 1988.
26. Newman KD, Bowman LM, and Eichelberger MR: The lap belt complex: Intestinal and lumbar spine injury in children. J Trauma 30:1133, 1990.
27. Bull MJ, Stroup KB, and Gerhart S: Misuse of car safety seats. Pediatrics 81:98, 1988.
28. Marchildon M: Unpublished data.
29. Barlow B, Niemirska M, and Gandhi R: Ten years of experience with falls from a height in children. J Pediatr Surg 18:509, 1983.
30. Roshkow JE, Haller JO, Hotson GC, et al: Imaging evaluation of children after falls from a height: Review of 45 cases. Radiology 175:359, 1990.
31. Selbst SM, Alexander D, and Ruddy R: Bicycle-related injuries. Am J Dis Child 141:140, 1987.
32. Sparnon AL and Ford WDA: Bicycle handlebar injuries in children. J Pediatr Surg 21:118, 1986.
33. Tepas JJ, DiScala C, Ramenofsky ML, et al: Mortality and head injury: The pediatric perspective. J Pediatr Surg 25:92, 1990.
34. Cooper A, Barlow B, DiScala C, et al: Mortality and thoracoabdominal injury: The pediatric perspective. J Trauma, in press.
35. Bickford BJ: Chest injuries in childhood and adolescence. Thorax 17:240, 1962.
36. Kilman JW and Charnock E: Thoracic trauma in infancy and childhood. J Trauma 9:863, 1969.
37. Smyth BT: Chest trauma in children. J Pediatr Surg 14:41, 1979.
38. Meller JL, Little AG, and Shermeta DW: Thoracic trauma in children. Pediatrics 74:813, 1984.
39. Rege VM and Deshmukh SS: Major thoracic trauma in children. J Postgrad Med 34:93, 1988.
40. Nakayama DK, Ramenofsky ML, and Rowe MI: Chest injuries in children. Ann Surg 210:770, 1989.
41. Peclet MH, Newman KD, Eichelberger MR, et al: Thoracic trauma in children: An indicator of increased mortality. J Pediatr Surg 25:961, 1990.
42. Haller JA: Injuries of the gastrointestinal tract in children: Notes on recognition and management. Clin Pediatr 5:476, 1966.
43. Selbst SM, Baker MD, and Shames M: Bunk bed injuries. Am J Dis Child 144:721, 1990.
44. Helfer RE, Slovis TL, and Black M: Injuries resulting when small children fall out of bed. Pediatrics 60:533, 1977.
45. Nimityongskul P and Anderson LD: The likelihood of injuries when children fall out of bed. J Pediatr Orthop 7:184, 1987.
46. Joffe M and Ludwig S: Stairway injuries in children. Pediatrics 82:457, 1988.
47. Barlow B, Niemirska M, Gandhi R, et al: Response to injury in children with closed femur fractures. J Trauma 27:429, 1987.
48. Rockwood CA, Wilkins KE, and King RE (eds): Fractures in Children, 3rd ed. Philadelphia, JB Lippincott, 1984.
49. Salter RB and Harris WR: Injuries involving the epiphyseal plate. J Bone Joint Surg 45A:587, 1963.
50. Trunkey D: Initial treatment of patients with extensive trauma. N Engl J Med 324:1259, 1991.
51. American Heart Association and American Academy of Pediatrics Working Group on Pediatric Resuscitation: Textbook of Pediatric Advanced Life Support. Dallas, American Heart Association, 1988.
52. American College of Surgeons Committee on Trauma: Advanced Trauma Life Support Student Manual. Chicago, American College of Surgeons, 1990.
53. American Academy of Pediatrics and American College of Emergency Physicians Joint Task Force on Advanced Pediatric Life Support: Advanced Pediatric Life Support. Elk Grove Village and Dallas, American Academy of Pediatrics and American College of Emergency Physicians, 1989.
54. Eichelberger MR and Randolph JG: Pediatric trauma: An algorithm for diagnosis and therapy. J Trauma 23:91, 1983.
55. Ruddy RM and Fleisher GR: Pediatric trauma: An approach to the injured child. Pediatr Emerg Care 1:151, 1985.
56. Harris BH, Latchaw LA, Murphy RE, et al: A protocol for pediatric trauma receiving units. J Pediatr Surg 24:419, 1989.
57. Schwaitzberg SD, Bergman KS, and Harris BH: A pediatric model of continuous hemorrhage. J Pediatr Surg 23:605, 1988.
58. Bohn D, Armstrong A, Becker L, et al: Cervical spine injuries in children. J Trauma 30:463, 1990.
59. Mattox KL, Bickell W, Pepe PE, et al: Prospective MAST study in 911 patients. J Trauma 29:1104, 1989.
60. Garcia V, Eichelberger M, Ziegler M, et al: Use of military antishock trouser in a child. J Pediatr Surg 16:544, 1981.
61. Velasco AL, Delgado-Paredes C, Templeton J, et al: Intraosseous infusion of fluids in the initial management of hypovolemic shock in young subjects. J Pediatr Surg 26:4, 1991.
62. Harris BH, Barlow BA, Ballantine TV, et al: American Pediatric Surgical Association: Principles of pediatric trauma care. J Pediatr Surg 27:423–426, 1992.
63. Tepas JJ, Mollitt DL, Talbert JL, et al: The pediatric trauma score as a predictor of injury severity in the injured child. J Pediatr Surg 22:14, 1987.
64. Champion HR, Sacco WJ, Carnazzo AJ, et al: Trauma score. Crit Care Med 9:672, 1981.
65. Anonymous: Field categorization of trauma patients (field triage). In: American College of Surgeons Committee on Trauma: Hospital and Prehospital Resources for Optimal Care of the Injured Patient and Appendices A through J. Chicago, American College of Surgeons, 1986, pp 15–18.
66. Jubelirer RA, Agarwal NN, Beyer FC, et al: Pediatric trauma triage: Review of 1,307 cases. J Trauma 30:1544, 1990.
67. Ebert RV, Stead EA, and Gibson JG: Response of normal subjects to acute blood loss. Arch Intern Med 68:578, 1941.

68. Cooper A, Floyd T, Barlow B, et al: Major blunt abdominal trauma due to child abuse. J Trauma 28:1483, 1988.
69. Oldham KT, Guice KS, Kaufman RA, et al: Blunt hepatic injury and elevated hepatic enzymes: A clinical correlation in children. J Pediatr Surg 19:457, 1984.
70. Synn AY, Mulvihill SJ, and Fonkalsrud EW: Surgical management of pancreatitis in childhood. J Pediatr Surg 22:628, 1987.
71. Lieu TA, Fleisher GR, Mahboubi S, et al: Hematuria and clinical findings as indications for intravenous pyelography in pediatric blunt renal trauma. Pediatrics 82:216, 1988.
72. Mukherji SK and Siegel MJ: Rhabdomyolysis and renal failure in child abuse. Am J Roentgenol 148:1203, 1987.
73. Fleisher AG, David I, Hilfer C, et al: Mediastinal hematoma mimicking aortic rupture. J Pediatr Surg 21:445, 1986.
74. Jewett TC: Chest and abdominal injuries. In: Ellerstein NS (ed): Child Abuse and Neglect: A Medical Reference. New York, John Wiley & Sons, 1981, pp 165–184.
75. Berger PE and Kuhn JP: CT of blunt abdominal trauma in childhood. Am J Roentgenol 136:105, 1981.
76. Karp MP, Cooney DR, Berger PE, et al: The role of computed tomography in the evaluation of blunt abdominal trauma in children. J Pediatr Surg 16:316, 1981.
77. Kaufman RA, Towbin R, Babcock DS, et al: Upper abdominal trauma in children: Imaging evaluation. Am J Roentgenol 142:449, 1984.
78. Mohamed G, Reyes HM, Fantus R, et al: Computed tomography in the assessment of pediatric abdominal trauma. Arch Surg 121:703, 1986.
79. Kane NM, Cronan JJ, Dorfman GS, et al: Pediatric abdominal trauma: Evaluation by computed tomography. Pediatrics 82:11, 1988.
80. Gorenstein A, O'Jalpin D, Wesson DE, et al: Blunt injury to the pancreas in children: Selective management based on ultrasound. J Pediatr Surg 22:1110, 1987.
81. Haftel AJ, Lev R, Mahour GH, et al: Abdominal CT scanning in pediatric blunt trauma. Ann Emerg Med 17:684, 1988.
82. Beaver BL, Colombani PM, Fal A, et al: The efficacy of computed tomography in evaluating abdominal injuries in children with major head trauma. J Pediatr Surg 22:1117, 1987.
83. Taylor GA and Eichelberger MR: Abdominal CT in children with neurologic impairment following blunt trauma: Abdominal CT in comatose children. Ann Surg 210:229, 1989.
84. Ben-Ami T, Rozenman J, Yahav, et al: Computed tomography in children with esophageal and airway trauma. J Pediatr Surg 23:919, 1988.
85. Sivit CJ, Taylor GA, and Eichelberger MR: Chest injury in children with blunt abdominal trauma: Evaluation with CT. Radiology 171:815, 1989.
86. Taylor GA, Eichelberger MR, O'Donnel R, et al: Indications for computed tomography in children with blunt abdominal trauma. Ann Surg 213:212, 1991.
87. Brick SH, Taylor GA, Potter BM, et al: Hepatic and splenic injury in children: Role of CT in the decision for laparotomy. Radiology 165:643, 1987.
88. Taylor GA, Fallat ME, Potter BM, et al: The role of computed tomography in blunt abdominal trauma in children. J Trauma 28:1660, 1988.
89. Hoelzer DJ, Brian MB, Balsara VJ, et al: Selection and nonoperative management of pediatric blunt trauma patients: The role of quantitative crystalloid resuscitation and abdominal ultrasonography. J Trauma 26:57, 1986.
90. Filiatrault D, Longpre D, Patriquin H, et al: Investigation of childhood blunt abdominal trauma: A practical approach using ultrasound as the initial diagnostic modality. Pediatr Radiol 17:373, 1987.
91. Harris BH, Morse TS, Weidenmier CH, et al: Radioisotope diagnosis of splenic trauma. J Pediatr Surg 12:385, 1977.
92. Howman-Giles R, Gilday DL, Venugopal S, et al: Splenic trauma—nonoperative management and long-term follow-up by scintiscan. J Pediatr Surg 13:121, 1978.
93. Karp MP, Jewett TC, Kuhn JP, et al: The impact of computed tomography scanning on the child with renal trauma. J Pediatr Surg 21:617, 1986.
94. Yale-Loehr AJ, Kramer SS, Quinlan DM, et al: CT of severe renal trauma in children: Evaluation and course of healing with conservative therapy. Am J Roentgenol 152:109, 1989.
95. Cass AS, Luxenberg M, Gleich P, et al: Clinical indications for radiographic evaluation of blunt renal trauma. J Urol 136:370, 1986.
96. Taylor GA, Eichelberger MR, and Potter BM: Hematuria: A marker of abdominal injury in children after blunt trauma. Ann Surg 208:688, 1988.
97. Stalker HP, Kaufman RA, and Stedje K: The significance of hematuria in children after blunt abdominal trauma. Am J Roentgenol 154:569, 1990.
98. Bass DH, Semple PL, and Cywes S: Investigation and management of blunt renal injuries in children: A review of 11 years' experience. J Pediatr Surg 26:196, 1991.
99. Kolihova E, Obenbergerova D, and Apetaurova B: Total severence of the renal pedicle caused by blunt trauma in children. Pediatr Radiol 1:59, 1973.
100. Barlow B and Gandhi R: Renal artery thrombosis following blunt trauma. J Trauma 20:614, 1980.
101. Powell RW, Green JB, Ochsner MG, et al: Peritoneal lavage in pediatric patients sustaining blunt abdominal trauma: A reappraisal. J Trauma 27:6, 1987.
102. Rothenberg S, Moore EE, Marx JA, et al: Selective management of blunt abdominal trauma in children—the triage role of peritoneal lavage. J Trauma 27:1101, 1987.
103. Kaufmann CR, Rivara FP, and Maier RV: Pediatric trauma: Need for surgical management. J Trauma 29:1120, 1989.
104. Haller JA: Emergency medical services for children: What is the pediatric surgeon's role? Pediatrics 79:576, 1987.
105. Beaver BL, Colombani PM, Buck JR, et al: Efficacy of emergency room thoracotomy in pediatric trauma. J Pediatr Surg 22:19, 1987.
106. Rothenberg SS, Moore EE, Moore FA, et al: Emergency department thoracotomy in children—a critical analysis. J Trauma 29:1322, 1989.
107. Boidon MP: Airway patency in the unconscious patient. Br J Anaesthesiol 57:306, 1985.
108. Safar P, Escarraga L, and Chang F: Upper airway obstruction in the unconscious patient. J Appl Physiol 14:760, 1959.
109. Levy JL: Management of crushing chest injuries in children. South Med J 65:1040, 1972.
110. Schwartz A and Borman JB: Contusion of the lung in childhood. Arch Dis Child 36:557, 1969.
111. Sladen A: Methylprednisolone: Pharmacologic doses in shock lung syndrome. J Thorac Cardiovasc Surg 71:800, 1976.
112. Wolfe JE, Bone RC, and Ruth WE: Effects of corticosteroids in the treatment of gastric aspiration. Am J Med 63:719, 1977.
113. Golladay ES, Donahoo JS, and Haller JA: Special problems of cardiac injuries in infants and children. J Trauma 19:526, 1979.
114. Tellez DW, Hardin WD, Takahashi M, et al: Blunt cardiac injury in children. J Pediatr Surg 22:1123, 1987.
115. Langer JC, Winthrop AL, Wesson DE, et al: Diagnosis and incidence of cardiac injury in children with blunt thoracic trauma. J Pediatr Surg 24:1091, 1989.
116. Ildstad ST, Tollerud DJ, Weiss RG, et al: Cardiac contusion in pediatric patients with blunt thoracic trauma. J Pediatr Surg 25:287, 1990.
117. Myers WO, Leape LL, and Holder TM: Bronchial rupture in a child with subsequent stenosis, resection, and anastamosis. Ann Thorac Surg 12:442, 1971.
118. Myers NA: Traumatic rupture of the diaphragm in children. Aust NZ J Surg 34:123, 1964.
119. Radhakrishna C, Dickinson SJ, and Shaw A: Acute diaphragmatic hernia from blunt trauma in children. J Pediatr Surg 4:553, 1969.
120. Holgersen LO and Schnaufer L: Hernia and eventration of the diaphragm secondary to blunt trauma. J Pediatr Surg 8:433, 1973.
121. Melzig EP, Swank M, and Salzberg AM: Acute blunt traumatic rupture of the diaphragm in children. Arch Surg 111:1009, 1976.
122. West K, Weber TR, and Grosfeld JL: Traumatic diaphragmatic hernia in childhood. J Pediatr Surg 16:392, 1981.
123. Meyer JA, Neville JF, and Hansen WG: Traumatic rupture of the aorta in a child. JAMA 208:527, 1969.
124. Meagher DP, Defore WW, Mattox KL, et al: Vascular trauma in infants and children. J Trauma 19:532, 1979.
125. Bergman K, Spence L, Wesson DE, et al: Thoracic vascular injuries: A post mortem study. J Trauma 30:604, 1990.
126. Eddy AC, Rusch VW, Fligner CL, et al: The epidemiology of traumatic rupture of the thoracic aorta in children: A 13-year review. J Trauma 30:989, 1990.

127. Schweich P and Fleisher G: Rib fractures in children. Pediatr Emerg Care 1:187, 1985.
128. Garcia VF, Gotschall CS, Eichelberger MR, et al: Rib fractures in children: A marker of severe trauma. J Trauma 30:695, 1990.
129. Harris GJ and Soper RT: Pediatric first rib fractures. J Trauma 30:343, 1990.
130. Thomas PS: Rib fractures in infancy. Ann Radiol 20:115, 1977.
131. Haller JA and Donahoo JS: Traumatic asphyxia in children: Pathophysiology and management. J Trauma 11:453, 1971.
132. Gorenstein L, Blair GK, and Shandling B: The prognosis of traumatic asphyxia in childhood. J Pediatr Surg 21:753, 1986.
133. Vock P, Kehrer B, and Tschaeppeler H: Blunt liver trauma in children: The role of computed tomography in diagnosis and treatment. J Pediatr Surg 21:413, 1986.
134. Karp MP, Cooney DR, Pros GA, et al: The nonoperative mangement of pediatric hepatic trauma. J Pediatr Surg 18:512, 1983.
135. Grisoni ER, Gauderer MWL, Ferron J, et al: Nonoperative management of liver injuries following blunt abdominal trauma in children. J Pediatr Surg 19:515, 1984.
136. Giacomantonio M, Filler RM, and Rich RH: Blunt hepatic trauma in children: Experience with operative and nonoperative management. J Pediatr Surg 19:519, 1984.
137. Cywes S, Rode H, and Millar AJW: Blunt liver trauma in children: Nonoperative management. J Pediatr Surg 20:14, 1985.
138. Bass BL, Eichelberger MR, Schisgall R, et al: Hazards of nonoperative therapy of hepatic injury in children. J Trauma 24:978, 1984.
139. Oldham KT, Guice KS, Ryckman F, et al: Blunt liver injury in childhood: Evolution of therapy and current perspective. Surgery 100:542, 1986.
140. Galat JA, Grisoni ER, and Gauderer MWL: Pediatric blunt liver injury: Establishment of criteria for appropriate management. J Pediatr Surg 25:1162, 1990.
141. Lackgren G, Lorelius LE, Olsen L, et al: Hemobilia in childhood. J Pediatr Surg 23:105, 1988.
142. MacGillivray DC and Valentine RJ: Nonoperative management of blunt pediatric liver injury—late complications: Case report. J Trauma 29:251, 1989.
143. Ein SH, Shandling B, Simpson JS, et al: Nonoperative management of the traumatized spleen in children: How and why? J Pediatr Surg 13:117, 1978.
144. Wesson DE, Filler RM, Ein SH, et al: Ruptured spleen: When to operate? J Pediatr Surg 16:324, 1981.
145. Pearl RH, Wesson DE, Spence LJ, et al: Splenic injury: A 5-year update with improved results and changing criteria for conservative management. J Pediatr Surg 24:121, 1989.
146. Ratner MH, Garrow E, Valda V, et al: Surgical repair of the injured spleen. J Pediatr Surg 12:1019, 1977.
147. Mishalany HG, Mahour GH, Andrassy RJ, et al: Modalities of preservation of the traumatized spleen. Am J Surg 136:697, 1978.
148. Buntain WL and Lynn HB: Splenorrhaphy: Changing concepts for the traumatized spleen. Surgery 86:748, 1979.
149. Cooney DR, Bearth JC, Swanson SE, et al: Relative merits of partial splenectomy, splenic reimplantation, and immunization in preventing postsplenectomy infection. Surgery 86:561, 1979.
150. vanWyck DB, Witte MH, Witte CH, et al: Critical splenic mass for survival from experimental pneumococcemia. J Surg Res 28:14, 1980.
151. Okinaga K, Giebink GS, Rich RH, et al: The effect of partial splenectomy on experimental pneumococcal bacteremia in an animal model. J Pediatr Surg 16:717, 1981.
152. Karp MP, Guralnick-Scheff S, Schiffman G, et al: Immune consequences of nonoperative treatment of splenic trauma in the rat model. J Pediatr Surg 24:112, 1989.
153. Velcek FT, Jongco B, Shaftan GW, et al: Function of the replanted spleen in dogs. J Trauma 22:501, 1982.
154. Velcek FT, Jongco B, Shaftan GW, et al: Posttraumatic splenic replantation in children. J Pediatr Surg 17:879, 1982.
155. Giebink JS, Folker JE, Kim Y, et al: Serum antibody and opsonic responses to vaccination with pneumococcal capsular polysaccharide in normal and splenectomized children. J Infect Dis 141:404, 1980.
156. Douglas RM, Paton JC, Duncan SJM, et al: Antibody response to pneumococcal vaccine in children younger than five years of age. J Infect Dis 148:131, 1983.
157. Jakse G, Putz A, Gassner I, et al: Early surgery in the management of pediatric blunt renal trauma. J Urol 131:920, 1984.
158. Mandour WA, Lai MK, Linke CA, et al: Blunt renal trauma in the pediatric patient. J Pediatr Surg 16:669, 1981.
159. Kuzmarov IW, Morehouse DD, and Gibson S: Blunt renal trauma in the pediatric population: A retrospective study. J Urol 126:648, 1981.
160. Ahmed S and Morris LL: Renal parenchymal injuries secondary to blunt abdominal trauma in childhood: A 10-year review. Br J Urol 54:470, 1982.
161. Cass AS: Blunt renal trauma in children. J Trauma 23:123, 1983.
162. Cass AS: Renal trauma in multiple-injured child. Urology 21:487, 1983.
163. Smith SD, Nakayama DK, Gantt N, et al: Pancreatic injuries in childhood due to blunt trauma. J Pediatr Surg 23:610, 1988.
164. Vane DW, Grosfeld JL, West KW, et al: Pancreatic disorders in infancy and childhood: Experience with 92 cases. J Pediatr Surg 24:771, 1989.
165. Dahman B and Stephens CA: Pseudocysts of the pancreas after blunt abdominal trauma in children. J Pediatr Surg 16:17, 1981.
166. Warner RL, Othersen HB, and Smith CD: Traumatic pancreatitis and pseudocyst in children: Current management. J Trauma 29:597, 1989.
167. Cobb LM, Vinocur CD, Wagner CW, et al: Intestinal perforation due to blunt trauma in children in an era of increased nonoperative treatment. J Trauma 26:461, 1986.
168. Pokorny WJ, Brandt ML, and Harberg FJ: Major duodenal injuries in children: Diagnosis, operative management, and outcome. J Pediatr Surg 21:613, 1986.
169. Grosfeld JL, Rescorla FJ, West KW, et al: Gastrointestinal injuries in childhood: Analysis of 53 patients. J Pediatr Surg 24:580, 1989.
170. Holgersen LO and Bishop HC: Nonoperative treatment of duodenal hematomata in childhood. J Pediatr Surg 12:11, 1977.
171. Winthrop AL, Wesson DE, and Filler RM: Traumatic duodenal hematoma in the pediatric patient. J Pediatr Surg 21:757, 1986.
172. Jewett TC, Caldarola V, Karp MP, et al: Intramural hematoma of the duodenum. Arch Surg 123:54, 1988.
173. Bryan WJ and Tullos HS: Pediatric pelvic fractures: Review of 52 patients. J Trauma 19:799, 1979.
174. Reichard SA, Helikson MA, Shorter N, et al: Pelvic fractures in children: Review of 120 patients with a new look at general management. J Pediatr Surg 15:727, 1980.
175. So SKS and Perry F: Injuries and mortality associated with pelvic fractures in children. J Trauma 22:641, 1982.
176. Torode I and Zeig D: Pelvic fractures in children. J Pediatr Orthop 5:76, 1985.
177. Musemeche CA, Fischer RP, Cotler HB, et al: Selective management of pediatric pelvic fractures: A conservative approach. J Pediatr Surg 22:538, 1987.
178. Garvin KL, McCarthy RE, Barnes CL, et al: Pediatric pelvic ring fractures. J Pediatr Orthop 10:577, 1990.
179. Barlow B, Rottenberg RW, and Santulli TV: Angiographic diagnosis and treatment of bleeding by selective embolization following pelvic fracture in children. J Pediatr Surg 10:939, 1975.
180. Brereton RJ, Philp N, and Buyukpamukcu N: Rupture of the urinary bladder in children: The importance of the double lesion. Br J Urol 52:15, 1980.
181. Merchant WC, Gibbons MD, and Gonzales ET: Trauma to the bladder neck, trigone, and vagina in children. J Urol 131:747, 1984.
182. Reda EF and Lebowitz RL: Traumatic ureteropelvic disruption in the child. Pediatr Radiol 16:164, 1986.
183. Bard JL and Klein FA: Ureteropelvic junction avulsion following blunt abdominal trauma. J Tenn Med Assoc 83:242, 1990.
184. Halsted CC and Shapiro SR: Child abuse: Acute renal failure from ruptured bladder. Am J Dis Child 133:861, 1979.
185. Sawyer RW, Hartenberg MA, and Benator RM: Intraperitoneal bladder rupture in a battered child. Int J Pediatr Nephrol 8:227, 1987.
186. Glassberg KI, Tolete-Velcek F, Ashley R, et al: Partial tears of prostatomembranous urethra in children. Urology 13:500, 1979.
187. alRifaei MA, Gaafar S, and Abdel-Rahman M: Management of posterior urethral strictures secondary to pelvic fractures in children. J Urol 145:535, 1991.
188. Glassberg KI, Kassner EG, Haller JO, et al: The radiographic approach to injuries of the prostatomembranous urethra in children. J Urol 122:678, 1979.
189. Cardin JM, Skandalakis JE, and Gray SW: Fat embolism following severe trauma in a child. J Med Assoc Ga 56:50, 1967.

190. Weisz GM, Rang M, and Salter RB: Posttraumatic fat embolism in children: Review of the literature and of experience in the Hospital for Sick Children, Toronto. J Trauma 13:529, 1973.

191. Nichols GR, Corey TS, and Davis GJ: Nonfracture-associated fatal fat embolism in a case of child abuse. J Forensic Sci 35:493, 1990.

192. Weisz GM, Schramek A, Abrahamson J, et al: Fat embolism in children: Tests for its early detection. J Pediatr Surg 9:163, 1974.

193. Barlow B, Niemirska M, and Gandhi R: Ten years' experience with pediatric gunshot wounds. J Pediatr Surg 17:927, 1982.

194. Barlow B, Niemirska M, and Gandhi R: Stab wounds in children. J Pediatr Surg 18:926, 1983.

195. Ordog GJ, Prakash AP, Wassenberger J, et al: Pediatric gunshot wounds. J Trauma 27:1272, 1987.

196. Selbst SM, Henretig F, Fee MA, et al: Lead poisoning in a child with a gunshot wound. Pediatrics 77:413, 1986.

197. DelGuercio LRM, Feins NR, Cohn JD, et al: Comparison of blood flow during external and internal cardiac massage in man. Circulation 31(S1):171, 1965.

198. vonHippel A: A Manual of Thoracic Surgery, 2nd ed. Anchorage, Stone Age Press, 1986.

199. Wesson DE, Ein SH, and Villamater J: Intraoperative autotransfusion in blunt abdominal trauma. J Pediatr Surg 15:735, 1980.

200. Heugham C, Grisles G, and Hunt TK: The effect of anemia on wound healing. Ann Surg 179:163, 1974.

201. Czer LS and Shoemaker WC: Optimal hematocrit value in critically ill postoperative patients. Surg Gynecol Obstet 147:363, 1978.

202. Menguy R and Masters YF: Gastric mucosal energy metabolism and "stress" ulceration. Ann Surg 180:538, 1974.

203. Hobbs CL, Mullen JL, Buzby GP, et al: The effects of nutrition on aspirin-induced mucosal ulceration in primates. Surgery 86:49, 1979.

204. Smale BF, Mullen JL, Hobbs CL, et al: Effect of acid secretion on aspirin-induced gastric mucosal erosions. Surg Forum 31:113, 1980.

205. Hastings PR, Skillman JJ, Bushnell LS, et al: Antacid titration in the prevention of acute gastrointestinal bleeding. N Engl J Med 298:1041, 1978.

206. Priebe HJ, Skillman JJ, Bushnell LS, et al: Antacid versus cimetidine in preventing acute gastrointestinal bleeding. N Engl J Med 302:426, 1980.

207. Simonian SJ and Curtis LE: Treatment of hemorrhagic gastritis by antacid. Ann Surg 184:429, 1976.

208. Athanasoulis CA, Baum S, Waltman AC, et al: Control of acute gastric mucosal hemorrhage. N Engl J Med 290:597, 1974.

209. Menguy R, Gadacz T, and Zajtchuk R: The surgical management of acute gastric mucosal bleeding. Arch Surg 99:198, 1969.

210. Lucas EC, Sugawa C, Riddle J, et al: Natural history and surgical dilemma of "stress" gastric bleeding. Arch Surg 102:266, 1971.

211. Richardson JD and Aust JB: Gastric devascularization: A useful salvage procedure for massive hemorrhagic gastritis. Ann Surg 185:649, 1977.

212. Wilkinson JD, Pollack MM, Ruttimann UE, et al: Outcome of pediatric patients with multiple organ system failure. Crit Care Med 14:271, 1986.

213. Kien CL, Young VR, Rohrbaugh DK, et al: Increased rates of whole body protein synthesis and breakdown in children recovering from burns. Ann Surg 187:383, 1978.

214. Winthrop AL, Wesson DE, Pencharz PB, et al: Injury severity, whole body protein turnover, and energy expenditure in pediatric trauma. J Pediatr Surg 22:534, 1987.

215. Whitesides TE, Haney TC, Morimoto K, et al: Tissue pressure measurements as a determinant of the need for fasciotomy. Clin Orthop 113:43, 1975.

216. Whitesides TE, Haney TC, Hirada H, et al: A simple method for tissue pressure determination. Arch Surg 110:1311, 1975.

217. Mubarak SJ, Hargens AR, Owen CA, et al: The wick technique for measurement of intramuscular pressure: A new research and clinical tool. J Bone Joint Surg 58A:1016, 1976.

218. Matsen FA: A practical approach to compartmental syndromes. Part I. Definition, theory, and pathogenesis. Am Acad of Orthop Surg Instructional Course Lectures 32:88, 1983.

219. Mubarak SJ: A practical approach to compartmental syndromes. Part II. Diagnosis. Am Acad Orthop Surg Instructional Course Lectures 32:93, 1983.

220. Rorabeck CH: A practical approach to compartmental syndromes. Part III: Management. Am Acad of Orthop Surg Instructional Course Lectures 32:102, 1983.

221. Haller JA, Shorter N, Miller D, et al: Organization and function of a regional pediatric trauma center: Does a system of management improve outcome? J Trauma 23:691, 1983.

222. Colombani PM, Buck JR, Dudgeon DL, et al: One-year experience in a regional pediatric trauma center. J Pediatr Surg 20:8, 1985.

223. Breaux CW, Smith G, and Georgeson KE: The first two years' experience with major trauma at a pediatric trauma center. J Trauma 30:37, 1990.

224. Pollack MM, Alexander SR, Clarke N, et al: Improved outcomes from tertiary center pediatric intensive care: A statewide comparison of tertiary and nontertiary facilities. Crit Care Med 19:150, 1991.

225. Ramenofsky ML and Morse TS: Standards of care for the critically injured pediatric patient. J Trauma 22:921, 1982.

226. Harris BH: Creating pediatric trauma systems. J Pediatr Surg 24:149, 1989.

227. Ramenofsky ML: Emergency medical services for children and pediatric trauma system components. J Pediatr Surg 24:153, 1989.

228. Anonymous: Planning pediatric trauma care. In: American College of Surgeons Committee on Trauma: Resources for Optimal Care of the Injured Patient. Chicago, American College of Surgeons, 1990, pp. 51–54.

229. Gausche M, Seidel JS, Henderson DP, et al: Pediatric deaths and emergency medical services (EMS) in urban and rural areas. Pediatr Emerg Care 5:158, 1989.

230. National Academy of Sciences: Accidental Death and Disability: The Neglected Disease of Modern Society. Washington, National Academy of Sciences, 1966.

231. Eichelberger MR and Stossel-Pratsch G: Pediatric Emergencies Manual. Baltimore, University Park Press, 1984.

232. Brownstein D, Monaghan S, Bennett R (eds): Pediatric Prehospital Care. Seattle, Washington State Emergency Medical Services for Children, 1989.

233. Simon JS and Goldberg AT: Pre-hospital Pediatric Life Support. St. Louis, Mosby-Year Book, 1989.

234. Elling R and Cooper A (eds): Pre-hospital Pediatric Care Course Student Manual. Albany, New York State Department of Health, 1991.

235. American Association for Automotive Medicine: The Abbreviated Injury Scale—1985 Revision. Arlington Heights, American Association for Automotive Medicine, 1985.

236. Baker SP, O'Neill B, Haddon W, et al: The injury severity score: A method for describing patients with multiple injuries and evaluating emergency care. J Trauma 14:187, 1974.

237. Wesson DE, Spence LJ, Williams JI, et al: Injury scoring systems in children. Can J Surg 30:398, 1987.

238. Mayer T, Matlak ME, Johnson DG, et al: The modified injury severity scale in pediatric multiple trauma patients. J Pediatr Surg 15:719, 1980.

239. Mayer T, Walker ML, and Clarke P: Further experience with the modified injury severity score. J Trauma 24:31, 1984.

240. Tepas JJ, Ramenofsky ML, Mollitt DL, et al: The pediatric trauma score as a predictor of injury severity: An objective assessment. J Trauma 28:425, 1988.

241. Ramenofsky ML, Ramenofsky MB, Jurkovich GJ, et al: The predictive validity of the pediatric trauma score. J Trauma 28:1038, 1988.

242. Kaufmann CR, Maier RM, Rivara RP, et al: Evaluation of the pediatric trauma score. JAMA 263:69, 1990.

243. Nakayama DK, Saitz EW, Gardner MJ, et al: Quality assessment in the pediatric trauma care system. J Pediatr Surg 24:159, 1989.

244. Ramenofsky ML, Luterman A, Quindlen E, et al: Maximum survival in pediatric trauma: The ideal system. J Trauma 24:818, 1984.

245. Tepas JJ, Ramenofsky ML, Barlow B, et al: National pediatric trauma registry. J Pediatr Surg 24:156, 1989.

246. Wesson DE, Williams JI, Salmi LR, et al: Evaluating a pediatric trauma program: Effectiveness versus preventable death rate. J Trauma 28:1226, 1988.

247. Zordludemir U, Ergoren Y, Yucesan S, et al: Mortality due to trauma in childhood. J Trauma 28:669, 1988.

248. Dykes EJ, Spence LJ, Bohn DJ, et al: Evaluation of pediatric trauma care in Ontario. J Trauma 29:724, 1989.

249. Eichelberger MR, Mangubat EA, Sacco WS, et al: Comparative outcomes of children and adults suffering blunt trauma. J Trauma 28:430, 1988.

250. Eichelberger MR, Mangubat EA, Sacco WJ, et al: Outcome analysis of blunt injury in children. J Trauma 28:1109, 1988.

Child Abuse and Neglect: A Critical Care Challenge

Mireille B. Kanda, M.D., and Lavdena A. Orr, M.D.

Child maltreatment is not a new problem: It can be traced through the history of most cultures and persists to this day. It has its roots in the way we have viewed children traditionally. Societies have often found it expedient to unburden themselves of the care of unwelcome or deformed infants through infanticide, children continue to be used as free labor in many countries, and the sexual exploitation of children is still prevalent (and increasingly evident).

It is relatively new to believe that children have rights and that they are entitled to experience their potential in a nurturing environment free of avoidable hazards. Society no longer condones overtly abusive behavior toward children, and there is now a widely shared belief that such activities are deviant and are appropriately under the sanction of the law.

Professionals in the field of child protection recognize the responsibility borne by primary caretakers (by definition, the parents) for the nurture and protection of children and thus define the three primary forms of maltreatment in terms of parental accountability:

1. *Physical abuse* is "the intentional, nonaccidental use of force on the part of the parent or other caretaker interacting with a child in his or her care (when said force is) aimed at hurting, injuring, or destroying that child."[1]
2. *Sexual abuse* is "the involvement of dependent, developmentally immature children and adolescents in sexual activities that they do not fully comprehend, to which they are unable to give informed consent, or that violate the social taboos of family roles."[2]
3. *Child neglect* has been defined as "the adverse consequences of inadequate or negligent parenting."[3]

The 2.4 million cases of child abuse reported nationally to child protective services in 1989 suggest the magnitude of the problem of child abuse and neglect. These reports represent only a fraction of the true number of maltreated children, as many never come to the attention of public systems either because they are not identified or because they are misdiagnosed.

Child victimization initially was viewed as a discrete problem primarily involving family dysfunction. Observers in the field have now realized that other societal problems—such as social isolation and alienation, domestic violence, substance abuse, and poverty—contribute to this scourge and exacerbate it. Thus, the current general consensus is that a multidisciplinary approach, involving close collaboration among professionals from many disciplines (medicine, nursing, social work, mental health, and law) is necessary for the successful management of child maltreatment.

Most children who are physically abused do not require medical intensive care. Patients whose injuries are serious, however, can seriously challenge the medical team's diagnostic and therapeutic acumen.

ESTABLISHING A BASIS OF SUSPICION

Certain patterns of injury (or a discrepancy between the explanation given and the nature of the injuries) lead to concerns about the true course of events preceding the hospitalization. It becomes the responsibility of the treating physician to address these inconsistencies and to consider the possibility that child abuse or neglect has occurred.

The value of obtaining a detailed history cannot be overstated. For the physician embarking on that task, many challenges emerge, including (1) interaction with the parents, (2) interaction with the patient, and (3) construction of a clear understanding of the circumstances leading to the hospitalization.

The Parents

The physical presentation of the parents does not necessarily correlate with the likelihood that the child may have been abused or that they may be the perpetrators. A wide range of often similar behaviors may be observed among perpetrators and nonperpetrators. Some adults react in a very dramatic manner to a child's injury or sudden illness, whereas others may be quite self-contained. Public displays of grief by parents, or conversely a lack of external manifestations of anxiety or sadness, should not be allowed to influence, either positively or negatively, the assessment process.

The parent should be approached in a nonjudgmental and open manner. No accusations should be made. The parents should be told of the difficulty in determining the cause of their child's condition, and their help should be enlisted in order to provide optimal care to the patient. It is important to remember that the physician is not an investigator or a fact finder but rather a medical professional gathering information for the purpose of treating a patient. The veracity of the parents' statements should not be challenged during the interview. Inconsistencies should, however, be carefully noted.

At the conclusion of the interview, the physician's legal obligation to refer the parents to the hospital child protection team should be explained to them. If there is no hospital team, the case must be reported to the appropriate legal authorities. (Failure to communicate clearly will result in a disruption in the relationship with the parents.) Some parents will become angry at this point, but in time they will work with the physician, particularly if the distinction between the roles of the practitioner and the investigator has been made clear to them. They should be told that it is not a matter of finger pointing but rather a need to clarify circumstances and ensure the safety of the patient.

The Child

These children may not be able to communicate verbally for a variety of reasons. They be unconscious, intubated, or otherwise unable to talk. When they can talk, there is still no guarantee that they will tell what really happened. The strange surroundings of the hospital and of unfamiliar faces may make these children unlikely to share information at least at first. In addition, these children may be afraid to talk, may feel somewhat responsible for their injuries, or may remain silent out of loyalty to the family.

Abused children may retain a strong attachment to the abusive parents and may not necessarily withdraw from them. However, behavioral changes and manifestations of fear or anger when family members visit should be duly noted. On occasion, after a variable period, these children may confide in a member of the medical team whom they have come to trust. Although it is important to pay close attention to the statements obtained from these children, leading questions suggesting a certain answer should be avoided, as they may taint the information received.

The Circumstances

The circumstances of the event leading to the child's injuries must be assessed. The medical provider should recognize the existence of a diverse range of child-rearing practices among socioeconomic groups and subcultures. No behavior should be discounted as unlikely to occur simply because it is outside the experience of the examiner—for example unusual injuries have re-

cently been observed that were caused while the parents were under the influence of drugs. There was no intent to harm the children, but nevertheless serious injury had resulted.

It may be difficult to ascertain the plausibility of the history given without a visit to the scene of the event. Such a visit is the responsibility of either police or child protective services, depending on the jurisdiction, and will take place during the course of the formal investigation.

The factual data to be gathered during the medical history are summarized in Table 86–1.

In settings in which there is no child protection team, the physician and the unit social worker may share the responsibility of gathering the historical information. Parent-child interaction at the bedside should be observed and documented in the chart in an objective and nonjudgmental manner. Statements made by the child that may bear on victimization should be recorded verbatim, and the treating physician should be made aware of this information.

Physical Examination

For forensic purposes, the physical examination ideally should take place as soon as the patient is received and before a number of diagnostic procedures have been performed. It becomes a challenge to assess a patient with bandages and a wide array of monitoring devices in place. It is most useful to have the first person who examines the patient carefully describe the external

Table 86–1. MEDICAL ASSESSMENT OF CHILD ABUSE AND NEGLECT HISTORICAL INFORMATION

Description of events preceding admission
    Exact time and location
    Individuals present
    Chain of events
Child's symptoms
    Immediately following acute event
    Progression over time
    Length of time elapsed between onset of symptoms and medical
      intervention
Past medical history
    Previous trauma and hospitalizations (location)
    Other illness, particularly of a chronic nature
    Immunization status (index of health supervision)
    Name of regular health care provider
    Brief developmental history
Review of systems
    Establish whether caretaker is aware of any other injury or
      symptom in addition to the ones under acute consideration
    Medication history past and present
Family psychosocial profile (may be brief and supplemented by
    social worker member of multidisciplinary team)
    Household composition
    Presence of siblings or other children in the home
    Primary caretakers (parents, sitters, and so on) and supervision
    Special stressors: poverty, poor housing, parental physical or
      mental illness, substance abuse, parental incarceration,
      domestic violence, recent family losses (death or other major
      events)
    History of previous involvement with child protective services or
      child welfare agencies

injuries. It is understood, of course, that lifesaving procedures take precedence over this documentation, but the documentation must be performed because of its legal value.

The examination must be complete and thorough. When head trauma is suspected, the head should be carefully palpated and inspected for evidence of bruises, lacerations, hematomas, and fractures. An ophthalmologic evaluation is recommended to document retinal hemorrhages and other traumatic ocular injuries suggestive of physical abuse. The ears should be examined, as should the mouth. Oral injuries are now recognized as evidence of abuse and may include hematomas and lacerations to the buccal mucosa and the tongue, tears of the frenulum, or avulsion of the teeth. The pharynx may show evidence of sexually transmitted diseases or acute lacerations or abrasions.

The examination of the chest and abdomen should be supplemented by appropriate radiologic procedures to exclude internal injuries.

The extremities should be palpated and inspected to detect the presence of fractures; this examination should also be supplemented by any indicated radiologic procedures.

The genitals deserve special attention, even if sexual abuse is not initially suspected. In boys, the external genitals should be examined for evidence of trauma and sexually transmitted diseases. Female genitals should be assessed for the size and shape of the vaginal introitus, the condition of the hymen, and evidence of trauma to the perineum, and to the vulva in particular. If at all possible, it is best to perform this evaluation without the presence of a Foley catheter.

The anus and rectum should be inspected for evidence of trauma, and any laxity of the anal sphincters should be noted.

A more detailed description of the genital examination follows in the discussion of sexual abuse.

The skin and soft tissues require a thorough examination, which should be repeated at regular intervals during the first few days to document the appearance and resolution of any bruises and hematomas that may not be clearly visible on admission.

Clinical Laboratory and Diagnostic Imaging Studies

The establishment of a suspicion of physical abuse is based on a constellation of data gathered through history taking and physical examination. Clinical laboratory and diagnostic imaging studies are useful in confirming injuries and in ruling out other medical causes that could be associated with the physical findings.

Clinical Laboratory Evaluation

If skin lesions such as petecchiae, bruises and ecchymosis of different ages and sizes, and abrasions are present, hemorrhagic diseases (pancytopenias and leukemia) can be excluded by obtaining a complete blood count and coagulation profile, which includes prothrom-

bin time, partial thromboplastin time, platelet count, bleeding time, and fibrinogen and fibrin split products determinations. The last two may be optional. Normal values can be used to rule out or confirm historical explanations such as "easy bruisability."

Serum electrolyte, glucose, amylase, blood urea nitrogen, and creatinine determinations may be useful if blunt abdominal trauma is suspected because of palpable abdominal masses or tenderness, hematuria, or lower rib fractures.

In addition to the previously mentioned blood studies, liver function and toxicology studies will help elucidate the cause of changes in mental status and acute neurologic deterioration.

When a child presents with severe failure to thrive, intensive care management may include hematologic tests and blood chemistry studies, as well as total protein and albumin determinations. The latter two values will confirm chronic and acute malnutrition.

Urine should be collected for urinalysis to screen for renal trauma, and urine toxicology screens can be used to assess exposure to environmental products, prescription drugs, and illegal substances in children who present with abnormal neurologic signs or seizures. All abnormal screening tests should be duly confirmed.

Diagnostic Imaging Evaluation

Imaging studies are strongly indicated in infants and young children with evidence of physical injury. These studies may reveal evidence of abuse in a child who is initially evaluated for a suspected natural illness or medical emergency.

The radiographic skeletal survey is the method of choice for skeletal imaging in cases of suspected abuse in children 2 years of age or younger.[4] Patients older than 2 years but less than 5 years of age must be assessed carefully and individually based on clinical indicators of abuse. At any age, however, when clinical findings point to specific injuries suggestive of abuse or nonaccidental trauma, a skeletal survey is useful in the evaluation of occult injuries that may be old or new. The skeletal survey must include anterior and posterior views of the long bones of both upper and lower extremities, as well as the feet, hands, pelvis, and skull. Lateral views of the skull and axial skeleton are required components of the survey. Radiologic findings may confirm patterns of injury associated with abuse—that is, metaphyseal lesions, scapular fractures, or other injuries that are specific for abuse.

Long bone x-ray studies are helpful in infants suffering from failure to thrive in order to exclude rickets and osteopenia.

Radionuclide bone scans may provide increased sensitivity for rib fractures, subtle shaft fractures, and areas of periosteal elevation.[5] Bone scans, however, are of more limited value in the detection of bilateral metaphyseal fractures and subtle spinal injuries.

Computed tomography (CT) is an important imaging study that is useful in assessing children with blunt or penetrating trauma to the chest or abdomen. The evaluation of pancreatic injury and duodenal hematoma, which are two characteristic findings associated with nonaccidental injury, is helped by CT.

Ultrasonography may be used to evaluate a patient with lesser signs of acute trauma or a constellation of nonspecific abdominal signs and symptoms without explanation. Ultrasonography produces reasonable studies of pancreatic injury, occult duodenal hematoma, or renal injury. Radionuclide scintigraphy is of value in the assessment of renal contusion and myoglobinuria.

Children and infants with signs and symptoms of intracranial injury must have cranial CT or magnetic resonance imaging (MRI) studies, or both. The presence of intracranial hemorrhage, cerebral contusion, edema or infarct without major explainable trauma is highly suspicious and usually diagnostic of nonaccidental injury. CT is a satisfactory imaging modality for evaluating head injuries and seems to detect subarachnoid hemorrhages better than does MRI. However, some investigators indicate that MRI provides better characterization of the age of the blood in areas of the brain. Furthermore, MRI is very good for depicting subdural hematomas over convexities, cortical contusion, and white matter injuries.[5] MRI is recommended for patients suspected of having intracranial injury when clinical findings are not explained adequately by CT.[6]

Laboratory Evaluation of Sexual Abuse

The suspicion of sexual abuse based on historical data and physical evidence (if present) is further strengthened by laboratory studies that are designed to identify venereal pathogens, exclude pregnancy, and confirm that sexual contact has taken place. The scope of the specimen collection depends on the history and physical examination findings, as well as on the time interval between the last episode of sexual contact and the medical evaluation. If sexual abuse has occurred within 72 hours of presentation, evidence of ejaculation may be present. If sexual abuse has occurred more than 72 hours prior to the medical examination, there may be no physical evidence; however, the child may be infected with one or more sexually transmitted diseases.

Tables 86–2 and 86–3 list the tests to be performed, depending on the timing of the suspected sexual activity and the age and gender of the patient.

COLLECTION AND DOCUMENTATION OF FORENSIC DATA

The collection, documentation, and clear presentation of forensic information may play a decisive role in the prosecution and legal outcome of child abuse cases. Public agencies involved in the investigation of these cases rely heavily on medical data to separate organic conditions and potentially accidental events from intentional injuries.

By dating fractures or establishing a time frame for the occurrence of head trauma, physicians can help investigators clarify a chain of events and even inculpate or exculpate a given suspect. In other cases, medical science is still unable to establish the precise timing of

Table 86–2. SEXUAL ABUSE FORENSIC TESTING LAPSE LESS THAN 72 HOURS

Site-Specimen	Test
Vagina-cervix	Gram stain (sperm identification)
	Swabs for seminal fluid (acid phosphatase, semen glycoprotein (P30), mouse antihuman sperm-5 (MHS-5) monoclonal antibody, DNA fingerprinting)*
	Gonorrhea culture†
	Chlamydia culture†
	Routine vaginal culture†
	Wet mount (STD§ and motile sperm)†
Rectum	Wet mount (STD and motile sperm)†
	Swabs for seminal fluid (as above)*
	Gonorrhea culture†
	Chlamydia culture†
Penile urethra	Gonorrhea culture†
	Chlamydia culture†
	Wet mount (STD)†
Oropharynx	Gonorrhea culture†
	Wet mount or Gram stain (sperm)†
	Saliva*
	Swabs for seminal fluid (as above)†
Blood	Serology test for†
	herpes,* syphilis, human immunodeficiency virus antibody,‡ hepatitis‡
	Typing*
Urine	Urinalysis†
	Urine culture†
	Pregnancy in postpubertal girls† (repeat in 2 wk)
Other	Clothing and debris collection*
	Fingernail scraping*
	Hair samples*

*Part of sex offense kit—give to investigators.
†Deliver to hospital laboratory.
‡As indicated.
§STD = sexually transmitted disease.

an event. If the child expires, the forensic pathologist may provide additional data from the postmortem examination.

The value of forensic data can be significantly strengthened by adhering to certain processes—that is, the use of protocols, chain of possession forms, medi-

Table 86–3. SEXUAL ABUSE FORENSIC TESTING LAPSE MORE THAN 72 HOURS

Specimen	Test
Urine	Urinalysis*
	Urine culture*
	Pregnancy in postpubertal girls (repeat in 2 wk)
Blood	Serology tests for human immunodeficiency virus antibody,* hepatitis*
Vaginal-cervical swabs	Gonorrhea culture
	Chlamydia culture
	Routine vaginal culture
	Wet mount (for STD†)
Pharyngeal swab	Gonorrhea culture
Penile urethral swab	Gonorrhea culture
	Chlamydia culture
	Wet mount (for STD†)
Rectal swabs	Gonorrhea culture
	Chlamydia culture

*As indicated.
†STD = sexually transmitted diseases.

colegal forms, sex offense kits, and photographic documentation.

The use of protocols ensures that child abuse evaluations are carried out in an orderly, organized, and predictable manner. Lapses in procedure are decreased, and all the professionals involved work together toward a joint goal. New and unusual issues can be discussed and responses developed prospectively.

Following the collection of specimens to be used for forensic purposes, it is most advantageous to use a chain of possession form to document their passage through the hands of the many individuals who must work with them. This process minimizes potential challenges from defense attorneys. A chain of possession form is essential for toxicology tests and for evidentiary material for sexual abuse cases.

Medicolegal forms are usually issued by police departments and are filled out by the physician examining the victim of alleged child abuse and neglect. Although the forms vary greatly in quality and in the amount of information required, their common purpose is to provide uniformity and consistency in the amount and type of information gathered for all cases investigated in a given jurisdiction. It is necessary to fill out these forms promptly and legibly and to retain a copy for documentation. The medicolegal forms do not replace the medical record, which must be completed concurrently.

Sex offense kits are available commercially and may also be issued by police departments. The kits allow a comprehensive and organized collection process. They are most useful when the suspected sexual contact has taken place less than 72 hours before the examination.

Photography is a useful adjunct to the documentation of physical injuries. It supplements the written word and provides a permanent visual record. Appropriate written consent should be obtained from the parent before photographs are taken.

INTERVENTION

The Multidisciplinary Approach

The complexity of the issues involved in cases of alleged child maltreatment requires a multidisciplinary approach. Physicians—in concert with social workers, psychologists, nurses, and other professionals—evaluate the patient and assess the overall situation. Interagency coordination is also paramount because both the family and the hospital-based professionals must interact with police, child protective services, the courts, and perhaps other child welfare agencies.

The importance of good communication among all parties cannot be overemphasized, nor can any of the professionals afford to forget to focus on the preeminent goal of all their efforts: to ensure that victimized children and their siblings are treated and protected. The corollary to this is that perpetrators will be brought to justice and will receive therapeutic intervention to prevent recidivism.

During the hospitalization of the child victim, the physician can serve as an advocate for the child and as

a liaison with the outside agencies. As discharge planning proceeds, delays in posthospitalization placement or services delivery can be minimized if all the professionals involved are aware of the child's specific needs.

Mental Health Intervention

In most cases of child abuse and neglect, intervention with the family is indicated. Mental health treatment, counseling, and parental skill development may be offered and begun while the child is still hospitalized. The child's medical condition, age, and development will dictate his or her own level of participation in the therapeutic process. The parents, even if they are the alleged abusers, will require support as well as therapy. If these services are not available, the parents should be helped to identify and tap resources in their own network. If the patient should die, the parents will need assistance in dealing with their grief. In these difficult cases, the medical team members should acknowledge their own feelings of sadness, anger, and revulsion. They must also beware of hasty judgments that may impair their efficacy as clinicians or advocates.

Reporting and Legal Issues

The treating physician is legally mandated to report a suspicion of child abuse and neglect. Failure to do so may result in civil or criminal liability or even malpractice litigation. Child abuse statutes, though varying somewhat from jurisdiction to jurisdiction, generally provide immunity from civil and criminal liability if a report is made in good faith, which implies both the presence of reasonable suspicion and the lack of malice.

The physician may be called to court to testify regarding the findings. Communication with the prosecutor (or defense attorney) prior to the trial will increase the likelihood that the physician's testimony will be most effectively used to clarify the presenting issues. The physician may be placed on call with the court to minimize disruptions to his or her schedule; a request to the court for "on-call" status, which is made through the attorney issuing the subpoena, is usually honored.

In addition to factual testimony, a physician may be asked to render an expert opinion about the possible mechanism of injury or the natural course of an illness. Although the ultimate decision is the province of the judge or jury, the physician may, when asked, make a statement about the likelihood that abuse or neglect has occurred. One must not, however, succumb to the temptation to designate an offender, though any statement made by the child about the identity of the perpetrator should be related to the court.

Even in the most hectic conditions, it is prudent for the physician to document any statement made to an attorney about the specifics of a case. Casual telephone conversations with attorneys (or anyone else) are better avoided, as words may be quoted—or misquoted—later when memories have faded.

Careful documentation will again prove its usefulness

after time has passed. It is always necessary to maintain clear, legible, and objectively written records.

When parents are the alleged offenders, questions may arise regarding their right to visit the hospitalized child. The physician should determine whether there is a court order restricting visitation; this information can be provided by the investigating agency.

Parental participation may also be an issue when important treatment decisions could conceivably have an impact on the outcome of the case. Termination of life support, for example, may shift a case from the realm of child abuse to that of homicide, which carries a much more serious legal penalty. In extreme cases, the help of the hospital's ethics committee might be sought. In other instances, a guardian might be appointed by the court to assist in determining the best interests of the child.

PHYSICAL ABUSE

The battered child syndrome, as described by Kempe and associates[9] more than 30 years ago, refers to the repeated abuse of infants and children, which is evidenced by objective indicia of healed and healing injuries involving the skin, viscera, or skeleton.[8] By conservative estimates, 1 to 2% of children in the United States are victims of nonaccidental or intentional injury. Reportedly 10% of injuries evaluated in hospital emergency departments in children less than 5 years of age result from abuse, and the victims are usually less than 2 years old.[9]

Severely injured children unfortunately require medical and surgical management in intensive care settings and often present difficult diagnostic challenges. Physicians must often distinguish inflicted injuries from other medical causes. Skillful diagnostic intervention includes thorough, nonjudgmental interviewing techniques; familiarity with normal child development; knowledge of objective clinical findings that are suggestive of physical abuse; and the use of laboratory procedures and other diagnostic data that can elucidate findings consistent with abuse.

Most often, clinical manifestations of physical abuse are represented by soft tissue injuries with involvement of trunk, arms, head, neck, and lower body. Usually, skin lesions most characteristic of abuse include bruises, ecchymoses, and lacerations. These lesions may be in various stages of healing, involve multiple body sites, or have distinctive patterns like loop marks, slap marks, pinch marks, bites, fingertip bruises, or grab marks. Typical sites for nonaccidental bruises include the buttocks, genitals, earlobes, frenulum of the tongue, and neck. The discoloration of a contusion or bruise to the skin may be useful in estimating the time of injury (Table 86–4).

Bite marks should raise suspicion of inflicted injury, depending on the location, size, shape, diameter, and number of tooth marks. If the intercanine distance is greater than 3 cm, the bite is consistent with permanent teeth or someone older than 8 years of age.

Physical examination may reveal ocular damage, in-

Table 86–4. AGE ESTIMATION OF CONTUSIONS*

Contusion Age	Discoloration
<24 hr	Red to blue or purple
1–5 days	Blue to purple
5–7 days	Green
10–14 days	Yellow to brown
2–4 wk	Resolution

*Modified from Wilson EF: Estimation of the age of cutaneous contusions in child abuse. Reproduced by permission of Pediatrics Vol. 60, p. 750. Copyright, 1977.

cluding hyphema, dislocated lens, detached retina, and retinal hemorrhage. Retinal hemorrhages may be a clue to head trauma, particularly subdural hematomas in infants and children with unexplained central nervous system findings. They may last from 3 to 21 days.

A challenging issue arises when an acutely ill child with no known history of trauma is found to have retinal hemorrhages following pulmonary resuscitation. Overzealous efforts by untrained individuals have been implicated as a possible cause. Bacon and colleagues[11] described this injury in a 2-month-old child in whom resuscitation was implemented with back slaps. The resuscitation was not witnessed, and abuse could not be proved. Kanter[12] investigated the possibility of the association of cardiopulmonary resuscitation (CPR) and retinal hemorrhage in a group of 54 children who underwent witnessed CPR. Six children had retinal hemorrhages, and all had conditions that could account for retinal hemorrhages—that is, four children had evidence of physical abuse, one was injured in a motor vehicle accident, and one was hypertensive. A prospective study of children undergoing resuscitation was conducted by Goetting.[14] It revealed that 2 of 20 patients (10%) who had no history or physical evidence of preceding trauma and no history of conditions associated with retinal hemorrhage had findings positive for retinal hemorrhage shortly after resuscitative efforts were completed. One child was a drowning victim and the other was diagnosed with sudden infant death syndrome. In both cases, a complete autopsy showed no evidence of trauma.[13]

Levin's[14] review of this subject re-emphasizes the necessity of ruling out the possibility of traumatic injury in any child admitted in cardiorespiratory arrest who is found to have retinal hemorrhage. This ophthalmologic finding should not be dismissed as being merely secondary to resuscitative efforts; it warrants a thorough evaluation for trauma after other medical conditions associated with retinal hemorrhages have been excluded.

Nonaccidental or inflicted head trauma may cause subdural hematomas, subarachnoid hemorrhages, scalp contusions, subgaleal hematomas, and traumatic alopecia. Guthkelch[15] and Caffey[16] were among the first to describe the shaken baby syndrome with its classic triad of intracranial injuries, retinal hemorrhages, and long bone fractures in young infants. Investigations by Duhaime and colleagues[17] demonstrated that in addition to shaking, a direct blow to the head was probably necessary to cause the extent of injury usually observed in these children. Usually these infants are less than 1 year of age; lack significant external stigmas of inflicted injury; and require intensive care management for coma, elevated intracranial pressure, seizures, or respiratory arrest. Helfer[18] and Billmire[19] and their colleagues have demonstrated the unlikely causation of severe head injury (i.e., subdural bleeding) by minor injury such as falls from cribs or beds. Children sustaining severe head injury from abuse may die or suffer permanent neurologic sequelae.

Blunt trauma to the abdomen is the most lethal form of physical abuse. These injuries include ruptured liver or spleen, intestinal perforation, duodenal hematomas, pancreatic injuries, and renal injuries. Since there may have been delay in seeking treatment, there may be no visible bruises or marks on the abdominal wall. Approximately 50% of these children who require inpatient care succumb to massive hemorrhagic shock from internal blood loss or septic shock.[20]

Nonaccidental skeletal injuries are a common manifestation of physical abuse. The type of fracture and the location, number, and age of injuries may be helpful in distinguishing accidental from nonaccidental trauma. A variety of skeletal injuries occurs in abused children, including metaphyseal lesions, diaphyseal fractures, dislocations, and periosteal new bone formation. The metaphyseal "corner fracture" or "bucket handle" lesion is virtually pathognomonic of infant abuse. Other skeletal injuries that are highly characteristic of nonaccidental trauma include posterior rib fractures, scapular fractures, sternal fractures, and spinous process fractures. Lateral and anterior rib fractures are suspicious injuries. Occasionally, the critical care specialist is required to decide whether a child's rib fractures are the result of abuse or CPR. The association between resuscitation and rib fractures is rare; it has been studied by several researchers,[11–14] and the subject is discussed earlier in this chapter.

A number of medical problems must be considered prior to making a firm diagnosis of child abuse. Some of these conditions may be life-threatening and require intense medical management. Conversely, some physical findings may be incidental and the result of medical folk practices or cultural beliefs.

A diagnosis of child abuse is not easily retracted, and it frequently leads to the involvement of the family with a number of public systems. Consequently, a careful exploration of diagnostic possibilities should establish a medical basis for unusual or challenging presenting problems, thus eliminating the need for an unnecessary investigation (Table 86–5).

SEXUAL ABUSE

Sexual abuse is usually not the presenting complaint in patients receiving intensive care. If the primary cause of injury is sexual abuse, it has usually been carried out in a violent manner and the assessment is obvious. The greater diagnostic challenge is posed by the child who is being treated for other problems and who is found, during the course of hospitalization, to have abnormal genital conditions or a sexually transmitted disease, or both. Thus, it is necessary for every child who is admit-

Table 86–5. DIFFERENTIAL DIAGNOSIS OF CHILD ABUSE BY ORGAN SYSTEM

Organ System	Differential Diagnosis
Integument and soft tissue	Impetigo
	Mongolian spots
	Cao Gao (coining)[23]
	Staph scalded skin syndrome
	Cupping[24]
	Moxibustion[25]
	Healed chickenpox marks
	Multiple nevi and café au lait spots
	Phytophotodermatitis
	Dermatorrhexis
	Ehlers-Danlos syndrome (type I)
	Idiopathic thrombocytopenia purpura
	Hemophilia
	von Willebrand disease
	Schönlein-Henoch purpura
	Vasculitis
	Erythema multiforme
Skeletal system	Osteogenesis imperfecta
	Congenital syphilis
	Leukemia
	Osteomyelitis
	Vitamin A intoxication
	Caffey disease
	Rickets
	Scurvy
	Osteopenia secondary to chronic illness
Ocular system	Coagulopathies
	Neoplasm
	Hypertension
	Infection (meningitis)
	Arteriovenous malformation
Gastrointestinal system	Peritonitis
	Meckel diverticulum
	Renal stone
	Torsion of spermatic cord
	Ovarian cyst
Central nervous system	Mollera caida (fallen fontanelle)[26]
	Infection
	Neoplasm
	Metabolic abnormalities

ted to an intensive care unit to have a thorough and comprehensive physical examination so that any unexpected findings will be detected before a succession of procedures takes place (e.g., catheterization, repeated rectal examinations, rectal temperature determinations, or enema administration) that might obscure the initial presentation.

If there is any question about the interpretation of the genital examination, the assistance of an experienced examiner should be sought to exclude normal anatomic variations or other genital conditions that might mimic sexual victimization. The physical examination should document the size of the hymenal opening (introitus) by measuring the horizontal and vertical diameters. The condition of the hymen should be stated, specifying tears, lacerations, irregularities, and sharpness or roundness of borders. The presence of scar tissue or a change in vascular pattern should be observed. Any vaginal or urethral discharge should be noted.

Bruises, scarring, fissures, skin tags, or genital warts should be described if present in the perianal area. Laxity of the anal sphincters should be noted. Any such laxity is a troubling finding: Although it may be observed in children who are paralyzed or in certain conditions with neurologic or gastrointestinal manifestations, its presence should alert the examiner to the possibility of sexual victimization and the need to intensify scrutiny for other potential findings. Sphincter laxity should be monitored and can be expected to resolve once the precipitating cause is no longer present.

The presence of genital warts (condyloma acuminata) should lead to a careful assessment because it raises concern about sexual contact. Although maternal transmission during childbirth may be the source of the infection in infants, this explanation does not apply to older children.

Whenever sexual abuse is suspected, the parents should be gently queried about any past history of gastrointestinal or genitourinary problems. It is important to strike a balance between gathering as much information as possible and creating undue anxiety in parents who may already be under considerable stress. Because child sexual abuse is usually accomplished by someone close to the child and carried out in a nonviolent manner, which very often causes minimal physical trauma, it is difficult to make the diagnosis without a history, particularly in the case of a severely ill child who may be subjected to a variety of procedures and attended by a number of professionals.

If any doubt remains or if antibiotics must be administered for other reasons, it is imperative to test the patient for sexually transmitted diseases, the presence of which can be a strong indicator of sexual abuse. Because there may be only one opportunity to retrieve the offending organisms, specimens should be obtained and handled through a chain of possession procedure, following the hospital's child sexual abuse protocol. Rapid diagnostic tests have no place in this process because they are not acceptable in court as incontrovertible evidence. Their lack of specificity may raise more questions than answers and may leave a lingering lack of resolution about issues deeply disturbing to both the family and the medical team.

The laboratory investigation includes tests for the most common sexually transmitted diseases. Specimens for gonorrhea culture should be obtained from the pharynx, the male urethra, the vagina, and the rectum. Even without a history of contact at multiple sites, it is not impossible to recover the organism at locations not mentioned initially by the victim of abuse.

Chlamydia cultures are useful for the vagina, urethra, and rectum. They must be carefully interpreted in children younger than 3 years of age to exclude the persistence of infection acquired at birth.

A wet mount of vaginal secretions will separate a yeast infection, trichomoniasis, and bacterial vaginosis from other entities. A routine vaginal culture will further identify nonsexual causes of vaginal discharges.

Herpes cultures are necessary to clarify the cause of ulcerative genital lesions. If similar lesions are present in the buccal mucosa, they should be cultured also.

Although serologic tests for hepatitis B and the human immunodeficiency virus may not be part of a routine evaluation for all cases of suspected child sexual abuse, these tests may be more advisable in the intensive care setting because of the frequent exposure of medical personnel to patients' body fluids. A decision to obtain these tests should be made after reviewing the data produced by the history and physical examination. The practice of universal precautions should minimize the risk of inadvertent transmission.

The results of the diagnostic tests must be reviewed with due caution. Nonsexual transmission of sexually transmitted diseases should be excluded in very young children who may have a persistent infection acquired at birth. Before proceeding with an official report, consultation should be sought with a child protection team or someone else familiar with victimization issues.

The subtleties of the diagnosis should not deter one from exploring the possibility that sexual abuse may have occurred. The great prevalence of this problem in the society at large argues for its presence in any patient population—regardless of class, race, or geography. One should not forego any opportunity to identify and be an advocate for a child at risk.

CHILD NEGLECT

Neglect represents the most common type of child maltreatment. Unlike suspicions of physical abuse, which are based on objective physical and laboratory data, concerns or suspicions of neglect may often emerge gradually during the course of interaction with a child and family. Manifestations of neglect may be interwoven with economic factors, cultural factors, and the educational limitations of the parents.

Although neglect takes many forms, the four presentations most likely to challenge the critical care specialist are (1) failure of supervision; (2) extreme, nonorganic failure to thrive; (3) medical neglect; and (4) abandonment.

Failure of supervision of children, especially infants and toddlers, may lead to serious or even fatal consequences. Children come to the intensive care unit because of near-drownings, falls, serious burns, fractures, or drug ingestions. Although there may have been no intent to cause or allow harm to the child, the seriousness of the situation must be presented to the parents and reported to the appropriate authorities for investigation. Confronting the possibility of maltreatment, and the subsequent reporting that initiates the process of investigation, is essential to prevent recurrence. Because it is so difficult to distinguish a moment of inattention from neglect or even abuse, the comprehensive multidisciplinary approach is very useful.

Extreme, nonorganic failure to thrive may present with symptoms of hypoglycemia, respiratory arrest, or electrolyte imbalance. In this patient population, suspicion should arise when there is no identifiable medical illness to explain the malnourished state of the child. The diagnosis is confirmed when treatment and adequate nutrition promptly resolve the symptoms.

Although starvation usually is associated with other signs of poor physical care in young children, it may also occur in an infant with a mother who provides hygienic care but has a distorted picture of her child.

Despite objective findings of a failure to maintain growth parameters, the mother may deny the problem and insist that the baby is doing quite well. In these instances, a mental health evaluation of the mother is indicated.

Medical neglect may present as a delay in seeking care or as a failure to give the child care or medications that have been prescribed for an acute or chronic condition—for example, the young diabetic child who is not receiving insulin, the asthmatic child who is admitted in respiratory failure after repeated visits to the emergency room showing a lack of blood levels of bronchodilators, or the epileptic patient who is admitted in status epilepticus for the third time without evidence of having been given anticonvulsants.

Assessments of medical neglect require a great deal of caution, and one must ascertain that the parental lapses are not due to financial inability to provide the needed medication or treatment. There must also be clear documentation of previous instructions to the parent. Occasionally, it does happen that poverty, parental cognitive limitations, or lack of communication between parent and health care providers are the cause of medical complications, and thus the situation is not one of neglect.

Abandonment is the ultimate form of child neglect. Although it is less commonly observed, from time to time an infant, usually a newborn, is found abandoned. The baby's condition may range from normal to critical, depending on climate, length of exposure, and degree of dehydration. Cases of abandonment usually create a great deal of public concern, and every effort is made to find the mother. In some circumstances, the infant and mother may be reunited under supervision; in others, the baby is placed out of the home.

OTHER FORMS OF CHILD VICTIMIZATION

Ingestions and poisonings represent a type of abuse or neglect that is difficult to assess. Whether occurring as accidents or as a result of neglect or even abuse, they challenge the critical care specialist.

Inadequate supervision of children or intentional acts may result in the ingestion of household products or over-the-counter or prescription drugs or in exposure to illegal substances.

Children who are felt to be at especially high risk of permanent or fatal consequences are the patients who present with repeated ingestions over a short time. Another group consists of children whose age and developmental level preclude the self-administration of the substance. In these two groups, the motivation of the caretakers and their ability to correct the neglectful behavior or the environment, or both, become essential and must be thoroughly evaluated.

Intentional drugging or poisoning refers to the practice of giving children medications or illegal drugs that are harmful or are not intended for them. These substances include (among others) alcohol, barbiturates, tranquilizers, antidepressants, crack cocaine, and phencyclidine piperidine (PCP).

School-aged children and adolescents who have symptoms of ingestion may be exhibiting suicidal behavior or drug dependency, a situation that is in contrast to clumsy experimentation. After their acute medical problems are resolved, these patients should not be released without an assessment of the circumstances leading to their hospitalization and an exploration of underlying issues such as victimization and depression.

Munchausen by proxy is a syndrome first described by Meadow in 1977.[26] It derives its name from the incredible and unlikely stories told by Baron Von Munchausen, a war veteran who is reputed to have greatly embellished his exploits. The syndrome that bears his name is a form of child abuse that occurs when a parent (usually the mother) creates a factitious illness in the child and thereby subjects the unfortunate victim to repeated diagnostic and therapeutic procedures in an elusive quest for the diagnosis and cure to an imaginary illness. Although initially thought to be a rarity, a number of cases of Munchausen by proxy syndrome have now been identified and described in the literature.[27, 28]

This bizarre condition has both fascinated and frustrated physicians because it is extremely difficult to diagnose and document. The child usually presents with a constellation of symptoms that do not fit any recognizable disease pattern. The medical staff, with characteristic vigor and tenacity, tries to identify the problem, subjecting the child to a variety of ever more invasive procedures. The mother is typically solicitous of the child and very involved with the medical staff, whom she befriends. The mother is usually quite comfortable in the hospital setting and is quite familiar with medical terminology and procedures. Her "model" behavior initially brings her much attention and appreciation from the staff.

Concerns usually arise after a number of tests have been performed without any clarity or definite progress in arriving at a diagnosis. Occasionally the mother's machinations are discovered accidentally (e.g., feeding her child unprescribed medication, falsifying tests, suffocating or other active provocation of life-threatening symptoms).

In a review of the literature, Rosenberg reported on 117 cases of Munchausen by proxy.[29] She found an even sex distribution and a mean age of 39.8 months ± 32.1 months. The mean time from onset of symptoms to diagnosis was 14.9 months ± 14 months. The children's ages ranged from birth to adolescence.

Although this condition might at first appear merely as an oddity, it carries sizeable long-term morbidity and a mortality rate of 9%. In Rosenberg's series, the symptoms prior to death included apnea, alteration in the state of consciousness, bleeding, seizures, and diarrhea. The children who died were all less than 3 years of age. In 20% of the cases, the diagnosis had been suspected prior to death, and the parents had been confronted. The children were subsequently sent home, only to die there in their parents' care.

Suspected cases of Munchausen syndrome by proxy require the same level of attention and concern as do other cases of child abuse. Even more than others, they require a multidisciplinary approach and legal intervention to protect the child.

CONCLUSION

Child maltreatment presents a serious and additional challenge to physicians caring for critically ill children. Although physicians may be tempted in the middle of the investigation to consider this issue the province of other disciplines, they should be aware of their vital role in identifying and intervening in this potentially life-threatening condition. Collaboration with other colleagues and use of a multidisciplinary approach will facilitate the task at hand and reduce the likelihood that cases will be missed or mishandled.

References

1. Gil D: Violence Against Children. Boston, Harvard University Press, 1970.
2. Kempe CH: Incest and other forms of sexual abuse. *In:* Kempe CH and Helfer RE (eds): The Battered Child. Chicago, Chicago University Press, 1980.
3. Schmidt BD: Child neglect. *In:* Ellerstein N (ed): Child Abuse and Neglect—a Medical Reference. New York, Churchill Livingstone, 1981.
4. Haller JO, Kleinman PK, Merten DF, et al: Diagnostic imaging of child abuse. Pediatrics 87:262, 1991.
5. Sato Y, Yuh WTC, Smith WL, et al: Head injury in child abuse: Evaluation with MR imaging. Radiology 173:653, 1989.
6. Kleinman P: Diagnostic imaging of child abuse. Baltimore, Williams & Wilkins, 1987.
7. Paradise J: The medical evaluation of the sexually abused child. Pediatr Clin North Am 37:4, 1990.
8. Kempe CH, Silverman FN, Steele FF, et al: The battered child syndrome. JAMA 181:17, 1962.
9. Schmitt BD and Kempe CH: Abuse and neglect in children. *In:* Behrman RE and Vaughan VC (eds): Nelson's Textbook of Pediatrics, 12th ed. Philadelphia, WB Saunders, 1983, p 100.
10. Wilson EF: Estimation of the age of cutaneous contusions in child abuse. Pediatrics 60:750, 1977.
11. Bacon CJ, Sayer GC, and Howe JW: Extensive retinal hemorrhages in infancy—an innocent cause. Br Med J 1:281, 1978.
12. Kanter RK: Retinal hemorrhages after cardio-pulmonary resuscitation or child abuse. J Pediatr 180:430, 1986.
13. Goetting M: Retinal hemorrhage after cardiopulmonary resuscitation in children: An etiologic reevaluation. Pediatrics 85:585, 1990.
14. Levin AV: Retinal hemorrhages after cardio-pulmonary resuscitation: Literature review and commentary. Pediatr Emerg Care 2:269, 1986.
15. Guthkelch AN: Infantile subdural hematoma and its relationship to whiplash injuries. Br Med J 2:430, 1971.
16. Caffey J: On the theory and practice of shaking infants. Am J Dis Child 124:161, 1972.
17. Duhaime AC, Gennarelli TA, Thibault LE, et al: The shaken baby syndrome: A clinical, pathological and biomechanical study. J Neurosurg 66:409, 1987.
18. Helfer RE, Slovis TL, and Black M: Injuries resulting when small children fall out of bed. Pediatrics 60:533, 1977.
19. Billmire EM and Myers PA: Serious head injury in infants: Accident or abuse? Pediatrics 75:340, 1985.
20. Wissow L: Child Advocacy for the Clinician. Baltimore, Williams & Wilkins, 1990, p. 75.
21. Feldman KW and Brewer DK: Child abuse, cardiopulmonary resuscitation and rib fractures. Pediatrics 73:339, 1984.
22. Yeatman GW, Shaw C, Barlow MJ, et al: Pseudo-battering in Vietnamese children. Pediatrics 58:616, 1976.
23. Asnes RS and Wisotsky DH: Cupping lesions simulating child abuse. J Pediatr 99:267, 1981.
24. Feldman KW: Pseudo-abusive burns in asian refugees. Am J Dis Child 138:168, 1984.
25. Guarnaschelli J, Lee J, and Pitts FW: "Fallen fontanelle" (Caida de mollera): A variant of the battered child syndrome. JAMA 222:1545, 1972.
26. Meadows R: Munchausen by proxy: The hinterland of child abuse. Lancet 2:343, 1977.
27. McGuire TL and Feldman KW: Psychologic morbidity of children subjected to Munchausen by proxy. Pediatrics 83:289, 1989.
28. Chan DA, Salcedo JR, Atkins DM, et al: Munchausen syndrome by proxy: A review and case study. J Pediatr Psychol 11:71, 1986.
29. Rosenberg DA: Web of deceit: A literature review of Munchausen syndrome by proxy. Child Abuse Neglect 11:547, 1987.

Burns in Children

Robert J. Attorri, M.D., Judson G. Randolph, M.D., and
Orrawin Trocki, M.S., R.D.

Thermal injuries afflict approximately 60,000 children each year in the United States. Nearly 2,000 of these children die, making burns the second leading cause of death in children 1 to 4 years of age, and the third leading cause of death in all children (after motor vehicle accidents and drownings).[1] Among survivors, burns result in a spectrum of anatomic, physiologic, psychologic, and social injuries, some of which may have devastating and lifelong consequences. Because of their potential severity and their protean effects, burns, more than any other traumatic injury, require a dedicated multidisciplinary team of health care providers for successful treatment and rehabilitation. Our care provider team for the burn patient includes surgeons, critical care physicians, nurses, nutritionists, psychiatrists, physical therapists, occupational therapists, social workers, and child life therapists.

More than 80% of all burns occur in the home; 84% of burn deaths result from house fires. More than one third of all fatal house fires are caused by cigarettes, including 15% of fires that kill children.[2] Scald burns are the most common type of burn in children and are especially prevalent in children less than 3 years of age. These burns are more likely to be partial-thickness than full-thickness injuries; but full-thickness skin injury is not uncommon in scalds, especially in scalds intentionally inflicted. Infants are usually burned by immersion in a tub or sink of hot water, unlike toddlers who are typically scalded by hot liquids that they spill or pull off of a hot surface. Flame burns are more common in children older than 3 years of age and account for the majority of full-thickness burns and burn mortalities. Young children tend to be burned by flames from matches, stoves, and cigarette lighters as a result of curiosity, whereas adolescents are burned by the use of matches in the proximity of gasoline or other flammable material.

Sadly, burns occurring as a result of child abuse account for 10 to 15% of all burns in children.[3] The overwhelming majority of inflicted burns are scalds, and nearly two thirds of injured children will have a typical immersion pattern of injury. These burns carry an alarming mortality rate of 30% (compared with 2% for accidental burns), and children who survive an intentional burn face a high risk for repeated injury. Consequently, recognition of the immersion burn pattern and identification of abuse cases is essential.

PREVENTION

Significant advances in the care of burned patients have been made, but the epidemiologic data point to the undeniable fact that the most plausible and effective means of burn management is prevention. Prevention consists mainly of eliminating the burn source but also includes alarms and extinguishing devices.

The great majority of burns are scalds, which usually occur in the home, frequently from the hot water source. The extent of burn injury is directly related to the water temperature and length of exposure (Fig. 87–1). The hot water temperature may be as high as 150°F in a home system, which can cause full-thickness injury in 1 to 5 seconds. By lowering the hot water temperature to 120°F, a temperature adequate for home use, the risk of scald burn injury can be largely eliminated, as only long exposure at this temperature (> 10 minutes) results in significant injury.[4]

Measures to prevent flame injuries are more complicated and more difficult to enact. Appropriate legislation has been enacted that mandates flame-retardant sleepware for children. This measure offers some protection but is inadequate in larger fires. The development of cigarettes that have little or no propensity to ignite furniture is technically possible and would save the lives of more than 100 children annually, but to date no law mandating such a development has been passed. Playing with cigarette lighters leads to 800 childhood burns and 120 deaths annually. Child-resistant lighters could be commercially available. The mandatory installation of home sprinklers and effective fire alarm systems has also been advocated, but usage is not widespread. It has already been demonstrated that the presence of properly functioning smoke detectors reduces the risk of dying in a fire by 50%. Effective and affordable residential sprinkler systems are available, but the cost of installation in existing structures is prohibitive, thus limiting the usefulness of this concept. Overall, as many as 75% of serious pediatric burns and burn deaths could be

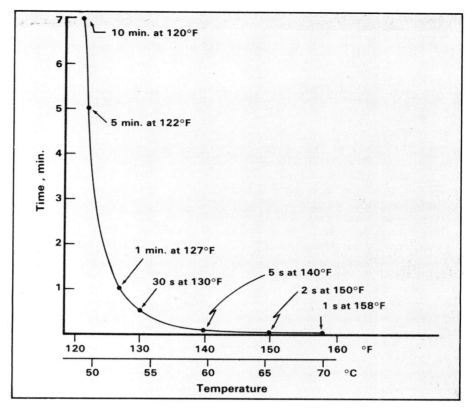

Figure 87–1. Necessary time of exposure with water of various temperatures to produce full-thickness burn. (Reproduced with permission from Katcher M: Scald burns from hot tap water. JAMA 246:1219, 1981. Copyright 1981, American Medical Association.)

prevented by a serious nationwide consensus on prevention.

INITIAL EVALUATION

Children have body proportions that are different from those of adults, and Lund-Browder charts are more practical guides in estimating the extent of injury than "the rule of nines."

The depth of burns is described as first, second, or third degree. Some authors prefer the designations partial- or full-thickness injury. First-degree burns are confined to the epidermis. They cause erythema, pain, and edema but heal spontaneously in 5 to 10 days without scarring. Second-degree burns are partial-thickness injuries that penetrate into, but not entirely through, the dermis. These burns are further classified as superficial or deep injuries, depending on the extent of dermal penetration. Superficial injuries are erythematous, have vesicle formation, and are very painful. If they do not become infected, they will heal completely in 2 to 4 weeks. Deep partial-thickness injuries may have a white, waxy appearance and may be difficult to distinguish from full-thickness or third-degree burns. In these deep second-degree burns, very little of the skin appendages remain, and healing may take as long as 6 weeks, often with permanent unsightly hypertrophic scars and severe wound contraction. Full-thickness burns penetrate the entire thickness of the skin and are insensate wounds that heal only by epidermal ingrowth from the edges of the wound or by the application of split-thickness skin

grafts. It is noteworthy that infants and young children have thinner skin than do older subjects and are therefore more likely to experience deep and full-thickness injuries.

Burn patients are initially evaluated and treated like any critically ill patient (i.e., with attention to airway, breathing, and circulation). Any patient with a compromised airway or hemodynamic status requires hospital admission. Many patients require admission on the basis of the extent or location of their skin injury (Table 87–1). Any child with a burn wound in excess of 10% of the total body surface area (TBSA) has sufficient wound care needs and risks of wound complication to warrant admission to a hospital. Additionally, in our institution, all children with burns to the face, hands, feet, or perineum are admitted even if the area of the burn is small. Any child who is the suspected victim of abuse is admitted regardless of the extent of burn injury, and the Child Protective Service is notified immediately.

Partial-thickness burns that become infected may develop into full-thickness injuries; therefore, it is essential to ensure an environment for proper wound care. Children whose home situation appears inadequate for appropriate wound care are admitted to the hospital.

Table 87–1. CRITERIA FOR ADMISSION TO CHILDREN'S HOSPITAL NATIONAL MEDICAL CENTER

1. >10%
2. Key areas—face, hand, foot, genitals
3. Possible child abuse
4. Inadequate home care

Because of the risk of full-thickness injury and possible permanent disability, hospital admission should be carried out in any questionable circumstance.

INHALATIONAL INJURY

Establishing an adequate airway and assuring sufficient ventilation are the crucial first steps during resuscitation of any patient. Attention to airway and breathing is of similar importance in the treatment of the burned child because of the injury that the thermal insult can inflict on the airway and lung parenchyma. Respiratory embarrassment is most commonly associated with direct inhalational injury. Signs, symptoms, and historical data characteristically associated with inhalational injury should be carefully sought during initial evaluation. Burns occurring in closed spaces lead to high concentrations of irritating and toxic combustion products and commonly cause inhalational injury.

Physical findings that should alert the examiner to the possibility of inhalational injury include burns to the head and neck region, evidence of upper airway mucosal injury, carbonaceous sputum, and altered mental status. Mucosal injuries appear as hyperemia with ulceration and blistering and almost always indicate damage to the distal airways and pulmonary parenchyma. Carbonaceous sputum is virtually pathognomonic for inhalational injury. An altered mental state can occur from carbon monoxide inhalation. Loss of consciousness suggests significant carbon monoxide intoxication, but headaches, confusion, visual changes, hallucinations, seizures, and coma are also typical symptoms of hypercarbia.

The pathophysiology of inhalational injury involves three mechanisms: (1) direct thermal injury, (2) chemical injury from noxious combustion products, and (3) carbon monoxide intoxication. Direct thermal injury affects primarily the upper airways, and inhaled vapors are effectively cooled to body temperature by the nasal mucosa and proximal airways. The products of combustion cause a chemical injury to the airway mucosa and can be inhaled deeply into the lungs, causing damage to distal airways and pulmonary parenchyma. Carbon monoxide, a byproduct of combustion, is responsible for most respiratory deaths following burns. It acts by depriving the blood of its oxygen-carrying capacity, which leads to asphyxia. Carbon monoxide has 200 times greater affinity for hemoglobin than does oxygen, and once bound to hemoglobin it forms carboxyhemoglobin, which impairs oxygen transport. Carbon monoxide also shifts the oxyhemoglobin dissociation curve to the left, which diminishes unloading of oxygen in the tissues. Carbon monoxide poisoning can bring about major neurologic changes and can even result in cardiopulmonary arrest and death. The most effective treatment of carbon monoxide poisoning is 100% oxygen (delivered in a hyperbaric oxygen chamber, if available), and we therefore provide 100% oxygen for our burned patients until carboxyhemoglobin levels and blood gas determinations have been obtained.

Patients in whom inhalational injury is strongly suspected should undergo bronchoscopy promptly. Evidence of mucosal injury will confirm the diagnosis, and the development of respiratory insufficiency can then be carefully monitored. Treatment is directed by the patient's symptoms, arterial blood gas determinations, and chest x-ray films. Some patients require only chest percussion and tracheal suctioning, whereas those with more severe distal injuries frequently require mechanical ventilation and positive end-expiratory pressure. Such patients usually require 7 to 10 days before their inhalational injury heals. The airway is maintained via nasotracheal or endotracheal intubation. Because of a high rate of complications in burned patients, tracheostomy is avoided except for patients in whom intubation is impossible and for those who require long-term ventilatory support.[5] Prophylactic antibiotics have not been demonstrated to be efficacious and may lead to emergence of highly resistant organisms. Cultures of respiratory secretions are monitored, and culture-proven infections are treated accordingly. Steroids have not been shown to be of value.

Cutaneous injury alone usually has little detrimental effect on pulmonary function, but fluid administration during the resuscitation phase may exacerbate pulmonary injury. Circumferential burns to the neck and thorax may severely impede ventilation and may require escharotomy.

FLUID MANAGEMENT

The skin is the largest organ of the body, composing 15% of total body weight, and it serves as a barrier to infection and as a means of homeostasis. In its role of thermal regulation, the skin permits heat loss via evaporation of free water. An intact cutaneous covering allows approximately 15 ml/m^2/hr of water loss, but with a deep partial-thickness or full-thickness burn, this rate may increase tenfold. Substantial intravascular volume can be lost not only by markedly increased evaporative losses but also by shifting of large volumes from the vascular to the interstitial space in the burn wound. During the first 24 hours following a burn, increased capillary permeability is accompanied by the egress of water, electrolytes, and serum proteins from the vascular compartments. A combination of evaporative loss and capillary leak can lead to catastrophic intravascular volume loss within a few hours in major burns. Thus, the recognition of these losses and reinstitution of intravascular fluid are vital in preventing shock, cardiac failure, acute renal insufficiency, and death.

Resuscitation of the burn victim begins immediately following the procurement of a secure airway and the establishment of adequate ventilation. Intravenous access is obtained in any burn exceeding 10% TBSA by the placement of at least one large intravenous (IV) line. Depending on the size of the burn and the size of the patient, more than one line may be needed. Although it is not preferred, initial IV access lines may be placed directly through the burned skin, because infection of the burn wound is not a problem until later in the period following injury.

The rate of fluid administration is based on the patient's weight and the calculated percentage of the burn[6] (Fig. 87–2). Newer formulas have been proposed, but it is important to remember that any formula serves only as an initial guide, and early and frequent adjustment of the rate of fluid administration is necessary (see also Chapter 58). Because of the capillary leak during the first 24 hours following a burn injury, no colloids are used. The Parkland formula is a handy guide for beginning therapy: 4 ml of lactated Ringer/kg/% burn area, with half of this amount given within the first 8 hours after the injury (not the first 8 hours of hospitalization) and the second half given during the following 16 hours. After the first 24 hours, colloids may be introduced to add an osmotic effect to fluid in the vascular space. Hypotonic saline and dextrose solution is useful to correct any volume deficit that remains.

Some workers advocate hypertonic solutions in the belief that adequate vascular volume can be maintained with less intravenous volume administration and less tissue edema. The superiority of this method has not been proved, and most burn care specialists continue to use isotonic fluid resuscitation, particularly in children. Once resuscitation has commenced, patient response must be carefully monitored. In victims with large burns in which hemodynamic changes occur, this includes electrocardiographic monitoring, blood pressure determinations, and urine output measurements. A Foley catheter is placed at the time of admission and output is recorded hourly. The IV fluid rate is adjusted to maintain 1 to 1.5 ml/kg/hr of urine output. Less than this amount can lead to poor renal perfusion, whereas greater amounts are often accompanied by undesirable tissue edema. Patients with hemoglobinuria or myoglobinuria require higher urine output in order to dilute these substances and avoid renal failure. Patients who have pigment in their urine should receive mannitol and additional sodium bicarbonate in the IV fluid in order to alkalize the urine and prevent precipitation of pigments.

In very sick patients and in those in whom peripheral access is difficult, a central venous catheter is promptly placed. This allows another important monitoring source, for central venous pressure of 8 to 12 cm H_2O usually indicates adequate fluid resuscitation. In addition to urine output, specific gravity, and central venous pressure, the peripheral circulation must be continually assessed.

Full-thickness burn injury combined with underlying tissue swelling can produce a tourniquet effect, rendering an arm or a leg pulseless and ischemic. This development represents a surgical emergency and escharotomy is performed on the affected part, whether it is a trunk or an extremity, as soon as vascular compromise is noted. This can be performed in the emergency department or at the child's bedside, because the eschar is insensate, and anesthesia is unnecessary. The incision is carried down deep enough to allow the burn wound edges to separate. In addition to vascular compromise, the onset of neurologic symptoms in an extremity is also an indication for decompressive escharotomy.

A nasogastric tube should be placed during the resuscitation phase in all patients with major burns, as ileus and gastric distention so frequently accompany these injuries. Gastric pH is monitored, and antacid therapy, usually in the form of cimetidine and an antacid, is used to maintain a gastric pH greater than 5.5.

Burn injuries can be extremely painful, and the frenzied events that often surround the event can exacerbate this pain, as well as cause substantial fear and anxiety. Once the patient is stabilized, a narcotic analgesic, usually morphine 0.1 ml/kg IV, and an antianxiety agent such as midazolam, 0.05 ml/kg IV, are useful.

WOUND CARE AND COVERAGE

Burn care begins with an inspection and size estimate in the emergency department. This takes place while the initial resuscitative measures are being performed.

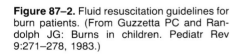

Figure 87–2. Fluid resuscitation guidelines for burn patients. (From Guzzetta PC and Randolph JG: Burns in children. Pediatr Rev 9:271–278, 1983.)

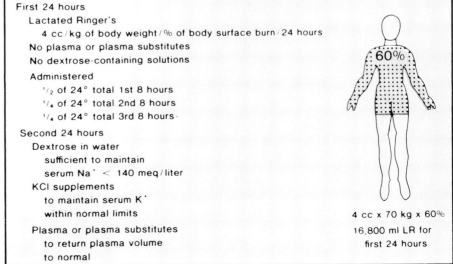

First 24 hours
  Lactated Ringer's
    4 cc/kg of body weight/% of body surface burn/24 hours
  No plasma or plasma substitutes
  No dextrose-containing solutions
  Administered
    1/2 of 24° total 1st 8 hours
    1/4 of 24° total 2nd 8 hours
    1/4 of 24° total 3rd 8 hours
Second 24 hours
  Dextrose in water
    sufficient to maintain
    serum Na^+ < 140 meq/liter
  KCl supplements
    to maintain serum K^+
    within normal limits
  Plasma or plasma substitutes
    to return plasma volume
    to normal

60%

4 cc × 70 kg × 60%
16,800 ml LR for first 24 hours

Sterile dressings soaked in cold saline solution reduce pain and can be left in place for 30 minutes to 1 hour. In small children, longer application may lead to hypothermia. The child's tetanus status is confirmed, and a booster is given if indicated. Antibiotics are not given routinely.

The wounds are débrided of loose tissue and blisters and then scrubbed with soap and water to which saline has been added. Leaching of sodium from the patient occurs if pure water is used, which can lead to clinically dangerous hyponatremia. Following débridement and washing, the wounds are gently dried and covered with silver sulfadiazine (Silvadene). Following this application, dry gauze dressings are applied and are wrapped with sterile gauze bandage followed by an elastic bandage. Burns of the face or ears are treated with antimicrobial ointment and covered with nonadherent dressing. Burned fingers and toes are individually dressed with gauze. Following the initial wound care, burns are débrided, cleansed, and dressed twice a day. The face is dressed three times daily. Between dressing changes, extremities are kept elevated, and joints involved with burn wounds are splinted in position of function to maintain maximum mobility. Superficial partial-thickness burns should heal with this regimen in about 10 to 20 days. Deeper wounds require up to 4 to 6 weeks to heal completely and may be more effectively cared for by excision and skin grafting. Such surfaces must be observed daily during the early period following burn injury, especially in children, for many apparently deep burns that initially appear unlikely to heal in fact may have dermal buds that grow and become covered with epithelium. All full-thickness burns and many deep partial-thickness burns will require excision and grafting.

The two most important factors that prevent successful burn wound healing are infection and poor nutrition, either of which can delay or halt healing.

An alternative to a prolonged course of dressing changes is the application of a skin substitute, such as porcine skin (xenograft) or artificial skin. This requires a very clean wound and no evidence of sepsis. At the first sign of wound sepsis, the skin substitute must be removed and dressing changes resumed.

Deep partial-thickness and full-thickness burns that will require more than 3 weeks to heal are usually best treated with split-thickness autografts. Coverage of deep burn wounds may be viewed as having two components, the first being the removal of burn eschar and preparation of the site for grafting and the second being actual closure (coverage) of the wound. In cases in which the burn size is less than 30% of TBSA, these components may be realized simultaneously, as there will be adequate skin available for complete coverage. Extensive burns usually require a staged approach.

Burn excision and graft site preparation are usually begun when the patient is hemodynamically stable.[7] Waiting longer than a few days allows the establishment of invasive infection in the wound with its attendant morbidity and mortality. Several methods for burn excision and site preparation are employed and include burn wound excision down to fascia, tangential excision, and enzymatic débridement. Spontaneous separation of eschar occurs in 2 to 3 weeks following the burn injury and leaves a bed suitable for grafting, but the risk of invasive burn infection is prohibitive, and some form of early excision is recommended for most children with deep burns.

Total excision involves all burn wounds, remaining dermis, and subcutaneous tissue down to underlying muscle fascia. It can be performed with relatively little blood loss and provides an acceptable site for immediate grafting. Because this involves the removal of subcutaneous tissue, there is major cosmetic deformity, and this method of excision is reserved for patients in whom survival is the primary objective rather than function or appearance. Conversely, tangential excision involves excision of only thin layers of the burn wound until viable tissue is reached. This method is more tedious than excision of fascia and results in substantial blood loss. Furthermore, it often leaves a bed for grafting of subcutaneous fat, which is less vascularized than muscle fascia. In children, however, this is usually a satisfactory site for grafting, with a high rate of graft success in experienced hands. Because of the significant blood loss, tangential excision is usually limited to 15 to 20% of TBSA at one time. The site of burn excision is determined by the extent of the burn and its location. In patients with very large burns in whom survival is the paramount goal, the first areas excised are usually those that represent the largest proportion of burn wound and offer the greatest likelihood of grafting success, namely, the chest, abdomen, and back. In large burns, we often elect excision of fascia in these locations so that blood loss can be minimized and further excision can be performed in a few days. In less extensive burns in which survival is more likely and function and appearance are of greater concern, burns of the extremities, hands, and face are usually excised first, and excision is almost always tangential.

Once the burn is excised, the remaining wound must be covered by an autograft (the patient's own skin), allograft (cadaveric skin), xenograft (skin from another species such as porcine skin), and most recently, cultured epithelium derived from the patient's own keratinocytes. Materials other than an autograft or cultured epithelium require ultimate replacement with the patient's own skin. The choice of skin replacement is usually dictated by the extent of the burn wound. Burns less than 40% of TBSA can often be closed entirely by an autograft, usually with 15 to 20% of surface area being covered at one time. Larger burns cannot initially be covered with an autograft, so an autograft is applied to part of the burn and other materials are used to close the remainder temporarily.

The patient's own skin is harvested, preferably from the thigh or buttock, but any unburned skin can be used. It is applied as a sheet if being used to cover the face or the hands, but for most other locations it is meshed. Meshing the graft serves three main purposes: (1) It increases the size of the graft 1½ to 3 times its original size, (2) it contours more precisely to irregular surfaces, and (3) the interstices allow egress of blood and serum that might otherwise collect underneath the graft, lifting it off its bed and leading to graft loss. The graft is applied to the clean, débrided wound and is fixed in place with either surgical staples or fine sutures. We attempt to cover the area evenly with as little gap as possible between grafts or between the graft and healed skin. Dry or impregnated gauze and Ace elastic wrapping are then applied. For grafted extremities, a splint is made to immobilize the graft site.

Allografts obtained from cadaveric donors are our most commonly used skin substitute when the size of the burn is too large for complete autografting. Allografts allow prompt closure of large burn wounds, thereby decreasing the complications of persistently open wounds (e.g., pain, electrolyte loss, and a persistent catabolic state). In addition, allografts decrease infections in these wounds and help prepare them for eventual autografting.

Although an allograft is initially accepted by the wound bed, it is usually rejected in 2 to 3 weeks. Because burned patients are immunosuppressed, these grafts may adhere for even longer periods. Eventually, however, almost all allografts require replacement with an autograft. Allografting usually provides coverage of sufficient duration to allow for donor site regeneration and replacement of the allograft with an autograft.

Xenografts are sometimes used as biologic dressings and temporary wound coverage following excision. We use them only when an autograft or allograft is unavailable. They perform similarly to an allograft, allowing early capillary ingrowth and wound adherence. Ultimately, however, these grafts are all rejected and require replacement with an autograft.

Skin substitutes may be used for temporary wound coverage. These synthetic polymer products will adhere to a wound and either allow healing or act as a dressing in anticipation of autografting.

Finally, the patient's own keratinocytes may be harvested and cultured into sheets of epithelium. When applied, the cultured keratinocytes appear as re-epithelialization but with no reconstitution of dermis. This may be lifesaving in very large burns, and we have experienced some early success with this technique.

INFECTION IN BURN WOUNDS

Infection is the leading cause of death from burns in children, with almost two thirds of burn deaths attributed to sepsis. The burn wound is the most common source of invasive infection, though the pulmonary tract is the most common location of active infection in the burned patient. The thermal injury removes the major barrier to infectious organisms and causes systemic immunosuppression in burn victims.

Immediately following a burn injury, the wound contains very few organisms. After 2 or 3 days, large numbers of gram-positive cocci colonize the wound, being replaced on day 5 or 6 by gram-negative rods and *Candida* organisms. The burn wound is most often the source of invasive infection because the nonviable eschar provides an ideal culture medium that is not affected by host immune defenses. Although topical antibiotics do not sterilize the burn wound, they limit bacterial density

and are the major modality for preventing burn wound infection.

Silver sulfadiazine (1% creme) is our topical antibiotic of choice. It has a wide bacteriostatic spectrum and can be applied twice daily to burn wounds with no discomfort or metabolic complications. It may cause neutropenia, thrombocytopenia, or a rash, all of which are resolved with cessation of use. Occasionally, resistant strains of *Pseudomonas* may emerge, requiring change to another agent.

Mafenide acetate is another topical creme that is applied twice daily. It also has wide bacteriostatic activity that penetrates deep burns and eschar far better than other agents. Its major disadvantages are pain on application, potent carbonic anhydrase inhibition leading to metabolic acidosis, and skin sensitivity.

Silver nitrate, 0.5% solution, remains a very useful topical antibacterial agent with a wide spectrum of activity. It is applied to dressings every 4 hours to keep them moist and is painless. It does not cause skin sensitivity, but it can leach electrolytes, causing hyponatremia, hypokalemia, hypochloremia, and hypocalcemia. It also causes dark discoloration of the wound, bed clothes, and anything else it contacts. We find silver nitrate especially useful in patients who experience sensitivity or resistance to silver sulfadiazene.

Topical antibiotics are used to limit burn wound colonization and prevent invasive infection, which is determined by quantitative wound culture or histologic examination of burn tissue. Arterial wound counts exceeding 10^5 organisms/g of tissue usually indicate invasive infection. Histologic examination of invasive infection reveals bacteria in normal tissue adjacent to the burn wound. Once invasive infection has been confirmed by either of these methods, excision of the burn wound is the only effective treatment. Subsequent application of topical antibiotics or biologic dressings are then used to prevent further infection.

Infection of the respiratory tract either by hematogenous spread from the burn wound or by airway transmission has become the leading type of septic complication in burned patients. The use of artificial airways has provided a common port of entry for infectious organisms, and inhalational injury further adds to the risk of infection by attenuating host defense mechanisms within the lungs. Hematogenous pulmonary infections are caused by organisms from the burn wounds, infected IV sites, or the gastrointestinal tract. They may present as infiltrative pneumonia or discrete lesions within the lungs. Culture specimens from the respiratory tract should be obtained and their results correlated with radiographic findings, as many patients will have airway colonization without parenchymal infection. The choice of IV antibiotics should be based on culture results. Excessive coverage will simply lead to more highly resistant organisms and opportunistic infections such as candidiasis.

Catheter sepsis and suppurative thrombophlebitis result from infection at IV access sites. These infections are especially common at cutdown sites, and frequent changes in these sites is the most effective means of prevention. Suppurative thrombophlebitis is a serious infection requiring surgical excision of the infected vessel.

Urinary tract colonization is common in patients whose urine output is monitored by catheterization. In the case of bacterial infection, appropriate IV antibiotics are given, but for fungal infections, bladder irrigations with amphotericin B are performed for 5 days. Prompt removal of bladder catheters is the best means of prevention, but for patients who require continued bladder drainage, changing catheters may help treat persistent urinary infection.

Bacterial endocarditis may complicate the clinical course, especially in patients who require central venous or pulmonary artery catheters. Bacterial endocarditis is usually suspected in patients with persistent fevers and no identified source or recognition of a new murmur. Echocardiography may facilitate this diagnosis, and most lesions are found on the right side of the heart. At least 3 weeks of intravenous antibiotics are required to treat these patients, and occasionally surgical valve replacement may be necessary.

Chondritis of the ear is an infectious complication of facial burns, which is usually noted several weeks following burn injuries. It is marked by swelling, erythema, tenderness, and protrusion of the pinna and is usually caused by *P. aeruginosa*. Because intravenous antibiotics are largely ineffectual for this problem, treatment consists primarily of meticulous local care, including washing, avoiding pressure, and application of mafenide acetate, which is particularly effective in penetrating into auricular cartilage.

NUTRITIONAL SUPPORT IN PEDIATRIC PATIENTS WITH BURN INJURY

Nutrition plays an integral role in the treatment of patients with burn injury. The provision of nutritional support to burned children poses a special challenge. Adequate energy and protein intake is required to meet the increased metabolic demand of the hypermetabolic state of the burn injury as well as normal growth and development. Prompt initiation of nutritional support is crucial to successful outcome and speedy recovery. Aggressive nutritional support has been associated with a reduction in the cost of hospitalization of severely burned patients.[8]

The goals of nutritional therapy in burned children are to preserve body stores, replace visceral and somatic protein losses, promote early wound healing, enhance immune functions, and allow normal growth and development.

Assessment of Caloric Requirements

Nutritional care in burned patients begins with determination of caloric requirements. Several formulas have been developed for estimating caloric requirements (Fig. 87–3). The clinical reliability of these formulas has been questioned because many factors known to influence metabolic expenditure, such as fever, sepsis, surgery,

Hildreth and Carvajal[9]	1800 kcal/m^2 + 2200 kcal/m^2 × % burn
Wolfe[10] wt < 20 kg	BMR × 1.75
wt > 20 kg	BMR × 2
Curreri Junior[11]	
0–1 yr	BMR + 15 kcal × % burn
1–3 yr	BMR + 25 kcal × % burn
3–15 yr	BMR + 40 kcal × % burn
Batchelor[12]	60 kcal × wt + 35 kcal × % burn
Watchel[13]	1.4 kcal (BMR × m^2 × 24 hr) + wt (growth + 0.6 × % burn)

m^2 = body surface area.
% Burn = body surface area burned.
BMR = basal metabolic rate.
Wt = weight (kg).

Figure 87–3. Examples of formulas for estimating energy needs in pediatric burned patients.

dressing changes, and activity, are not taken into account. Although underfeeding has a deleterious effect on wound healing, immunocompetence, and mortality, overfeeding can cause complications such as hyperglycemia, liver abnormalities, and respiratory dysfunction. Recently, Hildreth and associates[14] showed that the actual caloric intake required to maintain weight in pediatric patients with burns over greater than 30% of TBSA was significantly lower than the caloric requirement estimated by the formula used by Hildreth and Carvajal and the Curreri-Junior formula. Cunningham and coworkers[15] used indirect calorimetry to determine energy expenditure in severely burned children less than 3 years old. They reported that the Hildreth and Carvajal formula, Bachelor formula, and the Curreri-Junior formula all overestimated caloric requirements, whereas the Wolfe formula (basal metabolic rate ×2) closely estimated these requirements. Dietitians must be aware of the potential of overfeeding when mathematical formulas are used to predict caloric requirements.

At present, several burn centers are routinely using automated, portable direct calorimetry, which measures oxygen consumption and carbon dioxide production to determine resting energy expenditure. This is the most precise method to estimate energy expenditure because it accounts for fluctuations that occur with dressing changes, pain, fever, and activity. It is recommended that the patient's caloric goals be calculated at 120 to 130% of measured resting energy expenditure.

Macronutrients

Protein

Protein requirements in burned children are much higher than in normal children. In addition to increased loss of protein across the burn wound, there is a great demand for protein for wound healing, host defense, and gluconeogenesis as amino acids become a primary source of energy. Alexander and associates[16] reported beneficial effects of aggressive protein supplementation on the outcome of severely burned children, as evidenced by improved survival, decreased incidence of infection, and better immune function. They recommend that the optimal protein requirement for severely burned children is about 20 to 22% of calories as protein (2.5 to 4 g/kg) or a nonprotein calorie:nitrogen ratio of 100:1. Davis and Lilijedahl recommended the following formula for estimating the protein requirement in burned children: 3 g/kg + 1 g/% of TBSA burned. However, providing excessive protein to children less than 1 year of age should be avoided because they may not be able to tolerate high renal solute loads. No more than 4 g/kg protein should be given.

Even though branched-chain amino acid–enriched formulas are recommended for use in patients with stress, sepsis, and trauma, they have not been proved beneficial in burns.[17] In contrast, arginine supplementation has been shown to improve cell-mediated immunity and wound healing and to decrease morbidity and mortality in burns.[18]

Fat and Carbohydrate

Fat should be included in the nutritional support of the burned patient because it is a more concentrated source of energy than are carbohydrates, it provides essential fatty acids, and it is the carrier of fat-soluble vitamins. However, excessive fat intake has been associated with numerous complications, including diarrhea, cholestasis, hepatomegaly, coagulopathy and immunosuppression.[19] Long and colleagues[20] and Wolfe and coworkers[24] report that carbohydrate is more effective than fat in minimizing protein catabolism following burn injury. Mochizuki and associates[25] recommend that 5 to 15% of nonprotein calories should be provided as fat in the diet of the burned patient. A more recent experiment by Alexander and associates indicates that some deleterious effects of excessive fat could be related to a high content of linoleic acid, an ω-6 fatty acid that is the precursor of inflammatory and immunosuppressive dienoic prostaglandins.[26] They suggest that a diet relatively low in linoleic acid and high in ω-3 fatty acids would have a beneficial effect because of a reduction in immunosuppressive mediators after burn injury.

Micronutrients

To date, the vitamin and mineral requirements of burned children remain undefined. Body stores of vitamins and minerals in infants and small children are small. It is generally agreed that micronutrient requirements are elevated after burn injury. The increased demand is directly related to new tissue synthesis and wound losses. In order for the patient to efficiently use the increased protein and caloric intake, there must be an adequate supply of thiamine, riboflavin, niacin, and other B complex vitamins. Therefore, multivitamin supplementation at least equal to the Recommended Daily Allowance (RDA) is routinely prescribed to all pediatric patients with burn injury. Because of its role in wound healing and immune functions, vitamin C is often supplemented to 5 to 10 times the RDA, and vitamin A and zinc are supplemented to 2 times the RDA.[24] Routine therapeutic doses of iron should be avoided when there is associated infection and hypotransfer-rinemia because unbound iron seems to encourage bacterial and fungal growth.

Nutrition Delivery

Children less than 3 years of age with burns of less than 10% of body surface and older children with burns of less than 20% of body surface may be able to receive their nutritional needs by oral intake. High-protein, high-calorie foods, however, should be encouraged. Anorexia, anxiety, pain, repeated operative procedures, and wound care disruptive to mealtimes are among the numerous reasons that make children with larger burns incapable of voluntarily consuming the large amounts of foods needed to meet their elevated needs. The gastrointestinal tract is the preferred route for the supplementation of oral intake in burned patients. In addition to being safer, more economical, and more efficient in nutrient utilization than the parenteral route, enteral feeding preserves normal gastrointestinal function and mucosal integrity and decreases the incidence of hepatic steatosis and bacterial translocation.[28] In a prospective study of patients with burns covering more than 50% of TBSA, Herndorn and colleagues reported that early administration of parenteral nutrition for the first 10 days following injury had no beneficial effect on immune function, liver function, or survival.[21] In a follow-up study, they reported that the group of patients who received intravenous supplementation had twice the death rate of the enterally supplemented group during the first 14 days after burn injury.[22] These authors concluded that administration of intravenous supplementation decreases the amount of enteral calories that patients with burns can tolerate. Therefore, the use of intravenous supplemental nutrition in the early period following burn injury should be discouraged and its use limited only to nutritional support of patients whose enteral function has failed totally.

Enteral nutritional support should begin as soon as possible, preferably within 24 hours following the injury. Early enteral nutrition has been shown to reduce subsequent metabolic rate, decrease secretion of catabolic hormones, and decrease gut mucosal atrophy.[23] Nasogastric tube feeding can be used in the patient with a functioning gastrointestinal tract. Nasojejunal feeding is possible during gastric ileus following the burn injury. Continuous infusion over 10 to 24 hours using a feeding pump rather than intermittent boluses is recommended. Following medical stabilization, a feeding tube should be inserted for all children less than 3 years old with burns over more than 10% of TBSA and in older children with burns over more than 20% of TBSA.

Although numerous commercial enteral formulas are available, none is designed to meet the unique nutritional needs of burned children. Infant formulas or adult tube-feeding formulas must be modified in an attempt to increase their suitability for burned children. Recently, the Shriners Burns Institute at Cincinnati designed a modular tube-feeding formula for burned patients that is high in protein and low in fat and linoleic acid and is supplemented with arginine, ω-3 fatty acids, vitamin A, zinc, and ascorbic acid.

For infants less than 9 months old, commercial infant formulas can be used beginning with a standard dilution of 20 kcal/ounce. The concentration of the formula can gradually be increased as tolerated to 20 to 30 kcal/oz to meet protein and energy needs. For children 9 months and older, commercial adult tube-feeding formulas containing high protein and 1 kcal/ml may be used. Some high-protein, high-calorie products providing more than 1 kcal/ml may have to be diluted to reduce renal solute loads or to meet free water requirements. Since burned patients usually have normal digestive and absorptive capabilities, chemically defined elemental diets are not indicated. Most isotonic tube-feeding products can be started at full strength.

The initial infusion rate should be 1 to 2 ml/kg/hr and can be advanced as tolerated 5 to 20 ml/hr every 4 to 24 hours to the required volume. Gastric residuals should be monitored every 4 hours. The feeding rate can be advanced only when gastric residuals are within acceptable limits, usually half of the prescribed feeding amounts. If the residuals are greater than two times the hourly rate, tube feeding should be stopped.

Daily monitoring for gastrointestinal intolerance, including nausea, vomiting, abdominal pain, distention, diarrhea, and constipation, is essential.

Nutritional Monitoring

The adequacy and effectiveness of the nutritional therapy should be continuously monitored to identify potential complications and provide adjustments to meet the patient's changing needs. Nutritional monitoring begins by comparing the nutrient intakes obtained by daily calorie counts to the estimated requirements. The tube feeding rate may have to be increased or reduced occasionally to accommodate the oral intake.

Children should be weighed as soon as possible following burn injury. Thereafter, they should be weighed daily without dressings or splints. Nutritional support of burned children should at the very least be able to maintain preburn weight and preferably provide weight gain for normal growth and development. Other anthropometric measurements, such as midarm circumference and triceps skin-fold thickness, are also useful in monitoring the burned patient's fat and muscle reserves.

Serial measurements of albumin, transferrin, prealbumin, and retinol-binding protein can be used to assess the adequacy of protein provision. Reduction of these transport proteins can indicate an impairment of hepatic protein synthesis, as well as depletion of visceral protein stores. Serum albumin levels drop rapidly within a few days following the burn injury because of losses of albumin in the burn wounds. Transferrin is more sensitive than albumin in defining malnutrition in burned patients because of its shorter half-life. Low transferrin levels have been associated with an increased incidence of bacteremia in burns.[29] Retinol-binding protein and prealbumin concentrations have been reported to change earlier than albumin and transferrin levels and correlate better with nitrogen balance during nutritional therapy.[30]

The adequacy of protein intake to maintain lean body mass is commonly evaluated by a nitrogen balance study. However, the accuracy of the nitrogen balance study depends on the completeness of urine collection, which is very difficult to accomplish in infants and small children. It is also difficult to estimate. Nitrogen balance is neither useful nor practical in monitoring the protein status of burned children.

The protein and energy requirements of burned children should be reassessed frequently as the burn wound heals. Weekly measurement of the metabolic rate by indirect calorimetry will allow early detection of underfeeding or overfeeding and the tailoring of the patient's nutritional support.

RESULTS

The morbidity and mortality of burn wounds have decreased over the past 20 years, mainly because of prompt excision and grafting, improved antibiotics, and advancements in critical care techniques. The LD_{50} (lethal burn size area for 50% of patients) has increased steadily from approximately 40% 10 years ago to as high as 90% in recent reports, and survival appears to be similar across all age groups in the pediatric population. (Overall mortality in our burn unit and in other major burn centers is now 2 to 3%).

As previously discussed, the most common complications of burns are infections, and pneumonia is the leading cause of death in burned patients.

Gastrointestinal complications are also common and include gastric ulceration, pancreatitis, enterocolitis, and superior mesenteric artery syndrome. Stress ulceration of the stomach and duodenum (Curling ulcer) occurs to varying degrees in most patients following a serious burn and can be demonstrated endoscopically in 85% of patients within 72 hours after injury. Most of these ulcers heal spontaneously and without symptoms within 1 week. In 20% of patients, however, frank ulceration develops and may be compounded by hemorrhage or perforation. Antacid therapy has been clearly shown to prevent complications of Curling ulcer, and we administer antacids to maintain a gastric pH greater than 5.

Pancreatitis may also complicate large burns and may be manifested by abdominal pain, increasing fluid requirements, or intolerance to enteral feeding. Elevated serum or urinary amylase levels corroborate this diagnosis, and treatment is largely supportive, including nasogastric drainage, fluid resuscitation, and parenteral nutrition.

A form of enterocolitis is occasionally recognized in burn patients. These patients experience ulcerations in the ileum and colon, which may bleed or perforate. Colonic pseudo-obstruction may also develop and is most effectively treated by decompressive colonoscopy.

Superior mesenteric artery syndrome may occur in children who are very thin or who experience marked weight loss. The distal duodenum is compressed anteriorly by the superior mesenteric artery, and enteral feeding is impossible. Treatment consists of parenteral nutrition; as the child gains weight the duodenal obstruction is gradually relieved and enteral feeding can be reinstituted.

Renal dysfunction may complicate large burns. Inadequate renal perfusion and acute tubular necrosis may result from large intravascular fluid losses. Adequate resuscitation is the most effective means of prevention. Once established, acute tubular necrosis may require hemodialysis to clear excess metabolic waste.

Myoglobin and hemoglobin are both nephrotoxic hemochromogens that may be released following extensive burns. Large surface area burns can cause hemolysis, and very deep burns can lead to muscle necrosis and release of myoglobin. Brisk urine output and urinary alkalinization facilitate rapid excretion and prevent tubular precipitation of the pigments.

Finally, long-term wound and soft tissue complications may occur. Deep burns are prone to hypertrophic scar formation, which may be unsightly and debilitating. Early excision and grafting helps diminish the degree of scarring, and pressure garments will help flatten scars over time. Keloids are lesions that develop in burn wounds but then grow beyond the site of injury. They are much less responsive to pressure, and excision of keloids is associated with a 50% recurrence rate. Intralesional steroids are used with some success in the treatment of hypertrophic scars and keloids.

Rarely, chronic ulceration of old burn scars may lead to malignant degeneration. These Marjolin ulcers most often contain squamous cell carcinomas, and this malignancy may appear decades after the original injury. Chronic wound ulcers should be aggressively treated with excision and reclosure, and wide excision is indicated in the presence of malignancy.

Despite major advances in treatment and improved results, burns still represent a major cause of childhood morbidity and mortality. Prevention remains the most effective means of dealing with these injuries, but for those children who are burned, an aggressive, multidisciplinary approach to burn treatment and rehabilitation offers the best opportunity for a successful outcome and a long, useful life.

References

1. Guzzetta PC and Randolph JG: Burns in children: 1982. Pediatr Rev 9:271, 1983.
2. McLoughlin E and McGuire A: The causes, costs, and prevention of childhood injuries. Am J Dis Child 144:677, 1990.
3. Hobbs CJ: Burns and scalds. Br Med J 298:1302, 1989.
4. Feldman KW, Schaller, RT, Feldman, JA, et al: Tap water scald burns in children. Pediatrics 62:1, 1978.
5. Calhoun KH, Deskin RW, Garza C, et al: Long-term airway sequelae in a pediatric burn population. Laryngoscopy 98:721, 1988.
6. Graves TA, Cioffi WG, McManus WF, et al: Fluid resuscitation of infants and children with massive thermal injury. J Trauma 28:1656, 1988.
7. Tompkins RG, Remensnyder JP, Burke JF, et al: Significant reductions in mortality for children with burn injuries through the use of prompt eschar excision. Ann Surg 208:577, 1988.
8. Weinsier RL, Heimburger DC, Samples CM, et al: Cost containment: A contribution of aggressive nutritional support in burn patients. J Burn Care Rehab 6:436, 1985.
9. Hildreth M and Carvajal HF: A simple formula to estimate daily caloric requirements in burned children. J Burn Care Rehab 3:78, 1982.
10. Wolfe RR: Caloric requirements of the burned patient. J Trauma 21:712, 1981.
11. Day T, Dean P, Adams MC, et al: Nutritional requirements of the burned child: The Curreri junior formula. Proc Am Burn Assoc 18:86, 1986.
12. Batchelor ADR, Sutherland AB, and Colver C: Sodium balance studies following thermal injury. Br J Plast Surg 18:130, 1965.
13. Watchel TL, Yen M, Fortune JB, et al: Computer estimation and monitoring of nutrition programs for burned patients. J Burn Care Rehab 5:202, 1984.
14. Hildreth MA, Herndon DN, Desai MH, et al: Caloric needs of adolescent patients with burns. J Burn Care Rehab 10:523, 1989.
15. Cunningham JJ, Lydon MK, and Russell WE: Calorie and protein provision for recovery from severe burns in infants and young children. Am J Clin Nutr 51:553, 1990.
16. Alexander JW, MacMillan BG, Stinett JR, et al: Beneficial effects of aggressive protein feeding in severely burned children. Ann Surg 192:505, 1980.
17. Mochizuki H, Trocki O, Dominioni L, et al: Effect of a diet risk in branched chain amino acids on severely burned guinea pigs. J Trauma 26:1077, 1986.
18. Saito H, Trocki O, Wang S, et al: Metabolic and immune effects of dietary arginine supplementation after burn. Arch Surg 122:784, 1987.
19. Gottschlich MM and Alexander JW: Fat kinetics and recommended dietary intake in burns. J Parenter Enter Nutr 11:80, 1987.
20. Long JM, Wilmore AD, Mason AD, et al: The effect of carbohydrate and fat intake on nitrogen excretion during total intravenous feeding. Ann Surg 185:417, 1977.
21. Herndon DN, Stein MD, Rutan TC, et al: Failure of TPN supplementation to improve liver function, immunity and mortality in thermally injured patients. J Trauma 27:195, 1987.
22. Herndon DN, Barrow RE, Stein MD, et al: Increased mortality with intravenous supplemental feeding in severely burned patients. J Burn Care Rehab 10:309, 1989.
23. Jenkins M, Gottschlich MM, Alexander JW, et al: Enteral alimentation in the early postburn phase. In: Blackburn GL, Bell SJ, and Mullen J (eds): Nutritional Medicine: A Case Management. Philadelphia, WB Saunders, 1989.
24. Wolfe BM, Culebras AJ, Sim MR, et al: Substrate interaction in intravenous feeding. Ann Surg 186:518, 1977.
25. Mochizuki H, Trocki O, Dominioni L, et al: Optimal lipid content for enteral diet following thermal injury. J Parenter Enter Nutr 8:638, 1984.
26. Alexander JW, Saito H, Trocki O, et al: The importance of lipid type in the diet after burn injury. Ann Surg 204:1, 1986.
27. Gottschlich MM and Warden GD: Vitamin supplementation in patients with burns. J Burn Care Rehab 11:275, 1990.
28. Saito H, Trocki O, Alexander JW, et al: The effect of route of nutrient administration on the nutritional state, catabolic hormone secretion, and gut mucosal integrity after burn injury. J Parenter Enter Nutr 11:1, 1987.
29. Ogle CK, Alexander JW, and MacMillan BG: The relationship of bacteremia to levels of transferrin, albumin, and total serum protein in burn patients. Burns 8:32, 1981.
30. Winkler MF, Gerrior SA, Pomp A, et al: Use of retinol-binding protein and prealbumin as indicators of the response to nutrition therapy. J Am Diet Assoc 89:684, 1989.

Electrical Injuries in Children

Kurt Newman, M.D.

Because electrical burns are multisystem injuries with high morbidity and mortality, they require an intensive team approach to management. Downed power lines, exposed electrical cords, lightning, and electrical appliances are frequent causes of electrical injuries in children.[1] At the Children's National Medical Center, a regional pediatric trauma and burn center, approximately 400 children are admitted each year with burn injuries and 4% of these are due to electrical injury. We do not consider any electrical burn trivial, since over 1,500 deaths per year are attributed to electrical injury in the United States.[2]

PATHOPHYSIOLOGY

The high morbidity and mortality of electrical injury relate to the multisystem pathophysiology.[3] The observed skin wound is often only the tip of the iceberg. A hallmark of electrical injury is an extensive deep tissue injury that results from complex interactions between the tissue involved in the conducting pathway and the physical properties of electricity.[4] Electricity causes thermal injury to tissues as well as electrical disruption of cell membranes with resulting cell death.[5] In addition, the passage of current directly through organs, such as the heart, can cause pathologic changes (Fig. 88-1).

When caring for electrically injured children, obtaining an accurate history is important. The patterns of damage relate to the type of current (AC or DC), the resistance of the tissues involved, and the strength of the current (voltage).[6] Alternating current can produce prolonged muscular contraction, in essence paralyzing the involved muscles, and it is not uncommon for a victim to be frozen to the electrical circuit, with increased damage. The specific resistance of tissue varies: Bone is the most resistant, followed by fat, tendons, skin, blood vessels, and nervous tissue. Voltage refers to the strength of the current. Low voltages can produce injury, but high voltages produce the most explosive burns, with damage to muscles, vessels, nerves, and bones.[7] In addition, the path that the current takes through the body is quite important. Although the path of injury is often unpredictable, several studies have shown that a vertical pathway may be more likely to cause myocardial damage after high-voltage electrical

injury.[8] When these historical details are available, they are valuable in the initial evaluation of the child and establishment of a management plan.

TREATMENT

Emergency Management

Emergency treatment of the electrically injured child is crucial and begins in the field. When the child is removed from the electrical source extreme care must be taken to avoid injury to emergency personnel. Nonconductive clothing must be worn or used when separating the victim from the current. When indicated, cardiopulmonary resuscitation is begun.

On transfer to the emergency department, the airway is secured and ventilation is begun if respiratory arrest has occurred. Fluid resuscitation through large-bore intravenous lines should be initiated. Estimation of fluid requirements is difficult since the cutaneous manifestations do not accurately reflect the magnitude of injury.[9] A target of 1 to 2 ml/kg of urine output may be inadequate, especially if myoglobinuria is detected. Alkalinization of the urine and osmotic diuretics are useful adjuncts to the management of myoglobinuria.[10] An electrocardiogram (ECG) and creatine phosphokinase-myocardial band (CPK-MB) isoenzyme determinations are obtained. The patient should be monitored carefully to detect life-threatening cardiac rhythm disturbances. Tetanus prophylaxis is administered.

Long-Term Management

After the initial resuscitation, the long-term management issues relate to the magnitude of tissue destruction and to the care of these wounds.[11] Amputations are frequently necessary. Compartment pressure measurements may be useful in the early detection of compartment syndromes,[12] and elevation of the extremities and frequent monitoring of neurovascular status are required to prevent them. However, when in doubt, fasciotomies must be performed. Surface escharotomies are useful for circumferential injuries of extremities to restore the circulation. These can be done easily and safely in the

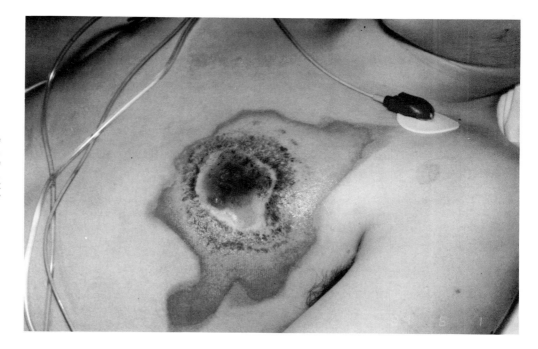

Figure 88–1. Exit wound on the chest due to high-voltage injury. The skin burn represents only the "tip" of an extensive deeper burn. The pathway of electrical current makes cardiac arrhythmias likely in this child.

intensive care unit. The amount of tissue necrosis is difficult to estimate clinically. Some centers have used ^{99}Tc radionuclide studies in the identification of devitalized muscle.

Controversy exists as to the best strategy for the management of soft tissue injury. In adults, early excision of necrotic tissue with split-thickness skin grafting has gained favor. However, in children an aggressive approach may lead to unnecessary removal of tissue. An appropriate balance between excision of devitalized

tissue and maintenance of healthy tissue is required. Serial sequential debridement with skin grafting has been used at our institution. However, early excision and coverage is important for specific injuries such as those to the hands so that early physical therapy and mobilization can begin (Fig. 88–2).

An electrical injury can involve almost any organ system. The cardiac manifestations of electrical burns are frequently rhythm disturbances. Serial ECGs and measurement of CPK-MB isoenzymes will reveal the

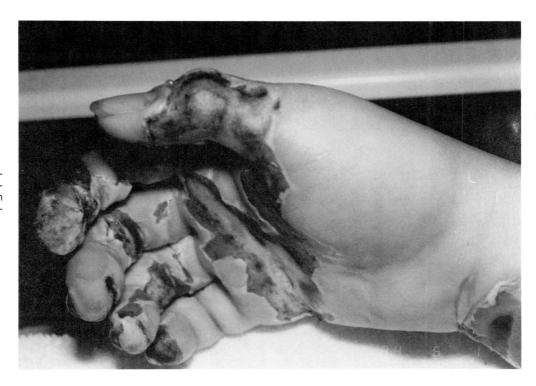

Figure 88–2. The typical appearance of a hand burned while grabbing a power line. Early excision and grafting of the hand are crucial to preserving function.

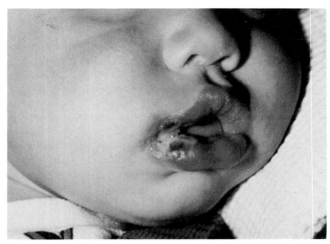

Figure 88–3. A burn to the lateral commissure from biting an electrical cord. Careful surgical attention is required to prevent a long-term cosmetic disaster.

injury. Sinus tachycardia, heart block, ventricular fibrillation and tachycardia, and supraventricular tachycardia are seen. Most rhythm disturbances will resolve spontaneously, but life-threatening arrhythmias require appropriate pharmacologic treatment (see Chapter 36).

Neurologic manifestations include seizures, coma, amnesia, spinal cord injuries, paralysis, and transverse myelitis. Peripheral nerve injuries result from vascular damage or from direct injury due to conduction of current through the nerves. The neurologic sequelae may be delayed and only come to attention years later. The prognosis for recovery is often poor with neurologic injury.

Renal damage from electrical injuries is similar to that seen in "crush" syndromes.[13] Other affected systems include ocular burns and cataracts, gastrointestinal bleeding and rupture, orthopedic injuries, including fractures and dislocations, and vascular complications due to arterial or venous occlusion. Associated injuries are common and must be sought since falls or blunt trauma often follows an electrical shock. Child abuse and neglect are factors in many electrical injuries (see Chapter 86).

Electrical burns to the lip are quite difficult to manage and require special attention. The burn is usually located laterally in the corner of the mouth and occurs when a child bites an exposed electrical cord (Fig. 88–3). These children are hospitalized, since the tissue may slough at 7 to 10 days, with resultant brisk bleeding. Prostheses have been useful in obtaining good cosmetic results in some centers. Excision with careful plastic closure may also give good aesthetic results.[14]

LIGHTNING INJURIES

A special category of electrical injury is that due to lightning. These injuries produce 500 to 600 deaths each year in the United States, many of which occur in children. There is often a characteristic spidery skin burn. Lightning current may pass through the brain, respiratory center, or heart and produce cardiac arrest. Cardiopulmonary resuscitation should be continued for long periods of time in children with lightning injuries, since there have been reports of complete response to prolonged resuscitation.

CONCLUSION

Electrical burn injuries in children are multisystem injuries, and optimum results are achieved by using a team approach with intensive monitoring and management until all potential problems are identified and resolved. Physicians caring for critically ill children must be conversant with the myriad patterns of electrical injury in children. A fundamental approach is that no electrical burn is minor—all must receive intensive investigation and care.

References

1. Frank DH and Fisher J: Complications of electrical injury. *In:* Greenfield LT (ed): Complications in Surgery and Trauma, 2nd ed. Philadelphia, JB Lippincott, 1990, pp. 26–38.
2. Mills W, Switzer WE, and Moncriet JA: Electrical injuries. JAMA 195:165, 1966.
3. Kobernich M: Electrical injuries: Pathophysiology and emergency management. Ann Emerg Med 2:633, 1982.
4. Wilkinson C and Wood M: High voltage electrical injury. Am J Surg 136:693, 1978.
5. Lee RC and Kolodnex MS: Electrical injury mechanisms: Electrical breakdown of cell membranes. Plast Reconstr Surg 80:672, 1987.
6. Solem L, Fische RP, and Strate RG: The natural history of electrical injury. J Trauma 17:487, 1977.
7. Hunt JL, Mason AD, Musterson TS, et al: The pathophysiology of acute electrical injuries. J Trauma 16:335, 1976.
8. Chandra NC, Siu CO, and Muster AM: Clinical predictors of myocardial damage after high voltage electrical injury. Crit Care Med 18:293, 1990.
9. Hunt JL, Sato RM, and Baxter CR: Acute electrical burns. Arch Surg 115:434, 1980.
10. Sances A, Carson SJ, Myklebust J, et al: Electrical injuries. Surg Gynecol Obstet 149:97, 1979.
11. Burke JF, Quinby WC, Bendouc C, et al: Patterns of high tension injury in children and adolescents and their management. Am J Surg 133:492, 1977.
12. Seffle JR, Zeluff GR, Werden GD, et al: Intramuscular pressures in the burned arm: Measurement and response to escharotomy. Am J Surg 140:825, 1980.
13. Artz CP: Electrical injury simulates crush injury. Surg Gynecol Obstet 125:1316, 1967.
14. Silverberg B, Banis JC, Verdi GD, et al: Microvascular reconstruction after electrical and deep thermal injury. J Trauma 26:128, 1986.

89

Disaster Management for Children

Peter R. Holbrook, M.D.

Disasters have taken the lives of over 3 million people in the last 20 years and have seriously affected the lives of over 800 million more.[1-3] While the natural disaster frequency is unchanged, the impact is more frequently felt as the world's population grows and the economic situation forces humans into inhabiting a greater percentage of the world's surface. Disasters created by humans are increasing in frequency as, for example, larger planes are developed, nuclear processing plants are utilized, and countries stockpile biologic or chemical weapons.

At the same time, the globe is shrinking with improved transportation at relatively lower cost. Geopolitical rearrangements, the end of the Cold War, the impact of the ecology movement, and greater global cooperation have resulted in, perhaps, an increased sense of the commonality of experience on the planet.

The United Nations has recognized the greater impact of disasters on society and the possibility of improving the situation by declaring the 1990s as The International Decade of Natural Disaster Reduction.[4]

Critical care medicine has also come of age in the last 20 years and has begun to be a major positive force in assistance in these issues.

Disaster is variously defined, but common to all definitions is a notion of widespread disruption of community functions with serious threat to the lives, health, or property of many people. A *medical disaster* may be further defined as a disaster that overwhelms the existing medical care system. The World Health Organization declares a natural disaster to be one of sufficient magnitude to require external assistance.[5-7]

ELEMENTS COMMON TO A DISASTER

Suddenness. There is usually no warning as in the case of tornadoes or avalanches, or when a building collapses. Even when advanced warning is given, as in floods and hurricanes, there is little time to plan, and the impact is felt all at once. Similarly, the event is usually over in a short time; the flood recedes, the tornado passes, and the earthquake ends. Casualties are suddenly produced. Although discovery may be delayed, in most disasters new casualties are not continuously produced. By implication, a response system must be immediate if it is to be beneficial.

Disruption. By definition, but also in reality, disasters are disruptive. The normal response systems will not work, either because they are overloaded or because they are directly affected by the disaster (e.g., the Mexican earthquake in 1985 leveled the Children's Hospital). Thus, new systems must be brought to bear on the problem. If disaster planning has not occurred, there will be further disruption.

Chaos. In the absence of the normal response to casualties, new systems will have to evolve quickly. Coordination is lost if the response to a situation is not rehearsed. Information is a casualty. Commonly, hospitals hear about a disaster when the first patient arrives. Similarly, a situation that is truly a disaster may not be recognized as such. An official must declare a disaster to exist in order to institute disaster plans. The official may not be on the scene or may not even be available.

ORGANIZATIONAL ISSUES

Because disasters come in all types and because there is no comprehensive plan for management in many communities, states, or nations, many organizations have expressed a desire to be involved in one or more aspect of disaster management. Each desire comes with a varying amount of commitment. Sorting through the maze of involved people is itself a challenge. Then, clarifying who has what responsibility is also a task. For example, the Red Cross, local ambulance companies, fire and rescue personnel, police, the National Guard, hospital-based emergency medical service (EMS) systems, and the local government office of emergency preparedness may all feel involved. If the federal government becomes involved, more than 100 organizations are added.

In the United States, an attempt has been made to coordinate the national disaster response system. By presidential decree, an Emergency Mobilization Preparedness Board (EPMB) has been established and a protocol for activating a federal response to a disaster has been created. The Federal Emergency Management Agency (FEMA) is the coordinator. This agency can draw on no fewer than 16 governmental or voluntary agencies to assist in various capacities.

The EMPB created the National Disaster Medical System (NDMS), which is intended to be a coordinated response system for domestic disasters. The United States has been divided into geographical regions, and for each region a Disaster Medical Assistance Team (DMAT) is recruited. This 29-member team consists of physicians (none are pediatricians), nurses, technicians, and support personnel. The DMAT is responsible for periodic training and education. They are provided with equipment from the NDMS and are intended to provide rapid response system.

Of interest is the recent evolution of specialized DMATs for specific functions. The Task Force on Disasters of the Society of Critical Care Medicine (SCCM) collected information on 800 of its members who expressed interest in disaster medicine. In January, 1991 the SCCM received a formal request from the Department of Defense to develop volunteer teams of critical care physicians to assist with anticipated casualties associated with Operation Desert Storm. Within 2 weeks 30 teams were organized and given credentials by the American Red Cross. Each team was prepared to go overseas for 2-week tours. Pursuant to this activity, the Task Force on Disasters has begun the development of pediatric DMATs to be available for pediatric assistance.

The current status of organizational issues is complex. It has been summarized by Dow and associates.[8]

ESSENTIAL ELEMENTS OF A DISASTER RESPONSE

Initial information exchange and assessment of the situation must be achieved. Coordination of communication frequencies, establishment of a resuscitation and staging area, and notification of receiving medical facilities are early goals. A skilled assessment of the scene to clear it for operations by the rescue team is essential. For example, loss of oxygen in a closed space, the presence of noxious fumes, or electricity hazards must be identified.

Search and rescue is now a sophisticated undertaking and should not be attempted by the novice. Suffice it to say that most lightly entrapped victims will be rescued

by local bystanders, that complex methods may be necessary for some, that medical care can begin prior to extrication in some cases, and that, despite the recognized principle of marked drop-off of survivors after the first 24 hours, exceptions do occur (e.g., in the survival of newborn infants after 1 week of entrapment in the Mexico City earthquake in 1985). Pediatric specific extrication principles have not yet evolved.

Initial care (EMS treatment) is given near the scene in the staging area. It is here that initial triage occurs, if necessary. A pediatric critical care physician or nurse can be of assistance in the triage of children.[9] For example, a screaming child will likely receive much attention, although he or she may be relatively healthy. Recognition of shock (see Chapters 6 and 7) may be difficult for the nonpediatric caregiver. Cardiopulmonary resuscitation, if necessary for cardiac arrest, will probably be fruitless.

Evacuation to a definitive care site may require the in-flight assistance of a skilled pediatric intensivist.

The incidence, anticipated medical conditions, and their implications for the pediatric disaster victim have been reviewed.[9] Highlights of that review include a relatively high incidence of pediatric victims in most disasters, the different impact of injury on the child, and the absence of systematic planning for the pediatric victims.

The basic steps in disaster management in the ICU are outlined in Table 89–1. ICU activities must be coordinated with the overall disaster situation to maximize effectiveness. If the regional pediatric ICU is to be the only effective critical care center for the immediate duration of the disaster, the principle of triage must be continued if there is to be the greatest benefit for the greatest number of casualties. If, on the other hand, other facilities can be relied on, then maximal, definitive care may be undertaken in the ICU. Close communication with the triage officers in the field is desirable.

As with all phases of the disaster response, the response in the ICU is best planned and rehearsed prior to implementation. "Dry runs" designed to locate extraordinary numbers of physicians, nurses, other personnel, equipment, and supplies are valuable. Review of roles in a situation of multiple casualties is better done by drill than on paper. Even a simulation of a possible

Table 89–1. ESSENTIAL ICU STEPS IN CRITICAL CARE DISASTER RESPONSE

Establish communications
  Field
  Emergency department
  Operating room
  Hospital communications system
Assess resources
  Medical care team
  Equipment
  Bed space
Transfer existing patients as possible
Receive patients
Continue triage as necessary
Perform care
Follow-up

triage scenario in which a mock patient is treated expectantly will allow surfacing of emotions and response patterns in advance of an actual disaster.

References

1. Guda-Sapir D and Lechat MF: Reducing the impact of natural disasters: Why aren't we better prepared? Health Policy and Planning 1:18, 1986.
2. National Research Council: Confronting Natural Disasters: An International Decade for Natural Disaster Reduction. Washington, DC, National Academy Press, 1987, pp. 1–67.
3. Office of US Foreign Disaster Assistance: Disaster History: Significant Data on Major Disasters Worldwide, 1900—Present. Washington, DC, Agency for International Development, 1990, pp.1–45.
4. U.N. General Assembly: International Decade for Natural Disaster Reduction: Report of the Secretary-General. 43 Session, Agenda items 86.A/43/723, 18 October, 1988.
5. Emergency care in natural disasters: Views of an international seminar. WHO Chronicles 34:96, 1980.
6. Pan American Health Organization: Emergency Health Management After Natural Disaster, Washington, DC, PAHO Office of Emergency Prepardness and Disaster Relief Coordination, Scientific Publication No. 407, 1981, pp. 1–76.
7. Wijkman A, and Timberlake L: Natural Disasters: Acts of God or Acts of Man. New York, Earthscan Paperback, 1984, pp. 1–178.
8. Dow AAC, Clark WE, Farmer JC, et al: Organizations and academic perspective. Crit Care Clin 7:2, 257, 1991.
9. Holbrook PR: Pediatric disaster medicine. Crit Care Clin 7:2, 463, 1991.

90

Pediatric Critical Care Transport

Carl B. Ramsey, M.D., and Peter R. Holbrook, M.D.

HISTORY

The history of the transport of critically ill patients can be traced to the Napoleonic wars in which horse-drawn vehicles were used to evacuate battle casualties.[1] In the early 1800s, a crude form of ambulance was used in parts of England to transport patients to hospitals.[2] The first aeromedical transport was performed during the Franco-Prussian War using hot air balloons to move wounded French soldiers over enemy lines to medical facilities.[3] Shortly thereafter, French scientists began to study the effects of altitude on human physiology.[4, 5] In World War I, the French and American armies used aeromedical evacuation. This form of transport was developed further during World War II, and reached fairly sophisticated levels during the Korean and Vietnam wars. Military transport systems are leaders in establishing policies and standard operating procedures that ensure the safety of their patients during transport. In one study of nearly 4,000 aeromedical evacuations from Vietnam, only 8 patients' conditions deteriorated during transport, with one death.[6]

The modern age for critical care transport can be traced to the 1950s when intensive care unit teams transported polio patients requiring ventilatory support to regional centers of care.[7] In 1970, Usher documented the value of regional centers in care of critically ill newborns.[8] His study examined the outcome of 32,000 infants and revealed a nearly twofold improvement in the mortality rate for critically ill infants cared for in regional centers, as opposed to those cared for in community hospitals.[8] The concept of regionalized critical care was promoted further by the well-documented safety of transport[9] and repeated studies showing improved outcome of critically ill infants transferred to regional centers.[10-18]

CURRENT ISSUES IN PEDIATRIC CRITICAL CARE TRANSPORT

General

Although pediatric critical care transport has reached a fairly sophisticated level, there are no universally accepted standards of care. The American Academy of Pediatrics Committee on Hospital Care published guidelines for air and ground transportation of pediatric patients in 1986.[19] In 1989, a national leadership conference was held on pediatric interhospital transport. A consensus was reached during this conference on various issues regarding transportation of critically ill pediatric patients.[20] Although there is a large volume of literature on critical care transport of adults and neonates, there has been little research on the transportation of older infants and children. This chapter will review studies of transportation of all age groups of patients from the scene, as well as studies of inter- and intrahospital transport.

Specific recommendations for transportation of critically ill pediatric patients are made when the literature is clear on an issue. It will be noted when recommendations made are based on information from pediatric or mixed pediatric and adult populations.

Transport from the Scene of Injury

Ground Versus Air Transport of Trauma Patients

The comparison of different transport methods for trauma patients can be performed by classifying anatomic injury in terms of severity and prognosis.[21, 22] The trauma score and injury severity score allow prediction of outcome for patients who have specific injury patterns. This method of scoring is known as TRISS and was validated in a multicenter trauma study.[23, 24, 29]

Baxt and Moody used trauma and injury severity scores for prediction of survival in patients with certain injury patterns caused by blunt trauma.[25] They compared equal numbers of patients with similar injury patterns who were transported by either standard paramedic-staffed, land-based vehicles or physician-manned helicopter transport. All patients studied were treated at the same tertiary referral center. A 52% reduction in predicted mortality was found in the physician-assisted air transport group.[25]

The study was repeated with other trauma centers in different locations.[26] The multicenter study showed a similar though less impressive result, with a 21% reduction in mortality in patients who had aeromedical evacuation. Other centers doing similar studies also documented the efficacy of flight physicians and aeromedical transport in decreasing mortality in patients who sustained injuries from blunt trauma.[27–35]

One exception to these findings was reported by Schiller and coworkers, who compared ground and air transport in an urban environment (Phoenix, AZ).[36] They found no difference in mortality in patients transported by these methods. Although the two groups had a similar number of head injuries and comparable trauma scores, injury severity scores were not calculated in the comparison populations. This precluded use of TRISS methodology to compare survival probabilities and could be an important omission, as the two groups may have differed. One must be careful in extrapolating the results of this study to areas of the United States where similar transport conditions may not exist.[37]

Helicopter transport of trauma patients from rural areas is less controversal and offers several advantages over ground transport.[27, 30, 32–35] The length of time it takes to transport patients via emergency medical support from rural areas gives air-transported patients a significant advantage. Also, the rural emergency medical support quality of care is often less sophisticated, with longer response and transport times.[37]

Boyd and associates reported data on physician interhospital transfer of rural trauma patients, comparing ground versus helicopter transport.[38] With two cohorts that differed only in mode of transport, they calculated probability of survival based on TRISS methodology. The patients transported by ground had the same mortality rate as predicted by TRISS calculations. The aeromedical transport patients had a 25% reduction in the predicted mortality rate. In this study, the time it took for the patient to receive definitive care at a trauma center was the only variable that was statistically significant between groups. Rapid transport may be the major factor contributing to improved survival in this study.

Helicopter transport is the most rapid form of travel for evacuation from rural scenes such as the ones described by Boyd and coworkers. Helicopter transport is not always the fastest mode of transport, especially in urban areas, but it is the transport method of choice if it brings more sophisticated care to the scene in a timely fashion.

Are Physicians Needed on Emergency Transports?

Is the reduction in predicted mortality seen with helicopter transports due to more rapid patient transfer by helicopters to regional trauma centers or to sophisticated treatment rendered earlier at the prehospital level by physicians? Although many studies favor physician-accompanied transport, most are based on subjective information.[39–42] Baxt and Moody[28] reported a prospective randomized study of blunt trauma patients transported by flight physician–flight nurse teams or flight paramedic–flight nurse teams. TRISS methodology was used to assess differences in outcome. The mortality rate in patients treated by the physician-accompanied team was 35% lower than that predicted and was significantly lower than that in the patients transported by nonphysician teams.

Based on these data, physician-accompanied teams appear to offer benefits over nonphysician teams. Yet a physician is not needed on every trauma or medical transport. It is also recognized that physician skill levels may vary widely. Providing aeromedical personnel with the level of skill appropriate for the clinical status of the patient may be a more important issue than the presence of a physician. When to send a physician and appropriate skill levels are areas of debate and the focus of much research in pediatric and adult transport programs. It will be discussed further in the section on interhospital transport.

Pre–Trauma Center Care: Helpful or Harmful?

Stabilization at the Scene or "Swoop, Scoop, and Run"? The role of prehospital advanced trauma life support for traumatized patients remains controversial in pediatric and adult medicine. Some recommend rapid transport of all patients to the nearest trauma center.[44–46] Several studies of the management of life-threatening injuries in the field have shown that time is often wasted by attempts to obtain vascular access and that definitive therapy is achieved only by rapid transport to the regional trauma center.[44–47] Others believe that advanced trauma life support by well-trained emergency medical support personnel in the field can be accomplished rapidly and efficiently, resulting in substantial hemodynamic improvement that translates into improved outcome.[48–53] The addition of intraosseous infusion techniques to the skills of field personnel may make a substantial contribution to the problem of intravenous access and the resultant time delay in the transport of younger children.[54] In general, procedures performed at the scene should be limited to the ABCs of resuscitation, aimed at maintaining adequate oxygen delivery and preserving cerebral function.[47]

Rapid transfer to regional trauma centers has proved to be the management method of choice over field stabilization in patients sustaining penetrating cardiac and thoracic injuries.[55, 56]

Hospital Care Prior to Transport to Level I Trauma Care. Most authorities in trauma care recommend that seriously injured patients be transported directly to a regional trauma center, even if nearby community hospitals are bypassed.[57–62] This recommendation is based on evidence that stopovers at community hospitals may delay lifesaving surgical intervention that is offered only at level I trauma centers.[63, 64] It is often argued that definitive data regarding this philosophy are still lacking and that patients who require immediate resuscitation may deteriorate during the extra time required to reach the more distant trauma center. There is evidence that pre–trauma center care in community hospitals is associated with prolonged hospitalization and higher costs.[65]

Sloan and associates reported the effect of community hospital bypass on prehospital transport times and subsequent level I trauma patient survival. Community hospital bypass made transport significantly longer but did not influence survival significantly.[64] It is important to know that the mean time from the injury event to arrival at the trauma center was 63 minutes, only 3 minutes longer than the time it took for the group that was taken to community hospitals. Comparison of trauma patient survival, using transport times of approximately 1 hour or less as a discriminator, may not be valid. It has been reported that the time taken to manage and transport hypotensive trauma patients to a level I trauma center is not related to an adverse outcome if the time from injury to arrival at the trauma center is 1 hour or less.[47, 66]

The first hour after injury seems to be an important recurring theme in the time it takes for transport issue and has been described by Cowley and colleagues as the "golden hour."[67] Definitive care during this time frame is associated with survival for trauma patients. Based on these data, it seems prudent to bypass community hospitals when the time from injury to the time of arrival at level I trauma centers is not expected to exceed 1 hour.

Triage in a Trauma Bay: When Is Early Transport to the Operating Room Indicated? Direct transport of trauma patients to the operating room has not affected survival.[68] There is evidence that early operative intervention is beneficial for patients who have sustained blunt abdominal trauma and are hypotensive during transport.[69, 70] This may be due to the shortened time between injury and definitive surgical repair of the source of bleeding.

Recommendations for Transport of Trauma Patients from the Scene of Injury and Rural Medical Centers. The following recommendations are based on studies of mixed pediatric and adult patient populations.

1. Physician-attended aeromedical transport from the scene of trauma is useful. It is especially useful in transport of trauma patients from rural areas. The determination of those transports in which physician attendance is essential is not currently possible.

2. Procedures performed at the scene should be limited to the ABCs of resuscitation.

3. Patients with penetrating thoracic or cardiac injuries should not receive prolonged resuscitation at the scene and should be transported immediately to a regional trauma center.

4. If the anticipated time from injury to arrival at a regional trauma center is 1 hour or less, community hospitals should be bypassed.

5. Early admission of trauma patients to operating rooms seems to be beneficial only in reducing mortality in patients who have blunt abdominal trauma and are hypotensive.

INTERHOSPITAL TRANSPORT

Team Composition, Staffing, and Triage

Determination of appropriate team composition to meet the needs of patients transported between hospitals

is one of the main issues in pediatric and adult transport systems. In 1986, the American Academy of Pediatrics Committee on Hospital Care published guidelines for air and ground transportation of pediatric patients[19] and recommended that specific criteria be developed for determining optimal team composition for any given transport. They also recommended team selection from a pool of individuals that includes physicians with at least 2 years of experience in pediatrics (a PL-III) and nurses and respiratory therapists with at least 1 year of experience in critical care pediatrics.

In 1988, McCloskey and Johnston conducted a survey to determine the standard of care regarding team composition and training, mobilization time, and vehicle use in pediatric critical care transport.[71] Responses from 30 pediatric referral centers revealed that 60% provide a critical care transport team. The average number of transports was approximately 300/year/program, and the response time ranged from 10 to 90 minutes. All teams included a physician all or most of the time, and all teams included a critical care nurse at all times. Half of the programs included a respiratory therapist on transport. Ambulances were used as the sole means of transport in approximately one fourth of the programs, with the remainder using a combination of ambulances, helicopters, and fixed-wing aircraft. It was concluded that there was no uniform provision of care for pediatric critical care transport in 1988. Furthermore, 40% of pediatric centers with critical care or emergency medicine fellowship programs had no method of transport designed to consistently institute pediatric intensive care intervention at the prehospital level. Only 28% of extant transport teams met the recommendation that the transport physician always be a PL-III or higher.[71]

Whether and when transport physicians are needed are major considerations in pediatric and adult critical care transport. These issues have extensive medical, legal, and financial implications. There are data indicating that a physician is not needed on all transports.[72] There have been several studies designed with the intent of determining the clinical criteria that identify patients who need physician-level skills on transport.[72–77] McCloskey and coworkers[72] reported a retrospective study of interventions performed by physicians in 191 interhospital transports. These transfers were performed by a pediatric critical care transport team that always included a physician. Physician-level procedures were performed in 9% of transports and the use of drugs that are commonly limited to the intensive care unit (ICU) occurred in 9% of transports. In approximately half of the transfers, the physician believed that his or her expertise was not needed for the successful completion of the transport.[72]

In another study of 148 transfers, McCloskey and coworkers used questionnaires before and after transport to determine whether the need for a physician could be predicted accurately by pretransport data obtained from the referring physician. In 73% of transfers, there was minimal change in the need for a physician between the pre- and post-transport assessments. In the transports in which the determination was significantly changed, most indicated a decreased need for a physician after completion of the transport. There was a significant increase in the perceived need for a physician in only 2% of cases. This study indicates that it may be possible to select in advance certain cases in which physician-level skills or judgment are not needed on transport.[73] There remains, however, the need to develop an objective clinical score based on pretransport data that will accurately predict the need for a physician.

Medical and financial issues in physician-accompanied transport were addressed in an interesting study by Rhee and coworkers.[78] This study assessed physician contributions to critical care transport by a questionnaire completed by the flight nurse after each flight. In the assessment by the flight nurse, the physician made a unique and important contribution to the care of the patient in 22% of patients transported. It is important to note that physician-level skills were cited as the unique contribution in only 1% of cases, whereas judgment was considered the important unique contribution by the physician in the remainder.

The cost of physician presence in that particular transport program was 7% of the annual budget of the program. The authors' conclusion was that the benefit of patients on 22% of transports outweighed the 7% cost for the physician's presence in the transport program.

Subjective and objective techniques have been used in an attempt to determine the need for physicians on transport, including questionnaires and clinical scoring systems such as PRISM and TRISS.[75–77] There are problems encountered with the use of these methods. PRISM was designed to predict mortality in a pediatric intensive care unit and has not been validated as useful in the main transport issues of morbidity and the need for technical intervention.[76, 79]

In order to use any clinical scoring system to accurately predict the need for physician-level skills in pediatric transport, the coordinator who determines team composition must receive a certain amount of accurate information as a baseline from the referring center. Herein lies the main problem in predicting the need for pediatrician-level skills in transport. Very basic information is often lacking from the centers requesting transport. This is usually due to lack of pediatric experience or lack of proper equipment, such as pediatric-sized blood pressure cuffs.

Orr and McCloskey reported that a complete set of vital signs is available only 33% of the time when the initial request for transport is made.[47]

These types of problems make it difficult to determine the need for a pediatric transport team and impossible to accurately predict patient needs regarding judgment and skill among team members. A possible solution to the question of the need for physician presence is to teach physician-level skills to members of the transport team.[80] Many feel that a well-trained and experienced team of nurses or nurse-paramedics could provide expertise at least comparable to a transport system in which a pediatric resident is team leader, as is the case in many programs. Lack of physician judgment is a pervasive concern among critics of nurse and nurse-paramedic programs. They argue that although skills can be taught to nonphysicians, the judgment that comes with medical training cannot be taught readily to the nonphysician. It is possible that judgment could be provided from a regional referral center if the physician coordinator is given complete and accurate information from the patient's bedside by experienced observers who are skilled to provide any invasive or intensive care needed.[20]

Tertiary Care Center and Transport Team Responsibility

The transport team is an extension of the regional center receiving hospital that it represents and should conform to the standard guidelines for resuscitation and protocols approved by the medical director. One recurring problem encountered by medical directors and team leaders of pediatric interhospital transport is the timing of transport from the hospital that is requesting transport (sending hospital).

When making interhospital transfers of unstable critically ill patients, the time to arrival at the regional center may not be as important in patient outcome as it is with patients who have acute life-threatening traumatic injuries. The more important factor is delivery of the regional center's expert care to the patient by the transport team. Often the pediatric patient, as opposed to the adult patient, has had inadequate initial resuscitation (such as intravenous access, fluid resuscitation, or definitive airway management) because of a lack of pediatric experience in the sending hospital's personnel or a lack of pediatric equipment. Therefore, the time spent with the patient by the transport team should be dictated by the condition of the patient on their arrival at the sending hospital.[47]

Regional flight teams and emergency medical support are focused on the adult problems of trauma and myocardial infarction—the major causes of morbidity in adult transports. They are trained to provide rapid response and minimal time at the scene. As a result, when adult-oriented teams respond to pediatric medical transport emergencies, they may feel pressured to leave the scene before adequate pediatric resuscitation is carried out. In addition, the referring physician may be accustomed to the "swoop, scoop, and run" philosophy of the adult-oriented transport teams and may pressure the pediatric team to leave the emergency department prematurely. If the team is only minutes away from the tertiary care center, the team leader may opt to minimize the time spent at the sending hospital and delay performance of procedures until arrival at the regional center.

Recommendations for Team Composition and Staffing

1. Each transport of a critically ill pediatric patient should be supervised by an attending physician experienced in pediatric critical care or emergency medicine.
2. Pediatric patients should be transported by staff

with the cognitive and technical skills needed for the particular patient. Transport staff should have sufficient ongoing experience to maintain those skills.

3. The time it takes to arrive at the tertiary care center may not be as important in medical transfers as is the delivery of the tertiary center's expert care through the transport team. The length of time spent at the referring hospital and the timing of transport should be the responsibility of the transport team coordinator and team leader.

INTRAHOSPITAL TRANSPORT

General

Research in critical care transport has been focused on prehospital and interhospital transport. Intrahospital transport has received less attention in spite of the occurrence of more intrahospital transports than any other type and the very high complication rates that accompany them.[20] Wallen and coworkers[81] reported a study in which 60% of pediatric intensive care patients undergoing intrahospital transfers had at least one major adverse event, including hypothermia (less than 36° C); a 20% change in heart rate, respiratory rate, or blood pressure; oxygen desaturation greater than 5% from baseline; endotracheal tube mishaps; medication errors; blood gas deterioration; and increased ventilator or inotropic support. Thirty-one per cent had more than one adverse event.[81] Indeck and coworkers reported a 68% incidence of significant physiologic changes of 5 minutes' duration in adult trauma patients who underwent intrahospital transport.[82] Another study of critically ill adults who had intrahospital transport from the operating room to the intensive care unit reported a 13% morbidity rate.[83] These data show a surprisingly high incidence of complications during the transfer of critically ill patients within the hospital. Complications may decrease if the quality of care provided during transport is in every way possible an extension of the care provided in the intensive care unit. The physician should always question the risk:benefit ratio of transfer for diagnostic or therapeutic procedures and limit transfers for tests or procedures that do not have a significant impact on patient care.

Personnel

A physician should either accompany the transport or be readily available to respond to an emergency. Although a consensus is lacking, many feel that a critical care physician should accompany any patient who is intubated and should accompany those who are unstable from a neurologic, cardiovascular, or respiratory standpoint.[47] A respiratory therapist should accompany the transport team if the patient is intubated or is unstable from a respiratory standpoint.

Concern for consistently safe intrahospital transport has given rise to the concept of intrahospital transport teams. If the volume of intrahospital transport warrants

it, this could be a team that is separate and distinct from the interhospital team. Otherwise, the interhospital team pool could be expanded, if necessary, and cross-trained for intrahospital transports.

Monitoring and Equipment

If a patient is being transferred from the ICU, all monitoring that was being performed in the ICU should be continued if at all possible. This includes cardiorespiratory monitoring via electrocardiography and impedance pneumography. Pulse oximetry should be continued if it was being used immediately prior to transfer or should be instituted if there is concern for respiratory compromise. If the patient is intubated, capnography should be used to monitor for effective ventilation.

An end-tidal carbon dioxide monitor outfitted with an alarm can be the earliest sign of endotracheal tube malposition or malfunction. Continuation of pulmonary arterial pressure monitoring may be necessary if the patient has labile pulmonary hypertension. Intravascular monitoring of blood pressure should be continued. Batteries for equipment should be checked regularly. Transport while the patient is on a mechanical ventilator is prohibitively cumbersome. It has been shown that manual ventilation during intrahospital transport is safe if the individual performing manual ventilation is well trained to approximate the ventilator-delivered minute ventilation.[84] Mechanical ventilation may be reinstituted when the patient is immobile for any significant period, (i.e., when undergoing computerized tomography scanning, and so on). Equipment carried on transport should include a "code kit" that contains medications used routinely in cardiopulmonary resuscitation and "crash" induction of anesthesia for tracheal intubations. An intubation kit containing all sizes of endotracheal tubes, stylettes, laryngoscopes, and suction catheters, and a valved ventilation bag with different-sized masks should be included. Evaluation of batteries, oxygen tanks, and the completeness and functioning of equipment should be performed routinely.

Special Units to Facilitate Transfer or Isolate Patients or Personnel

Specialized units for transport of the critically ill patient have been devised. Some have special attachment brackets to allow movement of pumps, monitors, and ventilators as a single mobile unit.[85–87] Other transport units have been devised for the patient who requires isolation or reverse isolation.[88, 89] Although many of these units have obvious advantages, no single transport unit has achieved widespread popularity.

SPECIAL CONSIDERATIONS

Aeromedical Transport

The main physiologic effects of aeromedical transport on patients involve changes in altitude, acceleration or deceleration, and noise and vibration from the transport vehicle. Physiologic changes associated with altitude changes are related to decreased atmospheric pressure with resultant decreased oxygen concentration and expansion of gases.

At sea level, the arterial oxygen saturation is greater than 97% and the PaO_2 is 110 mm Hg. Normally, the PaO_2 decreases linearly as altitude increases until 8,000 feet is reached. At 8,000 feet, the arterial oxygen saturation falls to 93% with a PaO_2 of 69 mm Hg. These decreases stimulate carotid chemoreceptors, with a resultant increase in ventilation. This lowers alveolar carbon dioxide, causing a further rise in alveolar and arterial oxygen tension. The degree of hyperventilation is proportional to the amount of hypoxia experienced by the chemoreceptors. Hypoxia causes a variety of mental changes: impaired judgment, drowsiness, dulled sensation to pain, euphoria, disorientation, loss of time sense, and headache.[90] Other physiologic effects of hypoxia are nausea, vomiting, tachycardia, and hypertension. It is difficult to assess patients for hypoxia in the transport environment because of poor lighting, noise, and movement of the transport vehicle. In addition, pulse oximetry can be unreliable because of movement artifacts during transport and poor perfusion. Supplemental oxygen should be administered or increased before aeromedical transport of patients.

Dysbarisms

Dysbarisms are disturbances in the body, excluding hypoxia, that result from a difference between ambient pressure and the pressure of gases within body cavities, tissues, and fluids.[91] The clinical significance of dysbarisms in aeromedical transport are realized in the patient who has abnormal accumulations of gas in closed spaces. Expansion of gases in closed spaces can be significant at relatively low altitudes. At a cabin altitude of 8,000 feet, air will increase in volume by approximately 30%.[92]

Any type of intestinal obstruction or malfunction can cause trapped intestinal air, which can expand at high altitudes. Intramural and intraluminal air expansion can impair bowel circulation or exert pressure on surgical anastomoses.

With pre-existent bowel gas and its subsequent expansion with increased altitude, abdominal distention can progress to the point at which ventilation is compromised. Therefore, gastric or rectal tubes, or both, should be used prophylactically in patients at risk. This does not always provide adequate decompression, and compromise of ventilation should be anticipated in these patients. This condition can be treated expectantly with endotracheal intubation and controlled ventilation if pressurized cabin or land transport is not feasible.

Even a small pneumothorax at sea level can become clinically significant at an increased altitude. Therefore, pneumothorax should be treated before transport. A chest tube should be attached to a Heimlich valve (a one-way flutter valve) or similar device that allows accumulating air or fluid to exit the pleural space.

Decompression Sickness

Decompression sickness is a general term for a group of effects that result from exposure to "high" altitude. This condition involves limb pain, skin and respiratory disturbances, central nervous system dysfunctions, and cardiovascular collapse (see also Chapter 43).[90, 91] The basic pathophysiology causing clinical symptoms is supersaturation of tissues with nitrogen. The rise in altitude results in subsequent nitrogen gas expansion that occurs faster than its vascular removal to the lungs, resulting in bubble formation (aeroembolism) in tissues.

Clinical symptoms will vary in type and severity depending on the location of the aeroembolism. Predisposing factors for decompression syndrome include increased age, obesity, fast rate of ascent, a high maximum altitude achieved, and increased tissue nitrogen levels prior to ascent.[93] Because of the possibility of increased tissue nitrogen levels before flight, it is recommended that divers do not fly within 24 hours of diving.[94] There are reports of symptoms when flying after diving at altitudes as low as 7,000 feet.[90] Patients with severe decompression sickness require transport to decompression facilities. When these patients are transported by air, they should be transported in fixed-wing aircraft only if transport can occur expeditiously with cabin pressures maintained at sea level. Reddick[96] reported worsening of symptoms in a group of these patients transported by helicopter when an altitude of 200 feet was exceeded. There was no worsening of symptoms at altitudes less than 200 feet, and transport was performed twice as quickly as was possible with ground transport. Rapid transport is very important, as Dully[95] has shown that delay of treatment can result in severe complications, even with relatively mild presenting symptoms of decompression syndrome.

Effects of Altitude on Equipment

Patient care can be affected by air expansion in equipment during aeromedical transport. During ascent or descent, pressure changes in intravenous solution containers can affect flow rates of fluids. This may be of special importance in smaller patients who are more susceptible to fluid changes or when intravenous solution containers and lines contain concentrated inotropic agents. Because of this, intravenous lines should be on volume-regulated pumps. Plastic intravenous fluid bags should be used, and glass should be avoided.[90]

Air expansion in endotracheal tube cuffs can be severe enough to cause tracheal mucosal damage. Cuff pressure should be low during ascent and should be normalized when constant altitude is reached. The cuff pressure should be rechecked during descent and on the ground to avoid excessive air leaks. Air splints should be avoided during transport, as they can become tight enough to impair limb circulation at altitudes as low as 2,000 feet.[94] Circulation should be assessed often when pneumatic trousers are used during transport. Other air-filled indwelling instruments should also be treated appropriately. Pulmonary artery catheter balloons should be deflated completely. Foley catheter balloons can be deflated or filled with water to prevent problems with air expansion.

Acceleration and Deceleration Changes

Acceleration and deceleration routinely occur during transport. One study using anesthetized dogs showed a 25 to 30% increase in saggital sinus pressure in dogs during take-off acceleration and ascent.[96] Most air ambulances exert only an additional 0.5 g during any type of flight maneuver. Therefore, the potential for problems appears to be minimal, except in the severely compromised patient.[90]

Vibration and Noise Interference

Noise during helicopter transport causes difficulty in communicating and hearing alarms on cardiorespiratory monitors. Pulse oximeters must be frequently checked visually and are often rendered nonfunctional by vibration. Even with fairly low-volume noise levels, auscultation may be difficult.

There are reports of pacemaker dysfunction during helicopter transport of unstable adult cardiac patients.[97, 98] Recommendations have been made for external transcutaneous pacers in a similar patient population.[99] Defibrillators may be used safely and effectively during transport.[100] The cause for this interference with the function of some electrical medical devices is unknown, though electromagnetic interference and routine vibration have been blamed.

There is evidence indicating that noninvasive blood pressure monitoring may be inaccurate in helicopter transports and that relying on noninvasive measures may lead to therapeutic mishaps.[101]

References

1. Jones DR: Aeromedical transportation of psychiatric patients: Historical view and present management. Aviat Space Environ Med 51:709, 1980.
2. Hart H: The conveyance of patients to and from the hospital, 1720–1850. Med Hist 22:397, 1978.
3. Johnson A: Treatise on aeromedical evacuation. Aviat Space Environ Med 48:546, 1977.
4. Hitchcock FA: Paul Bert and the beginnings of aviation medicine. Aerospace Med 42:1101, 1977.
5. Parsons CJ and Bobechko WP: Aeromedical transport: Its hidden problems. CMA J 126:237, 1982.
6. White MS, Chub RM, Rossing RG, et al: Results of early aeromedical evacuation of Vietnam casualties. Aerospace Med 42:780, 1971.
7. Cara M and Poisvert M: Premiers secours dans les détresses respiratoires. Paris, Mason, 1963.
8. Usher RH: The role of the neonatologist. Pediatr Clin North Am 17:199, 1970.
9. Hackel A and Wong R: The effect of interhospital transport variables on the survival of critically ill neonates with RDS. Pediatr Res 15:449, 1981.
10. Butterfield LJ: Regionalization for respiratory care. Pediatr Clin North Am 20:499, 1973.
11. Ferrara A: Transportation of sick neonates. Can Med Assoc J 110:1233, 1974.

12. Hackel A: A medical transport system for the neonate. Anesthesiology 43:258, 1975.
13. Pettet G, Merenstein GB, Battaglia FC, et al: An analysis of air transports: Results in the sick newborn infant. Pediatrics 55:774, 1975.
14. Segal S: Manual for the Transport of Sick Newborn Infants. Vancouver, Canadian Pediatric Society, 1972.
15. West JG, Trunkey DD, and Lim RC: Systems of trauma care: A study of two counties. Arch Surg 114:455, 1979.
16. Mackenzie CF, Shin B, Fisher R, et al: Two-year mortality in 760 patients transported by helicopter direct from the road accident scene. Am Surg 45:101, 1979.
17. Gill W, Champion HR, Long WB, et al: A clinical experience of major multiple trauma in Maryland. MD State Med J 25(1):55, 1976.
18. Duke JH Jr and Clarke WP: A university-staffed, private hospital-based air transport service: The initial two-year experience. Arch Surg 116:703, 1981.
19. Bergeson PS, Bushore M, Cravens JH, et al: Guidelines for air and ground transportation of pediatric patients. Pediatrics 78:943, 1986.
20. Day S, McCloskey K, Orr R, et al: Pediatric interhospital critical care transport: Consensus of a national leadership conference. Pediatrics 88:696, 1991.
21. Baker SP, O'Neil B, Haddon W, et al: The injury severity score: A method for describing patients with multiple injuries and evaluating emergency care. J Trauma 14:187, 1974.
22. Champion HR, Sacco WJ, Lepper RL, et al: An anatomic index of injury severity. J Trauma 20:197, 1980.
23. Boyd CR and Tolson M: Evaluating trauma care: The TRISS method. J Trauma 27:370, 1987.
24. Champion HR, Sacco WJ, Carnazzo AJ, et al: Trauma score. Crit Care Med 9:672, 1981.
25. Baxt WG and Moody P: The impact of a rotorcraft aeromedical emergency care service on trauma mortality. JAMA 249:3047, 1983.
26. Baxt WG, et al: Hospital-based rotorcraft aeromedical emergency care services and trauma mortality: A multicenter study. Ann Emerg Med 14:9, 1985.
27. Anderson TE, Rose WD, and Leicht MJ: Physician-staffed helicopter scene response from a rural trauma center. Ann Emerg Med 16:85, 1987.
28. Baxt WG and Moody P: The impact of a physician as part of the aeromedical prehospital team in patients with blunt trauma. JAMA 257:3246, 1987.
29. Baxt WG, Moody P, Cleveland HC, et al: Hospital-based rotorcraft aeromedical emergency care services and trauma mortality: A multicenter study. Ann Emerg Med 14:859, 1985.
30. Boyd CR, Corse KM, and Campell RC: Interhospital transport: Air vs ground. Presented at the 2nd Annual Eastern Association for the Surgery of Trauma Scientific Meeting. Oongboat Key, FL, January, 1989.
31. Fisher RP, Flynn TC, Miller PW, et al: Urban helicopter response to the scene of injury. J Trauma 24:946, 1984.
32. Leicht MJ, Dula DJ, Brotman S, et al: Rural interhospital transport of motor vehicle trauma victims: Cases for delays and recommendations. Ann Emerg Med 15:450, 1986.
33. Schiller WR, Knox R, Zinnecker H, et al: Effect of helicopter transport of trauma victims on survival in an urban trauma center. J Trauma 28:1127, 1988.
34. Urdaneta LF, Miller BK, Ringenberg, BJ, et al: Role of an emergency helicopter transport service in rural trauma. Arch Surg 122:992, 1987.
35. Urdaneta LF, Sandberg MK, Cram AE, et al: Evaluation of an emergency air transport service as a component of a rural EMS system. Am Surg 50:183, 1984.
36. Schiller WR, Knox R, and Zinnecker H, et al: Effect of helicopter transport of trauma victims on survival in an urban trauma center. J Trauma 28(8):1127, 1988.
37. Gabram SG and Jacobs LM: The impact of emergency medical helicopters on prehospital care. Emerg Med Clin North Am 8(1):85, 1990.
38. Boyd DR, Corse KM, and Campbell RC: Emergency interhospital transport of the major trauma patient: Air versus ground. J Trauma 29(6):789, 1989.
39. Carraway RP, Brewer ME, Lewis BR, et al: Why a physician?

Aeromedical transport of the trauma victim, abstracted. J Trauma 24:650, 1984.

40. Rhee KJ, Strozeski M, Burney RE, et al: Is the flight physician needed for helicopter emergency medical service? Ann Emerg Med 15:174, 1986.

41. Kaplan L, Walsh D, and Burney RE: Emergency aeromedical transport of patients with acute myocardial infarction. Ann Emerg Med 16:55, 1986.

42. Anderson TE, Rose WD, and Leicht MJ: Physician staffed helicopter scene response from a rural trauma center. Ann Emerg Med 16:58, 1986.

43. Pepe PE, Bickell WH, Wyatt CH, et al: Relationship between total prehospital time and outcome in patients with penetrating trauma. (Abstract) Ann Emerg Med 15:626, 1986.

45. Smith JP, Bodai BI, Hill AS, et al: Prehospital stabilization of critically injured patients: A failed concept. J Trauma 25:65, 1985.

46. Trunkey DD: Is ALS necessary for pre-hospital trauma care? J Trauma 24:86, 1984.

47. Orr RA and McCloskey KA: Mobilizing critical care for inter-hospital and intrahospital transport. In: Lumb PD and Shoemaker WC (eds): Critical Care: State of the Art, Vol 11. Fullerton, CA, Society of Critical Care Medicine, 1990, pp 303–320.

48. Aprahamian CA, Thompson BM, Towne JB, et al: The effect of a paramedic system on mortality of major open intra-abdominal vascular trauma. J Trauma 23:635, 1983.

49. Aprahamian CA, Dann JC, Thompson BM, et al: Traumatic cardiac arrest: Scope of paramedic services. Ann Emerg Med 14:583, 1985.

50. Copass MK, Oreskovich MR, Bladergroen MR, et al: Prehospital cardiopulmonary resuscitation of the critically injured patient. Am J Surg 148:20, 1984.

51. Fortner GS, Oreskovich MR, Copass MK, et al: The effects of prehospital care on survival from a 50-meter fall. J Trauma 23:976, 1983.

52. Jacobs LM, Sinclair A, Beiser, et al: Prehospital advanced life support: Benefits in trauma. J Trauma 24:8, 1984.

53. Pons PT, Honigman B, Moore E, et al: Prehospital advanced trauma life support for critical penetrating wounds to the thorax and abdomen. J Trauma 25:828, 1985.

54. Zimmerman JJ, Coyne M, and Logsdon M: Implementation of intraosseous infusion technique by aeromedical transport programs. J Trauma 29:687, 1989.

55. Gervin AS and Fischer RP: The importance of prompt transport in salvage of patients with penetrating heart wounds. J Trauma 22:443, 1982.

56. Ivatury RR, Nallathambi MN, and Roberge RJ: Penetrating thoracic injuries: In-field stabilization vs. prompt transport. J Trauma 27:1068, 1987.

57. Cales RH: Trauma mortality in Orange County: The effect of implementation of a regional trauma system. Ann Emerg Med 13:1, 1984.

58. Detmer DC, Moylan JA, Rose J, et al: Regional categorization and quality of care in major trauma. J Trauma 17:592, 1977.

59. Pepe PE, Stewart RD, and Copass MK: Prehospital management of trauma: A tale of three cities. Ann Emerg Med 15:1484, 1986.

60. Gervin AS and Fischer RP: The importance of prompt transport in salvage of patients with penetrating heart wounds. J Trauma 22:443, 1982.

61. West JG, Trunkey DD, and Lim RC: Systems of trauma care. Arch Surg 114:455, 1979.

62. West JG, Cales RH, and Gazzaniga AB: Impact of regionalization. Arch Surg 118:740, 1983.

63. Clemmer TP, Orme JF, Thomas FO, et al: Outcome of critically injured patients treated at level I trauma centers versus full-service community hospitals. Crit Care Med 13:861, 1985.

64. Sloan EP, Callahan EP, and Duda J: The effect of urban trauma system hospital bypass on prehospital transport times and level 1 trauma patient survival. Ann Emerg Med 18(11):1146, 1989.

65. Schwartz RJ, Lenworth MJ, and Yaezel D: Impact of pre-trauma center care on length of stay and hospital charges. J Trauma 29:1611, 1989.

66. Pepe PE, Wyatt CH, Bickell WH, et al: The relationship between total prehospital time and outcome in hypotensive victims of penetrating injuries. Ann Emerg Med 16:3 1987.

67. Cowley RS, Hudson F, and Scanlan E: An economical and proven helicopter program for transporting the emergency critically ill and injured patient in Maryland. J Trauma 13:1029, 1973.

68. American College of Surgeons Committee on Trauma: Hospital and pre-hospital resources for optimal care of the injured patient. Bull Am Coll Surg 71(10):4, 1986.

69. Law DK, Law JK, Brennan R, et al: Trauma operating room in conjunction with an air ambulance system: Indications, interventions, and outcomes. J Trauma 22:759, 1982.

70. Rhodes M, Brader A, Lucke J, et al: Direct transport to the operating room for resuscitation of trauma patients. J Trauma 29:907, 1989.

71. McCloskey KA and Johnston C: Pediatric critical care transport survey: Team composition and training, mobilization time, and mode of transportation. Pediatr Emerg Care 6:1, 1990.

72. McCloskey KA, King WD, and Byron L: Pediatric Critical Care Transport: Is a Physician Always Needed on the Team? Ann Emerg Med 183:247, 1989.

73. McCloskey KA and Johnston C: Critical care interhospital transports: Predictability of the need for a pediatrician. Pediatr Emerg Care 6:289, 1990.

74. McCloskey KA and King W: Variables Predicting the Need for Major Procedures During Pediatric Critical Care Transport. Presented at the meeting of the American Academy of Pediatrics, San Francisco, CA, October 21, 1989.

75. Kanter RK and Tompkins JM: Adverse events during interhospital transport: Physiologic deterioration associated with pre-transport severity of illness. Pediatrics 84:43, 1989.

76. Orr RA, Venkataraman ST, and Singleton CA: Pediatric risk of mortality (PRISM) score: A poor predictor in triage of patients for pediatric transport. Ann Emerg Med 18:450, 1989.

77. Mayer TA and Walker ML: Severity of illness and injury in pediatric air transport. Ann Emerg Med 13:108, 1984.

78. Rhee KJ, Strozeski M, Burney RE, et al: Is the flight physician needed for helicopter emergency medical services? Ann Emerg Med 15:174, 1986.

79. Pollack MM, Ruttimann UE, and Getson PR: Pediatric risk of mortality (PRISM) score. Crit Care Med 16:1110, 1988.

80. Smith DF and Hackel A: Selection criteria for pediatric critical care transport teams. Crit Care Med 57:699, 1986.

81. Wallen EA, Orr RA, Venkataraman ST, et al: Adverse events during intrahospital transport of critically ill children. Abstract Crit Care Med 19:S79, 1991.

82. Indeck M, Peterson S, Smith J, et al: Risk, cost and benefit of transporting ICU patients for special studies. J Trauma 28(7):1020, 1988.

83. Insel J, Weissman C, Kemper M, et al: Cardiovascular changes during transport of critically ill and postoperative patients. Crit Care Med 14(6):539, 1986.

84. Weg JG and Hass CF: Safe intrahospital transport of critically ill ventilator-dependent patients. Chest 96(3):631, 1989.

85. Petre JH, Bazaral MG, Estafanous FG, et al: Patient transport: An organized method with direct clinical benefits. Biomedical Instrumentation and Technology, p. 100, 1989.

86. Park GR and Selwyn J: A bed-mounted unit for the movement of critically ill patients. Anaesthesia 36:624, 1981.

87. Kondo K, Marty AT, and Henning RJ: Letters to the editor. Crit Care Med 13(12):443, 1985.

88. Talbot TL and Pizzo PA: Simple and microbiologically safe portable unit for patients requiring protected isolation. J Clin Microbiol 11:234, 1980.

89. Wilson KE and Driscoll DM: Mobile high containment isolation: A unique patient care modality. Am J Infect Control 15:120, 1987.

90. Lachenmyer J: Physiological aspects of transport. Int Anesth Clin 25:15, 1987.

91. Dhenin G: Aviation Medicine: Physiology and Human Factors. London, Tri-Med, 1978.

92. Harding RM and Mills FJ: Problems of altitude: I. Hypoxia and hyperventilation. Br Med J 286:1408, 1983.

93. U.S. Air Force: U.S. Naval Flight Surgeons's Manual, 2nd ed. Bethesda, MD: Naval Aerospace Medical Institute and Bio-Technology. Washington, DC, U.S. Government Printing Office, 1978.

94. Oxer HF: Aeromedical evacuation of the seriously ill. Br Med J 3:692, 1975.

95. Dully FE Jr: Central nervous system involvement following type I aviator's bends complicated by complacency. Aviat Space Environ Med 46:1186, 1978.
96. Reddick EJ: Aeromedical evacuation. Am Fam Phys 16:154, 1977.
97. French RS and Tillman JG: Pacemaker function during helicopter transport. Ann Emerg Med 18:305, 1989.
98. Sumchai A, Sternbach G, Eliastam E, et al: Pacing hazards in helicopter aeromedical transport. Am J Emerg Med 6:236, 1988.
99. Vukov LF and Johnson DQ: External transcutaneous pacemakers in interhospital transport of cardiac patients. Ann Emerg Med 18:738, 1989.
100. Dedrick DK, Darga A, Landis D, et al: Defibrillation safety in emergency helicopter transport. Ann Emerg Med 18:69, 1989.
101. Low RB and Martin D: Accuracy of blood pressure measurements made aboard helicopters. Ann Emerg Med 17:604, 1988.

91

Legal Considerations

Lee W. Doty, J.D.

This chapter answers the question: "What does the pediatric critical care physician need to know about the law in order to avoid a lawsuit or, at the very least, to provide a strong defense once involved in the almost inevitable lawsuit?" An effort is made to provide practical information of interest not to other lawyers, but to pediatric intensivists who are familiar with certain basic principles of tort law and consent law and who are wondering how such legal principles affect their daily practice. Since this subject matter is vast and space is limited, the basic principles will be reviewed briefly. Also, matters governed by specific state statutes, such as child abuse/neglect reporting and coroner's cases, which are generally handled through specific hospital policies, are not covered. Finally, since other chapters focus extensively on death and dying, these topics will not be addressed here.

The case law provides little guidance to the pediatric intensivist regarding professional liability since there are so few reported cases. One would hope that by simply practicing "good medicine," one would avoid professional liability. But relying upon this standard requires some caution, for the law does not generously hand out guarantees. For example, one might assume that a hospital's strict compliance with the Joint Commission on Accreditation of Healthcare Organization's (JCAHO) peer review standards would protect a hospital from liability for the acts of an incompetent physician, yet a California trial court held that the JCAHO peer review standards were deficient and therefore the hospital was liable.[1] But the opposite result was reached 6 years later in Georgia, when adherence to the JCAHO peer review standards allowed the hospital to avoid liability.[2] In another perhaps more dramatic case, the Washington Superior Court decided that, despite the customary practice of local ophthalmologists to wait until patients reached age 35 before administering a tonometer test for glaucoma, a more rigorous standard should be applied and the two defendant ophthalmologists were held liable for failing to adhere to this court-created standard.[3]

Fortunately, these counter-intuitive holdings are rare, but anyone who has ever been through a court proceeding understands that the outcome depends largely on the level of understanding and the biases of the judge and jury. A more cynical view is that the outcome, particularly in pediatric cases, is often influenced by the physical injuries and financial needs of the minor plaintiff. The pediatric intensivist must also recognize that the courtroom is not the only arena in which one must have a good defense. With the passage of the Health Care Quality Improvement Act of 1986,[4] a national practitioner data bank was established to receive information on a mandatory basis from hospitals regarding malpractice payments made on behalf of physicians. Hospitals are required to query the data bank when appointing and reappointing physicians to the medical staff, and physicians are called upon to defend their role in any malpractice claim that resulted in an indemnity payment. Another "trial" occurs during the years when the lawsuit is in progress. During this phase, which may be the most important, the physician's competence is scrutinized by lawyers, expert witnesses (who may be colleagues), hospital management, the hospital board of directors, and his or her peers. This "trial" and the credentialling process "trial" are won by the practice of "good medicine," perhaps better described as defensible medicine.

The following sections discuss what constitutes defensible medicine for the pediatric intensivist and, subject to some limitations, the law that defines it.

SPECIAL FEATURES OF THE PEDIATRIC CRITICAL CARE UNIT

The pediatric critical care unit (PCCU) is filled with critically ill or injured patients in need of 24-hour monitoring by full-time specialists with the skills and high-technology equipment to manage life support. To understand defensible medicine in the PCCU, it is helpful first to understand which of the unit's unique features are significant to a malpractice lawyer or risk manager and why

- Many of these ill patients were recently well. Now they are suffering from the failure of one or more organs or systems.
- Their parents are extremely fragile, worried, and watchful. They have never been in a PCCU and perhaps not even in a hospital. The awe-inspiring high-technology atmosphere and the multitude of specialists, coupled with the potential for tragedy, render many parents almost as needy as their sick children.
- The PCCU is like an ever-changing stage set. Patients are "stepped up" to the unit or "stepped down" from the unit, and this sequence can be repeated several times during one hospital admission because they are admitted to the unit based on their need, not their diagnosis. Meanwhile, a steady stream of pulmonologists, cardiologists, surgeons, and neurologists interact in the unit. It is not unusual for two specialists to treat a patient in the PCCU with the same problem differently, according to the specialist's own training. Furthermore, sometimes it is difficult to know which physician is ultimately responsible for the patient.
- The pediatric intensivist manages this ever-changing scene but also renders highly specialized care, which may itself cross specialty lines.
- The PCCU is a dangerous place. The risks of nosocomial infection and major tracheostomy complications, for example, are high. The monitoring equipment and invasive diagnostic procedures may themselves cause injury. One intensivist has compared the PCCU to the beltway around Washington, DC: If you are on it long enough, sooner or later you are going to get hit.
- Pediatric critical care is expensive. Serious cost/benefit studies for intensive care patients are underway,[5] and critical care rationing may result.
- Because the PCCU is designed to provide the closest monitoring of a patient within the hospital, there is the expectation that nothing will be missed and therefore nothing can go wrong.
- The PCCU is a training ground for new intensivists and other medical personnel.

These features of the PCCU make it fertile ground for claims of negligence, especially regarding medication-related error, equipment-related error, failure to diagnose, failure to supervise, delay in treatment, and failure to prevent complications.[6] One reason that pediatric intensivists have fewer claims than general surgeons is that PCCU patients are so closely monitored. By the same token, there is the expectation that sins of omission, in particular, should not occur in a unit where, by definition, the patient is closely monitored.

Understanding their unique environment and their peculiar vulnerability to claims of omission, intensivists can apply the principles of liability to better appreciate what practices will be defensible.

PRINCIPLES OF LIABILITY

In order for a patient to prove that the pediatric intensivist has committed malpractice, it must be shown that

- The intensivist owed that patient a duty to act in accordance with the standard of care;
- The duty was breached;
- The breach was the "proximate cause" of the patient's injury; and
- The patient suffered damage or harm.

Duty of Care

A special task for the intensivist is to understand *when* a duty to a particular patient arises, since so many different health care providers are involved in a PCCU patient's care. But even before a patient is admitted to the PCCU, the intensivist consults with other units to determine whether the patient should be "stepped up" to the PCCU. Thus, it could be argued that by examining the patient and determining that he is a candidate for the PCCU, the intensivist has already undertaken responsibility for the patient.

Henry v. Felici[7] illustrates the principle that a duty, like a ball, can be passed around, bounced, and dropped, but if the intensivist has sufficient information to warrant action on his part, then the ball is his. *Felici* involved the woefully prolonged transfer of a pediatric patient with a head injury from one hospital's intensive care unit to another hospital's unit that was equipped to perform computed tomography and neurosurgery. The parents sought to hold the doctors at the transferring hospital responsible for the 5½ hour delay (the transfer normally took 30 minutes), which resulted in a massive head bleed and eventual death of the child following surgery.

The delay occurred because the neurologists at the hospital to which the child was to be transferred were not made aware of the gravity of the child's condition. It was made worse by the unavailability, on this Saturday morning, of a transport nurse and an ambulance. The jury was asked to decide whether it was the duty of the physician or the transferring hospital staff to effect a prompt transfer. The jury agreed with expert testimony stating that once the doctor ordered a transfer, it became the hospital staff's responsibility to complete the transfer. It is standard medical practice for doctors to assume that their orders will be carried out, *unless they are informed otherwise*. If the hospital personnel did not tell the doctor that there was a problem with carrying out the order, the doctor was without fault. Conversely, if the doctor was made aware of the problem, then he had a duty to investigate and take the proper action. (The jury may have clung to this expert testimony in exonerating the physicians because, as soon as one of them did learn of the child's grave condition, he immediately drove to the hospital, gathered the instruments needed for the transport, and went on the transport himself.)

Therefore, while a physician may have an initial duty of care to a patient, he may discharge it and not assume it again unless other events put him on notice that his services are needed.

When an intensivist advises the primary physician that his patient should be admitted to the PCCU *immediately* and yet, 30 minutes later, the patient has not arrived, is the intensivist responsible for finding out why? The *Henry* case tells us that when the intensivist has reason to believe that his instructions (which have been agreed to) are not being carried out, he must act. If the intensivist instructs the unit clerk to expect cardiology patient John Jones and to prepare a monitored bed, and if John does not arrive and the unit clerk does not page the intensivist to let him know, then the intensivist is justified in assuming that the primary physician and hospital staff have carried out their responsibilities. If, on the other hand, the intensivist agrees to meet with John's parents in the PCCU in 30 minutes, then he will be in a position to know that the patient never arrived.

A slightly more difficult hypothetical situation occurs when the intensivist is evaluating a dangerously unstable patient for admission to the PCCU. Must the intensivist remain with the patient until he is admitted? Yes. When the likelihood that the patient will enter a crisis is so great that the intensivist is presumed to know that his special life support skills will be needed, then he must remain with the patient. The intensivist is under a duty to attend to his patient so long as the patient requires it or risk liability for abandonment.[8]

Even inside the PCCU, responsibility for the patient may shift from one physician to another. Hospital policy should clarify who will be the primary physician for patients admitted to the PCCU. In some hospitals, the intensivist will play this role for all but surgical patients, whose surgeons will continue to serve as the primary physicians in the PCCU. In that situation, the relationship between the intensivist and the surgeon may be one of cophysicians or primary and consulting physician. The titles are fairly unimportant, since the allocation of responsibility depends on the degree of involvement of the physician with the patient and on the tacit or written policy as to how responsibility will be apportioned. The standard practice may be that the surgeon, as primary physician, makes decisions and writes orders for his patients. This standard may be modified, however, by the degree of involvement of the intensivist. Because the intensivist is in a position to observe the patient, certain responsibilities will attach. For example, when the intensivist is aware that a surgical patient's endotracheal tube has remained in place longer than normal, has he discharged his duty by notifying the primary physician and making a note in the chart, or must he make sure that the tube is removed? Logic suggests that if the surgeon is made aware of the issue, but explains to the intensivist that it is his opinion that several more days will not harm the patient, then so long as other surgeons would agree, the intensivist's duty is discharged. More eloquently stated:

Where there is more than one recognized method of diagnosis or treatment, and no one of them is used exclusively and uniformly by all practitioners of good standing, a physician or

nurse is not negligent if, in exercising reasonable judgment, they select one of the approved methods, which later turns out to be a wrong selection or one not favored by certain practitioners.[9]

What often happens is that the intensivist will simply note the need for tube removal in the chart, along with the fact that the surgeon was notified. If the surgeon's response is not recorded, and the tube is not removed, the intensivist has probably discharged his duty. On the other hand, this situation may place both specialists in the hot seat before a jury because, from the jury's point of view, the patient was left in a precarious position that at least two physicians might have corrected. A better solution may be for the surgeon to briefly articulate in the chart his rationale for leaving the tube in place. When the intensivist doubts that any physician would leave the tube in so long, he should ask the appropriate department chairman to review the care plan or solicit the opinion of some other highly placed administrative physician. In other words, the intensivist may not be allowed to blindly accept the treatment plan of a cophysician when he has reason to believe the treatment is substandard.[10]

What about the director of the PCCU who is also the only intensivist in the hospital? What is the scope of his responsibility? Is he merely a consultant? Again, it will depend on (1) the relevant medical staff policies that assign responsibility and define when consultation with others is appropriate and (2) the degree of involvement with the patient. Some of the director's responsibilities are referenced in the JCAHO Accreditation Manual for Hospitals.[11] Briefly stated, the director is responsible for implementing medical staff policies, for making decisions for the disposition of a patient when patient load exceeds optimum operational capacity, and for assuring that the quality, safety, and appropriateness of patient care services provided within the unit are monitored and evaluated on a regular basis and that appropriate actions based on findings are taken. This list serves as general guidance on powerful evidence of the minimum responsibilities of a director of a PCCU.

Standard of Care and Breach of the Standard

Once the duty to a patient arises, the intensivist must conform to the standard of reasonable care in treating the patient. A jury first determines the standard of care based on the testimony of expert witnesses, who may be intensivists or other specialists, and then decides whether or not the standard was breached. In addition to expert testimony, the standard of care may be proven through reference to a statute, regulation, JCAHO standards, or hospital policy. Under certain circumstances, no expert testimony on the standard of care is necessary when common sense indicates what is substandard (for example, when a sponge is left inside a patient).

It should be noted that the standard of care owed a patient may differ depending on the circumstances under which treatment is given. Using an obvious example, the intensivist Good Samaritan at the roadside will not be held to as high a standard as the intensivist in the PCCU. The standard of care may also depend on a risk/benefit analysis of the proposed care. Clearly, the law does not ask medicine to guarantee results; if it did, all tests and therapies would have to be tried on every patient. The law allows and even requires a certain amount of analysis of whether a procedure's benefits outweigh its risks. If a diagnostic test is noninvasive, risk free, conclusive, inexpensive, and available and the chance of missing the diagnosis without it is great, the test should probably be performed.[3] If any of these characteristics is not present, then the physician will need to exercise good judgment.

Since professionals can and do differ on the standard of care, the jury will base its decision on the presentation and credibility of the experts. But when an institution has reduced the standard of care to a policy, and that policy is not followed, there is not much left to say. Policies are established because they promote good care. They are especially helpful in the PCCU because they impose a certain uniformity of practice on the part of physicians and ancillary professionals in a setting where they may not all report administratively through the same channels.

Case law informs us that hospitals often have good policies but fail to adequately communicate them to busy physicians, night-time personnel, Saturday float nurses, or first-year residents. This is a vulnerable point for intensivists in terms of liability and, more importantly, in terms of providing good medical care.

At one time, a majority of jurisdictions held that the relevant standard of care against which practitioners should be judged is that which is standard in the community (the so-called "locality rule"). But because plaintiffs had difficulty retaining local experts to prove their cases, the locality rule was replaced by a national standard; that is, the intensivist will be held to the standard of his profession as practiced nationally.

To what standard of care will the pediatric intensivist be held if he crosses specialty lines? Should he routinely cross specialty lines or must he often arrange for a consultation? The intensivist may have originally been trained and board certified as an anesthesiologist, pediatrician, surgeon, or internist. As noted previously, a surgically trained intensivist (or a surgeon in the PCCU) may manage a patient postoperatively quite differently from an intensivist trained as an anesthesiologist. The general rule is that the physician has a duty to exercise that degree of skill ordinarily possessed and exercised by the average member of the profession practicing in the field.[12] But which field? If the intensivist is performing a procedure that is within the scope of expertise of an intensivist (though performed just as often by general surgeons, anesthesiologists, and pediatricians), then he will be held to the standard of the average intensivist. If, however, he goes beyond his own field into one requiring a much greater depth of knowledge in a particular specialty, such as orthopedic surgery, then he will be held to the standard of an average orthopedic surgeon. Some intensivists ask themselves, might this patient enjoy better results through a consultation? If so, they make the referral.

Transport and telephone communication are other areas where the concepts of duty and standard of care become intertwined. The situation usually arises when a patient is being transferred from one hospital's emergency room or PCCU to another PCCU and the intensivist is being consulted as a specialist by the referring institution. Is there a physician-patient relationship giving rise to a duty between the intensivist and the patient when there is no physical proximity and no consent by the patient to accept the intensivist's services? Generally, a physician-patient relationship does not exist when the sole contact is a telephone call. But when the intensivist undertakes to provide advice on the safe transport of the patient, a duty does arise, and it requires that the intensivist ask the appropriate questions and, based on the answers, provide advice within the standard of reasonable care. Failure to ask the right questions is analogous to the failure to order appropriate tests before treating a patient. Before recommending a plan, a physician must have a sufficient factual basis upon which to base it.[13]

Causation and Damages

The third and fourth elements of the medical malpractice case involve correlating breach of the standard of care to the patient's injury. This is a problem for the intensivist because of the nature of his patient: with or without a breach of the standard of care, the child's condition is likely to worsen. Moreover, because the PCCU is "a dangerous place," the patient may suffer injuries not directly related to his illness.

Expert testimony is needed to prove that the injury complained of is the proximate result of the breach, but there are well-credentialed experts whose testimony will suffice to place the matter before the jury. In fact, the jury might well be instructed by the judge that the intensivist's negligence need not be the *only* cause of the injury, so long as there is a substantial possibility that his negligence caused the injury. Defense counsel is often afraid to try a case involving a critically ill child with long-term care needs, even though there is no causal relationship between the breach and the full spectrum of the child's injuries, because the jury may find that *all* aspects of the child's future care are the responsibility of the negligent physician who caused at least some of the damage.

While the jury may be expected to err on the side of the unfortunate child, the intensivist should strive to present his case in the best light. Already discussed was the need to document appropriately so that other caregivers, as well as a jury, will understand the thinking behind the decisions that were made. The intensivist whose patient's condition suddenly worsens should document fully the steps taken to address the crisis. Often, all aspects of the response to a crisis are not fully documented, in part because of the urgent circumstances and in part because, for the intensivist, such heroics are routine. But recall the *Henry* case where the physician, once aware of the delay in transport, rushed to the hospital and hopped into the ambulance to transport the patient. Defense counsel needs these kinds of facts to overcome a quite human bias toward an injured child.

Other loss control opportunities arise in the context of the consent process.

CONSENT LAW

General

Courts support the right of patients, or when they are legally incompetent, surrogate decision-makers, to make their own decisions with regard to medical and surgical treatment. In fact, a patient must give consent to any touching, whether or not the touching is invasive, or the physician may be guilty of a battery.[14] The extent of damages will depend on the outcome of the touching, though even a good outcome theoretically entitles the patient to nominal damages. The consent may be express (written or oral) or implied from the conduct of the patient. Failure to document the consent will unnecessarily increase the burden on the physician or the hospital to show that an appropriate consent was obtained.

There are a number of exceptions to the consent requirement, some of which deserve brief mention here. When the intensivist has been asked to remedy a condition, and not merely to perform a specific procedure, the scope of the original consent may be extended. Another exception arises when it is infeasible to obtain consent to correct an unanticipated problem, as when the patient is under general anesthesia and the parents cannot be located. On the other hand, good judgment and common sense should be the guide: if an organ or limb must be removed unexpectedly, another consent should be obtained.[15]

Emergency Exception

Consent is implied as a matter of law when the child's life is threatened or irreversible injury will result if treatment is delayed to obtain consent from the legal guardian. There may be a tendency in urban tertiary care hospitals to deem a situation an emergency when the child simply needs treatment but a competent parent is not available to make a timely and rational decision. Relying on the emergency exception under these circumstances to treat without consent may be acceptable when conscientious efforts are made to reach the guardian, when the procedure is of maximum benefit and relatively low risk, and when a second intensivist or another professional with similar qualifications also documents his belief that the patient will suffer harm from delay. A referral should eventually be made to the appropriate child protection agency so that the state can become the guardian if the parent still cannot be located. It is theoretically possible for the estranged parent to file suit on the child's behalf, alleging lack of proper consent, or for the child, once he reaches majority, to assert his own rights. However, since the child has been admitted to the PCCU, a certain degree of urgency must be presumed. It is a different matter, however, when the procedure poses high risks and there are treatment options. Proceeding with treatment without a court order under these circumstances violates the legal and ethical premise that the child is entitled to a surrogate decision-maker who is acting in his best interests, and the law does not allow the intensivist to act alone in that capacity.

Informed Consent

Consent for the hospital admission and for the performance of routine diagnostic tests and other routine procedures is obtained on a general admission form, the responsibility for which generally rests with hospital personnel. Consent is also required for special procedures that carry greater risk. Consent to such special procedures must be "informed," which means that the intensivist must disclose to the legal guardian the following elements:[16]

- The patient's diagnosis
- The nature and purpose of the recommended treatment
- The risks and consequences of the proposed treatment
- The probability of success
- The available alternatives
- The prognosis if consent is refused

In the past, the law required that the physician disclose only information that a *reasonable physician* would disclose under similar circumstances. However, today some states measure the adequacy of the consent against what would be material to the *reasonable patient* under like circumstances in reaching a decision.[14] Most states have hybrid disclosure standards. What is clear is that the proper content of the disclosure cannot be specified by case law or statute. There are simply too many variables for the court or legislature to presume to dictate an adequate disclosure under all circumstances. However, some generalizations can be made.

- A physician may not withhold risk information about the proposed treatment simply because the parent might refuse consent. Nevertheless, it is acceptable to urge the parent to agree to the recommended course.
- Guarantees about outcome are always inappropriate.
- When the physician has doubts about what or how much to disclose, consultation with a colleague, appropriately documented, is helpful to defend one's decision later on.
- Optimally, the informed consent process begins before the child reaches the PCCU. A suggestion that the child may obtain no benefit from a prolonged stay in the PCCU might serve to better prepare parents for the limitations of critical care medicine and for a change in treatment goals.
- In the multidisciplinary PCCU setting, regardless of who obtains the consent, the individual who performs the procedure will be called upon to prove that consent was obtained and that it was adequate.
- To present a parent with too much information is to

be uninformative. Focusing on factors that might make a difference to the parent in reaching a decision and that might make a difference to the intensivist in making a recommendation is a reasonable approach.

It may be difficult for the pediatric intensivist not to view the informed consent process as a confusing, threatening, and burdensome chore. But it can also be viewed as the opportunity to develop rapport with the family.

The critical variable in the filing of a malpractice claim is neither clinical error nor iatrogenic injury: it is the patient or the patient's family. . . . A small but growing body of research suggests an important correlation between poor physician and hospital staff communication with patients and malpractice claims filed by those patients. The implication is that the reason patients file malpractice claims is not only iatrogenic injury but also, and perhaps most importantly, the patient's negative perceptions of or hostility toward the hospital and physician.[17]

There are three characteristics common to most parents in the PCCU. First, they will be terrified that, through their own ignorance or silence, they will not be doing all that can be done for their child. They recognize quite dramatically and all at once that it is not within their power to make their child well. The parents reveal this anxiety in a variety of ways, but one way is through being demanding and behaving "unreasonably." Second, even under the best of circumstances, there will be a wide disparity between the family's understanding of medicine and the physician's. This difference may be pronounced in the multicultural, urban setting. Third, it is often difficult for parents to identify one physician in the PCCU who is available and who is familiar enough with their child to answer questions.

Understanding these realities is a first step. But mastery of communication techniques should be a mandatory second component. Such simple actions as making eye contact while speaking to the parent or shaking hands upon meeting can build bridges that last. Regardless of who is acting as the primary physician for the PCCU patient, there should be a knowledgeable intensivist to whom the parents can address questions about their child at any reasonable time.

Minor Consent

Sometimes a parent's consent to treatment may be unnecessary or inappropriate. State statutes generally specify the circumstances under which minors of any age can consent to their own treatment, such as for substance abuse, psychiatric problems, or sexually transmitted disease. States have also recognized that a minor will be considered emancipated and therefore able to give consent if he is living on his own and providing his own support (e.g., if he is married) or in the armed services. Generally, minors of any age can consent to treatment for their own child.

Refusal to Consent

The law allows parents great discretion to refuse consent to treatment (or, as may often occur in the PCCU, to the withdrawal of treatment), but it is not without limit.[18] If it is believed that the child will suffer significant harm, then the physician can seek court authority to treat the child over parental objection.[19] Where life is imminently threatened, then treatment can be rendered before the court order is obtained, but the legal process should be initiated as soon thereafter as possible, particularly if prolonged therapy, unapproved by the parent, is anticipated. This is often the case when parents object to life-saving blood transfusions on religious grounds. The legal proceeding is usually initiated under the state's child abuse/neglect statute. Critical to the court's decision to override the parent's refusal to consent is the physician's testimony that an emergency exists and that there are no viable options to the proposed therapy.

A court may be reluctant to rule against the parents when treatment is intended merely to improve the quality of life while subjecting the child to great risk, as in the case of cosmetic correction of a congenital deformity.[20] Courts have also declined to rule against the parents when the child has a terminal illness and the parents opt for unorthodox or experimental therapy.[21] An intensivist concerned about when court intervention is necessary should look for the following factors: (1) Is the child's life or well-being in imminent danger? (2) Is the withholding of consent based upon religious belief or on concerns related to the potential physical outcome? (3) Is it appropriate to wait until the child can assist in the decision-making, as when cosmetic surgery is needed? These same factors should be weighed in determining whether to allow the removal of a patient from the hospital against medical advice or to seek the assistance of security personnel, the police, legal counsel, or the courts to prevent the removal of the child.

Impaired Decision-Maker

Dealing with the rational surrogate decision-maker who withholds consent is easy compared to dealing with the impaired legal guardian. When there is any concern that the parent is incompetent to make a sound medical decision (because of substance abuse or mental illness, for example), a pre-existing protocol should be implemented under which social workers, nurses, legal counsel, and psychiatrists assist in the decision-making process. Before embarking on the informed consent session with an impaired legal guardian, the physician should determine whether the legal guardian appears rational and competent to understand him. If there is any doubt, a psychiatrist should be asked to assist in determining whether the legal guardian is able to make an objective medical decision that is in the best interests of the child (the "best interests" standard). The "substituted judgment" standard, whereby a surrogate attempts to identify subjectively what the patient would have wanted had the patient been able to consent for himself, does not apply when the patient was never legally competent to make such a decision, as in the case of a minor.[22] The competence assessment should be performed before the informed consent discussion begins, because the physician who later believes that the parent is incompetent to consent will be hard pressed to show that he has not reached this conclusion based upon the parent's refusal to consent to the recommended course of treatment. If it appears that the parent is incompetent to make a medical decision, the appropriate child protection agency should be asked to intervene on behalf of the child. Sometimes state agencies decline these cases, either because they believe the hospital and courts are better suited to sort through these questions or because their case load is too overwhelming for them to take on children who are, for the time being, in a safe environment. If the agency declines, direct court involvement is necessary because a consent obtained from the legal guardian would be considered legally invalid. The legal guardian may choose not to submit to a psychiatric evaluation, but the effort should be made before going to court.

The limitations of the courtroom are obvious, as the legal process is usually lengthy, inefficient, adversarial, and disruptive to the physician-parent relationship. The legal process can, however, help to eliminate the possibility that an inappropriate decision is being made or an appropriate decision is being made for the wrong reason. If nothing else, the legal process slows down the decision-making process enough to allow a review of all the relevant facts in an objective manner.

Perhaps the best solution is for the hospital and the concerned physician in the PCCU to seek the assistance of the court and the child protection agency in establishing a forum where the interests of the child can be considered in a swift but fair process, without the adversarial atmosphere of the courtroom. Bioethics committees might provide advice to such a forum, because they elicit facts from a multidisciplinary body with a wide variety of views, including nonmedical ones. But to date, the law has not allowed these committees to replace the legal guardians or the courts in the decision-making process.

CONCLUSION

A thorough understanding of the elements of professional liability and consent in the context of the PCCU will help to make the practice of defensive medicine unnecessary because the practice of defensible medicine will become second nature. Special features of defensible medicine in the PCCU include avoiding so-called sins of omission, recognizing when physician responsibility for a PCCU patient begins and ends, and being sympathetic to the position of the PCCU parent. Nowhere in a hospital is defensible medicine more essential than in the PCCU, a place that represents the only hope for many parents and patients.

References

1. *Gonzales v. Nork*, Cal. Super. Court. Mem. of Dec. No. 228566 (Nov. 19, 1973), *rev'd on other grounds*, 573 P.2d 478 (1978).
2. *Sheffield v. Zilis*, 316 S.E.2d 493 (Ga. Ct. App. 1984).
3. *Helling v. Carey*, 83 Wash.2d 514, 519 P.2d 981 (1974).
4. P.L. 99-660.
5. Jeannett B: Inappropriate use of intensive care. Br Med J 289:1709, 1984.
6. U.S. GAO/HRD 87–555 Medical Malpractice Closed Claims.
7. 758 S.W.2d 836 (Tex. App. 1988).
8. *Ascher v. Gutierrez*, 533 F.2d 1235 (C.A. D.C. 1976).
9. *Fraijo v. Hartland Hospital*, 160 Cal. Rptr.3d 246, 251 (Ct. App. 1979).
10. *Stovall v. Harms*, 214 Kan. 835, 522 P.2d 353 (1974).
11. Joint Commission on Accreditation of Healthcare Organizations: *Accreditation Manual for Hospitals*, Chicago, Joint Commission on Accreditation of Healthcare Organizations, 1990, pp. 245–258.
12. *Garcia v. Von Micsky*, 602 F.2d 51 (CA2, 1979); *Robbins v. Footer*, 553 F.2d 123 (C.A. D.C., 1977).
13. *Clark v. United States*, 402 F.2d 950 (CA4, 1968) (applying Virginia law).
14. *Canterbury v. Spence*, 464 F.2d 772 (D.C. Cir. 1972).
15. *Wells v. Van Nort*, 100 Ohio 101, 125 N.E. 910 (1919).
16. *Hospital Law Manual*. Rockville, MD, Aspen System Corp, 1989, p. 38.
17. Orlikoff JE, and Vanagunas AM: Malpractice Prevention and Liability Control for Hospitals, 2nd ed. Chicago, American Hospital Publishing, 1988.
18. *Prince v. Massachusetts*, 321 U.S. 158 (1944).
19. *Custody of a Minor*, 375 Mass. 733, 379 N.E.2d 1053 (1978); *Salz v. Perlmutter*, 362 So.2d 160 (Fla. Dist. Ct. App. 1978).
20. *In re Hudson*, 126 P.2d 765 (Wash. 1942).
21. *Matter of Hofbauer*, 65 App. Div. 2d 108, 411 N.Y.S.2d 416 (App. Div. 1978); 47 NY 2nd 648, 419 NYS 2d 936, 393 NE 2d 1009 (1979).
22. Sprung CL: Surrogate Decision-Making in Critical Care Medicine. *In* Critical Care—State of the Art. Fullerton, CA, The Society of Critical Care Medicine, Vol 11, p. 367 (1990).
23. President's Commission for the Study of Ethical Problems in Medicine and Biomedical and Behavioral Research: Deciding to Forgo Life-Sustaining Treatment, p. 132. New York, Concern for Dying, 1983.

Ethical Considerations

Jacqueline J. Glover, Ph.D., and
Peter R. Holbrook, M.D.

Perhaps nothing symbolizes more effectively the maturation of the specialty of pediatric critical care medicine than the coterminous evolution of ethical decision making in the pediatric intensive care unit (PICU). Gone are the days of the technologic imperative in which, "If it can be done, it should be done." In its place is the nearly constant struggle to provide the best care possible consistent with the likelihood of a positive outcome and consistent with the resources at hand. The discussion and debate over the concept of brain death seem mild compared with the problems relating to active euthanasia or the just allocation of scarce resources. The "Lone Ranger" physician making decisions exclusively, and based primarily on his or her own value system, is no longer the norm. Now families wield much more decision-making power (some would argue too much), and the number of people potentially involved in making decisions is prodigious. The questions that play out on a regular basis in the PICU number in the dozens.

The goal of this brief chapter is to provide a basic framework for ethical decision making and to illustrate its use with the analysis of two major issues confronting critical care practitioners: the limitation or withdrawal of therapy and the just allocation of health care resources.

FRAMEWORK FOR ETHICAL DECISION-MAKING

The goal of all decision-making in the PICU is to promote the well-being of the child. Both parents and practitioners share this responsibility. Parents are involved in decision making as an extension of their primary responsibility to care for and nurture their child. Professional responsibility necessarily includes making decisions about appropriate therapies.

An understanding of the child's well-being in its fullest sense includes the perspectives of both professionals and parents who work together in a therapeutic alliance. Given the stressful environment of the PICU, building such an alliance can be extremely difficult. Yet neither party can adequately serve as a surrogate for the other. Parents do not have the expertise to act as surrogate

health care professionals, but neither do professionals have the same strong bonds of affection and commitment to act as surrogate parents. One possible delineation of roles suggests that parents and professionals should agree about general treatment goals, but professionals should make decisions about which treatment modalities are necessary to advance these goals.[1] Exclusive control by one party or the other is undesirable since it does not adequately respect the fact that both parties have obligations to care for the child. When parents are absent, another surrogate must be found to represent the interests of the child, usually through some kind of court proceeding. Although judicial involvement may not be necessary or desirable from a theoretical perspective, courts have not yet recognized more informal mechanisms such as hospital ethics committees (see Chapter 91).

Two standards have emerged to help both parents and professionals evaluate whether alternative courses of action promote the child's well-being. The *best interest standard* weighs the benefits and burdens associated with proposed therapies.[2] On the face of it benefits seem fairly straightforward. Professionals and parents should assess the likelihood that a proposed therapy will prevent premature death and restore or maintain function. Yet positive outcomes are rarely gained without some kind of associated burden such as the pain and suffering associated with invasive procedures, fear, immobilization, prolonged hospitalization, and isolation from family and friends.

Complex questions arise about whether and how one should consider the burdens associated with therapy itself and the burdens associated with life after successful therapy. Present interests in being free from undue burdens must be weighed against all future interests.[3] Decisions are a complex amalgam of what the child's alternative futures will be like, how likely it is that these futures can be gained, and what the child has to endure to get there. It is obvious, given such complexity, that there is usually not *one* course of action that is in the best interest of the child, but rather a range of acceptable options. A decision-making process must maximize the likelihood that there is full consideration of all appropriate options and that unacceptable options are eliminated. A second standard, the *relational potential stan-*

dard, has been identified as a necessary adjunct to the best interest standard.[4] Some conditions, such as permanent loss of consciousness, render a child unable to experience either benefit or burden. Since such a child's interests are limited to the prolongation of mere biologic life and burdens cannot be cognitively experienced, a best interests standard seems inadequate. Rather than assume that any interests must be served when there are no corresponding burdens, many would argue that treatment may be limited or withdrawn if most of the reasons for that treatment are missing—better function, fewer symptoms, the opportunity for human relationships, or greater opportunity to achieve life's goals.[5]

Decision-Making Process

Any attempt to describe the complex process of professional/parent communication and decision making will be an oversimplification. What follows is an attempt to structure and thus highlight major features important to sound decision making, recognizing that the decision-making process is always fluid and ongoing.

1. The first step of the decision-making process is to identify and clarify the issue at hand. This initial step actually has two important elements—clarifying the medical facts and clarifying the value conflicts. Good ethics begins with good facts. In so far as possible, there should be general agreement among the attending and consulting physicians about the child's current condition, prognosis, and alternative courses of action.

The second element includes identifying any major value conflicts that are apparent among the alternative courses of action. The health care team should evaluate the appropriate goals of therapy and the range of options in meeting these goals. It is important to elicit information from all members of the health care team— nurses, social workers, and chaplains.

Conflicts arise most often when therapies are initiated without consideration of the goal they are meant to meet. Will they meet the goal? Is the goal an appropriate one? What trade-offs are appropriate among competing goals such as reducing suffering and preventing premature death?

2. The second step in the decision-making process is to sort out and rank the alternative courses of action. How does each measure up according to the best interest or relational potential standard? The attending physician, in consultation with other members of the team, will determine which options are to be recommended and which options, if any, are unacceptable even if preferred by the family.

3. Communication with the family around the specific decision to be made is the next step. All options should be outlined, and the consequences of each option discussed in a value neutral tone. The attending physician should also discuss which option or options he or she recommends and why. Some disagree and argue that the physician wields too much power and can manipulate the family with his or her stated recommendation. While this is a risk, it must be balanced against the risk that

the family will regard the decision as entirely their own and feel abandoned at this crucial time. As discussed previously, a decision does not rest solely with the family, for both professionals and parents have moral obligations to promote the well-being of the child.

4. A final step involves the resolution of conflicts. If the family has selected the "wrong" decision, each member of the health care team has to come to grips with the contrary decision. In most cases, the benefits of alternative positions can be re-evaluated and a mutually acceptable decision can be reached. It should be emphasized that the physician must truly accept the decision and not simply pay lip service while undermining it at every opportunity. An alternative would be to compromise. For example, a time-limited trial of therapy may be initiated before discussion is reopened. However, the physician must guard against constantly forcing the family to reconsider what is always a painful and difficult decision.

If the physician or other health care professional considers that he or she is morally compromised by the decision, then he or she must act accordingly. The issue may be taken to an external body such as the hospital ethics committee. If the conflict is still not resolved, legal action may be appropriate. If a legal resolution is not possible or satisfactory, the professional may withdraw from the case as long as steps are taken so that the patient is not abandoned.

Suggested procedure for withdrawing from a case*

1. Notify the patient or the patient's surrogates in writing of the physician's need to withdraw from the case and explain the reasons. Give the patient a reasonable period of time to find a new physician.

2. Provide a list of names, addresses, and telephone numbers of physicians who can deliver equivalent care.

3. Request that the patient or surrogates contact one of these physicians to request his or her participation in the care of the patient.

4. Provide all medical records, upon request approved by the patient or surrogate, to new physicians.

5. Continue medical care of the patient at the same level as that preceding notification.

6. Cooperate with the new physician as appropriate.

DECISIONS TO LIMIT OR WITHDRAW THERAPY

The most common conflicts among health care professionals or among professionals and parents concern a shift in the goal of therapy from the prolongation of life to the management of dying. Not only is there potential disagreement about when such a shift should occur but also there is disagreement about the level of involvement that persons should have in the dying process. Both professionals and parents share concern about their role in a child's death.

Concern is most often expressed as a desire not to be

---

*Adapted from Physician's Reference Guide on Medicolegal Matters. Washington, DC, DC Medical Society, 1988.

the cause of death. Persons are eager to draw a bright line between actions that cause death and omissions that simply allow a natural death to occur. A distinction is drawn between active euthanasia (injecting a lethal dose of potassium) and passive euthanasia (withdrawing a ventilator). The latter is permissible, whereas the former is not. One problem with relying on an active/passive distinction is that it is usually impossible to draw a bright line between the two. Injecting potassium is clearly an action, but so, it would seem, is turning off a ventilator. Also, some omissions are clearly culpable. Death that results from failure to provide a necessary drug is not justified on the basis that no action was taken. The moral weight of a decision must rest on something other than the active/passive distinction, namely the benefit and burden to the child.

Yet it is precisely on the basis of benefit to the child that some would argue that active euthanasia is permissible. Why is it preferable to withdraw therapy and thus prolong a burdensome dying process when a quick and burden free death is possible? Arguments against active euthanasia focus on three major consequences: the possibility of error, the possibility of abuse, and the likelihood of the erosion of trust in the professional-patient relationship. Since trust depends on the expectations of patients and their families, as social attitudes change, so too may the prohibition against active euthanasia.

The appropriate use of pain medication is closely associated with this debate about active euthanasia. Out of concern not to administer "the last dose," practitioners may be reluctant to provide adequate levels of pain-relieving medication. However, one might justify even levels high enough to suppress respiration according to a "double effect" reasoning that separates consequences that are intended from those that are merely foreseen. One intends to relieve pain, even though one can reasonably foresee that respirations may be suppressed. Although useful as a general guideline, there are obviously limits to the application of the principle of double effect. It is often difficult to separate one's own intentions quite so clearly, and it is even more difficult to provide evidence of them to others. Assuming that both the goals of relieving pain and avoiding active killing are important, professional standards are necessary to strike an appropriate balance.

A second distinction that health care professionals and parents often make is between decisions to withhold or to withdraw treatment. Once a therapy is begun, either or both may feel reluctant to stop it, reflecting some sense of commitment to the effort made or out of concern for the active/passive distinction discussed earlier. In an effort to avoid actions, some practitioners may agree not to escalate care but may be reluctant to withdraw care. It is important to note, however, that a refusal to withdraw care may prolong a burdensome dying process and thus may be inappropriate. Withdrawal of certain therapies does not mean that all care is withdrawn, and more invasive burdensome therapies can be replaced by activities that bring greater comfort and opportunity for interaction with family. Also, a reliance on this distinction between withholding and

withdrawing may make health care professionals reluctant to initiate possibly beneficial therapies out of concern that they cannot be withdrawn later. If one has sufficient justification not to initiate a therapy, then clearly one will have sufficient justification to withdraw it based on the knowledge of a limited trial.[6]

Parents and professionals also describe some therapies as *extraordinary* when they mean they can be withdrawn and *ordinary* when they mean that these therapies must be provided. Although such short-hand language can be useful, it can also be misleading. Too often people speak as though one can independently tell whether an intervention is extraordinary or ordinary and thus tell whether it ought to be provided. But what are the appropriate criteria for such independent judgment? Is cost, frequency of use, or invasiveness involved? None of these factors are clearly associated with the required use of a therapy independent of the assessment of benefit and burden. On the face of it, even costly and infrequently used invasive therapies ought to be provided if they provide sufficient benefit.

Distinctions like active and passive euthanasia, withholding and withdrawing therapy, foreseen but unintended consequences, and extraordinary and ordinary care can help to highlight important aspects of a decision, but none is complete or independent of the central analysis of burden and benefit. Decisions to limit or withdraw therapy, like all decisions, require the careful application of the best interests and relational potential standards. Examples follow of the application of these standards in a series of three cases and possible permutations.

CASE DISCUSSION

Terminal Illness

Consider the case of a 6-year-old boy with an underlying cancer who has been in the PICU for about 1 month following a bone marrow transplant. He is presently on a ventilator and is septic. His kidneys are beginning to shut down, and the question is raised about dialysis.

A decision favoring dialysis would be based on the benefit of prolonged life and on the reasonable possibility for a future transplant or an alternative therapy. If the chances for any future therapy are very small, then the benefits of a few weeks to months of life must be balanced against the burdens of this intervention and associated interventions.

A decision against dialysis would raise questions about the appropriateness of other therapies, including especially the ventilator. Discussions with the family focus on how the child will live until he dies and how he will die. Hopefully, the oncologist has laid the groundwork for this discussion in the PICU through previous discussions with the family.

▶ **First Permutation.** What would happen if the boy were 16 years old? A young adult may have preferences about the course of therapy. Although the boy is not legally able to give consent, the preferences of a 16-

year-old boy should carry weight. Minors should be involved in decision-making to the extent that their capacity allows. A general guideline would include a strong presumption favoring disclosure of information and discussion of important values. At either end of the spectrum, nondisclosure by the caregivers or unqualified authority for decisions by the patient, should occur in only the rarest circumstances.

▶ **Second Permutation.** What would happen if the boy has acquired immunodeficiency syndrome (AIDS) and he is in the PICU for an episode of pneumocystis pneumonia? No decision can be attached simply to a diagnosis, or even to the fact that a patient is terminally ill; after all, the line between terminal illness and mere mortality is in some respects arbitrary. Each of us is going to die at some point. However, the length of time until death is an important variable that people value differently. In either case, whether concerning cancer or AIDS, a decision will focus on the probable length of life, the quality of that life, and the value placed on both.

▶ **Third Permutation.** What would happen if the intervention proposed were an experimental drug protocol rather than dialysis? In terms of the decision-making process the only difference between accepted or experimental therapy is the difficulty in the consent process. In either case, parents should be aware of the possible risks and benefits. In the case of research, it takes a special effort to make it clear that the benefits are not well known. It is especially difficult in the case of a Phase 1 Drug Trial to make it clear that the intent of the research is not therapeutic. One proposal for consent for Phase 1 Drug Trials requires that the information be cohort specific so that the decision maker can more adequately weigh the level of risk and the possibility, however remote, of benefit. The later the cohort (i.e., the higher the dose) the greater will be the likelihood of both toxic and therapeutic levels of the drug.[7]

▶ **Severe Disability**

Consider the case of a 2-year-old girl with meningococcemia. After a difficult initial course of significant multisystem support, her condition is now beginning to stabilize. She requires less cardiac medication, her kidneys have improved, and she is beginning to respond. However, she remains on the ventilator after several unsuccessful weaning attempts. She also has significant tissue involvement amounting to the equivalent of 70% third-degree burns on all extremities and on her back and chest. She will also become blind with the imminent loss of her eyelids. There is no evidence of the loss of neurologic function. If she is to survive, amputations of all four extremities and debridement must begin immediately.

A decision against surgery would be based on the judgment that the burdens associated with repeated surgeries and a life of such severe disability and dependence on medical treatment would be greater than the benefits of the possible (although uncertain) chance of survival. A decision favoring surgery would be based on the judgment that life is valuable regardless of its quality or that the quality of life of a person without neurologic disability is acceptable despite severe physical disability.

▶ **First Permutation.** What would happen if the child did not depend on a ventilator? Even if the child were not ventilator-dependent, she would still be burdened with multiple surgeries. She would also be extremely difficult to rehabilitate. With blindness and the loss of all four extremities (assuming high amputations), she would most likely not be able to walk and would need to sit or lie on skin-grafted tissue. The high likelihood of breakdown would make further interventions necessary.

It is difficult to judge what weight should be given to the fact that she is not compromised neurologically. On one hand, she would be able to engage in all the intellectual activities that are highly valued despite her physical disabilities. On the other hand, she would be more acutely aware of her disabilities and the suffering entailed.

▶ **Second Permutation.** What if the level of disability were uncertain as well as her chances of survival? Some level of uncertainty always accompanies decision making in the PICU. But what is a reasonable course of action in the face of almost total uncertainty when the outcome and its likelihood are unknown? One possibility is to delay decision making until some information on which to base a prognosis can be gained. But this really is a decision of sorts to go forward. It is based on the presumption that any possible benefit is worth the burden of continued therapy until the benefit can be shown to be small. But what if the actual burdens are great? Is it reasonable to assume that actual burdens can never outweigh only possible benefits? If one answers yes, it is probably on the basis that not all benefits are only possible. As long as one is alive, there is always the actual benefit of that life. If one answers no, it is probably on the basis that actual burdens can be greater than any benefits, including the benefit of life now lived or in the future.

In a discussion of handicapped newborns, a recent President's Commision report argues that in the face of true uncertainty, parental decisions ought to be authoritative.[8] In this case, allowing the parents to refuse surgery would be to accept that there is a very high level of actual burden. But can the burdens of care in the PICU really be so great as to outweigh all benefits, even if only possible? To answer yes is to dramatically challenge presumptions about the value of such care that govern the development and expansion of critical care medicine.

▶ **Permanent Unconsciousness**

Consider the case of a 3-year-old girl who suffers a near-drowning event. She is on the ventilator and unresponsive. A repeat computed (CT) scan is consistent with severe anoxia.

A decision to withdraw the ventilator would be based on the judgment that the child has no potential to interact with her environment and to form relationships of any kind. Her life is devoid of all the qualities associated with living, except for certain biologic functions. A decision to continue the ventilator would be based on the judgment that life is valuable regardless of its quality.

▶ **First Permutation.** What should be done if she continues to breathe after the ventilator is removed? Given that the child does not die from the failure to protect her airway, a decision will have to be made about the provision of hydration and nutrition.

A decision not to provide hydration and nutrition is based on the judgment that this medical therapy can be limited. The appropriate use of this technology is judged like any other, according to the benefit offered to the patient. In this case, the child can experience neither benefit nor burden and has no potential for interaction of any kind.

Some would argue that the provision of hydration and nutrition is ordinary care that must always be provided. But to argue this way is to assume that it is always beneficial, as was discussed previously. However, there are clearly cases in which it is not (e.g., in the case of terminal illness in which it may cause discomfort and in cases in which it merely prolongs dying).[9] Benefit in this case is limited to the prolongation of mere biologic life.

Concerns are also raised about active euthanasia. There is such a clear association between withdrawal of feeding and death that withdrawal of feeding can be considered the cause of death. It is particularly abhorrent to "starve" a child to death. However, such language is misleading. Starvation is a cognitive experience that this child cannot have. Additionally, just as one can attribute death to the underlying neurologic deficit when a ventilator is removed, one can attribute death to this same deficit when it also renders a patient unable to eat.[10]

A decision to provide hydration and nutrition is based on the judgment that all life is valuable regardless of its quality or on the judgment that there is something so special about feeding that it must never be limited or withdrawn. Feeding is such a basic humane act that we cannot even claim to care and allow another to go hungry or thirsty. Feeding starving children is undeniably an act of caring that is morally required. Is the prolongation of the unconscious life of a child an equivalent act of caring?

FUTILITY

Discussions have emerged recently in the literature that challenge the framework for ethical decision making outlined in this chapter. Some would argue that a decision shared between parents and professionals is not appropriate when an intervention is considered futile. There is no moral obligation to provide futile therapy, which can be defined unilaterally by health care professionals.

Two definitions for futility have been proposed.[12] A quantitative definition is based on data expressing the probability of success. If a therapy has not worked in the last 100 cases, it can be considered futile. A qualitative definition is based on the quality of the life saved. An intervention that only serves to prolong a life of permanent unconsciousness or total dependence on intensive medical care can also be considered futile.

One can understand the circumstances that make a unilateral decision-making model desirable. Parents are often absent, unwilling, or unable to accept that an intervention has a very low probability of success. Children are burdened by the provision of such care, and health care professionals suffer as they are "forced" to provide it. Cardiopulmonary resuscitation (CPR) is a good example. Reconsider the three cases discussed earlier and the appropriateness of CPR in each? Very few professionals would think it appropriate to resuscitate in the case of the child dying of cancer and perhaps also in the case of a child with a severe disability and permanent unconsciousness.

Proposals include rewriting hospital policies to allow physicians to write Do Not Resuscitate orders without consent from the patient or surrogate.[13-15] Although such a policy would help in a few very difficult cases, it may also have several undesirable consequences. Futility is a very slippery concept. Without clear guidelines, it could be applied too liberally. One might also be concerned about the impact on communication patterns with families if unilateral decision making becomes an option. The search for a quantitative understanding of futility may lead to the false impression that decisions are more objective than they can be. As one author notes, the concept of futility may be an illusion.[16] The application of the term futile to certain qualitative states also exaggerates the level of agreement about the value of life of permanent unconsciousness or dependence on intensive medical care.

JUST ALLOCATION OF SCARCE RESOURCES

Cases that involve prolongation of death or of permanently unconscious life may also raise questions about the alternative uses of the resources expended. There are presently 35 million uninsured Americans, 25% of whom are children.[17] Questions are legitimate about the use of resources for interventions that offer little benefit compared with access to services of greater benefit.

Yet concerns about such reasoning at the bedside are also legitimate. In the absence of a broader social consensus, physicians' judgments may be idiosyncratic and inconsistently applied. Also, the American system (or nonsystem) does not readily allow for the transfer of resources. Even though one may soundly reason that money spent to maintain a comatose child is better spent on childhood immunizations, money cannot be transferred from a private insurance company to a government public health service.

What are the implications for pediatric critical care? One opinion is to regard questions of justice as somehow irrelevant to medical decision-making. Health care professionals ought to behave "as if" resources were unlimited and leave the allocation decisions to someone else. Although appealing on some levels, such a view has difficulties as well.

First of all, general allocation decisions cannot be so readily separated from bedside decisions. Choices about how much to spend on health care compared with other social goods and about how to spend health care dollars (allocation decisions) are linked inextricably with decisions about who gets what at the bedside (also called rationing). For example, the decision about the size of a PICU and the number of PICUs in a particular location will influence the kinds of decisions necessary at the bedside (see also Chapter 95).

Second, even if most decisions could be made by policy makers, the policies would still have to be applied by physicians. Policies that were made without adequate consideration of the reality of the patient's condition would also risk being seriously incorrect. It is true that if physicians were not involved in allocation decisions, they would never have to refuse any request made by their patients. But they would probably also lose any kind of authority to approve a patient's request.[18]

Finally, physicians who behave as if resources were unlimited also tend to leave that impression with patients and their families. But this is clearly not the case. Neither families nor practitioners can ignore the reality of scarce resources.

CASE DISCUSSION

Reconsider the cases previously described. A decision in each would have to determine how to weigh the issue of resources. For the dying child, it is ironic that resources are more likely available for dialysis than for hospice or home care.

For children with severe disability, either physical or neurologic, resources are a particularly difficult issue. Although funding is probably available for the hospital course, resources for chronic care are severely limited. In this era of fiscal restraint, government and private programs are being forced to cut back. Institutional placements are limited, as is the funding for home care. Despite the desire to make health care decisions only on some assessment of benefit the reality is that families may not be able to afford their decisions. What happens to them and their children when the funding runs out? Is it fair to them to pretend initially that resources are not an issue?

Questions of justice are unavoidable. Are these children and their families entitled to the services they need? Is it right to expend limited Medicaid dollars on a comatose child when the program was forced to raise its eligibility limit? Is it right to maintain a comatose child in the PICU when the PICU is full to capacity?

Questions of justice are also unavoidably frustrating—both practically and theoretically. Practically, there is no mechanism systematically to make trade-offs among alternative uses of resources. Theoretically, there are competing conceptions of justice that undergird the present system and are difficult to reconcile. All might agree that justice requires fair treatment, each receiving that to which he or she is entitled. But there is marked disagreement about what constitutes fairness. Egalitarians believe that each should receive some kind of equal share, usually construed as equal access to some adequate level of care. Libertarians believe that each should be free to spend his or her money without being forced to pay for the care of others.[19] Americans have firm commitments to both liberty and equality.

However, a kind of egalitarian consensus is emerging as efforts accelerate to provide access to health care for all. Even libertarians may have come to acknowledge that if the unrestrained access by some puts at risk the availability of resources for others, then limits may be placed. Libertarians may also have come to acknowledge that not all property is private and that health care is a common good that is appropriately supported by all.

But can a theory of justice be useful in the clinical setting? It depends on what is meant by useful. As a general guideline, an egalitarian conception of justice requires that people be treated equally. This has come to mean that decisions should be based on need rather than on merit or social worth, as policies for allocating organs and beds have come to reflect.

But there are also serious limitations to the application of a theory of justice in the clinical setting. A theory of justice necessarily requires consideration of the larger picture to compare the needs of all possible patients. A hospital may make judgments based only on need, but justice requires that consideration be given to patients outside the hospital as well. State policies may provide services to all citizens, but justice requires that comparisons even be made among countries.

Health care professionals obviously cannot engage in such far-reaching comparisons. But they can acknowledge the requirements of justice in two ways: by advocating for equal access to health care services and by helping to develop adequate allocation policies. The ethical framework outlined previously must be expanded in the future to reflect that decisions are a combination of what professionals recommend, what parents prefer, and what can be reasonably funded and still provide adequate services for all. This difficult work has only begun.

CONCLUSION

It is evident that the critical care practitioner must confront difficult ethical issues in the absence of broad social consensus. Often ethical debate may resolve once there is clear direction from academics, legislation, policy makers, and judges. Critical care practitioners must take an active role in working toward such consensus. But, even when policies seem clearly articulated, their application requires a thoughtful and comprehensive process of decision-making. There is really no easy ethical issue, and comfort is a rare companion to ethical decision making. A practitioner who becomes comfortable in his or her practice may not be allowing alternative approaches sufficient credibility or may be denying their suitable expression.

References

1. Rushton CH and Glover JJ: Involving parents in decisions to forego life-sustaining treatment for critically ill infants and children. AACN Clinical Issues in Critical Care Nursing 1:206, 1990.
2. Arras JD: Ethical principles for the care of imperilled newborns: Toward an ethic of ambiguity. *In:* Murray TH and Caplan AL (eds): Which Babies Shall Live? Clifton, NJ, Humana Press, 1985, pp. 83–135.
3. Buchanan AE and Brock DW: Deciding for others: The ethics of surrogate decision making. Cambridge, Cambridge University Press, 1989, pp. 215–260.
4. McCormick R: To save or let die: The dilemma of modern medicine. JAMA 229:172, 1974.
5. President's Committee for the Study of Ethical Problems in Medicine and Biomedical and Behavioral Research: Deciding to forego life-sustaining treatment. Washington, DC, US Government Printing Office, 1983, pp. 171–196.
6. President's Commission, pp. 43–90.
7. Freedman B: Cohort specific consent: An honest approach to phase I clinical cancer studies. IRB 12:5, 1990.
8. President's Commission, pp. 197–229.
9. Paris J and Fletcher J: Withholding of nutrition and fluids in the hopelessly ill patient. Clin Perinatol 14:367, 1987.
10. Miraie E and Mahowald M: Witholding of nutrition from seriously ill newborn infants: A parent's perspective. J Pediatr 113:262, 1988.
11. Paris JJ, Crone RK, and Reardon F: Physician's refusal of requested treatment: The case of baby L. N Engl J Med 322:1012, 1990.
12. Schneiderman L, Jecker L, and Jonsen A: Medical futility: Its meaning and ethical implications. Ann Intern Med 112:949, 1990.
13. Hackler C and Hiller FC: Family consent to orders not to resuscitate. JAMA 264:1281, 1990.
14. Tomlinson T and Brody H: Ethics and communication in do-not-resuscitate orders. N Engl J Med 318:43, 1988.
15. Younger S: Futility in context. JAMA 264:1295, 1990.
16. Lantos JD, Singer PA, Walker RM, et al: The illusion of futility in clinical practice. Am J Med 87:81, 1989.
17. Friedman E: Caring for the uninsured and underinsured: The uninsured from dilemma to crisis. JAMA 19:265, 1991.
18. Morreim EH: Clinicians or committees—who should cut costs? HCR 17:45, 1987.
19. Churchill LR: Rationing health care in America: Perceptions and principles of justice. Notre Dame, University of Notre Dame Press, 1987, pp. 43–103.

93

Death

Peter R. Holbrook, M.D.

Death is a fundamental part of the experience of any intensive care unit (ICU). It is the basic process against which intensive care specialists struggle and often lose. Death can move slowly: multiple organ system failure is the penultimate stage before death and often comes days or weeks after inciting events. It can also occur so rapidly that no meaningful medical care can be brought to bear (see Chapter 10).

In the last 10 to 20 years society's views toward death have changed: whereas it is still the usual enemy, it is increasingly considered as a more acceptable alternative to some states of life.

Research in critical care is often focused on complex, overwhelming processes such as shock or sepsis. Since these processes, if irreversible, lead to death, research into those conditions is research into death itself. It seems unlikely that unlocking the "secret" of death (which is also the secret of life) will be simple.

This chapter deals with the operational definitions of death, but preliminary observations are necessary.

SOCIETY AND DEATH

All persons have a vested interest in and will experience death. Thus, society owns the concept of death. Society gives portions of the concept to various groups. Physicians have been given the authority to deal with the operational aspects of death. This authorization by society is not a recognition that physicians know what death is, but rather that they can state when death has occurred. Physicians, although more familiar with death than many others, "own" only the operational aspects and are not authorized by society to range infinitely afield. For example, physicians are not allowed to define death in any other sense than an operational one. Even the ability to pronounce death is not absolute, and the physician must operate within accepted medical conventions, or society may censure him or her.

No definition of death is universally satisfying. Definitions commonly refer back to life (e.g., in "the cessation of life") or phrase the definition in religious terms, which may be acceptable only to a segment of the population. Everyone shares the same degree of ignorance.

In general, society considers death as the polar opposite of life, and, more specifically, assumes that there is no intervening condition. This bipolar nature is obvious in many areas. The living go about their activities, emotionally interact, and may carry life insurance, for example. The dead are immobile, are quickly put out of sight in most cases, do not emotionally interact, and have transferred the proceeds of life insurance to their heirs. Furthermore, the dying patient and the dead patient, although separated by only seconds, are treated in a completely different manner. There is no in-between state in the bipolar view. One doesn't lose life insurance benefits when dying, and one can't purchase it when dead.

Much of the ethical debate occurring throughout the critical care world now has to do with the fact that patients are, in fact, settling out "in between," and society doesn't know what to do with them (e.g., they do not go about their normal activities and may not emotionally interact). Society is struggling to give up the bipolar nature of life and death. If there evolves a conveniently defined "in between" state, the issues would be less debated and the ethical decision-making process will be easier (see Chapter 92).

OPERATIONAL DEFINITIONS OF DEATH

Since death is poorly defined, it may be viewed as a black box. Operational definitions of death are windows into the black box. If one has the training and experience (and, ultimately, the license) that authorizes a knowing look through the cardiovascular window, and one sees an arrested circulation, the physician is authorized to say "I don't know what death is, but this patient has it." In short hand, we say the patient is dead.

Until 1968 there was only one window, the cardiovascular one. Physicians then began the process of consensus building on a new window, namely, the brain death window. At first, a group of physicians published their opinions on what brain death was.[1] Subsequently, more than 1,000 medical papers were published on the concept and it has also been widely discussed by the lay population. As a result, almost all physicians have accepted that there is a new window, and now physicians can "see" death if brain death criteria are met. Importantly, the legal profession (to whom society has given the responsibility to write the laws regarding death) has recognized the existence of this new window by developing the Uniform Determination of Death Act. This act has been endorsed by the American Medical Association, The American Bar Association, the National Conference of Commissions on Uniform State Law, the President's Commission for the Study of Ethical Problems in Medicine and Biomedical and Behavioral Research, and the Special Task Force on Guidelines for the Determination of Brain Death in Children. It states:

> An individual who has sustained either (1) irreversible cessation of circulatory and respiratory functions, or (2) irreversible cessation of all functions of the entire brain, including the brain stem, is dead. A determination of death must be made in accordance with accepted medical standards.[2]

Other windows are possible. A certain panel of laboratory results could be considered diagnostic of death, if most physicians (and, ultimately, society) could be convinced of the validity of the findings. In addition, further modification of existing windows is possible. Society would leap to embrace a concept of death of the "sentient" brain, if it were convincing.

CARDIOVASCULAR DEATH

The operational definition of death, due to an arrested circulation, has been in existence for at least 4 centuries. All medical personnel have been exposed to it from the first days of training, and few register any difficulty with the concept.

But what exactly is "irreversible cessation of the circulatory and respiratory functions"? The irreversible adjective, which is clearly essential in the ICU setting, allows a great deal of judgment to enter the process. Sixty minutes of arrested circulation in the patient undergoing cardiovascular surgery in the operating room is not supposed to be irreversible, and indeed, is practiced regularly in most cardiovascular centers. In contrast, 60 minutes of arrest in the patient with sudden infant death syndrome is considered lethal. However, the recovery of a near-drowning patient after 60 minutes in icy water has been reported (see Chapter 9).

In fact, it is difficult to define the characteristics of irreversibility of the arrested cardiovascular and respiratory systems. Nonetheless, physicians rarely have difficulty with this concept. There are occasional difficulties when physicians go beyond the universally accepted conventions and use definitions that are controversial or when they confuse the inevitability of death with its occurrence. Nonetheless, the concept is well accepted and understood. However, because of all of the judgment that is required, it may not be appropriate to consider cardiovascular death as the "gold standard."

BRAIN DEATH

In 1968 the ad hoc committee of the Harvard Medical School published its observations on "A Definition of Irreversible Coma."[1] This landmark paper served as a lightning rod for comment and criticism from physicians and the lay public as well. Over the intervening years medical consensus has been reached on the basic elements of the hopelessly destroyed brain. More important society has become comfortable with the concept and allows physicians to utilize brain death determination readily. The authorizing mechanism is the local law, usually drawn from the Universal Determination of Death Act. As long as the physician performs within ordinary standards of medical practice, he or she will not be censured.

However, because fewer physicians are operationally comfortable with the ordinary standards of brain death determination, there is still considerable room for misunderstanding. No single set of criteria is universally accepted, although a set of modified Harvard Criteria is most widely used. Thus, any physician may use any set of criteria that he or she wishes, as long as he or she does not fall outside the ordinary standards of medical practice.

Brain Death and Children

What are the ordinary medical standards for children? Children were long excluded from the discussion on brain death, mostly because of an absence of widespread experience with neurologic death in small children. This has now changed. In 1987, a consensus group published its findings on brain death in children.[3] Although criticized by some,[4] the criteria serve as a reference point for practitioners. The elements are listed in Table 93–1. Several comments are in order.

First, the committee stated that there are no unique legal issues in determining brain death in children. It is clear that there are a number of social issues regarding children that differ from the issues involved regarding adults, but there are no legal issues.

Second, the criteria do not apply to premature infants (<38 weeks' gestation) or to children under 7 days of age, because of the considerable variability of findings among this group.[5]

Table 93–1. GUIDELINES FOR THE DETERMINATION OF BRAIN DEATH IN CHILDREN

History determines proximate cause of coma
Physical Examination
  Coexisting coma and apnea
  Absence of brain stem function
  Absence of hypotension or hypothermia
  Flaccid tone; absence of any movements (except spinal cord events)
  Persistence of examination findings throughout observation period

Observation Period
  Age 7 days to 2 months: 2 examinations, 2 EEGs 48 hours apart
  Age 2 to 12 months: 2 examinations, 2 EEGs* 24 hours apart
  Age 12 months to adulthood: 2 examinations† 12 hours‡ apart

*Second EEG obviated by negative flow study.
†Laboratory confirmatory tests are not necessary in usual cases.
‡The time should be extended to 24 hours if necessary (e.g., hypoxic ischemic encephalopathy with early first examination).
EEG = electroencephalogram.

Third, it is essential to have a reasonable cause for the child's condition to be certain that reversible conditions have been ruled out.

Fourth, the determination of apnea is the subject of some confusion. It is known that the rate of rise of $PaCO_2$ in the brain dead patient is less than in the non–brain dead patient.[6, 7] Further, it is known that the threshold for initiation of breathing may approach a $PaCO_2$ of 60 in adults.[8] Comparable data are not yet available for children. Until additional cases are reported, blood gas documentation of a $PaCO_2$ of more than 60 is necessary, regardless of how long the patient has been apneic.

Fifth, there are a few nuances that may aid the clinician in confusing cases. Stimulation of the vagus nerve (cranial nerve 10) causes heart rate slowing in normal patients. Atropine blocks this response, and since, in a child with brain activity, there is usually some tonic vagal tone, administration of atropine to a child will cause tachycardia—a response that is inconsistent with brain death.

Similarly, the brain dead child loses the normal beat-to-beat variation in pulse rate.[9] Thus, a monotonous unvarying heart rate may be suggestive evidence that brain death has occurred. Similarly, the brain dead patient will not show significant swings in pulse rate in the absence of volume or pressor rate infusion changes.

Finally, although the determination of brain death is no longer an ethical issue, but rather is a medical one, it should be noted that the concept is not a familiar one to many families. It is wise for the physician to allow considerable time for questioning by parents of the issues at hand while he or she proceeds with the diagnosis of brain death.

References

1. Ad Hoc Committee of the Harvard Medical School to Examine the Definition of Brain Death: A definition of irreversible coma. JAMA 205:337, 1968.
2. Guidelines for the Determination of Death: Report of the medical consultants on the diagnosis of death to the President's Commission for the Study of Ethical Problems in Medicine and Biomedical and Behavioral Research. Neurology 32:395, 1982.
3. Task Force on Brain Death in Children: Guidelines for the determination of brain death in children. Pediatrics 80:298, 1987.
4. Freeman JM and Ferry PC: New brain death guidelines in children: Further confusion. Pediatrics 81:201, 1988.
5. Volpe J: Brain death determination in the newborn. Pediatrics 80:293, 1987.
6. Rowland TW, Donnelly JH, and Jackson AH: Apnea documentation for determination of brain death in children. Pediatrics 74:505, 1984.
7. Outwater KM and Rockoff MA: Apnea testing to confirm brain death in children. Crit Care Med 12:357, 1984.
8. Schafer JA and Caronna JJ: Duration of apnea needed to confirm brain death. Neurology 28:661, 1978.
9. Kero P, Antila K, Ylitalo V, et al: Decreased heart rate variation in decerebration syndrome: Quantitative clinical criterion of brain death? Pediatrics 62:307, 1978.

94

Organ Donation

Carol Gannon Hartman, M.S.N., R.N., and
Elizabeth C. Suddaby, M.S.N., R.N., C.C.T.C.

Carrol's perfection of vascular anastomosis techniques in the early 1900s opened the field of transplantation research and led ultimately to today's clinical use of transplantation for end-stage organ failure. Early surgical attempts included a kidney transplant between identical twins at Peter Bent Brigham Hospital in 1954; Starzl's initial liver transplant at the University of Colorado in 1963; Hardy's first—albeit unsuccessful—lung transplant at the University of Mississippi in 1963; the world renowned heart transplant by Christian Barnard in South Africa in December 1967; and the first pancreas transplant at the University of Minnesota in 1966.

The use of transplantation as a treatment modality in pediatrics first occurred in New York in December 1967 with a heart transplant from an anencephalic donor to an infant with tricuspid atresia. Cooley's heart-lung transplant in an infant with an atrioventricular canal defect followed soon thereafter, as did the first successful liver transplant performed in 1967 by Starzl. The 18-month-old girl who received the liver transplant lived for 13 months before she died of a recurrent tumor. (The indications for different pediatric transplant procedures are shown in Tables 94–1 to 94–4) (see also Chapters 32, 55, and 56).

The growing demand for organ donors with the increase in transplant surgery has produced national legislation regarding organ donation. The statistics highlight the rising need for organ donors: approximately 20,000 patients per year need transplants, but there are only about 2,500 actual organ donors. Over 23,000 people, both children and adults, are currently on the national computer list awaiting transplants. Of those, nearly 18,592 people and more are waiting for new kidneys, more than 1,400 people are awaiting livers, and almost 2,000 are waiting for hearts. An additional 170 people and more are waiting for heart/lung transplants, and more than 479 people are waiting for lungs. More than 400 people are listed for pancreas transplants.[1, 32]

In the past, many families of potential donors were not even approached. As a result, many states as well as the federal government have passed required request/routine inquiry legislation that requires hospital administrators or their designee to ask the family of a suitable organ/tissue donor whether they would like their loved one to be a donor. The 1986 Omnibus Budget Recon-ciliation Act (OBRA) requires all hospitals that participate in Medicare/Medicaid to implement required request policies or risk loss of their Medicare/Medicaid funding.

State laws related to organ donation vary in content. Most state laws require hospitals to develop specific protocols covering organ and tissue donation. Some contain guidelines for obtaining consent. Some state laws identify specific individuals as "designated requestors" who can include hospital administrators, the chief executive officer (CEO), physicians, nurses, or personnel from organ procurement organizations (OPOs). Designated requestors should receive specialized training in how best to approach a potential donor's family. Laws in at least 23 states suggest or require such training. Many required request laws also grant immunity from civil/criminal action to those involved in implementing the law. This immunity does not cover negligence and is limited to actions performed in good faith.[2, 3]

CRITERIA FOR ORGAN AND TISSUE DONATION

Brain death is clearly the critical factor in identifying an organ donor. State laws vary on who may declare brain death. In some cases any licensed physician is adequate, but many states require two physicians to declare brain death. Other states require that at least one physician be a neurospecialist. State laws also differ in their requirements for confirmatory testing. In some states, clinical criteria are adequate to declare brain death. In others, confirmatory testing such as electroencephalograms (EEGs) or brain flow studies may be

Table 94–1. PEDIATRIC HEART TRANSPLANTATION

End-stage cardiomyopathy
Complex congenital heart defects
  Hypoplastic left heart syndrome
  Ebstein anomaly
  Pulmonary atresia with intact interventricular septum
Nonmalignant cardiac tumors
Life-threatening arrhythmias (resistant to treatment)

Table 94–2. PEDIATRIC LIVER TRANSPLANTATION

Biliary atresia
Metabolic disorders
  α_1-Antitrypsin disease
  Glycogen storage disease (types I and IV)
  Wilson disease
  Tyrosinemia
  Hemochromatosis
  Galactosemia
  Byler disease
  Blue histiocyte syndrome
End-stage hepatitis
Familial cholelithiasis
Budd-Chiari syndrome

Table 94–4. PEDIATRIC KIDNEY TRANSPLANTATION

Aplastic/hypoplastic/dysplastic kidneys
Obstructive uropathy
Focal segmental glomerulosclerosis
Systemic immunologic disease
Reflux nephropathy
Hemolytic uremic syndrome
Congenital nephrotic syndrome
Chronic glomerulonephritis
Agenesis of abdominal musculature syndrome
Familial nephritis

required. Some hospitals use confirmatory testing as a matter of policy.

To be declared clinically brain dead, a patient must show none of the following: response to external stimuli (prolonged, noxious stimuli such as nailbed or supraorbital pressure or sternal rub); reflexes (except those of spinal cord origin); pupillary response to light; corneal reflex; eye movement (as determined by oculocephalic [doll's eyes] and oculovestibular [cold calorics] testing). A brain dead patient will not demonstrate cough and gag reflexes, and the patient will be apneic despite the presence of adequate carbon dioxide stimulus.[4-9] A normal $PaCO_2$ is necessary before apnea testing can be conducted. To conduct the apnea test, the patient is preoxygenated with 100% O_2. The patient is then removed from the ventilator and placed on a 100% O_2 source, such as ambu bag or t-piece. The potential donor is observed for respiratory effort for up to 10 minutes, and arterial blood gases are taken at 1,3,5, and 10 minutes. A $PaCO_2$ of more than 60 without respiratory effort is considered a positive apnea test.[10] The patient should be normothermic (temperature >36°C) and free of any narcotic or other central nervous system (CNS) depressant drugs before testing. In many institutions testing in children is repeated at either 12- or 24-hour intervals (see Table 94–5 for clinical criteria; see also Chapter 93).

Assessing brain death in neonates is particularly difficult because of the immature cortical function and occult toxic and metabolic processes. There is no consensus on brain death criteria for children less than 7 days of age. If a child is under 7 days of age, some OPOs will call in as many as three physicians (including at least one neurospecialist) to perform two separate examinations, 24 to 36 hours apart. Each examination should include apnea, corneal reflex, higher reflex testing (i.e., nonspinal reflexes) as well as testing for cough and gag reflexes, and ocular, oculovestibular responses. To support the clinical diagnosis confirmatory testing is

recommended: two tests for cerebral blood flow, 24 to 36 hours apart, indicating total absence of cerebral blood flow (either four-vessel angiography or radioisotope scan), or 2 EEGs also 24 to 36 hours apart, demonstrating *absolute* electrocerebral silence for a minimum of 30 minutes. For infants over 7 days of age and less than 2 months, two physicians should test for the clinical criteria at least 48 hours apart, and confirmatory tests are again recommended. Children older than 2 months but less than 1 year should have two examinations 24 hours apart, and children older than 1 year should be examined at least 12 hours apart.[4,5]

The use of anencephalic infants as organ donors is a highly controversial and hotly debated issue in transplantation.[11,12] The unique difficulty in determining brain death in these patients has led many institutions to place a moratorium on the practice while testing of the anencephalic infant is studied. Shewmon, Holzgreve, and associates point out that currently the medical community even differs over the definition of anencephaly.[12,13] Beyond the question of declaring these infants brain dead is the issue of their suitability as donors. Because they tend to be premature, to have low birth weight, and to have associated anomalies—especially of the renal and cardiac systems—the potential for viable organs of suitable size or function for transplant is uncertain.[12,14,15]

In the process of establishing brain death, the medical team begins to assess the possibility for organ donation. Each potential donor is considered individually, and the donor's past and current medical history is evaluated. Most of the general criteria for organ and tissue donation relate to negative assurances; that is, a donor must not have:

1. Unresolved systemic infection (infection that has been treated for more than 72 hours, with decreased or normal temperature, lower or normal white blood cell

Table 94–3. PEDIATRIC LUNG OR HEART/LUNG TRANSPLANTATION

Primary pulmonary hypertension
Eisenmenger syndrome
Cystic fibrosis
End-stage chronic lung disease with cor pulmonale

Table 94–5. CLINICAL CRITERIA FOR BRAIN DEATH*

No response to external stimuli
No reflex activity unless of spinal cord origin
No pupillary response to light
No corneal reflex
No eye movement with caloric testing or doll's eye maneuver
No gag reflex
No cough reflex
Apnea in the presence of adequate carbon dioxide stimulus

*In the absence of intoxicant drugs and hypothermia.

count, and negative result of a blood culture, is acceptable)

2. Current extracranial malignancies, although primary brain tumors are not exclusionary. Organ donors are surgically explored for previously undetected malignancy, and a trunk autopsy is required for tissue donors.

3. Communicable diseases, e.g., human immunodeficiency virus (HIV), syphilis, or hepatitis. Each donor is evaluated for cytomegalovirus (CMV) in order to protect those recipients who are CMV negative. A positive result on a CMV titer would not exclude donation.

Organ specific criteria follow.

1. Kidneys. The age requirement is birth to 70 years. A patient who has been resuscitated from a cardiac arrest and has renal function is a viable candidate to donate kidneys. Trauma, especially blunt abdominal trauma, crush injuries, and electrical injuries must be evaluated for their impact on renal function. Other potentially damaging insults to the kidneys that should be worked up in the donor evaluation include infection, previous disease of the kidneys, periods of hypotension, and use of vasopressors. Kidney specific laboratory tests to evaluate the potential donor include blood urea nitrogen (BUN), creatinine, creatinine clearance if possible, complete blood count (CBC), and urine electrolytes. An intravenous pyelogram (IVP), renal scan, and arteriogram may be necessary to further evaluate an organ with marginal laboratory values.[16]

2. Liver. The age requirement is birth to 70 years. Patients who have been resuscitated from a cardiac arrest are considered as potential donors. As in the case of kidney donors, trauma to the abdomen must be carefully evaluated, along with previous medical conditions, infection, and drug history. Antibiotics, vasopressors, steroids, antiseizure medication, and birth control pills all affect liver function. Hepatic cells are particularly sensitive to hypotension and vasopressors. Because patient size is an important factor in placing a liver, the donor's height, weight, and build should be made available to the recipient center. Specific hepatic laboratory evaluation includes serum glutamic-oxaloacetic transaminase (SGOT), serum glutamic-pyruvic transaminase (SGPT), gamma glutamyltransferase (GGT), prothrombin time (PT), partial thromboplastin time (PTT), bilirubin, lactate dehydrogenase (LDH), and alkaline phosphatase.[16]

3. Pancreas. The age requirement is 1 year to 60 years. Patients who have been resuscitated from cardiac arrest are acceptable potential donors. Abdominal trauma must be carefully evaluated, as well as previous medical and social history. Alcoholism, diabetes, and pancreatitis are contraindications to donation. Laboratory tests to obtain in the evaluation of the potential pancreas donor are amylase, lipase, and glucose.[16]

4. Heart. The age range is from birth to 60 years. Even patients who have had a cardiopulmonary arrest and have been resuscitated may be candidates for donation. The acceptable period of time and extent of resuscitation are center specific. The evaluation of thoracic trauma is critical in the potential heart donor. The myocardium is highly sensitive to hypotension and va-

sopressors, making this valuable information to share with a recipient center. As with liver transplants, the weight and build of the donor are important for matching with potential recipients. Cardiac specific laboratory tests are creatine phosphokinase (CPK) isoenzymes with myocardial bundle (MB) fractions. If available, an echocardiogram (Echo) is an invaluable tool in evaluation of the heart; angiography may be necessary in those with inconclusive Echo results. A 12-lead electrocardiogram (ECG) is mandatory.[16, 17]

5. Lung. The age range is from birth to 60 years. The lung donor preferably has been intubated less than 24 hours, has no pulmonary injury, and has a negative result on a sputum culture and Gram stain. Centers vary on the acceptability of a donor who has been resuscitated after an arrest. Weight and build are very important in matching donor and recipient. (See Figure 94–1 for lung measurements.) Arterial blood gases (ABG), chest x-ray, tracheal aspirate, Gram stain, and chest measurements are the key evaluation tools for the potential lung donor.[16]

Tissue donors must be brain dead or cardiac dead and free of communicable disease and extracranial malignancies. Tissue specific criteria follow.

1. Eyes. The age requirement is newborn to 70 years of age for cornea transplants, but premature infants and donors older than 70 years can provide corneas for research. Transplantable tissue must be recovered within 6 to 8 hours of asystole. Previous medical history, with emphasis on eye diseases and trauma, should be evaluated. The donor's eyes should be flushed with sterile normal saline, closed, and covered with moist gauze. Because of the small sterile field involved, eye recovery

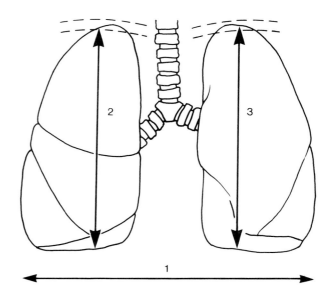

Figure 94–1. Lung measurements.
1. Horizontal measurement: Costophrenic angle to costophrenic angle
2. Right vertical: Peak of diaphragm to highest apical point on x-ray
3. Left vertical: Peak of diaphragm to highest apical point on x-ray*

*In centimeters.

can take place in the unit, the morgue, or the operating room (OR) if the patient is an organ donor or other tissue donor.[16]

2. Skin. Donors should be between 16 and 60 years old, weigh at least 120 lb (54.5 kg), and be free of dermatologic disorders, skin cancers, and infection. The donor's previous medical history should be evaluated for chronic medications. Skin may be recovered up to 24 hours after asystole. The body should be kept cool and delivered to the morgue ideally within 2 hours of death. Recovery must be in the OR under sterile conditions.[16]

3. Bone. Donors must be at least 16 years old. Only mature bone is transplantable, and by the time most people are 16 years of age, the epiphyseal plate has closed. The upper age limit is arbitrarily placed at 60 years of age, although some tissue banks set a lower age for postmenopausal women. An evaluation of trauma is key in the bone donor, because multiple fractures can rule out a donation as can previous bone disease or cancer history. Tendons, fascia, cartilage, and veins are procured at the time of bone recovery. Recovery must occur in the OR under sterile conditions.[16]

4. Heart Valves. A brain dead donor is preferred, but valves may be recovered up to 24 hours after asystole. Tissue banks vary on whether they will accept donors who have received cardiopulmonary resuscitation (CPR). In children, up to 30 minutes of CPR is generally acceptable for valve donation.[16]

REQUEST PROCESS

The need for improved organ recovery rates is manifest by the growing number of people on the transplant list. Thus, the request process is crucial. Approaching the family about organ and tissue donation requires a change in focus from the energy-consuming effort to save a life to the no less demanding task of converting the family's loss to the benefit of another patient. The first step is the identification of the requestor. The requestor's comfort level in offering the option of donation is based on his or her experience with death, as well as personal feelings about organ or tissue donation. It makes no sense to have a requestor whose own feelings about donation are ambiguous. In contrast, the requestor should be a person who believes in the organ donation process. The requestor, thus, need not be any specific member of the team (e.g., attending physician, house officer) but should be a person with the attitudes, experience, and sensitivity to maximize the likelihood of successful donation.

An assessment of the family's emotional and religious background can be helpful in determining how to approach them. This assessment includes the family's definition of death; their religion and depth of beliefs; what the patient means to them; what death means to the family; what the family has been told compared with what they have heard about the patient's condition; and what the family is asking.[18]

Timing is key to a successful request. It is vital that the family understand the concept of brain death and that they accept death before donation is requested. One of the most important aspects of the request for organ and tissue donation is the ability to clearly convey to the family that their child's death is a reality. This is the first step in the grief process. Many medical terms are confusing to the lay population including ventilator, brain death, life support, and the role of the brain in controlling body functions. For example, "life support" (usually the ventilator) is seen as "keeping the patient alive," therefore, when it is removed, the patient has been "killed." A better, alternative term is "organ support." An explanation that the ventilator supports lung function by providing oxygen and breathes for a patient who cannot do so unassisted may clarify misconceptions. Use of the term "brain death" itself can suggest a "special" kind of death that means the patient is not truly gone. Moving from the term "brain dead" to "dead" after the first presentation of the concept of brain death and the brain death evaluation may help. A description of the role of the brain may also be helpful.

In an ongoing research study, the Partnership for Organ Donation is finding that separating the discussion of brain death and the final pronouncement of death from the discussion of the organ donation option by a period of time (1 to 3 hours) results in a 40 to 60% greater consent rate.[19]

The setting of the request should be one of privacy, such as a consultation room, and ample time should be allowed for the family to ask questions and to express their grief. Providing comfortable seating and offering tissues or water may also help to demonstrate concern on the part of the health professional. The family's "saying good-bye" and telling others that the child is dead, as well as asking for information on the next steps, are signs of acceptance and readiness to hear about the organ donation option.

The requestor should be prepared to discuss a number of issues that commonly arise when organ and tissue donation are raised, including surgical procedures for recovery of the organ/tissue, use of organs/tissues, limitations, cost, and anonymity.

The family can be assured that an open casket service will be possible after donation. The family also needs to understand that no cost is associated with the donation. The OPO or transplant center takes over financial and medical responsibility from the time of consent. Explanations should include reassurance that anonymity on the part of the donor family and the recipient will be maintained.

To meet the requirements for informed consent, the medical team must include in their discussion the procedures completed to evaluate the donor, such as HIV testing and lymph node removal. Informed consent also requires a formal listing of all that is to be donated. This can be done sensitively, without its appearing to be a laundry list of organs, by interspersing descriptions of use and procedures.

No family should be denied the opportunity to donate a loved one's organs. Some medical personnel still express concerns about harming families and increasing their grief by discussing donation options. Based on responses to a written questionnaire sent to 41 donor families (34 responded) 6 weeks after the death of their family member, Bartucci determined that 89% of families agreed organ donation was a positive experience during their time of grief; 91% had no regrets about donating. The families generally had two reasons for wanting to donate: their loved one would have wanted to help, and donation offered something positive from their loss.[20] Buckley found that in a questionnaire sent to 102 donor families (53 responded) 26% were pleased, 21% were shocked, 19% needed time to think, and 6% expected the request. Of this group, 94% believed that they had made the right decision.[21]

Frauman and Miles explored the general population's response to organ donation before being faced with the situation through a random telephone survey of 585 adults. The 334 parents who responded were asked if they would donate their child's organs, and if not, why not? Forty-seven per cent of the respondents said that they would donate; 35% stated that they would not donate; and 19% said that they didn't know if they would donate. Those who said they would not donate offered a variety of reasons for their response: They found the idea bothersome; they had concerns about body mutilation; they thought that donation might interfere with survival; they didn't understand the procedure; and they believed that it was against their religion.[22] Proper presentation of the organ donation concept should address many of these issues.

DONOR MANAGEMENT

The goal of donor management is to obtain the best possible physiologic state in the donor prior to surgery for organ recovery. Achieving this objective requires management of the physiologic manifestations of brain death, which include the loss of respiratory control, vasomotor tone, electrolyte and hormonal balance, and temperature control, as well as the potential loss of blood from trauma patients. A retrospective review of derangements encountered and therapy administered in 26 pediatric organ donors is provided by Kisson and associates.[27]

The brain's control over body functions ends with brain death, when protective and homeostatic mechanisms are lost. The respiratory center, for example, no longer transmits the neurochemical message to breathe. Neither a lack of oxygenation nor hypercapnia creates any stimulating effect. Loss of the protective cough and gag reflexes also affect the respiratory system. Therefore, it is imperative to maintain an artificial airway and ensure ventilatory support. Maintenance of an adequate PaO_2 is vital for transplantable organs. An FIO_2 of less than 0.6 is preferable because of the potential for pulmonary oxygen toxicity in the potential lung donor. Positive end-expiratory pressure (PEEP) may be employed to increase alveolar ventilation. It should not be used at levels higher than 5 cm H_2O unless absolutely necessary, however, because of the potential for barotrauma and the negative impact on cardiac output. Tidal volumes of 10 to 15 ml/kg are usually satisfactory. Aggressive pulmonary toilet is critical in the potential

donor. Neurogenic pulmonary edema is possible in some donors. In these cases increased PEEP and FIO_2 may be required, as well as diuresis with furosemide. Close monitoring of the hemodynamic parameters is essential if diuretics are employed.[23]

The brain also directs the body to maintain vascular tone. When the brain ceases to give such direction, the vascular bed totally relaxes, resulting in pooling in the extremities and lungs. Hypotension, decreased preload, and extravasation of fluid into the airways must be reversed in order to maintain organ perfusion. The key to optimal perfusion of organs is the restoration and control of vasomotor tone. Maintenance of fluid and electrolyte balance is critical in this effort. The first step in donor management is to estimate fluid deficits/balance and to supplement those fluids to restore volume. The goal is a normal central venous pressure (CVP) 4 to 12 cm H_2O, urine output of 1 to 2 ml/kg, a hematocrit of 30, and stable vital signs. The child's heart (unless damaged) should be able to handle rapid fluid boluses, 10 to 20 ml/kg IV push, to restore volume.[23]

As volume is restored, the medical team should assess the continued need for vasoactive agents. Given the loss of neurologic control over vasomotor tone, inotropes may be required to obtain a normal blood pressure for age. Dopamine is the agent of choice because of renal vasodilatory effects at low doses. When dopamine or dobutamine are no longer effective for maintaining blood pressure, epinephrine or norepinephrine can be administered. Both have potent vasoconstrictive properties that can damage the donor's kidney, heart, and liver. Nonetheless, they may be necessary for short periods to stabilize the hemodynamic status. Some transplant surgeons will not accept an organ from a donor who has had epinephrine or norepinephrine drips or high doses of dopamine. More aggressive surgeons or those facing significant donor shortages will consider the organ based on present function.

A new approach in the armamentarium of the medical staff providing donor management is the T_3/T_4 infusion. To date, it has been found to have no detrimental effects on the donor while allowing the weaning of vasoactive drips. It is believed to supplement thyroid activity reduced by the loss of thyroid stimulating hormone from the hypothalamus.[23–25] Keogh and associates have found no abnormally low levels of TSH or T_4 in brain stem–dead donors, although T_3 was subnormal in 81%,[26] suggesting that further research is needed to determine this physiologic mechanism and to ensure that no detrimental effects occur in recipients. The T_3/T_4 infusion is begun after IV doses of glucose and insulin.

Brain death results in the destruction of the hypothalamus, which has significant effects on the donor's stability. The loss of antidiuretic hormone (ADH) follows the destruction of the supraoptic nuclei of the hypothalamus or its nerve tract to the posterior pituitary. The neurons of the supraoptic nuclei act as osmoreceptors that produce or withhold ADH in response to the concentration of the blood that supplies the hypothalamus. The nuclei also respond to stimuli from the atrial baroreceptors (indicating poor stretch, low preload, or hypovolemia) to cause marked vasoconstriction of the arterioles. The destruction of the supraoptic nuclei's control over fluid balance causes diabetes insipidus, resulting in an overwhelming loss of intravascular fluid through the renal/urinary system. Cardiovascular collapse can occur if this fluid loss is not controlled.

Urinary losses from diabetes insipidus should be replaced cc/cc every hour to half-hour and controlled by supplementing ADH. ADH (vasopressin) can be provided acutely by intramuscular or subcutaneous injection or through an IV drip. The IV drip, although rarely used in the pediatric setting, is the recommended procedure. Absorption occurs more quickly than with injection, and negative effects can be controlled more easily through titration of the drip. Vasopressin can produce anuria or significant hypertension. If either occurs, the drip can be titrated to a lower dose or discontinued. If discontinuation of the infusion does not reverse anuria or hypertension, treatment with diuretics or vasodilators may be necessary. Liver transplant surgeons prefer that vasopressin not be used, because it constricts the bile ducts. Therefore, if fluid replacement can keep up with losses, the use of vasopressin should be avoided.

The hypothalamus is also the temperature control center of the body. Without its input, the body temperature may fluctuate greatly from hypothermia to hyperthermia. To prevent damage to viable organs, normothermia must be maintained. Most donors become hypothermic, resulting in ECG abnormalities (J waves), dysrhythmias, decreased cardiac contractility, decreased glomerular filtration rate, and alterations in ABGs.[23] Prevention is the most effective form of intervention. If the head is covered, employing heating blankets and warmed O_2 and IV fluids at an early stage, problems in donor management can be avoided. Hyperthermia is also possible in a brain dead donor as a result of hypothalamic damage, infection, trauma, or dehydration. It is not uncommon to see extreme temperature elevations (104 to 108° F) just before brain stem herniation. The potential donor who manifests an elevation in temperature should be fully cultured, and cooling blankets and lukewarm sponge baths should be used to reduce body temperature. Acetaminophen may also be administered to help counter hyperthermia.

Compensating for the brain's lack of control clearly is a major part of donor management, but treatment of the underlying illness or injury and reversal of some of the medical efforts to preserve the brain may also be critical. Blood loss from major trauma, as well as fluid restriction and the use of osmotic diuretics to prevent cerebral edema, creates relative dehydration in the donor. Both must be addressed to promote adequate perfusion and oxygenation.

The potential for infection in the donor is great owing to the invasive lines and tubes required to maintain and monitor basic functions. Operative procedures and trauma that often precede donor management activity decrease the patient's immunocompetence. Moreover, the therapy in the intensive care unit (ICU) frequently sets the patient up for infection. Steroids given to decrease brain swelling alter the hematologic defense against infection, and antibiotics can promote growth of

viruses and resistant strains of bacteria. Aseptic technique is critical in all invasive procedures conducted as part of the donor's care. IV lines placed in the field should be replaced under sterile conditions. A nasogastric (NG) tube should be in place to avoid potential aspiration. Some centers also employ prophylactic antibiotics.

OPERATING ROOM MANAGEMENT

Continued support of the donor is essential throughout the OR course. Anesthesia personnel are needed to continue hemodynamic monitoring and support of vital signs (Table 94–6). Age-appropriate systolic blood pressure, CVP greater than 12, and urine output greater than 1 ml/kg/hour, adequate oxygenation (hematocrit >30%, FIO_2 of 100%) and control of excessive volume loss owing to diabetes insipidus must be maintained throughout the recovery procedure. Potential fluid needs include three units of packed red blood cells, 5 to 10 liters of crystalloid and colloid solutions, and 4- to 50-ml units of 25% albumin. Pretreatment of the donor with methylprednisolone is center specific; the dose is usually 25 mg/kg. After the aorta is clamped and flushing of the organs has begun, all supportive measures are discontinued including mechanical ventilation, IVs, and monitors. Circulating and scrub nurses are required as for any other abdominal or thoracic case (Fig. 94–2 for set up).[28]

The multiorgan procurement procedure is a systematic dissection of the thoracoabdominal organs. A midline incision from suprasternal notch to symphysis pubis is made, and the thoracic and abdominal cavities are explored for previously undetected disease and trauma. The order of dissection of organs is kidneys (en bloc), pancreas, liver, and finally heart/lung or heart and then lung. The heart and lungs are removed first, followed by the pancreas, liver, and kidneys.[28, 29]

Advances in preservation solutions and techniques based on principles of anaerobic metabolism have made organ sharing a reality today. The use of UW solution has increased cold ischemic storage of the kidney up to

---

Table 94–6. HEMODYNAMIC AND MONITORING SUPPORT IN OPERATING ROOM*

Anesthetist Functions
Arterial blood gas monitoring
Electrolyte monitoring and replacement
Drawing blood
Maintaining IV lines
Blood and crystalloid replacement of ongoing losses
Vasopressor administration
Administration of select preparatory drugs

Operating Room Drug Therapy
Mannitol, 25% 1 g/kg IV push 15 minutes after the incision
Furosemide, 2–4 mg/kg prior to heparinization near the end of the case (at the coordinator's request)
Heparin, 300 μm/kg IV push at the coordinator's request
Thorazine, 0.15 mg/kg IV if kidneys only are recovered

*Courtesy of Washington Regional Transplant Consortium.
IV = intravenous.

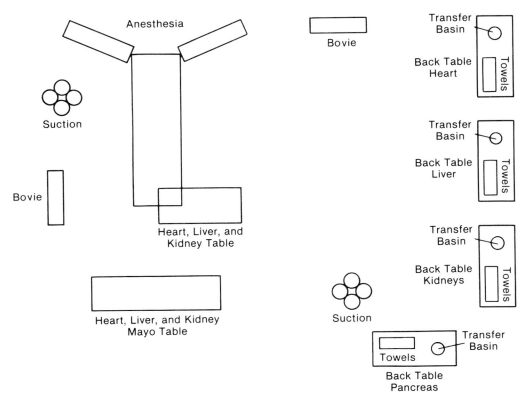

Figure 94–2. Operating room set-up.

72 hours; the liver can be preserved on ice in UW up to 24 hours; and the pancreas can be stored for up to 6 hours. Preservation solutions like UW are designed to minimize cell swelling and prevent intracellular acidosis as well as to avoid interstitial expansion during flush.[30, 31] Currently, most OPOs are employing hypothermic in situ flush with UW for kidneys, liver, and pancreas. The heart is flushed with cardioplegia, and the lungs are flushed with modified Euro Collins solution. Following flush and removal, the liver and pancreas may be re-flushed at the back table before being placed on ice for transport to the recipient center. Kidneys may also be reflushed at the back table and then either packed on ice or preserved on a continuous hypothermic perfusion pump.

ORGAN ALLOCATION

All organs are allocated according to United Network for Organ Sharing (UNOS) guidelines. UNOS, a federally designated organization with a central computer bank for matching donors and recipients, acts as the Organ Procurement Transplant Network. Allocation criteria for lifesaving organs such as heart and liver differ from those for quality-of-life–enhancing organs such as kidneys and pancreas. For the lifesaving organs, medical urgency plays an important role in the allocation process.[16]

Patients waiting for a heart who are in the ICU on inotropic agents or mechanical assist devices are classified as Status 1 (Table 94–7) and are offered an organ before a status 2 patient. Livers are allocated by blood group size and urgency. Least urgent patients are classified as status 1, most urgent status 4; patients may be classified as status 4 for 2 weeks at a time after which time their status must be reassessed. Kidneys and pancreas are allocated on a point system based on time on the list, blood group, and HLA matching (kidneys only). Organs are allocated on a local and regional basis first. OPOs serve distinct geographic areas, and organs procured within the jurisdiction of a particular OPO are allocated there if a suitable recipient can be found. If a local recipient is not available, a regional search will be made. If a suitable recipient is still not identified, a national offer is made through UNOS.[16]

Follow-Up

Contacting the donor's family members with recipient information is often very comforting to them. Some general information about each recipient gives them a view of how much good has come of their decision to donate and how many families have been helped. Providing autopsy results gives information regarding specific causes of death and can remove any doubt the family may have had by confirming the diagnosis. Both donor and recipient families should be assured that all information is kept strictly confidential and that no information will be released without their permission.

Debriefing of the staff after a donor experience and the provision of recipient information also bring the positive aspects of donation to them. The staff at hos-

Table 94–7. CARDIAC ALLOCATION GUIDELINES

Medical Urgency
All patients in Status 1 category = 20 points for urgency
All patients in Status 2 category = 0 points for urgency

ABO Compatibility
Recipient and donor in same blood group = 10 points
O donor and B recipient = 8 points
O donor and A recipient = 6 points
O donor and AB recipient = 5 points
A or B donor and an AB recipient = 5 points

Weight Considerations
If donor is within 20% of recipient's weight = 5 points
If donor is within 20% of recipient's weight AND the recipient
    weighs more than 90 kg and has any PVR OR if recipient weighs
    more than 80 kg and has a PVR of more than 5 = 10 points
If donor is not within 20% of the recipient's weight = 0 points

Time On List
Determine number of patients in the urgent category (n), and order
    patients by the date when they become urgent.
Divide the number of compatible patients in the urgent category into
    10.
Each patient gets a weighted multiple of this quotient based on his
    or her length of time on the list (e.g., the patient who has been
    listed in the urgent category for the longest time gets the full 10
    points; the patient in the urgent category for the shortest time gets
    the least number of points).
Repeat this process to assign points to the nonurgent patients.

CMV Status
CMV-negative candidates with a CMV-negative donor = 10 points
All other candidates = 0 points

*Courtesy of the Washington Regional Transplant Consortium.
CMV = cytomegalovirus; PVR = pulmonary vascular resistance.

pitals that do not perform transplants need to hear the positive aspects of organ donation and transplantation. The OPO coordinator can be a valuable resource in the feedback mechanism.

REFERENCES

1. UNOS: Number of patients waiting on UNOS waiting lists by organ needed and ABO blood group. UNOS Update 6:30, 1990.
2. American Hospital Association: Hospital responsibilities in requesting organ donations. AHA Technical Advisory Bulletin 12:1, 1986.
3. Public Law 98–507, National Organ Transplant Act, 1984.
4. Task Force for the Determination of Brain Death in Children: Guidelines for determination of brain death in children. Neurology 37:1077, 1987.
5. Freeman J and Ferry P: New brain death guidelines in children: Further confusion. Pediatrics 81:301, 1988.
6. Stephenson C: Brain death in children. Focus on Critical Care 14:49, 1987.
7. Zisfein J: Brain death in perspective. Hospital Physician 22:11, 1986.
8. Kaufman H and Lynn J: Brain death. Neurosurgery 19:850, 1986.
9. Report of the medical consultants on the diagnosis of brain death to the President's Commission for the Study of Ethical Problems in Medicine and Biomedical and Behavioral Research: Guidelines for determination of death. JAMA 246:2184, 1981.
10. Ropper A, Kennedy S, and Russell L: Apnea testing in the diagnosis of brain death. J Neurosurg 55:942, 1981.
11. Fost N: Organs from anencephalic infants: An idea whose time has not yet come. Hastings Cent Rep 18:5, 1988.
12. Shewmon D: Anencephaly: Selected medical aspects. Hastings Cent Rep 18:11, 1988.
13. Holzgreve W, Beller F, Bucholz B, et al: Kidneys transplanted from anencephalic donors. N Engl J Med 316:1069, 1987.
14. Giroud A: Anencephaly. In: Vinken PJ and Bruyn GW (eds): Handbook of Clinical Neurology, Vol. 30. New York, Elsevier North Holland, 1977, p. 176.
15. Cassady G: Anencephaly: A 6 year study of 367 cases. Am J Obstet Gynecol 103:1154, 1969.
16. UNOS: UNOS Coordinators Handbook. Richmond, UNOS, 1987.
17. Boucek M, Kanakriyeh M, Mathis C, et al: Cardiac transplantation in infancy: Donors and recipients. J Pediatr 116:171, 1990.
18. Gideon MD and Taylor PB: Kidney donation: Care of the cadaver donor's family. J Neurosurg Nurs 13:248, 1981.
19. Personal Communication: Partnership for Organ Donation, Boston, MA. July 12, 1990.
20. Bartucci MR: Organ donation: A study of the donor family perspective. J Neurosci Nurs 19:305, 1987.
21. Buckley PE: The delicate question of the donor family. Transplant Proc 21:1411, 1989.
22. Frauman AC and Miles MS: Parental willingness to donate the organs of a child. ANNA J 14:401, 1987.
23. Darby J, Stein K, Grenvik A, et al: Approach to management of heartbeating "brain dead" organ donor. JAMA 261:2222, 1989.
24. Zaloga G: Endocrine function after brain death. Crit Care Med 18:785, 1990.
25. Powner D, Hendrich A, Lagler R, et al: Hormonal changes in brain dead patients. Crit Care Med 18:702, 1990.
26. Keogh AM, Howlett TA, Perry L, et al: Pituitary function in brain-stem dead organ donors: A prospective study. Transplant Proc 20:729, 1988.
27. Kissoon N, Frewen TC, Bloch M, et al: Pediatric organ donor maintenance: Pathophysiologic derangements and nursing requirements. Pediatrics 84:688, 1989
28. NATCO: Coordinator's role in the operating room. NATCO Training Manual 4, 1989.
29. Cederna J and Toledo-Pereya L: Multiple organ harvesting. Contemp Surg 25:15, 1984.
30. Belzer F and Southard J: Principles of solid organ preservation by cold storage. Transplantation 45:673, 1988.
31. Belzer F: Principles of organ preservation. Transplant Proc 20:925, 1988.
32. UNOS: Expanded Donor Criteria Proposed by Ad Hoc Donations Committee. UNOS Update 8:1, 1992.

Clinical, Economic, and Political Implications of Critical Care

Allen I. Hyman, M.D., Raymond R. Arons, Dr. P.H., and
Brenda J. Milo, R.N.

As we approach the 21st century, critical care physicians must expand their scope of expertise to include knowledge of the politics and policies associated with the health care system. By taking a proactive role in this political process, physicians will have an effect on national health care policy, but by failing to become active participants in the shaping of health policies, key decision-making may be left to those with questionable qualifications, motives, and agenda.[1]

The aging population, poverty, crime-related trauma, substance abuse, premature births, the underinsured population, and the acquired immunodeficiency syndrome (AIDS) epidemic all contribute to the expenses and expansion of this nation's health care needs. As double-digit inflation continues to appear in the nation's cost of health care, the system becomes a prime target for budget reduction initiatives. Historically, health cost containment programs have focused on revisions of hospital and physician payment schemes. However, as we enter the 1990s, new approaches are being considered to deal with the cost-benefit issues of major medical advances, the application of life-sustaining technology, and the appropriateness of intensive care therapy.[2]

More than 15% of the nation's hospital health care dollars are expended in intensive care units (ICUs) across the United States yearly. In an era of cost cutting, it is anticipated that questions will be raised regarding the efficacy, necessity, and costs of ICUs and that they will become an obvious focus of cost-containment initiatives. With the advent of the Medicare Prospective Payment System in 1983, ICU patient days have not provided hospitals with additional reimbursement revenues, providing a strong incentive for both providers and regulators to limit duplication and unnecessary use of ICU services.[3]

It is clear that this decade's cost containment debate will focus on ICU usage and efficacy. Critical care physicians should play key roles in the political and policy-making process. This chapter presents not only the historical background and an economic overview of ICUs but also examines the crucial position of ICUs within the health care system in the United States, in order to prepare physicians to meet the professional challenges in the next decade.

NATIONAL HEALTH CARE EXPENDITURES

With the 1992 national budget deficit estimated to be over one third trillion dollars, future fiscal policy will require reduced spending and increased revenue.[4, 5] In 1990, the health care expenditures in the United States reached record levels of more than $666 billion, or 12.2% of the gross national product (GNP), and is expected to reach $1.5 trillion by the year 2000.[6] This was the third consecutive year in which the annual rate of health care inflation exceeded 10%. Per capita health expenditures in 1990 were $2,566 per person, representing more than 100% increase since 1980.[7] Almost forty per cent of the nation's health care expenses are attributed to hospital care, more than $250 billion annually.[8] Although health care expenditures continue to increase rapidly, a variety of unmet health needs have been identified; these include the lack of access to health care in rural areas, the uninsured and underinsured population, and the inadequate financing of long-term care.[9]

ICUs comprise 9.3% of the nation's 929,000 short-term hospital beds, and patients who require ICUs are estimated to account for 28 to 34% of total hospital costs (or $70 to $85 billion per year in 1990).[10–12] The physician and hospital reimbursement reforms of the 1980s will soon be supplemented with health care rationing programs to assist regulators in containing health care expenditures, considered by most to be out of control.[4, 13, 14] Reversal of the continuous upward spiral of public health expenditures is a clear way to reduce state and federal deficits.[9] As close scrutiny of health care expenditures continues,[15] the effective usage of the high-cost resources and technologies associated with the nation's critical care systems will undoubtedly be examined.

TRENDS IN HOSPITAL AND ICU BED SUPPLY

Hospital Growth

The Social Security Amendments of 1965 (Title XVIII and XIX), which created Medicare and Medicaid programs, provide the appropriate milestones with which to observe the supply trends of the nation's hospitals, hospital beds, and ICU beds over the last quarter of the century.[16] Hospitals (and the beds within these facilities) are hereafter identified in this study as short-term hospitals and include nonfederal, short-term general, and special facilities. Between 1965 and 1990, short-term hospitals represented more than 80% of all of the nation's hospitals.[17, 18]

Figure 95–1 presents the trends in numbers of short-term hospitals and short-term hospital beds between 1965 and 1990. As shown, there were 5,736 hospitals in 1965 which increased by 4.2% by 1975, to a maximum of 5,979 hospitals nationally. Since 1975, there has been a slow, but gradual, downward trend, which has resulted in a decline in the number of hospitals to a low of 5,728 by 1986, almost equal to the 1965 level. By 1990, the number of hospitals was further reduced to 5,420, 5.5% below the number of hospitals existing in 1965.

Bed Supply

Although the number of hospitals over the 25-year study period was reduced by 5.5%, the nation's bed supply increased by 25.5% during the same period. The number of short-term beds increased from 741,000 in 1965 to more than 1 million in 1983, an 18-year period of uninterrupted growth (Fig. 95–1). However, since

1983, the number of short-term beds has continued to slowly decline, reaching 929,000 in 1990.[10] This reduction can be attributed to several factors: the increased use of ambulatory surgery; home health care; the prevalence of out-patient high-technology diagnostic services; and lastly, hospitals closing as a result of poor fiscal performance.[9]

Growth of Intensive Care Units

With the introduction of mechanical ventilators in the late 1950s and the need for respiratory monitoring of polio and tetanus patients, ICUs were established, one of the first being in Massachusetts General Hospital.[11] When Medicare legislation was enacted in 1965, 27% of short-term hospitals had ICUs and 60% had premature nurseries.[19] Since the new Medicare program offered unprecedented hospital capital expense reimbursement, it is not surprising that within 5 years, the number of ICUs in 1970 nearly doubled to 2,628 units, 90% of which were cardiac care units (CCUs).[20, 21]

Despite the proliferation of federal and state cost containment regulations aimed at reducing health care expenditures, Figure 95–2 shows that the number of ICUs increased until they existed in over two thirds of hospitals in 1975.[22, 23] As subspecialty ICUs developed to meet the need of subspecialty areas of clinical medicine, almost 50% of the reported ICUs were in noncardiac clinical services with 3.3% of the nation's short-term hospital beds (or 31,699 beds) designated for intensive care therapy.[23]

Continued ICU growth stimulated the establishment of ICU resident training programs; the creation of national and international critical care societies; the introduction of Critical Care Medicine subspecialties by the American Boards of Anesthesiology, Internal Medicine, Pediatrics, and Surgery with the first Critical Care Medicine examinations given in 1986 and 1987; the need for and availability of ICU technology; and unabated favorable third-party reimbursement policies.[11, 24] By 1980, ICUs had grown to 6,243 units with 61,564 beds,

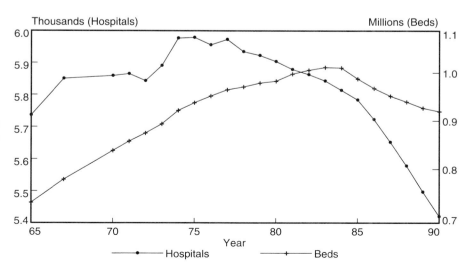

Figure 95–1. U.S. hospitals and bed supply (1965 to 1990): short-term, general, and other. (From the American Hospital Association.)

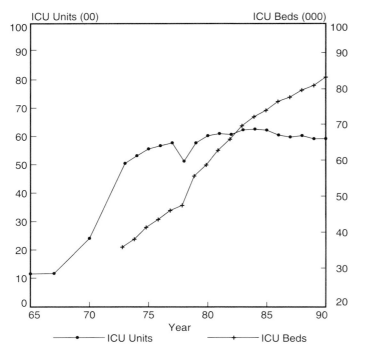

Figure 95–2. ICU beds and units (1965 to 1990): short-term, general, and other. (From the American Hospital Association.)

accounting for 6.2% of all hospital beds.[25] Although ICU growth continued between 1980 and 1990, the rate of increase per year (2,450 beds) was significantly slower than the rate experienced between 1975 and 1980 (3,460 beds per year). As also shown in Figure 95–2, by 1990 there were 86,000 ICU beds, representing 9.2% of all short-term hospital beds.[10]

Clinical Mix in the Intensive Care Unit

During the 1970s and 1980s, as the number of short-term hospitals and beds slowly trended downward, ICU units and their beds continued to increase. However, with this expansion, significant changes occurred in the clinical distribution of the ICUs in the United States. As previously indicated, 90% of ICUs in 1965 were CCUs. However, by 1990, only 18% of the 6,140 reported ICUs were designated CCUs. The remaining ICUs were distributed among pediatrics (5%), neonatal care (12%), and other clinical specialties (65%).[10]

Figure 95–3 presents the trends in subspecialty ICU beds between 1973 and 1990. (Clinical ICU subspecialty data have been reported only since 1979.) During this 11-year period, there was a 13.3% reduction in CCU beds (from 13,158 to 11,405). In contrast, there was a 68% increase in mixed or other clinical subspecialty ICU beds (36,878 to 59,588), a 54% increase in pediatric ICU beds (1,851 to 2,857), and a 76% increase in neonatal beds (6,483 to 11,405). What is most noteworthy is that by 1989 neonatal beds exceeded coronary care beds. Although neonatal ICU beds have had the largest percentage increase, the major expansion in the past decade has been in the number of beds assigned to

mixed or other clinical services. The American Hospital Association has yet to enumerate the clinical subspeciality distribution of this rapidly expanding "mixed" ICU category. To offer insight into the character of the mixed clinical ICU category, a review has been made of the ICU bed distribution in the Presbyterian Hospital in the City of New York at the Columbia Presbyterian Medical Center.

In 1990 this major urban medical center, with 1,479 total beds, had 107 designated ICU beds in seven ICUs, comprising 7.2% of the hospital's beds. Four of the seven ICUs fall into the American Hospital Association's mixed ICU category. They contain 54 beds, or 50%, of the total ICU beds and include a 16-bed surgical-anesthesia ICU; a 12-bed cardiac surgery ICU; a 14-bed medical ICU; and a 12-bed neuro/neurosurgery ICU. The remaining 53 ICU beds are divided among a neonatal ICU with 30 beds, a pediatric ICU with 9 beds, and a cardiac ICU with 14 beds. It should be noted that the CCU beds at Columbia Presbyterian Medical Center constitute 13% of the ICU bed compliment, closely reflecting the observed national percentage trends.[26]

NATIONAL INTENSIVE CARE UNIT EXPENDITURES

In 1990, hospital costs were reported to be 38% of the $666 billion in overall health care expenditures, or over $256 billion dollars.[7] A number of studies have attempted to place estimates on how much of these substantial hospital expenditures are made for ICU care.[12] Berenson's yet-to-be-duplicated definitive study

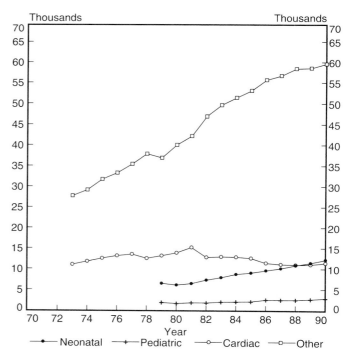

Figure 95–3. Intensive care beds: Clinical trends (1973 to 1990). (From the American Hospital Association.)

on critical care estimated that in 1979, 18% of all Medicare discharges included an ICU stay.[11] Knaus indicated that in 1981, the 66,000 hospital beds allocated to ICUs accounted for approximately 20% all hospital expenditures.[27] Berenson estimated that by 1982, the average ICU per diem rate was $408 compared with a $167 acute bed per diem rate. Furthermore, ICU costs were 14 to 17% of the total in-patient community hospitals' costs, or $13 to 15 billion, yielding a reported cost ratio for an ICU day and a regular care day in the United States ranging between 3.5:1 and 5:1.[11] In 1983, the National Institutes of Health (NIH) estimated that the cost of ICU care was in excess of 15% of all hospitals' costs, or 10 to 20 billion dollars per year.[28]

Several studies have examined costs specific for ICU care and services. Munoz studied 6,331 ICU patients discharged from Long Island Medical Center between 1985 and 1987. He found that the average cost per patient in the ICU was $18,332 (with an average reimbursement of $13,327), resulting in a net loss of $4,775 per patient; that the mean hospital cost per patient increased with the patient's age; and that the average length of stay for a patient in the ICU was 17.7 days.[29] Berenson estimated that, on average, the length of an ICU stay for nonsurvivors is 1.5 to 2 times longer than for survivors and that nonsurvivors accumulate up to two times more hospital charges than survivors. He also found that 65% of ICU costs are for labor and equipment (direct expenses) and 35% are for overhead (indirect expenses); and that ICUs use three times as many nursing hours as do general medical/surgical floors. In addition, the estimated 1982 national cost to charge ratio for ICUs for Medicare patients was 0.72.[11] The cost-to-charge ratio is a hospital financial measurement in which the cumulative charges generated by patients are sorted and compared to the actual (when available) operational costs of specific departments, such as ICUs, operating rooms, and laboratories. For example, if national Medicare claims submitted contained ICU charges of $20 billion, ICU costs would be estimated at (0.72 × $20 billion) $14.4 billion.

Rapoport and associates' study of patient cost data at Baystate Medical Center from 1987 to 1990 suggests that as the severity of illness rises, cost of care rises at a relatively lower rate and that the sickest patients are not necessarily the most costly. The most costly ICU patients were those with previous ICU admissions within a 6-month period; patients who were predicted to die but lived; and those who were predicted to live but died.[30] Deloitte and Touche indicated that days in intensive care in 1988 (including CCUs and burn units) reflected 8% of total hospital days, up from 7.2% in 1986. They attribute this to the increased complexity of a hospital's case-mix index. They also found that the number of days in the ICU in rural centers is lower than expected compared with the number of days in the ICU in major medical centers. One explanation for this is that smaller referral centers may designate a smaller proportion of ICU beds and as a result may treat some intensive care patients in general medical/surgical beds.[31]

THE PROSPECTIVE PAYMENT SYSTEM AND INTENSIVE CARE UNITS

In 1983, the Federal government initiated a health policy agenda aimed at controlling almost 2 decades of uncontrolled growth in Medicare expenditures. The linchpin of this cost control effort is the Prospective Payment System (PPS) used in hospital reimbursement based upon the Diagnosis-Related Group (DRG) scheme for classifying patients.[32-34] Public Law 98–21, entitled Social Security Amendments, mandated that hospitals caring for Medicare recipients receive an annually predetermined reimbursement for a hospital discharge. Contained within this law was a strategy that combined a hospital prospective payment system with a per case disease/diagnosis payment.[32]

Prior to the PPS, hospitals received payments through their retrospective per diem payment rates (based on expenditures from the prior year) for patients treated in an ICU setting. In no other area of hospital services have technical advances been accepted with so little documentation of efficacy as in the critical care environment.[35] Therefore, the objective of the PPS was to provide hospitals with the incentive to limit patients' lengths of stay and place controls on the usage of health care resources.[36] However, the Prospective Payment Assessment Commission (PROPAC), established by Congress to monitor the PPS program, reported to Congress in 1990 that over the first 7 years of PPS, cumulative payments per hospital discharge increased almost twice as rapidly as the market basket measure of inflation. In addition, it was reported that the costs per discharge increased even faster. PROPAC also commented that although teaching and other large urban hospitals appear to perform much better than rural facilities, PPS operating margins fell below zero in 1989 and that further reductions were expected in 1990.[9]

In the 1980s, per diem hospital rates were also replaced in a number of states, with all payer Prospective Payment Systems, which included Medicaid, Blue Cross, commercial insurers, and other third-party payers. Like Medicare, these third-parties also pay a predetermined reimbursement amount for each patient discharge regardless of the number of hospital days or resources needed by the patient over the course of an acute care hospital stay. If a patient uses fewer hospital services than provided by the disease-specific payment, the difference is considered a net gain. However, if the patient uses resources above the disease-specific payment, the balance of the hospital costs remains uncompensated. The system conditions hospital administrations to "reassess and modify [the hospital's] practices and the practices of the physicians utilizing the institution, or face the economic consequence of [financial] losses due to reduced reimbursements."[36]

Diagnosis-Related Groups

Diagnosis-related groups (DRGs), developed as a research tool at Yale University in the late 1970s, were originally intended to stratify hospital admissions for statistical purposes and hospital planning rather than to serve as a reimbursement methodology.[37] Presently, a patient is assigned a DRG based on the medical record coding of the principal discharge diagnosis, secondary diagnoses, and principal and secondary procedures according to the International Classifications of Diseases—Ninth Revision—Clinical Modification (ICD-9-CM).[38] These disease and procedure codes, along with other variables such as age and discharge status, are then assigned to a DRG based upon a flow chart (decision tree) or computerized program (DRG grouper) that determines the appropriate DRG assignment at the time a patient is discharged from a hospital.[39]

For example, in the New York State non–Medicare DRG grouper version 7.0, an infant (birthweight 2440 g) with a principal diagnosis of tetrology of Fallot (ICD-9-CM code 745.2) and secondary diagnoses of trisomy 13 (758.1) and hydronephrosis (753.2) who undergoes a principal procedure of cardiac catheterization (37.21) and secondary procedures of mechanical ventilation (93.92), echocardiography (88.72), and electrocardiography (89.52) would group into DRG 617, Neonate, Birthweight 2000–2499 grams W/O Significant O.R. Procedure with Multiple Major Problems.[40]

By 1990, the Medicare DRG system has reached its sixth revision and contained 477 DRG categories.[39] In New York State, one of the state's with an all payer DRG system, there are 603 valid DRGs in the 1990 seventh revision.[40] Some DRGs are disease or procedure generic; some specify a disease to be with (W) or without (W/O) complications or comorbidities (CC). Some DRGs are age specific, while others are age and complication specific. In addition, New York State currently has 30 neonatal DRGs specific for birthweights and 12 AIDS-related DRGs, which specify with or without opioid use. The only indication of resource usage in a DRG patient assignment lies within the resource or service intensity weight (SIW) that is given to each DRG.[39, 40]

Annually, Federal and state regulators develop relative weights (RWs) or SIWs from the charges on patient bills that are submitted for payment. They reflect the relative volume and types of diagnostic, therapeutic, and routine services required in the management of a particular diagnosis or treatment. SIWs are used to calculate the payment that a hospital will be reimbursed for any particular patient. For example, the 1990 New York State SIW for DRG 617 (cited previously) is 4.6704. The estimated reimbursement upon discharge would be $18,681 (based upon a hospital rate of $4,000 for a SIW equal to 1.000). Additional payments are provided on a per diem basis if a patient's length of stay exceeds a DRG specific length of stay (LOS), known as a trim point. The patient is identified as an outlier and additional payments are provided to hospitals at approximately 60% of the per diem rate.[9, 32]

Furthermore, SIWs are used as an overall indicator to determine the case-mix complexity of any given hospital. The term "case-mix index" (CMI) refers to the resource intensity demands that are placed upon a hospital by the clinical DRG population mixture that

exists within a given time period. From a clinical perspective, CMI refers to the range of patient conditions, complexities, and intensities of treatment. Hospitals, however, calculate their case-mix index to determine their revenues and to estimate the complexity of diseases being treated within their patient population. The overall CMI for any given hospital is the sum of the product of the number of patient discharges within each DRG category times the individual DRG SIW, divided by the total number of hospital discharges within any given time period.[32] This number will vary with changes in the complexity and intensity of the care provided and when modifications are made within the DRG system each year, including adjustments of SIWs, DRG additions or deletions, and reassignments of diagnoses and procedures within existing DRGs.

Diagnosis-Related Groups and Intensive Care Units

Compared with the preprospective payment era when hospitals received financial incentives to provide ICU services, the DRG system is "incentive unfriendly" in that there is no variable component within the system to differentiate between a general medical/surgical bed or an ICU bed.[39, 40] Therefore, ICU resource usage is not easily measured within a DRG system, concealing the utilization and costs of ICU care. Rapoport maintains that "simply singling out ICU patients in a DRG for higher reimbursement would not be workable, since it might create an economic incentive to use ICU resources inappropriately."[30] Others believe "there is no doubt that hospital administrators will cut costs, limit the use of ICUs, and reduce staffing and personnel costs by using lower-level nursing and technical personnel."[35]

In 1989, Hughes and colleagues examined Medicare's DRG system to determine if adequate allowances are made for severity of illness differences within DRGs. They found that there is a consistent and strong association between the type of medical procedures patients received in an ICU setting and the total charges in an ICU stay of Medicare inlier and outlier patients. Patients requiring either intubation or mechanical respiration assistance and patients with tracheotomies had average charges two to three times and four to five times higher, respectively, than patients without mechanical respiratory assistance. In addition, "the correlation of tracheotomy with outlier status was particularly striking."[41]

INTENSIVE CARE UNIT DESCRIPTORS

In 1983, the National Institutes of Health set forth the following guidelines for ICUs. Although their report does not include pediatric, neonatal, or burn units, it suggests that similarities are inherent and cannot be ignored. Generically, any ICU must be equipped with the following minimal technology: cardiopulmonary resuscitation equipment; airway management systems (endotracheal intubation and assisted ventilation); oxygen delivery systems with personnel to manage them; continuous electrocardiogram (ECG) monitoring; emergency, temporary cardiac pacing; easily accessible and rapid laboratory services; nutrition support services; titrated infusion interventions; portable life support systems; and any other equipment, personnel, or services needed for a specific ICU population.[28]

Hospitals have ICUs that are designated as either multispecialty or subspecialty units, usually described as level I, II, III, or IV. ICU criteria for staffing and services are specific and depend upon a hospital's capabilities and resources. A level I ICU is continuously physician directed with a nurse-patient ratio of 1:1. It can readily provide invasive and noninvasive therapy and is within a teaching or research environment. Level II can be a multipurpose or specific purpose unit, has an in-house available physician, and a nurse-patient ratio of 1:1 to 1:3. It must also provide invasive and noninvasive monitoring. Level III ICUs have limited ability to provide invasive monitoring and other therapeutic interventions. A physician director must be readily available with in-house coverage by a physician credentialed in life support. The nurse-patient ratio is 1:2 to 1:4. A level IV unit is described as a specialty care unit that does not meet the definition of an ICU. It can provide only noninvasive monitoring and basic cardiopulmonary resuscitation. There is a unit director who responds as needed. The nurse-patient ratio is 1:4 to 1:5.[28]

Intensive Care Unit Utilization*

There is a paucity of national data to describe ICU utilization in detail.[11] However, Berenson cites several ICU studies that provide descriptive statistics of ICU usage. For example, the male to female ratio is consistently 3:2; the mean LOS for Medicare patients is 4.2 days; the LOS for ICUs is one half that of CCU LOS; and ICU survivors have an average of 3.1 major diagnoses and nonsurvivors have an average of 6.09 diagnoses.[11] Knaus maintains that "historically, ICU utilization issues have not been raised very often because cost restraints have virtually been nonexistent."[27] However, with the advent of DRG reimbursements in 1983, closer scrutiny is being placed not only on ICU utilization but also on the costs associated with ICU care. Other studies indicate that because a small percentage of patients in CCUs have decreased mortality, analyses of benefit and efficacy are vital.[42]

Knaus states that patients are admitted to ICUs for one of three reasons: immediate need for one or more life support therapies; the perceived risk that a patient will be in need of these therapies; or the need for more nursing care. Also, once admitted to an ICU setting for aggressive therapy or monitoring, patients are thought to be at a higher risk for death. The point at which ICU care is deemed appropriate for a patient is usually left to the discretion of physicians and individual hospitals.[27] Silverstein views the ICU population as divided between two groups of patients: critically ill patients receiving intensive therapeutic intervention, and those with serious conditions who require intensive monitoring for life-threatening complications with immediate intervention available.[43]

The Society of Critical Care Medicine recommends that ICU patients be grouped into priority categories (I,II,III) depending on their clinical needs or conditions. Priority I is defined as "critically ill, unstable, requiring ventilator support and vasoactive drug infusion." Priority II is defined as "not critically ill but condition requires monitoring." Patients in these two categories are discharged from ICU care when the need for intensive treatment and monitoring is no longer present. Priority III is defined as "critically ill, unstable patients whose previous state of health, underlying disease, or acute illness, either alone or in combination, severely reduces the likelihood of recovery and benefit from ICU treatment." Discharge criteria is the same as for priorities I and II but with an additional criterion that priority III patients may be discharged from ICU care if it is determined that there is little to be gained from continued treatment.[44]

ROLE OF THE PHYSICIAN IN FUTURE PATIENT CARE MANAGEMENT

Does ICU care ever reach a point of diminishing return? Madoff and coworkers suggest that survival is inversely proportional to length of ICU stay and that elderly, debilitated patients, patients with renal failure, and patients with long ICU stays have poor long-term outcomes.[45] However, Cullen believes that despite its extremely high costs, ICU medical care for the surgical critical care patient does prolong life and can return the patient to a productive lifestyle.[46] Jennett and Wagner emphasize that ICU technology must be scrutinized carefully as the inappropriate use of aggressive therapy will lead to waste and lack of humanitarian interests; that equal results can be accomplished by simpler means; and that risks of complications can outweigh probable benefit.[47, 48] Jennett also states that ICU care should neither be unkind, in that the quality of life afterward is unacceptable; nor unwise, as precious resources may be diverted away from more useful activities (see also Chapter 96).[47]

Wanzer contends that physicians play a major role in the decision-making process for the hopelessly ill. Intense medical training and personal and professional beliefs can influence a physician's decision to proceed with heroic life-sustaining treatment or to withhold treatment, the latter being a far more difficult decision. However, all physicians must practice under certain guidelines to ensure that patients are (1) kept appraised of the scope of treatment at the onset and throughout their illness, (2) able to fully comprehend the course of treatment and give informed consent; and (3) kept emotionally as well as physically comfortable, especially when the decision to withhold treatment is made.[49]

Omenn cites a study of 42 hospitals in Massachusetts that indicated that the greater the physician's involvement in hospital decision-making, the lower the costs were per case. However, he warns that major infusions of tax revenue, cost sharing, and cost cutting will be necessary as large reductions in DRG pricing could lead to cost shifting, patient selection, and overuse of profitable treatments. Nationally, physician groups should advocate practical measures to determine severity of illness measurements within DRGs and units of payment tied to patients, not individual admissions. Patients should never be denied access to care because costs may exceed the DRG average payment.[50]

Patient selection, health care rationing, managed care, and the Canadian health care model are health care delivery methods that are receiving close attention.[51–53] As Callahan indicates, every cost containment effort has been negated by the rapid advances in technology and the increased demand for access. Therefore, clinical applications of treatment must be assessed before they become standards of care.[54] Kalb and Miller indicate that rationing of health care is an everyday occurrence in some hospitals and likely occurs to some extent in others. They suggest that current rationing practices are highly subjective and inequitable; that hospitals should either adopt formal rationing guidelines or make distinct efforts to avoid rationing by altering the supply of or the demand for ICU care.[12] "Until now [the courts] have not defined health care as a fundamental right but as an economic good. On that basis . . . rationing is legally permissible."[13] As Thompson underscores, neonatal health care is regulated by Federal laws that require doctors to begin treatment of all newborns except those who would clearly not benefit. No regulations exist to guide a physician's decision to stop treatment of a neonate.[55]

Relman points out that with increasing regulation and surveillance of physician decisions by third-party payers, de facto rationing of health care has become an intregal part of the medical care process.[56] According to Stanford ethicist Ernie Young, "To do cost-ineffective things, without being assured that the results will be beneficial, will be increasingly seen as irresponsible."[55] In Oregon, the goal of health care rationing is to distribute health care resources by establishing cost/benefit criteria by ranking each procedure and service based on three factors: the public's perception of value; effectiveness of outcome; and cost, with age as a strong indicator.[13] Opponents of an age criterion feel that allocation of resources should be based on the probability of benefit and that the noneconomic costs of restricting care to the elderly would be high.[57]

The ICU will increasingly be the arena where the physician's role and the physician's decision-making process will be closely observed. Berenson's 1984 list of ways to improve the environment for intensive care decision-making remains relevant. The areas cited for further study include:[11]

1. Expansion in research in development of accurate short- and long-term survival predictors for acute and chronic illnesses to provide hospital prognosis committees the ability to advise physicians, families, and patients on the likelihood of survival with ICU care.

2. The current DRG method of reimbursement for ICU care should be tested and modified to take sufficient account for severity of illness.

3. The need of the legal system to recognize the conflict between malpractice standards and the decision-making environment in which resources may be severely limited.

4. Health professionals, directly involved with the care of the critically ill, may benefit from further education in medical ethics and legal procedures and obligations.

5. The decision-making process relevant to the termination of life support may need further refinement and movement into a more decentralized forum to lift the burden of making difficult choices from individuals.

Fuchs asserts that the "pressure to control costs will raise explicitly the question of who gets how much care," a problem on which no one can agree.[52] He further believes that the divergence between what is good for the patient and what society believes to be efficient is the central conflict in health care spending. The responsibility for decision making and evaluation of costs versus benefits, development of new technology, and personnel training will undoubtedly be shared by the nation's practitioners, hospitals, and academic medical centers. This will inevitably reduce the individual power of the practicing physician.[52] Relman is convinced that the rationing of health care can be avoided if unnecessary services and facilities are eliminated, for if they are not "we will find our services to patients externally regulated and rationed as never before."[56] Callahan believes that what is needed is a restraint on our demands for unlimited medical progress, maximum choice, perfect health, profits, and income.[54] Bendixen supports the view that "the individual physician, in his efforts to save an individual patient, cannot, and cannot be expected to, consider the allocation of resources. Society, and its government, must accept this responsibility and the physician . . . must advise society and participate in the decision to limit investments in programs . . . if the cost-benefit ratio is less favorable than for competing programs."[58]

CONCLUSION

Nowhere in a modern hospital are our moral and ethical values tested more than in ICUs. ICUs bring the issues surrounding life and death into sharp focus. ICUs hold the resources to keep patients alive through extraordinary advances in technology and personnel management. Space age science has literally been brought to the bedside and has gradually been applied to patients within this special environment.

The social consequences have been even more revolutionary than the scientific developments. The ability to sustain life (or prolong death) indefinitely has created an enormous dilemma for the social responsibility, economics, and ethics of the medical profession today. Putting aside the obvious complex issues, such as right to life, the definition of death and death with dignity, the ethical question, as it applies to intensive care, is "Who shall live when not all can live?" Cost effectiveness issues have placed before the medical profession ethical problems in which life and death situations must be decided. Today, the bottom line of health care is not simply, "Is it necessary," but more to the point, "Can we afford it?" For the first time in history, the planned allocation of health care dollars brings the rationing of medicine to public attention and debate.

For too long, the prevailing view has been that everything possible must be done for everyone in need, regardless of who pays. Free health care (free in the sense of non–out-of-pocket expenses) has come to be viewed as a political right. Since we consume avidly, lavishly, and even wastefully what we perceive to be free, it should not be surprising that health care costs are rising more rapidly than any other element of our economy. The premise of Enoch Powell's law—the ultimate need for free health care for each person is infinite; the demand is everlasting and can never be met; the longer you live, the more you need, the more you get, the longer you live, and so on—leads to the inevitable conclusion that no matter how much we spend on health care, the demand will inevitably rise to exceed it.[59]

As the year 2000 approaches, difficult decisions must and will be made at every level of the health profession, industry, and government. ICUs embody and provide physicians the means to follow their basic inclination to do everything feasible for their patients. However, giving all to some may mean giving less to more. Rising ICU costs will inevitably put pressure on expenditures for other worthwhile, but less dramatic, hospital programs and will focus the economic spotlight on ICU resources and their utilization. What we may find is that too often patients with terminal disease and irreversible brain damage pass their last days tethered to life support systems, consume enormous amount of resources, and spend more health care dollars in their dying days than at any other time of their lives. The ultimate ethical questions will be "Who shall live, when not all can live" and "Who shall have the authority to decide"? Under our democratic system, each of us is responsible for determining the proportion of our economic output we wish to devote to medical needs. We must recognize and courageously face these challenges.

References

1. Shragg TA and Albertson TE: Moral, ethical, and legal dilemmas in the intensive care unit. Crit Care Med 12:62, 1984.
2. Demling RH: Assessing the critical care needs of the surgical patient. Bull Am Coll Surg 73:59, 1989.
3. Bloomfield RH and Moskowitz MA: Discharges decision-making in a medical intensive care unit: Identifying patients at high risk of unexpected death or unit readmission. Am J Med 84:863, 1988.
4. Kaden LB and Smith L: The Cuomo Commission on Trade and Competitiveness: The Cuomo Commission Report, A New American Formula for a Strong Economy. New York, Simon and Schuster, 1988.
5. The New York Times: Bush administration predicts increases in 1992 budget deficit, July 16, 1991.
6. The Nation's Health: Medical costs rising twice as fast as economy's average, November 12, 1991.
7. US Department of Health and Human Services: HHS News, Washington, DC, October 2, 1991.
8. Health Care Financing Administration, Bureau of Data Management and Strategy: 1991 HCFA Statistics. (HCFA Publication No. 03325)
9. Prospective Payment Assessment Commission: Medicare Prospective Payment and the American Health Care System: Report to the Congress. Washington, DC, 1990.
10. American Hospital Association: Hospital Statistics, 1991–1992 ed. A comprehensive summary of U.S. hospitals. (Data from the AHA 1990 Annual Survey, Chicago, IL).
11. Berenson RA: Intensive care units (ICUs): Clinical outcomes, costs, and decisionmaking. Health Technology Case Study 28, prepared for the Office of Technology Assessment, U.S. Congress, OTA-HCS-28, Washington, DC, November 1984.
12. Kalb PE, and Miller DH: Utilization strategies for intensive care units. JAMA 261:2389, 1989.
13. Southwick K: Ore. blazing a trail with plan to ration health care. Healthweek, March 12, 1990, pp. 30–33.
14. Ruffenach G: Debate grows over rationing medical care. Wall Street Journal, March 27, 1990.
15. Freudenheim M: Medicare's woes found worsening. The New York Times, September 6, 1990.
16. Hyman HH: Health Planning: A Systematic Approach. Germantown, Maryland, Aspens Systems Corporation, 1976.
17. US Department of Commerce: National Data Book and Guide to Sources, Statistical Abstract of the United States 1989. 109th ed. Washington, DC, US Department of Commerce, 1989.
18. US Department of Commerce: National Data Book and Guide to Sources, Statistical Abstract of the United States 1980. 101st ed. Washington, DC, US Department of Commerce, 1980.
19. American Hospital Association: Hospital, JAHA, Hospital Statistics. Chicago, American Hospital Association, 1966, pp. 466–467.
20. American Hospital Association: Hospital, JAHA Hospital Statistics. Chicago, AHA, 1971, p. 480.
21. Somers AR and Somers HM: Health and Health Care, Policies in Perspective, "Reasonable Costs" and "Reasonable Charges": Early Warning; Trouble Ahead. Germantown, Maryland, Aspen Systems Corporation, 1977, pp. 170–179.
22. Warner KR: Effects of hospital cost containment on the development and use of medical technology. Milbank Memorial Fund Quarterly/Health and Society 56(2):187–211, 1978.
23. American Hospital Association: Hospital Statistics. Chicago, American Hospital Association, 1976.
24. Grenvik A: Treating the critically ill: Planning for the next decade in critical care. In: Parrillo JE (ed): Critical Decisions: Key Issues in the Recovery of the Critically Ill. Toronto, BC Decker, 1988, pp. 77–87.
25. American Hospital Association: Hospital Statistics. Chicago, American Hospital Association, 1981.
26. The Presbyterian Hospital in the City of New York: Schedule of Rates, Section 170, March 24, 1990, pp. 1–2.
27. Knaus WA, Draper EA, and Wagner DP: Toward quality review in intensive care: The APACHE System. QRB 9:196, 1983.
28. National Institutes of Health. Office of Medical Applications: Critical care medicine. JAMA 250:798, 1983.
29. Munoz E, Josephson J, Tenenbaum N, et al: Economic aspects of critical care: Diagnosis-related groups, costs and outcome for patients in the intensive care unit. Heart & Lung 18:627, 1989.
30. Rapoport J, Teres D, Lemeshow S, et al: Explaining variability of costs using a severity-illness measure for ICU patients. Med Care 28:338, 1990.
31. Deloitte & Touche—National Health Care Group and Health Care Investment Analysts: The Sourcebook: The Comparative Performance of U.S. Hospitals, 3rd ed. Chicago, D&T and HCIA, 1989.
32. Arons RR: The New Economics of Health Care: DRGs, Case Mix and Length of Stay. New York, Praeger, 1984.
33. Department of Health and Human Services, Health Care Financing Administration: Medicare Program Prospective Payment for Medicare Inpatient Hospital Services: Interim Final Rule with Comment Period. Federal Register, September 1, 1983. Part IV: 48, No. 171–39752–39890.
34. Inglehart JK: Medicare begins prospective payment of hospitals. N Engl J Med 308:1428, 1983.
35. Downs, JB: Crisis and challenge. Crit Care Med 12:843, 1984.
36. Kasten BL: The Physician's DRG Handbook, 1987 ed. St. Louis, Mosby/Lexi-Comp, 1987.
37. Fetter RB, Shin Y, Freeman JL, et al: Case mix definition by diagnosis-related groups. Med Care 18(Suppl):1, 1980.

38. US Department of Health and Human Services: The International Classification of Diseases, 9th Revision, Clinical Modification, ICD-9-CM. 3rd ed, vol 1–vol 3. Washington, DC, US Government Printing Office, 1989.

39. Health Systems International: DRGs, Diagnosis Related Groups, Definitions Manual, 6th ed (No. 89–009 Rev. 00). New Haven, Health Systems International, 1989.

40. Bureau of Health Economics, Division of Health Care Financing, New York State Department of Health: Narrative Description of Proposed Changes to New State Version 7.0 DRG Grouper for 1990, 1989.

41. Hughes JS, Lichtenstein J, Magno L, et al: Improving DRGs—Use of procedure codes for assisted respiration to adjust for complexity of illness. Med Care 27:750, 1989.

42. Ron A, Aronne LJ, Kalb PE, et al: The therapeutic efficacy of critical care units: Identifying subgroups of patients who benefit. Arch Intern Med 149:338, 1989.

43. Silverstein, MD: Prediction instruments and clinical judgements in critical care. JAMA 260:1758, 1988.

44. Bekes CE: Task Force: On Guidelines, Society of Critical Care Medicine: Recommendations for intensive care unit admission and discharges criteria. Crit Care Med 16:807, 1988.

45. Madoff RD, Sharpe SM, Fath JJ, et al: Prolonged surgical intensive care: A useful allocation of medical resources. Arch Surg 120:698, 1985.

46. Cullen DJ, Keene R, Waternaux C, et al: Results, charges and benefits of intensive care for critically ill patients: Update 1983. Crit Care Med 12(No. 2), 102–106, 1984.

47. Jennett B: Inappropriate use of intensive care. Br Med J 289:1709, 1984.

48. Wagner DP, Draper EA, Abizanda Camposo R, et al: Initial international use of APACHE: An acute severity disease measure. Med Decis Making 4:297–313, 1984.

49. Wanzer SH, Adelstein SJ, Cranford RE, et al: The physician's responsibility toward hopelessly ill patients. N Engl J Med 310:955, 1983.

50. Omenn GS and Conrad DA: Implications of DRGs for clinicians. N Engl J Med 311:1314, 1984.

51. Schwartz H: The right medicine. National Review, March 10, 1989, pp. 26–28.

52. Fuchs VR: The "rationing" of medical care. N Engl J Med 311:1572, 1984.

53. Fuchs BC and Sokolovsky J: The Canadian health care system. CRS Report for Congress 90–95 EPW Feb 20, 1990, pp. 1–14.

54. Callahan D: Rationing medical progress: The way to affordable health care. N Engl J Med 322:1810, 1990.

55. Thompson D: Should every baby be saved? Time Magazine, June 11, 1990.

56. Relman AS: Is rationing inevitable? N Engl J Med 322:1809, 1990.

57. Levinsky NG: Age as a criterion for rationing health care. N Engl J Med 322:1813, 1990.

58. Bendixen HH: Costs, risks, and benefits of surgery. *In:* Bunker JP, Barnes BA, and Mosteller F (eds): The Cost of Intensive Care. New York, Oxford University Press, 1977.

59. Powell JE: A New Look at Medicine and Politics. London, Pitman, 1966.

Outcome Analysis

Murray M. Pollack, M.D.

Outcomes assessment, an important component of outcomes research, is concerned with the effects of diverse aspects of medicine such as technology, efficacy, therapies, process, and structure on outcome. This emphasis on outcomes research is generated by at least two major trends in American medicine. One is the general failure of quality assurance methods that concentrate on process and structure of care. Unfortunately, such evaluations often have no established validity and better reflect efficiency of care. By focusing on outcomes, improved validity of the quality assurance process may be achieved. The second major trend is the effort to control medical costs. Substantial efforts to identify practices that deliver quality care for fewer dollars are needed if the American health care system is to curtail its escalating costs. Outcomes assessment has made major contributions to both trends.

The intensive care unit (ICU) is an excellent hospital unit in which to both apply and conduct outcomes assessment research because quality and cost of care are so important. First, quality of care evaluations is relatively uncomplicated because outcomes such as survival and death are easy to assess. Second, economic ramifications of intensive care are huge (see also Chapter 95). Twenty per cent of hospital charges are generated by the ICU, and compared to routine hospital care, ICU bed charges may be five times higher and laboratory test use four times more frequent. With the introduction of prospective reimbursement systems, many ICUs will change from "profitable" hospital areas to "money losers." Therefore, monitoring the efficient utilization of ICUs is important.

PEDIATRIC INTENSIVE CARE UNITS AND PATIENTS TODAY

The application of outcomes research to organization and policy issues requires a knowledge of the similarities and differences among ICU patient populations. The Multi-Institutional Pediatric Intensive Care Study Group investigated characteristics of ICU patient populations and care in 1984 and 1985. Their data on patients in nine tertiary hospital ICUs with pediatric intensive care specialists provide the best assessment of *who* is cared

for in ICUs, *why* they are cared for, *what* types of care modalities are used, and *which* factors are associated with *outcome*.[1, 2] Since substantial changes have not occurred since these data were collected, they can be used to delineate our knowledge of ICUs and their patients.

Patients in the ICU were evaluated on admission for age, clinical service of primary responsibility, and chronic disease status to evaluate *who* receives care. Patients' ages were significantly different among the nine ICUs, with the median age, ranging from 14.5 months to 48 months, and the predominant age interval varied from infancy to children 12 years or older. The clinical services of primary responsibility for patient care also varied significantly among the ICUs. The medical/surgical distributions varied from 40 to 60% to 81 to 19% (Fig. 96–1). The largest percentage of medical admissions in all ICUs were the responsibility of the general medicine or ICU service. Of the clinical subspe-

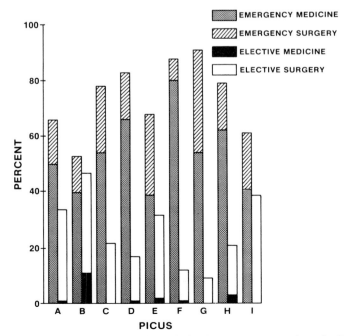

Figure 96–1. The distribution of elective/emergency and medical/surgical patients in nine intensive care units.

cialty services traditionally associated with ICUs, only cardiology and gastroenterology were responsible for at least 5% of admissions in any ICU. Neurology, pulmonary, hematology/oncology, and nephrology services were each responsible for fewer than 4% of admissions in all ICUs. The predominant clinical surgical services were relatively evenly distributed, with cardiovascular and general pediatric surgery the predominant surgical service in three ICUs each, neurosurgery in two ICUs, and orthopedic surgery in one ICU.

The long-term outcome of patients in the ICU may be linked more closely to their underlying conditions than to their acute conditions. The chronic disease status revealed that patients with severe chronic disease (life expectancy less than adult age or projected dependent functioning as an adult) were a significant proportion of the populations in all ICUs (Fig. 96–2). In eight of the nine ICUs, these patients accounted for more than 20% of admissions; the highest prevalence was 48%. Confirming the high prevalence of chronic disease, most ICU populations had a 6 to 12% prevalence of gross mental retardation and a 2 to 5% prevalence of chromosomal abnormalities.

The reasons necessitating a patient's admission to the ICU were evaluated on admission to determine *why* patients were admitted. Emergency admissions predominated in all ICUs and ranged from 53 to 91% (see Fig. 96–1). Emergency admissions were more likely to be medical than surgical patients while most surgical patients were elective admissions. No single diagnosis was prevalent enough to be important in all ICUs and even classification by physiologic system of primary dysfunction revealed no consistency among the ICUs.

Individual monitoring and therapeutic modalities were

Table 96–1. PREVALENCE OF MONITORING AND THERAPEUTIC MODALITIES*

Modality	Range (%)
Invasive Monitoring	
Arterial catheters	18–71
Cardiac output determinations	1–9
CVP catheters	9–64
ICP monitors	1–10
Noninvasive Monitoring	
Strict input/output	21–99
Hourly vital signs	58–99
≥ 4 *stat* studies/shift	23–68
ICU Therapies	
Mechanical ventilation	15–66
Continuous IV vasoactive agents	2–36
Potassium bolus	2–42
Nutritional support†	6–45
Non-ICU Therapies	
Antibiotics	40–83
Dialysis	1–4
Platelet transfusions	1–21

*Ranges from nine ICUs.[1, 2]
†Parenteral and enteral.

analyzed to determine *what* care modalities are given in ICUs. The use of invasive monitoring, noninvasive monitoring, ICU therapies, and non-ICU therapies differed widely (Table 96–1). For example, the frequency of use of arterial catheters ranged from 18 to 71%, central venous pressure catheters ranged from 9 to 64%, accurate input and outputs ranged from 21 to 99%, mechanical ventilation ranged from 15 to 66%, continuous vasoactive agent infusions ranged from 2 to 36%, and antibiotic use ranged from 40 to 83%.

Nonsurvivors were more likely than survivors to be medical service patients (nonsurvivors 74%, survivors 52%), emergency admissions (nonsurvivors 43%, survivors 27%), and younger (median age of nonsurvivors 18 months, survivors 24 months). The diagnostic categories revealed that 84% of nonsurvivors had medical disorders compared to only 51% of the survivors. Table 96–2 lists the diagnoses of the nonsurvivors. The most common primary diagnosis was cardiopulmonary arrest (total of 23) secondary to a variety of disorders. Septic

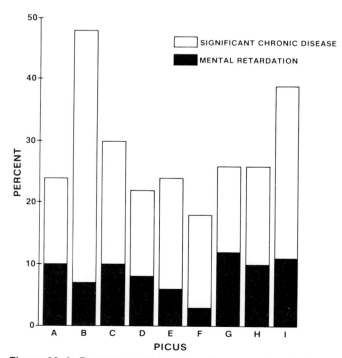

Figure 96–2. Percentages of patients with severe chronic disease and mental retardation in nine intensive care units.

Table 96–2. NONSURVIVOR* DIAGNOSES

Diagnosis	No. (%)
Cardiopulmonary arrest (multiple etiologies)	23 (15)
Septic shock	17 (11)
Cardiovascular surgery (multiple types of procedures)	17 (11)
Respiratory failures (including pneumonia)	16 (10)
Head trauma	13 (8)
Meningitis/encephalitis/encephalopathy	11 (7)
Cardiomyopathy/congestive heart failure (including congenital heart disease)	9 (6)
Liver failure (including Reye syndrome)	8 (5)
Intracranial bleeding (nontraumatic)	6 (4)
Oncologic problems	6 (4)
Drowning	5 (3)
Miscellaneous	24 (16)

*Nonsurvivors in nine pediatric intensive care units.[1, 2]

shock, cardiovascular surgery, and respiratory failure were the other predominant primary diagnoses in nonsurvivors. Resource utilization was also greater for nonsurvivors than survivors. The median duration of patient's stay in the ICU in the combined data base was longer for nonsurvivors than survivors, and most patients staying in for 7 days or more died. In the total data base, nonsurvivors comprised 8.5% of the sample but utilized 12.5% of the days of care and 18.5% of the Therapeutic Intervention Scoring System (TISS) points (Fig. 96-3). In total, nonsurvivors utilized approximately 3.3 times more resources per patient than survivors.

The survival rates in the ICU ranged from 82.4 to 97% (91.5% overall), and the hospital survival rates ranged from 79.1 to 97% (90.3% overall). The high prevalence of chronic and neurologic diseases indicate that prognosis for long-term survival and functional status for these children may be significantly worse than simple ICU or hospital survival rates would indicate. There are groups of pediatric patients in the ICU with very poor outlooks. In particular, patients remaining in ICUs for at least 2 weeks, although they constituted only 7% of the patients, utilized half of all ICU resources and, after 1 year, 58% had died or were severely disabled.[3]

This analysis demonstrates that the patient populations of pediatric ICUs and the frequencies with which various care modalities are used are diverse. This diversity was apparent in a group of university or university-affiliated tertiary care units with intensive care special-ists. Although it is widely believed that these types of units deliver the majority of pediatric intensive care, the number and composition of community hospital–based ICUs are currently unknown and analysis of these units would, presumably, add further variability. This suggests that the impact of social policy changes, reimbursement strategy changes, and advances in therapeutic and monitoring techniques will have different impacts on different ICUs.

The diversity demonstrated in this analysis indicates that the experience of a single ICU may not be applicable to other ICUs. The great variability in population characteristics, including chronic disease, age, and physiologic systems of dysfunction, poses important questions for outcomes assessment. If ICUs differ so widely, how can outcomes be compared? The variable that most successfully adjusts for these differences is severity of illness.

SEVERITY OF ILLNESS

Score Development

Conceptually, severity of illness is a continuous variable with extremes of outcomes (e.g., survival, death) occurring at low and high values; the threshold value determining outcome is unknown and may vary from one patient to another. Intermediate outcomes (e.g., severe neurologic dysfunction) can occur between the extremes at different points on the severity of illness scale. Clinical measurements are observable, and if taken in some combination, define severity of illness. In the early 1970s only indirect, general assessments of illness were used. Some were qualitative (e.g., Clinical Classification System) and others were objective but indirect (e.g., Therapeutic Intervention Scoring System).[4] In the 1980s, investigators realized that physiologic status was a direct and relevant reflection of intensive care mortality risk.

The clinical measurements of physiologic status used to assess severity of illness are generally tabulated in a "score" reflecting the overall extent of physiologic dysfunction. The strengths and limitations of scores can often be assessed by evaluating the methods used to create and validate them. There are two basic methods of score development, subjective and objective.[5] The subjective method relies on the opinions of experts to chose the important variables and decide how they should be quantified. Clinical scores using subjective development methods are often more acceptable to physicians because the thought processes involved in the selection of the variables are likely to be common to most physicians; that is, the content validity (see further on) is high. Examples of subjectively derived scores include the Glasgow Coma Scale (GCS), Apgar score, Physiologic Stability Index (PSI), and Acute Physiology and Chronic Health Evaluation (APACHE) score.[6, 7] These scores, although subjectively derived, may be improved by mathematical modeling after data bases of sufficient size have been acquired. Actually, the evolu-

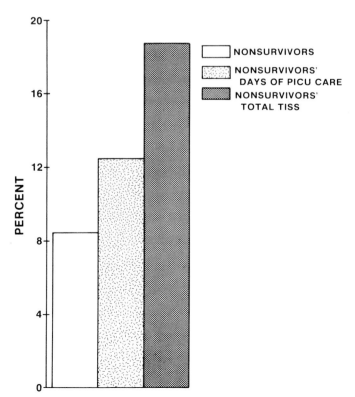

Figure 96–3. Resource consumption as a percentage of the total resources by nonsurvivors.

tion of scores is never complete, as continued recalibration to the changing status of care will be required.

The objective method uses formal statistical procedures (often unfamiliar to physicians), applied to (usually) large data bases to identify and quantify important variables. Objectively derived scores may have better statistical performance (construct validity) (see further on) because they have been derived by formal statistical methods, usually from large data bases. However, the same strength (objective derivation) may become their weakness; they are frequently mathematically more complex than subjective scores and, therefore, may be less acceptable to physicians. However, objectively derived scores may be quite acceptable to the physician. The Mortality Prediction Model (MPM), a mortality risk predictor for general adult ICU patients, was developed using objective methods.[8] It seems to have been acceptable to physicians because the variables included in the score are clinically relevant. Physician supervision of objective methods can help insure clinical relevance of the score. Other issues common to large data base collections may also be important to objective score development. For example, the data base may take so much time to collect that the data becomes outdated before it can be used. Also, the problems of missing data may be important, depending on the statistical methods used for score development.

In general, there are three criteria by which clinical scores should be judged: validity, reliability, and data requirements. At least two types of validity should be assessed: content validity and construct validity. Content validity is "what makes sense" to physicians, within a broad context. Construct validity is the ability of the score to do what it is supposed to do. Construct validity analyses involve statistical tests and frequently use mathematical models. Validity should be determined prospectively in data sets with dissimilar settings by correlating the score with (1) the outcome it proposes to measure, and (2) other indices that are correlated with the outcome measure. (Previous reviews have included statistical methods used to validate scores and are not presented in this chapter.[5]) Reliability should be assessed by evaluating the score for clear and appropriate definitions and maximum objectivity; inter-rater and intrarater reliability testing should be reported. Finally the data requirements should, to the extent possible, depend on routinely available information. This criterion is especially relevant if the score is to be routinely used or applied to large populations.

Severity of Illness Scores in the Pediatric Intensive Care Unit

There are a variety of commonly used ICU severity of illness scores, including the GCS, croup score, PSI, and Pediatric *Risk* of Mortality (PRISM) score.[9] The PSI and PRISM scores are the only mortality risk predictors calibrated and validated in large, multi-institutional studies. The PSI was developed using the subjective method. A panel of pediatric intensivists developed a consensus list of 34 physiologic variables from

the seven major organ systems and predetermined ranges of these variables. The variable ranges were based on the clinical importance of the abnormality but not necessarily on its deviation from the normal value. Of special importance to pediatric studies, unmeasured variables are assumed to be normal; therefore, extra tests are not required. The PSI was initially prospectively validated in one ICU by its relationship to mortality risk. As the data base expanded, the PSI score was improved using organ system weighting developed with multivariate logistic techniques. The performance of the PSI was then prospectively tested in eight other ICUs. Even though there was a sixfold difference in mortality rates among the ICUs, these differences could be explained by the differences in severity of illness distribution in the ICUs. The performance of the PSI was excellent. In all, 131 deaths in the ICU were observed, and 136.4 deaths were predicted. In all ICUs as well as the total data base, the outcome predictions were not different than expected using goodness-of-fit tests (discussed further on).

The revision of PSI is the PRISM score (Table 96–3). In brief, univariate and multivariate statistical techniques were applied to admission day PSI data (1,415 patients, four ICUs). As with the PSI score, the admission day is defined as that period of time lasting at least 8 hours in the admission day. If less than 8 hours of data are accumulated during the admission day, the time is rolled into the next day of care. Therefore, the admission day is a variable time period of 8 to 31 hours. This approach is effective because physiologic stability usually occurs very early in the ICU course. The resulting PRISM score consists of 14 routinely measured variables (reduced from 34) representing 23 variable ranges (reduced from 75). Each physiologic variable range is weighted to directly reflect its contribution to mortality risk on a logistic scale. All variables are either vital signs or routine blood tests. As with the PSI, variables not measured are assumed to be normal; therefore, extra tests are not required. The performance of the logistic function estimating ICU mortality risk from the PRISM score, age, and operative status was tested in a separate validation sample (1,227 patients, six ICUs). Goodness-of-fit test analyses comparing the observed numbers of outcomes in mortality risk categories to the predicted number of outcomes in each ICU separately, the total data base, and in major patient categories (operative, nonoperative, cardiovascular disease, respiratory disease, neurologic disease, and miscellaneous diseases) demonstrated excellent performance (Fig. 96–4). The number and distribution of outcomes in all comparisons were not different than predicted.

The evolution of severity of illness methods led to the development of serially updated predictors of acute (<24 hour) mortality risk based on daily PSI/PRISM scores.[10, 11] These predictors are unique in their ability to measure the changing status of disease and recovery with short-term mortality risks and have been important in expanding the uses of severity of illness methods in outcomes assessment research.

Table 96–3. PEDIATRIC RISK OF MORTALITY (PRISM) SCORE*

Variable	Age Restrictions and Ranges		Score
Systolic blood pressure (mm Hg)	Infants	Children	
	130–160/55–65	150–200/56–75	2
	>160/40–54	>200/50–64	6
	<40	<50	7
Diastolic blood pressure (mm Hg)	All ages		
	>110		6
Heart rate (beats/min)	Infants	Children	
	>160/<90	>150/<80	4
Respiratory rate (breaths/min)	Infants	Children	
	61–90	51–70	1
	>90/apnea	>70/apnea	5
Pao_2/Fio_2†	All ages		
	200–300		2
	<200		3
$Paco_2$‡ (mm Hg)	All ages		
	51–65		1
	>65		5
Glasgow Coma Scale§	All ages		
	<8		6
Pupillary reactions	All ages		
	unequal or dilated		4
	fixed and dilated		10
Prothrombin time/partial thromboplastin time	All ages		
	>1.5 × control		2
Total bilirubin (mg/dl)	>1 month		
	>3.5		6
Potassium (mEq/l)	All ages		
	3.0–3.5/6.5–7.5		1
	<3.0/>7.5		5
Calcium (mg/dl)	All ages		
	7.0–8.0/12.0–15.0		2
	<7.0/>15.0		6
Glucose (mg/dl)	All ages		
	40–60/250–400		4
	<40/>400		8
Bicarbonate‖ (mEq/l)	All ages		
	<16/>32		3
TOTAL	···		

Score only 1 abnormality/variable

P (ICU death) = exp(R) /(1 + exp[R]) where
  R = 0.207*PRISM$_a$ − .005*age (in months)
  − 0.433*operative status − 4.782.
operative status = 1 if postoperative,
  = 0 if not postoperative.

P (death within 24 hours) = exp(R)/(1 + exp[R])
where R = 0.160*PRISM$_a$ − 6.427 if only PRISM$_a$ is available or
  R = 0.154*PRISM$_t$ + 0.053*PRISM$_a$ − 6.791 if more than
    1 PRISM score is available.
  PRISM$_t$ = most recent PRISM score
  PRISM$_a$ = admission day PRISM score

*From Pollack MM, Ruttimann UE, and Getson PR: The pediatric risk of mortality (PRISM) score. Crit Care Med 16:1110, 1988. © by Williams & Wilkins, 1988.
†Cannot be assessed in patients with intracardiac shunts or chronic respiratory insufficiency. Requires arterial blood sampling.
‡May be assessed with capillary blood gases.
§Assessed only if there is known or suspected CNS dysfunction. Cannot be assessed in patients during iatrogenic sedation, paralysis, anesthesia, etc.
‖Use measured values.

USES OF SCORING SYSTEMS IN THE INTENSIVE CARE UNIT

Outcome-Based Quantitative Quality Assurance

The rigorous, multi-institutional evolution and validation of PSI/PRISM make them suitable for outcome-based quantitative quality assurance. Prior to development of these scores, performance evaluations of ICUs using crude mortality rates were extremely difficult because severity of illness and diagnostic distributions varied among ICUs. With the widespread availability of computer technology and appropriate software, the same rigorous validation methods can be readily used in single ICUs or regions to investigate quality issues of local or national interest. PRISM data can be collected in less than 10 minutes per patient.

The results of the multi-institutional studies of PSI/PRISM indicate that in most institutions, there is a consistent relationship between physiology-based predictors and outcome (mortality risk). The constancy of this relationship as demonstrated in the multicentered trials is the rationale for the use of these predictors for quality assurance purposes. If the observed number and distribution of outcomes are similar to the predicted number and distribution of outcomes, then the performance of the institution is equivalent to those institutions validating the predictor in the multicentered trial. If the performance of the institution is different than expected,

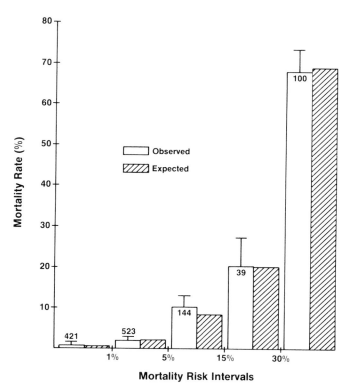

Figure 96–4. Observed and expected (based on the PRISM score) mortality rates in five severity of illness strata. The number of patients in each mortality risk group is shown as *insets*. The predicted outcomes were not different from the expected outcomes (chi square (5 df) = 0.80, p >0.95). (Reprinted with permission from Pollack MM, Ruttimann UE, and Getson PR: The pediatric risk of mortality [PRISM] score. Crit Care Med 16:1110, 1988. © by Williams & Wilkins, 1988.)

an explanation must be sought. Commonly used statistical evaluations include the Z-score and the goodness-of-fit test.[12, 13] The Z-score is based on the Z-statistic and compares the number of observed outcomes with the number of outcomes predicted by the score. It is less sensitive than the goodness-of-fit test to maldistributions of outcomes, but it is reliable with as few as five deaths in the sample. The goodness-of-fit test is a chi-square analysis that compares both the absolute number and the distribution of outcomes with the predicted number and distribution of outcomes.

Several studies demonstrate that this method of quality assurance, the comparison of observed and predicted numbers of outcomes, can be successful. In Oregon all children receiving critical care for 6 months were evaluated.[14] Evaluation of the observed and predicted death rates indicated that nontertiary pediatric critical care was associated with a mortality rate almost 40% higher than expected, whereas tertiary center pediatric critical care had accurately predicted mortality rates. Evaluations of specific therapies confirmed the conclusion that pediatric critical care is practiced differently at different resource levels. Tertiary level pediatric critical care used more technology-intensive monitoring and therapies while nontertiary level care used more personnel-intensive monitoring. Another pediatric study of a single institution demonstrated that severity of illness mortality

rates improved after an intensivist joined the staff.[15] In evaluating 13 adult medical center ICUs, Knaus and associates found that the actual mortality rate was well predicted by the APACHE II score in 11 of the 13 hospitals; however, in two hospitals, APACHE II did not accurately predict mortality rates. In an a posteriori analysis, the authors related their findings to the organizational structure of care delivery and concluded that the degree of coordination of care can significantly affect outcome.[16]

Trauma centers have been leaders in the use of severity of illness indices for quality of care evaluations. These centers have generally used the Trauma Score (TS) or Revised Trauma Score (RTS) combined with the Injury Severity Score (ISS), an anatomic index of injury severity.[17, 18] The TRISS method (an analysis combining the TS and the ISS) uses statistical comparisons of the numbers of observed and expected deaths and recommends subjective review of deaths that had a less than 50% mortality risk. TS and TRISS have been validated in one pediatric institution.[19] A separate Pediatric Trauma Score (PTS) has also been proposed and initial validation has been conducted.[20] The PTS's simplicity makes it an ideal triage score. Shackford and associates demonstrated the usefulness of the these trauma quality assurance methods. In their study, the outcomes controlled for severity of illness with the TS and ISS were compared before and after the regionalization of adult trauma care: after the regionalized trauma system was instituted, adult outcomes controlled for severity of illness were improved.[21]

Users of these quality assurance methods should be aware that the power to detect a performance deviation from predicted depends on the size of the sample and, especially, the number of deaths. The more deaths that are accumulated during a collection period, the greater the power to detect a deviation from expected. Preferably, at least 20 deaths should be accumulated. Small ICUs with low mortality rates may accumulate fewer deaths, but the power to detect a deviation from expected will be reduced.

The quantitative comparison of observed with predicted outcomes requires a follow-up process if problems are detected. Follow-up methods have not been formalized nor has a consensus been reached on the appropriate follow-up process. If the observed outcomes are similar to the predicted outcomes, then in-depth investigation of specific deaths in the ICU may not be required. However, if significant differences are noted between the observed and the predicted numbers of deaths, further investigation is needed. The TRISS method recommends this review for all deaths with predicted mortality risks less than 50%. When used in this way, the predictors are applied in a manner similar to that for a "sentinel health event," an occurrence that requires investigation. When possible, the investigation should be targeted to the deaths in the mortality risk strata that are most deviant. Other investigation methods have relied more on the evaluation of overall process than on individual deaths.

The investigation of "extra" deaths detected by the mortality predictors may or may not indicate that unnecessary events have occurred. There are legitimate explanations for "extra" ICU deaths. For example, if the ICU patient population is skewed toward diagnostic groups that have not been extensively tested (e.g., oncology patients, bone marrow transplant recipients), then the scores may not be applicable. In these patient groups, prognosis is more dependent on the underlying diagnosis than on the acute physiologic status. Subjective chart reviews may determine that the deaths were not unexpected. For example, a logical explanation for an underestimation of deaths in low severity of illness strata might be that many physiologically stable patients with terminal conditions were admitted. In pediatric intensive care, patients with degenerative neuromuscular disease sometimes present with respiratory failure, which is treated in the emergency room with intubation and ventilation. When these patients arrive at the ICU, they are physiologically stable and their physiology-based mortality risks are low. However, if care is withdrawn because of the terminal condition of these patients, their deaths would be unexpected (i.e., not predicted) but explainable.

It is also possible that fewer deaths than expected will be detected. Of course, this could indicate that the care delivered in the ICU is better than that delivered in the other institutions validating the score in its multicentered trial. However, other explanations must also be sought. An important possibility is that the resuscitative efforts made prior to arrival in the ICU were less complete than at other institutions. Therefore, some ICU admissions would have more treatable physiologic instability (and higher physiology scores) because of the less complete resuscitation. Improper use of the score may also explain the results. Data collectors should not be bedside caregivers to eliminate any possible bias in describing physiologic status.

As with any test, physicians using this type of quality assurance methodology will need to understand its strengths and limitations, causes of false-positive and false-negative results, confounding issues, and peculiarities of the method. This type of method is not designed to replace other quality assurance tasks such as evaluations of nosocomial infections and spontaneous extubations. However, it does provide a more objective and rigorous review than mortality conferences.

Cost Containment

Given the high costs of intensive care, it makes sense to attempt to use beds efficiently. Studies have documented that intensive care units are poorly utilized. For example, in a multi-institutional study of ICUs, efficiency rates varied from 55 to 89%; 30% of patients did not receive a unique intensive care therapy and were at very low (<1%) mortality risk (low-risk monitor patient) and another 20% could have been discharged earlier.[2]

Clearly, different institutions function with different efficiency rates, and therefore, improvements in efficiency can be accomplished at a substantial number of hospitals. Increased local efforts may be directed at documenting the current uses and abuses of intensive care utilization and improving ICU efficiency. Current methodology enables sophisticated evaluation of appropriate intensive care bed use. As noted in the previous section, evaluations of ICU utilization equivalent to those in this section can be done with widely available computer technology and software. The time requirements are greater, however. Evaluations of ICU utilization generally take 10 to 15 minutes for every patient day.

Since the primary purpose of intensive care is to treat patients with life-threatening physiologic dysfunction by using therapies that can only be provided in the ICU or to monitor and observe patients perceived to be at significant risk of dying, intensive care utilization can be evaluated by tabulating both therapies and severity of illness (risk of requiring a unique intensive care therapy). Therefore, evaluations of intensive care utilization require (1) a list of unique or active ICU therapies (therapies that are best accomplished in the ICU), and (2) a method of assessing severity of illness. Unique or active therapies are those that are delivered only in the ICU, such as mechanical ventilation, vasoactive agent infusion, dialysis for unstable patients, and treatment of life-threatening arrhythmias (cardioversion, defibrillation, antiarrhythmic infusions). In most studies, these therapies have been taken from the TRISS score; however, individual ICUs could easily determine their own list of active or unique ICU therapies. One such list is given in Table 96–4. Monitoring modalities generally carried out in the ICU (e.g., arterial catheterization) should not be included as unique therapies. Monitoring philosophies differ widely. In the context of utilization review, monitoring that does not lead to an active therapy or detect a threshold value of severity of illness (see later) was probably not required.

The second requirement for evaluation of ICU utilization is a measure of severity of illness. This is neces-

Table 96–4. UNIQUE PEDIATRIC INTENSIVE CARE UNIT THERAPIES*

Cardiac arrest and/or countershock
Mechanical ventilation
Balloon tamponade of varices
Continuous arterial infusion
Acute cardiac pacing
Hemoperitoneal or peritoneal dialysis/unstable patient
Induced hypothermia
Push or pressure activated blood transfusion for hypotension
G-suit
Emergency operative procedures (within 24 hours)
Lavage of acute gastrointestinal tract bleeding
Endotracheal intubation
Continuous positive airway pressure
Blind intratracheal suctioning
Frequent infusions of blood products (>20 ml/kg)
Vasoactive drug infusions
Continuous antiarrhythmic infusions
Emergency thoracenteses, pericardiocenteses, and paracenteses
Therapy for seizures or metabolic encephalopathy
Concentrated potassium infusion
Cardioversion for arrhythmias

*Adapted from Pollack MM, Getson PR, Ruttimann UE, et al: Efficiency of intensive care. A comparative analysis of eight pediatric intensive care units. JAMA 258:1481, 1987.

sary to counter the subjective impressions of physicians using ICU services that their patient is "too sick" to be cared for in a non-ICU area. Studies indicate that increasing physiologic instability correlates with increasing risk of requiring an active ICU therapy. The only suitable pediatric systems for these studies use mortality risk in the next 24 hours as an index for necessity of unique ICU therapy. An acute (<24 hour) mortality risk of less than 1% indicates a very low likelihood of requiring a unique therapy. The pediatric system is based on a modification of the PSI/PRISM system and is call the Dynamic Risk Index (DRI) for PSI-derived data and the Dynamic Objective Risk Assessment (DORA) for PRISM-derived data.[11, 12]

Using this information, the following new terms can be defined: Monitor patients are those who do not use an active or unique therapy during any portion of their ICU stay. Low-risk monitor patients are monitor patients who have daily mortality risks of less than 1% during every day in the ICU. Potential early-discharge patients did use a unique ICU therapy or had an acute mortality risk of more than 1% during the early portion of their ICU stay, but their last consecutive days of ICU stay extend into a period identical to low-risk monitor patients (no unique or active therapy and low risk). Efficiency is defined using days of care as follows:

$$\text{Efficiency} = (\text{[Total patient days of care]} - \text{[days of low-risk monitor patients]} - \text{[days of potential early discharge]})/ \text{(total patient days of care)}$$

Evaluations of inefficient use of intensive care services have not been designed for direct clinical use. Physician decision-making must incorporate many facts about the patient's disease, possibility of acute, life-threatening events, and the hospital's facilities and abilities outside of the intensive care unit. However, evaluations of efficiency will enable intensive care units to compare their performances to those of other institutions. If institutions are functioning in an inefficient manner, they can re-evaluate their admission and discharge policies and other hospital services to enable more efficient utilization of the ICU. If these units have too many low-risk monitor patients, potential early-discharge patients, or low efficiency rates, creation of an intermediate care unit emphasizing the services these patients used in the ICU may be helpful. This type of evaluation also would be beneficial prior to costly ICU bed expansion.

Predicting Death

Attempts to predict death with certainty using clinical scores have solicited numerous fears and concerns and a few advocates. Although infallible clinical scores have not been developed, the efforts to develop indicators with the potential to reliably predict outcome deserve evaluation. As society and physicians have become more open about discussing issues involving limitations of care, this prognostic research has been stimulated. For example, approximately 15% of adult patients in the ICU either have no likelihood of survival on admission,

progress to that state while in the ICU, or have, at best, only a chance for transient recovery. Some of the burdens of ICU-inflicted pain, suffering, and expense on the patient and family could be spared if decisions were made sooner. Since limiting care either through Do Not Resuscitate (DNR) orders or through treatment withdrawal is accepted by most physicians, aiding this decision-making with objective prognostic data while continuing the primacy of patient-family authority in this area would be beneficial. Prognostic scores could also prompt physicians to rethink their conclusion that therapy is futile and the outcome certain if this conclusion is based on acute physiologic status.

Even when predictors estimate a mortality risk of 100%, statistical analysis cannot conclusively state that the outcome will be death. For any statistical analysis, there is a confidence limit that depends on the number of patients assessed. When a data base indicates that no one has previously survived a certain set of physiologic events, the statistical conclusion is that, based on past experience, survival is unprecedented, not that survival is impossible. When approached in this manner, statistics are used "as a drunken man uses the lamppost—for support rather than illumination."[22] Objective, prognostic information may help the decision-making process, and experience indicates that a probability-based approach, using appropriate data, can aid clinical performance.

Pediatric efforts to evaluate the usefulness of clinical scores to predict death are only beginning. However, they will likely involve advanced modeling and statistical methods. While the acceptance of these methods by physicians is questionable, their potential application as an aid to decision-making is excellent.

Disease-Specific Scores

There are many disease- or condition-specific clinical scores to aid in the evaluation of severity of illness, prognosis, pathophysiology, or therapeutic needs. These indices come and go with rapidity. Scores that assess such parameters as upper airway obstruction, severity of asthma, or depth of coma are common. Users should be aware that the patient population size used for score development may be limited and that unmeasured factors specific to the institution that developed the score may be important. Therefore, the applicability of a disease- or condition-specific score to another institution, region, or locality may be limited. An excellent example of such limited applicability comes from the experience with extracorporeal membrane oxygenation (ECMO) for neonatal respiratory failure. To minimize the risks of ECMO, neonatologists sought to develop predictors to identify which neonates were at high risk of dying from respiratory failure, the group most likely to benefit from ECMO. However, many neonatologists were also hesitant to spend too much time developing and validating these predictors while a potential life-saving therapy was available. Therefore, retrospective data on limited numbers of patients were used to develop predictors. The variables used in the predictors included both physiologic and therapeutic data and little or no attempt was made to standardize the predictors for factors that might identify unique aspects of each population. The inclusion of therapeutic data raised the possibility that health care practices in individual institutions biased the predictor. Not surprisingly, when seven separate ECMO selection criteria were prospectively tested in two tertiary, neonatal ICUs, all seven predictors performed poorly in estimating risk of mortality and chronic lung disease.[23] This experience illustrates that predictors applicable to particular diseases or conditions require the same validation efforts as those described for clinical scores applicable to the general ICU population. Most important, they must be validated prospectively on different populations.

THE FUTURE

Clinical scoring systems are making an impact on critical care. Some states are now requiring outcome-based quality assurance programs, much as the Joint Commission on Accreditation of Hospitals and Organizations (JCAHO) has done. Geographic regions may mandate the collection of this type of data. The clinical scores discussed in this chapter or similar ones may be used to conduct these studies. Honest, dedicated physicians should not be averse to quality assurance programs that assess quality of care. The comparison of numbers of observed and expected outcomes is a reasonable and justifiable method to initiate quality assurance efforts. Results of outcome-based, objective, quality assurance studies need to be confirmed by evaluating the individual deaths in or the general functioning of the ICU, or both. Physicians understand laboratory tests—their strengths and limitations, false-positive and false-negative results, and the meaning of laboratory results under different circumstances. They understand when a laboratory test needs to be repeated or when circumstances invalidate the results. They may now need to understand the results of objective quality assurance studies in the same way.

Another area of concern is the financing of health care. Some are concerned that severity of illness methods may be used to limit ICU reimbursement. The methods discussed in this chapter will probably not be used for reimbursement purposes since they are too specific to the ICU. Methods applicable to all hospitalized patients are more likely to be used for general reimbursement because they assess severity of illness for all patients, not just those in the ICU. However, the methods discussed in this chapter have and will be used to evaluate ICU use. Since ICUs are expensive, ICU utilization deserves to be scrutinized. In some circumstances, the results may indicate overutilization. When information is negative, it will not be due to faults in the clinical scores but rather to problems in local health care systems.

Ethical problems in critical care medicine seem to be increasing as technology and knowledge enable more individuals to be kept alive, but without hope of meaningful or functional recovery. Prognostic scores will continue to evolve to help physicians and families make difficult decisions involving the withdrawal and limitation of care. It is amazing that physicians have been making these decisions without such aids for so long.

References

1. Pollack MM, Ruttimann UE, Getson PR, et al: Accurate prediction of the outcome of pediatric intensive care. A new quantitative method. Engl J Med 316:134, 1987.
2. Pollack MM, Getson PR, Ruttimann UE, et al: Efficiency of intensive care. A comparative analysis of eight pediatric intensive care units. JAMA 258:1481, 1987.
3. Pollack MM, Wilkinson JD, and Glass NL: Long-stay pediatric intensive care patients: Outcome and resource utilization. Pediatrics 80:855, 1987.
4. Keene AR and Cullen DJ: Therapeutic intervention scoring system: Update 1983. Crit Care Med 11:1, 1983.
5. Ruttimann UE: Severity of illness indices: Development and validation. In: Shoemaker WC, Ayres S, Grenvik A, et al (eds): Textbook of Critical Care. Philadelphia, WB Saunders, 1989, pp. 1442–1447.
6. Yeh TS, Pollack MM, Ruttimann UE, et al: Validation of a physiologic stability index for use in critically ill infants and children. Pediatr Res 18:445, 1984.
7. Knaus WA, Zimmerman JE, Wagner DP, et al: APACHE—acute physiology and chronic health evaluation: A physiology based classification system. Crit Care Med 9:591, 1981.
8. Teres D, Lemeshow S, Avrunin JS, et al: Validation of the mortality prediction model for ICU patients. Crit Care Med 15:208, 1987.
9. Pollack MM, Ruttimann UE, and Getson PR: The pediatric risk of mortality (PRISM) score. Crit Care Med 16:1110, 1988.
10. Ruttimann UE, Albert A, Pollack MM, et al: Development of a dynamic assessment of severity of illness in pediatric intensive care. Crit Care Med 14:215, 1986.
11. Ruttimann UE and Pollack MM: Dynamic objective risk assessment. Crit Care Med 19:474–483, 1991.
12. Lemeshow S and Hosmer DW: A review of goodness-of-fit statistics for use in the development of logistic regression models. Am J Epidemiol 115:92, 1982.
13. Flora JD: A method for comparing survival of burn patients to a standard curve. J Trauma 18:701, 1978.
14. Pollack MM, Alexander SR, Clarke N, et al: Improved outcomes from tertiary center, pediatric intensive care: A statewide comparison of tertiary and nontertiary care facilities. Crit Care Med 19:150–159, 1991.
15. Pollack MM, Katz RW, Ruttimann UE, et al: Improving the outcome and efficiency of pediatric intensive care. The impact of an intensivist. Crit Care Med 16:11, 1988.
16. Knaus WA, Draper EA, Wagner DP, et al: An evaluation of outcome from intensive care in major medical centers. Ann Intern Med 104:410, 1986.
17. Champion HR, Sacco WJ, Carnazzo AJ, et al: Trauma score. Crit Car Med 9:672, 1981.
18. Baker SP, O'Neill B, Haddon W, et al: The injury severity score: A method for describing patients with multiple injuries and evaluating emergency care. J Trauma 14:187, 1974.
19. Eichelberger MR, Mangubat A, Sacco WS, et al: Comparative outcomes of children and adults suffering blunt trauma. J Trauma 28:430, 1988.
20. Tepas JJ, Ramenofsky MI, Mollitt DL, et al: The pediatric trauma score as a predictor of injury severity: An objective assessment. J Trauma 28:425, 1988.
21. Shackford SR, Mackersie RC, Hoyt DB, et al: Impact of a trauma system on outcome of severely injured patients. Arch Surg 122:523, 1987.
22. Editorial. TPN and APACHE. Lancet 1:1478, 1986.
23. Cole CH, Jillson E, and Kessler D: ECMO: Regional evaluation of need and application of selection criteria. Am J Dis Child 142:1320, 1988.

XI Research in Critical Care

97

Research in Critical Care

Koteswara R. Chundu, M.D.

Research is crucially important in critical care medicine to reduce morbidity and mortality and also to contain health care cost by evaluation of intensive care cost effectiveness and utilization. A tremendous amount of research is being done in the natural history, risk, and outcome using various scoring systems.

The purpose of this chapter is to review the steps in the research process, including comments on organization and funding of a research project. Suggestions for critical reading of medical literature are offered. This chapter cannot cover the vast amount of the material on research in critical care; the intention is to give concise information and basic guidelines to early investigators in critical care medicine.

ORGANIZING AND PUBLISHING A RESEARCH PROJECT

Time for Research

Most of the academic pediatric critical care fellowships devote 16 to 20 months for research out of the total 36 months of required fellowship training. This short time period is optimally supplemented with at least 2 to 4 years in an extended fellowship or as a junior faculty member with protected time and financial resources. Although personal and financial consideration often hold sway, one should remember that the skills developed during training will be of great use throughout one's professional career.

Selection of the Laboratory

Although a research project should be inherently both interesting and fruitful, mastery of unique clinical skills or laboratory techniques are also valid goals. The novice should seek to be involved in a new and expanding area and to work under an individual with a reputation for

excellence. Selection of a supervisor is the most important decision that a research student will ever make. A good relationship with the mentor will make it easier for the beginning researcher to achieve goals. The ideal mentor encourages or constructively criticizes when the novice goes astray. It is essential to confer with the potential mentor and work out a mutually acceptable research topic and a plan in advance. The ideal selection process involves visiting a range of departments and research groups before selecting a mentor and topic.

Details of the Project

Once the topic is selected, a rough plan of research should be developed to fit within the allotted time frame. Because goals often take much longer than estimated to achieve, in research initial plans should be modest. The financing of the research must be planned before starting the project. A search and a critical evaluation of the literature pertaining to the research project is a crucial first step in planning the project.

Preparing for Studies

The basic outline of steps for a project appears in Table 97–1. Ideally, with a well-defined experimental aim, the design of a comprehensive research protocol is

Table 97–1. THE STEPS IN A RESEARCH PROJECT

1. Literature search
2. Identifying source of patients and controls
3. Developing goals
4. Developing statistical resources
5. Internal review board approval/obtaining appropriate consent
6. Collecting and analyzing data
7. Preparing for presentation of data
8. Manuscript preparation and choice of an appropriate journal
9. Answering criticisms and resubmissions

Millions

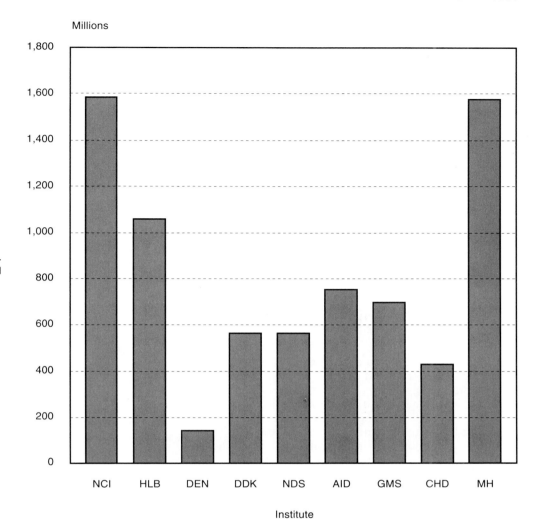

Figure 97–1. Appropriated funding to various Institutes of the NIH in 1988.

Institute

the next step. A good protocol takes a lot of worry out of the research project. Most hospitals have large computer-based research data processing facilities, and the appropriately trained personnel who can give the correct advice about using the right data base, data processing, and statistical analysis. Basic study design, subject numbers, subject selection, validation of methods, and recording the data are the cornerstones for the planning and execution of a well-done clinical study. After writing a feasible and practical protocol, the next step is to obtain institutional review board approval. Depending on the institution, this process might be a lengthy one, therefore activities should be planned accordingly. Collection and analysis of the data should then be exactly according to the protocol.

Collaborative research can yield excellent results, but such research can be time-consuming, cumbersome, and occasionally a sore point because of undecided questions of authorship or sharing of responsibilities. An early decision regarding the authorship of the final product is helpful.

Preparation of the manuscript, selection of the appropriate journal, submission of the manuscript, attention to the reviewer's criticisms, and resubmission of the manuscript complete the process.

RESOURCES AND FUNDING

The cornerstone of any project is money. Knowledge of where the money is, who gives it, and who gets it is the important first step in developing a grant and fundraising strategy. Three main grant-giving systems are in operation: the Federal Government and the Non-Governmental Granting System that includes individuals, foundations, and corporations and industrial support.

The Catalog of Federal Domestic Assistance (CFDA), published annually, describes more than 1,000 federal grant programs. This information is sent routinely to state agencies and educational institutes. There are two basic types of federal grants: project and formula. Project grants are awarded on a competitive basis to fund specific activities; formula grants are allocated according to statutory distribution guidelines for unspecified, ongoing activities. CFDA classifies all grants as either the formula type or the project type.

Figure 97–1 shows 1988 funding levels for various branches of the National Institutes of Health (NIH). The volume of approved applications has increased steadily so that the funding ratio has dropped to approximately 15 to 20% of the approved grants. Thus 4 to 5 grants must be written for each one funded. Large and prestigious centers have a disproportionate share of grants awarded from the NIH. Twenty pediatric departments received 64.7% of the total NIH pediatric rated funding in the last 5 years.

There are approximately 25,000 active grant-making foundations in the United States, and of these 17% have assets of 1 million dollars or more. In most cases proposals for foundations are relatively brief and have few rules compared with the lengthy, time-consuming NIH grant system.

The third grant system is the industrial support of drug and antibiotic testing and patentable applied research. There is a bibliography relating to grants at the end of this chapter.

Grant seeking is a cumbersome and time-consuming process for which the young trainees should be prepared during their fellowship.

UNDERSTANDING AND CRITICAL READING OF MEDICAL LITERATURE

It is imperative to keep abreast of new developments in the medical literature that could be incorporated into clinical practice or the research area. The medical literature contains reports of well done and poorly done studies. Although it is tempting to read the title, abstract, and conclusions and try to apply the new treatment or methodology, time must be spent critically reviewing the article in a systematic manner. This will help not only in the self-education process but also in avoiding costly errors by accepting the new findings in a hurried manner. Generally, high-quality peer-reviewed journals are likely to publish good, sensible, and solid reports of medical literature, but occasionally poor papers slip through. Some of the less established, newly founded journals are unlikely to have the same stringent peer review criteria as the older established journals, at least in the first few years. Thus, it is important that the young physicians learn how to critically assess the medical literature during their early training.

This subsection is divided into two parts. The first part deals with critical assessment of the medical report and the second part outlines the pertinent fundamentals of biomedical statistics.

Objective and Hypothesis

The pertinent starting point is an understanding of the investigator's objective. Even though the investigator is obligated to state the purpose of the study, sometimes this purpose gets lost or difficult to understand. Skilled researchers must formulate specific objectives and clean-cut hypotheses for testing. Mere collection of vast amounts of data does not guarantee an effective, meaningful publication. Lack of an understanding of objectives handicaps both the reader and the author in any assessment or interpretation of the results.

Study Design

To evaluate the study it is necessary to understand what is the research design and to know the various drawbacks of different study designs. The research design specifies the number of groups in a study and the timing of the interventions, including the order and frequency of the observations or measures. Three general questions discriminate among the major types of design:

1. Is there a planned treatment or intervention?
2. Will there be a control group comparison?
3. Is random assignment to groups possible?

If there is no planned treatment or intervention, but rather the study is a survey, the design is a *correlational* one. If there will be a control group comparison but random assignment to groups is not possible, the design is a *quasiexperimental* one. If there will be one or more control groups in the study and random assignment of participants to treatment and control groups, the design is an *experimental* one. Designs in health research are often mixed. Other design features include cross-sectional designs (single-shot) and longitudinal and prospective designs. Cross-sectional designs are the weakest but are more easily done. Prospective designs are difficult but provide the strongest potential for conclusions, especially when studying unpredictable and infrequent events.

Methodology and Observations

In the methodology section the author must clearly explain the definitions of the terms, including diagnostic criteria and criteria of the outcome and measurements made. Without a clear understanding of these definitions, it is impossible for the reader to assess not only that particular paper but also comparisons with other papers in the literature on a similar research topic. Classic critical care examples of unclear definitions are found in the area of catheter-related infections and adult respiratory distress syndrome (ARDS).

The reader must assess the methods of measurement to ascertain their consistency for all subjects in relation to the objectives of the investigation. The essential question is to assess whether inconsistencies in observation could have sufficient impact to influence the results of the study. The reader must also evaluate the reliability and reproducibility of the observations, even though it is a difficult task to do. When a subjective element enters the assessment area, a careful assessment of inter-rater and intra-rater variability is necessary. Assessment of outcome has particular relevance to critical care medicine. Life and death outcome definitions are clear-cut, but an assessment of morbidity, cost-effectiveness, and rationing of health care cost often are not.

Presentation of Results

Because of the frequency of numeric inconsistencies, it is a good idea to do some quick checks:

1. Columns and rows should add up to their indicated totals.

2. Percentages of mutually exclusive categories should add up to 100%.

3. Totals in various tables describing the same group or population should agree.

4. Numbers in tables and figures should agree with the text.

Finally, a graded assessment should be made of the importance of the final outcome.

Analyzing Data

There are two important aspects to analyzing data. The first one is looking for a bias that may be one of selection, observation, or analytic bias. The second aspect is looking at the appropriateness of the statistical testing and statistical significance of the presented data. The next subsection will help the reader to understand some of the basics in medical statistics.

Discussion and Conclusions

In the discussion section, the authors attempt to provide an interpretation of their findings and possible explanations for the results. Any differences with the literature should be explained. Three points need to be looked at critically in the discussion and conclusion area: (1) Are the conclusions relevant to the hypothesis and are there any unwarranted conclusions? (2) Does the sample size have enough power for the conclusions deduced? (3) How important are the significant conclusions? Statistical significance does not necessarily equate with clinical significance.

Basics of Biomedical Statistics

This section is not intended to substitute for textbooks in biomedical statistics but to present some basics in both descriptive and inferential statistics and hopefully stimulate the reader to pursue further study.

There are two distinct steps in the process of analyzing any data. The first one is to describe the data, using standard methods to determine average value, range of data around the average, and other characteristics known as *descriptive statistics*. The objective is simply to communicate the results without attempting to generalize beyond the sample of individuals to any other group. The second step is to *infer* the likelihood that the observed results can be generalized to other samples of individuals, which is known as *inferential statistics*. The goal of inferential statistics is to determine the likelihood that these differences could be explained by chance or could be real.

Descriptive Statistics

1. Means, medians, and modes: MEASURES OF THE MIDDLE. *Mean* is the arithmetic average; *median*

is the middlemost value, and *mode* is the most-frequently occurring value. Mean and median are frequently used whereas the mode is rarely used in clinical research. Figure 97–2 illustrates the mean, median, and mode. Note that this curve is asymmetric or "skewed," and the mean, median, and mode do not coincide. If there are two or more high points in the curve, it is referred to as a *bimodal* distribution.

2. *Measures of Variation:* RANGE, VARIANCE, and STANDARD DEVIATION. The most obvious measure of dispersion (highest minus lowest) is the *range,* which has a limited use for inference but may have importance clinically.

When the values of a set of observations lie close to their mean, the dispersion is less than when they are scattered over a wide range. *Variance* is the measure of dispersion relative to the scatter of the values about their mean.

Standard deviation (SD), which is a ubiquitous measure in clinical research, is defined as the square root of the variance.

$$SD = \frac{\sqrt{\text{sum of (individual value } - \text{ mean)}}}{\text{Number of values}}$$

3. *Normal (Gaussian) Distribution.* It has been observed that natural variation of many variables tend to follow a bell-shaped distribution (Fig. 97–3), with most values clustered symmetrically near the mean and a few values falling out on the tails. As noted in Figure 97–3, 68% of values are within 1 SD; 95% are within 2 SD; and 100% are within 3 SD. Empirically, the distribution of many quantitative measures fall in the normal distribution (e.g., weight, intelligence quotients). Unfortunately, many populations in critical care medicine do not follow the gaussian distribution. The importance of normal distribution is not only helpful in description per se but also plays a crucial role in the statistical inference.

Inferential Statistics

The goal of inferential statistics is to present a *p value* that characterizes the observed findings as "statistically

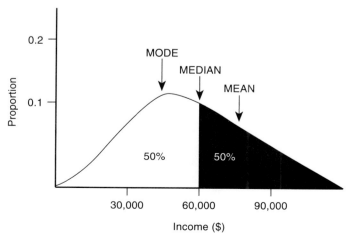

Figure 97–2. Graph of an asymmetric distribution illustrating the mean, mode, and median.

significant'' or ''not statistically significant.'' In other words, can an observed difference be reasonably assumed to represent a true difference? There are numerous personal computer–run software packages for calculation of the ''p values'' for various statistical tests.

Concept of Standard Error of the Mean (SEM)

Every measurement has some associated error because of sampling variation. If you apply this to an SD (which is a way to describe variation), the definition of standard error (SE) arises.

$$SE = \frac{SD}{\text{sample size}}$$

In some of the medical literature SD and SE are used interchangeably, and some authors believe that this somehow tightens the data because SE is a smaller number than that of the SD. The choice of mean ± SD or mean ± SE depends on the purported use of the data. If it is described to indicate variation of individual values about a mean, the choice is mean ± SD. If the intention is to indicate sampling variation of the mean and to perform a statistical inference regarding the mean, then the choice is mean ± SE.

Specifications for a Test of Significance

Three specifications are necessary to perform a test of significance.

1. *Null Hypothesis:* Assumes that the difference in population proportions is zero. For the comparison of two groups with quantitative data, the null hypothesis is that the mean in the underlying *''study''* and *''control''* population are identical or, alternatively, that the difference in population means is zero.
2. *Significance Level:* Setting a significance level is the *arbitrary* selection of a small enough chance for making a choice. By convention 0.05 or 5% and 0.01 or 1% are set as the levels of significance. Choice of 5% means that an event occurring only 1 time in 20 or less is sufficiently rare to risk drawing a conclusion that

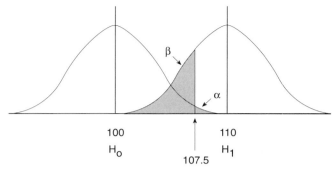

Figure 97–4. Illustration of α and β errors. See text for explanation.

excludes chance as a likely explanation of what was observed.

3. *One- or Two-Sided Test:* In the comparison of two groups one considers as alternatives to the null hypothesis only that the population mean in the study group may be higher than that in the comparison group, this is a *one-sided test.* If, however, one considers the possibility that the population mean in the study group may be higher or lower than that in the comparison group, this is a *two-sided test.* In practice, most of the statistical analyses use a two-tailed test.

Type I and Type II Errors (Fig. 97–4)

1. *Type I or α Error:* The probability of incorrectly rejecting the null hypothesis and the resultant error is called type I or α error. If you use a significance level of 0.05, that means that there is 1 chance in 20 of an α or type I error.
2. *Type II or β Error:* This is the probability of incorrectly accepting the null hypothesis when, in fact, the alternative hypothesis is true.
3. *Power:* Power of a statistical test is defined as 1 − β. Thus the power of a statistical test refers to the chance of correctly rejecting the null hypothesis when, in fact, the null hypothesis is false (i.e., the populations are different). Power is related directly to the sample size, since a larger sample size results in a smaller SE.

Parametric and Nonparametric Tests

Parametric Tests. These tests assume that sample population or populations are, at least, approximately **normally distributed.** An example of a parametric statistical test is a widely used t-test. Other tests included in the category are analysis of variance (ANOVA), regression analysis, analysis of covariance (ANCOVA), and time series analysis.

The *t-test* is used for measured variables, in comparing two means. The *unpaired* t-test compares the means of two independent samples. The *paired* t-test compares two paired observations on the same individual or on matched individuals.

$$t = \frac{\text{difference between means}}{\text{SE of the difference}}$$

ANOVA. This analysis allows comparison among

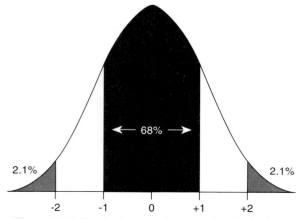

Figure 97–3. Graph of a normal or gaussian distribution.

more than two sample means. A one way ANOVA deals with a single categorical independent variable or factor. Factorial ANOVA can deal with multiple factors in many different configurations.

Regression Analysis. This analysis deals with the situations in which there is one measured dependent variable and one or more measured independent variables. The Pearson correlation and multiple correlation coefficient describe the strength of the relationship between the variables.

ANCOVA. This analysis combines both regression and ANOVA. There is one measured dependent variable. However, the independent variables can be both categorical factors and measured variables.

Time Series Analysis. This analysis allows us to look at data in which we make many repeated measurements on the same individual or organization over time.

Nonparametric Tests. A variety of statistical tests have been devised to examine the association between a single categorical independent variable and nominal (named category such as sex, marital status), ordinal (set of ordered categories such as cancer staging; pain rating) dependent variables. These are *distribution-free* statistics. The most frequently used nonparametric tests include the Chi-square, Fisher exact test, Mann-Whitney U test, the Kruskal-Wallis sign test, and Wilcoxon test.

Nonparametric Test for Nominal Data. Commonly used tests are Chi-square, the binomial and Fisher exact test for unpaired samples, and the McNemar tests for paired samples.

Nonparametric Tests for Ordinal Variables. Commonly used tests are the Mann-Whitney U test and the Kruskal-Wallis tests. There are other advanced and complicated nonparametric tests for various uses.

In summary, this chapter provides some basic ideas on how to plan, fund, organize, and publish a research project. A good student of this exciting field of both clinical and basic research will prosper in critical care medicine.

Bibliography

Daniel WW: Biostatistics: A Foundation for Analysis in the Health Sciences, 2nd ed. New York, John Wiley & Sons, 1978.

Levitan D: A Guide to Grants: Governmental and Nongovernmental, 2nd ed. Newton Center, MA, Government Research Publications, 1985.

Margolin JB: The Individual's Guide to Grants. New York, Plenum Press, 1983.

McGaghie WC and Fray JJ: Handbook for the Academic Physician. New York, Springer-Verlag, 1986.

XII Physician-Nurse Interaction in the Pediatric Intensive Care Unit

98

Physician-Nurse Interaction in the Intensive Care Unit

Mary Fran Hazinski, R.N., M.S.N., F.A.A.N.

The intensive care unit (ICU) "combines the capacity to provide needed care and technology with a potential to do great harm."[1] It can be an enormously stressful environment for physicians and nurses and a tremendously rewarding place to work.[2, 3] The opportunities for learning are enormous, yet the tolerable margin for error is small.

Critical care medicine is a multidisciplinary and multiprofessional medical-nursing field.[1] As a result, the relationship among physicians and nurses in the intensive care unit and the effectiveness of their communication will determine, to a great extent, the quality of the care provided in the unit. In fact, high levels of interdisciplinary collaboration and communication have been linked with improved patient survival in intensive care units.[4]

The physician-nurse relationship has changed significantly during the past 20 years and continues to evolve as a consequence of advances in medical technology and therapeutics, medical and nursing education, the litigious nature of our society, and the shortage of nurses. Although most physician-nurse interaction is positive, the relationship is not always ideal; there are multiple sources of real or perceived conflict. Certainly, some disagreements between nurses and physicians, when properly managed, can protect patients and improve patient care. However, unresolved conflicts can compromise the quality of patient care, and patient and family confidence in the health care team can suffer. The purposes of this chapter are to review the factors that influence physician-nurse interaction and affect staff nurse satisfaction and retention, to review aspects of

risk management in physician-nurse communication, and to present strategies to improve the interaction between the pediatric critical care physician and the nurse in the critical care unit.

RECENT DEVELOPMENTS IN HEALTH CARE AND EFFECTS ON PROFESSIONAL RELATIONSHIPS

The nature of medical and nursing care has changed dramatically during the past 20 to 30 years, as has the relationship between the nurse and physician. In the 1950s and 1960s, most physicians were male and occupied a relatively exalted and respected position in the community—in fact, the physician was viewed as omnipotent, kindly, caring, and reassuring.[5-7] Most nurses were women, viewed as the physician's right hand, serving the physician as much as the patient. The physician was considered to have total responsibility for patient care decisions, and the nurse served to provide "significant recommendations, but at the same time . . . [the nurse] must appear to be passive . . . to make her recommendations appear to be initiated by the physician."[5] Independent thought on the part of nurses, although frequent, was rarely expressed and was tacitly discouraged.

During the 1960s, when 80% or more of all nurses received diplomas at hospital-based schools,[8, 9] hospitals and physicians exerted a great deal of influence over the education of these nurses. If a physician was unhappy with the preparation of a nurse, that physician could theoretically walk down the hallway and suggest a change in curriculum to the nursing instructor. At that time, the nursing and teaching professions constituted the primary career opportunities available to women.

The 1960s were a time of unparalleled growth in hospital care. Medicare dollars funded hospital expansion and paid to keep patients in the hospital. Technology available to hospitals increased at an extraordinary rate, and the complexity of care provided in hospitals increased accordingly. Hospital administrators replaced physicians as directors of major medical centers and physicians no longer controlled hospital function, personnel, equipment, and budget.

In the early 1970s, in order to provide the high level of care required by their patients, more nurses attended schools of nursing in colleges and universities. By 1985, 60% of nurses graduating from nursing programs were college-educated with baccalaureate degrees, and by 1988, fewer than 15% of nurses were educated in hospital-based diploma programs.[7] As a result, hospitals and physicians no longer controlled the preparation of nurses. Early baccalaureate nursing education focused primarily on normal growth and development and psychosocial aspects of care, with little time devoted to physiology and assessment of organ system failure.

The 1970s and 1980s witnessed a curtailment of government-funded hospital expansion. During the 1980s, hospitals were forced to close beds and to compete for patients, and hospital occupancy rates decreased dramatically. Despite this, the number of nurses employed by hospitals grew by more than 55% between 1977 and 1984, because patient acuity rose, as did the complexity of patient illness and care.[8, 10, 11] In 1972, hospitals employed 50 nurses per 100 patients; by 1986, 91 nurses were employed per 100 patients.[8] This dramatic increase in the need for nurses occurred at a time when career opportunities expanded for women and enrollment in schools of nursing plummeted, two factors that contributed to the development of a significant nursing shortage in the United States. This shortage has focused attention on factors affecting nursing satisfaction and retention, which are discussed in subsequent sections of this chapter.

Critical care units have been particularly affected by the nursing shortage. In 1988, the American Association of Critical Care Nurses reported a 13.8% nurse vacancy rate in hospital critical care units and the expectation that the number of critical care units will double between 1988 and 2000.[12] In 1986, Ernst and Whinney predicted that during the next 50 years, hospitals will be converted into high-technology, critical care hubs, so the need for critical care nurses can only increase.[13] The National Association for Children's Hospitals and Related Institutions reports that the acuity of children on the floor in children's hospitals today is equivalent to the acuity of children in ICUs in 1988. Thus, even "ward" or "floor" nursing has evolved into critical care nursing. However, most undergraduate nursing education is designed to prepare the nurse as a "generalist," and little or no preparation for critical nursing care is provided.

Nursing faculty suggest that undergraduate nursing education should be compared to undergraduate medical education; both should provide only the theoretical basis for practice and must be paired with postgraduate hospital-based training before expertise is achieved. However, the quality and length of hospital-based nursing orientation varies widely from institution to institution, as few standards exist to determine the fundamental skills and knowledge requisite to critical care nursing. Standards for pediatric critical care nursing are even more difficult to find. In 1992, for the first time, the American Association of Critical Care Nurses will offer a Pediatric Critical Care nursing certification examination.

Our litigation-prone society has created an atmosphere of distrust between the patient (and patient family) and the health care team. Furthermore, difficult and often urgent ethical issues surrounding the care of complex medical problems have made management decisions difficult. The physician is no longer regarded as infallible; unavoidably, adverse patient outcomes are blamed on somebody. Any real or apparent inconsistency in information provided by nurses and physicians can provide grounds for litigation. This atmosphere has contributed to potential mistrust within the health care team itself, at a time when the team concept is more necessary than ever.

CONTRIBUTION OF THE NURSING PROFESSION TO POTENTIAL CONFLICT

The nursing profession is in transition and will continue to evolve as nurses seek to provide optimum care for complexly ill patients and their families. This transition has led to conflict within the nursing profession itself, as well as potential conflict with physicians and other health care professionals.

Educational Preparation

The nursing profession has been unable to develop consensus regarding the educational prerequisite for bedside nursing care. Since 1964, the American Nurses Association (ANA) has advocated that a baccalaureate degree be required for entry into nursing practice. However, since more than 60% of practicing nurses today have either associate degrees or diplomas, the ANA position has been opposed by many bedside nurses and has failed to change state licensing requirements.[12]

If baccalaureate degrees produce better preparation for bedside nursing care, then baccalaureate-prepared nurses should provide patient care that *is* measurably better than nurses with associate degrees or diplomas. This difference in care is difficult to prove, given the wide variety of clinical preparation provided in baccalaureate programs.

The college-educated nurse should possess a solid foundation in physiology and pathophysiology, psychology, and sociology. However, if the clinical faculty supervising the undergraduate students are not clinically competent, the student is likely to be inadequately prepared to provide bedside care. Many baccalaureate-prepared nurses complete their formal (undergraduate) nursing education with inadequate clinical nursing skills and are forced to acquire these skills after completion of their formal education. In order to convince nurses to obtain baccalaureate nursing education, and hospitals to preferentially hire baccalaureate-prepared nurses, the college or university should be able to guarantee that their graduates will be capable of providing skilled nursing care. Those graduates should be able, in turn, to command higher salaries.

The more educated and competent the bedside nurse is, the more valuable that nurse is perceived to be by the hospital (or employing institution).[16] If a nurse comes to the hospital with only 2 to 3 years of formal education, or with a college education and minimal clinical skills, that nurse will be viewed as unskilled and relatively replaceable by the hospital. Skilled nursing care can save the hospital money, since fewer experienced nurses may be required to provide care and the incidence of errors and complications may be reduced.[17, 18]

The controversy regarding nursing education includes advanced education for nurses. Many nurses seek a master's degree in nursing to increase their knowledge of physiology and pathophysiology and to develop an area of clinical specialization. The benefit of a master's degree in nursing and the contribution of the clinical nurse specialist to patient care have been questioned by some physicians and hospital administrators. This confusion results from the variability in the educational preparation of nurses with master's degrees, and the wide range of clinical expertise that these nurses bring to the clinical setting.

The term "clinical nurse specialist" implies that the nurse possesses an area of *clinical* expertise. However, the nursing profession utilizes this term to designate *educational* preparation, specifically a Master's degree in nursing, regardless of the nurse's level of clinical experience or expertise. "Clinical nurse specialist" is a misnomer when it is applied to a new master's graduate or a clinician with limited experience in clinical nursing care. It seems particularly confusing that a senior nurse with 25 years of experience in caring for postoperative cardiovascular patients cannot be called a clinical specialist (but must use other terms, such as nurse clinician), when a master's prepared nurse who has never cared for a cardiovascular patient may claim the title clinical specialist in cardiovascular nursing. It may be more reasonable for nurses to reserve the "specialist" title for experienced and expert clinicians. Designation of nursing education in a title may be appropriate, but the use of "*clinical* nurse specialist" should be earned through *clinical* as well as educational effort.

If a clinical nurse specialist (CNS) is active as a clinical teacher of patients and colleagues, the quality of care on that unit can improve. If, however, a CNS is unavailable for clinical problems, questions, teaching, and emergencies, that "specialist" may have no impact on the quality of care. A small number of studies suggest that units with a clinically involved CNS have decreased staff nurse stress, better documentation of systematic assessments and substantive patient care information, and reduced errors in nursing notes.[17–19] Studies such as these should be repeated to verify the effectiveness of the clinically involved CNS in ICUs today and to justify the expense of hiring these nurses. In addition, these studies should serve to encourage nurses who utilize the clinical nurse specialist title to become or remain actively involved in clinical practice, since such involvement can make tangible contributions to patient care.

Clinical Competence and Preparation

In general, nurses do have more years of preparation and education than in the past, yet many nurses acknowledge the fact that their education has left them inadequately prepared to provide patient care.[13] Physicians are frustrated with the lack of consistent nursing preparation and competence,[20] and the educational gap between nurses and physicians can contribute to poor communication and conflict.[21]

Nursing curricula have failed to keep pace with technologic advances in medical and nursing care and have not been physiologically based. Until recently, these curricula remained heavily weighted toward psychosocial and management areas, with inadequate preparation for the care of seriously ill or injured patients. Nursing faculty may be most comfortable with psychosocial issues since these aspects change less than the physiologic and technical aspects of care.

The content of current undergraduate pediatric nursing textbooks is still weighted heavily toward the care of the "normal" child; as much as 50% (or more) of the information contained in the most popular undergraduate pediatric nursing textbooks is related to normal growth and development, and only approximately 30% of the information is devoted to organ system dysfunction. These priorities should be re-evaluated.

A balance must be achieved during baccalaureate education between theory and clinical experience and between knowledge of the "norms" and understanding of abnormal physiology and complex illness. Nursing education should provide a solid scientific foundation, followed by ample opportunity to apply this science in the clinical setting.[21] The nursing faculty supervising the students in the clinical setting *must* be clinically expert; the faculty serve as role models of clinical practice and should also teach the students skills in multidisciplinary collaboration during patient care.

Following undergraduate education, hospital-based nurses require further education before they are able to care for acutely ill patients. An orientation program is provided (and paid for) by the employing hospital. If undergraduate nursing education continues to prepare nursing for only general practice, then schools of nursing should work with hospitals to develop formal "internships" to provide the necessary postgraduate education in acute care clinical nursing practice. Such internships have been successfully developed in many institutions. However, it is imperative that the internship be regarded as a commitment by *both* the nurse and the hospital to provide necessary education for the nurse. Since critical care is a medical-nursing specialty, physicians and nurses should be involved in teaching nurses about critical care. If the hospital, the medical staff, and the nursing staff invest in the education and preparation of the nurse, the nurse should be willing to make a commitment to the hospital. If the hospital pays the nurse a full salary during the internship, it is reasonable to expect that the nurse will remain at the hospital for several years.

As their educational level increases, nurses want and deserve to be accepted as full-fledged colleagues on the health care team. In the past, nurses were taught deference to physicians; now undergraduate nurses are taught to expect peer status with and respect from the physician. When nurses cite disagreements with physicians, lack of mutual trust and respect is most commonly reported.[20] While some physicians have always acknowledged this collegial relationship, other physicians fail to understand its need.

The shorter the educational preparation time of the nurse, the more expendable the nurse may be in the work force; conversely, the higher the level of preparation the nurse brings to the hospital, the greater will be that nurse's value to the hospital and the medical team. A diploma-prepared or inexperienced baccalaureate-prepared nurse is minimally trained and may be considered easily replaceable. Therefore, if the nurse wishes to become a valuable, contributing member of the hospital staff, he or she must bring a high level of educational and clinical expertise to the bedside.[16] In addition, the nurse must be able to delineate the unique contribution that nursing makes to patient care. Since many of the nurse's responsibilities include collaboration with physicians and following physicians' orders, it is difficult to elucidate the unique contribution of the nurse.

It is not surprising that nurses and physicians cannot agree on the professional responsibilities unique to physicians and nurses. Physicians indicate that they are responsible for assessing the patient, diagnosing the problem, and determining a plan of care. Yet, nurses believe that these responsibilities belong to the nurse. Neither physicians nor nurses are able to identify responsibilities that are unique to the nurse.[23] Physicians traditionally equate independence with the medical role, yet nurses are increasingly demanding credit for independent function.[23]

There is no question that a valuable and unique aspect of nursing care is psychosocial support. Nurses "are involved in the most private aspects of people's lives, and . . . do for others publicly what healthy persons do for themselves behind closed doors. Nurses, as trusted peers, are there to hear secrets, especially the ones born of vulnerability."[14] The nurse is the constant support in the hospital life of the child and family and "controls the environment of healing."[7] Although no one disputes the importance of the psychosocial support provided by the nurse, its value is difficult to measure. Hospitals can charge such tangibles as medications and dressings. Very often, psychosocial support is thought to be something the nurse provides while doing other things, and it is difficult to obtain reimbursement for or allow quantification of the time required for this support. Nurses must continue to assert the importance of psy-

chosocial support and its contribution in controlling the costs of hospital care. In addition, nurses must educate the public about the value of nursing care.

Nursing Salaries

Nursing salaries have not increased significantly during the past 20 years; in addition, the salary of the average experienced nurse is only approximately $7,000 more than that of a new graduate.[24] For the most part, nurses continue to accept hourly wages, rather than salaries. If nurses consider their care to be instrumental in supporting patient physical and emotional well-being and patient and family satisfaction, nurses should request to be paid a salary, with bonuses tied to staff nurse performance, seniority, and hospital profit. If nurses continue to be paid an hourly wage, they will continue to be dealt with as hourly employees, rather than as committed members of the hospital staff.

Nurse Managers

Until recently, most nurse managers were skilled bedside nurses who were promoted to administrative positions, and many lacked the preparation for and skill in motivating and managing adult employees. Unless or until the nurse acquires these skills, the efficiency of the unit may be compromised and nursing staff turnover may be higher than necessary. Too often, the only administrative role model available to the nurse manager is the hospital administrator. While the hospital (or any business) administrator can provide valuable insight about the management of budget and personnel in general, it is essential that the *nurse* administrator develop skills in the management and representation of and advocacy for *nurses*. If the nurse abdicates these skills, the hospital administration loses the mechanism to learn about the unique needs and motivation of the bedside nurses and the stimulus to maximize nursing competence and retention.

Definition of Nursing Contributions to Patient Care

As nursing grows as a profession, the specialized body of knowledge unique to nurses must be defined. This current period in the evolution of the nursing profession can be likened to the transition from adolescence to adulthood. The adolescent desires to gain independence from the parent; this is often accomplished through exaggeration and emphasis of differences between the parent and the adolescent. Nurses often attempt to demonstrate independence from physicians in an adolescent manner, by creating or emphasizing differences in scope of practice. An example of this emphasis on differences is the development of nursing diagnoses. Certainly some nursing diagnoses, such as "Potential decrease in cerebral perfusion" for the patient with head injury and increased intracranial pressure, clarify the challenges in patient care. However, some diagnoses, such as "Powerlessness related to total dependence on others secondary to disabling illness and perceived inability to influence current health status" are cumbersome, incomprehensible to physicians, irrelevant to patient care, and frequently ignored by nurses and physicians alike. The use of such diagnoses often causes physicians and other nurses to stop reading nursing notes, so communication is hindered rather than helped.

Nursing notes should communicate vital information about patient care and progress to members of the health care team. If nurses want nursing notes to be read, they must be concise and clear; extensive notes or those that appear to be written in "nursing code" will not be read by non-nurses and are best consigned to nurse-only correspondence. If nurses chart in the progress notes, this charting should be designed to clarify, not obfuscate, the plan of care.

With maturation, a self-confident adolescent is ultimately able to appreciate both similarities with and differences from the parent and to acknowledge both in a supportive manner. As nursing evolves as a profession, emphasis should be placed on collegial aspects of research and practice with physicians, as well as a mutual recognition of the substantial and relevant differences in scope of practice that exist.

Job Satisfaction

Nurses frequently cite a lack of positive feedback from physicians and administrators as a source of frustration.[25] Certainly, hospital administrators should realize that rewards given for a job well done can contribute to staff satisfaction and retention.[25] In addition, every member of the health care team should be conscious of the need for positive reinforcement; too often, we think that a colleague is doing a good job but never voice the thought. Typically, team members are more likely to make negative comments than positive ones.

Although positive feedback from colleagues is an important source of reinforcement, nurses should also be able to derive satisfaction from good nursing care. However, if any employee in any position requires constant positive feedback, that employee is bound to be dissatisfied. Nurses should learn objective self-appraisal during undergraduate education.

CONTRIBUTION OF THE MEDICAL PROFESSION TO POTENTIAL CONFLICT

The role of the physician in major medical centers is changing. The curtailment in government support of hospital care has led to potential competition for patient care dollars. For this reason, emphasis may be placed on funding of medical center physician salaries through research activities. In addition, academic appointment and promotion are often linked to research productivity. As a result, physicians in university-based medical centers may have very little time or incentive to teach residents or nurses. Thus, most of the medical care of the patients and the teaching provided to the nursing staff may come from the house officers. The attending physician becomes "an episodic presence in the life of a patient."[7]

In many instances, the experience and knowledge of the critical care nurse exceeds that of the junior house officer, yet the nurse must request orders from the house officer. If the house officer is unwilling to take suggestions from the bedside nurse, conflict arises and patient care can suffer.

Physicians frequently cite the importance of diplomacy and tactfulness, good clinical judgment, and helpfulness in ensuring good communication between physicians and nurses.[20] Surveyed physicians noted the need for nurses to "make . . . helpful suggestions . . . like trying to guide the ship without actually taking hold of the wheel."[20] Such indirect communication and responsibility can be extremely frustrating for the nurse, who feels competent enough to direct aspects of patient care. In addition, physicians may fail to use tact when communicating with the nurse; the very term "orders" provides insight into the nature of nurse-physician relationships of the past.

Since critically ill patients often have multisystem disease, many physician specialists may be involved in the care of each patient. If no one physician (e.g., the intensivist) controls the care of the patient, the nurse is often required to arbitrate differences among the recommendations and orders of the consulting services. When disagreements develop regarding patient care, the nurse may be caught in the middle, forced to choose among the orders. Such disagreements can be avoided if one physician and one nurse are clearly in charge of the patient's care. When several specialty teams are in charge of the patient's care, multidisciplinary, multispecialty rounds (including physicians and nurses from every service involved) should take place on a regular, if not daily, basis to determine the plan of care and planned response to potential patient deterioration. Each member of each team should be aware of the plan of care. When a physician writes an order to change that patient's care, that order should be discussed with the primary or bedside nurse, so the nurse has the opportunity to ask necessary questions or to clarify the order, if needed.

Admission of patients to the ICU is a frequent cause of nurse-physician conflict. If the unit is full when a physician calls about an admission, the charge nurse is often obligated to call other physicians until one of the existing patients in the unit can be transferred. Such last-minute conflict can be prevented if, on a daily basis, the director of the unit identifies the patients who should be transferred in the event of a new admission, and if an admitting house officer or physician is appointed to arbitrate disputes over available beds. Some intensive care units allocate a given number of beds to each major service; if a service fills the allocated beds, a physician from that service must negotiate for bed space with a physician from a service that has bed space available. Any of these plans appropriately removes the nurse from interphysician conflict and negotiation for bed space. The designation of an "admitting" house officer or physician can officially indicate the person responsible for bed allocation.

Physicians are both colleagues with the nurse in delivering patient care and customers of the hospital. If the physician is dissatisfied with the quality or type of nursing care provided at a hospital, he or she may well refer patients to another hospital. Thus, the nurse must be able to provide excellent care for the patient and maintain physician satisfaction; usually, these goals are mutually inclusive. Occasionally, however, the physician may demand attention or supplies that appear to be in excess of those needed to provide good patient care; at this point, the need to treat the physician as a customer may impede the development of a collegial relationship. It may also frustrate the nurse's sense of professional autonomy, harkening back to "handmaiden" days.[26]

Physicians frequently introduce new technology or therapy into the intensive care unit and the method of the introduction reflects the physician's opinion about the importance of nursing care. If the therapy or technology is introduced with little or no attempt made to include nurses in education and planning for changes in patient care, the physician effectively tells nurses that they are superfluous. If, on the other hand, the nurses are included in the early stages of planning, they will feel more committed to the success of the therapy and more essential to the patient care. A perfect example of the need for nursing involvement in the introduction of new technology is the use of extracorporeal membrane oxygenation (ECMO). If a patient suddenly returns from the surgical suite with an ECMO circuit in place, the anxiety level of the nurse increases dramatically. In actuality, the nurse will have no responsibility for the maintenance of the ECMO circuit (since a perfusionist is present at all times), but he or she will be responsible for dealing with the consequences of cannula dislodgement or separation or coagulopathy. If the nurses are involved in the preparation for ECMO therapy in the animal laboratory, the components, maintenance, and troubleshooting of equipment will be familiar from the moment the therapy is initially provided to a patient, so stress is minimized and collaboration is enhanced.

Finally, some physicians feel threatened by the desire of nurses for independence. Such physicians may think that nurses "have stopped wanting to 'do nursing'."[6] The author recalls the exasperated physician who remarked, "Nursing as a profession deteriorated when nurses began to worry about physiology and stopped rocking babies." These physicians must be educated by nurses and physicians alike about the responsibilities of nurses in the 1990s, and the contributions a skilled nurse can make to patient care.

The frustration of the medical profession with the nursing shortage was manifested in the 1988 proposal of the American Medical Association (AMA) for creation of a new class of hospital caregivers, the registered care technologist (RCT), to be educated and licensed by physicians. Amid a great deal of opposition from nursing organizations, the AMA Board of Directors in 1990 announced that they would cease recruitment of pilot

education sites for RCTs. Certainly, there were several problems with the proposed RCTs. Critical care units today need nurses with more rather than fewer skills. In addition, although physicians would ostensibly teach and license the RCTs, nurses would be responsible for their actions.

The AMA RCT proposal and the response to it are symbolic of the frustration of the medical profession and the lack of communication and cooperation that existed between the ANA and the AMA. Certainly, the nursing profession has not successfully eliminated the nursing shortage. Something definitely must be done to increase the number of nurses, the level of nursing preparation, and retention of nurses within the nursing profession. However, it would be much more constructive for the nursing and medical professions to look at this issue *together,* since both professions are involved in the problem and can aid in its solution. Ultimately, however, the nursing profession must be able to address the problems of the nursing profession.

The pediatric critical care nurse today must be knowledgeable about clinical assessment, hemodynamic monitoring, physiology, pathophysiology, pharmacology, and mechanical support of cardiopulmonary and renal function, while understanding pediatric nutrition, fluid and electrolyte balance, normal growth and development, and psychosocial support of the child and family. This body of knowledge is enormous and the nurse who masters this information should be well compensated. If the medical profession and hospital value this expertise and support the bedside nurse in its acquisition, the hospital and medical staff should be willing to continue the investment to keep that nurse practicing at the hospital. It is unreasonable to bemoan the fact that the new graduate of a nursing school is inadequately prepared, then expect the skilled nurse with 10 years of experience to work for a wage that is not much higher than that of the so-called "unskilled" new graduates. Hospitals and physicians should be willing to consider new ways of funding and rewarding good nursing care and seniority.

Nurse-physician conflict can arise if physicians attempt to provide hospital care for a patient without regard for the patient care organization. Physicians typically have autonomy in scheduling activities during the day and have more freedom in negotiating responsibilities for patient care within the physician team. The nurse does not have similar autonomy of scheduling and often is the recipient of "orders" and "assignments" (these very terms imply passivity) and must adjust a planned patient care schedule to the demands of diagnostic departments and physicians. During a given day, the nurse is also subject to demands for staff meetings or charge nurse responsibilities as designated by the unit nurse manager. It is not unusual for a nurse to be simultaneously responsible for assisting with a sterile procedure for one patient at the same time it is necessary to accompany a second patient to a diagnostic study. If physicians each schedule activities without consideration of additional and potentially conflicting schedules of other services, the nurse may spend more time on the telephone juggling schedules than providing nursing care.

FACTORS INFLUENCING NURSING SATISFACTION AND RETENTION

Nurses are the key element in critical care.[1] The function of the ICU and its integrity has, in a large part, more to do with the quality of the bedside nursing care than with any other factor.[27] The nursing shortage affects the ability of the ICU to provide care for critically ill patients. In fact, admission of patients during periods of short staffing is seen as one of the most common causes of nurse-physician conflict in the ICU.[28]

Sources of Satisfaction for Critical Care Nurses

Multiple studies of nursing satisfaction and stress have been reported, and their findings are remarkably consistent.[24, 29, 30–32] Since nursing salaries are typically lower than the salaries of most other college-educated professionals, nonmonetary rewards are very important to nurses.[33] Nurses tend to choose critical care nursing because of the nature of the direct patient care. Critical care nursing offers intellectual challenge, opportunities for learning, and the chance to give intensive care to a small number of patients. Nurses take pride in having responsibility for extremely ill patients, knowing that the skill of the nurse and the nurse's observations, knowledge, and support can contribute to the patient's survival and recovery. Approximately half of all nurses surveyed cited patient improvement, progress, recovery, and close patient contact as the sources of greatest satisfaction.[24]

Critical care nurses also cite the opportunity to develop proficiency in skills, to handle emergencies, and to be an effective member of a team as satisfying aspects of critical care. Variety and excitement increase the satisfaction of the critical care nurse.[24] In addition, the ability to function independently is very important to nurses surveyed. Interpersonal relationships are a potential source of satisfaction for nurses. Nurses express pride in being part of a skilled team, enjoying teamwork during crises, and appreciating peer recognition and support.[24] Critical care nurses also gain satisfaction from knowledge gained and the ability to demonstrate technical expertise in the fast-paced ICU. These nurses pride themselves on their ability to function well during emergencies.[24]

Reward systems and peer feedback can increase professional satisfaction for critical care nurses. Job security, tangible rewards for knowledge, skill, or education, and the support of colleagues are important.[24]

Sources of Stress for Critical Care Nurses

In several surveys of critical care nurses, consistent sources of stress have been cited.[24, 29, 30, 31] Ironically, many sources of satisfaction (e.g., relationships with colleagues, the fast-paced environment, constant opportunity to learn, need for technical expertise) can also introduce stress. The stressful factors most often cited by critical care nurses include interpersonal conflicts, the management of the unit, lack of administrative rewards, the nature of direct patient care, inadequate knowledge and skill, and the physical work environment.[24] Pediatric and neonatal intensive care unit nurses frequently cite the death of a child and the severity of the illness of the patients and potentially poor outcomes as sources of stress.[30, 31]

Interpersonal Conflicts

The major source of stress for the critical care nurse, according to most published studies, is interpersonal conflicts,[24, 29, 30–32] most frequently physician-nurse relationships. When conflict exists, characteristic attitudes can be documented among physicians and nurses alike. Physicians most frequently cite problems stemming from the nurse's lack of diplomacy or tactfulness, failure to use good clinical judgment, and lack of helpfulness as causes of negative interaction. These physicians value good communication from the nurse (including a nondemanding approach), willingness to help, and a high level of competence.

When stressful aspects of relationships with physicians are discussed by nurses, they most often cite a lack of respect for the nurse or the nurse's knowledge. Nurses, therefore, value mutual respect and trust most highly in relationships with physicians, and enjoy serving as a resource to physicians.[24] Nurses feel that they are a part of the team when the physician discusses the plan of care with the nurse and requests the nurse's input into that plan.[20, 23]

Unavailability of physicians was also cited by nurses as a potential cause of stress in nurse-physician relationships. The physician may be unavailable because of other commitments (e.g., cross-coverage of patients in other units or other emergencies). Physicians may also fail to come promptly when called if they are not convinced of the need to examine the patient. If the nurse does not convey important information, or if the physician fails to trust the information conveyed by the nurse, miscommunication will occur.

Nurse-nurse conflicts are additional sources of stress for the critical care nurse. Competitiveness and lack of camaraderie contribute to nurse-nurse conflict.[24]

Nurse-supervisor conflict is another source of stress cited by critical care nurses. If the nurse manager lacks administrative skills or fails to provide positive feedback, small problems can be magnified, and the nursing staff may become dissatisfied.

Management of the Unit

Management issues are frequently cited sources of stress for the bedside critical care nurse.[24] Often, critical care nurses cite in studies the absence of adequate staffing to provide care and the absence of competent staff. Inadequate ancillary services (transport, phlebotomy) increase the workload of the nursing staff and contribute to dissatisfaction.[24]

Nurses are versatile employees, so they often fill in when other hospital services are inadequately staffed (e.g., the nurse will do the work of an absent unit clerk when that position is eliminated). However, such use of nursing personnel is inappropriate and must cease. It is far better for the hospital to pay the wages of a unit clerk or a unit equipment manager than to utilize nursing personnel to answer the telephone, transcribe orders, and keep track of equipment and equipment charges. If adequate support personnel are present, nurses can be free to do what they are trained to do—care for patients.

Nature of Patient Care

Although the challenges and excitement of patient care can be extremely rewarding to the critical care nurse, certain aspects of patient care are universally stressful. Although flexibility and response to emergencies are necessary on a daily basis, emergencies can certainly be stressful, particularly if they cluster together or occur when staffing is inadequate.[24]

Prolongation of the life of an extremely ill or debilitated patient can be particularly problematic for the nurse and the physician. Although the physician can leave the unit periodically, the nurse must remain at the bedside and perform the procedures that are uncomfortable or painful. The nurse's position becomes difficult if the he or she feels the procedures are unnecessary or contrary to the wishes of the patient and family. Frequent nurse-physician, and multidisciplinary conferences with the patient (if age appropriate) and the family are needed to enhance communication and allow expressions of opinions until a decision is made. Input from the nurses must be actively considered during the decision-making process. If the nurse does not feel involved in the decision, yet must implement the plan of care, frustration and low morale may result.

Frustration can also arise if the nurse feels unable to meet the psychosocial needs of the patient and family. There are actually several potential sources of such feelings. First, unrealistic expectations of psychosocial support may be created during the undergraduate nursing education. Second, staffing patterns may be such that conversation with the patient and family must occur simultaneous with physical care. Some nurses are uncomfortable dealing with the emotional response of the child and family. Finally, the goals of nursing care, as stated by professional organizations, may be unrealistic. The ANA professional goal of care is to restore the patient to a complete state of mental, physical, emotional and social well-being. This may be an unattainable goal, so the nurse is destined to fail when trying to achieve it.

During undergraduate nursing education, the student typically cares for one patient. The needs of that single patient are thoroughly researched and the student's care is closely supervised and scrutinized, to ensure that comprehensive physical and psychosocial care is provided for the child and family. While this method of learning is good as an introduction, the student should eventually learn to provide excellent care to several patients and families simultaneously. It will be impossible to provide the same type and level of care to several patients and families as is provided to a single patient. Too often, the new graduate never learns to set realistic goals of care and so constantly feels that substandard care has been delivered.

The nurse should avoid separation of "technical care" time from "time for psychosocial support." Certainly, there are some occasions when the patient's physical needs must assume priority. However, the nurse must learn to communicate empathy, compassion, and receptiveness to the family at all times, so that psychosocial support is actually being provided even during silence. If the nurse is abrupt or aloof in communication style and posture while rendering physical care, it is unrealistic to expect that the patient and family will suddenly confide in the nurse when that nurse has "time" for psychosocial support.

Occasionally, a nurse may feel too emotionally exhausted to provide support to the child and family. This is particularly likely to occur if that nurse has recently been involved in the care of an extremely ill or dying patient. At rare times, the nurse may feel that a personality conflict interferes with effective care for the child and family. If the nurse is unable to render skilled and comprehensive care, another nurse must take over. The initial nurse may simply need a "break" before investing emotionally in the child and family.

Finally, interdisciplinary conferences and nursing care conferences should be utilized to set realistic goals for the care of the child and family. In many instances, physicians and nurses will not be able to restore a state of complete mental, physical, and emotional well-being for the child and family and so must determine the level of function that is achievable.

Inadequate Knowledge and Skills

Both new and experienced critical care nurses may feel that their knowledge of critical care pathophysiology and therapy is inadequate. For this reason, a structured orientation program must be followed by ongoing educational opportunities including both formal education (at conferences) and informal education at the bedside. Interdisciplinary bedside rounds will involve the bedside nurse in discussion of issues surrounding patient injury or illness and management. Nursing care rounds should also be utilized to enable nurses to share expertise acquired during patient care.

Nurses feel insecure when thrust into an unfamiliar patient care situation, knowing that an error can jeopardize the life of the patient. Therefore, inexperienced nurses should be paired with senior nursing staff or the clinical nurse specialist or head nurse during the care of the seriously ill patient. This enables the inexperienced nurse to gain experience and confidence without the risk of mistakes. Physicians and clinical resource nurses (including the clinical nurse specialist) should be available to teach the bedside nurse and answer questions.

Work Environment

The work environment is rarely cited as a major source of stress by critical care nurses. However, it can magnify existing stress, particularly on busy days. At those times, limited work space, the noise in the unit, and the lack of an uninterrupted break time for meals may all increase staff stress.

Administrative and clinical support nurses should be particularly sensitive to the need for break time from the unit and should offer to relieve the bedside nurse at regular intervals. Bedside nurses are likely to be intolerant of administrative or physician departmental "lunch meetings" when they must work an entire shift without any break time at all.

Physicians should be supportive of the nurse's need for a break from bedside care. The physician should offer to help the nurse move a patient out of the unit or change a dressing if it will enable the nurse to take a brief break. Too often, the nurse goes to the nursing lounge to eat a hurried lunch only to be called back to the bedside to assist in a (nonemergent) procedure that could be performed earlier or later in the day.

SOURCES OF PHYSICIAN STRESS AND SATISFACTION IN THE CRITICAL CARE UNIT

Very few studies have attempted to determine the factors that increase physician stress and satisfaction in the critical care unit. In adult ICUs, prolonged care of patients with poor prognosis has been cited as making the ICU more stressful than other units.[34] In the pediatric ICU, the death of a child was noted to be particularly stressful for house officers, because it is often viewed by the young physician as a failure (this sense of failure may be shared by nurses).[35] Other potential sources of stress for pediatric residents include interpersonal conflict, difficult decisions regarding the initiation and maintenance of sophisticated mechanized supports, apprehension about the quality of life that has been saved, frustration with the lack of measurable achievement despite significant investment of time and emotion, physical and emotional exhaustion, and feelings of inadequacy about knowledge and skill.[35] It is interesting to note that some pediatric resident physicians have difficulty dealing with their dependence on other members of the health care team during emergency situations.[34]

House officers assigned to the ICU were most likely to express anxiety about ignorance or experience during the early part of the ICU rotation.[35] These physicians are less likely to reflect on moral or ethical aspects of patient management decisions, since they have not yet mastered basic assessment and intervention skills, so attempts to involve them in patient care conferences will probably be unsuccessful. Anxiety regarding ethical decision-making is more likely to be expressed by pediatric house officers at the end of an ICU rotation.[35] These physicians would be more likely to participate in interdisciplinary care conferences regarding difficult patient management decisions.

Structured orientation and educational opportunities should be planned for new house officers assigned to the ICU. If the nursing staff is included in this orienta-

tion program, communication, cooperation, and camaraderie may be enhanced, particularly if nurses and physicians find that they share common stresses.

Potential sources of satisfaction for pediatric house officers in the ICU are remarkably similar to those cited by critical care nurses and focus on the challenges and rewards of patient care and interpersonal relationships. Physicians have noted an enormous sense of gratification following the recovery of an ill or injured child. Those who enjoy critical care medicine particularly like the opportunity to apply complex science and technology. In addition, the "elite camaraderie" in the pediatric ICU contributes to the rewards of caring for critically ill and injured children. This camaraderie may be enhanced through regularly scheduled physician-nurse discussion groups during which common concerns and questions may be addressed, and senior (attending) physicians and nurses can provide support to the inexperienced members of the health care team.[35]

RISK MANAGEMENT IN PHYSICIAN-NURSE COMMUNICATION

Communication between the physician and the nurse may be written or verbal but must always be precise. Misunderstandings and misstatements can compromise patient care and leave the health care team and the hospital vulnerable to legal action. Care must be taken in documentation, verbal communication, and team coordination. An excellent workbook that may be used to sharpen risk management skills is listed in the references.[36] Suggestions to improve nurse-physician communication and minimize risk are provided here.

Risk Management and Documentation

"The purpose of the medical record is to benefit the patient by preserving information."[36] Therefore, it should contain a complete yet concise record of examinations and observations that confirm a diagnosis or indicate a change in patient condition. In addition, conversations with the patient and family should be summarized. If standardized forms are used, all blanks and boxes should be filled out.[35]

Unusual occurrences, such as medical complications or mishaps, must be documented concisely and accurately, without judgmental language. The description should be limited to the event itself without explanation or rationalization; "the best record contains only information which is correct and needed for the care of the patient."[36]

Certain words assign blame or convey a judgment and should be avoided. Words such as "aberrant," "defective," "excessive," "faulty," "inadequate," "incorrect," "insouciant," "undesirable," "unsatisfactory," and "wrong" imply substandard performance or care. Words such as "accidental," "careless," "confused," "erroneous," "fault," "foolish," "inadvertent," "mistake," "negligent," "regretful," "terrible," and "unfortunate" appear to assign blame. These words should be used only after careful consideration.[36] Negative value judgments should not be included in the patient record, and speculative assignment of blame to personnel, the hospital, or economic factors is inappropriate—such information is better conveyed through incident reports. Inaccurate or deliberately misleading statements must be avoided.[36] Risk prevention actions (such as completion of an incident report) should not be included in the record, and these forms typically are not a part of the medical record.

Conversations with patients and families should be contemporaneously documented by health care personnel. Worries or concerns expressed by the patient or family should be recorded, and sources of information should be indicated. Information conveyed during informed consent should be included in the chart, but general information with notation of particularly important risks is usually preferable to long lists of potential complications. Such lists increase the likelihood of omission. When the nurse is asked to witness a signature on the consent form, he or she is attesting to the fact that the patient or family is providing informed consent, so the nurse should be present when the risks of the procedure or surgery are discussed. Instructions provided at discharge and telephone conversations should also be recorded. If the patient or family do not comply with the plan of care, this should be documented in the record.[36]

When charting about the patient, the family, or health care personnel, flippant or prejudicial expressions must be avoided. Comments about the presumed motives of another person have no place in the medical record.[36]

Physicians and nurses should read one another's notes and be aware of recommendations offered by members of the health care team. All notes should be legible and comprehensible; unclear terms or idiosyncratic terminology (e.g., unique to a unit) should be avoided.

If a recommendation made in the medical record is not followed, the record should document the reason. Open disagreement between members of the health care team should not be documented in the patient chart unless careful written explanation is offered. Whenever possible, recommendations should be noted with options, so that some flexibility in the carrying them out is possible.[36]

Risk Management in Verbal Communication

"It is human nature to forgive humility and punish arrogance."[36] Verbal communication in the presence of the patient and family must be precise and must consistently convey an attitude of concern; questions must be answered and information clearly provided. Only information that pertains to the patient's care should be discussed in the presence of the family; if family members hear informal conversation, they may assume that the physicians or nurses were distracted or unconcerned during care. Too often, in an attempt to relieve stress, staff members discuss personal information within the

hearing of the patient or family, and this practice should be discouraged.

Conflicting opinions and information should *not* be given to the patient and family. Nurses and physicians should avoid speculation about what another physician will or will not do. For example, if the family is told that "Dr. Summers always places two chest tubes during cardiovascular surgery," and only one chest tube is placed, the family may feel that their child received substandard care.

Members of the team should avoid value judgments about a particular procedure or therapy, since it may ultimately be used for the patient. For example, if the family is told that "radiation therapy is no longer provided as standard therapy for this form of tumor," and radiation therapy is prescribed, the family may feel that their child is receiving experimental or disproven therapy. If the plan of care is changed, careful explanation should be given to the family and noted in the chart.[36]

Members of the health care team should avoid overstating or understating the qualifications of members of the team. For example, if the family is told that "Dr. Smith is the only (or the best) physician qualified to deal with this problem" and Dr. Smith is out of town, the family may feel that they are in the care of an incompetent physician when Dr. Smith's partner is called. Negative opinions about the conduct or qualifications of another member of the health care team should never be made in the presence of the patient or family.[36] If the parents hear that "Dr. Armstrong is always irritable after a weekend on call," they may be alarmed when their child's surgery is scheduled for a Monday morning.

Unsolicited questions about patient care should be discussed in privacy, so they are not heard by the patient or family.[36] A relatively innocent question, such as, "Do you want to order a serum osmolality after the mannitol?" can be problematic. If the senior physician does not want such a test, the family may be left with the impression that the test should have been done, unless a lengthy explanation is provided. Disagreements about patient care must also be resolved in privacy. Too often, the family hears comments such as, "Dr. Jones told me to wean this patient, but your resident said we should maintain hyperventilation, and I don't know what to do," or, "Are you sure you want me to . . .?" Although some inconsistency in approach may be common in an ICU, its discussion can give family members the impression of conflict within the health care team.

Hospital problems should *never* be discussed with the patient and family. The author has frequently heard bedside nurses comment about short staffing in the presence of family members, and one mother (not a nurse, but an experienced parent of a chronically ill child) was asked, "Do you want to help staff the unit? We're two nurses short tonight." Comments about fatigue or delay in response or treatment (e.g., "I called Dr. Burger about your child's pain but he must have fallen back asleep," or "I told the nurses to give David plenty of pain medication, but it looks like they haven't gotten around to it yet," or "I know your child should have been suctioned quite a while ago, but we had another emergency") should also be avoided. Such comments leave the hospital vulnerable should a complication occur.

The patient or family should be notified of a mistake or mishap only after the attending physician has been apprised of the problem. If the mistake does not result in injury to the patient, it is not necessary to disclose it, unless the patient or family asks a direct question about the event.[36] Such disclosure may unnecessarily increase the anxiety of the patient and family. If injury does result from the mistake, the senior physician should be notified (if not already involved in the incident) and should give the patient and family a concise explanation.

The intensive care unit is a high-risk environment. The opportunity for miscommunication or failure to recognize a problem increases directly with the number of physicians and nurses involved in the care of the patient.[36] The attending physician is ultimately responsible for coordinating the actions, efforts, and assessments of the consulting services and the nursing staff. The primary nurse should also take responsibility for coordinating nursing care activities. The attending physician should be consulted if any conflicts or complications develop during the course of the patient's care, and the nursing staff should always ensure that the physician is aware of changes in the patient condition. If the nurse is dissatisfied with the medical care provided by a junior house officer, the nurse is obligated to contact the senior house officer. If satisfactory results are not obtained, the attending physician *must* be notified. If the patient, in fact, deteriorates as the result of substandard care and the nurse failed to notify senior physicians, the nurse is as responsible for the patient deterioration as the junior house officer.

SUGGESTIONS FOR IMPROVING PHYSICIAN-NURSE INTERACTIONS

Mutual respect, clear communication, flexibility, and collaboration are necessary to optimize physician-nurse interactions. The traditional physician-nurse attitudes of, respectively, dominance and deference should be put to rest.[37] The better the communication, collaboration, and cooperation among nurses and physicians, the better will be the quality of patient care provided in the intensive care unit.[4, 42–44]

Suggestions for Nurses

Nurses must acquire the best undergraduate baccalaureate education possible and must be committed to learning every day in the unit. If the baccalaureate education does not prepare the nurse adequately for patient care, he or she should communicate this information in no uncertain terms to the college alumni office (such information is particularly effective when provided in response to a request for a donation). If the scientific foundation and skills necessary to provide care for acutely ill or injured patients are lacking, the nurse must assume responsibility for acquiring them.

Nurses should develop mentors among both physician and nurse colleagues and learn from these role models. The nurse cannot practice in a vacuum; nursing participation in interdisciplinary rounds and formal continuing education is essential. If the bedside nurse continues to ask questions, bedside nursing care will continue to be challenging and rewarding. The nurse should always be aware of the plan of care and the planned response to a patient's deterioration. This plan should be discussed with the physician and nurse team at the end of each day.

Each nurse must be committed to the development of new skills and expertise. The more flexible and skilled the nurse, the more responsibility that nurse can command within the health care team.

Research is needed to document the cost-effectiveness of nursing care (such as patient and family teaching, and early recognition of potential complications). Nurses must be prepared to document improvements in patient outcomes following innovative nursing care strategies.

Nurses should also participate willingly in physician and nursing research. Such studies enable the nurse to be involved in the newest forms of therapy and to learn more about patient care. In addition, the nurse will be able to develop skills pertaining to new nursing techniques and technology; this will increase the value of the nurse to the hospital and to the health care team.

Nurses should be salaried employees of the hospital, and the nurse's salary should be commensurate with educational preparation, clinical experience, and clinical achievements and performance.[38] Clinical ladder systems may be useful in defining levels of nursing performance and relationship to salary. If sufficient salary is provided, the nurse must be willing to remain in the unit to help when emergencies arise and to come into the hospital for inservice education. Substantial differential salaries should be offered nurses working the evening and night shifts and weekends.

If staffing patterns are inadequate to maintain an appropriate standard of care, this information must be communicated to the physician director of the unit in an unemotional fashion. The nurse should avoid the use of the term "unsafe care" since this is an emotional term, and should use instead "substandard care" or "a level of care not consistent with the hospital standard."[39] The nurse should be prepared to document specific instances of compromise in the standard of care caused by inadequate staffing.

If the unit is absolutely inadequately staffed, the nurses should discuss the need for possible closure of beds with the physician director of the unit. However, nurses must also realize the economic cost to the hospital of empty beds and refusals of admissions. If referring hospitals are forced to develop alternative referral patterns, it may be difficult or impossible to regain the referrals once nursing staffing improves. Therefore, nurses must be committed to staffing beds if at all possible.[40]

Nursing staff retention is extremely important, and hospitals must be committed to keeping good nurses at the bedside. Creative staffing patterns (including self-staffing), job sharing, and incentive programs should be considered to keep good nurses. Since the cost of recruiting and educating a new nurse is estimated at approximately $30,000,[41] the hospital should consider provision of bonuses or profit sharing to nurses who remain longer than the average time.

Suggestions for Physicians

Physicians should be as involved as possible in patient care and must be committed to the education and continued development of the physicians and nurses within that unit. If nursing staffing is inadequate, the physician must be willing to consider closing of patient beds, even if this means cancellation of elective surgery.[4]

Nursing involvement in interdisciplinary morning rounds should be required, and nursing questions, comments, and suggestions should be specifically invited. At the end of the day, the physician should review the plan of care with the evening or night shift nurse and also review planned response to possible patient deterioration; then if the patient does deteriorate, everyone will know what to do.

Whenever possible, the physician should discuss written orders with the bedside nurse and explain the rationale for changes in therapy. The time taken for such communication will increase the nurse's knowledge of the patient and the plan of care and the involvement of the nurse in decision-making.

Flexibility should be demonstrated whenever possible. Certainly, emergency therapy should be provided on an emergent basis. However, elective procedures should be scheduled with consideration given to other demands on the time of the bedside nurse.

Unit management should represent a collaborative effort between physicians and nurses. Staff meetings and care conferences should be scheduled on a regular basis so that problems and issues in patient and family care can be aired before anger or resentment develops. The more involved nurses feel with decisions made in the unit and the more input they have in development of unit policies, the better the unit will function.[4] Collaborative patient care with good communication patterns has been shown to reduce the costs of patient care and increase patient satisfaction.[42-44] Absence of nurses from such interaction usually signals the presence of interdisciplinary problems that must be addressed and resolved.

Nurses should be included in planning for future developments in care and should be included in research conducted in the unit. In general, the more opportunity nurses are given to participate, the more committed they will be to the unit.

General Communication Style

Communication between physicians and nurses must be precise, and discussions of patient care issues should not be conducted in the presence of the patient or family. Compassion and empathy for colleagues will facilitate communication and camaraderie, and a sense of humor can often dissipate stress. Nurses and physi-cians alike should be aware of potential sources of satisfaction and stress for colleagues on the health care team and make an effort to provide sincere positive feedback for good patient and family care and support during stressful times.

Disagreements and problems should be aired in a constructive fashion away from the bedside. May[45] suggests some virtues to bring to professional disputes:

1. A measure of charity and good faith in dealing with an opponent
2. A good dose of caution in heeding a friend who approves only too quickly what we think and say
3. Humility before the powers we wield for good or for ill
4. The discipline to seek wisdom rather than to show off by scoring points
5. Sufficient integrity not to pretend more certainty than we have
6. Enough bravery to act even in the midst of uncertainty

References

1. Office of Medical Application of Research, National Institutes of Health, Critical care medicine: Concensus conference. JAMA 250:798, 1983.
2. Eisendrath SJ, Link N, and Matthay M: Intensive care unit: How stressful for physicians? Crit Care Med 14:95, 1986.
3. Mac Neil JM, and Weisz GM: Critical care nursing stress: Another look. Heart Lung 16:274, 1987.
4. Knaus WA, Draper EA, Wagner DP, et al: An evaluation of outcome from intensive care in major medical centers. Ann Intern Med 104:410, 1986.
5. Stein LI: The doctor-nurse game. Arch Gen Psychiatry 16:700, 1967.
6. Stein LI, Watts DT, and Howell T: The doctor-nurse game revisited. N Engl J Med 322:546, 1990.
7. Will GF: The dignity of nursing. Newsweek May 23, 1990.
8. Aiken LH and Mullinix CF: The nurse shortage: Myth or reality? N Engl J Med 317:641, 1987.
9. Nursing Data Review, 1985–1986. New York, National League for Nursing, 1986.
10. Department of Health and Human Services: The registered nurse population, Springfield, Virginia, National Technical Information Service, 1986 (DHHS publications number HRP 0906938).
11. Aiken LH and Mullinix CF: Recurring hospital nurse shortages: Explanations and solutions. Distinguished Scholar Lecture, Inaugurating the Center for the Advancement of Nursing Practice, Beth Israel Hospital, Boston, November 21, 1986.
12. Inglehart JK: Problems facing the nursing profession. N Engl J Med 317:646, 1987.
13. Levine and Associates: Summary and analysis of critical care nursing supply and requirements, Newport Beach, California, American Association of Critical Care Nurses, 1988.
14. Fagin C and Diers D: Nursing as a metaphor. N Engl J Med 309:116, 1983.
15. Goldsmith J: 2036: A health care odyssey. Hospitals 60:69, 1986.
16. Levin DL: Personal communication, June, 1991.
17. Georgopoulos BS and Jackson MM: Nursing kardex behavior in an experimental study of patient units with and without clinical nurse specialists. Nurs Res 19:196, 1970.
18. Georgopoulos BS and Christman L: The effects of clinical nursing specialization: A controlled organizational experience. New York, Edwin Mellen Press, 1991.
19. Brooten D et al: Early discharge and specialist transitional care. Image 20:64, 1988.
20. Prescott PA and Bowen SA: Physician-nurse relationships. Ann Intern Med 103:127, 1985.

PHYSICIAN-NURSE INTERACTION IN THE PEDIATRIC INTENSIVE CARE UNIT

21. Christman L: Nurse-physician communications in the hospital. JAMA 194:539, 1965.
22. Christman L and Kirkman RE: A significant innovation in nursing education. Peabody J Educ 50:1, 1972.
23. Weiss SJ: Role differentiation between nurse and physician: Implications for nursing. Nurs Res 32:133, 1983.
24. National Survey of Hospital and Medical School Salaries. Galveston, TX, University of Texas Medical Branch at Galveston, 1987.
25. Steffen SM: Perceptions of stress: 1800 nurses tell their stories. *In:* Claus KE and Bailey JT (eds): Living with Stress and Promoting Well-Being. Saint Louis, CV Mosby, 1980.
26. Luciano K and Darling LAW: The physician as a nursing service customer. J Nurs Administr 15:17, 1985.
27. Zaritsky A: Personal communication, June, 1991.
28. Banner W Jr: Personal communication, June, 1991.
29. Huckabay LMD and Jagla B: Nurses' stress factors in the intensive care unit. J Nurs Administr 9:21, 1979.
30. Hay D and Oken D: The psychological stresses of intensive care unit nursing. Psychosom Med 34:109, 1972.
31. Rosenthal SL, Schmid KD, and Black MM: Stress and coping in a NICU. Res Nurs Health 12:257, 1989.
32. Gramling L and Broome ME: Stress reduction for pediatric intensive care unit nurses. Clin Nurs Spec 1:185, 1987.
33. Mechanic D and Aiken LH: A cooperative agenda for medicine and nursing. N Engl J Med 307:747, 1982.
34. Eisendrath SJ, Link N, and Matthay M: Intensive care unit: How stressful for physicians? Crit Care Med 14:95, 1986.
35. Todres ID, Howell MC, and Shannon DC: Physician's reactions to training in a pediatric intensive care unit. Pediatrics 53:375, 1974.
36. Tennenhouse DJ and Kasher MP: Risk prevention skills: Communicating and record keeping in clinical practice, San Rafael, CA, Tennenhouse Professional Publications, 1989.
37. Kalisch BJ and Kalisch PA: An analysis of the sources of physician-nurse conflict. J Nurs Administr 7:51, 1977.
38. Maddox PJ: A novice-to-expert career ladder. *In:* French E and Lavandero R (eds): Nursing Recruitment and Retention, Strategies that Work. Newport Beach, CA, American Association of Critical Care Nurses, 1990, pp. 21–30.
39. Joy C: Personal communication, June, 1990.
40. Rudy EB: Nurse-managed special care units. *In:* French E and Lavandero R (eds): Nursing Recruitment and Retention, Strategies that Work. Newport Beach, CA American Association of Critical Care Nurses, 1990, pp. 51–58.
41. Minnick A: Rewards and retention. *In:* French E and Lavandero R (eds): Nursing Recruitment and Retention, Strategies that Work. Newport Beach, CA, American Association of Critical Care Nurses, 1990, pp. 39–48.
42. Koerner B and Armstrong D: Collaborative practice cuts cost of patient care: Study. Hospitals 58:52, 1984.
43. Koerner BL, Cohen JR, and Armstrong DM: Collaborative practice and patient satisfaction. Eval Health Prof 8:299, 1985.
44. Baggs JG and Schmitt MH: Collaboration between nurses and physicians. Image 20:145, 1988.
45. May WF: The virtues in a professional setting. The third annual memorial lecture of the Society for Values in Higher Education, Vassar College, August, 1984, Soundings, An Interdisciplinary Journal, 1985.

Index

Note: Page numbers in *italics* indicate illustrations; those followed by t indicate tables.